OBSTETRICS and GYNECOLOGY

OBSTETRICS and

Fifth Edition

with 86 authors

1097 illustrations

J. B. Lippincott Company   Philadelphia

London   Mexico City   New York

St. Louis   São Paulo   Sydney

GYNECOLOGY

Editors

David N. Danforth
PH.D., M.D., F.A.C.O.G., F.A.C.S.

Thomas J. Watkins Professor Emeritus of
Obstetrics and Gynecology
Northwestern University Medical School
Chicago, Illinois

James R. Scott
M.D., F.A.C.O.G.

Professor and Chairman, Department of Obstetrics and
   Gynecology
University of Utah School of Medicine
Salt Lake City, Utah

Associate Editors

Philip J. DiSaia
M.D., F.A.C.O.G.

Professor and Chairman, Department of Obstetrics and
   Gynecology
University of California at Irvine
School of Medicine
Los Angeles, California

Charles B. Hammond
M.D., F.A.C.O.G.

E. C. Hamblen Professor and Chairman, Department of
   Obstetrics and Gynecology
Duke University School of Medicine
Durham, North Carolina

William N. Spellacy
M.D., F.A.C.O.G., F.A.C.S.

Professor and Head, Department of Obstetrics and
   Gynecology
University of Illinois College of Medicine
Chicago, Illinois

Acquisitions Editor: Lisa A. Biello
Developmental Editor: Richard Winters
Manuscript Editors: Martha Hicks-Courant and Patrick O'Kane
Indexer: Barbara S. Littlewood
Art Director: Tracy Baldwin
Designer: Arlene Putterman
Production Coordinator: Charlene Catlett Squibb
Compositor: Tapsco, Inc.
Printer/Binder: Halliday Lithograph Corp.

Library of Congress Cataloging-in-Publication Data

Obstetrics and gynecology.

  Includes bibliographies and index.
  1. Gynecology. 2. Obstetrics. I. Danforth,
David N., 1912–   . II. Scott, James R., 1937–
[DNLM: 1. Genital Diseases, Female. 2. Obstetrics.
WQ 100 0145]
RG101.023 1986   618   86-2834
ISBN 0-397-50799-2

6   5   4   3

The authors and publisher have exerted every effort
to ensure that drug selection and dosage set forth in
this text are in accord with current recommendations
and practice at the time of publication. However, in
view of ongoing research, changes in government
regulations, and the constant flow of information
relating to drug therapy and drug reactions, the
reader is urged to check the package insert for each
drug for any change in labeled indications and
dosage and for added warnings and precautions.
This is particularly important when the
recommended agent is a new or infrequently
employed drug.

Authors

EZZAT I. ABOULEISH, M.B., Ch.B., D.A., D.M., M.D., F.S.A. (Egypt)
Chapter 34
Professor of Anesthesiology and Obstetrics and Gynecology, University of Texas Health
Science Center at Houston; Medical Director of Labor and Delivery, the Hermann
Hospital, Houston, Texas

KARLIS ADAMSONS, M.D., Ph.D., F.A.C.O.G.
Chapter 42
Professor and Chairman, Department of Obstetrics and Gynecology; Director of
Obstetrics and Gynecology, University Hospital of University of Puerto Rico, San Juan,
Puerto Rico

GEOFFREY ALTSHULER, M.B., B.S.
Chapters 43, 44
Professor of Pathology and Clinical Professor of Pediatrics, University of Oklahoma
Health Sciences Center, Oklahoma City, Oklahoma

RALPH C. BENSON, M.D., F.A.C.O.G., F.I.C.S.
Chapter 35
Professor and Chairman Emeritus, Department of Obstetrics and Gynecology, Oregon
Health Sciences University, Saint Vincent Hospital and Medical Center, Portland,
Oregon

MARC A. BERNHISEL, M.D.
Chapter 47
Assistant Professor of Obstetrics and Gynecology, Division of Reproductive
Endocrinology, University of Florida College of Medicine, Gainesville, Florida

ALFRED M. BONGIOVANNI, B.S., M.D., F.A.C.P.
Chapter 7
Professor of Pediatrics and Professor of Pediatrics in Gynecology and Obstetrics,
University of Pennsylvania School of Medicine; Director of Perinatal Endocrinology,
Pennsylvania Hospital; Staff, Children's Hospital of Philadelphia, Philadelphia,
Pennsylvania

SIDNEY F. BOTTOMS, M.D., F.A.C.O.G.

Chapter 38

Assistant Professor of Obstetrics and Gynecology, Wayne State University School of Medicine; Attending Obstetrician and Gynecologist, Hutzel Hospital, Detroit, Michigan

CAROLYN B. COULAM, M.D., F.A.C.O.G., F.A.C.S.

Chapter 6

Professor of Obstetrics and Gynecology, University of Pittsburgh; Chairman, Division of Reproductive Biology, Director, In Vitro Fertilization, Magee Women's Hospital, Pittsburgh, Pennsylvania

ROGER C. CRAFTS, Ph.D.

Chapter 3

Francis Brunning Professor Emeritus of Anatomy, University of Cincinnati, College of Medicine, Cincinnati, Ohio

WILLIAM T. CREASMAN, M.D., F.A.C.O.G.

Chapter 57

James Ingram Professor of Obstetrics and Gynecology and Director of Gynecologic Oncology, Duke University Medical Center, Durham, North Carolina

DWIGHT P. CRUIKSHANK, M.D., F.A.C.O.G.

Chapter 30

Professor of Obstetrics and Gynecology, Medical College of Virginia, Virginia Commonwealth University; Director of Obstetrics and Maternal-Fetal Medicine, Medical College of Virginia Hospitals, Richmond, Virginia

DAVID N. DANFORTH, Ph.D., M.D., F.A.C.O.G., F.A.C.S.

Chapters 29, 30, 31, 32, 33, 36, 38, 51

Thomas J. Watkins Professor Emeritus of Obstetrics and Gynecology, Northwestern University Medical School, Chicago, Illinois

JACK DAVIES, M.D.

Chapter 4

Professor of Anatomy and Surgery, Vanderbilt University School of Medicine, Nashville, Tennessee

RICHARD DEPP, M.D., F.A.C.O.G.

Chapter 41

Professor of Obstetrics and Gynecology, Northwestern University Medical School; Head, Section on Maternal-Fetal Medicine, and Director, Division of Obstetrics, Prentice Women's Hospital and Maternity Center of Northwestern Memorial Hospital, Chicago, Illinois

GUNTER DEPPE, M.D., F.A.C.O.G., F.A.C.S.

Chapter 56

Associate Professor of Obstetrics and Gynecology, Wayne State University School of Medicine; Director of Gynecologic Oncology, Hutzel Hospital; Vice-Chief of Gynecology, Harper Hospital, Detroit, Michigan

PHILIP J. DiSAIA, M.D., F.A.C.O.G., F.A.C.S.

Chapters 56, 62

Professor and Chairman, Department of Obstetrics and Gynecology, University of California, Irvine, Orange, California

WILLIAM L. DONEGAN, M.D., F.A.C.S.

Chapters 30, 60

Professor of Surgery, Medical College of Wisconsin; Chief, Department of Surgery, Mount Sinai Medical Center, Milwaukee, Wisconsin

BRUCE D. DOUST, M.D., F.R.A.C.R.

Chapter 61

Clinical Associate Professor of Radiology, Medical College of Wisconsin, Milwaukee, Wisconsin; Director of Radiology, Saint Vincent's Hospital, Sydney, Australia

WILLIAM DROEGEMUELLER, M.D., F.A.C.O.G.

Chapter 23

Professor and Chairman, Department of Obstetrics and Gynecology, University of North Carolina, School of Medicine; Attending Obstetrician and Gynecologist, North Carolina Memorial Hospital, Chapel Hill, North Carolina

LEO J. DUNN, M.D., F.A.C.O.G.

Chapter 39

Professor and Chairman, Department of Obstetrics and Gynecology, Medical College of Virginia, Virginia Commonwealth University, Richmond, Virginia

NITA J. DURHAM, M.B., B.S., F.R.C.R., M.R.A.C.R., D.D.U.

Chapter 61

Staff Radiologist, Saint Vincent's Hospital, Sydney, Australia

WILLIAM E. EASTERLING, Jr., M.D., F.A.C.O.G.

Chapter 40

Professor of Obstetrics and Gynecology and Associate Dean for Clinical Affairs, School of Medicine, University of North Carolina at Chapel Hill; Chief of Staff, North Carolina Memorial Hospital, Chapel Hill, North Carolina

DAVID A. ESCHENBACH, M.D., F.A.C.O.G.

Chapter 52

Professor of Obstetrics and Gynecology; Chief, Division of Gynecology, University of Washington; Attending Physician, University Hospital, Harborview Medical Center, Seattle, Washington

TOMMY N. EVANS, M.D., F.A.C.O.G., F.A.C.S

Chapter 49

Professor and Vice-Chairman of the Department of Obstetrics and Gynecology, University of Colorado; Chief of Gynecology, University of Colorado Hospital, Denver, Colorado

J. ANDREW FANTL, M.D., F.A.C.O.G.

Chapter 50

Associate Professor of Obstetrics and Gynecology, Medical College of Virginia, Virginia Commonwealth University, Richmond, Virginia

STEVEN G. GABBE, M.D., F.A.C.O.G.

Chapter 30

Professor of Obstetrics and Gynecology and Pediatrics, University of Pennsylvania School of Medicine; Director of Jerrold R. Golding Division of Fetal Medicine, Hospital of the University of Pennsylvania, Philadelphia, Pennsylvania

LAURA T. GOLDSMITH, Ph.D.
Chapter 8
Assistant Professor of Obstetrics and Gynecology, University of Medicine and Dentistry of New Jersey, New Jersey Medical School, Newark, New Jersey

DONALD PETER GOLDSTEIN, M.D., F.A.C.O.G., F.A.C.S., F.A.A.P.
Chapter 45
Assistant Clinical Professor of Obstetrics and Gynecology, Harvard Medical School; Chief, Division of Gynecology, The Children's Hospital; Director, New England Trophoblastic Disease Center, Brigham and Women's Hospital, Boston, Massachusetts

CLIFFORD P. GOPLERUD, M.D., F.A.C.O.G., F.A.C.S.
Chapter 25
Professor of Obstetrics and Gynecology, University of Iowa College of Medicine; Attending Obstetrician and Gynecologist, University of Iowa Hospitals and Clinics, Iowa City, Iowa

STUART C. GORDON, M.D.
Chapter 30
Clinical Fellow in Hepatology, Division of Hepatology, University of Miami School of Medicine, Miami, Florida

SAUL B. GUSBERG, M.D., D.Sc., F.A.C.O.G., F.A.C.S., F.R.C.O.G.(A.E.)
Chapter 56
Distinguished Service Professor and Chairman Emeritus, Department of Obstetrics and Gynecology, The Mount Sinai School of Medicine of the City University of New York; Consultant, The Mount Sinai Hospital, Mount Sinai School of Medicine, New York, New York

E. S. E. HAFEZ, M.D., F.A.C.O.G., F.A.C.S.
Chapter 4
Professor of Gamete Physiology and Andrology, Medical University of South Carolina, Charleston, South Carolina

CHARLES B. HAMMOND, M.D., F.A.C.O.G.
Chapters 47, 48
E. C. Hamblen Professor and Chairman, Department of Obstetrics and Gynecology, Duke University Medical Center, Durham, North Carolina

WILLIAM N. P. HERBERT, M.D., F.A.C.O.G
Chapter 40
Associate Professor of Obstetrics and Gynecology, School of Medicine, University of North Carolina; Attending Obstetrician and Gynecologist, North Carolina Memorial Hospital, Chapel Hill, North Carolina

ROBERT D. HILGERS, M.D., F.A.C.O.G., F.A.C.S.
Chapter 22
Professor of Obstetrics and Gynecology and Chief, Gynecologic Oncology Service, University of New Mexico, School of Medicine, Albuquerque, New Mexico

EDGAR O. HORGER III, M.D., F.A.C.O.G.
Chapter 30
Professor of Obstetrics and Gynecology and Director of Maternal-Fetal Medicine, Medical University of South Carolina, Charleston, South Carolina

STANLEY E. HUFF, M.D., F.A.D.A., F.A.A.D.
Chapter 30
Professor of Clinical Dermatology, Northwestern University Medical School; Senior Attending, Evanston Hospital, Evanston, Illinois

L. STANLEY JAMES, M.D., F.A.A.P.
Chapter 42
Professor of Pediatrics and Obstetrics and Gynecology, College of Physicians and Surgeons, Columbia University; Director, Division of Perinatal Medicine, Presbyterian Hospital (Babies Hospital), New York, New York

IRWIN H. KAISER, M.D., Ph.D., F.A.C.O.G.
Chapter 17
Professor of Obstetrics and Gynecology, Albert Einstein College of Medicine; Attending Obstetrician and Gynecologist, Albert Einstein College of Medicine Hospital, Bronx, New York

THOMAS C. KEY, M.D., F.A.C.O.G.
Chapter 18
Assistant Professor of Obstetrics and Gynecology and Director of Maternal-Fetal Medicine, University of California, San Diego, La Jolla, California

WILLIAM R. KEYE, Jr., M.D., F.A.C.O.G.
Chapter 10
Associate Professor of Obstetrics and Gynecology, University of Utah School of Medicine, Salt Lake City, Utah

ALLAN KILLAM, M.D., F.A.C.O.G.
Chapter 28
Professor of Obstetrics and Gynecology, Director of Obstetrics, and Co-Director of Perinatal Medicine, Duke University Medical Center, Durham, North Carolina

NEIL K. KOCHENOUR, M.D., F.A.C.O.G.
Chapters 20, 30
Associate Professor of Obstetrics and Gynecology, and Director of Maternal-Fetal Medicine, University of Utah School of Medicine, Salt Lake City, Utah

HOWARD P. KRIEGER, M.D., F.A.B.P.N.
Chapter 3
Professor of Neurology, Mount Sinai School of Medicine; Attending Neurologist, Mount Sinai Hospital, New York, New York

ROBERT J. KURMAN, M.D., F.A.C.O.G.
Chapter 59
Associate Professor of Pathology and Obstetrics and Gynecology, Georgetown University School of Medicine, Washington, DC

WILLIAM J. LEDGER, M.D., F.A.C.O.G., F.A.C.S.
Chapter 13
Professor and Chairman, Department of Obstetrics and Gynecology, Cornell University College of Medicine; Chief Obstetrician and Gynecologist, New York Hospital—Cornell, New York, New York

JOHN L. LEWIS, Jr., M.D., F.A.C.O.G., F.A.C.S.
Chapter 22
Professor of Obstetrics and Gynecology, Cornell University College of Medicine; Chief, Gynecology Service, Memorial Sloan-Kettering Cancer Center, New York, New York

STEVE N. LONDON, M.D.
Chapter 48
Assistant Professor of Medicine, Department of Obstetrics and Gynecology, Duke University Medical Center, Durham, North Carolina

HANS LUDWIG, M.D.
Chapter 4
Professor and Head of the Department of Obstetrics and Gynecology, University of Basel (Universitäts-Frauenklinik Basel), Basel, Switzerland

JOHN R. MARSHALL, M.D., F.A.C.O.G.
Chapter 7
Professor of Obstetrics and Gynecology, University of California, Los Angeles, School of Medicine, Los Angeles, California; Chairman, Department of Obstetrics and Gynecology, Harbor-UCLA Medical Center, Torrance, California

JAMES A. MERRILL, M.D., F.A.C.O.G.
Chapters 53, 56, 57, 58, 59
Clinical Professor of Obstetrics and Gynecology, University of Washington School of Medicine, Seattle, Washington

DANIEL R. MISHELL, Jr., M.D., F.A.C.O.G.
Chapter 14
Professor and Chairman, Department of Obstetrics and Gynecology, University of Southern California School of Medicine; Chief Professor, Services, Women's Hospital, Los Angeles County-University of Southern California Medical Center, Los Angeles, California

KAMRAN S. MOGHISSI, M.D., F.A.C.O.G., F.A.C.S.
Chapter 49
Professor and Associate Chairman, Department of Obstetrics and Gynecology, and Director, Division of Reproductive Endocrinology, Wayne State University School of Medicine; Chief of Obstetrics and Gynecology, Harper-Grace Hospitals; Vice-Chief of Obstetrics and Gynecology, Hutzel Hospital, Detroit, Michigan

JOHN C. MORRISON, M.D., F.A.C.O.G., F.A.C.S.
Chapter 30
Professor of Obstetrics and Gynecology and Director of Maternal-Fetal Medicine, University of Mississippi Medical Center, Jackson, Mississippi

SUE M. PALMER, M.D., F.A.C.O.G.
Chapter 30
Assistant Professor of Obstetrics and Gynecology, Division of Maternal-Fetal Medicine, University of Mississippi Medical Center, Jackson, Mississippi

ODETTE PINSONNEAULT, M.D., F.A.C.O.G., F.R.C.P.S.C.
Chapter 45
Assistant Professor of Obstetrics and Gynecology, University of Sherbrooke, Quebec, Canada; Attending Obstetrician and Gynecologist, Centre Hospitalier Universitaire de Sherbrooke, Sherbrooke, Quebec, Canada

ROY M. PITKIN, M.D., F.A.C.O.G.
Chapter 11
Professor and Head, Department of Obstetrics and Gynecology, University of Iowa College of Medicine, University of Iowa Hospitals and Clinics, Iowa City, Iowa

JOHN T. QUEENAN, M.D., F.A.C.O.G., F.A.C.S.
Chapter 9
Professor and Chairman, Department of Obstetrics and Gynecology, Georgetown University School of Medicine; Obstetrician and Gynecologist-in-Chief, Georgetown University Hospital, Washington, DC

ELIZABETH M. RAMSEY, M.D., Sc.D., F.A.C.O.G.(A)
Chapter 5
Research Associate, Department of Embryology, Carnegie Institution of Washington, Baltimore, Maryland

ROBERT RESNIK, M.D., F.A.C.O.G.
Chapter 18
Professor and Chairman, Department of Reproductive Medicine, University of California, San Diego, School of Medicine; Chief, Obstetrics and Gynecology, University of California, San Diego Medical Center, La Jolla, California

DANIEL H. RIDDICK, M.D., Ph.D., F.A.C.O.G.
Chapter 46
Professor and Chairman, Department of Obstetrics and Gynecology, University of Vermont College of Medicine; Chief of Service, Medical Center Hospital of Vermont, Burlington, Vermont

FELIX N. RUTLEDGE, M.D., F.A.C.O.G., F.A.C.S., F.R.C.O.G.
Chapter 54
Surgeon and Professor of Gynecology and Head of the Department of Gynecology, The University of Texas, System Cancer Center; M. D. Anderson Hospital and Tumor Institute, Houston, Texas

RUDY E. SABBAGHA, M.D., F.A.C.O.G.
Chapter 15
Professor of Obstetrics and Gynecology, Northwestern University Medical School; Director, Diagnostic Ultrasound Center at Northwestern Memorial Hospital, Chicago, Illinois

GLORIA E. SARTO, M.D., Ph.D., F.A.C.O.G., F.A.C.S.
Chapter 2
Professor and Chairman, Department of Obstetrics and Gynecology, University of Wisconsin at Milwaukee, Milwaukee, Wisconsin

EUGENE R. SCHIFF, M.D., F.A.C.P.

Chapter 30

Professor of Medicine, University of Miami School of Medicine, and Chief of the Division of Hepatology, Center for Liver Diseases; Chief, Hepatology Section, Veterans Administration Medical Center, Miami, Florida

JAMES R. SCOTT, M.D., F.A.C.O.G.

Chapters 12, 21, 24

Professor and Chairman, Department of Obstetrics and Gynecology, University of Utah School of Medicine, Salt Lake City, Utah

JOHN L. SEVER, M.D., Ph.D., F.A.A.P., F.A.C.E

Chapter 30

Professor of Pediatrics, Georgetown University Medical School, Washington, DC; Chief, Infectious Diseases Branch, Intramural Research Program, National Institute of Neurological and Communicative Disorders and Stroke, The National Institutes of Health, Bethesda, Maryland

HOWARD C. SHARP, M.D., F.A.C.O.G.

Chapter 30

Associate Professor (Clinical) of Obstetrics and Gynecology, University of Utah School of Medicine, Salt Lake City, Utah

JANNA S. SHERRILL, R.N., B.S.N.

Chapter 30

Perinatal Research Nurse, Division of Maternal-Fetal Medicine, Department of Obstetrics and Gynecology, University of Mississippi Medical Center, Jackson, Mississippi

MARY ANN SOUTH, M.D., F.A.B.P.

Chapter 30

Guest Worker, National Institutes of Health, National Institute of Neurological and Communicative Disorders and Stroke, Infectious Diseases Branch; Visiting Research Scientist, Gallaudet College, Bethesda, Maryland

HAROLD SPEERT, M.D., F.A.C.O.G., F.A.C.S.

Chapter 1

Assistant Attending Obstetrician and Gynecologist, Presbyterian Hospital, New York, New York; Consultant Gynecologist, Elizabethtown Community Hospital, Elizabethtown, New York

WILLIAM N. SPELLACY, M.D., F.A.C.O.G.

Chapter 27

Professor and Head, Department of Obstetrics and Gynecology, University of Illinois College of Medicine, Chicago, Illinois

ADOLF STAFL, M.D., Ph.D., F.A.C.O.G.

Chapter 56

Professor of Gynecology and Obstetrics, Medical College of Wisconsin; Senior Attending Gynecologist and Obstetrician, Milwaukee County Medical Complex, Milwaukee, Wisconsin

FATTENEH A. TAVASSOLI, M.D.
Chapter 59
Pathologist, Gynecologic and Breast Pathology Department, Armed Forces Institute of Pathology, Washington, DC

JOSEPH F. THOMPSON, M.D., M.P.H., F.A.C.O.G.
Chapter 16
Professor of Obstetrics and Gynecology, Indiana University School of Medicine, Indianapolis, Indiana

HAROLD M. M. TOVELL, M.D., F.A.C.O.G., F.A.C.S.
Chapters 51, 63
Professor of Clinical Obstetrics and Gynecology, College of Physicians and Surgeons, Columbia University; Senior Attending Obstetrician and Gynecologist, Saint Luke's Roosevelt Hospital, New York, New York

KENNETH F. TROFATTER, Jr., M.D., Ph.D.
Chapter 28
Assistant Professor of Obstetrics and Gynecology, Division of Perinatal Medicine, Duke University Medical Center, Durham, North Carolina

FREDERICK R. UELAND
Chapter 37
Research Technician, Stanford University Medical Center, Stanford, California

KENT UELAND, M.D., F.A.C.O.G.
Chapters 31, 37
Professor and Chairman, Department of Gynecology and Obstetrics, and Medical Director of Obstetrics, Stanford University Medical Center, Stanford, California

DAVID H. VROON, M.D.
Chapter 38
Associate Professor of Pathology, Emory University School of Medicine; Associate Chief of Pathology, Emory University Hospital/Grady Memorial Hospital, Atlanta, Georgia

EDWARD E. WALLACH, M.D., F.A.C.O.G.
Chapter 7
Professor and Chairman, Department of Gynecology and Obstetrics, The Johns Hopkins University School of Medicine; Gynecologist and Obstetrician-in-Chief, The Johns Hopkins Hospital, Baltimore, Maryland

GERSON WEISS, M.D., F.A.C.O.G.
Chapter 8
Professor and Chairman, Department of Obstetrics and Gynecology, University of Medicine and Dentistry of New Jersey, New Jersey Medical School, Newark, New Jersey

J. DONALD WOODRUFF, M.D., F.A.C.O.G.
Chapter 55
Richard W. Te Linde Professor of Gynecologic Pathology Emeritus and Professor of Gynecology and Obstetrics Emeritus, The Johns Hopkins Hospital, Baltimore, Maryland

RICHARD J. WORLEY, M.D., F.A.C.O.G.
Chapter 26
Associate Professor of Obstetrics and Gynecology, University of Utah School of Medicine, Salt Lake City, Utah

SAMUEL S. C. YEN, M.D., D.Sc., F.A.C.O.G., F.A.B.O.G., F.A.B.R.E.
Chapter 19
Professor of Reproductive Medicine and Director of the Division of Reproductive Endocrinology, University of California, San Diego School of Medicine, La Jolla, California

CHARLES J. ZALOUDEK, M.D.
Chapter 59
Associate Professor of Pathology, George Washington University Medical Center, George Washington University Hospital, Washington, DC

Preface

Many noteworthy advances have been made in obstetrics and gynecology since publication of the last edition of this book. Some of these are of major importance and have had profound impact on obstetric-gynecologic practice. Others have had more limited effects, but in sum they have greatly enlarged our horizons and have immeasurably improved our ability to deal with the problems that are inherent in the discipline of obstetrics and gynecology. As in earlier editions, a primary purpose of the new edition is to incorporate these advances so that this work will reflect our present knowledge of obstetrics and gynecology, and will serve as a modern, comprehensive textbook for students, residents, and practitioners.

In a volume of this kind, one of the editor's tasks is to be sure that the text is both current and inclusive. The previous editions offered no special problem, but it is now clear that this can be achieved only by utilizing the expertise of those who have special knowledge and talent both in our discipline as a whole, and in the subspecialties that are now an integral part of obstetrics and gynecology. I am pleased to welcome James R. Scott, who has provided inestimable help as co-editor of the new edition, and, as associate editors, Philip J. DiSaia, Charles B. Hammond, and William N. Spellacy, whose contributions to the subspecialties of obstetrics and gynecology are well known. Their active participation in the new edition has greatly strengthened the book.

The information in the fifth edition has been organized in much the same manner as in prior editions, but the revision is very extensive. Twenty-two chapters have been rewritten by new authors, and nine authors have written new sections dealing with medical and surgical complications of pregnancy. The existing chapters that have been retained from the last edition are updated to reflect current thought. We believe that the result is a balanced, modern text that will be useful to those for whom it is intended.

The reception accorded the previous editions of this book has been gratifying to all who participated in its writing and production. It is our hope that the new edition will also have an important position in the literature of obstetrics and gynecology.

It is again a pleasure to acknowledge the help of Rose Slowinski, librarian, and Linda Feinberg of the Evanston Hospital's Webster Medical Library. Their gracious help in obtaining obscure material, verifying references, and all other matters in which skilled library assistance was needed is greatly appreciated.

Finally, I wish to thank the J. B. Lippincott Company, and especially Richard Winters, for the meticulous attention they have given to all matters having to do with the preparation of this volume.

D.N.D.

Excerpts From the
Preface to the First Edition

A new textbook in a field already noted for the excellence of its literature needs a word of explanation of its background and objectives. In recent years the teaching in our field has been changing, and in all but two American medical schools obstetrics and gynecology are now combined in a single department and taught in a single sequence of courses by the same individuals. It seems a paradox that the student should require two separate books with their differing approaches and their repetition of material to help guide him through his course in the combined subject.

At teaching conferences it has been noted repeatedly that logic, convenience, and efficiency call for a single combined textbook in the interest of the student and the practitioner who require a reference to the basic essentials of the field. The new TEXTBOOK OF OBSTETRICS AND GYNECOLOGY is an attempt to meet this need.

It is designed to cover completely, in logical sequence and with maximum authority, the subject of obstetrics and gynecology in all the areas that are included in today's curriculum and it integrates the thinking of a faculty representing more than 30 medical schools in the U.S.A. and Canada. Each section has been written by an expert with special knowledge and experience in his assigned topic and this authority lends value to the text which could be achieved in no other way.

The scope of this text is wider than in most textbooks of either obstetrics or gynecology. This is deliberate and reflects the growth of knowledge in the field as well as the changing trends in medical education.

Because of the trend toward integrating the basic sciences with clinical problems throughout the medical curriculum, special emphasis is placed on chapters dealing with anatomy, physiology, endocrinology, embryology and genetics. These sections are intended to be sufficiently complete to serve as an authoritative reference source as well as a basis for the material that follows.

Documentation has been confined in most chapters to review articles, monographs, and other key references which will aid the reader in exploring areas of special interest.

Because of its distinguished authorship, and the breadth and detail of its content, it is hoped that the book will be of interest and use to the resident and practitioner as well as to the student. It should provide a central basic reference source around which the graduate can build a library of more specialized works in whatever direction his needs and inclinations may take him.

I am deeply indebted to each of the authors. It is their book and it is their work which has given the text its strength. Any omissions are the responsibility of the editor.

D.N.D.

Contents

Part II
NORMAL PREGNANCY

PART IV
NORMAL LABOR

PART V
ABNORMAL LABOR

PART I

General Considerations

Harold Speert

1

The special field of medicine known as obstetrics and gynecology boasts a background of unsurpassed drama. The discovery of the mammalian egg; the history of the obstetric forceps; the early cesarean sections; the conquest of puerperal fever; the controversy over obstetric anesthesia; the first successful abdominal operation, for ovarian cyst; and the cure of vesicovaginal fistula, one of the most distressing of woman's ills, form threads of a story with few equals in the annals of medicine. At least a superficial knowledge of the specialty's maturation is essential to the physician's general education as well as to an appreciation of his scientific heritage. The already crowded medical curriculum, however, provides scant opportunity for the pursuit of cultural interests beyond the expansive range of 20th-century science. This introduction to the history of obstetrics and gynecology is designed for the busy student with little time, and possibly little taste, for medical history. Contained herein are condensed accounts of a few of the major developments that have imparted to obstetrics and gynecology the specialty's distinctive character. The reader stimulated to further inquiry will find ample guidance in the recommended reading list at the end of this chapter.

EARLY MIDWIFERY

The history of obstetrics is the history of civilization itself. In biblical days, before the advent of physicians, labor and delivery were usually supervised by the midwives. These self-styled specialists of the obstetric art, usually without benefit of education or training, exercised a virtual monopoly over their craft until the 16th century or later. In 1552 Wertt, a physician in Hamburg, was burned at the stake for having posed as a woman in order to attend a patient in labor. The Old Testament records the role of the midwife in the second labor of

Rachel, wife of Jacob (Gen. 35:17) and in Tamar's delivery of twins (Gen. 38:27). During the period of the Hebrews' enslavement in Egypt, when their high birth rate began to pose a threat to Pharaoh's security, he ordered the midwives to destroy all the male children at birth. Not all obeyed, however, and when taken to task for their disobedience, the Egyptian midwives Shiphrah and Puah explained that "the Hebrew women . . . are lively, and are delivered ere the midwives come in unto them" (Exod. 1:15, 19).

The high standards of these Egyptian women did not characterize the practices of all midwives, however (Fig. 1-1); for centuries they were subjected to repeated vilification, and their calling was held in disrepute. At the fall of the Roman Empire, Eusebia, wife of the Emperor Constantius, jealous of her fecund sister-in-law Helen, the wife of Julian the Apostate, induced the midwife to murder Helen's child by allowing it to bleed from the umbilical cord.

As late as the 18th century, care of the pregnant woman was generally considered beneath the dignity of the physician, and false notions of modesty barred his participation in the delivery. As a result, the physician was usually summoned only in complicated and neglected cases. Mutilation of both mother and child often followed. The obstetrics of the Middle Ages has been characterized as neglect of normal cases and butchery of abnormal ones.

The first formal training for midwives was instituted by Hippocrates, in the 5th century B.C., but for several subsequent centuries efforts toward their education were halting and ineffectual. Self-taught or instructed by older midwives, most remained ignorant of the simple principles of obstetrics; many were careless, meddlesome, and dirty. Soranus (A.D. 98–138), the leading Greek authority on obstetrics and gynecology during the reigns of the emperors Trajan and Hadrian, made a noteworthy attempt to elevate the standards of midwifery with his

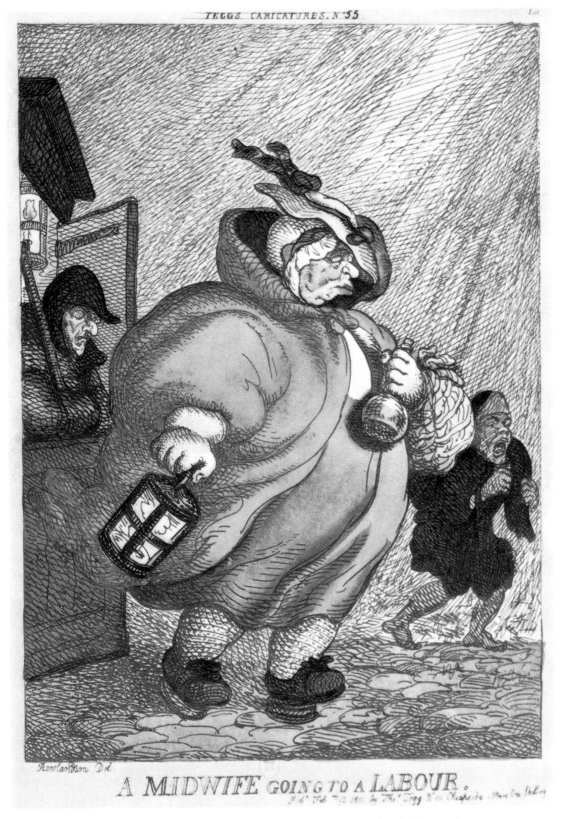

FIG. 1-1. Caricature of "midwife going to a labour"; holding in her right hand a lamp and in her left a flask of alcoholic refreshment, traditional accoutrements of midwives of 18th and 19th centuries. (Thomas Rowlandson, 1811)

celebrated text, but little improvement followed for 400 years. A new era in obstetric education was ushered in by the publication of Rösslin's *Der Schwangerenn Frawen und Hebammen Rosengarte* in 1513 (Fig. 1-2). Although it was based in large part on Soranus's *Gynecology* and contained little that was original, Rösslin's book had the great merit of being published in the vernacular German, which the midwives of his land could read and understand. It enjoyed the popularity of numerous editions, and its English translation, *The Byrth of Mankynde,* remained a best seller for 100 years.

Scipione Mercurio, who was born in the very year that *The Byrth of Mankynde* was published, soon introduced into Italy a similar work, *La Commare O'Raccoglitrice* (1595–1596), for the guidance of midwives. Like its German and English counterparts, this book received a warm reception and went into 20 editions. It is still remembered for its description of cesarean section and for the first mentioning of pelvic contraction as an indication for the operation. Obstetrics rapidly acquired the dignity of a clinical science with the pub-

lication of more scholarly treatises, outstanding among which were Mauriceau's *Traité des maladies des femmes grosses* (1668), Smellie's *Treatise on the Theory and Practice of Midwifery* (1752–1764), and Denman's *Introduction to the Practice of Midwifery* (1795).

The first obstetric publication in America was reprinted from a London pamphlet of 1663, entitled *A Present To Be Given to Teeming Women by Their Husbands or Friends, Containing Scripture-Directions for Women With Child.* The unhappy recipient was urged to ''prayer, repentance, reading of the Scriptures, meditation, resignation, and preparation for death.'' Samuel Bard's *Compendium of the Theory and Practice of Midwifery,* the first obstetric text by an American author, was published in 1807.

With the practice of obstetrics confined largely to midwives, a few achieved wide renown for their skill, writings, or devotion to their calling. Louise Bourgeois was selected by Henry IV in 1601 to deliver his wife, Marie de Medici, of their son, the future Louis XIII. The candle of this French midwife's fame was rapidly snuffed

FIG. 1-2. Title page of one of first texts for midwives (Heinrich Steiner's 1537 edition of Rösslins Rosengarte).

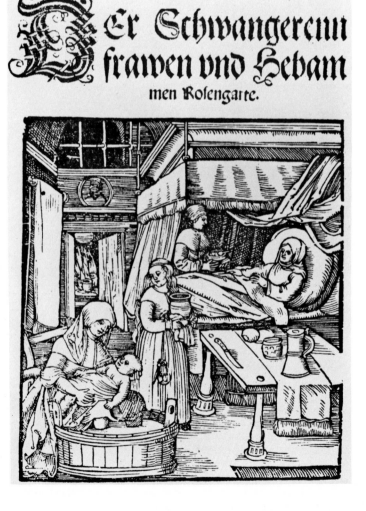

out, however, in 1627, when another of her fashionable clients, Madame de Montpensier, the Duchess of Orleans, tarnished her attendant's brilliant record by dying of puerperal infection. Perhaps most distinguished of all the French midwives was the scholarly Madame Boivin (1773–1841).

New Orleans was probably the first American community to license midwives, in 1722, but the unlicensed were permitted to practice their craft in the rest of Colonial America unhampered and unsupervised. Scarcely ever was a physician called to attend a woman in childbirth, except in dire emergency. As recently as 1920 no fewer than 4000 midwives were still practicing in North Carolina, where in one year they conducted 34,000 deliveries, one third of all births in that state. In New York City 3000 midwives handled 40% of the deliveries in 1909; in 1956 14 midwives performed a total of only 142 deliveries in the same city. The last of New York's licensed midwives retired in 1963, having attended her final patient in 1961. Superseding this unlamented obstetric guild is a growing corps of well-trained nurse–midwives, more than 2000 of whom were practicing in the United States at the end of 1983, the majority certified by the American College of Nurse–Midwives.

Early incursions of men into the obstetric domain were bitterly resisted by the women midwives. Their gradual acceptance and ultimate rise to a position of obstetric superiority have been credited to three developments: (1) Ambroïse Paré's popularization of podalic version in the second half of the 16th century; (2) the amorous intrigues and resultant obstetric activity in the Court of France during the 17th century, which required a high measure of secrecy; and (3) the introduction of the obstetric forceps. In Colonial America the prejudice against male midwives did not begin to melt away until the second half of the 18th century. First to penetrate this barrier was John Moultrie, who settled in Charleston, South Carolina, in 1733 and practiced obstetrics successfully there for the next 50 years. In 1765 William Shippen of Philadelphia began a course of lectures on midwifery, the first in America. Before the end of the 18th century a lying-in ward had been established in the New York Almshouse, the New York Lying-In Hospital had been organized, and obstetrics had achieved a respected place in American medicine. Yet not until 1813, more than six decades after its inception, did the medical school of the University of Pennsylvania make its course in obstetrics obligatory. At the Harvard Medical School, founded in 1782, no provision was made for instruction in obstetrics until 1815, with the appointment of Walter Channing as lecturer.

ANTENATAL CARE

Only in the present century has medical supervision during pregnancy achieved general acceptance. Earlier, the physician's role was limited to that of accoucheur at the woman's labor and delivery. He was called upon, in addition, when complications arose during pregnancy, but routine antenatal care as it is now understood was unheard of. As early as the 17th century, a few obstetricians recognized the importance of preventive midwifery. In Mauriceau's textbook, for example, we find the statement: "The pregnant woman is like a ship upon a stormy sea full of whitecaps, and the good pilot who is in charge must guide her with prudence if he is to avoid a shipwreck." From 1800 to 1840 in France alone no fewer than 55 doctoral dissertations were published on the hygiene of pregnant women, but most contained little that was original or scientifically valuable. A major advance in antenatal care was made in 1843, when the consistent occurrence of proteinuria in patients with eclampsia was noted. Another half century elapsed before the association of hypertension with this disorder was recorded, but not until almost 20 years later was elevated blood pressure accorded proper significance as a harbinger of eclampsia.

With the dawn of the 20th century obstetricians finally awoke to an appreciation of their expanding medical responsibility. In 1901 John W. Ballantyne, pleading for hospital facilities for pregnant women, succeeded in having one bed reserved for antenatal patients in the Royal Maternity Hospital in Edinburgh. With eloquence and perseverance he urged the medical supervision of obstetric patients throughout pregnancy rather than only when ill or in labor. Consultations for pregnant and nursing women were initiated in Paris about the same time. A great boon to antenatal care in the United States resulted from the affiliation of the Instructive District Nursing Association of Boston with the Boston Lying-In Hospital in 1901. In 1907 two teacher–nurses were engaged by the Association for Improving the Conditions of the Poor in New York City for the specific purpose of rendering antenatal care and instruction. The death rate among the infants born to the mothers who received this new type of supervision fell from 17.0% to 4.9%. The first maternity center in the United States was established one decade later, by the Women's City Club of New York, with the avowed objective of providing medical and nursing care of every woman in the district from the onset of pregnancy until one month postpartum. Physicians and clinics soon assumed responsibility for the complete medical care of expectant mothers. Obstetrics had gone beyond the confines of the delivery chamber and acquired the new dignity of preventive medicine.

THE BEGINNINGS OF EMBRYOLOGY

From the time of Aristotle, the development of the mammalian egg was believed to result from the admixture within the uterus of the menstrual blood and the male semen. The female seed was thought to contribute the substance of the embryo, the male the formative impulse to its growth. A somewhat different view was espoused by Galen. The female semen, he taught, originated in the ovarian vessels, and after being separated or strained in the ovaries, which were known in his day as the female testes, passed down the fallopian tubes and into the uterus. Contact with the male semen resulted in a frothy coagulum, from which the embryo evolved. For a thousand years the doctrine of preformation (*emboîtement*) prevailed, which regarded the fetus as the product of the female of the species. Each human being, in compressed form, lay encapsulated within the body of its mother, successive generations resulting from the mere unshelling and subsequent increase in size of the next order of individuals.

The rival theory of *epigenesis,* probably voiced first by Aristotle, was resurrected in the early 17th century by William Harvey, best known for his discovery of the circulation of the blood. This doctrine, which denied that the organism exists encased in a preformed state within the mother and which viewed embryogenesis instead as the gradual aggregation and building up of the body's component parts, received almost no attention, however, until revived in 1759 by Caspar Friedrich Wolff's celebrated *Theoria Generationis.* This work antedated Darwin's equally radical *Origin of Species* by exactly 100 years. Peering through his microscope into the chick embryo, Wolff saw no expanding of a preexisting form but instead a host of minute globules that produced the organs of the embryo by growth and multiplication. With the publication of Wolff's treatise the doctrine of *emboîtement* was dealt its final, crushing blow.

Meantime, the unsuccessful quest for the mammalian ovum, which was to engage man's attention for two millennia, continued. Between 1666 and 1672 Jan van Horne and Jan Swammerdam, working together in Leyden; the Danish anatomist Nils Stensen; and the Dutch Reinier de Graaf had developed the idea that the human female testes, like the ovaries of birds, produce eggs. While the others procrastinated and quibbled over priority, de Graaf published his own observations in a brilliant volume entitled *De Mulierum Organis Generationi Inservientibus,* which resulted in the eponymic association of his name with the ovarian follicles. De Graaf made the great mistake, however, of assuming the entire contents of the mammalian follicle to be the ovum, for when he immersed the ovaries of swine or cows in boiling water, the contents of the follicle coagulated into a white opaque mass, which when shelled out of the ovary, resembled the boiled albumen of the hen's egg. Another century and a half was to elapse before the actual discovery of the mammalian ovum in 1827.

Karl Ernst von Baer, studying the embryology of the dog, had departed slightly from the usual procedure of examining the embryos in sequential stages of development and was working backward instead, studying the later stages first in order to recognize the next earlier more easily. In this manner he had observed embryos of 24 days, next 12 days, then free blastocysts in the uterus, and finally tubal ova. He recounted:

It remained for me to ascertain the condition of the ova in the ovary, for it seemed clearer than light that the ova were not the very small Graafian vesicles expelled from the ovary, nor did I consider it likely that such solid little bodies had been coagulated in the tubes from the fluid of the vesicles. When I examined the ovaries before incising them, I clearly distinguished in almost all the vesicles, a whitish-yellow point which was in no way attached to the covering of the vesicle, but as pressure exerted with a probe on the vesicle indicated clearly, swam free in its liquid. Led on more by inquisitiveness than by hope of seeing the ovules in the ovaries with the naked eye through all the coverings of the Graafian vesicles, I opened a vesicle, of which, as I said, I had raised the top with the edge of a scalpel—so clearly did I see it distinguished from the surrounding mucus—and placed it under the microscope. I was astounded when I saw an ovule, already recognized from the tubes, so plainly that a blind man could scarcely deny it. It is truly remarkable and astonishing that a thing so persistently and constantly sought and in all compendia of physiology considered as inextricable, could be put before the eyes with such facility.

The origin of the mammalian ovum identified at last, the science of embryology found a new footing and was soon infused with the vigor of fresh discovery. Less than two decades after von Baer's recognition of the ovum, Martin Barry demonstrated a spermatozoon within the egg cell, and in 1875 Hertwig witnessed the actual union of male and female gametes.

THE OBSTETRIC PELVIS

Like the stumps of old trees, notions long cherished are hard to root out. For countless centuries practitioners of the obstetric art remained wedded to the erroneous concept that birth entails the self-propulsion of the fetus through a distensible pelvic girdle, whose bones separate to permit its passenger's easy egress. Difficulty in labor, it followed, resulted from faulty separation at the pelvic joints. This interpretation of the birth process was first challenged by Vesalius in 1543 and shortly thereafter by his pupil Arantius, but their protestations were ignored for more than a century, until the publication of Deventer's *Novum Lumen* in 1701. Deventer again insisted on the unyielding character of the pelvic inlet, but erred in his belief that the sacrum and coccyx are displaced backward during labor to permit the passage of the infant's head.

Pelvic mensuration was introduced by Levret in 1753, with his elaborate system of pelvic planes and axes, and gained clinical applicability the following year when Smellie proposed the diagonal conjugate as a simple, reliable index of the inlet's capacity. In addition to the impetus it gave clinical pelvimetry, Smellie's *Treatise on the Theory and Practice of Midwifery* is noteworthy for its lucid, accurate, and concise description of the labor mechanism, contained in the first chapter. In the New Sydenham Society's edition of this classic, A. H. McClintock comments that "had Smellie made no other contribution to midwifery than what is contained in this chapter, he would still have placed accoucheurs under a perpetual obligation."

Clinical pelvimetry achieved widespread acceptance and popularization following the publication of Jean–Louis Baudelocque's *L'Art des accouchemens* in 1781, but Baudelocque's best known contribution embodied an error that was to hinder obstetric practice for the next century and a half. The anteroposterior diameter of the pelvic inlet, he taught, could be estimated reliably by subtracting 3 inches from the external conjugate, measured "from the middle of the pubis to the tip of the spine of the last lumbar vertebra." Baudelocque's diameter, as it soon came to be known, could be measured with greater ease for the examiner and less discomfort for the patient than could the internal conjugate, and it rapidly overshadowed the latter in popularity. The obstetric unreliability of external pelvimetry was demonstrated repeatedly in the ensuing years, but so great was the appeal of this simple approach that obstetricians have finally renounced it only within the last two generations.

One of the first to stress the unreliability of the external conjugate as a measure of pelvic adequacy was Gustav Adolf Michaelis, in his monumental work, *Das Enge Becken* (1851). This book, based on the study of 1000 patients, provided the basis of modern clinical knowledge of the bony pelvis. It has been recognized as one of the most important contributions to obstetric literature; the late John Whitridge Williams was fond of saying that no obstetrician could pretend to understand contracted pelves until he had read it. *Das Enge Becken* was edited and published three years after Michaelis's death by his friend Carl Litzmann, but ironically its value was overlooked for several years. Indeed, only a few copies of the first edition were ever sold, the publisher marking the remainder as unsalable. Not until 1865 had the importance of the book attained sufficient recognition to warrant its reprinting.

Continuing and extending Michaelis's interest, Litzmann contributed another classic to the obstetric literature, *Die Formen des Beckens,* published in 1861. Its very first paragraph contains one of the most lucid and succinct interpretive descriptions of the female pelvis. Wrote Litzmann:

> The pelvis fulfills more extensive functions in the female body than in the male. In the female it forms not merely the bony foundation of the trunk . . . to which strong and numerous muscles are attached, but also shelters the largest part of the sexual apparatus in addition to the distal end of the intestinal canal and urinary passages, and thereby assumes great importance in reproduction. In addition to admitting the male organ during coitus, it has to provide space for the whole uterus at the beginning of pregnancy, and later for ex-

pansion of the lower uterine segment at least, and at birth a passageway into the outer world for the mature fetus together with its membranes. Nature has understood how to satisfy, in an amazing manner, the diverse and to some degree contradictory demands with which she is thus confronted. She has imparted the necessary firmness to the pelvis with maximal economy in bony substance by giving it an annular shape and supporting its joints with powerful ligaments, but amassing larger concentrations of bone only in the regions exposed directly to pressure. She has placed the canal that opens at the lowermost part of the trunk in such a position that the pelvis can maintain the burden of the abdominal viscera and provide support and purchase for the enclosed organs, by inclining the pelvis anteriorly at a sharp angle to the horizon, bending its axis in a curve convex posteriorly, and covering and finishing its walls with contractile and elastic soft parts; and in this way also achieving adequate capacity and dilatability for the act of birth. However, the space is so proportioned that even a relatively slight deviation from its normal size can interfere with delivery, insofar as a correspondingly more favorable condition in the remaining birth factors does not compensate for the difficulties.

Roentgen pelvimetry, the ultimate in precise mensuration, was introduced in 1897 in Germany by Albert and in France by Budin and Varnier.

THE OBSTETRIC FORCEPS*

The obstetric forceps, the sole surgical device reserved specifically for the obstetrician's use, has been characterized as "this noble instrument, which has done more to abridge human suffering, and to save human life, than any other instrument in the whole range of surgical appliances." Its origins lie buried in antiquity. A prehensile instrument equipped with teeth was probably used by Arabian physicians in the 11th and 12th centuries to extract the head of the dead fetus, for a device of this type is illustrated in an early manuscript of Albucasis, who lived at Cyropolis, a city of Media on the Caspian Sea. Even earlier evidence, from the 2nd or 3rd century, of the use of forceps for delivery of the living child was believed seen in a marble bas-relief said to have been discovered in the early 20th century in the vicinity of Rome (Fig. 1-3). This relief was recently adjudged fraudulent, however, and has been destroyed. The obstetric forceps for the delivery of living infants was introduced into clinical practice by the colorful Chamberlen family toward the close of the 16th century.

In 1569 William Chamberlen fled with his Huguenot family from Paris to Southampton to escape the persecution of Catherine de Medici. Two of his sons, curiously, were given the same name, Peter. These men,

---

* The material under the headings The Obstetric Forceps and Puerperal Fever is reprinted from Clin Obstet Gynecol 3:761, 788, 1960.

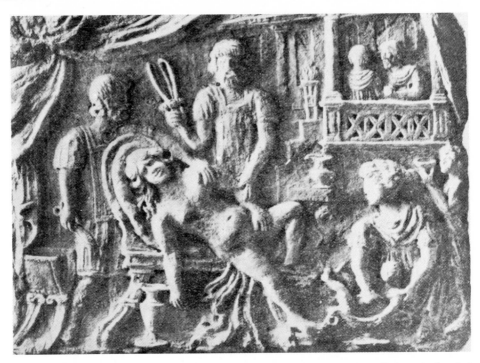

FIG. 1-3. Bas-relief of a birth scene depicting the obstetric forceps, allegedly from 2nd or 3rd century but now considered a fraud.

both of whom became barber–surgeons, were identified as Peter the Elder and Peter the Younger, and it is the former who invented, and probably constructed with his own hands, the instrument from which the modern obstetric forceps has evolved. Although consisting merely of two curved pieces of iron, shaped like spoons and united at a pivot joint, this invention remained a closely guarded secret, passed from one Chamberlen to another, for three generations and nearly 100 years.

The secret instrument was carried about in a massive wooden chest trimmed with gilt. Two men were required to lift it, and the Chamberlens are said to have used a special carriage for its transport. The eyes of the laboring patient were always blindfolded, lest the secret be discovered.

Peter the Elder achieved renown as a surgeon–midwife and attended both Queen Anne and Henrietta Maria, wife of Charles I. A third Peter Chamberlen, son of Peter the Younger, came to be known as Dr. Peter because of the medical degrees he acquired at Padua, Oxford, and Cambridge. Eccentric in all his activities, Dr. Peter was admitted to fellowship in the Royal College of Physicians on the condition that he "change his mode of dress" and accept "the decent and sober dress of its members." After establishing his reputation as an obstetric surgeon, Dr. Peter, in a manner reminiscent of the 20th century's labor leaders, attempted to organize the midwives of London. This enterprising Chamberlen, plying the female practitioners of his art with wine and promises of a variety of benefactions, proposed their

enrollment in a guild, to be taught and licensed by him. He, in turn, was to be paid a fee for each child they delivered and was to be summoned for consultation in all difficult cases. Only through the intercession of the Archbishop of Canterbury were the midwives able to emancipate themselves from the control of their self-styled benefactor.

The first effort to sell the family secret was made by Hugh Chamberlen, Senior, eldest son of Dr. Peter. While visiting Paris in 1670, he boasted of a device by which, he said, he could deliver any woman in 8 minutes and offered to sell it to the French government for a large sum. A consultation was arranged with Mauriceau, "the oracle of the obstetrics of his century." Mauriceau, coincidentally, had just been called to see a rachitic dwarf whose pelvis was so contracted that after several days of labor vaginal delivery appeared impossible. Chamberlen locked himself in a room with the hapless patient but after three hours of violent struggle emerged exhausted and unsuccessful. The patient died the following day, undelivered, her uterus ruptured. The Chamberlen invention, needless to say, remained unsold.

Hugh, Senior, enjoyed high political favor. He served as Physician in Ordinary to Charles II and attended Princess Anne of Denmark in childbirth. In Amsterdam he later sold a secret, but probably not the forceps, to Roger van Roonhuyze, a Dutch obstetrician. Roonhuyze, seeking to capitalize on his investment, achieved passage of a municipal law in 1747 requiring every practicing physician to purchase this secret under the pledge of silence. One recalcitrant, however, refused to pay this tribute to Roonhuyze and induced the latter's assistant to obtain a sketch of the instrument. The drawing, of a curved lever, was promptly sent to Paris, where a second lever was added by Jean Palfyn, this new instrument being known as the *mains de fer* (iron hands) for grasping the fetal head.

Not until 1813 was the actual instrument of the Chamberlen family revealed. In the house in which Dr. Peter died in 1683 and in which his descendants lived until 1715 when the residence was sold, a Mrs. Kemball, mother-in-law of a later owner of the property, happened upon a previously unknown trapdoor while rummaging one day in the attic. Between the floor and the ceiling she found a box containing a variety of oddments, including letters, fans, trinkets, a Bible dated 1695, and four pairs of obstetric forceps—undoubtedly the Chamberlen secret. These instruments are now in the possession of the Royal Society of Medicine in London.

The design of the obstetric forceps was first made public in 1733 in a book by Edmund Chapman. Since that date it has been modified and redesigned in new form and size probably more times than any other surgical instrument. Hundreds of models have been devised, each identified by the name of its inventor; until the mid-20th century, scarcely a year passed without the addition of at least one new instrument to the obstetrician's forceps arsenal.

PUERPERAL FEVER

Infection of the genital tract has ever been one of the leading causes of death from childbirth. Commonly known as childbed fever, this scourge was believed, from the time of Hippocrates, to result from suppression of the uterine discharge after delivery. Noting the failure of lactation among afflicted women, Hieronymus Mercurialis (1530–1606) concluded that the milk, instead of flowing to the breasts, localized in the uterus and produced the purulent discharge from this organ. "Milk fever" thus arose as an alternate name for the disorder. It assumed epidemic proportions with the establishment of lying-in hospitals, abetted by the frequent internal examinations by unwashed hands; contaminated instruments, dressings, and linens; crowding of patients; and lack of isolation facilities. The first recorded epidemic occurred in the Hôtel Dieu in Paris in 1646. Later statistics from the Allmänna Barnbördhuset in Stockholm reported one maternal death for every five women delivered. At the Allgemeines Krankenhaus in Vienna an epidemic beginning in 1821 and lasting 20 months took the lives of 829 out of 5139 parturients, a toll of almost one in six. From May 1 to May 10, 1856, 31 deaths occurred among the 32 patients delivered at the Maternité in Paris. The search for an understanding of this disease and the efforts to cope with it have produced some of the warmest debates and most colorful prose in the annals of medicine.

Among the first correctly to call attention to the mode of transmission of childbed fever was Dr. Alexander Gordon of Aberdeen, who wrote in 1795:

> This disease seized such women only, as were visited, or delivered, by a practitioner, or taken care of by a nurse, who had previously attended patients affected with the disease. . . . I arrived at that certainty in the matter, that I could venture to foretell what women would be affected with the disease, upon hearing by what midwife they were to be delivered, or by what nurse they were to be attended, during their lying-in: and almost in every instance, my prediction was verified. . . .
>
> In short I had evident proofs of its infectious nature, and that the infection was as readily communicated as that of the small pox or measles, and operated more speedily than any other infection, with which I am acquainted.
>
> . . . I had evident proofs that every person, who had been with a patient in the Puerperal Fever, became charged with an atmosphere of infection, which was communicated to every pregnant woman, who happened to come within its sphere. . . .
>
> It is a disagreeable declaration for me to mention, that I myself was the means of carrying the infection to a great number of women.

Several years later, Gordon's opinions were echoed by James Blundell, in his lectures on midwifery at Guy's Hospital in London:

> In my own family, I had rather that those I esteemed the most should be delivered, unaided, in a stable—by the manager side—than that they should receive the best help in the fairest apartment, but exposed to the vapours of this pitiless disease. Gossiping friends, wet nurses, monthly nurses, the practitioner himself, these are the channels by which, as I suspect, the infection is principally conveyed.

Others began to take up the cry. In 1842 Thomas Watson, professor of medicine in King's College, London, voiced

> the dreadful suspicion, that the hand which is relied upon for succour in the painful and perilous hour of child-birth, and which is intended to secure the safety of both mother and child, but especially of the mother, may literally become the innocent cause of her destruction: innocent no longer, however, if, after warning and knowledge of the risk, suitable means are not used to avert a castastrophe so shocking.

Stimulated by the force of Watson's writing, Oliver Wendell Holmes, then 34 years old, undertook a critical analysis of the recorded experience with childbed fever as published from several European centers. His resulting essay, "The Contagiousness of Puerperal Fever," was read before the Boston Society for Medical Improvement, February 13, 1843, and subsequently published in *The New England Quarterly Journal of Med-*

icine and Surgery. Although it contained little that was new or original, Holmes's essay has come to be regarded as one of the classics of American medicine, for by its incisive logic and brilliance of statement it roused the profession from its complacent acceptance of epidemics of infection as acts of Providence.

"The recurrence of long series of cases like those I have cited," Holmes wrote,

> reported by the most interested to disbelieve in contagion, scattered along through an interval of half a century, might have been thought sufficient to satisfy the minds of all inquirers that here was something more than a singular coincidence. But if on a more extended observation, it should be found that the same ominous groups of cases, clustering about individual practitioners, were observed in a remote country, at different times, and in widely separated regions, it would seem incredible that any should be found too prejudiced or indolent to accept the solemn truth knelled into their ears by the funeral bells from both sides of the ocean—the plain conclusion that the physician and the disease entered hand in hand, into the chamber of the unsuspecting patient.

With an eloquence rarely equaled in medical writing, Holmes emphasized the physician's role as a carrier of infection:

> It is as a lesson rather than as a reproach that I call up the memory of these irreparable errors and wrongs. No tongue can tell the heartbreaking calamity they have caused; they have closed the eyes just opened upon a new world of love and happiness; they have bowed the strength of manhood into the dust; they have cast the helplessness of infancy into the stranger's arms, or bequeathed it with less cruelty the death of its dying parent. There is no tone deep enough for regret, and no voice loud enough for warning. The woman about to become a mother, or with her new-born infant upon her bosom, should be the object of trembling care and sympathy wherever she bears her tender burden, or stretches her aching limbs. The very outcast of the streets has pity upon her sister in degradation when the seal of promised maternity is impressed upon her. The remorseless vengeance of the law, brought down upon its victim by a machinery as sure as destiny, is arrested in its fall at a word which reveals her transient claim for mercy. The solemn prayer of the liturgy singles out her sorrows from the multiplied trials of life, to plead for her in the hour of peril. God forbid that any member of the profession to which she trusts her life, doubly precious at that eventful period, should hazard it negligently, unadvisedly, or selfishly!

Holmes's conclusions were published in a journal with a small circulation and one that proved short-lived. Had they not been subjected to bitter attack by Charles D. Meigs and Hugh Lenox Hodge, professors of obstetrics in the Jefferson Medical College and the University of Pennsylvania, respectively, and the leading figures in

American obstetrics, probably little attention would have been drawn to the clinical speculations of this young anatomist. Meigs's bombastic denunciation of Holmes's theory, however, brought it into the full daylight of debate. Vigorously denying that the physician might be responsible for the transmission of disease, Hodge lectured:

> The mere announcement of such an opinion must strike one with horror, and might induce you, at once to abandon a pursuit fraught with such danger and involving such terrible responsibilities; for what rewards can possibly compensate the obstetrician, who has reason to believe that he has actually poisoned one of those valued and lovely beings who rested confidently and implicitly on him for safety and deliverance?

Many teachers of obstetrics continued to deny that puerperal fever was contagious, and as late as 1854 Meigs advocated copious bloodletting for its cure. In 1855, therefore, after he had been professor of anatomy at the Harvard Medical School for eight years and its dean for six, Holmes republished his original essay, together with additional remarks in answer to his adversaries. This pamphlet, entitled *Puerperal Fever as a Private Pestilence,* silenced most of the remaining opposition to his views and led to their final acceptance.

More dissimilar personalities would be hard to picture than the urbane, cultured, and self-possessed Holmes and his European counterpart in the conquest of puerperal fever, the irascible and emotionally unstable Ignaz Philipp Semmelweis, who ultimately became insane. The dedicated role of the latter, emphasized by the tragedy of his personal life, has doubtless gained in drama in the retelling.

In 1846 Semmelweis, a Magyar, was appointed assistant, under Professor Johann Klein, in the first obstetric division of the Vienna Lying-In Hospital, where the medical students received their training. The hospital's second division, identical to the first in all other respects, accepted no medical students, the deliveries being performed by midwives. In the six-year period 1841–1846, death from puerperal fever had been the lot of 1 woman of every 11 delivered on the first division; the corresponding mortality on the second division was 1 in 29. During 1846 the disparity grew even greater, until the death rate on the first division was ten times that on the second. But Semmelweis made the interesting observation that the mortality was negligible among the women assigned to his division who delivered before reaching the hospital (and hence without any internal examinations during labor).

Semmelweis struggled with the problem but made no progress toward its solution until the tragic death of his friend and colleague, Professor Kolletschka, who succumbed from a knife scratch accidentally suffered during an autopsy. The pathologic changes in Kolletschka's body, Semmelweis observed, were identical to those in the women dead of puerperal fever. He quickly concluded that the scourge of his clinic was caused by putrid material derived from living organisms and that the poison was transmitted from the dead body to the living patient by the examining finger. The students, who commonly went from the autopsy room directly to the parturient patient, were the obvious connecting link. Almost identical views, it will be noted, had already been voiced by others, but Semmelweis, unschooled in foreign languages and unfamiliar with the English literature, had reached his conclusions independently.

Fired with the elation of discovery, the impulsive Semmelweis promptly posted a notice on the door of his clinic, dated May 15, 1847, ordering every doctor and student to wash his hands thoroughly in a basin of chlorine water before entering the maternity ward. In 6 months, despite the grumbling of the students and the apathy of Professor Klein, the maternal mortality of the first division had dropped to one fourth its previous level and in 1848 attained a new low of 3%, surpassing the record of the midwives' division.

Like Holmes in America, Semmelweis soon came under the searing attack of reactionary authorities. Refused reappointment in the Vienna Lying-In Hospital, he returned, embittered, to his native Hungary. To Scanzoni, perhaps the outstanding figure in European obstetrics, who had stubbornly opposed the newfangled idea of contagion, the intemperate Semmelweis was goaded to write:

> Your doctrine, Professor, is based upon the corpses of parturient women murdered out of ignorance. If you think my theory wrong, I challenge you to communicate to me your reasons. . . . But should you continue, without having refuted my theory, to teach your pupils the theory of epidemic puerperal fever, I declare you a murderer before God and the world.

Disillusioned and frequently irrational, Semmelweis died August 13, 1865. Like his friend Kolletschka, he had developed septicemia from a cut on his finger.

In the very year of Semmelweis's death, two other principal actors in the drama of puerperal fever were making ready in the wings. Louis Pasteur had already begun his studies in fermentation, which led in 1879 to his demonstration of the villain in the piece, the hemolytic streptococcus. With the introduction of practical methods of asepsis by Joseph Lister, the specter of obstetric as well as surgical infection was laid to rest. The 20th century's antibiotics have brought a new air of tranquility to the obstetric scene. Puerperal infection still shows itself, but usually in subdued guise, rarely as a killer.

CESAREAN SECTION

Cesarean section, the most dramatic of all surgical operations, is also one of the oldest (Fig. 1-4). Earliest records trace its origins to the reign of Numa Pompilius (715–672 B.C.), a legendary king of Rome, who decreed that the child be excised from the womb of any woman who died late in pregnancy. Known initially as the *lex regia* (royal law), the requirement for postmortem section continued under the rule of the Caesars, when it acquired the name *lex caesarea*. As late as 1749, a Sicilian physician was condemned to death because of his failure to open the uterus of a recently deceased patient.

As an alternative explanation for the operation's

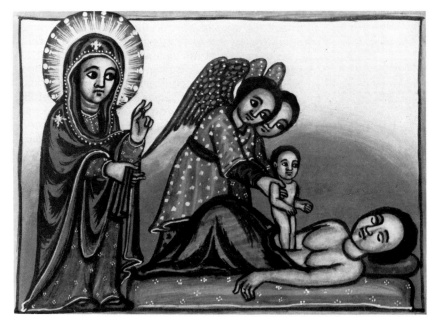

FIG. 1-4. Postmortem cesarean section, from old Ethiopian manuscript. Priest gives his blessing as archangels Michael and Gabriel extract infant from its dead mother's abdomen. Once infant was saved for baptism, purpose of operation was fulfilled. (British Museum, London)

name, some scholars have derived it from the Latin *caedere,* meaning to cut, an abdominal birth being termed *partus caesareus.* No valid basis can be found for the widely held belief that Julius Caesar, who was born about 100 B.C., was delivered by abdominal section and that the operation was named for him; indeed, this myth is controverted by all available evidence. The operation was performed then only on the dead or dying, and for many centuries thereafter was uniformly fatal when attempted on the living woman. Yet Caesar's mother survived his birth by many years, as proved by his letters written to her while he was engaged in his foreign wars. Others of similar or identical name antedated the great emperor; the name Caesar, therefore, could scarcely have been taken from his alleged mode of birth.

According to ancient belief, Buddha was delivered through the flank of his mother (about 563 B.C.), and Brahma is said to have emerged through the umbilicus. Abdominal delivery was also known to the ancient Jews. The Talmud prescribes laws of hygiene for survivors of the operation but provides no clear evidence that cesarean section was actually performed on a living woman.

The celebrated operation on Frau Nufer, in the year 1500, has been interpreted not as a true cesarean section but as a laparotomy for abdominal pregnancy. The patient's husband, a Swiss sowgelder, successfully delivered his wife of a living infant by cutting open her abdomen after 13 midwives and several barbers had failed in their vaginal attempts. Frau Nufer, we are told, lived to bear six more children, including twins.

The first documented, indubitably authentic cesarean operation on a living patient was performed on April 21, 1610, by two surgeons, Trautmann and Gusth. Their patient survived until the 25th postoperative day, longer than the vast majority of the hapless women who were subjected to cesarean section during the next two centuries. Most died either promptly, of hemorrhage, or within a week, of infection; they rarely recovered. From 1750 until the end of the 18th century the operation was carried out 24 times in Paris without a single maternal survival, according to Baudelocque. Denman reported a similarly bleak experience in England.

The first half of the 19th century saw a little improvement in the operation's record; in 1867 Nuyer reported a mortality of 54% among 1605 cases collected from the literature. In Paris, however, not one mother survived a cesarean section during the 90-year period from 1787 to 1876, and in Great Britain the maternal mortality was recorded at 85%. The American experience was scarcely more encouraging. By 1878 the operation had been carried out only 80 times in the United States, with a maternal mortality of 52.5%. At the Sloane Maternity Hospital (later renamed the Sloane Hospital for Women) not a single cesarean section was performed among the first 1000 confinements. Indeed, the operation was attempted but once from the hospital's founding in 1888 until 1897, and that case ended in disaster. In the entire city of Philadelphia, with a population of

800,000 in 1878, there had likewise been but one cesarean section in the preceding 40 years.

Harris, who reviewed the American cases in 1878, noted that the chances for success seemed greater when the operation was performed remote from the centers of civilization: 5 recoveries occurred among 9 rural patients who had operated upon themselves in desperation or had been gored by a bull, while in New York City during the same period only 1 of 11 survived who were operated upon by physicians. As an example of the former group, Harris cited the case of a woman, who in 1769, "actuated by a frenzied impatience, and violent of temper, to obtain relief in the quickest way, without regard to consequences," performed the operation with the hilt of a broken butcher knife, "cutting at one stroke through the abdominal and uterine walls, and making a two-and-a-half-inch incision into the thigh of the foetus." The mother's intestines were replaced and the wound was sutured by a plantation midwife, who failed, however, to remove the placenta. This was done by a surgeon, who reopened the wound and cleaned the blood and dirt from the peritoneal cavity, the original operation having been performed on the ground. The mother recovered and is said to have made preparations for a similar operation upon herself a year or two later, but was forced to submit to a natural delivery.

The first successful cesarean section in the United States, according to one version, was performed in 1794, in a cabin near Staunton, Virginia, by Dr. Jesse Bennett on his own wife. After Mrs. Bennett, a young primigravida, had labored for three days without result, consultation was obtained with Dr. Alexander Humphreys, a physician of greater experience, who confirmed Dr. Bennett's suspicion of contracted pelvis and the impossibility of a natural delivery, and proposed a destructive operation on the baby as the only means of saving the mother's life. Having already despaired of her own chances, Mrs. Bennett begged that a cesarean section be done for the sake of the child. This, however, Dr. Humphreys steadfastly refused, stating that he would not be the cause of his patient's death. Under the importunings of his suffering wife, Dr. Bennett thereupon announced to his older colleague that he himself would perform the operation and, if fate ordained, would assume the full responsibility for her death.

An operating table was improvised with two wooden planks, supported on barrels. Without anesthesia, and while two Negro women held his wife, Dr. Bennett rapidly incised her abdomen and uterus and extracted the living infant. To protect her against a recurrence of this ordeal, should she survive, he then quickly removed his wife's ovaries before closing her abdomen with linen thread. Both mother and child did indeed survive; but despite its successful outcome, Dr. Bennett never reported the case. When questioned years later concerning his reticence, Bennett replied: "No strange doctors would believe that the operation could be done in the Virginia backwoods and the mother live, and I'll be damn'd if I'd give them a chance to call me a liar."

The authenticity of the Bennett case has been questioned by some historians. Better documented as the first cesarean section in America is the operation by John Lambert Richmond of Newton, Ohio, in April, 1827.

To the mid-19th century, and even beyond, surgeons labored under the mistaken notion that the uterine wound at cesarean section required no treatment except cleansing. Sutures were held to be dangerous, leading to peritonitis. From 1769, when the Frenchman Lebas closed a uterine incision with three silk threads, the few attempts at uterine suture during the next century failed to dispel this fear of infection. The nonabsorbable sutures of silk or linen, left long and protruding from the wound to facilitate later removal, almost invariably led to the predicted, feared result. Following prolonged labor, on the other hand, with the uterine musculature lacking adequate retractile power, massive blood loss usually occurred from the edges of the incision if left unsutured. A satisfactory technique of closing the uterine wound therefore constituted one of the major improvements in the cesarean operation.

Silver wire was first used successfully for this purpose in 1852 by Frank E. Polin, a surgeon of Springfield, Kentucky. Although Polin did not bother to report his case, the experiences of less reticent surgeons of pioneer America soon found their way into the literature. Between 1867 and 1880 uterine sutures had been used in at least 16 cesarean sections in the United States. Only in 1882, however, with publication of Max Sänger's widely heralded monograph, was full recognition given to accurate coaptation of the wound edges as an essential part of the cesarean operation. Sänger's technique of longitudinal incision and suture of the uterine fundus has since been known as the classical cesarean section.

While the fundal incision has been largely superseded by approaches through the lower uterine segment, the cardinal features of Sänger's technique endure—hemostasis by suture and accurate approximation of the muscle edges. The cesarean operation of the mid-20th century, aided by the other advances of modern practice, has been shorn of its terror; many obstetric services can now boast of series of 1000 consecutive cases without a single maternal fatality.

The cesarean technique popularized by Sänger sharply reduced the hazard of hemorrhage, but the problem of infection remained. Even before the publication of Sänger's report, Edoardo Porro demonstrated a method of circumventing both dangers of abdominal delivery by the addition of a similarly formidable procedure, hysterectomy. Before 1863 abdominal hysterectomy had proved fatal in seven out of eight of the patients on whom it was attempted; only in three cases had it been performed successfully in the United States. The *London Medico-Chirurgical Review* of 1825 referred to it as "one of the most cruel and unfeasible operations that ever was projected or executed by the head or hand of man."

In Pavia, Italy, the 19th century record of cesarean section had been no better than elsewhere. Indeed, no woman had ever survived the operation in that city until the time of Porro. On April 27, 1876, a 25-year-old primigravid dwarf, Julia Cavallini, was referred to Porro's clinic in the university because of the suspicion of a malformed pelvis. She had all the bony stigmas of rickets, and the diagonal conjugate of her pelvis was markedly contracted, measuring only 7 cm. It was obvious to Porro that absolute disproportion existed, and he made elaborate preparations, long in advance, to carry out cesarean section at the time of labor and to amputate the uterus if hemorrhage proved threatening.

Fortunately unknown to Porro, cesarean hysterectomy had been attempted once previously, by Horatio Robinson Storer in 1869, with fatal outcome to both mother and child. Porro's patient went into labor on the morning of May 21, 1876. He had had four weeks for rehearsal of his plans. By midafternoon all was ready and cesarean section was carried out, with the delivery of a living female infant weighing 3300 g. Unable to control the bleeding from the cut edges of the uterus, Porro promptly proceeded according to plan. A wire snare was placed around the uterus and drawn tight at the level of the internal os; then the organ was rapidly excised, together with the left ovary. The patient made a complete recovery. During the ensuing years cesarean hysterectomy, which became known as the Porro operation, was adopted in many centers as the preferred method of abdominal delivery. Modern obstetricians continue to employ it, but with sharply modified indications.

ANESTHESIA FOR CHILDBIRTH

In 1591, so it is said, a gentlewoman of Edinburgh, Eufame Macalyane by name, was burned alive on Castle Hill by order of James VI. The lady's crime: she had secretly applied to the midwife for a potion to assuage the pangs of labor. Was this not a clear and flagrant violation of the scriptural injunction: "In sorrow thou shalt bring forth children" (Gen. 3:16)? Not until 1853, when Queen Victoria inhaled the vapors of chloroform during the birth of Prince Leopold, was opposition to pain relief for the parturient effectively silenced. The word "delivery," in the meantime, was used in a more restricted sense than in today's parlance. In the preanesthetic era, it was the mother who was delivered from her travail, at the moment of birth.

The introduction of anesthesia into obstetrics resulted from the efforts of one man, the gifted seventh son of the village baker of Bathgate, Scotland, James Young Simpson (1811–1870). Word had been received from America that sulfuric ether had been employed successfully during the excision of a neck tumor at the Massachusetts General Hospital on October 16, 1846. Quick to grasp the significance of this event which, in the minds of many, marks the greatest contribution to mankind in the entire history of medicine, and eager to adapt anesthesia to obstetric use, Simpson successfully employed ether on January 19, 1847, for version and extraction in a patient with a contracted pelvis.

The ensuing controversy over the use of pain-relieving drugs for childbirth has rarely been matched in fervor in the annals of obstetrics. Simpson's principal antagonists were the clergy, but they were ably abetted, on both sides of the Atlantic, by some of the most articulate and influential members of the medical profession. With a biblical knowledge equal to that of the prelates who attacked him, Simpson replied that the Book of Genesis also provided divine sanction for anesthesia. He called their attention to the 21st and 22nd verses of the second chapter, describing the creation of Eve from one of Adam's ribs. Did not the Lord prepare Adam for this ordeal by causing him to fall into a deep slumber?

Charles D. Meigs of Philadelphia, who had also opposed Holmes in the controversy over puerperal fever, referred to the pain of parturition as "physiological pain," insisted upon the serious dangers of anesthetics in labor, compared the unconsciousness resulting from them to the stupor of drunkenness, and asked whether any self-respecting woman could afford to submit to such an influence. Ashwell of London added that to use anesthesia in obstetrics constitutes "unnecessary interference with the providentially arranged process of healthy labour . . . sooner or later, to be followed by injurious and fatal consequences."

Simpson recalled the words of Galen, "pain is useless to the pained," and went on to provide scientific evidence of its mortal potential. Collecting by questionnaire the results of thigh amputations, he showed that ether anesthesia had nearly halved the mortality from this operation. "Bodily pain," he wrote,

> with all its concomitant fears and sickening horrors . . . is, with very few, if indeed any exceptions, morally and physically a mighty and unqualified evil. And, surely, any means by which its abolition could possibly be accomplished, with perfect security and safety, deserves to be joyfully and gratefully welcomed by medical science, as one of the most inestimable boons which man could confer upon his suffering fellow-mortals.

In a forceful, impassioned plea to his colleagues, Simpson urged the extension of anesthesia to obstetrics:

> Now, if experience betimes goes fully to prove to us the safety with which ether may, under proper precautions and management, be employed in the course of parturition, then . . . instead of determining . . . whether we shall be "justified" in using this agent . . . it will become, on the other hand, necessary to determine whether on any grounds, moral or medical, a professional man could deem himself "justified" in withholding, and *not* using any such safe means (as we at present presuppose this to be), provided he had the power by it of assuaging the agonies of the last stage of natural labour, and thus counteracting what Velpeau describes as "those piercing cries, that agitation so lively, those excessive efforts, those inex-

pressible agonies, and those pains apparently intolerable," which accompany the termination of natural parturition in the human mother.

As experience had begun to indicate to Simpson some of ether's shortcomings as an obstetric anesthetic, he set out in the autumn of 1847 in quest of a better agent. In collaboration with Drs. Thomas Keith and J. Matthews Duncan, Simpson conducted his experiments at the end of the regular day's work, seated at his dining room table. Countless agents, obtained from the local chemist, were tried. A small quantity of the test liquid was placed in a cup or tumbler, which was then immersed in hot water to increase the volatility. The intrepid trio then proceeded with their hazardous task of inhaling the vapors and recording the effects. In this manner they discovered, for the first time, the anesthetic properties of chloroform.

Exhilarated by the acquisition of this new agent, which appeared superior to ether, Simpson immediately substituted it for the latter in his obstetric practice. On December 1, 1847, with evangelic fervor, he sang the praises of the newly discovered chloroform to his Edinburgh colleagues:

> I do not remember a single patient to have taken it who has not afterwards declared her sincere gratitude for its employment, and her indubitable determination to have recourse again to similar means under similar circumstances. All who happen to have formerly entertained any dread respecting the inhalation, or its effects, have afterwards looked back, both amazed at, and amused with, their previous absurd fears and groundless terrors. Most, indeed, have subsequently set out, like zealous missionaries, to persuade other friends to avail themselves of the same measures of relief, in their hour of trial and travail. . . . All of us, I most sincerely believe, are called upon to employ it by every principle of true humanity, as well as by every principle of true religion. Medical men may oppose for a time the superinduction of anaesthesia in parturition, but they will oppose it in vain; for certainly our patients themselves will force the use of it upon the profession. The whole question is, even now, one merely of time. It is not—Shall the practice come to be generally adopted? but, When shall it come to be generally adopted?

After slowly gaining acceptance during the next few years, anesthesia became an integral part of obstetric practice. For three quarters of a century chloroform was employed almost exclusively. It has been supplanted gradually by other agents.

WOMAN'S FERTILITY AND ITS CONTROL

One of the foremost concerns of men and women has ever been their control of reproduction. Both fertility and sterility have been eagerly sought, each at its appointed time and in chosen circumstances. As stated by

Norman Himes in his *Medical History of Contraception,* "while women have always wanted babies, they have wanted them when they wanted them. And they have wanted neither too few nor too many."

Fertility Deities

Until about 6000 or 7000 years ago, man the hunter was probably hungry much of the time, living in daily competition with his fellow men for their dearly won food. With the adoption of an agrarian economy, competition gave way to cooperation. Now help was needed in cultivating the fields and tending the flocks. Fertility of family as well as soil became important. Specific deities were invoked to augment the family. Gifts were offered, amulets worn, and rituals performed. Ceremonies and deities were passed on from generation to generation as tribes migrated, nation conquered nation, and assimilation occurred. The gods and mythology of the early Greeks, for example, were acquired largely from the Egyptians, whose religious heritage had come, in turn, from the Sumerians and Chaldeans.

In the art of the ancients, deities were usually depicted in human form, similar to that of the worshiper; the fertility goddesses were most often shown in frontal view, with exaggerated breasts and pudenda.

With merging and changing of cultures the deities usually acquired new names. To the Semitic peoples of Mesopotamia, for example, the goddess of love, beauty, and fertility was known as Ishtar. To the Phoenicians she was Astarte. Others called her by still other names: Venus by the Romans and Aphrodite by the Greeks. The Egyptian goddess of fertility and love and protectress of women in the vicissitudes of life was Isis, daughter of Qêb and Nut, sister of Osiris, and mother of Horus. Isis was usually shown wearing a crown of two horns embracing a solar disc and often holding a papyrus scepter. After the 25th dynasty (663 B.C.), figures of Isis commonly portrayed her as a nursing mother, with Horus. When Christianity was introduced into Egypt, similarities were soon seen between the new religion and the moral system of the old cult, and many identified the Virgin Mary and her Child with Isis and Horus.

Not until relatively late in Egyptian history were animals worshiped, but they were always accorded a special status close to that of the gods because of their intimate knowledge of nature's laws. Toueris, Egyptian symbol of fecundity and protectress of the pregnant and parturient, was usually shown in the guise of a pregnant hippopotamus standing on her hind legs and holding the hieroglyph meaning protection in one paw, the sign for life in the other. Small figures of Toueris were popular as amulets.

Fertility Figures, Amulets, Votives, Dolls

As man conceived of his deities in human form, so did he likewise endow them with human emotions. Gods and goddesses, like men and women, would surely be flattered by figures in their image and influenced by gifts in their honor. Amulets to curry favor with the gods date back to prehistory; members of some primitive cultures still resort to them to enhance fertility. The Venus of Willendorf, a fertility goddess of the Old Stone Age (40,000–16,000 B.C.), unearthed in Austria in 1908, is believed to be one of the earliest known representations of the human form. Figures of the female torso and breasts, fertility symbols from the 7th millennium B.C., were uncovered in the early 1960s by James Mellaart at Catal Hüyük, a Neolithic city in Anatolia. Three prehistoric statuettes, probably used as amulets, depicting a fertility goddess in advanced pregnancy, were discovered in the caves of Grimaldi, Ventimiglia, in northwest Italy, the home of a negroid race of the late Paleolithic period (before 2500 B.C.). Perhaps most famous of all fertility figures is the marble statue of Artemis (Diana) of Ephesus, showing the goddess with her many breasts symbolizing her reproductive prowess (Fig. 1-5).

Votive tablets and free will offerings, usually in the form of the genital organs, together with torches and wreaths, were carried by the women of ancient Rome and Greece to their temples, beseeching fertility and easy delivery. Outlines of the uterus, as a fertility symbol, were included among the altar decorations of the temple of Babylon in addition to the forms of the deities. The Egyptians later placed the face of Hathor, their mother goddess, within this uterine form, which thus came to be known as Hathor's hairdress.

Fetishes, usually woodcarvings in human form, considered to be the seat of magic power or the abode of a spirit, are still worshiped in some primitive communities, particularly in Africa. The fetish was almost always endowed with an orifice into which the owner would place his or her own prayerful offerings. Amulets, worn as jewelry, were likewise endowed with magic properties, for example, the power to ward off evil such as infertility. Masks of clay, wood, and animal horns have been worn among the tribes of Africa, New Guinea, and South and Central America for the past 4000 years to dispel the spirits of sickness and death and bring the blessings of fertility. In ancient Mexico fertility figures were sometimes placed in graves as an offering to the dead, to ensure fertility to the living.

Among some African tribes, in which a woman's ability to bear children takes precedence over all other wifely functions, a doll was given to her when she was about to marry. Believed endowed with magic powers, the doll was sometimes worn as a necklace or bound to the woman's body to help her become pregnant. Fertility dolls of clay and beads still play an important role in the culture of certain tribes of South Africa. Copies of old beaded fertility dolls are now mass-produced there for sale to tourists.

Infertility

Until the physiological factors in reproduction began to be recognized, prayer remained the principal resort for relief from infertility. Barrenness was regarded as the

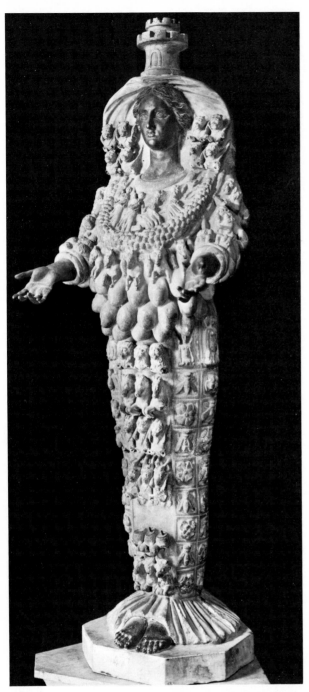

FIG. 1-5. Artemis (Diana) of Ephesus, Greek goddess of fertility. Marble statue with bronze head and hands. (Musei Capitolini, Rome)

supreme curse, as exemplified by Jeremiah's quotation of the Lord, "Write ye this man childless" (Jer. 22:30) and Rachel's entreaty to Jacob, "Give me children, or else I die" (Gen. 30:1). It was God who closed the wombs of Sarah (Gen. 16:2), Hannah (1 Sam. 1:6), Michal (2 Sam. 6:23), and the women in Abimelech's household (Gen. 20:18), while opening up the wombs of Leah (Gen. 24:31) and Rachel (Gen. 30:22). The early Greeks and Romans, in addition to appealing to their gods and goddesses for help in fulfilling their reproductive functions, resorted to theurgic devices including magic formulas, songs and incantations, and the laying-on of hands.

So long as the male partner could perform the conjugal act, infertility in a union was ascribed to the female. Male potency implied virility. Only when coitus could not be consummated because of impotence or anatomic aberration was the husband's role in the reproductive process impugned. The obvious resort was artificial insemination. This was first attempted in 1680, without success, by the Dutch anatomist Jan Swammerdam, with the eggs and sperm of fish. Ludwig Jacobi succeeded in 1742, but not until 1780 was artificial insemination successful in mammals. In that year the Italian anatomist Lazaro Spallanzani impregnated a bitch with the semen of a dog. At about the same time the illustrious John Hunter impregnated the wife of a man with hypospadias by vaginal injection of her husband's semen.

Attention was later focused on the importance of patency of the woman's reproductive tract. The diagnosis of patency or obstruction of the oviducts, however, depended on the clinical acumen of the examiner and was subject to frequent error. In 1919 the New York gynecologist I. C. Rubin introduced a nonsurgical insufflation test for tubal patency, using oxygen initially but switching later to the more rapidly absorbed and safer carbon dioxide.

Contraception

Twentieth-century humanity's unbridled fertility has produced perhaps its most urgent problem. Of the earth's 3 billion inhabitants, more than one third are sorely malnourished for lack of food. At the current rate of increase, the world's population will double in less than 35 years. Demographers, statesmen, theologians, physiologists, chemists, and physicians have joined hands at long last in a hopeful effort to stem this tide, which threatens to engulf mankind.

The Greeks were apparently the first to give serious thought to population control. Most of the early Greek philosophers considered a stable population essential, Plato placing the ideal population of the state at exactly 5040 inhabitants. Reproduction, he suggested, should be legally regulated, with overpopulation being checked by abortion and infanticide; underpopulation, by stimulating fertility and immigration.

In 1798 Thomas Robert Malthus, an English clergyman turned economist, in his *Essay on the Principle of Population,* called attention to the disparity between the geometric rate of population increase and the slower increase of the food supply. War and disease, he pointed out, as had Machiavelli three centuries earlier, were the only alternatives to voluntary limitation of family size in controlling excessive population. Extending the teaching of Malthus, Francis Place, an English sociologist, began to advocate contraception, beginning in the 1820s, as a restraint against population increase. Wrote Place:

Many young men who fear the consequences which a large family produces turn to debauchery, and destroy their own happiness as well as the happiness of the unfortunate girls with whom they connect themselves.

Other young men, whose moral and religious feelings deter them from this vicious course, marry early and produce large families, which they are utterly unable to maintain. . . . But when it has become the custom . . . to limit the number of children, so that none need have more than they wish to have, no man will fear to take a wife, all will be married while young—debauchery will diminish—while good morals, and religious duties will be promoted. . . .

If, above all, it were once clearly understood, that it was not disreputable for married persons to avail themselves of precautionary means as would without being injurious to health, or destructive to female delicacy, prevent conception, a sufficient check might at once be given to the increase of population beyond the means of subsistence.

Thus was the birth control movement launched, as a social issue.

The earliest known contraceptive formulas are found in the Petrie medical papyrus, an ancient Egyptian manuscript of three large pages from about 1950 B.C. Recommended among other prescriptions were contraceptive pessaries of crocodile dung and honey, and vaginal fumigations with minnis, an ancient drug. Some 2000 years later Soranus of Ephesus advocated, as a barrier to conception, mixtures of honey or cedar wood oil with figs or pomegranate pulp. Lucretius, the Roman poet, suggested violent body movements to shake the semen free after intercourse, while Pliny the Elder recommended wearing as an amulet the worms from the body of a hairy spider, as the most effective means for preventing conception. Blossoms of the palash flower, mentioned as an effective oral contraceptive in the *Kama-Sutra,* a 4th-century Hindu love manual, were tested on rats by the Indian Council for Medical Research in the 1960s and found to prevent conception in 80% of the animals.

In the years of the Crusades, when women were viewed as private property, men designed belts and girdles for their wives, mistresses, and unmarried daughters to be worn during their masters' absence, to frustrate the advances of other men. Known as chastity belts, they were made of metal, covered in part with leather, and worn in such a manner as to guard the entrance to the vagina and rectum. The chastity belt consisted of a waistband from which was suspended a metal plate, more often two, fore and aft, connected between the

wearer's legs by a joint. In each plate was a serrated opening that provided a portal of egress for the bladder, rectum, and uterus, but prevented the approach of a man. Secured with a lock, the plates could be removed only at the pleasure of the key holder. As recently as 1933 the League of Awakened Magyars advocated that every unmarried girl of age 12 or older be required to wear a chastity belt, the key remaining in the custody of her father or other competent authority.

A linen sheath for coitus, forerunner of the condom, was first described in 1564 by Gabriele Fallopio in his *De morbo gallico.* Penile sheaths were used initially for protection against venereal disease. Not until the 18th century did the membranous condom, usually fashioned from an animal's cecum, become popular for contraception. With the vulcanization of rubber in 1884, contraception achieved an explosive popularity because of the sudden cheapness of the new product. At mid-20th century the condom was the most widely used of all artificial contraceptives.

By 1880 a variety of chemical agents and mechanical devices, both intravaginal and intrauterine, were in use. Not enough, however, were the invention and improvement of these contraceptives, for traditional morality posed a formidable barrier to their distribution. Prominent among the opponents of contraception in the United States was Anthony Comstock, anti-sin crusader for whom the federal postal law of 1873 was named; this law prohibited the dissemination of birth control information and contraceptive materials through the mails. Later, as a special agent of the U.S. Post Office, he ordered the destruction of 160 tons of contraceptive literature, which he branded as "lewd, lascivious, and obscene." Not until 1965 did the Supreme Court make possible birth control clinics everywhere in the United States, when it declared unconstitutional Connecticut's law banning the dissemination of contraceptive advice.

Although rigidly opposed by the Catholic Church, the birth control movement received a tremendous boost in 1958 from the Lambeth Conference of Bishops of the Anglican Communion, which resolved:

The responsibility for deciding upon the number and frequency of children has been laid by God upon the consciences of parents everywhere . . . the means of family planning are in large measure matters of clinical and aesthetic choice . . . scientific studies can rightly help, and do, in assessing the effects and usefulness of any particular means; and Christians have every right to use the gifts of science for proper ends.

By the end of 1972 contraceptive advice was being offered by the International Planned Parenthood Federation in more than 100 countries, on every continent. In the United States during 1979 an estimated 4.5 million women received contraceptive services from Planned Parenthood affiliates and other organized family planning agencies, at 5195 locations. At the same time, however, about one third of the medically indigent women in the United States still lacked counsel in the principles and techniques of family planning.

GYNECOLOGY AS A SURGICAL SPECIALTY

Gynecology now seems securely wedded to the practice of obstetrics, but only after a prolonged succession of betrothals to other suitors. For many centuries the diseases of women lay within the province of general medical practice, the meager knowledge and techniques not justifying specialization. During the 18th and early 19th centuries gynecology, then a nonsurgical discipline, was commonly combined with pediatrics. Many of the textbooks of this era were devoted to "the diseases of women and children," and a large number of professorships were similarly designated. With the introduction of anesthesia and asepsis in the mid-19th century, gynecology abruptly changed in character. The surgeon laid claim to its practice, and in many teaching centers gynecology became a subdepartment of general surgery. Even though practiced in increasing measure by the obstetrician–gynecologist rather than the general surgeon, the specialty retains today its essentially, but not exclusively, surgical character.

Before the development of a truly rational system of gynecology, fad followed fad in the treatment of woman's ills. Toward the middle of the 19th century the Galenic doctrine was revived, attributing to uterine displacements and "uterine sympathies" virtually every sort of female complaint. As a result, the pessary school of gynecology began to flourish. Fortunes, it is said, were to be made by two groups of gynecologists of that day: those who inserted pessaries and those who removed them. This treatment, if not effective, was at least innocuous. Treatment, fortunately, was largely limited to such nonsurgical measures. From 1848 to 1851, for example, not a single gynecologic operation was performed at the New York Hospital. Shortly thereafter, however, when the surgeon learned how to open the peritoneal cavity with safety, a rash of suspension operations for uterine retroversion broke out, in which the round ligaments were, in the words of Fluhmann, "folded, ligated, plicated, shirred, plaited, planted, transplanted, replanted, drawn over, above, and through the broad ligaments and fastened to the back of the uterus." So popular had uterine suspension become by 1911 that when Mr. Alexander of Liverpool was asked to demonstrate the operation of his invention to a group of visiting surgeons, he was unable to comply. Four assistants, Alexander stated, were sent in quest of a patient, one into the north, one into the east, one into the west, and one into the south of Liverpool; but after diligent search, each returned with the report that in all of that great city he had been unable to find one woman who had not already had the Alexander operation.

Cervical cancer, one of the most important of gynecologic diseases, was attributed by Scanzoni, a leading figure of the mid-19th century, to immoderate coitus and excessive sexual stimulation. For cervical inflammation, leeches were often recommended. Mitchell gave the following instructions for their use:

> For the application of leeches, so often necessary in cases of inflammatory congestion of the cervix uteri, the patient should be placed in the same position as for labor, and a conical glass or metal speculum passed up to the uterus; care being taken that no part of the vagina is left around the rim of the instrument, as the bites of the leeches are not painful when the uterus only is wounded, but excessively so if the vagina is. Any adherent mucus is to be carefully wiped off, and the leeches put into the tube in the number required, eight or ten being the usual number. The mouth of the speculum is to be filled with lint, which requires to be pushed towards the extremity applied closely to the uterus, carrying the leeches along with it. In ten minutes the lint may be withdrawn, the speculum being allowed to remain in the vagina until the leeches fill, which will generally occupy from twenty minutes to half an hour. Occasionally, however, it is necessary to detach an odd one, which may readily be done by dipping a camel-hair pencil in a solution of common salt, and applying it to the head of the leech. . . . I think it is a good plan to apply the speculum so that the mouth of the uterus shall be external to its margin, as in one case I knew of troublesome symptoms arising from a leech crawling into the cervix uteri, and there adhering.

Like all branches of surgery, gynecology burst into flower when anesthesia and asepsis removed the stifling covers of pain and infection. Yet the mores of the times posed a major impediment to the full fruition of this new specialty. Vaginal examination was resorted to only on urgent indication, and even then, under protective drapes that effectively concealed the patient's genitalia from the examiner's eyes (Fig. 1-6). The vaginal speculum was regarded by some as an "instrument of unbridled indecency." Charles D. Meigs, with his characteristic knack for aligning himself on the wrong side of major issues, gave articulate expression to the prevailing puritanical attitudes in his "letters" to his students:

> I confess I am proud to say, that, in this country generally, certainly in many parts of it, there are women who prefer to suffer the extremity of danger and pain rather than waive those scruples of delicacy which prevent their maladies from being fully explored. I say it is an evidence of the dominion of a fine morality in our society.
>
> Even after we have been consulted, and where certain concessions are made, there often remains some degree of uncertainty, because we cannot, as we can in persons of our own sex, freely employ every means of research in exploring, and in repeating the explorations of their maladies.
>
> This difficulty is probably greater in this country than it is in Europe. I am rejoiced at it; because, however

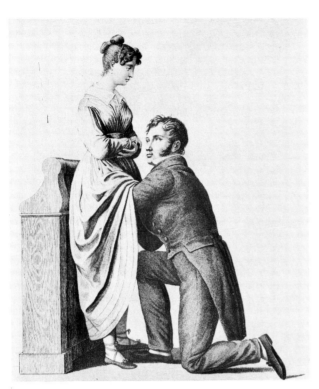

FIG. 1-6. Pelvic examination, early 19th century. Modesty precluded inspection. (Maygrier JP: Nouvelles démonstrations d'accouchemens. Paris, Béchet, 1822)

inconvenient, and however baffling in the particular instances of suffering, it is an evidence of a high and worthy grade of moral feeling. And I hope the day is far distant when the spectacle shall be seen in our hospitals, of troops of women, waiting in succession, for a public examination of their genitals, in presence of large classes of medical practitioners and students of medicine. I regard this public sentiment, as to the sanctity of the female modesty and chastity, as one of the strong safeguards of our spontaneous public polity;—for woman, and man's respect and love for her, are truly at the basis, and are the very corner-stone of civilization and order.

He is but the pander of vice who parades his thousands of uterine cases before the public gaze; and is himself an unchaste man, who ruthlessly insists upon a vaginal taxis in all cases of women's diseases that, however remotely, may seem to have any, the least connexion with the disorders of their reproductive tissues.

Meigs was not alone. In 1850 Dr. James P. White of Buffalo, bitterly attacked for conducting a delivery before a group of students, had to resort to legal action against one of his antagonists. The American Medical Association's Committee on Medical Information, commenting on the matter, stated that the only advantage that might accrue from exposing a patient during delivery was "a

somewhat greater facility in protecting the perineum," but held this to be insufficient compensation for "the obvious disadvantage." The committee stated further that a physician not prepared to conduct labor by the sense of touch alone was not competent to practice obstetrics.

Similar restrictions, based on a misguided concern for the patient's modesty, prevailed in Europe. Only in the examination of certain socially inferior groups, such as the prostitutes of Paris and the syphilitic women of Berlin, did a laxer attitude prevail toward inspection of the patient's genitals. It was in these groups, therefore, that the bluish coloration of the vagina as a diagnostic sign of pregnancy (subsequently designated Chadwick's sign) was first observed.

The modern era of gynecologic surgery began a few days before Christmas 1809, when Jane Crawford set out on her fateful ride to Danville, Kentucky—a ride that has since been compared with that of Paul Revere, Sheridan's from Winchester, and the charge of the Light Brigade for its historic significance and the courage it took. Dr. Ephraim McDowell's successful operation on Mrs. Crawford, Christmas morning, without anesthesia, marked the beginning of abdominal surgery.

Ovarian cysts had been regarded as incurable. In the few cases where excision had been attempted the result had been uniformly fatal. The only treatment that could be offered the hapless sufferer was temporary palliation by tapping, to withdraw the rapidly reaccumulating fluid.* In some cases this practice assumed staggering proportions, as in the patient reported by Heidrich, whose ovarian cyst (or peritoneal cavity) was tapped 299 times to remove 9867 lb of fluid. Physicians had been forced to an attitude of fatalism toward this disease.

McDowell's feat is best related by his own account, reported with two additional cases eight years later:

In December 1809, I was called to see a Mrs. Crawford, who had for several months thought herself pregnant. She was affected with pains similar to labour pains, from which she could find no relief. So strong was the presumption of her being in the last stage of pregnancy, that two physicians, who were consulted on her case, requested my aid in delivering her. The abdomen was considerably enlarged, and had the appearance of pregnancy, though the inclination of the tumor was to one side, admitting of an easy removal to the other. Upon examination, per vaginam, I found nothing in the uterus; which induced the conclusion that it must be an enlarged ovarium. Having never seen so large a substance extracted, nor heard of an attempt, or success attending any operation, such as this required, I gave

* Robert Houstoun successfully evacuated the contents of a large ovarian tumor, probably a mucinous cystadenoma, by laparotomy in August, 1701, but without removal of the ovary. The patient, aged 58, lived in good health until October 1714, when she died of an unknown cause (Philosophical Transactions 7:541, 1734).

to the unhappy woman information of her dangerous situation. She appeared willing to undergo an experiment, which I promised to perform if she would come to Danville (the town where I live), a distance of sixty miles from her place of residence. This appeared almost impracticable by any, even the most favourable conveyance, though she performed the journey in a few days on horseback. With the assistance of my nephew and colleague, James McDowell, M.D., I commenced the operation, which was concluded as follows: Having placed her on a table of ordinary height, on her back, and removed all her dressing which might in any way impede the operation, I made an incision about three inches from the musculus rectus abdominis, on the left side, continuing the same nine inches in length, parallel with the fibres of the above named muscle, extending into the cavity of the abdomen, the parietes of which were a good deal contused, which we ascribed to the resting of the tumor on the horn of the saddle during her journey. The tumor then appeared full in view, but was so large that we could not take it away entire. We put a strong ligature around the fallopian tube near to the uterus; we then cut open the tumor, which was the ovarium and fimbrious part of the fallopian tube very much enlarged. We took out fifteen pounds of a dirty, gelatinous looking substance. After which we cut through the fallopian tube and extracted the sack, which weighed seven pounds and one half. As soon as the external opening was made, the intestines rushed out upon the table; and so completely was the abdomen filled by the tumor, that they could not be replaced during the operation, which was terminated in about twenty-five minutes. We then turned her upon her left side, so as to permit the blood to escape; after which we closed the external opening with the interrupted suture, leaving out, at the lower end of the incision, the ligature which surrounded the fallopian tube. Between every two stitches we put a strip of adhesive plaster, which, by keeping the parts in contact, hastened the healing of the incision. We then applied the usual dressings, put her to bed, and prescribed a strict observance of the antiphlogistic regimen. In five days I visited her, and much to my astonishment found her engaged in making up her bed. I gave her particular caution for the future; and in twenty-five days, she returned home as she came, in good health, which she continues to enjoy.

On the heels of McDowell's triumph similar procedures were soon undertaken by others, especially in England, with encouraging results, and by the middle of the century ovarian excision, the archetype of abdominal surgery, was an established procedure.

Just as Ephraim McDowell was to be named the founder of abdominal surgery, James Marion Sims came to be known as the father of American gynecology because of his success in repairing vesicovaginal fistulas.

In 1835 Dieffenbach wrote this description of the plight of women with urinary fistulas:

A sadder situation can hardly exist than that of a woman afflicted with a vesicovaginal fistula. A source of disgust, even to herself, the woman beloved by her husband becomes, in this condition, the object of bodily revulsion to him; and filled with repugnance, everyone else likewise turns his back, repulsed by the intolerable, foul, uriniferous odor. As a result of the seepage from the opening, whether large or small, the usual retention of the urine in the vaginal folds makes it even sharper and more pungent. The labia, perineum, lower part of the buttocks, and inner aspect of the thighs and calves are continually wet, to the very feet. The skin assumes a fiery red color and is covered in places with a pustular eruption. Intolerable burning and itching torment the patients, who are driven to frequent scratching to the point of bleeding, as a result of which their suffering increases still more. In desperation many tear the hair, which is coated at times with a calcareous urinary precipitate, from the mons pubis. The refreshment of a change of clothing provides no relief, because the clean undergarment, after being quickly saturated, slaps against the patients, flopping against their wet thighs as they walk, sloshing in their wet shoes as though they were wading through a swamp. The bed does not soothe them, because a good resting place, a bed, or a horsehair mattress, is quickly impregnated with urine and gives off the most unbearable stench. Even the richest are usually condemned for life to a straw sack, whose straw must be renewed daily. One's breath is taken away by the bedroom air of these women, and wherever they go they pollute the atmosphere. Washing and anointing do not help; perfumes actually increase the repugnance of the odor, just as foul-tasting things become even worse when coated with sugar. This horrendous evil tears asunder every family bond. The tender mother is rejected from the circle of her children. Confined to her lonely little room, she sits there in the cold, at the open window on her wooden chair with a hole cut in its seat, and may not cover the floor with a carpet even if she could. Indifference overtakes some of these unfortunates; others give themselves over to quiet resignation and pious devotion. Otherwise they would fall victim to despair and would attempt suicide.

Physicians had struggled with vesicovaginal fistulas for centuries, exhausting their ingenuity on countless mechanical devices and surgical procedures, in their vain efforts to reclaim these social outcasts. J. Marion Sims, a young surgeon in Montgomery, Alabama, attacked the problem freshly in 1845, with experiments on the now legendary slaves, Anarcha, Betsy, and Lucy, sufferers from this dreaded affliction. After repeated attempts, about 40 in number, had ended in failure, the persistent Sims ultimately succeeded in developing a surgical technique for fistula repair, with the aid of the rediscovered knee–chest position, a vaginal speculum now named for him, and silver sutures.

Sims reported his success in his historic paper of

1852. The following year he moved to New York, where he founded, in 1855, a small hospital for women, the forerunner of the Woman's Hospital of the State of New York. Here Sims and his colleagues, Thomas Addis Emmet, E. R. Peaslee, and T. Gaillard Thomas, achieved a brilliant record for their fistula repairs and vaginal plastic operations. Gynecology had taken its place as a full-fledged surgical specialty.

REFERENCES AND RECOMMENDED READING

General

Fasbender HF: Geschichte der Geburtshilfe. Jena, Fischer, 1906

Graham H: Eternal Eve: The History of Gynaecology and Obstetrics. Garden City, NY, Doubleday, 1951

Irving FC: Safe Deliverance. Boston, Houghton Mifflin, 1942

Miller D: Res obstetrica in the Bible. J Obstet Gynaecol Br Emp 60:7, 1953

Ploss HH, Bartels M, Bartels P: EJ Dingwall (ed): Woman: An Historical, Gynaecological and Anthropological Compendium. London, Heinemann, 1935

Preuss J: Biblisch-talmudische Medizin, 3rd ed. Berlin, Karger, 1923. Rosner F (trans): New York, Sanhedrin Press, 1978

Ricci JV: Development of Gynaecological Surgery and Instruments. Philadelphia, Blakiston, 1949

Ricci JV: Genealogy of Gynaecology: History of the Development of Gynaecology Throughout the Ages. Philadelphia, Blakiston, 1950

Speert H: Obstetric and Gynecologic Milestones: Essays in Eponymy. New York, Macmillan, 1958

Speert H: Obstetrics and Gynecology in America: A History. Chicago, American College of Obstetricians and Gynecologists, 1980

Speert H: Iconographia Gyniatrica: A Pictorial History of Gynecology and Obstetrics. Philadelphia, FA Davis, 1973

Thoms H: Classical Contributions to Obstetrics and Gynecology. Springfield, IL, Thomas, 1935

Williams JW: Sketch of the history of obstetrics in the United States up to 1860. Am Gynecol 3:266, 340, 1903

Early Midwifery

Bancroft–Livingston G: Louise de la Vallière and the birth of the man–midwife. J Obstet Gynaecol Br Emp 63:261, 1956

Bard S: Compendium of the Theory and Practice of Midwifery, Containing Practical Instructions for the Management of Women During Pregnancy, in Labour, and in Childbed. New York, Collins & Perkins, 1807

Corner BC: William Shippen, Jr., Pioneer in American Medical Education. Philadelphia, American Philosophical Society, 1951

Denman T: Introduction to the Practice of Midwifery. London, Johnson, 1795

Heaton CE: Obstetrics in Colonial America. Am J Surg 45:606, 1939

Mauriceau F: Traité des maladies des femmes grosses et de celles qui sont accouchées. Paris, 1668. Chamberlen H (trans): London, Billingsley, 1673

Mercurio S: La Commare O' Raccoglitrice. Venice, Ciotti, 1595–1596

Rösslin E: Der Swangerenn Frawen und Hebammen Rosengarte. Strassburg, Flach, 1513

Smellie W: Treatise on the Theory and Practice of Midwifery. London, Wilson & Durham, 1752–1764. (Reprinted with annotations by AH McCintock, London, New Sydenham Society, 1876–1878)

Soranus of Ephesus: Gynecology. Temkin O, Eastman NJ, Guttmacher AF (trans): Baltimore, Johns Hopkins, 1956

Antenatal Care

Ballantyne JW: Plea for a pro-maternity hospital. Br Med J, April 6, 1901, p 813

Ballantyne JW: Visit to the wards of the pro-maternity hospital: A vision of the twentieth century. Am J Obstet 43:593, 1901

Taussig FJ: The story of prenatal care. Am J Obstet Gynecol 34:731, 1937

Embryology

von Baer KE: De Ovi Mammalium et Homini Genesi. O'Malley CD (trans): Leipzig, Voss, 1827

Corner GW: Discovery of the mammalian ovum. Lectures on the History of Medicine: A Series of Lectures at the Mayo Foundation, 1929–1932. Philadelphia, Saunders, 1933

de Graaf R: De Mulierum Organis Generationi Inservientibus. Corner GW (trans): Leyden, Hackiana, 1672

Wolff C: Theoria Generationis. Samassa (trans): Halle, Hendel, 1752

The Obstetric Pelvis

Baudelocque JL: L'art des accouchemens. Paris, Méquignon, 1781

van Deventer H: Operationes Chirurgicae Novum Lumen Exhibentes Obstetricantibus, quo fideliter manifestatur ars obstetricandi, et quidquid ad eam requiritur: Instructum pluribus figuris aeri incisis. . . . Leyden, Dyckuisen, 1701

Eastman NJ: Pelvic mensuration: A study in the perpetuation of error. Obstet Gynecol Surv 3:301, 1948

Levret A: L'Art des accouchemens, demontré par des principes de physique et de méchanique. Paris, Le Prieur, 1753

Litzmann CCT: Die Formen des Beckens, insbesondere des Engen Weiblichen Beckens, nach eigenen Beobachtungen und Untersuchungen, nebst einem Anhange über die Osteomalacie. Berlin, Reimer, 1861

Michaelis GA: Litzmann CCT (ed): Das Enge Becken nach eigenen Beobachtungen und Untersuchungen. Leipzig, Wigand, 1851

The Obstetric Forceps

Aveling JH: The Chamberlens and the Midwifery Forceps: Memorials of the Family and an Essay on the Invention of the Instrument. London, Churchill, 1882

Das K: Obstetric Forceps: Its History and Evolution. St. Louis, Mosby, 1929

Puerperal Fever

Blundell J: Severn C (ed): Lectures on the Principles and Practice of Midwifery. London, Masters, 1839

Gordon A: Treatise on the Epidemic Puerperal Fever of Aberdeen. London, Robinson, 1795

Hodge HL: On the Non-contagious Character of Puerperal Fever: An Introductory Lecture. Philadelphia, Collins, 1852

Holmes OW: Contagiousness of puerperal fever. N Eng Q J Med Surg 1:503, 1843. (Reprinted in Medical Classics 1: 211, 1936)

Holmes OW: Puerperal Fever as a Private Pestilence. Boston, Ticknor & Fields, 1855. (Reprinted in Medical Classics 1: 247, 1936)

Semmelweis IP: von Győry T (ed): Semmelweis' Gesammelte Werke. Jena, Fischer, 1905

Watson T: Lectures on the principles and practice of physic, delivered at King's College, London. London Med Gaz (NS) 1:801, 1842

Cesarean Section

Bixby GH: Extirpation of the puerperal uterus by abdominal section. J Gynaecol Soc Boston 1:223, 1869

Eastman NJ: Role of frontier America in the development of cesarean section. Am J Obstet Gynecol 24:919, 1932

Harris RP: Operation of gastro-hysterotomy (true caesarean section), viewed in the light of American experience and success; with the history and results of sewing up the uterine wound; and a full tabular record of the caesarean operations performed in the United States, many of them not hitherto reported. Am J Med Sci 75:313, 1878

King AG: America's first cesarean section. Obstet Gynecol 37: 797, 1970

Porro E: Dell' amputazione utero-ovarica come complemento di taglio cesareo. Ann Univ Med Chir 237:289, 1876

Sänger M: Der Kaiserschnitt bei Uterusfibromen nebst vergleichender Methodik der Sectio Caesarea und der Porro-Operation. Leipzig, Engelmann, 1882

Young JH: Caesarean Section: The History and Development of the Operation From Earliest Times. London, Lewis, 1944

Anesthesia for Childbirth

Simpson JY: Notes on the employment of the inhalation of sulphuric ether in the practice of midwifery. Monthly J Med Sci 7:721, 728, 1847

Simpson JY: Etherization in surgery. Monthly J Med Sci 8:144, 1847

Simpson JY: Account of a New Anaesthetic Agent, as a Substitute for Sulphuric Ether in Surgery and Midwifery. Communicated to the Medico-Chirurgical Society of Edinburgh at Their Meeting on 10th November, 1847. Edinburgh, 1847. Reprint. New York, 1848

Simpson JY: Priestley WO, Storer HR (ed): Obstetric Memoirs and Contributions of James Y. Simpson, MD, FRSE, Vol 2. Philadelphia, Lippincott, 1865

Watson BP: President's address: Sixty-first annual meeting of the American Gynecological Society. Am J Obstet Gynecol 32:547, 1936

Woman's Fertility and Its Control

Himes NE: Medical History of Contraception. New York, Gamut Press, 1963

Stopes MC: Contraception (Birth Control): Its Theory and Practice. London, Putnam, 1931

Wood C, Suitters B: The Fight for Acceptance: A History of Contraception. Aylesbury, Medical Technical, 1970

Gynecology as a Surgical Specialty

Clay C: Results of All the Operations for the Extirpation of Diseased Ovaria, by the Large Incision, from September 12, 1842, to the Present Time. Manchester, Irwin, 1848

Dieffenbach JF: Ueber die Heilung der Blasen-Scheiden-Fisteln und Zerreissungen der Blase und Scheide. Med Zeitung 5:117, 121, 173, 177, 1836

Fluhmann CF: Rise and fall of suspension operations for uterine retrodisplacement. Bull Johns Hopkins Hosp 96:59, 1955

Harris S: Woman's Surgeon: The Life Story of J. Marion Sims. New York, Macmillan, 1950

Heidrich CG: Diss. Sistens Casum Memorabilem Ascitae et Destructionis Ovariorum. Berlin, Brüsch, 1825

McDowell E: Three cases of extirpation of diseased ovaria. Eclectic Repertory Analyt Rev 7:242, 1817

Meigs CD: Females and Their Diseases: A Series of Letters to His Class. Philadelphia, Lea & Blanchard, 1848

Mitchell TR: Practical Remarks on the Use of the Speculum in the Treatment of Disease of Females. Dublin, Fannin, 1849

Peaslee ER: Ovarian Tumors, Their Pathology, Diagnosis, and Treatment. London, Lewis, 1873

Scanzoni FW: A Practical Treatise on the Diseases of the Sexual Organs of Women, 4th American ed. Gardner AK (trans): New York, De Witt, 1861

Sims JM: On the treatment of vesico-vaginal fistula. Am J Med Sci 23:59, 1852

Genetic Considerations

Gloria E. Sarto

2

Cytogenetic abnormalities have been found to be a major cause of multiple malformation syndromes, mental retardation, reproductive loss, and abnormal sexual development. Prenatal genetic diagnosis has become a common procedure. A variety of banding techniques and special cell culture media allow the diagnosis of an ever-increasing number of cytogenetic anomalies. These cytogenetic methods, coupled with recent advances in molecular genetics, have improved our ability to diagnose genetic disorders. Though all physicians encounter persons with genetic diseases, in no area of medicine has a knowledge of genetics become as important as in obstetrics and gynecology.

BASIC GENETICS

Molecular Genetics

DNA Replication

DNA (deoxyribonucleic acid) consists of two polynucleotide chains wound around each other in a double helix. There are four main nucleotides, each containing a deoxyribose residue, a phosphate group, and a purine base (adenine or guanine) or a pyrimidine base (thymine or cytosine). The bases are arranged such that adenine (A) always pairs with thymine (T) and guanine (G) with cytosine (C). The genetic code, the order of the bases, is on one polynucleotide chain; each consecutive three bases make up one codon and code for a specific amino acid (protein building block).

DNA is replicated during a specific part of interphase, the S (synthesis) period, with the aid of the enzyme DNA polymerase and several other enzymes. During replication the two strands of the DNA separate locally and each strand acts as a template for a new DNA strand by means of complementary base pairing (A with T and G with C). The new DNA strand is rapidly packaged with histones to form nucleosomes.

In higher organisms not all the DNA replicates simultaneously; some parts of chromosomes replicate earlier in the S period than others. Generally, regions that contain active genes replicate earlier, whereas inactive regions (which are often heterochromatic) replicate later.

Protein Synthesis

Transcription, the synthesis of RNA from a region of DNA, is catalyzed by the enzyme RNA polymerase. Three forms of this enzyme are found in higher organisms; each transcribes a different RNA with a specific function. Polymerase II transcribes messenger RNA (mRNA), which codes for most of a cell's proteins. Messenger RNA undergoes processing to eliminate nonprotein-coding regions. Polymerase III makes several small RNAs, including transfer RNA (tRNA) and small ribosomal RNA (rRNA). Polymerase I makes the large rRNA.

In the nucleolus or nucleoli within the nucleus, newly synthesized rRNA is packaged with ribosomal proteins to form the ribosomes. The nucleoli contain loops of DNA that code for rRNA. Such DNA loops are known as *nucleolus-organizing regions* (NORs). These regions are visible in condensed mitotic chromosomes as secondary constrictions in one or more chromosomes. In humans there are five pairs of chromosomes containing NORs; these are the heterochromatic short arms of the acrocentric chromosomes (13, 14, 15, 21, and 22).

During translation, which takes place in the cytoplasm, the ribosomes first bind to a specific site on the mRNA molecules. As the ribosome moves along the mRNA molecule, tRNA translates one codon at a time by adding amino acids to form a protein chain. When a ribosome reaches the end of the mRNA, it and the newly formed protein are released into the cytoplasm (Fig. 2-1).

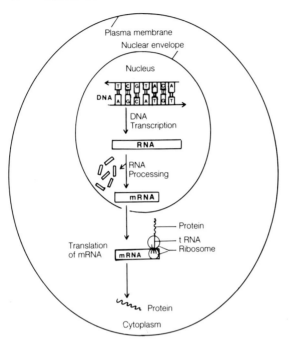

FIG. 2-1. Schematic representation of processes involved in protein synthesis.

Restriction Enzymes

Many bacteria produce enzymes, called *restriction endonucleases,* that possess recognition sites in the DNA for short, specific sequences of four to six nucleotides. These enzymes cleave DNA only where the specific sequences are found, resulting in series of DNA fragments known as *restriction fragments.* For example, the endonuclease EcoRI cleaves the normal α-globin gene at a specific site. Since in a mutant form of the gene this recognition site is changed, the enzyme cleaves the DNA not at this site but at a different site, resulting in an abnormally long DNA restriction fragment.

Electrophoresis of restriction fragments separates the fragments according to size as expressed in kilobases (Kb); they can then be hybridized to a DNA probe and an autoradiograph prepared. Application of this and the other molecular genetic technology has proven useful in the prenatal diagnosis of some hemoglobinopathies.

Cytogenetics

Chromosomes

A human cell contains several billion nucleotides of DNA, although only a small fraction is thought to code for essential proteins. The DNA is packaged into chromosomes for orderly cell division. The fundamental packaging unit, the nucleosome, consists of 146 base pairs of DNA wound around 8 histone molecules (two each of H2A, H2B, H3, and H4), plus about 60 nucleotides of linker DNA, which gives a "beads on a string"

appearance in the electron microscope. Together with another histone, H1, the nucleosome beads form a fiber that is 30 nm in diameter. This fiber is further packaged to form a chromosome that can be seen in the light microscope. Individual chromosomes are normally visible only during division; during the remainder of the cell cycle they are undergoing DNA replication and are actively transcribing mRNA.

Improvements in media and techniques for tissue culture and the use of colchicine to prevent spindle formation have made it possible to analyze cells in the metaphase stage of mitosis. The application of hypotonic solutions makes cells swell and thereby increases chromosome dispersement, and banding techniques permit identification of all the chromosomes.

Peripheral blood and fibroblasts are the most commonly studied tissues. The best way to obtain a large number of metaphases for analysis is to induce blood lymphocytes to divide by adding phytohemagglutinin. Phytohemagglutinin acts as an antigen and stimulates an immunologic response, transforming lymphocytes into blastlike cells capable of division in culture. Fibroblasts derived from skin biopsies or from other body tissues, including amniotic fluid, are grown on a glass surface and then subcultured. Usually about 15 to 24 hours after subculture there are a sufficient number of mitoses for analysis. Selected cells in metaphase can then be analyzed and photographed, and a karyotype can be prepared.

The relative size of a specific chromosome is stable within a species. However, chromosome size varies with stage of mitosis; for example, prophase chromosomes are longer and less coiled than metaphase chromosomes. It can also change with exposure to some environmental agents; treatment with colchicine, for example, shortens chromosomes.

CHROMOSOME IDENTIFICATION. Until 1970 only a limited number of chromosomes could be identified individually. They were grouped according to size and shape. Chromosome banding was introduced in 1970 when Caspersson and co-workers reported the use of fluorochrome stains and fluorescence microscopy for human chromosome identification (Fig. 2-2). Banding patterns are consistent from one tissue to another for all chromosomes, including meiotic chromosomes. Some variations in the intensity of certain bands are inherited; called *chromosome polymorphisms,* these variations have in certain circumstances been used to determine the parental origin of chromosomes.

Several techniques are used to induce banding. For Q banding the most common fluorescent stain used is quinacrine HCl (atebrine); unfortunately, the fluorescence technique requires expensive equipment, and the stain fades quickly. Another commonly used technique is one in which cells are pretreated and stained with Giemsa. It is termed *G banding;* the G bands correspond to the Q bands. The staining of the bands in R banding is the reverse of that in Q or G banding.

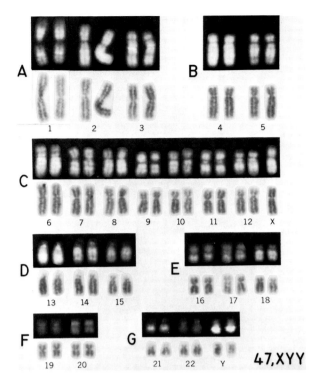

47,XYY

FIG. 2-2. 47,XYY karyotype stained with quinacrine mustard and photographed with ultraviolet light and fluorescence microscope. Each chromosome can be unambiguously identified.

Some stains identify only specific bands or structures. These include stains for heterochromatic bands (C bands), telomeric bands (T bands), and NORs. Autoradiography is used to identify the late-replicating inactive X chromosome(s) in a cell; the inactive X can also be identified by BrdU (5-bromodeoxyuridine), which changes the way in which chromosomes stain with Hoechst 33258 or acridine orange.

Methods exist to produce long chromosomes, such as those seen in prophase. With such chromosomes one can identify as many as 2000 bands. This technique, called *prophase* or *high-resolution banding,* is used primarily to identify small deletions.

CHROMOSOME NOMENCLATURE. The nomenclature for chromosome and banding patterns is very specific (Table 2-1). A document entitled *An International System for Human Cytogenetic Nomenclature (1978),* abbreviated *ISCN,* details all the major decisions about chromosome nomenclature that have occurred over the past several years.

Mitosis and Meiosis

Mitosis ensures that the genetic material replicated in the previous interphase is distributed equally to the two daughter cells. In meiosis the chromosome complement is halved. Abnormal chromosome constitutions

leading to abnormal growth and development can be caused by errors in either mitosis or meiosis.

MITOSIS. Mitosis and interphase make up the cell cycle. Interphase consists of the time between mitosis and the beginning of DNA synthesis (G_1), DNA synthesis (S), and the interval between the end of DNA synthesis and the beginning of mitosis (G_2). The total cell cycle in human cells is between 12 and 24 hours. DNA synthesis takes 7 to 7.5 hours, and mitosis takes 0.5 to 1.5 hours. Mitosis itself is divided into several phases: prophase, metaphase, anaphase, and telophase (Fig. 2-3).

PROPHASE. The chromosomes, each of which consists of two chromatids, contract and become more distinct. The nucleoli vanish, and the centrioles move to opposite sides of the nucleus.

METAPHASE. After the nuclear membrane has dissolved, a spindle is formed between the two centrioles. The centromeres, the primary function of which is to attach the chromosomes to the spindle fibers, lie in the metaphase plate equidistant from the two poles (equatorial plane). The centromeres become functionally double, and the daughter centromeres repel each other.

Table 2-1
Nomenclature Symbols, Chicago Conference, 1966

A–G	The chromosome groups
1–22	The autosome numbers (Denver system)
X,Y	The sex chromosomes
+	Indicates extra chromosome or part of a chromosome
−	Indicates missing chromosome
/	Separates cell lines in describing mosaicism
?	Questionable identification of chromosome or chromosome structure
ace	Acentric
cen	Centromere
del	Deletion
dic	Dicentric chromosome
dup	Duplication
end	Endoreduplication
h	Negative-staining region or secondary constriction
i	Isochromosome
inv	Inversion
inv (p+q−) or inv (p−q+)	Pericentric inversion
mar	Marker chromosome
mat	Maternal origin
p	Short arm of chromosome
pat	Paternal origin
q	Long arm of chromosome
r	Ring chromosome
s	Satellite
t	Translocation
tri	Tricentric

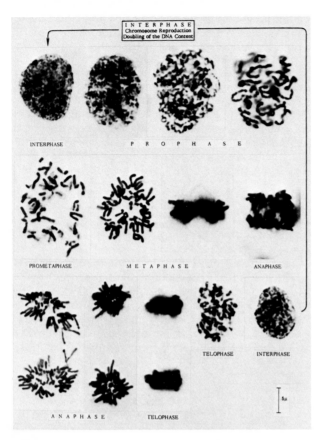

FIG. 2-3. Mitosis in human lymphocytes. (Therman E: Human Chromosomes. New York, Springer-Verlag, 1980)

ANAPHASE. The centromeres move to opposite poles with their attached daughter chromosomes.

TELOPHASE. A nuclear membrane is formed, and the nucleoli are reconstituted. The chromosomes revert to the interphase condition and lose their visible structure. At the end of telophase, the cytoplasm divides into two equal parts (cytokinesis).

MEIOSIS. Cells that are ready to enter meiosis are known as *primary oocytes* or *primary spermatocytes*. In meiosis homologous chromosomes are paired and cross over (Fig. 2-4). Because there are two cell divisions with only one duplication of chromosomes, the diploid number of chromosomes is halved. Meiosis brings about genotypic diversity by the independent segregation of chromosomes and recombination between homologous chromosomes.

PROPHASE I. Prophase of the first meiotic division (meiosis I) consists of the stages leptotene, zygotene, pachytene, diplotene, and diakinesis. Transition from one to the other is gradual and continuous. In leptotene the chromosomes appear as fine, single threads

throughout the nucleus, although they consist of two chromatids. During zygotene homologous chromosomes pair in a zipper fashion. At pachytene pairing is complete, and the number of pairs of homologous chromosomes (bivalents) is half the diploid number of chromosomes. Since each homolog is made up of two chromatids, the paired homologs (bivalents) consist of four chromatids. Diplotene is marked by contraction of the bivalents. The paired chromosomes separate, except where they are held together by one or more chiasmata (crossovers). In each crossover only two of the four chromatids are involved. During diakinesis the chromosomes become shorter and thicker, and the nucleolus disappears. The end of prophase I is marked by the division of the centriole and the disappearance of the nuclear membrane.

METAPHASE I. The bipolar spindle is formed. The centromeres of the paired chromosomes lie on opposite sides of the equatorial plate.

ANAPHASE I. The centromeres separate and move to opposite poles. When separation is complete, each pole has half the diploid number of chromosomes, each consisting of two chromatids. As a result of the crossover,

FIG. 2-4. Schematic diagram of meiosis. (After Therman E: Human Chromosomes. New York, Springer-Verlag, 1980)

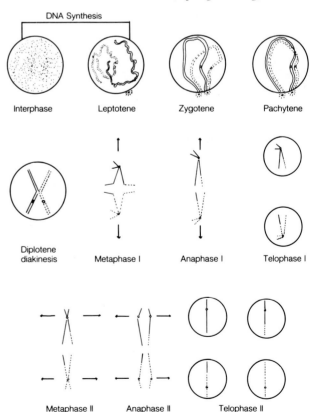

each chromosome has both maternal and paternal segments.

TELOPHASE I.   Cell division takes place, and a nuclear membrane is formed around each nucleus.

INTERPHASE I.   The chromosomes do not become extended during interphase I, which is very short. There is no reduplication of chromosomes. This phase is followed by the second meiotic division (meiosis II), which resembles a normal mitosis.

PROPHASE II.   The chromatids are widely separated but held together by the centromere.

METAPHASE II.   The nuclear membrane disappears and the spindle develops. The centromeres are lined up on the equatorial plate.

ANAPHASE II.   The centromeres divide and move to opposite poles, each with its attached chromatid.

TELOPHASE II.   The nuclear membrane is reformed, and subsequently the cell divides.

Numerical Abnormalities

ANEUPLOIDY.   Aneuploidy is the loss or gain of one or more chromosomes. It may be due to an error in mitosis or meiosis. Most forms of monosomy, a condition in which one chromosome of one pair is missing, are rare. Exceptions are X monosomy (which causes Turner's syndrome) and 21 monosomy. Several trisomies (in which there are three of a given chromosome instead of the usual pair) exist, each with a characteristic and relatively well defined phenotype.

One mechanism known to result in aneuploidy is *nondisjunction,* the failure of sister chromatids or chromosomes to pass to opposite poles of the spindle. Meiotic nondisjunction during gametogenesis can occur during the first or second meiotic division or both; it gives rise to gametes with one missing chromosome (nullisomic) or one extra chromosome (disomic) (Figs. 2-5 and 2-6).

Another cause of aneuploidy is *anaphase lag.* In this instance a chromosome does not move to its pole as readily as others and consequently is lost (Fig. 2-7).

POLYPLOIDY.   Triploidy, three haploid sets of chromosomes, can arise from any one of several errors in gametogenesis. For instance, failure of formation of the first or second polar body, with subsequent fertilization, results in fusion of three haploid sets of chromosomes (two maternal, one paternal). Double fertilization of a normally developed oocyte also causes triploidy (two paternal, one maternal chromosome sets). Fertilization of a normal oocyte by an unreduced sperm with a diploid set of chromosomes produces a triploid. Tetraploidy, four haploid sets of chromosomes, usually results from two chromosome replications without an intervening mitosis. Triploidy and tetraploidy are found frequently in plants but are not compatible with life in mammals; they are frequently found in abortuses. Several infants with triploid cells have survived; however, they have usually also had a diploid cell line.

MOSAICISM.   Chromosome mosaicism is the result of mitotic nondisjunction or anaphase lag in the embryo. Diagnosis is based on the presence of two or more cell types in different tissues and in successive cultures from the same tissues; the abnormalities should be consistent in all cultures. Sex chromosome mosaicism is much more common than autosome mosaicism.

FIG. 2-5.   Schematic diagram of spermatogenesis showing effects of meiotic nondisjunction.

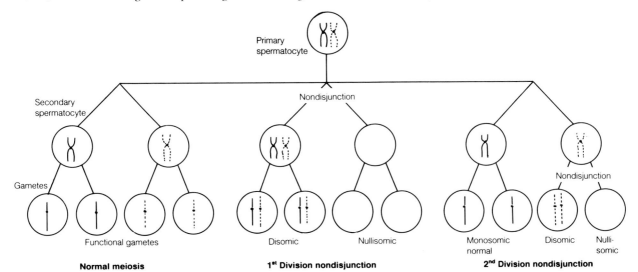

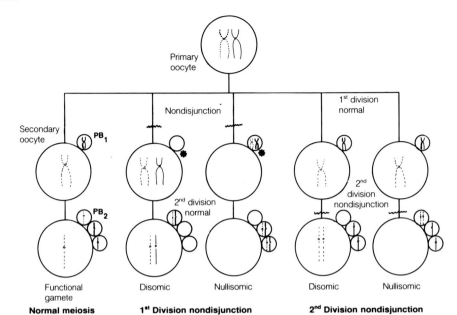

FIG. 2-6. Schematic diagram of oogenesis showing effects of meiotic nondisjunction. Corresponding types, such as those marked by asterisks, may not be equally frequent. This diagram shows division of first polar body.

CHIMERISM. Chimerism differs from mosaicism in that chimeric cells arise from two independent zygotes. The condition is thought to be most commonly due to an exchange of cells between dizygotic twins as a result of placental cross-circulation; such cross-circulation regularly occurs in cattle twins but only rarely in human twins.

Structural Abnormalities

CHROMOSOME AND CHROMATID BREAKS AND SISTER CHROMATID EXCHANGES. Chromosomes may break before or after they have replicated in interphase. If they break before, the result is chromosome breaks; if they

FIG. 2-7. Mitotic division showing failure of a chromosome to move to its pole (anaphase lag). (After Patau K: The origin of chromosomal abnormalities. Pathol Biol (Paris) 11:1163, 1963)

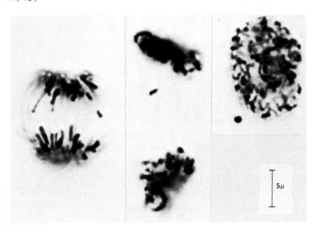

break after, the result is chromatid breaks. Broken chromosome ends may join with each other to form new chromosome configurations. Ionizing radiation and various chromosome-breaking substances greatly increase chromosome structural aberrations. The extent of sister chromatid exchange (SCE), the exchange of segments of DNA between sister chromatids, is often used to measure the effect of mutagenic substances. Certain recessive genes greatly increase the likelihood of such chromosomal abnormalities, leading to conditions such as Bloom syndrome, Fanconi anemia, and ataxia-telangiectasia.

INTRACHROMOSOMAL ABNORMALITIES. Breaks within the same chromosome may result in a deletion, a ring chromosome, or an inversion. *Deletions* can be terminal or interstitial; in an interstitial deletion two breaks occur, the intervening segment is lost, and the broken ends rejoin. A *ring chromosome* is caused by a break near the end of each arm of the chromosome and the rejoining of the broken ends. An *inversion* is the result of two breaks, with the segment between the two breaks becoming inverted. If the inverted segment does not involve the centromere, it is a *paracentric inversion;* if it includes the centromere, it is a *pericentric inversion.*

INTERCHROMOSOMAL REARRANGEMENTS. Breaks in two chromosomes may result in interchromosomal rearrangements. An exchange of chromosome segments between two chromosomes is a *reciprocal translocation.* If such a translocation is balanced—that is, if there is a mutual exchange with no loss of chromosome segments—there are usually no ill effects. If the translocation occurs between two acrocentric chromosomes, it is called *centric fusion* or a *Robertsonian transloca-*

tion. An individual with a balanced translocation is phenotypically normal; however, at meiosis the chromosomes may be rearranged and transmitted to the offspring in unbalanced form (Fig. 2-8). Depending on chiasma formation and segregation at meiosis, this can result in fetal loss, a malformed infant, a phenotypically normal individual with a balanced translocation, or a phenotypically and genotypically normal individual.

MISDIVISION OF THE CENTROMERE.   Transverse instead of the usual longitudinal division of the centromere results in an *isochromosome,* which has two identical arms. The most common isochromosome has the two long arms of the X.

Mendelian Genetics

Genes occur in pairs. Those occupying identical positions (*loci*) on a pair of chromosomes are *alleles.* A mutant gene may be inherited from one or both parents or, very rarely, may arise in the individual. The *genotype* is the genetic makeup of an individual. The *phenotype* is the sum total of all the morphologic and physiologic characteristics of the individual. If one of two alleles is mutant, the individual is *heterozygous* for that trait; if the alleles are identical, the individual is *homozygous*

FIG. 2-8. Schematic representation of possible zygotes from a 14/21 translocation.

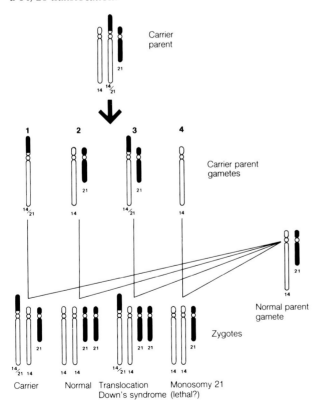

for that trait. If a disorder is inherited, probabilities of recurrence can be calculated according to mendelian laws (Table 2-2).

Autosomal Dominant Inheritance

An autosomal dominant disorder is brought about by a single mutant gene situated on an autosome. Characteristics of autosomal dominant inheritance include the following: (1) the trait is transmitted from one generation to the next from an affected person to an affected offspring; (2) on the average, half of the siblings and half of the children of an affected person are affected; and (3) the inheritance is usually independent of sex, *i.e.,* both sexes are equally affected. The potential risk for every child of a person with an autosomal dominant disorder is 50%. This assumes complete penetrance (described below). Family members who do not suffer from the defect cannot pass it to their offspring.

Autosomal Recessive Inheritance

An autosomal recessive disorder is manifested only when the affected individual inherits the mutant gene from both parents and thus is homozygous. Usually the parents are heterozygous for the mutant gene (*i.e.,* each one carries a mutant gene on one autosome and a normal allele on the other) and therefore are phenotypically normal. Autosomal recessive disorders are characterized by the following: (1) one quarter of the offspring of two heterozygotes are affected; (2) the children of an affected parent are not affected unless the other parent is a carrier (heterozygous for the mutant gene); and (3) usually all affected family members are in the same generation. Since the genes responsible for most autosomal recessive disorders are rare, the chances of two unrelated parents carrying the same mutant gene are small; parents of individuals with rare autosomal recessive disorders are often found to be blood relatives. Many metabolic disorders, such as phenylketonuria and cystic fibrosis, are inherited in this way.

X-Linked Inheritance

In X-linked inheritance, the mutant gene is on the X-chromosome. The characteristics of X-linked inheritance are different for dominant and recessive genes.

An *X-linked recessive* trait can be homozygous or hemizygous. Therefore, one's chance of manifesting the trait depends on one's sex. In the female an X-linked recessive disorder usually is not expressed, because a normal allele (gene) on one X chromosome counteracts the effect of the mutant gene on the other. In contrast, since the male has only one X chromosome, a single (hemizygous) recessive mutant gene on the X chromosome is expressed. Analyses of many pedigrees with X-linked recessive disorders show that the overwhelming majority of affected individuals are males, males inherit the disease through carrier mothers, and half of

Table 2-2
Approximate Recurrence Risks for Various Genetic Abnormalities

Abnormality	Risk of Recurrence
Mendelian Mutations	
Autosomal recessive	25%
Autosomal dominant	50% (unless there is a new mutation or unless penetrance is reduced)
X-linked for carrier females	25% overall; 50% males
X-linked for affected males	100% carrier daughters
	100% normal sons
Common Multifactorial Conditions	2–5% (increases with each affected child)
Chromosome Abnormalities	
Trisomy syndrome (Down)—parents chromosomally normal	1–2%
Balanced translocation in carrier parent*	2–100%

* See Table 2-5.

the brothers but none of the sisters of an affected male are affected. In the union of a carrier female and a normal male, half the sons are affected and half the daughters are carriers. All sons of an affected male are normal, since they inherit only the maternal X chromosome; all daughters of an affected male are carriers (heterozygous), since they inherit the paternal mutant X chromosome.

In *X-linked dominant inheritance,* both heterozygous females and hemizygous males manifest the abnormality. All sons of an affected male are unaffected; all the daughters are heterozygous, and since the mutant gene is dominant, are affected. It is sometimes difficult to differentiate between X-linked dominant and autosomal dominant modes of inheritance.

Y-Linked Inheritance

Theoretically, with Y-linked inheritance, only males are affected, and an affected male transmits the mutant gene to all of his sons and to none of his daughters. It has been claimed that several traits, including "hairy ears" and tall stature in males, are inherited in this way.

Multifactorial Inheritance

Many malformations are not inherited in a simple way. Rather, they are the result of the complex interaction of several genes at different loci. Anencephaly, spina bifida, cleft palate, and cleft lip are examples of such traits, which are considered multifactorial. In these conditions, genetic prognosis can be offered only in terms of empiric risks based on the analysis of many pedigrees. After the birth of one affected child, the risk to subsequent siblings is usually about 3% to 5%. After

the birth of two affected children, the risk increases. The exact risk of each disorder must be estimated from the literature.

Penetrance, Expressivity, Sex Limitation, Phenocopy, Genetic Heterogeneity

With some autosomal dominant inherited disorders, an individual may inherit a mutant gene from a phenotypically normal parent. This phenomenon is known as *incomplete penetrance;* the mutant gene is present but is not manifested. Penetrance is expressed statistically; for example, if 20 persons have the dominant gene but only 10 express the trait, it is said that the gene shows 50% penetrance. Obviously, to determine the degrees of penetrance for a particular mutant gene, it is necessary to study large pedigrees.

Some inherited disorders exhibit the phenomenon known as *varying expressivity.* In osteogenesis imperfecta, for example, some family members have blue sclerae, some have brittle bones, and some are deaf; others have two of the three and some have all three of these abnormalities, which are characteristic of the disorder. In such an instance, diagnosis can be difficult. A careful physical examination must be done on all possible affected family members. This variation in the expression of genes is probably due to the interaction of genes and the environment.

If a mutation is expressed in one sex only, it is termed a *sex-limited* disorder.

An environmental agent can cause an abnormality that phenotypically is very similar or identical to an anomaly caused by a gene mutation. Such a disorder is termed a *phenocopy* and is naturally not inherited.

Genetic heterogeneity exists when clinically, apparently identical diseases have different modes of inheritance. Data on genetic heterogeneity of a specific disorder must be obtained from the literature.

Sex Chromatin

X Chromatin (Barr Body)

The Lyon hypothesis was proposed in 1961. In general:

1. All X chromosomes in a cell except one are inactivated. Initially, inactivation is random, so that in some cells the paternal X and in others the maternal X is inactivated.
2. Once inactivation has occurred, the descendants of each X chromosome (active or inactive) behave like the parent X. The inactive X forms a sex chromatin and it is late-replicating during the synthesis period.
3. Inactivation of the genes on one X chromosome early in embryonic life offers an explanation for the phenomenon of dosage compensation for X-linked gene products.

The single active X hypothesis is supported by evidence from genetic and phenotypic studies involving X-linked genes and genes translocated to the X chromosome, by cytologic evidence, and by the results of biochemical studies of X-linked genes. For example, women heterozygous for two variants of glucose-6-phosphate dehydrogenase (G6PD) give rise to two types of fibroblast clones. Each clone expresses only one of the variants, indicating inactivation of the genes on the other X chromosome. There are exceptions to the inactivation hypothesis, however. For example, the Xg blood group locus and the steroid sulfatase gene do not undergo inactivation. Additional evidence indicating incomplete inactivation of the heteropyknotic X comes from the study of persons with abnormal numbers of X chromosomes. For example, if all except one X were inactivated, persons with 45,X and 47,XXX karyotypes would not be expected to differ from XX individuals or to have developmental anomalies, as they do. This is also true of males with XXXY and XXY sex chromosomes; XXXY is associated with a greater number of somatic anomalies than is XXY.

The X chromatin is a sex-specific heterochromatic body observed in the interphase nuclei of cells of mammalian females. The number of X-chromatin bodies in somatic cell nuclei is equal to the maximum number of X chromosomes minus one. Diploid interphase nuclei with two X chromosomes have a single X-chromatin mass, whereas cells with one X chromosome (45,X or 46,XY) have none. Though a correlation exists between the size of the X chromosome and the size of X chromatin, it should be emphasized that numerous factors affect the latter's size, density, shape, and deposition against the nuclear membrane, which make accurate assessment of its physical dimensions difficult. Although analyses of X chromatin in nuclei from buccal and vaginal smears have been used to screen for abnormalities of the X chromosome, such analyses are subject to errors in interpretation unless the smears are done with the greatest technical skill, and thus the procedure has limitations.

Y Chromatin (Y Body)

Y chromosomes are easily seen with Q banding; usually the distal part of the long arm in metaphase nuclei fluoresces brightly (see Fig. 2-2).

The human Y chromosome can be identified also in interphase nuclei as a bright fluorescent body (Fig. 2-9). Thus, with Q banding the Y chromosome can be identified in some of the same tissues as the X chromatin—buccal mucosa cells, amnion cells, and fibroblast cultures—and in spermatozoa. The number of Y bodies per nucleus equals the number of Y chromosomes.

Sex Determination

The development of normal male genitalia requires a fetal testis. Testosterone from the fetal testes stabilizes the wolffian ducts and permits differentiation of the vas deferens, seminal vesicles, and epididymis; müllerian-inhibiting factor causes the müllerian ducts to regress. Male differentiation of the external genitalia occurs under the influence of dihydrotestosterone, which requires α-reductase to convert testosterone to dihydrotestosterone. The major determinants responsible for testicular differentiation are located on the short arm of the Y chromosome. The manner in which these determinants act is not totally clear, but it appears that a cell surface antigen, H-Y antigen, is involved. Without H-Y antigen, the indifferent gonad develops into an ovary. The male sex determinants on the Y chromosome are so strong that testes develop even in individuals with an XXXY or even XXXXY constitution. However, the existence of several conditions in which a nonmosaic 46,XY chromosome constitution is associated with female or intersex external genitalia, with or without female internal

FIG. 2-9. Interphase nucleus from XYY individual showing two fluorescent Y bodies stained with quinacrine mustard and photographed with fluorescence microscope.

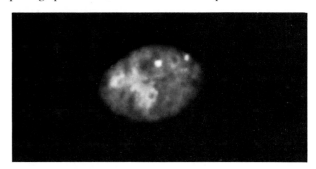

genitalia, indicates that gene mutations also influence sex determination and sex differentiation.

While the presence of a fetal testis is essential for male differentiation, the ovary is not essential for female differentiation; female internal and external genitalia differentiate even in the absence of ovarian tissue. Two intact X chromosomes seem to be necessary, however, for normal ovarian function. A loss of even a portion of one of the X chromosomes results in gonadal dysgenesis of varying degree. Again, the presence of gonadal streaks in some inherited 46,XX disorders indicates that both autosomal genes and genes located on the X affect ovarian differentiation.

CLINICAL GENETICS

Autosomal Abnormalities

Autosomal abnormalities include both numeric anomalies and structural rearrangements. The occurrence of abnormal chromosome constitutions in the newborn population is shown in Table 2-3. Structural aberrations are due to chromosome breakage and abnormal reunions resulting in deletions, rings, inversions, and translocations. All of these rearrangements are liable to produce total or partial trisomies or monosomies responsible for specific syndromes. Syndromes that can be reasonably described have been associated with total or partial trisomies or monosomies for chromosomes 4, 5, 6, 7, 8, 9, 10, 11, 12, 13, 14, 15, 18, 20, 21, and 22.

Table 2-3
Occurrence of Abnormal Chromosome Constitution in Newborn Population

Type	Incidence per 1000 Newborns	
Aneuploidy		
Sex chromosomes	1.65	
Autosomes	1.68	
Total		3.33
Unbalanced Rearrangements		
Centric fusion	0.07	
Other	0.12	
Total		0.19
Balanced Rearrangements		
Centric fusion	0.90	
Other	0.90	
Total		1.80
Other Structural Abnormalities		0.55
	Total	5.87

Numeric abnormalities consist primarily of trisomies. Although trisomies for all autosomes but number 1 have been found in spontaneous abortions, only three autosomal trisomies—21, 18, and 13 trisomy—are observed with any appreciable frequency at birth.

Clinical diagnosis of a chromosome disorder is often difficult, being based on a pattern of anomalies occurring together in an individual. No one anomaly is pathognomonic of a syndrome, since that anomaly not only may be associated with several different chromosome abnormalities but also may be found in normal individuals. A chromosome disorder should be considered when there are multiple anomalies with mental and growth retardation. Only the most common disorders are discussed here.

21 Trisomy (Down Syndrome)

Down syndrome was first described in 1886 by Langdon Down, who noted the association of mental retardation with mongoloid facies. In 1959 Lejeune made the significant discovery that Down syndrome is caused by trisomy for a G-group chromosome, now known to be 21.

Down syndrome, which occurs in approximately 1 in 700 liveborn infants (Table 2-4), remains the most common indication for chromosome analyses. The risk of having a child with Down syndrome increases with maternal age and perhaps even with paternal age greater than 55 years. Mean maternal age is 34.4 years. The risk for women in the 15- to 19-year-old age group is 1:2300, while the risk for women 45 years of age is 1:46.

About 95% of Down syndrome patients have trisomy 21; a translocation between chromosome 21 and another chromosome accounts for the remaining 5% of cases. The translocation usually involves 14 and 21 but may involve the other D-group chromosomes (Table 2-5). About 50% of the time, one of the two parents is a balanced translocation carrier. If the mother is a carrier of a 14/21 translocation, the risk of her having a child with Down's syndrome is approximately 10%. If the father is a carrier, the chance is about 2%. A carrier for a translocation between two 21 chromosomes produces gametes that are either disomic or nullisomic for chromosome 21. All liveborns from such a mating are trisomic and have Down's syndrome; the monosomic zygotes are aborted. Therefore, the risk of Down syndrome in a 21/21 translocation is 100%.

Down syndrome is characterized by mental retardation, oblique palpebral fissures with inner epicanthic folds, Brushfield spots on the irides, small or absent earlobes, flat occiput and flat nasal bridge, short broad hands with short fingers, and clinodactyly. The mouth is habitually open, with the tongue protruding. There is a wide space between the first and second toes. Affected children have marked hypotonia, and newborns lack the Moro reflex. Ventricular septal defects occur, so that individuals with Down syndrome are often troubled by respiratory illness. Dermatoglyphic examination

Table 2-4
Conditions Caused by Abnormal Chromosome Numbers

Type of Chromosomal Aberration*	Incidence per 1000 Newborns	Clinical Name	Remarks
Polyploidy			
Triploidy 69			Aborted (4% of spontaneous abortions), except for extremely rare liveborn diploid/triploid mosaics
Tetraploidy 92			Aborted (0.5% of spontaneous abortions)
Aneuploidy			
Gonosomal			
45,X	0.20	Turner syndrome	Typically short stature, undeveloped breasts, streak gonads (infertile)
47,XXX	0.45		Often normal and fertile; sometimes mentally retarded; children usually have normal chromosomes
47,XXY	0.50	Klinefelter syndrome	Typically tall, gynecomastic; testes small and histologically abnormal (infertile); sometimes retarded and/or psychotic
47,XYY	0.50		Typically tall, fertile; range from normal to psychotic and/or retarded; children usually have normal chromosomes
Others	Very rare		Generally abnormal and retarded
Autosomal			
47,+21	1.43	21 trisomy, Down syndrome	Mentally retarded; numerous anomalies, although individually variable, usually add up to a highly characteristic picture
47,+18	0.167	18 trisomy, Edward syndrome	Severely retarded; arches on three or more fingers (100%), micrognathia (97%), failure to thrive (97%), flexion deformity of fingers (94%), numerous other anomalies
47,+13	0.083	13 trisomy, Patau syndrome	Severely retarded; eye defect (94%), polydactyly (75%), cleft palate (72%), numerous other anomalies
Other trisomies			Practically always lethal
Any monosomy			Practically always lethal
Double aneuploidy	Very rare		For example, 48,XXY,+21

* Mosaicism (mixoploidy) excluded unless stated otherwise.

Table 2-5
Genetic Risk for Offspring of Carriers of Centric Fusion Disorders

Type of Translocation in Carrier	Liveborn Children of Carrier		Afflicted with Translocation Trisomy
	Phenotypically Normal		
	Chromosomally Normal	Carrier	
t(DqDq)*			
13/14 (usual)	About 2/5	About 3/5	<1%
13/15 (rare)			
14/15 (rare)			0
t(Dq21q)†			
Carrier: Mother	Almost 1/2	Almost 1/2	10%
Carrier: Father	Almost 1/2	Almost 1/2	About 2.4%
t(21q22q)‡			
Carrier: Mother	Almost 1/2	Almost 1/2	6.8%
Carrier: Father	Almost 1/2	Almost 1/2	<3%

* Incidence: 0.70/1000 births

† Incidence: 0.19/1000 births

‡ Very rare

shows simian palmar creases, distal axial triradius, and large numbers of loops instead of whorls and arches on the fingertips.

18 Trisomy (Edwards Syndrome)

The 18 trisomy syndrome was described in 1960. It is the second most common autosomal trisomy found among liveborn infants, occurring in 1 in 6000 live births (see Table 2-4). Trisomy 18 is usually due to meiotic nondisjunction; rarely, translocations occur, giving rise to various partial trisomies. Maternal age is not as clear a factor in 18 trisomy as in 21 trisomy; nevertheless, mean maternal age is slightly higher than normal, around 32 years. Females are 4 times as likely as males to have the disorder, possibly owing to the prenatal death of males.

Eighteen trisomy syndrome is characterized by failure to thrive, marked developmental retardation, occipital protuberance, low-set and malformed ears, micrognathia, and a shield-shaped chest with a very short sternum. A protrusion at the calcaneus produces feet that are described as "rocker bottom." A flexion deformity makes the fingers appear to be overlapping. Congenital heart disease, primarily ventricular septal defect and patent ductus, is common. Dermatoglyphic examination reveals a large number of arches on the fingertips. It is not uncommon for newborns with 18 trisomy to be postmature. Mean duration of pregnancy is 42 weeks, with decreased fetal activity, hydramnios, and small placenta; mean birth weight is less than 2300 g; mean survival time is about 70 days.

13 Trisomy (Patau Syndrome)

First described by Patau in 1960, 13 trisomy is the third most common trisomy syndrome known, occurring in 1 in 12,000 liveborns (see Table 2-4). As in most trisomy syndromes, the mean age of mothers of infants with 13 trisomy is somewhat higher than normal, around 32 years.

Some 75% of cases of 13 trisomy are caused by primary nondisjunction; about 20% are due to translocations, usually t(13q14q). The risk of recurrence is about 5%, regardless of the sex of the carrier parent. The risk of the disorder when one parent is a carrier of a t(13q13q) translocation is 100%.

Clinical characteristics of affected persons include low birth weight, developmental retardation, microcephaly, cleft palate and cleft lip (usually bilateral), microphthalmus, colobomas, malformed ears and presumed deafness, capillary hemangiomas, and polydactyly. Congenital heart defects, including atrial septal defect, patent ductus, and ventricular septal defect, occur in some 80% of the cases. Dermatoglyphic examination reveals a single palmar crease and distal axial triradius. The mean survival time of an infant with 13 trisomy syndrome is 130 days. Generally, the duration of pregnancy is normal. Mean birth weight is 2600 g.

5p– Syndrome (Cri-du-Chat)

The most common deletion syndrome, caused by deletion of part of the short arm of chromosome 5, was first described in 1963 by Lejeune and colleagues. The disease occurs in about 1 in 45,000 newborns. Clinical features include low birth weight, failure to thrive, developmental and mental retardation, microcephaly, ocular hypertelorism, epicanthic folds, hypotonia, round, moonlike facies, and strabismus. A distinctive, high-pitched cry at birth accounts for the name cat cry syndrome. The characteristic cry disappears later in life, at which time detection of the abnormality is based on physical appearance and profound mental retardation. Maternal age appears not to be a factor; generally, the mean ages of both parents are normal. In 88% of cases, the deletion occurs de novo; in 12%, the deletion is due to chromosomal rearrangement in a parent. Females are affected slightly more often than males, and affected infants are born at term.

Syndromes Caused by Partial Trisomy or Monosomy

Chromosomal structural abnormalities give rise to an almost unlimited variety of syndromes. Trisomy or monosomy for a chromosome segment causes mental retardation and multiple congenital anomalies, the particular combination of symptoms being characteristic for each chromosome segment.

Sex Chromosome Abnormalities

The frequency of sex chromosome anomalies in a population varies with ascertainment. The overall frequency of sex chromosome abnormalities in newborns, excluding mosaicism, is about 2 in 1000 (see Table 2-4). One fifth of all first-trimester abortions are 45,X. A woman with primary amenorrhea has about a 30% chance of possessing an abnormal sex chromosome constitution or one that disagrees with her phenotype.

Aneuploidy

45,X. The 45,X sex chromosome constitution is estimated to occur in 1 in 2500 phenotypic females. The diagnosis can be made at birth if there are significant nongenital somatic anomalies. If the diagnosis is not made at birth, it is frequently made during childhood on the basis of shortness of stature and associated anomalies. Without associated significant somatic abnormalities, the disorder may go undiagnosed until adulthood, at which time the affected individual consults a physician because of lack of secondary sexual characteristics.

The anomalies seen with a 45,X sex chromosome complement are those most commonly associated with Turner syndrome. Birth weight is lower than normal. Individuals are significantly short for their age; final height is 135 cm to 150 cm. Common somatic abnormalities include prominent ears, a narrow, highly arched palate, micrognathia, inner epicanthic folds, pterygium colli or short neck, a low posterior hairline, a broad chest with widely spaced nipples, cubitus valgus, and hand anomalies, including a short fourth metacarpal and transversely hyperconvexed fingernails. Frequently, there is a large number of pigmented nevi. Hypertension, thyroid deficiency, diabetes mellitus, and osteoporosis are common in persons with this disorder. Intelligence is usually normal. At puberty, secondary sexual development fails to occur. The external genitalia and müllerian ducts are normal female, though infantile. At birth the ovaries contain primordial follicles, but by puberty the gonadal tissue has usually been replaced by fibrous tissue devoid of germ cells. In a minority of cases (5–10%) spontaneous menses may occur, and a few affected women have had children. The children of these women (some 20 cases) have been chromosomally and phenotypically normal.

Estrogen levels of persons with a 45,X sex chromosome complement are low, and vaginal smears show an atrophic pattern. Pituitary gonadotropin levels are elevated after puberty. Growth hormone levels are normal.

In 78% of individuals with 45,X, the X is maternal in origin, indicating that the missing X was lost during paternal meiosis. There is no positive association between 45,X and parental age (maternal or paternal) or birth order.

47,XXX. The XXX chromosome constitution occurs in 1 in 1100 phenotypic females. Phenotypically, an XXX female commonly cannot be distinguished from a normal female. At birth only minor anomalies, such as clinodactyly and epicanthic folds, are seen. As adults, some affected women have primary and secondary amenorrhea; however, others have had children, the majority of whom have been chromosomally normal. A proportion of XXX women are mentally retarded or show psychotic tendencies.

45,X/46,XX; 45,X/47,XXX; 45,X/46,XX/47,XXX. Various phenotypes are associated with X-chromosome mosaicism; affected persons may have Turner syndrome or may be normal females capable of fertility. The phenotypic effects depend on the time of appearance of the 45,X cell line and on the proportion and distribution of the stemlines early in development. The physician should be alerted to the possibility of X-chromosome mosaicism by premature ovarian failure.

47,XXY. The most common chromosomal constitution of patients with Klinefelter syndrome is 47,XXY, which occurs in about 1 in 1000 phenotypic males. This syndrome is characterized by male internal and external genitalia, small testes, somewhat above average height with eunuchoid body proportions, little facial hair, and gynecomastia. Microscopic examination of the testes shows hyalinized seminiferous tubules lined by Sertoli cells. Leydig cells are clumped; spermatogenesis rarely occurs. Pituitary gonadotropin levels are usually elevated. Some 6% to 10% of oligospermic or azoospermic men may have variants of the XXY chromosome constitution.

Klinefelter syndrome with a 48,XXXY or a 49,XXXXY chromosome constitution is also found. The developmental abnormalities associated with the disorder are more severe as the number of X chromosomes increases. About 80% to 90% of individuals with Klinefelter syndrome are 47,XXY; mosaicism is seen in about 10% of cases. Mothers of XXY individuals are older than normal; fathers are not.

45,X/46,XY. A range of phenotypes is associated with Y chromosome mosaicism. Affected persons may be normal males capable of reproduction, may show incomplete masculinization manifested as intersexuality, or may have Turner syndrome.

The 45,X/46,XY sex chromosome constitution is most commonly manifested as mixed gonadal dysgenesis (sometimes called *asymmetric gonadal dysgenesis*). In this disorder internal genitalia consist of a uterus, usually with a dysgenetic testis on one side and a streak gonad on the other. Because of the possibility of neoplastic transformation, such gonads should be removed.

47,XYY. The 47,XYY chromosome constitution is found in about 1 in 1000 males. Noted in a disproportionate number of men in prisons and mental hospitals, it has been thought to be associated with deviant behavior. Males with the XYY karyotype indeed are more likely than normal to come into conflict with the law; however, the exact risk is not known, and many persons with XYY sex chromosome constitution appear normal. At birth this condition can be diagnosed only if chromosome studies are performed. A few individuals with 48,XYYY and 49,XYYYY chromosome constitutions have been reported. The greater the number of Y chromosomes, the more severe are the developmental defects. As adults, XYY individuals are generally taller than normal and may have poor coordination and mild facial asymmetry. Most have normal sexual development. Spermatogenesis is normal, as are children of XYY males.

Structural Abnormalities of the X Chromosome

Generally, the phenotypic expression of structural abnormalities of the X chromosome depends on which portion of the X is deleted. Whereas the loss of any segment of the arms of an X chromosome is associated with gonadal dysgenesis of varying degree, loss of a portion or all of the short arm is usually associated with the other symptoms of Turner syndrome. Though structural sex chromosome abnormalities can occur as a single cell line, often a 45,X cell line is also present, which makes phenotypic–karyotypic correlation difficult. Examples of structural abnormalities of the X chromosome are shown in Figure 2-10.

i(Xq) (Long Arm Isochromosome). The most common structural abnormality of the X chromosome is the long arm isochromosome, either as a single cell line or in combination with a 45,X cell line. The affected individual manifests many of the anomalies commonly seen with Turner's syndrome—short stature, skeletal abnormalities, and primary amenorrhea. As expected, the X-chromatin body is larger than normal.

Xp– (Short Arm Deletion). Deletion of the short arm of the X chromosome can occur as a single cell line but is commonly combined with a 45,X cell line. The individual with a nonmosaic short arm deletion is short and shows anomalies characteristic of Turner syndrome. Phenotypically, a person who lacks the entire short arm of one X chromosome or at least the distal part of Xp is indistinguishable from a 45,X individual. However, the former is more likely than the latter not to have primary amenorrhea.

Xq– (Long Arm Deletion). Deletion of the long arm of the X chromosome is less likely to be associated with Turner syndrome–like effects. Most affected persons have only gonadal dysgenesis. Turner syndrome anomalies, when present, may be due to an unidentified second 45,X cell line.

r(X) (Ring X Chromosome). The phenotypic effect of a ring X chromosome depends in part on the size of the missing segments and in part on whether the deletion affects primarily the long arm or the short arm.

X Translocations. Translocations between two X chromosomes and between an X and an autosome have been described. Though carriers of balanced translocations between two autosomes are phenotypically normal, individuals with balanced X/autosome translocations may have gonadal dysgenesis, particularly if the break involves the long arm of X.

FIG. 2-10. Structural abnormalities of the X chromosome, Q-banding. *a,* normal X chromosome; *b,* telocentric Xq; *c,* isochromosome Xq; *d,* deleted Xq; *e,* isodicentric Xq; *f,* isodicentric Xp.

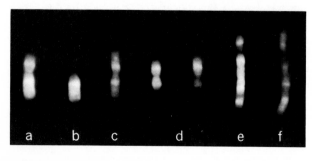

With unbalanced X/autosome translocations, the phenotype varies, depending on which portions of the X chromosome and autosome are deleted or duplicated. If autosomal material is deleted or duplicated, rather severe developmental defects are the result; the phenotype associated with X-chromosome deletion again depends on the size and location of the deleted segment.

X-Linked Mental Retardation

X-linked mental retardation associated with the fragile X chromosome is combined with a number of abnormalities, including large testes, delayed speech development, and certain facial features. The "marker X" was originally described by Lubs in 1969. However, it was not until seven years later that its connection to X-linked mental retardation became clear. Since then, over 90 families, including more than 250 affected males and 160 affected females and obligate carriers, have been described. The fragile X accounts for about one third of families with X-linked mental retardation and is probably the second most common chromosomal cause of mental retardation after Down syndrome. The gene responsible has variable penetrance, as demonstrated by siblings affected to different degrees and by transmission of the disorder by apparently normal males. Approximately one third of carrier females are mentally retarded. The degree of phenotypic expression in these females is extremely varied, perhaps owing to different proportions of cells in which the fragile X has been inactivated.

The fragile X chromosome has a constriction or break at the end of the long arm between regions q27 and q28; the appearance is often that of satellites on the end of Xq. Expression of the chromosome in cultured cells is dependent on culture conditions. Folic acid and thymidine inhibit expression, whereas folic acid antagonists such as 5-fluorodeoxyuridine induce expression. Disturbance of thymidylate synthesis may be the basis for the expression of the fragile site. Even under optimal culture conditions, the fragile X is seen in only 50% of cells in affected males and often not at all in some obligate heterozygotes. Prenatal diagnosis has been carried out with fetal blood and amniotic fluid cells, but genetic counseling is difficult because it is impossible to predict the degree of mental retardation that will result. It is not clear whether the fragile region itself or a closely linked gene is responsible for the syndrome.

Chromosome Breakage Syndromes

A number of inherited conditions are characterized by increased chromosome breakage and increased risk of cancer. Best known of these are Fanconi anemia, Bloom syndrome, ataxia telangiectasia, and xeroderma pigmentosum, each of which is caused by a different autosomal recessive gene.

Fanconi anemia (FA) patients have minor anatomic defects, mild mental and growth retardation, patchy brown skin pigmentation, and pancytopenia. Over 300 patients have been described. The most common cytogenetic features are chromatid breaks and chromatid translocations between nonhomologous chromosomes. Other aberrations are also present. It appears that a higher than normal proportion of FA patients develop leukemia and other cancers.

Bloom syndrome (BS) patients are small and have sun-sensitive telangiectatic skin lesions on the face. Approximately half of BS patients are of Jewish origin. The chromosome anomalies of BS differ from those of FA in several respects. In BS there is a greatly increased tendency toward homologous chromatid exchange, both sister chromatid exchanges and homologous chromatid interchanges (mitotic crossovers). Other types of chromosome breakage also occur with greater than normal frequency. Of the 103 patients in the BS registry, 25 have developed a total of 28 cancers at a mean age of 20.7 years. The most common malignancy is leukemia, but other types of carcinoma are also seen.

Ataxia telangiectasia (AT) patients have progressive cerebellar ataxia, telangiectasia of the eyes and skin, and severe immunodeficiency and are unusually sensitive to x-irradiation. Around 300 patients have been described. Chromosome breakage, especially translocations involving chromosome 14, is somewhat more frequent than normal among AT patients. The most common type of cancer in AT is lymphoma.

In xeroderma pigmentosum (XP), the associated biochemical defects are best understood. XP cells have a reduced ability to repair DNA damage, especially following ultraviolet irradiation. Some chromosome aberrations are seen in cultured cells. Cancers occur primarily in tissues that are likely to have been exposed to sunlight.

There are also a number of less well known chromosome breakage syndromes. Werner syndrome, also caused by a rare autosomal recessive gene, is characterized by short stature, premature aging, and early death. Chromosomal aberrations and the risk of cancer are increased with this syndrome. An increase in chromosome breakage has also been noted in several other syndromes, such as scleroderma and incontinentia pigmenti.

Mendelian Disorders Affecting Sexual Development

In addition to sex chromosome anomalies, abnormalities of sexual differentiation can occur in 46,XX and 46,XY individuals as a result of single gene mutations on an autosome or an X chromosome or on both. Though many of these patients show intersex genitalia, some have essentially normal female external genitalia. It is not uncommon for the latter group to go undiagnosed until puberty, at which time aberrant sexual development causes them to seek medical attention.

Complete Androgen Insensitivity (Testicular Feminization)

Testicular feminization is the most common and best known of the XY female syndromes. Except in those few individuals whose family histories suggest the condition or who are seen early in life with an inguinal hernia containing a testis, the disorder often is not diagnosed until puberty. There are no extragenital malformations. At puberty body proportions become eunuchoid. Breast development is excellent; axillary and pubic hair is usually absent or scanty. Primary amenorrhea is present in all patients. The external genitalia are female, but the vagina ends blindly at varying depths. There is no uterus. The testes, which may be located in the abdomen, inguinal canal, or labia, are accompanied by extremely hypoplastic wolffian duct structures. Though the testes may appear grossly and histologically normal in infants, spermatogonia gradually vanish, and tubular adenomas, with Leydig cell hyperplasia and degenerative changes of the tubular walls, become evident with increasing age.

An end-organ insensitivity to androgens accounts for the phenotypic expression of the disorder. Persons with testicular feminization are able to synthesize and maintain normal male levels of testosterone. Normal or slightly elevated amounts of 17-ketosteroids are excreted, and urinary estrogen levels are within the normal range for adult males.

The neoplastic potential of the testes increases with age and is sufficient to warrant orchiectomy. Because the risk of neoplasia is low in persons under 30 years of age, some physicians feel that the testes should not be removed until after feminization is complete. Others prefer to perform orchiectomy early in childhood; this approach mandates estrogen replacement therapy as the patient approaches puberty.

Affected individuals have a 46,XY chromosome constitution. "Sisters" and maternal "aunts" may also be affected. The disorder is inherited as an X-linked recessive mutation. Future apparent sisters of an affected individual have a one third chance of being XY.

Incomplete Androgen Insensitivity (Incomplete Testicular Feminization)

Incomplete testicular feminization is distinct from testicular feminization. At puberty individuals with the incomplete form feminize, *i.e.,* develop breasts, yet their external genitalia show evidence of virilization characterized by clitoral enlargement and partial labioscrotal fusion. Like patients with the complete form, these individuals have bilateral testes, no müllerian derivatives, a blindly ending vagina, and pubertal breast development. The disorder is inherited in X-linked fashion.

XY Pure Gonadal (Testicular) Dysgenesis (Swyer Syndrome)

Characterized by a female phenotype and normal chromosome constitution, pure gonadal dysgenesis has been described in both XX and XY individuals. The terms *XY pure gonadal (testicular) dysgenesis* and *Swyer syndrome* are used to refer to the condition in XY individuals. These persons have no unusual extragenital anomalies and are normally intelligent. They are usually of normal height with more or less eunuchoid body proportions. The disorder is characterized by severe early testicular dysgenesis, which results in streak gonads that are devoid of germ cells. The external genitalia are normal female. The vagina is normal, and a uterus is present. Hilar cells in the gonads may respond to gonadotropins with androgen production and subsequent clitoral enlargement. Urinary gonadotropin levels are increased after puberty. In patients with virilization, elevated urinary levels of testosterone and 17-ketosteroids have been documented.

Neoplastic change in the streak gonads has been reported in 20% to 30% of individuals with XY gonadal dysgenesis. It is recommended that the gonadal tissue be removed as soon as the diagnosis is established. Hormonal replacement is indicated to induce female secondary sexual characteristics; it may be given cyclically to induce regular uterine bleeding.

Two types of pure gonadal dysgenesis exist: that with and that without H-Y antigen. XY pure gonadal (testicular) dysgenesis usually occurs sporadically, but the syndrome has been reported in sisters and in several sibships of a single family. The disorder appears to be inherited either as an X-linked recessive or as an autosomal dominant gene limited in expression to the male sex, but genetic data do not exclude the possibility that it is caused by an autosomal recessive gene.

Other XY Syndromes

Other, very rare, XY syndromes show primary amenorrhea. An example is pseudovaginal perineoscrotal hypospadias (PPSH). Phenotypically, the syndrome is associated with few, if any, extragenital anomalies, but affected individuals have ambiguous external genitalia and undergo masculinization at puberty. The PPSH phenotype results from a deficiency of 5α-reductase, the enzyme required for the conversion of testosterone to dihydrotestosterone.

Another XY syndrome is true agonadism, or XY gonadal agenesis. This condition is characterized by female phenotype, female external genitalia, lack of secondary sexual characteristics, and lack of uterus, vagina, and gonads. It is extremely rare.

XX Pure Gonadal (Ovarian) Dysgenesis

Persons with XX pure gonadal (ovarian) dysgenesis show normal, though somewhat eunuchoid, growth; normal intelligence; no extragenital anomalies; lack of secondary sexual characteristics; normal external genitalia, uterus, and fallopian tubes; and streak gonads. The streak gonads are usually found at the time of laparoscopy or laparotomy during investigation for primary amenorrhea and lack of secondary sexual development.

Though most reported cases are sporadic, in some instances more than one member of a family has been affected. Available data suggest that the mode of inheritance is autosomal recessive.

True Hermaphroditism

True hermaphroditism entails the presence of both testicular and ovarian tissue. A true hermaphrodite may have a testis on one side and an ovary on the other side, an ovotestis bilaterally, or an ovotestis on one side and a testis or ovary on the other side. Some true hermaphrodites are reared as males, other as females. The external genitalia tend to be ambiguous. In most cases there is a uterus and a vagina, which may open into the perineum or into a urogenital sinus. The presence of an ovotestis or pure ovary on one side determines the extent of differentiation of the fallopian tube. At the time of puberty, virilization or feminization may occur. Therapy can then be directed toward inducing secondary sexual development to coincide with the sex of rearing. For a male this includes mastectomy; removal of uterus, fallopian tubes, and ovaries, if present; and efforts toward construction of male external genitalia. In a raised female, testicular tissue must be removed and external genitalia constructed.

The most common sex chromosome constitution found in true hermaphroditism is XX; a 46,XY chromosome constitution occurs in some. The finding of three 46,XX true hermaphrodites in one sibship suggests that, at least in some cases, true hermaphroditism is due to a gene mutation. Though XY true hermaphroditism is far less common than the XX type, one instance of familial occurrence has been reported.

Adrenogenital Syndrome

Adrenogenital syndrome in genetic females is the single most common cause of ambiguous genitalia. The mode of inheritance is autosomal recessive. The degree of virilization varies; an affected person may have clitoral hypertrophy or a phalluslike clitoris with a penile urethra. The disorder is caused by a deficiency of any one of several enzymes; however, 21-hydroxylase deficiency and 11β-hydroxylase deficiency are the most common causes. Diagnosis is based on measurement of specific steroids in the urine or serum. Elevated levels of urinary 17-ketosteroids and pregnanetriol are diagnostic, as are high serum levels of dehydroepiandrosterone and 17-hydroxyprogesterone. Therapy consists of steroid replacement; it is simple, may be lifesaving, and produces normal fertility.

Genetics of Spontaneous Abortion and Fetal Loss

First-Trimester Abortions

Approximately 10% to 15% of all clinically recognized pregnancies terminate in spontaneous abortion, usually during the first trimester. At least 50% to 60% of these abortuses are chromosomally abnormal. The earlier the gestational age at the time of abortion, the higher is the frequency of chromosome abnormalities.

Autosomal trisomy is found in approximately 50% of chromosomally abnormal abortuses. Trisomies for chromosome numbers 13, 16, 18, 21, and 22 are most common, but trisomy for every chromosome except number 1 has been observed. The trisomy most frequently found in abortuses is for number 16. Many of the trisomies observed in spontaneous abortions have not been observed in live births, presumably because they are incompatible with life. Monosomy for an autosome is rare among abortuses; a likely explanation for this is that such monosomy causes a genetic imbalance so severe as to be incompatible with development to any degree, leading the embryo to be lost at such an early stage as to go unnoticed. Monosomy X, however, occurs in about 25% of chromosomally abnormal abortuses; 45,X is the most common single chromosome complement found among abortuses.

Polyploidy accounts for 20% of chromosomally abnormal abortuses; triploidy is the most common. Most triploids abort early in pregnancy, and the gestational sac is usually empty. Associated with triploid abortuses is molar degeneration of the placenta, now referred to as *partial hydatidiform mole.* Two types of hydatidiform moles have been distinguished. The partial hydatidiform mole is characterized by hydropic degeneration of placenta with some fetal development and most often has a triploid karyotype; the complete hydatidiform mole generally is detected in the first or second trimester, has no fetal parts, and usually has a 46,XX karyotype.

Structural chromosome rearrangements account for 5% of all chromosomally abnormal abortuses; half of these are robertsonion translocations, which result in a duplication or deficiency of genetic material.

Second-Trimester Abortions

Second-trimester abortions have traditionally been considered more likely to be due to maternal than to fetal causes. Nevertheless, chromosome abnormalities have been detected in up to 35% of second-trimester abortions. Autosomal trisomies, monosomy X, and sex chromosome mosaicism are common among second-trimester abortuses; polyploidy is rare.

Stillbirths

Chromosome abnormalities are more frequent in antepartum or intrapartum stillbirths than in liveborns. Approximately 5% to 10% of antepartum or intrapartum stillborns have chromosome abnormalities, trisomy 18 being the most common.

Recurrent Spontaneous Abortions

Until the mid-1960s it was believed that the likelihood of a subsequent abortion after three spontaneous abortions was as high as 80% to 90%; the risks are now known to be much lower, around 15% to 30%, irrespective of the number of previous abortions. Investigations have shown that chromosome complements of two successive abortuses in a given family are likely to be either both normal or both abnormal. If a first abortus is chromosomally normal, the likelihood is about 80% that a second abortus will also have a normal karyotype. If the complement of a first abortus is abnormal, there is about a 70% chance that a second abortus will also be abnormal. Therefore, a couple with a history of trisomic fetuses, for example, should be considered for antenatal diagnosis in subsequent pregnancies.

Most chromosomal aberrations occurring in spontaneous abortuses are not heritable. Parents who carry structural rearrangements may have normal offspring, chromosomally abnormal offspring, or a greater than normal number of abortions. Among parents who have experienced repeated abortions, data indicate that the frequency of translocations is 3.4% in females and 1.6% in males; among those who have experienced both abortions and either a stillborn or an anomalous liveborn infant, the frequency of translocations is 16.4% in females and 4.2% in males. Many nongenetic causes for repetitive abortion have been postulated and should generally be ruled out before genetic investigations are instituted.

Prenatal Diagnosis of Genetic Disease

Amniocentesis, fetoscopy, and ultrasound techniques have dramatically increased our ability to detect fetal disorders antenatally. It is now possible to diagnose virtually all chromosome abnormalities, over 100 inborn errors of metabolism, biochemical and monogenic disorders, and an increasing number of structural abnormalities.

Amniocentesis

TECHNIQUES AND RISKS. Amniocentesis for the purpose of prenatal genetic diagnosis is best performed at 16 weeks' gestation. Most commonly, ultrasound is performed immediately before amniocentesis for determination of the position of the placenta, location of the amniotic fluid, determination of the presence of fetal cardiac activity and the number of fetuses, and confirmation of gestational age. Twenty-five to thirty-five milliliters of amniotic fluid are removed. For some disorders the amniotic fluid can be assayed directly, but in general the fetal cells are grown in tissue culture. Chromosome analysis or biochemical assay then follows.

Amniocentesis is associated with potential risks. The risks to the mother are very low. The incidence of amnionitis is about 0.1%, and minor maternal complications such as vaginal spotting or leakage of amniotic fluid occur in 2% to 3% of cases. In addition, Rh isoimmunization can occur if the mother is Rh negative and the fetus is Rh positive; therefore, Rho(D) immune globulin should be administered to Rh-negative women following amniocentesis. Potential fetal risks include bleeding and trauma. The major risk is fetal loss, the incidence of which is about 0.5%.

LIMITATIONS. Aberrations can occur *in vitro*. In "pseudo-mosaicism," which is of no clinical significance, a single cell contains an extra chromosome (most often a number 2 or X); this occurs in about 5% of amniotic fluid specimens. When an aberration is found in a culture, it is the responsibility of the laboratory to determine whether the aberration occurs in more than one flask or in more than one colony. Prediction of the phenotype is difficult when there is chromosomal mosaicism, a translocation, an inversion, or a small supernumerary chromosome. In these cases the parental chromosomes should be analyzed; if the identical abnormality is found in a normal parent, one can expect the offspring to be phenotypically normal. In contrast, if the abnormality has arisen *de novo,* the offspring has a 10% to 20% chance of being phenotypically abnormal.

CYTOGENETIC STUDIES. All chromosomal disorders are potentially detectable prenatally. Clearly accepted indications for cytogenetic studies include maternal age of over 35; a previous child with a chromosome abnormality, and a balanced translocation or inversion in a parent. Cytogenetic studies should also be performed to determine fetal sex if the child is known to be at risk for an X-linked disorder.

The most common indication for cytogenetic studies is advanced maternal age, which is generally considered to be 35 years or older. The likelihood of a mother having a child with trisomy 21 at age 35 is about 1 in 365; at age 39, the risk is 1 in 139; and age 45, the risk is 1 in 32. For women who have had a child with an autosomal trisomy, the risk of another liveborn having chromosome trisomy is around 1% to 2%. Antenatal diagnosis is warranted when there is a balanced translocation carrier parent. The risks vary with the chromosomes involved, the length of genetic material, and whether the mother or father carries the translocation. Empiric risk data for specific rare translocations are not available; however, with prenatal amniocentesis diagnoses can be made.

Determinaton of fetal sex for couples who are at risk for X-linked recessive disorders can be carried out by amniocentesis. Occasionally one can diagnose not only the sex, but also whether the fetus is affected. However, if one is unable to diagnose the disorder, the couple might want to limit their progeny to females.

A potential indication for cytogenetic studies is high paternal age, since it has been suggested that trisomy 21 may be associated with paternal age greater than 55. Other potential indications include previous stillborn births and a history of trisomic spontaneous abortions.

BIOCHEMICAL STUDIES. Antenatal diagnosis is now possible for more than 100 inborn errors of metabolism, biochemical abnormalities, and monogenic disorders.

Almost all such errors are transmitted in autosomal recessive fashion, although they may also be transmitted as X-linked recessive traits. Couples are usually identified as being at risk because of previously affected children. For parents who are diagnosed as being heterozygote carriers, as in Tay–Sachs disease, prenatal genetic diagnosis is indicated. In order for a metabolic error to be detected, the enzyme must be expressed in amniotic fluid fibroblasts. In each instance the amniotic fluid cells from the suspected case must be compared with amniotic fluid cells of the same gestational age from a normal gestation. Usually diagnosis takes 4 to 6 weeks because of the large number of cells required for analysis.

Mendelian disorders associated with chromosome breakage, such as Bloom syndrome and Fanconi anemia, have been diagnosed prenatally on the basis of a greater than normal rate of spontaneous chromosome breakage. X-linked mental retardation can be diagnosed prenatally by demonstration of the "fragile site" on the X chromosome.

MOLECULAR GENETIC STUDIES. It is possible antenatally to diagnose sickle cell anemia, α- and β-thalassemia, and other disorders of hemoglobin biosynthesis. Initially, diagnoses were made from fetal blood obtained either by aspiration from chorionic vessels under fetoscopic visualization or by direct placental aspiration. More recently, however, developments in molecular genetics have permitted the diagnosis of some hemoglobinopathies on amniotic fluid cells. Several techniques are employed. Usually the DNA is isolated from amniotic fluid cells for analysis. One method involves use of the group of enzymes called *restriction endonucleases.* Because most of the diagnoses made with this method are based on linkage analysis, the size of the DNA fragment to which the mutant gene is linked is first determined in the family under study, usually the parents and one other family member, before it is determined in the fetus. Another technique uses DNA probes that have been copied from an mRNA that codes for a specific protein. The probe hybridizes with the fragment of DNA containing the respective globin gene. The presence or absence of the nonmutant gene is then demonstrated with autoradiography. This technique is particularly applicable to disorders in which DNA is deleted, the most common example being α-thalassemia.

LINKAGE ANALYSIS. Linkage analysis can be used for the antenatal diagnosis of disorders for which neither metabolic assays nor other diagnosis techniques are available. Such analysis requires a measurable gene product of a marker gene that is closely linked to the mutant gene in question. The presence or absence of the mutant gene can then be inferred on the basis of the status of the marker gene.

This approach has been used to diagnose 21-hydroxylase adrenogenital syndrome. The gene for 21-hydroxylase deficiency and the HLA locus are tightly linked on chromosome 6. The inheritance pattern of the HLA haplotypes and the mutant gene in the parents and an affected child must be determined to establish the linkage. On the basis of this analysis it is possible to predict whether the fetus is affected by the disorder.

Because recombination can occur even between closely linked loci, diagnosis by linkage analysis is not absolute; however, as a more complete map of the human genome becomes available, linkage analysis probably will be increasingly useful in antenatal diagnosis. Other linkage relationships useful in antenatal diagnosis include hemophilia and G6PD, as well as myotonic dystrophy and the secretion of ABO antigens.

Neural Tube Defects

Antenatal diagnosis of neural tube defects can be accomplished by either ultrasonography or assay of the amniotic fluid for α-fetoprotein. Individuals who have had one affected pregnancy or who themselves are affected with a neural tube defect are at risk for recurrence. The recurrence risk after one affected pregnancy is 3% in an area of low population incidence such as the United States and 5% in an area with a high population incidence such as South Wales. After two pregnancies the recurrence risk increases to about 10%. Amniocentesis for determination of α-fetoprotein levels is the primary diagnostic test. Amniotic fluid false-negative tests in cases of open spinal defects are rare. False-negative results are more common in the case of closed neural tube defects, which account for 10% of affected pregnancies. False-positive elevations of amniotic fluid α-fetoprotein are more common than false-negative elevations, many being due to contamination of the amniotic fluid with fetal blood. False-positives may also be due to the gestational age and hence the α-fetoprotein level being different from what was expected. Other fetal defects have been associated with elevated amniotic fluid or maternal serum α-fetoprotein; they include omphalocele, gastroschisis, open skin defects, teratomas, Turner's syndrome, and the Finnish form of congenital nephrosis, which is associated with massive fetal proteinuria. Fetal demise also causes amniotic fluid α-fetoprotein levels to rise.

Since 90% to 95% of all affected children are born to parents who are not known to be at risk, a method for screening all pregnant women would be beneficial. In most such screening programs, maternal serum is obtained at about 16 to 18 weeks' gestation. If an elevated α-fetoprotein level is detected (in 7–8% of cases), a second sample is obtained. If the second level is elevated (in 4–5% of cases), ultrasound is indicated to rule out multiple pregnancies, underestimation of gestational age, and fetal demise. If the possibility of neural tube defect then persists, amniocentesis is performed (in 2–3% of the original population). Among patients in whom amniocentesis is performed, an elevated amniotic fluid α-fetoprotein level is found in approximately 10%. Overall, the risk of a fetal neural tube defect in women with a confirmed elevated serum α-fetoprotein level is 5% to 10%.

Ultrasonography

Ultrasound is becoming increasingly important in the diagnosis of fetal congenital abnormalities. Ultrasonography is used not only in association with other tests to assess fetal normality but also to diagnose fetal structural abnormalities. Anomalies of the central nervous system, including anencephaly, hydrocephaly, spina bifida, and meningocele, can be detected by ultrasound. Anomalies of the fetal gastrointestinal tract, including omphalocele, gastroschisis, intestinal obstruction, diaphragmatic hernia, and fetal ascites, may be seen as well. Renal dysplasia and renal agenesis have also been diagnosed by ultrasound, and the ultrasonic visualization of fetal limbs has been enhanced by the use of real-time imaging. Recently, diagnoses of cardiac arrhythmias and congenital heart disease have become possible.

Fetoscopy

Though in most instances midtrimester amniocentesis and ultrasonography are most commonly used to obtain information regarding fetal status, in some patients fetoscopy may be useful.

Fetoscopy is a method of direct visualization of the fetus and placenta with endoscopic instruments; it is best performed between the 17th and 20th week of gestation. Ultrasound is done before fetoscopy to diagnose multiple gestation, to locate the placenta, to verify gestational age, to determine fetal position, and to select the site of insertion of the fetoscope. Orientation within the amniotic cavity is usually difficult owing to a limited field of vision; therefore, ultrasonography during fetoscopy is useful in directing the endoscope toward specific anatomic landmarks of the fetus. If fetoscopy is performed for the purpose of obtaining fetal blood, a 25- or 27-gauge needle is directed through the trocar channel into a vessel on the placenta; if fetal skin biopsies are to be taken, a stationary area such as the fetal thorax or back is chosen.

Risks of fetoscopy include maternal or fetal infection, hemorrhage, and Rh isoimmunization; the major risk is spontaneous fetal loss, the incidence of which is 5% to 10%.

Chorionic Villous Sampling

Chorionic villous sampling is a relatively new technique that allows prenatal genetic diagnosis to be accomplished much earlier than is the case with amniocentesis and amniotic fluid cell culture. It is done between 8 and 12 weeks' gestation. Under ultrasonic visualization, a small catheter is passed into the uterine cavity and a sample of villi from the chorion, under the decidua capsularis, is obtained. The indications for chorionic villous sampling are the same as those for amniocentesis. Chromosome analysis can be performed on uncultured cells or after culture, and biopsied material can be used directly for DNA analysis. Metabolic disorders can be diagnosed by chorionic villous sampling. Though the technique is relatively new, there is increasing enthusiasm for it because of the short waiting period for results and the consequently lower risk associated with pregnancy termination, should it be necessary. Risks and limitations are still to be evaluated, but at present the risk of fetal loss appears to be about 5%.

Genetic Counseling

The aim of genetic counseling is to explain the risk of producing an affected child, to convey the prognosis, and to inform individuals seeking counseling of ways of dealing with the risk. Most persons seeking genetic counseling have already had an abnormal child, but as our ability to detect carriers increases, couples will increasingly seek counseling before pregnancy.

A correct diagnosis is the single most important prerequisite of genetic counseling. In some instances the diagnosis is obvious by physical examination; in others certain biochemical tests are needed; and in some the diagnosis is not readily made. Persons in whom no diagnosis can be established are commonly referred to a genetic counselor or counseling center. Often only such a center can make a diagnosis because of their diagnostic expertise in cytogenetics, pediatrics, neurology, ophthalmology, cardiology, and other syndrome identification. Some of the common indications for chromosome studies are multiple congenital anomalies with mental retardation; a phenotype indicative of a specific chromosome abnormality; X-linked mental retardation; abnormal sexual development; chromosome breakage syndrome (*e.g.,* Fanconi anemia); reproductive failure, including infertility, fetal demise, and abortions; and maternal age over 35. In addition, chromosome studies can be carried out for the prenatal diagnosis of balanced translocations.

With any disorder, once the diagnosis is known and the mode of transmission determined, recurrence risks can be determined (see Table 2-2). For disorders caused by single-gene mutations, risk of recurrence ranges from 25% for autosomal recessive disorders to 50% for autosomal dominant disorders (see Table 2-2). For common multifactorial conditions such as cleft lip, cleft palate, and anencephaly, empiric risks have been established on the basis of the analysis of a number of large pedigrees. Risk figures for specific disorders can be obtained from the literature; most are 2% to 5%, including that for the multiple congenital anomaly/mental retardation syndromes of the sporadic "idiopathic" type. Recurrence risks for chromosome abnormalities vary from approximately 1% to 2% for trisomy Down syndrome in families in which there is already a 21-trisomic child to 100% for a balanced 21/21 translocation from one parent. For rare balanced translocations, risk of recurrence is impossible to determine.

A couple's decision as to whether to take a risk depends to a great degree upon the burden—physical, emotional, and financial—that an affected child will be to the family. Thus, it is important for the adviser to convey the prognosis to the family, because it plays an important role in their decision.

CONCLUSIONS

Advances in biology and medicine that allow control of reproductive capabilities, both quantitatively and now qualitatively, are frequently a cause of concern. Though this seems particularly true in genetic counseling, screening for genetic diseases, and prenatal diagnosis, it is true in other areas of gynecology and obstetrics as well (*e.g.,* sterilization, artificial insemination, abortion, *in vitro* fertilization). In all of these areas, there is little need for concern if decision making remains an individual choice; when this choice is lost, all of humanity should be concerned.

REFERENCES AND RECOMMENDED READING

Alberts B, Bray D, Lewis J et al (eds): Molecular Biology of the Cell. New York, Garland Publishing, 1983

Borgoankar DS: Chromosomal Variation in Man: A Catalog of Chromosomal Variants and Anomalies, 4th ed. New York, Alan R Liss, 1984

Caspersson T, Zech L, Johansson C et al: Identification of human chromosomes by DNA-binding fluorescing agents. Chromosomes 30:215, 1970

de Grouchy J, Turleau C: Clinical Atlas of Human Chromosomes, 2nd ed. New York, John Wiley & Sons, 1984

Emery AEH, Rimoin DL (eds): Principles and Practice of Medical Genetics, Vols 1 and 2. New York, Churchill Livingstone, 1983

Fuhrmann W, Vogel F: Genetic Counseling, 2nd ed. New York, Springer-Verlag, 1976

Lejeune J, Lafourcade J, Berger R et al: Trois cas de délétion partielle du bras court d'un chromosome 5. C R Acad Sci Paris 257:3098, 1963

Makino S: Human Chromosomes. New York, American Elsevier, 1975

McKusick VA: Mendelian Inheritance in Man—Catalogs of Autosomal Dominant, Autosomal Recessive, and X-Linked Phenotypes, 6th ed. Baltimore, Johns Hopkins University Press, 1983

Sandberg AA (ed): Cytogenetics of the Mammalian X Chromosome. Part A: Basic Mechanisms of X Chromosome Behavior. Part B: X Chromosome Anomalies and Their Clinical Manifestations. New York, Alan R Liss, 1983

Schinzel A: Catalogue of Unbalanced Chromosome Aberrations in Man. Berlin, De Gruyter, 1984

Simpson JL, Golbus MS, Martin AO, Sarto GE: Genetics in Obstetrics and Gynecology. New York, Grune & Stratton, 1982

Stanbury JB, Wyngaarden JB, Fredrickson DS (eds): The Metabolic Basis of Inherited Disease, 5th ed. New York, McGraw-Hill, 1983

Therman E: Human Chromosomes: Structure, Behavior, Effects, 2nd ed. New York, Springer-Verlag, 1985

Vogel F, Motulsky AG: Human Genetics: Problems and Approaches. New York, Springer-Verlag, 1979

Gross Anatomy of the Female Reproductive Tract, Pituitary, and Hypothalamus

Roger C. Crafts
Howard P. Krieger

3

The Female Reproductive Tract*

Roger C. Crafts

The female reproductive tract consists of internal organs, located in the pelvic cavity, and the external genitalia, located in the perineum. The internal organs are the ovaries, uterine tubes, uterus, and vagina. The external genitalia consist of the mons pubis, labia majora, labia minora, the vestibule of the vagina, and related structures.

The international terminology, introduced in 1955 and periodically revised by the International Anatomical Nomenclature Committee, has been used in this chapter, with the terms formerly used placed in parentheses.

PELVIC CAVITY

Bony Structures

Before the pelvic cavity and perineum can be understood, it is mandatory that one be thoroughly familiar with the bones that form the pelvis. The bony pelvis is made up of the two coxal (innominate) bones, which are actually part of the lower limbs, and the sacrum and coccyx, which are parts of the axial skeleton.

Since the shape of a coxal bone is almost indescribable, the following description will be more comprehensible if a model of a bony pelvis is at hand. Care

* Portions of this chapter have been reprinted with permission from *A Textbook of Human Anatomy* by Roger C. Crafts, 3rd edition, published by John Wiley & Sons, Inc., 1985.

should be taken to hold the pelvis in the position found in the living human body.

Coxal Bones

The coxal bones are made up of three parts: *ilium, ischium,* and *pubis* (Fig. 3-1). The ilium is the wing-shaped superior portion of the coxal bone; the ischium, the short, blunt posteroinferior portion; and the pubis, the anterior inferior portion. These three bones come together at the *acetabulum,* the fossa that articulates with the head of the femur.

On the internal surface of the coxal bone, the *ilium* articulates inferiorly with the pubis and the ischium. This part of the coxal bone flares out into a thin, wing-like portion with a concavity on the medial surface. This concavity is the *iliac fossa.* Following this surface superiorly, one reaches the *iliac crest.* This crest starts anteriorly with the *anterior superior iliac spine* and proceeds posteriorly and laterally until it reaches the *posterior superior iliac spine;* it has an inner and outer lip and an intermediate line that serve for muscle attachment. In addition to these two superior spines, the ilium possesses an *anterior inferior iliac spine* and a *posterior inferior iliac spine.* The posterior inferior iliac spine is just posterior to the large surface of the ilium that articulates with the sacrum.

The superior end of the *ischium* is fused with the ilium and pubis. The ischium is the portion of the coxal bone upon which a person sits, and that roughened area located most inferiorly and posteriorly is known as the *ischial tuberosity.* Just superior to the ischial tuberosity is the *lesser ischiadic (sciatic) notch* and, separated from this notch by the *ischial spine,* the *greater ischiadic (sciatic) notch.*

The *pubis* articulates with the ilium and the ischium. This part of the coxal bone contains a medial portion—the *body*—and *superior* and *inferior rami.* The inferior

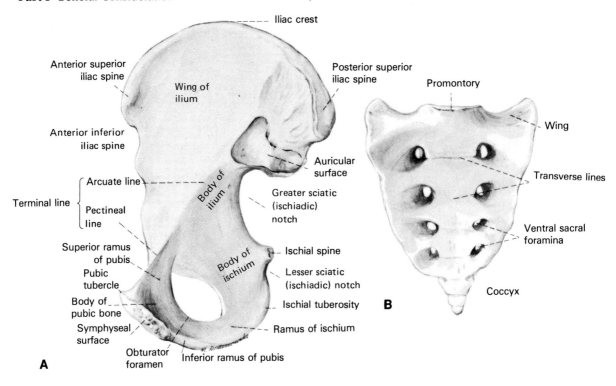

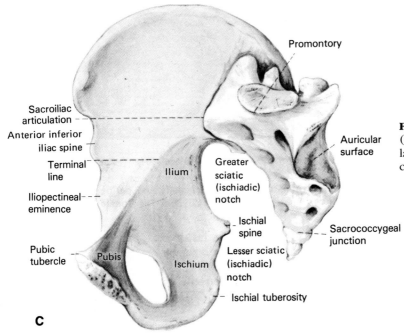

FIG. 3-1. (*A*) Coxal bone, medial aspect. (*B*) Sacrum, anterior aspect. (*C*) Articulated right coxal bone, sacrum, and coccyx, left oblique view.

ramus is the portion that joins the ischium, while the superior ramus joins the ilium and ischium at the acetabular notch. The superior surface of the body is smooth, while the inferior surface is quite rough because of the attachment of muscles. The articular surface is joined to the pubic bone of the other side by fibrocar-

tilage as well as ligaments. The *pubic crest* is that portion of the body of the pubis that is most easily felt and ends laterally in an elevation called the *pubic tubercle*. The superior surface of the superior ramus exhibits a sharp edge called the *pectineal line*. This line runs laterally from the pubic tubercle and joins the *arcuate line* to form the *terminal line*. The two rami of the pubic bone form partial boundaries of a large opening called the *obturator foramen*. The superior edge of this foramen exhibits an *obturator tubercle* and an *obturator sulcus* due to passage of vessels and nerves from the pelvis into the lower limb.

Sacrum and Coccyx

The sacral vertebrae are fused into one bone called the *sacrum* (Fig. 3-1*B*) that is broad superiorly and tapers inferiorly; it can be described as having a base superiorly and an apex inferiorly. It is concave anteriorly and convex posteriorly. On the anterior surface, a medial portion is separated from two lateral portions by four *foramina* on each side for passage of ventral rami of the sacral nerves and corresponding vessels. The median portion presents *transverse lines* that indicate the points of fusion of the five vertebrae. The lateral portions possess *articular surfaces* for articulation with the coxal bone. The vertebral canal continues through the sacrum. A *superior facet* serves for articulation with the fifth lumbar vertebra, and an *inferior facet* for articulation with the coccyx.

The *coccygeal vertebrae* (Fig. 3-1*B*) are usually fused into one bone also. The first vertebra is of some size but the remaining three are small rounded bones of various sizes and shapes. Extra bones may be found. The vertebral canal does not continue into these vertebrae.

Bony Pelvis as a Whole

The *pelvis* consists of the two coxal bones anteriorly and laterally and the sacrum and coccyx posteriorly (Fig. 3-2). It is divided into a *true* and *false pelvis*. The *inlet of the true pelvis* is superiorly placed and bounded by the sacral promontory posteriorly, the pubic symphysis anteriorly, and the terminal lines on the sides, the terminal lines being the pectineal lines anteriorly and the arcuate lines posteriorly; the *outlet* is the inferior end and is bounded from anterior to posterior by the pubic arch, inferior ramus of the pubis, ischial tuberosity, lesser ischiadic notch, ischial spine, greater ischiadic notch, and the sacrum and coccyx. As can be seen in Figure 3-2, ligaments actually form the boundaries of the outlet rather than the two notches mentioned. The *false pelvis* is that part above the inlet to the true pelvis.

The female pelvis differs from that of the male in several ways, although it is important to realize that there are many degrees of maleness and femaleness. Furthermore, there are racial differences that make measurements in a single sex quite variable.

Lines that have been established to measure the diameters of the pelvic inlet are shown in Figure 3-2. Anthropologists classify pelves into anthropoid, android, gynecoid, and platypelloid types. Figure 3-2 is a drawing of a gynecoid pelvis, typical of that found in most women. Anthropoid has a short transverse (C–D) diameter but a long anteroposterior diameter (E–F), while the platypelloid type is opposite to this, that is, it has a very long transverse (C–D) diameter and very short anteroposterior (E–F) diameter. Most males are anthropoid or android; most females are android or gynecoid, although mixed types occur with some frequency. The pelvic variations and their obstetric significance are discussed in Chapter 31.

In very general terms, the female pelvis, in comparison with the male pelvis, is lighter, the bones are more slender, and the markings made by the attachments of muscles are less pronounced. The ilium has a greater lateral flair, and the iliac fossa is slightly more shallow. The ischial spines to not project toward the center of the pelvis as they do in the male, and the same is true of the sacrum and coccyx; the promontory of the sacrum is less pronounced in the female. The ischial tuberosities are farther apart. The inlet to the true pelvis tends to be oval rather than heart-shaped as in the male. All of the above factors result in longer pelvic diameters in the female than in the male.

All of this is of interest to the anatomist or anthropologist, but the obstetrician is interested in comparing the size of the baby's head (fetal cephalometry) with the dimensions of the pelvic outlet (pelvimetry). Therefore, averages are not as important as the dimensions of the pelvic outlet on the particular patient giving birth to a baby. Additional measurements can be made between the pubic symphysis and the tip of the coccyx or the sacrococcygeal joint, transversely between the inside surfaces of the ischial tuberosities, and obliquely between the junction of the pubic and ischial rami anteriorly to the midpoint in the sacrotuberous ligament posteriorly. These are shown in Figure 3-3.

Joints and Ligaments of the Pelvis

A knowledge of the ligaments in this area, as well as a clear conception of the bony pelvis, is needed in order to understand the anatomy in this region.

The sacrum articulates with the fifth lumbar vertebra at the lumbosacral joint. The articulation of the coxal bones with each other in the pubic region (the pubic symphysis), and the articulation between the sacrum and these two coxal bones (the sacroiliac joints) remain. Furthermore, there are very important ligaments that connect the sacrum and coccyx to the ischial portion of the coxal bones, and some attention should be given to the articulation of the sacrum and coccyx, and to the obturator membrane.

Pubic Symphysis

A cartilaginous joint, the pubic symphysis is partially movable (Fig. 3-4*A*). The articular surfaces of each pubic bone are covered with hyaline cartilage, and between these two areas of cartilage is interposed a fibrocartilaginous lamina, the *interpubic disc*. This varies in thick-

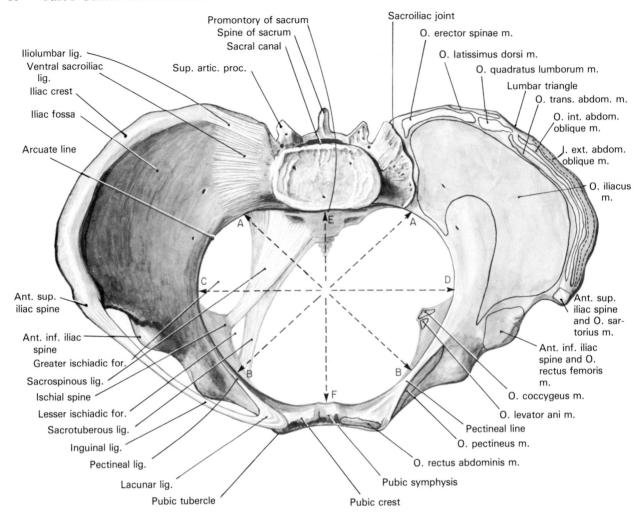

FIG. 3-2.   Female bony pelvis, with origins and insertions of muscles indicated on the *left* and the ligaments shown on the *right*. (*A*) Sacroiliac joint. (*B*) Iliopubic eminence. (*C*) and (*D*) Middle of pelvic brim. (*E*) Sacral promontory. (*F*) Pubic symphysis. (Crafts RC: A Textbook of Human Anatomy. Copyright © 1985. Reprinted by permission of John Wiley & Sons, Inc., New York)

ness in different areas and is a very dense and firm structure. In lower animal forms a hormone, relaxin, tends to soften this fibrocartilaginous material, allowing the pubic bones to spread apart during parturition. Although this occurs to a much lesser degree in the human being, it is thought that there is some softening of the fibrocartilage. This interpubic disc is aided by a *superior pubic ligament,* which connects the two pubic bones superiorly, and by the *arcuate pubic ligament,* a thick arch of ligamentous fibers that connects them inferiorly. The former ligament extends laterally as far as the pubic tubercles. The arcuate ligament forms the superior boundary of the *pubic arch* and continues laterally to be attached to the inferior rami of the pubic bones.

Sacroiliac Joint

Because they are required to bear great weight, the sacroiliac joints (Fig. 3-4*B*) are important. These joints are formed by the articulation between the sacrum and the iliac portion of the coxal bones. This joint is *partly cartilaginous* and *partly synovial* in type (Fig. 3-5). Some movement is allowed. Each articular surface is covered with a thin layer of cartilage, and between these cartilages is found a layer of fibrocartilage. The *ligaments* of this joint are the ventral sacroiliac, dorsal sacroiliac, and interosseous ligaments. The *ventral sacroiliac ligament* consists of several thin bands that connect the anterior surface of the sacrum to the anterior surface of

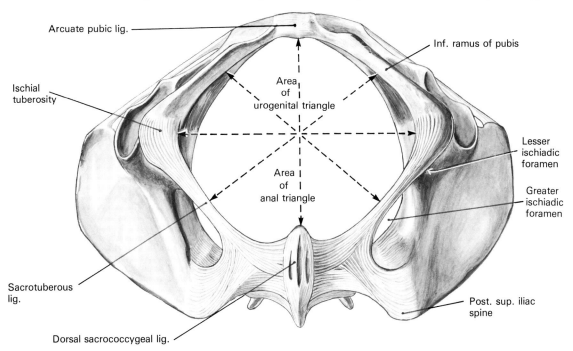

FIG. 3-3. Boundaries of the perineum. Note that a *line* drawn between the two ischial tuberosities divides this area into anterior urogenital and posterior anal triangles. *Dotted lines* represent measurements (pelvimetry) that can be compared with the baby's head (fetal cephalometry). (Crafts RC: A Textbook of Human Anatomy. Copyright © 1985. Reprinted by permission of John Wiley & Sons, Inc., New York)

the ilium. In contrast, the *dorsal sacroiliac ligament* is quite thick and forms the chief attachment of the sacrum and ilium. It consists of bundles that pass between the bones in several directions. The superior part is the *short dorsal sacroiliac ligament,* and the fibers take a nearly horizontal course. They pass between the first and second transverse tubercles on the posterior surface of the sacrum and the tuberosity of the ilium. The inferior part of this ligament—the *long dorsal sacroiliac ligament*— courses obliquely. It courses from the third transverse tubercle on the posterior surface of the sacrum and attaches to the posterior superior spine of the ilium. (This ligament is intermingled with the sacrotuberous ligament.) The *interosseous sacroiliac ligament* (see Fig. 3-5) is located deep to the posterior sacroiliac ligament just described. The fiber bundles are very short and connect the tuberosities of the sacrum and the ilium.

Several other ligaments serve to attach the coxal bones to the vertebral column. These are the iliolumbar, sacrotuberous, and sacrospinous ligaments. The *iliolumbar ligament* (Fig. 3-4 *B* and *C*) is attached superiorly to the transverse process of the fifth lumbar vertebra. It radiates inferiorly and laterally and is attached by two main parts to the coxal bone. The inferior portion courses toward the base of the ilium and blends with the ventral sacroiliac ligament. The superior portion is

attached to the crest of the ilium anterior to the sacroiliac articulation. The *sacrotuberous ligament* (Fig. 3-4 *B* and *C*) is a large, heavy ligament that attaches over a wide area to the posterior inferior spine of the ilium, to the fourth and fifth transverse tubercles of the sacrum, and to the inferior part of the lateral margin of the sacrum and the coccyx. It passes obliquely inferiorly and laterally, becoming narrower as it proceeds, to attach to the medial side of the ischial tuberosity. The *sacrospinous ligament* (see Fig. 3-4 *B* and *C*) is much shorter than the sacrotuberous ligament, but it is also triangular in form. Its medial attachment is to the lateral margins of the sacrum and coccyx, and its lateral attachment is to the spine of the ischium. It is anterior to the sacrotuberous ligament. These sacrotuberous and sacrospinous ligaments are in such a position that they make foramina out of the greater and lesser ischiadic notches. They also form part of the boundary of the inferior pelvic outlet.

Sacrococcygeal Junction

The cartilaginous joint formed between the inferior articular surface of the sacrum and the base of the coccyx is the sacrococcygeal junction; it is partially movable. In some cases, it is synovial in character, and consid-

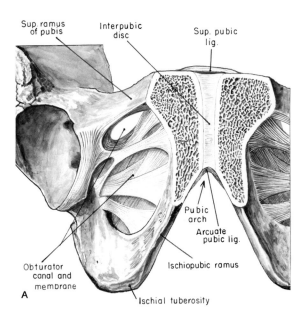

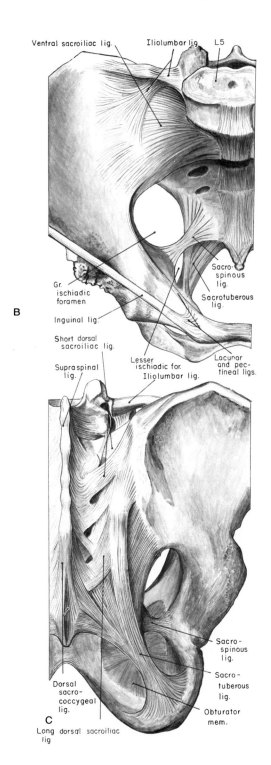

FIG. 3-4. (*A*) Pubic symphysis cut to show interpubic disc. (*B*) Anterior view of sacroiliac joints. (*C*) Posterior view of sacroiliac joints. (Crafts RC: A Textbook of Human Anatomy. Copyright © 1985. Reprinted by permission of John Wiley & Sons, Inc., New York)

erable movement is allowed. Its disc is much thinner than the discs in the rest of the vertebral column. It is supported by ligaments similar to those associated with the rest of the vertebral column. The one that corresponds to the anterior longitudinal ligament is the ventral sacrococcygeal ligament; those that correspond to the posterior longitudinal and supraspinal ligaments are the deep and superficial portions of the dorsal sacrococcygeal ligament. Lateral sacrococcygeal ligaments connect the transverse processes of the coccyx to the lower lateral angles of the sacrum.

Obturator Membrane

A thin but tough aponeurosis, the obturator membrane (see Fig. 3-4*A*) fills in the large bony obturator foramen, except for a small area superiorly for the passage of the obturator vessels and nerve, the *obturator canal.* The membrane, consisting of several interlacing bundles, most of which take a transverse direction, really should be considered part of the coxal bone; it serves for the attachment of the obturator internus and externus muscles that arise from the inside and outside surfaces, respectively, as well as from the surrounding bone.

General Description of Pelvic Cavity

If the pelvis is held in the correct position, it can be seen that it is not a bowl-like area that sits directly superiorly–inferiorly, nor is it one that has an anteropos-

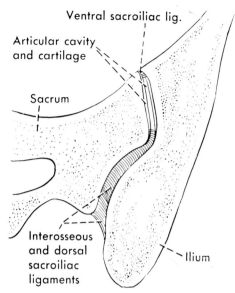

Ventral sacroiliac lig.

Articular cavity
and cartilage

Sacrum

Interosseous
and dorsal
sacroiliac
ligaments

Ilium

FIG. 3-5. Schematic horizontal section through sacroiliac joint. (Hollinshead WH: Anatomy for Surgeons, Vol 3. New York, Hoeber, 1958)

terior direction. As one looks inferiorly through the pelvis, one looks in an inferior–posterior direction. If the pelvic cavity is thought of as a bowl with several holes in the midline, the floor of this bowl resembles the floor of the pelvis (*pelvic diaphragm*), which is composed of muscles and their fascial layers. The area superior to this floor of the bowl or the pelvic diaphragm is the pelvic cavity proper; the part inferior and posterior to the bowl is the *perineum.*

The pelvic cavity is never empty (Fig. 3-6). That area that is not filled with the pelvic organs themselves contains the sigmoid colon, the cecum, and the ileum, the amount of sigmoid colon and cecum varying considerably.

The *sigmoid colon* continues into the pelvic cavity as the *rectum* and is just anterior to the promontory of the sacrum. The upper two thirds of the rectum is covered with peritoneum, making it a retroperitoneal organ. The uterus intervenes between the rectum and the urinary bladder and divides the pelvic cavity into two pouches, one in which the peritoneum reflects from the rectum to the posterior wall of the vagina and uterus and another in which the peritoneum is reflected from the anteroinferior (vesical) surface of the uterus to the urinary bladder. These pouches are the *rectouterine* and the *vesicouterine pouches,* respectively (Fig. 3-7). Note that, in spite of the name, the *rectouterine pouch* (pouch of Douglas) in reality is an area between the rectum and the superior end of the vagina (see Fig. 3-6). This is an important fact to realize since the very inferior end of the pelvic cavity is often a place where pus can collect as a result of infections of the peritoneum; it can be drained via the vagina.

The *uterine tubes* extend laterally from the fundus of the uterus as far as the lateral pelvic wall. The peritoneum does not simply reflect over the uterus itself, but is also reflected from the floor of the pelvis superiorly and anteriorly over the uterine tubes, and then back to the floor of the pelvis again (the *broad ligaments*). Therefore, the anteflexed uterus and its accompanying uterine tubes and layers of peritoneum cut the pelvic cavity in the female into an anterior and a posterior portion. The uterus bends anteriorly, so the posterior surface is actually a posterosuperior surface and the anterior surface an anteroinferior surface (see Fig. 3-6). This is the normal position for the uterus, and it is approximately at right angles to the direction taken by the vagina.

The fimbriated end of each uterine tube is in close approximation to an almond-shaped structure hanging onto the posterior–superior aspect of the broad ligaments (Fig. 3-8). These are the *ovaries,* which are suspended from the broad ligaments by two layers of peritoneum called the *mesovarium* (Fig. 3-9). In addition to this mesentery, the ovaries are attached medially to the uterus by a firm ligamentous structure, the *ligament of the ovary,* and laterally to the lateral pelvic wall by a *suspensory ligament* (*infundibulopelvic ligament*) consisting of a reflection of peritoneum over the vascular system entering the leaving the ovary. The broad ligaments can be divided into an area inferior to the mesovarium and an area superior to this structure (see Fig. 3-9). The superior area, between the mesovarium and the tube, is the *mesosalpinx* (mesentery of the tube); the inferior portion is the *mesometrium.*

The peritoneum around the rectum is distributed in such a manner as to form *pararectal fossae* (see Fig. 3-7). In this same area, two folds of peritoneum (*uterosacral folds*) stretch between the base of the uterus and the sacrum over the *uterosacral ligaments.* In addition, there are *paravesical fossae* on either side of the urinary bladder.

The midline structures, the structures on the lateral pelvic wall, and those on the anterior surface of the sacrum are all embedded in *subserous fascia* (see Fig. 3-8). Indeed, the subserous fascia in the abdominal cavity is directly continuous with similar fascia in the pelvis. It continues into the true pelvis, onto the deep fascia covering the muscles that form the floor of the pelvis, and thence onto the midline organs, where it blends with the capsule of each organ.

The *uterosacral ligaments* are condensations of this subserous fascia. Other condensations of this fascia occur at the point where the blood vessels leave the lateral pelvic wall to course along the floor of the pelvis to reach the uterus (the *cardinal ligaments* of the uterus) and anteriorly from the pubis to the bladder (*pubovesical ligaments*) and thence to the uterus (*uterovesical ligaments*). These ligaments are shown diagrammatically in Figure 3-10.

The *ureters* in the female cross the lateral pelvic wall and course inferior and posterior to the large ar-

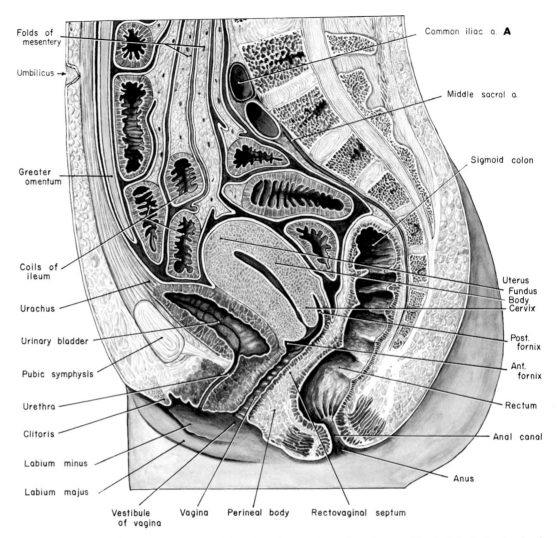

Folds of mesentery

Umbilicus →

Greater omentum

Coils of ileum

Urachus

Urinary bladder

Pubic symphysis

Urethra

Clitoris

Labium minus

Labium majus

Common iliac a. **A**

Middle sacral a.

Sigmoid colon

Uterus
Fundus
Body
Cervix

Post. fornix

Ant. fornix

Rectum

Anal canal

Anus

Vestibule of vagina   Vagina   Perineal body   Rectovaginal septum

FIG. 3-6. Sagittal section of female pelvic cavity and perineum. (Crafts RC: A Textbook of Human Anatomy. Copyright © 1985. Reprinted by permission of John Wiley & Sons, Inc., New York)

teries and veins of the uterus in this same layer of subserous fascia (Fig. 3-11). They also course to the lateral side of the vagina to reach the base of the bladder.

With the exception of the middle sacral artery, which is located on the anterior surface of the sacrum, the *arteries* entering the pelvis follow along the lateral pelvic wall and then the floor of the pelvis to reach the organs to be vascularized (see Fig. 3-11). The *veins* take a corresponding pathway in the opposite direction. In fact, the veins form a very profuse network on the floor of the pelvis. All vessels are located in the subserous fascia.

In addition to the vascular system, the *nerves* that form the visceral afferent and efferent systems are also found in this loose fascia. The hypogastric plexus, on the anterior surface of the sacrum, is made up of contributions from the sympathetic system as well as the

parasympathetic. These nerves form a very profuse network of fibers that follows the floor of the pelvis in this loose fascia and reaches the organs to be innervated in this manner. The two sympathetic chains can be seen to be prolonged into the pelvic cavity anterior to the sacrum in this same layer.

The deep fascia is called *parietal pelvic fascia* as a general term, but it also takes on the name of the particular muscle it covers (Fig. 3-12). If it is on the obturator internus muscle, it is called obturator fascia; if on the levator ani muscle, the supra-anal fascia; and so forth. This fascia is continuous with the transversalis fascia in the abdominal cavity.

The floor and sides of the pelvic cavity are covered by muscles and nerves (Figs. 3-12, 3-13, and 3-14). In the midline posteriorly is the sacrum, and just lateral and anterior to it are the many nerves that make up the

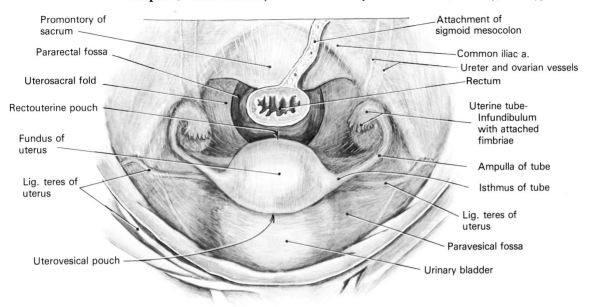

FIG. 3-7. Female pelvic cavity *in situ.* Note structures showing through peritoneum (exaggerated). (Crafts RC: A Textbook of Human Anatomy. Copyright © 1985. Reprinted by permission of John Wiley & Sons, Inc., New York)

FIG. 3-8. Female pelvic cavity. Peritoneum is intact on *left* and has been removed on *right* to show subserous fascia. (Crafts RC: A Textbook of Human Anatomy. Copyright © 1985. Reprinted by permission of John Wiley & Sons, Inc., New York)

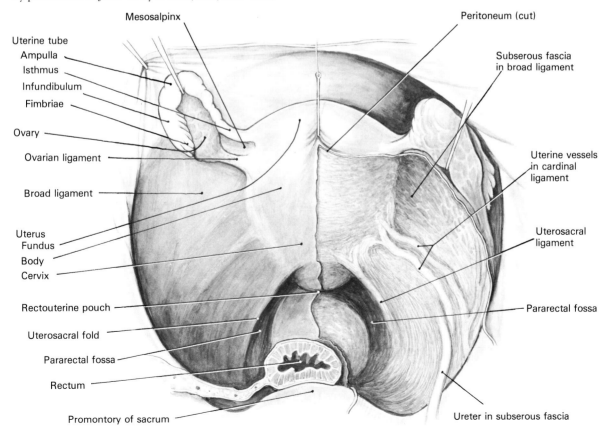

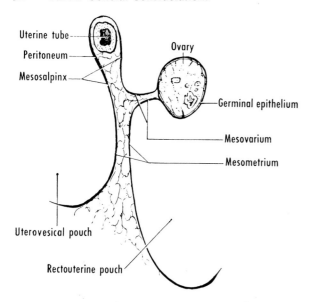

Uterine tube

Peritoneum

Mesosalpinx

Ovary

Germinal epithelium

Mesovarium

Mesometrium

Uterovesical pouch

Rectouterine pouch

FIG. 3-9.   Diagram of sagittal section showing broad ligament and its relations to ovary and uterine tube. Anterior aspect is on *left* side of diagram. (Gardner E, Gray DJ, O'Rahilly R: Anatomy: A Regional Study of Human Structure, 3rd ed. Philadelphia, WB Saunders, 1969)

sacral plexus. Just deep to these nerves is the *piriformis muscle,* arising from the sacrum and extending laterally to leave the pelvis through the greater ischiadic (sciatic) foramen (see Fig. 3-14). Anterior to this position, the *coccygeus muscle* extends from the ischial spine to the lateral surface of the coccyx. Anterior to that, the levator ani muscle arises from the pubis, lateral pelvic wall, and ischial spine, extending inferiorly in a funnel-shaped manner to blend with the organs in the pelvic cavity. This muscle can be divided into *pubovaginal, puborectal, pubococcygeal,* and *iliococcygeal portions* (see Fig. 3-12). The pubovaginal portion blends into the vagina. Some fibers of the puborectalis muscle not only blend with the rectum but also meet similar fibers from the opposite side in such a fashion as to form a sling for the rectum just posterior to it. This accounts for the change in direction at the rectoanal juncture. The pubococcygeal and iliococcygeal portions attach to the coccyx. The part of the levator ani muscle arising from the lateral pelvic wall is from the fascia on another muscle that helps to form the walls of the pelvis, the *obturator internus* muscle, and the fascia at this point forms a band called the *arcus tendineus.* The two muscles—the levator ani and the coccygeus muscles on each side—form the floor of the pelvis and are designated as the *pelvic diaphragm.*

FIG. 3-10.   Diagrammatic presentation of the condensations of the subserous fascia that have been called ligaments. (Crafts RC: A Textbook of Human Anatomy. Copyright © 1985. Reprinted by permission of John Wiley & Sons, Inc., New York)

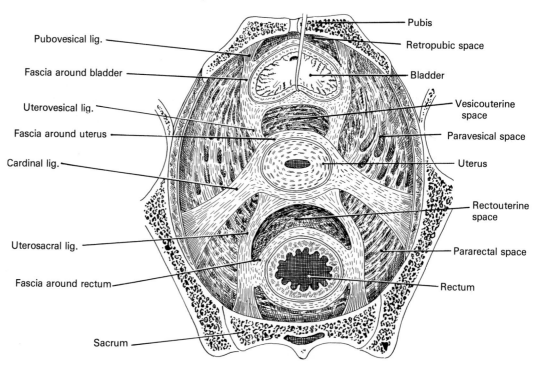

Pubovesical lig.

Fascia around bladder

Uterovesical lig.

Fascia around uterus

Cardinal lig.

Uterosacral lig.

Fascia around rectum

Sacrum

Pubis

Retropubic space

Bladder

Vesicouterine space

Paravesical space

Uterus

Rectouterine space

Pararectal space

Rectum

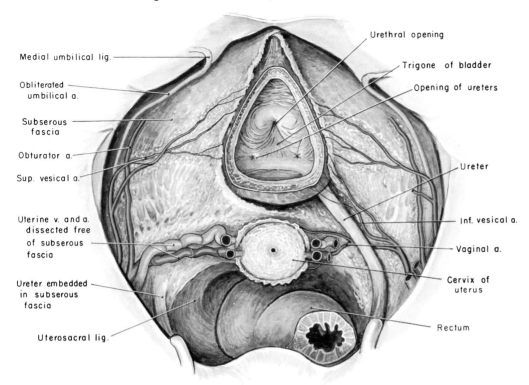

Medial umbilical lig.

Obliterated umbilical a.

Subserous fascia

Obturator a.

Sup. vesical a.

Uterine v. and a. dissected free of subserous fascia

Ureter embedded in subserous fascia

Uterosacral lig.

Urethral opening

Trigone of bladder

Opening of ureters

Ureter

Inf. vesical a.

Vaginal a.

Cervix of uterus

Rectum

FIG. 3-11. Female pelvic cavity. Uterine vessels have been dissected free of subserous fascia in which they course (cardinal ligaments) on *left* and have been removed on *right* to reveal course of ureter. Uterus has been removed to reveal urinary bladder, which has been cut to show its internal structure. (Crafts RC: A Textbook of Human Anatomy. Copyright © 1985. Reprinted by permission of John Wiley & Sons, Inc., New York)

In summary, the pelvic floor is formed by the levator ani and coccygeus muscles, with the sacrum located posteriorly and the pubic bones anteriorly; the obturator internus muscle is laterally placed while the piriformis muscle is located posteriorly in a position just lateral to the sacrum. These muscles are covered with parietal pelvic fascia that also covers the sacral nerves; the vessels, ureters, visceral nerves, and lymphatics are contained in a layer of subserous fascia; the organs, such as the uterus and vagina in the midline, are also covered with this same subserous fascia; and then the entire area is covered with peritoneum.

Arteries

The internal iliac (hypogastric) artery (Fig. 3-15) courses inferiorly into the pelvic cavity in a position posterior to the ureter and anterior to the corresponding internal iliac vein. The internal iliac artery usually divides into anterior and posterior divisions.

Although the branching of this artery is extremely variable, the following branches usually occur:

Branches of posterior division (PD)
1. Iliolumbar
2. Lateral sacral
3. Superior gluteal

Branches of anterior division (AD)
4. Umbilical and superior vesical
5. Uterine and vaginal
6. Middle rectal
7. Obturator
8. Internal pudendal
9. Inferior gluteal

The *posterior division* (PD), lying medial to the sacral plexus, terminates in the large *superior gluteal artery* (3), which exits from the pelvic cavity into the gluteal region through the greater ischiadic (sciatic) foramen in a position superior to the piriformis muscle. The *iliolumbar artery* (1) courses superiorly and laterally between the obturator nerve and the lumbosacral trunk. It is posterior to the common iliac artery. It divides into an iliac branch that ramifies in the iliac fossa and a lumbar branch that ascends superiorly in a position posterior to the psoas muscle. This latter branch sends a spinal

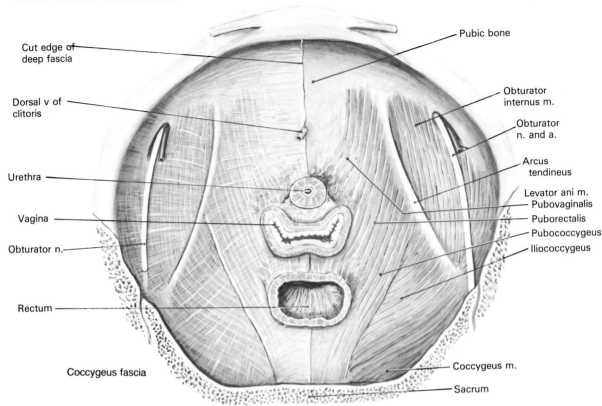

FIG. 3-12. Female pelvic cavity. The midline pelvic organs have been removed. The anterior part of the pelvic floor is seen, with deep fascia present on the *left* and removed on the *right*. Note that removing the subserous fascia has eliminated the blood vessels and the autonomic nerves. (Crafts RC: A Textbook of Human Anatomy. Copyright © 1985. Reprinted by permission of John Wiley & Sons, Inc., New York)

FIG. 3-13. Right half of pelvic diaphragm and sacral plexus, lateral view.

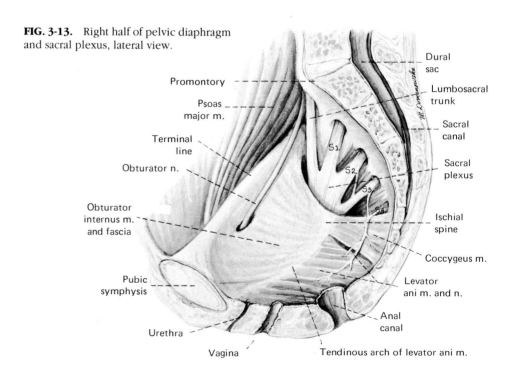

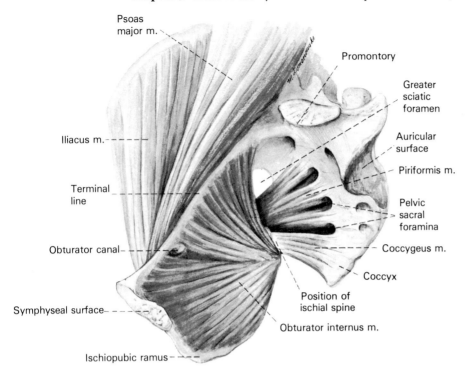

Psoas major m.

Promontory

Greater sciatic foramen

Auricular surface

Iliacus m.

Piriformis m.

Terminal line

Pelvic sacral foramina

Obturator canal

Coccygeus m.

Coccyx

Position of ischial spine

Symphyseal surface

Obturator internus m.

Ischiopubic ramus

FIG. 3-14. Muscles of right half of pelvic wall, anterolateral view.

branch into the vertebral canal through the lumbosacral intervertebral foramen. Two or more *lateral sacral arteries* (2) course inferiorly and medially, and enter the four anterior sacral foramina supplying structures in the sacral canal; they then emerge through the posterior sacral foramina and supply muscles and skin on the back of the sacrum.

The *anterior division* (AD) of the internal iliac artery continues inferiorly and divides into several branches. The pattern of the branching cannot be relied upon; it is quite variable. The *umbilical artery* and *superior vesical* (4) are usually combined into one stem. It continues along the side wall of the pelvis posterior to the obturator nerve and lateral to the ureter and the ligamentum teres. After giving off the superior vesical artery, it becomes the medial umbilical ligament. The *superior vesical arteries* (4) run medially from the umbilical arteries to supply the superior aspect of the bladder. The *uterine artery* (5) is of considerable size and courses anteriorly on the levator ani muscle to the base of the broad ligament. It then courses medially between the two layers of the broad ligament, superior to the ureter, and on the lateral fornix of the vagina. It supplies branches to the vagina and then continues on the lateral sides of the uterus, between the layers of the broad ligament, to the uterine tube; it gives off branches to these organs and anastomoses with the ovarian artery (Fig. 3-16). The inferior vesical artery in the female usually arises from this uterine artery. The *middle rectal artery* (6) courses medially on the lateral pelvic wall to reach the rectum. The *obturator artery* (7) courses inferiorly and anteriorly along the side wall of the pelvis in company with the obturator nerve. It leaves the pelvis

through the obturator canal. In approximately 40% of bodies, the artery may arise from the inferior epigastric branch of the external iliac (*abnormal obturator artery*). In this situation, it courses medially in a position posterior to the external iliac vein, and then courses over the brim of the pelvis to enter the obturator canal. It gives off branches to muscles on the lateral pelvic wall, to the bladder, and a *pubic branch* ramifies on the pelvic surface of the pubis. The *internal pudendal artery* (8) courses inferiorly and slightly posteriorly, and exits from the pelvic cavity into the gluteal region through the greater ischiadic (sciatic) foramen. It is very close to the ischial spine and enters the perineum by coursing through the lesser ischiadic (sciatic) foramen (see Fig. 3-30). The *inferior gluteal artery* (9) exits from the pelvic cavity into the gluteal region through the greater ischiadic (sciatic) foramen in a position inferior to the piriformis muscle.

Other arteries contribute to the supply of pelvic structures. The *middle sacral* emerges from the aorta just before it bifurcates, and this branch continues in the midline on the anterior aspect of the sacrum. The *superior rectal artery,* a branch of the inferior mesenteric, supplies the rectum, coursing just deep to the mucous membrane to anastomose finally with the *inferior rectal arteries* in the anal columns. The *middle rectal arteries* nourish the muscular walls of the rectum and thereby do not play a major role in the anastomosis of arteries on the rectum. The *arteries* to the ovary arise from the aorta just inferior to the origin of the renal arteries. They course retroperitoneally through the abdominal cavity, across the iliac vessels, and approach the ovaries from the lateral side, the peritoneum cov-

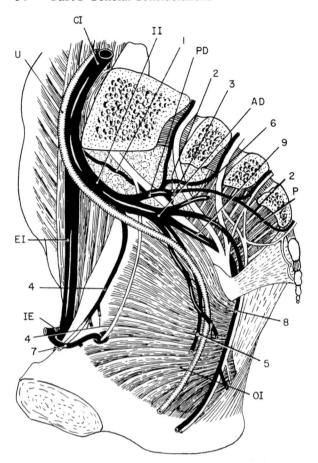

FIG. 3-15. Arteries of the pelvic cavity in the female. The pelvic floor (coccygeus and levator ani muscles) has been removed. Note relation of vessels to piriformis muscle (*P*) as they exit from the pelvic cavity through the greater ischiadic (sciatic) foramen. *AD,* anterior division; *CI,* common iliac; *EI,* external iliac; *IE,* inferior epigastric; *II,* internal iliac; *OI,* obturator internus muscle; *PD,* posterior division; *U,* ureter; *1,* iliolumbar; *2,* lateral sacral; *3,* superior gluteal; *4,* umbilical and superior vesical; *5,* uterine and vaginal; *6,* middle rectal; *7,* obturator arising from the inferior epigastric branch of the external iliac—the so-called abnormal obturator artery; *8,* internal pudendal; *9,* inferior gluteal. (Crafts RC: A Textbook of Human Anatomy. Copyright © 1985. Reprinted by permission of John Wiley & Sons, Inc., New York. Modified and redrawn after Jamieson)

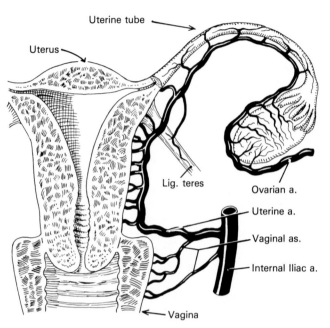

FIG. 3-16. Blood supply to the ovary, uterus, and vagina. (Crafts RC: A Textbook of Human Anatomy. Copyright © 1985. Reprinted by permission of John Wiley & Sons, Inc., New York)

Veins

The corresponding veins in the pelvic cavity (Fig. 3-17) form a profuse plexus before ending in the same branches as the arteries. The reproductive organs are surrounded by these plexuses, and parietal and visceral branches anastomose freely. They are located, as expected, in the subserous fascia. The umbilical and iliolumbar arteries have no corresponding veins. It should also be noted that the *deep dorsal vein of the clitoris* drains into the vesical plexus of veins. The *ovarian vein(s)* ascend along with the arteries and drain into the inferior vena cava on the right and the left renal vein on the left. It is important to realize that the *superior rectal veins* (part of the portal circulation) anastomose in the anal columns with the *inferior rectal veins* (systemic venous drainage); increased pressure in the portal circulation can lead to internal hemorrhoids at the point of this anastomosis. The *middle rectal veins* play a minor role, if any, in such hemorrhoids, since they are mainly concerned with the muscular walls of the rectum.

Lymphatics

The major groups of lymph nodes concerned with lymphatic drainage of the female reproductive organs lo-

ering these vessels forming the suspensory ligament of the ovary. The ovarian artery, after supplying the ovary itself, continues just inferior to the tube, between the layers of the broad ligament, supplying branches to the tube itself, and then anastomoses with the uterine artery (see Fig. 3-16). The ovarian artery sends branches to the ovarian ligament and to the proximal end of the ligamentum teres, as well as to these other structures.*

* Uncontrollable bleeding from the arteries supplying the uterus, vagina, superior aspect of the bladder, and midportion of the rectum can usually be stopped by ligating the anterior division

of the internal iliac artery just distal to its origin and proximal to the point where its first branch arises. In some cases, anastomosis with the ovarian artery is so rich that the suspensory ligament of the ovary (infundibulopelvic ligament) may also need to be tied. The collateral circulation is usually sufficient to prevent later disability from the loss of this blood supply.

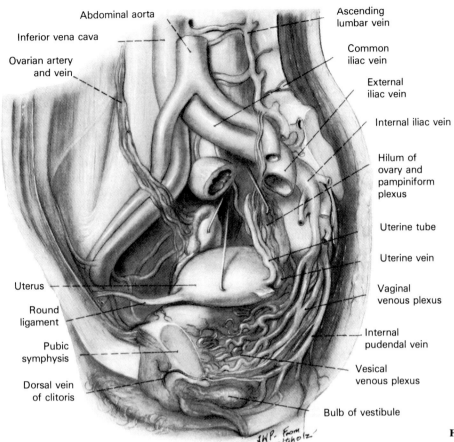

FIG. 3-17. Veins of female pelvic organs.

cated in the pelvic cavity include the external iliac, internal iliac, common iliac, and lumbar nodes (Fig. 3-18). These are arranged in general along the major arteries of the pelvic region. Sacral lymph nodes are found on the pelvic aspect of the sacrum, and scattered small nodes lie along parietal arteries (gluteal, pudendal, obturator) and in association with pelvic viscera (vesical, anorectal, parauterine, rectal). The course of lymph through these nodes leads eventually to lumbar nodes and to the thoracic duct.

Lymph vessels from the pelvic organs do not necessarily drain along the lines of the arterial pattern suggested by the arrangement of nodes mentioned above. Lymphatic vessels of the external genitalia, the anus, and the anal canal inferior to the pectinate line drain initially into the superficial inguinal nodes. The lymphatic vessels from the vagina may follow several routes. From the posteroinferior portion of the vagina the drainage may reach the sacral nodes. Other portions of the wall drain to internal, external, or common iliac nodes. The cervix drains to the external or internal iliac nodes and to the sacral nodes. The inferior portion of the body of the uterus drains mostly through the external iliac nodes. Lymphatic vessels from the superior body and the fundus pass principally with the ovarian lymphatics to the lumbar nodes. A few vessels, however,

go by way of the round ligament to the superficial inguinal nodes. Efferent vessels from the uterine tubes pass toward the ovary and reach the lumbar nodes. Lymphatic vessels from the ovary pass entirely out of the pelvis to the lumbar nodes.

The detailed lymphatic drainage as it is concerned in the spread of gynecologic cancer is considered in the appropriate sections.

Nerves

The nerves that supply the pelvis consist of fibers of several functional types. Striated muscles of the pelvic outlet and the skin of the perineum receive somatic motor and sensory fibers through branches of the lumbosacral plexus. The pelvic viscera are innervated by way of the autonomic plexuses, which convey sympathetic and parasympathetic motor and visceral sensory nerves to the organs. The spinal cord connections of these pathways include the lower thoracic and first lumbar segments, as well as the sacral and coccygeal levels.

Meninges and Spinal Cord

The walls of the vertebral canal, in which the spinal cord is lodged, are formed by the serially arranged ver-

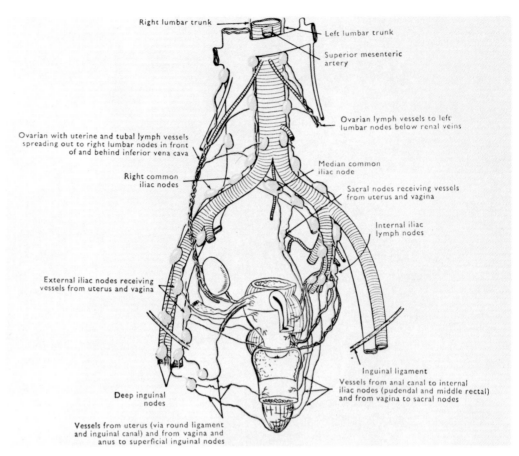

Right lumbar trunk

Left lumbar trunk

Superior mesenteric artery

Ovarian lymph vessels to left lumbar nodes below renal veins

Ovarian with uterine and tubal lymph vessels spreading out to right lumbar nodes in front of and behind inferior vena cava

Median common iliac node

Right common iliac nodes

Sacral nodes receiving vessels from uterus and vagina

Internal iliac lymph nodes

External iliac nodes receiving vessels from uterus and vagina

Inguinal ligament
Vessels from anal canal to internal iliac nodes (pudendal and middle rectal) and from vagina to sacral nodes

Deep inguinal nodes

Vessels from uterus (via round ligament and inguinal canal) and from vagina and anus to superficial inguinal nodes

FIG. 3-18.   Diagram of lymphatic vessels and lymph nodes of female genital organs. (Romanes GJ (ed): Cunningham's Textbook of Anatomy, 10th ed. London, Oxford University Press, 1964)

tebral arches of the individual vertebrae. Between adjacent vertebrae, the walls of the canal are completed by the ligamenta flava and interspinous ligaments posteriorly and by the intervertebral discs covered by the posterior longitudinal ligament anteriorly. The canal is continuous from the cranial cavity to the lower end of the sacrum, where it terminates as the hiatus of the sacral canal, an irregular opening covered by the superficial posterior sacrococcygeal ligament. The portion of the canal within the sacrum is known as the sacral canal.

The *dura mater* (Fig. 3-19) extends inferiorly as a closed tubular sac within the vertebral canal. The sac tapers rather abruptly to end opposite the body of the second sacral vertebra. A fibrous strand, the *filum terminale externum,* continues inferiorly from the sac to fuse to the coccyx. Several additional fibrous strands anchor the dura to the walls of the sacral canal. Sleevelike extensions of the dura also accompany the roots of the spinal nerves as far as the intervertebral foramina. The narrow epidural space (see Fig. 3-19) between the dural sac and the walls of the vertebral canal is occupied by fat, small arteries, and the internal vertebral venous plexus.

The thin *arachnoid* membrane (see Fig. 3-19) lines the inside of the dural sac and extends a short distance along the nerve roots. Spinal fluid fills the subarachnoid space between the arachnoid membrane and the pia mater covering the spinal cord.

The *pia mater* is the delicate inner layer intimately adherent to the surface of the spinal cord. Lateral fenestrated expansions of the pia mater, the *denticulate ligaments,* attach to the dura mater and help to anchor the spinal cord within the meninges.

The spinal cord (Fig. 3-19) extends inferiorly to the level of the body of the second lumbar vertebra, where it tapers to a cone-shaped termination (the *conus medullaris*), continuous inferiorly with a fibrous strand (the *filum terminale internum*), which extends caudally within the subarachnoid space to fuse with the terminal part of the dural sac.

Sacral and Coccygeal Nerves

The dorsal and ventral roots of the lower lumbar, sacral, and coccygeal nerves descend within the sub-

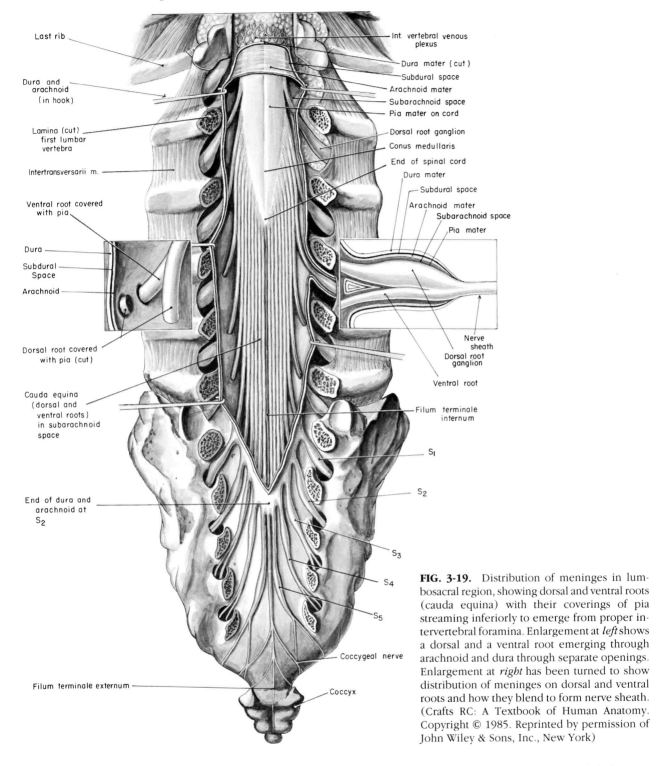

FIG. 3-19. Distribution of meninges in lumbosacral region, showing dorsal and ventral roots (cauda equina) with their coverings of pia streaming inferiorly to emerge from proper intervertebral foramina. Enlargement at *left* shows a dorsal and a ventral root emerging through arachnoid and dura through separate openings. Enlargement at *right* has been turned to show distribution of meninges on dorsal and ventral roots and how they blend to form nerve sheath. (Crafts RC: A Textbook of Human Anatomy. Copyright © 1985. Reprinted by permission of John Wiley & Sons, Inc., New York)

arachnoid space as elongated filaments known collectively as the *cauda equina* (see Fig. 3-19). Each set of roots penetrates the meninges as it approaches its level of exit from the vertebral canal, carrying an extension of the dura and arachnoid as far as the intervertebral foramen. The dorsal root ganglion is located close to the intervertebral foramen. Distal to the ganglion the dorsal and ventral roots join to form the spinal nerve. Each spinal nerve divides promptly into dorsal and ventral rami.

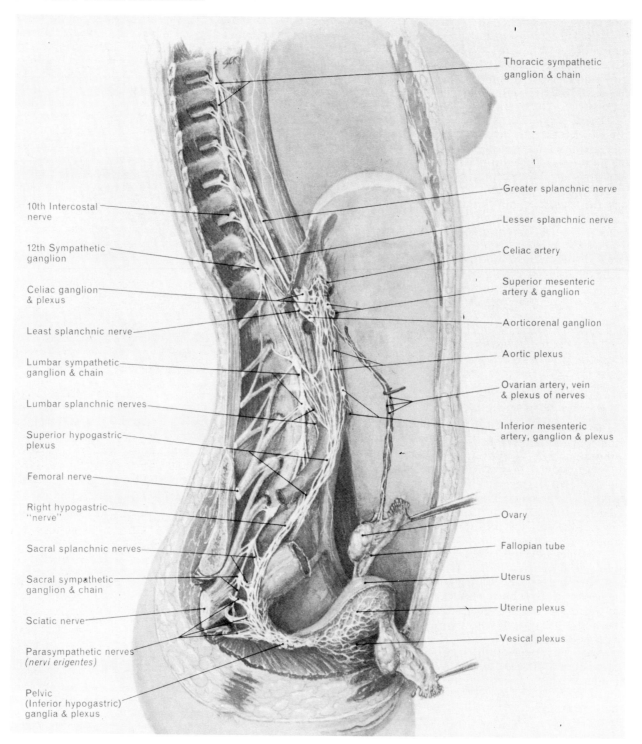

10th Intercostal nerve

12th Sympathetic ganglion

Celiac ganglion & plexus

Least splanchnic nerve

Lumbar sympathetic ganglion & chain

Lumbar splanchnic nerves

Superior hypogastric plexus

Femoral nerve

Right hypogastric "nerve"

Sacral splanchnic nerves

Sacral sympathetic ganglion & chain

Sciatic nerve

Parasympathetic nerves *(nervi erigentes)*

Pelvic (Inferior hypogastric) ganglia & plexus

Thoracic sympathetic ganglion & chain

Greater splanchnic nerve

Lesser splanchnic nerve

Celiac artery

Superior mesenteric artery & ganglion

Aorticorenal ganglion

Aortic plexus

Ovarian artery, vein & plexus of nerves

Inferior mesenteric artery, ganglion & plexus

Ovary

Fallopian tube

Uterus

Uterine plexus

Vesical plexus

FIG. 3-20.   Visceral nerves of female pelvis. Nervi erigentes is called *pelvic nerve* in text. (Bonica JJ: Atlas on mechanisms and pathways of pain in labor. What's New, No. 217, 1960)

The dorsal rami of the first three sacral nerves emerge through the dorsal sacral foramina to be distributed to the ligaments and periosteum of the sacrum, to the mutifidus muscle, and to the skin over the sacral region (middle cluneal nerves). The dorsal rami of the fourth and fifth sacral nerves and the coccygeal nerve are distributed to the skin posterior to the coccyx.

The ventral rami of the lumbar and sacral nerves

form the lumbosacral plexus; its branches are distributed to the pelvis and lower limbs. Except for parts of the lumbar plexus (obturator nerve, lumbosacral trunk) and the entire sacral plexus, which pass along the walls of the true pelvis and hence are anatomically related to the pelvic viscera, only certain components of these plexuses are directly involved in pelvic innervation.

The *sacral plexus* (see Fig. 3-13) is formed by the confluence of the lumbosacral trunk and the first, second, and third sacral nerves on the anterior aspect of the piriformis muscle. It is covered by the fascia of the piriformis and is, therefore, separated from the pelvic vessels and from the ureter. It is directed inferolaterally into the gluteal region through the greater ischiadic (sciatic) foramen. The superior gluteal nerve emerges from the pelvis superior to the piriformis muscle, whereas the inferior gluteal nerve, the ischiadic (sciatic) nerve, the posterior femoral cutaneous nerve, the nerve to the quadratus femoris, the nerve to the obturator internus, and the pudendal nerve course inferior to the piriformis. Small direct branches from the plexus supply the piriformis (S1 and S2), entering its anterior aspect. Branches to the levator ani and coccygeus muscles (S3 and S4) enter the pelvic surface of these muscles. Frequently a perineal branch from S4 passes independently to the sphincter ani externus.

Autonomic Innervation

The nerve plexuses associated with the pelvic organs contain sympathetic and parasympathetic motor pathways as well as numerous visceral sensory fibers (Fig. 3-20). Collections of nerve cells that form irregular ganglionic masses are scattered through these plexuses. Although the exact course of each of the fiber types is difficult to trace with certainty, the following outline indicates the principal pathways and connections of the autonomic nerves to the pelvis.

The ganglionated sympathetic trunks that lie on each side of the vertebral column pass into the true pelvis along the pelvic surface of the sacrum medial to the pelvic sacral foramina (see Fig. 3-20). Usually, four sacral ganglia are located along this part of each trunk. The trunks usually unite in front of the coccyx in the small ganglion impar.

Major autonomic plexuses associated with the aorta (celiac, superior mesenteric, aorticorenal, inferior mesenteric, and superior hypogastric) receive connections from the sympathetic trunks through splanchnic nerves. The superior hypogastric plexus (see Fig. 3-20) lies near the bifurcation of the abdominal aorta in close association with the inferior mesenteric plexus. It continues inferiorly in front of the promontory of the sacrum, where it divides into right and left portions. These strands pass inferiorly on either side of the rectum as the right and left hypogastric nerves. They diverge and swing anteriorly into the uterosacral folds, where an extensive inferior hypogastric plexus is present within which clusters of ganglion cells (pelvic ganglia) are located. The inferior hypogastric plexus (pelvic plexus) branches into subsidiary plexuses in relation to the sides of the rectum, uterus, vagina, and bladder. These are termed, respectively, the middle and inferior rectal plexus, the uterovaginal plexus, and the vesical plexus. The plexuses ramify along the blood vessels that reach the pelvic organs, including the ureter (see Fig. 3-20).

The cell bodies of sympathetic preganglionic fibers concerned with the innervation of the female reproductive tract lie in the intermediolateral cell column (lateral horn) of the spinal cord from the tenth thoracic to the first or second lumbar segments. Fibers from these cells pass through the ventral roots and white rami communicantes to the sympathetic trunks. The distribution of the fibers distally from the sympathetic trunks may follow two general pathways, with synaptic connections to postganglionic neurons possible in the ganglia of the sympathetic trunks or in the ganglia associated with the more peripheral plexuses.

1. Most of the sympathetic preganglionic fibers that supply the internal pelvic organs leave the sympathetic trunks through splanchnic nerves that pass to the aortic plexus. From this plexus delicate postganglionic fibers continue along the ovarian arteries to the ovaries, and a large collection of fibers extends downward as the superior hypogastric plexus described earlier.
2. Other preganglionic sympathetic fibers destined for the pelvic viscera enter the pelvis in the sympathetic trunks, synapse in the chain ganglia, and then pass to the pelvic plexuses directly through small sacral splanchnic nerves to reach the pelvic organs by means of blood vessels. Some fibers may not synapse until small ganglia in the hypogastric plexuses are reached.

The *preganglionic parasympathetic neurons* that supply the ovaries and at least the lateral portions of the uterine tubes arise in the dorsal motor nucleus of the vagus nerve; they accompany these nerves and then the ovarian plexuses to reach ganglia closely associated with these organs. Synapse occurs here, and postganglionic fibers continue to the ovaries and tubes. The preganglionic parasympathetic neurons that supply the remaining pelvic organs lie in the intermediolateral cell columns of the second, third, and fourth sacral segments of the spinal cord and send axons peripherally with the sacral nerves. As the nerves emerge from the pelvic sacral foramina, the parasympathetic fibers pass by way of pelvic nerves* (nervi erigentes) directly into the pelvic plexuses on each side. The prepostganglionic synapse occurs with cells in the pelvic ganglia or in the walls of the organ supplied. It should also be noted that sacral parasympathetic fibers ascend through the hypogastric nerves to reach the inferior mesenteric plexus for distribution to the descending colon and sigmoid colon.

---

* Others call these nerves "pelvic splanchnic nerves," but it seems better to restrict the term *splanchnic* to those nerves that leave the sympathetic chain, that is, greater, lesser, least, lumbar, and sacral splanchnics (see Fig. 3-20).

Visceral Sensory Innervation

The cell bodies of visceral sensory fibers, like those of somatic sensory fibers, are located in dorsal root ganglia. In areas reached by spinal nerves, visceral sensory fibers naturally follow the spinal nerves directly to the dorsal root ganglia. The situation is somewhat more complex in the case of sensory fibers from the pelvic organs not directly served by spinal nerves. In this case, the afferent nerves must necessarily follow autonomic plexuses either to reach the sympathetic trunk (ascending to enter spinal nerves T10 to L2 through white rami communicantes) or possibly to enter the sacral nerves through pelvic nerves that also carry parasympathetic fibers.

Relatively little is understood of the anatomic details of the visceral afferent pathways from the reproductive tract. It is known, however, that the ovary, uterine tube, fundus, and perhaps the body of the uterus send afferent fibers that carry pain impulses upward through the ovarian plexuses to reach the spinal cord at the level of T10, T11, and T12. Sensory fibers from the cervix ascend through the hypogastric plexuses to enter the spinal cord also at T11 and T12. Pain is likely to be referred to the skin innervated by these particular nerves as indicated in Figure 3-21.

Internal Reproductive Organs

Ovaries

In the nullipara, the ovaries are smooth, pink, and the shape and size of a large almond. In the elderly woman, they are small and quite roughened in appearance. The ovaries are located between the uterus medially and the lateral pelvic wall laterally, and, as mentioned previously, they are suspended from the posterior–superior surface of the broad ligaments by the mesovarium (see Fig. 3-9). The ovary is attached to the uterus by a derivative of the gubernaculum; this short ligament is the *ligament of the ovary.* The ovary is also suspended laterally from the pelvic wall by the *suspensory ligament of the ovary* which is made up of peritoneum covering the vascular system entering and leaving this organ. The mesenteries forming the mesovaria are continuous with the germinal epithelial layer on the ovaries themselves.

Since either the ileum or the colon fills in the pelvic cavity, the ovaries are in definite *relation* to either one of these two organs. Each ovary is also close to the lateral pelvic wall and separated only by peritoneum from the umbilical artery, obturator vessels, and nerve on the obturator internus muscle.

The arterial supply, venous and lymphatic drainage, and nerve supply were described starting on page 53.

Uterine Tubes

Approximately 4 inches long and ¼ inch in diameter, the *uterine tube* (see Figs. 3-7, 3-8, 3-22, and

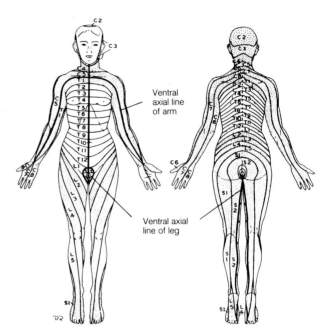

Ventral axial line of arm

Ventral axial line of leg

FIG. 3-21. Dermatome chart of the human body. (Keegan JJ, Garrett FD: The segmental distribution of the cutaneous nerves in the limbs of man. Anat Rec 102:409, 1948. Courtesy of the Wistar Institute of Anatomy and Biology)

3-23) is attached to the fundus of the uterus. The tube extends laterally, enters the free edge of the broad ligament, and curls around the ovary to end in approximation with it on the medial surface of that organ. The abdominal end is the funnel-shaped *infundibulum* that ends in many fingerlike processes called *fimbriae,* one of which is attached to the ovary (*fimbria ovarica*). The middle portion of the tube, the *ampulla,* is considerably smaller and is slightly coiled. The medial portion is narrow and straight and is called the *isthmus.* Although the isthmus attaches to the uterus, the lumen penetrates the uterine wall (*interstitial portion of tube*) to join the uterine cavity. It is obvious that the uterine tube forms a direct connection between the peritoneal cavity at one end and the uterine cavity at the other.

The uterine tube is also related to the ileum and to the cecum. The latter relationship causes confusion between pathology of the appendix and the uterine tube.

The uterine tube contains *smooth muscle* and is lined with a *ciliated columnar epithelium.* At the time of ovulation, the fimbriated end of the tube picks up the ovum; by a combined ciliated action and muscle contraction, the ovum is pushed down the tube toward the waiting uterus.

The area of the broad ligament between the mesovarium and the tube (*mesosalpinx*) contains several minor tubules (*epoophoron;* see Fig. 3-23) that correspond to structures in the male. These tubules are remnants of the mesonephric tubules and correspond to the ducts of the testes and to the lobules of the epididymis.

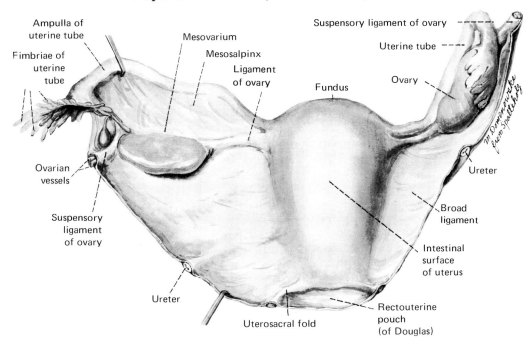

FIG. 3-22. Excised uterus, uterine tubes, and ovaries, posterior aspect.

They end in a horizontal tubule called the duct of the *epoophoron,* the latter being a remnant of the mesonephric (wolffian) duct and corresponding to the canal of the epididymis. It continues as Gartner's duct. Note that *vesicular appendices* can occur (see Fig. 13-23). The *paroophoron* (not shown in Fig. 3-23) consists of a few microscopic tubules that lie nearer the uterus; these are derived from the mesonephros and correspond to the paradidymis. Abnormal growth can occur in these structures.

The arterial supply, venous and lymphatic drainage, and nerve supply were described starting on page 53.

Uterus

Usually described as a pear-shaped organ, the uterus (see Figs. 3-6 through 3-8, 3-22, and 3-23) has a comparatively narrow *cervix,* which extends into the vagina, and a wider *body* or *corpus,* which ends superoanteriorly as the *fundus* to which are attached the uterine tubes. The cervix is divided into vaginal and supravaginal portions, and the point of juncture between it and the body of the uterus is often called the *isthmus.* That part of the vaginal cervix that is anterior to the ostium is the anterior labium; that part posterior, the posterior labium (Fig. 3-23). The normal uterus of an adult weighs 60 g to 80 g.

The uterus is a hollow organ, and the lumina of the uterine tubes are directly continuous with the *lumen* inside the uterus (see Fig. 3-23). This, in turn, opens into the vagina through the cervix. The lumen inside the uterus has a different shape in different parts (see Fig. 3-23). In the cervix it is a fairly small, narrow opening approximately 2.5 cm in length. Its distal end is called the *ostium* of the uterus. The cavity in the body of the uterus is approximately 4 cm in length and is triangular in shape. The wall of the corpus is rather thick and made up of peritoneum (perimetrium), smooth muscle (myometrium), and a glandular lining on the inside (endometrium). The wall of the cervix, however, is composed almost entirely of dense fibrous connective tissue. The transition from fibrous cervix to muscular corpus is usually abrupt and occurs at about the level of the internal ostium.

The uterus, located between the rectum and the bladder, overhangs the bladder anteriorly (see Fig. 3-6). As mentioned earlier, it is normally bent anteriorly and forms approximately a right angle to the vaginal canal. Its vesical surface is in direct relation to the bladder, and the peritoneum on this surface does not cover the entire uterus. The intestinal surface of the uterus is completely covered with peritoneum and is in direct relation to the ileum. It should be noted that the appendix can hang down into the pelvic cavity very close to the uterus.

The *uterus* has five paired ligaments. The *broad ligaments* (see Fig. 3-22) are extensions of the peritoneum from the margins of the uterus to the lateral pelvic walls; these two layers stretch over the uterine tubes from the floor of the pelvis. In addition to the uterine tube, these folds of the broad ligament, as just described, enclose embryonic remnants, the ovarian ligament, vessels, lymphatics, and nerves. The *round ligaments* (see Fig. 3-7) of the uterus (ligamentum teres uteri) extend

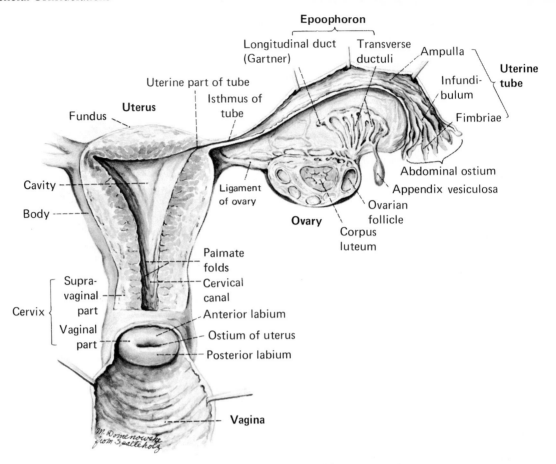

FIG. 3-23. Sectioned female reproductive organs, anterior view.

laterally from the fundus between the folds of the broad ligament to the lateral pelvic wall, and finally leave the abdominal cavity through the internal ring of the inguinal canal. They terminate in the labia majora attached to the diverticular process as indicated in Figure 3-25. Occasionally these ligaments are accompanied by a persistent processus vaginalis (canal of Nuck). The two *cardinal ligaments* (see Figs. 3-8 and 3-10) extend from the lateral pelvic wall to the cervix of the uterus and are condensations of subserous fascia around the uterine blood vessels. The *uterosacral ligaments* are also condensations of subserous fascia that extend from the sacrum, around the rectum, to the cervix of the uterus. (Similar condensations have been described extending anteriorly from the uterus to the base of the urinary bladder as seen in Figure 3-10; these are *uterovesical ligaments.*) The uterosacral and cardinal ligaments are by far the most important of the ligaments of the uterus. Without these, the uterus tends to prolapse into the vagina. The round ligaments are of little value, and the reflections of the peritoneum are equally unimportant. The broad ligaments probably do serve a purpose in holding the uterus in position.

The arterial supply, venous and lymphatic drainage,

and nerve supply were described starting on page 53. The intimate relation of the ureters to the uterine vessels—posteroinferior to the vessels (water flows under the bridge)—should be recalled.

Vagina

The copulatory and birth canal in the female, the *vagina,* starts as an opening in the external genitalia posterior to the urethra and anterior to the rectum (see Fig. 3-6). The opening to the vagina in the virgin is usually guarded by a *hymen,* folds of mucous membrane that extend into the lumen of the vagina. The hymen may take the form of a complete membrane, which has to be severed at the first menstruation; it may be a sieve-like structure; or there may be no hymen at all. After rupture, the fragments of the hymen persist as small nodules designated as *hymenal caruncles.*

The *vagina proper* extends from the hymen to the cervix of the uterus. It traverses a muscular layer in the perineum—the urogenital diaphragm—and then goes through the pelvic diaphragm by passing the inferior edges of the levator ani muscles. These diaphragms are diagrammed in Fig. 3-29 (see p. 72). Since the cervix extends into the anterior aspect of the superior end of the vagina, the anterior wall is shorter than the posterior. The anterior wall is approximately 8 cm long, while the posterior wall is 9 cm to 10 cm long (see Fig. 3-6). The clefts produced by the cervix projecting into the vagina are called *fornices;* there are anterior, posterior, and two lateral fornices, the posterior being by far the deepest. The posterosuperior part of the vagina is covered by peritoneum, but the anterior wall makes no contact with it.

The *relations* of the vagina are important, for many structures in the pelvic cavity can be palpated via this canal. These relations are as follows:

Anterior—bladder and urethra
Posterior—the inferior end of the pelvic cavity, small intestine, rectovaginal septum, rectum, and perineal body (a point in the midline between the vaginal and anal openings)
Lateral—broad ligaments, ureters, uterine vessels, pelvic surface of the levator ani muscle, muscles in the deep space of the perineum, greater vestibular glands, and bulbospongiosus muscles

Thus, any structure in the inferior part of the pelvic cavity can be palpated through the vagina, particularly if bimanual palpation is used (one hand on the anterior abdominal wall). Structures contained in the broad ligaments can be felt, and when the ovary is increased in size from any pathologic condition, it can be felt from the vagina as well. Naturally, the cervix of the uterus is also palpable.

The *walls of the vagina* are in contact with each other except where the cervix intervenes. They are made up of smooth muscle and are lined with stratified squamous epithelium. Ridges (vaginal rugae) are found on the anterior and posterior walls, and several transverse folds around the walls of the vagina connect these ridges. During sexual excitement, the vagina elongates in the area of the posterior fornix, it produces a clear fluid by transudation, and the distal third undergoes a vasocongestion, all parasympathetic actions. The vestibule of the vagina has two *greater vestibular* or *bulbourethral glands* that empty just inferior to the hymenal caruncles (see Fig. 3-27); they provide lubrication and are also under control of the parasympathetic system. Several small mucous glands, the *lesser vestibular,* open on the side walls of the vestibule.

The *arteries* to the vagina branch from the uterine arteries, from the internal iliac artery directly, and from the middle rectal; the inferior end derives its blood supply from branches of the internal pudendal artery (see Figs. 3-27 and 3-28).

The vagina obtains its *sympathetic nerve supply* from the hypogastric plexus (L1–L3) and its *parasympathetic* from the sacral region of the cord through the pelvic nerve. The inferior end of the vagina is more sensitive than the superior end, receiving its *sensory branches* from the pudendal nerve.

The *lymphatics* drain to glands on the rectum and along the iliac arteries, but some of the lymphatics from the inferior end of the vagina may drain into the inguinal glands in the femoral triangle.

Ureters

In its *course,* the ureter enters the pelvic cavity by crossing the external iliac artery near its branching from the common iliac (see Fig. 3-7) and follows along the lateral pelvic wall just deep to the peritoneum. It is anterior to the internal iliac artery and vein. Lateral are the psoas major muscle, the obturator internus muscle, and the levator ani. As the ureter approaches the floor of the pelvis, the vessels entering the broad ligament pass superior and medial to the ureter, as does the broad ligament itself (see Fig. 3-8). The ureter continues inferiorly and after passing deep to these uterine vessels enters the bladder by passing close to the lateral fornix of the vagina (see Fig. 3-11). Although the ovary is not in immediate relation, it is very close to the ureter, being anterior and medial to it. The ureters penetrate the bladder wall in an oblique slanting fashion; this is important in preventing reflux of urine into the ureters when the bladder is distended.

The ureters receive small *arteries* from the renal, ovarian, vesical, and middle rectal arteries.

The ureters receive autonomic innervation from the *sympathetic* nervous system, fibers originating in T12–L2 spinal cord segments. The vagus contributes the *parasympathetic fibers* to the upper part; the pelvic nerve, to the lower part. The ureter can function without a nerve supply; peristalsis will occur. Spasm is induced by stimuli of an unusual nature. *Sensory fibers* return to segments T12–L2.

The *lymphatics* end in glands closest to it in the pelvis and in the abdominal cavity.

Urinary Bladder

Although the urinary bladder is not a reproductive organ, its intimate relation to the reproductive tract warrants its being included in any description of the pelvic cavity. The urethra assumes a similar importance in the perineum.

The *urinary bladder* occupies the anterior portion of the pelvic cavity and is just superior and posterior to the pubic bone (see Figs. 3-6 and 3-11). When the bladder is empty, it is said to have an *apex,* a *superior surface,* two *inferolateral surfaces,* a *base* or posterior surface, and a *neck.* The *apex* reaches to a short distance superior to the pubic bone and ends as a fibrous cord, which is a derivative of the urachus (a canal in the fetus that connects the bladder with the allantois). This fibrous cord extends from the apex of the bladder to the umbilicus between the peritoneum and the transversalis fascia; it raises a ridge of peritoneum called the median umbilical ligament. The *superior surface* is the only surface of the bladder covered by peritoneum; it is in relation with the uterus and ileum in the female. The *base* of the bladder faces posteriorly and is separated from the rectum by the uterus and vagina. The *inferolateral* surfaces on each side of the bladder are in relation with the pubic bone, and with the levator ani and obturator internus muscles, but the bladder is actually separated from the pubic bone by the retropubic space, which contains fat. The *neck* of the bladder is the most inferior part next to the urethra. The bladder is a dilatable structure; when filled with urine, the neck remains in position but the superior part rises into the pelvic cavity.

The loose *subserous fascia* of the pelvic cavity is continuous superiorly over the pelvic organs, and this is true for the bladder as well. Condensations of this fascia form attachments for the bladder, and those running from the levator ani muscle and the pubic bone to the bladder are called the *pubovesical ligaments.*

The *bladder wall* consists of a partial covering of peritoneum, the subserous fascia, a muscular coat made up of intermingling longitudinal and circular fibers of smooth muscle, a submucous layer of connective tissue, and a layer of transitional epithelium.

The interior of the bladder (see Figs. 3-6 and 3-11) is wrinkled except at the *trigone,* that area between the openings of the ureters and the opening of the urethra. When the bladder is dilated, all walls become equally smooth in appearance. A ridge is found between the openings of the ureters—the *interureteral ridge.* The trigone of the bladder is an important area in that infections tend to persist at this particular point.

The muscular component of the wall of the bladder—the *detrusor muscle*—consists of three layers of smooth muscle—outer and inner longitudinal layers and a circular layer between them. These layers are not distinct entities, for they tend to form an intermingling meshwork. However, the outer longitudinal layer is continuous with a layer of muscle blended with the vagina. The circular and inner longitudinal layers are continued into the urethra. There seems to be no internal sphincter; in fact, the muscle arrangement at the neck of the bladder is such as to cause an opening of the urethra rather than a constriction. A considerable amount of *elastic tissue* is found at the neck of the bladder, however, and this is arranged in such a manner as to aid in keeping the urethra closed.

The *nerves* to the bladder are part of the nerve plexuses found in the pelvic cavity; they follow the arteries to get to the bladder. The *sympathetic* fibers arise in the last thoracic and the first and second lumbar segments of the spinal cord. They innervate the trigone, the ureteral orifices, and the blood vessels. They also carry pain fibers from the bladder. The *parasympathetic* fibers arise in the second, third, and fourth sacral segments. These fibers innervate the detrusor muscle. Afferent fibers from the bladder wall start as stretch receptors. A full bladder stimulates these receptors, and the impulses follow the pelvic nerve back to the sacral region of the spinal cord.

The *arteries* to the bladder are the superior and inferior vesical branches of the internal iliac artery (see Fig. 3-15). There are corresponding *veins* that form a profuse plexus near the base of the bladder; this plexus drains into the internal iliac veins (see Fig. 3-17).

PERINEUM

The *perineum* is the most inferior end of the trunk; it is the region between the thighs and between the buttocks. It is *bounded* anteriorly by the pubic arch; laterally by the pubic and ischial rami combined, the ischial tuberosity, and the sacrotuberous ligament; and posteriorly by the sacrum and coccyx (see Fig. 3-3). Its *superior limit* is the pelvic diaphragm, consisting of levator ani and coccygeus muscles. If a line is drawn transversely through the point between the anus and the posterior end of the vagina, it will extend laterally to the ischial tuberosities. This line, which bisects the *central perineal tendon (perineal body),* divides the perineum into a posterior *anal triangle* and an anterior *urogenital triangle.*

Anal Triangle

The *anal opening* is located in the anal triangle (Fig. 3-24). The sphincter muscles of the anus keep the opening closed, and there are bundles of smooth muscle in the superficial fascia around the anal opening that radiate from the margins of the anus and are attached to the skin around it. This gives the anus a puckered appearance. The smooth muscles are the *corrugator cutis ani* muscles. A layer of fatty fascia, which is the same as the fatty layer of superficial fascia located in the abdominal wall, lies under the skin of the anal triangle. It is also continuous with a similar fatty layer in the urogenital triangle. This fat fills in a large wedge-shaped area on either side of the anus—the *ischioanal (ischiorectal) fossa* (see Figs. 3-25 and 3-26).

The *boundaries* of the ischioanal fossa are as follows:

Anterior—the transverse muscles of the perineum and the fascia that covers them. (If the finger is pushed anteriorly in the ischioanal fossa, it can be seen that the finger will be superior to the urogenital diaphragm; this is the anterior recess of the ischiorectal fossa.)
Posterior—the sacrotuberous ligament and the overlying gluteus maximus muscle
Lateral—the obturator internus muscle with its covering of deep fascia
Medial—the levator ani and external sphincter muscles covered with deep fascia—the inferior fascia of the pelvic diaphragm

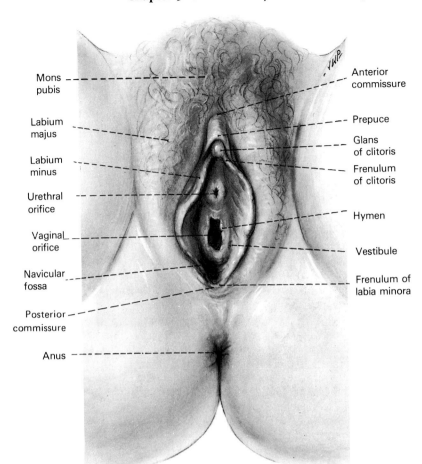

Mons pubis

Labium majus

Labium minus

Urethral orifice

Vaginal orifice

Navicular fossa

Posterior commissure

Anus

Anterior commissure

Prepuce

Glans of clitoris

Frenulum of clitoris

Hymen

Vestibule

Frenulum of labia minora

FIG. 3-24. Surface view of female peri neum and vulva. Labia have been spread apart.

The *inferior rectal arteries* and *nerves* stream from the lateral superior aspect of the ischioanal fossa toward the rectum and anus (Fig. 3-25). These nerves and blood vessels supply innervation and vascularity to the inferior end of the anal canal, the circularly arranged external sphincter ani muscle that surrounds the anal opening, and the skin around the anus. These nerves are important, for incontinence results if they are cut. These nerves and arteries are branches of the *pudendal nerve* and *internal pudendal artery* that course in the layer of fascia on the obturator internus muscle. This canal of fascia is the *pudendal canal* (Fig. 3-26).

In addition to the inferior rectal nerve, a very small branch, the *anococcygeal nerve,* can be found close to the posterior part of the external sphincter muscle of the anus close to where this muscle attaches to the coccyx. This is a sensory nerve to the skin over the coccyx.

The *sphincter ani externus muscle* is divided into subcutaneous, superficial, and deep parts (see Fig. 3-26). The *subcutaneous part* completely encircles the anus in a position just deep to the skin. The *superficial portion* has attachments posteriorly to the coccygeal ligament and to the coccyx, and anteriorly to the perineal

body, a central fibrous point just anterior to the anus to which several muscles attach. The *deep portion* completely encircles the anal canal (see Fig. 3-27); this portion is intimately fused with the puborectal portion of the levator ani muscle. The latter two parts—superficial and deep—are just lateral to the internal sphincter, which is made up of smooth muscle (see Fig. 3-26). The external sphincter is skeletal muscle under voluntary control; *nerve supply,* as mentioned earlier, is from inferior rectal branches of the pudendal nerve.

(Abscesses occur in the ischioanal fossa, and these can spread to the opposite side since the fat pads are continuous both anterior and posterior to the anus. They heal poorly because of the scanty blood supply; they can penetrate the rectum or anal canal between the internal and external sphincter muscles.)

Urogenital Triangle

The urogenital triangle in the female contains the *external genitalia* or *vulva* (see Fig. 3-24). There is a pad of fat called the *mons pubis* anterior and inferior to the

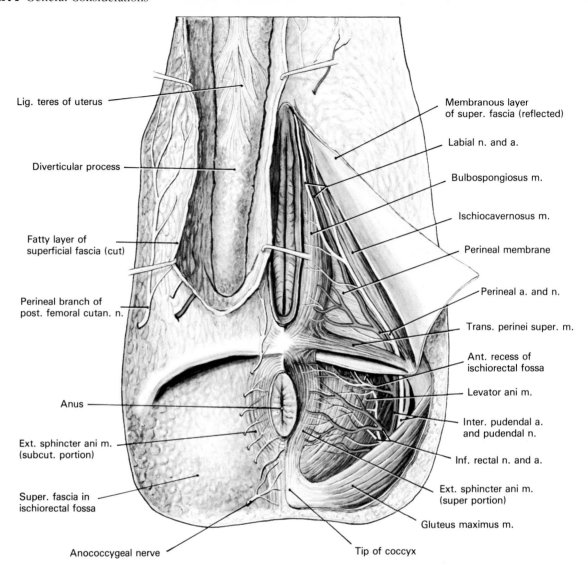

Lig. teres of uterus

Diverticular process

Fatty layer of
superficial fascia (cut)

Perineal branch of
post. femoral cutan. n.

Anus

Ext. sphincter ani m.
(subcut. portion)

Super. fascia in
ischiorectal fossa

Anococcygeal nerve

Membranous layer
of super. fascia (reflected)

Labial n. and a.

Bulbospongiosus m.

Ischiocavernosus m.

Perineal membrane

Perineal a. and n.

Trans. perinei super. m.

Ant. recess of
ischiorectal fossa

Levator ani m.

Inter. pudendal a.
and pudendal n.

Inf. rectal n. and a.

Ext. sphincter ani m.
(super portion)

Gluteus maximus m.

Tip of coccyx

FIG. 3-25. Perineum in the female. The fatty layer of superficial fascia is intact in the anal triangle on the *right* side of the body, but has been incised in the labium majus to reveal the diverticular process. The fatty layer of superficial fascia has been removed on the *left* side to reveal the contents of the ischioanal fossa, and the membranous layer of superficial fascia cut and reflected to show contents of the superficial space. (The deep fascia has been removed from the muscles in this space and from the pudendal canal.) (Crafts RC: A Textbook of Human Anatomy. Copyright © 1985. Reprinted by permission of John Wiley & Sons, Inc., New York)

pubic bone. After puberty, this area is covered with hair. This pad of fat can be followed posteriorly to two large lips—the *labia majora.* The point where the lips come together anteriorly is the *anterior labial commissure,* and the region where they come together posteriorly, the *posterior labial commissure.* These labia majora are also covered with hair. Medial to the labia majora are two fleshy small lips called the *labia minora.* These lips are devoid of hair and are usually in contact with one another. The point where the labia minora come to-

gether posteriorly is the *frenulum of the labia,* while the point where they come together anteriorly is designated as the *frenulum of the clitoris.* The head or glans of the *clitoris* can be seen just at the anterior end of the labia minora, and the fleshy fold just anterior to the glans of the clitoris is the *prepuce of the clitoris.* The space between the labia minora is the *vestibule of the vagina.* This has two openings: (1) the opening of the urethra, which is located about 2.5 cm posterior to the head of the clitoris and appears puckered in the living state, and

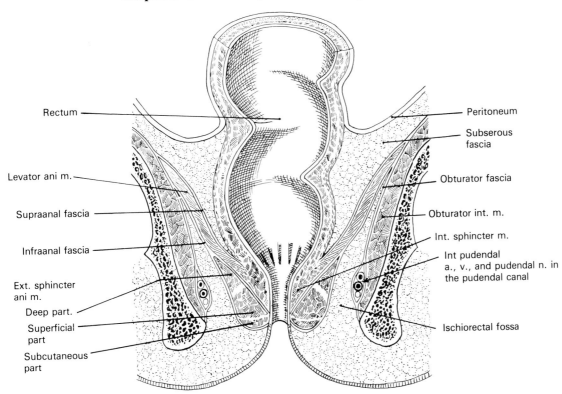

Rectum

Levator ani m.

Supraanal fascia

Infraanal fascia

Ext. sphincter
ani m.

Deep part.

Superficial
part

Subcutaneous
part

Peritoneum

Subserous
fascia

Obturator fascia

Obturator int. m.

Int. sphincter m.

Int pudendal
a., v., and pudendal n. in
the pudendal canal

Ischiorectal fossa

FIG. 3-26.   Diagram of a frontal section through the anal triangle of the perineum. (Crafts RC: A Textbook of Human Anatomy. Copyright © 1985. Reprinted by permission of John Wiley & Sons, Inc., New York)

(2) posterior to that the opening to the *vagina.* If a *hymen* is present, it guards the entrance into the vagina from the vestibule. Just inferior to the hymen on either side are the openings of the *greater vestibular glands.* These glands provide lubrication for the medial sides of the labia minora, being aided in this by small *lesser vestibular glands* opening on the medial sides of these labia.

The labia majora contain an organized process of fat called the *diverticular process* (see Fig. 3-25). This is continuous with the fat over the mons pubis and is the structure to which the round ligament of the uterus is attached. The *membranous layer of the superficial fascia* lies deep to the fat and diverticular process; it is exactly the same layer of fascia as found in the abdominal wall. It is attached posteriorly to the posterior edge of the perineal membrane at the line that divides the urogenital triangle from the anal triangle and laterally to the deep fascia on the thigh. Because of these attachments, any matter contained in the area deep to this fascia (the superficial space) is confined to the urogenital triangle, the mons pubis, and the anterior abdominal wall.

In the *superficial space of the perineum,* on either side of the labia minora, are the *bulbospongiosus mus-*

cles; these muscles cover the *vestibular bulb,* which is made up of erectile tissue (Fig. 3-27). Each bulb continues anteriorly and actually joins with that of the opposite side near the head of the clitoris. The *greater vestibular glands* are located just posterior to each bulb. Laterally in the superficial space (see Fig. 3-25) the *ischiocavernosus muscles* are attached to the ischiopubic rami; these muscles cover the *crura of the clitoris,* which also consist of erectile tissue. Two small muscles run transversely from the perineal body to the inferior pubic rami—the *transversus perinei superficialis muscles.* The bulbospongiosus muscles (see Fig. 3-25) form a sort of sphincter around the inferior end of the vagina, the ischiocavernosus muscles may serve to keep the clitoris erect during sexual excitement by compressing the venous return in the crura, and the action of the transversus perinei superficialis muscles is to tense the central point of the perineum, thus aiding in the action of the other muscles.

If the two bulbs and their covering muscles, the two crura with their ischiocavernosus muscles, and the transversus perinei superficialis muscles are removed (see Fig. 3-27), the superficial space is seen to be bounded superiorly by a heavy layer of fascia, called the *perineal membrane,* which stretches across the uro-

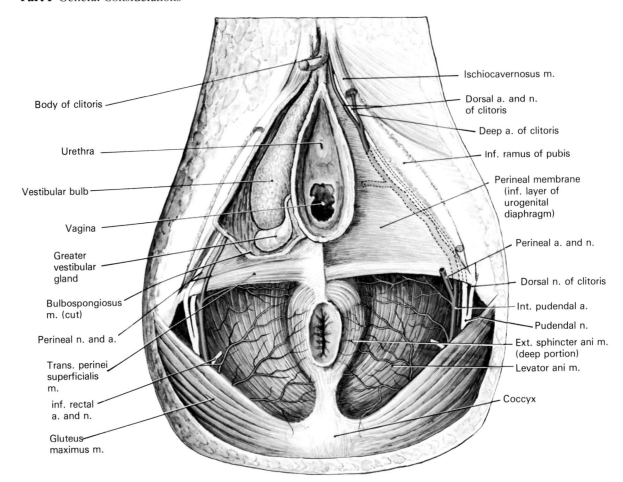

Body of clitoris

Urethra

Vestibular bulb

Vagina

Greater
vestibular
gland

Bulbospongiosus
m. (cut)

Perineal n. and a.

Trans. perinei
superficialis
m.

inf. rectal
a. and n.

Gluteus
maximus m.

Ischiocavernosus m.

Dorsal a. and n.
of clitoris

Deep a. of clitoris

Inf. ramus of pubis

Perineal membrane
(inf. layer of
urogenital
diaphragm)

Perineal a. and n.

Dorsal n. of clitoris

Int. pudendal a.

Pudendal n.

Ext. sphincter ani m.
(deep portion)

Levator ani m.

Coccyx

FIG. 3-27.　Perineum in the female. The bulbospongiosus muscle has been incised on the *right* side to reveal the vestibular gland and duct, and the bulb. The ischiocavernosus muscle has been removed from the crus of the clitoris. On the *left* side of the body the entire contents of the superficial space have been removed. (Crafts RC: A Textbook of Human Anatomy. Copyright © 1985. Reprinted by permission of John Wiley & Sons, Inc., New York)

genital triangle between the two inferior pubic rami. This is penetrated by both the urethra and vagina (see Fig. 3-30).

If the perineal membrane is removed, the contents of the deep space are revealed (Fig. 3-28). The muscles located in this space are in the form of a thin sheet of muscle tissue that is divided into several parts. *Compressor urethrae muscles* arise from the pubic rami and the fascia surrounding the vessels and nerves in those areas, and proceed anteriorly toward the midline to reach a position anterior to the urethra. They blend with muscle tissue that completely surrounds the urethra (*sphincter urethrae muscle*). Other portions surround the vagina as well as the urethra and have been designated as the *sphincter urethrovaginalis muscles;* they meet in the midline at the perineal body. In addition, there are a few muscle fibers coursing transversely and inserting on the vagina (*transverse vaginae muscle*). The remaining tissue is mainly smooth muscle; the so-

called transverse perinei profundus muscle is difficult to find. It should be noted that the sphincter urethrae muscle is not confined to the deep space; it continues superiorly through the midline opening in the pelvic diaphragm to reach the neck of the bladder.

If these muscles in the deep space are removed (see Fig. 3-28), a layer of *deep fascia* that is continuous with the fascia on the obturator internus muscle (Fig. 3-29) is found. If this deep fascia, in turn, is removed, the inferior surface of the levator ani muscle is seen.

The layers of the urogenital triangle are, therefore, as follows:

1. Skin
2. Fatty layer of superficial fascia
3. Membranous layer of superficial fascia
4. Muscular layer in the superficial space
5. Perineal membrane

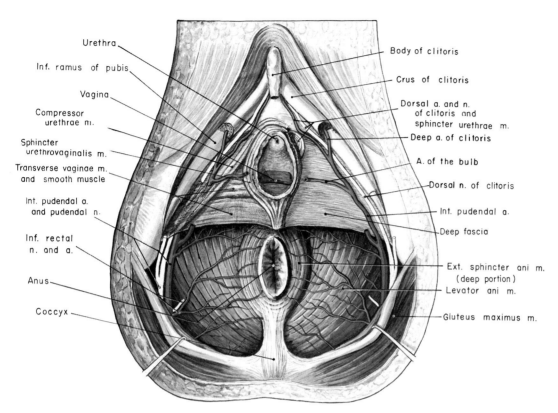

FIG. 3-28.   Perineum of the female. The perineal membrane has been removed on the *right* to reveal the muscles found in the deep space: the compressor urethrae, sphincter urethrovaginalis, and transverse vaginal muscles. On the *left,* these muscles have been removed to reveal the deep fascia that covers the superior surface of these muscles and the circularly arranged fibers of the sphincter urethrae muscle that follows the urethra superior to the urinary bladder. (Crafts RC: A Textbook of Human Anatomy. Copyright © 1985. Reprinted by permission of John Wiley & Sons, Inc., New York)

6. Muscular layer in the deep space
7. Deep fascia on the superior side of these muscles

These are shown in Figure 3-29. The *superficial space* is the area between layers 3 and 5 in this list, while the *deep space* is between 5 and 7. The perineal membrane, the muscle layer in the deep space, and the deep fascia superior to this muscle (5, 6, and 7) form what has been called for many years the *urogenital diaphragm.* Therefore, another name for the perineal membrane is the *inferior layer of the urogenital diaphragm,* and another name for the fascia of layer 7 is the *superior layer of the urogenital diaphragm.** This urogenital diaphragm fills

* As a result of the finding by T. M. Oelrich (Anat Rec 205: 223, 1983) that the muscles in the deep space are continued into the pelvic cavity, the concept of the "sandwich-like" urogenital diaphragm has been questioned.

the opening in the pelvic diaphragm between the two levator ani muscles and supports the pelvic organs.

Clitoris

The *clitoris* (see Figs. 3-24 and 3-28) has a structure very similar to that of the penis except that it is much smaller and does not contain the urethra. It is composed of three portions—the *two corpora cavernosa* and the *corpus spongiosum.* The former two arise from the crura of the clitoris in the perineum, and the corpus spongiosum is an anterior continuation of the bulbs in the superficial space of the perineum. The corpus spongiosum, as in the male, ends in a dilated head or *glans.* The organ is erectile in nature. It has a *suspensory ligament* that suspends the clitoris from the pubic symphysis. The clitoris, which is about 2.5 cm long, takes a sharp bend at the point where the suspensory ligament

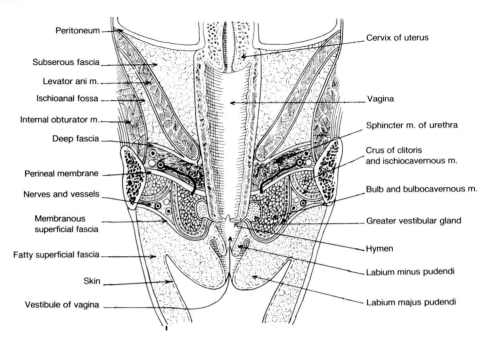

Peritoneum

Subserous fascia

Levator ani m.

Ischioanal fossa

Internal obturator m.

Deep fascia

Perineal membrane

Nerves and vessels

Membranous
superficial fascia

Fatty superficial fascia

Skin

Vestibule of vagina

Cervix of uterus

Vagina

Sphincter m. of urethra

Crus of clitoris
and ischiocavernous m.

Bulb and bulbocavernous m.

Greater vestibular gland

Hymen

Labium minus pudendi

Labium majus pudendi

FIG. 3-29. Frontal section of the urogenital triangle of the female. The layers, from inferior to superior, are skin, fatty superficial fascia, membranous superficial fascia, superficial space and its contents, perineal membrane, deep space and its contents, and deep fascia that is continuous with that on the free edge of the levator ani muscle as well as with the obturator fascia. The muscle surrounding the urethra in the deep space extends superiorly into the pelvic cavity to reach the neck of the urinary bladder. (Crafts RC: A Textbook of Human Anatomy. Copyright © 1985. Reprinted by permission of John Wiley & Sons, Inc., New York. Modified after Jamieson)

is attached and heads posteriorly and inferiorly. The loose fold of skin over the clitoris is the *prepuce* of the clitoris.

The nerve and blood supply to the clitoris is discussed below.

Urethra

The urethra in the female is about 4 cm long (see Fig. 3-6). It courses inferiorly and slightly anteriorly from the neck of the bladder through the urogenital diaphragm to end in the vestibule of the vagina between the labia minora approximately 2.5 cm posterior to the glans of the clitoris. It is anterior to the opening of the vagina, and its external orifice has firm raised margins. Very small glands open at the sides of the external urethral orifice.

The smooth muscle of the urethra is under control of the *parasympathetic nervous system* (S2, S3, and S4). The external sphincter (sphincter urethrae, compressor urethrae, and sphincter urethrovaginalis muscles) is under voluntary control after infancy.

Vessels and Nerves

The *blood and nerve supply* to the urogenital triangle is by branches of the *internal pudendal artery*

and *pudendal nerve* (see Fig. 3-25), aided by the *perineal branch of the posterior femoral cutaneous nerve* and branches from the *ilioinguinal* and *genitofemoral nerves*. Although the main role of the *posterior femoral cutaneous nerve* (S2 and S3) is to provide sensory innervation to the posterior surface of the thigh, its *perineal branch* is possibly more important. Because it provides cutaneous innervation to a large part of the perineum (see Fig. 3-25), it must be considered in anesthesia of this area. The *ilioinguinal* and *genitofemoral nerves* supply the mons pubis and the anterior part of the labia majora.

The internal pudendal artery and the pudendal nerve arise from the internal iliac artery and the sacral plexus (S2, S3, and S4), respectively, course inferiorly on the inside surface of the piriformis muscle, leave the pelvic cavity through the greater ischiadic (sciatic) foramen in a position inferior to the piriformis muscle to enter the gluteal region, wind around the ischial spine, and enter the lesser ischiadic (sciatic) foramen to become located in the perineum *because they now course inferior to the pelvic diaphragm*. The vessel and nerve continue anteriorly and inferiorly on the obturator internus muscle in a fascial canal—the *pudendal canal*. The first branch of this nerve and artery is the *inferior rectal,* which courses medially through the fat in the ischioanal fossa to reach the inferior part of the anal canal (see Fig. 3-25).

While the internal pudendal artery and pudendal nerve are in the pudendal canal, a *perineal branch* is given off that penetrates the posterior aspect of the membranous layer of the superficial fascia and therefore enters the superficial space (see Fig. 3-25). This perineal nerve and artery immediately divide into *muscular branches* to innervate and give blood supply to the muscles already mentioned and into *labial branches,* which carry on to innervate the skin of the posterior surface of the labia and give this area a blood supply. In addition, branches of this perineal nerve enter the deep space to innervate the muscles contained therein, entering the space at its posterior edge.

Returning to the main internal pudendal artery and pudendal nerve, the branching differs after this point. The artery continues anteriorly and enters the deep space, where it occupies a lateral position (see Fig. 3-28). In addition to *branches to the muscles* contained in this pouch, an *artery to the bulb* emerges, courses medially in the deep space, and then turns inferiorly and penetrates the perineal membrane to terminate in the vestibular bulb. The internal pudendal artery continues anteriorly, divides into *deep* and *dorsal* arteries of the clitoris, which then penetrate the perineal membrane to reach this structure. These two vessels course on the dorsum of the clitoris (dorsal branch) and enter the corpora cavernosa of the clitoris (deep branch).

The *pudendal nerve,* in contrast to the artery, terminates before entering the deep space by dividing into the *perineal branch* already mentioned and the *dorsal nerve of the clitoris.* Therefore, the nerve in the deep space is this latter nerve, which then penetrates the perineal membrane to course on the dorsum of the clitoris (see Fig. 3-28).

Figure 3-30 is presented as an aid in visualizing the course taken by the internal pudendal artery (as well as the accompanying veins and the pudendal nerve).

The *external pudendal* arteries also supply perineal structures. These vessels are branches of the femoral artery and supply the mons pubis and the more anterior aspect of the labia majora.

Veins of the perineum accompany arteries usually as double or plexiform vessels. However, the *deep vein of the clitoris,* unpaired, empties directly into the vesical plexus by passing superiorly between the urogenital diaphragm and the pubic arcuate ligament. *Superficial dorsal veins* of the clitoris as well as *anterior labial veins* are tributaries of the femoral veins.

The perineal membrane is a relatively thick structure that joins with the pelvic fascia anteriorly and posteriorly to form an enclosed space. The anterior edge of this membrane is called the *transverse perineal ligament* (see Fig. 3-3); it does not reach the pubic symphysis. This opening is utilized by the dorsal vein of the clitoris to reach the plexus of veins in the pelvic cavity.

The body of the clitoris, the vestibular bulbs, the crura of the clitoris, and the blood vessels in the perineum are innervated by the autonomic nervous system. The sympathetic fibers arise in the upper lumbar segments and ultimately follow the pudendal nerve and internal pudendal arteries to gain their destination. The parasympathetic fibers from S2, S3, and S4 also follow the pudendal arteries and are concerned in erection of these tissues, causing more blood to enter than leaves the erectile tissue.

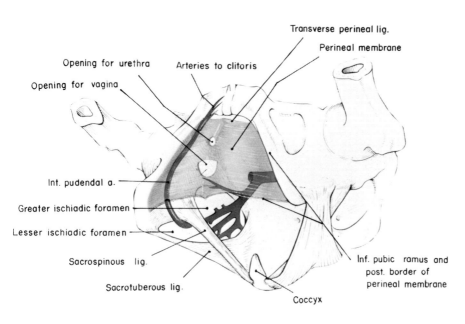

FIG. 3-30. The perineal membrane and the course taken by the internal pudendal artery (and the veins and pudendal nerve) to reach the perineum from the pelvic cavity. (Courtesy of the Ohio Regional Audiovisual Consortium, Columbus, OH)

Transverse perineal lig.

Perineal membrane

Opening for urethra

Arteries to clitoris

Opening for vagina

Int. pudendal a.

Greater ischiadic foramen

Lesser ischiadic foramen

Sacrospinous lig.

Sacrotuberous lig.

Coccyx

Inf. pubic ramus and post. border of perineal membrane

Lymphatics

Lymphatics from all structures in the perineum drain into the inguinal nodes.

REFERENCES AND RECOMMENDED READING

Langman J: Medical Embryology. Baltimore, Williams & Wilkins, 1981

Nomina Anatomica, 5th ed. Baltimore, Williams & Wilkins, 1983

Warwick R, Williams PL (eds): Gray's Anatomy, 35th British ed. Philadelphia, WB Saunders, 1973

The Hypothalamus and Pituitary

Howard P. Krieger

HYPOTHALAMIC–PITUITARY INTERRELATIONS

The pituitary, once considered the master gland, is now known to be functionally dominated by the hypothalamus. The hypothalamus, in turn, is essentially an inte-grator of influences that arise from the cerebrum (especially the limbic system), from the brain stem (especially the reticular activating system), from the spinal cord, and from the endocrine end organ products carried in the bloodstream.

The functional relations among the nervous structures in the complex system are synaptic. The relation between the hypothalamus and the posterior pituitary is synaptic and secretory (Fig. 3-31). The last synapse in the mechanism is at the supraoptic or paraventricular nuclei, which lie in the anterior part of the hypothalamus. The axons of the neurons in these nuclei collect to form the supraoptic–hypophyseal tract, which traverses the hypothalamus and the pituitary stalk and ends in the posterior pituitary. Here the axon terminals abut upon blood vessels instead of other neurons. The products of these neurons are formed in the nuclei, migrate down the axons, and are secreted into the bloodstream. These neurons are thus a classic example of hypothalamic secretory neurons. The secretory products in this case are antidiuretic hormone and oxytocin (or possibly their precursors).

The anatomic arrangement in the case of the anterior pituitary is basically the same. Neurons from the central nervous system synapse with the axons of neurons of various nuclei of the hypothalamus. The axons end upon blood vessels into which their products are

FIG. 3-31.   Interconnections of hypothalamus with remainder of central nervous system. (Krieger DT, Hughes JC (eds): Neuroendocrinology. New York, HP Publishing, 1980)

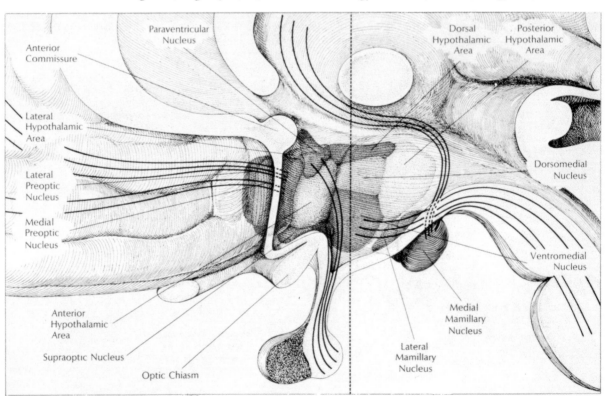

secreted. The hypothalamic–anterior pituitary relation is special because these products are secreted into a portal system (Fig. 3-32), the hypothalamic–pituitary portal system, which arises in the floor of the hypothalamus essentially in the midline just above the pituitary stalk, a region called the median eminence. This portal system descends in and about the pituitary stalk and breaks up into its second capillary system within the anterior pituitary itself. Thus, the products of the hypothalamic secretory neurons (which may be either releasing or inhibiting factors) are delivered from the hypothalamus directly to the pituitary cells. This arrangement allows a very high concentration of these products to enter the anterior pituitary before becoming diluted in the general circulation. Whether the products of small

regions of the hypothalamus are selectively delivered to special regions of the anterior pituitary has not been settled, but it seems unlikely. Although there are many nuclei within the hypothalamus and some may have delineated functions, it is still not known whether a given neuron produces only one secretory product (releasing or inhibiting). It also seems that the various functional cell types are not absolutely limited to specific nuclei.

Thus, the basic anatomic plan of the hypothalamus is like that of the rest of the nervous system. The hypothalamic secretory neuron is analogous to a lower motor neuron (*e.g.,* an anterior horn cell of the spinal cord). Both types of neurons are integrators of neuronal information from cerebrum, brain stem, and spinal cord. The result of this neural integration is the production

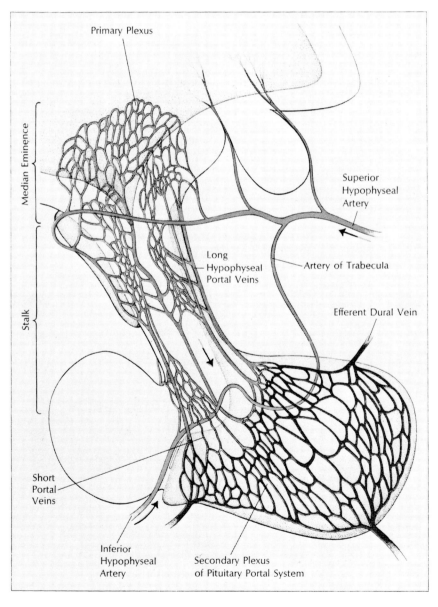

FIG. 3-32. Main features of unusual circulation that connect hypothalamus and pituitary. *Arrows* indicate direction of blood flow. Blood passing into hypophyseal portal veins from median eminence area is distributed to anterior pituitary through secondary capillary plexuses before draining into general venous circulation; hence, virtually all afferent blood supply of anterior pituitary has first been in contact with hypothalamic median eminence area. (Krieger DT, Hughes JC (eds): Neuroendocrinology. New York, HP Publishing, 1980)

Primary Plexus

Median Eminence

Stalk

Superior Hypophyseal Artery

Long Hypophyseal Portal Veins

Artery of Trabecula

Efferent Dural Vein

Short Portal Veins

Inferior Hypophyseal Artery

Secondary Plexus of Pituitary Portal System

of a secretory factor and its delivery to an effector; in the case of the hypothalamic secretory neuron, the product is delivered either to the anterior pituitary by means of the portal system or to the kidney or the uterus by means of the systemic bloodstream from the posterior pituitary; in the case of the lower motor neuron, the secretory product (acetylcholine) is delivered to a motor end plate across a synaptic cleft.

Although the total pathway is long and complex, the effects can occur with astonishing speed. For example, in the case of cortisol, the original stimulus may arise in the temporal lobe; thereafter, the route is from the temporal lobe through the limbic system to the hypothalamus, over the portal system to the anterior pituitary, and through the bloodstream to the adrenal. In the cat, a stimulus to the temporal lobe is reflected in a rise in blood 17-hydroxycorticosteroids within 1 minute. Thus, it appears that the neuroendocrine system is a very rapid organizer of behavioral and physiological response.

In addition to the central nervous system–pituitary end organ interrelations, the endocrine end organ products act upon the central nervous system. The sites of action are numerous, as can be demonstrated by labeling the cell nuclei that take up hormones made radioactive (Fig. 3-33). The limbic system of the temporal lobe (hippocampus and amygdala), which projects into the hypothalamus, is a major site of cortisol uptake. The hypothalamic preoptic area is a major site of estradiol uptake, but this hormone is also significantly taken up by nuclei of the amygdala and hippocampus. These receptor sites act as sensors of the blood level of the end organ product. The sensors act to excite or dampen hypothalamic and thus pituitary activity. The various endocrine end organ products probably also act directly on the pituitary. In any case, the anatomicophysiologic system is such that endocrine activity can be quickly integrated into the total behavioral response at any time by means of feedback mechanisms and multiple nervous system pathways leading to the hypothalamus.

Clearly, sensory stimuli from essentially the entire body have potential neuroanatomic access to the hypothalamic–pituitary system. The generally accepted relation of the breast, cervix, and vagina to oxytocin release serves as an example. Although some of the details are not clear, it is suggested that sensory stimuli arising from the nipple, the cervix, or the vagina travel along peripheral nerves to the spinal cord, up to the brain stem, and finally to the hypothalamus, to reach the paraventricular nuclei in the anterosuperior aspect of the hypothalamus. There oxytocin or its precursor is formed and transported along the neurons of the supraoptic–hypophyseal tract to the posterior pituitary, where it is released into the bloodstream. It is then transported to the breast and uterus. Some of the oxytocin is probably also released into the median eminence and carried over the portal system to the anterior pituitary, where it triggers production of prolactin, which is also carried to the breast. Alterations in the menstrual cycle illustrate the effect of psychic and first cranial nerve stimuli that reach the cerebrum and then are relayed to the hypothalamus–pituitary system. Psychic effects upon the menstrual cycle are well known. Perhaps less well known is the fact that a group of cycling females living together, as in a dormitory, may soon have coinciding cycles. In the case of rats, this has been shown to require an intact olfactory nerve and to depend upon pheromones or substances carried through the air from one organism to another.

PITUITARY–JUXTAPITUITARY INTERRELATIONS

A different set of pituitary–hypothalamic–nervous system relations reflects the anatomic juxtaposition of parts of

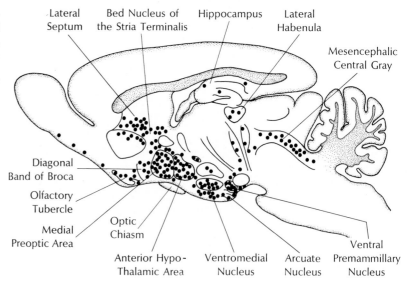

FIG. 3-33. Estrogen-binding sites in hypothalamic and limbic structures demonstrated by uptake of injected radioactive estradiol in rat. *Black dots* show areas of radioactivity. (McEwen BS: In Krieger DT, Hughes JC (eds): Neuroendocrinology, p 36. New York, HP Publishing, 1980)

Lateral Septum

Bed Nucleus of the Stria Terminalis

Hippocampus

Lateral Habenula

Mesencephalic Central Gray

Diagonal Band of Broca

Olfactory Tubercle

Medial Preoptic Area

Optic Chiasm

Anterior Hypo-Thalamic Area

Ventromedial Nucleus

Arcuate Nucleus

Ventral Premammillary Nucleus

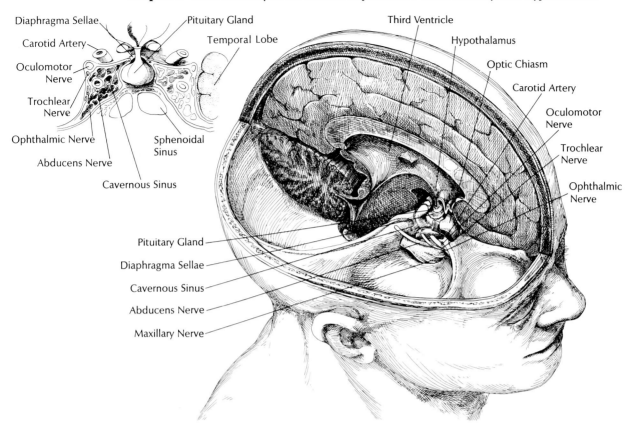

FIG. 3-34. Relation of contents of sella turcica to surrounding structures. Disease processes here can compromise optic function, affect nearby cranial nerves, and derange neuroendocrine functions. (Krieger HP: In Krieger DT, Hughes JC (eds): Neuroendocrinology. New York, HP Publishing, 1980)

these areas rather than a physiological relation. Figure 3-34 shows the relations among the hypothalamus, chiasm, pituitary, sella turcica, cavernous sinuses and their contents, sphenoid sinus, and temporal lobes. For the most part, the anatomic juxtaposition of these structures becomes clinically important only in disease. Thus, neoplasms in this region (whether they arise in the pituitary, hypothalamus, neighboring meninges, or sphenoid sinus), as well as large aneurysms (such as occur in the carotid artery as it passes lateral to the sella), produce a clinical picture compounded of pituitary–hypothalamic dysfunction (either hypofunction or hyperfunction) and dysfunction (ischemic or destructive) of neighboring neurologic structures. When a mass develops in this region, the most commonly affected nervous system structure is the optic chiasm (producing typically a bitemporal hemianopsia), but any other neighboring structure may be affected. The older literature indicates that during pregnancy the pituitary swells and can produce a visual field defect secondary to chiasmatic compression. We have never seen such a case, and it must be very rare. Temporal lobe seizures are also rare.

Various types of third, fourth, and sixth nerve palsies, as well as rupture of the floor of the sella and extension of its contents into the sphenoid sinus, are also uncommon in disease in this area. When masses arise in the hypothalamus, a combination of hypofunction and hyperfunction may occur in conjunction with destruction of chiasmatic function.

REFERENCES

Krieger DT: The hypothalamus and neuroendocrinology. In Krieger DT, Hughes JC (eds): Neuroendocrinology, p 3. New York, HP Publishing, 1980

Krieger HP: Sellar and juxtasellar disease: A neurologic viewpoint. In Krieger DT, Hughes JC (eds): Neuroendocrinology, p 275. New York, HP Publishing, 1980

Krieger HP, Krieger DT: Chemical stimulation of the brain: Effect on adrenal corticoid release. Am J Physiol 218(6): 1632, 1970

McEwen BS: The brain as a target organ of endocrine hormones. In Krieger DT, Hughes JC (eds): Neuroendocrinology, p 33. New York, HP Publishing, 1980

Microscopic Anatomy of the Female Reproductive Tract and Pituitary

Jack Davies
E. S. E. Hafez
Hans Ludwig

4

Histology

Jack Davies

The female reproductive system includes the ovaries, the prime purpose of which is to produce the female germ cells (eggs); the sexual ducts (uterine tubes, uterus, vagina); and the external genitalia. Associated with the latter are certain glandular structures that collectively form the accessory organs of reproduction. The female reproductive system, unlike that of the male, shows cyclic alterations in structure coincident with the phases of the menstrual cycle, which are in turn dependent upon the activities of the estrogenic and progestational hormones of the ovaries. It also shows striking modifications in structure and function during pregnancy.

THE OVARIES

The ovaries are bilateral structures attached to the posterior leaf of the broad ligament in relation to the lateral pelvic wall. Their epithelial covering, or *germinal epithelium* (Fig. 4-1), is a modified area of the celomic lining, which, in the embryo and fetus, gives rise by proliferation to the germinal and supporting elements of the ovary. It is a cuboidal or low columnar epithelium continuous at the hilum with the flat squamous mesothelium of the peritoneal cavity; the transition between the two epithelia is abrupt and marked by Farre's white line. The postnatal origin of the germ cells from the germinal epithelium is disputed, but the weight of evidence is against it. It is probable that the full comple-

ment of eggs (estimated as at least 150,000 in the two ovaries) is present at birth and that no further formation of eggs occurs after birth. If this is true, some of the eggs must lie dormant within the ovary for 40 years or more before they complete their maturation in the ovulatory cycle or degenerate. Of this large number of eggs, only about 400 may be successfully ovulated during the sexual life of the woman; the rest degenerate. It is also important to understand that the "eggs" present in the postnatal ovary are primary oocytes, that is, they have already entered upon the maturation cycle and are arrested in the prophase of the first maturation division (see Fig. 4-1).

The ovary is customarily described as having a cortex and a medulla. The *medulla,* or central core of the ovary, is continuous with the connective tissue of the broad ligament at the hilum, through which the blood vessels and lymphatics penetrate the organ. Here also are found vestiges of the rete ovarii, homologous with the rete testis of the male, as well as epithelial remnants of the mesonephros (wolffian body) that form the epoophoron.

The ovarian *cortex* in prepubertal and early sexual life contains large numbers of primary oocytes embedded in a highly cellular connective tissue. During sexual life there are also graafian follicles in varying stages of development. The cortical stroma is condensed beneath the germinal epithelium into a tunica albuginea. The germinal epithelium is said not to rest on a basement membrane. This may be true in fetal life, when the germinal epithelium is actively proliferating; however, in the adult ovary, a thin basement membrane can always be demonstrated by electron microscopy.

Several stages in the maturation of the primary oocytes and of the graafian follicles may be studied in Figure 4-1, which is from a section of the rabbit ovary; the sequence of events is essentially the same in the human

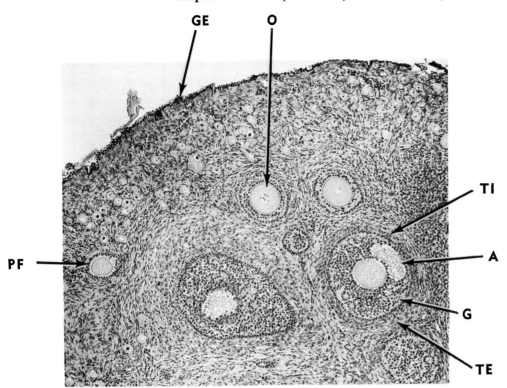

FIG. 4-1. Cortex of ovary of virgin rabbit. Surface germinal epithelium (*GE*) is cuboidal. There is a thin tunica albuginea deep to germinal epithelium. Primary oocytes (*O*) lie embedded in superficial cortex and are surrounded by fibroblastic cells; nuclei of oogonia are in prophaselike state. Primordial follicles (*PF*) lie deeper in cortex. Here also oocyte is larger than in superficial layer and is surrounded by layer of cuboidal granulosa cells. Other follicles are in later stages of development. A follicle with beginning antrum formation (*A*) is shown to right. External to thick layer of granulosa cells (*G*) in larger follicles is theca interna (*TI*), external to which is theca externa (*TE*). A thin zona pellucida is present in oocyte to *right.* (H&E, ×220)

ovary. A group of primary oocytes begins to mature at the beginning of each menstrual cycle under the influence of pituitary gonadotropins, probably chiefly follicle-stimulating hormone (FSH). What factors are involved in the selection of one group of follicles rather than another are unknown and present an important problem for solution. It is interesting that the number of maturing follicles in any cycle is constant (Lipschutz's law of follicular constancy); if one ovary is removed, the number of maturing follicles in the remaining ovary is approximately doubled.

Development of the Graafian Follicle

A *primordial follicle* (see Fig. 4-1) consists of a primary oocyte enclosed by a single layer of cuboidal cells derived from the surrounding stroma. The oocyte and the follicular (nurse) cells around it grow *pari passu* until the oocyte is about 80μ and the follicle is about 0.2 mm in diameter. Thereafter, the follicle grows more rapidly

than the oocyte. In a fully mature follicle the oocyte is about 120μ in diameter, and the follicle may reach a diameter of 5 mm to 10 mm. The cells surrounding the oocyte increase in number by mitosis, and when the follicle is about 0.2 mm in diameter a fluid-filled space (*antrum*) appears. The fluid (*primary liquor folliculi*) is metachromatic at a neutral pH and stains with the periodic acid-Schiff (PAS) method, indicating the presence of neutral or weakly acidic mucopolysaccharides. A secondary liquor folliculi of gelatinous consistency is also described in the antrum of larger follicles. A more watery tertiary liquor folliculi accumulates rapidly within the antrum of a follicle that is destined to rupture at ovulation; it is probably secreted by the lining cells. This preovulatory swelling of the mature follicle is believed to depend upon the action of pituitary luteinizing hormone (LH), which is released into the blood just before ovulation.

In the mature graafian follicle (see Figs. 4-1 and 4-2), the cells surrounding the antral cavity are known as the *granulosa cells* or the *membrana granulosa.* The mature oocyte lies within a localized mound of granulosa cells, the *discus proligerus* or *cumulus oophorus* (Fig. 4-2), which is oriented toward the medulla of the ovary. The granulosa cells are avascular and are several layers in thickness; the basal layer of cells rests on a well-marked basement membrane that stains strongly with the PAS method. The stromal elements of the ovary are condensed around the follicle in two layers, the theca interna and the theca externa (see Fig. 4-1). The *theca externa* is relatively avascular and forms a con-

nective tissue capsule around the follicle. The *theca interna* is vascular, and its cells undergo marked hypertrophy as the follicle matures (Fig. 4-3). The cells become rounded and epithelial in appearance and sudanophilic droplets appear within their cytoplasm. As ovulation approaches, the hypertrophied thecal cells resemble the luteal cells of the corpus luteum (Fig. 4-4) but are smaller. The luteal hypertrophy of the theca interna probably results from the action of pituitary LH. In some animals, such as the cat, a striking preovulatory

FIG. 4-2. Portion of wall of mature human graafian follicle. Primary oocyte is surrounded by zona pellucida (*Z*). Oocyte is embedded in cumulus oophorus (*CO*). Antral cavity filled with liquor folliculi lies at *top* of picture. *N,* nucleus; *NL,* nucleolus. (Grollman A: Essentials of Endocrinology, 2nd ed. Philadelphia, Lippincott, 1941)

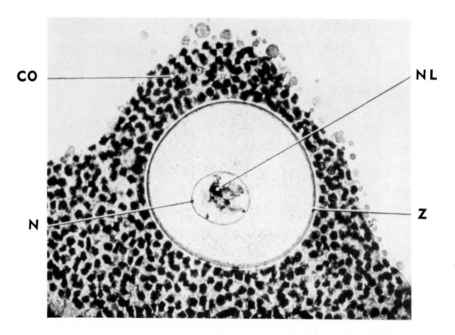

FIG. 4-3. Portion of wall of mature human graafian follicle at about 17th day of cycle, *i.e.,* just before ovulation. Antral cavity at *top* contains coagulated liquor folliculi. Granulosa cells (*G*) form layer five or six cells in thickness; they have small dark nuclei with very little cytoplasm. Basement membrane of granulosa cells is not demonstrated by this stain. External to latter is theca interna (*TI*), made up of epithelium-like cells and containing many blood vessels. Theca externa (*TE*) of condensed connective tissue lies external to theca interna. (H&E, ×100)

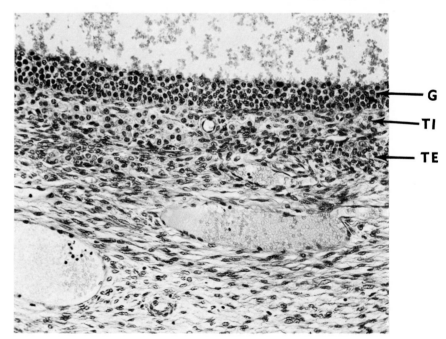

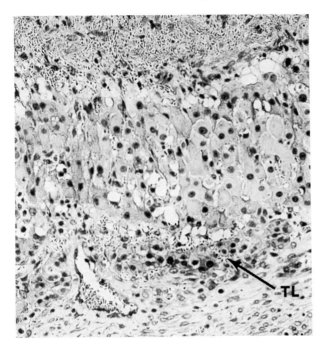

FIG. 4-4. Early stage in luteal transformation of ruptured graafian follicle. Antral cavity at *top* contains organizing fibrinous material. Granulosa cells are hypertrophied and show marked increase in amount of cytoplasm that is acidophilic. Clusters of theca granulosa cells; cells are smaller than granulosa lutein cells. Vessels have grown into modified granulosa layer and are beginning to invest luteal cells with sinusoidal capillary vessels. *TL,* theca lutein cells. (H&E, ×220)

luteal hypertrophy of these cells occurs. This may also occur under certain circumstances in the human ovary.

The changes in the primary oocyte during the maturation process are complex. An initial *growth phase,* coincident with the proliferation of the granulosal and thecal elements of the follicle, is followed by a *maturation phase,* in which the growth rate is reduced and in which there is an active synthesis of cytoplasmic proteins and yolk droplets. The nuclei of the oocytes remain in a peculiar prophaselike state both in the dormant phase within the primordial follicle (see Fig. 4-1) and during the preliminary phase of maturation. Mitochondria appear in abundance within the cytoplasm, and there is a well-marked Golgi region. When the oocyte has reached a diameter of about 80μ, a highly refractile membrane (*zona pellucida*) appears between the granulosa cells and the oocyte. It may be a secretory product of the granulosa cells, which show increased cytoplasmic complexity in the electron microscope. Microvilli from the surface plasma membrane of the granulosa cells and from that of the oocyte (*vitelline membrane*) are found within the zona pellucida and may make contact with each other, suggesting a possible avenue of transmission of materials between them. The zona pellucida stains strongly with the PAS method and is meta-chromatic at a low pH, suggesting the presence of strongly acid mucopolysaccharides. Between the zona pellucida and the oocyte is a perivitelline space, which may be exaggerated as an artifact of fixation and dehydration.

A fully mature graafian follicle may reach a size of 5 mm to 10 mm in the human ovary. Just before ovulation, the mature occyte completes the first reduction division, in which the diploid number of chromosomes (46) is halved to the haploid number (23); the smaller daughter cell forms the *first polar body* and lies within the perivitelline space. The egg is now a *secondary oocyte* and is in this stage when ovulation takes place. The second reduction division does not occur until after fertilization of the oocyte in the upper reaches of the uterine tubes. Following sperm penetration, the *second polar body* is formed. This second division of the oocyte nucleus is, however, comparable to a mitotic process with a reduced number of chromosomes, and there is no further alteration in the haploid number.

The secondary oocyte with its polar body enclosed within the zona pellucida is shed at ovulation by rupture of the graafian follicle. The process has been observed by cinephotography in rodents. As ovulation approaches, an area of the follicular wall underlying the germinal epithelium becomes thinned and avascular. The wall then ruptures at this point, and a mixture of gelatinous and fluid liquor folliculi spurts through the hole. The egg may emerge first or may follow the initial spurt of follicular fluid. The egg carries with it a cluster of cells of the cumulus oophorus (*corona radiata*). It is then carried by fluid currents and ciliary action into the infundibulum of the uterine tube.

Follicular Atresia

A phenomenon of great importance is *follicular atresia.* Of the six or more follicles that begin the growth and maturation process at each cycle, only one as a rule undergoes the preovulatory swelling and ruptures at ovulation. The remaining follicles of the group fail to swell and undergo a degenerative change known as atresia. There is degeneration and nucleus pyknosis of the granulosa cells, beginning in the cells nearest to the antrum. The follicular fluid becomes inspissated, and the entrapped egg degenerates. The zona pellucida may persist for an extended time as a highly refractile, strongly PAS-positive band. The granulosa cells degenerate completely, and the antrum becomes filled with organizing fibrinous material. The basement membrane of the granulosa layer becomes thickened and highly refractile, forming the *glassy membrane;* it also may persist for an extended time as a crumpled refractile homogeneous band. The follicle collapses, and the theca interna and externa are also modified. In some instances, the theca interna may show only fibrotic changes, whereas in others, perhaps depending on whether an effective luteinizing stimulus is present or not, the theca interna may undergo a luteal hypertrophy. The cells become epithelial and store lipid droplets, and in all respects except size they resemble the luteal cells of the corpus luteum. Such a luteinized follicle is called a *corpus luteum atreticum* and is not to be confused with a true corpus luteum, which is formed only after ovulation. Corpora lutea atretica, as well as atretic follicles in general, are formed in increased numbers in pregnancy in women and in animals with prolonged gestation periods such as the horse. Their appearance in pregnancy may be associated with powerful luteinizing effects emanating from the placenta, which produces human chorionic gonadotropin (hCG) in women and pregnant mare serum gonadotropin (PMSG) in the mare. The rate of follicular atresia is also markedly increased in the postovulatory stage of the menstrual cycle in women and primates and of the estrous cycle in animals, as well as after the administration of progestational compounds. The significance of follicular atresia and the hormonal significance of corpora lutea atretica remain two of the most important unsolved problems of reproductive physiology.

Development of the Corpus Luteum

Following ovulation, the follicle is converted into a true *corpus luteum.* In animals with multiple ovulations, like the rabbit, there are multiple corpora lutea, and their number correlates to a striking degree with the number of viable fetuses at a later stage. Only one, corresponding to the ovulation occurring in that cycle, is present in the human ovary. In rats, which have very short estrous cycles of four to five days, there are several generations of corpora lutea, and it may be difficult to identify the ones corresponding to the most recent ovulation.

The manner of formation of the corpus luteum from the follicular elements has been debated for many years. In some animals, such as the rabbit, it is clear that only the granulosa cells are involved in the luteal transformation of the follicle. In the human ovary there are two types of luteal cells, the *granulosa lutein cells* and the *theca lutein cells,* the latter being derived from the theca interna. The cells differ only in size, the theca lutein cells being much smaller in the earlier stages. Later in the development of the corpus luteum it is impossible to identify the two types of cells. Following the rupture of the follicle, the antral cavity collapses and may contain a little extravasated blood. Hemorrhagic cystic follicles without ovulation and associated with theca luteinization are common in animals, such as the rabbit, following coitus or a large dose of a luteinizing preparation. Theca lutein cysts are found in the ovaries of newborn and adult human beings, but their pathogenesis and hormonal basis are poorly understood.

After collapse of the antral cavity following ovulation, the granulosa cells proliferate by mitosis and undergo a steady hypertrophy and growth. The basement membrane of the granulosa layer is broken in several places, and there is an invasion of capillary sprouts and connective tissue from the theca interna into the granulosa layer (see Fig. 4-4). Under the continuing luteal stimulus, both the granulosa cells and the smaller theca cells become slowly transformed into luteal cells, and the two types of cells become closely intermingled. Within two to three days the corpus luteum becomes organized into a spherical body in which the luteal cells are arranged in more or less radial cords around the central remnant of the antral cavity. There are coarse septa of connective tissue separating the principal cords of luteal cells that contain the larger vessels, and there are delicate capsules of reticular tissue and capillaries around the individual luteal cells and groups of cells. The structure is highly vascular and bleeds profusely on cutting, so that it may be a source of serious intraabdominal bleeding.

The luteal cells resemble cells of the adrenal cortex in appearance under both light and electron microscopes. These steroid-secreting cells share fine structural characteristics that may tentatively be identified with their function as producers of steroid hormones such as the estrogens and progestational compounds. The mitochondria are rounded and tend to have tubular cristae rather than the usual lamellar type. The cytoplasm is occupied by a honeycomb of small sacs and short tubules of the endoplasmic reticulum. Between these sacs and tubules are numerous ribonucleoprotein granules (ribosomes). There are large lipid inclusions enclosed in membranous sacs, probably representing sites of hormone deposition or synthesis. The droplets of lipid are acetone soluble, doubly refractile, and autofluorescent; they also give the Schultz reaction for cholesterol and other histochemical reactions considered typical of the ketosteroids, though not specific for them.

Degeneration of the luteal cells is accompanied by changes in the solubility and refractility of the lipid droplets. The droplets also tend to coalesce and form large sudanophilic masses. There are also droplets of the wear-and-tear pigment *lipofuscin;* its presence in the degenerating corpus luteum of the human ovary caused earlier observers to note its yellow color and so to give it its name.

The corpus luteum is formed during the first three days after ovulation under the predominant influence of pituitary LH. Thereafter a luteotropic influence is pituitary in origin in the luteal phase of the menstrual cycle. The corpus luteum declines and becomes functionless a few days before the next menstrual cycle, presumably owing to the withdrawal of the luteotropic stimulus. In the pregnant woman, however, the corpus luteum of menstruation fails to degenerate and increases in size, forming the *corpus luteum of pregnancy.* Its continued life and function depend upon a new luteotropic stimulus, this time emanating from the placenta. This stimulus is probably hCG, which has been identified in the trophoblast soon after implantation and appears in the urine at a slightly later stage. Its effects in animals are predominantly luteinizing; in women large doses have been shown to be luteotropic also. The corpus luteum functions throughout the first third of pregnancy but declines thereafter and has degenerated by the last third. New ovulations with the production of accessory corpora lutea, as in the mare, are not known to occur in women. The final stages in the degeneration of the human corpus luteum of menstruation may last up to a year. They consist of shrinkage and hyalinization of the luteal cells and the intercellular connective tissue and conversion of the corpus luteum into a hyalinized mass (*corpus albicans*). Figure 4-5 diagrams this sequence of events.

Interstitial Cells

Interstitial cells of the ovary are abundant in the rabbit, in which they form an interstitial gland and appear to be a source of estrogen and progestational compounds. They are inconspicuous in the human ovary but may be found in considerable numbers in the medulla in the region of the hilum; they are increased in number in the ovary of the patient with the Stein–Leventhal syndrome. Their microscopic appearance is similar to that of the steroid-secreting cells described earlier, and it is reasonable to suppose that they also may be a source of

steroid hormones, including estrogenic, progestational, and androgenic compounds.

THE UTERINE TUBES

The oviducts (uterine tubes) are about 10 cm in length. They are bilateral structures that pierce the wall of the uterus at the lateral margins of the fundus on either side. They are divided into three parts: the ampulla, the isthmus, and the intramural part. The uterine tube communicates with the peritoneal cavity close to the ovary through the infundibulum. The margins of the opening are expanded into tentaclelike structures (*fimbriae*) that become turgid at the time of ovulation and closely applied to the rupturing follicle, thereby decreasing the chance of loss of the egg into the peritoneal cavity. The *ampulla* is the relatively dilated lateral half of the tube. Its lumen is wider than the isthmic portion, and the lining mucosal folds are more complex. It is in this portion of the tube that fertilization of the oocyte takes place and in which it completes its second maturation division and later segmentation. The *isthmic portion* of the tube is very narrow, and its lumen is difficult to enter with a probe. The *intramural portion* is about 1 cm in length and penetrates the muscular wall of the uterus.

FIG. 4-5. Diagram of ovary, showing sequence of events leading to maturation and rupture of follicles, luteinization, and involution of corpus luteum. Nonruptured follicles undergo atresia. (Patten BM: Human Embryology. New York, Blakiston, 1946)

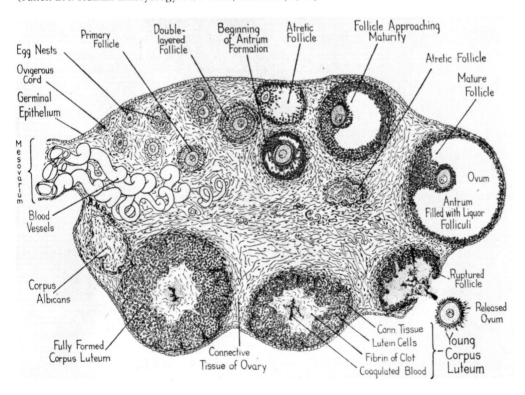

The epithelium lining all parts of the uterine tube is simple or pseudostratified columnar (Fig. 4-6). Many of the cells are ciliated, while others appear to be secretory or absorptive in type. The ciliated cells occur singly or in islands. The nuclei of the secretory cells show a characteristic tendency to lie close to the lumen of the tube, causing the apical part of the cell to bulge into it. Evidence for the secretory activity of the cells is provided in some animals, such as the rabbit, in which an albuminous coat is added to the zona pellucida during the passage of the fertilized egg through the uterine tube. During estrus in many rodents, large amounts of fluid accumulate within the uterine tubes.

The fundamental importance of the secretions of this part of the reproductive tract in the successful passage and nourishment of the dividing egg and blastocyst in animals and women is only slowly becoming recognized, and much remains to be learned about the nature of these secretions. Of equal importance is the muscular wall of the oviduct, which is responsible for its motility. The tubal transport of the fertilized egg toward the uterus and of the spermatozoa in the opposite direction is poorly understood and appears to depend upon precise patterns of motility of the tube as well as on the presence of fluid currents and ciliary activity. The cilia beat in the direction of the uterus. The bundles

FIG. 4-6. (*A*) Transverse section of uterine tube at level of ampulla. (*B*) Details of epithelium of ampulla of uterine tube. Ciliated cells are shown at *arrow.* Other cells are secretory in type and there are some narrow peglike cells with dark nuclei. (H&E, approximately ×500) (*C*) Isthmus. Note that folding of mucosa is less marked and muscle is thicker. (Leeson TA, Leeson CR (eds): Histology, 2nd ed. Philadelphia, WB Saunders, 1970) (*D*) Interstitial or intramural segment of tube. (Greep RO (ed): Histology, 2nd ed. New York, McGraw-Hill, 1966)

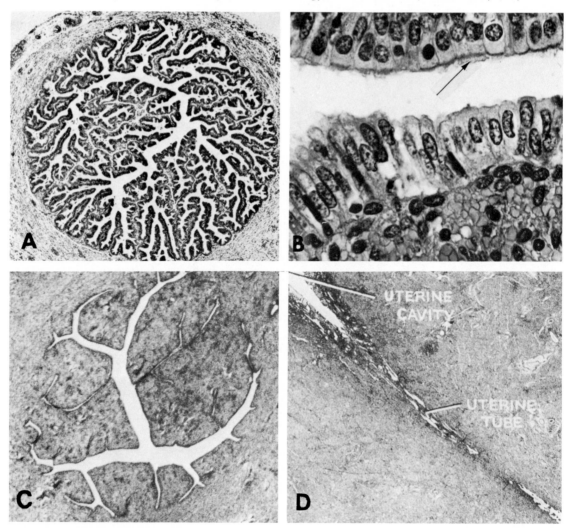

of smooth muscle in the wall of the uterine tube consist of mingled outer longitudinal and inner circular and spiral bands.

A thick lamina propria of vascular connective tissue lies between the epithelial and the muscular layer (see Fig. 4-6); it is especially dense and tough in the isthmic portion and causes the mucosa to pout from within the smooth muscle of the wall when the tube is cut transversely. External to the muscular layer is a layer of visceral peritoneum, the epithelium of which is a typical flattened mesothelium and is separated from the muscle by a loose subserous layer of connective tissue rich in blood vessels and lymphatics. Changes in the epithelium have been described in the different phases of the menstrual cycle, but such changes are less evident than in other parts of the reproductive tract.

THE UTERUS

The uterus is a pear-shaped organ lying in the midline enclosed between the two layers of the broad ligament. It consists of a fundus, a body (corpus uteri), and a neck (cervix uteri).

The Corpus Uteri

The wall of the uterus consists of three layers: an inner endometrium, a middle myometrium, and an external peritoneal (serous) coat. The endometrium undergoes cyclic changes governed by the interplay of hormones of pituitary and ovarian origin that underlie the menstrual cycle and is profoundly modified in pregnancy. The myometrium also shows cyclic changes, but the most striking changes occur in pregnancy.

FIG. 4-7. Endometrium in proliferative phase of cycle. Glandular epithelium is tall columnar and shows marked cytoplasmic basophilia. There are numerous mitotic figures in epithelium. Stroma is richly cellular. (H&E, ×220)

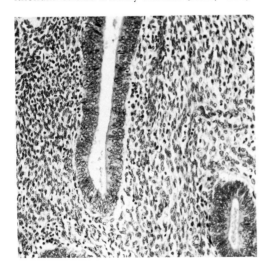

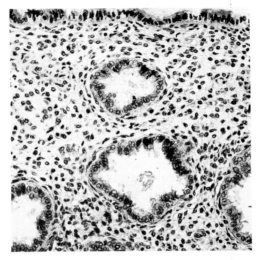

FIG. 4-8. Endometrium at midcycle, approximately at time of ovulation. Surface epithelium is columnar. Glands are dilated and lined by irregular columnar epithelium showing evidence of secretory activity. These cells have lost cytoplasmic basophilia of early proliferative phase. Stroma is edematous, fibroblasts being more widely separated than in early stage (compare Fig. 4-7). (H&E, ×220)

Endometrial Changes During the Menstrual Cycle

A menstrual cycle associated with cyclic bleeding from the endometrium is found only in women and primates. The first day of the cycle is considered to be the first day of external vaginal bleeding. The bleeding phase lasts from several days to a week in normal women and occurs approximately every 28 days. The sequence of events in the cycle is briefly summarized as follows. Under the influence of FSH, several follicles in the ovary begin to grow. The initial maturation of the follicle, up to the early stage of antrum formation, may not be dependent on pituitary gonadotropins, since it occurs in hypophysectomized animals. The later stages of follicular growth and preovulatory swelling are, however, dependent upon the pituitary. As the follicles grow, estrogen is produced from either the thecal or granulosal elements, and this estrogen in turn affects the endometrium. There is a thickening of the endometrial mucosa and an increase in the number and complexity of the glands (Fig. 4-7). This is the *follicular (proliferative) phase* of the cycle. The glands and surface epithelium show intense mitotic activity. The epithelial cells, which are tall columnar cells, show a marked cytoplasmic basophilia that is abolished by ribonuclease and so is due largely to cytoplasmic ribonucleoprotein (RNP). The stroma becomes vascular and edematous toward the middle of the cycle. Ovulation probably occurs 11 to 14 days before the next menstrual period, that is, on about the 17th day of the cycle (Fig. 4-8). The preovulatory swelling of the follicle is associated with the release of LH from the pituitary. There is also good evidence for the production of progestational substances by the follicle before its rupture, probably from the cells of the hypertrophied theca interna.

Ovulation initiates the *luteal (secretory) phase* of the menstrual cycle, which is dependent upon the presence of a functional corpus luteum and the production of progestational hormones. In this phase, the endometrial glands become tortuous and their walls become sinuous, presenting a characteristic sawtooth pattern (Fig. 4-9). The lining cells show evidence of secretory activity, and the glandular lumen becomes distended with secretion that gives a strong PAS reaction and is probably mucopolysaccharide in nature. Glycogen also appears in the glandular epithelium, in the glandular secretion, and in the fibroblastic cells of the endometrial stroma. The latter may show an early decidual reaction in the late secretory (premenstrual) phase of the cycle.

The decline of the corpus luteum of menstruation and the withdrawal of progestational influences from the endometrium are correlated with the involution of the latter and the onset of menstrual bleeding. This phenomenon has been studied in endometrial grafts in the anterior chamber of the eye in monkeys. A day or so before menstrual bleeding, the endometrial transplant shrank markedly (the ischemic phase), presumably because of the withdrawal of water. Throughout the cycle, but most markedly before menstruation, there was a rhythmic contraction and relaxation of the endometrial arterioles, which produced an alternate blushing and blanching of the graft. Small petechial hemorrhages then appeared beneath the epithelial surface and were shortly followed by bleeding from the graft. The changes in the vascular tone of the endometrial vessels are clearly of great importance and may be associated with an increasing dominance of estrogen over progesterone as the corpus luteum declines.

The human endometrium in the late luteal phase or in early pregnancy has three layers, beginning at the luminal surface: a *zona compacta* in the region of the mouths of the glands, a deeper *zona spongiosa* in which the glands are tortuous and dilated, and a *zona basalis* adjoining the myometrium. The zona compacta and zona spongiosa are often combined as the *zona functionalis* since they are shed at menstruation. There are two sets of arteries supplying the endometrium (Fig. 4-10). Arteries of one type supply only the zona basalis. This zone accordingly remains intact after menstruation, and the endometrial lining is regenerated from it by the outgrowth of epithelium from the glands. Arteries of the second type are the spiral arterioles, which pursue a tortuous course through the zona functionalis and supply it. These vessels show the alternate constriction and relaxation described in the terminal (ischemic) phase of the cycle. They also play an important role in the pregnant uterus.

Endometrial Changes in Pregnancy

If the egg is fertilized, it undergoes a series of mitotic divisions, resulting in a ball of cells (*morula*). A cavity then appears within the morula, converting it into the *blastocyst.* The outer wall of the blastocyst (*trophoblast*) consists of ectodermal cells, which are directly involved in the implantation process and in the later formation of the placenta. Implantation takes place about the seventh day after ovulation.

The presence of the blastocyst within the uterus is directly or indirectly responsible for the transformation

FIG. 4-9. Two sections of endometrium in late luteal or premenstrual phase of cycle. (*A*) Surface epithelium is tall columnar (compare Fig. 4-8). Deep to epithelium is zona compacta. (*B*) Glands in deeper layers of endometrium (zona spongiosa) are dilated and show characteristic sawtooth pattern. Glandular lumen contains secretion material. Fibroblasts of stroma are hypertrophied but show no decidual change. There is considerable stromal edema. (H&E, ×220)

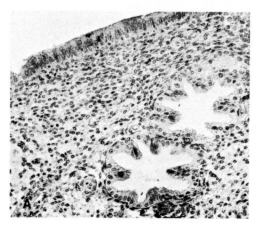 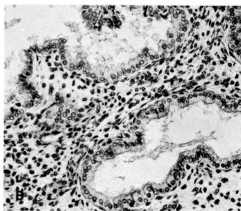

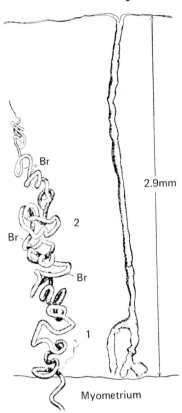

2.9mm

Br

2

Br

Br

1

Myometrium

FIG. 4-10. Diagram of spiral arteriole and gland from endometrium at about fourth day. A small branch (type 1) supplies zona basalis close to myometrium. Spiral vessels (type 2) supply zona functionalis. (Daron SH: The arterial pattern of the tunica mucosa of the uterus in Macacus rhesus. Am J Anat 58: 349, 1936)

of the corpus luteum of menstruation into the corpus luteum of pregnancy, probably because of a luteotropic hormone emanating from the trophoblast. As a result, there is an enhanced output of progestational substances from the corpus luteum, and the endometrium undergoes further transformations. The endometrial stroma shows a *decidual reaction.* Beginning about the 12th day, the stromal cells become enlarged and epithelial in appearance, and there is a deposition of cytoplasmic lipid and glycogen. This is illustrated at the fifth month of pregnancy in Figure 4-11. This decidual bed forms an ideal pabulum for the implanted ovum and may also in some way modify or restrain the invasive activities of syncytiotrophoblast. Following the establishment of the mature placenta, there is a complex *junctional zone* between the peripheral trophoblast and the myometrium, consisting of intermingled trophoblastic and decidual cells. A *zone of separation* is later formed in this area, and the placenta separates through this zone at parturition. The spiral arterioles of the zona functionalis are the first vessels to be encountered by the invading

trophoblast. They are ruptured, and the maternal blood floods into the lacunae within the trophoblastic shell.

Another apparently specific but atypical response of the endometrium to the presence of viable trophoblast is the so-called *Arias–Stella reaction* (Fig. 4-12). In one study, the reaction was found in only five of many specimens studied from the Hertig collection at the Carnegie Institution of Washington and was first observed at the 17th day of gestation. It consists of irregular hyperplasia of the superficial epithelial and glandular cells with large, irregular, hyperchromatic nulcei; proliferative appearances in the glands, consisting of villuslike foldings of the cells into the lumen with piling up of cells; and secretory appearance in the glands associated with hyperplasia and cytoplasmic vacuolation. The reaction is usually focal and occurs independently of inflammation.

The Myometrium

The smooth muscle of the wall of the uterus is very thick and is arranged in bundles separated by cellular connective tissue that contains vessels. The inner layers are dispersed in a sphincterlike manner around the intramural portions of the uterine tubes. The intermediate layer is thick and irregularly dispersed with many large venous channels, giving it a spongy texture. The outer layer consists of intermingled longitudinal and circular fibers. There is a serous coat external to the myometrium, except laterally in relation to the attachment of the broad ligament.

FIG. 4-11. Decidual reaction in endometrium at fifth month of pregnancy. Superficial and glandular epithelia appear atrophic. (H&E, ×220).

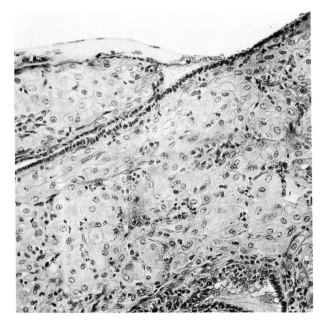

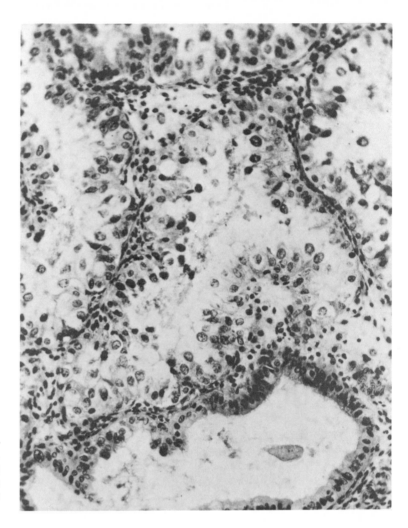

FIG. 4-12. Arias–Stella reaction. Gland at *center* shows proliferative and secretory activity. Some nuclei are about three times as large as those seen in adjacent gland. (Oertel YC: The Arias–Stella reaction revisited. Arch Pathol Lab Med 102:651, 1978)

The myometrium shows great hypertrophy in pregnancy. Individual smooth muscle fibers may increase in length from 50μ to 500μ, and there may be new formation of muscle fibers.

The Cervix Uteri

The cervix forms a short transition zone between the corpus uteri and the vagina. A portion of it lies above the level of the vaginal vault (*supravaginal cervix*), and a portion lies exposed inferiorly within the vagina and is covered by epithelium of vaginal type (*portio externa*). The cervical lumen is constricted and encroached upon by folds of the mucosal lining that in the virgin form the *plicae palmatae*.

In cross section the cervical lumen presents a complex branching configuration (*arbor vitae*). The *endocervical canal* is about 1 inch long in average women but shows great variation. It is lined by a columnar or pseudostratified columnar epithelium, which is variably mucified (Fig. 4-13). There are deeply penetrating

glands of a tubular branching type, which are also lined by columnar epithelium. The stroma of the cervix is composed mainly of collagenous connective tissue with a small amount of elastic tissue and occasional smooth muscle fibers. The stroma becomes very vascular during pregnancy.

Mucification of the endocervical epithelium is the salient reaction of this part of the female reproductive tract to cyclic changes in hormone secretion and is maximal just before ovulation, when estrogen is at a high level and progesterone begins to appear. An increase in the amount of mucus at the vaginal introitus is commonly observed by women and appears to coincide more or less closely with ovulation. Ferning of the cervical mucus at about this time is described in Chapter 49, Infertility.

Basally, the endocervical epithelium rests on a continuous basement membrane that is too thin to be resolved by the light microscope. Staining of the basement membrane by such techniques as the PAS method is probably due to polysaccharide materials associated with the basement membrane rather than to the membrane

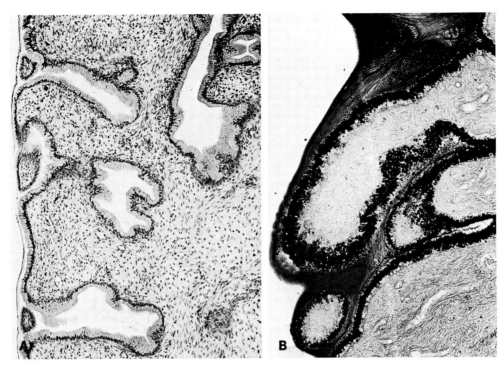

FIG. 4-13. Glands of endocervix at 17th day of cycle. Glands are simple branching in type and are lined by tall clear columnar epithelium (*A*) (×90), which is mucified (*B*) (×220). (*A*, H&E; *B*, PAS)

itself. Studies with the electron microscope are essential if statements are to be made with respect to the integrity or lack of integrity of the basement membrane in pathologic processes involving the endocervix or the portio externa. Electron-microscopic studies confirm the virtual absence of smooth muscle from the cervical stroma.

The transition from the columnar epithelium of the endocervix to the stratified squamous epithelium of the portio externa is usually abrupt (Fig. 4-14). The columnar epithelium, however, may extend outside the external os onto the vaginal aspect of the cervix, a common feature of the cervix of the newborn infant and the pregnant woman; it is frequently referred to as physiological erosion or ectropion. Chronic inflammatory changes are common in the region of the external os and are often associated with an actual loss of the epithelium around the external os (*true erosion*) and with an encroachment of stratified squamous epithelium into the endocervical canal. Blocking of the mouths of the cervical glands near the external os may result in the formation of clear cysts (*ovula nabothi*).

The region of the external os is one of the most important junctional regions in the body, comparable to such mucocutaneous junctions as the red margin of the lips and the anus. It shares with these areas a marked predisposition toward cancer. This tendency is enhanced in the case of the cervix by the extreme lability of the junction between the two epithelia involved and by the responsiveness of these to hormonal stimulation.

Other common histologic changes in the region of the cervix are illustrated in Figure 4-15. They are the decidual transformation of parts of the endocervical stroma and the squamous metaplasia of the columnar epithelium. The latter is common in normal cycling women and is almost universal in pregnancy. The nature and significance of this squamous metaplasia have aroused much controversy. Since it often occurs in the depths of the mucosal folds and crypts of the endocervix, far removed from the external os, it cannot result from an invasion of stratified squamous epithelium from the portio externa. It has been regarded by some as a true metaplasia of the columnar epithelium; by others, as a proliferation of indifferent (reserve) cells lying in the deep layer of the epithelium close to the basement membrane. It is enhanced in the endocervix of the newborn infant, where it appears to be correlated with the intense estrogenic stimulation of the reproductive tract at the time of birth, and in rodents and monkeys receiving large doses of estrogen. It does not appear to be a premalignant change.

THE PORTIO EXTERNA CERVICIS

The portio externa of the cervix is covered by a stratified squamous epithelium identical with that lining the vagina. The reaction of these two identical epithelia to estrogenic stimulation differs fundamentally from that

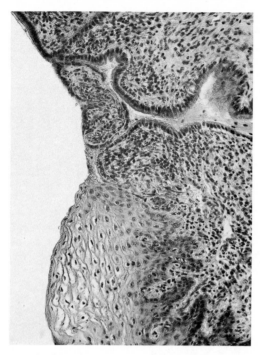

FIG. 4-14. Region of external os of cervix at 17th day of cycle. Transition from columnar epithelium of endocervix to stratified squamous epithelium of vaginal type of portio externa is abrupt. Cervical stroma near external os is infiltrated with leukocytes. (H&E, ×220)

of the endocervical epithelium. The stratified squamous epithelium reacts by thickening and by cornification of the superficial cells; the endocervical epithelium reacts by mucification.

The stratified squamous epithelium of the portio externa (Fig. 4-16) is made up of several layers conventionally described as basal, parabasal, intermediate, and superficial. The *basal layer* consists of a single row of cells and rests on a thin basement membrane. The cells are basophilic, the basophilia being enhanced in pregnancy. The *parabasal* and *intermediate layers* together constitute the prickle cell layer analogous to the same layer in the epidermis. The cells of the parabasal layer show cytoplasmic basophilia that is less in degree than that of the basal layer and decreases toward the intermediate layer. The intermediate layer is vacuolated, largely because of the presence of glycogen that is not stained or dissolved out in the preparation of the sections. The *superficial layer* varies in thickness, depending upon the degree of estrogenic stimulation. It consists of flattened cells that show an increasing degree of cytoplasmic acidophilia in the direction of the surface. The desquamation of surface cells goes on constantly, and the epithelium is replenished by mitotic division of cells in the basal layer and to a lesser extent in the parabasal layer.

The superficial and intermediate layers of the epithelium contain a large amount of glycogen (Fig. 4-17*A*). This glycogen serves an important function in main-

FIG. 4-15. Two patterns of cellular metaplasia in endocervix at 5th month of pregnancy. (*A*) Decidual transformation of endocervical stroma. (*B*) Squamous metaplasia of columnar epithelium of endocervical glands. (H&E, ×220)

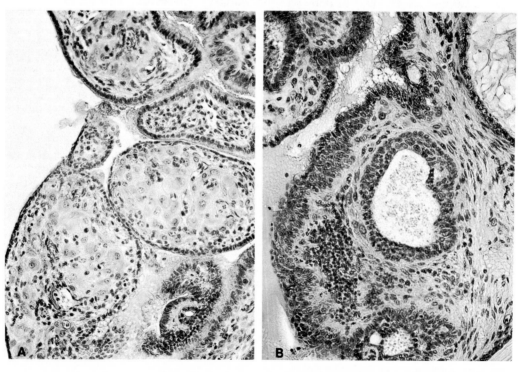

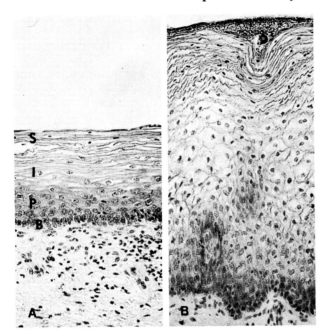

FIG. 4-16. Stratified squamous epithelium of portio externa cervicis following amenorrhea of several months' duration (*A*) and at fifth month of pregnancy (*B*). *B,* basal layer; *I,* intermediate layer; *P,* parabasal layer; *S,* superficial cornified layer. Thickening of all layers in pregnancy are striking. (H&E, ×220)

taining the acid *p*H of the vaginal contents. The glycogen is released by the cytolysis of the desquamated cells and is then acted upon by the glycolytic bacterial flora of the vagina, forming lactic acid. Both the thickness of the epithelium (see Fig. 4-16) and the glycogen content of the epithelium are increased following estrogenic stimulation, thus accounting for the therapeutic effect of estrogens in atrophic vaginitis. The staining of glycogen in the normal epithelium of the portio externa is the basis of the Schiller test. Following the removal of glycogen by salivary digestion (Fig. 4-16*B*), the intercellular regions stain intensely with the PAS method; the same areas are also sudanophilic. Histochemical studies indicate that the staining material may consist of mucopolysaccharide associated with some kind of lipid. Glycogen is easily identified in the superficial layers.

The superficial cells are desquamated into the vaginal lumen but retain their nuclei, unlike the desquamating cells of a heavily cornified epithelium such as thick skin. There is no stratum granulosum containing electron-dense granules of keratohyalin, as in the epidermis. However, the epithelium of the portio externa and that of the vagina must probably be considered nonkeratinizing epithelia comparable to that of thin skin. The process of cornification is enhanced following estrogenic stimulation, and there seems to be no reason to doubt that cornification of the vaginal epithelium and keratinization of the epidermis are similar processes differing only in degree. Under abnormal circumstances, for example, prolapse of the uterus in which the vaginal mucosa and vaginal portion of the cervix are exposed to irritation, there is more complete keratinization of the exposed surfaces.

THE VAGINA

The vagina is lined by a stratified squamous, nonkeratinizing epithelium identical in origin, histology, and fine structure with that covering the portio externa of the cervix. It rests on a basement membrane and on a lamina propria of mixed collagenous and elastic connective tissue rich in blood vessels and lymphatic vessels. The lamina propria intrudes into the basal layer of the epithelium in the form of papillae similar to the dermal papillae of the skin. Lymphocytes, singly or in aggregates, are common in the lamina propria and may occasionally be observed migrating through the epithelium. Polymorphonuclear leukocytes are also common in the epithelium and vaginal lumen at certain stages of the cycle. There are no glands in the vaginal mucosa, which is kept moist by the transudation of moisture through the epithelium and by the drainage of mucus from the cervix. As in the portio externa, the epithelium shows changes in thickness in different physiologic states and pathologic conditions. It undergoes thickening under the influence of estrogen and in pregnancy (see Fig. 4-16). It is thicker in women who regularly have intercourse than in those who do not. Keratinization of the superficial layers may occur in abnormal circumstances such as excessive exposure to irritation caused by prolapse of the uterus, or in other poorly understood dyskeratotic conditions.

The muscular wall of the vagina consists of bundles of smooth muscle disposed in interlacing circular and

FIG. 4-17. Two sections of portio externa cervicis at 17th day of cycle, stained with PAS method before treatment of section with saliva (*A*) and after such treatment (*B*). Note large amount of glycogen revealed in superficial layers of epithelium (*A*). Following removal of glycogen (*B*), intercellular areas stain intensely with PAS stain. Basement membrane also stains strongly. (×200)

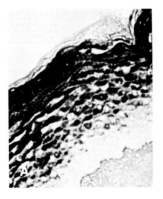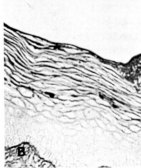

longitudinal layers. These interlace inferiorly with fibers of striated muscle of the levator ani, which forms the principal sphincter of the vagina. External to the muscular layer of the vagina is an adventitial coat of loose connective tissue rich in blood vessels, nerves, and lymphatic vessels. The dead space of the pelvis around the uterus and vagina and other pelvic viscera consists of a richly cellular areolar connective tissue (*parametrium*) that is highly susceptible to infection.

The *hymen* consists of a perforated fold of mucous membrane between the lower end of the vagina and the vestibule. It is covered by stratified squamous epithelium on both its vaginal and vestibular surfaces and encloses a thin lamina of connective tissue in which may be found vestiges of the duct of the mesonephros (*Gartner's duct*).

Vaginal Smear

The changes that occur in the epithelium of the portio externa of the cervix and the vagina under the influence of estrogenic and progestational hormones of the menstrual cycle are reflected in the cells found in the vaginal lumen. Cells derived by exfoliation from the vagina, cervix, endometrium, or even the uterine tube are obtained from the vaginal fornix by aspiration, or from the external os, endocervix, or endometrial lumen by gently scraping or curetting. They are spread on a glass slide, fixed for about 15 minutes in alcohol–ether, and then stained with Harris's hematoxylin (for nuclei and cytoplasmic basophilia) and counter-stained with a mixture containing either light green or orange G with phosphotungstic acid (for cytoplasmic structures and inclusions).

The interpretation of the cytologic picture requires expert training and judgment, but such a smear can tender valuable information about the hormonal status of the patient, with particular respect to estrogen, and, especially when done sequentially, about the presence of premalignant or malignant changes. Smears are classified in various ways, for example, that of Papanicolaou: grade I, no atypical or abnormal cells; grade II, atypical cells but no evidence of malignancy; grade III, suggestive but not conclusive of malignancy; grade IV, strongly suggestive of malignancy; grade V, conclusive of malignancy. Criteria of malignancy or premalignancy are as follows:

1. Nuclear changes: variation in size (pleomorphism), hyperchromasia, aberrant patterns of chromatin, enlargement of or increase in number of nucleoli, multinucleation, mitosis, thickening of the nuclear membrane, degenerative changes including vacuolation
2. Cytoplasmic changes: pronounced basophilia or acidophilia and vacuolation
3. Changes of the whole cell: enlargement and variation in size, aberrant and bizarre forms, degenerative or necrotic changes, dyskeratotic changes affecting the process of keratinization
4. Interrelations of cells: irregular patterns of clumping, variations in size within cell clusters (anisokaryosis and anisocytosis), dense grouping and crowding of cells, engulfment of cells one by another, pronounced stratification

Leukocytic inclusions within cells may be normal, and histiocytes or macrophages with engulfed leukocytes are also not uncommon in normal smears. Intense acidophilia with orange G may be a normal concomitant of keratinization, as in the patient taking high doses of estrogen.

Analysis of the types of cells in vaginal smears or smears of exfoliated cells from the endocervix or uterine body requires an understanding of the normal histology of these areas and their response to sex hormones. These essential details have been illustrated earlier (*e.g.,* Fig. 4-16). Cells of strictly vaginal origin, as well as those from the ectocervix, consist of parabasal, intermediate or navicular, and superficial more or less cornified cells (see Fig. 4-16). Parabasal cells are rarely shed, being the germinative layer. When they are shed, the parabasal cells are rounded, having lost their intercellular spiny processes when shed. They contain glycogen in proportion to the level of estrogenic stimulation (Fig. 4-18) and have relatively large nuclei. Intermediate cells, including the more superficial cells that contain keratohyaline granules, are best developed in high estrogenic states. They are moderately flattened, are smaller than parabasal cells, and may contain keratohyalin. Their general acidophilia or orangeophilia (with orange G) is a measure of their keratinization; complete keratinization is rare in normal females. The cells from the more superficial zone are flattened with pyknotic nuclei. In high estrogenic states, the keratinized cells appear as squames or scales, intensely acidophilic and lacking nuclei.

Cells derived from the endocervix reflect the normal mucosal pattern of this area, namely, a columnar surface epithelium (simple, mucified, or ciliated) and tubular glands lined by columnar epithelium (Fig. 4-19). Mucification can be identified by appropriate stains. Ciliated cells are rare but increase in low estrogenic states. Mucified cells are more common in the late luteal phase of the cycle and in pregnancy.

Cells of endometrial origin again reflect the histology of this area (Fig. 4-20). Mucification is rarely seen. Ciliation is very rare but again is more common in postmenopausal women and in low estrogenic states. The cells are smaller than those of endocervical origin and tend to occur in more compact groups. Rarely, glands or portions of them may be seen. Changes coincident with the menstrual cycle are not of reliable significance in women; in contrast, the vaginal smear in rodents reflects accurately the preovulatory, postovulatory, and resting phases of the estrous cycle. The corpus luteum is short-lived in rodents so that the luteal phase is ab-

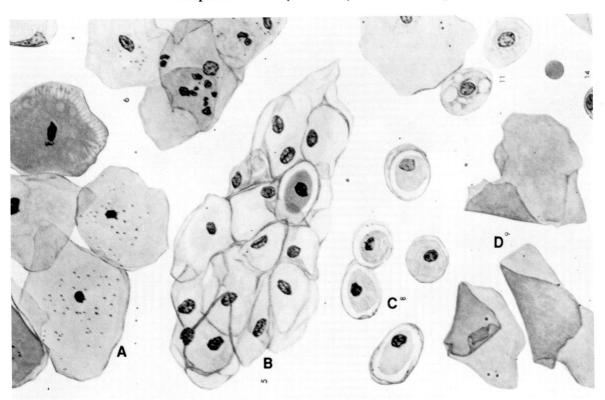

FIG. 4-18. Normal cells in vaginal and cervical aspiration or swab smears. (*A*) Superficial squamous cells (late follicular or preovulatory stage of menstrual cycle), stained for glycogen. (*B*) Cells of intermediate or navicular type (parabasal), stained for glycogen. (*C*) Parabasal cells from ectocervix from patient taking estrogen, stained for glycogen. (*D*) Superficial squamous cells showing complete keratinization from 48-year-old woman. (Approximately ×500) (Papanicolaou G: Atlas of Exfoliative Cytology. Cambridge, MA, Harvard University Press, 1954)

breviated, whereas in women the prolonged luteal phase and the extended action of progesterone causes its own effects on vaginal smear morphology. In particular, the character of the mucus that appears in the smear and emerges from the external os reflects the action of progesterone. It is watery and of low viscosity in the period of high estrogenic activity, that is, during the follicular phase, and tenacious and sticky during the late luteal stage. During pregnancy there is abundant tenacious mucus and many navicular cells of parabasal type with rather thick cellular walls. Showers of polymorphonuclear cells may appear transiently in the normal smear by the time of ovulation and again in the later luteal phase.

THE EXTERNAL GENITALIA

The *labia minora* are covered by a thin epidermal layer of stratified squamous epithelium continuous with that of the vestibule. The papillae of the submucosal layer are richly developed, and the epithelium may also contain a large amount of pigment. There are scattered glands of the sebaceous type but no hair follicles. The glands secrete a material called *sebum.*

The *labia majora* are covered by thick skin that contains coarse hair follicles and well-developed sweat and sebaceous glands. These glands and the hair follicles are influenced by the sex hormones of the ovary at the time of puberty.

Associated with the vestibule are glandular structures; their principal function is lubrication. The most important of these are the greater vestibular (Bartholin's) gland and the paraurethral (Skene's) glands. The glands are of the compound tubuloalveolar type, and the alveoli are lined by mucus-secreting columnar cells. The duct of the greater vestibular gland is lined by stratified squamous epithelium continuous with that of the vestibule.

Surrounding the vestibule are certain modifications of the connective tissue that comprise the erectile tissue of the area: the bulbs of the vestibule, the clitoris, and the pars intermedia. The bulbs of the vestibule are homologous with the corpus spongiosum penis. The crura and glans clitoridis are homologous with the corpora cavernosa and glans penis. The erectile tissue of these

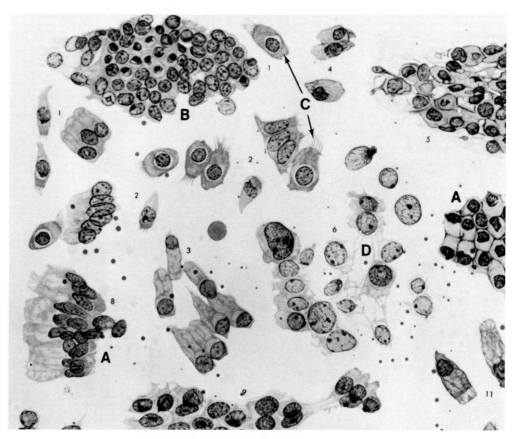

FIG. 4-19. Normal cells in cervical and endocervical smears. (*A*) Endocervical mucous columnar cells shown from side and from their basal surfaces. (*B*) Cluster of columnar cells from endocervical aspiration (mucous and ciliated). (*C*) Ciliated cells. (*D*) Endocervical columnar cells showing variation in nuclear size (anisokaryosis) and cytolysis. (Approximately ×500) (Papanicolaou G: Atlas Exfoliative Cytology. Cambridge, MA, Harvard University Press, 1954)

organs consists of a spongelike system of vascular spaces lined by endothelium and separated by delicate fibroelastic septa containing blood vessels. The arteries and veins supplying the erectile spaces are so arranged that blood is allowed to enter the spaces while the venous drainage is temporarily obstructed. The erectile tissue is richly supplied with sympathetic and parasympathetic nerves (nervi erigentes).

PITUITARY–HYPOTHALAMIC SYSTEM

The pituitary gland and its vascular and nervous connections with the hypothalamus are remarkably constant in structure and function throughout the vertebrate phylum, reflecting their fundamental role in the regulation of sexual, metabolic, and osmotic function. The pituitary develops in two parts, both of ectodermal origin: the pars distalis and the pars nervosa. The pars distalis arises as an upgrowth (Rathke's pouch) from the roof of the stomatodeum, or embryonic mouth, which becomes apposed to a downgrowth from the floor of the diencephalon (infundibular process). The pars distalis includes the pars anterior (anterior lobe) and the pars intermedia (intermediate lobe); in some forms, but not in humans, there is a remnant of the stomatodeal cleft between the two. The pars anterior extends up toward the base of the brain as the pars tuberalis, where it forms a small mass of pituitary tissue that partially encircles the infundibular stalk and median eminence. The pars posterior is essentially a downgrowth of the brain and is connected to the hypothalamus by a leash of nerves, constituting the hypothalamohypophyseal tract.

Pars Distalis

The pars distalis stands in intimate relation with the hypothalamus by means of a vascular portal system. The anterior lobe is supplied by superior hypophyseal arteries from the internal carotid, which forms a primary vascular plexus within the hypothalamus. From this

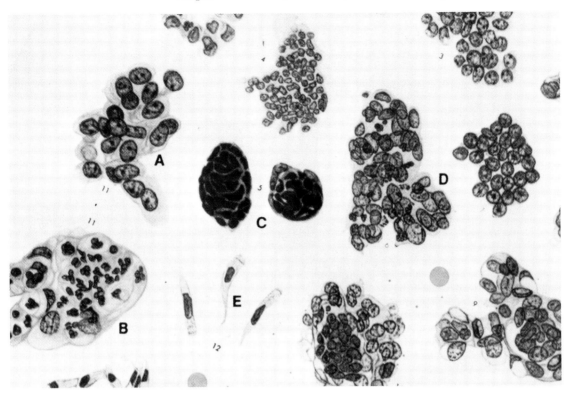

FIG. 4-20. Normal cells in vaginal smear of endometrial origin. (*A*) Clusters of endometrial cells, early menstrual cycle. (*B*) Cluster of endometrial cells with leukocytic infiltration. (*C*) Cluster of endometrial cells showing clumping, shrinkage, and nuclear pyknosis. (*D*) Cluster of endometrial cells, late menstrual cycle. (*E*) Ciliated and mucous cells, from 55-year-old woman with hyperplasia of endometrium. (Approximately ×500) (Papanicolaou G: Atlas of Exfoliative Cytology. Cambridge, MA, Harvard University Press, 1954)

plexus a leash of vessels descends into the anterior lobe, forming the hypophyseoportal system. It breaks up within the anterior lobe, where it forms a secondary vascular plexus. This arrangement of vessels, which permits blood to reach an anterior lobe only after it has passed through the hypothalamic plexuses, is remarkably constant throughout the vertebrate phylum. The direction of blood flow has been shown by direct observation. It is now known that regulatory substances (*releasing factors*) are manufactured within the hypothalamic neurons and are transported via the portal vessels to the pars distalis, where they cause the release of hormones. Such releasing factors have been demonstrated for thyroid-stimulating hormone (TSH), adrenocortex-stimulating hormone (ACTH), lactogenic hormone (prolactin), growth hormone (somatotropin, STH), and the gonadotropins (LH and FSH). In some instances the releasing hormones have been isolated and synthesized. They act in exceedingly minute amounts and will have increasing clinical significance.

The general types of cells within the pars distalis are illustrated in Figure 4-21. Classically, they are described within the anterior lobe as of three types: acid-

ophils (40%), basophils (10%), and chromophobes (50%). The acidophils, which are most numerous posteriorly within the anterior lobe, have granules that stain intensely with acid dyes, that is, they are themselves basic. They are thought to be the site of growth hormone and prolactin production. Acidophilic adenomas are associated with giantism (acromegaly). The basophils, at least in the rat, are of two types. One group stains with both the PAS and the aldehyde fuchsin methods. These cells are thyrotropes, that is, they secrete TSH. A second type stains with the PAS but not the aldehyde fuchsin method. These are the site of gonadotropic secretion (FSH and LH). In humans, the secretion of ACTH appears to be associated with the basophils, and following ACTH or adrenocorticoid administration, these cells undergo a degenerative change (Crooke's hyaline change). The acidophils increase in pregnancy and lactation, probably associated with prolactin production.

The pars intermedia is poorly developed in humans. It appears to be a source of melanocyte-stimulating hormone (MSH), which causes dispersal of melanin in amphibians. Its role in the human is unclear; injection, however, produces hyperpigmentation.

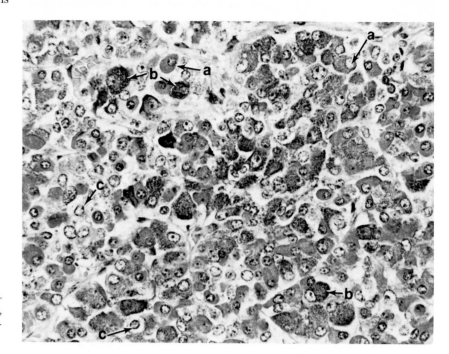

FIG. 4-21. Human pituitary (pars distalis), showing principal cell types. *a,* acidophils; *b,* basophils; *c,* chromophobes. (Halmi, ×300)

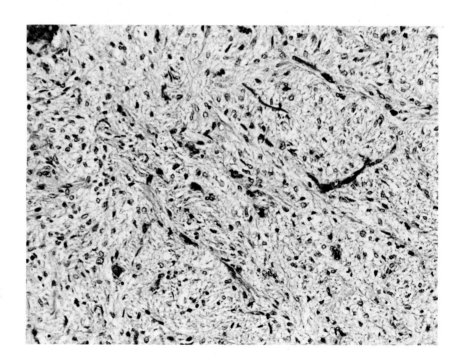

FIG. 4-22. Human pituitary (pars nervosa), showing dense feltwork of glial cells (pituicytes) and nerve fibers with abundant blood vessels. (Halmi, ×300)

Pars Nervosa

The pars nervosa or posterior lobe (Fig. 4-22) is made up of clusters or nests of pituicytes, which appear not to have a secretory role in themselves. It now appears certain that the hypothalamohypophyseal tract of nerves is the path by which secretory material of hypothalamic origin reaches the posterior lobe. The "neurosecretory material" that may be observed in the axons of this tract may be shown experimentally to dam up proximal to a point of constriction. It is manufactured within the specialized neurons of the supraoptic and paraventricular nuclei. It is then transferred by axoplasmic flow to the posterior lobe, where the hormones (antidiuretic hormone [ADH] and oxytocin) are released. These materials, which are polypeptides, then enter the perivascular spaces, where they apparently lose their staining properties and are carried into the bloodstream. Vasopressin is identical with ADH and the latter name is preferable. Both the hypothalamic neurons and the posterior lobe cells are influenced to release ADH by changes in the osmolality of the blood. Destruction of the hypothalamohypophyseal tract or lesions in the paraventricular and supraoptic nuclei result in an uncontrolled excretion of large volumes of very dilute urine, a condition known as *diabetes insipidus.* Oxytocin has a contracting effect on the uterus and also causes ejection of milk from the milk ducts.

REFERENCES AND RECOMMENDED READING

Arias–Stella J: Atypical endometrial changes associated with presence of chorionic tissue. Arch Pathol 58:112, 1954

Bamforth J: Cytological Diagnosis in Medical Practice. Boston, Little, Brown & Co, 1966

Daron SH: The arterial pattern of the tunica mucosa of the uterus in Macacus rhesus. Am J Anat 58:349, 1936

Fluhman F: The Cervix Uteri and Its Diseases. Philadelphia, WB Saunders, 1961

Greep RO, Weiss L (eds): Histology, 3rd ed. New York, McGraw-Hill, 1973

Hafez ESE, Blandau RJ (eds): The Mammalian Oviduct. Chicago, University of Chicago Press, 1969

Hafez ESE (ed): Human Reproduction, 2nd ed. Hagerstown, Harper & Row, 1980

Ham AW: Histology. Philadelphia, JB Lippincott, 1974

Harris GW, Donovan BT (eds): The Pituitary Gland. Berkeley, University of California Press, 1966

Markee SH: Menstruation in intraocular endometrial transplants in the rhesus monkey. Contrib Embryol 28:219, 1940

Naeb ZM: Exfoliative Cytology. Boston, Little, Brown & Co, 1970

Noyes RW, Hertig AH, Rock J: Dating the endometrial biopsy. Fertil Steril 1:3, 1950

Odell WD, Moyer DL: Physiology of Reproduction. St Louis, CV Mosby 1971

Oertel YC: The Arias–Stella reaction revisited. Arch Pathol Lab Med 102:651, 1978

Papanicolaou GN: Atlas of Exfoliative Cytology. Cambridge, MA, Harvard University Press, 1954

Reid DS, Ryan KJ, Bernirschke K: Principles and Management of Human Reproduction. Philadelphia, WB Saunders, 1972

Reynolds SRM: Physiology of the Uterus, 3rd ed. New York, Hoeber, 1949

Shearman RP (ed): Human Reproductive Physiology. Oxford, Blackwell Scientific Publications, 1972

Williams RH (ed): Textbook of Endocrinology. Philadelphia, WB Saunders, 1974

Woodruff JD, Pauerstein CJ: The Fallopian Tube: Structure, Function, Pathology and Management. Baltimore, Williams & Wilkins, 1969

Wynn RM: Cellular Biology of the Uterus. New York, Appleton-Century-Crofts, 1967

Zuckerman S (ed): The Ovary. New York, Academic Press, 1962

Scanning Electron Microscopy of Human Reproduction

E. S. E. Hafez
Hans Ludwig

Scanning electron microscopy (SEM) has been used extensively to study the physiomorphology and pathophysiology of human reproduction. Unlike transmission electron microscopy, scanning electron microscopy can be used to investigate the organization of tissues and to observe large, intact surface areas with high resolution and depth of field.

Techniques have to be developed to measure results obtained by scanning electron microscopy, which is most widely used with the secondary electron imaging technique. As several biologic cellular structures have similar surface ultrastructures, complementary techniques can be more discriminative and measure more easily and more accurately than scanning electron microscopy alone. Back-scattered electron imaging can be used to locate subsurface structures with the help of element contrast. In combination with scanning electron microscopy, immune and other surface-labeling techniques can be successfully applied to several problems of basic cell research. The high resolution of scanning electron microscopy permits the application of very small markers like gold or ferritin, eventually in combination with x-ray microanalysis. Several other techniques can be used in conjunction with scanning electron microscopy, including energy loss spectrometry, laser microprobe mass analysis, secondary ion mass spectrometry, proton microprobe, and x-ray microanalysis. These promising techniques have introduced new functional elements into scanning electron microscopy investigations, the significance of which still awaits elucidation.

FEMALE REPRODUCTIVE TRACT

There are remarkable morphologic differences in the tissue organization of the mucosa of different segments of the female reproductive tract. Under the low magnification (×200) of the scanning electron microscope, the cells of the oviduct and uterus appear uniform in shape and are closely packed, showing a "cobblestone" pattern. In some instances the borders of the cells are ill defined and covered with short microvilli and residual mucus. Under high magnification (×2000–20,000), two basic epithelial cell types are observed: ciliated cells and nonciliated secretory cells (Fig. 4-23).* Ciliated cells are covered by kinocilia, which overlap the surface

---

* All specimens shown in this section have been fixed in 2.5% glutaraldehyde solution, processed by critical point drying, and gold coated by the sputtering technique.

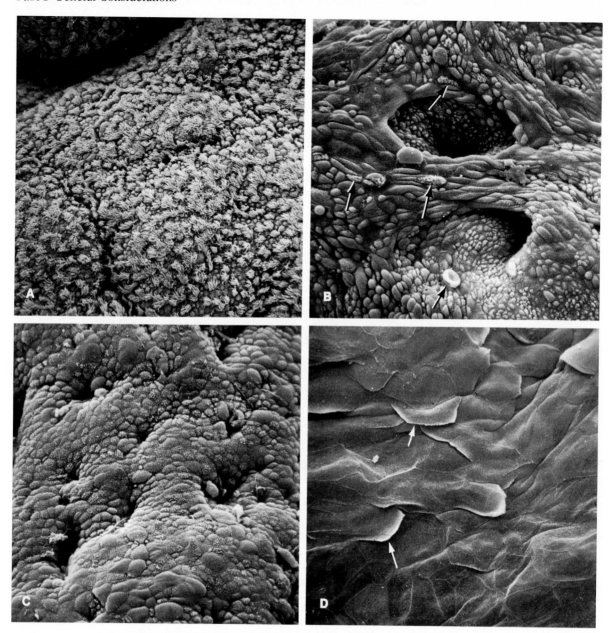

FIG. 4-23. Scanning electron micrographs showing surface ultrastructure of human female reproductive tract during 1st week of menstrual cycle. Note differences in tissue organization and cell characteristics and differentiation of different organs at same magnification. (*A*) Oviduct, ampullar portion. Note ciliated cells surrounding small clusters of secretory cells. (×500) (*B*) Endometrium. Note openings of endometrial glands (50–60 m), extended ciliated cells with short cilia (*arrows*), and bulging tops of secretory cells. The erythrocyte (*arrow*) gives an idea of size relations. (×500) (*C*) Cervix. Note regular size of cylindric epithelium and small glandular openings. Ciliated cells resemble those in endometrium. (×500) (*D*) Ectocervix. Flat and homogeneous layer of vaginal epithelium, with some cells in process of exfoliation (*arrows*).

of secretory cells that have a dome-shaped surface covered with microvilli. Ciliated cells are found singly or in groups, arranged in rows or a mosaic pattern.

The percentage of ciliated calls in the tubal epithelium varies in different parts of the tube. The maximum number of ciliated cells is found in the fimbriae, where they are so closely packed it is impossible to distinguish their boundaries. The proportion of ciliated cells decreases gradually from the ampulla to the isthmus, reaching 50% near the ampullary–isthmic junction.

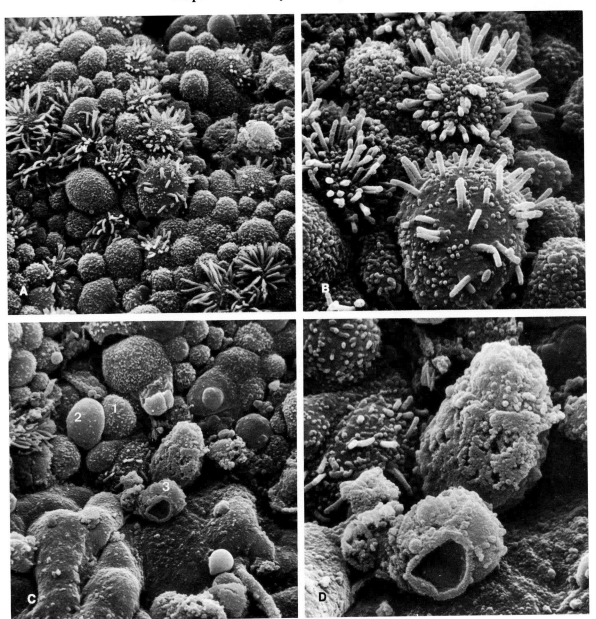

FIG. 4-24. Scanning electron micrographs of human endometrium during midcycle showing superficial characteristics of individual endometrial cells. (*A*) Ciliated and secretory endometrial cells. Note ciliated cells with short cilia of irregular number, unlike those in oviduct. Note microvilli covering secretory cells. (×2000) (*B*) Detail of *A*. Apical portion of some ciliated cells may be succulent, so that microvillous pattern of surface disappears. (×5000) (*C*) Secretory endometrial cells in different stages of activity: (1) cell with normal superficial cell membrane, proliferating; (2) cell with intact superficial cell membrane but of extreme tension before release of secretory material; (3) cell with ruptured superficial cell membrane and clumped secretory material near ruptured surface. (×2000) (*D*) Two secretory cells, one with ruptured cell membrane, after release of secretory material. Note difference between normal microvilli (*left* ciliated cell) and secretory material attached to apical cell membrane (*middle*). (×5000)

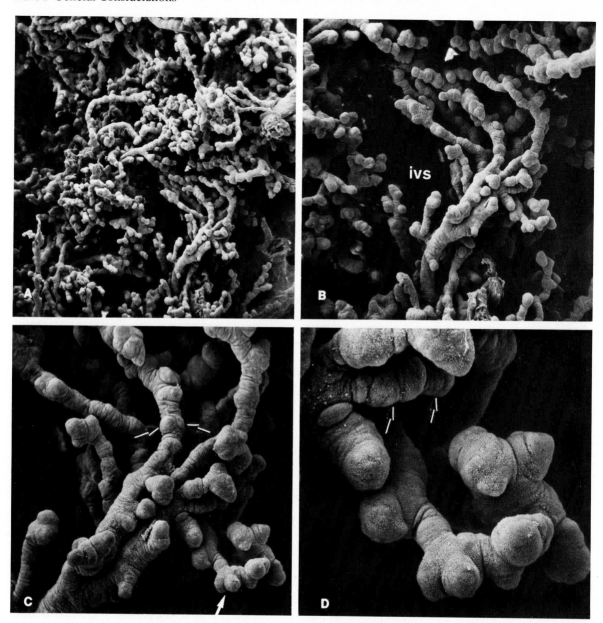

FIG. 4-25.   Scanning electron micrographs of normal human term placenta taken after normal pregnancy and spontaneous delivery. Figures 4-25 and 4-26 show 8 degrees of magnification (×50–20,000). (*A*) Placental villi with equal shapes and diameters, but with various depths and widths of intervillous space. (×50) (*B*) Ramification of single villous branches. Note terminal subdivisions of villi and various widths of intervillous space (*ivs*). (×100) (*C*) Placental villi are continuously covered with velvety layer of syncytiotrophoblast. Note terminal ramification of terminal villi (*large arrow*) and placental knots (*small arrows*). (×200) (*D*) Note homogeneity of surface of normal syncytiotrophoblast, which consists of numerous microvillous protrusions. Nuclear areas along flanks create bulging areas (*arrows*) of villous branches. (×500)

The kinocilia in the female reproductive tract beat rhythmically toward the vagina, creating a directional flow of luminal fluids for the transport of particles and gametes. Two types of ciliary motility are recognized: an effective stroke and a recovery stroke. In the effective stroke, the cilia bend near the basal body, and the degree of bending proceeds as a slow wave toward the tip. In the oviduct, cilia beat some 1200 times per minute. Ciliary activity is responsible for the movement of ova into the ostium of the fimbriated tip and through the upper

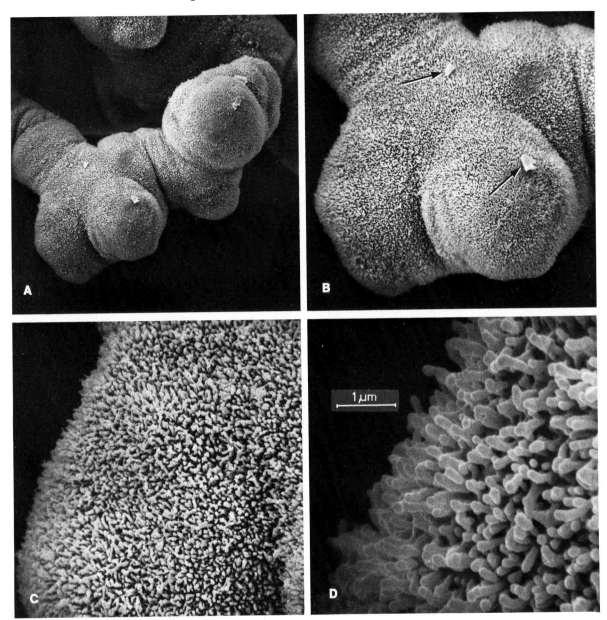

FIG. 4-26. Scanning electron micrographs of surface of placental syncytiotrophoblast from normal human term placenta (continued from Fig. 4-25). (*A*) Top of terminal placental villi floating in intervillous space, showing homogeneous layer of syncytiotrophoblast. (×1000) (*B*) Syncytiotrophoblast surface consists of a microvillous turf. Note deposits of nonstructured material (*arrows*). (×2000) (*C*) Microvilli of syncytiotrophoblast are slender and homogeneous in length and thickness. (×5000) (*D*) Single microvilli measure average of 0.65 μm in length and 0.15 μm in thickness. (×20,000)

ampulla. Concomitant with this is a sharp increase in the intensity of muscular contractions at the time of ovulation and during preliminary migration of the ovum through the tube.

The cilia may facilitate the release of secretory material from the adjacent secretory cells and the distri-
bution of secretions within the lumen. Infection of the oviduct is associated with the loss of ciliated cells in the oviduct and the accumulation of oviductal fluid and inflammatory exudate, which may contribute to the development of salpingitis. Oviducts taken from patients with endogenous or exogenous estrogenic stimulation

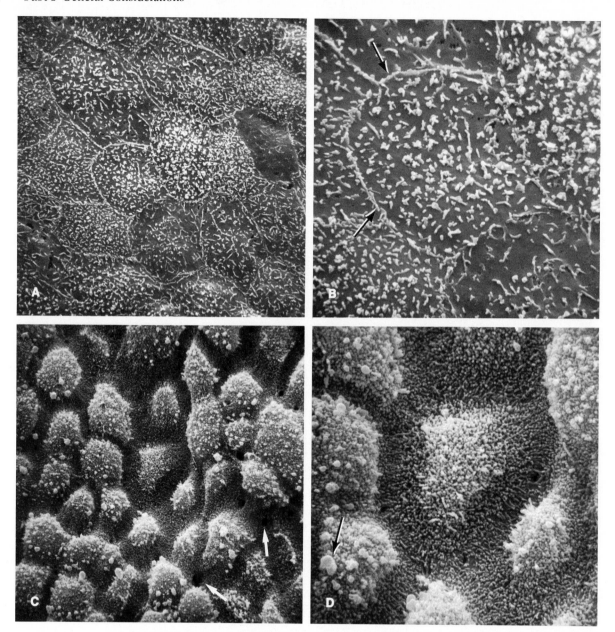

FIG. 4-27. Scanning electron micrographs of human amniotic epithelium, showing development of surface differentiation from first trimester to term pregnancy. (*A*) First trimester. Note polygonal, flat epithelial cells and variations in density of microvillous relief. (×2000) (*B*) Detail of *A*. Cell borders shown by *arrows*. Note structure of microvilli. (×5000) (*C*) Term pregnancy. Succulent amniotic epithelial cells with dense microvillous pattern. Cell borders lie in smooth intercellular spaces. Note secretory material (granules) above microvillous relief and openings of intercellular channels (*arrows*). (×2000) (*D*) Detail of *C*. Whole cell area, including intercellular space, is covered by microvilli. These are standing densely together in area of cellular nucleus. Secretory granules are shown by *arrow*. (×5000)

possess comparatively more ciliated cells in the ampulla and fimbriae than in the isthmus.

The tubal fluid plays a major role in the transport and maturation of the gametes. The peak of tubal secretory activity coincides with the time of ovulation, in-dicating that oviductal secretion is mediated by the ovarian hormones of the ovulatory and early postovulatory phases. After menopause the oviducts become atrophic and the ciliated cells decrease in number.

The surface epithelium of the endometrium un-

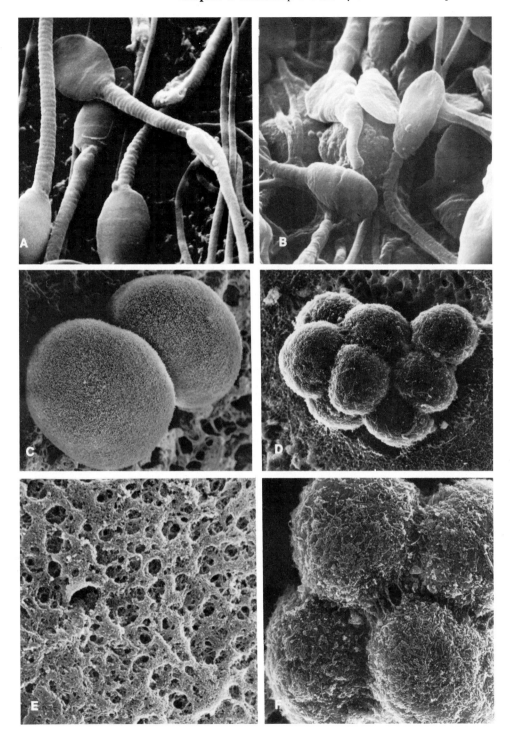

FIG. 4-28. Scanning electron micrographs of mammalian gametes. Species differences in surface ultrastructure are more remarkable in spermatozoa than eggs. (*A*) Epididymal spermatozoa from macaque. Note cytoplasmic croplet along midpiece. (×6400) (*B*) Human spermatozoa. (×11,000) (*C*). Two-cell egg from rat after removal of zona pellucida. Note abundance of microvilli. (×1000) (*D*) Morula of baboon after removal of zona pellucida. (×800) (*E*) Zona pellucida of rat egg. Note irregular surface. (×8000) (*F*) Morula of baboon (same as *D*) after removal of zona pellucida. Note connections between blastomeres. (×2000) (Micrographs courtesy of JE Flechon, ESE Hafez, and D Kraemer)

dergoes cyclic alterations in cell shape, apical microvilli, ciliation, and secretory activity (Fig. 4-24). These changes are hormone dependent; lack of estrogens leads to a loss of cilia and cessation of secretory activity, both of which can be restored by exogenous administration of estrogens. Similar cyclic changes occur in the epithelium of the endocervical mucosa and the cervical crypts.

The normal squamous epithelium of the lower vagina is relatively smooth, with very little undulation of the surface. The cells appear flat and polygonal, with thin-edged interdigitating borders.

The multilayered cells overlap each other irregularly, similar to layers of shingles on a roof. The cell edges roll back and lift their borders during the process of exfoliation. Most vaginal cells exhibit delicate interlacing microridges with a pattern resembling that of fingerprints. When the exfoliated cells dry, they appear wrinkled and the surface microridges become obscured.

PLACENTA

The primary villi of the human placenta arise from the syncytium of the intervillous space. As soon as mesenchyme develops and invades the primary villi, the features of secondary villi become apparent. The identifying sign of tertiary villi is the presence of fetal vessels in the villous stroma. Quarternary villi are subdivisions of tertiary villi at later stages of pregnancy, when the cytotrophoblastic layer has disappeared. Tertiary and quarternary villi are sometimes referred to as *resorptive villi.*

As pregnancy advances, there is a decrease in the length and thickness of these microvilli (except for some luxuriant forms that are of extreme length), but their density rises sharply. Clumping of microvilli occurs within marginal zones where basal and chorionic plates are close together. In the term placenta, clumping of microvilli associated with protrusions of trophoblastic sprouts indicates maturity (Figs. 4-25 and 4-26).

During the seventh week of gestation, the main villus branches into secondary and tertiary villi that show remarkable variability in size and length. During the 14th week of gestation, the surface of the secondary and tertiary terminal villi are covered with a dense microvillous turf. The microvilli, regular in shape, are more evenly distributed than those that were present 4 weeks before. At this stage the microvillous pattern is highly differentiated, and there are protrusions on a syncytiotrophoblast. During the 28th week of gestation, the villous tree is covered by an uninterrupted layer of syncytiotrophoblast differentiated into microvilli.

The cells of the amniotic membrane undergo ultrastructural changes throughout gestation (Fig. 4-27). The changes are adaptive physiologic mechanisms to accommodate the growing fetus and the accumulation of amniotic fluid.

SPERMATOZOA

Epididymal spermatozoa undergo cytologic changes that involve dehydration and migration of the cytoplasmic droplet toward the end of the middle piece, narrowing of the neck, and reduction of marginal thickening of the acrosomal region (Fig. 4-28).

Unlike those of other mammalian species, human spermatozoa show remarkable heterogeneity in the size and shape of sperm heads and mitochondria. There are also significant regional differences in the membrane structure of spermatozoa. Normal ejaculated spermatozoa are ovoid with slight dorsoventral flattening. The anterior and equatorial segments are not clearly demarcated, and a shallow circumferential groove of variable depth is observed between the acrosome and postacrosomal region. The acrosome contains proteolytic enzymes, which probably facilitate sperm penetration in cervical mucus and in luminal fluids in the uterus and the zona pellucida. Closely apposed mitochondria that have flattened surfaces and are of variable sizes are arranged in a regular or irregular pattern.

Abnormal spermatozoa are observed in all ejaculates of fertile and infertile men. Abnormalities of the head include large, deformed spheroid formations or duplicated rudimentary heads. Amorphous spermatozoa have structural defects in the shape or size of the head. Oval, large, small, tapering, and bicephalic forms are also common. Abnormalities of the midpiece include parts of thin and constricted midpieces, enlargement, breakage, and duplication. Morphologic anomalies may result from trauma, illness, or the use of antispermatogenic agents.

CLINICAL CONSIDERATIONS

Scanning electron microscopy, used in combination with other modern techniques (such as immunoelectron microscopy and x-ray dispersive analysis), is a valuable technique for the clinical study of human reproduction, diagnosis of female and male infertility, detection of certain types of gynecologic carcinoma and several andrologic and gynecologic disorders, chromosome analysis, and development of new contraceptives. Surface characteristics of amniotic fluid cells (renal epithelium, sebaceous fat cells, pneumonocytes) may be of clinical value comparable to that of biochemical parameters in monitoring fetal maturity.

REFERENCES AND RECOMMENDED READING

Ferenczy A, Richart RM: Scanning Electron Microscopy: Female Reproductive System, Dynamics of Scanning and Transmission Electron Microscopy, p 213. New York, John Wiley & Sons, 1974

Hafez ESE (ed): Human Reproduction: Conception and Contraception, 2nd ed. New York, Harper & Row, 1980

Hafez ESE (ed): Reproduction in Farm Animals, 4th ed. Philadelphia, Lea & Febiger, 1980

Hafez ESE (ed): Scanning Electron Microscopy of Human Reproduction. Ann Arbor, Ann Arbor Science, 1978

Hafez ESE (ed): Scanning Electron Microscopical Atlas of Mammalian Reproduction. New York, Springer-Verlag, 1975

Hafez ESE, Barnhart MI, Ludwig H et al: Scanning electron microscopy of human reproductive physiology. Acta Obstet Gynecol Scand, Suppl 40, p 21, 1975

Hafez ESE, Evans TN (eds): Human Vagina. Amsterdam, Elsevier, 1978

Hafez ESE, Kanagawa H: Scanning electron microscopy of human, monkey, and rabbit spermatozoa. Fertil Steril 24: 1776, 1973

Hafez ESE, Kenemans P (eds): Atlas of Human Reproduction by Scanning Electron Microscopy. Lancaster, England, MTP Press, 1982

Hafez ESE, Ludwig H: Scanning electron microscopy of the endometrium. In Wynn RW (ed): Biology of the Uterus. New York, Plenum, 1977

Hafez ESE, Ludwig H, Metzger H: Human endometrial fluid kinetics as observed by scanning electron microscopy. Am J Obstet Gynecol 122:929–938, 1975

Hafez ESE, Thibault C (eds): Biology of Spermatozoa: Maturation, Transport and Fertilizing Ability. Basel, S Karger, 1975

Ludwig H, Metzger H: The Human Female Reproductive Tract. A Scanning Electron Microscopic Atlas. New York, Springer-Verlag, 1976

Embryology and Developmental Defects of the Female Reproductive Tract

Elizabeth M. Ramsey

5

Familiarity with the embryology of the female reproductive system is as necessary a part of the obstetrician and gynecologist's armamentarium as are surgical instruments. The notorious "difficulty" of the subject need be no deterrent to attainment of this useful familiarity, for confusion can be minimized if the following four underlying factors are recognized at the outset.

1. There is a close relation between the primitive urinary and reproductive systems. Various structures initially formed for excretory functions alone are subsequently used jointly by the two systems or are diverted to reproductive tract use exclusively.
2. Although the sex of the future individual is settled at the time of the union of the nuclei of egg and sperm, reproductive tract structures first appear in a sexually undifferentiated form. During subsequent development most of the tract is modified to conform to the genetic sex of the individual, yet remnants of structures appropriate to the opposite sex persist.
3. Development, particularly of the excretory system, occurs in consecutive but often overlapping waves, each commencing high in the abdominal cavity and progressing toward the pelvis. It thus comes about that structures of quite different stages of developmental maturity may exist simultaneously.
4. The external genitalia owe their origin in part to modification of the primitive cloaca, or joint urinary–intestinal–reproductive receptacle, which is derived at a very early stage from the hindgut.

The chronologic relations between developmental events in the four systems involved in genital tract formation are shown, in capsule form, in Figure 5-1. The interrelations and interchanges among elements of the systems are indicated by arrows. The text takes up the systems one by one and carries each from inception to birth. Reference to this chart will make it possible to envisage another dimension, that of relative time, including the sequence or simultaneity of events.

PRIMORDIAL GERM CELLS

In the embryos of lower vertebrates, birds, and mammals (including humans), certain distinctive cells appear at a very early somite stage as discrete clumps in the wall of the yolk sac (Fig. 5-2). These primordial germ cells subsequently migrate through the mesoderm surrounding the hindgut and take up a position within the paired genital ridges from which the gonads are formed (Figs. 5-3 and 5-4).

In gonads that become testes, the primordial germ cells are incorporated into the developing testicular stroma and come to lie in the sex cords. These cords, when subsequently canalized, form the seminiferous tubules, and the germ cells there undergo continuous proliferation and maturation into spermatogonia throughout reproductive life.

In gonads that become ovaries, the primitive germ cells are similarly incorporated in the developing stroma. According to one school of thought (the preformation theory), they and their descendants form the definitive ova of the ovarian follicles. Adherents to a second school of thought (the neoformation theory) accept that distinctive primitive cells migrate from the yolk sac to the ovary but deny that these have any kinship with the definitive ova. The latter they regard as products of cyclic proliferation of the coelomic epithelium that originally covers the genital ridges and that in adult life becomes the germinal epithelium on the surface of the ovary.

Extensive experimental testing of both theories (Blackler, Mossman and Duke, and Witschi) has failed

AGE	GLANDS	URINARY TRACT	♂ DUCTS ♀	EXTERNAL GENITALIA
3-4 weeks	PRIMORDIAL GERM CELLS	PRONEPHROS (nonfunctional) Tubules and Ducts	PRONEPHRIC	
4-9 weeks		MESONEPHROS or WOLFFIAN BODY (temporary function) Tubules and Ducts	MESONEPHRIC or WOLFFIAN	CLOACA
5th week	UROGENITAL RIDGE			
6th week	INDIFFERENT GONAD: GERMINAL AND CORE EPITHELIUM	METANEPHROS or KIDNEY (permanent) Tubules and Ducts	PARAMESONEPHRIC or MÜLLERIAN	CLOACA SUBDIVIDES — — — GENITAL TUBERCLE
7th week	MALE TYPE CORDS			ANAL AND URETHRAL MEMBRANES RUPTURE
8th week	TESTIS AND OVARY			URETHRAL AND
9th week			MÜLLERIAN DUCTS FUSE AT TUBERCLE	LABIOSCROTAL
10th week			MÜLLERIAN DUCTS DEGENERATE / WOLFFIAN DUCTS DEGENERATE	FOLDS,
11th week			SEMINAL VESICLES, EPIDIDYMIS, VAS DEFERENS	PHALLUS AND GLANS
12th week	OVARY DESCENT COMPLETE		SEMINAL VESICLES, EPIDIDYMIS, VAS DEFERENS / WALLS FORM	SEX DISTINGUISHABLE
5 months	TESTIS AT INGUINAL RING		SINUS EPITHELIUM GROWS IN VAGINAL CLEFT	
8 months / TERM	TESTIS DESCENT COMPLETE		RAPID UTERINE GROWTH	

FIG. 5-1. Chart showing interrelations and time sequence of events in development of genitourinary system.

to produce conclusive evidence of neoformation. The preformation theory is the one currently accepted.

Certain experimental studies have revealed features of practical importance. For example, if genital ridge tissue of mice is excised and transplanted before the primordial cells have reached it in their migration, no sex cells are formed, although genital ridge derivatives appear normally. Conversely, if sex cells are present in the ridge tissue when it is transplanted, fully typical gonads form. An additional and more subtle relation is reflected in the following observation: if the primordial sex cells are totally destroyed, the genital ridges themselves do not develop; if, on the other hand, the genital ridges are destroyed before the sex cells reach them, the sex cells undergo degeneration upon arrival at the area. This reciprocal, inductive relation has important implications in certain types of congenital anomalies. In similar fashion, the possibility that ovarian tissue cannot produce new ova in adult life must be borne in mind when ovarian surgery is contemplated.

DEVELOPMENT OF THE OVARY

The Indifferent Gonad

Development of the gonads starts a little later in fetal life than that of the structures giving rise to the reproductive ducts. The first signs occur during the fifth week of embryonic life, when the second of the fetal kidneys has already begun to form. At this time a thickening of the coelomic epithelium occurs on each side of the midline of the dorsal wall. Beneath the epithelium, the mesenchyme also proliferates, and the organ thus formed, the indifferent gonad, bulges into the coelomic cavity at the level of the midportion of the mesonephros. A common mesentery suspends the gonad and the mesonephros from the dorsal body wall. At this time the gonad and the mesonephros bear the joint name *urogenital ridge*. The growth of the gonadal component outstrips that of the mesonephros. Indeed, the latter commences to degenerate fairly soon. In consequence,

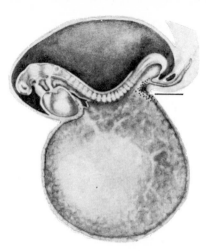

FIG. 5-2. Reconstruction of 25.5-day embryo, showing primordial germ cells (*black dots*) in anterior wall of hindgut and adjacent regions of yolk sac. (Carnegie No. 8005, ×22) (Witschi E: Migration of the germ cells of human embryos from the yolk sac to the primitive gonadal folds. Contrib Embryol 32:67, 1948)

deep grooves appear in the urogenital ridge, and by the seventh week the gonad has become quite independent, attached to the ridge only by a new mesentery of its own, the *mesorchium* or *mesovarium,* as the case may be, which persists to maturity.

Meanwhile, the thickening of the surface epithelium continues, and fingerlike sprouts begin to penetrate the mesenchymal core of the gonad. The primordial germ cells that had reached the gonadal site just before the epithelial thickening commenced are carried down into the core by the epithelial sprouts and at the same time undergo rapid proliferation of their own (Figs. 5-5 and 5-6).

Sexual Differentiation

Early in the seventh week in the gonad that will become a testis, the epithelial sprouts assume the form of clearly demarcated epithelial cords with intervening mesenchymal stroma. At the same time, the primordial germ cells disappear from the surface (germinal) epithelium, all of them becoming incorporated in the sex cords. A dense fibrous layer, the *tunica albuginea,* forms beneath the epithelium, separating the sex cords from it (Fig. 5-7).

Distinctive changes in the female gonad do not appear quite as early as those in the male, so that, as Gillman says, "the young ovary is identified chiefly by the fact that it is not a testis." Throughout the seventh week the epithelial sprouts grow more cordlike (Pflüger's cords), though less dramatically so than in the male (Fig. 5-8). By the end of the seventh week, these break up into discontinuous clumps of cells that become grouped into the *primordial ovarian follicles,* each containing a primordial sex cell (Fig. 5-9). Nothing analogous to the tunica albuginea of the testis separates

FIG. 5-3. Part of transverse section through 7-week embryo, showing thickening of coelomic epithelium and condensation of underlying mesenchyme that form genital ridge. (Carnegie No. 6524, Sect. 48-3-4, ×250) (Gillman J: Development of gonads in man, with consideration of the role of fetal endocrines and the histogenesis of ovarian tumors. Contrib Embryol 32:81, 1948)

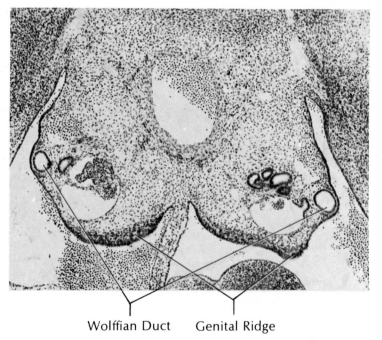

Wolffian Duct   Genital Ridge

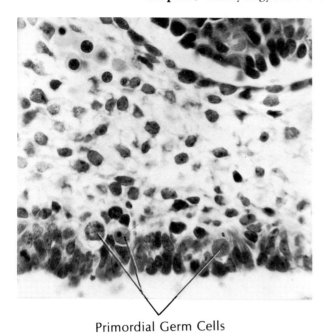

Primordial Germ Cells

FIG. 5-4. Genital ridge of 7-week embryo. (Carnegie No. 8098, Sect. 10-5-4, ×800)

FIG. 5-5. Part of frontal section through 7-week embryo, showing genital ridge at stage slightly more advanced than those shown in Figures 5-3 and 5-4. (Carnegie No. 6516, Sect. 11-1-4, ×500) (Gillman J: Development of the gonads in man, with consideration of the role of fetal endocrines and the histogenesis of ovarian tumors. Contrib Embryol 32:81, 1948)

Sex Cord

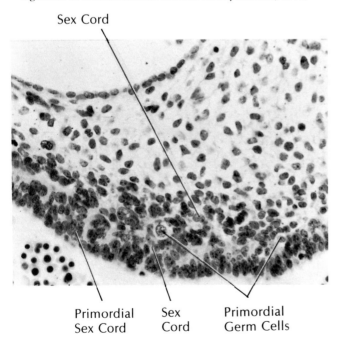

Primordial Sex Cord   Sex Cord   Primordial Germ Cells

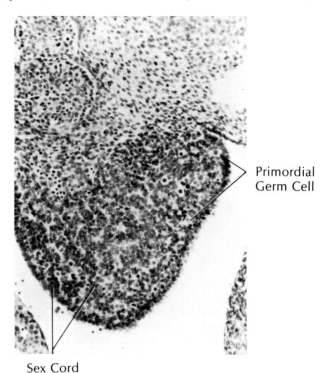

Primordial Germ Cell

Sex Cord

FIG. 5-6. Frontal section of gonad in undifferentiated stage (7th week). (Carnegie No. 6507, Sect. 11-1-5, ×100) (Gillman J: Development of the gonads in man, with consideration of the role of endocrines and the histogenesis of ovarian tumors. Contrib Embryol 32:81, 1948)

the germinal epithelium of the ovary from the underlying tissue.

The Rete Complex

Differentiation of the sex cords occurs essentially within the future cortex of the gonads, but the epithelial strands continue their growth into the medulla, forming the interlocking networks of the *rete testis* and *rete ovarii,* respectively. The former grows through the mesorchium into the contiguous tissue of the mesonephros and joins the persisting mesonephric tubules. The strands become canalized in the fourth month and establish contact through the mesonephric (wolffian) duct with the exterior.

The rete ovarii is less fully formed. Its union with mesonephric tubules is normally sporadic and imperfect, and there is no systematic canalization. The consequent lack of a route to the exterior necessitates the more complicated process of ovarian follicle rupture into the abdominal cavity and transport of ova thence through the lower reproductive tract. The ovarian rete usually disappears during the course of fetal develop-

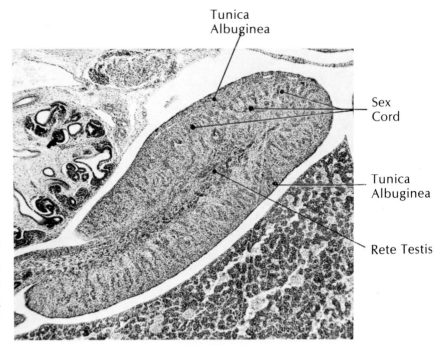

Tunica Albuginea

Sex Cord

Tunica Albuginea

Rete Testis

FIG. 5-7. Section through testicle of 9-week embryo, showing early tubules connected in part with rete testis. (Carnegie No. 5621a, Sect. 97-1-2, ×60) (Gillman J: Development of the gonads in man, with consideration of the role of endocrines and the histogenesis of ovarian tumors. Contrib Embryol 32:81, 1948)

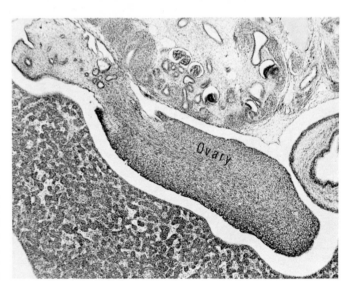

Ovary

FIG. 5-8. Section through ovary of 9-week embryo. Compare ill-defined rete and very cellular cortex without distinct tubules with condition of testis shown in Figure 5-7. Note that magnifications are same. (Carnegie No. 4304, Sect. 66-3-2, ×60) (Gillman J: Development of the gonads in man, with consideration of the role of endocrines and the histogenesis of ovarian tumors. Contrib Embryol 32:81; 1948)

ment, leaving only rudimentary vestiges at the ovarian hilum.

Maturation of the Ovary

Although by the 17th week the ovary and testis can be readily differentiated, numerous developments must yet take place before the fetal ovary resembles the adult organ. These changes occur in a series of steps, and their sequence is important. First comes encapsulation of the primitive ova by primitive granulosa cells (pre-granulosa cells), transforming the disorganized cell clumps that were derived from the sex cords into primary ovarian follicles. Coincident with this, the ova swell. Next comes a proliferation of the fetal stroma and its widespread penetration throughout the organ. If these two steps are reversed, the unprotected ova disintegrate upon contact with the stroma.

There is evidence from histologic and biochemical studies that this stroma is the precursor of the theca that surrounds the follicles and provides a rich source of estrogens. It follows that the theca is to be regarded as a mesenchymal derivative, whereas the granulosa cells,

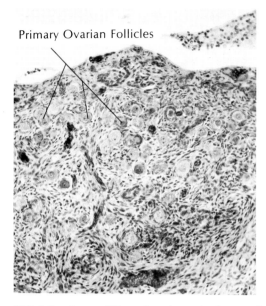

Primary Ovarian Follicles

FIG. 5-9. Ovary of 30-week embryo. Fetal stroma has invaded throughout cortex. (Carnegie No. Forbes 12-30, ×200)

descendants of the cells composing the sex cords, are of epithelial origin. This concept does much to dispel previous confusion about the origin of the two types of cells, but it must be noted that some authorities continue to contend that granulosa cells as well as theca cells are derived directly from the mesenchyme.

About the time these alterations are completed (seventh month), proliferation of granulosa occurs in many follicles throughout the ovary, with formation of antra in which fluid collects (*graafian follicles*). The implication seems clear that the ovary has become responsive to maternal gonadotropic hormones. Thus, at birth a small proportion of follicles presents a surprisingly adult appearance (Fig. 5-10), but this normal condition should not be mistaken for a pathologic one. When deprived of maternal hormone stimulation after birth, the follicles regress until puberty.

Descent of the Ovary

The gonads of both sexes develop high in the abdominal cavity retroperitoneally. They descend into the pelvis, late in fetal life, by different routes; the testes by slipping along the posterior body wall behind the peritoneum, the ovaries by sagging into the peritoneal cavity. In doing so, the ovaries pull the tubes with them, stretch the broad ligaments, and cause an angulation in the round ligaments. These relations are illustrated in Figure 5-11.

The ligaments themselves are formed essentially as a result of the bulging of the ovaries and müllerian ducts into the peritoneal cavity, since they carry a double fold of peritoneum with them. Connective tissue is deposited between the layers, a particularly large amount in the

broad ligament, where the mesonephros was originally located. The round ligament is a carryover from the inguinal ligament of the mesonephros, which attached the inferior pole of that organ to the lower margin of the body cavity. The pull of these various ligaments upon the ovaries prevents them from pursuing the same path of descent as the testes.

THE DUCTS

In a brief review of the early development of the urinary tract to make clear its relation with the development of the reproductive system, prime interest focuses upon those urinary tract components that later become functional portions of the reproductive tract, namely, the ducts.

In the development of the mammalian excretory system, three successive kidneys are formed, all of them bilaterally paired. The first, the *pronephros*, probably does not function in the human being. Its first segments appear high in the abdominal cavity during the third week, and development proceeds downward. The organ is composed of tubules whose medial ends meet and fuse to form a common *pronephric duct*. This grows toward the cloaca, into which it eventually opens. As development of the pronephros progresses, the highest tubules commence to degenerate, even before the lowest ones are formed, but the duct does not degenerate.

FIG. 5-10. Ovary of full-term fetus. Maternal hormones have stimulated development of two of the follicles shown. (Carnegie No. Forbes 12-14 ×100)

Primitive Follicles

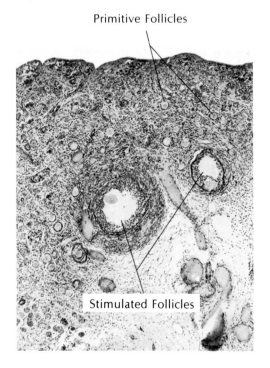

Stimulated Follicles

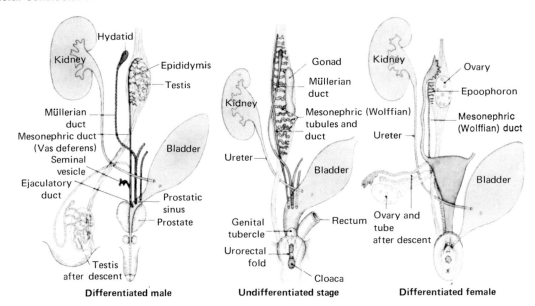

FIG. 5-11. Schematic diagrams showing plan of development of definitive male and female urogenital systems from primitive, undifferentiated state. (Patten BM: Human Embryology, 2nd ed. Philadelphia, Blakiston, 1953)

The second kidney, the *mesonephros,* begins to replace the pronephros in the subdiaphragmatic location in the fourth week. It is composed of tubules similar to those of its predecessor, but instead of elaborating a duct of its own, it appropriates the pronephric duct, which thereafter is known as the *mesonephric duct* or by the more familiar eponym, the *wolffian duct.* There is evidence that the mesonephros, unlike the pronephros, does have at least rudimentary function for a time, but like the pronephros, it degenerates. The definitive kidney, the *metanephros,* supplants it. The tubules of this final excretory organ form a little lower in the abdominal cavity than those of the previous kidneys and first appear in the sixth or seventh week. Its duct originates as an outpouching of the lower end of the mesonephric duct, the *ureteric bud,* which grows upward, eventually invaginating the metanephros and connecting with the metanephric tubules. The connection of the ureter with the mesonephric duct is interrupted at an early stage by differential growth processes that give the two ducts separate entrances to the urogenital sinus. It is important to emphasize the close association between the definitve urinary tract and those parts of the reproductive tract that are derived from the mesonephric duct. Note in particular the common origin of their lining epithelium.

The foregoing developments are common to both male and female in the early "neuter" stage. With the assumption of all excretory functions by the metanephric complex, the mesonephric duct is used by the male exclusively as the channel through which the sex cells

are conducted from the testis to the exterior. Its further course in the male is shown in Figure 5-11. In the female it gradually degenerates and disappears, except for occasional rests.

The female reproductive duct, the *paramesonephric* or *müllerian duct,* is made afresh for the purpose. It originates during the sexually indifferent period, early in the sixth week, and is therefore present in the future male as well as the future female. In the former it degenerates about the tenth week, at approximately the time when the mesonephric duct is degenerating in the female. The müllerian duct originates as an invagination of coelomic epithelium lateral to the upper end of the mesonephric duct. The epithelium in the base of the small pit so formed proliferates to form a solid, blind cord that grows downward toward the pelvis. This later becomes canalized. This mechanism, which results in a lining coelomic epithelium, contrasts with the bulging of the gonads into the body cavity, which produces a covering of coelomic epithelium. The müllerian ducts of both sides grow toward each other, crossing over the wolffian duct anteriorly to meet and fuse in the midline during the ninth week. The medial walls of the fused ducts gradually disappear, producing a single uterovaginal cavity (Fig. 5-12). The upper portions of the ducts, which do not fuse, remain as the paired uterine (fallopian) tubes, each with a persistent ostium to the peritoneum at its tip (see Fig. 5-11). When the lower end of the fused müllerian ducts makes contact with the urogenital sinus, the cell cords are still solid (Fig. 5-12). They merge with the endodermal cells growing

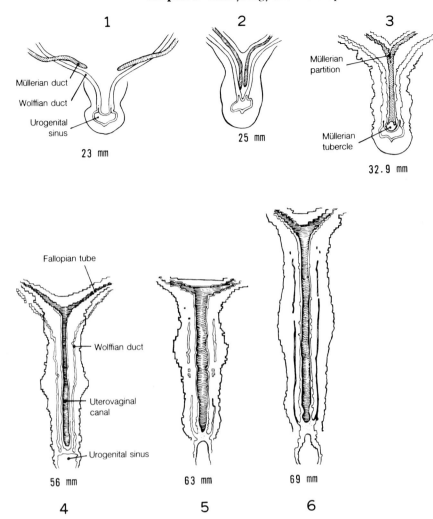

FIG. 5-12. Reconstructions of müllerian and wolffian ducts in female embryos at 8 to 14 weeks of development. (After Koff AK: Development of the vagina in the human fetus. Contrib Embryol 24:59, 1933)

back from the sinus to form a temporary barrier between the uterovaginal cavity and the urogenital sinus, the *müllerian tubercle*.

DERIVATIVES OF THE UROGENITAL SINUS

The *cloaca,* the primitive receptacle into which reproductive, excretory, and intestinal tracts open, is the blind end of the hindgut. Hence, the cloaca and its derivatives are lined with endoderm. In the sixth week, the urorectal septum divides the cloaca, separating intestinal and genitourinary compartments. The latter, the *urogenital sinus,* opens exteriorly shortly thereafter as the result of rupture of the urogenital (urethral) membrane, and the urogenital duct system thus acquires access to the outside (Fig. 5-13). Previously, certain landmarks appeared in the future perineal region, preeminently a midline protuberance; the *genital tubercle,* precursor of the phallus; the *genital folds;* and the *labioscrotal swellings* lateral to them. The depression between the genital folds is the *primitive urethral groove* (Fig. 5-14). In the female this becomes the outer part of the vestibule, and the rupture of the urethral membrane occurs in its depth. Since this rupture creates a large orifice, the whole urogenital sinus is converted into an open trough that forms the inner portion of the vestibule. The junction between perineal ectoderm and urogenital sinus endoderm occurs on the inner aspect of the genital folds, which become the labia minora.

The opening of the ureter, via its terminal segment, the urethra, occurs in the deep endodermal portion of the vestibule, as does the opening of the uterovaginal cavity. The latter, however, is not entirely simple. Not until the fifth month does sinus epithelium (endodermal in origin) penetrate the wall of the urogenital sinus in the müllerian tubercle where the fused müllerian ducts ended blindly. Subsequent canalization of this barrier

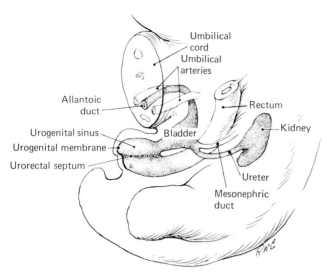

FIG. 5-13. Relations of cloaca and its derivatives.

opens the vaginal canal into the vestibule. A residue of the barrier still persists in attenuated form as the *hymen*. Thus, the lower portion of the vagina is lined with epithelium tracing its ancestry to gut endoderm, whereas the upper portion, derived from the müllerian duct, originated in coelomic epithelium. The müllerian epithelium becomes columnar and forms a characteristic mucosa. The vaginal epithelium becomes stratified squamous. The junction between the two types, occurring at the site of the future cervix uteri, is not abrupt, and the interaction between the two epithelia is the basis of a number of important pathologic processes that may occur in the adult.

For comparison between male and female development, it may be noted that, although the clitoris is homologous to the penis, the urethral groove at its base is rudimentary only and does not normally deepen or close over in the manner of the penile urethra. Bartholin's glands provide another such comparison between the sexes. They are homologs of the male bulbourethral (Cowper's) glands and, like them, arise by budding from the endodermal epithelium of the portion of the urogenital sinus that forms the urethra.

THE EXTERNAL GENITALIA

Accurate determination of the sex of embryos is a duty of the obstetrician that may have social, legal, and statistical importance. Such determination may be achieved by study of the sex chromatin complement of embryonic cells obtained by amniocentesis, buccal smear, and so on, but these methods are used in relatively few instances; the responsibility for the most part still rests on the obstetrician. In many cases this is not easy. The dif-

ficulty lies in the fact that the phallus of a female embryo and of an embryo of undifferentiated sex is as prominent as that of a true male and in consequence may be mistaken for a penis. Altogether different landmarks must be used for accurate determination.

The genetic sex of the embryo is determined at the time of fertilization, but some weeks of development must pass before what Novak calls "the impress of sex" is made upon various portions of the genital tract. Before the sixth week the determination can be made only by the genetic studies mentioned above. From the seventh to the tenth weeks differentiation must be based on the histologic characteristics of the developing gonads (see Fig. 5-14). In certain cases a slightly earlier decision on the basis of external genitalia may appear possible, but this appearance should be distrusted, as relative retardation may occur in males. Since, as indicated (see Fig. 5-1), the müllerian ducts of the female commence to fuse in the ninth week, gross inspection of the abdominal organs may be of some help in differentiation at about this time. Caution must be observed, however, for entirely male wolffian ducts may lie so closely side by side in the pelvis that they will be mistaken for müllerian ducts about to fuse to form a uterus.

During the 11th week, a series of diagnostic changes in the external genitalia commences, as illustrated in Figure 5-15. In the top row of photographs, showing specimens of the 11th week, male and female can be differentiated. If the phallus, which is similar in the two, is disregrded, it will be noted that in the male the urogenital outlet has become smaller and has apparently migrated toward the tip of the phallus. Actually, the process is a covering over of the lower portion of the prim-

FIG. 5-14. Perineal region of $6\frac{3}{7}$-week embryo (24.5 mm) showing undifferentiated precursors of external genitalia. (Carnegie No. 6263)

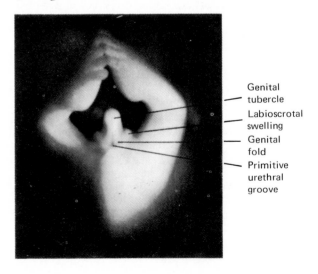

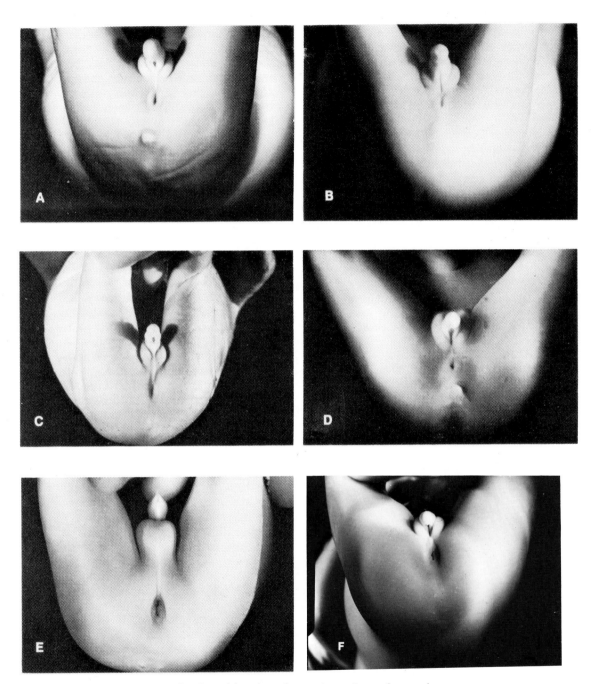

FIG. 5-15. External genitalia of male and female embryos. Carnegie numbers and ages are as follows: (*A*) 7589, 44 mm, $10\frac{3}{7}$ weeks. (*B*) 5622, 41.5 mm, $10\frac{1}{2}$ weeks. (*C*) 9917, 50 mm, 11 weeks. (*D*) 9426, 59 mm, 12 weeks. (*E*) 6214, 92 mm, $14\frac{1}{2}$ weeks. (*F*) 9745, 96 mm, 15 weeks.

itive urethral groove by fusion of the genital folds. In the female the urogenital opening remains large and continues to be at the base of the phallus. A slight depression separates the posterior ends of the labio-scrotal swellings. The closing over of the inferior portion of the outlet in the male brings the scrotolabial folds together in a distinctive band of connective tissue, the scrotal raphe. Since when diagnosing an individual specimen the obstetrician does not always have an example of the opposite sex at the same stage at hand for comparison, an absolute criterion of sex is more useful than relative ones. The scrotal raphe is perhaps the most reliable such landmark. It is absent in the female at all stages but is detectable early in the male.

By the stage illustrated in the specimens in the middle row of Figure 5-15 (13th week), there is no serious diagnostic difficulty if the foregoing differential points are borne in mind and if, most importantly, the genitalia are examined from the perineal aspect. Diagnosis of the specimens illustrated in the bottom row of photographs, which are of an even later stage (15th week), is equally clear-cut, again provided it is made on the basis of perineal examination. Figure 5-16 shows, however, that confusion and error may still result if examination is restricted to the anterior aspect. Here the phallus is the most conspicuous feature and may easily be mistaken for a penis. A characteristically female bending of this organ toward the anus, which is often described, may be obscured by fixation artifact. Even the labial swellings resemble a scrotum if the separation of the posterior ends of the labia at the commissure is not observed. The female phallus normally becomes recognizable as a clitoris in the fourth month.

Two small practical points that facilitate diagnosis may be mentioned: (1) it is essential to have a good source of illumination when examining the specimen, if possible a focused beam; and (2) a dissecting microscope or other means of magnification should be employed whenever a case is in doubt.

ANOMALIES

In the transformations and interactions that take place in the course of prenatal growth and development, there are certain points of weakness, certain areas of stress, where departures from the normal course of development may most readily occur.

The result of these aberrations may be relatively simple (*e.g.,* extra digits) or exceedingly complicated, with abnormalities occurring at various sites and overlapping confusingly (*e.g.,* exstrophy of the bladder with anomalies of external genitalia). Even so, it is possible to formulate certain generalizations grouping female genital malformations according to their embryologic history as follows:

1. Breakdown in time schedule
2. Failure of primordium to appear
3. Anomalies of fusion
4. Failure of transitory structures to disappear
5. Reduplication of structures
6. Anomalies of position
7. Multiple anomalies

These types of anomaly occur in otherwise normal, healthy individuals. Excluded are those types known to be based on chromosomal aberrations, endocrinologic abnormality, intrauterine infection, or the action of toxic substances and mechanical interference, which are dealt with elsewhere in this book. Still, one must keep an open mind about the types of anomaly listed; although the initiating factors for a given deviation may be unknown at present, new information may require reallocation to one of the specific categories, such as chromosomal aberration.

The anomalies in categories 1, 2, 5, and 6 are more common in other organ systems than the genitourinary, and when they do involve the genital tract, they are frequently associated with anomalies elsewhere in the

FIG. 5-16. Two views of external genitalia of female embryo shown in Figure 5-15F, demonstrating masculine appearance of anterior view (*A*) and emphasizing necessity of examination of perineal aspect (*B*) of all specimens. (Carnegie No. 9745, 96 mm, 15 weeks)

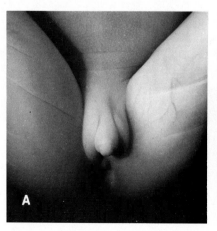
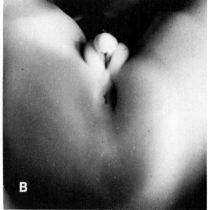

body. These rare and complicated cases are best studied in texts primarily dealing with malformations.

Closely related to the topic of this chapter, however, are anomalies of categories 3, 4, and 7.

Anomalies of Fusion of Müllerian Ducts

At any stage during the course of normal müllerian duct fusion, an impediment may occur. Resultant conditions range from the extreme case of double uterus and double vagina (Fig. 5-17*G*) to an inconspicuous notching of the fundus of the uterine cavity (Fig. 5-17*E*) with or without accompanying notching of the uterine wall (Fig. 5-17*A*). The clinical importance of the various forms of bicornuate uterus lies in the effect they may have on the course of pregnancy. The milder degrees of the condition are not uncommon and are often unrecognized clinically unless radiologic study is carried out for some coincidental reason. The more complete partitioning is rare and may present complications. Double pregnancy in two separate cavities with term deliveries at separate times has been reported. Unsuspected cases of this rare circumstance may form the basis of some cases regarded as superfetation.

Figure 5-17*D* illustrates a different type of failure of fusion: failure not, in this instance, of two like structures to fuse (*e.g.,* two müllerian ducts), but of two unlike structures to fuse (müllerian ducts and urogenital sinus). The designation *failure to fuse* is perhaps more descriptive of what actually takes place in such cases than the term *atresia*. An anomaly of this sort, of course, precludes pregnancy.

A different sort of müllerian duct anomaly is now thought to underlie the occurrence of adenoma, a condition in which larger or smaller nodules of glandular tissue stud the vagina and cervix. Some of these nodules may undergo malignant transformation.

In 1971 a connection was reported between the occurrence of clear cell adenocarcinoma of the genital tract in young women and the use of diethylstilbestrol (DES) by their mothers during pregnancy. The early reports of this condition were often confusing and contradictory, but evidence is now gradually falling in place, particularly since the initiation in 1974 of the National Diethylstilbestrol Adenosis (DESAD) Project, which is funded by the National Cancer Institute and with which numerous medical research facilities throughout the country are affiliated. Definitive studies have dealt with the incidence of DES sequelae in male and female offspring of treated mothers, with the nature of the lesions and malignant changes in them, with spontaneous regression of symptoms, and with treatment. The clinical evaluation and management of the condition are considered elsewhere in this book. Pertinent to the present discussion are two special features: (1) the time and dose relationship of drug administration and (2) the probable life history of the lesions.

It has been established that 90% of the lesions occurred when the drug was administered in large doses early in pregnancy (*i.e.,* between the 8th and 16th weeks). This time interval corresponds with the period of active formation of the lower genital tract and bears out the concept of "time and points of stress." Further, the specific origin of the lesions (cervical extropion,

FIG. 5-17. Schematic diagrams of various types of abnormal uteri. (Patten BM: Human Embryology, 3rd ed. Philadelphia, Blakiston, 1968)

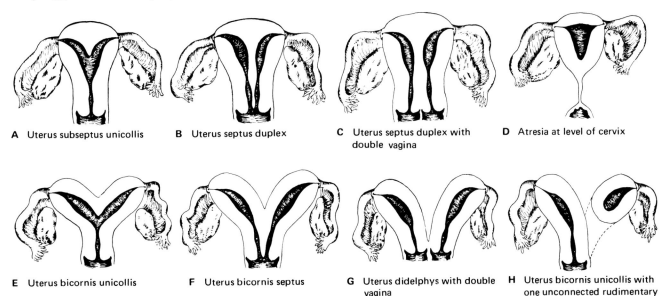

A Uterus subseptus unicollis

B Uterus septus duplex

C Uterus septus duplex with double vagina

D Atresia at level of cervix

E Uterus bicornis unicollis

F Uterus bicornis septus

G Uterus didelphys with double vagina

H Uterus bicornis unicollis with one unconnected rudimentary horn

adenoma formation, transverse ridging) seems to be due to a failure of normal upgrowth of urogenital sinus epithelium to replace the müllerian duct epithelium covering the vagina and cervical portio. DES has also been shown to affect the sensitive stroma of the tract that is developing at this time, resulting in deformities.

It may be noted that no malignant change has been reported in males whose mothers took DES, but alterations in duct structure is frequent, and anomalies of spermatogenesis have been reported.

Failure of Mesonephric Tubules and Ducts to Disappear

The persistence of vestigial remnants of wolffian ducts and tubules in the female, either with or without symptoms, is more common than anomalies of müllerian duct fusion. The most frequent locations in which these rests occur are the mesovarium and the broad ligament. In the former site they form the epoophoron (if located high) or the paroophoron (if lower in the ligament). These are often referred to as *hydatids of Morgagni,* and they occur so regularly that they can hardly be classed as abnormal. Their clinical significance lies in their propensity to cystic dilation and infection, with attendant symptoms. The remnants of the wolffian duct in the broad ligament bear the additional eponym of Gartner's duct. Other, less common residual segments of these ducts occur in the walls of the vagina, in the labia minora close to the clitoris, and around the urethra. All are subject to the same clinical symptoms as the cysts of the epoophoron.

Multiple Anomalies

The intimate association of the urinary and reproductive tracts gives rise to a number of malformations in which both are involved. These are among the most complex of all anomalies. As classic examples may be cited persistent cloaca, which occurs when the urorectal septum fails to form, and exstrophy of the bladder and attendant anomalies of the external genitalia, which results from defective closure of the anterior abdominal wall. Beyond this brief notation, it is recommended that combined anomalies be studied, as occasion arises, in specialized texts and reviews.

Ovarian Tumors

Related to the congenital malformations of the female genital tract, though not properly described as anomalies, are the special ovarian neoplasms (see Chapter 59, Lesions of the Ovary). These tumors may be composed of one or more of the cell types normally occurring in the gonad at any stage of its development. If derived from cells of the sexually indifferent stage, the tumor cells may differentiate along the male or the female path,

regardless of the fact that the patient's normal gonad became an ovary. A firm grasp of the basic steps of the embryologic development of the gonads renders the complexity of ovarian tumors less baffling. The following points should be noted:

1. Totipotent primordial germ cells migrate from the primitive yolk sac through the gut mesentery to the site of gonad formation. Query: Could a cell, sidetracked during migration, remain viable but dormant until subsequent stimulation to proliferation? Could this account for ovarian type tumors in ectopic locations?
2. The epithelial lining of the müllerian ducts, and therefore of all structures derived from it, originates from the coelomic epithelium. It is unknown at what stage the multipotency of this epithelium ceases or whether subsequent stimulation of any sort can reactivate it. This consideration is allied to the problem of the cause of endometriosis and may be implicated in the histogenesis of certain ovarian tumors, since the germinal epithelium of the ovary has the same origin in coelomic epithelium.
3. Although granulosa cells and theca cells are probably of different origins and not interchangeable, there is evidence that the granulosa cell, at a particular stage of development, induces the differentiation of theca cells from the stroma. Breakdown of the normal time schedule or imbalances in mutual influence might have pathologic consequences.

In conclusion, it may be reiterated that familiarity with the normal development of the reproductive tract and appreciation of the general ways in which developmental processes can go awry are of greater assistance in an understanding of the complexities of congenital anomalies than the memorizing of individual examples. The multiplicity of eponyms should not be a matter of concern, for once the anatomic definition of a condition is determined, the nature and origin of that condition can be comprehended against the background of normal developmental processes. Such analyses are useful because anomalies frequently are multiple, involving various systems, and it is important to know for what unsuspected condition any given patient should be examined.

REFERENCES AND RECOMMENDED READING

General

Arey LB: Developmental Anatomy, 7th ed rev. Philadelphia, WB Saunders, 1974
Corlis CE: Patten's Human Embryology. New York, McGraw-Hill, 1976
Greep RO (ed): Handbook of Physiology, Vol II, Endocrinology. Washington, DC, American Physiological Society, 1975
Hamilton WJ, Mossman HW: Human Embryology, 4th ed. Baltimore, Williams & Wilkins, 1972

Jones HW, Jones GS: Novak's Textbook of Gynecology, 10th ed. Baltimore, Williams & Wilkins, 1981

Langman J: Medical Embryology, 4th ed. Baltimore, Williams & Wilkins, 1981

Ramsey EM: Malformations of the female genital tract. In Fox H (ed): Haines and Taylor's Textbook of Gynaecological and Obstetrical Pathology, Chap 2. Edinburgh, Churchill Livingstone, in press

Origin of Primordial Germ Cells

Blackler AW: Transfer of primordial germ cells between two subspecies of *Xenopus laevis*. J Embryol Exp Morphol 10: 641, 1962

Mossman HW, Duke KL: Comparative Morphology of the Mammalian Ovary. Madison, University of Wisconsin Press, 1973

Saxen L: Embryonic induction. Clin Obstet Gynecol 18:149, 1975

Witschi E: Migration of the germ cells of human embryos from the yolk sac to the primitive gonadal folds. Contrib Embryol 32:67, 1948

Development of the Ovary

Gillman J: Development of the gonads in man, with consideration of the role of fetal endocrines and the histogenesis of ovarian tumors. Contrib Embryol 32:81, 1948

Mossman HW, Duke KL: Comparative Morphology of the Mammalian Ovary, Madison, University of Wisconsin Press, 1973

VanWagenen G, Simpson ME: Embryology of the Ovary and Testis: *Homo sapiens* and *Macaca mulatta*. New Haven, Yale University Press, 1965

Ducts

Gruenwald P: The relation of the growing müllerian duct to the wolffian duct and its importance for the genesis of malformations. Anat Record 81:1, 1941

Hunter HR: Observations on the development of the female genital tract. Contrib Embryol 22:91, 1930

Koff AK: Development of the vagina in the human fetus. Contrib Embryol 24:59, 1933

O'Rahilly R: The embryology and anatomy of the uterus. In International Academy of Pathology, Monograph No 14. Baltimore, Williams & Wilkins, 1973

Witschi E: Embryology of the uterus: Normal and experimental. Ann NY Acad Sci 75:412, 1959

Derivatives of Urogenital Sinus

Forsberg JG: Estrogen, vaginal cancer and urogenital development. Am J Obstet Gynecol 113:83, 1972

Shikinami J: Detailed form of the wolffian body in human embryos of the first eight weeks. Contrib Embryol 18:49, 1926

External Genitalia

Corliss CE: Patten's Human Embryology, Chap 19. New York, McGraw-Hill, 1976

Koff AK: Development of the vagina in the human fetus. Contrib Embryol 24:59, 1933

Spaulding MH: Development of the external genitalia in the human embryo. Contrib Embryol 13:67, 1921 (to be read in conjunction with Gillman, who modifies certain of Spaulding's conclusions)

Anomalies

General

Bransilver BR, Ferenczy A, Richart RN: Female genital tract remnants. Arch Path 96:255, 1973

Czernobilsky B, Lancet M: Broad ligament adenocarcinoma of Müllerian origin. Obst Gynecol 40:238, 1972

Dougherty CM, Spencer R: Female sex anomalies. Hagerstown, Maryland, Harper & Row, 1972.

Gruenwald P: Relation of the growing müllerian duct to the wolffian duct and its importance for the genesis of malformations. Anat Rec 81:1, 1941

McKelvey JL, Baxter JS: Abnormal development of the vagina and genitourinary tract. Am J Obstet Gynecol 29:267, 1935

Marshall FF, Beisel DS: Association of uterine and renal anomalies. Obstet Gynecol 51:559, 1978

Warkany J: Congenital Malformations. Chicago, Year Book Medical Publishers, Inc. 1972

Wilson JG: Environment and Birth Defects. New York, Academic Press, 1973

Young HH: Genital Abnormalities, Hermaphroditism and Related Adrenal Diseases. Baltimore, Williams & Wilkins, 1937

DES-Associated

Bibbo M, Gill WB et al: Follow-up study of male and female offspring of DES-exposed mothers. Obstet Gynecol 49:1, 1977

Burke L, Antonioli D, Rosen S: Vaginal and cervical squamous cell dysplasia in women exposed to diethylstilbestrol in utero. Am J Obstet Gynecol 152:537, 1978

Forsberg JG: Cervicovaginal epithelium: Its origin and development. Am J Obstet Gynecol 115:1025, 1973

Hanoy AF, Hammond MG: Infertility in women exposed to diethylstilbestrol *in utero*. J Reprod Med 28:851, 1983

Johnson LD, Driscoll SG et al: Vaginal adenosis in stillborns and neonates exposed to diethylstilbestrol and steroidal estrogens and progestins. Obstet Gynecol 53:671, 1979

Noller KL, Townsend DE, Kaufman RH et al: Maturation of vaginal and cervical epithelium in women exposed *in utero* to diethylstilbestrol (DESAD Project). Am J Obstet Gynecol 146:279, 1983

Prins RP, Morrow P: Vaginal embryogenesis, estrogens and adenosis. Obstet Gynecol 48:246, 1976

Robboy SJ, Kaufman RH et al: Pathologic findings in young women enrolled in the National Cooperative Diethylstilbestrol Adenosis (DESAD) project. Obstet Gynecol 53:309, 1979

Scully RE, Robboy SJ: Pathology and pathogenesis of diethylstilbestrol-related disorders of the female genital tract. In Herbst AL (ed): Intrauterine Exposure to Diethylstilbestrol in the Human. Proceedings of Symposium on DES, 1977. Chicago, American College of Obstetricians & Gynecologists, 1978

Ulfelder H, Robboy SJ: The embryologic development of the human vagina. Am J Obstet Gynecol 126:769, 1976

Cyclic Ovarian Function and Its Neuroendocrine Control

Carolyn B. Coulam

6

The periodic release of gametes (oocytes) is the primary responsibility of the ovary. In the human, egg production is cyclic and the periodicity of oocyte liberation is monthly. In the process of oogenesis, the ovary secretes various hormones cyclically. Both gametogenesis and hormone production are the result of the continuous repetitive process of follicle maturation, ovulation, and corpus luteal formation and regression. The control of follicular development and hence steroidogenesis involve the cyclic influence of the pituitary gonadotropins, especially follicle-stimulating hormone (FSH) and luteinizing hormone (LH). The pituitary gland does not have innate cyclicity but is stimulated to release gonadotropins by cyclic incitement from the hypothalamus as well as by the ovarian hormones themselves. Mature hypothalamic function is characterized by hourly (every 60–120 minutes) pulses of gonadotropin-releasing hormone (GnRH). While pulsatile stimulation of hypothalamic GnRH is required by the pituitary gland for the synthesis of gonadotropins, ovarian estrogen determines the cyclic pattern of FSH and LH as they occur in the normal cycle. Thus, the menstrual (monthly) cycle is the result of circhoral (hourly) stimulation by the central element of the hypothalamic–pituitary–ovarian system.

This chapter examines the mechanisms by which the hypothalamic–pituitary–ovarian system functions to allow cyclic gametogenesis by defining the role of each of the elements involved in the system: the hypothalamus, the site of hourly release of GnRH; the pituitary, the site of translation of hypothalamic signals into gonadotropic stimuli; and the ovary, a cyclic organ that releases ova monthly. The ovary not only provides cyclic feedback control signals to the hypothalamic–pituitary complex but also operates as a local feedback system, performing critical control functions within itself.

NEUROENDOCRINE CONTROL

The reciprocal relationships of the hypothalamus, pituitary, ovary, and endometrium are diagrammed in Figure 6-1. The major influence of the two pituitary gonadotropins, FSH and LH, within the ovary is on the ova-containing follicles. As a consequence of the action of FSH, granulosa cells proliferate, estrogen synthesis is stimulated, antral fluid is accumulated, and LH receptors are induced. All of these events lead to the formation of a graafian follicle, which secretes large quantities of estrogen into the circulation. The increase of estrogen in the blood triggers the release of LH, which causes rupture of the follicle, expulsion of the egg, and formation of the corpus luteum. When the effect of LH on the corpus luteum regresses, the production of steroid hormone declines and endometrial shedding (menstruation) occurs (Fig. 6-1). The cyclic secretion of FSH and LH from the anterior pituitary gland each month relies on the cyclic stimulation of the pituitary gonadotrope by the hypothalamic hormone GnRH. Each hour the pulsatile release of GnRH is mediated by catecholamines and can be modified by gonadal steroids and endorphins. Thus, the mechanism of the neuroendocrine control of cyclic ovarian function involves the interaction of the hypothalamus and the pituitary gland.

Hypothalamus

Gamete production is a consequence of a gradual orderly process that is dependent on the development of the central nervous system, specifically the hypothalamus. The hypothalamus has two anatomically distinct nervous systems. One consists of the nonmyelinated nerve fibers that originate in the hypothalamus; these are the peptidergic neurons that synthesize the hypothalamic peptides, such as GnRH and the tubohypophyseal dopamine system. The second involves the myelinated nerve fibers, with cell bodies outside the hypothalamus and only axons within the hypothalamus. These axonal synapses transmit noradrenergic or serotonergic impulses into the peptidergic neurons for an increase or decrease in the synthesis of peptide hormones. The functional hypothalamic unit consists of

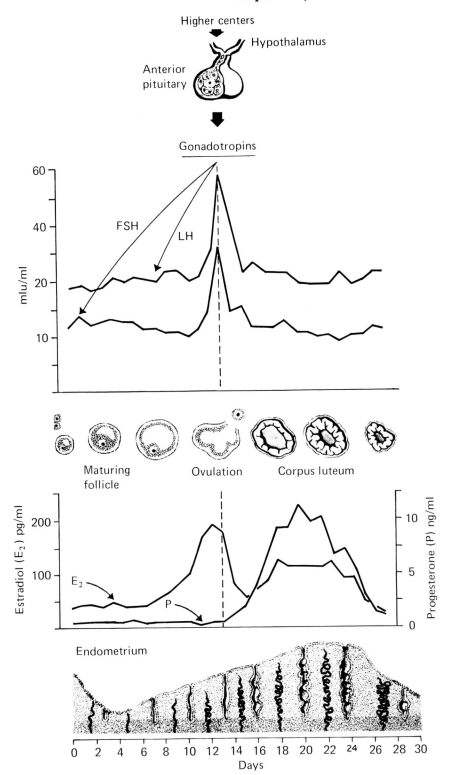

FIG. 6-1. Diagrammatic representation of events of pituitary, ovarian, and menstrual cycles. Note that plasma estradiol peaks about day 12, plasma FSH and LH about day 13, and ovulation about day 14.

peptidergic neurons that synthesize GnRH, axonal neurons that secrete neurotransmitters to regulate the synthesis of hypothalamic peptides by both stimulus and inhibition, and neurons with axon–axonal junctions that initiate the release of hormones. This third set of neurons comprises the tubohypophyseal dopamine system.

Hypothalamic Function

The peptidergic neurons of the hypothalamus control the vegetative nervous system that regulates food intake, fluid balance, temperature, sleep, respiration, circulation, growth, and reproduction. The peptidergic neurons control reproduction by pulsatile release of the hypothalamic hormone GnRH, which stimulates the synthesis and release of FSH and LH from the anterior pituitary gland. The release of GnRH, which reaches a maximum at 30 minutes, affects FSH to a lesser degree than LH. Frequent sampling techniques have demonstrated that gonadotropins are released in rapid, rhythmic pulses superimposed on a low level of continuous secretion. The pulsatile release occurs every hour (60–120 minutes) and is dependent on hypothalamic control. In castrated animals with hypothalamic lesions that eliminate endogenous GnRH, the characteristic hourly secretions of LH can be reproduced by the hourly administration of GnRH. Circhoral pulses of GnRH, which are dependent on stimulation by catecholamine, have been detected in the peripheral plasma of women. The synthesis of GnRH occurs in neurosecretory cells of the hypothalamus, which receive input from higher centers in the central nervous system and receive feedback signals from the developing follicle. GnRH is transported down the axon to its terminal in the region of the median eminence, where it is secreted into the portal capillary venous network that bathes the anterior pituitary gland. GnRH secretion reflects a balance of the actions of noradrenergic excitement and dopaminergic inhibition.

Control of Hypothalamic Function

The ability to reproduce is under hypothalamic control, which in turn is dependent on maturation of the central nervous system. Specifically, ability to reproduce involves the concentration of neurotransmitters within the hypothalamus. The neurotransmitters concerned with reproduction—norepinephrine, dopamine, and serotonin—are concentrated in the hypothalamus from their source of synthesis in the cortex and sensory organs. The noradrenergic nervous system is the only part of the nervous system that has the ability to grow postnatally. Ruf has hypothesized that, when the adrenergic neurons reach the limit of their growth potential, puberty is initiated by adult adrenergic neurons synapsing with hypothalamic peptidergic neurons that produce GnRH.

The serotoninergic pathway, although important in the corticotropin system, does not seem to play a sig-

nificant role in the control of GnRH. However, in the pineal gland, serotonin is converted to melatonin and its derivative, which may decrease GnRH secretion. The levels of melatonin in blood decrease in children entering puberty. However, the serotonin/melatonin pathway does not seem to play an important role in the day-to-day regulation of the adult cycle. In contrast, the concentration of catecholamines in the hypothalamus increases with increasing age and is significantly involved in the menstrual cycle. Evidence implicates dopamine as a direct inhibitor of a broad spectrum of hypothalamic functions. It not only inhibits GnRH, thereby reducing the secretion of FSH and LH, but also reduces corticotropin and thyroid-stimulating hormone by hypothalamic suppression as well as by suppression of prolactin. Norepinephrine has a stimulatory effect on GnRH secretion. While adrenergic neurons synapse with the GnRH-secreting body, dopaminergic neurons exert their influence on gonadotropin secretion through axon–axonal communication in the area of the median eminence. In this relationship GnRH secretion reflects a balance of noradrenergic excitation and dopamine inhibition.

Appreciation of the role of catecholaminergic neurotransmitters, combined with evidence of estrogen feedback, has stimulated interest in the idea of a potential mechanism for their interaction. Investigation of estrogen metabolism in the brain has revealed that the hypothalamus is rich in 2-hydroxylation activity. The enzymatic addition of a hydroxyl group to carbon 2 of the steroid nucleus gives estrogen remarkable structural similarity to the neurotransmitters norepinephrine and dopamine (Fig. 6-2). The enzyme responsible for the degradation of these catecholamines, catechol-O-methyl-transferase, also metabolizes the catechol estrogens; in addition, it exhibits a greater affinity for catechol estrogens than for catecholamines, thus providing catechol estrogens with the capacity to alter the effective

FIG. 6-2. Structural similarities among estrogen, catechol estrogen, and catecholamines. The enzyme catechol-O-methyl-transferase metabolizes both norepinephrine and 2-hydroxyestradiol, rendering them biologically inactive.

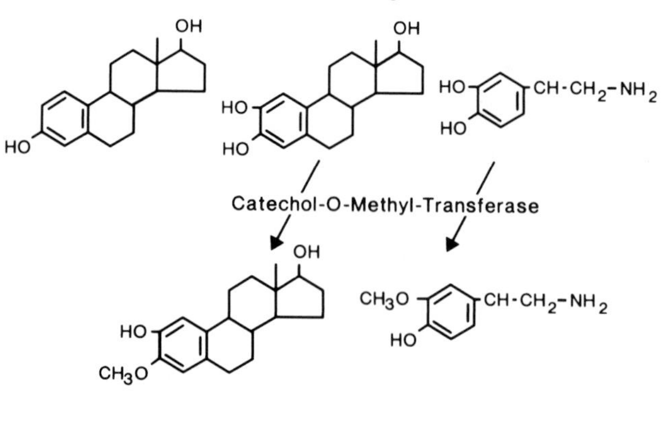

hypothalamic concentrations of neurotransmitters. Alternatively, the catechol estrogens may exert actions directly through catecholamine or estrogen receptor mechanisms.

Modulation of Hypothalamic Function

Hypothalamic function is modulated in four ways: by steroid feedback (the long loop), by pituitary feedback (the short loop), by hypothalamic feedback (the ultrashort loop), and by endorphins.

STEROID FEEDBACK. Within the established monthly pattern, gonadotropins are secreted in a pulsatile fashion with a frequency and magnitude that vary with the phase of the cycle (Fig. 6-3). The frequency of gonadotropin release is every 60 to 120 minutes throughout most of the cycle but only every 3 to 4 hours during the midluteal phase. Pulse amplitude is greatest during the midcycle surge and least in the late follicular phase. Both the amplitude of the pulse and the frequency of the gonadotropin secretion change throughout the cycle, and the pulsatile pattern of gonadotropin

release from the pituitary gland is causally related to pulsatile stimuli from hypothalamic GnRH, all of which suggests that steroid modulation occurs at least in part at the level of the hypothalamus. Estrogen receptors are present in the hypothalamus. When estradiol is infused into the central nervous system, the neurosecretion of GnRH declines. The gonadal steroids exert their feedback effects on gonadotropin secretion by modulating the magnitude and frequency of GnRH secretion. Estrogen appears to be most effective in dampening the amplitude of gonadotropin pulses, more of FSH than of LH. An increase in estrogen from the preovulatory follicle may signal the decline in pulsatile amplitude that is observed during the late follicular phase. The lower levels of circulating estrogen allow higher peaks of LH during the midcycle surge. Feedback from increasing levels of progesterone has been implicated in the reduction in pulse frequency noted during the midluteal and luteal phases.

PITUITARY FEEDBACK. The mechanism by which GnRH secretion is terminated is unknown. An increase in the concentration of pituitary LH within the hypo-

FIG. 6-3. Serum LH and FSH concentrations (mean ± 1 SD) before and after administration of 150 μg luteinizing hormone–releasing hormone (LHRH) during different phases of the cycle, studied serially. *Arrow* indicates time of injection of LHRH. It has been suggested that a change in gonadotropin release during the cycle is due to effects of varying levels of ovarian hormones on the pituitary. (Yen SSC, Vandenberg G, Rebar R et al: Variation of pituitary responsiveness to synthetic LRF during different phases of the menstrual cycle. J Clin Endocrinol Metab 35: 931–934, 1972)

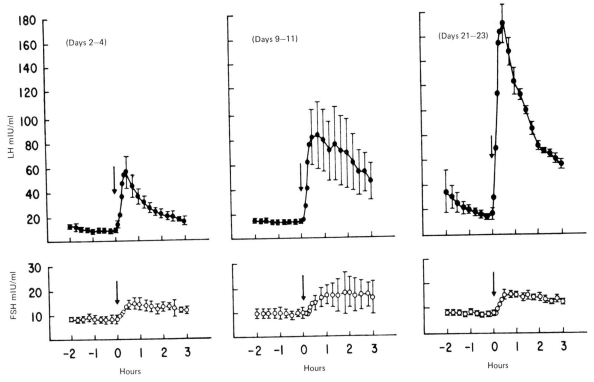

thalamus is associated with a decrease in the secretory activity of the GnRH neurons. Pituitary gonadotropins can reach the hypothalamus in concentrations much greater than those observed in the peripheral circulation through retrograde portal blood flow. LH can decrease GnRH by its stimulatory effect on levocystine arylamidase, an enzyme that destroys GnRH. Given that this enzyme is activated by estrogen, it is not present in high concentrations in postmenopausal women, in whom gonadotropin secretion therefore continues to rise.

HYPOTHALAMIC FEEDBACK. GnRH can desensitize its own receptors on the pituitary gonadotropic membrane. An abrupt decrease in pituitary GnRH receptor content occurs coincidentally with the ovulatory surge of gonadotropins. Evidence suggests that there is a preovulatory increase in GnRH in portal blood and peripheral plasma, which increase could promote the rapid decline in receptor concentration observed at midcycle by inducing an acute down-regulation of its own pituitary receptor.

ENDORPHINS. Endorphins also appear to modulate GnRH secretion. The infusion of naloxone, an opiate (endorphin)-receptor antagonist, during the luteal but not the early follicular phase of the menstrual cycle raises both the frequency and the amplitude of pulsatile LH levels, apparently as a result of an increase in GnRH secretion. The direct intravenous injection of β-endorphin during the early follicular phase promptly elevates prolactin levels and leads to an eventual decline in LH concentrations. Thus, the response of gonadotropin to the administration of an opiate-receptor antagonist varies with the phase of the cycle. These observations suggest that endogenous opiate peptide may inhibit GnRH neuronal activity directly or indirectly through suppression of noradrenergic neurons. Alternatively, endorphins may affect gonadotropin secretion through their action on dopaminergic neurons. A reduction in dopaminergic activity might initially stop the inhibition of GnRH secretion while stimulating the secretion of prolactin, thus prompting a rebound increase in dopamine release and suppression of GnRH. Indeed, a transient increase in LH content has been observed before the eventual decline after β-endorphin injection. In any event, endorphins affect both prolactin and gonadotropin secretion.

Hypothalamic Hormones

The hypothalamus synthesizes and releases a number of peptide hormones that control the release of anterior pituitary trophic hormones. The hypothalamic factor that is responsible for the control of anterior pituitary gonadotropin synthesis and release has been isolated in animals and identified as a decapeptide (Fig. 6-4), synthesized, and designated GnRH. It has also been called *luteinizing hormone-releasing hormone (LHRH), luteinizing-releasing hormone (LRH),* and *lubibern.* GnRH is not species specific. As stated, its release is

$$\text{Pyro} \atop \text{Glu} - \text{His} - \text{Trp} - \text{Ser} - \text{Tyr} - \text{Gly} - \text{Leu} - \text{Arg} - \text{Pro} - \text{Gly} - \text{CONH}_2$$

FIG. 6-4. Structure of the decapeptide gonadotropin-releasing hormone.

pulsatile, occurring every 60 to 120 minutes, and is dependent on catecholamine stimulation. The half-life of GnRH is between 2 and 4 minutes.

As mentioned earlier in this chapter, GnRH is associated with the synthesis and release of LH and, to a lesser degree, FSH. The release effect of GnRH reaches a maximum at 30 minutes and is associated with calcium ions. GnRH induces the synthesis of the carbohydrate fractions of the gonadotropic glycoproteins, therefore stimulating gluconeogenesis rather than protein synthesis. This synthetic function, which is associated with the accumulation of cyclic adenosine monophosphate, requires 2 to 8 hours for initiation and maximal response on the gonadotropic cell membrane.

In addition to isolating GnRH, recent experiments in the rat have identified an undecapeptide that is synthesized in the neurons of the suprachiasmatic nucleus and that inhibits the action of GnRH on pituitary gonadotropin release in animals under estrogen stimulation. This peptide has been called *substance P.* It has been postulated that substance P stabilizes the gonadotropic cell membrane and is itself inhibited by estrogen.

The hypothalamus contains two hormone carrier peptides: estrogen-sensitive neurophysin, which carries GnRH through the pituitary portal system, and nicotine-sensitive neurophysin, which is the carrier protein for oxytocin and vasopressin. A third group of hypothalamic peptides from the amino precursor uptake and decarboxylation series has also been identified; its functions are less well understood.

Pituitary Gland

The pituitary gland as an isolated unit has little, if any, reproductive function. It is dependent on hypothalamic input, and the resultant output by the gonadotropes is determined by the frequency and magnitude of the hypothalamic stimulus. The cyclicity of pituitary gonadotropin secretion is modulated largely by the ovarian steroids by way of the long-loop feedback mechanism, as well as by the short-loop feedback of pituitary LH to the hypothalamus through countercurrent blood flow.

Pituitary Function

The major influence of the two pituitary gonadotropins, FSH and LH, is on the ova-containing follicles within the ovary. FSH stimulates the ovarian granulosa cells to synthesize estrogen receptors. Estrogen receptor interaction promotes replication of granulosa cells; stimulates aromatase enzyme activity, thereby increasing estrogen synthesis; stimulates the secretion of muco-polysaccharides (glycosaminoglycans), the ground substances for the follicular fluid, the basement membrane of the follicle, and the zona pellucida of the oocyte; stimulates the production of a protein hormone inhibitor that regulates FSH feedback; and stimulates the formation of LH receptors on both the granulosa and the theca cells. Thus, in the female, in contrast to the male, LH action is dependent on prior FSH stimulation.

When FSH stimulation has induced the production of LH receptors, steroidogenesis is activated by LH stimulation. Androgen is synthesized by theca cells and converted to estrogen by granulosa cells. Estrogen triggers the LH surge, which in turn affects luteinization of the granulosa cells, production of progesterone, and formation of the corpus luteum. The 14-day luteal span is maintained by minimal stimulation of LH. In addition to initiating and maintaining the production of progesterone by the corpus luteum, the LH surge may be important in the maturation of oocytes and the completion of meiosis.

An understanding of the coordination of gonadotropin secretion with events in the ovary is essential to elucidation of the mechanism of cyclic pituitary function (Fig. 6-1). An estrogen peak precedes the LH surge by 24 hours. After an initial stimulatory phase associated with the LH surge, a desensitization of LH receptors occurs. This "down-regulation" results in a refractory stage during which there is diminished steroidogenesis, lack of cyclic adenosine monophosphate accumulation, and a decrease in both the number and the sensitivity of LH receptors. This desensitization process is necessary for ovulation, which is inhibited by high levels of cyclic AMP; it also explains the decreased synthesis of estrogen after the LH surge (see Fig. 6-1).

Thus, the pituitary's role in the reproductive process is to synthesize and release FSH and LH. FSH rescues the ovarian follicle from atresia and promotes follicular growth and maturation. LH induces ovulation, maturation of oocytes, and luteinization of the follicle.

Control of Pituitary Function

The pituitary secretion of both FSH and LH requires the activation and stimulation of the pulsatile release of GnRH. In the fetal pituitary, before development of the hypophysiotropic portal system, the primitive gonadotrope secretes FSH and prolactin. When these primitive gonadotropic cells are studied in culture, they respond to the addition of GnRH by release of FSH only. After the establishment of the portal system, fetal gonadotropes secrete LH as well as FSH. Still, more FSH than LH is released in response to the addition of GnRH. Thus, the gonadotrope seems to induce FSH synthesis and release, while LH production appears to depend on hypothalamic hormonal stimulation.

Like GnRH, FSH and LH are secreted in pulsatile fashion. The initiation of the pulsatile pattern of gonad-otropin secretion occurs at puberty, with nighttime elevations in LH level. After puberty pulsatile secretion is maintained throughout the 24-hour period but varies in both amplitude and frequency. The pulsatile secretion of gonadotropins is due to the pulsatile release of GnRH into the portal system. Once released into the portal circulation, the gonadotropins increase in concentration in the hypothalamus through retrograde portal blood flow. The pronounced increase in gonadotropin concentration in the hypothalamus terminates the secretion of GnRH from peptidergic neurons and thus serves the short-loop feedback system for the release of GnRH. Thus, the ontogenetic sequence for the appearance of FSH and LH appears to be determined by GnRH, but ovarian steroids and inhibin also have roles in modulating the secretion of FSH and LH by the gonadotrope.

Modulation of Pituitary Function

The activity of the pituitary gonadotropes at any given time is determined by the control of direct input by GnRH and by the modulation of feedback impact by ovarian factors.

ESTROGEN EFFECTS. Variation in the amount of prior exposure to estrogen influences the pituitary response to any given dose of GnRH. With increasing amounts of circulating gonadal steroids, especially estradiol, there is preferential inhibition of the release of FSH and paradoxic augmentation of the secretion of LH. This differential action of estrogen on the release of FSH and LH is consistent with the reduction of the FSH:LH ratio during sexual maturation and the initiation of the menstrual cycle. When exposed to increasing levels of estradiol in a manner similar to that observed during the late follicular phase, the pituitary gland responds to a GnRH challenge with a prolonged and augmented pattern of gonadotropin release. In contrast, short-term exposure to preovulatory levels of estradiol blunts the response of the pituitary gland to a bolus of GnRH. Low levels of estradiol have no effect on pituitary sensitivity to GnRH, whereas higher concentrations given for the same amount of time augment GnRH-induced release of gonadotropin.

It has been proposed that estradiol may modulate pituitary sensitivity to GnRH and subsequent gonadotropin secretion by altering the GnRH receptor content of the gonadotrope. However, pituitary responsiveness to GnRH does not always reflect the GnRH concentration of tissue receptor. During estrogen priming, the content of the GnRH receptor increases steadily with increasing duration of estrogen exposure, and GnRH-induced release of LH is initially suppressed. Pituitary responsiveness to a GnRH challenge is positively correlated with receptor concentrations only when there is positive estrogen feedback. These findings suggest that, although the positive feedback mechanisms may involve an increase in GnRH receptor concentration, the negative component of estrogen feedback operates through a different mechanism.

Controversy exists as to the sites at which estradiol exerts its feedback effects to modulate the release of gonadotropins. There is evidence that, in addition to having an inhibitory effect at the level of the hypothalamus, estrogen can modulate the secretion of gonadotropin at the level of the pituitary gonadotrope. Autoradiographic studies have revealed estrogen receptors in the anterior pituitary gland. When infused directly into the pituitary gland, estradiol decreases the responsiveness of gonadotropins to GnRH stimulation. However, the most convincing evidence in support of the idea that estrogen acts on the pituitary comes from experiments performed on castrated monkeys with hypothalamic lesions. The secretion of endogenous GnRH was eliminated in these animals and gonadotropin secretion then reestablished by a pulsatile infusion of GnRH. Neither the positive nor the negative feedback effects of estrogen administration were affected as a result. Surges of estrogen-induced gonadotropin have been observed before and after pituitary stalk sectioning and placement of a Silastic barrier between the severed ends. On the basis of these observations, it has been suggested that GnRH has only a permissive, although obligatory, role in the control of gonadotropin secretion and that feedback modulation of gonadal steroids, acting directly on the pituitary gland, produces the cyclic pattern of gonadotropin secretion observed in the menstrual cycle.

The idea that the hypothalamus exerts only a passive influence on gonadotropin secretion has been based on the assumption that the experimental designs employed eliminated any hypothalamic input. However, questions have been raised about the completeness of separation of the hypothalamus and pituitary, and Silastic barriers have been shown to be permeable to GnRH. Results of various experiments are consistent with the view that a "specific hypothalamic message" may be required for the preovulatory gonadotropin surge.

Other recent experiments by Kerdelhué and coworkers and by Vijayan and McCann indicate that substance P inhibits the action of GnRH on pituitary LH and FSH release in animals under estrogen stimulation. It has been proposed that substance P is inhibited by estrogen and stabilizes the gonadotropin cell membrane. A working hypothesis is that, in the absence of a high-estrogen environment, the gonadotropic membrane is stable and the gonadotrope accumulates both FSH and LH. As the estrogen level increases and the critical level of estrogen exposure is attained, the membrane stabilizer is inhibited, the now permeable gonadotropic membrane releases its accumulated LH, and the preovulatory LH surge occurs. Thus, positive estrogen feedback is believed to be the result of an inhibition of an inhibition, representing a double-negative effect. This positive estrogen feedback effect depends on the critical stimulation of estrogen over an exposure period of from 36 to 75 hours. Such a time lag, in combination with the finding that the effect of estradiol in pituitary cell cultures is to stimulate cell synthesis but not release of LH, argues against the idea that estrogen exerts a direct effect on the pituitary.

PROGESTERONE EFFECTS. The feedback actions of progesterone also appear to be directed at the pituitary gland as well as at the hypothalamus. Progesterone, at low levels and in the presence of estrogen, augments the pituitary secretion of LH and elicits a surge of FSH in response to GnRH stimulation. Administration of luteal levels of progesterone during the follicular phase does not prevent estrogen-induced surges of gonadotropin on pulsatile GnRH replacement in monkeys with arcuate lesions. In intact animals, injection of estrogen fails to produce the acute release of gonadotropin; in contrast, the ability of progesterone to augment an estrogen-induced release of gonadotropin remains intact. Thus, it appears that progesterone may inhibit gonadotropin release at the hypothalamic level and facilitate the midcycle surge through action at the pituitary level.

ANDROGEN EFFECTS. Testosterone may act preferentially in the potentiation of GnRH-mediated release of FSH. Testosterone added to pituitary cells in culture inhibits GnRH-mediated release of LH but potentiates GnRH-mediated release of FSH. This finding indicates that testosterone has a direct feedback effect on the pituitary gland, independent of the aromatization process and the effect of estrogen.

INHIBIN. The effect of ovarian factors, other than steroids, on the differential feedback regulation of FSH and LH release should be considered. A nonsteroidal testicular factor has been shown selectively to inhibit the secretion of FSH without affecting the release of LH. This factor, called *inhibin*, has recently been demonstrated to be present in follicular fluid. Follicular inhibin may exert its effect at the pituitary level, selectively inhibiting the secretion of FSH.

Pituitary Hormones

Both FSH and LH have been isolated from human material and characterized as glycoproteins, each with a molecular weight of about 30,000. The amino acid composition and carbohydrate content have been described for both gonadotropins, and partial degradation studies have revealed the essential role played by the sugar moieties attached to the protein.

FSH and LH can be isolated from the human pituitary gland, since the gonadotropins do not autolyze at death. In addition, high levels of gonadotropin excreted in the urine of postmenopausal women (owing to lack of the negative feedback mechanism) can also be extracted and purified for human use.

FSH and LH are available for patients who do not ovulate spontaneously as a result of pituitary or hypothalamic defects. When FSH and LH are administered in a pattern approximating the normal cycle, follicular development occurs and ovulation can be induced by injection of a "surge" level of either LH or human chorionic gonadotropin, an LH-like hormone produced by the placenta. Such treatment occasionally results in multiple ovulation.

Although a specific luteotropic hormone that maintains the corpus luteum has been described in certain animals, such a hormone has not been described in human or primate reproduction. In humans LH itself appears to exert this luteotropic action. The role of prolactin in control of the human cycle remains to be determined. Patterns of LH secretion during the midcycle surge, as determined by radioimmunoassay and bioassay, are different from those at other times, suggesting that the LH released at midcycle may be a more biologically active molecule than that secreted at other times in the cycle. It has been suggested that the feedback effects of gonadal steroids may include modulation of sialylation and subsequent size and activity of the gonadotropins released.

CYCLIC OVARIAN FUNCTION

The monthly release of oocytes from the ovary is the result of the cyclic secretion of gonadotropins, which requires hourly hypothalamic stimulation. However, the major controller of gonadotropic cyclicity is ovarian estrogen. Evidence has been presented that ovarian hormones not only provide feedback signals to the hypothalamic–pituitary complex but also operate as a local feedback system performing critical control functions within the ovary.

Local Feedback

Cyclic ovarian hormones are produced as a consequence of follicular maturation. The ovulatory cycle of steroid production can be described in three phases: the follicular phase, ovulation, and the luteal phase.

Follicular Phase

During the follicular phase of the ovulatory cycle, which occurs over a 10- to 14-day period of primordial follicle growth, differentiation of the primary, secondary, and tertiary follicles occurs. In addition to the morphologic changes described in Chapter 4, each of these events is associated with endocrinologic manifestations that are responsible for the cyclicity of the ovarian cycle.

The event that triggers the initial growth of the primordial follicle is not known, but it does not appear to be dependent on gonadotropins, since gonadotropin receptors are not present in the granulosa cells of the primordial follicle and the follicle can achieve growth and differentiate into a primary follicle without pituitary support. Once follicular growth is initiated, the granulosa cells begin to proliferate and the primordial follicle differentiates into a primary follicle. Whereas the granulosa cells of the primordial follicle do not possess receptors for FSH, the cell membrane of the primary follicle does. The interaction of FSH and its receptor exerts a mitogenic effect on granulosa cells, stimulates the proliferation of granulosa cells, increases the concentration of its own receptor on granulosa cells, and induces the aromatase enzyme system. The aromatase enzyme system, which converts androgens to estrogens, appears to limit ovarian estrogen production. Thus, the more FSH there is, the more FSH receptor there is; the more FSH-receptor-induced activity there is, the more aromatase activity there is; and the more aromatase activity there is, the more estrogens are produced. An estrogenic microenvironment is necessary for follicular growth.

Estrogen combines with its receptor to stimulate mitosis and the proliferation of granulosa cells as well as to increase the synthesis of FSH receptor; the more estrogen there is, the more FSH receptor is produced. Together, FSH and estrogen promote the rapid accumulation of FSH receptor, which results in both an increase in the number of granulosa cells and a change in the receptor density of individual cells.

In addition to estrogen receptors, specific androgen receptors have been identified in the cytoplasm of granulosa cells. The actions of androgen within the granulosa cell are divergent. At low concentrations androgens enhance aromatase activity; at high levels they cause the follicles to become atresic. Enhancement of the activity of aromatase due to low levels of androgens can be blocked by prevention of translocation of the androgen receptor complex from the cytoplasm to the nucleus. Although androgens at low levels serve as a substrate for FSH-induced aromatization, they do not do so when present at high levels in granulosa cells from primary follicles; under these conditions androstenedione is converted to 5α-reductase, which reduces androgens, making them unable to convert to estrogens and perhaps inhibiting aromatase activity. Thus, the role of androgens in early follicular development is complex, and the fate of the primary follicle is dependent on its hormonal environment.

As the granulosa cells undergo proliferation, the theca layer begins to organize from the surrounding stroma. Whereas FSH receptors are detectable only on granulosa cells, LH receptors are present on theca cells at all stages of follicular development. The major product of theca cells is androstenedione. *In vitro* studies of both isolated and recombined granulosa and theca tissues have demonstrated a cooperative effect in estrogen production and have led to the two-cell theory of ovarian steroidogenesis: in response to LH, theca tissue is stimulated to produce androgens; these androgens are then converted to estrogens by the granulosa cells through FSH-induced aromatization. Early in follicular growth, limited development of the theca layer may minimize the amount of androgen available to be preferentially converted by 5α-reductase to more potent androgen, thus diminishing atresia. It is believed that follicles will develop only if growth begins when FSH content is high and LH level is low.

Follicular fluid is produced and accumulates in the intercellular spaces of the granulosa layer under the influence of estrogen and FSH. Eventually, the fluid coalesces to form a cavity or antrum, producing a secondary follicle called an *antral follicle*. In addition to producing follicular fluid, the granulosa cells of the secondary follicle demonstrate LH, prolactin, and prostaglandin receptors. Because each fluid-filled antrum is separate from other antra, each follicle resides in its own unique hormonal microenvironment. The follicular fluid contains the protein hormone inhibin, which is probably produced by the granulosa cells and which suppresses the production of FSH preferentially over that of LH. Neither FSH nor LH is detectable in follicular fluid unless gonadotropin levels are elevated in plasma. The steroids present in antral fluid reflect the activity of the surrounding granulosa and theca cells and can be found in much higher concentrations here than in plasma. Secondary follicles with the highest estrogen concentrations and lowest androgen:estrogen ratios display the greatest rates of granulosa cell proliferation and are most likely to contain maturing oocytes. As intrafollicular androgen levels increase, degenerative changes in the oocytes and follicular atresia ensue. Thus, follicular growth and maturation depend on the presence in follicular fluid of estrogen produced by FSH-induced aromatization. Such interaction between estrogen and FSH may also play a role in the selection of the follicle destined to ovulate.

Selection of an ovulable follicle is at least a two-step process. First, a follicle growing in the presence of gonadotropins is "recruited" from a pool of cohorts and, when exposed to sufficient gonadotropic stimulation, may progress to ovulation. Second, a number of growing follicles are chosen by the process called *selection* to continue their maturation, their ultimate destiny being ovulation rather than atresia.

Asymmetric ovarian function is inherent to maturation of the selected (dominant) follicle. The dominant follicle dictates the course of events in the ovaries, both temporally and spatially, for the duration of the cycle. Asymmetry in ovarian estrogen production, presumably an expression of the emerging dominant follicle, can be detected in ovarian venous effluent as early as cycle days 5 to 7. Exogenous estrogen administered after selection of the dominant follicle disrupts preovulatory development and induces atresia. By cycle day 7, after removal of the dominant follicle, no follicles still retain the ability to respond to exogenously administered gonadotropins. Similarly, if the dominant follicle is ablated by cauterization, the expected midcycle surges of estradiol and LH are abolished. The next preovulatory surges appear 12 to 14 days after cautery, which time interval approximates the length of a typical follicular phase.

Thus, it appears that no other follicle can substitute for the cauterized follicle to accommodate an ovulation during that cycle; instead, the next follicle to ovulate is the product of a new cohort of follicles that develops after cautery. It also appears that the dominant follicle inhibits follicular growth at the level of the ovaries. When steroid hormone concentrations in ovarian venous effluents are compared, the intraovarian progesterone level emerges as the most likely local regulator of folliculogenesis during recruitment and selection of the dominant follicle in the ovarian cycle. Progesterone displays antifollicular action at the ovarian level.

Secondary follicles with the highest concentration of estrogen in their follicular fluid display the greatest rates of granulosa cell proliferation. A high rate of granulosa cell proliferation gives the dominant follicle the advantage of great FSH receptor content. As a result, the stimulus for aromatization increases and the selected follicle develops a capacity for estrogen production exceeding that of the other follicles. The large mass of granulosa cells is accompanied by advanced development of the vasculature within the theca interna, allowing amplified exposure of FSH to its receptor. These events may account for the ability of the dominant follicle to continue to grow despite increases in intraovarian progesterone concentrations.

In addition to stimulating aromatization and proliferation of granulosa cells, FSH induces LH receptors on the granulosa cells of secondary follicles. Estrogen controls the rate of appearance of LH receptor; accelerated estrogen production by the dominant follicle promotes further induction of LH receptor. The secondary follicle acquires receptor activity other than LH receptor. FSH induces specific prolactin receptors on granulosa cells. Prolactin concentrations within follicular fluid progressively decrease during folliculogenesis and are lowest in the preovulatory cycle. What influence prolactin exerts at the ovarian level during folliculogenesis remains unclear. High concentrations of prolactin in tissue cultures of granulosa cells decrease progesterone production by these cells. The appearance of prostaglandin receptors is the final event in the differentiation of the secondary follicle.

During the preovulatory stage, the granulosa cells of the tertiary follicle enlarge and acquire lipid inclusions. These cells, which are associated with the increasing production of steroid hormones, preferentially metabolize androgens to estrogens; in contrast, granulosa cells in primary follicles exhibit a tendency *in vitro* to convert androgens from the theca layer to the more potent 5α reduced form. Serum estrogen concentrations increase rapidly, with peak levels occurring approximately 24 to 36 hours before ovulation. An increase in progesterone production can be detected in the venous effluent on the ovary containing the tertiary follicle 24 to 48 hours before ovulation, and a significant increase in circulating levels of progesterone occurs 12 to 24 hours before ovulation.

Reduction of the mitotic index and atresia of granulosa cells are observed when preantral granulosa cells are placed in an androgen-rich environment *in vitro*. As androgen levels increase within follicular fluid, degenerative changes within the follicle become more apparent. Thus, whereas an estrogenic environment within the follicle stimulates proliferation of granulosa cells, responsiveness of FSH, and aromatization, an androgenic milieu antagonizes estrogen-induced granulosa cell proliferation and ultimately leads to degenerative changes in the oocyte. Granulosa cells of the primary and early secondary follicles exhibit an *in vitro* tendency to convert androgens to the more potent 5α reduced form. Consequently, the relative balance between the enzymatic activities of aromatase and reductase early in follicular development determines whether that follicle will generate an estrogenic environment and grow or generate an androgenic milieu and become atretic.

Ovulation

The tertiary follicle initiates its own ovulatory stimulus through the increasing elaboration of estradiol, which triggers an LH surge from the anterior pituitary gland. Ovulation occurs approximately 10 to 12 hours after the LH peak. The LH surge appears to be necessary for completion of the first meiotic division and initiation of the second meiotic division in the oocyte, luteinization of granulosa cells, and synthesis of prostaglandins—events essential for follicular rupture. The preovulatory LH surge and the consequent production of progesterone and prostaglandin also affect the mechanism of ovulation.

Luteal Phase

After ovulation the granulosa cells that have been left behind in the ruptured follicle enlarge and accumulate lipid. The size and number of lipid droplets in luteal cells accurately reflect the level of progesterone production throughout the luteal phase. Progesterone production, which is dependent on the actions of several hormones, including LH, human chorionic gonadotropin, and prolactin, is thus a measure of the functional capacity of the corpus luteum.

LUTEINIZATION OF THE CORPUS LUTEUM. Continuous tonic levels of LH are necessary for corpus luteum function. When LH engages its receptor on the membrane of the luteal cell, cyclic adenosine monophosphate is activated; this stimulates the cleavage of cholesterol from its ester, making it available for mitochondrial conversion to pregnenolone, which in turn is metabolized to progesterone. In addition, progesterone production appears to be dependent on circulating levels of low-density lipoprotein as a source of cholesterol. The lack of availability of low-density lipoprotein–cholesterol in the avascular granulosa cell has been suggested as the factor that limits the synthesis of progesterone in the preovulatory follicle. After ovulation vascularization of the corpus luteum allows low-density

lipoprotein–cholesterol to reach the luteinized granulosa cell and be used in progesterone biosynthesis. Levels of progesterone normally increase sharply after ovulation, peaking approximately eight days after the LH surge (see Fig. 6-1).

A local function of progesterone is to suppress new follicle growth. If luteectomy is performed follicular growth resumes, but there is an interval between luteectomy and the next LH surge of the same duration as that between cautery of the dominant follicle and ovulation, indicating that interruption of dominance during either phase of the cycle is followed by essentially the same response. Further, progesterone alone administered exogenously after luteectomy inhibits the growth of new follicles and delays the next ovulation. When ovarian vein effluents are monitored for progesterone levels after removal of the corpus luteum, there is greater secretion of progesterone from the luteectomized ovary than from the contralateral ovary. However, this difference is apparent for only one day after luteectomy. Thus, the luteectomized ovary is not at a clear disadvantage compared with the contralateral ovary with respect to new follicle growth. If only one ovary exists, intraovarian progesterone levels decrease rapidly enough to allow a subsequent cycle. In monkeys the side of ovulation is neither completely random nor reliably alternating; ovulation occurs in alternating ovaries about 70% of the time.

LH cannot extend the luteal phase with progressively increasing LH exposure. Unless pregnancy intervenes, degeneration of the corpus luteum is inevitable. Chorionic gonadotropin, the only luteotropin known in humans, maintains luteal function until placental steroidogenesis is well established. Luteectomy usually induces abortion in humans if carried out before seven weeks' gestation. Human chorionic gonadotropin binds to LH receptor and significantly augments progesterone production. In addition, human chorionic gonadotropin inhibits prostaglandin synthesis. After 8 to 10 weeks of gestation, the corpus luteum becomes refractory to the trophic effects of human chorionic gonadotropin. This refractoriness is believed to be due to prolonged exposure to high concentrations of chorionic gonadotropin, leading to down-regulation of LH–gonadotropin receptors. Only the corpus luteum appears to be unresponsive to trophic hormone stimulation, as evidenced by the fact that ovulation can be induced with exogenously administered gonadotropins during pregnancy. Some evidence suggests that the corpus luteum becomes activated again late in gestation. Reactivation of the corpus luteum appears to be independent of pituitary influence but may require placental support.

The role of prolactin as a luteotropic agent in humans is not clear. Specific binding sites for prolactin are present in luteal tissue. Evidence from tissue culture experiments suggests that prolactin at physiologic concentrations permits luteal function. The level of progesterone produced by human granulosa cells maintained in culture is significantly reduced when prolactin present in the culture medium is neutralized with specific antiserum. When present at higher concentrations, prolactin may inhibit the synthesis of progesterone.

LUTEOLYSIS OF THE CORPUS LUTEUM. After reaching a peak about eight days after the LH surge, progesterone levels gradually return to basal values. As the corpus luteum becomes progressively less sensitive to LH stimulation, LH receptor binding decreases, paralleling the secretion pattern for progesterone. The mechanism of decrease in LH receptor binding is unclear but is known to be associated with a nonsteroidal LH receptor binding inhibitor, estradiol, and prostaglandins.

Once formed, the corpus luteum regresses by the luteolytic action of its own estrogen production. This luteolytic action is mediated by an alteration in local concentrations of prostaglandin. As the corpus luteum undergoes luteolysis, the production of progesterone decreases, permitting new follicular growth, and circulating levels of estrogen decline, allowing an increase in FSH. With increasing concentrations of FSH, the next cycle is initiated. The coordination of this system involves the transmission of messages by ovarian hormones, allowing interplay between the ovarian follicle and its neuroendocrinologic controls in the brain.

Ovarian Effects on Neuroendocrines

Once the hypothalamic–pituitary unit assumes the operative state characterized by the hourly pulsatile secretion of GnRH, the ovaries, facilitated by the dominant follicle, dictate the course of events that result in the monthly ovarian cycle. The 28-day menstrual cycle is not determined by independent events in the hypothalamus or pituitary gland but rather by the ovaries. As follicles are recruited and a dominant follicle is selected within the ovary, ovarian steroids are secreted into the circulation and provide feedback at the level of the hypothalamus–pituitary unit.

Follicular Phase

The beginning of the menstrual cycle is initiated by an increase in FSH level, which occurs in response to the decline in estradiol content in the preceding luteal phase. Peripheral levels of estradiol begin to increase significantly by cycle day 7, shortly after the dominant follicle has been selected. Estradiol maintains follicular sensitivity to FSH by increasing the follicle's content of FSH receptor. Derived primarily from the dominant follicle, estradiol levels increase steadily and, through negative feedback at both the hypothalamic and pituitary levels, exert an increasingly suppressive influence on FSH release. While causing a decline in FSH levels, the midfollicular increase in estradiol level exerts a positive influence on the release of LH. As the dominant follicle emerges, the increasing production of estrogen initiates

a shift from suppression to stimulation of LH release. LH levels increase steadily during the late follicular phase, stimulating the production of androgen in the theca layer. FSH-induced aromatization allows androgen to be used as a substrate by the granulosa cells to further accelerate the production of estrogen. At high local concentrations, estradiol enhances the follicular response to LH by working synergistically with FSH to induce the LH receptors on granulosa cells. As the LH levels increase, the granulosa cells begin to secrete progesterone into the bloodstream. The process of luteinization is inhibited by the presence of the oocyte; this suppresses progesterone secretion, ensuring that only low levels of progesterone reach the pituitary gland. Low levels of progesterone in the presence of estrogen augments the pituitary secretion of LH.

Ovulation

Enough estrogen is produced in the preovulatory follicle to achieve and maintain peripheral threshold concentrations to induce the LH surge at both the hypothalamic and pituitary levels. The preovulatory increase in progesterone facilitates the positive feedback action of estrogen and elicits the FSH surge in response to GnRH. With the LH surge, levels of progesterone in the preovulatory follicle continue to increase up to the time of ovulation. The progressive increase in progesterone levels during the periovulatory period may act to terminate the LH surge, since negative feedback is exerted at high concentrations. The LH surge stimulates completion of the reduction division in the oocyte, the luteinization of the granulosa cells, and the synthesis of progesterone and prostaglandins. The progesterone-dependent midcycle increase in FSH serves to free the oocyte from follicular attachments and induce sufficient LH receptors to ensure adequate progesterone production in the subsequent luteal phase.

Luteal Phase

After ovulation, luteinization is accompanied by a large increase in progesterone levels which, in the presence of estrogen, exert strong negative feedback to suppress the secretion of gonadotropin. This action of progesterone occurs at the hypothalamic level to decrease GnRH secretion and at the pituitary level to suppress response to GnRH stimulation. During the luteal phase of the cycle, the pulse frequency of gonadotropins decreases from every 60 to 90 minutes to every 3 to 4 hours. As the corpus luteum regresses, circulating levels of ovarian steroids diminish, causing a central negative feedback effect. FSH levels then increase and rescue the next cohort of developing follicles.

In summary, the gonadal steroids appear to exert their feedback effects directly on both the pituitary and the hypothalamus through modulation of the pulsatile pattern of GnRH secretion. They may also influence the degree of sialylation and subsequent biologic activity of the gonadotropins.

Ovarian Hormones

The ovary secretes three general classes of steroid hormones: estrogens, androgens, and progestins. All steroid hormones have a common carbon ring structure, the fundamental differences among them being the number of carbon atoms present and the substituents attached. In the numbering sequence illustrated in Figure 6-5, estrogens have 18 carbons, androgens 19 carbons, and progestins 21 carbons (consisting essentially of a 19-carbon androgen molecule with a 2-carbon side chain attached to carbon 17).

Biosynthesis of Ovarian Steroids

The parent compound from which all steroid hormones can be derived is cholesterol, which has a carbon structure identical to that of the steroid hormones but with a longer side chain. Cleavage of a portion of this side chain in endocrine tissue results in the formation of pregnenolone, the immediate precursor of progesterone (Fig. 6-6). All steroid hormones, as well as cholesterol, are ultimately derived from the simple 2-carbon compound acetate. The cholesterol side chain is partially split off to form the C-21 compound pregnenolone, which is readily converted to progesterone by oxidation of the hydroxyl group at position 3 and rearrangement of the double bond. The C-21 compounds, progesterone and pregnenolone, are converted to androgens by the complete removal of the side chain to form the C-19 series; finally, the C-19 androgens are aromatized to form estrogens.

Estrogen biosynthesis entails the following sequential steps: (1) acetate to cholesterol; (2) cholesterol to pregnenolone; (3) pregnenolone to progesterone or, bypassing progesterone, to 17-hydroxypregnenolone; (4) progesterone to 17-hydroxyprogesterone and then to androstenedione and testosterone, or 17-hydroxypregnenolone to dehydroepiandrosterone and then to androstenedione and testosterone; and (5) testosterone to estradiol, or androstenedione to estrone.

FIG. 6-5. Cyclopentenophenanthrene ring system. Each ring is identified by a letter from *A* to *D*. Carbon atoms are numbered in the sequence shown.

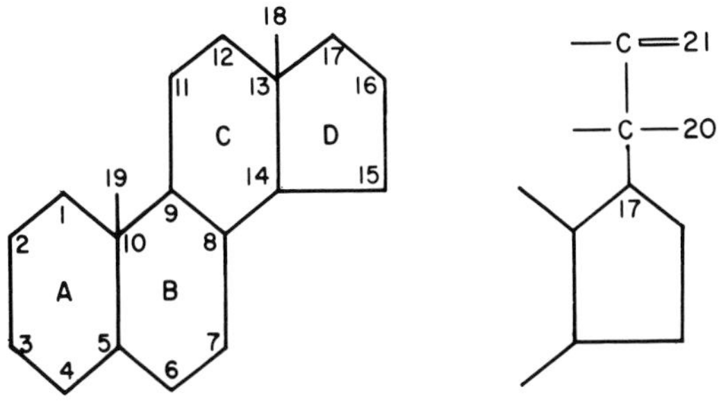

Metabolism of Ovarian Steroids

Estradiol is readily converted to estrone by peripheral tissue and thence to estriol in the liver. In addition, modifications in the orientation of the substituents at carbons 17 and 16 result in as many as four stereoisomeric forms of estriol. Estriol or its epimers may also be oxidized at position 16 or 17 to form five ketolic steroids. Any of the estrogens may also be hydroxylated at carbons 2, 6, 11, and 16, resulting in a myriad of metabolites. Most of these metabolic products do not have biologic activity, and their biologic function, if any, is unknown. At present they are used simply as a measure of estrogen catabolism.

Progesterone is metabolized by reduction of the double bond in ring A and total or partial reduction of the keto groups at positions 3 and 20. These reactions lead to several stereoisomeric forms of pregnanediols and pregnenolones. The compound usually measured in urine as pregnanediol (5-pregnane-3,20-diol) represents only about 20% of the progesterone metabolites, but it suffices as a guide to the extent of progesterone secretion. The 20-keto group of progesterone may be reduced to form a compound (20-hydroxy-4-pregnen-3-one) with some progestational activity, but most metabolites are devoid of recognizable hormone function. Progesterone may also be hydroxylated at position 17, producing a metabolite that ultimately gives rise to the pregnanetriols found in the urine during the ovarian cycle and in pregnancy.

Androgen metabolism consists essentially of reduction of the ring-A double bond. Although various isomers are possible, the major excretory products are the 17-ketosteroids, androsterone, and etiocholanolone. Given that dehydroepiandrosterone and testosterone give rise to androstenedione, the metabolites for all three are similar. The major portion of the 17-ketosteroids in urine is derived from adrenal, not ovarian, precursors. As noted earlier, androgens also can be converted to the potent metabolites dihydrotestosterone and estrogens.

Progesterone, estrogen, and androgen metabolites are usually conjugated with either glucuronic or sulfuric acid, rendering them more water soluble. In addition, the parent hormone or metabolite can be bound in dissociable form to plasma proteins that influence both blood levels and clearance from the body. The hormonal metabolites may also find their way into the biliary system, from which they are excreted into the intestinal tract for either elimination or reabsorption into the bloodstream. The metabolism of both estrogens and progesterone is extremely rapid, occurring largely in the liver, although other peripheral tissues may also be involved.

Production Rates and Blood Levels of Ovarian Steroids

During the peak of the follicular phase and again in the midluteal phase, estradiol production has been

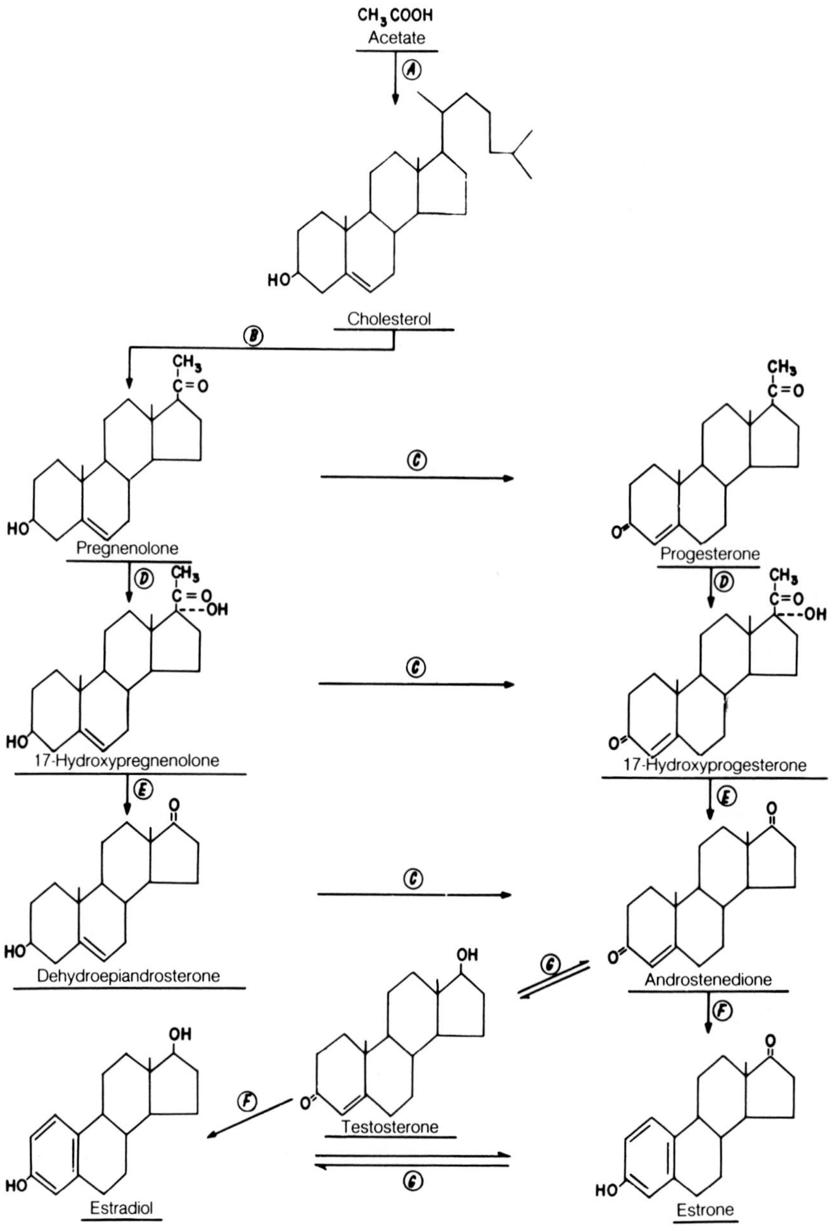

FIG. 6-6. Pathways for biosynthesis of ovarian hormones from acetate and cholesterol. Note alternate routes on *left* and *right* sides of diagram from pregnenolone or progesterone to androgens and estrogens. (Smith OW, Ryan KJ: Estrogen in the human ovary. Am J Obstet Gynecol 84:141–153, 1962)

estimated at 200 μg to 500 μg per day, with peripheral blood levels of 100 pg to 200 pg/ml.

Progesterone production is 3 mg per day in the follicular phase and 22 mg per day at the peak of the luteal phase. The plasma progesterone concentration is approximately 0.1 μg/dl when the corpus luteum is present.

The androstenedione level in blood is higher in the female than in the male, at a concentration of 0.1 μg/dl. The production rate of androstenedione is 3.4 mg per day; production of testosterone is one tenth that of androstenedione. The adrenal gland is the major source of these hormones.

REFERENCES AND RECOMMENDED READING

Adams TE, Norman RL, Spies HG: Gonadotropin-releasing hormone receptor binding and pituitary responsiveness in estradiol-primed monkeys. Science 213:1388–1390, 1981

Ball P, Knuppen R, Haupt M et al: Interactions between estrogens and catechol amines. III. Studies on the methylation of catechol estrogens, catecholamines and other catechols by the catechol-O-methyltransferase of human liver. J Clin Endocrinol Metab 34:736–746, 1972

Bolton RA, Coulam CB, Ryan RJ: Specific binding of human chorionic gonadotropin to human corpora lutea in the menstrual cycle. Obstet Gynecol 56:336–338, 1980

Carr BR, Sadler RK, Rochelle DB et al: Plasma lipoprotein regulation of progesterone biosynthesis by human corpus luteum tissue in organ culture. J Clin Endocrinol Metab 52:875–881, 1981

Clark JR, Dierschke DJ, Wolf RC: Hormonal regulation of ovarian folliculogenesis in rhesus monkeys. III. Atresia of the preovulatory follicle induced by exogenous steroids and subsequent follicular development. Biol Reprod 25:332–341, 1981

DiZerega GS, Marut EL, Turner CK et al: Asymmetrical ovarian function during recruitment and selection of the dominant follicle in the menstrual cycle of the rhesus monkey. J Clin Endocrinol Metab 51:698–701, 1980

Ferin M, Rosenblatt H, Carmel PW et al: Estrogen-induced gonadotropin surges in female rhesus monkeys after pituitary stalk section. Endocrinology 104:50–52, 1979

Fritz MA, Speroff L: The endocrinology of the menstrual cycle: The interaction of folliculogenesis and neuroendocrine mechanisms. Fertil Steril 38:509–529, 1982

Grant LD, Stumpf WE: Localization of ^{3}H-estradiol and catecholamines in identical neurons in the hypothalamus (abstract). J Histochem Cytochem 21:404, 1973

Hillier SG, De Zwart FA: Evidence that granulosa cell aromatase induction/activation by follicle-stimulating hormone is an androgen receptor-regulated process *in vitro*. Endocrinology 109:1303–1305, 1981

Hodgen GD: The dominant ovarian follicle. Fertil Steril 38:281–300, 1982

Kerdelhué B, Valens M, Langlois Y: Stimulation de la sécrétion de la LH et de la FSH hypophysaires après immunoneutralisation de la substance P endogène chez la Ratte cyclique (abstract). C R Acad Sci [D] (Paris) 286:977–999, 1978

Knobil E, Plant TM, Wildt L et al: Control of the rhesus monkey menstrual cycle: Permissive role of hypothalamic gonadotropin-releasing hormone. Science 207:1371–1373, 1980

Krieger DT, Liotta AS, Brownstein MJ et al: ACTH, β-lipotropin, and related peptides in brain, pituitary, and blood. Recent Prog Horm Res 36:277–344, 1980

Marut EL, Williams RF, Cowan BD et al: Pulsatile pituitary gonadotropin secretion during maturation of the dominant follicle in monkeys: Estrogen-positive feedback enhances the biological activity of LH. Endocrinology 109:2270–2272, 1981

McCann SM: Effect of progesterone on plasma luteinizing hormone activity. Am J Physiol 202:601–604, 1962

McNatty KP, Hunter WM, McNeilly AS et al: Changes in the concentration of pituitary and steroid hormones in the follicular fluid of human graafian follicles throughout the menstrual cycle. J Endocrinol 64:555–571, 1975

McNatty KP, Makris A, Reinhold VN et al: Metabolism of androstenedione by human ovarian tissues *in vitro* with particular reference to reductase and aromatase activity. Steroids 34:429–443, 1979

McNatty KP, Sawers RS, McNeilly AS: A possible role for prolactin in control of steroid secretion by the human graafian follicle. Nature 250:653–655, 1974

McNeill TH, Sladek JR Jr.: Fluorescence-immunocytochemistry: Simultaneous localization of catecholamines and gonadotropin-releasing hormone. Science 200:72–74, 1978

Quigley ME, Yen SSC: The role of endogenous opiates on LH secretion during the menstrual cycle. J Clin Endocrinol Metab 51:179–181, 1980

Richards JS, Midgley AR Jr.: Protein hormone action: A key to understanding ovarian follicular and luteal cell development. Biol Reprod 14:82–94, 1976

Ruf KB: How the brain controls the process of puberty. Z Neurol 204:95–105, 1973

Vijayan E, McCann SM: *In vivo* and *in vitro* effects of substance P and neurotensin on gonadotropin and prolactin release. Endocrinology 105:64–68, 1979

Yen SSC, Tsai CC, Vandenberg G et al: Gonadotropin dynamics in patients with gonadal dysgenesis: A model for the study of gonadotropin regulation. J Clin Endocrinol Metab 35:897–904, 1972

Other Aspects of the Endocrine Physiology of Reproduction

Edward E. Wallach
Alfred M. Bongiovanni
John R. Marshall

7

ADRENAL CORTEX

Biochemistry and Physiology

The adrenal cortex consists of three distinguishable zones and produces three distinct types of steroids. Each of the three zones functions as a separate endocrine structure. The outer zone, the *zona glomerulosa,* produces aldosterone, a mineralocorticoid that affects salt and water metabolism and in excess amounts can lead to sodium retention, potassium loss, and hypertension. The middle zone, the *zona fasciculata,* produces hydrocortisone. This glucocorticoid affects carbohydrate, protein, and lipid metabolism. The overall action of glucocorticoids is catabolic; however, in the liver glucocorticoid has an anabolic influence on gluconeogenesis. Hydrocortisone also suppresses the inflammatory reaction and the body's resistance to infection. The inner zone, the *zona reticularis,* produces sex steroids, predominantly androgens.

The biochemical pathways for adrenocortical hormones are illustrated in Fig. 7-1. Adrenocortical steroids are synthesized from either 2-carbon acetate molecules or from cholesterol, both of which can be extracted directly from the circulation. The metabolic pathway then proceeds through pregnenolone, the common precursor of all adrenal steroids. This rate-limiting step in steroid synthesis is accomplished through cleavage of the cholesterol side chain by way of 2-hydroxylating enzymes (20-hydroxylase, 22-hydroxylase) and a desmolase. Most of the biochemical reactions occur in the cellular mitochondria and microsomes. The enzyme systems present in each zone determine the specific steroids produced by that zone. The enzyme systems also differentiate steroid production in the adrenal cortex from that in the ovary and testis. The enzyme 17α-hydroxylase is contained in the zona fasciculata and zona reticularis, as well as in the ovary and testicle, but is deficient in the zona glomerulosa. 11β-Hydroxylase is found almost exclusively in the adrenal cortex and is present in all three zones. 18-Hydroxysteroid dehydrogenase is found only in the zona glomerulosa, which accounts for the exclusive production of aldosterone in that zone. A deficiency of any of these enzymes results in overabundance of precursor steroids and frequently produces elevated serum concentrations of steroids that can be diagnostic for the specific enzyme deficiency.

Adrenal control mechanisms play an essential role in the normal function of the adrenal cortex. Adrenocorticotropic hormone (ACTH) regulates cortisol production in the zona fasciculata by attaching to cell surface receptors and activating adenylate cyclase. The control mechanism for aldosterone is also through a negative feedback loop but is otherwise entirely different, involving the renin–angiotensin system. Control mechanisms for the androgenic steroids produced by the zona reticularis are poorly understood, but they may be regulated differently from the other two.

Corticotropin-releasing factor (CRF) is produced in the median eminence of the hypothalamus and ultimately released into the hypophyseal portal vascular system. CRF is a polypeptide that acts on the basophilic cells of the anterior pituitary to effect the release of ACTH, a 39-amino-acid polypeptide that acts on the adrenal cortex to effect the production and release of cortisol. A negative feedback loop controls cortisol production. When circulating levels of cortisol are low, CRF release increases; this results in an increase in ACTH release, which in turn brings about an increase in cortisol production. When cortisol levels are high, CRF release by the hypothalamus is normally low. This simple servomechanism is adequate for routine control but can be overridden by extrahypothalamic neural stimuli. For example, during severe stress CRF secretion is increased

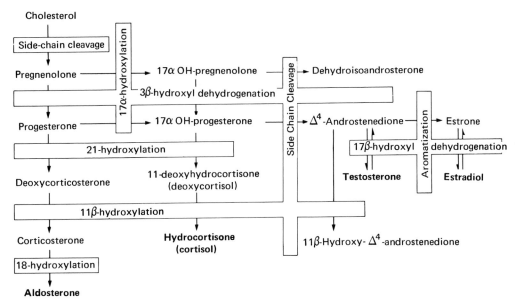

FIG. 7-1. Biochemistry of adrenal corticosteroids. Significant biosynthetic steps are demonstrated by horizontal and vertical bars. (Ezrin C, Godden JO, Volpe R, Wilson R (eds): Systemic Endocrinology. Hagerstown, Harper & Row, 1973)

even when circulating plasma cortisol levels are high. This response cannot be blocked even by the administration of massive doses of glucocorticoids.

Normally, ACTH and cortisol secretion are episodic. However, overlying these episodic fluctuations is a recognizable circadian pattern. Peak values of both ACTH and cortisol occur between 4 AM and 8 AM; lower concentrations are noted in the afternoon and evening. Disturbances in the normal diurnal variation may be important in the genesis of Cushing's syndrome.

The precise mechanism of action of ACTH on the adrenocortical cell is not known; however, it is clear that ACTH is necessary for significant adrenocortical output. ACTH probably acts on the outer cell membrane to activate the adenylate cyclase system within the inner cell membrane. Adenylate cyclase converts adenosine triphosphate (ATP) to $3'5'$-adenosine monophosphate (cyclic AMP), which in turn stimulates protein synthesis, resulting in steroidogenic conversion of acetate or cholesterol to cortisol.

All corticosteroids are relatively insoluble in water and circulate in the blood reversibly bound to an α_2-globulin called *transcortin* or *corticobinding globulin* (CBG). This glycoprotein also has a high affinity for progesterone. Roughly 15% of plasma cortisol is loosely bound to albumin; approximately 75% of serum cortisol is closely, but reversibly, bound to CBG; the free 10% of cortisol is the active form of the steroid. CBG is always almost entirely saturated so that a rapid release of corticosteroids from the adrenal results in a rapid increase in free cortisol. Total plasma cortisol is increased in the presence of estrogen by virtue of an increase in serum concentration of CBG, but the concentration of free or active cortisol remains relatively unchanged. Androgens tend to decrease serum CBG concentrations.

Tests of Adrenal Function

The level of adrenal function can be readily evaluated by measurement of blood levels of corticosteroids and certain androgens. The development of highly sensitive and specific protein-binding assays and radioimmunoassays has provided good tools for the assessment of endocrine function in general; and these assays may be applied to each of the specific adrenal steroids.

Urine Tests

Measurement of urinary *17-hydroxycorticosteroids* (17-OHCS) by means of the Porter–Silber chromagen reaction is quite specific for metabolites of cortisol and cortisone. This color reaction depends on the presence of 17,21-dihydroxy-20-ketone groups. The normal excretion rate of 17-hydroxycorticosteroids by nonpregnant adults ranges from 4 mg to 12 mg per 24 hours.

Measurement of *urinary 17-ketosteroids* (17-KS) is a time-honored method of estimating adrenal androgen production using the Zimmermann reaction. This colorimetric test measures predominantly the urinary metabolites of dehydroepiandrosterone, dehydroepiandrosterone sulfate, and androstenedione. Normal values range between 7 mg and 20 mg per 24 hours. The test is of value as a screening procedure, particularly for congenital adrenal hyperplasia and androgen-producing adrenal tumors, in which values are markedly elevated. Measurements of 17-KS cannot always be used to identify tumors that produce predominantly testosterone, however. Structurally testosterone, the most potent androgen, is not, per se, a 17-KS. Although about 50% of its metabolites are 17-KS, the microgram quantities of these materials that are produced each day are relatively insignificant when compared with the milligram quantities of the other constituents of the 17-KS pool. Thus, marked increases in serum testosterone concentrations result in only minimal increases in 17-KS excretion. Moreover, both the adrenal gland and the ovary also produce steroids that are excreted as 17-KS, so that 17-KS measurement alone cannot reliably identify the source of any increased androgen production. However, 11-oxygenated derivatives of androsterone and etiocholanolone, which are the most abundant of the 17-KS and are exclusively of adrenal origin, can be fractionated by chromatography and specifically measured.

Measurement of *urinary 17-ketogenic steroids* (17-KGS) is even less specific and less useful than measurement of the other urinary steroids.

Serum Tests

Specific assays are now available for virtually every steroid involved in adrenal steroidogenesis. These tests, which are sensitive and specific, require only small quantities of blood. They have largely supplanted tests that use urine for the diagnosis and management of patients with adrenal problems.

Suppression and Stimulation Tests

Adrenal suppression and stimulation tests provide information about the hypothalamic–pituitary–adrenal axis that cannot be obtained by the static measurement of either urinary excretory products or serum concentrations of specific steroids. Such tests can determine adrenal reserve, ACTH secreting potential, and pituitary–adrenal suppressibility.

The *dexamethasone suppression test* is based on the principle that exogenous glucocorticoids suppress ACTH stimulation; lack of ACTH stimulation in turn results in diminished endogenous adrenal glucocorticoid production. Dexamethasone is used because it is an exogenous corticosteroid that can suppress ACTH yet does not interfere with the assays used to assess endogenous adrenocortical function. Dexamethasone is customarily administered according to two dosage schedules. A low dose, 0.5 mg given 4 times daily for 2 days, suppresses the normal but not the hyperplastic adrenal gland (Table 7-1). Consequently, within 2 days the 24-hour 17-OHCS excretion rate falls to 3 mg or less. A higher dose of dexamethasone, 2 mg given 4 times a day for 2 days, is usually required to suppress the hyperplastic adrenals of Cushing's syndrome. Adrenocortical tumors are usually not suppressed by any dosage. Thus, significant suppression of adrenocorticosteroids with dexamethasone practically eliminates the possibility of an adrenocortical tumor.

Interpretation of the dexamethasone suppression test can be facilitated by information about ovarian and adrenal contributions to circulating steroid levels. As shown in Table 7-2, the relative contributions may vary during the menstrual cycle; in general, however, the adrenal cortex contributes 50% to total peripheral levels of testosterone, dihydrotestosterone, and androstenedione, and 80% to 95% to dehydroepiandrosterone and its sulfate. While the adrenal cortex contributes 100% of the circulating deoxycortisol, the ovary contributes 100% of the estradiol and most of the circulating pro-

---

Table 7-1

Response of Adrenal Cortex to Dexamethasone Suppression and Metopirone Stimulation Under Various Conditions

Condition	Suppression by Dexamethasone		Positive Response to Metopirone
	2 mg/day	8 mg/day	
Normal adrenal glands	+	+	+
Bilateral adrenal hyperplasia			
Without demonstrable pituitary tumor	−	+	+
With benign pituitary tumor	−	Variable	
With malignant pituitary tumor	−	−	−
Secondary to ectopic ACTH-producing tumor	−	−	−
Adrenal adenoma	−	−	−
Adrenal carcinoma	−	−	−

Table 7-2
Ovarian and Adrenal Contributions to Peripheral Androgens

| | Ovarian Contribution | | | |
Steroid	Early Follicular Phase	Midcycle	Late Luteal Phase	Adrenal Contribution
Testosterone				
Contribution (ng/ml)	0.1	0.3	0.1	0.2
Percent contribution	33	60	33	40–66
Dihydrotestosterone*				
Contribution (ng/ml)		0.1		0.1
Percent contribution		50		50
Androstenedione				
Contribution (ng/ml)	0.5	1.5	0.8	0.6
Percent contribution	45	70	60	30–55
Debydroepiandrosterone*				
Contribution (ng/ml)		0.8		3.2
Percent contribution		20		80
Debydroepiandrosterone Sulfate				
Contribution (ng/ml)	80	200	80	2000
Percent contribution	4	10	4	90–96

* Ovarian contribution not influenced by phase of menstrual cycle.

(Abraham GE: Ovarian and adrenal contributions to peripheral androgens during the menstrual. J Clin Endocrinol Metab 39:340, 1974. © 1974, The Endocrine Society)

gesterone and 17-hydroxyprogesterone that are present during the luteal phase.

The *Metopirone* (*metyrapone*) test assesses pituitary reserve by means of direct adrenal suppression. Metopirone inhibits 11β-hydroxylation and thereby decreases the conversion of 11-deoxycortisol to hydrocortisone. Through negative feedback, this treatment in turn results in increased pituitary ACTH secretion, which in normal subjects produces a twofold increase in urinary 17-OHCS and causes elevation of other adrenal steroids (see Table 7-1). The usual dosage of Metopirone is 500 mg to 750 mg administered every 4 hours for 24 hours. Before it is concluded that a lack of response to Metopirone is secondary to pituitary disease, adrenocortical status should be assessed with an ACTH stimulation test. If the adrenal cortex responds appropriately to ACTH but fails to respond to Metopirone, adrenal insufficiency due to pituitary or hypothalamic malfunction can be assumed.

The *ACTH stimulation test* measures adrenal response to the administration of ACTH. Several dosage schedules are in use. In a typical schedule, 0.25 mg synthetic ACTH is infused intravenously in 500 ml saline over an eight-hour interval beginning at 8 AM. A baseline 24-hour urine sample is collected beginning 24 hours before the onset of the test. This first sample serves as a control for comparative purposes. If adrenal function is normal, the second 24-hour urine sample, the collection of which begins at the onset of the ACTH infusion, should demonstrate a three- to fivefold increase in 17-OHCS excretion. Similar increases in serum cortisol are found if this substance is measured by radioimmunoassay. There are numerous modifications of this test, one of which entails the intramuscular administration of ACTH. In this test synthetic ACTH (Cortrosyn) is administered in a single dose of 25 μg, and plasma cortisol is measured both before administration and 60 minutes after the injection. In the normal patient a rise in cortisol of 10 μg/dl to 20 μg/dl should be anticipated.

Disorders of Adrenal Function

Primary disorders of the adrenal cortex involving aldosterone do not usually affect the reproductive system and are not usually managed by the obstetrician–gynecologist. In contrast, disorders in which glucocorticoids and androgens are deficient or excessively produced influence reproductive function.

Hyperfunction

The term *Cushing's syndrome* is generally used to describe any clinical entity associated with excessive and prolonged action of glucocorticoids. The syndrome, described by Harvey Cushing in 1932, was originally thought to be due to "pituitary basophilism." It is now recognized that the syndrome of adrenocortical excess can result from a number of conditions that lead to increased secretion of cortisol.

Approximately 75% of patients with Cushing's syndrome have bilateral adrenocortical hyperplasia, probably secondary to an abnormality of the mechanisms controlling the hypothalamic–pituitary–adrenal axis. The first change appears to be disruption of the normal diurnal rhythm of cortisol secretion with loss of the usual afternoon decline in serum cortisol concentrations. Eventually, plasma cortisol levels remain elevated throughout the entire day. At this stage of the disease, the adrenal gland retains its ability to respond to stress with an increased elaboration of cortisol and continues to be suppressible. With further progression of the disorder, this responsiveness is lost.

Ectopic secretion of ACTH can also give rise to Cushing's syndrome. Certain nonendocrine tumors that produce polypeptides immunologically and biologically similar to ACTH can also cause bilateral adrenal hyperplasia. Oat cell carcinoma of the lung is the most common nonendocrine cause of Cushing's syndrome secondary to ectopic ACTH secretion.

Benign adrenocortical adenomas are responsible for Cushing's syndrome in 10% to 15% of patients. Malignant tumors account for 5% to 10% of cases. Adenomas are bilateral in approximately 10% of cases and are occasionally associated with adenomatous hyperplasia of the adrenal. Both benign and malignant adrenal tumors secrete cortisol independently of pituitary–hypothalamic control, and accordingly, diurnal variability is lost. Moreover, prolonged hypercorticism results in diminished pituitary secretion of ACTH and functional atrophy of the remaining, normal adrenal tissue. Occasionally the adenomas also produce excessive androgens, causing precocious puberty or virilization. Excessive androgen production occurs more frequently with adrenal tumors than with Cushing's syndrome secondary to pituitary abnormalities.

The signs and symptoms of Cushing's syndrome result from an excess of glucocorticoids. The classic features of the syndrome are central obesity, buffalo hump, moon facies, purple cutaneous striae, abnormal glucose tolerance, hypertension, osteoporosis, muscle wasting, and heightened susceptibility to infection. Oligomenorrhea, amenorrhea, infertility, and hirsutism are also common. The biologic effects of cortisol excess due to different causes are listed below:

Related to Protein Metabolism
Red striae
Demineralization and loss of bone matrix
Muscle wasting and weakness
Capillary fragility and bruising
Thinning of skin

Related to Lipid Metabolism
Central fat distribution
Moon facies

Related to Carbohydrate Metabolism
Decreased glucose tolerance
Overt diabetes

Related to Hematopoiesis
Eosinophilia
Lymphopenia
Polymorphonuclear leukocytosis
Erythrocytosis

Related to Electrolyte Balance
Sodium retention/potassium loss
Hypertension
Hypervolemia

Other
Hypercalcuria and renal calculi
Gastric ulcer
Impaired immunologic competence
Emotional disturbance/psychosis
Susceptibility to infection

Diagnosis of Cushing's syndrome involves verification of excess corticosteroid production and determination of the cause. The simplest initial screening test consists of measurements of serum cortisol taken at 8 AM and 4 PM of the same day. Normal cortisol levels and the presence of abnormal diurnal variation rule out Cushing's syndrome. If results are equivocal, an overnight dexamethasone suppression test may be performed: 2 mg dexamethasone is administered at 11 PM, and a blood specimen for serum cortisol measurement is drawn at 8 AM the following morning. Cortisol levels of less than 4 μg/dl are considered normal, levels of greater than 20 μg/dl are indicative of Cushing's syndrome, and intermediate values are of limited diagnostic value. *Cushing's disease* is the designation used for those cases of Cushing's syndrome that are clearly secondary to inappropriate pituitary secretion of ACTH. *Cushing's syndrome* is a more broadly used term referring generically to chronic excess of glucocorticoids.

Further evaluation and treatment are best carried out in conjunction with an endocrinologist. Bilateral adrenal hyperplasia secondary to pituitary hyperstimulation can be treated by transsphenoidal resection of the pituitary microadenoma, if present, or by pituitary irradiation. Severe disease may require bilateral total adrenalectomy, which is associated with a very low five-year survival rate. Treatment involves excision, if possible, and subsequent treatment with adrenolytic drugs.

Hypofunction

Adrenocortical insufficiency may exist in either a primary or a secondary form. The primary condition,

Addison's disease, involves insufficiency of the hormones secreted by all zones of the adrenal cortex, with deficiency of mineralocorticoids, glucocorticoids, and androgens. Primary adrenal insufficiency is an extremely rare disease resulting from bilateral tuberculosis (the major cause in Addison's original description), amyloidosis, mycotic infections, or possibly an autoimmune phenomenon. An idiopathic form of adrenal atrophy also occurs. Secondary adrenocortical insufficiency may occur as a consequence of hypothalamic or pituitary disease, trauma, surgery, or suppression following a course of exogenous corticosteroid administration.

Adrenocortical insufficiency should be suspected whenever a patient who is hypotensive and has darkly pigmented skin complains of weakness and tiredness. The pigmentation is secondary to increased secretion of melanocyte-stimulating hormone. Chronic adrenal insufficiency results in salt wasting with decreased serum sodium and increased serum potassium values. The signs and symptoms of primary adrenocortical insufficiency are listed below:

Weakness
Skin pigmentation
Weight loss
Hypotension
Anorexia
Nausea and vomiting
Abdominal pain
Constipation
Diarrhea
Syncope
Vitiligo

An acute, life-threatening episode of adrenal insufficiency (addisonian crisis) consists of weakness, syncope, hypotension, rapidly progressing pyrexia, vascular collapse, shock, and death. It can occur secondary to the stress of infection or trauma or following the abrupt cessation of adrenocortical therapy in a patient deficient in adrenocortical reserve. Salt and cortisol replacement are urgently required. Treatment of an addisonian crisis is best handled by the prompt administration of 100 mg hydrocortisone intravenously, followed by intravenous infusion over an 8-hour period of 100 mg of hydrocortisone contained in 1 liter of normal saline. Several liters of saline may be required because of the contracted body fluid compartments.

Less urgent forms of primary adrenocortical insufficiency are diagnosed on the basis of an inability of the adrenal cortex to respond to ACTH stimulation. The diagnosis of secondary adrenocortical insufficiency is usually suggested by the finding of other, more visible, pituitary tropic hormone deficiencies. Afflicted patients are normally unable to excrete a water load but promptly do so following administration of a small dose of cortisol. Additional tests involve insulin stimulation of ACTH production and the Metopirone stimulation test.

Failure to respond appropriately to these tests confirms the diagnosis of pituitary insufficiency with secondary adrenal insufficiency.

Treatment of chronic adrenal insufficiency requires the replacement of both glucocorticoids and mineralocorticoids if the adrenal insufficiency is primary, but replacement only of cortisol if it is secondary. Cortisol requirements range from 15 mg to 30 mg per day. Because aldosterone is ineffective orally, fluorocortisone, about 0.1 mg per day, can be used as mineralocorticoid replacement. The appropriate dosage can be calculated on the basis of body weight, blood pressure, and edema.

Congenital Adrenal Hyperplasia

The essential problem with congenital adrenal hyperplasia is a deficiency, but not complete lack, of one or more of the enzymes required for normal steroidogenesis. The defect most often results in deficient cortisol production, which in turn leads to increased adrenal stimulation through enhanced ACTH secretion. In mild cases, enough cortisol is produced to maintain life. However, because of an enzyme deficiency, excessive adrenal stimulation by ACTH results in an overproduction of steroids in the metabolic pathway immediately preceding the enzyme deficits. In most cases these steroids serve as precursors for conversion to adrenal androgens, which are in turn converted peripherally to testosterone, with resultant hirsutism or virilization.

When the enzyme deficiency is profound, disturbed steroid production will have begun during fetal life and manifestations of the disorder are apparent at birth. In less severe enzymatic defects, often referred to as *attenuated* forms, clinical features are deferred until menarche or even later. In severe cases, the defects are incompatible with life and adrenal crisis occurs within a few days of birth. Congenital adrenal hyperplasia is most often seen in infancy or childhood. When the milder forms of the disorder appear during adolescence, they are often manifested as oligomenorrhea, hirsutism, or both. Several years later infertility may also supervene. The sites of severe enzyme deficiencies are illustrated in Figure 7-1.

Newborns with defective side-chain cleavage (deficiency of 20,22-desmolase) produce no steroids and do not survive. At autopsy, the adrenal glands of these infants are found to be large and laden with fat.

Newborns with a 3β-hydroxysteroid dehydrogenase deficiency usually do not survive. This enzyme is essential for the restructuring of rings A and B in the steroid configuration. The disorder was originally recognized in newborn males with ambiguous genitalia who were unable to produce sufficient testosterone *in utero* to bring about full male development, as well as in newborn females who were mildly virilized at birth. Such infants are unable to convert pregnenolone to progesterone, 17-hydroxypregnenolone to 17-hydroxyprogesterone, or dehydroepiandrosterone to androstenedione.

Serum concentrations of pregnenolone, 17-hydroxy-pregnenolone, and dehydroepiandrosterone are elevated. This entity is manifested in a variety of ways. An apparently common attenuated late-onset form that resembles polycystic ovarian disease is diagnosable by an increase in 17-hydroxypregnenolone levels in response to Cortrosyn.

Females with 17-hydroxylase deficiency survive and have primary amenorrhea. The defect, which is present in both the adrenal cortex and the ovary, precludes formation of adequate amounts of both androgens and estrogens. Hydrocortisone production is diminished; deoxycorticosterone and corticosterone production are increased. The weak glucocorticoid effects of these two steroids substitute for that of hydrocortisone, but their mineralocorticoid effects result in sodium retention, potassium loss, and hypertension.

The most common enzymatic defect is a 21-hydroxylase deficiency, an autosomal recessive disorder that occurs more often in females than in males; it is found in approximately 1 of every 5000 liveborn infants. This defect limits both glucocorticoid and mineralocorticoid production. Elevated serum levels of progesterone and 17-hydroxyprogesterone give rise to increased urinary excretion of pregnanediol and pregnanetriol. 17-Hydroxypregnenolone concentrations are also high. Serum 17-hydroxyprogesterone is the most significantly elevated steroid. Because the precursors are converted to the androgens dehydroepiandrosterone and androstenedione, their increased levels result in virilization and increased excretion of urinary 17-KS.

The degree of 21-hydroxylase deficiency may vary. Mild deficiency results in androgenic effects manifested at puberty as mild hirsutism, amenorrhea, and poor breast development. An intermediate defect is most common. A female with an intermediate deficiency is born with an enlarged clitoris; if the disorder is not treated, she will precociously develop a male habitus, pubic hair, and a deep voice, and at puberty she will not experience menarche. Severe 21-hydroxylase deficiency, present in about one third of affected patients, results in severe virilization and mineralocorticoid insufficiency, with sodium wasting, hypotension, and dehydration. Newborns with this severe form do not survive without treatment. In the attenuated, or late-onset, form, clinical manifestations are limited and baseline values of 17-hydroxyprogesterone may be normal. As a consequence, adrenal stimulation with ACTH is necessary to establish the diagnosis. Serum 17-hydroxyprogesterone rises beyond normally expected levels in response to ACTH stimulation.

Patients with an 11β-hydroxylase deficiency are unable to produce hydrocortisone, corticosterone, or aldosterone. Consequently, they produce an excess of deoxycorticosterone; virilization, salt retention, hypertension, and hypokalemia ensue. The defect is similar to 21-hydroxylase deficiency except for the tendency toward hypertension.

Diagnosis of all of the congenital defects in adrenal steroid biosynthesis must be based on the measurement of steroid levels in either serum or urine. The specific steroids measured in serum are dehydroepiandrosterone sulfate and 17-hydroxyprogesterone, and in urine 17-KS and pregnanetriol.

Therapy consists of prompt replacement of the necessary steroids and subsequent maintenance throughout life. Drugs commonly used in treatment of adrenocortical disorders are listed in Table 7-3. With adequate replacement therapy, patients can anticipate a normal life as well as fertility. However, the effects of increased androgens on the external genitalia may ultimately require reconstructive surgery.

THYROID

Because the thyroid gland influences fertility, pregnancy, and general well-being, an understanding of thyroid function is essential for the obstetrician–gynecologist.

The thyroid gland was the first endocrine gland to evolve in the vertebrate. In lower animals, thyroid hormones have profound effects. In frogs and toads they are responsible for the metamorphosis from tadpole to adult. In humans they are largely responsible for control of the general level of metabolism. They stimulate calorigenesis, potentiate epinephrine, and are essential for normal central nervous system development. Calcitonin, also secreted by the thyroid, plays a role in calcium and phosphorus metabolism.

The thyroid develops from an invagination of the pharynx at the base of the tongue and is well differentiated by the 15th week of fetal life, at which time thyroid function is initiated.

Table 7-3
Drugs Commonly Used in Diagnosis and Treatment of Adrenocortical Disorders

Drug	Form Supplied
Hydrocortisone	20-mg tablet
Cortisone	30-mg tablet
Hydrocortisone sodium succinate	100 mg/ml
Prednisone	5-mg tablet
Prednisolone	5-mg tablet
Dexamethasone	0.25-mg to 0.75-mg tablet
Florinef (9α-fluorohydrocortisone)	0.1-mg tablet
Deoxycorticosterone	5 mg/ml
ACTH (synthetic B1-24)	0.25 mg
Metopirone	250-mg capsule

(Ezrn C, Godden JO, Volpe R, Wilson R [eds]: Systematic Endocrinology. Hagerstown, MD Harper & Row, 1973)

Physiology and Biochemistry

The thyroid gland, like the adrenal, ovary, and testis, functions under the feedback control of the hypothalamus and pituitary. In the median eminence, thyrotropin-releasing hormone (TRH), a compound composed of three amino acids, is produced, passes through the hypothalamic–hypophyseal portal vessels in the pituitary stalk, and brings about the secretion of thyrotropin, or thyroid-stimulating hormone (TSH), from the pituitary. TSH in turn controls iodine uptake and release of the two major thyroid hormones, thyroxine (T_4) and triiodothyronine (T_3), from the thyroid gland. Serum concentrations of T_4 control TRH release by the hypothalamus and resultant stimulation of the thyroid. This internal control mechanism tends to maintain a homeostatic level of thyroid function.

TSH is thought to act on the thyroid gland by attaching itself to the cell membrane and stimulating the formation of adenylate cyclase, which catalyzes the formation of cyclic AMP, the intracellular "second messenger."

Thyroid biosynthesis can be considered in four steps: (1) iodide transport and trapping, (2) iodination of tyrosine, (3) coupling and storage, and (4) release and secretion of thyroid hormones. Inorganic iodides absorbed from the small intestine are carried in the circulation and trapped by the thyroid gland against a 20:1 gradient. The inorganic iodide is converted in the thyroid to organic iodine, which then combines with tyrosine to form monoiodotyrosine (MIT) and diiodotyrosine (DIT). One molecule of MIT plus one molecule of DIT forms T_3; two molecules of DIT form T_4. T_3 and T_4 combine with thyroglobulin for their storage as colloid contained in the thyroid follicles. As stated, release of T_3 and T_4 from the colloid is under the control of TSH; T_3 and T_4 are split from the thyroglobulin, which is recycled within the thyroid cell, and are released into the thyroid venous circulation.

In the blood, T_3 and T_4 are transported bound to three carrier proteins: thyroxine-binding globulin (TBG), which carries 60% of the bound hormones; a thyroxine-binding prealbumin, which carries 30% of the bound hormones; and an albumin, which carries 10% of the bound hormones. More than 99% of the total circulating T_3 and T_4 is bound to these three proteins. However, the less than 1% that is unbound or free is the only metabolically active thyroid hormone.

The serum concentrations of these thyroid-binding proteins are increased at least twofold in pregnant women as well as in patients on estrogen therapy. This phenomenon profoundly affects the results of thyroid function tests.

T_3 is 3 to 4 times more potent than T_4 on a weight basis. Approximately half of T_4 is converted to T_3. The half-life of T_3 is 1 day or less, whereas the half-life of T_4 is approximately 6 to 8 days. Approximately 30% of the total body pool of T_4 is in the liver. Both T_3 and T_4 are deactivated by deiodinization and are excreted in the feces.

Thyroid Function Tests

Thyroid function tests fall into five main categories: (1) measurement of peripheral effect, (2) measurement of serum-binding protein concentration, (3) measurement of circulating thyroid hormone, (4) measurement of serum thyrotropin, and (5) measurement of thyroidal iodine uptake. Values of the useful thyroid function tests are summarized in Table 7-4. Exact values may vary according to the laboratory performing the test.

Tests of peripheral effect include basal metabolic rate, serum cholesterol, and Achilles reflex tests. They are relatively insensitive and inaccurate and have little place in modern clinical medicine.

Serum unsaturated binding protein (TBG) concentration is measured by the resin uptake of T_3 labeled with iodine 131. In this *in vitro* test, T_3 is added to serum that contains radioactive iodine, and the unbound radioactive iodine is then picked up by a resin and counted. The test results can be reported as a percentage of normal.

Tests of circulating thyroid hormones can measure either T_3 or T_4 and either total (bound plus free) or free hormones. Tests can be either positively associated with or independent of binding protein concentrations. Because many situations in clinical obstetrics and gynecology are concerned with changes in estrogen concentrations and, consequently, with changes in TBG concentrations, it is necessary to consider the influence of binding protein concentrations on specific tests. The ideal test for determining thyroid hormone concentration would be one independent of binding protein concentration.

Tests positively associated with TBG concentrations include the measurement of protein-bound iodine (PBI), the assessment of T_3 by radioimmunoassay, and the assessment of T_4 by the Murphy–Pattee technique or displacement analysis. Increased TBG concentrations result in increased values in each of these tests. The PBI test measures all protein-bound iodine, including organic and inorganic iodine from previously administered radiopaque dyes; however, this test has been replaced by more specific tests. Measurement of T_3 by radioimmunoassay uses specific antisera. It is an accurate but sometimes difficult test to perform and not as readily available as other tests. Measurement of T_4 by the Murphy–Pattee technique involves the progressive displacement of T_4 from protein-binding sites that measure only T_4; it is not influenced by other iodoproteins. This test is relatively easy to perform and readily available.

Tests independent of TBG concentration measure free T_4, free T_4 index, and effective T_4. Measurement of free T_4 is a difficult technique and not commonly performed. The test measures only the less than 1% of T_4

Table 7-4
Thyroid Function Studies

Test	Normal	Hypothyroidism	Hyperthyroidism	Pregnancy
Measurement of Unsaturated Serum-Binding Protein Concentration				
T_3 resin uptake as percentage of uptake (T_3RU)	25–35	Decreased	Increased	Decreased
T_3 resin uptake as percentage of unity (T_3RU%)	0.8–1.2	Decreased	Increased	Decreased
Measurement of Circulating Thyroid Hormones				
Positively associated with protein concentration				
PBI (μg/dl)	4–8	Decreased	Increased	Increased
T_4 Murphy–Pattee (T_4) (μg/100 ml)	4–11	Decreased	Increased	Increased
T_3 RIA (T_3) (ng/dl)	50–150	Decreased	Increased	Increased
Independent of binding protein concentration				
Free T_4 (μg/dl)	0.6–1.7	Decreased	Increased	
Free T_4 index (ng/dl)	1–3.5	Decreased	Increased	Normal
Measurement of Thyrotropin				
TSH by radioimmunoassay (uU/ml)	0–10	Increased	Decreased	Normal
Measurement of Iodine Uptake				
RAI uptake (%)	10–35	Decreased	Increased	Contraindicated

that is unbound in serum, and the information it provides is not of sufficient clinical value to compensate for the difficulty involved in performing it.

The free T_4 index (FTI) is calculated by multiplication of the T_4 value obtained by the Murphy–Pattee procedure times the T_3 value calculated by resin uptake. This test uses the TBG value obtained from resin uptake of T_3 labeled with radiolabeled iodine to compensate for alterations in T_4 level secondary to changes in TBG.

The effective T_4 (ET_4) test utilizes the same Murphy–Pattee measurement of T_4 and the same resin uptake value to compensate for binding. However, T_3 resin uptake is reported as a percentage of normal, and this percentage is what is used in the calculation. Normal values for this test are the same as those for the usual measurement of T_4 and are not influenced by the effects of estrogen or pregnancy on TBG serum concentrations. This test is ideal for following thyroid function in pregnant women or in patients receiving an estrogen preparation (*e.g.,* oral contraception).

Indirect measurement of TSH yields information about effective circulating thyroid hormone levels. TSH is measured by radioimmunoassay using the patient's serum. The test is particularly effective in identifying hypothyroidism, because low levels of circulating thyroid hormones result in compensatory elevations of serum TSH. Normal TSH concentrations are 0 μU to 10 μU/ml. Values greater than 20 μU/ml are usually indicative of hypothyroidism. The normal range is unaffected by pregnancy.

Measurement of iodine uptake determines the ability of the thyroid gland to bind administered radioactive iodine. This ability is decreased in hypothyroidism and increased in hyperthyroidism. Results can be recorded either as percentage of uptake or through a scan of the thyroid gland as differential uptake. Iodine uptake is an effective and useful indicator of thyroid function; however, iodine uptake tests are contraindicated in pregnancy because of placental passage and uptake by the fetal thyroid of the radioactive iodine.

Clinical evaluation of thyroid function for the obstetrician–gynecologist involves a careful history, physical examination, and appropriate laboratory tests. Laboratory evaluation should include measurement of T_4 by the Murphy–Pattee method or of T_3 by radioimmunoassay. If TBG is thought to be elevated, or if increased T_4 or T_3 values suggest the possibility of TBG elevation, a T_3 resin uptake test (indicative of TBG concentrations) should be performed. The FTI or ET_4 can then be calculated from the T_4 and the T_3 resin uptake values. If the diagnosis of hypothyroidism is being entertained, serum TSH determination is indicated. Measurement of radioactive iodine uptake may be helpful in the nonpregnant patient.

Disorders of Thyroid Function

Nontoxic goiters, benign or malignant thyroid neoplasms, and thyroiditis are not usually treated by the obstetrician–gynecologist. However, the gynecologist occasionally sees patients with hyperthyroidism and hypothyroidism, because these disorders can result in reproductive abnormalities.

Hyperthyroidism

Hyperthyroidism occurs in approximately 0.1% of the general population but in only 0.04% to 0.075% of the pregnant population. The manifestations of hyperthyroidism are always due to excess circulating levels of T_3 and T_4.

There are three basic types of hyperthyroidism. *Iatrogenic hyperthyroidism* is due to excess administration of thyroid substances, either because of presumed need or for weight reduction.

The more common endogenous form of hyperthyroidism, *Graves' disease* or diffuse exophthalmic goiter, usually occurs in women under 50 years of age. The hypersecretion of T_3 and T_4 originates from a diffusely hyperplastic gland. The disease is associated with frequent spontaneous remissions and exacerbations and is commonly accompanied by exophthalmos and pretibial myxedema. Excess circulating levels of long-acting thyroid stimulator (LATS) are most commonly noted in patients with exophthalmos and pretibial myxedema.

LATS is a 7S γ-globulin frequently present in the serum in patients with Graves' disease. It appears to arise from lymphocytes as an antibody to one or more components of thyroid cells, but its exact mode of action is unknown. Although it has been cited as a possible cause of the hyperthyroidism itself, as well as of the exophthalmos and neonatal hyperthyroidism frequently associated with Graves' disease, there is a distinct lack of unanimity in these opinions.

The second form of endogenous hyperthyroidism, Plummer's disease or toxic nodular goiter, usually occurs in women over 50 years of age. Thus, it is seldom seen in pregnant women. Hypersecretion of T_3 and T_4 originates from one or more hyperplastic and autonomous areas of the nodular goiter. Signs and symptoms are associated with excess quantities of thyroid hormones, but exophthalmos is rarely present. This disease is usually of insidious onset and slowly progressive.

The clinical signs and symptoms of hyperthyroidism are nonspecific and independent of the cause of the hyperthyroidism. Tachycardia, weight loss, fatigue, and heat intolerance are each seen in more than 80% of patients. Muscle weakness is fairly common but sometimes difficult to demonstrate; it is usually present in the proximal muscles of the trunk and lower limbs. During pregnancy, weight loss may be obscured by the physiologic weight gain of pregnancy. Symptoms of hyperthyroidism are listed below:

Related to Catecholamines
Nervousness
Palpitations
Tachycardia
Tremor

Related to Increased Metabolism
Diaphoresis
Heat intolerance
Fatigue
Increased appetite
Weight loss

Related to Gastrointestinal Tract
Hypermotility
Diarrhea

Related to Muscular Effects
Weakness or paralysis
Dyspnea

Other
Personality changes/psychosis
Decreased central nervous system efficiency
Menstrual irregularities
Symptoms of congestive heart failure
Hair loss
Eyelid retraction
Exophthalmos
Lid lag

In nonpregnant patients, therapy for hyperthyroidism can consist of administration of radioactive iodine or thyroid-blocking agents, or thyroidectomy. Radioactive iodine treatment must not be used during pregnancy. During pregnancy hyperthyroidism should be treated with propylthiouracil, 100 mg 3 times a day, to gain control; this is followed by a diminished dose (usually 100 mg propylthiouracil daily) to maintain slight hyperthyroidism. Although thyroidectomy can be considered in the second trimester or postpartum, it is frequently unnecessary; approximately 50% of patients who continue propylthiouracil therapy for one year postpartum experience permanent remission.

Since both propylthiouracil and methimazole block synthesis of T_4 but not release of T_4 from the gland, the clinical effects of these agents are not realized until after stored hormone has been utilized. Clinical response can be followed by measurement of T_4. Although the most common complication of propylthiouracil and methimazole treatment is a rash, agranulocytosis occurs in 0.6% of patients. Therapy with these antithyroid drugs requires monitoring with leukocyte counts before and during treatment. The patient should be instructed to report promptly to the physician fever or sore throat, which may signify agranulocytosis. Both drugs cross the placenta when given in high doses and can cause fetal goiter. Lower doses do not appear to affect fetal thyroid function. Although some authors recommend concomitant administration of thyroid hormone when these blocking agents are given during pregnancy, there is little evidence to support this practice.

Thyroid storm is a rare, life-threatening, acute worsening of all symptoms of severe hyperthyroidism. Fever, tachycardia, and severe dehydration are common, and death occurs in about 25% of instances. Storm occurs most often in patients with poorly controlled or undiagnosed disease who are subject to a stress such as labor, cesarean section, or infection. Treatment consists of administration of 1 g intravenous sodium iodine to block T_4 secretion, large doses of propylthiouracil, 2 mg to 4 mg propranolol to control tachycardia, intravenous cortisol, fluid replacement, and hypothermia.

Hypothyroidism

Hypothyroidism, which is about one tenth as common as hyperthyroidism, most frequently occurs in women between the ages of 30 and 60. Most cases occur in women beyond the age of childbearing. Medical treatment, thyroidectomy, and administration of radioactive iodine are the most usual causes. End-stage thyroiditis can also result in hypothyroidism.

Clinical signs and symptoms of mild disease consist of paresthesias, cold intolerance, constipation, cool dry skin, coarse hair, irritability, and inability to concentrate. Severe disease is manifested by myxedema, periorbital edema, enlarged tongue, and a hoarse voice. Severe disease is rare during pregnancy. Because so many of the symptoms of mild disease are difficult to distinguish from symptoms of anxiety or depression, the best evidence of hypothyroidism is elevation of serum TSH concentration. Values are unaffected by pregnancy and are usually less than 3 μU/ml. Values of greater than 10 μU/ml suggest hypothyroidism. Other thyroid function tests are generally less sensitive indicators of hypothyroidism but may be useful for both diagnosis and monitoring of therapy.

Treatment of hypothyroidism consists of replacement of thyroid hormones. Appropriate therapy enables serum TSH concentrations to return to normal. Available agents are desiccated thyroid, levothyroxine, liothyronine, and a fixed combination of the last two. Desiccated thyroid is the time-honored pharmacologic form of thyroid hormone. It is inexpensive, but its potency depends on protein rather than T_3 or T_4 content, so that its effectiveness can vary considerably depending upon the lot. Levothyroxine (Synthroid) is synthetic T_4. It is inexpensive and its potency consistent, but administration in doses sufficient to treat hypothyroidism raises serum T_4 levels above the normal range. Thus, measurement of serum T_4 cannot be used to monitor patients taking levothyroxine. Liothyronine (Cytomel) is synthetic T_3. It acts quickly but for a short time only and thus is not as useful for long-term therapy as is levothyroxine. Patients who are euthyroid on T_3 therapy have subnormal serum T_4 concentrations. Synthetic T_4 and T_3 combined in a 4:1 ratio is marketed as Euthroid. It is expensive and has no advantage over T_4 alone except that administration does not result in distortion of serum T_4 concentrations. Hypothyroid patients who receive thyroid replacement during pregnancy may need increased doses except toward term, when requirements may decrease.

Thyroid and Reproduction

The effects of hyperthyroidism on reproductive functions are variable. There is little solid evidence that fertility is affected by the condition. Although menstrual irregularities are fairly common and no particular pattern predominates, there is disagreement in the literature as to associated fetal wastage and mortality. Mild to moderate hyperthyroidism apparently has no significant effect on pregnancy, but severe disease may be associated with increased fetal wastage.

The effects of hypothyroidism on reproduction are also varied. Menstrual irregularities, polymenorrhea, oligomenorrhea, and hypermenorrhea are associated with mild disease, and amenorrhea is encountered in 70% of patients with myxedema. Although some reports suggest that women with hypothyroidism have a higher than normal incidence of spontaneous abortion and others attempt to show that hypothyroidism is associated with congenital defects in the neonate and undifferentiated developmental retardation, several reports detail patients with untreated myxedema who have carried apparently normal babies to term.

Pregnancy itself has particular and recognizable effects on thyroid function. Maternal TBG level rise by four weeks of gestation and remain elevated for one to two months postpartum. Physiologic enlargement of the maternal thyroid gland is associated with pregnancy, as is an increase in the basal metabolic rate. The latter phenomenon reflects the presence of the fetus rather than a metabolic dysfunction. Serum TBG values, total serum T_3 and T_4 values, iodine uptake, and renal clearance of iodide are all increased in pregnancy. Serum concentrations of TSH, free T_3, and free T_4 remain unchanged. Assessments of thyroid function during pregnancy must be based on measured levels of TSH and on calculated FTI or ET_4.

The placenta selectively passes materials important in thyroid physiology. Iodine and antithyroid blocking agents readily cross the placenta. T_3 and T_4 traverse the placenta very slowly, and TSH does not cross at all. LATS traverses the placenta and can affect the newborn. Human chorionic gonadotropin (hCG) secreted by the trophoblast possesses TSH-like activity that can result in clinical hyperthyroidism. This is especially apparent in certain patients with trophoblastic neoplasia and very high serum concentrations of hCG.

Maternal thyroid secretions appear to be required for maintenance of early pregnancy. After 12 weeks of gestation, the fetal thyroid gland traps iodine and begins to secrete T_3 and T_4. T_4 appears necessary for the development of the fetal central nervous system but not for fetal growth. The T_4 supplied by the fetal thyroid appears adequate for this purpose.

PINEAL

The pineal is a small organ located superior to the entrance of the cerebral aqueduct at the posterior aspect of the third ventricle. Historically, it was once thought to be the seat of the soul and to control the flow of conscious thought. Recently it has been recognized as an intricate and sensitive biologic clock that converts nervous impulses generated by environmental light into endocrine function.

The pineal originates in the brain of the developing embryo, but it loses its direct nerve connections to the brain soon after birth. Ultimately innervation of the pineal comes from the superior cervical ganglion by way of the sympathetic nerves that follow the blood vessels through the cranium. Anatomically, this arrangement is similar to that found in the adrenal medulla, where sympathetic nerve fibers end in contact with medullary cells.

The pineal gland is the only organ capable of synthesizing melatonin. The human pineal contains high concentrations of melatonin's precursor, serotonin, as well as the methoxylating enzyme o-methyltransferase.

In rats and other lower animals, the pineal is important in control of the secretion of gonadotropic hormones. In these animals melatonin acts to inhibit hypothalamic release of gonadotropin-releasing factor. In rats, for example, melatonin lowers the incidence of estrus and slows ovarian growth. Light impulses from the optic nerves stimulate the sympathetic fibers of the superior cervical ganglion. These impulses are then transmitted through the sympathetic chain to the pineal gland, where they inhibit melatonin production. As levels of melatonin decrease, so do its inhibitory effects on the hypothalamus, resulting in increased basal secretion of gonadotropin-releasing factor and gonadotropins. This subsequently causes stimulation of the ovaries and increased estrogen production. The net result is the persistent estrus seen in rats under constant illumination. However, when pineal extracts are implanted directly into the median eminence or reticular formation in rats, they inhibit release of luteinizing hormone.

The role of the pineal in humans is even less well understood. Boys with tumors that originate from pineal supporting tissues or teratomas near the gland demonstrate precocious puberty. True pineal tumors result in delayed puberty. Girls blind since birth would be expected to show retarded sexual development; instead, surprisingly, they experience menarche at an earlier age than girls with normal vision, regardless of the cause of their blindness. Although data suggest that the pineal may play some role in the onset of puberty in humans, no abnormalities of adult reproductive function have yet been ascribed to this gland. There is also no evidence to support the idea that blindness has any effect on long-term fertility.

PROSTAGLANDINS

In 1933 Goldblatt and von Euler independently isolated a potent vasopressor and smooth muscle–stimulating lipid from human seminal plasma and sheep vesicular gland; von Euler named it *prostaglandin*. In 1959 Bergstrom identified the basic chemical structure as a 20-carbon derivative of prostanoic acid, which contains a five-member ring. The four basic families, prostaglandins A (PGA), B (PGB), E (PGE), and F (PGF), are further subdivided according to chemical structure. The different prostaglandins have strikingly different physiologic and pharmacologic effects. PGE and PGF appear to be most important in obstetrics and gynecology.

Prostaglandins can arise from virtually all tissues of the body, but they are present in unusually high concentrations in the male and female reproductive tracts. They appear to be synthesized in the microsomes from arachidonic acid, an unsaturated fatty acid. Their release from tissues is enhanced by nervous, humoral, chemical, and physical stimulation; the mere handling of tissue can cause prostaglandin release. The extremely efficient clearance of prostaglandins by the lungs, 90% in a single passage, accounts for their short half-life, measured in seconds to minutes; because of this short half-life, changes in serum or plasma concentrations in antecubital vein blood cannot be measured following release of prostaglandins into the uterine venous circulation.

Prostaglandins affect the gastrointestinal and respiratory tracts, the cardiovascular and central nervous systems, the kidneys, connective tissue, and the female reproductive system. Particular effects are determined by the tissue, the specific prostaglandin, and the dose. Prostaglandins can cause smooth muscle contraction or relaxation, tachycardia, hypotension, nausea, vomiting, diarrhea, bronchodilation, or bronchoconstriction. In the central nervous system they appear to potentiate polysynaptic transmission. In connective tissue they are potent inflammatory agents and pyrogens. Aspirin and indomethacin are potent inhibitors of prostaglandin synthesis.

Prostaglandins have multiple effects on the female reproductive tract. Because most studies of prostaglandins have been conducted in animals, the role of prostaglandins in human reproduction remains unclear, yet considerable data have accumulated implicating them in reproductive processes at various levels. Prostaglandins may act as central nervous system transmitters, mediating the effects of hypothalamic releasing hormones on the pituitary either by altering vascular permeability or by modifying intracellular concentrations of cyclic AMP. $PGF_{2\alpha}$ increases the pituitary content of luteinizing hormone, and both indomethacin and aspirin can block ovulation by blocking the release of luteinizing hormone from the pituitary, presumably by suppressing prostaglandin synthesis. Evidence indicates that $PGF_{2\alpha}$ is involved in the mechanics of follicle disruption following the luteinizing hormone surge. PGF and PGE levels increase within the follicle as ovulation approaches. Prostaglandin synthesis inhibitors block ovulation induced by exogenous gonadotropins; ovulation can be restored by administration of $PGF_{2\alpha}$, indicating that this prostaglandin has a direct effect at the ovarian level. Furthermore, in the extracorporeal perfused rabbit ovary, $PGF_{2\alpha}$ alone, without gonadotropins, can cause follicle rupture.

Prostaglandins may also play a role in ovarian steroidogenesis, particularly in the production of progesterone, as well as in luteolysis. Prostaglandins incubated with mammalian ovarian tissue slices cause increased production of progesterone. Prostaglandin inhibitors block not only the effects of PGE_1 and PGE_2 but also the effect of luteinizing hormone on cyclic AMP and progesterone production. It has been suggested that luteinizing hormone may act on the cell membrane by stimulating prostaglandin synthesis and subsequent activation of adenylate cyclase and cyclic AMP, resulting in steroid production. Prostaglandins have a luteolytic effect in some animals by virtue of their direct action on the corpus luteum or by changes in ovarian blood flow. In sheep, for example, prostaglandins originating in the uterus are delivered to the ovary by way of the utero-ovarian circulation and thereby cause luteolysis. Extirpation of the uterus following ovulation in ewes results in persistence of the corpus luteum. Prostaglandins may also serve as the intermediary in estradiol-inducing luteolysis in animals. However, no such effect has been found in humans when prostaglandins are administered during the luteal phase. In such circumstances, uterine bleeding appears to be induced through a direct effect of the prostaglandins on the endometrium, possibly by means of the endometrial vasculature.

PGE, the prostaglandin present in particularly high concentrations in seminal fluid, causes contraction of the proximal portion and relaxation of the distal portion of the fallopian tube. These effects may be important in tubal ovum transport and retention, as well as in sperm transport. PGF causes contraction of the entire fallopian tube. Prostaglandins have also been implicated in infertility associated with minimal endometriosis. The postulated effects are either in the ovaries, interfering with follicular or luteal function, or in the fallopian tubes.

The effects of prostaglandins on the uterine musculature have had the most therapeutic usefulness. $PGF_{2\alpha}$, which increases resting uterine tone and amplitude of myometrial contractions, reaches its highest concentrations in menstrual endometrium and may be associated with uterine contractions during menstruation. It has been suggested that patients with dysmenorrhea produce a higher proportion than normal of PGF compounds and that these compounds are responsible for these patients' increased uterine contractility, spasm, and pain.

Prostaglandins are thought to be involved in the uterine contractions that follow the intra-amniotic infusion of hypertonic saline. It is postulated that saline disrupts the prostaglandin-containing decidual lysosomes, and since $PGF_{2\alpha}$ has a destabilizing effect on lysosomal membranes, the contractile process may be self-perpetuating. The delay in contractions associated with administration of indomethacin in patients under-

going abortion with hypertonic saline and the increase of $PGF_{2\alpha}$ concentrations in amniotic fluid associated with the onset of labor support the idea that prostaglandins play a role in saline-induced abortion.

It has also been postulated that prostaglandins play a part in eclampsia. According to this hypothesis, PGA is responsible for maintaining reduced resistance to flow through the uteroplacental vascular bed. If this were the case, decreased prostaglandin levels would be associated with hypertension. The recent finding of significantly lower than normal PGA levels in patients with essential hypertension and renal artery stenosis supports this hypothesis. If it is indeed true, PGA might be of therapeutic benefit in eclampsia. Agents that inhibit prostaglandin synthesis (such as indomethacin, which has been used to prevent premature labor), cause *in utero* closure of the ductus arteriosus.

Prostaglandins are readily absorbed by the vagina after they have been introduced for induction of labor or abortion, or from semen following coitus. Prostaglandin-induced uterine contractions may be the source of the lower abdominal crampy postcoital discomfort noted by some women.

The major clinical usefulness of prostaglandins in obstetrics and gynecology is in the induction of abortion in midtrimester pregnancy. In approximately 80% of patients, intra-amniotic administration of PGF induces uterine contractions that result in cervical dilatation and subsequent delivery of the fetus. Compared with amnioinfusion of hypertonic saline, prostaglandin amnioinfusion is associated with a shorter interval from instillation to delivery, no reported occurrence of maternal disseminated intravascular coagulation, and no other recognized life-threatening maternal side-effects. The disadvantages of prostaglandin amnioinfusion are an increased frequency of nausea and vomiting, the occasional delivery of a live fetus, and the rare development of a uterovaginal fistula. Prostaglandins are also under investigation as a medication to induce uterine contractions at term.

The position of prostaglandins in the normal initiation of labor is discussed on page 589.

REFERENCES AND RECOMMENDED READING

Adrenal

Abraham GE: Ovarian and adrenal contributions to peripheral androgens during the menstrual. J Clin Endocrinol Metab 39:340, 1974

Bongiovanni AM: Acquired adrenal hyperplasia with special reference to 3 β-hydroxysteroid dehydrogenase. In Wallach EE, Kempers RD (eds): Modern Trends in Infertility and Conception Control, p 89. Philadelphia, Harper & Row, 1982

Bongiovanni AM: The response of several adrenocortical steroids to the administration of ACTH in hirsute women. J Steroid Biochem 18:745, 1983

Cooke CW, McEvoy D, Bulaschenko H, Wallach EE: Adreno-cortical and ovarian function in the hirsute female. Am J Obstet Gynecol 114:65, 1972

Hardling BW: Synthesis of adrenal cortical steroids and mechanism of ACTH effects. In DeGroot LJ et al (eds): Endocrinology, p 1131. New York, Grune & Stratton, 1979

Krieger DT: Plasma ACTH and steroids. In DeGroot LJ et al (eds): Endocrinology, p 1139. New York, Grune & Stratton, 1979

Nelson DH: Synopsis of diagnosis and treatment diseases of the adrenal cortex. In DeGroot LJ et al (eds): Endocrinology, p 1235. New York, Grune & Stratton, 1979

West CD, Meikle AW: Laboratory tests for the diagnosis of Cushing's syndrome and adrenal insufficiency and factors affecting those tests. In DeGroot LJ et al (eds): Endocrinology, p 1157. New York, Grune & Stratton, 1979

Thyroid

DeGroot LJ: Synopsis of diagnosis and treatment of thyroid conditions. In DeGroot LJ et al (eds): Endocrinology, p 545. New York, Grune & Stratton, 1979

DeGroot LJ: Thyroid physiology. In DeGroot LJ et al (eds): Endocrinology, p 373. New York, Grune & Stratton, 1979

Gibson M, Tulchinsky D: The maternal thyroid. In Tulchinsky D, Ryan KJ (eds): Maternal–Fetal Endocrinology, p 115. Philadelphia, WB Saunders, 1980

Pineal

Wurtman RJ: The pineal organ. In DeGroot LJ et al (eds): Endocrinology, p 95. New York, Grune & Stratton, 1979

Prostaglandins

Arrata WS, Tsai AY: Prostaglandins in reproduction. J Reprod Med 20:84, 1978

Challis JRG, Mitchell BF: Hormonal control of pre-term and term parturition. Semin Perinatol 5:192, 1981

Liggins GC: Fetal influences on myometrial contractility. Am J Obstet Gynecol 16:148, 1973

Niebyl JR: Prostaglandin synthetase inhibitors. Semin Perinatol 5:274, 1981

Ramwell PW, Leovey EMK: Prostaglandins and humoral regulation. In DeGroot LJ et al (eds): Endocrinology, p 1711. New York, Grune & Stratton, 1979

Speroff L: Physiologic and pharmacologic roles for prostaglandins in obstetrics. Clin Obstet Gynecol 16:109, 1973

Speroff L: Toxemia in pregnancy. Am J Cardiol 32:582, 1973

Wallach EE, de la Cruz A, Hunt J et al: The effect of indomethacin on HMG-HCG induced ovulation in the rhesus monkey. Prostaglandins 9:645, 1975

Wiquist N, Widholm O, Nillius SJ et al: Dysmenorrhea and prostaglandins. Acta Obstet Gynecol Scand (Suppl) 87, 1979

Puberty, Adolescence, and the Clinical Aspects of Normal Menstruation

Laura T. Goldsmith
Gerson Weiss

8

PUBERTY

Puberty is defined as the period between childhood and the adult state during which the individual attains sexual maturity and the capacity to reproduce. This developmental period is characterized by profound somatic changes:

1. Development of secondary sexual characteristics (development of the breasts, pubic hair, and axillary hair and maturation of the genitalia)
2. Acceleration of linear growth (the adolescent or pubertal growth spurt)
3. Bone maturation
4. Relative changes in body composition.

These changes are required for normal adult function.

Somatic Development

Secondary Sexual Characteristics

Although there is wide individual variation among normal girls, detailed studies on the progression of physical changes during puberty allowed Tanner to classify the specific stages that occur and describe the temporal relations among thelarche (development of the breasts), pubarche (development of pubic hair), the growth spurt, and menarche (the onset of periodic vaginal bleeding).

The stages that occur during *breast development* are classified as follows (Fig. 8-1):

Stage 1—Preadolescent: Areola not pigmented; elevation of papilla only
Stage 2—Breast bud stage: Elevation of breast and papilla in a small mound; enlargement of areola diameter

Stage 3—Further enlargement of the breast and areola with no separation of their contours
Stage 4—Projection of areola and papilla to form a secondary mound above the levels of the breast
Stage 5—Mature stage: Projection of the papilla only, due to recession of the areola to the general contour of the breast.

Neither breast size nor shape is considered a factor in determination of maturational stage; rather, these parameters are influenced by the genetic and nutritional status of the individual.

Development of the breast and the modified areolar apocrine glands is primarily under the control of ovarian estrogens. Although optimal development of the breast requires the coordinated action of many hormones (prolactin, estrogen, progesterone, adrenal steroids, insulin, growth hormone, glucocorticocoids, and thyroid hormone), a simplified summary view is that estrogen promotes primarily duct growth, whereas prolactin and progesterone are necessary for lobuloalveolar development and prolactin governs lactation.

The multiple rudimentary mammary ducts found beneath the nipple in infancy grow and branch slowly during the prepubertal years. Under the influence of estrogens, the nipples grow, duct branching progresses, and fatty stromal growth increases. The other hormones mentioned above play a permissive role. Lobulation appears at menarche with branching of the terminal ducts into multiple blind saccular buds. These effects are thought to be due to the presence of progesterone. Full alveolar development occurs during pregnancy under the influence of additional progesterone and prolactin. Prolactin does not affect breast development or growth without the influence of estrogen and progesterone.

The stages of *development of pubic hair* are classified as follows (Fig. 8-2):

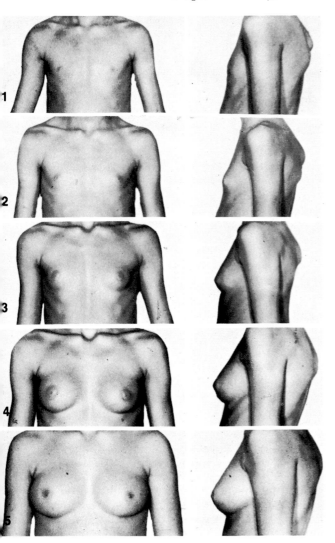

FIG. 8-1. Standards for evaluating breast development. (Tanner JM: Growth at Adolescence, 2nd ed. Oxford, Blackwell Scientific, 1962)

Stage 1—Preadolescent: No pubic hair
Stage 2—Sparse growth of long, slightly pigmented, downy hair appearing chiefly along the labia
Stage 3—Considerably darker, coarser, and curlier hair spread sparsely over the junction of the pubis
Stage 4—Adult-type hair, covering a smaller area than in the adult, with no spread to the medial surface of the thigh
Stage 5—Adult type and quantity of hair, distributed to the medial surface of the thigh but not up to the linea alba or above the base of the inverse triangle (normal female escutcheon).

The growth of pubic and axillary hair is mainly under the influence of androgens secreted primarily by the adrenals. Estrogens have a modest stimulating effect on sexual hair growth, which may be due to induction of androgen receptors by estrogen.

Although there is marked individual variation in age of onset at and duration of these stages, normal development requires passage through each stage. Rarely does an individual skip a stage or revert to a previous stage.

There are as yet no defined standards for genital development in girls. However, considerable information about pubertal development can be obtained by inspection of the labia and vagina for evidence of an estrogen effect. During the prepubertal period, the labial and vulvar membranes are bright red owing to thinness of the epithelial layer (the labia minora have sharp edges, and their secretions are watery). An early sign of estrogen stimulation is thickening of the labia minora, the presence of a mucoid vaginal secretion, and change in coloration from bright red to pink. Estrogen secretion can be confirmed during physical examination by the finding of uterine enlargement. The onset of periodic vaginal bleeding (menarche) in the human female is the best evidence that normal development is progressing.

Development of the breasts is usually the first external manifestation of puberty; breast changes are usually well under way and may even have reached stage 4 before pubic hair appears. However, pubic hair development occasionally reaches stage 3 or 4 before there is any development of the breasts. Completion of maturation of the breasts before the appearance of pubic hair is uncommon, as is completion of pubic hair development before initiation of breast development; these events would suggest abnormal development. As a rule, growth of axillary hair begins about the time the breasts reach stage 3 or 4 of development.

Some sign of puberty is seen in normal girls between 8.5 and 13 years (mean, 11 years) of age. Since all reports in the literature give standard deviations of about 1 year for the age at which each stage of puberty is reached, the appearance of secondary sexual characteristics before 7.5 years of age should be considered precocious, and puberty should be considered delayed if physical changes are not apparent before 14 years of age. The interval from the first sign of puberty to complete maturity varies from 1.5 years to over 6 years.

In the majority of normal girls, menarche occurs during breast development stage 3 or 4, but in some, menstruation does not occur until the breasts are fully mature. Breast development reaches the mature stage between the ages of 11.8 and 18.9 years. The mean interval from the first signs of puberty (breast development stage 2) to menarche is about 2.3 years (range, 6 months to 5.75 years). Mean age at menarche is 12 to 13. That 2.3 (±1) years is the mean interval required from the first detection of puberty to the time of menarche suggests that a girl whose breast development begins at 14 years might not experience the onset of menses before 17 years.

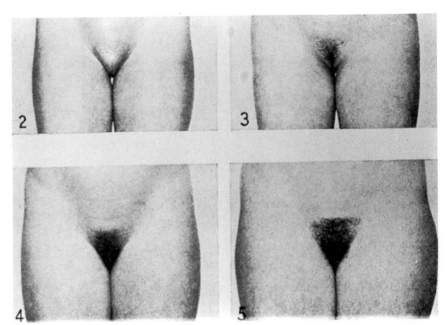

FIG. 8-2. Standards for evaluating pubic hair development. Numbers refer to stages. (Tanner JM: Growth at Adolescence, 2nd ed. Oxford, Blackwell Scientific, 1962)

It is important to recognize that the relationship between the different events of puberty are a more significant index of normality than the chronologic age at which they occur. For example, a 17-year-old girl who has not yet menstruated but is growing rapidly and whose breasts and pubic hair development have just reached stage 3 could be regarded as an example of a normal but slow-developing adolescent. Menarche could be expected in the near future. However, a girl who has not yet menstruated but whose breasts and pubic hair reached the mature stage two or three years earlier should be evaluated to determine if an abnormality exists.

Acceleration of Linear Growth

The *spurt in height* that occurs during normal puberty in girls occurs early during the developmental process, usually during breast stage 2 or 3. Growth is fastest at the mean age of 12.1 years. All studies on this subject report that the peak of this height spurt is passed before menarche; thus, the tall girl who has reached menarche at an early age can be assured that her growth is now slowing down. In contrast, in boys the growth spurt peaks on average nearly two years later than in girls; it is also unusual for boys to reach the peak of their growth spurt until their genitalia are quite well developed. Growth of the testes, the first sign of puberty in the male, usually occurs about six months later than the first change in girls, which is usually breast development.

Girls grow a mean of 25 cm during the growth spurt (between the time of take-off and cessation of growth),

and boys grow a mean of 28 cm. Thus, the average mean height difference of 10 cm between men and women is due more to the height difference at age of take-off (which in turn is due to a longer period of preadolescent growth in boys) than to growth during the spurt. Furthermore, the extremities grow faster than the trunk during the prepubertal period (resulting in greater leg length in males), whereas trunk growth is relatively greater during puberty.

Both growth hormone and gonadal sex steroids play a major role in the adolescent growth spurt; adrenal androgens are less important. The growth spurt is either minimal or absent in children with severe primary or secondary hypogonadism; a normal growth spurt is seen in children with deficient adrenal androgen secretion. Patients deficient in both gonadotropins and growth hormone do not have a growth spurt when growth hormone only is replaced; gonadal sex steroids must also be given. Thus, steroids allow for the growth-promoting effects of growth hormone. The precise mechanisms of pubertal growth are poorly understood.

Bone Maturation

Osseous maturation is assessed by comparison of radiographs of hand, knee, or elbow to standards of maturation in a normal population. The radiographic atlas of skeletal development by Greulich and Pyle is often used for such standards. Assessment of bone age can be useful in evaluation of the developmental process. Bone age more closely correlates with menarche than does chronologic age. Bone age, height, and chronologic age can be used for the prediction of final adult height from the Bayley–Pinneau tables (Table 8-1). Separate standards are used for boys and girls, since osseous maturation is more advanced in females than in males of the same chronologic age.

Body Composition

The development of secondary sexual characteristics and increased secretion of steroid hormones during puberty are accompanied by marked changes in *body composition*. Lean body mass, skeletal mass, and body fat mass are about equal in prepubertal children. However, adult males have about 1.5 times the lean body mass, muscle mass, and skeletal mass of women, and women have twice as much body fat as men. Adult males have twice as many muscle cells as females, and the size of each muscle cell in the male is larger.

A summary of the sequence of events that occurs in girls at puberty is shown in Figure 8-3.

Endocrine Development

Adrenal

The first well-defined endocrine event of puberty is an increase in adrenal androgen production, a developmental process termed *adrenarche*. The major androgens secreted by the adrenal cortex are androsterone and the weaker, less potent dehydroepiandrosterone (DHA) and its sulphate (DHAS). DHA and DHAS are secreted in much higher concentrations than androsterone. The source of these steroids is the zona reticularis.

The progressive increase in androgen secretion in girls, which starts at 7 or 8 years of age and continues to 13 to 15 years, occurs about 2 years before the increase in gonadotropin and gonadal sex steroid secretion. It is not associated with increased sensitivity of the pituitary to gonadotropin-releasing hormone (GnRH) or with sleep-associated luteinizing hormone (LH) secretion. Neither the control of adrenarche nor the role it plays in puberty is clearly understood. Adrenal androgens are required for normal development of pubic and axillary hair.

The temporal relationship between adrenarche and maturation of gonadal function (gonadarche) prompted the hypothesis that adrenal androgens play a role in the onset of puberty. However, although precocious puberty may occur in young children who have been exposed to excessive androgens from either an endogenous or an exogenous source, individuals who reach puberty at an early chronologic age are most frequently of pubertal bone age. No compelling evidence has been provided to suggest that adrenarche and gonadarche are causally related; rather, it appears that they are independent events, controlled by separate mechanisms, and that adrenarche is not essential for the onset of gonadarche.

Prepubertal children with congenital or acquired chronic adrenal insufficiency (Addison's disease), who consequently have deficient or absent adrenal androgen secretion, usually have normal onset of and progression through puberty when given appropriate glucocorticoid and mineralocorticoid replacement therapy. Furthermore, most patients with premature adrenarche who secrete excessive amounts of adrenal androgens for their age enter puberty and experience menarche within the normal age range. Thus, early activation of adrenal androgen secretion does not lead to precocious puberty, nor is deficient or absent androgen output associated with delayed puberty.

Administration of LH to agonadal patients does not increase plasma levels of adrenal androgens. The mechanism responsible for the control of adrenal androgen secretion is undefined. Patients with either gonadal dysgenesis or isolated gonadotropin deficiency demonstrate both normal onset of adrenarche and adrenal androgen levels appropriate for their bone age, suggesting that neither estrogens nor gonadotropins play an important role in the control of adrenal androgen secretion.

It has been suggested that adrenocorticotropic hormone (ACTH) is responsible for stimulation of adrenal androgen secretion during development, since it increases DHA production and since DHA secretion is suppressed by the administration of dexamethazone. Although no change in the rate of ACTH secretion is observed at adrenarche, evidence suggests that the adrenal secretory response to ACTH changes with maturation. The postulation that a distinct pituitary adrenal androgen–stimulating hormone is responsible for adrenarche has been supported by meager data. Elucidation of the mechanisms responsible for adrenarche have also been hampered by the paucity of appropriate animal models; although many mammalian species have been examined, only the chimpanzee exhibits an increase in adrenal androgen production similar to that seen in humans.

Hypothalamic–Pituitary–Gonadal Axis

The menstrual cycle in the mature adult female is characterized by specific hormone secretion patterns that are controlled by established regulatory mechanisms and are integral to successful reproduction. The decapeptide GnRH, which is synthesized within neurons in the medial basal hypothalamus, reaches the pituitary by way of the hypothalamic–pituitary portal system, where it controls pituitary synthesis and release of both LH and follicle-stimulating hormone (FSH). GnRH has also been localized in other parts of the brain, where it may function as a neurotransmitter.

Table 8-1

Prediction of Adult Height from Correlation of Skeletal Age and Proportion of Adult Stature Achieved *

Skeletal Age (years)	6-0	6-3	6-6	6-10	7-0	7-3	7-6	7-10	8-0	8-3	8-6	8-10	9-0	9-3	9-6
Percent of Mature Height	72.0	72.9	73.8	75.1	75.7	76.5	77.2	78.2	79.0	80.1	81.0	82.1	82.7	83.6	84.4
Present Height (inches)															
37	51.4														
38	52.8	52.1	51.5												
39	54.2	53.5	52.8	52.0	51.5	51.0									
40	55.6	54.9	54.2	53.3	52.8	52.3	51.8	51.2							
41	56.9	56.2	55.6	54.6	54.2	53.6	53.1	52.4	51.9	51.2					
42	58.3	57.6	56.9	55.9	55.5	54.9	54.4	53.7	53.2	52.4	51.9	51.2			
43	59.7	59.0	58.3	57.3	56.8	56.2	55.7	55.0	54.4	53.7	53.1	52.4	52.0	51.4	
44	61.1	60.4	59.6	58.6	58.1	57.5	57.0	56.3	55.7	54.9	54.3	53.6	53.2	52.6	52.1
45	62.5	61.7	61.0	59.9	59.4	58.8	58.3	57.5	57.0	56.2	55.6	54.8	54.4	53.8	53.3
46	63.9	63.1	62.3	61.3	60.8	60.1	59.6	58.8	58.2	57.4	56.8	56.0	55.6	55.0	54.5
47	65.3	64.5	63.7	62.6	62.1	61.4	60.9	60.1	59.5	58.7	58.0	57.2	56.8	56.2	55.7
48	66.7	65.8	65.0	63.9	63.4	62.7	62.2	61.4	60.8	59.9	59.3	58.5	58.0	57.4	56.9
49	68.1	67.2	66.4	65.2	64.7	64.1	63.5	62.7	62.0	61.2	60.5	59.7	59.3	58.6	58.1
50	69.4	68.6	67.8	66.6	66.1	65.4	64.8	63.9	63.3	62.4	61.7	60.9	60.5	59.8	59.2
51	70.8	70.0	69.1	67.9	67.4	66.7	66.1	65.2	64.6	63.7	63.0	62.1	61.7	61.0	60.4
52	72.2	71.3	70.5	69.2	68.7	68.0	67.4	66.5	65.8	64.9	64.2	63.3	62.9	62.2	61.6
53	73.6	72.7	71.8	70.6	70.0	69.3	68.7	67.8	67.1	66.2	65.4	64.6	64.1	63.4	62.8
54		74.1	73.2	71.9	71.3	70.6	69.9	69.1	68.4	67.4	66.7	65.8	65.3	64.6	64.0
55			74.5	73.2	72.7	71.9	71.2	70.3	69.6	68.7	67.9	67.0	66.5	65.8	65.2
56				74.6	74.0	73.2	72.5	71.6	70.9	69.9	69.1	68.2	67.7	67.0	66.4
57						74.5	73.8	72.9	72.2	71.2	70.4	69.4	68.9	68.2	67.5
58								74.2	73.4	72.4	71.6	70.6	70.1	69.4	68.7
59									74.7	73.7	72.8	71.9	71.3	70.6	69.9
60										74.9	74.1	73.1	72.6	71.8	71.1
61												74.3	73.8	73.0	72.3
62														74.2	73.5
63															74.6
64															
65															
66															
67															
68															
69															
70															
71															
72															
73															
74															

* Predicted adult height in inches is read off directly at point of intersection of skeletal age and present height. Table shown is for average girls with skeletal age within 1 year of chronologic age. Other tables, presented in original article, are to be used if skeletal age is either accelerated or retarded 1 or more years. (Bayley N, Pinneau SR: Tables predicting adult height from skeletal age: Revised for use with the Greulich-Pyle hand standards. J Pediatr 40:432, 1952)

Studies from the laboratory of Knobil have demonstrated that a pulsatile pattern of secretion of GnRH is fundamental to the control of gonadotropin secretion. These studies were carried out with adult female rhesus monkeys, in whom radiofrequency lesions were used to destroy the arcuate nucleus of the medial basal hypothalamus, abolishing endogenous GnRH production and consequently pituitary gonadotropin secretion. In these animals, regardless of the infusion rate, continuous administration of GnRH failed to sustain gonadotropin secretion, whereas a GnRH replacement regimen given as an intermittent, pulsatile infusion (at a frequency of

9-9	10-0	10-3	10-6	10-9	11-0	11-3	11-6	11-9	12-0	12-3	12-6	12-9	13-0	13-3	13-6	13-9	14-0
85.3	86.2	87.4	88.4	89.6	9.6	91.0	91.4	91.8	92.2	93.2	94.1	95.0	95.8	96.7	97.4	97.8	98.0
51.6	51.0																
52.8	52.2	51.5															
53.9	53.4	52.6	52.0	51.3													
55.1	54.5	53.8	53.2	52.5	51.9	51.6	51.4	51.2	51.0								
56.3	55.7	54.9	54.3	53.6	53.0	52.7	52.5	52.3	52.1	51.5	51.0						
57.4	56.8	56.1	55.4	54.7	54.1	53.8	53.6	53.4	53.1	52.6	52.1	51.6	51.1				
58.6	58.0	57.2	56.6	55.8	55.2	54.9	54.7	54.5	54.2	53.6	53.1	52.6	52.2	51.7	51.3	51.1	51.0
59.8	59.2	58.4	57.7	56.9	56.3	56.0	55.8	55.6	55.3	54.7	54.2	53.7	53.2	52.7	52.4	52.1	52.0
61.0	60.3	59.5	58.8	58.0	57.4	57.1	56.9	56.6	56.4	55.8	55.3	54.7	54.3	53.8	53.4	53.2	53.1
62.1	61.5	60.6	60.0	59.2	58.5	58.2	58.0	57.7	57.5	56.9	56.3	55.8	55.3	54.8	54.4	54.2	54.1
63.3	62.6	61.8	61.1	60.3	59.6	59.3	59.1	58.8	58.6	57.9	57.4	56.8	56.4	55.8	55.4	55.2	55.1
64.5	63.8	62.9	62.2	61.4	60.7	60.4	60.2	59.9	59.7	59.0	58.4	57.9	57.4	56.9	56.5	56.2	56.1
65.7	65.0	64.1	63.3	62.5	61.8	61.5	61.3	61.0	60.7	60.1	59.5	58.9	58.5	57.9	57.5	57.3	57.1
66.8	66.1	65.2	64.5	63.6	62.9	62.6	62.4	62.1	61.8	61.2	60.6	60.0	59.5	58.9	58.5	58.3	58.2
68.0	67.3	66.4	65.6	64.7	64.0	63.7	63.5	63.2	62.9	62.2	61.6	61.1	60.5	60.0	59.5	59.3	59.2
69.2	68.4	67.5	66.7	65.8	65.1	64.8	64.6	64.3	64.0	63.3	62.7	62.1	61.6	61.0	60.6	60.3	60.2
70.3	69.6	68.7	67.9	67.0	66.2	65.9	65.6	65.4	65.1	64.4	63.8	63.2	62.6	62.0	61.6	61.3	61.2
71.5	70.8	69.8	69.0	68.1	67.3	67.0	66.7	66.4	66.2	65.5	64.8	64.2	63.7	63.1	62.6	62.4	62.2
72.7	71.9	70.9	70.1	69.2	68.4	68.1	67.8	76.5	67.2	66.5	65.9	65.3	64.7	64.1	63.7	63.4	63.3
73.9	73.1	72.1	71.3	70.3	69.5	69.2	68.9	68.6	68.3	67.6	67.0	66.3	65.8	65.1	64.7	66.4	64.3
	74.2	73.2	72.4	71.4	70.6	70.3	70.0	69.7	69.4	68.7	68.0	67.4	66.8	66.2	65.7	65.4	65.3
		74.4	73.5	72.5	71.7	71.4	71.1	70.8	70.5	69.7	69.1	68.4	67.8	67.2	66.7	66.5	66.3
			74.7	73.7	72.9	72.5	72.2	71.9	71.6	70.8	70.1	69.5	68.9	68.3	67.8	67.5	67.3
				74.8	74.0	73.6	73.3	73.0	72.7	71.9	71.2	70.5	69.9	69.3	68.8	68.5	68.4
						74.7	74.4	74.1	73.8	73.0	72.3	71.6	71.0	70.3	69.8	69.5	69.4
									74.8	74.0	73.3	72.6	72.0	71.4	70.8	70.6	70.4
											74.4	73.7	73.1	72.4	71.9	71.6	71.4
												74.7	74.1	73.4	72.9	72.6	72.4
														74.5	73.9	73.6	73.5
															74.9	74.6	74.5

1 pulse per hour) maintained pituitary gonadotropin secretion and resulted in normal ovulatory menstrual cycles.

Additional studies in both monkeys and humans (as well as studies of several other species) have established the pulsatile nature of the secretion of both LH and FSH, thought to be a consequence of a corresponding pattern of intermittent GnRH discharge by the brain. Although direct evidence for a tightly coupled temporal relationship between endogenous GnRH and LH release has yet to be provided (owing to the overwhelming difficulty of collecting portal blood without interrupting the neu-

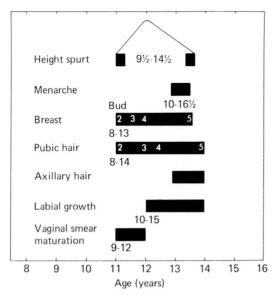

FIG. 8-3. Sequence of events that occurs in girls at puberty. Numbers under each event are normal range of ages within which event may occur. (Tanner JM: Growth at Adolescence, 2nd ed. Oxford, Blackwell Scientific, 1962)

rovascular link to the pituitary gland), nevertheless indirect evidence supports this concept. In women the frequency of LH pulses is once every 1 to 2 hours during the follicular phase and somewhat less often during the luteal phase. No doubt, normal ovarian function requires specific GnRH and gonadotropin secretion pulse frequency. Evidence from monkeys with arcuate nucleus radiofrequency lesions demonstrates that even small reductions in the frequency of GnRH stimulation have profound effects on the quality of follicular development.

Although GnRH plays an important role in the normal synthesis and secretion of pituitary gonadotropins, the major regulator of circulating gonadotropin concentrations is ovarian steroid secretion, principally estradiol. During the early and midfollicular phases, peripheral estradiol concentrations are relatively low. These low concentrations of estradiol exert a negative feedback effect upon the pituitary, maintaining LH and FSH at relatively constant basal concentrations. With appropriate gonadotropin input, ovarian follicular growth occurs, resulting in increasing estradiol secretion. FSH induces both granulosa cell proliferation and aromatase activity, such that increased estradiol production results both from greater production by each cell and from an increase in cell number. Furthermore, this process is self-perpetuating, since estradiol enhances the mitogenic effect of FSH on granulosa cells. When estradiol levels rise above a certain concentration (200–300 pg/ml) for several days, a positive feedback effect occurs, causing the midcycle outpouring of gonadotropins, the LH/FSH

surge. Both the amount and the duration of estradiol secretion are critical to this positive feedback response. Data suggest that high levels of estradiol have a stimulatory effect on gonadotropin synthesis and storage whereas lower amounts have an inhibitory effect. However, the evidence is not definitive.

In response to the LH surge, the graafian follicle ruptures, the ovum is expelled, and the corpus luteum is formed. Progesterone secretion increases as the corpus luteum develops; in humans sizable quantities of estradiol are secreted as well. During the luteal phase, progesterone blocks the ability of estradiol to exert a positive feedback effect. The precise locus of the feedback effects of gonadal steroids is not defined; studies suggest the primary locus of estrogen action is the pituitary whereas effects of progesterone appear to be exerted at higher levels in the brain. An increase in the secretion of progesterone causes transformation and hyperplasia, resulting in a secretory endometrium. Spontaneous regression of the corpus luteum (luteolysis) occurs in the absence of pregnancy with a concomitant decline in steroid hormone secretion to levels insufficient to maintain the endometrium, resulting in menstruation. The specific mechanisms that limit the life span of the corpus luteum are unknown.

With this review of the basic principles of how the adult hypothalamic–pituitary–gonadal system functions, we can now examine the developmental sequence of events that allows for normal adult reproductive function.

PREPUBERTAL PERIOD. FSH and LH are detectable in the human fetal pituitary gland by 10 weeks of gestation, and pituitary gonadotropin content increases sharply until 25 to 29 weeks. The fetal pituitary is capable of secreting these hormones by 11 to 12 weeks. Subsequently, plasma concentrations of LH and FSH in the fetus rise until midgestation, then fall toward term. That FSH levels are generally higher in female than in male fetuses is thought to be due to lower plasma testosterone levels in females.

During the first year or two after birth, gonadotropin levels fluctuate greatly, occasionally reaching adult concentrations. Thereafter, however, FSH and LH concentrations remain low until just before puberty. Even the low amounts of gonadotropins secreted in prepubertal children are secreted in a pulsatile fashion.

GnRH has been detected in the human fetal hypothalamus by about 6 weeks' gestation. Fetal pituitary gonadotropes are responsive to GnRH. The release of LH following administration of exogenous GnRH is minimal in prepubertal children beyond infancy, increases strikingly in children in the peripubertal period and at puberty, and is greater still in adult males and females (depending upon the phase of the menstrual cycle); this suggests that pituitary sensitivity to GnRH increases with development. In contrast, FSH release after administration of GnRH is similar in prepubertal, pubertal, and adult males, as well as in prepubertal, pubertal, and adult females. Prepubertal and pubertal females release more FSH in response to GnRH than males at all stages of sexual maturation. It is thought that testosterone inhibits the FSH response to GnRH stimulus in males.

In the female fetus throughout gestation, plasma estrogen concentrations are extremely high owing to placental conversion of fetal and maternal C19 steroids. Fetal estrogen levels plummet immediately after delivery and remain very low throughout infancy and childhood until puberty. Evidence suggests that the negative feedback mechanism of estradiol is operative in prepubertal children (probably from infancy); in contrast, positive feedback cannot be demonstrated before middle or late puberty.

PUBERTY. At some point shortly before somatic signs of puberty can be detected, gonadotropin secretion begins to increase during sleep. Augmentation of LH and FSH secretion during sleep is very apparent by the time puberty is at midstage (Tanner stage 2–3), yet daytime (waking hour) levels of LH and FSH may be undistinguishable from prepubertal values. By late puberty, increased LH and FSH secretory activity is detected during sleep and waking hours; however, nighttime (sleep) activity is still greater than daytime (waking) activity until the adult pattern is achieved.

During puberty, augmentation of FSH secretion generally precedes that of LH, such that FSH levels reach the adult range earlier during pubertal development than LH. Rising FSH levels may be detected during Tanner stage 2, whereas an increase in LH may not be detected until well into stage 3. Figures 8-4 and 8-5 dem-

FIG. 8-4. Serum LH (*A*) and FSH (*B*) concentrations in girls of different ages and in adult women. *Shaded area* represents limit of sensitivity of assay. ●, prepubertal; ▲, premenarchal; ○, postmenarchal; *LMP,* last menstrual period. (Winter JSD, Faiman C: Pituitary–gonadal relations in female children and adolescents. Pediatr Res 7:948, 1973)

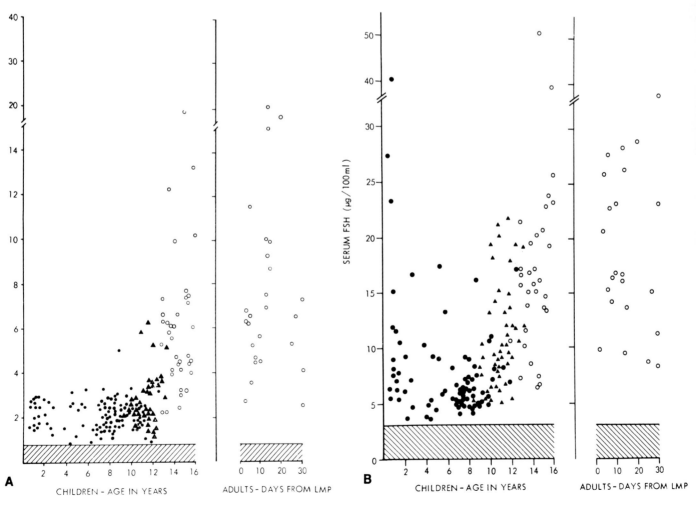

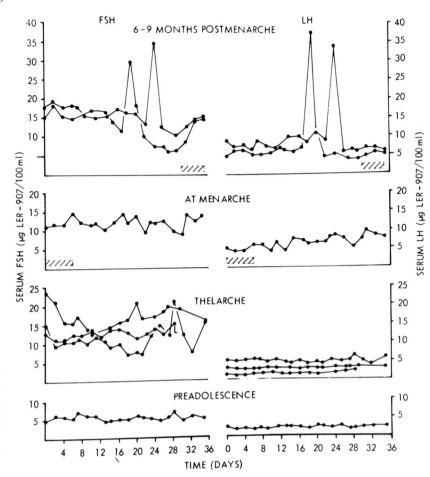

FIG. 8-5. Serum FSH and LH values at 2- to 3-day intervals in seven perimenarchal girls. Each line represents values from a separate individual. The hatched bars denote menses. (Winter JSD, Faiman C: The development of cyclic pituitary–gonadal function in adolescent females. J Clin Endocrinol Metab 37:714, 1973)

onstrate the changes in gonadotropin secretion that occur as development progresses. In girls estradiol rises steadily throughout the stages of puberty until maturity.

Prolactin

Studies of cultures of the human fetal pituitary gland suggest that this organ synthesizes prolactin as early as five weeks' gestation, and detectable levels of prolactin have been found in sera of fetuses from 88 days of gestation. Concentrations increase substantially late in gestation (after about 29 weeks), presumably owing to stimulation by placental estrogen. In the neonate, plasma prolactin levels remain elevated during the first day of life, then decrease within seven days by about 30%. Concentrations remain at this level for about the first six weeks of life before decreasing to normal prepubertal levels (<15 ng/ml). During puberty prolactin levels increase in both girls and boys; however, a greater increase is seen in girls, probably reflecting the increased estrogen secretion in girls. In concert with other hormones, prolactin is required for normal breast development and function. No other function has been attributed to this hormone in humans.

GROWTH HORMONE AND SOMATOMEDINS. Linear growth during normal development requires the coordinated action of a variety of hormones and growth factors. Growth hormone, required for normal skeletal and muscle growth and growth of most body organs, is among the most important of these. However, there is not always a good correlation between growth velocity and growth hormone levels; the correlation is much stronger between growth velocity and serum somatomedin levels (which mediate the growth-promoting actions of growth hormone). The somatomedins, a family of low-molecular-weight peptides similar in structure to insulin, are known to be involved in the growth process (as is insulin). However, it is not known what exact role is played by each of these molecules.

Mechanisms Initiating Puberty

The precise mechanisms responsible for the onset of puberty have yet to be established. Studies by Foa dating back to 1900, the pioneering work of Harris and Jacobsohn, and a large body of experimental and clinical studies have established that neither the gonads nor the anterior pituitary gland is a rate-limiting factor in the process of sexual maturation. It has thus been assumed that puberty results from a developmental process within the brain, the nature of which remains to be elucidated.

One hypothesis is that there is an alteration in the sensitivity of certain brain areas to the negative feedback effect of gonadal steroid hormones. This concept, originally proposed by Hohlweg and Junkmann, holds that the brain of a young animal is highly sensitive to the negative feedback effect exerted by the small amounts of sex steroids produced by the immature gonads, so that gonadotropin secretion from the pituitary proceeds at a minimal rate. As puberty approaches, these small amounts of steroid hormones become less efficient at suppressing pituitary secretion, and the "gonadostat" is reset at a new level such that gonadotropin secretion and, consequently, steroid production are greatly increased.

The concept that puberty in humans results from increased secretion of pituitary gonadotropins due to a gradual decrease in sensitivity of the hypothalamic "gonadostat" to gonadal steroid inhibition has been largely supported by the studies of Grumbach and colleagues. These investigators administered the antiestrogen clomiphene citrate (Clomid) and the potent synthetic estrogen ethinyl estradiol to children at various stages of pubertal development. In adults Clomid stimulates gonadotropin secretion, presumably by inhibiting estradiol binding to receptors in the hypothalamus and pituitary and thus blocking negative feedback mechanisms. However, when Clomid was administered to prepubertal children (in doses that would stimulate gonadotropin secretion in adults), no such effect was detected. Rather, suppression of gonadotropins occurred, which was attributed to the weak estrogenic properties of Clomid. Similarly, prepubertal children given ethinyl estradiol exhibited suppression of gonadotropin secretion. Children in midstages of puberty demonstrated slight or no suppression, nor was suppression seen in children at late puberty. These studies suggest that there is decreased sensitivity to steroid feedback with progression of puberty. It is also possible that this differential sensitivity to estrogen is due to differences in the metabolic clearance rates of gonadotropins or sex steroids between prepubertal children and adults.

Several other investigators think it is unnecessary to invoke the gonadostat hypothesis to explain the onset of puberty. The same pattern of elevation of gonadotropin secretion is seen at the appropriate time during development both in women with gonadal dysgenesis and in neonatally ovariectomized rhesus monkeys, neither of whom has ovarian estradiol. Knobil has provided evidence that puberty may normally be initiated by the activation of hypothalamic mechanisms that control the pulsatile release of GnRH; precocious puberty was induced in immature female rhesus monkeys by administration of a pulsatile infusion of GnRH. Terasawa has

demonstrated an increase in LH pulse amplitude but no changes in pulse frequency occur with progression of puberty in the rhesus monkey; similar results have been demonstrated in humans by Kelch and associates. These investigators have therefore concluded that puberty is controlled by maturation of the hypothalamus facilitating release of GnRH rather than by changes in steroid hormone feedback.

Recently, controversy has arisen regarding the role of body weight and composition in the onset of puberty. Several clinical observations suggest a relationship between body weight and the onset of menarche: (1) moderately obese girls experience menarche at a relatively young age; (2) malnourished girls show a delay in menarche; (3) girls with anorexia nervosa or severe weight loss due to other conditions show changes in gonadotropin secretion and amenorrhea; and (4) young, thin ballet dancers show delayed menarche.

Prompted by studies by Kennedy and Mitra on the influence of body size and food intake on the onset of puberty in the rat, Frisch and Revelle measured the height and weight of normal, healthy girls at menarche. Mean weight range at menarche was found to be 47.2 kg to 48.7 kg regardless of age, leading the authors to conclude that attainment of a critical body weight is required for initiation of regular menstrual function. The researchers further hypothesized that attainment of this critical weight causes a change in metabolic rate, which in turn reduces the sensitivity of the hypothalamus to estrogen, altering ovarian–hypothalamus feedback.

Frisch calculated total water and lean body weight as correlates of metabolic rate and ratios of total body water to body weight as an index of fatness in girls between the beginning of their adolescent growth spurt and menarche. Finding a large increase in fat (120%) from the time of spurt initiation to the time of menarche, as compared with a 44% increase in lean body weight, Frisch postulated that a particular ratio of fat to lean mass is necessary for menarche. He also hypothesized that a minimal fatness level of about 22% of body weight is necessary to maintain regular ovulatory cycles. Human female adipose tissue can aromatize androgens to estrogen, suggesting that adipose tissue may be a source of extragonadal estrogen, which may in turn precipitate the pubertal process.

This critical body composition hypothesis has been severely criticized by several investigators, including Trussell, Cameron, and Billewicz, who suggest mathematical or statistical inaccuracies in Frisch's studies. Johnston and colleagues have presented data from normal girls who attained menarche at body weights significantly different from the 47-kg to 48-kg range. That weight and body composition change during sexual maturation is not under question; however, epidemiologic data for a relationship between body weight and puberty have yet to be supported by any physiologic mechanisms, nor has any causal relationship between the two been demonstrated. The fact that menstruation starts again in anorexic girls who have gained sufficient weight cannot be viewed as evidence that body weight plays a role in menarche, since the trigger that leads to the first menstruation may not be the same as that which causes its resumption after starvation amenorrhea.

In a similar vein, Steiner and Bremner and colleagues have proposed a metabolic theory for the onset of puberty in primates. Studies associating metabolic disturbances with reproductive impairment suggested to them a possible link between abnormal puberty and a "fasting" metabolic state involving low insulin levels and alterations in circulating levels of amino acids and free fatty acids. These researchers found that plasma insulin levels were significantly higher in adult than in prepubertal monkeys. Further experiments designed to determine the effects of a chronic carbohydrate stimulus or essential amino acids on gonadotropin secretion demonstrated no effects from carbohydrate only; in contrast, a sustained increase in both plasma amino acids and dextrose caused markedly stimulated LH secretion in a prepubertal animal that would not normally have exhibited such an increase until the normal time of puberty 12 to 18 months later. These results suggest that metabolic cues may initiate an increase in GnRH secretion and hence the onset of puberty in primates. This idea is supported by the finding that insulin binds to specific receptors in the hypothalamus arcuate nucleus and median eminence, as well as by some indirect evidence relating insulin to neurotransmitter activity. However, much additional information is required before this concept can be considered tenable.

In an attempt to reconcile the several hypotheses being proposed to explain the onset of puberty, Ruf has suggested that functional maturation of adrenergic neurons is a key factor in the initiation of puberty. On the basis of the data of Wurtman suggesting that central adrenergic neurons are sensitive to steroids, Ruf has proposed that the resetting of the gonadostat is caused by an increase in the hypothalamic drive for the activation of the pituitary gonadal axis due to an increase in terminal arborization of adrenergic neurons synapsing with neurons elaborating GnRH. It is also possible that the number of GnRH neurons increases with maturity.

Evidence has led several investigators to propose that the pineal gland plays an important role in human puberty. A few reports have described declining serum concentrations of melatonin with advancing development in boys from ages 11 to 14. Also in boys, tumors of the pineal gland have been associated with abnormal puberty. Other investigators, however, find no evidence of marked changes in blood melatonin concentrations either during normal development or in precocious puberty; furthermore, precocious puberty associated with central nervous system tumors appears to be due to pressure of these growths on the hypothalamus. Therefore, it is possible that the etiology of pineal tumors associated with abnormal puberty is pressure related. In addition, the time of first detection and the subsequent time course of an increase in circulating gonad-

otropin concentrations were similar in male orchiectomized rhesus monkeys whose pineal glands had been removed prepubertally and in control male orchiectomized monkeys, which finding suggests that the pineal gland does not play a role in puberty in higher primates. Certainly the evidence available does not support the idea that melatonin and the pineal gland play a significant role in puberty.

MENSTRUATION

Menstruation is the episodic shedding of the endometrium that is the hallmark of the reproductive years. Normal menstruation is the shedding of a secretory endometrium after an ovulatory menstrual cycle. Periodic anovulatory bleeding due to estrogen decrease or withdrawal from a proliferative endometrium should be differentiated from normal menstruation. However, this differentiation may be difficult to make by history alone. Menses associated with ovulatory cycles are usually preceded by breast swelling, fluid retention, and cramps. However, some normal ovulatory cycles are not preceded by any symptoms.

Characteristics of the Menstrual Cycle

The accepted standard cycle length is 28 days. This is highly arbitrary, however; normal cycles lasting as few as 23 days and as many as 35 days are not uncommon. By convention, the first day of the cycle is considered to be the first day of bleeding, and the last day of the cycle is the last day before the beginning of the next bleeding episode. The follicular phase of the menstrual cycle is usually more variable than the luteal phase, which is usually 14 days long, plus or minus 2 days. Most menstrual cycle lengths vary little in the same woman.

The duration of normal menstrual flow is usually two to seven days. Rybo found that only 1.5% of a population of normal women had flow longer than seven days; 19.2% of the women had flow of two to three days, 57.5% flow of four to five days, and 21.8% flow of six to seven days.

Irregular menstrual cycle length associated with anovulatory cycles is common the first year after menarche and the last years of reproductive life. However, it is not unusual for otherwise normal women to occasionally have an anovulatory cycle of a different length than her usual cycles. Such a cycle may be associated with illness, stress, travel, exercise, or weight loss.

The amount of blood lost during a menstrual cycle is normally between 60 ml and 80 ml. The mean blood loss in 476 women studied by Hallberg and colleagues was 43.4 ml. Different age groups generally lost similar quantities of blood; however, 15-year-olds tended to have the smallest loss, and 50-year-olds the largest loss. Blood loss averaged 38.5 ml in women who considered their cycles to be normal. If women with iron deficiency anemia were excluded, mean blood loss was 33.2 ml.

Characteristics of Menstrual Blood

Menstrual blood is generally dark red. Many patients consider the color important and report changes to their physicians. Generally, black flow or dark brown flow is old menstrual blood that has been acted on by proteolytic enzymes. Bright red flow generally indicates a rapid loss of blood that has not been affected by enzymes or diluted with other menstrual blood components such as cervical mucus or vaginal contents. The endometrium is shed as part of the menstrual flow. This contains the superficial layers, including most of the spongiosa.

Generally, the small "clots" that pass during menses do not contain fibrin but are a coagulum that forms in the vagina and contains red cells and mucoid substances. The reason menstrual blood does not form a true fibrin clot is that menstrual flow is rich in plasminogen activator, which causes rapid fibrinolysis and fibrinogenolysis. There is also a striking difference between the amount of plasminogen and the amount of plasmin inhibitor in menstrual blood sampled from the uterine cavity and vaginal pool; this shows that cervical mucus provides an active proteolytic system. In contrast, the blood in abnormally brisk uterine bleeding is clotted because proteolytic enzymes have not had a chance to act on it.

Possible Mechanism of Menstruation

The mechanism of menstruation is not fully understood. Endometrial function is controlled by the local interplay between estrogen and progesterone. The endometrium produces many substances, including prolactin, relaxin, and a multitude of endometrium-specific proteins. However, the roles of these substances and their interaction are not yet understood.

In the late secretory and early menstrual phases, there is variable acid hydrolase activity in the intercellular spaces of the stromal and epithelial layers. The hydrolases gradually spread between adjacent endothelial cells and the swollen arteriolar membranes. The acid hydrolases are derived from lysosomes, on which progesterone has a stabilizing effect. Progesterone withdrawal in the late secretory phase may initiate the destabilization of lysosomes and the escape of lysosomal enzymes, resulting in cellular digestion and endometrial tissue necrosis.

Endometrial prostaglandin production is under the control of sex steroids. During the secretory phase prostaglandins accumulate in the endometrium. During the menstrual phase they may contribute to menstrual bleeding by causing local vasoconstriction of arterioles. This may result in local hypoxia, a destabilizing influence on lysosomes. In addition to causing the release of acid hydrolases, vasoconstriction of arterioles may result in the release of phospholipase A2 and a resultant increase in prostaglandin synthesis, thus maintaining the effects of prostaglandins.

Menstrual bleeding is minimized by vasoconstriction in the ruptured vessels and by the rapid formation of platelet plugs providing hemostasis. By the second day of the cycle, re-epithelialization occurs, resulting in cessation of bleeding. Additionally, the residual glandular epithelium spreads over and covers the denuded areas. This repair can occur in the absence of sex steroids.

DYSMENORRHEA

The term *dysmenorrhea,* as commonly used, refers to painful menstruation. Some discomfort is normal during menstruation in ovulatory cycles; the term *dysmenorrhea* is reserved for pain perceived by the patient as burdensome. About half of menstruating women are affected by dysmenorrhea. Untreated, 10% of menstruating women are incapacitated by dysmenorrhea for one to three days. Dysmenorrhea is the most frequent cause of absenteeism from work and school among young women.

Dysmenorrhea is classified as primary if it is not related to detectable pelvic pathology. It is considered secondary if it is due to pelvic disease such as endometriosis, uterine polyps, liomyomata, or pelvic inflammatory disease.

Primary dysmenorrhea usually occurs in ovulatory cycles. In some women, whether a cycle is ovulatory or anovulatory can be determined by the presence or absence of menstruation-related symptoms. Primary dysmenorrhea usually appears some months after menarche, once ovulation has been established. Pain commences any time from several hours before to after the onset of the menstrual flow. The pain is cramplike and can be mild to incapacitating. It is generally felt in the suprapubic area and sometimes radiates to the back or upper thighs. The pain is frequently accompanied by other symptoms, the most common of which are nausea with occasional vomiting, fatigue, diarrhea, headache, and backache. The symptoms usually last from a few hours to a day and may occasionally last even longer than two days.

Physical examination should normally be performed, although the uterus may be tender during crampy episodes. The diagnosis of primary dysmenorrhea is made on the basis of the clinical features, which include ovulatory cycles, short duration of symptoms (rarely longer than 72 hours), pain beginning before or just after the start of menstrual flow, cramplike character of the pain, and absence of significant physical findings. The diagnosis is usually confirmed by appropriate response to drug therapy.

The causes of primary dysmenorrhea have been defined fairly well in recent years. Psychologic factors had been implicated in the etiology of this disorder. However, this formulation was derived from a lack of data rather than from supportive evidence. Although pain perception has psychologic determinants, there is no convincing evidence that the causes of primary dysmenorrhea are psychologic. Primary dysmenorrhea is related both to diminished blood flow to the uterus and to uterine hyperactivity. The available evidence indicates that excess prostaglandin F2α is responsible for dysmenorrhea. Prostaglandin F2α stimulates uterine contractions and is present in menstrual blood, and its concentration is greater in the menstrual blood of women with dysmenorrhea than in the menstrual blood of women without dysmenorrhea. Furthermore, infusion of prostaglandin F2α can induce the symptoms of dysmenorrhea in sensitive women. The levels of prostaglandin F2α in the endometrium are determined by the hormonal milieu of the woman. Levels are highest at the end of the ovulatory cycle.

There are two major effective drug modalities for primary dysmenorrhea treatment. Combination oral contraceptives, which reduce menstrual fluid prostaglandin concentrations, are effective in treating primary dysmenorrhea and are the drug of choice for women also desiring oral contraceptives. Prostaglandin synthetase inhibitors are the other class of agents effective in the treatment of primary dysmenorrhea. These agents reduce the amount of endometrial prostaglandins released by inhibiting cycloxygenase, a component of the prostaglandin synthetase enzyme system. Ibuprofen (Motrin), mefenamic acid (Ponstel), naproxen sodium (Anaprox, Naprosyn) and indomethacin (Indocin) are all effective in relieving dysmenorrhea. Aspirin is not effective because the concentrations of its active metabolites are not high enough. Indomethacin is associated with a higher incidence of unpleasant side-effects than the other agents. Contraindications to these agents include hypersensitivity to aspirin, nasal polyps, and gastric or duodenal ulcers. The major side-effect is gastric upset. In patients with nasal polyps, an acute asthmatic reaction may occur. Frequently, if one agent is ineffective, a different agent or dosage will result in relief. Because these agents take several hours to be effective, treatment should begin at the very onset of menstruation or symptoms. It is rarely necessary to continue treatment for more than two or three days.

If drug therapy is ineffective in relieving the symptoms of dysmenorrhea, it is possible that the dysmenorrhea is secondary to endometriosis or chronic salpingitis. Diagnostic laparoscopy may be used to determine the presence of pelvic pathology.

Secondary dysmenorrhea usually occurs many years after the menarche. The symptom complex may significantly differ from the typical pattern of primary dysmenorrhea. The diagnosis is frequently revealed by pelvic examination in conjunction with appropriate diagnostic testing, including blood count, erythrocyte sedimentation rate, ultrasonography, and occasionally hysterosalpingography or laparoscopy. Therapy is then directed at the underlying cause.

PREMENSTRUAL SYNDROME

The symptom complex of premenstrual syndrome (PMS) includes headache, breast swelling and tenderness, abdominal bloating, peripheral edema, fatigue, irritability, tension, and depression. Increased thirst and appetite, constipation, and acne may also occur. Dysmenorrhea is not a part of PMS, although the two conditions may exist in the same woman. PMS can occur in both ovulatory and anovulatory cycles, though it is much more common in ovulatory cycles. It is most prevalent in women in their twenties and thirties. The symptoms begin at midcycle or a few days before menses. They increase premenstrually and are relieved by the menstrual flow. Most PMS patients have only a few symptoms, the most annoying and unpleasant of which are the behavioral symptoms. Sufferers complain of marked irritability and report yelling at their spouses, children, and associates while simultaneously recognizing that they are overreacting. Many patients become tearful and cry with only minor provocation. Others complain of marked depression, even suicidal ideation. Sufferers feel that these manifestations are not their normal behavior but rather a temporary aberration due to their condition.

The cause of PMS is not known. In fact, various aspects of the syndrome may have different causes. For instance, edema may be due to different causes than depression. Research on PMS is limited by the lack of specific syndrome markers or animal models. The syndrome seems to follow a pattern of response to a substance that is increased in the late menstrual cycle and decreased during menses; however, this substance has not been identified and is not even positively known to exist. Many theories have been proposed to explain the syndrome. Attempts have been made to relate PMS to excessive or abnormal levels of estrogen or progesterone secretion; however, the syndrome is most severe when the concentrations of these hormones are falling. Hypoglycemia and vitamin deficiencies have been proposed as causes, but there is little reproducible supporting evidence. Prostaglandins have been implicated in PMS, also without much supporting data. Endorphins have recently been implicated as a contributor to PMS, but additional data are needed to support this hypothesis.

As is the case with many poorly understood conditions of unknown cause, there are many suggested treatments for PMS, all empirical and none universally accepted. Mild cases may respond to simple physician reassurance. Diuretic therapy is appropriate for the treatment of edema and swelling. Spironolactone, an aldosterone inhibitor, is effective either alone or in combination with phenothiazides in decreasing edema; some patients report relief of other symptoms as well. A number of women report relief of premenstrual breast pain by the elimination of coffee and caffeine from their diets.

Recently, progesterone or synthetic progestins have been widely prescribed for the treatment of PMS, but few appropriate controlled prospective studies have been carried out on their effectiveness. There is little agreement as to the best progestin to use, the dose, or the duration of therapy. Some patients' symptoms are relieved by prolonged progestin treatment starting before midcycle. Whether the beneficial effects are due to placebo effect, a nonspecific alteration of the menstrual cycle, or a specific therapeutic effect is not known.

REFERENCES AND RECOMMENDED READING

Puberty

Bayley N, Pinneau SR: Tables predicting adult height from skeletal age: Revised for use with the Greulich-Pyle hand standards. J Pediatr 40:432, 1952

Belchetz PE, Plant TM, Nakai Y et al: Hypophysial responses to continuous and intermittent delivery of hypothalamic gonadotropin-releasing hormone. Science 202:631, 1978

Billewicz WZ, Fellowes HM, Hytten CA: Comments on the critical metabolic mass and the age of menarche. Ann Hum Biol 3:51, 1976

Boyar R, Finkelstein J, Roffwarg H et al: Synchronization of augmented luteinizing hormone secretion with sleep during puberty. N Engl J Med 287:582, 1972

Cameron N: Weight and skinfold variation at menarche and the critical body weight hypothesis. Ann Hum Biol 3:279, 1976

Cutler GB, Glenn M, Bush M et al: Adrenarche: A survey of rodents, domestic animals and primates. Endocrinology 103:2112, 1978

Cutler GD, Loriaux DL: Adrenarche and its relationship to the onset of puberty. Fed Proc 39:2384, 1980

Fernstrom JD: In Kreiger DT (ed): Endocrine Rhythms, pp 89–122. New York, Raven Press, 1979

Foa C: La greffe des ovaires en relation avec quelques questions de biologie générale. Arch Ital Biol 34:43, 1900

Frisch RE: Pubertal adipose tissue: Is it necessary for normal sexual maturation? Evidence from the rat and human females. Fed Proc 39:2395, 1980

Frisch RE: Critical weight at menarche. Initiation of the adolescent growth spurt and control of puberty. In Grumbach MM, Grave GD, Mayer FE (eds): Control of the Onset of Puberty, p 403. New York, John Wiley & Sons, 1974

Frisch RE, Revelle R: Height and weight at menarche and hypothesis of critical body weights and adolescent events. Science 169:397, 1970

Greulich WW, Pyle SI: Radiographic Atlas of Skeletal Development of the Hand and Wrist, 2nd ed. Stanford, Stanford University Press, 1959

Grumbach MM, Richards GE, Conte FA, Kaplan SL: Clinical disorders of adrenal function and puberty: An assessment of the role of the adrenal cortex in normal and abnormal puberty in man and evidence for an ACTH-like pituitary adrenal androgen stimulating hormone. In James VHT (ed): The Endocrine Function of the Human Adrenal Cortex, p 583. London, Academic Press, 1978

Grumbach MM, Roth JC, Kaplan SL, Kelch RP: Hypothalamic–pituitary regulation of puberty in man: Evidence and concepts derived from clinical research. In Grumbach MM (ed): Control of the Onset of Puberty, p 115. New York, John Wiley & Sons, 1974

Harris GW, Jacobsohn D: Functional grafts of the anterior pituitary gland. Proc R Soc Lond (Biol) 139:263, 1952

Hohlweg W, Junkmann K: Die hormonal-nervöse Regulierung der Funktion des Hypophysenvorderlappens. Klin Wschr 11:321, 1932

Johnston FE, Roche AF, Schell LM, Wettenhall NB: Critical weight at menarche: Critique of a hypothesis. Am J Dis Child 129:19, 1975

Kelch RP, Marshall JC, Sauder S et al: Gonadotropin regulation during human puberty. In Norman R (ed): Neuroendocrine Aspects of Reproduction, p 229. New York, Academic Press, 1983

Kennedy GC, Mitra J: Body weight and food intake as initiating factors for puberty in the rat. J Physiol 166:408, 1963

Klein DC: Melatonin and puberty. Science 224:6, 1984

Knobil E: The neuroendocrine control of the menstrual cycle. Rec Prog Horm Res 36:53, 1980

Marshall WA, Tanner JM: Variations in pattern of puberty changes in girls. Arch Dis Child 44:291, 1969

Nakai Y, Plant TM, Hess DL et al: On the sites of the negative and positive feedback actions of estradiol in the control of gonadotropin secretion in the rhesus monkey. Endocrinology 102:1008, 1978

Plant TM, Zorub DS, Moossy J: Effect of pinealectomy on the developmental pattern of gonadotropin secretion in the rhesus monkey. Fed Proc 40:389, 1981

Pohl CR, Richardson DW, Hutchison JS et al: Hypophysiotropic signal frequency and the functioning of the pituitary ovarian system in the rhesus monkey. Endocrinology 112:2076, 1983

Ramirez DV, McCann SM: Changes in hypothalamic luteinizing hormone secretion in immature and adult rats. Endocrinology 72:452, 1963

Reynolds EL, Wines JV: Individual differences in physical changes associated with adolescence in girls. Am J Dis Child 75:329, 1948

Rich BH, Rosenfield RL, Lucky A et al: Adrenarche: Changing adrenal response to adrenocorticotropin. J Clin Endocrinol Metab 52:1129, 1981

Ross JL, Loriaux DL, Cutler GB: Developmental changes in neuroendocrine regulation of gonadotropin secretion in gonadal dysgenesis. J Clin Endocrinol Metab 57:288, 1983

Ruf KB: How does the brain control the process of puberty? J Neurol 204:95, 1973

Silman RE, Leone RM, Hooper RJ, Preece MA: Melatonin: The pineal gland and human puberty. Nature 282:301, 1979

Sklar CA, Kaplan SL, Grumbach MM: Evidence for dissociation between adrenarche and gonadarche: Studies in patients with idiopathic precocious puberty, gonadal dysgenesis, isolated gonadotropin deficiency and constitutionally delayed growth and adolescence. J Clin Endocrinol Metab 51:548, 1980

Steiner RA, Cameron JL, McNeill TH et al: Metabolic signals for the onset of puberty. In Norman R (ed): Neuroendocrine Aspects of Reproduction, p 183. New York, Academic Press, 1983

Styne DM, Grumbach MM: Puberty in the male and female: Its physiology and disorders. In Yen SSC, Jaffe R (eds): Reproductive Endocrinology, p 189. Philadelphia, WB Saunders, 1978

Tanner JM: Growth at Adolescence, 2nd ed. Oxford, Blackwell, 1962

Terasawa E, Nass TE, Yeoman R et al: Hypothalamic control of puberty in the female rhesus monkey. In Norman R (ed): Neuroendocrine Aspects of Reproduction, p 149. New York, Academic Press, 1983

Trussell J: Menarche and fatness: Reexamination of the critical body composition hypothesis. Science 200:1506, 1978

Van Houten M, Posner BI, Kopriwa BM, Brawer JR: Insulin-binding sites localized to nerve terminals in rat median eminence and arcuate nucleus. Science 207:1081, 1980

Wildt L, Hutchison JS, Marshall G et al: On the site of action of progesterone in the blockade of the estradiol-induced gonadotropin discharge in the rhesus monkey. Endocrinology 109:1293, 1981

Wildt L, Marshall G, Knobil E: Experimental induction of puberty in the infantile female rhesus monkey. Science 207:1373, 1980

Winter JSD, Faiman C: Pituitary-gonadal relations in female children and adolescents. Pediatr Res 7:948, 1973

Winter JSD, Faiman C: The development of cyclic pituitary-gonadal function in adolescent females. J Clin Endocrinol Metab 37:714, 1973

Wurtman RJ: Brain monoamines and endocrine function. Neurosci Res Prog Bull 9:172, 1971

Menstruation

Beller FK: Observations on the clotting of menstrual blood and clot formation. Am J Obstet Gynecol 111:535, 1971

Beller FK, Weiss G: The fibrinolytic enzyme system in cervical mucus. Fertil Steril 17:654, 1966

Hallberg L, Hogdahl AM, Nilsson L et al: Menstrual blood loss—A population study. Acta Obstet Gynaecol Scand 45:320, 1966

Henzl MR, Smith RE, Boost G et al: Lysosomal concept of menstrual bleeding in humans. J Clin Endocrinol Metab 34:860, 1972

McLennan CE, Rydell AH: Extent of endometrial shedding during normal menstruation. Obstet Gynecol 26:605, 1965

Rybo G: Clinical and experimental studies on menstrual blood loss. Acta Obstet Gynaecol Scand 45 (Suppl 7), 1966

Schwarz BE: The production and biologic effects of uterine prostaglandins. Semin Reprod Endocrinol 1:189, 1983

Dysmenorrhea

Chan WY, Dawood MY, Fuchs F: Relief of dysmenorrhea with the prostaglandin synthetase inhibitor ibuprofen: Effect on prostaglandin levels in menstrual blood. Am J Obstet Gynecol 135:102, 1979

Larkin RM, Van Orden DE, Poulson AM et al: Dysmenorrhea: Treatment with an antiprostaglandin. Obstet Gynecol 54:456, 1979

Ylikorkala O, Dawood MY: New concepts in dysmenorrhea. Am J Obstet Gynecol 130:833, 1978

Premenstrual Syndrome

Reid RL, Yen SSC: Premenstrual syndrome. Am J Obstet Gynecol 139:85, 1981

Ruble DN: Premenstrual symptoms: A reinterpretation. Science 197:291, 1977

The Patient

John T. Queenan

9

THE PHYSICIAN–PATIENT RELATIONSHIP

More than is true of most obstetrician–patient dialogues, that during a woman's initial visit to the gynecologist's office can be fraught with anxiety, concern, and even humiliation. Whatever her age, social background, or previous experience—and all these influence her reaction—she usually expects the encounter with the gynecologist and the examination to be uncomfortable both emotionally and physically. Unfortunately, misapprehensions about the experience are all too common; rumor and hyperbole often heighten a young patient's fears. Even more unfortunately, previous experiences may have given this anxiety a very real foundation. It is the physician's responsibility to allay undue apprehension, dispel false impressions, and make the visit as comfortable and informative as possible so that the patient leaves the office calm and in an improved frame of mind. This is best achieved by an understanding attitude and a matter-of-fact approach. Condescension and domination have no place in the physician–patient relationship.

Even under the best of circumstances, the patient is likely to find the visit disagreeable. Soon after entering the office or clinic, she is asked to discuss her most personal problems, which she has mentioned to few, if any, others. Then, after verbally exposing herself, she must undress, put on the most unappealing of garments, and be examined by a complete stranger. No wonder the visit to the gynecologist for an annual checkup or for help with a pressing problem is rarely anticipated with enthusiasm. Indeed, subsequent visits are usually as trying as the first.

The patient is sensitive to subtle nuances in the physician's words or facial expression, a fact rarely appreciated by the busy practitioner. The physician's demeanor is extremely important in allaying the patient's anxiety and in establishing rapport; the physician who appears abrupt, preoccupied, hurried, hesitant, embarrassed, or flippant can destroy the possibility of a satisfactory physician–patient relationship. Frivolity and lightheartedness rarely have a place in the initial evaluation. The seriousness of the moment for the patient should be foremost in the physician's mind. Propriety of address and composure are qualities all patients appreciate and respect. The physician should express sincere concern in a friendly, direct atmosphere.

There are other rules for the relationship of an obstetrician–gynecologist with the patient. Many women have expressed resentment toward physicians who address their patients by first names, or by familiar terms such as "dear." Use of surnames also has a practical value, for a midnight call from "Janet" may be recognized less quickly than a call from "Janet Henderson" or "Mrs. Henderson." While conducting the examination the physician should not "think out loud," articulating possible diagnoses, for needless and disturbing explanations may be required later. Finally, the physician should evaluate the patient's mien and attitude, and make every effort to adjust to it. Patients will not alter or adjust their personalities to conform to the wishes of the physician; any adjusting that is needed must be done by the physician.

Today, women are more curious and more knowledgeable about anatomy and physiology than ever before. Voluminous data, both accurate and inaccurate, are readily available to them. Lay periodicals abound in articles on contraception, sexual function, abortion, obstetric practices, and gynecologic operative procedures. The physician must often correct misinformation and educate. A forthright dialogue with full explanation of the diagnosis and rationale for therapy is essential to effective physician–patient communication. An explanation of what medications are being prescribed and why, and a straightforward discussion of anticipated surgical procedures, duration of hospital stay, potential

163

complications, and possible sequelae constitute the minimum information a gynecologist owes the patient.

The physician must be honest and forthright in answering the probing questions asked by today's woman. If the physician is not familiar with certain matters, it is acceptable to admit the lack of knowledge and to express a willingness to obtain the appropriate information. A vague answer or avoidance of the question altogether is unacceptable.

Every patient is a combination of anatomic, physiologic, endocrinologic, and psychologic components. In evaluating her condition, the physician must not let the parts obscure the whole patient. The patient can well appreciate that one component is diseased, but it is the whole person who wishes to know what is happening, what is to be done, and what the results will be. This is the minimum information she deserves.

THE HISTORY

When large numbers of patients are involved, as in a clinic setting or in a very busy office, certain basic information (*e.g.,* age, ethnic background, marital status, obstetric history, and whatever the patient may wish to divulge about the problem for which she consults the physician) is often obtained by interview with an office nurse or by a questionnaire the patient is asked to fill out. Although these devices are sometimes considered essential, it is astonishing how little time they really save; by obtaining these data personally, the physician provides a logical opening for the interview and establishes a preliminary rapport with the patient. In addition, the manner in which she answers these mundane questions may alert the physician to areas that should be probed more deeply.

The setting for the history taking is important. A quiet area where distractions (telephone calls, interruptions) can be kept to a minimum and where privacy is ensured promotes a comfortable dialogue between physician and patient. The foundation for rapport in a continuing relation can be established during these 15 to 30 minutes of the initial history taking. This is perhaps the most critical time the physician spends with most patients.

History of the Obstetric Patient

The patient's initial obstetric visit does not usually pose a diagnostic problem. She may have been referred by another physician who has already confirmed her pregnancy, or she may have made the diagnosis herself on the basis of a home pregnancy test kit. The obstetrician, however, should review recent events and confirm the probability of pregnancy, the current status of the pregnancy, the patient's general well-being, and her feelings about the pregnancy. The obstetrician should never accept another's diagnosis. While the occasion would certainly be uncommon, the patient's presumption of pregnancy can be in error—based merely on an overdue period coupled with the fear of or desire for a pregnancy.

The obstetric history should include the following information:

History of current pregnancy
    Date of last menstrual period
    Bleeding, spotting, or staining since last normal period
    Pelvic cramps noted since last period
    Documentation of positive result on pregnancy test
    Findings of previous pelvic examinations during this pregnancy and relative uterine size
    Whether this pregnancy was planned
    Patient's attitude to the pregnancy
    Occupation
History of menstrual function
    Age of menarche
    Regularity of menstrual cycle
    Frequency of menstrual flow
    Use of contraceptives, in particular birth control pills, and how long since these were discontinued
    Whether pregnancy immediately followed discontinuance of oral contraception or progesterone withdrawal
    History of dysmenorrhea
Past obstetric history
    Number of pregnancies
    Number of living children
    Number of abortions, spontaneous or induced
    History of preceding pregnancies (duration of pregnancy, antepartum complications, duration of labor, type of delivery, anesthesia employed, intrapartum complications, postpartum complications, hospital, physician, time when deliveries occurred)
    Perinatal status of fetuses (birth weights, comments pediatricians may have made, and perhaps comments about early growth and development of children, including feeding habits, growth, and overall well-being)
Previous gynecologic history
    Date of pelvic examinations, uterine size
    Vaginal infections
    Previous pelvic surgery
    Abnormal results of cytologic examinations
    Treatment of cervical disease (cauterization, cryosurgery, conization)
    Use of hormone agents, including birth control pills and fertility pills, and when discontinued
    Treatment for sexually transmitted disease
Current medical history
    Medications currently taken (sedatives, hypnotics, psychotropic agents)
    Allergy to medications and specific reactions to them, environmental allergens
    Potential teratogenic events during this pregnancy (viral infections, roentgenographic examinations, medications)

Past medical history
    Conditions for which physician treatment or hospitalization has been required
    Surgical history (type of operation, anesthesia employed, problems related to anesthesia, postoperative complications)
    Bleeding disorders or tendency
    Requirement for blood transfusions (blood type and Rh status, if known)
Review of systems
    Neurologic disorders
    Pulmonary disorders
    Cardiac disorders
    Gastrointestinal disorders (nausea, vomiting, constipation, diarrhea, melena)
    Genitourinary disorders (frequency, nocturia, dysuria, incontinence)
    Cardiovascular symptoms (edema, leg cramps, history of phlebitis, fainting, other signs of vascular instability)
Social history
    Exercise
    Drug use
    Smoking habits
    Alcohol use
Family history
    Preeclampsia, diabetes, hypertension, hematologic disorders
    Occurrence of twins, impression of weights of babies in family
Dietary history
    Maternal food ingestion, fads, cravings
    Vitamin ingestion

History taking should be a dialogue conducted with a minimum of stress. The physician should use terms the patient can understand. He or she should not assume that the patient understands the relevance of the questions and should follow questions with explanations, when needed, of why they are asked. Professional people, nurses, and physicians should be treated the same way. The obstetrician must not assume that they know what to mention. If it appears that the questions are not clearly understood, they must be rephrased. The more questions asked during the course of the interview, the more answers and data are accumulated.

History of the Gynecologic Patient

There can be no set pattern for the gynecologic history taking. Certain obvious medical data should be obtained in a straightforward manner. However, appreciation of subtle aspects of the patient's history, social circumstances, and functioning requires time and subsequent visits.

The patient's own description of her primary symptoms is the first matter for discussion. It is wise for the physician to say as little as possible and allow the patient to elaborate. General questions can be asked to help her expand on a subject, but judgmental comments should not be made. The physician should not exhibit amazement no matter how bizarre the information unearthed by the history. Neither should practices that do not conform to the physician's own moral code be criticized, unless they are detrimental to the patient's health, in which case their unsuitability should be explained in these terms.

Duration, severity of the disorder, frequency of occurrence, and what aspect is most bothersome to the patient constitute the basic information that can be elaborated on by guided questioning. After the patient has had her say, the physician should pursue pertinent questions, not only to complete the clinical picture but also to demonstrate concern for the patient. The comfort and confidence that can be established in the history taking can make the examination easier and more productive.

The gynecologic history should include the following information:

Chief complaint
    The primary problem
    Duration
    Severity
    Occurrence in relation to other functions (menstrual cycle, coital activity, gastrointestinal activity, voiding, or other pertinent functions)
    Any previous similar symptom and its diagnosis and management
    Change in normal lifestyle resulting from the complaint
Menstrual history
    Contraception
    Date of onset of last menstrual period
    Frequency of menstrual periods
    Duration of flow
    Degree of discomfort
    Menarche
    Regularity of menstrual flow
    Quantity of menstrual flow (number of pads used per day)
    Premenstrual tension
Obstetric history
    Number of pregnancies
    Abortions
    Obstetric problems
    Response to pregnancies
Gynecologic history
    Last Pap smear
    Galactorrhea
    Findings of previous gynecologic examinations
    Previous gynecologic surgery, including details
    Vaginal infections, abnormal results of cytologic examinations
    DES exposure
    Sexually transmitted disease
Medical history
    Medical symptoms for which care was required

Surgical history
    Any operative procedures
Review of systems
    Pulmonary disorders
    Cardiac disorders
    Gastrointestinal disorders
    Genitourinary disorders
    Vascular disease, especially circulatory defects affecting extremities
    Leg cramps
    Phlebitis
Social history
    Exercise
    Drug use
    Alcohol use
    Smoking habits
    Marital status
    Number of years married
    Coital activity (libido, dyspareunia, orgasm)
Family history
    Significant medical and surgical disorders in family members
Nutrition
    Assessment of dietary habits, affection for fad diets
    Use of vitamins
Medications taken
    Hormone pills, birth control pills, fertility pills
    Medications employed on a long- or short-term basis, especially sedatives, hypnotics, psychotropic agents

The history provides information about the total patient and is perhaps the most important part of the gynecologic evaluation. It enables the patient to become acquainted with the physician in a nonthreatening situation. In most cases, it gives the physician data to establish a tentative diagnosis before the physical examination. In many respects, the gynecologist who takes a history is like the detective who keeps the various clues that are pertinent and discards those that are deliberately or inadvertently misleading. If the gynecologic history is sufficiently penetrating, it should in almost all cases permit the physician to narrow the likely possibilities to one, or most two, probable diagnoses. This preliminary opinion may not always be correct, but the history-taking session should not be ended until a tentative diagnosis has been made.

Like a hospital chart, the office history is a legal, as well as a medical, record. As such, it is subject to subpoena, and whatever is recorded in it may at some future date need to be defended in court. It should not contain extraneous or casually written material, and the notes should be sufficiently complete that the case can be readily reconstructed.

TYPES OF PATIENTS

The *neonate* is occasionally brought to the gynecologist's office because of vaginal discharge or bleeding.

The true patient is not the infant, who is responding physiologically to the withdrawal of maternal estrogen, but an anxious and justifiably apprehensive mother who needs reassurance.

The *young child* is frequently brought to the office because of a mother's concern about a genital problem, such as pruritus or discharge, that she cannot explain. In dealing with a young child, the gynecologist's primary responsibility is to avoid creating fear or apprehension. Gentleness is mandatory, but the examination should never be compromised because of the child's possible sensitivity. On rare occasions significant pathology, such as sarcoma botryoides, may be present. Pelvic evaluation under anesthesia may be required, but in the long run this will be far less traumatic than examining a frightened child in the office.

Today, an increasing number of mothers are bringing an *adolescent* daughter to the gynecologist for her first examination. Simple problems of breast development, vaginal discharge, irregularity of menses, and painful menstruation should be discussed openly and treated appropriately. Reassurance is important, regardless of the findings. Minutes spent in such education and preparation of the maturing adolescent can do much to establish a healthy attitude toward reproductive functions and should set the stage for good gynecologic care in the future.

Occasionally, a teenager is brought to the gynecologist in the hope that responsibility for sex education can be shifted from parents to physician. While this is certainly not the ideal approach, the responsibility for sex education cannot be ignored. In such a case it is appropriate for the physician, in the quiet atmosphere of a discussion (preferably without a parent present), to explain such matters as menstrual function, the physiology of maturation, pregnancy, and contraception. There may also be opportunity to discuss venereal disease and, in some cases, the psychologic maladjustments that can result from the new freedom of sexual expression. Adolescence is not the time to correct educational and cultural maladjustments that have been established over the years, but it is of great value for the teenage girl to have access to a person who is knowledgeable and concerned about her well-being.

The *mature woman* does not have the identical complaints of her adolescent counterpart, although some of the symptoms may be similar. She does require, however, the same care and consideration. It is a mistake to presume that, because a woman is sexually active, has borne children, seems familiar with contraceptive agents, and has undergone multiple gynecologic evaluations, she will be at ease with the present examination. When the physician undertakes the pelvic examination as a perfunctory procedure, the patient immediately senses it and her response is quite negative.

Some of the problems of the *postmenopausal woman,* notably hot flashes and atrophic vaginitis, are the direct result of estrogen deficiency. But it is a serious error to presume that all emotional and physical problems that arise in this age group are "due to the change."

Of special importance are depression, irritability, and anxiety. Sometimes they result from the woman's conviction that the menopause marks the onset of senility and that her years of attractiveness and femininity are past. Reassurance and an explanation of the positive and rewarding aspects of the menopausal years can be of much help. Emotional problems are often the direct result of the stresses that commonly beset women of this age group: responsibility for aging parents, sons and daughters whose attitudes seem unacceptable, and marital problems that may be compounded by the demands of the patient's or her husband's employment. In a few cases, the stage is already set for mental illness, and the menopause is a nonspecific precipitating factor. It is, of course, idle to presume that problems such as these can be solved by prescribing estrogens, and it is axiomatic that physical and emotional disorders arising in the menopausal or postmenopausal years should be investigated on their own merits. Problems of patients in this age group deserve the same consideration accorded problems of younger patients.

Perhaps no single condition is responsible for more obstetric and operative morbidity than obesity. Our culture accepts overweight as a fact of life. In no other nation is obesity more of a problem. It is truly remarkable that, even though so many medical disorders are related to obesity, an intensive effort has not yet been made to combat overweight. For the gynecologic as well as the obstetric patient, obesity predisposes not only to simple problems of hygiene and a greater frequency of vaginitis, but also to more significant intraoperative and postoperative complications. The physician should suggest a weight reduction program and a program of physical activity for such a patient. Here, as in few other circumstances in medicine, a potentially hazardous clinical problem must be approached aggressively.

OFFICE OPERATIONS

Today, many procedures heretofore considered hospital practices are performed in the physician's office. Cervical biopsy, endometrial aspiration, colposcopically directed biopsies, and cryosurgery for conditions such as mild cervical dysplasia are now routinely done in the gynecologist's office. It is common for amniocentesis to be performed in the office. These procedures involve equipment unfamiliar to most patients. The purpose of the procedure and the functioning of the equipment should be explained to the patient.

SEXUALITY

Major cultural changes in recent years have allowed women to express their individuality more freely. The women's movement is one aspect of this change. Some women today resent and distrust men who are in positions of authority. The male gynecologist is in just such a position, and he must learn not only to respect his

patient's individuality but also to deal with his own discomfort in the face of her hostility.

Cultural change has also sanctioned greater sexual freedom for women and a code of sexual morality that may conflict with traditional values. Though the patient may not specifically refer to sexual attitudes, it is safe to assume that many young women experience serious anxiety in this area. The physician's role is never to judge. It is to counsel and educate—forthrightly if the patient asks, tactfully if she only hints at questions.

The enormous amount of popular writing about sex and sexuality may be the source of the patient's questions. The gynecologist should be prepared to discuss masturbation, orgasm, coital positions, and sexual techniques—topics once rarely mentioned but now commonplace.

In addition, the gynecologist is often the first physician whose advice is sought regarding marital and sexual problems. For the busy practitioner this is time-consuming and frustrating. The physician's degree of involvement, of course, is related to interest and time available, but a request for help must not be passed off with the suggestion that the problem will take care of itself in time. The gynecologist should be versed in basic counseling and questioning techniques and should be able to offer some elementary recommendations. He or she must be prepared to evaluate the severity of such problems and to direct the troubled patient or couple to another physician or an appropriate agency for help.

THE PHYSICAL EXAMINATION

It is important for the obstetrician–gynecologist to know the physical condition of the patient. In the case of the obstetric patient, a complete physical examination and appropriate laboratory tests should be performed at the first visit. A complete physical examination may or may not be a part of the first or subsequent office vist of the gynecologic patient. For the woman in good health who has consulted an internist recently or is under the care of an internist for some ongoing disorder, such as hypertension or diabetes, a complete physical examination is not needed. For the woman with an endocrine disorder, a complete physical examination clearly should be a part of the gynecologist's evaluation. The designation of the obstetrician–gynecologist as a "primary physician for women" is variously interpreted by the practitioners of this discipline. An important part of this responsibility is referral to other physicians for such special examinations as may be needed, including referral to a family practitioner or an internist for periodic physical appraisal. Except for the breasts, which should be examined at every gynecologic visit, the detail of the physical evaluation of gynecologic patients varies according to the circumstances.

Upon entering the examining room, the physician should make some brief comment to put the patient at ease, but to expect the patient to "relax" is probably out of the question. During the physical examination another woman participant, usually a nurse or aide, must be present. Not only can this woman assist the physician, but she lends an element of psychologic support to the patient. Her presence is also of legal importance to the physician as a guard against accusations that may be initiated by an unscrupulous or disturbed patient. The dialogue between physician and patient should continue during the examination. Distracting conversation with the nurse or aide tends to influence the patient adversely and detracts from the physician–patient rapport.

Evaluation of General Appearance

A general impression should be recorded of the color, texture, and coarseness of the patient's skin; of birth marks; of the condition of her fingernails; and of her state of nutrition.

Examination of the Head and Neck

The patient's hair should be examined for cleanliness, texture, and scalp health. Eye examination should include funduscopy to detect retinal aberrations. The patient's nose, throat, and teeth should be checked. Otoscopy should be performed, and the anterior cervical, posterior cervical, and supraclavicular nodes should be palpated. The thyroid gland should be palpated both in the direct anteroposterior position and with the patient's head turned.

Examination of the Chest

From the back, the vertebral column can be assessed and degree of curvature noted. The chest should be percussed and auscultated, and the breasts examined (see Chap. 60). The heart should then be percussed and auscultated.

Examination of the Abdomen

The patient should be positioned supine, with her arms against her body, in order to relax the abdominal musculature. The knees should be elevated and flexed, also to decrease abdominal wall tone. In methodical and consistent fashion, all quadrants of the abdomen should be examined, percussed, and palpated. Relaxation of the abdomen to evaluate a suspected mass can be assisted by having the patient breathe deeply and then exhale. After all quadrants have been examined, the inguinal nodes should be palpated. Abdominal scars should be discussed; even though the surgery has been noted during history taking, new information may be learned at this time.

Examination of the Lower Extremities

Examination of the lower extremities supplies important information regarding the cardiovascular system. The presence of significant varicosities, for example, would be a disturbing finding in a multigravida. Peripheral pulses should be checked.

Examination of the Pelvis

The pelvic examination consists of inspection and palpation. To allow adequate exposure, the patient should be placed in the lithotomy position. She should be reasonably comfortable and properly draped.

Except in special circumstances, a deftly performed bimanual pelvic examination should not be painful. Special circumstances might involve the patient who is virginal and has not used tampons for menstrual protection and the woman with an inflammatory or other painful condition. Such a patient should understand in advance the nature of the information needed and the probability that the examination will be uncomfortable. In some cases sufficient information can be obtained by using the index finger only for the bimanual examination instead of inflicting the discomfort of the more customary index and middle fingers.

The vulva should be examined for general state of hygiene, growth of hair, regions of ulceration, rash, discoloration, labial abnormalities, excessive vaginal discharge, evidence of perineal trauma from previous deliveries, and evidence of rectal disease such as hemorrhoids. Bartholin's and Skene's glands can be inspected and palpated. The labia should be spread apart for inspection of the labia minora as well as the urethra. Severe vesicovaginal or rectal prolapse can be appreciated at this point. Having the patient strain down may allow better assessment of anatomic distortion.

The physician should prepare the patient for any pelvic manipulation by warning her in advance of examining fingers and speculum. This is important not only because the patient cannot see what is going on but also because the area to be examined is extremely sensitive, both psychologically and physically.

A Graves or Pederson bivalve speculum is employed for visualization of the vagina and cervix. Several points of technique should be remembered. If material is to be obtained for cytologic examination, the speculum should be rinsed in warm water; if not, the instrument should be lubricated. By spreading the labia and placing some tension on the posterior fourchette, the speculum can be gently inserted downward at an angle of about 45 degrees to avoid the urethra. This angled insertion is necessary because, with the patient in a supine position, the vagina is not horizontal. The speculum should be completely inserted and rotated to the horizontal plane. In most patients, it should now lie inferior to the cervix. With the gentle opening of the speculum, the valves separate and the cervix can be visualized.

The cervix should be inspected for color, erosion, degree of discharge, evidence of trauma, and presence of lesions. Two smears are usually taken: (1) a scraping from the region of the squamocolumnar junction of the cervix and (2) a collection of cells from the posterior fornix. Each is smeared on a glass slide and fix-dried by an aerosol spray. When the vaginal sidewalls have been examined, the speculum may be gently rotated to get a more complete view of the superior and inferior surfaces of the vaginal vault.

In the patient with severe vaginitis, when immediate microscopic assessment is desirable, the secretions that have pooled in the inferior valve of the speculum can be used as the sample for microscopic study; otherwise, a vaginal aspirate may be obtained. The speculum should then be withdrawn over the cervix and slowly removed; during withdrawal the walls of the vagina can be visualized and the supporting structures assessed for cystocele and rectocele. Incontinence may be demonstrated by asking the patient to cough after the speculum has been removed, provided the bladder contains sufficient urine. Usually, however, the patient has voided before the examination and this assessment is not possible.

Various authors describe different techniques for the bimanual examination. One method is illustrated in Figures 9-1 through 9-5. Generally, the physician should acquire proficiency with the index and middle fingers of one hand and then always use that hand for the vaginal

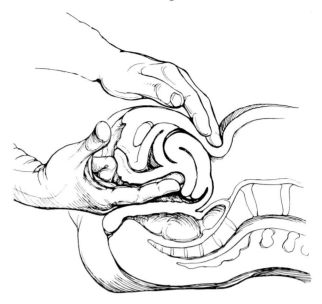

FIG. 9-2. Bimanual examination, *second step.* Vaginal fingers are moved into the anterior fornix to permit palpation of the uterine corpus. If the abdominal wall is thin and well relaxed, it is possible by this maneuver to define even minor irregularities in the contour or consistency of the uterus. *Third step:* With vaginal fingers still in the anterior fornix and with the aid of the abdominal hand, the uterus is moved gently toward a retroverted position and then from side to side to determine its mobility and presence or absence of pain on movement of the uterus. (Figure drawn by G McHugh)

FIG. 9-1. Bimanual examination, *first step.* Vaginal fingers first feel consistency and symmetry of the cervix and its axis in relation to the axis of the vagina. They then elevate the uterus toward the abdominal wall so the total length of the uterus can be determined. (After Duncan AS. In Bourne A: British Gynaecological Practice, 1st ed. Philadelphia, FA Davis, 1955. Figure drawn by G McHugh)

FIG. 9-3. If the fingertips of the abdominal and vaginal hands come together in carrying out step 2, it can be concluded that the uterus is retroverted; the vaginal fingers are then moved to the posterior fornix to outline symmetry, consistency, and mobility of the retoverted corpus. (Figure drawn by G McHugh)

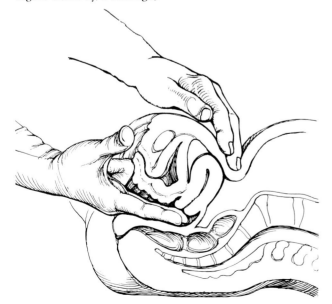

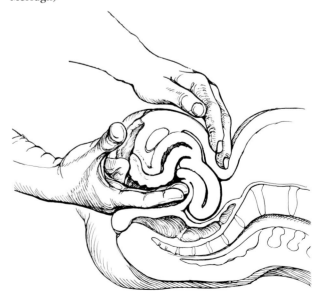

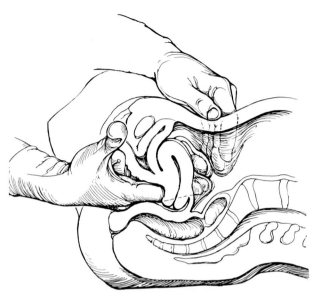

FIG. 9-4. Bimanual examination, *fourth step.* To outline the adnexa, the vaginal fingers are moved to the right fornix, and the examiner attempts to bring the abdominal and vaginal fingers together at a point presumed to be superior to the tube and ovary. (Figure drawn by G McHugh)

examination. After the speculum has been withdrawn, the physician should gently insert the index and middle fingers along the posterior wall of the vagina. It is helpful to place a stool at the base of the examining table and support the examining arm and elbow during the examination. This support of the elbow allows greater sensitivity in the examining fingers. At the same time, a second dimension is added by pressing on the patient's abdomen with the other hand. The first palpable structure is the cervix. Next is the anteriorly placed uterine fundus. The bimanual technique can outline its position, size, shape, consistency, and degree of mobility. Uterine or cervical mobility can be further assessed by placing the fingers on one side of the structure and moving it to the contralateral side. This can be done on both right and left sides to detect chronic or acute inflammatory changes and fixation. The abdominal hand is then placed on one lower quadrant and slowly worked inferiorly and medially to meet the examining fingers of the vaginal hand. In this way, adnexal structures on that side can be appreciated. The degree of adherence of an adnexal structure to the uterus can be ascertained. Enlargement, consistency, and position of ovaries and tubes can be noted. Expressions of pain and discomfort should be heeded. The ovary is a sensitive structure, and patients differ in tolerance to palpation. The contralateral side should be similarly examined.

A third dimension in the bimanual examination is the rectovaginal examination. A fresh glove is donned, and the lubricated middle finger is inserted in the patient's rectum and the index finger in the vagina. Hem-

orrhoids, sphincter tone, and perineal integrity are evaluated. The pouch of Douglas is checked for masses. Uterosacral ligaments can be palpated for tone and nodularity. This examination permits palpation a little higher than is possible in vaginal bimanual examination and should be employed in almost all patients, repeating the steps noted earlier.

When the patient is apprehensive and difficult to examine, the procedure is sometimes facilitated by having the patient place her hands on her abdomen, inhale deeply, and then exhale completely. Hyperventilation must be avoided, however. Any additional mechanisms to promote relaxation are helpful.

After the examination is completed, the physician should assist the patient to a sitting position and leave the examining room.

The information gained from the pelvic examination can be recorded in the following outline form:

Perineum
    Old lacerations
    Lesions
External genitalia
    Stage of development
    Color
    Evidence of lesions
    Bartholin's glands
Vestibule
    Skene's glands
    Urethral orifice
    Hymenal ring

FIG. 9-5. Bimanual examination, *fifth step.* When the fingers of the abdominal and vaginal hands are quite close together (it is desirable, but not always possible, to approximate these fingers), they are then moved gently toward the examiner so the adnexa slip between the fingers and can so be outlined. (Figure drawn by G McHugh)

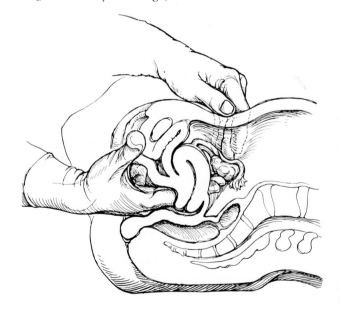

Vagina
    Presence of leukorrhea
    Color
    Lesions
    Tone
    Rugae
Cervix
    Shape
    Consistency
    Mobility
    State of parity
    Lesions
Uterus
    Position
    Mobility
    Size
    Shape
    Consistency
Adnexa
    Position and mobility of ovaries and tubes
    Presence of masses or tenderness
Results of rectovaginal examination
    Degree of confirmation of previous findings
    Statement about additional pathology

When the patient rejoins the physician in the consultation room, diagnosis and findings should be explained in terms she can understand. The implications of the findings should be carefully detailed. It is occasionally helpful to have the patient paraphrase what the physician has said to make certain she understands. This is especially relevant when surgery is contemplated, for the nuances of an operation and its results may be unclear to the patient. At this time, the use of medications and the duration of their use must be explained. The physician should also carefully explain the symptoms that may be expected after any treatment given during the office visit (*e.g.,* heavy leukorrhea following cryosurgery or bleeding following cervical biopsy). Advice against coitus should be given when appropriate, and the duration of abstinence should be made clear. The importance of a follow-up examination should be stressed. Prescriptions for hormones should be adequately detailed and restrictions on refills explicitly stated.

RAPE*

Many gynecologists are reluctant to become involved in cases of alleged rape because the time required for courtroom procedures infringes on their other professional duties. Nevertheless, as physicians, their primary responsibility is the care of their patients, and when this care extends outside the hospital and into a court of law, the responsibility remains.

Rape is a legal rather than a medical diagnosis. The

* See also ACOG Technical Bulletin #52 (November, 1978).

physician can testify about the findings at the time of examination, but the court must decide whether rape occurred. The record of the examination of a rape victim, whether emergency room record or physician's office chart, should be complete in every respect. It is the responsibility of the physician to document fully the state of the patient, from her emotional composure to her physical appearance. Data should be recorded as fact; allegations should be recorded as allegations, since the legal status of the situation is undefined at the time of the examination.

History

A thorough history of the episode should include locale, time, description of the assailant, and description of the alleged assault with particular reference to penetration and ejaculation. While this interrogation will probably have been done earlier by police authorities, the physician's interview supplies corroborating evidence in a court of law.

Physical Examination

The record should note the patient's overall appearance and the state of her clothing, composure, and attitude. Physical examination should include a search for evidence of trauma and recent injury. Pertinent negative points should be noted. All data, from vital signs to the findings of a thorough physical examination, should be documented. The record of the pelvic examination should include all findings that support the allegation of rape, such as evidence of trauma and lacerations.

Laboratory Data

In some cities, local crime laboratories have attained great expertise in the processing of evidence in cases of rape and have prepared detailed instructions for obtaining the materials for analysis. When appropriate, they wish to have and are equipped to take photographs that can later be used as evidence. If specimens are sent to the crime laboratory, duplicates should also be submitted to the hospital laboratory.

Laboratory evaluations should include a complete blood count, a serologic test for syphilis, blood typing, Rh determination, and blood tests for alcohol and drugs. Vaginal aspirate should be studied for motile sperm, acid phosphatase, and ABO antigens. Cervical and vaginal material should be cultured for gonorrheal organisms. Slides should be obtained for permanent fixation to show the presence of sperm. Other specimens that should be obtained including clippings and washings from pubic hair, debris from beneath fingernails, and washings of blood or foreign material obtained from clothes.

Treatment

Treatment consists of medication to prevent pregnancy. Common prescriptions are diethylstilbestrol, 25 mg twice daily for 5 days; conjugated estrogen, 20 mg per day for 5 days; or conjugated equine estrogen, 50 mg injected intravenously (see p. 247). The oral medication should be prescribed with an antiemetic. Prophylactic penicillin or other antibiotic must be employed according to the apparent need, depending on the circumstances of the incident and the physician's judgment. Since many persons are allergic to this agent, its routine use is not recommended.

The physician should be aware that many, perhaps most, women involved in assault episodes require comfort, understanding, and emotional support. These should be supplied initially by the physician, but many victims also need the help of a crisis counselor, an appropriately trained social worker, or a psychiatrist.

Follow-Up

A repeat examination of the patient should be performed approximately six weeks after the episode to ensure resumption of menstrual function. At this visit, the serologic test for syphilis and culture of cervical material for *Neisseria gonorrhoeae* should be repeated.

Counseling in Obstetrics and Gynecology

William R. Keye, Jr.

10

Although most obstetrician–gynecologists do not think of themselves as counselors or psychotherapists, almost every gynecologic or obstetric patient either requests or would benefit from counseling. This is not surprising for several reasons. First, most gynecologists' patients are young and healthy; thus, when confronted by illness, they are often surprised, frustrated, angry, or depressed. Second, almost all obstetric and gynecologic conditions have psychosexual overtones, since by definition they involve either the breasts or genital organs. Third, the physical and endocrinologic changes that accompany puberty, the normal menstrual cycle, pregnancy, and the climacteric may have profound effects on emotions, behavior, and body image. Finally, many obstetric and gynecologic disorders have an impact on social relationships because they are the result of sexual interaction.

Most obstetrician–gynecologists provide more counseling than they believe they do. During the course of an active clinical practice, a typical obstetrician–gynecologist may help an adolescent patient adjust to the physical changes of puberty, choose an appropriate form of contraception, or deal with an unplanned pregnancy. He may help the young adult patient understand the implications of such problems as herpes vulvitis, acute salpingitis, infertility, or endometriosis and may help the older patient deal with a malignancy or menopause. Clearly, almost all of an obstetrician–gynecologists's patients receive some form of counseling in addition to drug or surgical therapy.

Unfortunately, many patients express displeasure with the patient–physician relationship. It has become apparent that there is a greater need than ever for physicians, especially obstetrician–gynecologists, to practice humanistic medicine, combining an understanding of the psychosocial aspects of disease with effective counseling and communications skills.

This chapter consists of three parts. The first pre-

sents a discussion of the psychosocial reactions to disease and the factors that determine such reactions. Armed with an understanding of these reactions, the astute physician will find it much easier to interpret patient behavior and offer constructive suggestions for coping with illness. The second section reviews the principles of effective communication and counseling using the model of human relations developed by Robert Carkhuff. Finally, the third part applies these principles to the common but often difficult areas of sexual dysfunction and premenstrual syndrome.

PSYCHOSOCIAL REACTIONS TO DISEASE

Although the terms *disease* and *illness* are often used interchangeably, they denote quite different phenomena. *Disease* refers to pathophysiologic conditions often associated with objective anatomic deformities caused by infections, toxic agents, trauma, or degenerative processes. Since the Flexner report of 1910, medical education has focused almost exclusively on the diagnosis and treatment of disease, with an emphasis on the scientific aspects of medical care. Although this emphasis has led to important and exciting therapeutic and technologic advances, such preoccupation with the scientific and technical aspects of medicine has in part been responsible for erosion of the patient–physician relationship. Students of medical sociology suggest that the growing dissatisfaction in our country with physicians is due in large part to physicians' preoccupation with disease and neglect of the patients' illnesses.

By contrast, *illness* is the personal and subjective distress a person experiences as a result of either real or perceived disease. Thus, the term *illness* takes into account the altered self-image, decreased functional capacity, and personal suffering of the patient. In reality, although disease and illness almost always accompany one another, the patient often is more concerned with the illness than with the underlying disease. Most persons want to be healthy but define *health* as the absence of illness, not the absence of disease. They desire first to be free of suffering and second to be free of disease. To understand this important distinction between disease and illness is to better understand the feelings and behavior of patients and thus to be in a position to be a more effective physician–counselor.

To counsel effectively, the physician must be aware of the broad range of psychosocial reactions to disease and the fact that each patient has her own reaction. The final form of the reaction is determined by the patient's symptoms, her knowledge of and beliefs about the underlying disease, and the messages she receives from her physicians, family, and friends. In turn, the patient's psychosocial response may influence for better or worse the ultimate course and outcome of the disease.

For most patients, a disease is perceived in one or more of the following ways: as a loss, as a challenge or threat, as a gain, or as a punishment.

1. Loss—Many patients view their disease as a loss, a loss that may be real or symbolic. Real loss may involve the loss of a body part or bodily function. Symbolic loss may include loss of self-esteem, loss of independence, loss of security, loss of pleasure, or loss of personal or physical attractiveness. Patients who lose self-esteem or independence often develop depression as a result. Depression that results from the loss of self-worth often is superimposed on the depression that results from the burden of serious or chronic disease. A patient who perceives her disease as a loss may experience a grief reaction characterized by surprise, denial, anger, guilt, sadness, brooding, an inability to experience joy and pleasure, and a lack of interest in her environment. However, depression is the most common psychiatric reaction to disease. Patients who view disease as a loss often cope with their grief and depression through withdrawal, hostile confrontation, helpless attention seeking, noncompliance, or even suicide.
2. Punishment—Patients may regard their disease as either a just or an unjust punishment for real or imaginary transgressions. A common example is the woman who feels her infertility is a just punishment for a previously induced abortion or tubal infection with gonorrhea. When the disease is judged by the patient to be just, she may surrender to it, accepting it as her lot in life and making no attempt to seek medical evaluation or treatment. In contrast, if she views her disease as an undeserved punishment, she may react with anger and bitterness directed at her family, friends, or physician. Paranoid, hostile, or litigious behavior may result.
3. Threat—When a patient views her disease predominantly as a threat, she is likely to respond with feelings of anxiety, fear, or anger. As a result, she may

see the disease as the enemy and attempt to achieve victory over it, or she may deny the threat and ignore it. Alternatively, she may regard her disease as the work of evil forces or people and become angry, hostile, or frankly paranoid. Finally, she may become paralyzed with fear, failing to act or make necessary decisions.
4. Gain or relief—For some, disease represents a socially acceptable way out of difficult social, economic, or interpersonal situations or obligations. Others may use disease to rationalize personal failures or inadequacies. Often, this occurs at an unconscious level and is not recognized by the patient as readily as it is by persons close to the patient. A patient who views her disease as a means of providing relief or gain may be inappropriately indifferent or even cheerful when faced with a serious disease or disability. Such a patient is likely to be noncompliant with treatment and may cling to the sick role, causing her physician to feel helpless and ineffectual. In this case an ambivalent, if not overtly hostile, relationship may develop between doctor and patient.
5. Challenge—A patient who views her disease as a challenge may accept the challenge and attempt to overcome it by any available means. Such a patient usually minimizes her symptoms or discomfort and does not manifest excessive or maladaptive emotional symptoms. She aggressively seeks medical care, complies with treatment programs, attempts to educate herself, compensates for impaired or lost function, and approaches her disease in a rational and flexible way. Obviously, such a view of disease and the behavior that follows is constructive and should be encouraged.

Factors Influencing Reactions to Disease

Lipowski has proposed that four major factors influence psychosocial reactions to disease: intrapersonal, interpersonal, disease-related, and sociocultural–economic.

One intrapersonal factor that influences a patient's reaction to disease is the patient's personality, that is, her characteristic manner of responding to life's events. For example, a person who habitually responds to life's events by intensifying them is likely when sick to experience more intense pain and distress than someone who tends to minimize the intensity of life's events. In addition, a patient's unique combination of needs, goals, defense mechanisms, self-esteem, and tendency to experience anxiety, guilt, or depression also influence her reaction to disease. For example, a woman whose self-esteem is derived largely from intellectual or physical achievement is likely to perceive disease as a threat or a loss and to experience decreased self-esteem, anxiety, or depression. Finally, a patient's previous experience with illness may also influence her reaction to a new disease. Patients who have experienced secondary gain with a previous illness may perceive a new disease in much the same way.

Interpersonal factors also influence a patient's reaction to disease. A patient who has a good patient–physician relationship is more likely to view a disease as a challenge than as a loss or overwhelming threat. The physician can often influence the patient's response to her disease by encouraging her to view it as a challenge and offering to assist her in becoming victorious in her fight against it.

Disease-related factors are the nature of the disease and its effects on body parts or bodily function. If the gynecologic patient values highly her sexuality and therefore her reproductive organs, she is more likely to feel as a major threat or loss a gynecologic disease than a nongynecologic disease, even though the nongynecologic disease may be medically more serious. For example, a woman may be more devastated by an early carcinoma of the breast requiring mastectomy than by incurable diabetes or heart disease.

Coping with Disease

In one fashion or another, every patient attempts to cope with her disease through cognitive or behavioral strategies. Two major cognitive coping styles described by Lipowski are minimization and vigilant focusing. Individuals who cope by minimization habitually play down the emotional impact and personal significance of their disease. In contrast, those who use vigilant focusing respond to disease with purposeful and rational (at times even exaggerated and obsessive) attention and concern.

A patient may cope behaviorally in one of three ways: by actively dealing with the disease, by submitting to the disease, or by denying the disease. Some coping strategies may be helpful in dealing with disease, whereas others may be maladaptive and interfere with recovery.

Summary

In order to become an effective therapist and counselor, it is essential that the physician remember that "doctors do not treat disease; they treat patients who have diseases." Therefore, an effective physician–counselor considers not only the biomedical aspects of the disease but also the personal, social, and psychologic aspects, of the patient's illness. Although illness is not easily quantified, it is important to the course of the disease.

PRINCIPLES OF EFFECTIVE COUNSELING

In this age of rapidly expanding medical knowledge, the development of simpler, safer, and more effective techniques of diagnosis and treatment, and an emerging emphasis on preventive health care, it is ironic that there is widespread dissatisfaction with the doctor–patient relationship. It appears that the origin of this dissatisfaction is multifactorial. "High-tech" procedures dehumanize medical care; threats of malpractice, an increasing load of paperwork, and regulations imposed by those who finance medical care often distract physicians; and patients who have come to accept the "miracles" of laser surgery, artificial hearts, and *in vitro* fertilization as routine often have unrealistic expectations of treatment and a low tolerance for unpredictable or suboptimal response to therapy. Furthermore, there is increasing evidence that the attitude of the physician influences not only patient compliance but even the ultimate effect of therapy. These factors suggest that physicians, in addition to counselors who provide psychotherapy, sex therapy, or marital therapy, must possess an understanding of the techniques of effective communication.

Armed with these skills, the physician is more likely to be viewed by peers as well as by patients as caring and warm. Since most patients are not in a position to evaluate the technical competence of their physicians, they usually base their judgment on their interpersonal relationships with their physicians and their perceptions of the physicians' respect, understanding, and concern. Once a sense of trust and affection has developed between a physician and a patient, the patient is more likely to follow the physician's advice, pay bills promptly, demonstrate trust in the physician's competence, and speak highly of and recommend the physician to friends and acquaintances.

Goals of Counseling

Carkhuff defined three goals of effective counseling: to encourage self-exploration, to facilitate understanding, and to direct action on the part of the patient. These goals are based on his model of problem solving, according to which self-exploration leads to a better understanding of the problem, which makes possible an appropriate and successful course of action. The action taken by the patient should have the effect of increasing her understanding of the problem, which in turn should lead her to further alter her course of action. The patient repeats this cycle of self-exploration, understanding, and action as many times as necessary to achieve the desired goal. This method of problem solving works for most persons who are motivated and in contact with reality.

The first of these three goals, self-exploration, can be achieved through exploration of the problem and all of its ramifications. Through the process of defining the problem, the patient and physician will gain insight into it. A common error made by physicians without well-developed counseling skills is giving advice without exploring the problem fully. Such advice is often inappropriate and based on too little information, and frequently the patient has already considered and tried the course being advised and found it to be ineffective. Therefore, a good counselor usually refrains from giving advice until the patient has explored the problem in detail.

The second goal of effective counseling is to help the patient better understand herself as well as the problem. The physician should strive to help the patient make some sense out of the problem and its many facets.

The final, and often most difficult, step is to devise a plan of action to resolve the problem. In determining an appropriate course of action, the physician and patient should consider alternative plans and the possible consequences of each. Sometimes a single physician cannot help the patient plan the entire course of action but must be satisfied with playing a small role in a broad plan growing out of the patient's interactions with several physicians or health care professionals.

Characteristics of an Effective Counselor

The first step in achieving the goals defined by Carkhuff is the establishment of a good relationship with the patient. Research in human relations has demonstrated that a rapport is most readily established if the physician possesses and displays certain qualities, including empathy, respect, nonpossessive warmth, genuineness, nonjudgmental acceptance, kindness, and interest. These qualities are common to all effective counselors and can be learned by most.

Empathy, perhaps the most important of these characteristics, is the attempt to understand someone else's feelings; it is described as "putting yourself in someone else's shoes" or "seeing things through someone else's eyes." Whereas to sympathize with a patient (*i.e.,* actually feel the patient's pain, frustration, or depression) could interfere with the physician's ability to counsel the patient, to empathize (*i.e.,* understand without feeling) facilitates effective counseling. However, the physician as counselor must not just understand the patient's feeling but also be able to verbalize that understanding. This act of empathetic communication convinces the patient that the physician is listening and really understands what she wants to have understood. It also convinces the patient that her physician is giving her his full attention and thinks she is important. Unfortunately, the phrases "I understand" and "I know what you mean" are often ineffective in communicating empathy, and therefore should be avoided.

The next most important quality of the effective counselor is respect; the physician should believe in the worth and potential of the patient and have confidence in the patient's ability to help herself. Studies of the physician–patient relationship have demonstrated that patients are more often described by their physicians as competent if they believe their physicians take a personal interest in them and treat them with concern. It also means the physician does not show disrespect by

suggesting that a patient's complaint is insignificant or unfounded. Obviously, arguing with the patient, making fun of the patient's feelings, dismissing the patient's feelings as unimportant or wrong, or glibly offering superficial and simple suggestions for complex problems interfere with the communication of respect for the patient.

Warmth is the degree to which the physician communicates a caring about the patient. It is usually communicated together with empathy and respect by a variety of nonverbal and verbal messages. For example, warmth may be shown by gestures, tone of voice, facial expression, or touch. However, warmth that is not genuine can usually be detected by the patient, for if verbal and nonverbal messages do not agree, the patient usually believes the nonverbal ones.

To be genuine is to be authentic, sincere, and believable. When the patient perceives a genuine quality about her physician, she is more apt to disclose deep and threatening feelings that must be revealed before effective counseling can occur.

The remaining qualities of an effective counselor, those of nonjudgmental acceptance, kindness, and interest, are to some extent included in the qualities described above. To express these characteristics is to convey empathy, respect, warmth, and genuineness.

Effective Communicating Styles

Merely possessing the qualities described above is not enough; the physician must be able to communicate them to the patient through both verbal and nonverbal messages. For example, the physician conveys empathy and respect by listening intently and giving the patient his undivided attention. The physician reinforces these qualities by summarizing his understanding of the patient's problem in a tone of voice analogous to that of the patient and in terms that the patient can understand.

Communication of warmth, kindness, and interest is for the most part nonverbal. Examples of nonverbal communication that convey these qualities include the following:

Maintaining eye contact
Having a relaxed, open posture
Facing the patient
Leaning forward toward the patient
Showing a facial expression consistent with the patient's
    predominant emotion
Having a modulated, nonmechanical tone of voice

Forced or excessive expressions of warmth during the early stages of the patient–physician relationship may be counterproductive.

Once the physician has developed the qualities described above and has learned to communicate them, he must put them together to become an effective counselor. The steps involved in doing this include those listed below:

1. Effective listening
2. Creating a nonthreatening atmosphere in which the patient feels free to express herself
3. Creating a relationship based on mutual trust and caring
4. Responding to the patient in verbal and nonverbal ways that convey empathy, respect, and warmth by:
   a. Reflecting accurately and fully the patient's feelings
   b. Communicating acceptance of the patient as a person
   c. Showing attentiveness and caring through nonverbal behavior
5. Defining and agreeing with the patient about the exact role of the physician in the counseling situation

Difficult Counseling Situations

The Angry Patient

Every physician has had the experience of being verbally attacked by an angry patient without warning, perhaps for no apparent reason. Such an angry outburst usually stems from a remote condition or conditions unrelated to the precipitating incident. Examples of such conditions include unhappiness with oneself, with one's anger toward oneself being directed outward, or failure to achieve a life goal, causing frustration. Alternatively, anger can be an immature attempt on the part of the patient to demonstrate strength and maintain control, a defensive maneuver to keep the physician at a comfortable emotional distance, or a desperate effort to get the full attention of the physician when less dramatic cries for help have gone unheeded.

In order to respond appropriately, the physician must recognize his response (*e.g.,* anger) and avoid immediate "gut" reactions, which may not only be ineffective but may also be distorted or misinterpreted by the patient. In addition, the physician must realize that the patient's attack is probably not personal but rather the result of an unrelated situation or condition. The physician can often diffuse the patient's anger by showing the patient that he is trying to understand the remote condition behind the outburst.

The first step to take in dealing with the angry patient is to listen, letting the patient vent all of her angry feelings. Often the anger dissipates soon after the patient has finished her outburst. Although the physician may not agree with the patient's reasons for being angry, he should accept her right to be angry and continue to respect her and to convey that respect. When the patient is ready, the physician should communicate empathy, demonstrating to the patient that he recognizes how important the situation is to her and that he wants to

understand how she feels and why she feels that way. If the physician is or has been part of the problem, he should admit it fully and willingly and act to correct the situation. If he has not been part of the problem, he should offer to act on behalf of the patient or help the patient develop a response that will correct the perceived or real problem.

The Grieving Patient

Many physicians find it difficult to deal with a grieving patient or the grieving family of a patient who is critically ill or who has died. An appropriate, helpful response requires keen perception and a carefully formulated plan. Unfortunately, many physicians are inhibited by the taboos surrounding a discussion of death and dying. Furthermore, most physicians experience a complex set of emotions in response to the situation—grief, sadness, inadequacy, guilt, helplessness, or anger—which emotions may interfere with effective communication and counseling.

In order to effectively help the grieving patient or family, the physician must understand his own attitudes and feelings as well as those of the grieving. Kubler-Ross has described five stages of grieving: denial, anger, bargaining, depression, and acceptance. Specific responses can be formulated according to the stage of grieving the patient or family is going through. In general, the physician needs to be fully accepting of the greving patient and her behavior, sincere in offering help and support, supportive without reinforcing unrealistic expectations, willing to give some control to the patient or family, and available.

Other Difficult Counseling Situations

In addition to dealing with angry or grieving patients, physicians may have to deal with other difficult interpersonal situations, including patients who are passive, dependent, seductive, demanding, hypochondrial, antisocial, self-destructive, or noncompliant. Although effective counseling requires a different strategy for each patient and situation, the common principle underlying all situations is that the counselor needs to recognize his own emotional and behavioral response to the patient. The effective physician does not react with derision, rejection, or avoidance to his feelings of impatience, frustration, or anger with the patient. Instead, he is aware of his emotional responses to his patients and recognizes the role of those emotions and responses in the outcome of therapy.

SEXUAL COUNSELING

Sexual dysfunction is a frequently overlooked but common problem among women seeking care for gynecologic disorders. In a recent study of well-adjusted, happily married couples selected from the community, 63%

of the women admitted to a sexual dysfunction, and 77% indicated that they experience sexual difficulties. Because sexual problems are so common, a question or two about the quality of the patient's sexual relationship should be a routine part of every gynecologic history. Unfortunately, some physicians may not ask questions because they are uncertain about what to do if a patient responds positively. Therefore, the physician should have in mind a logical approach to asking about and responding to questions about sexual problems. Armed with a basic understanding of sexual dysfunction and the principles of sexual counseling, the gynecologist can screen for sexual problems and when appropriate either counsel or refer patients.

Sexual problems can be arbitrarily categorized in a variety of ways. In general, however, most sexual problems are a result of either disruptions in the sexual response cycle or disordered sexual relationships. Examples of sexual dysfunctions include inhibited sexual desire, orgasmic dysfunction, vaginismus, dyspareunia, and generalized sexual inhibition. Dissatisfaction with sexual relationships can stem from disagreement between partners regarding the frequency or timing of sexual relations, the varieties of sexual activity, the initiation or refusal of sexual advances, the techniques of sexual activity, and the interpersonal feelings that accompany a sexual relationship.

Taking a Sexual History

Although there are many models for sexual histories, most are not appropriate for the nonpsychiatric physician or in the setting of a brief office visit. However, a model for office practice has been developed and detailed by Munjack and Oziel, who describe two types of sexual histories: a screening history and a problem-oriented history. The screening history is brief and is suited for inclusion in the comprehensive medical history that is often part of a patient's first visit to her gynecologist. The problem-oriented history is more detailed and is designed to investigate those problems identified by the screening history.

The screening history is designed to determine whether there are any major sexual difficulties that need in-depth evaluation and therapy, and whether the physician can deal with the problem or whether it should be referred elsewhere for more intensive evaluation. In an attempt to put the patient at ease, the physician can begin the sexual history by prefacing his questions with statements such as "Most people experience . . ." or "Because sexual problems can develop as part of other gynecologic problems, ..." In addition, if the physician can convey a willingness to help, the patient is more likely to discuss with him any problems she may have. Finally, the screening history should begin with a discussion of topics that are unlikely to provoke anxiety. For example, questions about the occurrence of pain during intercourse are less likely to cause anxiety

than questions about orgasmic function or noncoital sexual practices.

With these principles in mind, the gynecologist can begin with a general question such as, "Are you having any sexual problems?" If the physician receives a noncommital response, a more specific question, "Are you satisfied with the frequency of sexual relations?", can be posed. Once a problem is identified, the gynecologist can proceed to the problem-oriented sexual history and ask about the following: date of onset, severity, previous evaluation and treatment and the results of such treatment, conditions that diminish or exacerbate the problem, the patient's response to the problem, and the effect of the problem on the patient's relationship with her spouse. To conclude the screening history, the physician should invite the patient to bring up any concerns that have not been covered by the screening history. Even if the patient denies having any problems, the screening history is of value, since it demonstrates the willingness of the physician to discuss sexual problems.

As suggested above, the problem-oriented history is designed to differentiate organic from psychogenic sexual problems, determine the complexity of the problem, determine the need for referral of the patient to a more sophisticated sexual counselor, and provide information for the formulation of a treatment program if the gynecologist elects to treat the patient. The problem-oriented sexual history should include the following topics:

Onset of the problem
Course of the problem
Conditions that decrease or increase the severity of the problem
Previous evaluation of the problem and the results of such evaluation
Previous treatment of the problem and the results of such treatment
Severity of the problem
Patient's reaction to the problem
Impact of the problem on the patient's sexual relationships
Patient's sexual attitudes and upbringing
Patient's sexual practices
Quality of patient's sexual and/or marital relationship

A rational treatment or referral plan can be formulated on the basis of discussion of these and related questions.

Rapid Treatment of Sexual Problems by the Non-Sex Therapist

Annon devised one of the most useful approaches to the rapid treatment of sexual problems, known as the *PLISSIT approach. PLISSIT* is an acronym made up of the initial letters of the words *p*ermission, *l*imited *in*formation, *s*pecific *s*uggestions, and *i*ntensive *t*herapy— the four increasingly deep levels of therapeutic intervention proposed by Annon. The PLISSIT model is applicable to the majority of sexual concerns, can be used by therapist and nontherapist alike, can be tailored to the degree of competence of the physician, and is suitable when time is limited.

The first level of this model is that of *permission:* giving permission to the patient to experience certain attitudes, feelings, or behaviors. Concerns about masturbation, sexual fantasies, or nudity can often be eliminated by an explanation that such activities or thoughts are normal. Such an explanation enables the patient to give herself permission to think, act, or feel in particular ways and thereby relieves her of guilt.

Limited information refers to the provision to the patient of specific factual information that is relevant to her sexual concerns or perceived problem. Concerns about genital anatomy, breast size, physiologic reactions to sexual stimulation, or noncoital sexual activities often disappear when the patient learns that she is normal and her sexual activities are common.

To give appropriate *specific suggestions,* the physician must first obtain a problem-oriented history. Examples of specific suggestions include sensate focus exercises and proscriptions regarding coitus or new sexual activities. Obviously, the appropriateness (and therefore the value) of the suggestions increases as the physician becomes more familiar with the patient's specific sexual problem, any antecedents it may have, the role of sex in her life, and her attitude toward her problem and her own sexuality.

Finally, *intensive therapy* is indicated when the first three levels of the PLISSIT model have not been successful. At this point, most gynecologists will refer the patient to a bona fide sex therapist or a psychologist with skills in sex therapy. Intensive therapy is indicated when, for example, the sexual problem is secondary to significant psychopathology or when it is causing marital discord.

Referral of the patient is indicated in several situations. First, the patient should be referred if the physician does not have the time or skill to deal with her particular sexual problem. Second, most physicians refer a patient with a sexual problem if the problem is only part of a much larger psychologic problem or problem with the patient's relationship with her partner. Third, referral is indicated if therapy is failing or if new complications (*e.g.,* serious marital problems) have developed during the course of therapy. Finally, the patient should be referred if the physician has personal feelings toward the patient that interfere with an appropriate professional relationship (*e.g.,* dislike, lack of interest, or sexual feelings).

PREMENSTRUAL SYNDROME

Another common clinical condition that often requires counseling by the obstetrician–gynecologist is the premenstrual syndrome (PMS). Estimates of the prevalence of PMS have ranged from near 40% to over 90%. This wide range is at least in part the result of differences in the definition of PMS and the interpretation of symptoms. Despite the fact that PMS was first described over 50 years ago, it is still only vaguely defined as the presence of recurrent emotional, physical, or behavioral symptoms during the two weeks before the onset of menses. This vague definition and the large number of symptoms reported (over 150) have led some clinicians and researchers to even question the existence of PMS. Nonetheless, distress and discomfort in the luteal phase of the menstrual cycle is very real and a major source of emotional and social problems for many women.

Although several hypotheses have been suggested to account for PMS, no single hypothesis is universally accepted. It is likely that premenstrual symptoms result from a variety of medical and psychologic conditions that are associated with the luteal phase of the menstrual cycle. In addition, a subgroup of women who experience premenstrual symptoms may suffer from a unique, and as yet undefined, disease that is either hormonal in nature or modulated by the cyclic changes of hormones during the menstrual cycle.

Clinical Features

Typically, women with moderate or severe premenstrual symptoms report the onset of those symptoms either during adolescence or during the puerperium and following postpartum depression. They frequently do not seek care while the symptoms are mild but wait until age 30 to 40, when the symptoms become more severe and prolonged.

The symptoms experienced by women with PMS are physical, emotional, and behavioral. The most common of the physical symptoms are fatigue, headache, abdominal bloating, breast tenderness and swelling, acne, joint pain, constipation, and recurring herpetic or yeast infections. Although these physical symptoms are often uncomfortable, most women with moderate or severe PMS complain most about their premenstrual emotional symptoms, especially depression, anxiety, hostility, irritability, rapid mood changes, altered libido, and sensitivity to rejection. In addition, women with PMS may also experience a variety of behavioral symptoms, including physical or verbal abuse of self or others, a craving for or intolerance of alcohol, a craving for sugar or chocolate, and binge eating.

Only recently have investigators recognized that long-standing or severe PMS can cause psychologic or social problems that may be as disruptive as the primary premenstrual symptoms listed above. Psychologic reactions to PMS include guilt, shame, decreased self-esteem, unassertiveness, decreased self-confidence, a negative body image, and a sense of hopelessness. In addition, many women with long-standing PMS report that their recurrent emotional and behavioral symptoms have eroded their relationships with friends, husbands, children, and co-workers. Finally, PMS has been an un-recognized factor in poor work records or failed educational pursuits for many women.

Evaluation and Treatment

The evaluation of women with premenstrual complaints consists at least of a medical and PMS history, a physical examination, and the prospective charting of their symptoms. For those with severe or long-standing symptoms, psychosocial evaluation is an important addition to the workup. The purposes of the evaluation are to determine the presence of premenstrual symptoms, to rule out underlying physical or emotional diseases the symptoms of which are present or most severe only during the premenstrum, and to identify any psychosocial problems the patient may have developed in response to years of recurrent premenstrual symptoms.

A review of the literature reveals a long list of suggested treatments. High-protein–low-carbohydrate diet, exercise, vitamins, diuretics, oral contraceptives, progestins, bromocriptine, progesterone, tranquilizers, lithium, and psychotherapy have all been recommended in the past decade. Unfortunately, none of these treatments has consistently withstood the test of double-blind, placebo-controlled studies; furthermore, even controlled studies are suspect, for there are no universally accepted diagnostic criteria for PMS, methods for grading responses, or criteria for categorization of subjects into groups. Thus, no single treatment for PMS is universally accepted or recommended.

In view of these confusing and contradictory findings, it is not surprising that most physicians are frustrated in their attempts to offer a rational approach to the treatment of PMS. Unfortunately, there is no way to predict which form of therapy will be most effective for a specific patient. Therefore, until a large, multiagent, double-blind, placebo-controlled study utilizing uni-versally accepted diagnostic criteria and measures of severity and response is performed, physicians are left with a "trial and error" approach to therapy, striving to provide effective treatment with the safest, most simple therapy at the lowest possible cost.

SUMMARY

To be an effective counselor, the obstetrician–gynecologist must become familiar with the principles of human relations, sexuality, counseling, and communication. The physician who is well trained in these areas of counseling will not only encourage the discussion of personal and sexual problems by the patient but will also be able to respond to such problems appropriately and effectively.

REFERENCES AND RECOMMENDED READING

Annon JS: The Behavioral Treatment of Sexual Problems: Brief Therapy. New York, Harper & Row, 1976

Carkhuff RR: Helping and Human Relations. A Primer for Lay and Professional Helpers, Vols. I and II. New York, Holt, Rinehart & Winston, 1969

Cassell EJ: The relief of suffering. Arch Intern Med 143:522, 1983

Gazda GM, Walters RP, Childers WC: Human Relations Development. Boston, Allyn & Bacon, 1975

Gorlin R, Zucker HD: Physicians' reactions to patients: A key to teaching humanistic medicine. N Engl J Med 308:1059, 1983

Kubler-Ross E: Death: The Final Stage of Growth. Englewood Cliffs, NJ, Prentice-Hall, 1975

Lipowski ZJ: Psychosocial reactions to physical illness. Can Med Assoc J 128:1069, 1983

Munjack DJ, Oziel LJ: Sexual Medicine and Counseling in Office Practice: A Comprehensive Treatment Guide. Boston, Little, Brown, 1980

Nutrition in Obstetrics and Gynecology

Roy M. Pitkin

11

Nutrition exerts important influences on the course and outcome of pregnancy and has implications for lactation and hormonal therapy as well. This chapter examines the role of diet and nutrition in all of these reproductive events.

Important concepts underlie the terms *requirement* and *allowance* as used with respect to diet and nutrition. Though related to one another, the terms are not synonymous. *Requirement* refers to the minimum amount of a specific nutrient necessary to prevent a deficiency state (*i.e.,* maintain normal health and function). For any nutrient the requirement varies considerably from individual to individual and even within the same individual from time to time. Moreover, methods of estimating requirements are often necessarily indirect and imprecise. One derives the *allowance* for a particular nutrient by increasing the average requirement proportionately to account for individual variations in need, absorption, and utilization, thereby arriving at a value applicable to a population as opposed to an individual. In the case of nearly all nutrients, the allowance is set somewhat above the requirement.

The National Research Council periodically publishes its Recommended Dietary Allowances (RDA), which are defined as "the levels of intake of essential nutrients considered . . . to be adequate to meet the known nutritional needs of practically all healthy persons." Table 11-1 lists the current RDA for women of reproductive age as well as the additions for pregnant and lactating women.

PREGNANCY

During gestation, the maternal organism undergoes a remarkable series of physiologic adjustments in order to provide for the growth and development of the conceptus and at the same time preserve maternal homeo-stasis. Concomitantly, exchange between mother and fetus occurs across the placenta, and the fetus modifies its own development through its maturing regulatory processes. Many aspects of these complex, integrated physiologic systems are nutritional in nature or are directly related to diet.

Energy, Weight, and Weight Gain

Energy Requirements

More energy than usual is needed during pregnancy to support development of the conceptus and growth of certain maternal tissues. The total energy cost of pregnancy, estimated from the amounts of protein and fat accumulated in maternal and fetal compartments and the metabolic additions incurred by these tissue accretions, approximates 75,000 kcal.

The additional caloric expenditure of pregnancy is not evenly distributed throughout gestation, nor does it parallel fetal growth. It is minimal during the first few weeks following conception, increases sharply near the end of the first trimester, and remains essentially constant through the remainder of gestation. During the second trimester, the added caloric cost of pregnancy reflects principally growth in the maternal compartment (*i.e.,* expansion of blood volume, growth of uterus and breasts, and accumulation of fat stores), whereas third-trimester expenditures are required mainly for fetal and placental growth.

Because energy expenditure throughout most of gestation is relatively constant, albeit for differing reasons, the daily incremental need attributable to pregnancy can be estimated by division of the total cumulative caloric cost (75,000 kcal) by duration (250 days). This approach, used in arriving at the RDA (see Table 11-1), yields a value of 300 kcal per day. This value

Table 11-1
Recommended Dietary Allowances—National Research Council, 1980

Nutrient	Female 15–18	Female 19–22	Female 23–50	Pregnancy	Lactation
Energy (kcal)	2100	2100	2000	+300	+500
Protein (g)	46	44	44	+30	+20
Vitamin A (μg RE)	800	800	800	+200	+400
Vitamin D (μg)	10	7.5	5	+5	+5
Vitamin E (mgα-TE)	8	8	8	+2	+3
Vitamin C (mg)	50	60	60	+20	+40
Thiamin (mg)	1.1	1.1	1	+0.4	+0.5
Riboflavin (mg)	1.3	1.3	1.2	+0.3	+0.5
Niacin (mg NE)	14	14	13	+2	+5
Vitamin B_6 (mg)	2	2	2	+0.6	+0.5
Folacin (μg)	400	400	400	+400	+100
Vitamin B_{12} (μg)	3	3	3	+1	+1
Calcium (mg)	1200	800	800	+400	+400
Phosphorus (mg)	1200	800	800	+400	+400
Magnesium (mg)	300	300	300	+150	+150
Iron (mg)	18	18	18	*	*
Zinc (mg)	15	15	15	+5	+10
Iodine (pg)	150	150	150	+25	+50

* Iron supplementation, in amounts providing 30 mg to 60 mg of ferrous iron daily, is recommended during pregnancy and for 2 to 3 months postpartum.

represents the amount needed for pregnancy per se and does not take into account other variables, such as body size, physical activity, ambient temperature, and growth requirements unrelated to gestation (as in the pregnant adolescent).

Weight Gain

Normal or optimal weight gain during pregnancy is extraordinarily difficult to determine because of intrinsic methodologic problems. First, it varies with how the "baseline" weight is regarded; some studies have employed weight at first antenatal visit (which of course depends on the timing of that visit and ignores any changes that have already occurred), whereas others have used patient recollection of preconceptional weight (which is subject to errors of memory and variations in scale accuracy). Moreover, populations from which averages are derived may include a large number of persons who make deliberate efforts to manipulate their weight, on the basis of either medical advice or their own initiative, making applicability to the "natural" state problematic.

The American College of Obstetricians and Gynecologists has identified a range of 10 kg to 12 kg as the average value for total weight gain during pregnancy. This range is that of average, as opposed to optimal (*i.e.,* the level associated with best outcome for mother and infant); nevertheless, most authorities find that the lowest frequency of obstetric complications seems to occur at about these mean values, so that average and optimal values are similar.

More important than the amount of gain is the pattern by which weight accumulates. Unfortunately, information relating outcome to various patterns is limited. However, the pattern generally assumed to be normal consists of minimal change during the first trimester followed by a steady, progressive rate of gain, averaging 0.4 kg per week, through the last two trimesters.

Figure 11-1 portrays the pattern and components of pregnancy weight gain. Of the mean total value of 11 kg at term, the maternal compartment contains 6 kg and the fetal compartment 5 kg. However, accumulation in

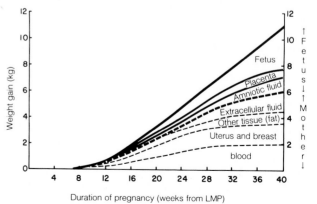

FIG. 11-1. Pattern and components of weight gain during pregnancy. *LMP,* last menstrual period. (Pitkin RM: Nutritional support in obstetrics and gynecology. Clin Obstet Gynecol 19: 489–513, 1976. Reproduced with permission)

the two compartments varies with duration of gestation. During the second trimester most of the weight gain reflects maternal growth, whereas during the third trimester most of it results from growth of the intrauterine contents.

Relationship to Birth Weight

Although many questions about the relationship of nutrition and pregnancy outcome remain unresolved, the association between maternal size, both preconceptional and during gestation, and infant size at birth is reasonably clear. In virtually all populations examined, weight before conception and gain during gestation have been found to correlate significantly with birth weight. These two influences, which are independent and additive, generally rank second only to gestational age as determinants of birth weight. Thus, in a pregnancy of any given duration, birth weight will reflect maternal prepregnant weight and weight gain during gestation.

The epidemiologic evidence linking maternal and infant weight has been confirmed by certain "natural experiments" in human malnutrition. Studied particularly thoroughly was the Dutch famine that occurred during the late stages of world War II. This famine involved severe protein–caloric malnutrition, which was suddenly imposed and then abruptly relieved a few months later. In women subjected to the famine at various stages of pregnancy, it was found that caloric intakes below 1500 kcal per day led to decreases in infant weight (averaging 250 g), length, and head circumference, as well as placental weight. No further effects were observed with starvation in either early or late gestation; women starved only in early pregnancy produced infants of normal size, confirming the prediction based on Figure 11-1 that the effect of maternal weight gain on birth weight is largely a third-trimester phenomenon.

Additional evidence for a relationship between maternal energy intake and birth weight comes from intervention studies in which women with known or presumed deficient nutritional status are provided with a supplement of calories and in some cases protein. The results of these studies have varied. Some, usually conducted in developing countries with severely malnourished populations, have revealed a substantial effect of maternal energy intake on birthweight (e.g., mean increases of 250–300 g with resultant lowering of the prevalence of low-birth-weight infants from 25–30% to 5–6%). Others, particularly those conducted with impoverished populations in developed countries, have recorded less impressive results; for example, an analysis of the U.S. Government Supplemental Program for Women, Infants, and Children (WIC) estimates an increase in birth weight of 30 g to 50 g resulting from participation in that program. This discrepancy in the effect of suplemental feeding on birth weight in different populations is probably due to the varying severity of the underlying or baseline deprivation.

In spite of a reasonably well documented relation-

ship between pregnancy weight gain and fetal growth, other effects of maternal diet on the fetus, particularly those on long-term outcome, are more difficult to determine. Studies in experimental animals, particularly rats, have revealed that maternal dietary restriction affects various morphologic aspects of brain development. These results have given rise to concern about the possible relevance of maternal diet to neurologic, behavioral, and cognitive development. However, the few available long-term follow-up studies suggest that normal infant development occurs across a wide range of pregnancy weight gains.

Deviation in Weight and Weight Gain

Although standard definitions for deviation in preconceptional weight and weight gain during pregnancy are lacking, the following are suggested as reasonable guidelines:

Underweight—Prepregnant weight 10% or more below standard (Table 11-2)
Overweight—Prepregnant weight 20% or more above standard (Table 11-2)
Inadequate gain—Gain of 1 kg or less per month during the second and third trimesters
Excessive gain—Gain of 3 kg or more per month

The hazards presented by the underweight pregnant woman have generally been underappreciated. Such a woman has a high risk of delivering a low-birth-weight infant, and some studies have suggested that she is likely to develop preeclampsia as well.

Table 11-2
Women's Height and Weight Table

Height		Weight (lbs) by Body Frame Size		
Feet	Inches	Small	Medium	Large
4	10	102–111	109–121	118–131
4	11	103–113	111–123	120–134
5	0	104–115	113–126	122–137
5	1	106–118	115–129	125–140
5	2	108–121	118–132	128–143
5	3	111–124	121–135	131–147
5	4	114–127	124–138	134–151
5	5	117–130	127–141	137–155
5	6	120–133	130–144	140–159
5	7	123–136	133–147	143–163
5	8	126–139	136–150	147–167
5	9	129–142	139–153	149–170
5	10	132–145	142–156	152–173
5	11	135–148	145–159	155–176
6	0	138–151	148–162	158–179

1979 Build Study, Society of Actuaries and Associates of Life Insurance Medical Directors of America.

The overweight woman faces several risks during pregnancy, notably those related to hypertensive disorders and diabetes mellitus. She is also likely to give birth to a larger than average infant. Any unfavorable outcome of pregnancy is probably due to coincidental medical complications; it seems unlikely that obesity per se exerts an adverse influence. It is generally agreed that weight loss during pregnancy is ill advised; however, what constitutes proper dietary counseling for obese gravidas is a matter of controversy. Some physicians advise a diet moderately restricted in energy to limit weight gain (*e.g.*, to 6–8 kg) so that the woman will conclude the reproductive cycle with a net lowering of weight. Others question the advisability of any dietary restriction on grounds that (1) nutrients other than energy may inadvertently be affected, (2) optimal protein utilization depends on adequate enrgy intake, and (3) fat catabolism releases ketone bodies, which may adversely affect fetal development.

The gravida whose weight gain is less than normal is at increased risk for delivering a low-birth-weight infant. She requires careful dietary counseling and close follow-up to normalize her weight gain pattern.

Excessive weight gain during pregnancy was long thought to predispose to a number of obstetric complications. Several generations of United States physicians were taught that restriction of weight gain, sometimes to very small amounts, is important in antenatal care. It is now clear that, except for having a modest effect on fetal growth, excessive weight gain per se has no influence on the course or outcome of pregnancy. However, if the weight is not lost following parturition, it will contribute to the long-term development of obesity.

As mentioned previously, preconceptional weight and pregnancy weight gain are independent but additive influences on birth weight. Thus, one may operate to overcome an adverse effect exerted by the other. For example, an underweight woman who gains little weight has a very high risk of delivering a low-birth-weight infant; if she gains the average amount of weight, the risk is lower, and if she gains more than average, the risk can be minimized.

Protein

Requirements

More protein than usual is needed by the pregnant woman for tissue synthesis in the expanding maternal compartment and in the products of conception. The magnitude of the increased need may be estimated in two ways. A theoretical estimate is derived from the known sites of protein storage (illustrated in Figure 11-1), which total approximately 1 kg at term. Division of this figure by the duration of gestation and then correction of the daily increment for variability in biologic quality and efficiency of conversion of dietary to tissue protein yields an estimate of approximately 10 g per day

as sufficient to provide for the additional needs of gestation.

The experimental approach to estimating nutritional requirements utilizes balance studies in which all intakes and losses are measured assiduously across a range of dietary intakes and the point of shift from negative to positive balance is taken as the requirement. Nitrogen balance studies in pregnant women have fairly consistently indicated values 2 to 3 times theoretical predictions. The reason for this discrepancy is unclear, but most authorities regard balance studies as systematically tending to overestimate requirements and, therefore, theoretical estimates as more accurate. Nevertheless, because of uncertainties about protein storage in pregnant women, the tendency at present is tentatively to accept the higher value. Thus, the RDA provides for an addition of 30 g per day during gestation; this translates to a total intake of 1.3 g per kg of body weight per day in the mature woman, 1.5 g per kg of body weight per day in the adolescent aged 15 to 18, and 1.7 g per kg of body weight per day in the adolescent under age 15.

The complex metabolic relationship between energy and protein makes it necessary for the two nutrients to be considered together in any estimation of requirements or determination of effects on pregnancy outcome. Given that energy needs take first priority in metabolism, optimal protein utilization presupposes adequate energy supply.

Relationship to Pregnancy Outcome

Protein is of course an essential nutrient, but some seem to regard it as an almost magical determinant of pregnancy outcome. However, the morphologic, biochemical, and developmental effects of dietary protein restriction seen in experimental animals, principally rats, cannot be applied directly to humans.

In humans the relationship between dietary protein and birth weight is particularly problematic. In a critical review Zlatnik concluded that all reported studies of the question suffer from serious methodologic inadequacies, including failure to take into account preconceptional weight or pregnancy weight gain, conscious or unconscious manipulation of diet, selection bias (due to subjects' being volunteers), and the inherent inaccuracy and subjectivity of dietary survey data.

A potential relationship between dietary protein and preeclampsia has long been a subject of speculation. It used to be believed that excessive intake was the cause of the disease, but more recently it has been hypothesized that deficient intake levels limit plasma volume expansion and that this in turn leads to a hypertensive state. Several retrospective studies have associated low protein intake (determined by diet history) with preeclampsia, but any cause–effect relationship is far from clear because of confounding by socioeconomic status, race, marital status, age, and parity.

Production of urea, the end product of metabolism, varies directly with protein intake levels. This relationship may be used to develop a simple, objective index of dietary ingestion. Population screening by repeated measurements of urinary urea excretion (expressed as the ratio of urea to cretinine) has confirmed the expected relationship between maternal weight and birth weight; however, no correlation has been found between protein intake and infant weight, length, head circumference, ponderal index, or preeclampsia. These observations seem to indicate that, at least as far as effects evident at birth are concerned, a relatively wide range of maternal dietary protein intake is compatible with normal pregnancy outcome. Of course, the possibility that adverse effects of a subtle nature may exist or become evident later cannot be excluded.

In spite of the many uncertainties regarding the influence of dietary protein on pregnancy outcome, protein is clearly an important nutrient for the pregnant woman and should be ingested in adequate amounts. All available evidence indicates that the RDA (1.3 g per kg of body weight for the mature gravida and somewhat larger amounts for the adolescent) is an appropriate guideline and may even be something of an overestimate. Nevertheless, many clinicians regularly recommend intakes in excess of this amount, often 2 g per kg of body weight or more. Some caution in this regard is warranted in view of observations of an increase in perinatal mortality, due principally to increased frequency of preterm labor, among women given a protein-rich supplement during gestation.

Iron and Folate

One of the most striking physiologic adjustments of pregnancy is the expansion of maternal blood volume, illustrated in Figure 11-2. Plasma volume begins to increase in the first few weeks after conception and con-

tinues to expand at a relatively rapid rate until the early third trimester, when its growth slows and then effectively ceases. At its maximum, at 34 to 36 weeks, plasma volume averages 50% above the nonpregnant level. Erythrocyte volume also increases but, in contrast to the sigmoidlike shape of the plasma curve, its pattern is much more nearly linear and the final extent only half as much. These gestational changes in blood volume have direct implications with respect to iron and folate, the two micronutrients most directly involved in hematopoiesis.

Requirements

The extent of increase in erythrocyte mass during pregnancy depends in large part on the availability of iron. Without iron supplementation, total red cell mass increases by an average of only 250 ml; in contrast, if iron is supplemented, the augmentation approximates 400 ml. The difference between these two values is equivalent to 500 mg of elemental iron, the amount the bone marrow uses in the augmented erythropoiesis of pregnancy if iron is available in ample amounts. The fetus and placenta require an additional 300 mg of iron. Although further iron is expended in the blood lost at parturition, this may be disregarded in calculations, since the augmented volume more than compensates for the loss. A "saving" of iron of approximately 120 mg may be projected from the amenorrhea that accompanies pregnancy, but this may also be disregarded as roughly equivalent to obligatory losses in urine, stool, and sweat. Thus, the total iron "cost" of pregnancy averages about 800 mg.

Folate requirements also increase substantially with gestation. Given that folate is an essential co-enzyme in purine and pyrimidine metabolism, needs for the vitamin are especially high during rapid growth of tissues. Thus, gestational augmentation in maternal erythropoiesis, trophoblastic growth and proliferation, and obligatory placental transfer account for a substantial increase in the pregnant woman's need for folate. The precise magnitude of the pregnancy requirement is not known with certainty. The RDA is 800 μg, double that for the nonpregnant woman. It is likely that actual needs more than double; if so, the difference between requirement and allowance (*i.e.,* the "safety factor") is narrower in the gravid than in the nongravid patient.

Effects of Deficiency and Place of Supplementation

To meet the projected total iron need of approximately 800 mg above normal requirements, the gravida has two potential sources available: diet and stores. The usual mixed diet contains 10 mg to 15 mg of elemental iron, of which 10% to 15% is absorbed under normal conditions; thus, dietary sources may be expected to provide roughly 400 mg over the course of gestation. Iron stored in the reticuloendothelial cells of the bone

FIG. 11-2. Plasma and erythrocyte volume changes during pregnancy. (Pitkin RM: Nutritional support in obstetrics and gynecology. Clin Obstet Gynecol 19:489–513, 1976. Reproduced with permission)

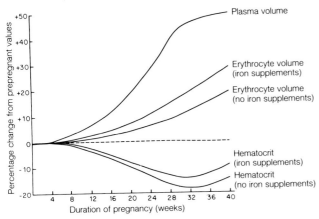

marrow averages 300 mg in women of reproductive age, but as many as one third of healthy females have little or no stored iron. Thus, diet and stores are often insufficient to meet the projected iron need of the gravida; as a result, there is a decline in hemoglobin–hematocrit levels during the course of pregnancy.

Anemia, defined as hemoglobin–hematocrit values of less than 11 g/dl and 33%, respectively, is seen in a third or more of pregnant women at some time during gestation, usually during the late second or early third trimester. Although the anemia is typically microcytic and hypochromic, these findings are not necessarily diagnostic. To confirm iron deficiency as the cause of anemia in an anemic gravida, other biochemical–morphologic findings (*e.g.,* low serum iron, low percentage saturation of transferrin, low serum ferritin, and no histochemical iron stores) are needed. Table 11-3 lists these diagnostic findings.

Anemia is a risk factor for adverse pregnancy outcome. The anemic gravida is ill prepared to tolerate hemorrhage and therefore more likely than normal to suffer complications from blood loss with or after parturition. She is also probably less able than normal to cope with infections and is thus at increased risk for urinary tract infection or puerperal sepsis. Prevention of anemia is therefore desirable, and in view of the fact that dietary and storage iron sources are often inadequate to meet the projected needs of pregnancy, most authorities recommend routine iron supplementation during at least the last half of gestation and for two or three months postpartum. Supplements should be in the form of simple iron salts providing 30 mg to 60 mg of elemental iron per day (Table 11-4). Numerous studies have documented that this approach virtually eliminates iron deficiency anemia as a complication of pregnancy. However, the concept of routine iron supplementation is not universally accepted. According to a contrary view, particularly prevalent in Britain, the iron-induced augmentation of erythrocyte mass is a pharmacologic effect and not desirable unless actual deficiency is documented.

In subjects placed on a folate-free diet, the earliest observed effect (generally seen in 2–3 weeks) is a low

Table 11-3
Findings in Iron Deficiency Anemia

Substance	Level
Hemoglobin	<11 g/dl
Hematocrit (packed cell volume)	<33%
Mean corpuscular volume	<80 μ^3
Mean corpuscular hemoglobin	<30%
Serum iron	<50 μg/dl
Percentage saturation transferrin	<15%
Serum ferritin	<10 μg/ml
Histochemical iron in bone marrow	<1+

Table 11-4
Elemental Iron Content of Supplements

Supplement	Content (%)
Ferrous fumarate	33
Ferrous sulfate (exsiccated)	30
Ferrous sulfate (nonexsiccated)	20
Ferrous gluconate	11

serum folate concentration. Next in the sequence of morphologic and biochemical effects of folate deprivation is neutrophil hypersegmentation (6–8 weeks) followed in turn by elevated foriminoglutamic acid excretion (12–14 weeks), low erythrocyte folate level (16–18 weeks), megaloblastic bone marrow (17–19 weeks), and finally anemia (20 weeks). The prevalence of folate deficiency varies widely among populations. In developed countries megaloblastic anemia is relatively unusual. However, serum folate levels fall with gestation, and low values (*i.e.,* < 3 ng/ml) are seen in as many as 20% of otherwise normal pregnancies.

Whereas the association between folate deficiency and megaloblastic anemia is clear, the clinical significance of preanemic indices of deficiency is uncertain. Early reports, mainly retrospective in nature, suggested an association between folate deficiency and various obstetric complications (*e.g.,* spontaneous abortion, fetal malformation, preeclampsia, and abruptio placentae), but more recent prospective investigations cast doubt on the existence of any such relationship. Fetal malformation may be an exception; drugs that impair folate metabolism (*e.g.,* methotrexate) have been found to be teratogenic, and several clinical trials have suggested that periconceptional supplementation with folate, either alone or in combination with other vitamins, has a beneficial effect in patients at high risk for fetal neural tube defects.

In view of the evidence suggesting that a woman's need for folate is substantially increased with pregnancy, some authorities advocate routine folate supplementation of all gravidas. The situation is not quite analogous to that with iron, since it is possible to meet the gestational needs for folate from diet alone. However, average dietary folate intake tends to be marginal, and losses of the active vitamin with cooking are substantial. If supplements are not given to all women, they should still be used in cases of chronic hemolytic anemia, multiple gestation, anticonvulsant drug therapy, and low intake that cannot be corrected by dietary means. The recommended level of supplementation is 400 μg per day, although supplemental preparations designed for use in pregnancy typically contain somewhat higher levels, such as 1 mg.

Anemia due to either iron or folate deficiency exerts surprisingly little recognizable effect on the offspring. Infants born to even severely anemic women typically have normal hemoglobin levels and storage indices, presumably reflecting the highly efficient parasitic nature of the fetus.

Calcium and Vitamin D

The additional calcium accumulated during pregnancy totals slightly less than 30 g, almost all of it in the fetus. Given that most of this accumulation occurs during the last 3 months or so of gestation, coincident with mineralization of the fetal skeleton, the daily increment averages 250 mg to 300 mg per day over the last trimester. Calcium absorption increases during gestation and urinary excretion tends to fall. The serum level of total calcium declines in parallel with the fall in serum albumin concentration.

The RDA for calcium in pregnancy is 1200 mg, an increase of 400 mg over the allowance for the nonpregnant adult. Because it is virtually impossible to reach this level with natural foods other than diary products, milk is considered by many physicians a highly desirable food for the pregnant woman. The 1200-mg daily allowance is contained in 1 quart of milk. Women who do not consume milk or milk products require calcium supplementation.

The essential roles of vitamin D in calcium metabolism are mediated by its active metabolite, 1,25-dihydroxycholecalciferol, levels of which increase substantially during pregnancy. Calcium absorption is facilitated by intestinal calcium-binding protein, promoting a positive calcium balance. Vitamin D also acts in conjunction with parathyroid hormone in regulating the dynamics of bone formation and resorption. The placenta transfers the intermediate metabolite 25-hydroxycholecalciferol to the fetus, where 1α-hydroxylation takes place in the fetal kidney and probably also in the placenta itself. For all of these reasons, the RDA for vitamin D is increased by 5 ng (200 IU) in the pregnant woman.

Some years ago, it was suggested that leg cramps in pregnant women might be associated with calcium–phosphorus metabolism. According to this theory, leg cramps result from transient hypocalcemia and can be prevented or relieved by any of several measures: curtailment of milk intake (since milk contains large quantities of phosphate as well as calcium), ingestion of nonphosphate salts of calcium, and ingestion of aluminum hydroxide antacids (to form insoluble aluminum phosphate salts in the gut). However, clinical trials testing these various modalities have yielded conflicting results, and the relationship between leg cramps and milk, calcium, or phosphate remains unclear.

In populations in which milk is not consumed after the age of weaning, pregnancy outcome seems not to be remarkably affected. Presumably needs for calcium during gestation are subsidized by maternal skeletal stores. Repeated pregnancies with only short intervals in between in patients with inadequate calcium–vitamin D status have been observed to diminish maternal bone density and, in extreme instances, to cause osteomalacia. Additionally, studies indicate a direct correlation between bone density in the newborn and maternal calcium intake during gestation, suggesting that the fetus may not be an effective parasite with respect to this mineral.

Certain drugs, notably heparin and phenytoin compounds, inhibit renal 1α-hydroxylation of vitamin D. When long-term treatment with these drugs is necessary in the pregnant woman, supplemental 1,25-dihydroxycholecalciferol may be advisable to prevent bone loss.

A possible association between maternal calcium–vitamin D status and early neonatal hypocalcemia is suggested by several observations. A seasonal incidence of this complication, with peak incidence when late pregnancy coincides with time of least sunlight, has been observed. Low serum calcium levels during the first 2 days of life have been associated with deficient maternal calcium and vitamin D status.

Evidence suggests that intake of calcium in pregnancy may play a role in preeclampsia. Epidemiologic data imply a potential relationship between deficient intake of the mineral and pathogenesis of the disease. This relationship requires further study, however.

Other Vitamins and Minerals

Water-Soluble Vitamins

Maternal blood levels of water-soluble vitamins generally decline during gestation, presumably reflecting expanded extracellular fluid volume, increased urinary excretion, and transfer of vitamins to the fetus. As a result, the proportion of gravidas exhibiting low or deficient values (as judged by standards for nonpregnant populations) is high, but whether this circumstance represents true deficiency states is uncertain. Vitamin supplementation generally has little if any effect on the falling blood levels, a relationship more suggestive of physiologic adjustment than of actual deficiency.

Placental transfer of water-soluble vitamins occurs against a concentration gradient, making fetal blood levels regularly higher than maternal blood levels. Maternal overdosage can thus potentially cause fetal toxicity, as will be discussed later.

The RDA for ascorbic acid (vitamin C) in pregnancy is 80 mg, an increase of 20 mg over the allowance for the nonpregnant adult woman. Association of vitamin C deficiency with premature rupture of the membranes has been suggested but remains unconfirmed.

Vitamin B_6 (pyridoxine) has been the subject of much speculation because of laboratory findings suggesting that deficiency is common in normal pregnancy. Blood levels of the vitamin regularly decline with gestation, and there is marked accumulation of xanthurenic acid, an intermediary compound catalyzed by pyridoxal phosphate to the next step in the metabolism of tryptophan to serotonin. These metabolic effects are thought to reflect estrogen-induced corticosteroid stimulation of tryptophan oxygenase activity, although the possibility that they reflect actual deficiency of the vitamin cannot be excluded. Current dietary allowances reflect this uncertainty; the RDA is 2 mg per day plus an additional 0.5 mg during gestation, although the latter amount is substantially below what would be necessary to "normalize" the biochemical findings in pregnancy.

Studies of blood and urinary thiamine levels and erythrocyte transkelolase activity all indicate an increased need for thiamine with gestation. Similarly, urinary thiamine excretion and results of the erythrocyte glutathione reductase activation test imply an increased need for riboflavin as well. Little is known about niacin requirements during pregnancy, but some increase seems likely, since ingestion of this vitamin correlates with energy intake. An increase in vitamin B_{12} intake is necessary to support augmented maternal erythropoiesis as well as to provide for fetal transfer. Blood levels and urinary excretion of pantothenic acid have been observed to decline in pregnant teenagers with "normal" intake levels, suggesting a need for supplementation.

Fat-Soluble Vitamins

Blood levels of vitamin A generally tend to increase in accordance with the hyperlipemic effect of pregnancy, with additional influences exerted by season, age, parity, and social class. To provide for increased maternal levels and for transfer to the fetus, the RDA is 200 retinol-equivalents (1000 IU) higher than normal during pregnancy. Placental permeability for vitamin A is limited, so that fetal levels of the vitamin are generally lower than maternal levels, but the potential still exists for toxicity with maternal overdosage, as summarized later.

Trace Elements

Trace elements are nutrients, usually minerals, that are consumed in small amounts and that serve essential roles as cofactors in various metabolic processes. The trace mineral that has received the greatest attention, particularly with respect to reproduction, is zinc. Zinc deficiency is teratogenic in several animal species and, as suggested by epidemiologic evidence, perhaps in humans as well. Zinc levels in amniotic fluid correlate with antimicrobial activity, suggesting that zinc plays a role in protecting against intrauterine infection. To meet the increased need associated with pregnancy, the RDA for zinc is increased from 15 mg to 20 mg.

Levels of zinc in both plasma and hair (the latter is probably a better index of nutritional status than the former) decline progressively with gestation. The fall may be ameliorated but is not prevented by zinc supplements. In some studies an inverse correlation between plasma zinc levels and iron levels has been noted, suggesting that iron supplementation may adversely influence zinc nutriture.

Iodine needs increase with gestation; the RDA goes from 150 μg to 175 μg. Goiter due to iodine deficiency used to be a relatively common occurrence, particularly in the "goiter belt" of the upper midwestern region of the United States. However, widespread iodization of salt has virtually eliminated this complication.

It has been suggested that supplemental fluoride during pregnancy protects against dental caries in the offspring. However, fluoride exerts its anticaries effect by replacing calcium in hydroxyapatite; the fact that the pre-eruptive tooth bud of the fetus contains only small amounts of calcium makes such protection unlikely.

Plasma copper levels increase consistently during pregnancy, presumably reflecting estrogen-induced ceruloplasmin synthesis. Whether this implies increased dietary need is unclear.

Sodium

Several gestational physiologic adjustments have implications with respect to maternal sodium balance. Glomerular filtration increases by as much as 50%, resulting in an additional filtered sodium load of at least 5000 mEq per day. This natriuretic effect is augmented by progesterone and posture. Compensatory mechanisms, notably activation of the renin–angiotensin–aldosterone system, are necessary to promote tubular reabsorption and preserve maternal homeostasis.

Ideas about sodium metabolism in pregnancy have changed markedly in recent years. The traditional view is that pregnant women have an insidious tendency to retain sodium, increasing vascular reactivity and predisposing to development of preeclampsia. An obvious implication of this hypothesis is that dietary salt should be restricted and diuretics used freely to promote excretion of sodium. A more modern theory, based on physiologic evidence that pregnancy resembles a chronic salt-losing state, holds that inadequate sodium intake in the face of excessive losses leads to hypovolemia and in turn to compensatory vasospasm. Which of these two views is correct cannot be stated with certainty, but no convincing rationale supports sodium restriction in normal gestation. The most resonable course seems to be to advise patients to neither restrict nor increase dietary sodium but rather to use salt to taste and rely on the physiologic functioning of the renal tubule to ensure proper sodium balance.

The evidence is considerably clearer with respect to agents that promote sodium excretion. Thiazide diuretics, in spite of early speculations to the contrary, are of no benefit in preventing preeclampsia. Maternal complications of these drugs include hypokalemia, hyperglycemia, hyperuricemia, and pancreatitis; in the fetus, hyponatremia and thrombocytopenia can occur. Since they do no good and may cause harm, diuretics should not be used by normal obstetric patients.

The foregoing considerations apply specifically in normal gestation. For patients with coincidental illnesses that would otherwise be treated by sodium restriction or administration of diuretics, proper management during pregnancy cannot be stated dogmatically. Perhaps the clearest case is that of cardiac disease with threat of congestive failure, in which sodium restriction and diuretics offer considerable potential benefit.

Alternative Dietary Practices

Vegetarianism

The term *vegetarianism* is used rather loosely to describe customs and practices ranging from little ingestion of red meat to total avoidance of all foods of animal origin. The two most common patterns are those of the lacto-ovo vegetarian (who avoids red meat, poultry, and fish but consumes milk products and eggs) and the vegan (who consumes no animal foods whatsoever).

The amount, type, and frequency of animal food consumption is important to determine, since it influences nutritional status with respect to several essential nutrients, the most evident of which is protein. Animal proteins (including milk and eggs) tend to be of higher biologic quality than proteins of vegetable origin, which generally lack one or another of the essential amino acids. It is of course possible to design an entirely satisfactory diet by using different vegetable proteins to complement one another with respect to amino acid composition, but some degree of knowledge and considerable motivation is required for such a diet to be successful.

A related problem derives from the generally low nutrient density of vegetarian diets. Chronically low energy intake will be reflected in low preconceptional weight and pregnancy weight gains. Additionally, any difficulties arising from protein quality will be exaggerated in inadequate energy intake.

Willingness to use vitamin–mineral supplements is of critical importance. Even women who eat meat, a righ source of iron, face problems with iron nutriture during pregnancy. These problems are magnified in the vegetarian gravida, for whom iron supplementation is therefore especially important. Flesh foods are also relatively high in zinc, and as their consumption decreases and that of cereals (which are rich in phytates and fiber) increases, zinc intake may become a problem.

The lacto-ovo vegetarian presents no particular nutritional problems during pregnancy, with the possible exceptions of those related to iron and zinc. The vegan, however, requires special nutritional support first during gestation and later during lactation. Among the nutrients requiring specific attention, in addition to those mentioned previously, are calcium, vitamin D, vitamin B_{12}, and riboflavin.

Pica

Pica refers to the compulsive ingestion of nonfood substances with little or no nutritive value. The practice most commonly involves clay (geophagia) or starch (amylophagia); other substances (ice, gravel, charcoal, and hair) are less frequently involved. Although it is probably most likely to be seen during pregnancy, this disorder is not specific to the gravid state. Pica seems to be particularly prevalent among blacks in the southern portion of the United States, where surveys indicate that as many as half or more of pregnant women consume starch or clay regularly. However, the practice is not limited to any specific geographic region, race, or culture.

The medical implications of pica are not well understood. In theory, it could result in the displacement of essential nutrients from the diet and, if the substance ingested provides calories (*e.g.,* starch), might lead to obesity as well. One possible negative effect is cation exchange interfering with mineral absorption; this mechanism would explain the finding in several studies of an association between pica and low hemoglobin levels. It has also been suggested that pica may be cured by iron administration, raising the possibility that the abnormal craving might itself be a manifestation of iron deficiency.

Physicians need to be aware that pica is not uncommon, especially among low-income black women of rural southern background. Few are willing to volunteer information on pica, so careful questioning is necessary to uncover the practice.

Megadose Nutrients

The term *megadose* refers to nutrient intakes of 10 or more times the RDA. Some individuals believe ingestion of large amounts of certain nutrients to have various types of health benefits. However, there is little scientific evidence to support such a practice; moreover, a distinct potential for toxicity exists.

At least three features of the maternal–fetal relationship could theoretically predispose to fetal toxicity with maternal ingestion of excessive levels of essential nutrients. First, it is a general rule of biology that susceptibility to damage is greater the earlier in development the noxious influence is applied. Second, the placental characteristic of transporting certain substances (*e.g.,* amino acids, water-soluble vitamins) from mother to fetus against a concentration gradient could result in fetal exposure to unusually high levels with maternal overdosage. Finally, the fetus possesses a limited capacity for excretion of potentially toxic compounds.

Vitamin A has been demonstrated to be teratogenic in a wide variety of animal species, and several anecdotal reports about humans have described nervous system and urinary tract malformations in infants whose mothers ingested 25,000 IU to 150,000 IU of the vitamin daily during early gestation. Large doses of vitamin D given to rabbits have produced hypercalcemia and cardiovascular lesions similar to those seen in the severe form of infantile hypercalcemia. However, treatment of hypoparathyroid pregnant women with 50,000 IU to 100,000 IU of vitamin D per day has not been associated with any neonatal abnormalities.

A suggestion that chronic overdosage of vitamin C (taken as prophylaxis against the common cold) during pregnancy might predispose to infantile scurvy comes from anecdotal reports in humans and from experiments in guinea pigs. It has also been suggested that excessive intake of vitamin B_6 during gestation might lead to a pyridoxine-dependency state in the offspring, although extensive observations in both humans and other animal species have failed to confirm a relationship.

Very high intake of iodides, ingested as expectorants in the treatment of asthma and other respiratory diseases, has led to congenital goiter in the offspring. Whether this may also occur with dietary iodine sources such as kelp tablets is unknown.

Summary

Pregnancy is characterized by increased needs for virtually all nutrients. Energy requirements increase by approximately 300 kcal per day, and a caloric intake sufficient to support a weight gain averaging 0.4 kg per week through the last two thirds of gestation should be maintained. Additional protein intake of 30 g per day, for a total allowance of 1.3 g per kg of body weight per day, is adequate to meet nutritional needs during pregnancy. Iron occupies a unique position among nutrients in that gestational iron needs cannot be met by dietary sources; supplementation with simple ferrous salts providing 30 mg to 60 mg of iron daily is recommended throughout the last half or two thirds of gestation and for two to three months postpartum. Folate supplements should be given in some circumstances, if not routinely. Supplementation with other vitamins and minerals, although widely practiced, is probably neither helpful nor harmful. Sodium is an essential nutrient, and there is no valid reason to restrict its intake in normal gestation. Certain alternative dietary practices, such as vegetarianism, pica, and ingestion of megadose nutrients, require careful assessment and attention.

LACTATION

Throughout nearly all of human existence, nutrition of the infant has depended entirely on breast milk from the mother. Beginning in the first half of the 20th century, the frequency of breastfeeding declined markedly, particularly in developed nations, as formulas for infant feeding were developed and widely popularized. This pervasive trend seems to have been reversed over the last decade, and current data indicate that half or more of newborn infants in the United States are fed, partially or completely, with human milk.

The return to breastfeeding is particularly prevalent among members of the upper social and educational strata, precisely the same classes that initiated the trend away from the practice two generations earlier. It is motivated by both physiologic and psychologic benefits known or presumed to accompany breast feeding.

As a general rule, milk volume and composition seem to be affected amazingly little by fairly wide variations in maternal nutritional status; only with severe deprivation are alterations in the gross indices of quantity and quality observed. Nevertheless, adequate nutritional support of the nursing mother is important for optimization of the lactation process for both her and her infant. In most instances it is possible to estimate maternal dietary needs from milk composition and volume.

Energy

Human milk has a caloric content of approximately 0.7 kcal/ml. Assuming an efficiency of conversion of dietary to milk energy of 80%, approximately 90 kcal are required for production of each 100 ml of milk produced. Thus, 850 ml of milk, a reasonable approximation of the average amount produced daily during established lactation, requires approximately 750 kcal.

The RDA for energy in the lactating woman is 500 kcal in addition to the basic allowance. The difference between this amount and the projected need of 750 kcal can be met by catabolism of maternal fat stores. An average of 3 kg of fat is stored during pregnancy, and this fat may be mobilized postpartum to provide an additional 250 kcal per day for 3 months. By the end of three months of lactation, it is likely that maternal fat stores will have been exhausted. Of course, these are generalizations that apply only to women whose preconceptional weight was within the normal range and whose pregnancy weight gain was at least 12 kg.

The amount and source of energy intake have some influence on milk composition. With caloric restriction, the fatty acid composition of human milk comes to resemble that of depot fat, presumably reflecting mobilization of fat stores. Increased energy intake in the form of carbohydrate results in higher content of lauric and myristic acids, whereas a diet high in polyunsaturated fats yields milk with a high level of polyunsaturated fats.

Protein

The protein content of human milk tends to decline during lactation. Assuming an average protein content of 1 g/dl, an efficiency of conversion of dietary to milk protein of 70%, and an average daily milk production of 850 ml, the amount of protein needed in the maternal diet would average 12 g per day. The RDA is 20 g, the difference being intended to provide for individual variation.

Neither the amount nor the type of protein in milk seems to be affected much by maternal protein ingestion. However, data suggest that the levels of certain essential amino acids are low in milk from women on protein-deficient diets, which may affect the nutritional quality of the milk produced.

Calcium

The calcium content of human milk averages 30 mg/dl. An average milk daily output of 850 ml would therefore require a calcium intake of approximately 250 mg per day. The RDA for calcium in the lactating woman is 1200 mg per day, an increase of 400 mg over the allowance for the nonpregnant, nonlactating individual. Considering humans' adaptive ability to increase absorption and decrease urinary excretion when needed, this allowance should provide an adequate amount unless milk production is extraordinarily high.

The calcium content of milk appears to be maintained quite well in spite of intakes substantially below the RDA, a phenomenon presumably related to the availability of a relatively large reservoir of calcium stored in the maternal skeleton. Studies using various methods of assessing bone density have suggested that lactating women mobilize approximately 2% of skeletal calcium over 100 days of nursing.

Vitamins

Levels of water-soluble vitamins in milk generally correlate closely with blood levels, which in turn reflect dietary intake. Thus, maternal diet influences milk composition with respect to these nutrients. Ingestion of large doses, as occurs with supplements, produces transient but significant elevations in milk levels. At the other extreme, deficiencies in maternal intake can result in deficiency states in the infant, as evidenced by reports of beriberi in infants nursed by women with the disease.

By contrast, levels of fat-soluble vitamins in milk are independent of blood levels and thus unrelated to dietary intake. Appreciable levels of vitamin A and E are found in human milk, but the vitamin D content is low, so that rickets has been observed occasionally in breastfed infants.

Other Nutrients

Concentrations of trace elements in human milk are generally low and unrelated to maternal intake. Iron supplementation is advised for all puerperal women, whether lactating or not, for replenishment of iron stores depleted during pregnancy. Iron saturation of lactoferrin seems to decrease the antimicrobial properties of this milk constituent *in vitro,* but clinical studies have not indicated any such adverse effect *in vivo* with maternal iron supplementation. Maternal iron administration does not influence milk levels of the mineral, so many pediatric nutritionists advise routine iron supplementation of the breastfed infant as well as for prevention of iron deficiency anemia later in infancy.

Fluoride levels in milk are unrelated to maternal intake; in order to provide protection against dental caries, some authorities advocate fluoride supplementation for infants consuming only breastmilk.

The sodium content of human milk is closely related to maternal sodium intake.

Summary

Whereas severe and chronic maternal malnutrition can adversely affect lactation performance, milk production seems to be maintained surprisingly well across a relatively wide range of maternal diets. Certain aspects of lactation, such as the quantity of milk produced and the protein and calcium content, appear to be relatively independent of maternal nutritional status, whereas others, such as amino acid, fatty acid, and water-soluble vitamin composition, vary with maternal intake.

Compared with the nonpregnant woman, the nursing mother requires substantially more energy, protein, and calcium, as well as somewhat higher amounts of most other nutrients. She should receive careful nutritional counseling, using the guidelines provided by the RDA. Maternal iron supplementation is advisable for two or three months postpartum; vitamin supplementation is also reasonable.

HORMONAL THERAPY

The nutritional and metabolic implications of treatment with sex steroid hormones are of considerable current interest, given the widespread use of oral contraceptives and the finding of biochemical effects suggesting an alteration in need for certain nutrients. However, almost all published observations related to oral contraceptives and the extent to which they apply to natural hormones, such as those used in estrogen treatment during and after menopause, is conjectural.

Vitamin B_6

Increased urinary xanthurenic acid excretion after ingestion of a test dose of tryptophan, the classic laboratory finding of vitamin B_6 deficiency, is observed fairly consistently in women taking oral contraceptives. This effect, which seems to be related to the estrogenic component of birth control pills, is similar to that seen in pregnant women but more marked in that the level of vitamin B_6 supplementation required for "normalization" is greater. For example, supplements of 30 mg pyridoxine hydrochloride (25 mg vitamin B_6) are necessary to consistently suppress xanthurenic acid excretion in oral contraceptive users, compared with 10 mg pyridoxine hydrochloride (8.3 mg vitamin B_6) in pregnant women. These values represent 12 times and 4 times, respectively, the RDA for vitamin B_6 in the non-pregnant adult woman.

The clinical significance of these metabolic changes is uncertain. Most of the concern currently focuses on a possible relationship with mental depression. It has been demonstrated that patients who become depressed while taking oral contraceptives have particularly marked derangements of vitamin B_6 metabolism and respond with symptomatic relief to supplemental vitamin B_6. Though routine pyridoxine supplementation for oral contraceptive users probably is not indicated, it seems reasonable to consider vitamin B_6 deficiency in the differential diagnosis of patients who become clinically depressed while taking synthetic sex steroid compounds. If appropriate laboratory studies confirm vitamin B_6 deficiency, supplementation with pyridoxine may prove beneficial.

Folate

Oral contraceptives are thought to interfere with absorption of polyglutamates, the principal food form of folate, and some (but not all) studies have found low values for serum or erythrocyte folate in oral contraceptive users. However, although folate-responsive megaloblastic anemia has been reported in several patients taking oral contraceptives, this has been an infrequent finding. Routine folate supplementation is probably not justified, but some attention to hematologic status in oral contraceptive users is warranted.

Other Nutrients

Several observations suggest that vitamin C needs may be higher in oral contraceptive users than in nonusers. Estrogen increases the rate of ascorbic acid metabolism, apparently by raising levels of ceruloplasmin, a known catalyst of ascorbic acid oxydation. In several studies, plasma, platelet, and leukocyte levels of ascorbic acid have been found to be lower than normal in patients taking oral contraceptives.

Low serum vitamin B_{12} levels have been found in approximately half of all women taking oral contraceptives. However, other tests of vitamin B_{12} status, such as the Shilling test and methylmalonate excretion, are typically normal. Therefore, the effect is believed to represent a lower level of binding protein rather than a true deficiency state. In any event, serum vitamin B_{12} levels in oral contraceptive users need to be interpreted with caution.

Biochemical findings suggest mild deficiencies of thiamine and riboflavin in oral contraceptive users. The significance of these observations is uncertain.

Serum iron levels and total iron-binding capacity are increased moderately in oral contraceptive users, effects apparently related to the progestational component of the contraceptives. The volume of menstrual bleeding is typically reduced with oral contraceptive treatment, suggesting that iron requirements may be lowered by contraceptive steroid usage. Absorption of iron, as well as that of copper and zinc, does not seem to be affected by hormonal contraceptives.

Summary

Synthetic sex steroid hormone administration is associated with biochemical changes suggesting altered need for several nutrients. Except for a possible relationship between vitamin B_6 and depression, the clinical significance of these laboratory findings is uncertain.

REFERENCES AND RECOMMENDED READING

Guidelines for Perinatal Care. Washington, DC, American Academy of Pediatrics and American College of Obstetricians and Gynecologists, 1983

Hambidge KM, Krebs NF, Jacobs MA et al: Zinc nutritional status during pregnancy: A longitudinal study. Am J Clin Nutr 37:429, 1983

Hemminki E, Stanfield B: Routine administration of iron and vitamins during pregnancy: Review of controlled clinical trials. Br J Obstet Gynaecol 85:404, 1978

Laurence KM, James N, Miller MH et al: Double blind, randomized, controlled trial of folate treatment before conception to prevent recurrence of neural tube defects. Br Med J 282:1509, 1981

Lindberg BS: Salt, diuretics and pregnancy. Gynecol Obstet Invest 10:145, 1979

Miranda R, Saravia NG, Ackerman R et al: Effect of maternal nutritional status on immunological substances in human colostrum and milk. Am J Clin Nutr 37:632, 1983

National Research Council: Alternative Dietary Practices and Nutritional Abuses in Pregnancy. Washington, DC, National Academy of Sciences, 1982

National Research Council: Laboratory Indices of Nutritional Status in Pregnancy. Washington, DC, National Academy of Sciences, 1978

National Research Council: Recommended Dietary Allowances, 9th ed. Washington, DC, National Academy of Sciences, 1980

Pitkin RM: Nutritional support in obstetrics and gynecology. Clin Obstet Gynecol 19:489, 1976

Pitkin RM: Calcium metabolism in pregnancy and the perinatal period: A review. Am J Obstet Gynecol 151:99, 1985

Prentice AM, Watkinson M, Whitehead RG et al: Prenatal dietary supplementation of African women and birth-weight. Lancet 1:489, 1983

Report to the Committee on Agriculture, Nutrition, and Forestry, United States Senate: WIC Evaluations Provide Some Favorable but No Conclusive Evidence on the Effects Expected for the Special Supplemental Program for Women, Infants and Children. Washington, DC, U.S. General Accounting Office, 1980

Rush D, Stein Z, Susser M: A randomized controlled trial of prenatal nutritional supplementation in New York City. Pediatrics 65:683, 1980

Soltan MH, Jenkins DM: Maternal and fetal plasma zinc concentration and fetal abnormality. Br J Obstet Gynaecol 89:56, 1982

Standards for Obstetric–Gynecologic Services, 5th ed. Washington, DC, American College of Obstetricians and Gynecologists, 1982

Stein Z, Susser M: The Dutch famine, 1944–1945, and the reproductive process. I. Effects on six indices at birth. Pediatr Res 9:70, 1975

Stein Z, Susser M: The Dutch famine, 1944–1945, and the reproductive process. II. Interrelations of caloric rations and six indices at birth. Pediatr Res 9:76, 1975

Stein Z, Susser M, Rush D: Prenatal nutrition and birth weight: Experiments and quasi-experiments in the past decade. J Reprod Med 21:287, 1978

Tavris DR, Read JA: Effect of maternal weight gain on fetal, infant, and childhood death and on cognitive development. Obstet Gynecol 60:689, 1982

Taylor DJ, Lind T: Haematological changes during normal pregnancy: Iron induced macrocytosis. Br J Obstet Gynaecol 83:760, 1976

Theuer RC: Effect of oral contraceptive agents on vitamins and mineral needs: A review. J Reprod Med 8:13, 1972

Thomas MR, Sneed SM, Wei C et al: The effects of vitamin C, vitamin B_6, vitamin B_{12}, folic acid, riboflavin, and thiamin on the breast milk and maternal status of well-nourished women at 6 months postpartum. Am J Clin Nutr 33:2151, 1980

Van Eijk HG, Kroos MJ, Hoogendoorn GA et al: Serum ferritin and iron stores during pregnancy. Clin Chim Acta 83:81, 1978

Varma TR: Maternal weight and weight gain in pregnancy and obstetric outcome. Int J Gynaecol Obstet 22:161, 1984

Zlatnik FJ: Dietary protein and human pregnancy performance. J Reprod Med 22:193, 1979

Zlatnik FJ, Burmeister LF: Dietary protein in pregnancy: Effect on anthropometric indices of the newborn infant. Am J Obstet Gynecol 146:199, 1983

Immunobiologic Aspects of Obstetrics and Gynecology

James R. Scott

12

The obstetrician is in a unique position to observe the only natural grafting of tissue from one person to another—pregnancy. Since tissue grafts exchanged between mother and infant following delivery are doomed to failure, the immunobiologic mechanism that allow the maternal–fetal parabiotic relationship to prosper for nine months are all the more intriguing. Nevertheless, interest in immunology developed relatively slowly in obstetrics and gynecology until the field was legitimized by the understanding, treatment, and finally the remarkably effective prophylaxis against Rh immunization (see Ch. 24). This disorder demonstrated to physicians for the first time that maternal–fetal immunology was of more than academic interest and suggested that other problems in obstetrics and gynecology should be studied from the immunologic standpoint. Although still in its infancy, reproductive immunology has now become a rapidly changing and expanding area of investigation and clinical application.

FUNDAMENTAL IMMUNOBIOLOGY

It is important to place the entire field of immunology in proper perspective. There has been a tendency to attribute all disorders of unknown cause to abnormal immunologic responses or mechanisms; however, it is doubtful that they are responsible. Moreover, thousands of new articles on immunology appear each month, and it is not possible for one individual to remain current on all new developments. Consequently, recent textbooks on basic immunology and immunologic diseases are usually the most practical reference sources for the nonimmunologist and busy clinician.[1,2]

The principal function of the host immune system is to maintain the body's integrity by repelling and destroying invaders or antigens of extrinsic origin. However, abnormal cells, foreign tissues, and organs vary in their ability to withstand rejection by a host with an intact immune system, depending on such properties as inherent antigenicity or, in the case of grafted tissue, the ability of the tissue to endure ischemia and the type of vascular and lymphatic anastomosis developed at the graft site. Even more important is the genetic relationship between donor and recipient; a major role of the immune system is to distinguish, in a biologic sense, "self" from "nonself." If the ability to distinguish self from nonself antigens is disturbed, autoimmune disease can result.

Autografts, in which the recipient receives a graft of his or her own tissue, and syngeneic grafts exchanged between monozygotic twins or members of inbred strains of animals survive indefinitely. Conversely, allografts, which are those exchanged between genetically dissimilar members of the same species, are ultimately rejected after a transient period of viability. The antigens of the human leukocyte antigen system (HLA antigens) are products of a gene complex located on the short arm of chromosome 6 and constitute the major histocompatibility system in humans (Fig. 12-1). These antigens, associated with certain diseases that appear to have immunologic overtones, are cell membrane–associated glycoproteins of 45,000 molecular weight expressed by all nucleated human cells (Table 12-1).

The characteristic cells of the immune system are derived from undifferentiated stem cells that originate in the fetal yolk sac, whence they migrate to the fetal thymus (T cells) or to bursa-equivalent structures (B cells). (The term *bursa-equivalent* takes its origin from the bursa of Fabricius, a primary lymphoid organ in the avian hind gut that mediates humoral immunity in birds. In the human, this term refers to such tissues as bone marrow, liver, spleen, Peyer's patches, and the pharyngeal tonsils.) After partial maturation in thymus or bursa-equivalent areas, the cells migrate to the secondary lymphatic structures, where they undergo further mat-

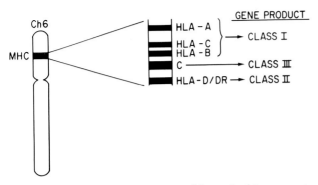

FIG. 12-1. Chromosomal location of the major histocompatibility complex (*MHC*). Within the complex are genes that encode as follows: for class-I antigens (HLA-A, HLA-B, and HLA-C); for several components of the complement cascade; and for class-II antigens (HLA-D/DR). (Scott JR, Rote NS (eds): Immunology in Obstetrics and Gynecology, p 35. Norwalk, CT, Appleton-Century-Crofts, 1985)

uration and differentiation when they are confronted by an antigen.

Normal Immune Reactions

Primary allograft rejection and elimination of foreign cells of any origin require three essential processes that occur in sequence and involve chiefly the lymphatic system (Fig. 12-2): (1) the action of the afferent limb, (2) central processing, and (3) the action of the efferent limb. In the *afferent limb,* the foreign antigens are identified by tissue macrophages, and some of the alien antigenic material is carried to the draining lymph nodes.

The antigen provokes a reactive response in the lymphoid organs, and clones of small lymphocytes divide and differentiate for certain specialized functions. Differentiation proceeds along two general lines, producing either "sensitized" lymphocytes (T cells) or plasma cells (B cells). This is central processing.

T cells are involved principally in *cellular response.* They represent roughly 60% to 80% of the lymphocytes in the peripheral blood and characteristically bind sheep red blood cells to form rosettes that can be seen by light microscopy and readily counted (Fig. 12-3). At least five categories of T cells, differing from one another both in function and in cell surface features, have been identified:

1. *Effector cells* are an immunologically specific population of lymphocytes activated and generated predominantly in regional lymph nodes. It is thought that effector cells may be the precursors of the other categories of T cells.
2. *Killer cells,* which destroy foreign cells by elaboration of a cytotoxin, are largely responsible for allograft rejection.

3. *Memory cells* provide the cellular basis for anamnestic ("remembered") responses, by which an antigen that was introduced in the past is quickly recognized if it is reintroduced.
4. *Suppressor cells* are regulatory cells that modify or suppress the formation of humoral antibody by B cells, thus modulating the humoral antibody response. This is one of the ways in which there is interdependence between B cells and T cells.
5. *Helper cells* promote the formation of antibody by enabling the B cells to respond to antigens that they would otherwise not recognize.

B cells are plasma cells that produce large amounts of surface immunoglobulins (Ig). These immunoglobulins circulate in the blood and other body fluids and can be detected with fluorescent anti-immunoglobulin serum. It is these cells that give rise to the *humoral antibody response.* Also, some B cells are specialized, having been modified by the action of helper T cells so that they can recognize a reintroduced antigen.

In the *efferent limb,* the specially committed small lymphocytes leave the node through the efferent lymphatics, where they migrate to and infiltrate the parenchyma of the foreign tissue or confront invading organisms; they initiate the mechanism of destruction

Table 12-1
Association of Specific Diseases and HLA Antigens in Caucasians

Disease*	HLA	Relative Risk (%)†
Ankylosing spondylitis	B27	87
Subacute thyroiditis	Bw35	14
Immunologic thrombocytopenic purpura	DR2	10
Sjogren's syndrome	Dw3	10
Insulin-dependent diabetes	DR3/DR4	33
Early onset	DR4	6
Late onset	DR3	3
Addison's disease	B8	4
Systemic lupus erythematosus	DR2	4
Grave's disease	Dw3	4
Myasthenia gravis	B8	3
	DR3	3
Rheumatoid arthritis—adult onset	DR4	3
Rheumatoid arthritis—juvenile	DR5	2
	DR8	2

* Many of these diseases are most frequently seen in women of reproductive age.

† Relative risk is calculated by:

$$\frac{\% \text{ of patients with specific HLA antigen} \times \% \text{ of controls without}}{\% \text{ of patients without specific antigen} \times \% \text{ of controls with}}$$

(After Scott JR, Rote NS (eds): Immunology in Obstetrics and Gynecology, p 43. Norwalk, CT, Appleton-Century-Crofts, 1985)

Afferent	Central	Efferent

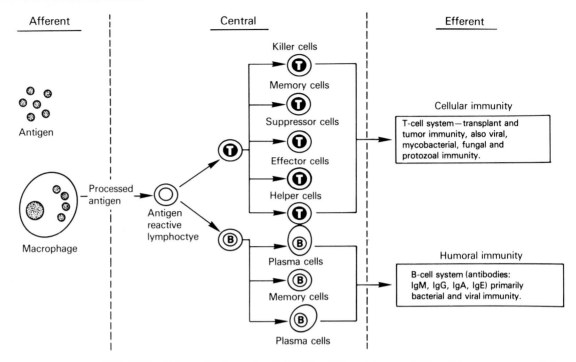

FIG. 12-2. Schematic view of cellular (T cells) and humoral (B cells) components of the immune system.

FIG. 12-3. Scanning electron micrograph of a rosette between a T lymphocyte and sheep erythrocytes. (Scott JR, Rote NS (eds): Immunology in Obstetrics and Gynecology, p 22. Norwalk, CT, Appleton-Century-Crofts, 1985)

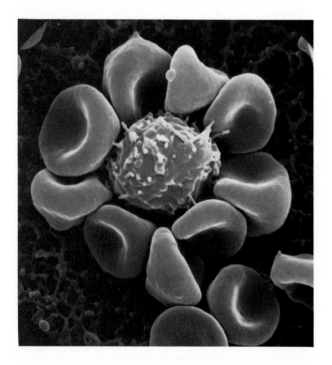

by direct binding with target cells, production of lymphotoxin, and secretion of soluble factors that activate macrophages and cause them to accumulate. The plasma cells, on the other hand, produce specific antibody that circulates through the bloodstream and destroys target cells, usually in concert with complement.

The primary humoral antibody response to an antigen in the adult is in the IgM fraction, which is soon superseded by a predominantly IgG response. Because the lymphoid system is capable of remembering its first contact with the antigen, a second exposure results in an accelerated and intensified anamnestic response. Antibodies themselves are heterogenous proteins composed of several different classes of immunoglobulins (Table 12-2). Four different subclasses of human IgG, each with slightly different properties, can be distinguished on the basis of differences in the heavy polypeptide chain of the Ig unit. In addition, human immunoglobulins carry highly specific labels, termed *allotypic markers,* that can be used to analyze the genetic control of immunoglobulin structure. Because antigens usually have multiple determinants, most humoral immune responses are polyclonal and contain a mixture of antibodies produced from multiple clones of lymphocytes. It is anticipated that one of the most significant advances in clinical and reproductive immunology will be the diagnostic and therapeutic uses of monoclonal antibodies, which can now be produced in hybridoma cell lines (Fig. 12-4).

Table 12-2
Comparison of Properties of Various Immunoglobulins

Immunoglobulin Class	Cross Placenta?	Molecular Weight	Primary Location	Serum Concentration (mg/dl)	Antibody Activity
IgG	Yes	146,000–165,000	Intravascular	1000–1500	Most antibodies to bacterial and viral infections; major part of secondary response; Rh isoagglutinins; lupus erythematosus factor
IgM	No	970,000	Intravascular	50–110	First antibody formed; ABO isoagglutinins; rheumatoid factor
IgA	No	160,000–385,000	Seromucous	170–300	Major antibodies of external secretions—milk, colostrum, saliva, and secretions of gastrointestinal, reproductive and respiratory tracts
IgD	No	184,000	Interstitial membrane–bound	0.3–40	Antibody activity rarely demonstrated; found on lymphocyte surfaces
IgE	No	190,000	Skin and epithelium	0.01–0.07	Reaginic antibodies

Immunologic Unresponsiveness

It is obvious that the human being has a very elaborate and efficient immune system. Nevertheless, tumors grow, allografts are accepted, patients die of infections, and immunologic attack on the fetus is apparently infrequent. These dichotomies indicate that the immune apparatus is capable of responses ranging from sensitization to complete tolerance; the specific response depends on such variables as the strength, dose, physical form, route of administration, and age of the host at the time of antigen exposure. At times, the humoral mechanism may obstruct cell-mediated destruction of allogeneic cells through the production of blocking antibodies or formation of antigen–antibody complexes. This mechanism of immunologic enhancement may involve (1) the afferent limb, if the antibody binds with the antigen and inhibits its antigenicity; (2) the central processing, if antibodies react with and inhibit the immunologically competent cells; or (3) the efferent limb, if antibodies coat target antigens and prevent interaction with the lymphoid cells. Host suppressor T cells and their factors can also undermine effective immune responses. These thymus-derived cells can inhibit antibody synthesis by B lymphocytes, exert a suppressive or restraining influence on mixed lymphocyte reactions, promote tumor cell proliferation, and establish unresponsiveness to certain antigens when adoptively transferred.

REPRODUCTIVE IMMUNOLOGY

Morphology of Lymphoid Tissue in the Female Genital Tract

There is a marked contrast between the highly organized lymphoid tissue in the gut and lung mucosa and the sparse lymphoid content in the much less studied female reproductive tract. The lymphatic drainage and main regional lymph nodes potentially involved in local and systemic immune responses in the human female genital tract are shown in Figure 12-5.

Although IgA and IgG immunoglobulins have been detected in vaginal secretions, it has been difficult to ascertain their origin. In view of the paucity of immunocompetent tissue in the vaginal epithelium and the constant contamination of the vagina by cervical secretions, it is likely that vaginal immunoglobulins are products of the cervix and endometrium. In cervical mucus, the ratios of IgA to IgG appear to be much higher than those observed in the serum, and variations in immunoglobulin levels have been demonstrated during the menstrual cycle. The concept of local synthesis of antibodies is supported by reports showing the presence of IgA and IgA-containing cells in cervical tissues.[3] IgA and IgG have also been found in the human endometrium during the proliferative, secretory, and decidual phases. The immunoglobulins are distributed in the stroma between the glands and along the basement

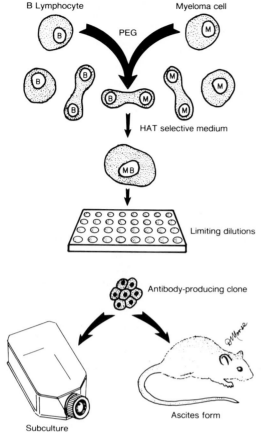

FIG. 12-4. Production, selection, and maintenance of hybridoma cell lines. Splenic B lymphocytes are fused with myeloma cells by polyethylene glycol (*PEG*). The cellular products potentially include unfused and autofused B lymphocytes and myeloma cells, as well as hybrid fusions of lymphocytes and myeloma cells. Unfused and autofused B lymphocytes die in tissue culture within a few days. Unfused and autofused myeloma cells, which would normally overgrow the culture, are selected against by their sensitivity to hypoxanthineaminopterin-thymidine (*HAT*) in the medium. Aminopterin provides a metabolic block in the synthesis of purine and pyrimidine bases. This block can be bypassed in normal cells by the incorporation and utilization of hypoxanthine and thymidine from the medium. The myeloma cell lines used in this procedure are mutants that cannot utilize exogenous hypoxanthine or thymidine and eventually die during tissue culturing. The surviving hybridoma cells are separated and cloned by limiting dilutions. Then the hybridomas can either be maintained in tissue culture or, because they are now tumerogenic, grow as an ascites in the peritoneal cavity of a mouse. (Scott JR, Rote NS (eds): Immunology in Obstetrics and Gynecology, p 34. Norwalk, CT, Appleton-Century-Crofts, 1985)

FIG. 12-5. Lymphatic drainage system and regional lymph nodes of female genital tract.

membrane of glandular epithelium. Although various tissues from the human genital tract are capable of *in vitro* synthesis of secretory immunoglobulins, IgG predominates in all endometrial specimens. Immunoglobulins in tubal fluid are also thought to be derived from serum.

Fetoplacental Antigenicity

The processes of fertilization and implantation constitute the two essential and specific acts of immunologic recognition between genetically dissimilar cells. The fertilized ovum undergoes fundamental changes in organization that render it potentially vulnerable to a maternal immune reaction, since minor and major transplantation antigens transiently appear on oocytes and early embryos.[4,5] There is evidence, however, that early embryonic tissue is functionally hypoantigenic: ectopic pregnancies in many different sites are normally successful for considerable periods, even in presensitized hosts, and small grafts of pure trophoblastic tissue obtained from ectoplacental cones are invulnerable to transplantation immune reactions.

Further evidence that trophoblast becomes an immunologically privileged tissue comes from studies on plasma membranes prepared from human placentas that

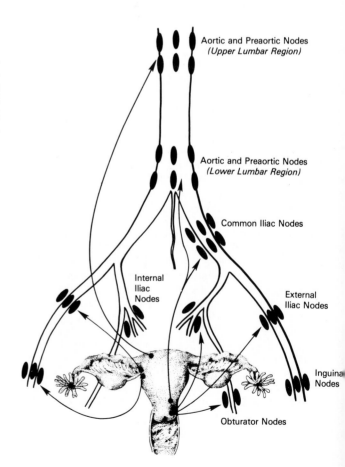

express very low levels of inherited HLA antigens. Investigations on mature human placentas have failed to reveal HLA-A, -B, or -C antigens, B2 microglobulins, or Ia antigens on the plasma membranes of syncytiotrophoblast.[5,6] By contrast, the mesenchymal cells and vascular endothelial cells within the chorionic villi do express HLA antigens. The once popular belief that a thick sialomucin glycocalyx associated with trophoblast plays an antigen-quarantining role has failed to withstand critical tests.[6,7]

It is essential to mention that, although antigenic peculiarities are associated with trophoblastic tissue, gestating mothers normally respond immunologically to the presence of allogeneic fetuses in their uteri, as evidenced by the production of circulating cytotoxic antibodies. Definite Rh antigens have been found on human embryonic red cells by the 38th day of life, the embryo possesses a number of iso- and autoantigens by at least 6 weeks, and fetal tissues implanted outside the uterus are rejected.[8]

Fetal Immunocompetence

During the second and third weeks of gestation in the human fetus, pluripotential yolk sac stem cells form the precursors of all the blood cell series.[9,10] The thymus develops at about 6 weeks' gestation, and lymphocyte differentiation proceeds in the complete absence of foreign antigens. Small lymphocytes appear in the peripheral blood at about 7 weeks and in connective tissue around lymphocyte plexuses by 8 weeks. Primary lymph node development and lymphopoeisis do not occur until at least 12 weeks, but as early as 13 weeks' gestation, T cells capable of responding to mitogens and recognizing histoincompatible cells begin to appear. In the spleen, lymphocyte aggregates form at 14 weeks, and by 20 weeks' gestation the human fetus can respond to congenital infections with the production of plasma cells and antibody.

The fetus generally enjoys a high degree of protection from infectious organisms in its isolated intrauterine environment and is not often called upon to demonstrate its immunologic capabilities, but immunologic maturation proceeds in preparation for exposure to a highly contaminated world. The transition of the fetus from immunologically incompetent to immunologically competent has a profound influence on disease processes. Immunologic immaturity and susceptibility of organizing fetal tissues are factors that make first-trimester congenital rubella infection such a severe teratogenic process as compared with the relatively benign adult disease. Conversely, an active fetal immune response can actually contribute to the pathologic process in certain situations. For example, the changes caused by *Treponema pallidum* after it has crossed the placenta and gained access to the fetus are probably not due to adverse effects of the organism on fetal cells but rather to widespread inflammatory responses. Thus, the infec-

tion may occur at a much earlier stage but follow a benign course until the fetal host develops the capacity to respond to the organism during the fifth month of gestation.

In contrast to the response in an adult, the dominant humoral antibody response in the fetus is the IgM immunoglobulin fraction. Indeed, the presence of circulating IgM of fetal origin in umbilical cord blood assists in the clinical diagnosis of such congenital infections as rubella, toxoplasmosis, syphilis, and cytomegalovirus. Since the large IgM molecule does not cross the placenta and immunoglobulins are not synthesized before antigenic stimulation, IgM is usually not detected in the fetal circulation or amniotic fluid in normal pregnancies. Conversely, the smaller IgG molecule, by virtue of its Fc fragment, is specifically selected for placental transfer (Fig. 12-6). Fetal IgG, usually about 10% of adult levels by the middle of the first trimester, gradually increases throughout pregnancy, and a significant number of newborns have IgG levels higher than those of the mother (Fig. 12-7).

Thus, adequate humoral immunity in the newborn period depends on the circulating maternal antibodies that have crossed the placenta. However, fetal blood levels of IgG tend to reflect maternal levels, and specific antibody protection in turn depends on the mother's own total antigenic experience. Moreover, maternal IgG

FIG. 12-6. The transport of maternal IgG across the trophoblast and into the fetal circulation is an active process. Maternal IgG binds to Fc receptors on the surface of the trophoblast and is internalized into vacuoles. These receptors are specific for the Fc portion of IgG and do not bind other classes of immunoglobulins. The interaction of IgG with the receptors probably protects the antibody from digestion during the transport of the vacuole across the cell. On the fetal side, IgG is released into the fetal circulation. (Scott JR, Rote NS (eds): Immunology in Obstetrics and Gynecology, p 70. Norwalk, CT, Appleton-Century-Crofts, 1985)

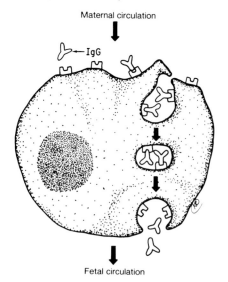

Maternal circulation

IgG

Fetal circulation

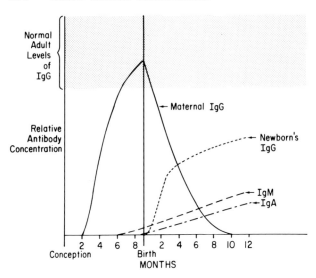

FIG. 12-7. Levels of antibody in the cord blood and neonatal circulation. Early in gestation, maternal IgG crosses the placenta and enters the fetal circulation. At the time of birth, the fetal circulation normally contains a near-adult level of IgG, which is almost exclusively maternal, and small amounts of fetal IgM and IgA. After delivery of the child, maternal IgG is rapidly catabolized while neonatal IgG production increases. (Scott JR, Rote NS (eds): Immunology in Obstetrics and Gynecology, p 69. Norwalk, CT, Appleton-Century-Crofts, 1985)

antibodies, in addition to their primary role of protecting the neonate from infections, can result in disease syndromes such as neonatal thrombocytopenia, hyperthyroidism, and erythroblastosis fetalis.

Maternal Immunologic Reactivity

It is at once apparent that the placenta implanted on the maternal endometrium is in many respects analogous to a skin graft (Fig. 12-8), but it is also clear that the fetoplacental unit does not behave like most other conventional allografts. Of the many theories that have been put forward over the years to account for survival of the conceptus,[11] none appears to explain it completely. The fetus and its placenta with self-protecting properties are not a vascularized intercommunicating graft and may not sensitize the host in the usual way, but the uterus is endowed with a vascular supply and lymphatic drainage system capable of eliciting classic transplantation immunity. Thus, most recent studies have focused on the possibility that maternal serum contains nonspecific or immunologically specific factors that protect the fetus from rejection.

During pregnancy there is increased production of adrenocortical steroid, ovarian, and placental hormones, as well as a temporary involution of some of the maternal lymphoid tissues. It is now generally agreed that placental protein hormones, fetal embryonic antigens, and

sex steroids in the maternal blood can at best provide only a weak ancillary protective mechanism for prevention of maternal alloimmunization. A more attractive hypothesis is that some of the hormones produced in high concentrations by the trophoblast may have a local immunosuppressive effect, preventing immunologically significant interactions between maternal lymphocytes and trophoblast. Although there is a wide variation in placental architecture and intimacy of encounter of the trophoblast with the uterus among different mammalian species, a common theme shared by all is progesterone production by the trophoblast during some portion of gestation. Recent studies support the concept that local suppression of the maternal cellular immune responses by high tissue concentrations of progesterone may contribute to acceptance of the conceptus.[6]

It has been shown *in vitro* that the maternal host can develop sensitized T cells capable of destroying embryonic cells, but the lymphocytes are prevented from interacting with the fetal cells by blocking antibody, excess antigen, or antigen–antibody complexes suggestive of immunologic enhancement.[6,12] In humans, IgG eluted from placentas has complement-dependent cytotoxic effects on lymphocytes that are capable of inhibiting mixed lymphocyte culture reactions and prolonging the survival of skin allografts. These antibodies may protect the conceptus by binding to receptors on

FIG. 12-8. Anatomic differences between a skin allograft and the placental allograft.

Skin allograft

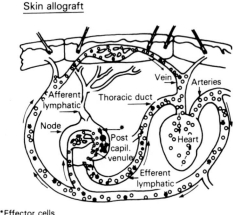

*Effector cells
°Small lymphocytes

Placenta

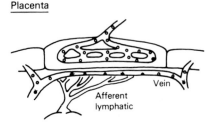

the trophoblast cells, but a relationship between the suppressor T-cell system and the success of the fetus as an allograft must also be considered. Several populations of suppressor cells are found in the circulation and in the decidua of pregnant animals.[13-15]

Even the stimulus for maternal unresponsiveness to fetoplacental antigens is not known. It is possible that the unique method by which "transplantation" antigens are presented to the host in pregnancy might determine the type of reaction they evoke. Spermatozoa phagocytosed in the reproductive tract could cause the initial stimulus. Moreover, in a fertilized ovum there is only a minute quantity of antigenic material foreign to the host, and exposure to those antigens is not only gradual as fetal tissue grows but is also extended over a long period of time. Trophoblasts are demonstrable in maternal circulation as early as 10 to 14 days after implantation; since the intravenous route is the most efficient way to induce either sensitization or tolerance, this could also be important in the production of maternal blocking factors or suppressor T cells.

In summary, the mechanisms that prevent rejection of the fetus are extremely complex, but the most important of them seem to be (1) decreased antigenicity of trophoblast at the maternal–fetal junction, (2) separate maternal and fetal circulations and lymphatic drainage systems, and (3) the maternal production of blocking factors or suppressor T cells.

POTENTIAL IMMUNOBIOLOGIC DISORDERS

Infertility

Approximately 15% of married couples in the United States have an infertility problem, and the standard infertility workup identifies the cause (*e.g.,* male, tubal, or hormonal abnormalities) in the vast majority of cases. It has often been stated that in about 15% of infertile couples no definite cause is found for the problem; the incidence is now probably less than 5%, however, because of the development of laparoscopy and more sophisticated methods of evaluation. Largely by the clinical process of exclusion, immunologic mechanisms have been suspected or implicated in these patients.

Theoretically, immunologic factors could operate at any stage in the human reproductive process, but there is little evidence that a host response to the ovum or maternal hormones, tissues, or secretions plays a significant role in infertility. If women commonly developed an immune response to gonadotropins or ovarian steroids, it is assumed that the ensuing menstrual abnormalities and anovulation would have more resistance to standard treatment regimens than usually occurs (see Ovarian Failure, page 875).

Through sexual activity, the female reproductive tract is repeatedly inoculated with millions of immunogenetically alien spermatozoa. Whole semen chemically and physiologically is a very complex material that contains a variety of antigens variously distributed in the sperm head, acrosome, tail, and seminal fluid. Introduction of spermatozoa directly into the uterine cavity of rodents elicits regional node hypertrophy, transplantation immune reaction, and a local hypersensitivity reaction.[16] Consequently, it is curious that allergic reactions occur so infrequently in women. After degradation, spermatozoa are presumably processed in a manner that involves the afferent, central, and efferent pathways, providing the basis for a local or systemic immune response on the part of the female host (Fig. 12-9).[17]

Many, but not all, workers have described varying degrees of reduced fertility in female animals following immunization with seminal or testicular material. Nevertheless, the relevance of many of these studies to the human situation can be questioned because adjuvants are virtually always necessary to produce this effect, and parenteral routes are used for injection.[18] Without the use of adjuvants, infertility is rarely produced in female animals by sensitization to male antigens. The establishment of an association between immune phenomena

FIG. 12-9. Elicitation and expression of systemic and local immune responses following local challenge of the reproductive tract of the female with a foreign antigen. (Beer AE, Neaves WB: Antigenic status of semen from the viewpoints of female and male. Fertil Steril 29:3, 1978)

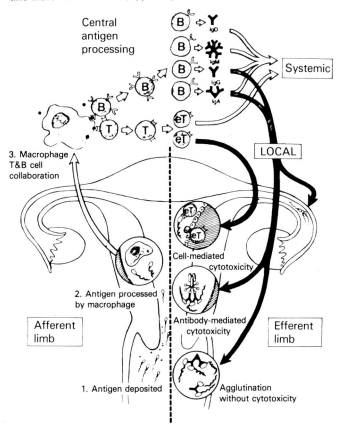

and infertility in humans has been hampered by the lack of definition of the antigen–antibody or cell-mediated immune systems involved and by the lack of standardization or refinement of techniques used for assessing the alleged immune reactions in infertile subjects.

By chance alone, about 20% of couples could be expected to be ABO incompatible; if erythrocyte antibodies were important in the etiology of this problem, these couples would be infertile. However, most studies on infertile married couples have failed to reveal any excess of ABO incompatible matings. Although blood typing of husband and wife is still being performed in some infertility evaluations, this practice is of doubtful value. Since HLA differences between husband and wife are the rule rather than the exception, it can safely be predicted that histoincompatibility must be an extremely rare cause of infertility.

There have been many attempts to measure serum antibody to sperm antigens, but the results have been inconclusive.[19,20] The controls have usually been pregnant patients because of their proved fertility, but the immunologic alterations that occur during gestation may make them less than optimum subjects. There are marked differences in the results, and only the sperm immobilization test seems to have no false-positives. Proponents of sperm antibody testing maintain that these discrepancies can be explained by flaws in technique, study design, or interpretation. However, it has been reported that the Franklin–Dukes method measures a lipoprotein–steroid conjugate rather than true antibody, which casts some doubt on the significance of follow-up pregnancy rates in couples studied only by this method. The other tests measure an IgG or IgM antibody, but which of the multiple antigens present in semen provokes the antibody response is not well understood. It is even possible that current sperm antibody tests may have no relationship to infertility but simply assay "nonspecific immunologic noise" from repeated exposure to sperm, somewhat analogous to the development of clinically insignificant HLA antibodies in many multiparous females. It has also been suggested that sperm antibodies as presently measured are simply cross-reacting antibodies to various bacteria commonly found in the vaginal flora and that they merely reflect exposure to these organisms.[20] Possibly women who do develop isoimmunity to spermatozoa may represent a genetically determined subgroup of individuals prone to the development of immunity to specific antigens.

Since the tissues and secretions of the female reproductive tract contain antibodies, antibody-forming cells, macrophages, and T lymphocytes, the possibility of local immunity at the site at which spermatozoa are deposited and processed is potentially more relevant than systemic immunity. This is supported by the poor correlation between serum sperm antibody levels and antibody activity in cervical mucus or postcoital tests. It should be noted, however, that the status of the postcoital test and its role in infertility investigations is in question, since sperm can be recovered from the peritoneal cavity in most patients with a negative or poor postcoital test. Unfortunately, studies to date on sperm antibodies in cervicovaginal secretions are no more revealing than those done on serum from infertile women. Moreover, the complement cascade components necessary for antibody-mediated sperm cytotoxicity are normally absent from cervical mucus, and semen itself has properties that are markedly inhibitory to the elicitation and expression of local immune responses.

Investigation of cell-mediated immunity has been relatively neglected in infertility problems, particularly in view of the fact that spermatozoa are cellular transplants analogous to those of a kidney graft or tumor cells. Although cell-mediated immunity of peripheral blood lymphocytes to sperm antigens correlates poorly with the presence of sperm antibodies, too few studies have been done to determine whether cell-mediated immunity has any association with infertility.

Immunologic causes of infertility remain speculative at the present time, and no consistently reliable diagnostic tests have yet emerged from numerous investigations. It is intriguing that the fertilization process is so successful in the vast majority of cases and that there is no evidence that fertility decreases with multiparity. Treatment modalities currently in use are nonspecific and of uncertain clinical value, and this will remain the case until evidence is collected that definitely implicates immune mechanisms as a cause of infertility.

Abortion

Since the immunologic mechanisms that allow a mother to tolerate her fetus are incompletely understood and alloantigens are only weakly expressed on preimplantation embryos, it is difficult to assess to what extent the failure of one of these factors might be responsible for spontaneous abortion. Despite the general resistance of fetuses to rejection, there are some indications from experimental animal studies that implantation and fetal survival can be influenced by the maternal immune response.[8,21] In exaggerated maternal–fetal incompatibility models, illustrated by the transfer of fertilized sheep ova into a goat uterus, implantation occurs but the gestation usually fails by the 60th day of pregnancy. The death of the embryo and associated infiltration of adjacent maternal tissues by lymphocytes have been interpreted as evidence for a local immunologic response by the mother that is initiated by organ-specific or species-specific antigens of the trophoblast. Further evidence for this concept has come from studies in which abortion has been artificially produced in rodents and primates by active or passive immunization against a variety of placental antigens.

It has been reported that women with recurrent abortions lack an immunologic "blocking factor" that is present in the sera of women who have had successful pregnancies (Chapter 21).[12] The blocking factor was shown to be an immunoglobulin, almost certainly IgG, and could be specific for antigens coded at the HLA-D locus, a gene exerting some control over immune response. Primigravidas were not tested, and it is possible that the presence of the blocking factor is the result rather than the cause of a successful pregnancy. Nevertheless, if blocking antibody is found to be important in the prevention of abortion, this would provide new therapuetic possibilities for women with recurrent pregnancy wastage.

An immunologic cause of intraspecies abortion is not shown in all studies. T- and B-cell levels, lymphocyte blast transformation, and response to mutogens are not altered in these patients. Several authors have disputed the evidence that either ABO or HLA incompatibility is relevant to the abortion problem.[8] The most recent information indicates that antigen incompatibility between the parents within the ABO, HLA, Rhesus, MN, S, Lewis, Kell, P, and Duffy systems is not of signficance. Indeed, one investigator has found that a higher percentage of couples with repeated abortion have common HLA antigens, suggesting an increased incidence of homozygotic fetuses in these cases. Animal studies also point toward a more successful pregnancy outcome in hybrid matings as compared with more compatible inbred matings, and successful pregnancies also follow the transfer of eggs of maximal immunogenetic disparity to foster mothers. These pregnancies proceed normally even when the foster mother has been presensitized with skin grafts from both the father and mother of the transferred ovum.[11] It is therefore difficult to attribute abortions exclusively to immunologic factors, since many studies have shown that the majority of such conceptuses are chromosomally abnormal.

Preeclampsia

Although the frequency and risks of preeclampsia have been reduced through modern obstetric care, the etiology of this disease, which occurs only in humans and only during gestation, is still poorly understood, thereby precluding specific treatment or effective prevention. An immunologic cause has long been suspected, but because of the broad clinical spectrum of hypertensive diseases of pregnancy, it is more likely that both immunogenetic and nonimmunologic factors are involved (see Chapter 26 for discussion).

SPECIFIC CLINICAL IMMUNOLOGIC PROBLEMS

Transplant Patients

More physicians are now being confronted with disorders encountered in allograft recipients. For example, over 50,000 kidney transplants have been performed, and the number is rapidly increasing (Fig. 12-10).

Disorders of the reproductive tract in nonpregnant transplant patients, although more frequent, have not attracted the same publicity nor received the same emphasis in the literature as have the pregnancies in female renal allograft recipients. These women may have any gynecologic disease that afflicts the general population, but a number of problems are specifically related to the immunosuppressive drugs they receive (Table 12-3). The physician caring for these patients is therefore wise to review the side-effects of the drugs to determine whether they can account for the symptoms the patients

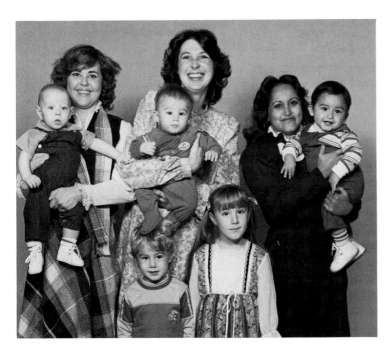

FIG. 12-10. Three women who have had successful pregnancies following renal transplantation pictured with their children. The patient in the middle recently delivered her fourth child. (Scott JR, Rote NS (eds): Immunology in Obstetrics and Gynecology, p 203. Norwalk, CT, Appleton-Century-Crofts, 1985)

Table 12-3

Properties of Immunosuppressive Agents Commonly Used in Renal Transplantation

	Prednisone	*Azathioprine (Imuran)*	*Cyclophosphamide (Cytoxan)*	*Cyclosporin A (Cyclosporine)*
Class	Corticosteroid	Purine antimetabolite	Alkylating agent	Fungal metabolite
Principal action	Anti-inflammatory	Decreases primary immune response	Decreases ongoing immune responses	Affects lymphocyte function
Maintenance dose per day	5–25 mg	75–150 mg	50–150 mg	6–8 mg per kg of body weight
Hazards				
Immunosuppression	Infection Neoplasia (?)	Infection Neoplasia	Infection Neoplasia	Neoplasia(?)
Other activities	Fluid and electrolyte disturbances, myopathy, osteoporosis, peptic ulcer, impaired wound healing, carbohydrate intolerance, cataracts, glaucoma, negative nitrogen balance	Bone marrow depression, mutagenesis, anorexia	Bone marrow depression, mutagenesis, teratogenesis, hemorrhagic cystitis, gonadal suppression, alopecia, anorexia	Nephrotoxicity, hepatotoxicity, hirsutism, CNS toxicity, gingival hyperplasia, hypertension
Idiosyncracy hypersensitivity	Pancreatitis	Drug fever, rash, myopathy, arthralgia pancreatitis, hepatic cholestasis or fibrosis	Inappropriate antidiuretic hormone secretion	Hemolytic anemia, thrombocytopenia

are experiencing or whether they will affect the management plan.

Menstrual abnormalities are common in women with chronic renal disease, and amenorrhea usually occurs when the serum creatinine rises to 5 mg to 10 mg/dl. Amenorrhea often persists during hemodialysis treatment, and the most common serum gonadotropin pattern is a normal concentration of follicle-stimulating hormone (FSH) and a moderately elevated level of luteinizing hormone (LH) similar to the tonic profile found in males and in females with polcystic ovarian disease.[22] More of a problem to the physican are women who develop dysfunctional uterine bleeding, specifically hypermenorrhea, while they undergo dialysis treatment and are markedly anemic. Although no hormonal regimens are completely successful, oral contraceptives or intramuscular medroxyprogesterone can be used to decrease the frequency and quantity of menstrual bleeding, produce therapuetic amenorrhea, and prevent hemorrhagic dysfunctional ovarian cysts, a troublesome syndrome in women taking anticoagulants and undergoing intermittent dialysis.[23] Following renal transplantation, resumption of ovulatory cycles and regular menses correlates relatively closely with level of renal function.[24] With less successful transplants, many women continue to have amenorrhea or irregular menses. Nevertheless, effective contraception is necessary in all women who have received a renal transplant.

The incidence of cancer in renal transplant patients taking immunosuppressive drugs is approximately 100 times greater than that observed in the general population in the same age range.[25] The most common gynecologic neoplasms in these patients have involved the cervix, and it has been estimated that the risk of intraepithelial cervical carcinoma is increased nearly 14-fold over that of the general population. Therefore, all women receiving immunosuppressive drugs should have regular pelvic examinations and Pap smears.

More than 500 women with renal allografts from living or cadaver donors (plus two liver allograft recipients and six women with bone marrow transplants) have now become pregnant.[26] Although the general tone in the literature is one of optimism, this is a high-risk situation that requires expert obstetric and pediatric care in addition to superior perinatal facilities. The 50% to 60% long-term graft survival rate makes the prognosis for these women somewhat guarded. It is likely that some transplant recipients may not live long enough to raise their children to adulthood and may leave their surviving spouses the problem of raising the children. There is unanimous agreement that a good graft is essential before pregnancy should be considered. For adequate assessment of renal function, the patient must be followed for at least one to two years after transplant. Pregnancy should probably not be attempted in any patient with serum creatinine above 2.0 mg/dl. Other medical problems such as diabetes mellitus, recurrent infections, or serious side-effects from the immunosuppressive drugs also make pregnancy inadvisable.

Early diagnosis of pregnancy is important so that

meticulous antepartum care can be given and an accurate date of delivery can be calculated, because intervention may be necessary should complications arise. The following prenatal care regimen is suggested for renal transplant patients:[27]

I. First antepartum visit
   A. Routine prenatal history
   B. Physical and pelvic examination: Establish estimated date of confinement and compatibility of uterine size with date of last menstrual period
   C. Record of weight
   D. Baseline laboratory values
      1. Urinalysis
      2. Urine culture
      3. Total protein (24-hour urine specimen)
      4. Creatinine clearance
      5. Complete blood count
      6. Blood type and Rh
      7. Test for venereal disease
      8. Serum Na, K, Cl, CO_2, blood urea nitrogen (BUN), creatinine, glucose, serum glutamic-oxaloacetic transaminase (SGOT), alkaline phosphatase, bilirubin
      9. Cervical cytology
II. Subsequent visits at least every 3 weeks until 28 weeks' gestation, then weekly
   A. General health and evaluation of any infections
   B. Weight, blood pressure, urinary protein, and glucose
   C. Fundal height and fetal heart tones
   D. Periodic creatinine clearance and urine culture
   E. Ultrasound for placental localization and biparietal diameter of fetal head in midtrimester; repeat for biparietal diameter at 32 and 36 weeks
   F. Cervical cultures for viruses at 28 weeks
   G. Repeat complete blood count, cervical cytology at 32 weeks
   H. Fetal maturity studies and hospitalization as necessary

Immediate hospitalization should be considered if any complications arise.

Normal pregnancy is associated with an elevated glomerular filtration rate (GFR), which is observed at about 8 to 10 weeks and persists until term. Very few transplant patients have shown even a moderate increase of the GFR; in most it has decreased during the third trimester, although this deficit has been reversible after delivery except in a few cases. Preeclampsia, preterm delivery, small-for-gestational-age infants, and premature ruptured membranes have been the most common obstetric complications in these women.[26] Figure 12-11 illustrates the week of delivery and the birth weight of the infants of mothers with renal allografts. Of 57 pregnancies that progressed to the third trimester, the percentage of preterm births (before the 37th week) was 35%. Excluding three sets of twins, 48 (89%) of the infants were below the 50th percentile for weight, and 26

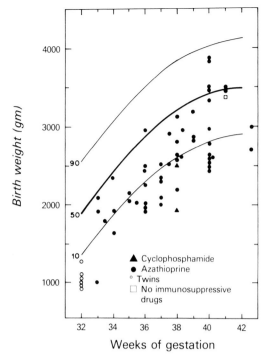

FIG. 12-11. Birth weight and week of gestation of infants born to mothers taking azathioprine or cyclophosphamide throughout pregnancy. All azathioprine-treated women were renal transplant patients, and the two mothers treated with cyclophosphamide had multiple myeloma and Hodgkin's disease, respectively.

(48%) below the 10th percentile were small for their gestational age. Although animal experiments suggest that immunosuppressive drugs decrease both placental and fetal weight,[26] it is not clear in humans whether the drugs or the underlying maternal disease is responsible for this phenomenon.

The position of the kidney in the pelvis is not usually a major obstacle to normal vaginal delivery, nor is the kidney damaged. If the fetal head is not engaged when labor begins, the possibility of soft tissue dystocia can be assessed by ultrasound. Indications for cesarean section must be studied on a case-by-case basis and the decision made primarily on the basis of obstetric factors.

Despite studies in animals showing anomalies in offspring secondary to ingestion of corticosteroids and azathioprine, no statistical increase in congenital anomalies in humans has been attributed to these agents. However, single cases of pulmonary artery stenosis, diaphragmatic hernia, and pyloric stenosis have occurred in infants delivered from mothers who took these drugs during pregnancy.[26] Chromosomal changes, adrenocortical suppression, and infection with hepatitis and cytomegalovirus have also been observed.[26] Since the incidence of infections and neoplasms is increased in association with primary immunologic deficiencies and administration of immunosuppressive drugs, it is imperative that any child exposed to these agents *in utero* have a careful evaluation of the immune system and long-term follow-up.

Autoimmune Diseases in Pregnancy

Autoimmunity is the process by which a humoral or cellular response is directed against a specific component of the host. Cells that are capable of recognizing self-antigens and producing an immune response seem to be present in all normal people, but they are actively regulated by a process involving antigen–antibody complexes or suppressor T cells. *Autoimmune diseases apparently result from a breakdown in this regulatory mechanism, leading to the inability to discriminate between self and nonself and the formation of endogenous antibodies, antigen–antibody complexes, or sensitized lymphocytes that react with the host's own cells or tissues.* Since these disorders have a predilection for women in their reproductive years, associations with gestation are not uncommon. Pregnancy may affect the disease process; in turn, some of the disorders adversely influence the course of pregnancy or are detrimental to the fetus (Table 12-4).

Systemic Lupus Erythematosus

A chronic multisystem inflammatory disease, systemic lupus erythematosus (SLE) is one of the most frequent serious disorders affecting women of child-bearing age. Despite the general impression that the disease is rare, more than 250,000 persons are known to have SLE, and an estimated 50,000 new cases are diagnosed each year. Although the etiology remains unknown, it has been established that the development of antibody to autologous DNA and other cell components leads to the deposition of antigen–antibody complexes and resultant inflammatory responses in target tissues. The frequency of SLE among identical twins and familial

aggregations, as well as abnormal distributions of HLA antigens in these patients, also strongly implicates genetic factors. With an increased awareness of the disease, more sophisticated diagnostic methods, and improved drug therapy, the outlook for these patients has greatly improved. The ten-year survival rate for SLE now appears to exceed 90%.[28]

CLINICAL CHARACTERISTICS. The disease is easily overlooked because it may begin with such mild symptoms as fatigue and is characterized by protean manifestations with periods of exacerbation and remission. In 1982 the American Rheumatism Association proposed a revised set of criteria for SLE to incorporate new immunologic knowledge and improve disease classification. Four or more of the following criteria are required for the diagnosis of SLE:

1. Malar rash
2. Discoid lupus
3. Photosensitivity
4. Arthritis
5. Antibody to DNA, Sm cells, or lupus erythematosus cells, or false-positive serologic test for syphilis
6. Proteinuria, 0.5 g per day, or cellular casts
7. Pleuritis and pericarditis
8. Oral ulcers
9. Psychosis or seizures
10. Hemolytic anemia, leukopenia, or thrombocytopenia
11. Abnormal antinuclear antibody titer

The most common clinical manifestations include arthralgia or arthritis (90%), dermatologic involvement (70%–80%), renal disease (46%), hematologic abnormalities (50%), and cardiovascular disease (30%–50%).[29]

SLE AND PREGNANCY. The cause of flares and remissions remains unknown, and in general, the clinical course of the disease is not adversely influenced by

Table 12-4
Autoantibodies in Pregnancy and Their Effect on the Fetus

Autoimmune Disorder	Cross Placenta	Fetal Effect	
		Clinical Manifestations	*Frequency*
Systemic lupus erythematosus	++++	Discoid lupus, anemia, neutropenia, thrombocytopenia, congenital heart block	+
Rheumatoid arthritis	0	None	—
Hyperthyroidism	+	Thyrotoxicosis	+
Myasthenia gravis	++	Weak cry, suckling, facial muscles; respiratory problems	++
Immunologic thrombocytopenic purpura	+++	Thrombocytopenia; petechiae; gastrointestinal, genitourinary, intracranial bleeding	+++

pregnancy. In the past, most maternal deaths occurred during the puerperium, but more recent studies show little or no increase in disease activity postpartum.[30,31] This may be related to greater experience with steroid therapy and a greater general awareness of SLE. Maternal complications correlate most closely with the activity of the disease and with cardiac or renal involvement. Diffuse proliferative lupus glomerulonephritis carries a risk of renal failure, hypertension, and superimposed preeclampsia. In fact, superimposed preeclampsia is sometimes difficult to differentiate clinically from a lupus flare.

Spontaneous abortion, preterm delivery, fetal growth retardation, and stillbirths are frequent in SLE patients. The lupus anticoagulant was first described in SLE patients and more recently has also been implicated in patients with recurrent abortion and fetal deaths.[32] This acquired immunoglobulin is detected by a prolonged activated partial thromboplastin time (APTT) and tissue thromboplastin inhibition test (TTI) and is associated with a paradoxic tendency toward thrombotic episodes. The decidua and placenta in affected pregnancies show progressive thrombosis and infarction, but delivery of live infants has been achieved by treatment throughout pregnancy with prednisone, 40 mg to 60 mg per day, and aspirin, 75 mg per day.[33] Corticosteroids theoretically suppress autoantibody synthesis and inhibit antigen–antibody interaction, and low-dose aspirin is used to restore the normal prostacyclin–thromboxane balance. However, even with this regimen careful surveillance is necessary, since severe fetal growth retardation, thrombocytopenia, and preeclampsia are common.

Fetal loss is also related to disease activity and renal status. A maternal serum creatinine level of greater than 1.5 mg/dl is associated with a 50% fetal loss rate,[30] and proteinuria and decreased creatinine clearance further increase pregnancy wastage to 80%.[34] However, in patients with SLE renal disease who are in remission before conception, the rate of successful live births is over 90%.[35]

MANAGEMENT OF PREGNANCY. Most patients should be counseled to postpone conception until at least one to two years after the diagnosis of SLE when the disease is in good control with low doses of corticosteroids. Diaphragm, condom, and sterilization are the preferred methods of fertility regulation. Although elective termination of pregnancy should be an option, induced abortions exert little if any positive influence on the subsequent clinical course.[36] There is little evidence that therapeutic abortion alone is "therapeutic" in a flare.[37]

The mainstay of therapy for active SLE is corticosteroids. An initial regimen of prednisone, 60 mg to 100 mg daily, induces remission in most patients. With a satisfactory response, the dosage can usually be gradually tapered over several weeks to 10 mg to 15 mg per day. Intravenous hydrocortisone, 100 mg every 8 hours

during labor and delivery, and continuation of adequate corticosteroid treatment during the first two months postpartum, are recommended to limit the chances of exacerbation. Dialysis,[34] plasmapheresis,[38] or azathioprine therapy may occasionally be needed in seriously ill patients, but cyclophosphamide should be avoided because of its significant teratogenicity in the human. In contrast, adverse fetal effects from maternal corticosteroid administration are rare. However, it is important that the relationship between corticosteroids (and other immunosuppressive drugs) and infection be appreciated, because infection is now a leading cause of death among SLE patients.[39]

Clinical precautions in pregnancies associated with SLE are similar to those required for other high-risk pregnancies. In addition to routine obstetric laboratory work, periodic urinalysis, serum creatinine, creatinine clearance, and total urinary protein assays are useful in the monitoring of renal status. Because a fall in complement levels may herald the onset of an exacerbation, a complement assay has been advocated by some as a useful indicator of disease activity.[36] Efforts should be made early in pregnancy to establish dates should intervention become necessary. Serial ultrasonography and antepartum and intrapartum fetal heart rate monitoring are useful in the diagnosis of fetal growth retardation and reduction of the risk of stillbirth. The route of delivery should be based on appropriate obstetric indications; SLE per se is not an indication for cesarean section.

SLE EFFECTS ON INFANTS. Antinuclear antibodies and SLE cells can be found in the blood of infants born to women with SLE. The maternal autoantibodies disappear after several weeks, and the infants are usually asymptomatic. The two most common manifestations of neonatal SLE are dermatologic and cardiac in nature. Neonatal lupus and discoid skin lesions are erythematous, scaly, and atrophic, usually involve the face and upper thorax, and disappear by 12 months of age.[40]

Cardiac involvement is usually in the form of a congenital complete heart block (CCHB). The mother may or may not have clinical evidence of SLE at the time of delivery of the affected child; 30% to 60% of mothers of children with CCHB show or will eventually show evidence of the disease.[40] Among infants with no other defects the mortality rate is low, but the condition is sometimes associated with other congenital heart defects and cardiomyopathies.

The pathologic changes in the conduction system of infants with CCHB include lack of a myocardial connection between the atrial conduction system and atrioventricular node, a node entrapped in excessive fibrous tissue, degeneration of the nodal structure, and lesions of the atrioventricular bundle.[41] Endomyocardial fibrosis or fibroelastosis has been the most common pathologic finding in children with CCHB whose mothers have SLE.

In recent years, autoantibodies to the Ro(SS-A)-La(SS-B) antigen system (tissue ribonucleoproteins) have been found in certain patients with SLE. Such antibodies cross the placenta and are associated with CCHB in infants.[42] Screening of all mothers with SLE for Ro and La may be justified, since presence of the antibody alerts the physician to the possibility of disease in the fetus. Furthermore, if the diagnosis of CCHB is established *in utero* and the fetus' condition not mistaken for fetal distress, a needless cesarean section can be avoided by careful fetal monitoring. Fetal echocardiographic monitoring may also alert the physician to the presence of associated congenital heart disease, as well as confirm the well-being of the fetus. A pacemaker can be made ready for early use should the infant be distressed.[44] Infants with CCHB who survive the neonatal period usually do well; the condition is a permanent but presumably nonprogressive insult.[45]

Because CCHB is relatively specific for maternal SLE and rare in infants born to normal women, a search for maternal SLE should be made if the disorder is found in an infant delivered from an asymptomatic woman. In some cases maternal SLE has become clinically evident only months or years after delivery of such an infant.[46]

Rheumatoid Arthritis

Rheumatoid arthritis is a chronic inflammatory process that can affect several organ systems but primarily involves synovia-lined joints, which become swollen and painful.[47] The following criteria must be met to establish the diagnosis of rheumatoid arthritis (seven criteria for classic rheumatoid arthritis, five criteria for definite rheumatoid arthritis, three criteria for probable rheumatoid arthritis, and two criteria for possible rheumatoid arthritis):

1. Morning stiffness
2. Pain, tenderness in at least one joint
3. Swelling of at least one joint
4. Swelling of at least one other joint
5. Symmetric joint swelling
6. Subcutaneous nodules
7. X-ray changes typical of rheumatoid arthritis
8. Positive test for rheumatoid factor
9. Poor mucin precipitate of synovial fluid
10. Characteristic histologic changes of synovium
11. Characteristic histologic changes of nodules

Fortunately, most cases are mild and require little or no medical treatment; in others, however, the disease is characterized by an intermittent course with ultimate progression over many years to typical joint deformities and the findings listed previously. Since the disease affects 1% of adults and exhibits a threefold female preponderance, rheumatoid arthritis is a common complication of pregnancy.

The signs and symptoms gradually improve in the majority of pregnant patients, which may be related to increased blood levels of free cortisol or to enhanced phagocytosis of immune complexes. The rheumatoid

factors (IgM antibodies against autologous IgG) do not cross the placenta, and there is no fetal or neonatal involvement.

Proper management of rheumatoid arthritis during pregnancy includes an appropriate balance of rest and exercise, heat and physical therapy, and salicylates, 3 g to 6 g per day as tolerated. Despite some concerns, such as mild hemostatic changes in the infant and an increase in the average length of gestation attributed to maternal ingestion of large doses, aspirin probably remains the safest and most useful anti-inflammatory drug in these patients. Systemic corticosteroids can reduce the inflammatory response, but because of the complications associated with chronic use, their place in rheumatoid arthritis is limited to acute situations in which other methods are ineffective.

Other Rheumatic (Collagen Vascular) Diseases

Disorders of undetermined etiology, characterized by inflammation of various tissues, have usually been termed *systemic rheumatic* or *collagen vascular diseases*. More recently, many have been classified as autoimmune disorders because of their association with the production of autoantibodies and other immunologic aberrations. This group includes mixed connective tissue disorder (MCTD), Sjogren's syndrome, polyarteritis nodosa, dermatomyositis, and scleroderma; their significance in pregnancy is similar to that of SLE. The risk of both maternal and perinatal death is particularly high in patients with polyarteritis nodosa and scleroderma.[48,49]

Hyperthyroidism

Although disorders of thyroid function are covered more completely in Chapters 7 and 30, it should be mentioned here that hyperthyroidism is unique among autoimmune diseases in that it frequently involves immunoglobulins that have biologic effects similar to those of thyrotropin. There is now considerable evidence implicating both cellular and humoral immunity in hyperthyroidism and Hashimoto's thyroiditis.[50] Both have familial associations, and many patients have demonstrable antibodies to a variety of thyroid antigens. This suggests that the two diseases are primarily due to genetic defects in immunologic surveillance, resulting in an inability to destroy or control a specific clone of lymphocytes that arises by random mutation.

Long-acting thyroid stimulator (LATS) and thyroid-stimulating antibody (TS Ab) are immunoglobulins frequently present in the sera of patients with autoimmune thyroid disease, and the transplacental passage of such immunoglobulins can have a significant impact on the fetus. It is now recognized that mothers who have thyrotoxicosis during pregnancy may give birth to infants who have manifestations of the disease. Likelihood of hyperthyroidism in the neonate can be predicted by antepartum observations of the fetal heart rate for tachycardia and by tests for circulating maternal thyroid-stimulating immunoglobulins. A reasonable approach is to obtain LATS and TS Ab levels in pregnant women with hyperthyroidism, to obtain serum thyroxine (T_4) and thyroid-stimulating hormone (TSH) levels from cord blood immediately after delivery, and on day 2 of life to follow infants carefully for signs of thyrotoxicosis.[51] The neonate with this condition is a jittery, underweight baby with tachycardia, tachypnea, goiter, and diarrhea. The duration of the neonatal disease is almost always less than three months, and most affected infants recover without incident.

MYASTHENIA GRAVIS. Myasthenia gravis is a chronic neuromuscular autoimmune disease characterized by fatigue and weakness, typically of the extraocular, facial, pharyngeal, and respiratory muscles. It is worsened by exertion and relieved by rest and anticholinesterase drugs. Antibodies to human acetylcholine receptors (AChR) are detectable in up to 90% of myasthenic patients.[52] The anti-AChR antibodies are involved in complement-dependent destruction of the postsynaptic membrane of the myoneural junction resulting in decreased nerve impulse transmission.[53] In addition, the disorder is often accompanied by a thymoma, thymic hyperplasia, or other autoimmune diseases. The functional abnormalities associated with the disease are similar to those induced by curare. The course during pregnancy is variable, although there is a tendency for relapse during the puerperium.

The cholinesterase inhibiters and their equivalent doses most commonly used to alleviate symptoms are (1) 0.5 mg intravenous neostigmine, (2) 1.5 mg subcutaneous neostigmine, (3) 15 mg oral neostigmine, (4) 60 mg oral pyridostigmine, and (5) 5 mg oral ambenonium. Drugs are adjusted to the dose at which the patient's muscle strength is optimal with a minimum of cholinergic side-effects. Excessive cholinergic medication results in unpleasant side-effects such as abdominal cramps, flatulence, diarrhea, nausea and vomiting, and excessive secretion of saliva and tears. Advanced effects include muscle weakness and respiratory failure, which can mimic myasthenic crises and may be fatal. Treatment with high-dose corticosteroids has also been used successfully in some patients. Regular rest periods with limited physical activity should be prescribed for the pregnant myasthenia gravis patient, and aggressive treatment of any infections is indicated, since infections appear to exacerbate the disorder. Some antibiotics, such as the aminoglycosides, may produce a myasthenic crisis and should be avoided.

Careful plans should be made for drug therapy during pregnancy, labor, delivery, and the postpartum period. Labor typically progresses normally or even more rapidly than usual, since smooth muscle is unaffected. Vaginal delivery is the rule; cesarean section is reserved for obstetric reasons. Assisted ventilation should be available in the event of respiratory difficulty. During labor, the patient's oral dose of anticholinesterase should be discontinued and replaced with an intramuscular equivalent. Myasthenic patients are often very sensitive to sedatives, analgesics, tranquilizers, and especially narcotics. Muscle relaxants should be avoided, if possible; local or regional anesthesia is preferable. It should also be noted that magnesium sulfate is contraindicated, since the drug diminishes the acetylcholine effect and has been known to induce a myasthenic crisis.

Approximately 12% to 20% of infants born to myasthenic women exhibit neonatal myasthenia, which lasts from a few hours to several days.[54] The manifestations are due to the transplacental transfer of acetylcholine-blocking factor. Interestingly, neonatal myasthenia may not occur in all infants of the same myasthenic patient. The classic features of neonatal myasthenia gravis differ from those seen in the adult form. Usually, the symptoms do not develop until the first or second day of life, probably because of some protection to the baby from the maternal blood levels of anticholinesterase agents. It is clinically important to recognize this phenomenon, since a baby who appears healthy at birth may later develop respiratory failure with asphyxia. The involved infant shows generalized muscular weakness and hypotonic limbs and is limp and motionless. The Moro reflex is often weak or absent, and there may be a feeble cry, inability to suck, and associated difficulty in swallowing and breathing. Arthrogryposis (joint contractures) which may develop as a result of reduced intrauterine movement, has been reported in several infants of myasthenic mothers.[54]

Immunologic Thrombocytopenia Purpura

The most common autoimmune hemolytic disorder encountered during pregnancy is thrombocytopenic purpura (ATP). Platelets form complexes with endogenous antiplatelet antibodies and are sequestered and destroyed in the reticuloendothelial system at a rate that exceeds the compensatory ability of the bone marrow. This results in the hemorrhagic consequences of abnormally low platelet levels in peripheral blood. The diagnosis is based on (1) a platelet count repeatedly less than 100,000/mm³ with or without megathrombocytes on the peripheral smear, (2) a bone marrow aspirate with normal or increased numbers of megakaryocytes that are otherwise normal, and (3) exclusion of other diseases or drugs associated with thrombocytopenia. Corticosteroids are the mainstay of drug therapy, but splenectomy is used for those patients who fail to respond to or develop serious complications from steroid therapy.

The overall course of ATP does not differ in pregnant and nonpregnant women. Gestation appears to exert little influence on the disease. The principal maternal risk is that of bleeding from lacerations of the birh canal, episiotomy, or cesarean section.

The most serious clinical problem regarding the obstetric management of these patients involves the transplacental passage of the maternal antiplatelet antibody, which results in a platelet count of less than 100,000/mm³ in approximately 50% of infants born to these women. Unfortunately, it is impossible to predict which baby will be thrombocytopenic, but those with low platelet counts often have clinical bleeding manifestations such as purpura, hematuria, melena, or intracranial bleeding (which is also the most common cause of perinatal death).

Largely because of the unpredictable nature of fetal thrombocytopenia and the suspected but not proven relationship between neonatal intracranial hemorrhage and the trauma of vaginal delivery, the optimum method of delivery for these women has become controversial.[50] If, as some authors have proposed, universal cesarean section is used to avoid trauma to the fetal head during vaginal delivery,[55] the operation will be performed unnecessarily in the 50% of cases in which the infant platelet count is normal. If, as others have suggested, the decision for cesarean section is based on a maternal platelet count less than 100,000/mm³,[56] a significant number of infants delivered abdominally will have normal platelet counts (Fig. 12-12). Despite reports to the contrary, we have not found the fetal platelet count to correlate closely enough with maternal platelet–associated IgG (PAIgG),[57] circulating antiplatelet antibody levels,[58] splenectomy,[59] or corticosteroid treatment[60] to justify use of these parameters to determine the safest route of delivery for an individual patient (Figs. 12-13 and 12-14). Moreover, unless there is a definite benefit to the infant in each case, cesarean section cannot be advised lightly in any patient with a coagulopathy because of the risk of maternal bleeding at the time of surgery.

FIG. 12-12. Relationship of maternal and infant platelet counts in pregnant patients with immunologic thrombocytopenic purpura from a series of patients managed at the University of Utah Medical Center and the University of Iowa Hospitals.

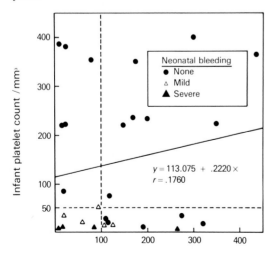

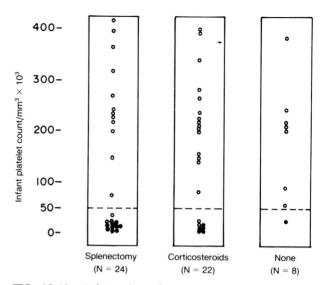

FIG. 12-13. Relationship of maternal treatment to infant platelet counts. Eight mothers had previously had a splenectomy and were also receiving corticosteroids. The *solid dots* represent infants who had purpura, petechiae, or symptomatic bleeding. (Scott JR, Rote NS, Cruikshank DP: Antiplatelet antibodies and platelet counts in pregnancies complicated by autoimmune thrombocytopenic purpura. Am J Obstet Gynecol 145:932, 1983)

In a retrospective review of the literature, it was found that no infant with a platelet count greater than 50,000/mm³ developed a significant bleeding problem.[62] Consequently, direct platelet counts from fetal scalp blood have been proposed as a method for determining the safety of vaginal delivery.[62,63] At the time of amniotomy for induction of labor or very early in labor, scalp blood is obtained in a manner similar to that used for scalp blood pH determinations. If the fetal platelet count is below 50,000/mm³, the infant is delivered by cesarean section; if it is above 50,000/mm³, the infant is delivered vaginally. In those few cases in which it is impossible to obtain a scalp sample because of an undilated cervix or a high presenting part, it may be necessary to perform a cesarean section. No abnormal bleeding has occurred from the puncture site in the scalp of thrombocytopenic infants when pressure has been carefully applied with a gauze sponge through two subsequent uterine contractions. This approach is considerably more accurate than a decision based on any other parameter, and it safely allows vaginal delivery in the majority of patients while sparing the thrombocytopenic fetus the possible hazards of vaginal birth. Regardless of the method of delivery, whole blood, platelets, and fresh-frozen plasma should be available for the mother, and a pediatrician or neonatologist should be present to provide prompt treatment for any hemorrhagic complications in the neonate.

Isoimmune thrombocytopenic purpura (IITP) should be suspected in thrombocytopenic infants of mothers with normal platelet counts. The disorder is

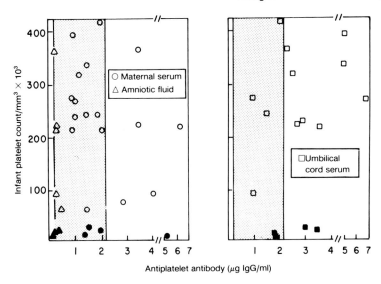

FIG. 12-14. Relationship of maternal serum, amniotic fluid, and umbilical cord serum antiplatelet antibody concentrations to infant platelet counts. Normal values are indicated by the *shaded areas;* the *solid symbols* represent infants who had purpura, petechiae, or symptomatic bleeding. (Scott JR, Rote NS, Cruikshank DP: Antiplatelet antibodies and platelet counts in pregnancies complicated by autoimmune thrombocytopenic purpura. Am J Obstet Gynecol 145:932, 1983)

the result of maternal isoimmunization by a platelet antigen (usually PlA1) that is lacking on her own platelets, similar to neonatal hemolytic diseases caused by maternal–fetal incompatibility.[61] In contrast to Rh immunization, IITP is seen about half the time in infants of primiparas not previously exposed to the sensitizing stimulus or to blood transfusions, and the diagnosis is not usually made until after delivery.[50] Future siblings of an infant with IITP have approximately a 75% chance of also having the disorder. Although the etiologies of IITP and ATP are different, the bleeding problems in affected infants are similar. Therefore, the same obstetric management, consisting of cesarean section or fetal scalp blood sampling for platelet counts, is indicated. However, in IITP, in contrast to ATP, platelet concentrate from the mother or another known PlA1-negative donor should be available for possible transfusion.

Tumor Immunology

Oncologists have long hoped for a screening test for cancer, a means to assess the patient's condition more precisely after definitive treatment, and an effective immunologic method for eradicating malignant tissue. Most investigations of the immunologic reaction against cancer cells have been based on the belief that some unique factor distinguishes a cancer cell from a normal cell and that this difference can be recognized by the body's immune system. Tumors induced in animals by chemical carcinogens generally have cell surface antigens (Fig. 12-15) that are specific for a given tumor, whereas viruses produce common antigens even when different organs or tissues are involved. In humans the occurrence of tumor-specific transplantation antigens is more difficult to establish because of histocompatibility differences between patients, but their existence is suggested by a number of studies.[64] The concept of immunologic surveillance attributes the evolution of

adaptive immunity and the host's ability to recognize nonself antigens to the need to detect cells with a malignant potential, which may arise as a result of somatic mutation. Such cells may then be eliminated by immunologic mechanisms. Escape mechanisms not yet understood and failure of the immune response on the part of the host undoubtedly play a role in the development of some human neoplasms. For example, in patients with immunodeficiency disorders and in transplant patients receiving immunosuppressive drugs, the incidence of cancer is markedly higher than normal.

FIG. 12-15. Tumor-specific antigens that appear on the surface of most and perhaps all cancer cells as a consequence of the malignant transformation. Like the transplantation antigens on both normal and cancer cells, the tumor-specific antigens are thought to be complexes of protein and carbohydrate that have been synthesized within the cell and inserted into the cell membrane. (Old LJ: Cancer immunology. Sci Am 236:64, 1977)

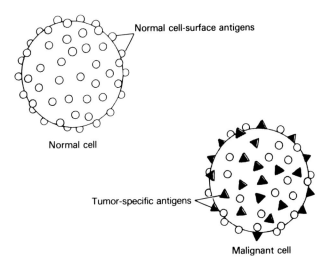

Immunodiagnosis

Because of the difficulty in early diagnosis and effective therapy of ovarian carcinoma once signs and symptoms occur, most investigations into the antigenicity of tumors and immunocompetence of the host have been in patients with this disease.[64] The detection of tumor-specific or tumor-associated antigens must fulfill several criteria to be clinically useful: (1) the antigens must pass from the tumor into body fluids, (2) they should be cancer-specific and, ideally, site- or tumor-specific, (3) they should decline in amount with successful therapy and rise again with recurrence, and (4) they must be readily measurable by routine methods.

None of the substances for which assays are currently available completely meets these criteria. Although the development of radioimmunoassay procedures provides a laboratory technique for the assessment of *carcinoembryonic antigen* and *α-fetoprotein,* neither is sufficiently specific for gynecologic neoplasms to be ideal as a routine screening procedure. A review of work to date, in which both heterologous antibody and human antibody have been used, suggests that the common epithelial ovarian tumors produce at least one surface-specific antigen. However, purification and characterization of the antigen are necessary before it can be used in radioimmunologic studies.

If the theoretic model of immunosurveillance in which cellular mechanisms destroy tumors is valid, then clinical recognition of a malignant tumor of the reproductive tract implies abrogation of the cell-mediated immunity of the host. Studies of response to multiple skin test antigens have shown that lack of immunity is associated with a poor prognosis. An unsolved dilemma is the demonstration of apparently normal cell-mediated immunity to specific tumor antigens in some patients with progressive tumors. Answers may come from more detailed examination of the components in the cellular immune response, particularly as new information becomes available about effector cells, suppressor cells, and the mechanisms involved with tumor kill and cell migration.

Immunotherapy

Although immunotherapy in gynecologic oncology is still in the experimental stage, enthusiasm for such a concept is based on the presumption that the immunologic attack could be directed specifically against the malignant cells without the attendant damage to normal tissues that is inherent to all other forms of cancer therapy.[65] The possible forms of immunotherapy are the following:

1. *Specific*
   a. *Active*—Inoculation with tumor cells, extracts, or chemically modified tumor antigens
   b. *Passive*—Administration of antitumor sera of allogeneic or xenogeneic origin
   c. *Adoptive*—The use of allogeneic or xenogeneic sensitized lymphocytes, immune RNA, transfer factor
2. *Nonspecific*
   a. *Active*—Nonspecific stimulation of immune responsiveness with bacille Calmette Guérin, (BCG), *Corynebacterium parvum,* or levamisole
   b. *Passive*—Employment of nonspecific serum factors such as properdin or interferon
   c. *Adoptive*—Transfer of normal lymphoid cells from allogeneic or xenogeneic donors or removal of blocking factors by plasmapheresis

Assessment of the value of immunotherapy is difficult, since in most instances it has been employed only in cases of advanced malignancy. It should be noted that a theoretic danger with immunotherapy is that it could produce immunologic enhancement, which could actually enhance tumor growth. A recent development is the concept of *immunochemotherapy,* whereby cytotoxic drugs are coupled with specific antitumor antibodies to direct the chemotherapeutic agent more precisely to tumor cells. At present it seems doubtful that immunotherapy is capable of producing a cure when there is a large volume of tumor in the host, but it may be able to stimulate the host's immune response to eliminate small numbers of malignant cells once the tumor mass has been reduced by conventional measures, such as surgery, radiation, or chemotherapy.

Choriocarcinoma

The unique importance of choriocarcinoma from an immunologic standpoint is that it links two apparent anomalies. The first is that many neoplasms have been demonstrated to have tumor-specific antigens and are therefore antigenically different from the rest of the host's tissues, but an effective immune response to them does not appear to occur in the host. The second is that malignant trophoblastic tissue of fetal origin derives half of its genetic material from the father and is therefore foreign to the mother, but it also escapes immune rejection. However, it seems somewhat pointless to argue that choriocarcinoma should be immunologically rejected when it is not known exactly why normal trophoblastic tissue is not rejected in the usual pregnancy. Patients with choriocarcinoma have not been reported to have impaired responses to other antigens, and the development of this tumor can be attributed to a maternal immunologic failure only with caution. Nevertheless, complete cure with chemotherapy and the association of choriocarcinoma with occasional spontaneous regression has suggested that the host's immune mechanism might be involved.[66]

Since choriocarcinoma is abnormal placental tissue, at least partially paternal in origin, it must possess tissue antigens similar to those of other allografts. Direct evidence of HLA antigens on choriocarcinoma cells is at present restricted to one reported case, but HLA antibodies against the antigens present on the paternal lymphocytes have been found in women with persistent trophoblastic disease following a first pregnancy with a hydatidiform mole. Choriocarcinoma also appears to contain a tumor-associated antigen that is missing from normal placental tissue, as demonstrated by immunoelectrophoresis, immunodiffusion, and a cytotoxic effect of the antiserum on choriocarcinoma cells cultured *in vitro.*

The hypothesis that progressive tumor growth is dependent on tumor–host histocompatibility has been substantiated by some studies but not confirmed by others.[67] Recent large series of patients have shown no association of HLA or ABO compatibility with the occurrence of gestational trophoblastic neoplasia. About 2% sharing of paternal haplotypes is estimated for a random mating of Caucasians. This represents a 1:50 incidence of compatibility, yet the incidence of trophoblastic neoplasia is 1:12 to 1:40,000. Recent investigations, however, have correlated the morbidity of trophoblastic disease with maternal antibody to particular HLA phenotypes.

To date, reports of immunotherapy in patients with advanced trophoblastic disease that is resistant to multiple drug therapy reveal only transient successes in small numbers of patients.[67] Paternal lymphocytes, paternal skin grafts, and the use of nonspecific stimulants of cell-mediated immunity such as *C. parvum* and BCG have produced variable results. Nevertheless, it seems possible that a potent heterologous antiserum directed against tissue-specific antigens and trophoblast- or tumor-specific antigens in malignant trophoblastic tissue might eventually be developed.

Maternal Neoplasms and the Fetus

Immunologic competence is greatest during young adulthood when neoplasms are uncommon; as immunologic competence decreases with age, the incidence of cancer increases. Nevertheless, the incidence of malignancy in the 25 to 35 age group is approximately 0.06%, and this is not altered by pregnancy. Gestation does not change the five-year survival rates of women with leukemia, Hodgkin's disease, and various solid tumors, even when the malignancy is one that is frequently affected by the endocrine milieu, such as carcinoma of the breast.

Relatively little attention has been focused on the possibility of fetal–placental metastasis in pregnant women with common types of malignancies because it has never become a clinical problem. For example, carcinoma of the cervix occurs once in every 2000 to 6000 pregnancies, but there has never been a verified report of placental or fetal invasion by this tumor. Although leukemia and Hodgkin's disease are not uncommon in women of reproductive age and as many as 1 in every 35 patients with carcinoma of the breast is pregnant, transmission of these malignancies to the fetus is also exceedingly rare. This is particularly surprising in the case of hematologic malignancies in which there are relatively large numbers of malignant stem cells in the maternal bloodstream. There is a possibility that diseases such as leukemia are oncogenic viral diseases and that the virus is occasionally transmitted early in fetal life.

Although the spread of cancer to the placenta is unusual, it can occur, as illustrated by cases, listed in Table 12-5, in which the placenta and fetus were studied in detail.[8] It is apparent that the representation of melanoma is out of proportion to its incidence, but the reason for this phenomenon is unknown. Careful histologic observation in pregnant women with malignancies has shown that tumor cells may be present in the intervillous spaces, but only rarely is there invasion of the villi. Moreover, in the extremely unusual instances of congenital neoplasia such as neuroblastoma, melanoma, or leukemia, the tumor does not spread from the fetus to the mother. The placental villus thus appears to be an effective barrier to the spread of tumor cells from the maternal to the fetal circulation, as well as in the opposite direction. Once malignant tumor cells enter the fetal bloodstream, however, they can be disseminated throughout the entire fetus and are usually sequestered in the liver.

Since fetal and maternal tissues are genetically dissimilar, maternal–fetal metastasis can logically be considered an allograft or the transplantation of foreign cells. The rare cases of fetal dissemination of maternal malignant disease may be isolated examples of acquired tolerance in which fetuses were exposed to maternal antigen before the development of immunologic competency and as a result did not recognize the maternal tumor cells as foreign. Conversely, those cases in which maternal malignant melanoma has widely metastasized to the fetus and then regressed spontaneously after birth

Table 12-5

Reported Cases of Metastasis of Neoplastic Disease to Placenta or Fetus

Malignancy	Total Number	Placental Metastasis	Fetal Metastasis
Malignant melanoma	15	9	6
Hepatic carcinoma	2	1	1
Sarcoma	2	1	1
Leukemia	7	5	2
Hodgkin's disease	1	0	1
Bronchial carcinoma	3	3	0
Breast carcinoma	6	6	0
Gastric carcinoma	2	2	0
Pancreatic carcinoma	1	1	0
Ethmoid carcinoma	1	1	0
Adrenal carcinoma	1	1	0
Ovarian carcinoma	1	1	0
Totals	40	31	11

are probably examples of true allograft rejection. This phenomenon could also explain what may be under-diagnosed cases of placental transmission of other maternal malignant diseases, particularly during the latter half of pregnancy, after the establishment of fetal immunocompetence.

REFERENCES

1. Sampter M (ed): Immunological Diseases, 3rd ed. Boston, Little, Brown, 1978
2. Lachman PJ, Peters DK (eds): Clinical Aspects of Immunology, 4th ed. Boston, Blackwell Scientific Publishers, 1982
3. Vaerman JP, Ferin J: Local immunological response in the vagina, cervix and endometrium. Acta Endocrinol (Suppl) 194:281, 1973
4. Heyner S: Alloantigen expression on mouse oocytes and early embryos. In Wegman TS, Gill TJ (eds): Immunology of Reproduction, p 77. New York, Oxford University Press, 1983
5. Faulk WP, Saunderson AR, Temple A: Distribution of MHC antigens in human placental villi. Transplant Proc 9:1379, 1977
6. Billingham RE: Immunobiology of the maternal–fetal relationship. In Gleicher N (ed): Reproductive Immunology, p 63. New York, Alan R Liss, 1981
7. Gill TJ, Repetti CF: Immunological and genetic factors influencing reproduction. Am J Pathol 95:465, 1979
8. Scott JR: Reproductive immunology. In Wynn RM (ed): Obstetrics and Gynecology Annual, p 101. New York, Appleton-Century-Crofts, 1974
9. Siegel I, Gleicher N: Development of the fetal immune system. In Gleicher N (ed): Reproductive Immunology, p 31. New York, Alan R Liss, 1981
10. Rote NS: Maternal–fetal immunology. In Scott JR, Rote NS (eds): Immunology in Obstetrics and Gynecology, p 55. Norwalk, CT, Appleton-Century-Crofts, 1985
11. Beer AE, Billingham RE (eds): The Immunobiology of Mammalian Reproduction. Englewood Cliffs, NJ, Prentice Hall, 1976
12. Rocklin RE, Kitzmiller JL, Carpenter CB et al: Maternal–fetal relation: Absence of an immunologic blocking factor from the serum of women with chronic abortions. N Engl J Med 295:1209, 1976
13. Chaouat G, Voisin GA: Regulatory T cell subpopulations in pregnancy. I. Evidence for suppressive activity of the early phase of MLR. J Immunol 122:1393, 1979
14. Clark DA, McDermott MR: Impairment of host vs graft reactions in lymph nodes draining the uterus. J Immunol 121:1389, 1978
15. Slapsys R, Clark DA: Active suppression of host-versus-graft reaction in pregnant mice. V. Kinetics, specificity, and *in vivo* activity of non–T suppressor cells localized to the genital tract of mice during first pregnancy. Am J Reprod Immunol 3:65, 1983
16. Beer AE, Billingham RE: Host responses to intra-uterine tissue, cellular and fetal allografts. J Reprod Fertil (Suppl) 2:59, 1974
17. Urry RL, Caudle MR, Rote NS: Autoimmune infertility and recurrent abortion. In Scott JR, Rote NS (eds): Immunology in Obstetrics and Gynecology, p 77. Norwalk, CT, Appleton-Century-Crofts, 1985
18. Lande IJ, Scott JR: Immunology and the infertile female. Curr Probl Obstet Gynecol 1(4):3, 1977
19. Jones WR: Immunological aspects of infertility. In Scott JS, Jones WR (eds): Immunology of Human Reproduction, p 375. London, Academic Press, 1976
20. Beer AE, Neaves WB: Antigenic status of semen from the viewpoints of female and male. Fertil Steril 29:3, 1978
21. Clark DA, Slapsys R, Croy A et al: Regulation of cytotoxic T cells in pregnant mice. In Wegman TG, Gill TJ (eds): Immunology of Reproduction, p 341. New York, Oxford University Press, 1983
22. Strickler RC, Woolever Ca, Johnson M et al: Serum gonadotrophin patterns in patients with chronic renal failure of hemodialysis. Gynecol Invest 5:185, 1974
23. Thaysen JH, Olgaard K, Jensen HG: Ovarian cysts in women on chronic intermittent hemodialysis. Acta Med Scand 197:433, 1975
24. Merkatz IR, Schwartz GH, David DS et al: Resumption of female reproductive function following renal transplantation. JAMA 216:1749, 1971
25. Penn I: The incidence of malignancies in transplant recipients. Transplant Proc 7:323, 1975
26. Scott JR: Transplantation in obstetrics and gynecology. In Scott JR, Rote NS (eds): Immunology in Obstetrics and Gynecology, p 197. Norwalk, CT, Appleton-Century-Crofts, 1985
27. Scott JR: Gynecologic and obstetric problems in renal allograft recipients. In Buchsbaum HM, Schmidt J (eds): Gynecologic and Obstetric Urology, 2nd ed, p 547. Philadelphia, WB Saunders, 1982
28. Schur PH: Clinical Management of Systemic Lupus Erythematosus, p 7. New York, Grune & Stratton, 1983
29. Budman DR, Steinberg AD: Hematologic aspects of systemic lupus erythematosus. Ann Intern Med 86:220, 1977
30. Syrop CH, Varner MW: Systemic lupus erythematosus and pregnancy. Clin Obstet Gynecol 26:547, 1983
31. Gimovsky ML, Montoro M, Paul RH: Pregnancy outcome in women with systemic lupus erythematosus. Obstet Gynecol 63:686, 1984
32. Carreras LO, Vermylen J, Spitz B et al: Lupus anticoagulant and inhibition of prostacylcin formation in patients with repeated abortion, intrauterine growth retardation and intrauterine death. Br J Obstet Gynaecol 88:890, 1981
33. Lubbe WF, Butler WS, Palmer SJ et al: Fetal survival after prednisone suppression of maternal lupus-anticoagulant. Lancet 1:1361, 1983
34. Fine LC, Barnett EV, Danovitch GM et al: Systemic lupus erythematosus in pregnancy. Ann Intern Med 94:667, 1981
35. Hayslett JP, Lynn RI: Effect of pregnancy in patients with lupus nephropathy. Kidney Int 18:207, 1980
36. Devoe L, Taylor RL: Systemic lupus erythematosus in pregnancy. Am J Obstet Gynecol 135:473, 1979
37. Zuluran JI, Talal N, Hoffman GS et al: Problems associated with the management of pregnancies in patients with systemic lupus erythematosus. J Rheumatol 7:37, 1980
38. Hubbard HC, Portney B: Systemic lupus erythematosus in pregnancy treated with plasmapheresis. Br J Dermatol 101:87, 1979
39. Dubois EL, Wierychowiecki M, Cox MB et al: Duration and death in systemic erythematosus—An analysis of 249 cases. JAMA 227:1399, 1974
40. Draynini TH, Esterly NB, Fureu N et al: Neonatal lupus erythematosus. J Am Acad Dermatol 1:437, 1983
41. Vetter VL, Rashkind WJ: Congenital complete heart block and connective tissue disease. N Engl J Med 309:237, 1983

42. Scott JS, Maddison PJ, Taylor PV et al: Connective-tissue disease, antibodies to ribonucleoprotein, and congenital heart block. N Engl J Med 309:209, 1983

43. Scott JS: Systemic lupus erythematosus and allied disorders in pregnancy. Clin Obstet Gynecol 6:461, 1979

44. McCue C, Mantakas M, Tingelstad JB: Congenital heart block in newborns of mothers with connective tissue diseases. Circulation 56:82, 1977

45. Garsenstein M, Pollak V, Karls R: Systemic lupus erythematosus and pregnancy. N Engl J Med 165:267, 1962

46. Reid RL, Panchaw SR, Kean WF et al: Maternal and neonatal implications of congenital complete heart blocks in the fetus. Obstet Gynecol 54:470, 1979

47. Thurnau GR: Rheumatoid arthritis. Clin Obstet Gynecol 26:558, 1983

48. Pitkin RM: Polyarteritis nodosa. Clin Obstet Gynecol 26:579, 1983

49. Goplerud CP: Scleroderma. Clin Obstet Gynecol 26:587, 1983

50. Scott JR: Immunologic diseases in pregnancy. In Scott JR, Rote NS (eds): Immunology in Obstetrics and Gynecology, p 165. Norwalk, CT, Appleton-Century-Crofts, 1985

51. Hollingsworth DR: Graves disease. Clin Obstet Gynecol 26:615, 1983

52. Lindstrom J: An assay for antibodies to human AChR in serum from patients with myasthenia gravis. Clin Immunol Immunopathol 7:36, 1977

53. Newsom-Davis J, Vincent A: Myasthenia gravis. In Lachman PJ, Peters DK (eds): Clinical Aspects of Immunology, 4th ed, p 1032. Boston, Blackwell Scientific Publishers, 1982

54. Plauche WC: Myasthenia gravis: The disease and its relationship to pregnancy. Clin Obstet Gynecol 26:592, 1983

55. Murray JM, Harris RE: The management of the pregnant patient with idiopathic thrombocytopenia purpura. Am J Obstet Gynecol 126:449, 1976

56. Territo M, Finklestein J, Oh W et al: Management of autoimmune thrombocytopenia in pregnancy and the neonate. Obstet Gynecol 41:579, 1973

57. Kelton JG, Inwood MJ, Barr RM et al: The prediction of thrombocytopenia in infants of mothers with clinically diagnosed thrombocytopenia. Am J Obstet Gynecol 144:449, 1982

58. Cines DB, Schrieber AD: Immune thrombocytopenia: Use of Coombs' antiglobin test to detect IgG and C3 on platelets. N Engl J Med 300:106, 1979

59. Carlos HW, McMillan R, Crosby WH: Management of pregnancy in women with immune thrombocytopenic purpura. JAMA 244:2756, 1980

60. Karpatkin M, Porges RF, Karpatkin S: Platelet counts in infants of women with autoimmune thrombocytopenia. N Engl J Med 305:936, 1981

61. Pearson HA, Shulman NR, Marder UJ et al: Iso-immune neonatal thrombocytopenic purpura: Clinical and therapeutic considerations. Blood 23:154, 1964

62. Scott JR, Cruikshank DP, Kochenour NK et al: Fetal platelet counts in the obstetric management of immunologic thrombocytopenic purpura. Am J Obstet Gynecol 136:495, 1980

63. Scott JR, Rote NS, Cruikshank DP: Antiplatelet antibodies and platelet counts in pregnancies complicated by autoimmune thrombocytopenic purpura. Am J Obstet Gynecol 145:932, 1983

64. Barber HRK, Dorsett B: The immune system in gynecologic malignancies. In Gleicher N (ed): Reproductive Immunology, p 357. New York, Alan R Liss, 1981

65. Jolles CT, Beeson JH: Reproductive tumor immunology. In Scott JR, Rote NS (eds): Immunology in Obstetrics and Gynecology, p 221. Norwalk, CT, Appleton-Century-Crofts, 1985

66. Deligdisch L: Trophoblastic disease: A bridge between pregnancy and malignancy. In Gleicher N (ed): Reproductive Immunology, p 323. New York, Alan R Liss, 1981

67. Patillo RA: Histocompatibility antigens in pregnancy, abortions, infertility, preeclampsia, and trophoblastic neoplasms. In Gleicher N (ed): Reproductive Immunology, p 259. New York, Alan R Liss, 1981

Obstetric and Gynecologic Infections: General Considerations and Antibacterial Therapy

William J. Ledger

13

There has been an explosion of new information in the past decade on the nature of bacterial infections in women. Practitioners must struggle with the significance of such new and unfamiliar microinvaders as anaerobic bacteria, chlamydia, and mycoplasma in pelvic infections. As in any period of rapid change, a new and broader data base must be assimilated, and new therapeutic strategies that reflect the new realities must be formulated. Much has been learned, but much is still unclear about the pathophysiology of pelvic infections.

MICROBIOLOGY OF PELVIC INFECTION

There has been a complete change in our understanding of the microbiology of pelvic infection. The emphasis in the early years of bacteriology was on a single bacterial pathogen. Because the development of any new medical science, whether cell biology or microbiology, can be justified only by its significance in the understanding of disease, there is little wonder that early workers like Koch and Pasteur focused on individual bacterial species to demonstrate the importance of microbiology. These investigators isolated bacterial species from the site of recognized clinical infections, cultured these isolates in artificial media, and showed that the bacteria could reproduce pathologic states when reinoculated into animals or human volunteers. The concept that single bacterial species, pathogens, caused diseases became the dominant theme of microbiology.

This model closely represented many clinical entities. Infections, including pneumococcal pneumonia or an *Escherichia coli* pyelonephritis, became the model for the therapeutic approach to all bacterial infections. One pathogenic species caused a disease, and the selection of an appropriate antibiotic effective against this one species would result in a cure for that disease. It was a simple, straightforward model of infection; how-

ever, both laboratory and clinical studies in the last few years have shown the limitations of this concept when applied to such soft tissue pelvic infections as the infected abortion, salpingo-oophoritis, postpartum endomyometritis, and postoperative pelvic infection. These infections have a diffuse microbiologic etiology with multiple bacterial isolates, and anaerobic bacteria are present in most of the patients.

Many aspects of these mixed bacterial soft tissue infections are not completely understood. Many fear that anaerobic bacteria do not fulfil Koch's postulate. When injected alone, *Bacteroides fragilis* without a capsule do not produce disease in animals. Is it a nonsignificant contaminant? That is unlikely, for these same organisms combined with an enterococcus or a gram-negative aerobe result in an overwhelming infection. The confusion about the pathophysiology of these infections is not limited to research in animal models. Clinical cures can be seen in patients who are treated with antibiotics that are not effective against all of the bacterial isolates obtained from the site of infection. In contrast, therapeutic failures can be seen in women with a pelvic abscess who fail to respond to antibiotics, despite the presence of bacteria within the abscess that are susceptible to the antibiotics employed. In the latter case, local environmental changes such as pH or protein binding of antibiotic may prevent antibacterial activity.

A major drawback in the clinical evaluation of infectious disease in obstetrics and gynecology has been the paucity of accurate microbiologic data. The standard investigations of the impact of antibiotics on bacterial infection have used microbiologic data to help in the assessment of clinical results. The antibiotic susceptibility of the bacteria isolated from the site of infection and the bloodstream is measured, and a test of the apparent clinical cure is the elimination of the bacterial pathogen from the infection site. Such microbiologic data can seldom be obtained for the evaluation of pelvic infections in women because these infections are internal and attempts at bacterial sampling must traverse the abundant surface bacterial contamination of the lower genital tract. Attempts to distinguish the bacteria on the surface of the endometrial cavity of noninfected postpartum women from the bacteria similarly recovered from women with a diagnosis of postpartum endomyometritis have not been successful. The same kinds of bacteria have been isolated in both infected and noninfected women.

The only reliable microbiologic data on pelvic infection are obtained from women who fail to respond to systemic antibiotic therapy and require operative intervention for the drainage or removal of an abscess. Although these cases provide excellent bacteriologic information, since large amounts of purulent material can be obtained directly, this patient population is small and unique. These women represent the infrequent treatment failures and are not representative of the majority of women with pelvic infections, who respond to antibiotic therapy. When there have been difficulties with the collection of human data, one approach commonly employed to gain insight has been the use of an animal model of infection.

A popular model of intra-abdominal infection in the rat has been developed by Gorbach and Bartlett. Pooled rat feces and barium sulfate were encased in a gelatin capsule and used as the bacterial inoculum. These capsules were inserted into the peritoneal cavity of rats. As the gelatin dissolved, there was a uniform response to the presence of the feces, with huge bacterial counts of both aerobes and anaerobes in the peritoneal cavity. All of the animals developed peritonitis; when their bloodstreams were sampled, gram-negative aerobic organisms were recovered. This peritonitis and the associated bacteremia were lethal to approximately 40% of the rats, and none of those that died had abscesses. The survivors appeared better for one to two days and then developed symptoms of an intra-abdominal infection. Sacrificed, they were found to have intra-abdominal abscesses in which anaerobes were the predominant organisms. Gorbach and Bartlett postulated a biphasic response to this mixed bacterial insult, *i.e.,* early-onset sepsis in which gram-negative aerobes predominated and late-onset abscess formation in which anaerobes predominated. The major appeal of the model was the reproducibility of the results.

The next step in experimental design was to determine if this response could be modified by the use of systemic antibiotics. When an aminoglycoside such as gentamicin, which has antibacterial activity against gram-negative aerobes, was given systemically at the time of the bacterial insult, the early-onset phase was largely eliminated, but the survivors later developed intra-abdominal abscesses. When an antibiotic with antibacterial activity against anaerobes, clindamycin, was given at the time of the bacterial insult, there was no impact on the early-onset phase, but the late-onset development of intra-abdominal abscesses was largely eliminated. These observations influenced many infectious-disease experts to recommend a combination of clindamycin and gentamicin for the treatment of soft tissue pelvic infections in humans.

There are distinct variations between the animal model and human experience that must be accounted for in any prospective judgment about appropriate antibiotics. The animal model involves a massive bacterial insult that is seldom reached in human infection. Deaths from sepsis were seldom seen on obstetric–gynecologic services in the 1970s, and patients with intra-abdominal abscesses are a small proportion of the total population of women with pelvic infections. These differences do not negate the lessons of the animal model but suggest that individual risk factors must be considered in each of the human infections that require treatment.

COMMUNITY-ACQUIRED INFECTIONS

Infected Abortion

Patients with infected abortion are a much less common problem for the obstetrician–gynecologist in the 1980s than they were in the 1960s. Not only is the number of patients with infected abortion lower, but also death from sepsis occurs far less frequently than in previous decades. Center for Disease Control statistics indicate a dramatic drop in the number of maternal deaths from sepsis after a termination of pregnancy.

There are several obvious influences on these encouraging statistics. One was the development of better contraceptive methods in the late 1960s and early 1970s. These new and better methods of contraception were rapidly introduced into clinical practice. In addition, considerable effort was put into the delivery of contraceptive care to populations at high risk for an unwanted pregnancy; family planning for the urban poor became a reality. These developments gave a greater proportion of sexually active women more control over their reproductive destinies. There was also a breakthrough in the availability of definitive care for the woman with an unwanted pregnancy. Pregnancy termination by licensed physicians became legal. Although no termination technique is free of complications, the incidence of difficulties is, of course, lower when abortion procedures are performed by qualified medical personnel. Because of the availability of legal abortion, patients sought confirmation of pregnancy at an early date; unwanted pregnancies were terminated early, when complications occur much less frequently. The net result has been a dramatic decrease in both the number of women with pelvic infection following abortion and the number of women with life-threatening infection. Despite all this, some women with infected abortions will be seen by the obstetrician–gynecologist.

Evaluations of infected abortions in the 1970s indicate that this is a low-risk infection. Generally, these women respond rapidly to medical and surgical therapy

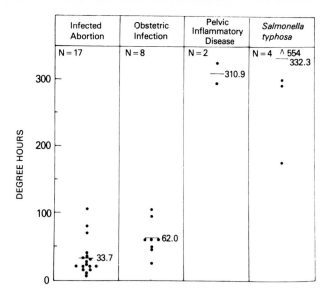

FIG. 13-1. Fever indices in degree hours of patients with bacteremia from a community infection. *Salmonella typhosa* refers to patients with an enterocolitis. The mean fever index is indicated for each group. (Ledger WJ, Kriewall TJ, Gee C: The fever index: A technique for evaluating the clinical response to bacteremia. Obstet Gynecol 45:603, 1975)

and recover without serious complications. Figure 13-1 shows the fever index of patients hospitalized with a community-acquired infection and an associated bacteremia. In general, bacteremia characterizes those patients on an obstetric–gynecologic service who are most seriously ill with infection, so this analysis includes only a small group of the total number of women with infection. The fever index is a quantitative measure of patient response to infection, and the clinical response of patients with infected abortion is usually the least

serious of the responses to all the major categories of community-acquired infections.

Treatment

Patient responses to infected abortion differ from responses to most other pelvic infections. Patients usually respond rapidly to medical and operative therapy. One study by Chow and colleagues indicated that curettage was a more important component in the cure than systemic antibiotics. This is probably related to the efficient bacteria-clearing mechanism of the pregnant uterus. Successful responses to therapy, based on microbiologic data, are seen in situations in which an inappropriate antibiotic was used. Many women with a *B. fragilis* bacteremia become afebrile and are cured despite the use of systemic antibiotics that do not cover this microorganism. This is an important observation, for Rotheram and Schick have shown that *B. fragilis* is the second most common bloodstream isolate in patients with infected abortion. If cures could not be achieved without specific antibiotic coverage, there would be more widespread use of such agents as clindamycin and chloramphenicol in these patients. These potentially toxic agents are seldom needed; in one woman with infected abortion and an associated *B. fragilis* bacteremia, however, chloramphenicol was necessary to achieve a cure (Fig. 13-2). Usually, these women can be treated with a single agent, such as a cephalosporin, or a combination of penicillin and an aminoglycoside. If they fail to respond to this or are critically ill on admission, clindamycin or chloramphenicol should be prescribed as initial therapy.

Factors That Impose Special Risk in Infected Abortion

Some situations increase the risk of serious infection for patients with infected abortion. Identification of

FIG. 13-2. Infected abortion, *B. fragilis* bacteremia. Chloramphenicol was required for cure. (Ledger WJ: Anaerobic infection. Am J Obstet Gynecol 123:111, 1975)

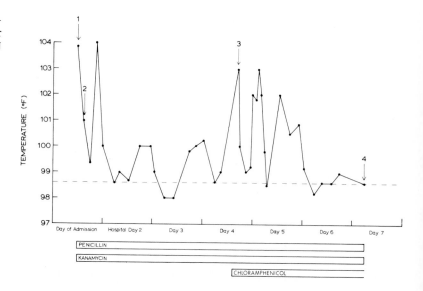

these possibly serious problems is an indication for more aggressive antibiotic and operative therapy. Any evidence of infection beyond the limits of the uterus puts the patient in a high-risk category. This is usually secondary to damage to the uterus, particularly perforation at the time of induced abortion, and it provides a setting in which the patient is more likely to develop a pelvic abscess. In these women, antibiotics that are effective against both gram-negative aerobes and anaerobic organisms should be ordered to prevent abscess formation.

Another subgroup at high risk is those women with a clinical picture of endotoxic shock. In these clinical situations, therapy should be directed primarily toward gram-negative aerobic organisms, since these are most frequently the culprits. On occasion, however, the only isolate from the bloodstream is an anaerobe. Therefore, antibiotic coverage effective against anaerobes should be employed at the initiation of therapy. Even in these high-risk patients, the clinical prognosis is still more favorable than it is in other serious infections seen on an obstetric–gynecologic service. Figure 13-3 documents the fever index response of seriously ill patients treated with a combination of antibiotics and either

clindamycin or chloramphenicol as coverage for *B. fragilis.* Again, uncomplicated posttreatment courses were seen in patients with infected abortion, and none of these women developed a pelvic abscess that required operative drainage.

A final group of high-risk patients includes women who are critically ill, with evidence of myometrial gas formation and an "onion skin" appearance on roentgenographic examination, which is pathognomonic of a *Clostridium perfringens* infection. Infections of this type can be lethal because of the toxins produced by these organisms, and they require an aggressive operative approach when they are extensive. The recovery of *C. perfringens* per se from a site of infection or the identification of gram-positive rods in the purulent exudate is not an indication for hysterectomy. There should be clinical evidence of extensive infection with intravascular hemolysis and renal failure or roentgenographic evidence of extensive pelvic infection before hysterectomy is performed. In these critically ill patients, antibiotic coverage should be directed against gram-positive and gram-negative aerobes as well as all anaerobes. Curettage is important, with hysterectomy reserved for those patients whose condition continues to deteriorate after the curettage. However, this aggressive approach is not universally accepted for critically ill patients with renal failure following pregnancy termination. In one series of cases from England, 17 of 19 women with this problem survived with treatment limited to antibiotics and supportive measures while awaiting return of renal function. These results are far superior to the usually quoted mortality rate of nearly 100% when these patients are treated without surgery. Although these medical treatments represent an advance, the goal in therapy is to avoid death, and, in some cases, this may be best accomplished by appropriate operative intervention with the removal of infected pelvic tissue.

Salpingo-oophoritis

There is currently much controversy about the etiology and treatment of salpingo-oophoritis. The microbiologic basis for the syndrome of salpingo-oophoritis has not been firmly established. In the past decade, the nongonococcal nature of many cases of salpingo-oophoritis has become increasingly clear, but not all the potentially causative organisms have been identified. For example, one Swedish study established a major role for *Chlamydia* nongonococcal salpingitis, and this has been confirmed in investigations by Sweet and coworkers. Some of the clinical bases for the diagnosis of salpingitis have been challenged. Afebrile salpingitis is reported to be common, particularly in the woman with an intrauterine device in place. It may be difficult to differentiate afebrile salpingitis from other noninfectious causes of pelvic pain, particularly if *culdocentesis,* a commonly employed diagnostic technique, cannot be performed. All reported treatment regimens represent best guesses;

FIG. 13-3. Fever index response to clindamycin and chloramphenicol in patients seriously ill with *B. fragilis* infection. (Ledger WJ, Moore DE, Lowensohn RI et al: A fever index evaluation of chloramphenicol or clindamycin in patients with serious pelvic infections. Obstet Gynecol 50:523, 1977)

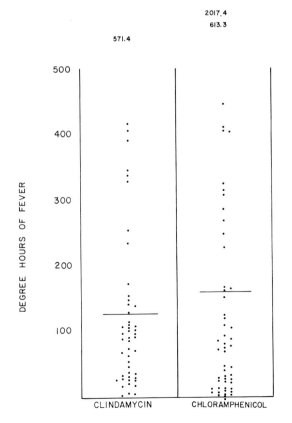

they are not based on firm scientific data. Should patients with salpingitis be treated as outpatients? This controversy can be resolved only by a careful prospective treatment study to determine the effectiveness of an inpatient versus an outpatient treatment regimen.

There are no data available on the most important aspect of medical care—the future fertility of the woman. Westrom has shown the impact of repeated episodes of salpingitis upon future fertility (Table 13-1). These data make the dangers of salpingitis obvious. None of the many alternative therapeutic regimens currently employed has been evaluated for this important end point. Until this is done, any treatment recommendations remain empirical. This is an important fact to acknowledge, since a rapid clinical response does not necessarily indicate better tubal function in the future. For example, in Falk's study patients treated with steroids plus antibiotics had a better initial clinical response than did patients treated with antibiotics alone; they became afebrile more rapidly, and pelvic tumors regressed in size more rapidly. However, on follow-up laparoscopic examination, the incidence of adhesion formation and blocked tubes did not differ in the two treatment groups. Future studies of drug therapy will require evaluation of future tubal function as a definitive measure of the effectiveness of therapy. This will require laparoscopy or long-term follow-up measuring subsequent fertility.

Classification

Any acceptable method of classification of salpingo-oophoritis should be based on methods that are both reproducible and available to all clinicians. Monif has championed the concept of endometritis–salpingitis–peritonitis (ESP), but a classification based on (1) the presence or absence of a pelvic mass and (2) the recovery or nonrecovery of *Neisseria gonorrhoeae* from the endocervical culture seems preferable. In addition,

Table 13-1
Fertility Following Salpingitis

Type of Infection	Incidence of Involuntary Sterility with Tubal Occlusion (%)
Gonococcal	6
Nongonococcal	17
Number of Episodes of Salpingitis	
One	13
Two	35
Three	75

(After Westrom L: Effects of acute pelvic inflammatory disease on fertility. Am J Obstet Gynecol 121:707, 1975)

such a classification can be used as a guide to therapy. Before the initiation of therapy, a pelvic examination should be performed to determine whether the patient has a pelvic mass. This information is important because women with a pelvic mass are in a higher risk category and may require an operation for the drainage of a pelvic abscess. Total agreement on the significance of a pelvic mass has not been reached; for example, an ultrasound study by Spaulding and colleagues did not show any poorer outcomes in women with a fluid-filled pelvic mass. However, since such a mass may be a pelvic abscess with anaerobes, particularly *B. fragilis,* as the predominant organisms, therapy should be initiated with either clindamycin or metronidazole to cover these organisms, as well as an antibiotic effective against gram-negative aerobes. Even so, many patients fail to respond to medical therapy and for cure require operative intervention in the form of drainage or extirpation of the abscess.

For those women who do not have a pelvic mass before the initiation of therapy, another factor is important—regardless of whether *N. gonorrhoeae* can be recovered from the endocervical culture. Women who have an infection that involves this microorganism become afebrile more rapidly with antibiotic therapy, rarely develop abscesses, and have a more favorable prognosis for future fertility. The male partner should be treated before the patient resumes sexual activity.

It is difficult for the clinician to differentiate between gonococcal and nongonococcal salpingitis on the first examination of the patient. Some have suggested that this diagnosis can be made on the basis of a Gram stain of an endocervical smear, *i.e.,* that a positive smear correlates with a positive culture. The difficulty lies with the patient with a negative smear, since a positive culture can be obtained in some women with a negative smear. In addition, others found poor correlations between both positive and negative smears and cultures. It is hoped that some fluorescent staining technique will be developed to identify women with gonococcal salpingitis. In any event, women with no pelvic masses have a favorable response to therapy; few go on to develop a pelvic abscess that requires operative drainage.

Treatment

The widely divergent treatment regimens employed in patients without a pelvic mass are a good indication that a controlled study to demonstrate immediate and long-term effectiveness of specific regimens has not yet been done. Outpatient studies in which the effectiveness of ampicillin was compared with that of a standard tetracycline showed similar results with both gonococcal and nongonococcal salpingitis. An inpatient study that evaluated ampicillin and doxycycline in gonococcal and nongonococcal salpingitis showed a better response, as indicated by the fever index, in the women treated with doxycycline.

A major problem in the evaluation of the antibiotic treatment of salpingo-oophoritis is the lack of microbiologic information about this disease. The internal anatomic location of the fallopian tubes and ovaries makes it difficult to obtain culture material. Since peritoneal fluid is sterile in the asymptomatic woman, any bacteria recovered from the peritoneal fluid aspirate are assumed to be the same as those causing the inflammation in the endosalpinx. Unless the cul-de-sac is not free, this procedure should be done in afebrile women with pelvic pain who are suspected of having salpingitis. Some physicians are reluctant to diagnose salpingitis unless there is evidence of infection, *i.e.,* bacteria and white blood cells in the peritoneal fluid smear, although Monif in his ESP classification would classify the disease of the patient with negative peritoneal fluid as simply endometritis–salpingitis (ES). Unfortunately, there seem to be major limitations in the microbiologic evaluations of fluid obtained by culdocentesis. Using direct aspiration of peritoneal fluid at the time of laparoscopy, Sweet and colleagues have found poor correlation between the bacteria recovered from the peritoneal fluid and that recovered from the endosalpinx fluid obtained from the fimbria.

There is increasing evidence that chlamydia are important in salpingo-oophoritis. Clinically, chlamydia appear to be important because of the favorable response of patients with salpingitis to doxycycline, which is effective against chlamydia. Mardh and colleagues, using fimbrial biopsy through laparoscopy, recovered chlamydia from 30% of women with nongonococcal salpingitis. Sweet and co-workers recovered chlamydia from the endometrial biopsy cultures of patients with salpingitis.

The intrauterine contraceptive device (IUD) affects both the frequency and the type of pelvic infection seen in nonpregnant women. A number of studies done in the past few years indicate that women who use the IUD for contraception have a higher frequency of pelvic infection, particularly if they are young and unmarried, than women who do not. In addition, there is evidence that the host response to infection is altered when an IUD is present. Pelvic infections due to *Actinomyces bovis* are much more frequently seen in IUD users than in nonusers. The unilateral tubo-ovarian abscess occurs more frequently than normal in IUD users, and the pathophysiology of this unilateral problem resembles that of the ovarian abscess more than it resembles the ascending types of infection seen with salpingitis. IUDs do not always cause a more severe infection. An evaluation of the response to triple antibiotic therapy for salpingo-oophoritis showed no difference between patients who were using an IUD and patients who were not (Fig. 13-4).

Operative treatment of patients with salpingo-oophoritis remains an important component of therapy. Women who have clinical evidence of a ruptured tubo-ovarian abscess, such as diffuse peritonitis and a

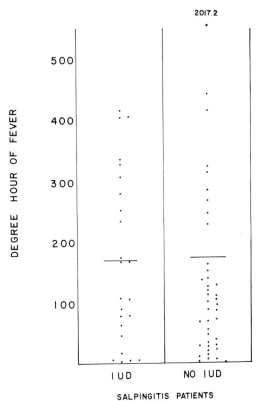

FIG. 13-4. Response to triple antibiotic therapy for salpingo-oophoritis in patients with and without an IUD. (Ledger WJ, Moore DE, Lowensohn RI et al: A fever index evaluation of chloramphenicol or clindamycin in patients with serious pelvic infections. Obstet Gynecol 50:523, 1977)

tachycardia out of proportion to their temperature, are critically ill. Failure to operate could be fatal, and the operation should include hysterectomy and bilateral salpingo-oophorectomy for cure. The problem is not as simple in women who fail to respond to antibiotic therapy and show no signs of a tubo-ovarian abscess rupture. For years, physicians have been reluctant to perform surgery in the acute phase of infection because of the increased incidence of complications and mortality associated with surgery at this time. In recent years, however, it has been shown that operations can be performed in the acute phase of infection without serious complications. This is undoubtedly related to the availability of antibiotics that are effective against the organisms involved in these acute infections. Although the operations can be performed, they are seldom necessary and should be reserved for patients who fail to respond within 72 hours to antibiotic therapy that includes clindamycin or chloramphenicol. Figure 13-5 shows the recovery of anaerobes in such situations and indicates the reason for the recommendation of 72 hours of medical therapy to eliminate anaerobes from the site of infection.

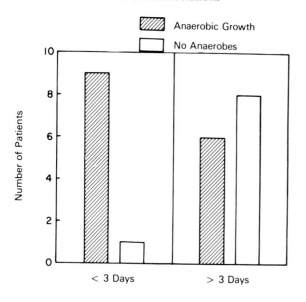

FIG. 13-5. Isolation of anaerobes from abscesses, depending on the length of preoperative exposure to clindamycin or chloramphenicol. Increase in the recovery of anaerobes is significant when preoperative duration of therapy is three days or less. $P < 0.01$ by the Fisher exact test. (Ledger WJ, Gee C, Pollin P et al: The use of pre-reduced media and a portable jar for the collection of anaerobic organisms from clinical sites of infection. Am J Obstet Gynecol 125:677, 1976)

HOSPITAL-ACQUIRED INFECTIONS

Hospital Personnel

Despite continued emphasis on the importance of asepsis, some of the standard hospital rules are repeatedly disregarded. Shoe covers, caps, and masks should be discarded immediately when the wearer leaves the operating or delivery room. Scrub suits should not be worn outside the operating rooms and delivery rooms except in special circumstances, and the wearer must change to a fresh scrub suit before reentering an aseptic or controlled area. Abundant facial hair can be a collector, and a shedder, of bacteria, especially the gram-positive, coagulase-positive type; men with beards or mustaches should use an antistaphylococcus shampoo regularly and should exercise special care in the use of operating room caps and masks. Medical attendants who develop skin infections, even if they are hidden from view, should not be directly involved in patient care. One hospital outbreak of group-A β-hemolytic streptococcal infections was traced to an anesthesiologist who was an asymptomatic anal carrier of this organism. One series of coagulase-positive staphylococcal wound infections was related to a surgical resident's contamined beard; another, to a pustule on the hand of an anesthesiologist.

Infection After Pregnancy Termination

With the liberalization of abortion laws in the 1960s, infection following pregnancy termination became an entity to be addressed by the practicing obstetrician-gynecologist. A number of observations about these infections seem universal. The later in pregnancy the termination occurs, the more frequently the infections occur, but serious infections following therapeutic abortion are rare. Because of the infrequency of infection following pregnancy termination before 12 weeks' gestation, there has been little enthusiasm for the use of prophylactic antibiotics; however, one study showed that tetracycline was effective when used in this manner. A more logical approach would be to screen patients for *N. gonorrhoeae* before curettage; those whose test results are positive should be treated with antibiotics, since this population has increased postoperative morbidity. The most serious infections, which have resulted in disseminated intravascular coagulation and death, have occurred after hysterotomy in women over 38 years of age. Therefore, hysterotomy has been largely abandoned as a termination procedure. Recently, evacuation of the uterus by suction curettage has been used in women beyond 12 weeks' gestation. Although this technique compares favorably with prostaglandin and saline abortion techniques, serious soft tissue injury and subsequent serious pelvic infection are possible.

In all women with a postabortion infection, the basic therapeutic approach is the same: antibiotic coverage followed by operative intervention to remove any retained products of conception. If there is evidence of infection beyond the confines of the uterus, antibiotics that are effective against *B. fragilis* should be used, and laparotomy should be performed in the patient who fails to respond to therapy or shows any evidence of clinical deterioration.

Puerperal Endomyometritis

The most problematic of hospital-acquired infections on the obstetric–gynecologic service in the 1980s is puerperal endomyometritis. These infections occur frequently and may become the most serious infections seen on the inpatient service. Because of their importance, the clinican should have a clear view of the risk factors, modes of prevention, and treatment of these infections. The clinical features of puerperal endomyometritis are considered in Chapter 40.

The established risk factors for patients with puerperal endomyometritis are few in number. There is good evidence that both the rate and severity of infection are greater following cesarean section than following vaginal delivery (Fig. 13-6). Other factors that influence puerperal infections are not as obvious. There is evidence that the incidence of puerperal endomyometritis following cesarean section increases as the time interval

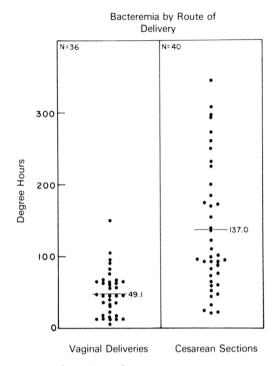

Bacteremia by Route of Delivery

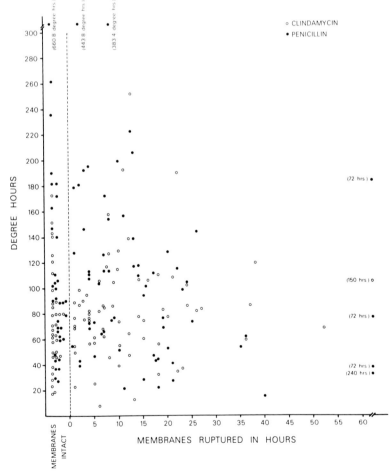

between membrane rupture and delivery lengthens, but these longer time intervals are not associated with more severe infections (Fig. 13-7). The relationship of the invasive intrauterine monitoring catheter and postpartum infection is also unclear. Several studies have suggested that there is no correlation between intrauterine monitoring and the rate of infection, but two studies with private patients demonstrated a greater frequency of infection when this technique was used. It is possible that the multiple factors associated with infection in a low socioeconomic population prevent discrimination of individual factors.

The high risk of infection following cesarean section, particularly when the procedure is performed on a woman in labor, has generated a great deal of interest in prophylactic antibiotics. Clinical experience with prophylactic antibiotics in vaginal hysterectomy has

FIG. 13-6. Fever indices in degree hours of patients with puerperal bacteremia, comparing patients with a vaginal delivery with patients delivered by cesarean section. The mean is indicated. (Ledger WJ, Kriewall TJ, Gee C: The fever index: A technique for evaluating the clinical response to bacteremia. Obstet Gynecol 45:603, 1975)

FIG. 13-7. Scattergram of patient's febrile response to endomyometritis after cesarean section compared with the length of time of membrane rupture. (DiZerega G, Yonekura L, Roy S et al: A comparison of clindamycin–gentamicin and penicillin–gentamicin in the treatment of post–cesarean section endometritis. Am J Obstet Gynecol 134:238, 1979)

been favorable. Almost without exception, therapeutic results with prophylactic antibiotics have been better than those with a placebo. The same is true for cesarean section. Despite this, there are still concerns about the best use of prophylactic antibiotics to prevent infections. A most important concern is the timing of the antibiotic administration. In prior clinical evaluations of prophylactic antibiotics, the medication has been given just before the operative procedure. In cesarean section, this produces therapeutic levels of antibiotics in the fetus. Since mothers at high risk for infection also deliver babies with a greater than usual chance for infection, the presence of measurable levels of antibiotic in the fetus complicates evaluation of the blood culture in the infant with suspected sepsis. The administration of antibiotics after cord clamping may produce results similar to those obtained by the more standard preoperative adminis-

tration. This avoids any dosage to the fetus, but intravenous administration of antibiotic to an anesthetized patient may not be the most acceptable approach to the problem; two deaths have been reported with this technique. An alternative prophylactic strategy is antibiotic lavage.

A different approach to this problem has been extraperitoneal cesarean section. This does not avoid postoperative infection, but it transforms an intraperitoneal infection to an extraperitoneal infection, which is better tolerated by the human host. Although a whole generation of obstetrician–gynecologists lacks experience with the technique, it remains a viable alternative.

Another approach has been to employ different therapeutic strategies in the treatment of patients with puerperal endomyometritis following cesarean section. DiZerega and colleagues found that a clindamycin–

Table 13-2
Comparison of Clindamycin–Gentamicin Regimen with Penicillin–Gentamicin Regimen

	Clindamycin–Gentamicin	Penicillin–Gentamicin	Significance
Number of Patients	100	100	N.S.
Therapy Completed, No Problems	86	64	$p < 0.001$
Poor Clinical Results			
No response—third antibiotic	5	29	$p < 0.001$
Abdominal wound infection	8	16	N.S.
Operative drainage only	6	4	N.S.
Prolonged febrile course after drainage	2	12	$p < 0.02$ (Fisher's exact test)
Serious Problems	0	4	$p < 0.06$
Pelvic abscess, total abdominal hysterectomy, bilateral salpingo-oophorectomy	0	1	
Wound evisceration	0	1	
Heparin	0	2	
Reaction During Antibiotics	4	3	N.S.
Rash	2*	2	
Hematuria	0	1†	
Diarrhea	2	0	
Indirect Measures of Morbidity			
Hospital days	7.4	8.7	$p < 0.01$ (Mann–Whitney U test)
Fever index in degree hours			
Median	77.3	91.3	$p < 0.02$
Mean	81.2	110.7	
±SD	±40.6	±89.6	
±SE	±4.06	±9.0	

N.S., not significant; *SD,* standard deviation; *SE,* standard error.

* Drug continued, rash disappeared, one patient.

† Drug continued, hematuria stopped.

(DiZerega G, Yonekura L, Roy S et al: A comparison of clindamycin–gentamicin and penicillin–gentamicin in the treatment of post–cesarean section endometritis. Am J Obstet Gynecol 134:238, 1979) gentamicin combination produced more favorable results than did a penicillin–gentamicin combination (Table 13-2). Although not statistically significant, the prevention of serious infection would seem to be the most important result of the study. The 4% rate is exactly the same as that reported by Gibbs and colleagues in patients treated with penicillin–kanamycin. The same results were seen when clindamycin–gentamicin was compared with cephalothin–gentamicin in a study from Newark. In making the final judgment on the use of this regimen, the physician must weigh the potential toxicity of clindamycin against the possibility of preventing serious infection in a small percentage of patients. Similar favorable results with post–cesarean section endomyometritis have been achieved with the newer cephalosporins and penicillins.

Although they occur infrequently, serious infections following cesarean section can be devastating to the patient. A pelvic abscess that develops after cesarean section is distressing. Not only must these patients endure a protracted hospital stay and treatment that may have unpleasant side-effects, but also they are subjected to the risks of a second operation. If they are fortunate, they need only vaginal drainage of a pelvic abscess. If there is an extensive uterine infection or tubo-ovarian abscesses are present, extirpation of the pelvic organs is required. This invariably results in a cure but leaves the patient with no hope for future childbearing.

Treatment of the patient with puerperal endomyometritis following vaginal delivery is much simpler than that for a patient with the same condition following cesarean section. There is no need for frequent use of the first-line agents used so successfully in post–cesarean section patients. Those who develop infection after vaginal delivery usually respond favorably to single-antibiotic treatment such as ampicillin, cephalothin, or metronidazole. Rarely are additional antibiotics necessary for cure.

Postoperative Infections

The surgical technique has much to do not only with the postoperative course in general, but with infection in particular: the longer the operative procedure, the greater the incidence of postoperative infection. As Victor Bonney noted many years ago, "an operation rapidly yet correctly performed has many advantages over one technically as correct, yet laboriously and tediously accomplished." Until the time of their retirement, surgeons should strive continuously to improve the precision of their technique and to reduce their operating time, not by increased speed of action, but by avoiding unnecessary movements that do not advance the procedure and can significantly prolong it.

Hospital-acquired infections are frequent problems following gynecologic operations. The abundant bacterial flora of the lower genital tract may multiply and invade the crushed and necrotic tissue that remains after a pelvic operation. Many of the operative procedures in gynecology involve sites close to the urinary tract, often necessitating the use of a catheter to maintain bladder drainage. This markedly increases the risk of a urinary tract infection. All of these factors make a knowledge of infection control and treatment important for the obstetrician–gynecologist.

Urinary Tract Infection

A frequent source of postoperative complications is the urinary tract infection. In order to deal properly with this problem, the physician must have a knowledge of techniques for both the prevention and treatment of infection. The prevention of urinary tract infection in the postoperative gynecologic patient must be focused on the care of the catheter. A catheter should be inserted only when necessary and then with meticulous care. A closed drainage system not only decreases the total number of urinary infections, but also delays the entry of bacteria into the urinary tract. This is an important consideration for the gynecologist who frequently uses short-term bladder drainage in postoperative patients. Despite these precautions, urinary tract infections still occur, particularly when the catheter must remain in place for longer than 48 hours. In postoperative patients who are likely to have the catheter removed by the fourth or fifth postoperative day, there is evidence that the systemic use of nitrofurantoins as prophylaxis dramatically reduces the subsequent incidence of urinary tract infection.

Women who develop a postoperative urinary tract infection should be approached by the physician in a logical, structured way to acquire the necessary diagnostic information before therapy is begun. Urine should be obtained for culture and susceptibility testing before a systemic antimicrobial agent is prescribed. Since there is a good correlation between the presence of bacteria on high-power magnification of centrifuged urine and subsequent bacterial colony counts of greater than 10^5/ml, this evaluation should be done immediately. If any postoperative patient complains of costovertebral angle pain, an intravenous pyelogram should be taken to determine the possibility of operative ureteral damage with obstruction rather than to assign a diagnosis of pyelonephritis. When the evaluation is complete, the patient should be treated with drugs such as the sulfas or the nitrofurantoins. These drugs are as effective as oral penicillin or cephalosporin, and their antibacterial activity is limited to the urinary tract. Broad-spectrum agents may mask symptoms of infection and make it impossible for the physician to delineate the infection site clinically. The most important evaluation of treatment is the urine culture obtained after 36 to 48 hours of therapy. If this is free of bacteria, the patient should not have prolonged difficulties with recurrent infection.

If bacteria are present, susceptibility testing should be carried out to determine whether alternative agents should be employed.

Respiratory Tract Infections

Postoperative respiratory tract infections are relatively infrequent problems for the gynecologist. Most elective operative procedures are done on women in good health, and the incidence of postoperative respiratory difficulties is understandably lower after pelvic operations than after operations that require an upper abdominal incision (*e.g.,* cholecystectomy). The major concern in postoperative patients is aspiration, which is usually recognized immediately or within 24 hours of the operation. Such patients may require supportive respiratory measures if a large amount of material was aspirated. Other patients may develop a postoperative pneumonia because of difficulty in establishing a normal breathing pattern postoperatively. Since there is an increase in the gram-negative aerobic respiratory flora of hospitalized patients, antibiotic therapy should include agents effective against these aerobes.

Pelvic Infections

Postoperative pelvic infections occur with some frequency, and therapy usually prolongs the patient's stay in the hospital. These pelvic infections may take many forms with different prognoses. An infected collection of material in the vaginal cuff after hysterectomy can often be treated by simple operative drainage alone. A diffuse pelvic cellulitis always requires systemic antibiotics; heparin is required if the infection progresses to septic pelvic thrombophlebitis. Postoperative pelvic abscesses can be lethal if they rupture into the peritoneal cavity. If this occurs, immediate laparotomy must be performed to remove the infected pelvic organs. Patients with unruptured abscesses usually do not respond to medical therapy and require operative intervention, with all of the risks of a second anesthetic and major operation, for drainage or removal of the abscess.

Widely diverse techniques have been employed to prevent postoperative pelvic infections. The most popular technique has been systemic antibiotic prophylaxis, particularly in the premenopausal woman undergoing vaginal hysterectomy. A wide variety of antibiotics has been used successfully in this situation, including penicillin, cephalosporin, tetracycline, and metronidazole. There is evidence that a short course of prophylaxis limited to the day of the operation is just as effective as therapy for three to five days postoperatively. In fact, one study of vaginal hysterectomy in which patients were given only 1 g cefazolin intramuscularly just before the operation showed outstanding results. All of these prophylactic regimens have been associated with a reduction in the number of postoperative pelvic infections.

There are alternative methods of prevention of postoperative pelvic infection, however. Using closed-suction T-tube drainage of the space between the peritoneum and vaginal cuff in abdominal and vaginal hysterectomy, Swartz and Tanaree have shown a marked reduction in postoperative pelvic infections. The addition of systemic antibiotic prophylaxis to the closed suction drainage system did not result in further lowering of the postoperative infection rate. A very different approach to the prevention of infection was championed by Osborne and colleagues. By performing hot conization of the cervix just before hysterectomy to remove the potential bacterial contamination from the endocervix, they demonstrated a sharp reduction in the number of postoperative pelvic infections.

The patient with a postoperative pelvic infection requires careful evaluation before therapy is instituted. A pelvic examination should be performed to determine the location of the infection. If purulent material can be aspirated directly from the vaginal cuff, it should be cultured for aerobic and anaerobic bacteria. If there is a suggestion of a pelvic mass, ultrasonography may be a helpful diagnostic tool to determine whether there is a fluid-filled mass in the pelvis. Several antimicrobials have been successfully employed in patients with pelvic cellulitis. These include the newer cephalosporins and penicillins, tetracyclines, or clindamycin and an aminoglycoside. If there is evidence of a widespread infection on the initial examination or if the patient shows no response after 48 to 72 hours of the initial therapy, then metronidazole should be added to the regimen for coverage of *B. fragilis.*

If the patient continues a febrile course after antibiotics effective against *B. fragilis* have been given, then the possibility of either septic pelvic thrombophlebitis or a pelvic abscess should be considered. There are no specific diagnostic techniques to confirm the presence of septic pelvic thrombophlebitis, but a tentative diagnosis can be made if the patient has a persistent fever and no evidence of a pelvic mass. Such a patient should be treated with intravenous heparin by continuous pump infusion; dosage should be determined by pretreatment and intratreatment coagulation studies. The continuous infusion method should be employed instead of intermittent bolus therapy because it decreases the risk of serious bleeding in these postoperative patients. In the patient who remains febrile after 36 to 48 hours of heparin therapy or who has a pelvic mass, the diagnosis to be considered is a pelvic abscess. Operative drainage or removal is indicated.

Abdominal Wound Infections

The drainage of an infected abdominal wound not only is a distressing psychologic event for a patient, but also prolongs her stay in the hospital. A serious infection with synergistic bacteria may result in necrotizing fasciitis and death, while badly infected abdominal wounds may progress to dehiscence and evisceration. This serious problem of abdominal wound infection requires knowledge of techniques of prevention as well as a reasoned clinical approach.

Methods of prevention have been detailed by Cruse and Ford, whose studies have implicated a series of pre- and intraoperative rituals with an increase in the abdominal wound infection rate. They showed that a prolonged preoperative stay in the hospital, shaving the incision site the day before the operation instead of the day of the operation, and using an electrocautery knife, plastic wound drapes instead of towels, and a wound drain through the abdominal wound all resulted in a higher than normal number of postoperative wound infections. Elimination of these factors, as well as other preventive techniques, may decrease the number of abdominal wall infections. In the very obese patient or the patient with massive intraoperative bacterial contamination, delayed primary closure of the wound with reapproximation of the subcutaneous tissue and skin three days after the operation has been associated with a low abdominal wound infection rate. Another variation in preventive care of the massively obese woman who requires laparotomy has been the use of closed-suction drainage of the wound site, with the drainage tube exiting away from the operative incision.

Despite all of these attempts to prevent operative site infections, some abdominal wound problems are seen. The first task of the physician attending a woman with an infected abdominal wound is to establish drainage and determine that the fascial incision is intact. Careful assessment is necessary to be certain that the drainage is not secondary to an evisceration, rather than to the supposed infection. Antibiotics are rarely needed for the treatment of an abdominal wound infection, but they should be prescribed whenever inflammation of the skin appears to be spreading. Since a coagulase-positive *Staphylococcus* may be involved in this event, the use of a cephalosporin is preferable to the use of a penicillin in these women. Women with evidence of skin inflammation should be carefully monitored because rapid spread may denote a necrotizing fasciitis that necessitates operative debridement for cure.

Superficial Thrombophlebitis of the Upper Extremity

The long-term use of intravenous infusion lines is responsible for a relatively new syndrome, superficial thrombophlebitis of the upper extremity, which may give rise to fever on the third postoperative day. A simple preventive measure is prohibition of the use of intravenous infusion lines for longer than 48 hours after surgery.

ANTIBIOTICS

The basic judgment every physician must make when prescribing a drug is whether the benefits of the agent outweigh its dangers. To make an intelligent choice among antibiotics, a physician must know the antibacterial spectrum of activity, the organisms most frequently involved in the infection to be treated, the appropriate route of administration, and the toxicity of the drugs.

The Penicillins

The penicillins are still the most valuable single group of antibiotics. Because of the vast difference between therapeutic levels and toxic levels, these antibiotics have a wide range of safety. In addition, they have not been specifically prohibited from use in obstetric patients. Also, they are the drugs of choice for the treatment of infections due to *N. gonorrhoeae* and *Treponema pallidum*. One of the great developments in applied research has been the discovery of new congeners of penicillin that have broadened its spectrum of activity. Penicillin G is primarily effective against gram-positive aerobes, although it has some gram-negative aerobic rod coverage when very high doses are given intravenously. Problems with penicillin-resistant coagulase-positive staphylococci have been largely eliminated by the introduction of the new semisynthetic penicillin. The introduction of ampicillin in the early 1960s provided better coverage of gram-negative aerobes, and the later development of carbenicillin, ticarcillin, piperacillin, and mezlocillin improved the coverage of *Pseudomonas aeruginosa*. All of the penicillins are effective against anaerobes. This broad spectrum of activity makes the various penicillins attractive as therapy for the obstetric–gynecologic patient with a bacterial infection.

The penicillins are versatile drugs because of the varied routes of administration that can be used. The intravenous route should be used for the hospitalized patient with an infection, although intramuscular therapy can be used for either an inpatient or an outpatient. The oral forms of penicillin are especially helpful for the patient who requires prolonged outpatient therapy. They have not been shown to be more effective than either the sulfa drugs or nitrofurantoins in the treatment of lower urinary tract infections, however, and the nitrofurantoins remain the drugs of choice for this condition because they have a more limited effect on bowel flora than does ampicillin.

There are a number of toxic reactions to penicillin. Such reactions may be allergic, or they may be directly related to toxic effects of the drugs. The allergic reactions are most easily categorized as either immediate or late. Immediate reactions, *i.e.*, anaphylaxis, are the most feared, for they can result in the death of the patient. Late reactions, such as a maculopapular eruption, are not life threatening, but they prolong the patient's discomfort and distress. Ampicillin is the penicillin that is most likely to produce these late-appearing skin eruptions, although such reactions are usually related to some substance in the ampicillin other than the penicillin molecule itself.

The toxic reactions to penicillin vary with the form employed. Very high doses of intravenous penicillin, in excess of 40 million units per day, may produce very high serum levels in elderly patients with reduced renal function and may result in convulsions because of the increased excitability of the central nervous system in these patients. Intravenous methicillin may result in nephropathy. Ampicillin caused fatal pseudomembranous enterocolitis in one patient following abdominal hysterectomy. The high dosages of intravenous carbenicillin therapy can be associated with many serious side-effects. The huge sodium load with these megadoses may be poorly tolerated by a cardiac patient. Hypokalemia can occur in up to 20% of women who have received a high dosage of intravenous carbenicillin therapy. In addition, carbenicillin affects platelets, and administration of the drug may be accompanied by unexpected bleeding. The physician must be aware of these side-effects and be on the alert for their appearance.

The Cephalosporins

Although introduced primarily as alternative bactericidal antibiotics for the penicillin-allergic patient, the cephalosporins have been widely used by obstetrician–gynecologists as primary therapeutic agents. There are a number of reasons for this popularity. The cephalosporins have a broad spectrum of antibacterial activity, similar in many respects to that of the penicillins. They are effective against the coagulase-positive *Staphylococcus* and all gram-positive aerobes except the enterococci. They are also effective against gram-negative aerobes, especially *Klebsiella,* which is often resistant to ampicillin, but they have not been effective against *P. aeruginosa.* Against the anaerobes, their action is very similar to that of penicillin, but they are much less effective against *B. fragilis* than is carbenicillin. These are versatile drugs, for they can be given intravenously, intramuscularly, and orally. The oral form has no advantages over sulfa or nitrofurantoin in the treatment of urinary tract infection. Despite these favorable activities, potential toxicity prevents the cephalosporins from being the drugs of choice for single infections in obstetrics–gynecology if other drugs are appropriate. Cephalosporins are commonly prescribed as prophylaxis in elective pelvic operations.

Second and third generations of cephalosporins have been approved by the Food and Drug Administration (FDA). In general, these provide broader coverage of gram-negative aerobic organisms. Cefoxitin, a cephamycin, has the distinct advantage of good activity against *B. fragilis* and is similarly effective in the treatment of soft tissue infections. It is unique among the cephalosporins currently available because of its activity against *B. fragilis.* Clinical studies of patients with soft tissue pelvic infections have demonstrated a high degree of effectiveness.

Despite clinicians' widespread interest in the cephalosporins, there can be toxic side-effects. Immediate reactions can occur, and death due to cardiovascular collapse after the intravenous administration of a cephalosporin has been reported. Anaphylaxis is a possibility, and there is danger of cross-reactivity in the woman with a history of penicillin anaphylaxis. Late reactions range from a mild allergic skin reaction to death from pseudomembranous enterocolitis, probably from alterations in the bacterial flora of the gut. Renal toxicity has been reported, particularly with cephaloridine, but all of the cephalosporins have this potential, especially when used in combination with aminoglycosides.

The Aminoglycosides

A valuable family of antibiotics for the obstetrician–gynecologist, aminoglycosides are highly effective against gram-negative aerobes, particularly the more resistant ones found in hospitalized patients. This is really the sole reason for their use. However, their use presents many problems. They are the least versatile of the classes of antibiotics discussed thus far because they can be given only intravenously and intramuscularly. In addition, the range between therapeutic levels and toxicity both to the eighth cranial nerve and to the kidney is quite narrow. Predictions of serum levels based on the patient's weight are not always accurate, and up to 40% of young women have subtherapeutic levels with standard dosing. To avoid serum levels so high that toxicity results or so low that therapy is ineffective, peak and trough levels should be obtained in patients undergoing a therapeutic course. These complicated safeguards make it necessary to limit the use of aminoglycosides to seriously ill, hospitalized patients.

TREATMENT OF SOFT TISSUE INFECTIONS

An awareness of the importance of anaerobes, particularly *B. fragilis,* in pelvic infections has led to the use of many agents, some unfamiliar, in the treatment of soft tissue infections.

The tetracyclines are a unique group of antibiotics. They are the drugs of choice for only a few exotic infections, but they are second-line drugs for many common obstetric–gynecologic infections. Because of their toxicity to pregnant women when given intravenously for pyelonephritis, with maternal death from fatty liver, they are contraindicated in pregnancy. In the laboratory, the newer tetracyclines are more active against all anaerobic strains than is standard tetracycline. In addition, all of these agents are highly effective against *Chlamydia.* Because of these factors, the most frequent infection to be treated with tetracycline is nongonococcal salpingitis. Generally, the therapeutic results have been favorable in this population.

Clindamycin is one of the most popular drugs for the treatment of anaerobic infections, particularly those due to *B. fragilis*. It is highly effective and can be administered intravenously or orally. There are problems related to the use of this drug, however, particularly in the gastrointestinal tract, where pseudomembranous enterocolitis can develop. The cause of this reaction has now been determined. The enterocolitis is caused by a specific strain of *Clostridium difficile,* which is resistant to clindamycin and produces an enterotoxin. This strain of clostridia is susceptible to vancomycin, and it is hoped that treatment with vancomycin will diminish the severity of the gastrointestinal effects of clindamycin. It is important for the physician prescribing clindamycin to be alert to any changes in the patient's gastrointestinal function. Consequently, every patient taking the drug should make a daily record of her bowel movements. If she has more than five, the drug should be stopped, and in this way, progression of the gastrointestinal difficulties may be halted. If diarrhea persists, then sigmoidoscopy should be performed.

Chloramphenicol is a valuable drug for the treatment of anaerobic infections. It is highly effective against anaerobes involved in pelvic infections, particularly *B. fragilis*. Since there is no evidence that chloramphenicol is superior to clindamycin in serious pelvic infections, the decision regarding which drug to use must be based on the physician's concern about the toxicity of the two agents. An occasional patient, somewhere between 1 in 20,000 and 1 in 100,000 of those receiving chloramphenicol, will develop an aplastic anemia that may be fatal. This complication is not dose dependent and cannot be prevented by pretreatment laboratory screening. This rare event is devastating when it occurs. Although it does not absolutely prevent the problem, intravenous chloramphenicol for the total length of therapy is preferable because it appears to be associated with a lower incidence of aplastic anemia than oral chloramphenicol. This complication is rare, but its severity has led many physicians to use clindamycin in all patients except those with preexisting gastrointestinal difficulties.

Metronidazole is another effective anaerobic antibiotic. It is the most bactericidal to *B. fragilis* of any agent in the laboratory, and it has been successfully employed clinically in soft tissue pelvic infections. The drug shows great promise, and the intravenous form has been well tolerated in clinical studies. Metronidazole also presents problems, however. It should be used with other antibiotics, since an increasing number of gram-positive anaerobes show resistance to it; its lack of activity against gram-negative aerobes means that a second and third antibiotic will be necessary for the treatment of seriously ill patients. In addition, although this has not been demonstrated to date in humans, the drug is carcinogenic in animals and mutagenic for bacteria. These are disturbing findings that mandate continued observation of women who have received the drug in the past.

REFERENCES AND RECOMMENDED READING

Bartlett JG, Chang TW, Taylor NS et al: Colitis induced by *Clostridium difficile*. Rev Infect Dis 1:370, 1979

Burkman RT, Tonascia JA, Atienza MG et al: Untreated endocervical gonorrhea and endometritis following elective abortion. Am J Obstet Gynecol 126:648, 1976

Chow AW, Marshall JR, Guze LB: A double-blind comparison of clindamycin with penicillin plus chloramphenicol in treatment of septic abortion. J Infect Dis 135:535, 1977

Collins CG, Nix FG, Cerha HT: Ruptured tubo-ovarian abscess. Am J Obstet Gynecol 72:820, 1956

Cruse PJF, Ford R: A five-year prospective study of 23,649 surgical wounds. Arch Surg 107:206, 1973

Cunningham FG, Hauth JG, Strong JD et al: Tetracycline or penicillin–ampicillin for pelvic inflammatory disease. N Engl J Med 296:1380, 1977

Dawood MY, Birnbaum SJ: Unilateral tubo-ovarian abscess and an intrauterine contraceptive device. Obstet Gynecol 46:429, 1975

Dineen P, Druzin L: Epidemics of postoperative wound infections associated with hair carriers. Lancet 2:1157, 1973

DiZerega G, Yonekura L, Roy S et al: A comparison of clindamycin–gentamicin and penicillin–gentamicin in the treatment of post–cesarean section endometritis. Am J Obstet Gynecol 134:238, 1979

Eschenbach DA, Harnisch JP, Holmes KK: Pathogenesis of acute pelvic inflammatory disease: Role of contraception and other risk factors. Am J Obstet Gynecol 128:838, 1977

Falk V: Treatment of acute non-tuberculous salpingitis with antibiotics alone and in combination with glucocorticoids. Acta Obstet Gynecol Scand (Suppl 6) 44, 1965

Gibbs RS, Jones PM, Wilder CJ: Antibiotic therapy of endometritis following cesarean section. Obstet Gynecol 52:31, 1978

Gibbs RS, Listria HM, Read JA: The effect of internal fetal monitoring on maternal infection following cesarean section. Obstet Gynecol 48:653, 1976

Gibbs RS, Weinstein AJ: Bacteriologic effects of prophylactic antibiotics in cesarean section. Am J Obstet Gynecol 126:226, 1976

Golde SH, Israel F, Ledger WJ: Unilateral tubo-ovarian abscess: A distinct entity. Am J Obstet Gynecol 127:807, 1977

Goldman P: Drug therapy: Metronidazole. N Engl J Med 303:1212, 1980

Gorbach SL, Thadepalli H: Clindamycin in the treatment of pure and mixed anaerobic infections. Arch Intern Med 134:87, 1974

Gordon HR, Phelps D, Blanchard K: Prophylactic cesarean section antibiotics: Maternal and neonatal morbidity before and after cord clamping. Obstet Gynecol 53:151, 1979

Hagen D: Maternal febrile morbidity associated with fetal monitoring and cesarean section. Obstet Gynecol 46:269, 1973

Hawkins DF, Levitt LH, Fairbrother PF et al: Management of septic chemical abortion with renal failure: Use of a conservative regimen. N Engl J Med 282:722, 1975

Kaplan AL, Jacobs WM, Ehresman JB: Aggressive management of pelvic abscess. Am J Obstet Gynecol 98:482, 1967

Kunin CM, McCormack RC: Prevention of catheter-induced urinary tract infection by closed sterile drainage. N Engl J Med 274:1155, 1966

Ledger WJ: Anaerobic infection. Am J Obstet Gynecol 123:111, 1975

Ledger WJ, Gee CL, Lewis WP: Bacteremia on an obstetric–gynecological service. Am J Obstet Gynecol 121:205, 1975

Ledger WJ, Gee C, Lewis WP: Guidelines for antibiotic prophylaxis in gynecology. Am J Obstet Gynecol 121:1038, 1970

Ledger WJ, Gee CL, Lewis WP et al: Comparison of clindamycin and chloramphenicol in treatment of serious infections of the female genital tract. J Infect Dis 135:530, 1977

Ledger WJ, Gee CL, Pollin P et al: The use of pre-reduced media and a portable jar for the collection of anaerobic organisms from clinical sites of infection. Am J Obstet Gynecol 125:677, 1976

Ledger WJ, Kriewall TJ, Gee C: The fever index: A technique for evaluating the clinical response to bacteremia. Obstet Gynecol 45:603, 1975

Ledger WJ, Lewis W, Golde S et al: The use of metronidazole in obstetric and gynecologic infections. Proceedings of the International Metronidazole Conference, Montreal, Canada, p 356. Excerpta Medica, 1976

Ledger WJ, Moore DE, Lowensohn RI et al: A fever index evaluation of chloramphenicol or clindamycin in patients with serious pelvic infections. Obstet Gynecol 50:523, 1977

Ledger WJ, Sweet RL, Headington JT: The prophylactic use of cephaloridine in the prevention of pelvic infection in premenopausal women undergoing vaginal hysterectomy. Am J Obstet Gynecol 115:776, 1973

Mardh PA, Ingerselv HJ et al: Endometritis caused by *Chlamydia trachomatis.* Brit J Ven Dis 57:191, 1981

Mardh PA, Ripa T, Svensson L et al: Role of *Chlamydia trachomatis* infection in acute salpingitis. N Engl J Med 296:1377, 1977

Monif GRG, Welkos SL, Baer H et al: Cul de sac isolates from patients with endometritis–salpingitis–peritonitis and gonococcal endocervicitis. Am J Obstet Gynecol 126:158, 1976

Morrow PJ, Hernandez WL, Townsend DE et al: Pelvic celiotomy in the obese patient. Am J Obstet Gynecol 127:335, 1977

Onderdonk AB, Kasper DL, Cisneras RL et al: The capsular polysaccharide of *Bacteroides fragilis* as a virulence factor: Comparison of the pathogenic potential of encapsulated and unencapsulated strains. J Infect Dis 136:82, 1977

O'Neill RT, Schwarz RH: Clostridial organisms in septic abortions. Obstet Gynecol 35:458, 1970

Osborne NG, Wright RC, Dubay M: Pre-operative hot conization of the cervix. Am J Obstet Gynecol 133:374, 1979

Rotheram EB, Schick SF: Non-clostridial anaerobic bacteria in septic abortion. Am J Med 46:80, 1969

Rudd EG, Long WH, Dillon MB: Febrile morbidity following cefamanadole nafate intrauterine irrigation during cesarean section. Amer J Obstet Gynecol 141:12, 1981

Schultz JC, Adamson JS, Workman WW et al: Fatal liver disease after intravenous administration of tetracycline in high dose. N Engl J Med 269:499, 1963

Sen P, Apuzzio J, Reyelt C et al: Prospective evaluation of combination of antimicrobial agents in cesarean section endometritis. Surg Obstet Gynecol 151:89, 1980

Simpson FF: The choice of time for operation for pelvic inflammation of tubal origin. Surg Gynecol Obstet 9:45, 1909

Spaulding LB, Gelman SR, Wood SO et al: The role of ultrasonography in the management of endometritis/salpingitis/peritonitis. Obstet Gynecol 53:442, 1979

Spruill FG, Minelte LJ, Stumer WC: Two surgical deaths associated with cephalothin. JAMA 229:440, 1974

Subbagha RE, Hyashi TT: Disseminated intravascular coagulation complicating hysterectomy in elderly gravidas. Obstet Gynecol 38:844, 1971

Swartz WH, Tanaree P: Suction drainage as an alternative to prophylactic antibiotics for hysterectomy. Obstet Gynecol 45:305, 1975

Sweet RL, Ledger WJ: Cephoxitin: Single-agent treatment of mixed aerobic–anaerobic pelvic infections. Obstet Gynecol 54:193, 1979

Sweet RL, Mills J, Hadley MK et al: Use of laparoscopy to determine the microbiologic etiology of acute salpingitis. Am J Obstet Gynecol 134:69, 1979

Weinstein WM, Onderdonk AB, Bartlett JG: Antimicrobial therapy of experimental sepsis. J Infect Dis 132:282, 1975

Weinstein WM, Onderdonk AB, Bartlett JG et al: Experimental intra-abdominal abscesses in rats: Development of an experimental model. Infect Immun 10:1250, 1974

Westrom L: Effects of acute pelvic inflammatory disease on fertility. Am J Obstet Gynecol 121:707, 1975

Westrom L, Bengtsson LP, Mardh PA: The risk of pelvic inflammatory disease in women using intra-uterine contraception devices as compared to non-users. Lancet 2:221, 1976

Wong R, Gee CL, Ledger WJ: Prophylactic use of cefazolin in monitored obstetric patients undergoing cesarean section. Obstet Gynecol 51:407, 1978

Zashe DE, Cipolle RJ, Strate RG, Malo JW, Koszalka MF, Jr: Rapid gentamicin elimination in obstetric patients. Obstet Gynecol 56:559, 1982

Control of Human Reproduction: Contraception, Sterilization, and Pregnancy Termination

Daniel R. Mishell, Jr.

14

The term *family planning* implies that the birth of each child is planned and desired by the parents. To prevent unplanned or unwanted children, couples can use *contraception* (the temporary avoidance of pregnancy), *sterilization* (the permanent prevention of pregnancy), or *induced abortion* (voluntary evacuation of the fetus from the uterus before it has attained viability).

An ideal method of contraception has not yet been developed. All existing contraceptive techniques have advantages and disadvantages. Therefore, the physician's advice about contraception should include an explanation of the advantages and disadvantages of each method so that the patient is fully informed and can rationally choose the method most suitable for her. If there are medical reasons for not using certain methods, the physician should inform the patient and offer her alternatives. Except for the condom, no acceptable method has been developed for use by the male. Therefore, the physician usually discusses contraceptive methods with the female partner.

CONTRACEPTIVE USE

The use of contraceptives has steadily increased in the United States since 1960. By 1982, of the 55 million women in the United States aged 15 to 44, about 19 million had never been pregnant, and of the remaining 36 million women, all but 3 million were using a method of contraception. The most frequently used methods to prevent conception were male and female sterilization. Of the nonsurgical methods of contraception, oral contraceptives were most popular, followed by the condom, IUD, spermicides, diaphragm, withdrawal, and rhythm (Table 14-1). Overall, of women practicing contraception, 27% used oral contraception, this method's greatest popularity being among women under 30; of women under 25 using contraception in 1982, almost half (48%)

used oral contraception. For women over 35, the condom was the most popular method of nonsurgical contraception. Overall, 8% of women exposed to the risk of unwanted pregnancy (more than 3 million women in the United States) did not practice any form of contraception.

The use of sterilization increased from 7.8% in 1965 to 18.6% in 1976 among married U.S. women, and by 1982 to 21% among all U.S. women aged 15 to 44. Oral contraceptive use among all married couples in the United States aged 15 to 44 increased from 15.3% in 1965 to a high of 25.1% in 1973 and then declined to 22.5% in 1976. In 1975 U.S. pharmacy purchases of oral contraceptives began declining; by 1982 oral contraceptives were used by only 18% of all U.S. women in this age group. Likewise, use of the IUD increased from 0.7% in 1965 to 6.7% in 1973 and then declined to 6.3% in 1976 among married women and to 4% by 1982 among all U.S. women aged 15 to 44. Thus, since 1976 use of sterilization and of the less effective barrier methods of contraception has increased, while use of the two most effective nonsurgical methods of contraception has declined.

CONTRACEPTIVE EFFECTIVENESS

It is difficult to determine the effectiveness of various methods of contraception because of the large number of factors that affect contraceptive failure. The terms *method effectiveness* and *use effectiveness* (or *method failure* and *patient failure*) have been used to differentiate between conception occurring with correct use (method failure) and conception occurring with incorrect use (patient failure) of the contraceptive method. In general, methods that are used at the time of coitus, such as the diaphragm, condom, foam, rhythm, and withdrawal, have much greater method effectiveness

231

Table 14-1

Exposure to the Risk of Unintended Pregnancy and Method of Contraception Currently Used in U.S. Women Aged 15 to 44

Exposure to Risk	Number (in 000s)	Percentage
Exposed and using a method	33,425	61
Sterilization	11,643	21
Tubal	(6783)	(12)
Vasectomy	(4860)	(9)
Pill	9996	18
IUD	2307	4
Condom	4475	8
Spermicide	1463	3
Diaphragm	1908	3
Withdrawal	930	2
Rhythm	553	1
Douche and other	150	*
Exposed and not using a method	3053	6
Not exposed	18,137	33
Total	54,615	100

* Less than 0.5%.

(Forrest JD, Henshaw SK: What U.S. women think and do about contraception. Fam Plann Perspect 15:162, 1983)

than use effectiveness. With methods in which coitus-related activities are not required, such as oral contraceptives and the IUD, there is less of a difference between method effectiveness and use effectiveness, so that the overall effectiveness of these methods is greater than that of coitus-related methods.

The overall value of a contraceptive method as used by a couple (correctly or incorrectly) is determined by calculation of actual effectiveness as well as by the continuation rate. Actuarial methods such as the log-rank life table method, not the less accurate Pearl index, should be used to determine these rates. Even with the use of these excellent statistical techniques, however, it is difficult to determine the effectiveness of the various methods in actual practice. Most studies undertaken to determine effectiveness of a contraceptive method are carefully controlled clinical trials during which frequent contact with supportive clinic personnel results in lower failure rates and higher continuation rates than occur in actual use in the field. Furthermore, these clinical trials are infrequently performed in a comparative, randomized manner, so clinicians cannot compare the results of a trial of one type of contraceptive method with the results of a trial of another type. In addition, failure rates of prospective studies are consistently lower than those of retrospective interview studies.

Several factors influence contraceptive failure rates. One of the most important is motivation of the couple. Contraceptive failure, especially for coitus-related

methods, is more likely to occur among couples seeking to delay a wanted pregnancy than among couples seeking to prevent pregnancy altogether. Age of the woman has a strong negative correlation with failure of a contraceptive method, as do socioeconomic class and level of education. Thus, many variables must be considered in an evaluation of the effectiveness of any method of contraception for an individual patient.

First-year failure rates according to data obtained from questionnaires used in the 1973 and 1976 National Surveys of Family Growth were lowest for oral contraceptives, 2.5%, and highest for rhythm, 18.8% (Table 14-2). With all methods, failure rates were lower among women wishing to prevent a pregnancy than among women wishing to delay a pregnancy, lower among women aged 35 to 44 (1.4%) than among women aged 15 to 24 (10.7%), and inversely related to education and income (socioeconomic class). The least variation in failure rates occurred with oral contraceptives, and the greatest with rhythm. Theoretically, the method failure rate should be the lowest failure rate found in the subgroup of women who wish to prevent a pregnancy, have the highest income, and are over 30. In this group the first-year failure rates were 0.8% for oral contraceptives and 1.5% for the IUD. Further data from these surveys indicate that one-year continuation rates for the various contraceptive methods were highest for the IUD and oral contraceptives and lowest for the diaphragm, condom, and spermicides.

VAGINAL FOAMS, CREAMS, AND SUPPOSITORIES

Vaginal foams, creams, and suppositories all contain a spermicidal ingredient, usually nonoxynol 9, that im-

Table 14-2

Contraceptive Failure During the First Year of Use in Married Women Aged 15 to 44, United States, 1970–1975

Contraceptive Method	All Women	Women over 30 with Annual Income >$15,000 Wishing to Prevent Pregnancy
Sterilization	0	0
Pill	2.5	0.8
IUD	4.8	1.5
Condom	9.6	0.9
Diaphragm	14.4	6.4
Foam, cream, jelly, suppository	17.7	6.1
Rhythm	18.8	8.3
Other	11.5	4

(Data from Grady WR, Hirsch MB, Keen N, Vaughan B: Contraceptive failure and continuation among married women in the U.S., 1970–75. Stud Fam Plann 14:9, 1983; Schirm AL, Trussell J, Menken J, Grady WR: Contraceptive failure in the United States: The impact of social, economic and demographic factors. Fam Plan Perspect 14:68, 1982)

mobilizes or kills sperm on contact; they also provide a mechanical barrier to sperm and therefore need to be placed into the vagina before coitus. There are no data comparing the efficiency of the various types of vaginal spermicides, but as noted above, their effectiveness increases with age of the user and is similar to that of the diaphragm for all age and income groups. The increased effectiveness of vaginal spermicides in older women is probably due to increased motivation. Furthermore, acts of coitus are more likely to be less spontaneous and to occur less frequently in older than in younger women, making spermicides easier to use. A spermicide-treated vaginal sponge, which was recently approved for use in the United States, can be left in place for 24 hours and therefore does not need to be inserted before each coital act. However, in clinical trials it has been associated with slightly higher failure rates than the diaphragm. Although two studies have indicated that contraceptive failure with spermicides may be associated with a higher than normal incidence of congenital malformations, this finding has not been confirmed by numerous other studies.

DIAPHRAGM

The diaphragm must be carefully fitted by the physician or nursing personnel. The largest size that does not cause discomfort or undue pressure on the vaginal epithelium should be used. After the fitting, the patient should remove the diaphragm and reinsert it herself. She should then be examined to make sure the diaphragm is covering the cervix. When the woman is wearing the diaphragm, she should not be aware of its presence or have any discomfort. The diaphragm should be used with contraceptive cream or jelly and should be left in place for at least 8 hours after the last coital act.

Data from the Oxford Family Planning Association Study indicate that among women who use a diaphragm successfully for at least several months, it is very effective. In this study of married women over 25 who had been using a diaphragm for at least five months, the failure rate was only 2.4/100 woman-years. Therefore, prospective new users should be informed that the diaphragm is an effective method of contraception after the first few months of use.

CERVICAL CAP

Various types of plastic and rubber devices that are cup-shaped and fit around the cervix have been used as barrier contraceptives for decades, mainly in Britain and Europe. Each type of device is manufactured in different sizes and should be fitted to the cervix by a clinician. The cervical cap should not be left in place more than 72 hours because of possible problems of ulceration, odor, and infection. Although these devices are not currently approved for general use in the United States,

they are a popular method of contraception among a segment of the population. Clinical trials with cervical caps among motivated women report first-year failure rates of about 9%.

CONDOM

The use of condoms should be encouraged among individuals with multiple sexual partners, since this method of contraception is most effective in preventing transmission of sexually transmitted disease. The condom should not be applied tightly. The tip should extend beyond the end of the penis by about 0.5 inches to collect the ejaculate. Care must be taken upon withdrawal not to spill the ejaculate. In the Oxford Family Planning Study, all condom users had previously used another method, mainly oral contraception. During 12,497 woman-years of exposure, 449 unplanned pregnancies occurred for a use-pregnancy rate of 3.6/100 woman-years. The pregnancy rate increased linearly over time. This study is one of the largest for which findings have been published, and the results are consistent with those of several older studies, which show a similar high level of effectiveness for the condom when used by couples with enough motivation for the wife to attend a family planning clinic. In the U.S. survey discussed above, the first-year condom failure rate was only 0.9% among women over 30 who wanted to prevent further pregnancies and had an annual income of more than $15,000.

RHYTHM

The Roman Catholic church officially proscribes all methods of contraception other than rhythm, or periodic abstinence. The rationale for the rhythm method is based on three assumptions: first, the human ovum is capable of being fertilized for only about 24 hours after ovulation; second, spermatozoa can retain their fertilizing ability for only 48 hours after coitus, and finally, ovulation usually occurs 12 to 16 days (14 ± 2 days) before the onset of the subsequent menses. The woman who is going to use the rhythm method should first record the length of her cycles for several months and then establish her fertile period by subtracting 18 days from the length of her shortest cycle and 11 days from the length of her longest cycle. Then, in each subsequent cycle, the couple abstains from coitus during this calculated fertile period.

The use effectiveness of this calendar method of periodic abstinence is poor. Failure rates have been reported to vary between 21 to 47 per 100 woman-years. In the U.S. surveys, the first-year failure rate of the rhythm method was 18.8%. The reasons for this lack of success as summarized by Mastroianni are numerous, despite advances in knowledge of human reproductive physiology. First, there is no good evidence that the three assumptions on which the rhythm method is based have scientific validity. Second, there is great irregularity in menstrual cycle length, so that women with normally regular cycles occasionally show marked variation in cycle length. Cycle irregularity is particularly common in perimenarchal and perimenopausal women, two groups among whom most pregnancies are unwanted. Third, because a woman is menstruating during several of the nonfertile days of her cycle and most couples do not have coitus during this time, the period of abstinence is frequently longer than the time during which sexual relations may be practiced.

To increase the effectiveness of the rhythm method, instead of relying solely on the calendar method described above, it is advisable also to measure one's basal body temperature every day. Ovulation is associated with an increase in progesterone levels, which in turn causes an increase in basal body temperature. If the couple abstains from intercourse from the start of menses until at least 48 hours after the rise in basal body temperature (two days after ovulation), sexual relations will take place only after the ovum is no longer capable of being fertilized. Data from several sources indicate that the use of daily basal temperature for determining the days of periodic abstinence increases the effectiveness of the rhythm method. One British study reported a failure rate of only 6.6 per 100 woman-years among women practicing the temperature method for determining the time of periodic abstinence.

Recently there have been reports that women can detect changes in the quality and quantity of their own cervical mucus and can be taught to use these changes to predict the time of ovulation. Although enthusiasts have reported extraordinary success with this method, careful analysis of their results suggests that the actual effectiveness of this modification is substantially less than claimed.

Thus, periodic abstinence, or the rhythm method, requires a high degree of motivation, communication, and sophistication. Even with these qualities, the rhythm method of family planning is associated with a high failure rate.

ORAL STEROIDS

There were originally three major types of oral steroid contraceptive formulation: combination, sequential, and daily gestagen. The combination is the most widely used and the most effective type. It consists of tablets containing both an estrogen and a gestagen given continuously for 3 weeks. The original sequential type, which is no longer marketed, consisted of a regimen of estrogen alone given for about 2 weeks followed by a combination of estrogen and gestagen given for 1 week. Recently, combination formulations that contain two or three different amounts of the same estrogen and gestagen have been marketed. Each of the tablets containing one of these various dosages is given for intervals varying from 7 to 11 days during the 21-day medication period.

These formulations have been described as biphasic or triphasic and are generally known as multiphasic. The idea behind this type of formulation is to administer a low total dose of steroid without increasing the incidence of breakthrough bleeding. With combination oral contraceptives, usually no pills are taken for 1 week out of 4 to allow withdrawal bleeding to occur. The third type of contraceptive formulation consists of a tablet of gestagen without any estrogen. This formulation is ingested daily without a steroid-free interval.

Pharmacology

Oral contraceptives presently being used are formulated from synthetic steroids and do not contain natural estrogens or gestagens. There are two major types of synthetic gestagens: (1) derivatives of 19-nortestosterone and (2) derivatives of 17α-acetoxyprogesterone. The latter group are C-21 gestagens, consisting of steroids such as medroxyprogesterone acetate and megestrol acetate; they are not used in present contraceptive formulations. In contrast to 19-nortestosterone derivatives, C-21 gestagens have been associated with a higher than normal incidence of mammary cancer when given in high doses to female beagle dogs. Because of this carcinogenic effect, contraceptives with these gestagens are not marketed. All oral contraceptive formulations now available in the United States consist of varying dosages of one of the following five 19-nortestosterone gestagens: norethynodrel, norethindrone, norethindrone acetate, ethynodiol diacetate, and norgestrel (Fig. 14-1). With the exception of two daily gestagen formulations, the gestagens are combined with varying dosages of two estrogens, ethinyl estradiol and ethinyl estradiol-3-methyl ether (also known as *mestranol*) (Fig. 14-2). All the synthetic estrogens and gestagens in oral contraceptives have an ethinyl group on the 17 position. The presence of this ethinyl group enhances the oral activity of these agents, causing their essential functional groups to be more slowly hydroxylated and conjugated as they pass through the liver by way of the portal system than the essential functional groups of orally ingested natural sex steroids. The synthetic steroids thus have greater potency per unit weight than the natural steroids when both are ingested orally.

The differences in chemical structure of the different synthetic gestagens and estrogens also alter their biologic activity. Therefore, one cannot compare the pharmacologic activities of the various gestagens or estrogens present in a particular contraceptive only on the basis of the amount of steroid present in the formulation. The biologic activity of each steroid must also be considered. Established tests for progestational activity in animals have revealed that an equivalent weight of norgestrel is several-fold more potent than the same weight of norethindrone. Studies in humans using delay of menses as an end point, or endometrial histologic alterations such as subnuclear vacuolization, also conclude that

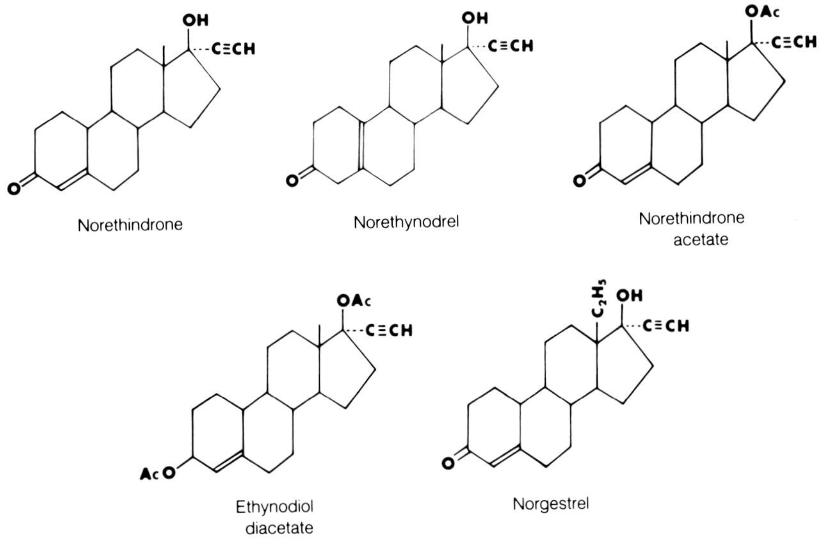

FIG. 14-1. Formulas of the five gestagens used in combination oral contraceptives.

norgestrel is 3 to 5 times more potent than an equivalent weight of norethindrone. Norethindrone acetate and ethinyldiol diacetate are metabolized in the body to norethindrone. The human studies using the parameters of progestational activity described above, as well as other studies comparing the effects of steroids on serum lipids, indicate that all of these three gestagens have approximately equal potency per unit weight.

The two types of estrogenic compounds present in oral contraceptives, ethinyl estradiol and mestranol, also have different biologic activities in the human. Mestranol does not bind to estrogen cytosol receptors, so to become biologically effective, it has to be demethylated to ethinyl estradiol. The degree of conversion of mestranol to ethinyl estradiol varies among individuals; some are able to convert it completely, others convert only a portion of it. Thus, in some individuals a weight of mestranol is as potent as the same weight of ethinyl estradiol, whereas in others it is only about half as potent. With human endometrial response and effect on liver corticosteroid-binding globulin (CBG) production used as end points, it has been estimated that a quantity of ethinyl estradiol is about 1.7 times as potent as an equivalent weight of mestranol. Thus, it is important to evaluate the biologic activity as well as the quantity of steroid components when comparing the potency of various formulations.

Using radioimmunoassay, Brenner and colleagues measured daily serum levels of levonorgestrel, follicle-stimulating hormone (FSH), luteinizing hormone (LH), estradiol, and progesterone in three women taking combination oral contraceptives containing 500 μg dl-norgestrel and 50 μg ethinyl estradiol. Daily measurements were taken 3 hours after ingestion of the pill, as well as during the intervening pill-free interval, for two consecutive treatment cycles. Daily levels of levonorgestrel rose during the first few days of medication, plateaued thereafter, and declined after ingestion of the

last pill of the cycle (Fig. 14-3). Nevertheless, substantial amounts of levonorgestrel remained in the serum for at least the first three to four days after the last pill had been ingested. These levels of steroid were sufficient to suppress gonadotropin release, so that follicle maturation, as evidenced by low estradiol levels, did not occur during the pill-free interval. It seems reasonable to conclude from these data that accidental pregnancies during oral contraceptive therapy probably do not occur owing to failure to ingest one or two pills more than a few days after treatment is initiated but rather because initiation of the next cycle of medication is delayed for a few days, thus lengthening the pill-free interval sufficiently that pill protection is lost. Therefore, it is very important that the pill-free interval be limited to no more than 7 days. This is best accomplished by administration either of a placebo or of an iron pill daily during the steroid-free interval (the so-called 28-day package). If the 21-pill package is used, treatment should be started on the first Sunday after menses begins instead of the fifth day of the cycle. It is easier to remember to start each cycle on a Sunday than to have to calculate it anew each time. Patients should be warned that the most important pill not to forget to ingest is the first one.

FIG. 14-2. Formulas of the two estrogens used in combination oral contraceptives in the United States.

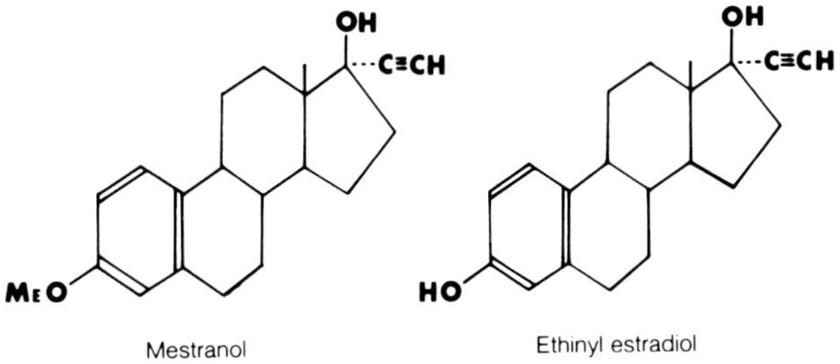

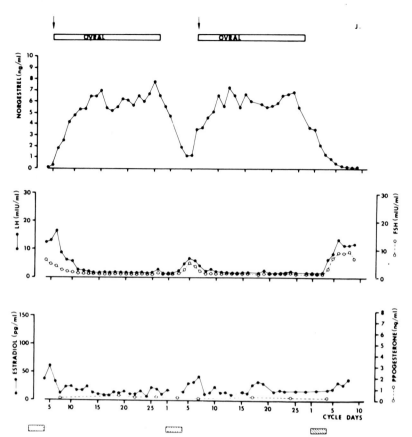

FIG. 14-3. Serum d-norgestrel, FSH, LH, estradiol, and progesterone levels in a subject during and following oral administration of 500 μg dl-norgestrel and 50 μg ethinyl estradiol for two subsequent 21-day periods interrupted by a pill-free interval of 6 days. (Brenner PF et al: Serum levels of d-norgestrel, luteinizing hormone, follicle-stimulating hormone, estradiol, and progesterone in women during and following ingestion of combination oral contraceptives containing dl-norgestrel. Am J Obstet Gynecol 129:133, 1977)

Physiology

Mechanism of Action

Combinations of estrogen and gestagen are the most effective type of oral contraceptive formulation; these preparations consistently inhibit the midcycle gonadotropin surge, thus preventing ovulation. These drugs act on other aspects of the reproductive process as well. They alter the cervical mucus, making it thick, viscid, and scanty in amount, which retards sperm penetration. They alter the motility of the uterus and oviduct, thus altering the transport of both ova and sperm. They also alter the endometrium, so that its glandular production of glycogen is diminished and less energy is available for the blastocyst to survive in the uterine cavity. Finally, they may alter ovarian responsiveness to gonadotropin stimulation. Nevertheless, neither gonadotropin production nor ovarian steroidogenesis is completely abolished, and levels of endogenous hormones in the peripheral blood during ingestion of combination oral contraceptives are similar to levels in the peripheral blood during the early follicular phase of the normal cycle.

The daily gestagen preparations without estrogen do not consistently inhibit ovulation, and their effectiveness is therefore significantly lower than that of the combination oral contraceptives. Because a low dose of gestagen is used in these formulations, it is important that they be ingested at the same time each day to ensure that blood levels do not fall below the contraceptive effective level.

Although no significant difference in clinical effectiveness has been demonstrated among the various combination formulations currently available in the United States (Table 14-3), the formulations containing only 20 μg ethinyl estradiol may be slightly less effective than the other preparations. Provided no tablets are omitted, the pregnancy rate with all combination formulations is less than 0.2% per year.

Metabolic Effects

Oral contraceptives have other metabolic effects in addition to their effects on the reproductive axis (Table 14-4). The incidence of adverse effects has steadily decreased as the dose of steroids in the formulations has decreased. Fortunately, in most instances these adverse effects have been relatively mild. The majority are produced by the estrogenic component of the formulation, while the rest are produced by the progestin component alone or by a combination of estrogen and progestin. The most frequent symptoms produced by the estro-

Table 14-3
Composition of Oral Contraceptives Currently Marketed in the United States

Product	Type	Progestin Content	Estrogen Content	Manufacturer
Brevicon	Combination	0.5 mg norethindrone	35 μg ethinyl estradiol	Syntex
Norinyl 1+35	Combination	1 mg norethindrone	35 μg ethinyl estradiol	Syntex
Norinyl 1+50	Combination	1 mg norethindrone	50 μg mestranol	Syntex
Norinyl 1+80	Combination	1 mg norethindrone	80 μg mestranol	Syntex
Norinyl 2	Combination	2 mg norethindrone	100 μg mestranol	Syntex
NOR-Q.D.	Progestin only	0.35 mg norethindrone		Syntex
Tri-Norinyl 7/	Combination-triphasic	0.5 mg norethindrone	35 μg ethinyl estradiol	Syntex
9/		1 mg norethindrone	35 μg ethinyl estradiol	Syntex
5/		0.5 mg norethindrone	35 μg ethinyl estradiol	Syntex
Demulen 1/35	Combination	1 mg ethynodiol diacetate	35 μg ethinyl estradiol	Searle
Demulen 1/50	Combination	1 mg ethynodiol diacetate	50 μg ethinyl estradiol	Searle
Ovulen	Combination	1 mg ethynodiol diacetate	100 μg mestranol	Searle
Enovid E	Combination	2.5 mg norethynodrel	100 μg mestranol	Searle
Enovid-5	Combination	5 mg norethynodrel	75 μg mestranol	Searle
Enovid-10	Combination	9.85 mg norethynodrel	150 μg mestranol	Searle
Loestrin 1/20	Combination	1 mg norethindrone acetate	20 μg ethinyl estradiol	Parke-Davis
Loestrin 1.5/30	Combination	1.5 mg norethindrone acetate	30 μg ethinyl estradiol	Parke-Davis
Norlestrin 2.5/50	Combination	2.5 mg norethindrone acetate	50 μg ethinyl estradiol	Parke-Davis
Norlestrin 1/50	Combination	1 mg norethindrone acetate	50 μg ethinyl estradiol	Parke-Davis
Lo/Ovral	Combination	0.3 mg norgestrel	30 μg ethinyl estradiol	Wyeth
Nordette	Combination	0.15 mg levonorgestrel	30 μg ethinyl estradiol	Wyeth
Ovral	Combination	0.5 mg norgestrel	50 μg ethinyl estradiol	Wyeth
Ovrette	Progestin only	75 μg norgestrel		Wyeth
Tri-Phasil 6/	Combination-triphasic	50 μg levonorgestrel	30 μg ethinyl estradiol	Wyeth
5/		75 μg levonorgestrel	40 μg ethinyl estradiol	Wyeth
10/		125 μg levonorgestrel	30 μg ethinyl estradiol	Wyeth
Ovcon-35	Combination	0.4 mg norethindrone	35 μg ethinyl estradiol	Mead Johnson
Ovcon-50	Combination	1 mg norethindrone	50 μg ethinyl estradiol	Mead Johnson
Modicon	Combination	0.5 mg norethindrone	35 μg ethinyl estradiol	Ortho
Ortho-Novum 1/35	Combination	1 mg norethindrone	35 μg ethinyl estradiol	Ortho
Ortho-Novum 1/50	Combination	1 mg norethindrone	50 μg mestranol	Ortho
Ortho-Novum 1/80	Combination	1 mg norethindrone	80 μg mestranol	Ortho
Ortho-Novum 2	Combination	2 mg norethindrone	100 μg mestranol	Ortho
Ortho-Novum 10/	Combination-biphasic	0.5 mg norethindrone	35 μg ethinyl estradiol	Ortho
11/		1 mg norethindrone	35 μg ethinyl estradiol	Ortho
Micronor	Progestin only	0.35 mg norethindrone		Ortho
Ortho-Novum 7/	Combination-triphasic	0.5 mg norethindrone	35 μg ethinyl estradiol	Ortho
7/		0.75 mg norethindrone	35 μg ethinyl estradiol	Ortho
7/		1 mg norethindrone	35 μg ethinyl estradiol	Ortho

genic component are nausea, breast tenderness, and fluid retention, the latter of which usually does not exceed 2 kg of body weight.

Ethinyl estradiol, the synthetic estrogen used in oral contraceptives, causes an increase in hepatic production of several globulins, the amount of the increase being related to the dose of estrogen in the formulation. An increase in globulins involved in the blood clotting process may cause a hypercoagulable state and then thrombosis. Increased levels of one globulin, angiotensinogen, may cause an increase in angiotensin II levels, which may in turn result in the development of hypertension. However, only a small percentage of women taking oral contraceptives develop high blood pressure,

Table 14-4
Metabolic Effects of Contraceptive Steroids

Affected Structure	Effects	
	Chemical	Clinical
Estrogen–Ethinyl Estradiol		
Proteins		
Albumin	↓	None
Amino acids	↓	None
Globulins	↑	
Angiotensinogen		↑ Blood pressure
Factors VII and X		Hypercoagulability
Carrier proteins (CBG, TBG, transferrin, ceruloplasmin)		None
Carbohydrates		
Plasma insulin	None	None
Glucose tolerance	None	None
Lipids		
Cholesterol	None	None
Triglycerides	↑	None
HDL–cholesterol	↑	None
LDL–cholesterol	↓	None
Electrolytes		
Sodium excretion	↑	Fluid retention
		Edema
Tryptophan metabolism	↓	Depression
		Mood changes
		Sleep disturbances
Vitamins		
B-complex	↓	None
Ascorbic acid	↓	None
Vitamin A	↑	None
Skin		
Sebum production	↓	Less acne
Pigmentation	↑	Chloasma
Target tissues		
Breasts	↑	Breast tenderness
Endometrial receptors	↑	Hyperplasia
Gestogens–19-Nortestosterone Derivatives		
Proteins	None	?
Carbohydrates		
Plasma insulin	↑	None
Glucose tolerance	↓	None
Lipids		
Cholesterol	↓	None
Triglycerides	↓	None
HDL–cholesterol	↓ ⎫	
LDL–cholesterol	↑ ⎬	? ↑ CV disease
Nitrogen retention	↑	↑ body weight
Skin—Sebum production	↑	↑ Acne
Androgens	↑	Nervousness
Endometrial receptors	↓	↓ Endometrial cancer

and this elevation is temporary, disappearing when the medication is stopped; there is no evidence that oral contraceptive use produces permanent hypertension.

Estrogen's diversion of tryptophan metabolism from its minor pathway in the brain to its major pathway in the liver causes a decrease in levels of the end product of tryptophan metabolism, serotonin, in the central nervous system; low serotonin levels in turn can produce depression in some women and sleepiness and mood changes in others. Fortunately, this is a relatively uncommon, reversible symptom that disappears when oral contraceptives are stopped.

The incidence of all these estrogenic side-effects is much lower now than it was a decade ago because the formulations in use today contain only one fifth as much estrogen as the formulations that were used in the 1960s.

The gestagens, which are structurally related to testosterone, have certain androgenic effects, including weight gain, acne, amenorrhea, and a symptom perceived by some women as nervousness. Considerable weight gain during use of oral contraceptives is produced by the anabolic effect of the progestin component. Alterations in glucose metabolism, which are produced by the gestagen component, are of small magnitude and of no clinical importance; these minor alterations are temporary and disappear when oral contraceptive use is discontinued. While estrogens decrease sebum production, gestagens increase sebum production and can cause acne to develop or worsen. Thus, patients who have acne should be given a formulation with a low gestagen:estrogen ratio. Another symptom produced by the gestogenic component is amenorrhea. Because the progestins decrease the number of estrogen receptors in the endometrium, endometrial growth is decreased; in some women this causes withdrawal bleeding not to occur. Although this symptom is not important medically, it is desirable to have some amount of periodic withdrawal bleeding during the days the woman is not taking steroids. Finally, estrogen and the gestagens can act together to produce irregular bleeding or chloasma. Breakthrough bleeding, which is usually produced by not enough estrogen or too much gestagen or a combination of the two, as well as amenorrhea, can be alleviated by an increase in the amount of estrogen in the formulation or by a more estrogenic formulation. The symptom of chloasma, pigmentation of the malar eminences, is accentuated by sunlight and usually takes a long time to disappear after oral contraceptives are stopped.

The effects discussed above are relatively common; however, oral contraceptives are also associated with rarer, more serious problems that can lead to death or severe complications. Although the incidence of cholelithiasis is about twofold higher than normal in women who have used oral contraceptives for four years or less, data from a Royal College study indicate that the incidence decreases to lower than normal after four years of oral contraceptive use. Thus, oral contraceptives appear to accelerate the process of cholelithiasis but do not increase its overall incidence. The risk of deep vein thrombophlebitis is increased 3 to 4 times by oral contraceptive use, as is the risk of thromboembolism. However, the absolute annual incidence of these disorders, which are not necessarily related (*i.e.,* patients with thromboembolism do not necessarily have clinical symptoms of thrombophlebitis) is in the order of 1 in 10,000 users for thrombophlebitis and 1 in 30,000 users for thromboembolism. Oral contraceptives appear to increase the incidence of hemorrhagic and possibly thrombotic stroke, although the epidemiologic data are conflicting; it seems that the increased risk of stroke in oral contraceptive users is mainly limited to women with underlying vascular disorders like hypertension and to older women who smoke. Although the risk of stroke may be 3 times higher than normal in oral contraceptive users, the incidence remains quite low, about 1 in 20,000 to 1 in 30,000 a year. There is also epidemiologic evidence that oral contraceptive users over 35 who smoke or have other associated risk factors, such as hypertension or hypercholesterolemia, have an increased risk of developing myocardial infarction; however, the incidence of myocardial infarction in this group is also low, about 1 in 5000 a year. Benign liver adenomas occur rarely in oral contraceptive users, the estimated frequency being 1 in 30,000 to 1 in 50,000 a year; the incidence is higher in women who have used the formulations for more than five years.

Major Concerns

Women have three major concerns about oral contraceptives: (1) an increased risk of developing cancer, (2) problems with future childbearing, and (3) an increased chance of developing heart attacks and stroke. These concerns are mostly unwarranted.

Cancer

A thorough review of the literature of the last 22 years reveals only scant evidence that use of oral contraceptives increases the risk of any type of cancer, including breast cancer, cancer of the uterus, cancer of the cervix, and cancer of the liver. Three large prospective studies of oral contraceptive users were started in 1968, two in Great Britain (the Royal College of General Practitioners Study [RCGP] and the Oxford Family Planning Study) and one in the United States (the NIH-sponsored Walnut Creek Study). Each of these studies compared large groups of women using oral contraceptives with similar numbers of control women using other methods of contraception. To date, none of these studies has established an increased risk of any type of cancer associated with oral contraceptive use. The Oxford investigators found an increased risk of cervical cancer, but this appears to have been due to confounding factors. Data from the Walnut Creek study indicate that women who use oral contraceptives and are exposed to large amounts of sunlight may have an increased risk of melanoma, but this association has not been found in other studies.

BREAST CANCER. At present, women using oral contraceptives in these prospective as well as other retrospective epidemiologic studies do not have a higher incidence of breast cancer than a control group of women of similar age using other methods of contraception. In fact, because oral contraceptives contain a gestagen, which counteracts the stimulatory action of estrogen on target tissues, women ingesting oral contraceptives have a lower incidence of nonmalignant cystic disease of the breast than do controls.

The Cancer and Steroid Hormone study (CASH), a large, multicenter epidemiologic study performed by the Centers for Disease Control in Atlanta, has established no increased risk of breast cancer in oral contraceptive users, including the various high-risk subgroups such as women with a family history of breast cancer, women with benign breast disease, and women who started using oral contraceptives before a first pregnancy. Furthermore, the study has revealed no change in risk of breast cancer with increasing duration of oral contraceptive use or time since last oral contraceptive use (Table 14-5). Data from this and other studies indicate no increased risk of breast cancer with any specific type of oral contraceptive formulation or with long-term use at an early age.

ENDOMETRIAL CANCER. There is no evidence that the incidence of carcinoma of the endometrium is higher than normal in oral contraceptive users. In fact, data from several epidemiologic studies, including the CASH study, indicate that women who use combination oral contraceptives are less likely to develop cancer of the endometrium than are women who do not use oral contraceptives. This finding is probably due to the effects of the gestagens as well as the estrogen contained in the formulations. Gestagens inhibit the synthesis of estrogen receptors and thus, when given with an estrogen, prevent estrogen's growth-promoting activity.

CERVICAL CANCER. Evidence from the Oxford study suggests that users of oral contraceptives have a high incidence of cancer of the cervix. In this and other studies, oral contraceptive users have been found to have a higher incidence of dysplasia of the cervix (including carcinoma *in situ*) than controls using other methods of contraception. Dysplasia, as well as epidermoid cancer of the cervix, has also been linked with onset of sexual intercourse at a young age and with multiple sexual partners. In other studies in which oral contraceptive users were found to have a higher incidence of dysplasia than controls, it was also found that oral contraceptive users had more sexual partners and had started intercourse at a younger age than had the controls who used other methods of contraception. These studies indicate that the increased incidence of dysplasia is most likely due to factors other than oral contraceptive use, including large number of sexual partners and frequent cytologic screening. It is also possible that members of the control groups were protected from dysplasia by their use of diaphragms or condoms.

LIVER CANCER. Cancer of the liver is uncommon in young women, and women who use oral contraceptives do not have a greater than normal chance of developing it. Women who use oral contraceptives for more than five years appear to have a greater chance than normal of developing benign liver adenomas. These tumors, which occur in only about 1 in 50,000 oral contraceptive users, gradually decrease in size and eventually disappear after the oral contraceptives are discontinued.

Pregnancy After Discontinuation of Oral Contraceptives

Although after discontinuing the use of oral contraceptives, both nulligravid and nulliparous women may experience a delay of a few months in return to fertility, eventually the percentage of women who conceive after stopping the pill is the same as the percentage of women who conceive after stopping any other method of birth control. As reported by Vessey in the Oxford Family Planning Study, after a two- to three-year interval, fertility rates were the same among former oral contraceptive users and former users of other methods of contraception (Fig. 14-4).

Table 14-5
Relative Risk* of Breast Cancer† with Oral Contraceptive Use

Time Since First OC Use (Years)	*Duration of OC Use (Years)*					
	<2	*2–5*	*6–7*	*8–10*	*≥11*	*All Ever-Users*
<10	0.7	2.0	2.8	0.8	—	1.4
10–12	1.2	2.0	0.3	0.9	1.2	1.2
13–15	0.9	1.0	1.2	0.8	1.1	1.0
≥16	0.9	1.0	0.8	0.7	0.8	0.9
All	0.9	1.2	1.0	0.7	0.9	0.9

* Relative to never-users of oral contraceptives. None of the figures are statistically significant.

† By time since first oral contraceptive use and according to duration of oral contraceptive use; excludes 53 women with unknown duration of oral contraceptive use.

OC, oral contraceptive.

(After Centers for Disease Control Cancer and Steroid Hormone Study: Long-term oral contraceptive use and the risk of breast cancer. JAMA 249:1591, 1983)

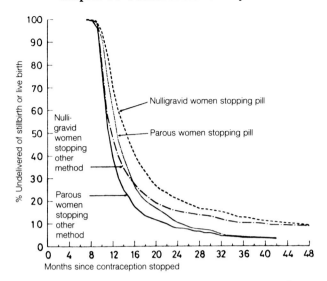

FIG. 14-4. Fertility in women who have stopped different methods of contraception in order to conceive. (Vessey MP, Wright NH, McPherson K et al: Fertility after stopping different methods of contraception. Br Med J 1:265, 1978)

Because the return of ovulation is delayed after oral contraceptives are stopped, it is difficult to estimate expected date of delivery in cases in which conception takes place before spontaneous menses resume. Therefore, a woman who stops taking oral contraceptives in order to conceive should probably continue to use a barrier method until her regular cycles resume. If she does conceive before spontaneous menses resume, gestational age should be estimated by serial sonography.

Spontaneous abortion rates are the same in women who conceive after stopping oral contraceptives as in the general population or in women who conceive after stopping other contraceptive methods. One study reported a high incidence of lethal chromosomal abnormalities in abortuses of women who conceived within a few months of stopping oral contraceptives. However, more recent studies have established that the incidence of chromosomal abnormalities is the same in abortuses of women who have not used oral contraceptives.

There have been several large studies of babies born to women who conceived after stopping oral contraceptives. These studies show that such infants have no greater than normal chance of being born with any type of birth defect. The incidence of congenital anomalies is the same in babies born to women who previously used oral contraceptives as in babies born to women who previously used other methods of contraception or women who did not use any method of contraception. In the largest of these studies, which contained data from the Walnut Creek Study, the rate of major malformation was 173 in 100,000 in infants born to women who had used oral contraceptives before conception, compared with rates of 150 and 201 in 100,000 in infants

born to women who had used other methods or no method, respectively. These differences were not significant. In this study, women who conceived within one month of stopping oral contraceptives had fewer malformed babies than those who conceived one to five months later.

Cardiovascular Disease

Retrospective case control epidemiologic studies performed to determine the risk of drug-associated disease provide a figure called a *relative risk* or *"times"* rate. This figure can be misleading and is therefore problematic. For example, in studies of oral contraceptives it has been stated that myocardial infarction occurs 3 times more frequently in oral contraceptive users than nonusers. However, because young women rarely develop myocardial infarctions, the absolute risk of any one woman developing the disease is extremely low. Although the relative risk figure may be frightening, the absolute-risk figure is more important. The three prospective studies of oral contraceptive users mentioned above, which have been going on for more than ten years, indicate that the absolute risk of any oral contraceptive user's developing cardiovascular disease is very low. In the United States and Britain, the incidence of death due to heart attack has decreased in women aged 20 to 45 over the past 15 years, a period during which oral contraceptive use has increased dramatically. (This decrease in heart attack death rates in these countries has been similar for men and women.) Results from the three prospective oral contraceptive studies indicate that a woman who uses oral contraceptives is at significant risk of developing cardiovascular disease only if she is over 35 years of age and smokes or if she is of any age and also has some type of preexisting vascular disease, such as hypertension, diabetes, or hypercholesterolemia (Tables 14-6 and 14-7). There is no reliable evidence that nonsmokers under age 45 and smokers under 35 who use oral steroids have an increased chance of dying from a heart attack, provided they do not have preexisting vascular diseases.

A few years ago analysis of mortality data from the RCGP Study suggested that women who had used oral steroids for more than five years were at increased risk of dying from cardiovascular disease. However, recent data from the same study indicate that this concern was not valid, since the incidence of death from cardiovascular disease has not increased with increased duration of oral contraceptive use. This information, together with data from many other epidemiologic studies showing no increase in mortality from myocardial infarction in former users of oral contraceptives, indicates that the cause of myocardial infarction or stroke in oral steroid users is arterial thrombosis, not atherosclerosis. Thus, despite data indicating that certain oral contraceptive formulations lower high-density lipoprotein (HDL)–cholesterol and raise low-density lipoprotein (LDL)–cholesterol levels (changes that theoretically could be

Table 14-6
Circulatory Disease Mortality by Age, Smoking Status, and Oral Contraceptive Use

	Mortality Rate (per 100,000 Woman Years)		Relative Risk (95% Confidence Limits)
Age	Ever-Users (Number of Deaths)	Controls (Number of Deaths)	Ever-Users vs. Controls
15–25			
Nonsmokers	0 (0)	0 (0)	—
Smokers	10.5 (1)	0 (0)	—
25–34			
Nonsmokers	4.4 (2)	2.7 (1)	1.6
Smokers	14.2 (6)	4.2 (1)	3.4
35–44			
Nonsmokers	21.5 (7)	6.4 (2)	3.3
Smokers	63.4 (18)	15.2 (3)	4.2*
45 and up			
Nonsmokers	52.4 (4)	11.4 (1)	4.6
Smokers	206.7 (17)	27.9 (2)	7.4*

* Significantly different.

(After Royal College of General Practitioners' Oral Contraception Study: Further analysis of mortality in oral contraceptive users. Lancet 1:541, 1981)

Table 14-7
Walnut Creek Study: Diseases of the Circulatory System

	Standard Rates			Relative Risk	
Disease	Never	Current	Past	Current	Past
Acute myocardial infarction	0.23	0.27	0.2	1.1	0.8
Ischemic heart disease	0.79	1.09	0.9	1.4	1.1
Subarachnoid hemorrhage	0.04	0.43	0.1	10.1*	2.3*
Cerebral thrombosis	0.24	0.53	0.29	2.2*	1.2
Arterial thrombosis	0.24	0.76	0.24	3.2*	1
Pulmonary embolism	0.38	0.22	0.29	0.6	0
Thrombophlebitis	0.51	0.42	0.48	0.8	1.8

(After Ramcharan S, Pellegrin FA, Ray RM, Hsu J-P: The Walnut Creek Contraceptive Drug Study: A Prospective Study of the Side Effects of Oral Contraceptives, Vol. III, NIH Publication #81-564. Washington, DC, United States Government Printing Office, 1981)

* Not significantly different overall; significantly different only in smokers over 40 years of age.

atherogenic), there is no evidence that long-term use of oral steroids produces a permanent harmful effect on the blood vessels such as development of atherosclerosis. Furthermore, the lipid alterations produced by some formulations, especially those with high gestagen potency, are small and within the normal range, and there is no evidence that such small alterations lead to atherosclerosis. Thus, women can take oral contraceptives for an unlimited time no matter how old they are when they start taking them. In addition, there is no evidence that there is need for a rest period after a few years of oral contraceptive use.

Other Concerns

Various other concerns about oral contraceptives have also proven to be untrue. It is not the case that oral steroids produce vitamin deficiency; they do lower blood levels of the B-complex vitamins and vitamin C, but low levels of these vitamins are not accompanied by any clinical evidence of vitamin deficiency, so vitamin supplementation is not necessary. It is also not true that use of oral contraceptives in young teenagers will cause permanent changes in the hypothalamic–pituitary–ovarian axis and produce premature epiphyseal closure, causing growth to stop; oral contraceptives may be used by women of any age who have started to have regular menstrual cycles. Finally, there is no evidence that women with adenosis or other genital tract changes due to antenatal diethylstilbestrol (DES) exposure are at increased risk for cancer or other harmful alterations if they take oral contraceptives.

Contraindications to Oral Contraceptive Use

Oral contraceptives can be prescribed for the majority of women of reproductive age; however, there are certain absolute contraindications to their use. These include a present or past history of vascular disease, including thromboembolism, thrombophlebitis, atherosclerosis, and stroke; a present or past history of systemic vascular disease, such as lupus erythematosus or hemoglobin SS disease; hypertension; diabetes mellitus with vascular disease; and hyperlipidemia. One of the contraindications for oral steroid use listed by the United States Food and Drug Administration (FDA) is cancer of the breast or endometrium, although there are no data indicating that oral contraceptives are harmful in women with this condition. Patients who are pregnant should not ingest oral steroids because of the masculinizing effect of the gestagens on the external genitalia of the female fetus. Concerns that ingestion of oral contraceptives during pregnancy produces other deleterious effects on the fetus, such as limb reduction defects and heart defects, have not proven to be valid. As shown by Wilson and Brent, data linking ingestion of progestational agents in pregnancy to an increased incidence of congenital abnormalities has mostly been obtained from women having threatened abortions, and bleeding in pregnancy in itself is associated with a higher than normal number of anomalies. Furthermore, the incidence of anomalies has not decreased since gestagens have stopped being used for treatment of threatened abortion. Patients with heart disease should not use oral contraceptives, since the fluid retention produced by these agents could produce congestive heart failure. Finally, patients with active liver disease should not receive oral steroids, since steroids are metabolized in the liver. However, patients who have had liver disease in the past, such as viral hepatitis, but whose liver function tests have returned to normal can receive oral contraceptives.

Relative contraindications to oral contraceptive use include heavy cigarette smoking, migraine headaches, amenorrhea, and depression. Migraine headaches can be made worse by use of oral steroids, and an increased incidence of headaches of the migraine type, fainting, loss of vision or speech, or paresthesias may precede a stroke. Development of any of these symptoms in an oral contraceptive user is therefore an indication that the steroids should be stopped. Patients who are amenorrheic for a cause other than polycystic ovarian syndrome should probably not receive oral contraceptives; these steroids mask the symptoms of both amenorrhea

and galactorrhea, which may be produced by enlargement of the adenoma. Anyone who develops galactorrhea while taking oral contraceptives should discontinue their use and after two weeks have her serum prolactin level measured. If the prolactin level is elevated, further diagnostic evaluation, such as x-ray films of the sella turcica, is indicated. However, a recent National Institutes of Health study reported by the Pituitary Adenoma Study Group confirmed the conclusion of other studies that oral contraceptives do not produce prolactin secretory pituitary adenomas.

Beginning Oral Contraceptives

In Adolescents

In deciding whether the pubertal, sexually active girl should use oral steroids for contraception, the clinician should be more concerned about compliance than about possible physiologic harm; provided the postmenarchal girl has demonstrated maturity of the hypothalamic–pituitary–ovarian axis by having had at least three regular, presumably ovulatory, cycles, it is safe to prescribe oral contraceptives without being concerned about permanent damage to the reproductive process. It is probably best not to prescribe oral contraceptives to any woman with oligomenorrhea, a condition most frequently seen in adolescents, because of the association of this disorder with postpill amenorrhea; the only exception to this rule is women with oligomenorrhea and polycystic ovarian syndrome. One need not be concerned about accelerating epiphyseal closure in postmenarchal females; their endogenous estrogens already initiated the process a few years before menarche, and contraceptive steroids will not hasten it.

Following Pregnancy

There is a difference in return of ovulation and bleeding between the postabortal woman and the woman who has had a term delivery. The first episode of menstrual bleeding postabortion is usually preceded by ovulation. The first episode of bleeding following a term delivery is usually anovulatory. Ovulation usually occurs between two and four weeks after an abortion; in contrast, after a term delivery ovulation is usually delayed beyond six weeks, though it may occur as early as four weeks after delivery in a woman who is not breastfeeding.

Thus, after spontaneous or induced abortion of a fetus of less than 12 weeks' gestation, oral contraceptives should be started immediately to prevent conception following the first ovulation. For patients who deliver after 28 weeks and are not nursing, combination pills should be initiated 2 weeks after delivery. If termination of the pregnancy occurs between 21 and 28 weeks, contraceptive steroids should be started 1 week later. The reason for the delay in the latter instances is that the normally increased risk of thromboembolism occurring postpartum may be further enhanced by the hypercoagulable state associated with contraceptive steroid ingestion. Given that the first ovulation is delayed for a period of at least four weeks after a term delivery, there is no need to expose the patient to this increased risk.

It is probably best for women who are nursing not to use combination oral contraceptives; their use may diminish the amount of milk produced, since estrogen inhibits prolactin's action on the breast. Women who are breastfeeding every 4 hours, at night as well as during the day, do not ovulate until at least ten weeks after delivery and thus do not need contraception before that time. Since only a small percentage of breastfeeding women ovulate while they continue full nursing and most remain amenorrheic, either a barrier method or an oral contraceptive containing a gestagen only can be used. The latter does not diminish the amount of breast milk produced.

In All Patients

At the initial visit, after a history and physical examination have determined that there are no medical contraindications to the use of oral contraceptives, the patient should be informed about the benefits and risks of birth control pills. It is a good idea to have the patient sign a written informed consent as well as to note on her medical record that the benefits and risks have been explained to her.

Types of Formulation

It is best initially to prescribe a formulation with 30 μg or 35 μg ethinyl estradiol. In a study performed in Great Britain, Meade and associates reported that the incidence of total deaths as well as of deaths due to arterial causes alone was significantly lower among patients using formulations with 30 μg ethinyl estradiol than among patients using formulations of 50 μg ethinyl estradiol (Table 14-8). The incidences of ischemic heart disease

Table 14-8
Ratio of Observed to Expected Events by Estrogen Dose

Events	50 μg ethinyl estradiol	30 μg ethinyl estradiol
Venous deaths	1.4	0.65
Nonvenous deaths	1.52	0.53*
Ischemic heart disease	1.48	0.54*
Stroke	1.2	0.8
Pregnancy	0.62	1.33*

* Significant.

(After Meade TW, Greenberg G, Thompson SG: Progestogens and cardiovascular reactions associated with oral contraceptives and a comparison of the safety of 50- and 30-μg estrogen preparations. Br Med J 1:1157, 1980)

and stroke were also significantly decreased in women using the lower dose estrogen formulations. Because levels of serum globulins, including angiotensinogen as well as serum globulins involved with coagulation, are related to the dose of estrogen administered, it is reasonable to conclude that low doses of estrogen would not cause as great or frequent increases in blood pressure or venous thrombosis as would higher doses of estrogen. With rare exceptions, there is no need to prescribe formulations with more than 50 μg of estrogen. There is some indication from the Royal College and other studies that the incidence of total arterial disease in oral contraceptive users is directly related to the dose of gestagen ingested; it would therefore appear reasonable to use formulations with the lowest possible dosage of gestagen. The FDA has stated that the product prescribed should be one that contains the least possible amount of estrogen and progestin while simultaneously having a low failure rate and being compatible with the needs of the individual patient. Until large-scale studies are performed to compare different marketed formulations, the clinician has to decide what formulations to use according to which have the least adverse effects among his patients. There is no evidence that some patients do better with formulations that are more estrogenic while other patients do better with formulations that are more gestagenic.

The contraceptive formulations containing gestagens without estrogen have a lower incidence of adverse metabolic effects than the formulations containing estrogen. The incidence of thromboembolism in women ingesting gestagen-only compounds is probably not higher than normal, nor do these compounds affect blood pressure, cause nausea or breast tenderness, or lead to changes in milk production or quality. However, gestagen-only agents are associated with a high frequency of intermenstrual and other abnormal bleeding patterns, including amenorrhea, and a lower rate of effectiveness than compounds that also contain estrogen. The actual use failure rate of these preparations has been reported to vary between 2% and 8% per year, and a relatively high percentage of these pregnancies are ectopic. The major disadvantages of gestagen preparations are minimized for nursing mothers, who have reduced fertility and are amenorrheic. Furthermore, insofar as these preparations do not affect milk production and quality, they seem ideal for nursing women. A small portion of these synthetic steroids have been detected in breast milk but do not appear to have any effect on infants who ingest the milk.

Follow-Up

In a patient who has no contraindications to oral contraceptive use, the only routine laboratory tests indicated are a complete blood count, urinalysis, and Pap smear. At the end of three months the patient should be seen again; at this time a nondirected history should be obtained and the patient's blood pressure measured. After this visit the patient should be seen annually, at which time a nondirected history should again be taken, blood pressure and body weight measured, and a physical examination, including a breast, abdominal, and pelvic examination (including a Pap smear), performed. It is important to perform annual Pap smears on oral contraceptive users, since they are at relatively high risk for the development of cervical neoplasia. The routine performance of other laboratory tests is not indicated unless the patient is over 35 or has a family history of diabetes or vascular disease. For patients over 35 who wish to continue taking oral contraceptives, it is advisable to obtain a lipid panel, including HDL– and LDL–cholesterol, total cholesterol, and triglycerides. If lipid levels are abnormal, another method of contraception may be safer. In addition, because of the increased incidence of diabetes among persons over age 35, a 2-hour postprandial blood glucose test should be performed. If the level is elevated, a full glucose tolerance test should be performed, and if the results of this test are abnormal, the oral contraceptives should probably be stopped. Routine use of these tests in women under 35 is not indicated because the incidence of positive results is extremely low. However, if a patient under 35 has a family history of vascular disease, such as myocardial infarction occurring in family members under the age of 50, it is advisable to obtain a lipid panel before and after oral contraceptives are started, and if the patient has a family history of diabetes or evidence of diabetes during pregnancy, a 2-hour postprandial blood glucose should be obtained before and after oral contraceptives are started. A patient who has a past history of liver disease should have a liver panel done to ensure that her liver function is normal before she starts oral steroids.

Drug Interactions

Although synthetic sex steroids can retard the biotransformation of certain drugs, such as phenazone and meperidine, owing to substrate competition, such interference is not important clinically. Oral contraceptives have not been shown to inhibit the action of other drugs. However, some drugs can clinically interfere with the action of oral contraceptives by inducing the production of liver enzymes that convert the steroids to more polar and less biologically active metabolites. Other drugs have been shown to accelerate the biotransformation of steroids in humans; these include barbiturates, sulfonamides, cyclophosphamide, and rifampicin. Several investigators have reported a relatively high incidence of oral contraceptive failure in women ingesting rifampicin, so these two agents should not be given concurrently. The clinical data concerning oral contraceptive failure in users of other antibiotics, analgesics, and barbiturates, are less clear. A few anecdotal studies have appeared in the literature, but there is no reliable evidence that these drugs have a clinical inhibitory effect.

Nevertheless, until controlled studies are performed, it would appear prudent when any of these agents is given to a woman on birth control pills to suggest use of a barrier method in addition to the oral contraceptives. In addition, women with epilepsy requiring medication are best given a 50-μg-estrogen formulation; an unusually high incidence of accidental pregnancy has been reported in these women with the use of low-dose estrogen formulations.

Noncontraceptive Health Benefits

In addition to being the most effective method of contraception, oral steroids provide several health benefits due to the effects of the estrogens and gestagens they contain.

Both natural progesterone and synthetic gestagens inhibit the proliferative effect of estrogen; this is called the *antiestrogenic effect*. Estrogens increase the synthesis of both estrogen and progesterone receptors, while progesterone decreases their synthesis. Thus, one mechanism whereby progesterone exerts its antiestrogenic effect is by decreasing the synthesis of estrogen receptors. Relatively little gestagen is needed to do this; the amount present in oral contraceptives is sufficient. Another way progesterone produces its antiestrogenic action is by stimulating the activity of the enzyme estradiol-17β-dehydrogenase within the endometrial cell. This enzyme converts the more potent estradiol to the less potent estrone, reducing estrogenic action within the cell.

Benefits from the Antiestrogenic Action of Progestins

As a result of the antiestrogenic action of the progestins in oral contraceptives, the height of the endometrium is less than in an ovulatory cycle, and there is less proliferation of the glandular epithelium. These changes produce several substantial benefits for the oral contraceptive user. One is a reduction in the amount of blood lost at the time of endometrial shedding. In ovulating women mean blood loss during menstruation is about 35 ml; in women ingesting oral contraceptives it is only 20 ml. This decreased blood loss makes the development of iron deficiency anemia less likely. Data from the RCGP study showed that oral contraceptive users are about half as likely to develop iron deficiency anemia as are women who do not use oral steroids. This effect seems to hold true even in women who used to use oral contraceptives and then stopped, probably because an increase in iron stores obtained during oral steroid use remains for several years after the drug is discontinued.

Given that oral contraceptives produce regular withdrawal bleeding, it would be expected that oral contraceptive users would have fewer menstrual disorders than controls. This idea was confirmed by the results of the RCGP study, which showed that oral contraceptive users are significantly less likely than nonusers to develop menorrhagia, irregular menstruation, or intermenstrual bleeding. As a result, oral contraceptive users are also less likely to require curettage, which is frequently used to treat these disorders.

Because gestagens inhibit the proliferative effect of estrogens on the endometrium, it is not surprising that women who use oral contraceptives have been found to be significantly less likely than normal to develop adenocarcinoma of the endometrium. Data from three retrospective case comparison studies, including the CASH study, indicate that the relative risk of developing endometrial cancer among combination oral contraceptive users is only half that among nonusers. The protective effect seen in these studies increased the longer the agents were used, and the reduced risk of endometrial cancer persisted for at least five years after treatment had been discontinued.

Estrogen exerts a proliferative effect on breast tissue, which also contains estrogen receptors. Gestagens probably inhibit the synthesis of estrogen receptors in this organ as well as elsewhere, exerting an antiestrogenic effect on the breast. Several studies have shown that oral steroids reduce the incidence of benign breast disease, and two prospective studies have indicated that this reduction is directly related to the amount of gestagen in the compounds.

Users of oral contraceptives in the Oxford study had an 85% reduction in the incidence of fibroadenomas and a 50% reduction in the incidences of chronic cystic disease and nonbiopsied breast lumps compared with controls using IUDs or diaphragms. The risk of developing these three diseases decreased with increased duration of oral steroid use and persisted for about one year following discontinuation of oral contraceptives, after which no reduction in risk was observed.

Benefits from the Inhibition of Ovulation

Other noncontraceptive medical benefits of oral contraceptives result from their main action, inhibition of ovulation. Some disorders, such as dysmenorrhea and premenstrual tension, occur much more frequently in ovulatory than anovulatory cycles. Inhibition of ovulation by exogenous steroids has been used as therapy for severe dysmenorrhea for decades. The 1974 report of the RCGP study showed that oral contraceptive users had 63% less dysmenorrhea and 29% less premenstrual tension than controls.

Another serious adverse effect of ovulatory menstrual cycles is the development of functional ovarian cysts, particularly follicular and luteal cysts, which frequently require laparotomy because of enlargement, rupture, or hemorrhage. When ovulation is inhibited, functional cysts do not usually develop. In a survey performed by the Boston Collaborative Drug Surveillance Program, under 2% of women with a discharge diagnosis of functional ovarian cysts were taking oral steroids, in contrast to 20% of controls. However, 20% of women with nonfunctional cysts were taking oral contraceptives, an incidence similar to that observed in controls.

Another disorder linked to incessant ovulation is ovarian cancer. Several case control studies have shown that the risk of developing ovarian cancer decreases as the number of pregnancies increases, and it has been reported that the incidence of ovarian cancer correlates inversely with the number of children born. The trauma to the ovarian surface epithelium produced by incessant ovulation may in some way contribute to the development of ovarian cancer. Data from a case control study reported by Casagrande and associates indicate that the relative risk of ovarian cancer decreases as the number of live births and incomplete pregnancies as well as oral contraceptive use increases. When the anovulatory years from all three factors are added, the decreased relative risk is statistically significant. These investigators found that 12 months of oral steroid use is protective to about the same degree as one pregnancy and live birth. Three recent case control studies, including the CASH study, reported that oral contraceptive users have only about half the risk of developing ovarian cancer as nonusers and that this protection persists for at least ten years after the oral contraceptives are stopped.

Other Benefits

The RCGP study showed that the risk of rheumatoid arthritis among oral contraceptive users is only about half that among nonusers. Another benefit is protection against salpingitis, commonly referred to as *pelvic inflammatory disease (PID)*. There have been at least 11 published epidemiologic studies estimating the relative risk of PID among oral steroid users. In seven of these studies, in which oral contraceptive use was compared with no use of any contraception, the relative risk of PID among oral contraceptive users was generally found to be about 0.5.

It has been estimated that between 15% and 20% of women with cervical gonorrheal infection develop salpingitis. In a study from Sweden by Ryden and colleagues, all cases of suspected salpingitis were confirmed by laparoscopic visualization one day after admission of the patients. Of patients with cervical gonorrhea who used contraception other than the IUD and oral steroids, 15% developed salpingitis; in contrast, of patients with cervical gonorrhea who used oral contraceptives, only 8.8% developed salpingitis. The results of this study indicate that oral steroids reduce the clinical development of salpingitis in women infected with gonorrhea. This protection may be related to the decreased duration of menstrual flow, which permits a smaller number of gonococcal organisms to ascend to the upper genital tract and allows the body's defenses to eliminate them more easily. One of the sequelae of PID is ectopic pregnancy, a condition that has tripled in incidence in the last decade. Oral contraceptives reduce the risk of ectopic pregnancy by more than 90%

in current users and may also reduce the incidence in former users by decreasing their chance of developing salpingitis.

Ory estimated that for every 100,000 oral contraceptive users in the United States per year, use of the formulations prevents iron deficiency anemia in 320, rheumatoid arthritis in 32, and PID not requiring hospitalization in 450. In addition, 150 fewer women are hospitalized for PID, 235 fewer for breast disease, 35 fewer for ovarian tumors, and 117 fewer for tubal pregnancy per 100,000 oral contraceptive users (Table 14-9). Ory estimates that each year about 1 of every 750 women taking oral contraceptives will not develop a serious disease that she would have developed had she not been taking oral steroids. He also estimates that use of oral contraceptives prevents 50,000 women in the United States from being hospitalized each year. It is unfortunate that the infrequent adverse effects of oral contraceptives have received widespread publicity, while information about the more common noncontraceptive health benefits has attracted little attention.

INJECTABLE STEROIDS

Four injectable steroid contraceptive formulations have undergone extensive clinical trials, but none has been approved for use in the United States. Depomedroxyprogesterone acetate (DMPA), a microcrystalline suspension administered in a dosage of 150 mg every 3 months, is marketed in many countries, including Sweden and the United Kingdom. Studies have also been undertaken with 300 mg of DMPA administered every 6 months; norethindrone enanthate (NET-EN), 200 mg every 2 months or every 12 weeks; combinations of dihydroxyprogesterone acetofenide and estradiol enanthate; and medroxyprogesterone acetete (MPA) and estradiol cypionate, administered monthly. NET-EN is formulated in an oily suspension, and its duration of action is shorter than that of DMPA. It is marketed as a contraceptive in some European countries. Although these injectable formulations are very effective, they produce a high incidence of abnormal bleeding patterns and amenorrhea. Following use of DMPA, there is a delay of several months until ovulation resumes. Nevertheless, this effective contraceptive is appropriate for use in certain individuals.

PREGNANCY INTERCEPTION (POSTCOITAL CONTRACEPTION)

Morris and van Wagenen suggested in 1973 that high doses of estrogen given in the early postovulatory period can prevent implantation in women. Morris has suggested that the term *interception* be used for what is commonly called the *morning-after pill*. The estrogen compounds that have been used by various investigators for interception include diethylstilbestrol, 25 mg to 50 mg per day; diethylstilbestrol diphosphate, 50 μg per day; ethinyl estradiol, 1 mg to 5 mg per day; and conjugated estrogens, 20 mg to 30 mg per day. Treatment is continued for 5 days and is most effective if begun within 72 hours after an isolated midcycle act of coitus. If more than one episode of coitus has occurred, or if treatment is initiated more than 72 hours after coitus, the method is much less effective. Failure rates are usually reported to be 0.3% to 0.7%. Side-effects associated with this therapy are nausea and vomiting, breast soreness, and menstrual irregularities. In one study it was found that if treatment was begun two days after coitus, the pregnancy rate was 1.7-fold greater than if it was begun the day after coitus. Thus it is best to start treatment within 24 hours of coitus.

Because the side-effects of high-dose estrogen lead some women not to complete the 5-day course, a regimen of 4 tablets of ethinyl estradiol, 0.05 mg, and dl-norgestrel (Ovral), 0.5 mg, ingested as 2 tablets on 2 occasions 12 hours apart has been widely used in Canada and elsewhere. The effectiveness of this regimen is comparable to that of the high-dose estrogen regimen, and the duration of adverse symptoms is shorter. Yuzpe and co-workers summarized their experience with this regimen among 692 women treated in 24 clinics. There were 11 pregnancies (1.6%), but 4 of the pregnant subjects had had unprotected intercourse more than 72 hours before treatment and therefore should not have been included in the study. Excluding those 4 subjects, the pregnancy rate was 1%. About half of the subjects (42.4%) had no side-effects; 51.7% experienced nausea

---

Table 14-9
Hospitalizations Prevented Annually by Use of Oral Contraceptives According to Disease, United States*

Disease	Rate (per 100,000 pill users)	Number
Benign breast disease	235	20,000
Ovarian retention cysts	35	3000
Iron deficiency anemia†	320	27,200
Pelvic inflammatory disease (first episodes)		
Total episodes†	600	51,000
Hospitalizations	156	13,300
Ectopic pregnancy	117	9900
Rheumatoid arthritis†	32	2700
Endometrial cancer‡	5	2000
Ovarian cancer‡	4	1700

* Except where noted, figures refer to hospitalizations prevented among the estimated 8.5 million current users of oral contraceptives in the United States.

† Episodes prevented regardless of whether hospitalization occurred.

‡ Based on an estimated 39 million U.S. women who have ever used oral contraceptives.

(Ory HW: The noncontraceptive health benefits from oral contraceptive use. Fam Plann Perspect 14:182, 1982).

or vomiting. Other side-effects, such as mastalgia and menorrhagia, were infrequent, occurring in under 1% of the women. Thus, the effectiveness of this method appears to be similar to that of higher dosages of estrogen alone and results in a lower incidence of abnormal and delayed menses. Because the side-effects of this regimen appear to be less severe and because treatment takes only one day, patient compliance should be greater with this technique. If a patient continues to need contraception after the cycle in which interception is used, one of the conventional contraceptive methods should be utilized.

INTRAUTERINE DEVICES

IUDs are highly effective and have no associated systemic metabolic effects, and their long-term use requires only a single act of motivation. These characteristics, as well as the fact that discontinuation of the method requires a visit to a health care facility, account for the fact that IUDs have the highest continuation rate of all currently available reversible methods of contraception. Barrier techniques have higher use failure rates than method failure rates; in contrast, the method effectiveness and use effectiveness rates for IUDs are similar. First-year failure rates are generally reported to range from 2% to 3% but vary with the skill of the clinician inserting the IUD. Correct high fundal insertion, which is most likely to be performed by an experienced clinician, is associated with a low incidence of partial or complete expulsion and, as a result, with a low pregnancy rate. Furthermore, the annual incidence of accidental pregnancy decreases steadily after the first year of IUD use. Among women who have used the loop for six years, the cumulative failure rate is less than 1% per year. In addition, the incidence of all major adverse events with IUDs, including pregnancy, IUD expulsion, and IUD removal for bleeding or pain, steadily decreases

with increasing age; the pregnancy rate of women over 35 using the loop is less than 2% in the first two years of use (Table 14-10). Thus, the IUD is especially suited for older parous women who wish to prevent further pregnancies.

Mechanism of Action

It is generally accepted that the contraceptive action of the IUD is due to production of a local sterile inflammatory reaction caused by the presence of the foreign body in the uterus. There is nearly a 1000% increase in the number of leukocytes present in uterine washings of the human endometrial cavity from before IUD insertion to 18 weeks after IUD insertion. The tissue breakdown products of these leukocytes are toxic to all cells, including sperm cells and the blastocysts. Small IUDs do not produce as great an inflammatory reaction as larger devices. Therefore, small IUDs are associated with higher pregnancy rates than larger devices of the same design. The addition of copper increases the inflammatory reaction. The short phase of sperm transport from the cervix to the oviduct is markedly impaired in women wearing IUDs; thus, very few if any sperm reach the oviducts and ova usually do not become fertilized in these women. Further evidence that IUDs affect sperm transport was found in a study in which oviductal flushings were performed in 54 women with and without IUDs who were sterilized by salpingectomy soon after ovulation and had had unprotected sexual intercourse shortly before ovulation. Normally cleaving ova were found in the tubal flushings of about half of the women not wearing IUDs, whereas no normally cleaving ova were found in the oviducts of the women wearing IUDs. If fertilization does occur, copper ions, as well as the locally released prostaglandins, probably alter the normal process of implantation, increasing the contraceptive effectiveness of the method.

Table 14-10
Two-Year Net Cumulative Event Rates with the Loop D per 100 Women

| Events | Age at Insertion | | | |
	15–24	*25–29*	*30–34*	*35–49*
Pregnancy	5.8%	4.7%	2.8%	1.5%
Expulsion	17.4%	9.8%	7.1%	5.4%
Removal for bleeding or pain	18%	17.7%	16.8%	16.2%
Continuation	58%	66.7%	72%	75.4%
Number of first insertions	2753	2082	1397	1187
Woman-months of use	41,758	34,574	23,874	19,912

(Tietze C, Lewit S: Evaluation of intrauterine devices: Ninth progress report of the Cooperative Statistical Program. Stud Fam Plann 1(55):27, 1970. Reprinted with the permission of the Population Council)

Upon removal of both copper-bearing and non-copper-bearing IUDs, the inflammatory reaction rapidly disappears and resumption of fertility occurs at the same rate as following discontinuation of use of barrier methods of contraception.

Vessey and associates reported that the pregnancy rate among women who discontinue use of an IUD after one or two years are similar to that among women who discontinue use of a barrier method after one or two years; the only exception is among women who discontinue use of the IUD for medical problems, including infection, who have a slightly lower pregnancy rate at two years.

Types of IUD

In the last 15 years, numerous models of IUDs have been designed and used clinically. Although many of these devices are available for use in Europe, Canada, and other countries, at present only five types of IUD, all of which have a monofilament tail, are available for general unrestricted use in the United States (Fig. 14-5). These types of IUD are the barium-impregnated plastic loop, the copper-bearing Copper 7, the Copper T 200B, the Copper T 380 Ag, and the progesterone-releasing T-shaped device. There is little evidence of any significant difference in rates of occurrence of major adverse events among the IUDs currently available in the United States.

However, because of the constant dissolution of copper, the daily amount of which is less than that in-

FIG. 14-5. IUDs currently approved for use in the United States. From *left* to *right:* Copper T 200B, loop, progesterone-releasing IUD, Copper T 180 Ag, and Copper 7.

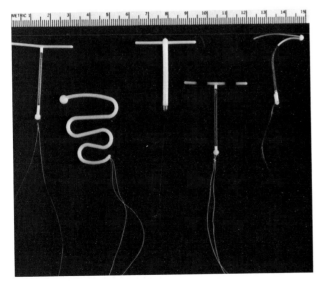

gested in the normal diet, copper IUDs have to be replaced at periodic intervals. The necessary interval was originally estimated to be two to three years but is now believed to be four to five years. Several published studies have indicated that the annual pregnancy rates with the Copper 7 and Copper T 200 IUDs do not increase in the fourth and fifth years after insertion, and the World Health Organization stated in 1982 that the Copper 7 is safe and effective for at least four years. The Copper T 200B is now approved for use for four years in the United States. The device can then be removed and a new one inserted during a single clinic visit.

Addition of a reservoir of progesterone to the vertical arm increases the effectiveness of the T. The presently marketed progesterone IUD releases 65 μg of progesterone daily; this amount is sufficient to prevent pregnancy by local action in the endometrial cavity but is not enough to cause a measurable increase in peripheral serum progesterone levels. The currently approved model of the progesterone-releasing IUD needs to be replaced annually, since the reservoir of progesterone becomes depleted after about 18 months of use.

There is no need ever to change a plastic IUD unless the patient develops increased bleeding after the IUD has been in place for more than a year. Calcium salts are slowly deposited on the plastic, and their roughness can cause ulceration and bleeding of the endometrium. If increased bleeding develops after a non-copper-bearing plastic IUD has been in the uterus for a year or more, the old IUD should be removed and a new one inserted.

The copper and progesterone-releasing IUDs are tolerated better by nulliparous women than are the larger plastic devices. Multiparous women tolerate all types of IUD equally well, so in their case the advantages of less blood loss with a medicated IUD must be weighed against the disadvantages of necessary periodic replacement. Until randomized comparative studies demonstrate that a particular device is superior to all others, the decision as to which device to use in a multiparous woman should be made by the physician and patient after they have considered the relative advantages and disadvantages of the medicated and the nonmedicated devices.

Time of Insertion

Although it is widely believed that the optimal time for insertion of an IUD is during menses, data indicate that if a woman is not pregnant the IUD can be safely inserted on any day of the cycle. White and colleagues found that rates of adverse effects are similar no matter what day of the cycle the device is inserted. It has also been recommended that following a pregnancy an IUD not be inserted until more than three months have elapsed. However, rates of adverse effects of Copper T IUDs inserted between four and eight weeks postpartum and more than eight weeks postpartum are similar, indicating that Copper T IUDs can be safely inserted at the time of the routine postpartum visit. A withdrawal technique of insertion should be used to avoid perforation, since the perforation rate has been reported to be higher in lactating than in nonlactating women.

Incidence of Adverse Effects

In general, in the first year of use IUDs are associated with about a 2% pregnancy rate, a 10% expulsion rate, and a 15% rate of removal for medical reasons, mainly bleeding and pain. The incidence of each of these events, especially expulsion, diminishes steadily in subsequent years.

The continuation rate of the loop after use for six years is 42.4%. A total of 5.4% of the terminations that occur during the six years are due to pregnancy, a little less than 1% per year. Thus, although the pregnancy rate in the first year of use of the IUD is greater than that with oral contraceptives, over a longer time period the use-pregnancy rates with IUDs and combination oral contraceptives are similar. About half of all women who discontinue use of the loop after six years do so because of bleeding, pain, or other medical reasons or a combination of these factors.

In a five-year experience with the Copper T 200, despite a high proportion of young users, the net pregnancy rate was 5.8%, about 1% per year, the discontinuation rate for expulsion was 7.2%, and the rate of removal for bleeding and pain was 23.7%, similar to rates with the loop. Another copper T device, the Copper T 380A, which has copper on both the horizontal and the vertical arms and was recently approved for use in the United States, is also associated with a very low pregnancy rate; Sivin and Tatum reported that the net cumulative pregnancy rate with this device at the end of four years was only 1.9%. Thus, the addition of copper on the horizontal arm appears to lower the pregnancy rate as well as increase the estimated duration of action to four years or more.

Types of Adverse Effects

Uterine Bleeding

Nearly all medical reasons for IUD removal involve one or more types of abnormal bleeding: heavy menses, prolonged menses, or intermenstrual bleeding. The IUD does not influence follicular maturation, the time or incidence of ovulation, or corpus luteum function; however, it does exert a local effect upon the endometrium, causing menses to start about two days earlier than normal, when steroid levels are higher than in control cycles. This early onset of menses may be produced by a premature and increased rate of release of prostaglandins brought about by the presence of the intrauterine foreign body. The stimulation of uterine contractions

by excessive prostaglandin levels may prolong the duration of the menstrual flow, which is significantly longer in women wearing IUDs than in women not wearing IUDs.

The amount of blood lost in each menstrual cycle is also significantly greater in women wearing inert as well as copper-bearing IUDs than in nonwearers. In a normal cycle the mean amount of menstrual blood loss (MBL) is about 35 ml; after insertion of a loop IUD the mean MBL increases to 70 ml to 80 ml. The increase is less with copper-bearing devices. With the Copper 7 the mean MBL has been found to vary from 50 ml to 55 ml, and with the copper T 200 the mean MBL varies from 50 ml to 60 ml. In contrast, with the progesterone-releasing IUD, the amount of blood loss per cycle is only about 25 ml.

Some investigators report that the increase in MBL with copper-bearing IUDs is greatest in the first cycle after IUD insertion, after which it declines steadily; however, others report that the increase in MBL persists for one year after copper IUD insertion. Guillebaud has shown that a greater than normal percentage of women wearing copper-bearing as well as inert IUDs have MBL in excess of 80 ml, which can produce severe iron deficiency. However, the decrease in mean hemoglobin level as well as the incidence of anemia are less dramatic in women using the Copper 7 than in women using the loop. A sensitive, noninvasive indicator of tissue iron stores is measurement of serum ferritin levels. Several studies have shown that women wearing both copper-bearing and inert IUDs have a significant decrease in serum ferritin levels, and in some the levels even drop to less than 16 μg/liter), indicating an absence of iron in bone marrow. Low serum ferritin levels are a good predictor of the development of anemia. Therefore, it is best that both ferritin and hemoglobin be measured annually in all non-steroid-releasing IUD wearers. If either parameter decreases significantly, the patient should receive supplemental iron.

Excessive bleeding in the first few months after IUD insertion should be treated with reassurance and supplemental oral iron. The bleeding may diminish with time as the uterus adjusts to the presence of the foreign body. Excessive bleeding that continues or develops several months or more after IUD insertion may be treated by systemic administration of one of the prostaglandin synthetase inhibitors such as mefenamic acid. If bleeding continues despite this treatment, the IUD should be removed. After a one-month interval another device may be inserted if the patient still wishes to use an IUD for contraception. If the original device was nonmedicated, the new device should be a copper- or a progesterone-releasing IUD; these smaller devices are associated with less blood loss than the larger, plastic devices.

Perforation

Although it is uncommon, one of the potentially serious complications associated with use of the IUD is perforation of the uterine fundus. Perforation initially occurs at insertion and can best be prevented by straightening of the uterine axis with a tenaculum and then a probe of the cavity with a uterine sound. IUD insertion is then best performed by the withdrawal technique. Sometimes only the distal portion of the IUD penetrates the uterine muscle at insertion, and then uterine contractions over the next few months force the IUD into the peritoneal cavity. IUDs correctly inserted entirely within the endometrial cavity do not wander through the uterine muscle into the peritoneal cavity. The incidence of perforation is generally related to the shape of the device and the amount of force used during its insertion, as well as to the experience of the clinician. The perforation rate with the loop and the copper IUDs has been reported to be about 1 in 1000 insertions. The clinician should always suspect that perforation has occurred if a patient states that she cannot feel the appendage but has not noticed the device being expelled. In this case one should not assume that an unnoticed expulsion has occurred. Frequently, the device has rotated 180 degrees and the appendage has withdrawn into the cavity. In this situation, after a pelvic examination has been performed and the possibility of pregnancy excluded, the uterine cavity should be probed. In a study of 100 patients who had no IUD appendage visible at the time of a routine examination, 69 had the IUD *in utero* with the strings drawn up into the endometrial cavity, 17 had had an unnoticed expulsion, and 10 had a uterine perforation. If the device cannot be felt with a uterine sound or biopsy instrument, an x-ray film or sonography should be ordered. It is best to obtain x-ray films of both anteroposterior and lateral views with contrast medium or a uterine sound inside the uterine cavity. The IUD may be located in the cul de sac, and the diagnosis may be missed if only an anteroposterior film is obtained.

If the IUD is found to be outside the uterus, it should be electively removed as soon as possible after the diagnosis of perforation is made, since complications such as adhesions and bowel obstruction have been reported with IUDs located intraperitoneally. Unless severe adhesions have developed, most intraperitoneal IUDs can be removed by means of laparoscopy, avoiding the necessity of laparotomy.

Perforation of the cervix has also been reported to occur with devices having a straight vertical arm, such as the Copper T and Copper 7. The incidence of downward perforation of these types of IUD into the cervix has been reported to range from about 1 in 600 to 1 in 1000 insertions. When follow-up examinations are performed on patients wearing these devices, the cervix should be carefully inspected and palpated; frequently, the perforation does not extend completely through the ectocervical epithelium. Cervical perforation is not a major problem, but devices that have perforated downward should be removed through the endocervical canal with uterine packing forceps, since such downward displacement is associated with reduced contraceptive effectiveness.

Infection

In the 1960s, despite great concern among gynecologists, there was little evidence that use of the IUD was associated with a marked increase in the incidence of salpingitis. In this decade the IUD was mainly inserted into parous women, and the incidence of sexually transmitted disease was not as high as it is now. Mishell and associates prepared aerobic and anaerobic cultures of endometrial homogenates obtained transfundally at varying intervals after insertion of a loop. In the first 24 hours following insertion of a loop, they found that the normally sterile endometrial cavity was consistently infected with bacteria; however, the body's natural defenses destroyed these bacteria within 24 hours in 80% of instances. In this study the endometrial cavity, the IUD, and the portion of the thread within the cavity were found to be consistently sterile when transfundal cultures were obtained more than 30 days after insertion (Fig. 14-6). These findings indicate that development of salpingitis more than one month after insertion of the loop type of IUD is of venereal origin and is unrelated to the presence of the IUD.

These findings agree with the incidence of PID found clinically in a group of 23,977 mainly parous women wearing IUDs who were analyzed by Tietze and Llewit in 1970. When PID rates were computed according to how long the IUD had been in place, they were found to be highest in the first two weeks after insertion and to steadily diminish thereafter. Rates after the first month were in the range of 1 to 2.5 per 100 woman-years (Table 14-11). The results of both these studies provide evidence that one should not insert an IUD in a patient who may recently have been infected with a pathogen such as *Gonococcus,* since insertion of the device would transport the pathogen into the upper genital tract. If the clinician suspects the existence of a gonococcal or chlamydial endocervicitis, cultures

FIG. 14-6. Relation of incidence of positive endometrial cultures to duration of use of IUD prior to hysterectomy. (Mishell DR Jr. et al: The intrauterine device: A bacteriologic study of the endometrial cavity. Am J Obstet Gynecol 96:119, 1966)

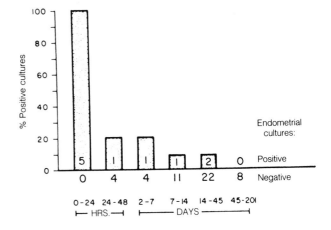

Table 14-11
*Rate of Pelvic Inflammatory Disease
by Period of Diagnosis*

Period	Cases	Woman-Years	Rate Per 100 Woman-Years (95% Confidence Limits)
1–25 days	75	969	7.7 (6–9.5)
26–30 days	34	913	3.7 (2.5–5)
2–12 months	421	16,144	2.6 (2.4–2.9)
13–24 months	236	10,588	2.2 (1.9–2.5)
25–36 months	94	6068	1.5 (1.2–1.9)
37–72 months	40	4420	0.9 (0.6–1.2)

(Tietze C, Lewit S: Evaluation of intrauterine devices: Ninth progress report of the Cooperative Statistical Program. Stud Fam Plann 1(55):22, 1970. Reprinted with the permission of the Population Council)

should be obtained and the IUD not inserted unless the results are negative. It is not cost effective to administer systemic antibiotics routinely during the time period of IUD insertion, but the insertion technique should be performed as aseptically as possible.

Following introduction and widespread use of the shield, particularly among nulliparous women, in whom IUDs had previously been inserted only occasionally, several studies suggested that use of IUDs significantly increases the relative risk of salpingitis and PID. There are several problems with these studies. One is that the guidelines used for the diagnosis of salpingitis and PID were not uniform. Differences in the criteria used to establish the diagnosis of salpingitis may have increased the frequency of the diagnosis among IUD wearers. Furthermore, patients with lower abdominal pain who had only minimal or no elevation in temperature may have been more often diagnosed as having salpingitis if they were using an IUD. A second problem is the evidence that oral contraceptives, condoms, and diaphragms provide protection against the development of salpingitis; data from numerous studies indicate that both febrile and nonfebrile PID occur about half as frequently in women using oral contraceptives and barrier methods as in women using no method of contraception. In the Oxford Family Planning Study, the incidences of PID requiring hospitalization were similar for these two methods of contraception. In many of the studies performed in the 1970s, a high percentage of women with IUDs were using the shield, which is more likely than other devices to have a causal relationship with salpingitis. Tatum and colleagues carefully examined the sheaths of the appendages of new shields, in their sterile packages, and the sheaths of shields removed from patients; they found that 34% of the former and 9% of the latter had breaks around the knot attaching the sheath to the device. Such breaks would allow bacteria continuous access from the vagina into the endometrial cavity and thus increase the risk of upper genital

tract infection. Finally, none of these studies differentiated between episodes of salpingitis developing in the first few months after IUD insertion, which have been shown to be related to insertion of the IUD, and episodes developing a few months after insertion. Recently, Lee and associates reported results from a multicenter case control study of the relationship of the IUD and PID. They found that the overall risk of PID in IUD users compared with noncontraceptive users is 1.9. Shield users had a risk of 8.3; users of other IUDs had a risk of only 1.6. When the PID risk of IUD users (other than users of the shield) was correlated with duration of use, it was found to be significantly increased only for the first four months after insertion (Table 14-12). Thus, this study is in agreement with the earlier studies mentioned above indicating that salpingitis occurring more than a few months after insertion of the loop or copper devices is most likely due to a sexually transmitted disease and is not related to the IUD.

The populations at high risk for PID include women with a prior history of PID, nulliparous women under 25 years of age, and women with multiple sexual partners. The FDA has recommended that women with these characteristics be advised about the risks of salpingitis with use of an IUD and the possibility of subsequent loss of fertility. They should be told to be alert for early symptoms of PID so that treatment can be started before complications occur. At present it would appear prudent for nulliparous women who wish eventually to conceive to avoid use of an IUD.

Symptomatic salpingitis may be successfully treated by antibiotics; the IUD should not be removed until the patient becomes asymptomatic. In patients who have

Table 14-12
Duration of Current IUD Use (Excluding Use of the Dalkon Shield) in Women With and Without PID

Duration of Use of Current IUD*	Women with PID†	Controls†	Relative Risk‡
≤1 month	27	17	3.8 (2.1–6.8)
2–4 months	22	32	1.7 (1.1–3.1)
5–12 months	33	90	1.1 (0.7–1.7)
13–24 months	32	81	1.2 (0.7–1.8)
25–60 months	23	62	1.2 (0.7–2)
>60 months	13	40	1.4 (0.7–2.7)
No method	250	763	1 (Referrent)

* IUD used in the three months before interview.

† Limited to women who reported no past history of pelvic inflammatory disease.

‡ Relative risk adjusted for age, marital status, and number of sexual partners within the previous six months; 95% confidence intervals in parentheses.

PID, pelvic inflammatory disease.

(Lee NC, Rubin GL, Ory HW, Burkman RT: Type of intrauterine device and the risk of pelvic inflammatory disease. Obstet Gynecol 62:1, 1983. Reprinted with permission from The American College of Obstetricians and Gynecologists)

clinical evidence of a tubo-ovarian abscess or who have a shield in place, the IUD should be removed after a therapeutic serum level of appropriate parenteral antibiotics has been reached and, preferably, after a clinical response has been observed. An alternative method of contraception should be used in patients who develop salpingitis with an IUD in place and in patients who have a past history of salpingitis. There is evidence that IUD users are at increased risk of colonizing *Actinomyses* organisms in the upper genital tract. The relationship of actinomycosis to salpingitis is unclear, but at present it would appear best to try to identify these organisms on the routine annual cytologic smear; if the organisms are present, the IUD should be removed and left out until they disappear, at which time a new device can be safely inserted. The use of antibiotics in asymptomatic women with actinomycosis is unnecessary.

Complications Related to Pregnancy

Congenital Anomalies

When pregnancy occurs with an IUD in place, implantation occurs away from the device, so the device is always extra-amniotic. Although there is a paucity of published data on the subject, there appears to be no evidence of an increased incidence of congenital anomalies in infants born of mothers with IUDs *in utero*. In Poland's study of aborted tissue from women who had had spontaneous abortions, 21% of the fetuses of women who had conceived with an IUD *in situ* had evidence of embryonic abnormalities. This was considerably less than the 44% incidence of abnormalities found in abortuses from women who had been using no contraception and was similar to the incidence of embryonic abnormalities found in abortuses of women who had had induced abortions. This study suggests that the presence of the IUD has no influence on embryonic development and that the higher than normal incidence of spontaneous abortion in IUD users is not due to a higher than normal incidence of abnormalities of the embryo.

Of 166 conceptions that occurred in women wearing intrauterine copper T IUDs and that progressed to a size large enough for examination for anomalies, only one infant was found to have a congenital anomaly, a fibroma of the vocal cords. Guillebaud reported that of 167 babies born to women with the Copper 7 in place, 159 were normal. No details were given regarding three infants, and the remaining five had a variety of anomalies. The incidence of congenital defects, 3%, was the expected rate. Thus, there is no evidence from these studies to indicate that the presence of copper in the uterus exerts a deleterious effect on fetal development. Although only few infants have been born to women with progesterone-releasing IUDs in place, careful examination of these infants has also revealed no increased incidence of cardiac or other anomalies.

Spontaneous Abortion

In all series of pregnancies among women with any type of IUD *in situ,* the incidence of fetal death has not been significantly higher than normal; however, the incidence of spontaneous abortion has been consistently increased. Results of three separate studies indicate that if a patient conceives with an IUD in place and the IUD is not removed, the patient's chance of having a spontaneous abortion is about 55%, approximately 3 times greater than the chance of a patient who conceives without an IUD.

If after conception the IUD is spontaneously expelled, or if the appendage is visible and the IUD is removed by traction, the incidence of spontaneous abortion is reduced to about 20%. Thus, if a woman conceives with an IUD *in situ* and wishes to continue the pregnancy, her IUD should be removed if the appendage is visible. If the appendage is not visible, the uterine cavity should not be probed; probing may increase the chance of abortion as well as of sepsis.

Septic Abortion

Evidence suggests that the risk of septic abortion may be higher than normal if an IUD in a woman who has conceived remains in place. Most of this evidence comes from women who conceived with the shield type of IUD, which had a multifilament tail. Bacteria were able to enter the spaces between the filaments of the tail underneath the sheath; when the shield device was drawn upward into the uterus as gestation advanced, the bacteria within the tail could cause a severe and sometimes fatal uterine infection. However, the shield type of IUD is no longer on the market, and bacteria cannot enter the monofilament tails of the devices that are now available. There is no conclusive evidence that a patient conceiving with an IUD with a monofilament tail has a risk of septic abortion higher than that associated with spontaneous abortions due to any cause; about 2% of all abortions become septic. If intrauterine infection does occur with an IUD in the pregnant uterus, the endometrial cavity should be evacuated after a short interval of appropriate antibiotic treatment, similar to the treatment of uterine sepsis without an IUD in place.

Ectopic Pregnancy

The IUD prevents intrauterine pregnancy more effectively than it prevents ectopic pregnancy, although use of an IUD reduces the overall incidence of ectopic pregnancy by 60% compared with use of no method of contraception. Nevertheless, a pregnancy that occurs with an IUD in place has a greater chance of being ectopic than a pregnancy that occurs with no IUD in place. If a patient conceives while wearing an IUD, her chances of having an ectopic pregnancy range from 3% to 9%. This incidence is about 10 times greater than that for total births in similar populations, 0.3% to 0.7%.

Thus, if a patient conceives with an IUD in place,

her physician should be alert to the possibility of ectopic pregnancy. The frequency of ectopic pregnancy is higher with use of the progesterone-releasing IUD than with use of other IUDs, so patients who conceive while wearing the former device should have sonography performed early in gestation. The possibility of ovarian pregnancy should also be considered. Patients wearing an IUD who have a clinical diagnosis of ruptured corpus luteum may in fact have an unrecognized ovarian pregnancy. If any patient with an IUD has an elective termination of pregnancy, the evacuated tissue should be examined histologically to establish that the gestation was intrauterine.

Prematurity

Several studies indicate that the rate of preterm delivery is higher than normal among women who keep their IUDs in place throughout gestation. If it is not possible to remove the IUD and the patient wishes to continue her gestation, she should be warned of the risk of prematurity in addition to the risk of spontaneous abortion. She should also be informed about the risk of ectopic pregnancy and septic abortion and told to report to her physician any signs of pelvic pain or fever. There is no evidence that pregnancies with an IUD *in utero* are associated with an increased incidence of other obstetric complications; there is also no evidence that prior use of an IUD is associated with a higher than normal incidence of complications in subsequent pregnancies.

Overall Safety

Several long-term studies have indicated that the IUD is not associated with a higher than normal incidence of carcinoma of the cervix or endometrium. Jain estimated that IUD users have an annual mortality rate of 3 to 5 deaths per 1 million women, most of the deaths being due to infection. He also demonstrated that with respect to mortality, the IUD is as safe as or safer than other methods of contraception, including sterilization, and safer than no contraception at all for women of any age. Use of the IUD may produce complications requiring hospitalization; the main causes of hospitalization among IUD users are complications of pregnancy, uterine perforation, hemorrhage, and pelvic infection. However, despite the relatively high morbidity rates associated with the IUD, the actual incidence of problems has been low and is probably lower still now that the shield is no longer being used and physicians are aware of the potential complications associated with use of the IUD in pregnancy. The IUD is a particularly useful method of contraception for women who do not want any more children but do not wish to undergo sterilization, as well as for older women, in whom the risks associated with oral contraceptives may be increased.

STERILIZATION

In 1982 one partner had been sterilized in each of about one third of all married couples in the United States who had been using a method of contraception. Sterilization was the most popular method of preventing pregnancy if the wife was over 30, if the couple had been married more than 10 years, and if the couple desired no further children. In contrast to the other methods of contraception, which are reversible or temporary, sterilization should be considered permanent. Although reanastomosis following vasectomy or tubal ligation is possible, the reconstructive operation is much more difficult than the original sterilizing procedure, and the results are variable. Pregnancy rates following reanastomosis of the vas range from 45% to 60%, and those following oviduct reanastomosis range from 50% to 80%, depending on the amount of tissue damage associated with the original procedure as well as on the technical competency of the surgeon.

Voluntary sterilization is legal in all 50 states. The decision to be sterilized should be made solely by the patient in consultation with the physician. Since all sterilization procedures entail surgery, patients who request sterilization should be counseled regarding both the risks and the irreversibility of the procedures. It is advisable to fully inform the patient, and the spouse if possible, of the benefits and risks of these voluntary surgical procedures. A woman requesting sterilization who is less than 25 years of age and has fewer than three living children, or who is of any age and has no children, should see more than one counselor before undergoing the procedure.

Reversibility

The reason for the careful scrutiny of young candidates for sterilization is that such candidates are more likely than older candidates to change their minds and have less fixed attitudes, and they face a longer period of reproductive life during which divorce, remarriage, or death among their children can occur. About 1% of sterilized women subsequently request reversal. In the United States, approximately 7000 women request reversal each year.

The most effective, least destructive, most easily reversed method of tubal occlusion is the most desirable in younger patients. The effective laparoscopic band techniques or the modified Pomeroy technique (Fig. 14-7) should be used in patients who are less than 25 years of age. Reversal of this method of sterilization is followed by pregnancy in about 75% of cases, a rate that is higher than that reported following reversal of most laparoscopic fulgurations, in which more tube is destroyed. So little viable tube remains after laparoscopic fulguration that most patients who have undergone this type of sterilization are not candidates for reversal.

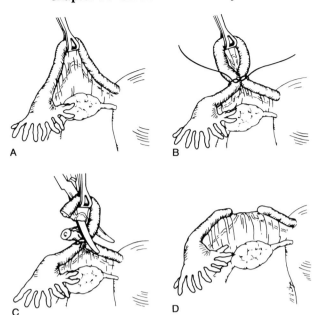

FIG. 14-7. Modified Pomeroy technique of female steriliza-tion. (Sciarra JJ: Surgical procedures for tubal sterilization. In Sciarra JJ, Zatuchni GI, Daly MJ: Gynecology and Obstetrics, Vol 6. Philadelphia, Harper & Row, 1984)

Male Sterilization

Sterilization of the male is accomplished by vasectomy, an outpatient procedure that takes about 20 minutes and requires only local anesthesia. In this procedure the vas deferens is isolated and cut and the ends of the vas are closed, either by ligation or by fulguration, and are then replaced in the scrotal sac. Then the incision is closed. Complications of vasectomy include hematoma (in up to 5% of subjects), sperm granulomas (inflammatory re-sponses to sperm leakage), and spontaneous reanasto-mosis (if this is to occur, it usually does so a short time after the procedure). Hematoma is best prevented by ligation of all small vessels in the scrotal wall. The oc-currence of sperm granuloma is minimized by cauter-ization or fulguration, instead of ligation, of the ends of the vas. After the procedure the man is not considered sterile until he has produced two sperm-free ejaculates; this usually requires about 15 to 20 ejaculations. Semen analysis should be performed one and two months after the procedure. Although in the United States requests for reversal range from 6% to 7%, vas reanastomosis is a difficult procedure that requires meticulous surgical technique. Reversal of vasectomy has a success rate of about 50%.

Female Sterilization

Sterilization of the female is more complicated, requir-ing a transperitoneal incision and, usually, general

anesthesia. In postpartum sterilization a small infraum-bilical incision is made and the fallopian tubes ligated with either a Pomeroy or a modified Irving technique. This simple, rapid procedure can be performed either in the delivery room immediately after delivery or in the operating room the following day without prolong-ing the patient's hospital stay. The same operative tech-niques can be used for female sterilization at times other than the puerperium, but for such "interval sterilization" additional procedures are also required. Ligation of the oviducts by the Pomeroy technique can be easily and rapidly performed through a small abdominal incision; this has been termed a *minilaparotomy*. On occasion a colpotomy incision may also be used, but this incision is associated with a higher incidence of postoperative infection than an abdominal incision.

The development of fiberoptic light sources has made laparoscopy a popular gynecologic operative technique. By using various accessories in addition to the laparoscope, the operator can fulgurate and cut the oviducts without making an intraperitoneal incision other than one or two small punctures. Most gynecol-ogists find the two-puncture technique for laparoscopy sterilization easier to learn and perform than the single-puncture technique. General anesthesia is usually used for laparoscopic sterilization, but overnight hospitaliza-tion is unnecessary. The failure rate following this tech-nique is about 1 per 1000 procedures. Given that the pregnancy rate following fulguration and transection is similar to that following fulguration alone, it is recom-mended that the oviducts not be cut following fulgura-tion. The incidence of complications following lapa-roscopic fulguration ranges from 1% to 6%; major com-plications (hemorrhage, puncture or cautery of bowel) occur in about 0.6% of cases.

Bipolar forceps were developed to replace the uni-polar apparatus and thereby eliminate the problem of bowel injury. In the unipolar system the current passes through a grounding plate attached to the patient; in the bipolar system the current passes into one prong of the forceps, through the tissue, and out the other prong, thus producing limited coagulation with destruction of a small segment of the oviduct. After coagulation, if di-vision is to be performed, scissors are introduced to cut the oviduct. If division is not to be performed, some operators perform contiguous burn coagulation on each oviduct to ensure adequate obliteration of the lumen. When the unipolar apparatus is used, a single 1-cm burn on each oviduct is sufficient. However, even with this small amount of coagulation, local tissue damage is ex-tensive, and attempts at reanastomosis have a very low rate of success. Bipolar coagulation not only is safer but also is associated with a higher success rate following reanastomosis; therefore, this technique is now the rec-ommended form of oviduct fulguration.

Because of the problems associated with electro-coagulation, efforts have been made to develop safer methods that destroy less tissue. Nonelectrical tubal oc-clusion may be performed through the laparoscope with tantalum, plastic, and spring-loaded clips, with a Silastic band, or with a Falope ring. All of these techniques involve a modification of conventional laparoscopy, and their performance requires special training. The failure rate for the clip and band techniques averages about 2 per 1000 procedures, the range being 1 to 6 per 1000.

INDUCED ABORTION

When contraception or sterilization is not used or fails, abortion may now be legally performed in the United States and many other countries. Each state of the United States may regulate the abortion procedure for second- and third-trimester abortions in ways that are reasonably related to maternal health.

From 1973 to 1980 the number of legal abortions performed in the United States steadily increased, but since then the abortion rate has remained stable. In 1982 there were an estimated 1.6 million legal abortions; in the same year, 26% of all pregnancies were terminated by induced abortion, a rate of 29 per 1000 women between the ages of 15 and 44, and 300 abortions were performed for every 1000 live births plus abortions. In 1982 about 3% of all women of childbearing age in the United States underwent an abortion. About one third of these abortions were in women under the age of 20, and another third were in women aged 20 to 24. One fourth of these abortions were obtained by married women. About 90% of abortions were performed at eight weeks' gestation or less. About 85% of abortions were performed by suction curettage, 10% by surgical curettage, and 5% by saline infusion. Under 2% were terminated by administration of prostaglandins.

Methods

There are three major methods of termination of pregnancy: instrumental evacuation by the vaginal route, stimulation of uterine contractions, and major surgical procedures.

Vaginal Evacuation

Vaginal evacuation by either dilatation and curettage or vacuum aspiration (suction) is mainly limited to abortion in the first trimester. In the first few weeks of gestation, endometrial aspiration, sometimes misnamed *menstrual extraction,* can be done with a small, flexible plastic cannula without dilatation or anesthesia. Abortions performed eight or more weeks after the onset of the last menses may require dilatation of the cervix and general or local paracervical anesthesia. The need for mechanical dilatation of the cervix can often be avoided by use of laminaria tents, which swell after placement in the cervical canal. Usual practice is to allow them to remain in place for several hours before evacuation of the uterus. Use of these tents is particularly helpful in

the nulliparous woman, and their routine use allows the majority of first trimester abortions to be performed without anesthesia. Beyond 12 to 13 weeks, it is advisable to evacuate the uterus in the operating suite, but overnight hospitalization is usually not necessary.

Suction curettage used to be largely restricted to cases in which gestation was less than 13 weeks. However, recent studies have shown that dilatation and evacuation can be performed in the second trimester: dilatation is achieved by means of either graduated dilators or preinsertion of several laminaria; use of a large suction cannula may suffice, and ovum forceps may also be used. At 12 to 16 weeks' gestation, dilatation and evacuation is safer, more rapid, and less expensive than the infusion technique or surgery. Between 16 and 20 weeks' gestation, the incidence of minor complications associated with this method is probably similar to that associated with saline or prostaglandin infusion, but the incidence of major complications, such as uterine and bowel perforation, is probably greater. Disadvantages include the great technical expertise that is required, the emotional trauma to participating physicians and paramedical personnel, and the possible long-term effects of cervical trauma.

Stimulation of Uterine Contractions

Second-trimester abortion is usually initiated by the stimulation of uterine contractions. The most commonly used method is the replacement of 100 ml to 200 ml of amniotic fluid with up to 200 ml of 20% saline solution. Labor usually starts within 12 to 24 hours after the instillation, and evacuation of the uterine contents usually follows 12 to 24 hours later. The delay can usually be shortened by the concomitant use of oxytocin; however, the addition of oxytocin increases the incidence of complications, especially consumption coagulopathy and cervical rupture, that may result in cervicovaginal fistula.

Intra-amniotic administration of 40 mg prostaglandin $F_{2\alpha}$ is also used to stimulate uterine contractions in the second trimester. This technique has a slightly higher success rate (90–95%) than saline instillation (85–90%), and the infusion-to-abortion time interval is somewhat shorter.

Other solutions that have been injected into the amniotic fluid to induce abortion are urea and hypertonic glucose. The former is frequently used in Great Britain, but the latter is associated with a high incidence of infection and its use is not recommended.

Transvaginal extra-amniotic administration of prostaglandin $F_{2\alpha}$ and placement of a metreurynter into the lower uterine segment are also used to initiate uterine contractions in the second trimester. These procedures are usually recommended for use early in the second trimester, at 12 to 16 weeks' gestation, when it is easiest to avoid the amniotic sac.

Two additional prostaglandins have been approved for abortion. These are vaginal suppositories of prostaglandin E_2 (20 mg) and intramuscular 15 methyl prostaglandin $F_{2\alpha}$. Both are noninvasive techniques associated with few complications (the most common complication is infection) and ease of administration. They should not be used in patients who have asthma or who have undergone uterine surgery, but in all other patients they have a success rate greater than 95% with an abortion time of just 8 to 12 hours. Repeated insertion or injection is necessary in both techniques. Both are associated with a high incidence of gastrointestinal side-effects, primarily nausea, vomiting, and diarrhea, which can usually be controlled by appropriate premedication. The E_2 suppositories also cause a chilly sensation and elevation of body temperature. These newly approved methods are the recommended method for termination of pregnancy between 12 and 18 weeks' gestation. After 18 weeks' gestation intra-amniotic saline is probably the method of choice.

Hysterectomy or hysterotomy can be performed in both the first and second trimesters. Hysterotomy is associated with a high incidence of complications and should therefore be avoided if possible. Hysterectomy has the advantage of sterilizing the patient while eliminating the possibility of subsequent uterine or menstrual disorders. Abortion hysterectomy has been performed with low morbidity both abdominally and vaginally in both the first and early second trimesters in relatively large numbers of patients.

Complications

The possible immediate complications of evacuation of the uterus include perforation of the uterus, hemorrhage, and cervical laceration. Hypertonic saline may cause consumption coagulopathy with severe hemorrhage, as well as adverse central nervous system effects. Complications of prostaglandin administration include hypertension, tachycardia, bronchoconstriction, nausea, vomiting, and diarrhea, as well as development of slow-healing cervicovaginal fistulas. The possible delayed complications of all therapeutic abortions include retention of a portion of the placenta causing bleeding problems, infection, thrombophlebitis, preterm labor in subsequent pregnancies, RH sensitization in RH-negative women, and sterility, especially in patients who develop infection and perhaps in others who develop intrauterine synechiae.

Complication rates are 3 to 4 times higher for second-trimester abortions than for first-trimester abortions. By technique, complication rates are lowest for vacuum aspiration, followed in order by dilatation and curettage, hypertonic saline, hysterotomy, and hysterectomy. The complication rate for abortion by hysterotomy is 2 to 3 times higher than the usual rate for second-trimester abortion by other methods, which is already high.

In young women, the incidence of both serious complications and death is higher for abortion than for any method of contraception. For this reason, contraception or sterilization is the preferred method of preventing unwanted pregnancy; therapeutic abortion should be reserved for cases in which these safer techniques fail.

REFERENCES AND RECOMMENDED READING

Alvior GT Jr.: Pregnancy outcome with removal of intrauterine device. Obstet Gynecol 41:894, 1973

Anderson ABM, Haynes PJ, Guillebaud J et al: Reduction of menstrual blood loss by prostaglandin synthetase inhibitors. Lancet 1:774, 1976

Boston Collaborative Drug Surveillance Program: Oral contraceptives and venous thromboembolic disease, surgically confirmed gallbladder disease, and breast tumors. Lancet 1:1399, 1973

Brenner PF et al: Serum levels of d-norgestrel, luteinizing hormone, follicle-stimulating hormone, estradiol, and progesterone in women during and following ingestion of combination oral contraceptives containing dl-norgestrel. Am J Obstet Gynecol 129:133, 1977

Casagrande JT, Louie EW, Pike MD et al: "Incessant ovulation" and ovarian cancer. Lancet 2:170, 1979

Centers for Disease Control Cancer and Steroid Hormone Study: Long-term oral contraceptive use and the risk of breast cancer. JAMA 249:1591, 1983

Dixon GW, Schlesselman JJ, Ory HW, Blye RP: Ethinyl estradiol and conjugated estrogens as postcoital contraceptives. JAMA 244:1336, 1980

Forrest JD, Henshaw SK: What U.S. women think and do about contraception. Fam Plann Perspect 15:162, 1983

Garcia C-R, Huggins GR, Rosenfeld DL et al: Postcoital contraception: Medical and social factors of the morning after pill. Contraception 15:445, 1977

Grady WR, Hirsch MB, Keen N, Vaughan B: Contraceptive failure and continuation among married women in the U.S., 1970–75. Stud Fam Plann 14:9, 1983

Guillebaud J: Copper IUCDs and pregnancy (letter). Br J Fam Plann 7(3):88, 1981

Jain AK: Safety and effectiveness of intrauterine devices. Contraception 11:243, 1975

Klein TA, Mishell DR Jr.: Gonadotropin, prolactin and steroid hormone levels after discontinuation of oral contraceptives. Am J Obstet Gynecol 127:585, 1977

Layde PM, Beral V, Kar CR: Further analyses of mortality in oral contraceptive users. Royal College of General Practitioners' Oral Contraceptive Study. Lancet 1:541, 1981

Lee NC, Rubin GL, Ory HW, Burkman RT: Type of intrauterine device and the risk of pelvic inflammatory disease. Obstet Gynecol 62:1, 1983

Lehfeldt H, Tietze C, Gorstein F: Ovarian pregnancy and the intrauterine device. Am J Obstet Gynecol 108:1005, 1970

Lewit SL: Outcome of pregnancies with intrauterine devices. Contraception 2:47, 1970

Liedholm P, Sjöberg N-O, Astedt B: Increased bleeding and increased fibrinolytic activity in the endometrium in women using the copper T. In Hefnawi F, Segal SJ (eds): Analysis of Intrauterine Contraception, p 391. Amsterdam, Elsevier–North Holland, 1975

Luukkainen T, Allonen H, Nielsen N-C et al: Five years' experience of intrauterine contraception with Nova-T and Copper-T-200. Am J Obstet Gynecol (in press)

Mastroianni L Jr.: Rhythm: Systematized chance-taking. Fam Plann Perspect 6:209, 1974

Meade TW, Greenberg G, Thompson SG: Progestogens and cardiovascular reactions associated with oral contraceptives and a comparison of the safety of 50- and 30-μg estrogen preparations. Br Med J 1:1157, 1980

Millen A, Austin FJ, Bernstein GS: Analysis of 100 cases of missing IUD strings. Contraception 8:485, 1978

Mishell DR Jr.: The effects of contraceptive steroids on hypothalamic–pituitary function. Am J Obstet Gynecol 128: 60, 1977

Mishell DR Jr., Roy S: Copper intrauterine contraceptive device event rates following insertion 4 to 8 weeks postpartum. Am J Obstet Gynecol 143:29, 1982

Mishell DR Jr. et al: The intrauterine device: A bacteriologic study of the endometrial cavity. Am J Obstet Gynecol 96: 119, 1966

Morehead JE, Matthews A, Guillebaud J, Bonnar J: Menstrual blood loss in users of an IUD. In Hefnawi F, Segal SJ (eds): Analysis of Intrauterine Contraception, p 381. Amsterdam, Elsevier–North Holland, 1975

Morris JM, van Wagenen G: Interception: The use of postovulatory estrogens to prevent implantation. Am J Obstet Gynecol 115:101, 1973

Nash HA: Depo-provera: A review. Contraception 12:377, 1975

Oral Contraceptives and Health: An Interim Report from the Oral Contraceptive Study of the Royal College of General Practitioners. New York, Pitman Publishing, 1974

Ory HW: The noncontraceptive health benefits from oral contraceptive use. Fam Plann Perspect 14:182, 1982

Pike MC, Henderson BE, Krailo MD et al: Breast cancer in young women and use of oral contraceptives: Possible modifying effect of formulation and age at use. Lancet 2: 926, 1983

Pituitary Adenoma Study Group: Pituitary adenomas and oral contraceptives: A multicenter case-control study. Fertil Steril 39:753, 1983

Poland B: Conception control and embryonic development. Am J Obstet Gynecol 106:365, 1970

Porter JB, Hunter JR, Danielson DA et al: Oral contraceptive and nonfatal vascular disease—Recent experience. Obstet Gynecol 59:299, 1982

Ramcharan S, Pellegrin FA, Ray RM, Hsu J-P: The Walnut Creek Contraceptive Drug Study: A Prospective Study of the Side Effects of Oral Contraceptives, Vol III, NIH Publication #81-564. Washington, DC, United States Government Printing Office, 1981

Royal College of General Practitioners' Oral Contraception Study: Further analysis of mortality in oral contraceptive users. Lancet 1:541, 1981

Royal College of General Practitioners' Oral Contraception Study: Mortality among oral contraceptive users. Lancet 2:727, 1977.

Ryden G, Fahraeus L, Molin L et al: Do contraceptives influence the incidence of acute pelvic inflammatory disease in women with gonorrhea? Contraception 20:149, 1979

Schirm AL, Trussell J, Menken J, Grady WR: Contraceptive failure in the United States: The impact of social, economic and demographic factors. Fam Plann Perspect 14:68, 1982

Schwallie PC, Assenzo JR: Contraceptive use—Efficacy study utilizing medroxyprogesterone acetate administered as an intramuscular injection once every 90 days. Fertil Steril 24:331, 1973

Schwallie PC, Assenzo JR: The effect of depomedroxyprogesterone acetate on pituitary and ovarian function, and the return of fertility following its discontinuation: A review. Contraception 10:181, 1974

Scott JA et al: Comparison of the effects of contraceptive steroid formulations containing two doses of estrogen on pituitary function. Fertil Steril 30:141, 1978

Sivin I, Tatum HJ: Four years of experience with the T Cu 380A intrauterine contraceptive device. Fertil Steril 36:159, 1981

Swyer GIM: Potency of progestins in oral contraceptives—Further delay of menses data. Contraception 26:23, 1982

Tatum HJ, Schmidt FH, Jain AK: Management and outcome of pregnancies associated with the copper T intrauteirne contraceptive device. Am J Obstet Gynecol 126:869, 1976

Tatum HJ, Schmidt FH, Phillips DM: Morphological studies of Dalkon Shield tails removed from patients. Contraception 11:465, 1975

Tietze C, Lewit S: Evaluation of intrauterine devices: Ninth progress report of the Cooperative Statistical Program. Stud Fam Plann 1:55, 1970

Vessey MP et al: A long-term follow-up study of women using different methods of contraception—An interim report. J Biosoc Sci 8:373, 1976

Vessey MP, Lawless M, McPherson K, Yeates D: Fertility after stopping use of intrauterine contraceptive device. Br Med J 286:106, 1983

Vessey MP, Wright NH, McPherson K et al: Fertility after stopping different methods of contraception. Br Med J 1:265, 1978

Westrom L: Incidence, prevalence and trends of acute pelvic inflammatory disease and its consequences in industrialized countries. Am J Obstet Gynecol 138:880, 1980

White MK, Ory HW, Rooks JB, Rochat RW: Intrauterine device termination rates and the menstrual cycle day of insertion. Obstet Gynecol 55:220, 1980

Williams P, Johnson B, Vessey M: Septic abortion in women using intrauterine devices. Br Med J 4:253, 1975

Wilson JG, Brent RL: Are female sex hormones teratogenic? Am J Obstet Gynecol 141:567, 1981

World Health Organization Expanded Programme of Research Development and Research Training in Human Reproduction: Task force on long-acting systemic agents for the regulation of fertility. Contraception 15:513, 1977

Yuzpe AA, Smith RP, Rademaker AW: A multicenter clinical investigation employing ethinyl estradiol combined with dl-norgestrel as a postcoital contraceptive agent. Fertil Steril 37:508, 1982

Ultrasound in Obstetrics and Gynecology

Rudy E. Sabbagha

15

PRINCIPLES

The use of ultrasound for diagnostic purposes is based on two technologies. The first is concerned with the transmission of high-frequency sound waves through interfaces between tissues of different densities. The second pertains to the display of the echoes produced at these interfaces on a cathode ray tube (crt) or television monitor. The sound waves used in ultrasound imaging are transmitted and received by a piezoelectric crystal or crystals housed within a transducer. Transducers can be of varying shapes (Fig. 15-1). The transducer is electrically pulsed at a rate of approximately 600 to 1000 times per second. The piezoelectric crystal also receives echoes and transforms the sound into electrical energy. The thickness of the piezoelectric crystal determines the frequency of the emitted beam: thinner crystals produce higher frequencies. The frequencies commonly utilized in obstetric and gynecologic imaging range from 2 to 5 million vibrations (MHz) per second.

Velocity

The velocity of ultrasound is determined by the elastic properties and density of the medium it traverses. The average speed of ultrasound in soft tissue is 1540 meters per second (m/sec). This constant has practical applications because it is used as a basis for defining the centimeter scale printed on echograms (Fig. 15-2) and for calibrating the distance between electronic measuring calipers.

The size of fetal structures and pelvic masses is gauged in relation to the centimeter scale or the electronic calipers. For example, when measured ultrasonographically, the biparietal diameter (BPD) used in estimating fetal size is the product of the time taken by the echo to traverse the distance between leading edges of the strongest echoes of the head and the speed of ultrasound (Fig. 15-2). If the time taken is 0.0000585 seconds, for example, and the average ultrasound tissue velocity is 1540 m/sec, then the machine automatically makes the calculation as follows:

$$BPD = 0.0000585 \times 1540 = 0.09 \text{ m or } 9.0 \text{ cm}$$

BPDs measured in this way represent the outer-to-inner (O–I) dimension of the fetal head. However, if a velocity of 1600 m/sec is used, the BPD is transformed into an anatomic outer-to-outer (O–O) dimension. Thus, in the example cited the calculation is changed to:

$$BPD = 0.0000585 \times 1600$$
$$= 0.0935 \text{ m or } 9.35 \text{ cm}$$

The increase of 0.35 cm is equivalent to the thickness of the distal skull and scalp.

In some European countries a tissue velocity of 1600 m/sec is deliberately used in the calibration of electronic calipers to produce anatomic outer to outer BPD measurements. The BPD charts produced in this way are larger than those employed elsewhere by a factor of 1600/1540, or 1.039.

Depth of Penetration

As ultrasound passes through interfaces between tissues of different density, energy is reflected, scattered, refracted, and absorbed. Thus, the ultrasound beam reaching posterior structures of the body is attenuated. The rapidity of attenuation is directly related to the frequency used. For example, ultrasound at a frequency of 5 MHz is more rapidly attenuated than ultrasound at a

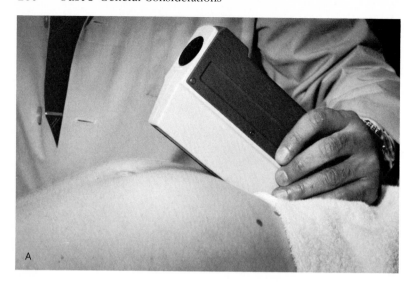
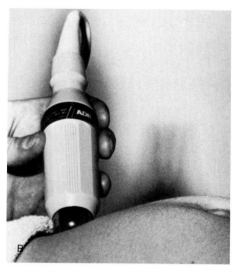

FIG. 15-1. (*A*) A linear dynamic transducer cannot be appropriately angled to show the uterus. Partial contact with the skin is lost in both sagittal and transverse planes because of interference from the symphysis pubis and lateral aspect of the pelvis, respectively. (*B*) A sector transducer with a small scanning head can be easily angled toward adnexal areas (here shown pointing to the left side) and is therefore suitable for use in gynecologic imaging.

frequency of 3 MHz. The degree of attenuation is measured in decibels (db), which are units expressing the ratio between the strengths or amplitudes (A) of two signals. In soft tissue the degree of attenuation (attenuation coefficient) is in the neighborhood of 0.5 to 1.0 db/cm/MHz. Echoes produced by attenuated beams are weak and must be amplified to produce images of good quality. This amplification is accomplished by a time gain control mechanism.

Time Gain Control

A time gain control (TGC) mechanism is incorporated in all ultrasonic equipment. Its function is to decrease the amplitude of echoes from structures close to the transducer and increase the strength of weak posterior signals. In this way a more uniform image is produced and resolution is improved. Near and far gain controls can be adjusted manually or automatically to produce the desired effect.

Wavelength and Image Resolution

The relationship among wavelength, speed of sound, and frequency is governed by the formula:

$$Wavelength = speed\ of\ sound/frequency$$

Thus, wavelength is inversely proportional to frequency. At high frequencies, the wavelength of the sound beam is shorter and resolution of two reflectors or structures

within the path of the sound beam can be achieved (Fig. 15-3). In other words, at higher frequencies the wavelength of the beam is shorter and images are sharper. However, this improvement in resolution mainly occurs in the near field of the transducer because there is increasing attenuation and diversion of the sound beam distally, in the far field.

The overall resolution of any ultrasonic system both axially (along the path of the beam) and laterally (perpendicular to the path of the beam) is dependent on frequency and wavelength. Ideally, the transducer should utilize a frequency high enough to produce a narrow or focused beam but a wavelength long enough to enable penetration to the desired depth.

B-Mode (Brightness Mode) Display

In the B-mode format, echo signals are used to form a two-dimensional image of the anatomic structures being examined. Gray-scale sonography has enhanced B-mode imaging; in this technology a scan converter with a solid-state semiconductor device is used to recognize and store echo signals with different amplitudes. Digital circuitry is then used to instantaneously transform these signals to a television image in which the strongest echoes are depicted as white and the less strong as varying shades of gray. In this way all echoes, weak or strong, are represented and little information is lost.

The B-mode format also includes dynamic or *real-time imaging,* in which a variety of linear and sector transducers with different focusing mechanisms are used to enhance image resolution; in this format the monitor

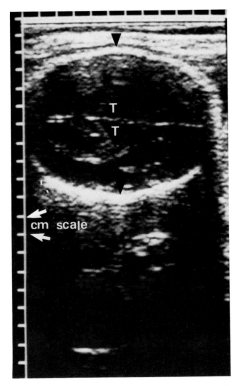

FIG. 15-2. Echogram of fetal head at the plane showing both thalamic bodies (*T*). Such an echogram is used for measuring the biparietal diameter (BPD), occipitofrontal diameter (OFD), and head circumference (HC). The BPD, used to estimate dates and fetal growth, is measured from the leading edge of the strongest echoes (*arrows*). It is an outer-to-inner measurement rather than an anatomic measurement. The HC can be measured directly with a digitizer or estimated from the following formula: (BPD + OFD/2) × 3.14. The cephalic index is obtained from the formula BPD/OFD × 100. The outer-to-outer BPD and OFD are used in calculating the HC or the cephalic index.

display is continually updated to depict motion in the structures being examined. In dynamic equipment the transducer is attached to a flexible cord and can readily be moved to different planes and angles until the sought-after structure or target (for example, the mitral valve or the femur) is perfectly imaged. Thus, real-time equipment permits targeted dynamic imaging (TDI). TDI is particularly applicable to obstetric sonography because the fetus is a moving target. Within the obstetric context TDI appreciably shortens scanning time and provides clear sonographic images that can be photographed or videotaped.

Acoustic Energy

The acoustic energy generated by ultrasound is measured in watts. Acoustic power per unit area is the acoustic intensity. For example, if the acoustic power of a transducer with a radius of 1 cm is 10 milliwatts (mW) the spatial average intensity I(SA) at the surface of the transducer is:

$$10 \text{ mW/area} = 10 \text{ mW/}\pi r^2$$
$$= 10 \text{ mW/3.14 cm}^2 = 3.2 \text{ mW/cm}^2$$

The spatial peak intensity of sound, referred to as I(SP), is the highest intensity in an ultrasound beam at a specified distance from the face of the transducer. If the ultrasonic beam is unfocused the I(SP) is three or four times greater than the I(SA). On the other hand if the ultrasonic beam is focused—that is, narrow—the I(SP) can be greater than the I(SA) by a factor of 10 or more.

Intensity of sound is also measured temporally and is dependent on the *duty factor,* which is the duration of an ultrasonic pulse divided by pulse repetition frequency. The instantaneous peak intensity or I(IP) of a pulse can be greater than the time-averaged intensity or I(TA) by a factor of 1000. The relationship can be expressed as:

$$I(IP) = I(TA)/\text{duty factor}$$

In calculating acoustic energy for the study of biologic effects of ultrasound investigators must consider both spatial and temporal intensities of sound in tissues. The following acronyms are used:

I(SATA) for spatial average and time average intensity
I(SPTA) for spatial peak and time average intensity
I(SPIP) for spatial peak and instantaneous peak intensity

Typical values of I(SATA) are 1.0 to 60 mW/cm² and of I(SPTA) are 1.0 to 200 mW/cm². In pulsed Doppler devices the intensity levels may be much higher. Manufacturers of ultrasound equipment introduced into U.S. commerce are required to report these outputs to the Food and Drug Administration (FDA).

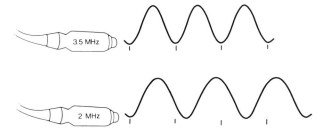

FIG. 15-3. High-frequency transducers (*e.g.,* 3.5 MHz) produce small wavelengths capable of separating two reflectors or interfaces. As a result, their resolution is superior to that of transducers with lower frequencies; the latter emit wide wavelengths and fail to resolve reflectors situated close to each other.

Biologic Effects

A number of epidemiologic studies tend to support the safety of ultrasound in humans. However, many of these studies do not adequately address a number of important questions about issues such as the following.

1. Dosimetry. Dose is related to the length of the ultrasound examination or exposure time, and this can vary markedly.
2. Possible interaction between ultrasound and agents or events that may influence cell development, such as drugs, ionizing irradiation, and hypoxia.
3. Long-term status of exposed infants, as evaluated by randomized clinical trials.

Teratologic effects have been observed in some experimental animals at energy levels higher than those used clinically, and these may be attributable to significant tissue hyperthermia. Biologic effects, such as reduction in immune response, change in cell membrane function, and increase in sister chromatid exchanges, have also been produced *in vitro*. However, none of these effects has been independently reproduced. Furthermore, the results of these experiments cannot be meaningfully extrapolated to human subjects.

In 1984 a National Institutes of Health panel consisting of 26 members published a consensus report concerning the safety and usefulness of ultrasound in pregnancy. The panel concluded that:

1. Some of the reported biologic effects cannot be entirely overlooked, despite their lack of applicability to the human fetus.
2. Additional controlled studies dealing with biologic effects in the human fetus are desirable.
3. Diagnostic ultrasound for pregnant women improves patient management and outcome when there is an accepted medical indication.

The panel listed 28 clinical situations in which diagnostic ultrasound imaging had been shown to be useful (Table 15-1). In the course of this chapter these indications will all be addressed, though not in the order presented in Table 15-1.

THE ULTRASONIC EXAMINATION

A great deal of information about the pregnant uterus can now be obtained sonographically. In particular, a number of fetal anomalies can be recognized. Thus, questions about the amount of data gathered at each examination, the length of exposure to ultrasound, and the extent of physician involvement in scanning have become important. They have also generated some controversy.

Physicians who do not advocate the routine use of ultrasound for detection of all fetal anomalies in low-risk pregnancies are concerned about a variety of issues including the following:

Table 15-1

Indications for Use of Diagnostic Ultrasound Suggested by National Institutes of Health Consensus Conference

Estimation of gestational age for patients with uncertain clinical dates	Suspected abruptio placentae	Suspected ectopic pregnancy
Evaluation of fetal growth	Adjunct to external version from breech to vertex presentation	Adjunct to special procedures
Vaginal bleeding of undetermined etiology in pregnancy	Estimation of fetal weight and/or presentation in premature rupture of membranes and/or premature labor	Suspected fetal death
Determination of fetal presentation		Suspected uterine abnormality
Suspected multiple gestation	Abnormal serum alpha-fetoprotein value	Intrauterine contraceptive device localization
Adjunct to amniocentesis	Follow-up observation of identified fetal anomaly	Ovarian follicle development surveillance
Significant uterine size/clinical dates discrepancy	Follow-up evaluation of placental location for identified placenta previa	Biophysical evaluation for fetal well-being after 28 weeks of gestation
Pelvic mass	History of previous congenital anomaly	Observation of intrapartum events
Suspected hydatidiform mole	Serial evaluation of fetal growth in multiple gestation	Evaluation of fetal condition in late registrants for prenatal care
Suspected polyhydramnios or oligohydramnios	Adjunct to cervical cerclage placement	

(Diagnostic Ultrasound Imaging in Pregnancy. Report of the Consensus Development Conference, National Institute of Child Health and Development. NIH Publication No 84-667. Washington, DC, Government Printing Office, 1984)

1. The fact that tests can be administered by nonphysician professionals (sonographers) or by physicians with little experience in the use of ultrasound for the diagnosis of anomalies;
2. The fact that routine use of ultrasound leads to long exposure to ultrasound that is unnecessary for the general population;
3. The fact that cost-to-benefit ratio is poor, as reflected in the low yield of positive results in low-risk pregnancies;
4. The fact that single ultrasound studies performed at 16 to 18 weeks of gestation (an interval commonly used for initial scans) are unable to detect a number of anomalies, including microcephaly, late-onset hydrocephaly, intestinal obstruction, polycystic renal disease, and some forms of skeletal dysplasia, such as heterozygous achondroplasia.

The difficulties arising from the complexity of ultrasound examinations were first addressed by the participants of the Third International Genetic Conference, held in 1980 at Scarborough, Maine. The concept of a two-tier system in the form of stage-I and stage-II ultrasound examinations was introduced then; these stages have evolved into what is now known as basic or standard ultrasound studies and targeted imaging for fetal anomaly (TIFFA) studies.

The standard ultrasound study is used to define gestational age and fetal number, assess growth, and examine the pregnancy to determine presence of fetal heart motion, presentation, qualitative amniotic fluid volume, and placental position and texture. In addition, fetal anatomy is surveyed for gross anomalies, such as anencephaly.

A Standard study is essential for the interpretation of an abnormal level of maternal serum alpha fetoprotein (MS/AFP). For example, if a fetus is ultrasonically determined to be more mature than was estimated clinically on the basis of menstrual history, an apparently abnormal elevation in MS/AFP can be reinterpreted. Additionally, elevated levels of MS/AFP associated with twin pregnancies or undiagnosed intrauterine fetal death can be explained. Follow-up studies of women with abnormally elevated MS/AFP values have shown that in approximately 50% the reason for the elevation is clarified by the findings of a basic ultrasound examination.

TIFFA studies are performed on women at high risk for birth defects. In this way the yield in terms of anomalies found is increased, and the test becomes cost-effective. Examinations involving TIFFA are best done by very experienced sonologists, in a hospital setting where interaction with specialists in perinatal medicine and genetics is possible.

Standard Study

Gestational Age

In obstetrics the terms *gestational age* and *fetal age* refer to the length of pregnancy from the first day of the last menstrual period (LMP) and not from the time of ovulation. A *term pregnancy* is defined as one that progresses until 38 to 42 menstrual weeks. Fetuses who deliver prior to 38 weeks and after 42 weeks are considered preterm and postterm, respectively.

Clinical assessment of gestational age is fraught with error because the LMP is uncertain in 20% to 40% of gravidas. Sabbagha found that even when the LMP is reported with certainty, in 15% of pregnancies the clinically assessed gestational age will vary by at least 3 weeks from the age assigned to the newborn by careful pediatric examination. Anderson also reported that the LMP, even if known with certainty, is predictive of gestational age to within a margin of 3 weeks and with only 90% confidence. Further, Hertz showed that in women with certain menstrual dates the pregnancy should be carried to 42 weeks to assure the physician with 90% confidence that term has been reached.

Similarly, the pelvic examination is unreliable as a method for dating. In the first trimester, under ideal conditions, such as normal pregnancy, average body build, and anteverted uterus, fetal age can be assessed by pelvic examination to within ±2 weeks. That is, a 6 to 8 week pregnancy can be differentiated from one at 8 to 10 weeks. However, if the uterus is retroverted, as it is in approximately 30% of women, the accuracy of fetal age determination deteriorates to ±4 weeks.

In the second trimester, when the fundal height is used to estimate the length of pregnancy at least three factors complicate the dating process:

1. In tall or short women, the distance between the symphysis pubis and the umbilicus is increased or decreased and, as a result, the standard distance of 16 cm is inapplicable.
2. Conditions such as large fetal size, multiple pregnancy, polyhydramnios, uterine myoma, ovarian cyst, and hydatidiform mole make the fetus appear more mature than its true age.
3. Oligohydramnios, intrauterine growth retardation, and undiagnosed intrauterine fetal death lead one to believe that the fetus is less mature than it is.

Knowledge of dates is essential in the management of pregnancy because gestational age forms the X-coordinate of many graphs pertaining to the evaluation of fetal status. For example, the level of α-fetoprotein in either maternal serum (MS/AFP) or amniotic fluid (AF/AFP) cannot be interpreted without accurate definition of fetal age (Fig. 15-4).

Accurate information about maturity is needed by the obstetrician deciding whether to prematurely abbreviate a pregnancy, for example, or perform a repeat cesarean section. Errors in clinical judgment concerning pregnancy dates have contributed to the development of respiratory distress syndrome (RDS) in the newborn with a resultant increase in perinatal morbidity and mortality. In a collaborative study Benson and colleagues reported that 8.5% of neonates delivered by re-

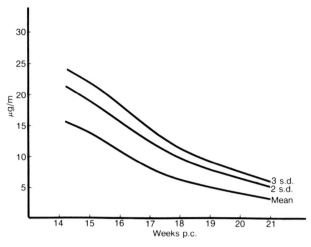

FIG. 15-4. Graph showing levels of α-fetoprotein (AFP) in amniotic fluid. In a pregnancy assumed to be 17 weeks, an AFP level of 15 μg is abnormal. However, if ultrasound reveals the pregnancy instead to be 16 weeks, the AFP level is considered normal. (Cowchock FS: Use of alpha-fetoprotein in prenatal diagnosis. Clin Obstet Gynecol 19:871, 1976)

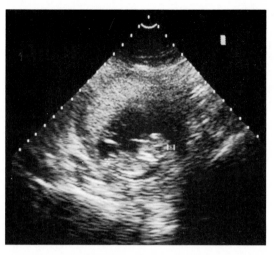

FIG. 15-5. Echogram shows fetal crown-rump (CRL) of 5.5 cm, consistent with a mean gestational age of 12+ weeks.

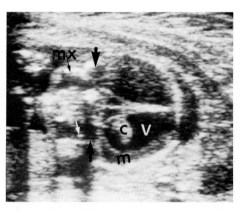

FIG. 15-6. Dynamically obtained image of fetal head showing hydrocephalus. The choroid plexus (*c*) is seen floating in the dilated cerebral venticle (*v*). The cerebral mantle (*m*) is only 0.5 cm in thickness. The fetal face, pointing to the left side of the photograph, shows the maxillary bone (*mx*), the orbits with the lens in one eye (*small arrow*), and the biocular distance (*large arrows*).

peat cesarean section weighed under 2500 g. In two other studies, one performed by Goldberg and the other by Hack, 12% to 15% of cases of RDS were attributed to untimely physician intervention.

In 1979 a task force assigned by the National Institutes of Health (NIH) placed the national annual cost of iatrogenic prematurity at approximately $50,000,000. The investigators also emphasized the fact that in addition to financial cost, the families in question experienced a great deal of emotional stress as they followed the uncertain progress of their babies in intensive care units. The NIH consultants issued guidelines for assessment of fetal maturity; these guidelines are incorporated in the following discussion.

Ultrasonic Assessment of Gestational Age

Gestational age can be predicted from a variety of ultrasonically derived fetal parameters. The most accurate of these are fetal crown-rump length (Fig. 15-5); biparietal diameter (BPD), measured singly or serially; femur length (FL); head circumference (HC); and abdominal circumference (AC). In some cases, when there is doubt about the normality of any of these parameters, determination of fetal age may be based on the length of a long bone other than the femur, such as the humerus, or on the binocular distance (Fig. 15-6). However, estimates of fetal age based on these measurements are less accurate.

In ultrasonic determinations of gestational age one fact clearly stands out: the variability related to mean estimates in weeks is much smaller in the first 26 weeks. Because of this, the charts used in the estimation of fetal age are presented in two tables. Table 15-2 pertains to

the mean estimates of dates prior to 26 weeks and Table 15-3 to the mean estimates in the last part of gestation. In the latter chart the confidence limits are clearly displayed to remind the physician of the wide variation involved.

BPD.   The ultrasonically derived BPD used for estimating dates should represent the largest measurement of the head between the outer and inner parietal echo complexes (see Fig. 15-2). The largest BPD is obtained from a plane that shows either the thalamic bodies or

Table 15-2

Mean Gestational Age in Weeks Relative to Fetal Crown Rump Length (CRL), Biparietal Diameter (BPD), Femur Length (FL), Head Circumference (HC), and Abdominal Circumference (AC) in the First Two Trimesters of Pregnancy

Wk/CRL	Length (cm)	Wk/BPD	Wk/FL	Wk/HC	Perimeter (cm)	Wk/AC
7+	1.0–1.2			14–	8.5	
8–	1.3		14–	14	9.0	
8	1.4–1.5		14	14+	9.5	
8+	1.6–1.7		15–	15–	10.0	16–
9–	1.8		15	15	10.5	16
9–	1.9		15+	15+	11.0	16+
9–	2.0		16–	16–	11.5	17
9–	2.1		16	16	12.0	17+
9	2.2		16+	16+	12.5	18–
9+	2.3–2.4		17–	17–	13.0	18
9+	2.5		17	17	13.5	19–
9+	2.6	13+	18–	17+	14.0	19
10–	2.7	14–	18–	18–	14.5	20–
10–	2.8	14	18	18	15.0	20
10–	2.9	14+	19–	18+	15.5	20+
10	3.0	14+	19–	19–	16.0	21–
10+	3.1	15–	19	19	16.5	21
10+	3.2	15	20–	20–	17.0	22–
10+	3.3	15+	20–	20	17.5	22
10+	3.4	16–	20	20+	18.0	23–
11–	3.5	16	21–	21–	18.5	23
11–	3.6	16+	21	21	19.0	24–
11–	3.7	17–	21+	22–	19.5	24
11–	3.8	17	22–	22	20.0	25–
11–	3.9	17+	22	22+	20.5	25
11	4.0	18–	22+	23	21.0	25+
11+	4.1	18	23–	23+	21.5	26–
11+	4.2	18+	23	24–	22.0	26
11+	4.3	19–	24–	24+	22.5	27–
11+	4.4	19	24	25	23.0	
11+	4.5	19+	24+	25+	23.5	
12–	4.6	20–	25–	26	24.0	
12–	4.7	20	25	26+	24.5	
12–	4.8	20+	26–			
12–	4.9	21–	26			
12–	5.0	21	26+			
12	5.1	21+				
12	5.2	22–				
12+	5.3	22–				
12+	5.4	22				
12+	5.5	22+				
12+	5.6	23–				
12+	5.7	23				
13–	5.8	23+				
13–	5.9	24–				
13–	6.0	24				
13–	6.1	24+				
13–	6.2	25–				
13–	6.3	25				
13	6.4	25+				
13+	6.5	26–				
13+	6.6	26				
13+	6.7	26+				

Note: BPD values represent composite means: Plus sign = +1 to +3 days; minus sign = −1 to −3 days: Range for CRL = +/−5 days (2SD), for BPD = +/−10 days (2SD) and for FL = +/−10 days (2SD).

(Adapted from Robinson HP, Fleming JEE: A critical evaluation of sonar CRL measurements. Br J Obstet Gynaecol 82:702, 1975; Sabbagha RE, Hughey M: Standardization of sonar cephalometry. Obstet Gynecol 52:405, 1978; Hadlock FP, Harrist RB, Deter RL et al: Fetal femur length as a predictor of menstrual age. Am J Radiol 138:875, 1982; Hadlock FP, Deter RL, Harrist RB, et al: Fetal head circumference: Relation to menstrual age. Am J Radiol 138:649, 1982; Hadlock FP, Deter RL, Harrist PB, et al: Fetal abdominal circumference: Relation to menstrual age. Am J Radiol 138:649, 1982)

Table 15-3
Mean (M) and Range* (R) of Gestational Age (Menstrual Dates) in Weeks Relative to Fetal Biparietal Diameter (BPD),† Femur Length (FL), Head Circumference (HC), and Abdominal Circumference (AC) in the Third Trimester of Pregnancy

| Wk/BPD | | Length | Wk/FL | | Wk/HC | | Perimeter | Wk/AC | |
R	M	(cm)	M	R	R	M	(cm)	M	R
		5.1	27	±3			22.5	27−	±2
		5.2	27+	±3			23.0	27	±2
		5.3	28−	±3			23.5	28−	±2
		5.4	28	±3			24.0	28	±2
		5.5	29−	±3			24.5	29−	±2
		5.6	29	±3	±2.1	27−	25.0	29	±2
		5.7	30−	±3	±2.1	27	25.5	30−	±2
		5.8	30	±3	±2.1	28	26.0	30	±3
		5.9	30+	±3	±3.0	28+	26.5	31−	±3
		6.0	31	±3	±3.0	29	27.0	31	±3
		6.1	31+	±3	±3.0	30−	27.5	32−	±3
		6.2	32	±3	±3.0	30	28.0	32	±3
		6.3	32+	±3	±3.0	31	28.5	33−	±3
		6.4	33−	±3	±3.0	32−	29.0	33	±3
		6.5	33	±3	±3.0	32	29.5	34−	±3
		6.6	34−	±3	±3.0	33−	30.0	34	±3
		6.7	34	±3	±3.0	33	30.5	35−	±3
±2	27−	6.8	35−	±3	±3.0	34	31.0	35	±3
±2	27+	6.9	35	±3	±3.0	35	31.5	36−	±3
±2	27	7.0	36−	±3	±3.0	36−	32.0	36	2.5
±2	27+	7.1	36	±3	±3.0	36	32.5	37−	2.5
±2	28	7.2	37−	±3	±2.5	37	±33.0	37	2.5
±2	28+	7.3	37	±3	±2.5	38−	33.5	38−	2.5
±3	29−	7.4	38−	±3	±2.5	38	34.0	38	2.5
±3	29	7.5	38	±3	±2.5	39	34.5	39−	2.5
±3	29+	7.6	39−	±3	±2.5	40	35.0	39	2.5
±3	30−	7.7	39	±3	±2.5	41−	35.5	40−	2.5
±3	30	7.8	40−	±3	±2.5	42−	36.0	40	2.5
±3	30+	7.9	40	±3	±2.5		36.5	41−	2.5
±3	31	8.0							
±3	31+	8.1							
±3	32	8.2							
±3	32+	8.3							
±3	33−	8.4							
±3	33	8.5							
±3	33+	8.6							
±3	34	8.7							
±3	35−	8.8							
±3	35+	8.9							
±3	36	9.0							
±3	36+	9.1							
±3	37−	9.2							
±3	38−	9.3							
±3	39	9.4							
±3	40	9.5							

* Range: confidence interval for BPD is 90% and for femur length, HC, and AC is 95%

† BPD value represents menstrual dates relative to *composite* Mean BPD values.

Plus sign = +1 to +3 days; minus sign = −1 to −3 days.

(Adapted from Sabbagha RE, Hughey M: Standardization of sonar cephalometry. Obstet Gynecol 52:405, 1978; Hadlock FP, Harrist RB, Deter RL et al: Fetal femur length as a predictor of menstrual age. Am J Radiol 138:875, 1982; Hadlock FP, Deter RL, Harrist RB, et al: Fetal head circumference: Relation to menstrual age. Am J Radiol 138:649, 1982. Hadlock FP, Deter RL, Harrist PB, et al: Fetal abdominal circumference: relation to menstrual age. Am J Radiol 138:649, 1982) the septum cavum pellucidum. This plane is slightly inferior to that of the lateral cerebral ventricles.

Because fetal populations at or near sea level do not show a statistically significant variation in BPD, particularly from 14 to 26 weeks, the American College of Obstetricians and Gynecologists has recommended the use of a composite mean BPD chart derived from several studies (see Table 15-2).

PAIRED BPDs. Animal and human studies have found that in 90% of normal fetuses, BPD growth from approximately 20 to 33 weeks is maintained within one of three percentile subgroups. These are defined as large (>75th percentile), average (25th to 75th percentile), and small (<25th percentile). Thus, in some pregnancies it may be beneficial to use two BPD measurements to determine BPD growth rank. The first, taken at 20 to 26 weeks, is used for an initial estimate of gestational age; the second, taken at 31 to 33 weeks, is used to place BPD in a specific growth bracket. For example, if the second BPD is large (Table 15-4), the fetus is likely to be less mature than was estimated on the basis of the first BPD measurement (Fig. 15-7). Similarly, if the BPD is small, the fetus is likely to be more mature than was suggested by the first BPD measurement.

Once fetal BPD is placed in one of three percentile ranks, fetal age can be estimated to within ±3 days with 90% confidence. The method of dating pregnancies by analysis of paired BPD growth is known as *growth adjusted sonar age* (GASA). The clinical use of this and other means of determining fetal age is discussed in Chapter 41.

Table 15-4
Growth-Adjusted Sonographic Age (GASA) Assignments Based on Second Soner Determinations of Biparietal Diameter Ranges

Fetal Age (wk)	Average Fetus (25th to 75th percentile)	Large Fetus (75th to 95th percentile)	Small Fetus (5th to 25th percentile)
29	7.4–7.7	7.8–8.3	6.8–7.3
29+	7.5–7.8	7.9–8.4	6.9–7.4
30−	7.6–7.8	7.9–8.5	7.0–7.5
30	7.7–7.9	8.0–8.6	7.1–7.6
30+	7.8–8.0	8.1–8.7	7.2–7.7
31−	7.8–8.0	8.1–8.7	7.2–7.7
31	7.9–8.1	8.2–8.8	7.3–7.8
31+	8.0–8.2	8.3–8.9	7.4–7.9
32−	8.0–8.2	8.3–8.9	7.4–7.9
32	8.1–8.3	8.4–9.0	7.5–8.0
32+	8.2–8.4	8.5–9.0	7.6–8.1
33−	8.3–8.4	8.5–9.1	7.6–8.2
33	8.4–8.5	8.6–9.1	7.7–8.3
33+	8.5–8.6	8.7–9.2	7.8–8.4
34−	8.5–8.7	8.8–9.2	7.8–8.4
34	8.6–8.8	8.9–9.3	7.9–8.5
34+	8.7–8.9	9.0–9.4	8.0–8.6
35−	8.7–8.9	9.0–9.5	8.1–8.6
35	8.8–9.0	9.1–9.6	8.2–8.7
35+	8.9–9.0	9.2–9.6	8.2–8.8
36−	8.9–9.1	9.3–9.6	8.2–8.8
36	9.0–9.2	9.3–9.7	8.3–8.9
37	9.1–9.3	9.4–9.8	8.4–9.0
38	9.2–9.4	9.5–9.9	8.5–9.1
39	9.3–9.5	9.6–10.0	8.7–9.2
40	9.5–9.6	9.7–10.1	8.9–9.4

BPD = biparietal diameter, measured from outer to inner aspects of fetal head; + = plus 1–3 days; − = minus 1–3 days.

* First sonar is done prior to 26 weeks because of small variation in fetal age of ± 11 days. Second sonar: 1) must be done between 30–33 weeks because of maximal variation in fetal BPD size in this interval and prior to onset of IUGR in most cases; 2) must be done at least 6 weeks after first BPD. The second sonar BPD places a fetus in a large or average or small growth bracket and a growth-adjusted sonographic age (GASA) is used.

(Sabbagha RE, Hughey M, Depp R: Growth-adjusted sonographic age: A simplified method. Obstet Gynecol 51:383, 1978)

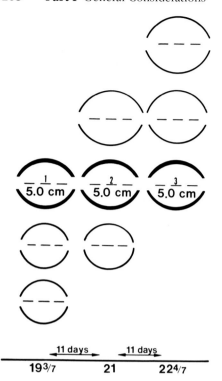

FIG. 15-7. Three fetuses with the same biparietal diameter are not of the same gestational age. However, they are all assigned a mean age of 21 weeks if only one biparietal diameter is obtained for each. Fetus 1 has a large biparietal diameter for its age of 19+ weeks. If its growth pattern is subsequently revealed by a second biparietal diameter obtained at 31 to 33 weeks, estimation of its gestational age can then be reduced by up to 11 days. Similarly, if the biparietal diameter of fetus 3 is found by a second measurement to have been small, estimation of its gestational age can be advanced by up to 11 days.

FEMUR LENGTH. The shaft of the femur is the easiest fetal long bone to visualize and measure (Fig. 15-8). However, the accuracy of estimating dates from femur length is still in question. In independent studies, Queenan, Hohler, and Hadlock found the confidence interval for estimates derived from femur length to be smaller in the second trimester than in the third trimester of pregnancy (Tables 15-2 and 15-3). By contrast, Jeanty has reported a confidence interval of ±2.8 weeks (2SD) throughout pregnancy.

HEAD CIRCUMFERENCE (HC). Head circumference is less accurate than the BPD as a predictor of fetal age prior to 26 weeks (Table 15-2). It is also more difficult than either BPD or femur length to measure with precision. The perimeter is obtained in one of two ways. In the first a light pen or digitizer is used and the actual circumference is calculated as described in Figure 15-2. In the second the outer-to-outer occipitofrontal (OFD) and biparietal diameters are measured in the

same plane and the approximate head circumference is derived by applying the formula:

$$HC = [(BPD + OFD)/2] \times 3.14$$

ABDOMINAL CIRCUMFERENCE (AC). Although the abdominal circumference is less accurate than BPD, femur length, or head circumference as a predictor of dates prior to 24 weeks, it is the most useful measurement for evaluations of fetal growth. The abdominal circumference should be derived from a plane that is perpendicular to the fetal longitudinal axis just below the cross-sectional view of the heart and that shows one or more of the following structures: fetal stomach, ductus venosus, bifurcation of the main portal vein, small segment of the umbilical vein, and gall bladder. The methods of measuring the abdominal circumference are similar to those used for the head circumference (Fig. 15-9).

CHOICE OF PARAMETERS. In some situations the physician will be forced to rely on only one fetal parameter in estimating dates. For example, the femur should be used in the following circumstances:

1. Occiput posterior position of the fetal head, which prohibits accurate measurement of BPD or head circumference.
2. Side-to-side flattening of the fetal head, or dolichocephaly, a condition that artificially reduces the BPD but that rarely occurs before 26 weeks of gestation.
3. Hydrocephaly or microcephaly.

On the other hand, the BPD or head circumference should be used when the femur cannot be imaged properly or when it is abnormally small, as in fetuses with limb dysplasia. These circumstances should be borne in mind when BPD and femur data are being interpreted. Some sonologists routinely use the ratio of BPD to femur length or the BPD/OFD ratio (cephalic

FIG. 15-8. Echogram of diaphysis of femur (*arrows*).

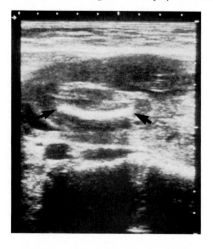

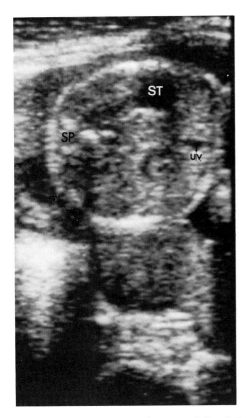

FIG. 15-9. Cross-sectional image of the abdominal circumference at the level of the umbilical vein (*uv*) and stomach (*ST*). The abdominal circumference can be measured by a digitizer or estimated from two outer-to-outer diameters. The first is measured from the spine (*SP*) to the anterior abdominal wall; the second is either perpendicular or tangential to the first. The formula used is (D1 + D2/2) × 3.14.

index) to ensure that the limb or cephalic dimensions can be reliably used for dating. (See Fig. 15-2 and Table 15-5.)

MULTIPLE PREDICTORS. As previously discussed, fetal CRL, BPD, and possibly femur length are the most accurate indicators of fetal age before 26 weeks of gestation. When menstrual dates by clinical history predict a similar mean fetal age or at least fall within the confidence limits of any of these methods, the probability of the accuracy of the clinical history is increased. As a result, the physician can assign dates by accepting the ultrasound estimates or by using an average of clinical and sonar dates. If menstrual dates fall outside the normal confidence limits of these parameters, the ultrasonic estimates of length of pregnancy should be accepted as definitive. Thus, in the first situation ultrasound is used to confirm clinical dates; in the second it is used to establish dates.

Some investigators have suggested that estimations of gestational age could be improved if several ultrasonic

predictors were used. This translates into averaging all estimates or using multiple linear regression techniques, in the hope of deriving a more accurate result. However, indiscriminate averaging of ultrasonic estimates of dates is unlikely to be helpful and may even be detrimental. It is essential that the obstetrician evaluate each fetus independently and link the findings to clinical circumstances before deciding when and what to average. The following are specific considerations.

First, the biologic variation and measurement error for each of the ultrasound parameters is independent of the others. For example, in a particular fetus a BPD of average size will by itself correctly predict mean gestational age. However if the true mean date is averaged with an estimate based on a long femur, which falsely advances dates, the result is less accurate. In such an example the contribution of the best predictor or the BPD is diluted by introduction of the femur. Furthermore, because the accuracy of the femur length as a predictor of dates in the second trimester of pregnancy is still in question, the confidence limits may be much greater than those derived from the BPD in the same interval of pregnancy. Thus, by giving the BPD and the femur equal weight, the error in the estimate of dates is compounded.

Selection of the correct parameter is crucial in the presence of altered fetal growth. In symmetric intrauterine growth retardation (IUGR) all the fetal dimensions are reduced in size, and averaging all parameters will in no way improve the accuracy of dating.

In a fetus with asymmetric IUGR, the head circumference should be relied upon because in the presence of dolichocephaly the BPD will be small, as will the abdominal circumference because of loss of subcutaneous tissue. In addition, the femur may be shortened. If all parameters are averaged in an infant with asymmetric IUGR, the effect of the best predictor, head circumference, is diluted.

Table 15-5
Normal Ratio of Fetal Femur Length to BPD and BPD to Occipitofrontal Diameter

Ratio	*Normal Range (%)*	
FL/BPD*	73–86	90% CI
BPD/OFD†	74–83	(1 SD)

BPD = biparietal diameter; OFD = occipitofrontal diameter; FL = femur length.

* When the ratio is 73% or 86%, the sonologist is alerted to one of the following possibilities: skeletal dysplasia, hydrocephaly, microcephaly, or dolichocephaly (side-to-side flattening of the fetal head).

† When the ratio is 74%, the diagnosis of dolichocephaly is made. If the ratio is 83%, the diagnosis of brachycephaly (wide BPD) is made. In either case the BPD should not be used to predict dates.

(After Hohler CW, Quetal TA: Comparison of ultrasound femur length and biparietal diameter in late pregnancy. Am J Obstet Gynecol 141:759, 1981; Estimating fetal age: Effect of head shape on BPD. AJR 137:83, 1981. © 1981, American Roentgen Ray Society)

Table 15-6

Accuracy of Biparietal Diameter (BPD) in the Prediction of Intrauterine Growth Retardation (IUGR)

BPD	IUGR	Normal	Total
<25th percentile	37	34	71
25th–95th percentile	24	368	392
Total	61	402	463

Predictive value of abnormal = 37/71 (52%)
Predictive value of normal = 368/402 (94%)
Sensitivity = 37/61 (60%)
Specificity = 368/402 (91%)

(Sabbagha RE: Intrauterine growth retardation: Antenatal diagnosis by ultrasound. Obstet Gynecol 52:252, 1978. Reprinted with permission from The American College of Obstetricians and Gynecologists)

Fetal Growth

In the area of fetal growth, the physician is mainly interested in the detection of intrauterine growth retardation (IUGR) and macrosomia. Both conditions are associated with an increase in perinatal morbidity and mortality and with long-term central nervous system deficits. The diagnosis in these altered states of growth is based on birth weight relative to gestational age. In IUGR the birth weight falls below the 10th or even the 5th percentile; in macrosomia it exceeds the 90th percentile.

Both IUGR and macrosomia are difficult to diagnose on clinical grounds. For example, it is estimated that only 30% to 40% of pregnancies complicated by IUGR can be recognized by monitoring uterine growth. Part of the difficulty stems from the fact that dates may be erroneous in a substantial number of these women.

By comparison, a diagnosis of altered growth can

Table 15-7

BPD Percentile Ranges and Measurements from 16 to 40 Weeks for Black and White Fetuses

Fetal Age (weeks)	BPD Percentiles							N
	5	10	25	50	75	80	95	
16	3.1	3.2	3.4	3.7	4.0	4.1	4.5	12
17	3.4	3.5	3.7	4.0	4.3	4.4	4.7	15
18	3.7	3.8	4.0	4.3	4.5	4.6	4.9	22
19	3.9	4.2	4.3	4.5	4.8	4.9	5.1	33
20	4.2	4.5	4.6	4.7	5.0	5.1	5.3	39
21	4.5	4.8	4.9	5.0	5.3	5.4	5.5	40
22	4.9	5.0	5.2	5.3	5.6	5.7	5.8	48
23	5.2	5.3	5.5	5.6	5.9	6.0	6.2	57
24	5.5	5.6	5.8	5.9	6.2	6.3	6.6	50
25	5.8	5.9	6.0	6.2	6.5	6.6	7.0	47
26	6.1	6.2	6.3	6.6	6.8	6.9	7.3	43
27	6.4	6.5	6.7	6.9	7.1	7.2	7.6	51
28	6.6	6.7	7.0	7.2	7.4	7.5	7.9	51
29	6.8	6.9	7.3	7.5	7.8	7.9	8.3	53
30	7.1	7.2	7.6	7.8	8.0	8.2	8.6	50
31	7.3	7.4	7.8	8.0	8.2	8.4	8.8	48
32	7.5	7.6	8.0	8.3	8.4	8.6	9.0	47
33	7.7	7.8	8.3	8.5	8.6	8.8	9.1	50
34	7.9	8.0	8.5	8.7	8.9	9.1	9.3	50
35	8.2	8.3	8.7	8.8	9.1	9.3	9.6	49
36	8.3	8.5	8.9	9.0	9.3	9.4	9.7	48
37	8.4	8.8	9.0	9.2	9.4	9.5	9.8	43
38	8.5	8.9	9.1	9.3	9.5	9.6	9.9	42
39	8.7	9.0	9.2	9.4	9.6	9.7	10.0	29
40	8.9	9.3	9.4	9.5	9.7	9.8	10.1	15

(From Sabbagha RE, et al: Sonar biparietal diameter II: Predictive of three fetal growth patterns leading to a closer assessment of gestational age and neonatal weight. Am J Obstet Gynecol 126:485, 1976) either be excluded or verified by ultrasound in approximately 95% and 85% of cases, respectively. These figures indicate that ultrasound, like other tests used to assess biologic function, is more specific in predicting the unaffected fetus than it is sensitive in the diagnosis of IUGR or macrosomia.

Ultrasonic criteria used in the assessment of growth include:

1. Biometry (BPD, head circumference, abdominal circumference, and femur length)
2. Estimation of fetal weight
3. Determination of amniotic fluid volume
4. Dynamic assessment of fetal activity
5. Blood flow studies

BPD AND HEAD CIRCUMFERENCE. The methods of measuring the BPD and head circumference are discussed elsewhere. In terms of growth, the predictive accuracy, specificity, and sensitivity of the BPD is shown in Table 15-6. Notice that when the BPD remains in a normal percentile bracket (25th percentile to 95th percentile) the predictive probability of a normal outcome exceeds 90%. By contrast, a small BPD (<25th percentile) accurately predicts only 52% of growth-retarded fetuses.

The limitations in using BPD to evaluate growth are related to brain sparing, which is evident in asymmetric IUGR, and the occurrence of side-to-side flattening of the fetal head, or dolichocephaly, which is mainly observed in twin pregnancies or following premature rupture of the membranes during the third trimester.

Because of the possibility of dolichocephaly, head circumference must be measured in fetuses with small BPDs (<25th percentile) before the possibility of IUGR is considered. The percentile growth brackets of the BPD and head circumference are presented in Tables 15-7 and 15-8.

ABDOMINAL CIRCUMFERENCE. In growth-retarded fetuses the liver and the layer of subcutaneous tissue in the area are diminished in size. Conversely, in the presence of macrosomia, the liver is large and the subcutaneous layer is thick. The abdominal circumference, measured at the appropriate plane, as previously discussed, reflects the changes described in altered fetal growth. The percentile growth brackets of the abdominal circumference are shown in Table 15-9.

In the overall assessment of growth, BPD, head circumference, and abdominal circumference should be considered. If each of these measurements is placed in a specific percentile bracket (large, average, or small), nine fetal growth patterns emerge, as shown in Figure 15-10. Note that growth patterns 3 and 6 indicate a high risk for asymmetric IUGR and pattern 9 indicates a high risk for symmetric IUGR. Further, macrosomic fetuses fall in growth patterns 1 and 4; most of these fetuses are characterized by an abdominal circumference above the

Table 15-8
Mean Head Circumference (HC) Values at Specific Weeks in Gestation

Menstrual Age (weeks)	Number of Fetuses	Mean HC (cm)	SD (cm)
15	5	11.4	0.38
16	15	12.2	1.23
17	18	13.4	0.69
18	10	14.8	0.66
19	17	16.0	1.14
20	17	17.7	1.16
21	15	18.2	0.85
22	16	19.3	1.16
23	13	20.8	1.07
24	21	22.1	0.78
25	10	23.9	1.34
26	13	24.1	1.21
27	14	25.6	1.04
28	9	27.1	1.51
29	12	27.3	1.15
30	10	27.7	0.80
31	12	28.1	1.12
32	12	29.2	0.71
33	12	30.2	1.13
34	17	30.9	1.00
35	8	31.7	1.23
36	11	32.2	0.94
37	8	33.0	1.16
38	32	33.6	0.76
39	44	34.0	0.90
40	25	34.5	0.81
41	4	35.4	0.98

(Hadlock FP, Deter RL, Harrist RB, Park SK: Fetal head circumference: Relation to menstrual age. AJR 138:649, 1982. © 1981, American Roentgen Ray Society)

95th percentile (Fig. 15-11). The predictive value of each abnormal growth pattern in the diagnosis of IUGR and macrosomia is still under investigation. Preliminary results suggest that the sensitivity is approximately 75% to 80%.

RATIO OF HEAD CIRCUMFERENCE TO ABDOMINAL CIRCUMFERENCE. Prior to term the ratio of head circumference to abdominal circumference is greater than 1.0, indicating that in premature fetuses the cephalic dimension is larger than the abdominal girth. By contrast, past 36 weeks the fetus rapidly accumulates subcutaneous tissue in the abdominal area. As a result, the abdominal circumference increases in size at a faster rate than the head circumference, and the ratio is reversed (see Table 15-10).

When the ratio of head circumference to abdominal circumference is greater than 1.0, prematurity and IUGR can be distinguished only when gestational age is accurately known. When the ratio of head circumference

Table 15-9
Fetal Abdominal Circumference at Different Gestational Ages

Weeks of Gestation	Percentile									No
	2.5	5	10	25	50	75	80	95	97.5	
18	9.8	10.3	10.9	11.9	13.1	14.2	14.5	15.9	16.4	3
19	11.1	11.6	12.3	13.3	14.4	15.6	15.9	17.2	17.8	10
20	12.1	12.6	13.3	14.3	15.4	16.6	16.9	18.2	18.8	24
21	13.7	14.2	14.8	15.9	17.0	18.1	18.4	19.8	20.3	26
22	14.7	15.2	15.8	16.9	18.0	19.1	19.4	20.8	21.3	28
23	16.0	16.5	17.1	18.2	19.3	20.4	20.7	22.1	22.6	30
24	17.2	17.7	18.3	19.4	20.5	21.6	21.9	23.3	23.8	28
25	18.0	18.5	19.1	20.2	21.3	22.4	22.7	24.1	24.6	18
26	18.8	19.3	19.9	21.0	22.1	23.2	23.5	24.9	25.4	11
27	20.4	20.9	21.5	22.6	23.7	24.8	25.1	26.5	27.0	9
28	22.0	22.5	23.1	24.2	25.3	26.4	26.7	28.1	28.6	2
29	23.6	24.1	24.7	25.8	26.9	28.0	28.3	29.7	30.2	15
30	24.1	24.6	25.2	26.3	27.4	28.5	28.8	30.2	30.7	24
31	24.7	25.2	25.8	26.9	28.0	29.1	29.4	30.8	31.3	48
32	25.4	25.9	26.5	27.6	28.7	29.8	30.1	31.5	32.0	51
33	25.7	26.2	26.8	27.9	29.0	30.1	30.4	31.8	32.3	34
34	26.8	27.3	27.9	29.0	30.1	31.2	31.5	32.9	33.4	28
35	28.9	29.4	30.0	31.1	32.2	33.3	33.6	35.0	35.5	18
36	30.0	30.5	31.1	32.2	33.3	34.4	34.7	36.1	36.6	14
37	31.1	31.6	32.3	33.3	34.4	35.5	35.8	37.2	37.7	18
38	32.4	32.9	33.5	34.6	35.7	36.8	37.1	38.5	39.0	37
39	32.6	33.1	33.7	34.8	35.9	37.0	37.3	38.7	39.2	34
40	32.8	33.3	33.9	35.0	36.1	37.2	37.5	38.9	39.4	23
41	33.8	34.3	34.9	36.0	37.1	38.2	38.5	39.9	40.4	3

(Tamura, Sabbagha RE: Percentile ranks of sonar fetal abdominal circumference. Am J Obstet Gynecol 138:475, 1980)

FIG. 15-10. Nine fetal growth patterns are determined by use of percentile growth ranks of biparietal diameter (*BPD*), head circumference (*HC*), and abdominal circumference (*A-C*). *L,* large; *A,* average; *S,* small.

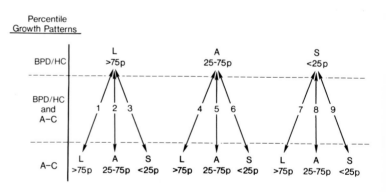

to abdominal circumference is less than 1.0 in a pregnancy known to be at term, IUGR can be virtually ruled out, and the differential diagnosis can be narrowed to a normal versus a microcephalic fetus.

In approximately 70% of asymmetrically undergrown fetuses the ratio of head circumference to abdominal circumference is greater than 2SD above the mean (see Table 15-10). In symmetric or near-symmetric IUGR, the predictive value of the ratio is very low.

FEMUR LENGTH. Fetal length can be extrapolated from the size of the diaphysis of the femur, which can be ultrasonically measured (see Fig. 15-8). Fetal length is one of the major determinants of fetal weight. Several studies clearly demonstrate the contribution of the crown-heel-length to birth weight (Table 15-11). Careful attention to weight versus length (ponderal index) will enhance the accuracy of predictions of birth weight. The percentile growth brackets of the femur in pregnancy are shown in Table 15-12.

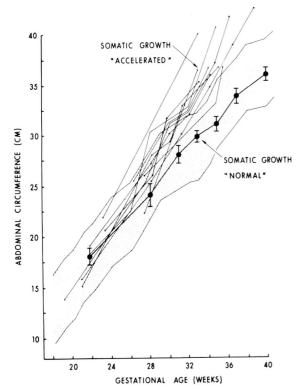

FIG. 15-11. The abdominal circumferences of macrosomic fetuses of diabetic mothers exceed the 95th percentile as early as 28 to 32 weeks' gestation. (Ogata ES, Sabbagha RE, Metzger BD et al: Serial ultrasonography to assess evolving fetal macrosomia. Studies in 23 pregnant diabetic women. JAMA 243: 2405, 1980. Copyright 1980, American Medical Association)

Table 15-10
Ratios Between Head Circumference and Abdominal Circumference at Different Gestational Ages

Gestation (weeks)	H/A Ratio	
	Mean	±2SD
28	1.13	1.21
32	1.08	1.17
34	1.04	1.13
36	1.02	1.12
38	0.99	1.06
40	0.97	1.05

(Campbell S, Thomas A: Ultrasound measurement of the fetal head to abdomen circumference ratio in the assessment of growth retardation. Br J Obstet Gynecol 84:165, 1977)

Table 15-11
Birthweights for Given Percentiles in Babies of Different Crown-Heel Lengths

Birthweight Percentiles	Crown-Heel Length (cm)		
	48.0	51.0	55.0
95	3.16	3.79	4.76
90	3.05	3.66	4.59
75	2.95	3.54	4.45
50	2.81	3.37	4.21
25	2.67	3.19	4.04
10	2.56	3.08	3.86
5	2.45	2.94	3.69

(Adapted and reproduced with permission from Miller HC, Merritt TA: Fetal Growth in Humans. Copyright © 1979 by Year Book Medical Publishers, Inc., Chicago)

Birth Weight

The birth weight predicted from fetal cephalic and abdominal parameters falls within 12% to 15% (2SD) of actual weight. The accuracy is related to the size of the fetus. Thus, the absolute error is small (150 g) in a fetus weighing 1000 g and large (600 g) in one weighing 4000 g.

When the fetus is of average size (*e.g.,* 3000 g) the difference between predicted and actual birth weight can be 450 g, a difference large enough to lead either to a false abnormal or a false normal diagnosis of IUGR at term. Because of this poor relationship in the fetus of average size, it is important that birth weight estimates and growth profile (see Fig. 15-10) be used together in the evaluation of the normality of fetal growth.

Shepard and co-workers developed a formula for estimating birth weight from BPD and abdominal circumference. Because the formula is derived from fetuses with a wide range in birth weight, it is applicable to any gestational age regardless of whether growth is normal or altered and whether the ratio of head circumference to abdominal circumference is greater or less than 1.0.

Recently Weiner and co-workers derived a more ac-curate formula incorporating head circumference, abdominal circumference, and femur length measurements from fetuses who were delivered prematurely:

$$BW = 94.593 \ (HC) + 34.227 \ (AC) - 2134.616$$

This formula is targeted to low birth weight fetuses, premature or growth retarded. In fetuses with long or short bones (>75th percentile or <25th percentile) the birth weight estimated by this formula is then multiplied by the ratio of actual femur length to 50th percentile femur length for the dates in question. When used for its targeted group, the formula is more accurate than that of Shepard and co-workers. The mean error per kg is 98.7 g with 95% confidence limits ranging from 66 g to 127 g.

Antenatal prediction of birth weight has proven to be especially useful in the management of women at

Table 15-12
The Number of Measurements Taken and the Mean Length ± 2 SD of the Ultrasound Femur Length from 14 Weeks of Gestation to Term

Weeks of Gestation	No. of Measurements	Arithmetic Mean (mm)	±2 SD (mm)
14	31	16.6	2.5
15	28	19.9	2.3
16	28	22.0	3.0
17	35	25.2	2.9
18	30	29.6	3.1
19	32	32.4	3.1
20	27	34.8	2.5
21	29	37.5	4.1
22	23	40.9	3.9
23	33	43.5	3.6
24	38	46.4	3.5
25	33	48.0	4.6
26	39	51.1	5.0
27	37	53.0	3.2
28	39	54.4	4.1
29	28	57.3	4.3
30	48	58.7	3.8
31	50	61.5	4.5
32	52	62.8	4.2
33	41	64.9	4.6
34	41	65.7	4.4
35	59	67.7	4.8
36	56	69.5	4.6
37	51	70.8	4.3
38	46	71.8	5.6
39	34	74.2	5.1
40	28	75.4	5.6

(O'Brien GD, Queenan JT: Growth of the ultrasound fetal femur length during normal pregnancy. Part I. Am J Obstet Gynecol 141:833, 1981)

high risk for premature delivery. The reason is related to the fact that in approximately 35% of preterm infants exceeding 1000 g, clinical estimates of weight can be quite low, leading the physician to assume falsely that the chances of survival for the fetus are minimal. At present, accurate determination of birth weight even in the range of 750 g to 1000 g is important because the perinatal outcome of very low birth weight infants managed in modern intensive care neonatal centers has markedly improved.

Calculating birth weight from ultrasonically derived fetal parameters has enhanced our understanding of fetal growth, particularly in relation to premature births. Using birth weight estimates derived from BPD and abdominal circumference, Tamura and co-workers showed that fetuses born preterm after spontaneous labor or rupture of membranes are diminished in growth when compared to those who progress to term. Ott found that *in utero* birth weights published in the literature (and derived from actual birth weights of premature babies)

are smaller than those calculated from the BPD and abdominal circumference using Shepard's formula. Weiner and co-workers reached the same conclusion using a formula based on fetal head circumference and abdominal circumference. These two studies indirectly confirm Tamura's finding.

OLIGOHYDRAMNIOS AND IUGR. The data in the literature concerning a connection between oligohydramnios and IUGR are controversial. Manning and co-workers found that in approximately 90% of pregnancies suspected of growth retardation, amniotic fluid volume is diminished. Diminished fluid volume was defined as presence of a fluid compartment measuring 1 cm or less in a vertical axis.

Hoddick and co-workers were not able to confirm Manning's findings. In a retrospective study of pregnancies with known growth retardation they showed that the predictive value of the "1-cm sign" of oligohydramnios (amniotic fluid pockets less than 1 cm in diameter) is poor, namely 7.7%.

Philipson and co-workers reported that in an unselected population, oligohydramnios was present in only 16% of growth retarded fetuses, that is, the sensitivity of the test is poor. However, their data suggested that 40% of pregnancies with oligohydramnios are complicated by IUGR (*i.e.,* the predictive value of oligohydramnios is 40%). They defined oligohydramnios as paucity of fluid in the uterus associated with fetal crowding.

In general, when IUGR is suspected on the grounds of clinical assessment, abnormal biometry, or both, the presence of oligohydramnios assumes significance.

Fetal Activity

Ultrasound has been used as a tool for the observation of a number of fetal biologic functions including fetal breathing movements, fetal body motion, hiccups, swallowing, micturition, and eye movements. Collection of data pertaining to all these functions is difficult and time consuming. Further, the data, so far, even when quantified lack accuracy in the prediction of fetal hypoxia and IUGR. To date the most extensively investigated area is that of fetal breathing movements.

FETAL BREATHING MOVEMENTS. Pharmacologic modulation of fetal breathing movements has been qualitatively examined in human pregnancy. An increase in fetal breathing movements is observed following administration of central nervous system stimulants, such as caffeine, B-agonists, and nicotine. Conversely, a decrease is noted when diazepam, barbiturates, and morphine are administered.

In the uncompromised fetus, fetal breathing movements appear to be modulated by maternal glucose level. A significant increase occurs 1 hour after peak maternal glucose levels and approximately 2 hours after maternal oral glucose intake. The mechanism for this increase in fetal breathing movements is not clear, but it is believed to result from excesses in carbon dioxide (produced by increased glucose oxidation) within the fetal brain which stimulate medullary chemosensitive receptors. Of importance in this area is that in normal pregnancies inhalation by the mother of 5% carbon dioxide induces a significant increase in fetal breathing movements whereas when fetal hypoxia is present the response is blunted. Potentially, once safety in this area is established, tests of this nature may assume significance in the detection of the hypoxic fetus.

Patrick and others have shown that normal fetuses have periods of apnea extending up to 2 hours. Additionally, a prolonged significant increase in the incidence of fetal breathing movements is noted between 1 A.M. and 7 A.M. when the mothers are asleep, suggesting a circadian rhythm of fetal breathing activity. All of these observations point to the difficulty of using fetal breathing movements for accurate prediction of IUGR.

Biophysical Profile

Manning and co-workers used dynamic ultrasound imaging to evaluate fetal health by observing, for a period of approximately 30 minutes, five variables: fetal breathing movements; fetal body movements; fetal tone (shown, for example, when the fetus exhibits extension of any extremity with quick return to the flexed position); amniotic fluid volume; and response to nonstress testing. They referred to these variables as a fetal biophysical profile.

The investigators assigned a score of 2 for each variable when normally present and a score of 0 when it was absent. They showed that the perinatal mortality of fetuses with a score of less than 6 was significantly greater than those with a higher score.

Research in this area is continuing in order to define the threshold at which each component can be considered abnormal and to structure the test so that certain prerequisite criteria relating to the circadian rhythm of fetal breathing movements and to maternal glucose level are standardized. The use by the mother of any medication known to inhibit the fetal central nervous system should be carefully investigated prior to testing.

It would appear that the biophysical profile test, particularly if standardized, will be useful in the decision-making process regarding the most appropriate time for delivering the IUGR fetus. Whether its use will enhance formulation of this decision beyond that reached from electronic fetal monitoring (the nonstress test and the contraction stress test) remains to be elucidated.

Blood Velocity Studies

A number of fetal vessels, such as the aorta and the umbilical artery and vein, can be localized by two-dimensional imaging, and blood velocity can be determined by the use of pulsed or continuous wave ultrasound. This is possible because echoes from a moving target (e.g., blood flowing in an artery) are changed in frequency. The echo frequency is decreased if the ultrasonic beam travels the vessel in the direction of blood flow and is increased if its path is against the flow. This change in frequency is known as the Doppler shift (DS). It is measured in kilohertz (KHz). For example, if the frequency of the emitted sound wave is 3 MHz and that of the returning wave is 3.003 MHz, the difference will be 3 KHz. Because the frequency falls within the range of audibility, the shift can be well appreciated by the sonographer.

The Doppler shift (DS) is directly proportional to the product of blood velocity (BV), ultrasound frequency (UF), and angle of incidence of the ultrasound beam (Cos ϕ). It is indirectly proportional to ultrasound velocity (UV) in soft tissue. The relationship is expressed as

$$DS = BV \times 2UF \times Cos\ \phi/UV$$

Because the Doppler shift can be measured, the unknown in the equation—blood velocity—can be determined as follows:

$$BV = DS \times UV/2UF \times Cos\ \phi$$

CHANGES IN BLOOD VELOCITY. Blood velocity continually changes throughout the cardiac cycle. As a result, the Doppler shift changes in frequency. These changes can be processed through a Fast Fourier system and either fed into a computer terminal for complex analysis of the spectrum, yielding maximum, mean, and time-averaged frequencies, or presented in real time as a velocity waveform or Doppler sonogram on a television screen (Fig. 15-12).

In the fetus the blood velocity waveform obtained from the aorta or one of the umbilical arteries (Fig.

FIG. 15-12. Fetal arterial velocity wave. Peak systole/end diastole or A/B ratio is increased as normal pregnancy advances because end-diastolic velocity is high and resistance at the placental bed is low. By contrast, the A/B ratio is decreased in intrauterine growth retardation (*IUGR*) because diastolic velocity comes to a halt secondary to high resistance in the placental bed.

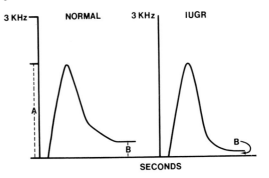

15-12) can be used to derive information about the rate of acceleration and deceleration of blood during cardiac systole and diastole, and information about end diastole, which reflects peripheral resistance to flow in the placental vascular bed.

The extent of peripheral resistance may be quantified by the degree of pulsatility of the arterial velocity wave, which can be expressed in a number of ways. One of these is the ratio between peak systole and end diastole (Fig. 15-12). A pulsatility index can be used to eliminate the effect of the angle of incidence between the ultrasonic beam and the vessel wall, since this angle is the same during systole and diastole.

Studies to date show that in normal pregnancy, pulsatility is low and diastolic velocities are high in the fetal aorta and umbilical arteries, which indicates that resistance in the placental bed is low.

By contrast, high pulsatility and low diastolic velocities are noted in such abnormal states as premature rupture of membranes and IUGR, suggesting that resistance in the placental bed is higher than normal.

Recent studies also show that when uteroplacental perfusion is impaired, the velocity wave forms in the arcuate arteries within the myometrium reflect an increase in placental bed resistance; in other words, pulsatility is increased and end-diastolic velocity is decreased. Preliminary data suggest that in such abnormal pregnancies the increase in pulsatility can be appreciated during the second trimester of pregnancy.

BLOOD FLOW. Inferences about resistance in the placental bed are based on the arterial velocity wave form. However, velocity should not be mistaken for flow, which is directly proportional to the cross-sectional area of the vessel lumen as well as the blood velocity.

Assessment of fetal status by inference from blood flow is difficult. First, the diameter of fetal blood vessels cannot always be measured accurately. Second, the scenario is complicated because arterial blood flow is also dependent on viscosity of blood and on the compensatory mechanisms that come into play when blood flow slows; namely, an increase in blood pressure and an increase in the extraction of oxygen and substrate by the fetus.

Multiple Pregnancy

Ultrasound can provide grounds for suspicion of multiple pregnancy early in the first trimester of pregnancy by providing evidence of two or more gestational sacs. However, in such cases the actual diagnosis of twins should be postponed for one or two weeks until two fetuses are clearly identified (Fig. 15-13).

A diagnosis of twins based only on the presence of two pregnancy sacs can be misleading because in many cases, one of these structures will be abnormal. Specifically, the second sac may contain nothing more than accumulation of blood at the site of the trophoblast in a single pregnancy. Even if the circular structures actually represent a twin gestation, one sac may be anembryonic and will be gradually resorbed.

Recent data suggest that growth of the BPD and abdominal circumference in twin pregnancy normally falls short of that in singletons. Socol and associates

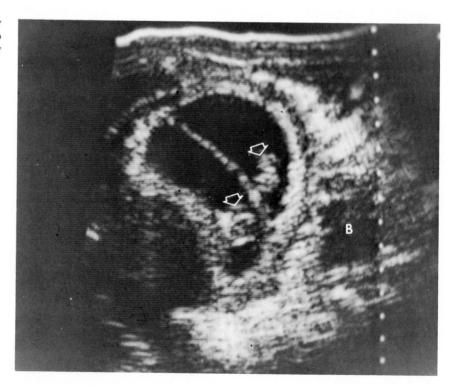

FIG. 15-13. Twins as indicated by two separate gestational sacs and two fetuses (*arrows*). *B,* bladder. (Courtesy of BD Doust, M.D.)

published a chart reflecting the progression in size of these parameters (Table 15-13).

The Placenta

Examination of placental position, texture, and abnormalities is one of the requirements of a basic or standard ultrasound scan.

POSITION. In approximately 15% to 20% of second-trimester asymptomatic pregnancies the placenta is seen in the lower uterine area, covering the location of the internal os of the cervix. However, in almost all of such pregnancies (99.5%), the position of the placenta changes with advancing maturity so that by term implantation is back to normal. The mechanism of this change is not fully understood, but it is believed that the uterine fundus grows at a much faster rate than the placenta in the third trimester of pregnancy; in so doing it favors growth of the placenta toward the fundus. Regardless of etiology, serial examination of women with low placentas is mandatory for identification of pregnancies with placenta previa.

Ultrasonic diagnosis of placenta previa is quite accurate (Fig. 15-14). As a result the need for obstetricians to perform a double set-up examination in symptomatic women with vaginal bleeding has markedly decreased and is limited to situations in which the lower part of the placenta cannot be imaged well. In the absence of placenta previa, vaginal bleeding is usually attributed to placental abruption. Although large retroplacental clots secondary to abruption can be ultrasonically visualized, in most cases clots do not form a recognizable interface to allow for direct diagnosis of abruption.

TEXTURE. Placental texture changes with advancing pregnancy and has been classified into four grades. In grade 0 through grade II, the placenta changes from having a homogeneous appearance to showing an increase in undulations from the basal plate and internal echogenic densities.

In grade-III placenta the undulations reach the basal plate and divide the organ into distinct compartments, the cotyledons (Fig. 15-15). The importance of a grade-III placenta is related to the fact that it is predictive of pulmonary maturity in 91% to 100% of normal pregnancies. However, grade-III placentas are noted only in approximately 15% of pregnancies with pulmonically mature fetuses. Thus, the clinical utility of the test in the diagnosis of lung maturity is poor.

Table 15-13
Growth Percentiles for Biparietal Diameters and Abdominal Circumferences in Twin Pregnancies

Week	Biparietal Diameter (cm)				Abdominal Circumference			
	25th	50th	75th	N	25th	50th	75th	N
17	3.7	4.0	4.1	12	12.5	12.9	13.2	5
18	3.9	4.1	4.1	8	15.1	15.1	15.7	3
19	4.2	4.4	4.5	4	15.0	16.6	17.7	4
20	4.2	4.5	4.8	6	16.0	16.3	16.7	4
21	4.9	5.1	5.2	4	16.2	17.2	17.9	6
22	5.2	5.3	5.5	15	18.1	19.0	20.2	12
23	5.4	5.8	5.9	5	18.0	18.5	20.3	5
24	5.5	5.9	6.1	6	18.7	21.6	22.4	6
25	6.2	6.5	6.7	10	21.3	22.5	22.6	7
26	6.1	6.4	6.8	11	21.4	22.0	24.0	10
27	6.6	6.9	7.2	6	23.3	24.2	25.5	6
28								
29	7.0	7.4	7.8	8	25.6	26.2	27.2	8
30	7.6	7.9	7.9	14	25.9	26.9	29.4	14
31	7.1	8.0	8.2	6	25.6	27.2	28.5	6
32	7.8	7.9	8.1	34	28.0	29.2	30.3	36
33	8.1	8.4	8.8	16	28.2	29.6	31.4	19
34	8.0	8.2	8.7	13	27.8	29.3	31.4	14
35	8.2	8.8	8.9	20	29.5	30.9	32.5	21
36	8.6	8.7	9.0	11	31.0	32.5	33.7	13
37	8.7	8.9	9.2	13	31.3	33.4	33.7	13

N = number of measurements.

(Socol ML, Tamura RK, Sabbagha RE et al: Diminished biparietal diameter and abdominal circumference growth in twins. Obstet Gynecol 64:235, 1984. Reprinted with permission from The American College of Obstetricians and Gynecologists)

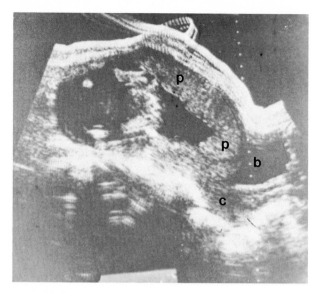

FIG. 15-14. Placenta previa. Placenta (*p*) in lower uterine area covers internal os of the cervix (*c*), which is situated posterior to the junction of the base and posterior walls of the bladder (*b*). (Courtesy of BD Doust, M.D.)

Preliminary data also suggest that in the presence of diabetes mellitus a grade-III placenta may not be very reliable in predicting pulmonary maturity and that in IUGR a grade-III placenta can be seen prior to 35 weeks of gestation.

PLACENTAL ABNORMALITIES. A number of placental abnormalities can be ultrasonically detected *in utero,* including excessive thickness in Rh disease, large size in some pregnancies complicated by maternal diabetes mellitus, chorioangioma, succenturiate lobe, or hydatidiform mole.

Abnormalities of Early Pregnancy

In all the conditions discussed in this section—molar pregnancy, missed abortion, anembryonic gestation, and ectopic gestation—the examiner is much more likely to arrive at the correct diagnosis if the history, pelvic examination, laboratory data, and ultrasound findings are carefully correlated.

The presenting sign in most of these abnormal pregnancies is vaginal bleeding and the role of ultrasound is to differentiate normal from abnormal pregnancy. Of interest in this area is the finding of Jouppila and coworkers that when a live fetus is ultrasonically visualized at 9 weeks of gestation, the chance that the pregnancy will continue to term is approximately 90%. This finding also, indirectly, means that pregnancy loss in the form of missed abortion occurs earlier than 9 weeks.

MOLAR PREGNANCY. In partial moles ultrasound shows a classic image, in which the uterus is filled with uniform echoes produced by the large number of small villi. A living fetus, albeit a stunted one with abnormal karyotype, is sometimes present and can be visualized ultrasonically.

Approximately 25% of molar pregnancies are complete: that is, the villi are of various sizes, some being quite large (Fig. 15-16). The ultrasonic image produced by a complete mole can be mistaken for missed abortion, large myomas, and even some ovarian tumors that secrete human chorionic gonadotropin (hCG), such as dysgerminoma.

MISSED ABORTION. In missed abortion the fetus and placenta are usually not distinguishable from each other. The image produced is of a nonspecific mass of central echoes resembling molar pregnancy and even uterine myoma.

ANEMBRYONIC PREGNANCY. The typical finding in anembryonic pregnancy is a large gestational sac (8–14 weeks) in which no fetus, or only a remnant of a fetal pole, is seen (Fig. 15-17). Jouppila and associates showed that ultrasound is more useful than hCG titer in establishing the diagnosis of anembryonic pregnancy because in 50% of cases the hCG titer remains normal until 11 weeks.

ECTOPIC PREGNANCY. In about 5% to 10% of ectopic pregnancies, the diagnosis can be made readily because the uterine cavity appears empty and the products of conception are clearly visualized outside the uterus. In other cases a cystic or complex mass is noted in one of the adnexal areas or in the cul-de-sac.

FIG. 15-15. Cotelydons (*C*) are readily noted in grade-III placenta, suggesting pulmonary maturity in 91% to 100% of cases.

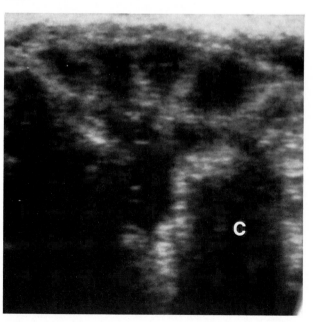

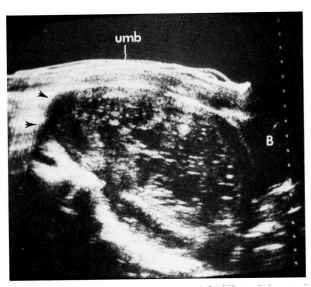

FIG. 15-16. Sagittal section of a hydatidiform mole at 11 weeks' gestation. The fundal height is at the umbilicus (*arrows*). Note the large cystic areas characteristic of a complete mole. *umb,* umbilicus; *B,* bladder. (Courtesy of BD Doust, M.D.)

In the majority of women clinically suspected of having an ectopic pregnancy, however, the only ultrasonic finding is an empty uterine cavity. In such cases, and if clinical exigencies permit, additional evaluation is necessary, as follows:

Step 1: A repeat scan should be done in 3 to 5 days to determine if a gestational sac has become apparent in the uterus. If a sac is indeed seen it should also be differentiated from a pseudogestational pregnancy. The latter resembles an early pregnancy but is formed by thick decidua surrounding a small clot of blood. The mean diameter of a pseudogestational sac is usually 6 mm or less. If it is still not possible to rule out ectopic pregnancy, the physician should proceed to Step 2.

Step 2: A baseline titer for the β-subunit of hCG should be obtained. If the titer is at or greater than the discriminatory zone (6500 mIU) and the gestational sac is not visualized ultrasonically, the diagnosis of ectopic pregnancy can be made with certainty. On the other hand if the titer is less than 6500 mIU, the measurement should be repeated in 48 hours. In a normal intrauterine pregnancy the titer is expected to double every other day.

Ultrasound As a Secondary Test

Ultrasound is an essential adjunct in the following areas:

Amniocentesis—ultrasound allows for safer removal of amniotic fluid without traversing the placenta or in-

juring the fetus. In multiple pregnancy, imaging of each sac permits safe removal of fluid from each compartment.

Fetoscopy—ultrasound is used to orient the fetoscope for sampling of umbilical cord blood or for biopsy of skin in suspected lethal conditions of the integument, such as harlequin ichthyosis.

Chorionic villi sampling—ultrasound is used in early pregnancy to orient insertion of a catheter to the placenta for sampling villi. The villi samples are used for DNA analysis, chromosome mapping, and enzymology.

Facilitation of in utero *procedures*—ultrasound is used to guide insertion of a needle and a catheter to shunt fluid to the amniotic cavity in some cases of fetal hydrocephalus or of obstruction to the urethra (see Anomalies).

Rh-disease monitoring—the use of ultrasound enhances interpretation of the ΔOD at 450 mu by defining gestational age, allows for close monitoring of the increase in the size of the fetal abdomen, a sign of fetal deterioration in worsening erythroblastosis fetalis, and delineates the fetal abdomen, facilitating insertion of a needle into the fetal peritoneal cavity when intrauterine transfusion is indicated. Monitoring pregnancies complicated by Rh-disease is of particular importance in women with twins, premature rupture of membranes, and sensitization to the Kell system. When sensitization to the Kell system has occurred, changes in the bilirubin pigment in amniotic fluid may not reflect the severity of sensitization because the hemolytic process may be very rapid.

External version of a fetus in breech presentation at term and version/extraction of second twin—ultrasound permits safer execution of these procedures.

Monitoring of ovarian follicle development—ultrasound is used in conjunction with estrogen level to help

FIG. 15-17. Large gestational sac (*S*) is seen within the uterus, but no fetal echoes are noted, indicating anembryonic pregnancy.

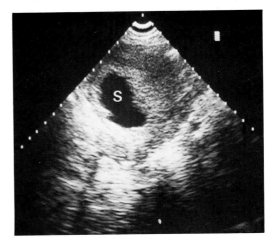

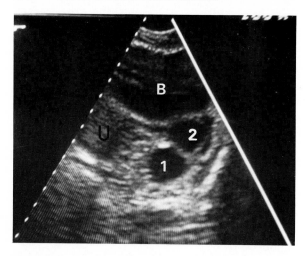

FIG. 15-18. Cross-sectional scan showing bladder (*B*), uterus, (*U*), and two mature follicles (*1* and *2*), each measuring 2 cm.

the physician decide when to administer hCG to induce ovulation in women who received follicle stimulating hormone. Research data indicate that ovulation is much more likely when a maturing follicle reaches 2 cm in size (Fig. 15-18). Ultrasound is also used to determine the number of follicles developing in response to "fertility drugs." If three or more follicles appear mature (mean diameter 2 cm), hCG is withheld to avoid triplet or quadruplet pregnancies. Finally, ultrasound is used in *in vitro* fertilization.

Cervical cerclage—ultrasound is used to evaluate fetal development and establish the best timing for the procedure. In some cases it is used to assist in the proper placement of the suture.

Intrauterine device (IUD) location—ultrasound is used to localize or assist in the removal of IUDs. A pregnancy occurring with an IUD in place is at increased risk for complications. In such circumstances the IUD is best removed under direct dynamic imaging to reduce the risk of pregnancy loss.

Pelvic abscess or hematoma drainage—ultrasound is used to guide drainage of such masses.

Targeted Imaging for Fetal Anomaly

Congenital Anomalies

TIFFA studies are pivotal in the care of women at high risk for fetal anomalies. First, if the defects are surgically remediable, ultrasound enables the physician to consider antenatal therapy by a team of specialists; to decide about the time, place, and mode of delivery; and to arrange for immediate transfer of the care of the infant to a group of neonatologists familiar with the defect and prepared to handle ensuing complications.

Second, TIFFA studies are an essential component of counseling because they allow the parents to learn about the severity of the lesion and whether it is compatible with life; the extent to which it is associated with other anomalies; and the degree to which surgical correction is possible both *in utero* and during the neonatal period.

The indications for TIFFA studies include elevation of AFP levels in amniotic fluid, hydramnios or oligohydramnios, history of a previous defect, suspicion of an anomaly on a standard ultrasound examination, presence of maternal diabetes mellitus, and presence of other pregnancy conditions, such as IUGR and breech presentation, at term. These indications are discussed individually.

α-Fetoprotein Levels

Elevation of α-fetoprotein in amniotic fluid is a marker not only for neural tube defects but also for a number of other abnormalities, such as omphalocele, duodenal atresia, cystic hygroma, Rh disease, and fetal death. More important, elevated levels of α-fetoprotein (even if acetylcholinesterase activity is also detected by gel electrophoresis) can be associated with a normal fetus. Within this context normal TIFFA studies can result in the salvage of a number of fetuses that otherwise will probably be aborted because of falsely positive biochemical markers.

Polyhydramnios/Oligohydramnios

The incidence of abnormalities is increased in the presence of oligohydramnios and polyhydramnios. It is estimated that abnormalities occur in 25% of pregnancies complicated by polyhydramnios. Some conditions associated with polyhydramnios, such as endocardial fibroelastosis, tracheoesophageal fistula, and chromosomal aberrations, cannot be ultrasonically visualized.

Anomalies Suspected on "Standard Examinations"

In a recent study it was reported that 40% of anomalies suspected on standard or basic ultrasound examinations were found not to exist on subsequent detailed TIFFA studies. Thus, physicians should verify preliminary abnormal findings by obtaining second opinions in the form of detailed TIFFA studies.

Other Complications

TIFFA is indicated in such conditions: pregnancy in diabetic women, IUGR, and breech presentations at term. In all these conditions, the frequency of anomalies is increased and the presence of anomalies influences the mode of management.

NEURAL TUBE DEFECTS. A number of neural tube defects can be diagnosed ultrasonographically, including anencephaly, microcephaly, meningocele, hydrocephalus, and spina bifida. The overall predictive accuracy of ultrasound in this area exceeds 95%.

Anencephaly can be suspected when fetal crown-rump appearance is abnormal. The diagnosis can be verified by 14 weeks of gestation.

In microcephaly, it is mandatory to assess the normality of the head circumference rather than just the BPD. The reason is that in this anomaly the occipito-frontal diameter is reduced more than the BPD. Further, the BPD should not be used to define dates in fetuses examined for microcephaly because if the condition is present, the maturity of the fetus will be underestimated and the defect will be missed.

A meningocele can be differentiated from cranial or craniocervical masses (*e.g.*, hygroma colli, teratoma) or even fetal edema by its variable shape and very thin wall. In an encephalocele, neural tissue is usually noted within the defect.

Hydrocephalus has a varied etiology. In some cases a specific diagnosis such as Dandy-Walker syndrome can be made following visualization of hypoplastic cerebellar hemispheres in conjunction with a posterior fossa cyst. In general, however, the diagnosis of hydrocephalus is based on dilatation of the cerebral ventricles (see Fig. 15-6). After the 18th week of pregnancy, the width of the lateral ventricles should not exceed 30% to 50% of that of the cerebral hemispheres. A diagnosis of hydrocephalus cannot be made before 18 weeks of gestation.

The possibility and efficacy of *in utero* treatment for progressive hydrocephalus is being examined at many centers. Michejda and Hodgen reported benefit from placement of *in utero* ventriculoamniotic shunts in monkeys with induced hydrocephalus. On the strength of these results *in utero* shunting of progressive hydrocephaly is being carried out in some centers when the diagnosis is made prior to 32 weeks of gestation.

An accurate diagnosis of spina bifida can be made in about 90% of cases. The defect is easier to identify in the presence of a skin-covered meningocele, a lesion that may not affect maternal or serum α-fetoprotein levels.

ABNORMALITIES OF THE FETAL CHEST. Cross-sectional views of the chest will clearly show the fetal lungs and heart. Tumors of the lung (*e.g.*, adenomatoid malformation) or masses such as diaphragmatic hernias can be visualized.

The four-chamber image of the heart can be located (Fig. 15-19*A*). When an electronic cursor is placed over specific areas of the heart, an M-mode tracing, outlining cardiac chamber size and rhythm is produced (Fig. 15-19*B*). Echocardiography can be used in making a number of diagnoses, including primum and secundum atrial septal defects, single atrium or ventricle, hypoplastic ventricles, and large ventricular septal defects.

ABNORMALITIES OF THE FETAL ABDOMEN. A variety of gastrointestinal (GI), renal, and pelvic fetal abnormalities can be appreciated on ultrasound examination. However, in some of these defects, for example, bowel obstruction and polycystic renal disease, the process may not become apparent until the third trimester of pregnancy.

Intestinal obstruction is diagnosed when large dilated loops of bowel with thin walls are seen. Duodenal atresia characteristically is indicated by two cystic areas

FIG. 15-19. Four-chamber view of the heart. *Spine* is on the right side. The interventricular septum is clearly noted between the two ventricles. The foramen ovale is closed (*arrow*). *lv*, left ventricle; *la*, left atrium; *rv*, right ventricle; *ra*, right atrium. (*B*) M-mode tracing of fetal heart from area traversed by electronic cursor (*white line*) shows premature contractions (*arrows*).

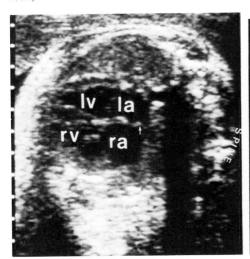 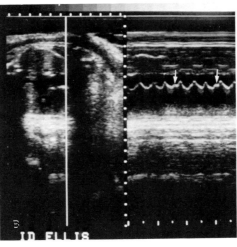

(double bubble sign) representing a dilated stomach and the proximal portion of the duodenum; 30% of such fetuses also have trisomy 21. Esophageal atresia should be considered in the absence of stomach and bowel echoes from the abdomen.

Omphalocele can be differentiated from gastroschisis. In the former, the umbilical cord is seen attached to the apex of the sac. Both anomalies are surgically correctable in the infant. However, in 50% of infants with omphalocele, other abnormalities involving the fetal heart and karyotype are noted.

Polycystic and multicystic renal dysplasias can be differentiated from each other. Fetuses with urethral obstruction may be salvaged if urine can be successfully shunted to the amniotic cavity early in pregnancy.

A number of skeletal dysplasias can be diagnosed ultrasonically. Detection is possible because limbs are short and cephalic size is large. In thanatophoric dwarfism, a condition not compatible with life, the chest is also very small.

Pelvic Sonography

The normal pelvis is readily imaged by dynamic sector ultrasound (Fig. 15-20). Because the procedure can be performed in a relatively short period, Campbell and associates in Europe are investigating in a pilot study the "pick-up rate" of ovarian cancer in women over the age of 40 years.

Even if a pelvic mass is first detected on bimanual examination, ultrasound is still useful because it helps in (1) delineating the size of a mass objectively; (2) differentiating some ovarian cysts from uterine myomas;

FIG. 15-20. Cross-sectional view of lower pelvis showing bladder (*B*), uterus (*U*), and ovaries (*O*).

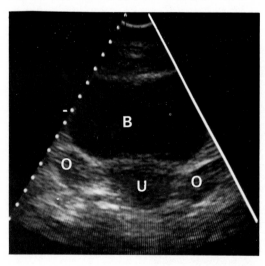

(3) defining the nature of a tumor, that is, whether it is cystic, solid, or complex; (4) assessing the degree of resolution, if any, of a hematoma or pelvic abscess; and (5) draining pelvic abscesses.

Ultrasound is also useful in the diagnosis of such conditions as uterus didelphys, uterus bicornuate unicollis, and vaginal atresia. Because the reproductive organs are closely linked to the renal system embryologically, malformations of the uterus and vagina are frequently associated with congenital anomalies of the kidney and ureters. It is therefore important to image the renal system when a uterine anomaly is noted.

In all these conditions sonography serves as a second opinion and allows the patient to appreciate visually the extent of the disease process. Furthermore, the procedure is an excellent teaching tool for both residents and students.

BIBLIOGRAPHY

Campbell S: Ultrasound in obstetrics and gynaecology: recent advances. Clin Obstet Gynecol 10:475, 1983

Cousins L: Congenital anomalies among infants of diabetic mothers: Etiology, prevention, prenatal diagnosis. Am J Obstet Gynecol 147:333, 1983

Cruikshank DP, Guest ED: Antepartum fetal surveillance. Clin Obstet Gynecol 25:719, 1983

Garris J, Kangarloo H, Sarti D, et al: The ultrasound spectrum of prune-belly syndrome. J Clin Ultrasound 8:117, 1980

Hadlock FP, Deter RL, Harrist RB, et al: Fetal head circumference: Relation to menstrual age. Am J Radiol 138:649, 1982

Hobbins JC, Winsberg F, Berkowitz RL: Ultrasonography in Obstetrics and Gynecology, 2nd ed. Baltimore, Williams & Wilkins, 1983

Hoddick WK, Callen PW, Filly RA, et al: Ultrasonographic determination of qualitative amniotic fluid volume in intrauterine growth retardation: Reassessment of the 1 cm rule. Am J Obstet Gynecol 149:758, 1984

Jassani MN, Gauderer MWL, Fanaroff AA, et al: A perinatal approach to the diagnosis and management of gastrointestinal malformations. Obstet Gynecol 59:33, 1982

Manning FA, Hill LM, Platt LD: Qualitative amniotic fluid volume determination by ultrasound: Antepartum detection of intrauterine growth retardation. Am J Obstet Gynecol 139:254, 1981

Manning FA, Platt LD, Sipos L: Antepartum fetal evaluation: Development of a fetal biophysical profile. Am J Obstet Gynecol 136:787, 1980

Michejda M, Hodgen G: In utero diagnosis and treatment of non-human primate fetal skeletal anomalies. I: Hydrocephalus. JAMA 246:1093, 1981

Milunsky A, Alpert E, Kitzmiller JL, et al: Prenatal diagnosis of neural tube defects. VIII: The importance of alpha-fetoprotein screening in diabetic pregnant women. Am J Obstet Gynecol 142:1030, 1982

Milunsky A, Sapirstein VS: Prenatal diagnosis of open neural tube defects using the amniotic fluid acetylcholinesterase assay. Obstet Gynecol 59:1, 1982

O'Brien GD, Queenan JT: Growth of the ultrasound fetal femur length during normal pregnancy. Am J Obstet Gynecol 141:833, 1981

Ogata ES, Sabbagha RE, Metzger BD, et al: Serial ultrasonography to assess evolving fetal macrosomia: Studies in 23 pregnant diabetic women. JAMA 243:2405, 1980

Paul RH, Koh KS, Monfared AH: Obstetric factors influencing outcome in infants weighing from 1,001 to 1,500 grams. Am J Obstet Gynecol 133:503, 1979

Philipson EH, Sokol RJ, Williams T: Oligohydramnios: Clinical associations and predictive value for IUGR. Am J Obstet Gynecol 146:271, 1983

Sabbagha RE: Diagnostic Ultrasound Applied to Obstetrics and Gynecology. Philadelphia, Harper & Row, 1980

Sabbagha RE: Intrauterine growth retardation: Antenatal diagnosis by ultrasound. Obstet Gynecol 52:252, 1978

Sabbagha RE, Barton FB, Barton BA: Sonar biparietal diameter. I: Analylsis of percentile growth difference in two normal populations using same methodology. Am J Obstet Gynecol 126:479, 1976

Schulman H, Fleischer A, Stern W, et al: Umbilical velocity wave ratios in human pregnancy. Am J Obstet Gynecol 148:985, 1984

Smith DW: Recognizable Patterns of Human Malformation. Philadelphia, WB Saunders, 1976

Socol ML, Tamura RK, Sabbagha RE, et al: Diminished biparietal diameter and abdominal circumference growth in twins. Obstet Gynecol 64:2, 1980

Stuart B, Drumm DE, Fitzgerald D, et al: Fetal blood velocity wave forms in normal pregnancy. Br J Obstet Gynaecol 87:780, 1980

Tamura RK, Sabbagha RE, Depp R, et al: Fetuses born preterm after spontaneous labor or premature rupture of membranes show diminished growth. Am J Obstet Gynecol 148:1105, 1984

The Vital Statistics of Reproduction

Joseph F. Thompson

16

Traditionally, the obstetrician–gynecologist's concern has been with the patient as an individual and with her particular medical problem. Public health agencies, through their function of analyzing routinely collected vital data, have fostered an awareness of gynecologic and obstetric problems of population groups identified by certain common racial, ethnic, socioeconomic, geographic, or reproductive characteristics. The health facts of an individual patient are described in terms of single events: a birth, a death, an abortion, a diagnosis, a cure, a five-year survival. Health facts describing populations are presented as rates, ratios, and percentages. This is necessary because populations differ in number. To compare data from one year with those from the next, or from one group with those from another, the number of events in question per unit of population must be determined. For rates, ratios, and percentages to be meaningful, the original data, gathered from year to year or in two areas simultaneously, must be obtained through comparable methods and with similar diligence and identical definitions.

The gathering of health data about the obstetric and gynecologic problems of groups has created an awareness of similar and dissimilar trends of disease, morbidity, and mortality rates among groups studied. This knowledge has had several important, highly practical effects on the community and public health aspects of medicine. It has demonstrated that certain patients, because they are members of characteristic groups, have a greater or lesser probability of a particular obstetric or gynecologic insult than other patients do. It has also shown that certain diseases are more important than others in contributing to morbidity or mortality, and it has provided a basis for accurate prediction of and effective preparation for expected events in future years. Moreover, it has demonstrated that there are adverse environmental factors affecting medical events that can-

not be completely neutralized by intensifying medical care.

This knowledge has led to effective methods of prevention and treatment, to research directed toward disabling problems, and to intensified care in areas or groups showing the most need or the poorest results.

The purpose of this chapter is to indicate the kinds of information that can be obtained from local, state, and federal health agencies and to discuss the trends of recent years.

VITAL DATA AND THEIR COLLECTION

Vital records include certificates of birth, death, stillbirth, marriage, and divorce. In the United States, legal responsibility for the collection of such data rests with the states. In all states it is the responsibility of the person who attends the birth or death to report the event to the legal authority. Certain additional data are required, including information about age, residence, cause of death, and length of gestation. The reporting of information such as the legitimacy of the pregnancy, the number of living children, and the date of the last delivery is not required in all states. There are other variations. For example, not all states use the same measure for gestation period for registration purposes. In some states gestation is measured in weeks; in some, by weight. In most, however, gestations exceeding 20 weeks' duration or 500 g in weight are reported.

Fortunately most states use the same basic definitions of stillbirth and live birth. These definitions, recommended by the World Health Organization in 1950, are:

> *Live birth* is the complete expulsion or extraction from its mother of a product of conception, irrespective of

the duration of pregnancy, which after such separation, breathes or shows any other evidence of life such as beating of the heart, pulsation of the umbilical cord, or definitive movement of voluntary muscles, whether or not the umbilical cord has been cut or the placenta is attached; each product of such a birth is considered liveborn.

Fetal death [*stillbirth*] is death prior to the complete expulsion or extraction from its mother of a product of conception, irrespective of the duration of pregnancy; the death is indicated by the fact that after such separation, the fetus does not breathe or show any other evidence of life such as beating of the heart, pulsation of the umbilical cord, or definite movement of voluntary muscles.

In 1972 the American College of Obstetricians and Gynecologists modified this definition to exclude from the livebirth category those births in which the infant exhibits only transient heartbeats or fleeting respiratory efforts.

After the certificate of registration is completed and signed by the attendant, it is sent to the local health department, either city or county, where certain data are recorded and a copy of the certificate may be retained. The original is then forwarded to the state health department, which in most states has the legal responsibility and authority for collecting and storing the data. In 1902 Congress authorized the Bureau of the Census to begin collection of individual birth and death data from the states. The states had to fulfill certain accuracy and reliability requirements before the federal government would accept their data. All states met these requirements by 1933. The National Center for Health Statistics of the Public Health Service now has the responsibility for gathering state data on individual births

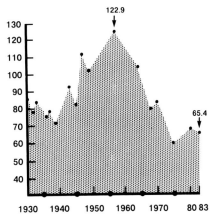

FIG. 16-2. Fertility rates (births per 1000 women aged 15–44 years), United States, 1930 to 1983. (Vital Statistics of the United States, 1930–1983, Vol 1. Washington, DC, US Department of Health and Human Services)

and deaths. It is also a source of a great deal of other health data, which it gathers directly.

REPRODUCTIVE RATES

The *birth rate* is the number of live births per 1000 population for a particular unit of time, usually one year. For birth rates to be comparable, the definitions of "births" (*i.e.,* whether live births only or live births plus stillbirths) must be the same, and there must also be agreement on the minimum period of gestation necessary for the designation of birth in contradistinction to abortion. Accurate birth data covering almost all the states have been available only since 1930, when 46 states were included in the birth registration program. The birth rate during this period has varied from a high of 26.6 in 1947 to a low of 14.8 in 1976. In 1983 the birth rate was 15.5 (Fig. 16-1).

The *fertility rate* is the number of live births per 1000 women aged 15 to 44 per year. This is a more accurate index than the birth rate for comparing the reproductive results of two different groups. For example, if the two populations to be compared contain markedly different percentages of women aged 15 to 44, they might well exhibit marked differences both in birth rate and in actual number of births, but have a similar fertility rate. The fertility rate also makes it possible to compare data within a single population group that over a period of years has experienced a change in the percentage of women of childbearing age. Since 1930 the fertility rate has varied from a high of 122.9 in 1957 to a low of 65.4 in 1983 (Fig. 16-2).

The accurate forecast of the approximate number of births in any geographic area 2 or 3 or even 15 or 20 years in advance was at one time quite simple because fertility rates were reasonably predictable and basic

FIG. 16-1. Birth rates (births per 1000 population), United States, 1930 to 1983. (Vital Statistics of the United States, 1930–1983, Vol 1. Washington, DC, US Department of Health and Human Services)

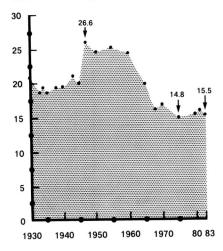

census trends were stable. However, changing life-styles, unexpected migration of women of childbearing age because of changing environmental or economic conditions, increased availability and reliability of contraception, acceptance of legal abortions, and the prevalence of sterilization had led modern demographers to be cautious in predicting the number of births that will occur in the future. In Marion County, Indiana, for example, the 1970 fertility rate was 90. Based on a predicted population in 1990 of 300,000 women aged 15 to 44 and using this fertility rate, the number of births expected to occur in 1990 was 26,000. In 1983, however, there were 13,010 births in a population of 185,959 women aged 15 to 44, making the fertility rate 70 and casting doubt on the 1970 prediction of the number of births to be expected in 1990.

OBSTETRIC AND GYNECOLOGIC MORBIDITY RATES

Hospital Morbidity Rate

The classic definition of hospital morbidity is the elevation of body temperature above 100.4°F on two occasions 24 hours apart in the postoperative or postpartum period after the first 24 hours. The American College of Obstetricians and Gynecologists defines *puerperal morbidity* as an oral temperature above 38°C (100.4°F) on any of the first ten postpartum days, excluding the first 24 hours, with the temperature taken at least four times daily.

Morbidity rate is computed as a percentage of the total patients in each of the groups defined above and is used to compare the occurrence of operative or puerperal infection in different institutions or in the same institution over a period of time. With the introduction of routine prophylactic antibiotics, the importance and usefulness of this rate has declined. However, the hospital morbidity rate is a figure in which local health departments maintain continuing interest.

Preterm Delivery

Attempts are now being made to introduce for routine use comparable and more accurate methods of identifying physiological immaturity. The most generally accepted, easily defined, error-free measure of physiological immaturity is the weight of the newborn at birth. Newborns weighing less than 2500 g (5 lb 8 oz) are identified as preterm. The use of such a simple method excludes some physiologically immature newborns and includes some physiologically mature newborns, but the definition is useful for the evaluation of a large number of newborns. The American College of Obstetricians and Gynecologists defines a preterm neonate as one born at any time up to the end of the 37th week of gestation (259 days).

A refinement developed by Yerushalmey and colleagues over 20 years ago is still germane. These authors divided all newborns into five groups according to length of gestation and weight (Table 16-1). This classification identifies those newborns with different intrauterine growth rates but comparable periods of gestation. When this is done, differences in prognosis, as shown by relative mortality, become evident. The effect of weight alone (intrauterine growth) on gestations of similar length can be seen by comparing the relative mortality of group III with that of group V and the relative mortality of group II with that of group IV. The effect of gestation length alone can be seen when group II is compared with group III and group IV with group V. This classification also tends to group newborns with major congenital anomalies in group III, because they characteristically exhibit intrauterine growth retardation, and to group newborns born to diabetics and isoimmunized newborns in group IV, because they are pathologically excessive in size and weight for the length of their gestation.

Congenital Anomaly Rate

The congenital anomaly rate is usually computed as a percentage of total births. Not every state has a reporting

Table 16-1
Relationship of Birth Weight, Length of Gestation, and Mortality

Classification	Birth Weight (g)	Gestation (wk)	Relative Mortality
Group I	Less than 1588	All gestations	139.6
Group II	1617 to 2500	Less than 37	19.9
Group III	1617 to 2500	More than 37	6.4
Group IV	More than 2524	Less than 37	2.9
Group V	More than 2524	More than 37	1

(Yerushalmey J, van den Berg BJ, Erhardt CL, Jacobziner H: Birth weight and gestation as indices of "immaturity." Am J Dis Child 109:43. Copyright 1965, The American Medical Association)

mechanism for congenital anomalies, and, as a result, these data are neither complete nor routinely published. Major inaccuracies in comparability arise because of variation in definitions, in methods of classification, in diligence in examining the neonate, and in the time period over which examinations are made, and because of the selective termination of some pregnancies complicated by anomalous fetuses in the second trimester before a birth would have been recorded. Similarly, there are no good methods of reliable collection of data on the incidence rates of cerebral palsy, central nervous system damage, or birth trauma.

SOCIAL MORBIDITY RATES

The concept of measuring social morbidity on the basis of vital data is relatively new to obstetricians and gynecologists. Information about the legitimacy of a pregnancy, a social fact, is required on birth certificates by 40 states and the District of Columbia. Other data from the certificate that may be used to indicate social morbidity associated with the birth are maternal age, previous pregnancy loss, date of previous delivery, address, number of prenatal visits, month of first prenatal visit, and educational attainment of the mother. The variable accuracy and completeness of the reporting greatly affect the comparability of specific items. However, such information is important as an index of social morbidity associated with birth and death.

Illegitimacy may be measured as a rate (number of births per 1000 unmarried women aged 15 to 44) or as a ratio (number of illegitimate births per 1000 live births). It is difficult to draw conclusions from such data because of inaccuracy in collection and reporting. Figure 16-3 illustrates some of the possible errors in reporting that may occur from the time the population at risk is identified (at the base of the pyramid) and a conception out of wedlock occurs until the illegitimate birth is cor-

rectly recorded. Illegitimacy data, as they are presently gathered, probably more accurately indicate the variable environmental pressures upon geographically, socio-economically, and racially identified groups than the occurrence of conception among unmarried women.

Figure 16-4, showing total births and recorded illegitimate births according to maternal age and parity, gives some idea of the extent of this problem in urban areas, in this case, Marion County, Indiana. These data show that the illegitimate birth ratios are still increasing but the percentage of illegitimate births among young women and those pregnant for the first time is decreasing.

MORTALITY RATES

Maternal Mortality

The American College of Obstetricians and Gynecologists defines *maternal death* as death from any cause, during pregnancy or up to 42 days after pregnancy terminates. A direct maternal death is one resulting from an obstetric complication, an indirect death is one resulting from a preexisting disease or illness that is aggravated by pregnancy, and a nonmaternal death is one in which the cause of death is unrelated to medical illness or obstetric complications.

The *maternal mortality rate* was the number of maternal deaths per 10,000 live births. Because the national rate is in the range of 0.8 to 1.0, the National Center for Health Statistics now uses a base of 100,000 live births to give the number more realistic variation. Presently, most states have a committee that reviews the facts surrounding maternal deaths. Deficiencies, responsibilities, and preventability in relation to each death are studied. These state committees were first established in the 1930s and have been instrumental in bringing preventable factors associated with maternal

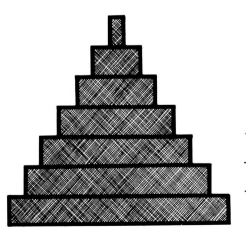

Those identified correctly as to race, age, geographic location, etc.

Those not falsifying marital status

Those not undergoing abortion

Those not getting married

Those getting pregnant

Those having intercourse

All unmarried women aged 15—44 years

FIG. 16-3. Illegitimacy: possible errors affecting comparability of reporting.

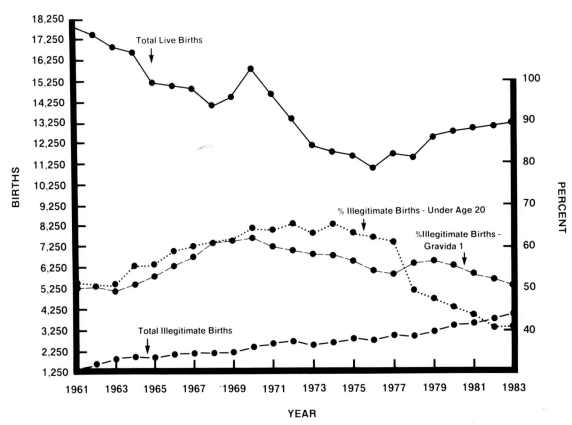

FIG. 16-4. Illegitimacy, Marion County, Indiana, 1961 to 1983. (Annual Reports, Health and Hospital Corporation of Marion County)

death to the attention of the medical community. The maternal mortality rate has gradually decreased over the years (Fig. 16-5), and in 1981 in the United States there were 8.5 maternal deaths for each 100,000 live births.

This decrease has resulted largely from the emergence of obstetrics and gynecology as a recognized specialty, the increased use of hospitals for delivery, the recognition and special care of pregnant women at high risk, the availability of antibiotics to combat infection and of blood for transfusions, the use of postpartum recovery units, improvement in the quality of anesthesia, and the intensive study of the preventable causes of maternal death. Recent data from large urban areas, in which excessive numbers of maternal deaths resulted from infected illegal abortions, show a considerable decrease in maternal deaths. This decline has been attributed to the availability of safe legal abortions.

In 1963 201 maternal deaths resulted from septic abortion; in 1971 there were 99 such deaths, in 1977 there were 27, and in 1979 the figure decreased to 16 abortion-related maternal deaths.

Hemorrhage and preeclampsia—eclampsia are still the most common causes of death among pregnant women. The leading causes of maternal death in the United States in 1979 are listed in Table 16-2.

Abortion

The termination of pregnancy before the 20th week of gestation is termed abortion in most states. *Spontaneous abortion* identifies those pregnancies that terminate as a result of abnormal fetal development or other frequently unidentifiable or unknown uterine, fetal, or maternal conditions. A fetus may or may not be involved or identified; in some cases the pregnancy may have been so abnormal that a fetus did not exist. There are no routinely collected vital data concerning spontaneous abortions. On the basis of hospital records from the Illinois Department of Health, it seems that about 10% of known pregnancies terminate in hospitals as incomplete or complete abortions. Shapiro and colleagues, in a study of members of a prepayment medical insurance group, found that 11.5% of known pregnancies terminated by the end of the 20th week of gestation. In the United States data concerning trends, socioeconomic variation, and geographic differences in spontaneous abortion ratios are almost nonexistent.

Pregnancies that terminate prior to the 20th week of gestation when the fetus weighs about 500 g almost never produce a surviving infant. While some infants weighing less than 500 g at birth have survived, this

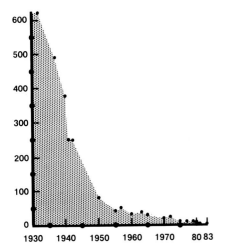

FIG. 16-5. Maternal mortality rates (deaths per 100,000 live births), United States, 1930 to 1983. (Vital Statistics of the United States, 1930–1983, Vol 2. Washington, DC, US Department of Health and Human Services)

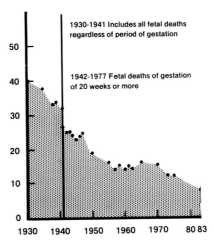

FIG. 16-6. Stillbirth rates (fetal deaths per 1000 live births), United States, 1930 to 1983. (Vital Statistics of the United States, 1930–1983, Vol 2. Washington, DC, US Department of Health and Human Services)

Table 16-2

Causes of Maternal Death in Women of All Ages, United States, 1979

Cause	Total Number of Deaths
Complications of the puerperium	96
Complications of labor and delivery	65
Hypertension	49
Ectopic pregnancy	45
Antepartum hemorrhage	28
Abortion	16
Hyperemesis	1
Other complications of pregnancy	10
Other medical illness	10
Unknown	16
Rate/100,000 live births	9.6

(Vital Statistics of the United States, 1979, Vol 2. Washington, DC, US Department of Health and Human Services, 1982)

medical curiosity is disregarded for the purposes of routine data collection.

Legal abortion identifies those pregnancies that are terminated legally by physicians or other health professionals using mechanical or pharmacologic means. Some authors have further subdivided legal abortions into therapeutic and elective, the former denoting pregnancies terminated because of complicating medical factors that compromise the life or health of the mother and the latter denoting those terminated upon request of the patient for socioeconomic or other environmental reasons. An *illegal abortion* is a procedure performed by the woman herself or by someone unlicensed to practice medicine, or without the supervision of a person who is licensed.

The *abortion rate* is the number of abortions computed as a percentage of total pregnancies. Since the total number of pregnancies in a geographic area is almost impossible to determine accurately, the *abortion ratio* is used. This is the number of abortions per 1000 live births. The spontaneous abortion ratio is usually given as a percentage of live births, while legal abortions are reported as a ratio of the number of legal terminations per 1000 live births. Most, but not all, states require the reporting of legal abortions. The completeness of the reporting is unknown and may be variable. In some states, all legal abortions must take place in a licensed health facility, while in others this is not a requirement. Unless there is a pathologic examination, the presence of a conceptus at the time of "menstrual extraction" would in some instances be unknown. Calculated from available data, the legal abortion ratio for the United States in 1981 was 358 abortions per 1000 live births.

Stillbirth

An infant born after the 20th week of gestation who shows no sign of life at birth is termed *stillborn*. The *stillbirth rate* is the number of stillborn infants per 1000 live births. Although there are notable exceptions, the almost universal acceptance of the World Health Organization definition of stillbirth has done much to permit international comparison of rates. In the United States the stillbirth rate has shown a decreasing trend (Fig. 16-6), reaching an all-time low of 8.9 in 1981. A further decline in stillbirths can be expected because the use of tests for antepartum fetal evaluation and the acceptance of intrapartum fetal monitoring is increasing.

Table 16-3
Causes of Stillbirth, Indiana, 1983

Cause	Total Number of Stillbirths
Complications of placenta, cord, or membranes	242
Fetal oxygenation problems	66
Complications of pregnancy	44
Congenital anomalies	33
Gestational growth problems	30
Maternal illness	24
Complications of labor and delivery	16
Other	26
Unknown	146

(Indiana Vital Statistics, 1983, Indiana State Board of Health)

The major causes of stillbirth in Indiana in 1983 are listed in Table 16-3.

Newborn Mortality

The *infant mortality rate* is the number of liveborn infants who die within the first year of life per 1000 live births. The *neonatal mortality rate* is the number of liveborn infants per 1000 live births who die within the first 28 days of life. The *hebdomadal death rate* is the number of liveborn infants who die within the first seven days of life per 1000 live births.

Newborn mortality rates are computed from death certificates. In many cases, additional information is obtained by studying the birth certificate along with the death certificate. Formal committees for the study of the facts surrounding a stillbirth or the death of a newborn came into existence shortly after the formation of committees to investigate maternal death. Because of the openness of the deliberations and the practicality of each hospital having such a committee, these groups, frequently termed perinatal mortality committees, became valuable sources of continuing education for all who participated. Such committees also were instrumental in raising the standards of care of the pregnant woman and the newborn child. Data for 1983 reveal an infant mortality rate of 10.9 and a neonatal mortality rate of 6.9 (Fig. 16-7).

The major causes of infant death are postnatal asphyxia and atelectasis, immaturity (unqualified), congenital malformations, influenza and pneumonia (including pneumonia of the newborn), and maternal complications. Infants do not die at a uniform rate during the first year of life; also, the leading causes of death in one period may vary from those in another. For the purposes of study, the first year may be divided into the first 24 hours, the remainder of the first week, the remainder of the first month, and the remainder of the

first year. About 40% of infant deaths occur within the first 24 hours of life. At this time, the leading cause of death is unqualified immaturity. About 25% of infant deaths occur during the remainder of the first week, when the leading causes are postnatal asphyxia and atelectasis. During the remainder of the first month, another 8% die; during the subsequent 11 months, the final 27% die. The leading causes of death for each period are given in Table 16-4. These data are compiled from death certificates on a nationwide basis.

The causes of death are not exclusive of other associated or underlying causes. Variability in accuracy, interest, and diagnostic criteria may affect these data.

After the first year of life and up to about the 40th year, accidents are the leading cause of death.

Perinatal Mortality

The number of stillbirths plus the number of neonatal deaths per 1000 live births is the *perinatal mortality rate*. There are numerous variations in this rate. In some cases the denominator comprises total births, while the numerator may be restricted by weight exclusions (below 1000 g) or time of death after birth (7 days rather than 28 days). The logic of such a rate becomes apparent when it is considered that an obstetric complication in its severest form may kill both the mother and her unborn child and, in lesser degrees of severity, may result in a stillborn infant, a preterm liveborn infant who dies, a preterm liveborn infant with disabling central nervous system damage, or a term infant with minimal central nervous system impairment. Yankhauer must be given credit for pointing out the amount of life lost during the period extending "from the 20th week of gestation to

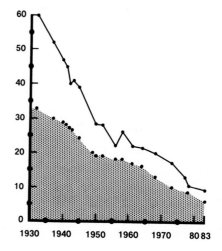

FIG. 16-7. Infant and neonatal mortality rates (deaths per 1000 live births), United States, 1930 to 1983. (Vital Statistics of the United States, 1930–1983, Vol 2. Washington, DC, US Department of Health and Human Services)

Table 16-4
Causes of Death During First Year of Life, in Order of Frequency for Each Period

Under 1 Day	1 to 6 Days	7 to 27 Days	28 Days to 11 Months
Immaturity (unqualified)	Postnatal asphyxia and atelectasis	Congenital malformation	Influenza and pneumonia*
Postnatal asphyxia and atelectasis	Immaturity (unqualified)	Influenza and pneumonia*	Congenital malformation
Birth injuries	Maternal complications	Maternal complications	Accidents
Maternal complications	Congenital malformation	Immaturity (unqualified)	Residuals of accidents
Congenital malformation	Birth injuries	Postnatal asphyxia and atelectasis	Gastrointestinal infections

* Including pneumonia of the newborn.
(Infant and Perinatal Mortality in the United States. National Center for Health Statistics, Series 3, No 9, p 17. Washington, DC, US Department of Health, Education, and Welfare, 1965)

the seventh day of life.'' He states that there are more lives lost during this period than in the next 40 years.

Pregnancy Wastage

It seems logical to combine the stillbirth rate with the neonatal mortality rate to arrive at a figure that represents pregnancy loss between the 20th week of gestation and the 28th day of life. It is just as logical to start routine data collection on pregnancies that terminate prior to the 20th week and to add these pregnancy losses (abortions) to the perinatal rate. From a combination of such data, *total pregnancy wastage* can be ascertained. This concept is shown in Figure 16-8. Figure 16-9 gives an example of the numbers of total pregnancy wastage from known conception to completion of the first year of life. This figure is a hypothetical cohort of 1000 known conceptions, their spontaneous or legal termination, and the resultant infant survival at the end of the first year of life. It assumes a 10% spontaneous abortion ratio, a legal abortion ratio of 358, a stillbirth rate of 9, a neonatal mortality rate of 8, and a postneonatal mortality rate of 4. Pregnancy wastage from conception to the first missed menses has not been considered, although new preg-

nancy tests that use monoclonal antibodies and are capable of detecting β-subunit chorionic gonadotropin at extremely low levels (1–50 mIU) should provide additional information about pregnancy wastage occurring between implantation and the first missed menses.

EPIDEMIOLOGY OF PREGNANCY MORBIDITY AND MORTALITY

The identifying characteristics used in classic descriptive epidemiology are time, place, and person.

Time

As noted, the secular trends of morbidity and mortality rates show a progressive decrease over time. This probably results from improved medical care and an increase in the general resistance of the population to obstetric health hazards. This increase in the general resistance has been facilitated by improvements in the health environment and in the nutritional status of the population, which have also lowered many other morbidity and mortality rates.

FIG. 16-8. Total pregnancy wastage.

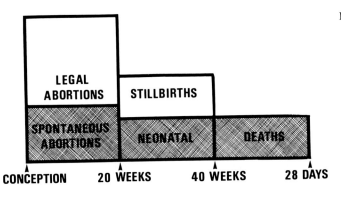

CONCEPTION   20 WEEKS   40 WEEKS   28 DAYS

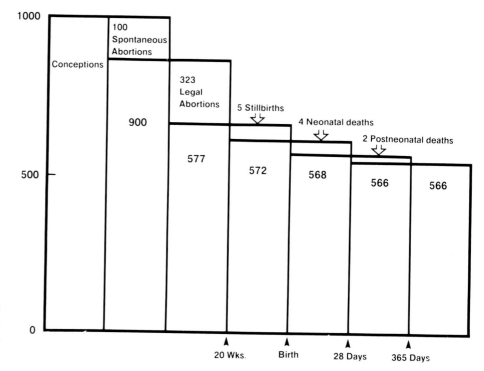

FIG. 16-9. Life table of 1000 known conceptions from conception to 1 year of postnatal life.

Place

Making comparisons of the reproductive rates of geographically identifiable populations, along with assumptions and explanations for the differences noted, has become a common pastime. It is important to remember, however, that for data to be meaningful they must be obtained using comparable methods, similar diligence, and identical definitions.

International Differences

The neonatal and infant mortality rates of the United States and some other countries are presented in Table 16-5. These rates are based on live births. Although the differences probably reflect actual differences in the numbers of neonatal and infant deaths occurring in each country, there are several reasons why they cannot be taken absolutely at face value. In a special study in Sweden in 1956, 17% of "stillborn" infants breathed and therefore should have been classified as liveborn infants who died, thus raising Sweden's infant and neonatal mortality rates. In many western European countries, it is the responsibility of the parents to report the birth. In the Netherlands, birth weight is not reported; the extent of underreporting is unknown, and registration of fetal death is required only for gestations of 28 weeks or more. In Norway, birth registration is an ecclesiastical function.

These are examples of some differences in methods, diligence, and definitions. However, those who have

studied these discrepancies conclude that more is concerned than differences in the collection of data. These matters are discussed at length in *International Comparison of Perinatal and Infant Mortality,* published by the U.S. Department of Health, Education, and Welfare.

Table 16-5

Neonatal and Infant Mortality Rates in Various Countries, 1980

	Neonatal Mortality Rate (%)	Infant Mortality Rate (%)
Sweden	4.9	6.9
Japan	4.9	7.5
Finlnd	—	7.6
Norway	5.1	8.1
Denmark	5.6	8.4
Netherlands	5.7	8.6
Switzerland	5.9	9.1
France	5.6	10.0
Canada	6.7	10.4
Spain	—	11.1
Ireland	—	11.2
Hong Kong	—	11.8
United States	8.4	12.5

(World Health Statistics Annual, Vol I. Geneva, World Health Organization, 1983)

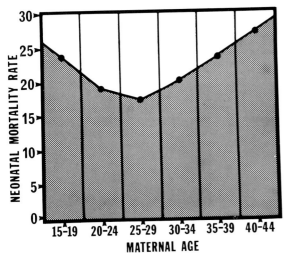

FIG. 16-10. Maternal age and neonatal mortality rate. (Infant and Perinatal Mortality in the United States, Series 3, No 4, p 77. Washington, DC, US Department of Health, Education, and Welfare, 1965)

Urban–Rural Differences

Arranging identifiable geographic areas according to population density and then studying the associated pregnancy wastage rates can also provide insight into the relation between environment and reproductive loss. Strong positive associations between preterm delivery and population density and between perinatal mortality and population density have been demonstrated.

Person

For purposes of epidemiologic investigation, the patient may be identified by personal characteristics such as age, race, socioeconomic status, previous pregnancy loss, and interval since last delivery, and the pregnancy may be identified by such factors as breech presentation, premature rupture of membranes, repeat cesarean section, or labor in excess of 18 hours. Figure 16-10 shows the relationship of neonatal mortality to one of these parameters, maternal age. These data indicate that reproductive wastage is lowest among gravidas who are in the third decade of life.

REFERENCES AND RECOMMENDED READING

Abortion Surveillance: 1976. US Department of Health, Education, and Welfare. Washington, DC, Center for Disease Control, 1978

The Facts of Life and Death, p 6. Washington, DC, US Department of Health, Education, and Welfare, 1965

Fielding JE: Adolescent pregnancy revisited: Trends in births to adolescents. N Engl J Med 299:893, 1978

International Comparison of Perinatal and Infant Mortality, Series 3, No 6. Washington, DC, US Department of Health, Education, and Welfare, 1967

Shapiro S, Jones E, Densen P: A life table of pregnancy terminations and correlates of fetal loss. Milbank Mem Fund Q 40:1, 1962

State Definitions of Livebirths, Fetal Deaths, and Gestation Periods at Which Fetal Deaths Are Registered, p xii. Washington, DC, US Department of Health, Education, and Welfare, 1966

Statistical Abstract of the United States. Washington, DC, US Bureau of the Census, 1978

Thompson J: Some observations on the geographic distribution of premature births and perinatal deaths in Indiana. Am J Obstet Gynecol 101:43, 1968

Yankhauer A: The public health aspect of perinatal mortality. NY State J Med 57:2499, 1957

Yerushalmey J, van den Berg BJ, Erhardt CL et al: Birth weight and gestation as indices of "immaturity." Am J Dis Child 109:43, 1965

World Health Statistics Annual, 1983, Vol I. Geneva, World Health Organization, 1983

PART II

Normal Pregnancy

Fertilization and the Physiology and Development of Fetus and Placenta

Irwin H. Kaiser

17

EVENTS SURROUNDING FERTILIZATION

The anatomy and physiology of ovulation are discussed in Chapters 4 and 6. The events of ovulation, fertilization, and implantation are diagramed in Figure 17-1.

The ovum, with the mass of surrounding granulosa cells that form the cumulus oophorus, is shed into the fimbriated end of the tube. Muscular and ciliary activity move it into the ampulla, where it encounters the spermatozoa that have ascended through the uterus. The mobility of ovaries and tubes enables an ovum from one ovary to enter the opposite tube. It is unknown whether sperm can migrate from one tube to the other.

Spermatogenesis (Fig. 17-2) occurs in the tubules of the testis under the influence of both follicle-stimulating hormones and the testosterone formed by the adjacent Leydig cells, which are under the influence of luteinizing hormones. Secretion of these hormones is essentially continuous after pubarche. The maturation from spermatogonium to spermatozoan involves several distinct stages—spermatocyte and spermatid—during which reduction division is accomplished, so that the spermatozoan has a haploid number of chromosomes. The nuclear mass becomes the head of the sperm. X-bearing sperm are minutely heavier than Y-bearing sperm. The cytoplasm of the spermatid makes up the spiral midpiece and the elongated tail of the mature sperm.

A spermatozoan has an outer plasma membrane and an outer coat that may contain antigenic material. The acrosome, a minute structure, is situated at the tip of the head of the sperm and contains the hyaluronidase that initiates the dispersion of cells surrounding the ovum. It may also contain an enzyme that causes the zona pellucida to become readily permeable to the head of the sperm and its chromosomal material.

Behind the head of the sperm is the coiled helix of the midpiece, which consists of mitochondria. These generate most of the energy responsible for tail motion. The tail consists of two long longitudinal fibers surrounded by nine pairs of shorter fibers. These are the contractile units that generate both forward motion and rotation. This motion is essential to fertilization.

A spermatozoan is able to maintain motility for as long as a week in the fallopian tube, but it is probably actually fertile for less than half that time. It cannot repair damage, having lost its ribonucleic acid (RNA), and its energy systems are needed only to maintain motility. Once the stored adenosine triphosphate is exhausted, cell death ensues. There are some intracellular lipids, but extracellular substances, principally fructose, are essential to support glycolysis. When the sperm is immobile, its energy consumption is virtually nil, and it can therefore survive for several weeks in the male reproductive tract after release from the seminiferous tubule.

The suspending material for the sperm, the seminal plasma, is derived from epididymis, vas deferens, seminal vesicle, prostate, and urethral glands. It has a characteristic odor because of unique amines, and it contains considerable fructose. It also contains prostaglandins, whose physiological function is still unclear, and considerable amounts of amino acids.

In coitus, 2 ml to 4 ml semen is deposited in the vagina at the cervix. It contains more than 50 million sperm. In healthy fertile specimens, more than 75% of these spermatozoa are of normal morphology and more than half of these are motile. Of the motile sperm, more than half exhibit forward motion and rotation.

If the cervical mucus is favorable, as it is at midcycle, some of these sperm penetrate and ascend the female tract at a rate of about 5 mm to 6 mm/minute. It is thought that uterine contractions assist in sperm progress, but nonmotile sperm do not reach the fallopian

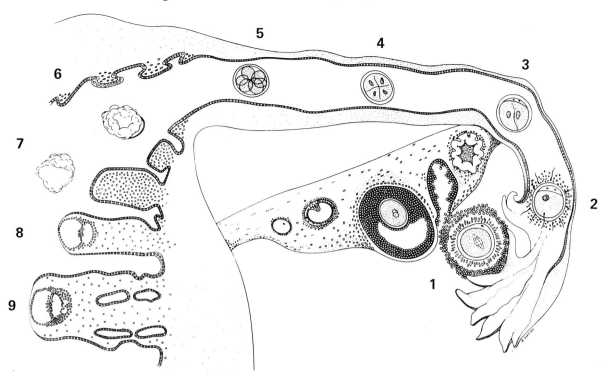

FIG. 17-1. Schematic representation of events of ovulation, fertilization, and implantation. *1.* Extrusion of ovum, with first polar body and cumulus oophorus, which then forms corona radiata. *2.* Cells of corona have become loosened, sperm has penetrated zona pellucida and entered ovum, and second polar body has formed. *3.* Cleavage of fertilized ovum has begun, and ovum has moved well into fallopian tube. *4.* Further cleavage proceeds. About 24 hours have elapsed since fertilization. *5.* By 48 hours, many cells are present and zona begins to fragment. *6.* At 72–84 hours, zona has fallen away and ovum has entered uterine cavity. Central cavity begins to form in ovum. *7.* By 120 hours, there is distinct cell mass on one side of ovum, which is still free in uterine fluid. *8.* At 7 days, implantation has taken place. Ovum is promptly covered over by surface epithelium. Trophoblast burrows into endometrial stroma and starts to form syncytiotrophoblast. Primitive amniotic and chorionic cavities have begun to form, and germ disk is recognizable. *9.* By 9 days, lacunae have begun to appear in syncytiotrophoblast. They will form intervillous space. Germ disk is well formed, as is amnion. (After Dickinson RL: Human Sex Anatomy, 2nd ed. Baltimore, Williams & Wilkins, 1949)

tubes. The fluid in the uterus or tubes enables the sperm to fertilize an ovum. This process is called *capacitation* and requires some hours. One of the major problems in achieving *in vitro* fertilization has been the production of artificial capacitation.

When the spermatozoan and ovum meet in the tube, syngamy takes place. It is known that a number of sperm can make contact with the cumulus and corona radiata and penetrate to the zona pellucida (Fig. 17-3). In some species, the zona consists of two layers, and sperm must penetrate both to enter the cytoplasm of the ovum. Once one sperm has entered, a reaction occurs in the zona that renders it impervious to other sperm. A diploid chromosome number is reestablished, and mitotic cell division of the fetus can begin.

TIMING OF PREGNANCY

In the precise timing of pregnancy, the initial event is considered to be ovulation, and physicians may refer to *ovulation age.* When the time of fertile coitus is known, especially with laboratory animals, this time may be used as well and is stated in hours, days, or weeks.

Clinically, however, pregnancy is dated from the first day of the last menstrual period, when this is known. From this, an expected date of labor or confinement (EDL or EDC) is calculated by assuming a duration of 280 days. Nägele's rule, by which 3 is subtracted from the original number of the month and 7 is added to the date, is based on this estimate. Since in an idealized cycle ovulation occurs on the 14th day, the actual du-

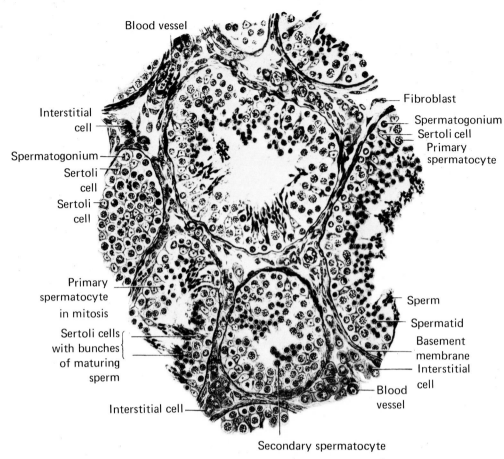

Blood vessel

Interstitial cell

Spermatogonium

Sertoli cell

Sertoli cell

Primary spermatocyte in mitosis

Sertoli cells with bunches of maturing sperm

Interstitial cell

Fibroblast

Spermatogonium

Sertoli cell

Primary spermatocyte

Sperm

Spermatid

Basement membrane

Interstitial cell

Blood vessel

Secondary spermatocyte

FIG. 17-2.   Section of human testis. Transected tubules show various stages of spermatogenesis. (×170) (Bloom W, Fawcett DW: A Textbook of Histology, 9th ed. Philadelphia, WB Saunders, 1968)

ration of pregnancy is 266 days. When cycles are very irregular or artifically induced, timing must be based on a presumed date of ovulation or fertilization and 266 days added.

Although actually the duration of pregnancy may vary by several weeks, these estimates of expected duration are accurate enough for clinical use. The embryologist and reproductive endocrinologist prefer the more precise statement, however.

THE FERTILIZED OVUM

The Hertig–Rock Series

Information about human pregnancy is obviously difficult to obtain, and most of our present knowledge is based upon what is referred to as the Hertig–Rock series of ova. A large number of women who were awaiting hysterectomy for gynecologic disease, but who were normally fertile and within the reproductive epoch, were asked to report their menstrual and coital dates to these

researchers. At the time of hysterectomy, meticulous study of the uteri and fallopian tubes was made for evidence of early ova. A remarkably large number were recovered and were described in great detail in a series of publications in the *Contributions to Embryology* of the Carnegie Institution of Washington. Because the women studied were all essentially normal from a reproductive standpoint, great reliance can be placed on the normality of these data, in contrast to data obtained at the time of spontaneous abortion or uterine curettage for bleeding.

Early Fetal Loss

The unusually high fetal loss originally observed in the pig (*i.e.,* a greater number of corpora lutea in the pig's ovary than viable fetuses in the uterus) has been found, on the basis of the Hertig–Rock series, to apply to the human as well. Too few ova have been examined prior to implantation to allow generalization, and indeed it is difficult to adduce entirely satisfactory criteria of nor-

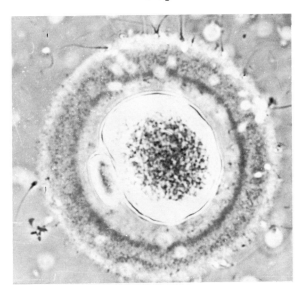

FIG. 17-3. Human ovum. Polar body is on *left*. Many spermatozoa are visible in and around zona pellucida. (Shettles LB: Ovum Humanum. New York, Hafner, 1960)

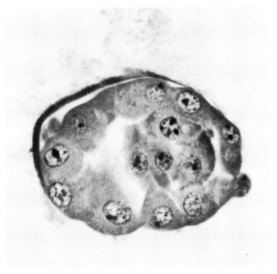

FIG. 17-5. Section of fixed, stained 58-cell human conceptus found in uterine cavity within 4 days of conception. Zona pellucida is intact, and cells appear to be differentiating into outer and inner group. (Carnegie No. 8794, ×600) (Hertig AT, Rock J, Adams EC, Mulligan WJ: On preimplantation stages of human ovum: Description of 4 normal and 4 abnormal specimens ranging from second to fifth day of development. Contrib Embryol 35:199, 1954)

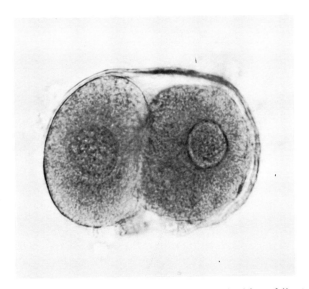

FIG. 17-4. Two-cell human conceptus, washed from fallopian tube within 36 hours of conception. Polar body can be seen *below*, still within zona pellucida. (Carnegie No. 8698, ×500) (Hertig AT, Rock J, Adams EC, Mulligan WJ: On preimplantation stages of human ovum: Description of 4 normal and 4 abnormal specimens ranging from second to fifth day of development. Contrib Embryol 35:199, 1954)

mality in such a group. However, if consideration is restricted to implanted ova recovered up to the 14th day following ovulation (obtained, therefore, from patients who had no way of knowing they were pregnant), major disturbances of differentiation of the germ disk or of implantation or proliferation of the trophoblast are ob-

served in more than 40%. Those ova with marked hemorrhage at the implantation site or marked deficiency in the formation of trophoblast and villi are probably lost at the time of the next menstrual period, and the mother would never know that she had been pregnant. The remainder probably account for the greater portion of abortions that result from defective germ plasma, which include most spontaneous abortions.

Early Development and Transport of Ovum

After fertilization, mitotic division begins, slowly at first but gradually increasing in speed. During its life in the fallopian tube, the ovum undergoes considerable growth, more in terms of the number of cells than in actual size, although the latter also increases (Figs. 17-4 and 17-5). During most of the period when it exists in the tube, the fertilized ovum is a solid mass of cells. Blastocyst formation begins at about the fifth day. On the fifth or sixth day, the blastocyst (Fig. 17-6) enters the uterine lumen, where it continues a free-floating existence for at least 24 hours. The outermost layer of the blastocyst is one or two cells thick, with a central cell mass located somewhere on the inner surface. This central mass consists of cells that are not much more differentiated than those elsewhere in the blastocyst. Some investigators believe that the fertilized ovum spends three to four days in the uterine cavity; however, the fact that Hertig and Rock failed to find a substantial

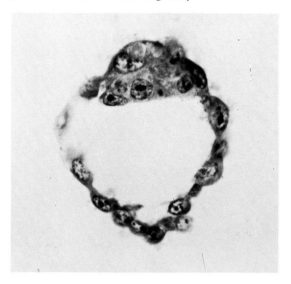

FIG. 17-6. Section of 107-cell human blastocyst approximately 1 day older than embryo in Figure 17-5. This embryo was also found in uterine cavity. Zona pellucida is now gone, and differentiation into inner cell mass, which will form embryo, and outer layer, which forms trophoblast, has taken place. (Carnegie No. 8663, ×600) (Hertig AT, Rock J, Adams EC, Mulligan WJ: On preimplantation stages of human ovum: Description of 4 normal and 4 abnormal specimens ranging from second to fifth day of development. Contrib Embryol 35:199, 1954)

number of unattached ova in that location makes this unlikely.

Implantation of Ovum

The formation of the corpus luteum in the ovary and the consequent secretion of progesterone in large quantities begin to alter the endometrium in preparation for implantation. Since the uterine cavity is only potential at this time and, for practical purposes, consists only of an anterior and a posterior wall, the initial implantation of the ovum tends to take place on one of these two surfaces of the endometrium. Implantation most often occurs at about the middle of the roughly triangularly shaped uterine wall, but the reason for this is not completely understood. There are deviations from the pattern, but implantation does not appear to be entirely random.

Implantation ordinarily takes place on the surface epithelium at a point equidistant from a series of openings of endometrial glands, that is, directly over endometrial stroma (Fig. 17-7). At this point in the development of the endometrium, the coiled arteries approach closer and closer to the surface, and capillary sprouts, which extend from the distal ends of the arteries, reach up almost to the epithelial lining. Thus, the area in which implantation takes place is likely to have, on a microscopic scale, an immediately available blood supply. Up to this point the ovum has been leading a relatively anaerobic existence and probably does not experience any sudden increase in requirements for gas exchange. On the other hand, it has probably begun to approach the limits of its ability to continue to exist and grow as a free-floating organism, so it can be assumed that implantation improves the metabolic condition of the ovum. If the trophoblast invades the blood vessels prematurely, however, the effect is deleterious; hematomas are likely to form under the implantation site and, consequently, implantation is defective. It is also noteworthy that decidual alteration of endometrial stroma, which is greatest in the vicinity of the coiled arteries, appears after, rather than before or simultaneous with, implantation.

Within 24 hours the blastocyst apparently burrows into the endometrium, and the surface epithelium of the endometrium has begun to proliferate over top of the blastocyst. By 7.5 days after ovulation, this implantation, which is referred to as interstitial because the blastocyst burrows into the endometrium, is complete. Shortly thereafter the surface epithelium heals over the blastocyst. As can be seen from Figures 17-5 and 17-6, the blastocyst tends to bulge above the normal surface of the epithelium, and the implanted ovum can be seen under the dissecting microscope and, in favorable conditions, with the naked eye.

Development of Primitive Placenta

The advancing trophoblast, which consists almost entirely of syncytiotrophoblast at this stage, is being provided with ready gas exchange and, in the glycogen-rich endometrium, a ready source of energy, and begins to develop rather rapidly into the primitive placenta (Figs. 17-8 and 17-9). This consists of large masses of syncytiotrophoblast, among which spaces begin to form. These are the primitive lacunae, which are destined to form the intervillous space. Columns of trophoblast, the primary villi, then form, and some attach themselves to the decidua as anchoring villi. In these villi, central cores of connective tissue develop to give rise to the secondary villi.

On about the 11th day, the advancing cytotrophoblast penetrates a maternal capillary and initiates a flow of blood into the lacunae of the primitive placenta (Fig. 17-10). The circulation in this early placenta is necessarily sluggish and the pressure of blood extremely low. This is desirable because penetration of an arteriolar structure by the early trophoblast would presumably release blood into this primitive placenta at a pressure that might dislocate the ovum. The perforation of maternal blood vessels by the syncytiotrophoblast also allows human chorionic gonadotropin to be directly injected into the maternal circulation. Within the next few days human chorionic gonadotropin converts the corpus luteum in the ovary into a corpus luteum of pregnancy,

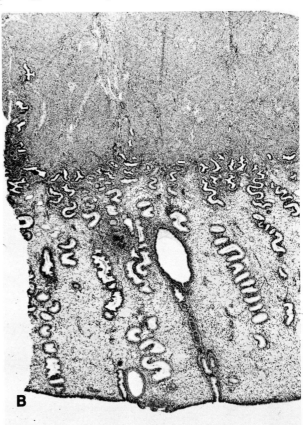

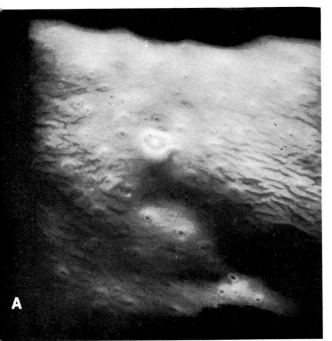

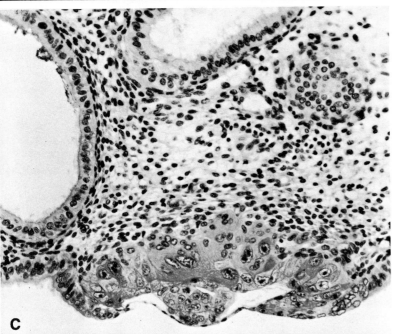

FIG. 17-7. Human conceptus 6.5 to 7 days old. (*A*) Surface view of collapsed blastocyst attached to endometrium. Note position away from gland mouths and clearly seen inner cell mass. (*B*) Low-power view of perpendicular fixed and stained section directly through conceptus. Condition of endometrium and superficial location of implantation are clear. (*C*) Higher power view of same section as in *B*. Bilaminar nature of germ disk is evident, as is variegated nuclear morphology of advancing syncytiotrophoblast. Surface epithelium is not complete over embryo. Endometrial stroma directly under trophoblast is more compact than deeper. (Carnegie No. 8020. *A*, ×22; *B*, ×30; *C*, ×250) (Hertig AT, Rock J: Two human ova of previllous stage, having developmental stage of about seven and nine days, respectively. Contrib Embryol 31:65, 1945)

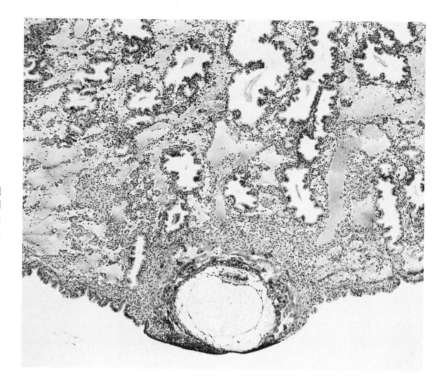

FIG. 17-8.   Human conceptus, estimated age 12 days. Trophoblast has now formed lacunae that contain maternal blood from sinusoid on *right*. Endometrium is much more advanced. Trophoblast has differentiated into cytotrophoblast and syncytiotrophoblast. Germ disk is formed, and several extraembryonic structures such as extracelomic membrane and amnion have differentiated. Compare with Figures 17-7 and 17-9. (Hertig AT, Rock J: Two human ova of previllous stage, having ovulation age of about 11 and 12 days, respectively. Contrib Embryol 29:127, 1941)

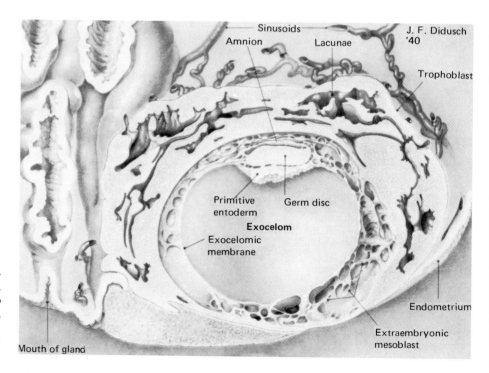

FIG. 17-9.   Artist's reconstruction of Carnegie No. 7700. (×160) (Hertig AT, Rock J: Two human ova of previllous stage, having ovulation age of about 11 and 12 days, respectively. Contrib Embryol 29:127, 1941)

thereby preventing the withdrawal of hormonal support from the endometrium and allowing the continuation of the pregnancy. This, of course, results in failure to menstruate, one of the obvious signs of early pregnancy.

The proliferation of syncytiotrophoblast can con-tinue throughout the entire surface of the sphere of the blastocyst. However, there is very little growth on the surfaces that are most remote from maternal circulation; the greatest growth is toward the endometrium. This growth differential, which is apparently determined

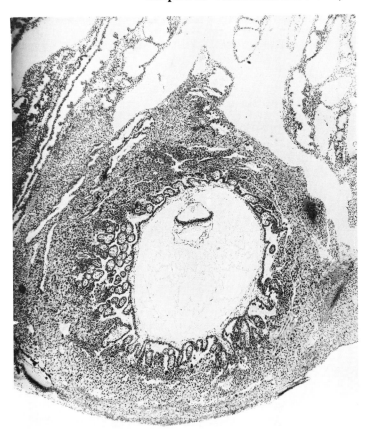

FIG. 17-10. Human conceptus about 16.5 days old. Note formation of primitive villi around much of periphery of trophoblast. Further development in germ disk has produced much larger amnion and early yolk sac. (Carnegie No. 7802, ×30) (Heuser CH, Rock J, Hertig AT: Two human embryos showing early stages of definitive yolk sac. Contrib Embryol 31:85, 1945)

largely by the availability of nutrients, sets the stage for the development of the definitive placenta at the site of implantation. Because implantation is interstitial in humans, ordinarily there is only one placenta at the site of implantation. The healing of surface epithelium over the ovum effectively keeps the trophoblast from contacting the opposite uterine wall in the course of its further growth and development, and hence the placenta forms on only one side.

By about the 18th day, as a result of local angiogenesis, capillaries have developed within what are now the tertiary villi. The primitive heart of the embryo is simultaneously forming, along with islands of hematopoiesis, and together these establish the fetal side of the placental circulation.

As pregnancy advances, the endometrium almost entirely changes into decidua. Although the term *decidua* means that which is shed, areas of decidua are retained within the uterus, both at the placental site and elsewhere, and are later the source of relining of the uterine cavity by endometrium at the conclusion of pregnancy. The gradual expansion of the membranes flattens the decidua into a layer to which the chorion is rather loosely attached. Scattered throughout this area there may be remnants of the villi that at one time covered the entire surface of the chorion as the chorion frondosum (Fig. 17-11).

THE DEFINITIVE PLACENTA

Location

The definitive placenta tends to form and to delimit itself in the area where blood supply is most satisfactory. In the corpus, this is under the developing embryo at the site of the original interstitial implantation. When implantation takes place in the lowermost portion of the uterus, which almost certainly is the anatomic antecedent of placenta previa, the blood supply is not as efficient as in the corpus, and the placenta ordinarily is much larger in area and less in thickness. Since, however, the entire surface of the chorion is, in its primitive stages, covered with placental villi that participate in the fetal circulation and then are lost secondarily, it is possible for the placenta to form almost anywhere (Fig. 17-11). It is undoubtedly in this fashion that separate small islands of placenta, known as *placenta succenturiata*, are formed. In rare instances, placental tissue covers almost the entire surface of the chorion; this is known as *placenta membranacea*.

Insertion of Cord

The factors that determine the site of insertion of the umbilical cord on the placenta are not entirely known.

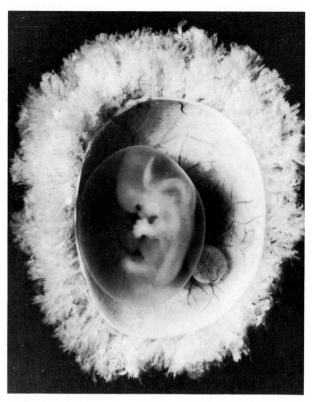

FIG. 17-11. Well-differentiated human embryo, approximately 40 days old, with portion of chorion frondosum dissected away to show amnion and yolk sac. Formation of villi over entire surface is evident. (Carnegie No. 8537A, ×1.5)

The primitive germ disk differentiates with what is destined to be the dorsal surface of the fetus closest to the uterus so that the ventral surface, which eventually differentiates the umbilical cord, is directed toward the uterine cavity. Rotation of the germ disk or the embryo

takes place as the amnion differentiates. If the orientation of the embryo within its membranes influences the direction of the umbilical cord, failure of the embryo to achieve a 180-degree rotation might direct the umbilical cord to a point other than what will become the center of the definitive placenta. It seems equally possible that such an event is result rather than cause and that the site of insertion of the umbilical cord on the amnion in relation to the placenta is an entirely random event, since some length of umbilical cord is necessary for the growth and development of the fetus and insertion of the umbilical cord must occur. In the case of twins, one of the cords ordinarily inserts near the margin of one of the placentas or the main placenta, and in the placenta associated with placenta previa there is also a higher than ordinary incidence of marginal insertion. In rare circumstances, the cord may insert away from the placenta, a *velamentous* insertion, so that the vessels run along the membranes from the site of cord insertion to the surface of the placenta. When the insertion of the cord is over the cervix, a condition known as *vasa praevia,* rupture of the membranes prior to delivery may disrupt the blood vessels and cause fetal hemorrhage. This is a rare event that is almost impossible to diagnose and treat.

Size

Early in the second trimester, the placenta approximately equals the size of the infant; as pregnancy advances, it becomes relatively smaller, although it continues to grow until term (Fig. 17-12). The placenta eventually attains a size approximately 15 cm in diameter and 2 cm in thickness. At term the ratio of its weight to that of the fetus is about 1:6 but may vary from 1:2 to 1:10 (Fig. 17-13). The weight of the membranes and cord is trivial, but smaller placentas are associated with smaller infants. At term the placenta may weigh 300 g to 1200

FIG. 17-12. Placental growth by weeks of gestation, based on over 11,000 births at University Hospitals of Cleveland, 1956 to 1962. *Solid line,* mean; *dashed line,* ±1 standard deviation; *dotted line,* 12 standard deviations. (Hendricks CH: Patterns of fetal and placental growth: The second half of pregnancy. Obstet Gynecol 24:360, 1964)

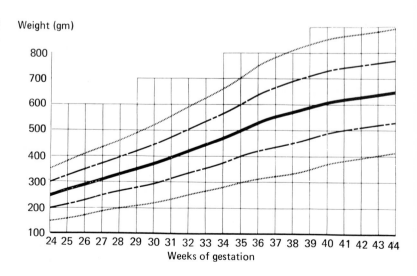

Weeks of gestation

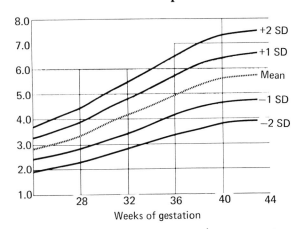

FIG. 17-13. Ratio of fetal to placental weight, based on over 11,000 births at University Hospitals of Cleveland, 1956 to 1962. *SD*, standard deviation. (Hendricks CH: Patterns of fetal and placental growth: The second half of pregnancy. Obstet Gynecol 24:361, 1964)

g. Extensive placental infarction is not responsible for any striking decrease in weight of the placenta. Placental edema, however, sometimes causes an increase in weight, as well as alteration in color.

The observation that the placenta continues to increase in size leaves unsettled one curious but clinically important point. It is clear that the fetus depends on the growth of the placenta for its welfare and that the growth of the placenta must keep pace with that of the fetus. Should the placenta fail, the fetus must either be delivered or experience intrauterine starvation or asphyxiation. There is little question that in unusual instances the placenta does fail to grow sufficiently to meet the needs of the infant, and the result is either a wizened, malnourished-looking newborn devoid of subcutaneous fat and obviously mature beyond its size or a stillborn fetus. There is, however, little evidence that placental growth is limited under normal conditions or that such limitation restricts fetal growth.

Morphology

Normally, the placenta consists of blood vessels and vascular spaces, with a small amount of supporting connective tissue and a relatively transparent endothelium on the surface of the villi. The maternal surface of the placenta has the dark red color of venous blood while the fetal surface is shiny and consists of large opaque-walled blood vessels coursing on the dense opalescent surface of the thickened chorion. The pale color of the edematous placenta is enhanced on the fetal surface because many conditions that produce placental edema are also associated with fetal anemia.

On the maternal surface, the placenta is usually divided ordinarily into 12 to 20 subdivisions, referred to as *cotyledons.* There is no consistent pattern of anchoring villi or connective tissue septa that establishes the cotyledon arrangement. A further, functional subdivision has been demonstrated by angiography and dissection. (Fig. 17-14). The arborizing fetal vessels eventually are distributed to small units of the placenta, each of which is irrigated by a coiled artery on the maternal side. The jet of maternal blood enters the middle of the unit and spreads from there. There are about 50 such lobules in the human placenta.

Histology

Changes in the microscopic appearance of the placenta occur with time. The primitive villi are replaced by villi that contain blood vessels and a relatively large amount of connective tissue. Their surface is covered by a double layer of epithelium, the innermost being the cytotrophoblast (Langhans' layer) and the outer the syncytiotrophoblast. There is now overwhelming evidence that the syncytiotrophoblast is entirely derived from the cytotrophoblast; presumably, this may still be true even late in pregnancy when the cytotrophoblast can no longer be readily identified in microscopic sections. Some of the villi extend downward to the decidua basalis, and their connective tissue cores become the anchoring areas of the placenta. Others form main stems through which large fetal blood vessels travel and from which secondary and tertiary branching occurs. As pregnancy proceeds, the villi contain relatively less and less connective tissue; toward term, the outermost villous twigs consist of little more than fetal capillaries surrounded by the syncytiotrophoblast, which is equivalent to the endothelial lining of the intervillous space.

Two cells that may be found in the connective tissue are worthy of special mention. One of these is the plasma cell, which ordinarily is quite rare but which has been identified beyond question in an instance of maternal agammaglobulinemia. The other is the Hofbauer cell, which has a varied appearance depending on the type of preparation in which it is seen. Most of the time, it contains a small amount of eosinophilic cytoplasm and a dense basophilic nucleus. It stands in contrast to the ordinary connective tissue cells of the villus, which contain very little cytoplasm and have smaller, more pyknotic nuclei. The Hofbauer cell is a phagocyte and has been shown to have IgG surface receptors.

As pregnancy advances, the trophoblast is more thinly spread over the surface of the villi, and its nuclei tend to accumulate in localized areas (Fig. 17-15). This gives rise to what is referred to as a *syncytial knot.* In the face of injury, the trophoblast tends to revert to a more primitive type, and with fetal disease, the cytotrophoblast may occasionally be readily seen. A more common event, however, is the deposit of maternal fibrin on the surfaces of villi. Apparently, it is possible for this to build up, perhaps by interfering with the flow in the intervillous space, so that eventually large areas of a

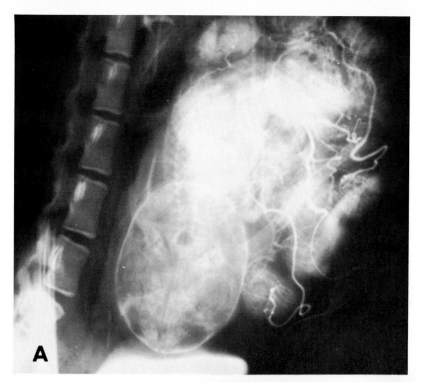

FIG. 17-14. Lateral radiographs of 152-day pregnancy in a macaque. Fetal head and spine can be readily seen. *A* was taken 3 seconds after injection of radiopaque material into an interplacental (umbilical) artery to display fetal side of placental circulation. Note several well-filled fetal cotyledons. *B* was taken 2 seconds after injection of radiopaque material into maternal uterine arteries. It can be seen that there are functional cotyledons without functional maternal arterial entry tracts, and vice versa. (Ramsey EM, Martin CB, Jr, Donner MW: Fetal and maternal placental circulations. Am J Obstet Gynecol 98:419, 1967)

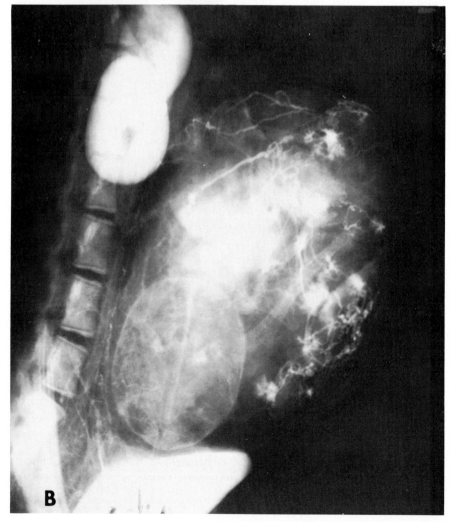

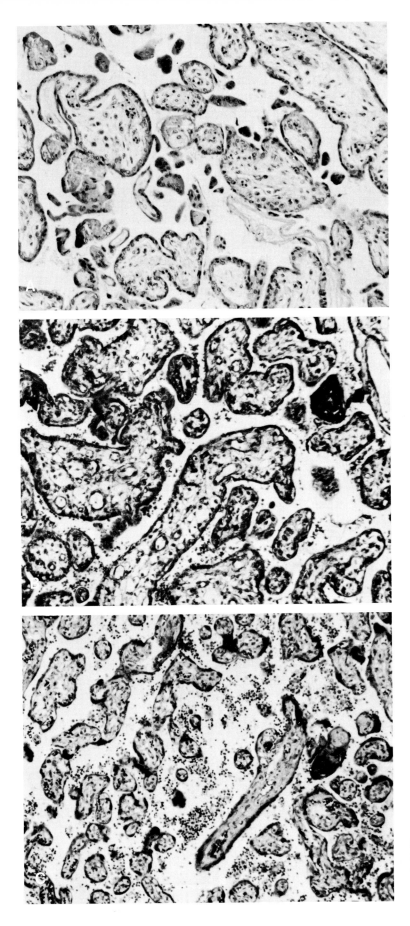

FIG. 17-15. Photomicrographs, at same magnification, of villous substance of placenta (*A*) at 6 weeks, (*B*) at 6 months, and (*C*) at term. (×200). (Wilkin P: Pathologie du Placenta. Paris, Masson, 1965)

cotyledon may be deprived of normal maternal circulation. This, in turn, appears to be followed by a shutdown of activity on the fetal side, and eventually a large inactive area of placenta that is slowly undergoing involution can be seen.

Area Available for Exchange

In the presence of all these changes, the area available for diffusion increases slowly but steadily, at least until the last few weeks of pregnancy. Regardless of the gross size or weight of the placenta, fetal welfare depends on the area available for diffusion. Such processes as intervillous fibrin deposition and the calcification that occurs within the intervillous space under these circumstances reduce the area for diffusion, but whether the net effective area of normal placenta is reduced is unknown.

The concept of *aging of the placenta* has been based in part upon anatomic evidence. In addition, studies of placental exchange have shown some decreases in exchange near term. There is some question about whether enough data have been obtained from these studies to permit the generalization that there is a diminution in function, comparable to senescence, which is a simple consequence of placental age. Nevertheless, this concept, which suggests an increasing precariousness of intrauterine life as term approaches, has great appeal, and the concept of placental senescence as a basis for clinical management still dominates a good deal of thinking. It may be correct, but most of the evidence for it is still intuitive.

Circulation

The circulation through the placenta on the fetal side is simply described. The umbilical arteries divide as the umbilical cord reaches its attachment to the membranes, and they subdivide continuously to supply arterial blood to all portions of the placenta. The arteries proceed down intervillous stems into precapillary arterioles and then into the capillaries traversing the villi themselves. These capillaries then empty into venules, which join to form veins and eventually give rise to the umbilical vein. There are also arteriovenous anastomoses that permit bypass of villous capillaries.

On the maternal side, the circulation comes from the capillary extensions of the endometrial arterioles. As the placenta grows and as placental circulation becomes more complex, the rather sluggish capillary circulation through the trophoblastic lacunae is succeeded by a circulation arising from the endometrial arterioles themselves. This is, of course, under greater pressure because it empties into venules without the intervention of a capillary bed. As shown in Figure 17-16, blood enters the intervillous space under the pressure of maternal arterial systole. Blood almost certainly enters the inter-

villous space continuously, but under much greater force and at a greater speed during systole. The blood thus injected through the open tips of the arterioles mixes in the intervillous space and leaves the placenta through veins at the base of the cotyledons. Some of the blood in the intervillous space mixes just under the fetal surface of the chorion in the subchorionic lake and, indeed, may flow transversely across the placenta to enter the marginal vein at its edge.

There is some evidence that not all endometrial arterial jets function at all times and that the rate of flow from each endometrial artery is under some form of local control, either by the muscles in the wall of the artery itself or by localized contraction of the myometrium, through which the artery must pass before reaching the intervillous space. Therefore, it is likely that under normal conditions the entire placenta is not in a state of maximum function at any single time. Furthermore, because intrauterine pressure during uterine contractions may approach or even exceed maternal systolic pressure, there are periods when there is no inflow to the placenta. Very little is known about the venous outflow from the placenta; there is evidence that this outflow is also influenced by uterine contractions (Figs. 17-17 and 17-18).

The biochemical characteristics of the blood in the portions of the intervillous space near the inflow tracts are necessarily different from those of the blood in the outflow tracts. Thus, the composition of intervillous-space blood is not uniform, but varies from place to place within the intervillous space and from time to time, depending on changes in local vascular control and in uterine contractility. There is an average value, but from a practical standpoint, there is no possibility of obtaining blood samples that will assuredly represent it.

Since villi are present in immense numbers in the intervillous space, where they serve as baffles, it is by no means unusual for fragments of trophoblast, or even whole villi, to break off and enter the maternal circulation. Some of these are trapped in blood vessels within the uterine wall; indeed, this is where they are most commonly found when suitable material is available for examination. However, a trophoblast fragment can reach the maternal lungs, where it may be found at autopsy performed on an otherwise normal pregnant woman who has died suddenly. When the placenta is normal, this trophoblast apparently does not have the capacity to implant in or invade the structures of the lung.

Maternal–Fetal Blood Exchange

It is possible for maternal blood to enter the fetal circulation or for fetal blood to enter the maternal circulation when gross breaks in the placenta occur. In view of the pressure relations involved, the latter event is more likely, but it is also more difficult to prove. The fetus must lose a relatively large amount of blood into

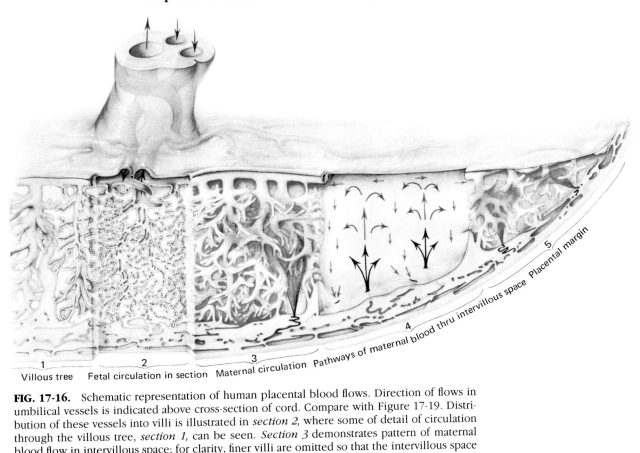

1 Villous tree   2 Fetal circulation in section   3 Maternal circulation   4 Pathways of maternal blood thru intervillous space   5 Placental margin

FIG. 17-16. Schematic representation of human placental blood flows. Direction of flows in umbilical vessels is indicated above cross-section of cord. Compare with Figure 17-19. Distribution of these vessels into villi is illustrated in *section 2,* where some of detail of circulation through the villous tree, *section 1,* can be seen. *Section 3* demonstrates pattern of maternal blood flow in intervillous space; for clarity, finer villi are omitted so that the intervillous space appears more empty than it is in fact. *Section 4* shows maternal intervillous space flow schematically, making clear that outflow proceeds through subchorionic lake and through basal veins. *Section 5* depicts these same arrangements at margin of placenta. Marginal sinus is inconstant feature of widely varying size. (Ramsey EM, Davis RB: Carnegie Institution of Washington Year Book 61. Washington, DC, Carnegie Institution, 1962)

its mother's circulation before analysis of the concentration of fetal hemoglobin in maternal blood or differential blood typing can determine that this exchange has taken place.

It is likely that the incidence of fetomaternal exchange has been exaggerated on the basis of the frequently observed increased concentration of hemoglobin F in the circulation of the pregnant woman. In supposing that this event proves the presence of fetal blood in the maternal circulation, many authors have overlooked the fact that increased maternal production of hemoglobin F is a response to a high chorionic gonadotropin concentration, combined with the stress on the bone marrow caused by the need to keep up with the drainage of iron by the fetus. It is noteworthy that the highest concentrations of hemoglobin F observed in the pregnant woman have occurred in the presence of hydatidiform mole, in which case there is no fetal erythropoiesis and the hemoglobin F must arise from the woman's own bone marrow.

For the perfusion of any sizable amount of blood from fetus to mother, the break in the fetal circulation must occur in the fetal arteriole. This does take place; there are now a large number of unquestionably demonstrated instances of fetomaternal transfusion, proven because, among other things, a severely anemic infant was born. This may account for a certain number of otherwise unexplained stillbirths as well.

There is also a substantial body of evidence supporting the transmission of maternal erythrocytes, leukocytes, and platelets to the fetus, so there can be no doubt about the transfer of solutes such as antibodies from mother to fetus.

Transfer of formed fetal blood elements to the mother in immunologically significant amounts is most likely to occur at the time of placental separation. For this reason, the administration of anti-D (anti-Rh) globulin to prevent D sensitization in an unsensitized D-negative mother who has borne a D-postive child is undertaken in the early puerperium.

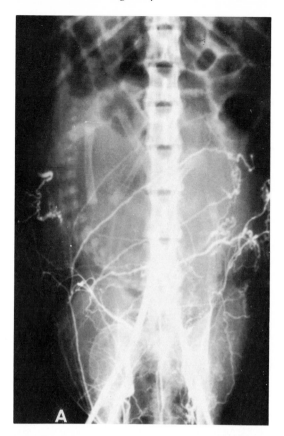

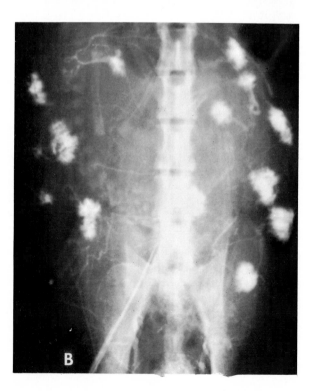

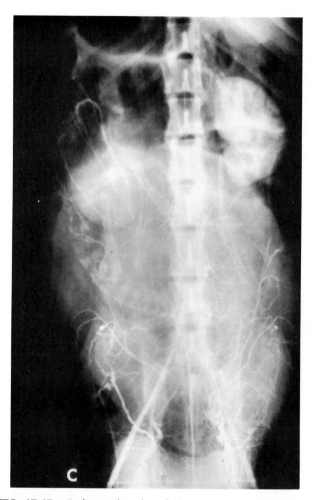

FIG. 17-17. Radiographs taken following injection of radi-opaque material into aorta of macaque on 130th day of pregnancy. Fetal spine and extremities are clearly seen. *A* and *B* were taken 2 and 6 seconds, respectively, after injection during uterine relaxation. In *A,* femoral and uterine arteries are well opacified, and many small uterine arterial branches to both placentas can be seen. In *B,* spurts of material into intervillous space are clearly shown. In *C,* taken 4 seconds after injection during a strong uterine contraction, spurts previously seen are no longer visible. (Courtesy EM Ramsey and Carnegie Institution of Washington)

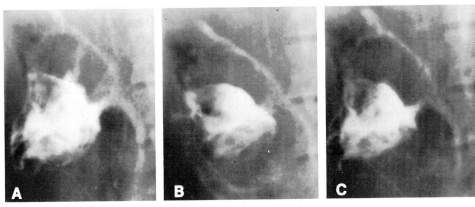

FIG. 17-18. Radiographs taken after slow injection of radiopaque material into intervillous space of macaque placenta on 99th day of pregnancy. In *A,* several drainage channels can be seen. In *B,* taken during uterine contraction, size of intravillous space pool has changed little, but drainage tracts are emptied. In *C,* taken as uterus relaxed, drainage tracts are restored. (Ramsey EM, Martin CB, Jr., McGaughey HS et al: Venous drainage of the placenta in rhesus monkeys: Radiographic studies. Am J Obstet Gynecol 95:948, 1966)

Exchange Across the Placenta

Ever since it was established that the maternal and fetal circulations are separate, the phenomenon of exchange across this intact membrane has fascinated investigators. Many analogies between exchange across the lung and exchange across the placenta, particularly in regard to the transfer of gases, have been made. The difference lies primarily in the fact that in the placenta the exchange occurs in a water-to-water system, whereas in the lung the exchange occurs in an air-to-water system. It is also highly probable that the functions of lung and placenta are different. Since it has been proven that exchange across the lung takes place by passive diffusion in proportion to gradients, it is tempting to extend this without argument to the placenta; in fact, this mechanism does apply for a number of substances. The placenta, however, is a more complex structure than the lung, and the exchange process is not the same for all substances. Page has suggested that placental exchange be discussed in terms of four groups of substances discussed below.

Group I: Substances That Maintain Biochemical Homeostasis or Protect Against Sudden Fetal Death

For these substances the rate of transfer is measured in milligrams per second, and the predominant mechanism is rapid diffusion. This category includes electrolytes, water, and respiratory gases. In regard to oxygen, the gradient on each of the placenta's two sides is considerable, corresponding to a very rapid rate of exchange. On the other hand, although the gross exchange of water is immense, the gradient is quite small because the net exchange is relatively small. The best estimate is that the gross transfer of water in one direction across the placenta is in excess of 500 ml/second. Carbon dioxide, which is more soluble in water than in oxygen, has a very small gradient but a very large gross transfer. An electrolyte such as sodium travels at its peak rate at about 1 mg/second, so the range of transfer in this class of substances is rather large. Finally, because some substances that are probably exchanged at these rates are metabolized in the placenta, the net transfer appears to be negligible. Examples are 5-hydroxytryptamine and possibly epinephrine, which can be affected by the very high concentration of monoamine oxidase in the placenta.

Group II: Substances That Maintain Fetal Nutrition

Exchange of these substances is measured in milligrams per minute. They are primarily moved by carrier systems, although the process of diffusion is also involved. Examples are the amino acids, sugars, and most of the water-soluble vitamins. For some substances there may be carrier systems operating equally in both directions; this appears to be the case, in some species, in regard to glucose, because the transfer of this substance is far in excess of what can be accounted for by diffusion alone. Some materials, such as the amino acids, are found in greater concentrations in fetal rather than maternal plasma; these substances are probably moved by carrier systems that operate against a concentration gradient. A third type of material is exemplified by riboflavin. The total content of riboflavin in fetal blood is 20% higher than in maternal blood, whereas the free riboflavin content is 300% greater. There appears to be, therefore, an unequal distribution of these substances, with some sort of alteration of the riboflavin molecule or its precursor during active transport across the placenta.

Group III: Substances That Modify Fetal Growth and Maintain Pregnancy

Transfer of these substances is measured in milligrams per hour. The predominant mechanism of transport is probably slow diffusion of relatively large molecules. Most of the hormones are included in this group. The most satisfactory information currently available relates to labeled thyroxine and estrogen and progesterone.

Group IV: Substances of Immunologic Importance Only

Transfer of these substances is measured in milligrams per day and may occur by leakage through large pores in the placenta or by droplet transfer through pinocytosis. There is evidence that particles as large as red cells can traverse the placenta through breaks in its membrane. There is also, however, some evidence that this is not normal, and using group-IV substances to illustrate exchange under physiologic conditions might be questioned. Also included in this group are plasma proteins, which may be exchanged by means of droplets in the vesicles, which have been observed in the placental epithelium under the electron microscope.

Placental Hormone Production

The role of the placenta as an important endocrine gland is considered in Chapter 19.

Placental Metabolism

The placenta is endowed with an incredible variety of enzyme systems, which have been studied mainly *in vitro*. It is a safe generalization that, given appropriate conditions in a Warburg apparatus and given a substrate and suitable cofactors, living placenta will manifest almost any enzymatic reaction that has been observed in other tissues. The conclusions to be drawn from this and related observations are limited.

The intrinsic metabolic activity of the placenta is rather low. There is good evidence that most of the activity of the placenta in the genesis of hormones and the exchange of materials resides in the trophoblast and that the connective tissue stroma and the walls of the fetal blood vessels are inactive. Under these circumstances, the energy consumption of the placenta is not great, although, like the lung, it has an immense blood flow. So far there is little evidence to suggest a correlation between any known abnormality of pregnancy and change in placental metabolism. Because intervillous fibrin and infarcts are undoubtedly metabolically inert, activity per gram is low when they make up a sizable fraction of placental weight. It is, therefore, difficult to determine the metabolic activity of the living fraction of placenta.

One placental enzyme, diamine oxidase, which is actually a histaminase, is found in steadily increasing amounts in the maternal plasma as pregnancy proceeds. Its concentration has been used, along with other findings, as an indicator of fetoplacental well-being.

Pregnancy-Specific β-1 Glycoprotein

Pregnancy-specific β-1 glycoprotein (PSβG) is produced by the trophoblast and is secreted primarily into the intervillous space, quickly reaching both the maternal bloodstream and the amniotic fluid. The substance can be detected in maternal serum as early as seven days after ovulation, and thereafter it increases very rapidly in the various body fluids (Table 17-1). Its function is not known; but, because PSβG is of placental origin, it has been suggested that the body fluid levels may provide an index of placental function. The serum level has been correlated with fetal weight, indicating a possible application in the diagnosis of intrauterine growth retardation. Because PSβG is unique to pregnancy and appears very early, it can be used as a simple, rapid, specific test for pregnancy.

Table 17-1
PS/βG Concentrations in Various Body Fluids During Pregnancy

Body Fluid	Concentration (μg/liter)
Maternal Blood	
21–24 days postovulation	50–100
10–11 weeks	10,400 ± 3100
20 weeks	33,500 ± 970
20–21 weeks	53,000 ± 16,900
38 weeks	166,000 ± 46,000*
Amniotic Fluid	
15–22 weeks	616 ± 180†
27–40 weeks	300–3800
Term	1200*
Cord Blood	
17–22 weeks	116 ± 65
25 weeks	66
27–40 weeks	100–600
Term	300*
Breast Milk	
Colostrum 25 weeks	135
Term	160
Urine	
3–8 weeks postovulation	0–400*
Early pregnancy	0–4000
Late pregnancy	0–30,000
Term	0–8000

* Mean values from 4 studies. See Horne-Towler article for references.

† Figures given here were calculated from data shown graphically.

(From Horne CHW, Towler CM: Pregnancy-specific beta₁ glycoprotein: A review. Obstet Gynecol Surv 33:761, 1978)

THE UMBILICAL CORD

Location

The umbilical cord runs from the infant's umbilicus to the point of its insertion in the membranes or placenta. The origin of the umbilical cord from the umbilicus is subject to few variations; the most common is *omphalocele*. In this condition, the ring of connective tissue of the anterior abdominal wall at the point of the umbilicus fails to close, and a certain portion of the intestinal contents are not in the abdomen but in the sac, which is lined with peritoneum and covered by a thin layer that resembles amnion. This sac joins the infant's skin at the level of the anterior abdominal wall. The cord ordinarily inserts on the apex of this mass, and the vessels then run along the mass between the two thin covering layers. This does not seem to interfere with the function of the umbilical cord during intrauterine life.

Anatomy and Histology

The cord itself consists of the umbilical vessels, usually two arteries and one vein. A small amount of connective tissue, within which is distributed a gelatinous material known as *Wharton's jelly,* supports these structures. All of this is covered by a thin layer of amnion.

The microscopic appearance of the umbilical cord varies according to whether it has been fixed in the distended or collapsed state (Fig. 17-19). If the cord is clamped while in a state of distention and then fixed, it is clear that the vessels are huge relative to the connective tissue, Wharton's jelly, and amnion. On the other hand, in cross-sections of the collapsed umbilical cord, which are the kind typically studied in the pathology laboratory, the vessels look rather trivial.

The arteries have characteristic arterial walls. The vein has more than the expected amount of connective tissue and muscle in its wall. The stroma contains very few cells, and these contain little cytoplasm. Occasionally, on the surface of the cord, the cells of the amnion are slightly piled up, which creates the appearance of small squamous plaques. In contrast to the fetal villi, there are ordinarily no wandering cells in the stroma of the umbilical cord.

Length

Umbilical cords have been observed to vary from 20 cm to 150 cm in length. The normal length is in the range of 50 cm to 70 cm. As the umbilical cord reaches a greater length, the incidence of complications, such as cord obstruction due to wrapping of the cord around the infant's neck or over the extremities and prolapse of the cord, increases. Such complications are still relatively infrequent, however. The umbilical cord, being an erectile structure maintained in a state of turgor dur-

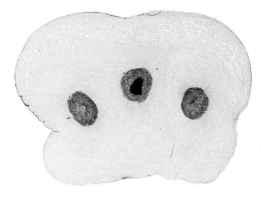

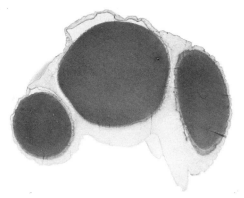

FIG. 17-19. Cross-sections of umbilical cord fixed after collapse (*above*) and in distended state (*below*). Vein is between two arteries here. Cord is distended during function *in utero.* (Reynolds SRM: The proportion of Wharton's jelly in the umbilical cord in relation to distention of the umbilical arteries and vein, with observations on the folds of Hoboken. Anat Rec 113:368, 1952)

ing normal intrauterine life, does not tend to fall loosely from one place to another as it does after delivery. If its blood flow is obstructed, the cord may become flaccid and more liable to accident; possibly, cord abnormalities result from primary interference with cord circulation. However, the presence of cord wrapped around the neck, one, two, three, or more times is not presumptive evidence of fetal difficulty and may cause no trouble at all.

An unusually short cord may be responsible for dystocia, since it may literally restrict the descent of the fetus, much as a dog is restricted by the length of the chain attached to its collar.

Distribution of Blood Vessels

Within the umbilical cord, the distribution of blood vessels is subject to a number of variations. One reason for this is that the vessels tend to coil around one another. Although it is generally supposed that the vein is interposed between the two arteries, this ordinarily is not the case. The vein is subject to more twists and turns than the arteries and may produce rather complex structures in which it is coiled upon itself, producing what is called a *false knot*. The thickness of the arterial walls and the greater force of blood flowing through them apparently endow the umbilical arteries with greater resistance to this kind of reduplication. Although from time to time it has been proposed that the pulsatile flow through the umbilical arteries may have some influence in maintaining flow through the umbilical vein in the opposite direction, the complexities of the umbilical vein provide so many exceptions to the anatomic relationships between it and the umbilical arteries that the general proposition is probably incorrect. False knots are, of course, of no clinical consequence. On the other hand, if the cord is long, it is possible, particularly in the middle trimester of pregnancy, for the infant to pass through a loop of the cord and thereby create a *true knot*. In fact, this may occur more than once, and several true knots may be encountered in the cord. Since the cord is an erectile structure, it is unusual for a true knot to be pulled tight enough to produce irreversible cord obstruction.

Blood Flow

Total blood flow through the umbilical cord has been estimated at approximately 125 ml per kg of body weight per minute, or approximately 500 ml/minute in the average human fetus at term. In the fetus the umbilical arteries are the main branches of the dorsal aorta, arising from the external iliacs just beyond the bifurcation of the common iliac arteries and constituting their major branches. The systolic pressure in the umbilical arteries is about 60 mm Hg and the diastolic about 30 mm Hg. There is a pressure drop across the placental capillary bed such that the pressure in the umbilical vein is about 20 mm Hg and is not pulsatile. As blood enters the abdominal wall of the fetus through the umbilical vein, it enters the liver, where it can flow either into the substance of the liver or directly into the inferior vena cava. The ductus venosus, which contains a sphincteric mechanism that is at least partly under nervous control, is interposed between the umbilical vein and the inferior vena cava. Under certain circumstances contraction of the ductus venosus diverts blood into the substance of the liver, which returns it to the systemic circulation through the hepatic vein. Under other circumstances the ductus relaxes and allows blood to flow directly into the right atrium. This structure, therefore, is located in a position that has a regulatory influence on the pressure in the umbilical vein. As mentioned earlier, the umbilical vein must have an elevated blood pressure, since the blood vessels in the villi have to be maintained in a state of patency while within the intervillous space, which is itself under pressure greater than the venous pressure of the mother. Under steady-state conditions, dilation of fetal umbilical and placental arteries and ar-

terioles is near maximal, as is placental blood flow. Stroke volume and heart rate are reciprocal. The fetus therefore cannot materially increase placental blood flow under stress. There is only inferential evidence of major vascular shunts within the fetus.

THE FETAL MEMBRANES

Anatomy and Histology

In the ordinary course of events, the fetal membranes line the uterine cavity and completely surround the fetus. The chorion, the outer membrane, forms a good deal of the connective tissue thickness of the placenta on its fetal side and is the structure through which the major branching umbilical vessels travel on the surface of the placenta. The remnants of the yolk sac are found resting on top of the chorion, usually near the insertion of the umbilical cord. Occasionally, small fluid-containing cysts are formed by duplications of the chorion on the placental surface. When felt grossly, this membrane is quite thin but is obviously more than a single layer of cells in thickness.

The outer side, which is typically applied to the decidua reflexa (the area of the altered endometrium that is not the site of the implantation of the placenta), is somewhat rough and may be adherent in areas in which an extraordinary degree of villous penetration by the chorion frondosum took place. The chorion does not usually have a fetal blood supply, except in cases of velamentous insertion; even then, the fetal blood vessels do not have branches to the chorion, and it is reasonable to suppose that the vascular support of the chorion is provided primarily by blood vessels arising from the decidua. On its inner (fetal) side, the chorion is juxtaposed to the outer layer of amnion (Figs. 17-20 and 17-21).

These two membranes slide upon each other readily; indeed, there is little connective tissue attachment between the two. This looseness of attachment between amnion and chorion not only may provide some safety features for the fetus in the course of its growth but also may permit differential sliding if the chorion ruptures while the amnion remains intact in the course of labor and delivery. The inner surface of the amnion has a smooth, slippery lining and is shiny in appearance under normal circumstances. The strength of the membranes is imparted by the layer of dense connective tissue to which the amnion epithelial cells are attached.

Membranes in Multiple Pregnancy

In multiple pregnancy, the membranes may be duplicated; the ultimate number of amnion and chorion layers depends on the number of eggs from which the multiple pregnancy was derived. In the case of monozygotic (derived from a single egg) twins, it depends on the stage

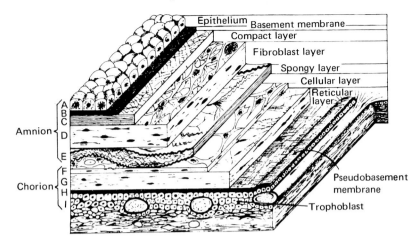

Epithelium ̶ Basement membrane
Compact layer
Fibroblast layer
Spongy layer
Cellular layer
Reticular layer

Amnion { A B C D E

Chorion { F G H I

Pseudobasement membrane

Trophoblast

FIG. 17-20. Composite diagram showing relation of layers of amnion and chorion. (Bourne GL: The microscopic anatomy of the human amnion and chorion. Am J Obstet Gynecol 79:1070, 1960)

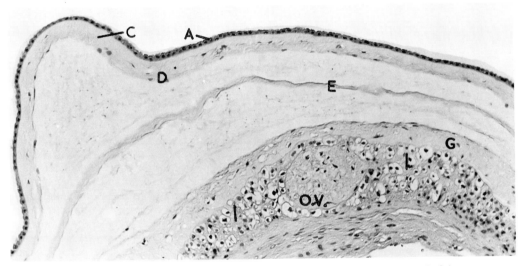

FIG. 17-21. Human amnion and chorion. *A*, epithelium; *C*, compact layer composed of dense connective tissue; *D*, fibroblast layer; *E*, spongy layer; *G*, reticular area; *I*, trophoblast; *OV*, obliterated villus. (×90, reduced) (Reproduced by permission from Bourne G: The Human Amnion and Chorion. London, Lloyd-Luke Medical Books, 1962)

of gestation at which splitting took place. Since secondary resorption of some of the layers can also occur, dizygotic twins (derived from two separate eggs) are occasionally found lying within a single chorion but, of course, separate amnions. Examination of the membranes can be considered conclusive proof of monozygotic twinning only when both infants are found within a single amniotic sac. If each infant is found within a single chorion, it is likely that they are monozygotic twins. When chorion and amnion are both unquestionably duplicated, it is likely that the twins are dizygotic, but this again is not conclusive (see Chap. 43).

Function

The principal functions of the membranes appear to be to retain the amniotic fluid and to assist in its formation. This provides for the growth and development of the fetus in a stable, mechanically buffered environment and in a state of relative weightlessness, because the specific gravity of the infant is, for practical purposes, the same as the specific gravity of the amniotic fluid. Growth and development of the extremities are therefore unimpeded, and resistance to fetal muscular activity is diminished compared with what would be present in the uterus without an interposing buffer of fluid. The amniotic sac is also repository for a number of secretions and excretions from the fetal urinary, respiratory, and alimentary tracts. Exchange of materials between the fetus and amniotic fluid is essentially rather sluggish, but there is rapid transfer of water between the amniotic fluid and the mother, presumably across the amnion and chorion in the large surface area applied to the decidua.

During most of gestation, amniotic fluid is similar

to plasma in total osmolarity and electrolyte content, although it has a relatively low protein content. Near term it becomes hypotonic relative to plasma. A decrease in the concentration of electrolytes accounts for virtually all of the decrease in osmolarity. However, the cause of these events is not known. Fetal urine undoubtedly contributes to, but hardly accounts for, the observed hourly water turnover of 350 ml to 600 ml. The exchange of water may occur by simple diffusion, but there is a characteristic differential in the transfer rate of certain tagged substances. In the rat, there are differences in protein fractions between amniotic fluid and maternal serum, which suggests that the exchange process is neither by transudation nor by the ultrafiltration of plasma. The demonstration of special amnion cells that overlie the placenta and are believed to have secretory properties (Fig. 17-22) suggests that the membranes themselves play an important role in amniotic fluid formation.

THE AMNIOTIC FLUID

Amniotic fluid is derived from maternal and fetal sources. The major portions are a maternal plasma filtrate and a fetal urinary contribution. Exchange of water takes place from the cavity across the amnion and chorion into the maternal decidua and into the placenta itself. Some exchange occurs across the umbilical cord. There is a flow of fluid into and out of the respiratory passages, and the fetus swallows a considerable fraction. Thereafter, exchange takes place across fetal mucous membranes. All the components of amniotic fluid are simultaneously being exchanged in the intervillous space between fetus and mother. This has been idealized and studied as a three-compartment system, as illustrated in the classic figure described by Hutchinson and co-workers (Fig. 17-23).

At term, the gross exchange of water between fetus and mother is about 3500 ml/hour in each direction. Between fetus and amniotic fluid, it is about 225 ml/

hour in each direction. The normal fetus is believed to swallow about 20 ml fluid an hour, but exchange in the respiratory tree of the fetus is still unmeasured. The gross exchange between amniotic fluid and maternal decidua, presumably directly across the membranes, is also about 225 ml in each direction. In normal pregnancy at term, the net turnover of fluid is probably no more than 10 ml/hour. The total volume at term is variable but generally is less than 1 liter.

In the first half of pregnancy, the fluid is similar to maternal plasma, but the osmolarity declines steadily to term. This is attributed to dilution with increasing amounts of fetal urine, since the concentrations of urea and creatinine rise and those of sodium, potassium, and chloride fall. The exchange rates appear to be specific for each solute.

Various clinical observations, some of which have been confirmed by experimental study, have shed light on this most complex relation. Fetuses lacking kidneys have virtually no amniotic fluid. When a fetus has no hypothalamus, excessive fluid is present. Hydramnios is common in diabetic pregnancy. In severe hemolytic disease, hydramnios may accompany hydrops fetalis and placental edema. This is usually due to fetal hypoproteinemia and cardiac failure. The hydramnios and hydrops may occur without fetal hemolysis and are then of unknown cause.

Amniotic fluid has an odor and a distinct faint yellow or greenish yellow color; the nature and source of the responsible substances are not known. Near term, the fluid becomes opalescent, probably because of the presence of vernix caseosa, a fatty material coating the skin, principally over the vertex, back, and extremities.

The pH of the fluid is 7.22 early in pregnancy and falls to 7.11 at term. Carbon dioxide pressure correspondingly rises from 41 mm Hg to 51 mm Hg, while the bicarbonate concentration falls slightly. Oxygen pressure is always quite low, usually below 10 mm Hg. Bilirubin is present at midpregnancy but gradually decreases to almost nil at 36 weeks. Protein follows a similar course.

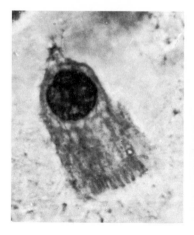
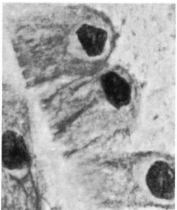

FIG. 17-22. Isolated cells from placental surface of amnion. Brush type border is evident in cells, canalicular apparatus in focus in one cell. (Original mag. ×323) (Danforth DN, Hull RW: Microscopic anatomy of the fetal membranes with particular reference to the detailed structure of the amnion. Am J Obstet Gynecol 75:541, 1958)

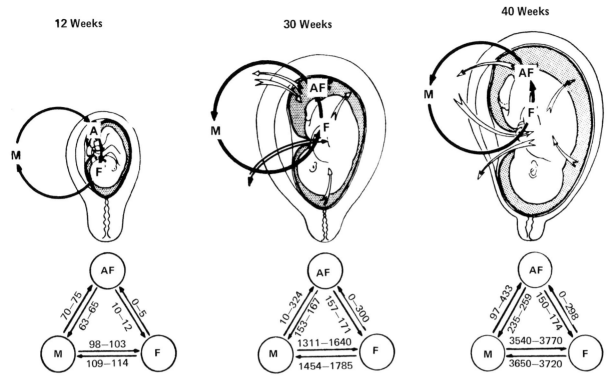

FIG. 17-23. Schematic representation of water exchange among mother (*M*), fetus (*F*), and amniotic fluid (*AF*) in pregnancy. *Arrows* in the lower diagrams indicate directions; *numbers,* hourly gross transfer in milliliters. *Heavy circles on left* of upper diagrams indicate direction of net transfer. (Hutchinson DL, Gray MJ, Plentl AA et al: The role of the fetus in the water exchange of the amniotic fluid of normal and hydramniotic patients. J Clin Invest 38:979, 1959)

The formed elements are all of fetal origin. Viable cells can be cultured and stained for genetic studies. As the fetus grows, however, laboratory culture is less successful. As term approaches, increasing amounts of fat are derived from the fetus's vernix caseosa. Occasionally several millimeters thick, vernix caseosa is vigorously antibacterial.

There is no known physiologic or pharmacologic means of affecting amniotic fluid volume. Early in pregnancy, the ratio of fluid to fetus is large. At about 20 weeks, it is approximately 3:2. Thereafter, the rate of fetal growth exceeds that of fluid accumulation, and at term there is usually no more than a few hundred milliliters. The volume of amniotic fluid at the different stages of pregnancy is shown in Figure 17-24.

THE FETUS

The somatic growth and development of what eventually will be the newborn infant can be divided into three major stages. The first is the period of differentiation, which begins at the time of fertilization and ends when the last structure destined to be present at birth has formed. Streeter devoted the latter years of his distin-

guished career as an embryologist to the delineation of events during this period and was satisfied that the final structure to make its appearance in the human fetus is the nutrient artery of the humerus, which appears toward the end of the 11th week after ovulation.

In the second period, a time of rapid growth that extends from the 11th to approximately the 27th week after ovulation, the fetus reaches a weight of approximately 850 g but still has not developed to the point where it would be likely to survive if born. Few fetuses in this age range survive birth.

From the 27th week after ovulation until term, although the rate of growth necessarily decreases, the absolute growth increases rapidly to an eventual term size of approximately 3300 g; with increasing physiological maturity, survival becomes increasingly likely (Figs. 17-25 and 17-26). Among the factors concerned in fetal growth, insulin appears to have an important role. This is supported by the finding of very high concentrations of high-affinity receptors for insulin on fetal cells.

Differentiation

Streeter's greatest contribution was the delineation of what he referred to as the *horizons of embryonic de-*

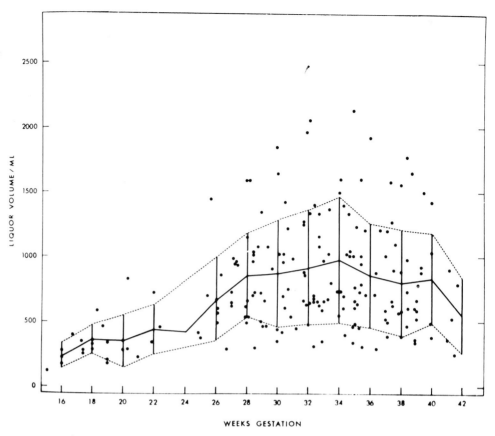

FIG. 17-24. Range of normal volumes of amniotic fluid plotted against weeks of gestation. (Queenan JT, Thompson W, Whitfield CR et al: Amniotic fluid volumes in normal pregnancies. Am J Obstet Gynecol 114:34, 1972)

FIG. 17-25. Fetal growth by weeks of gestation, based on over 11,000 births at University Hospitals of Cleveland, 1956 to 1962. *Heavy solid line* = mean; *dashed line* = 1 standard deviation; *light solid line* = 12 standard deviations. Compare with Figure 17-13. (Hendricks CH: Patterns of fetal and placental growth: The second half of pregnancy. Obstet Gynecol 24:358, 1964)

FIG. 17-26. Mean daily fetal growth in grams during previous week of gestation, based on same data as Figure 17-25. (Hendricks CH: Patterns of fetal and placental growth: The second half of pregnancy. Obstet Gynecol 24:358, 1964)

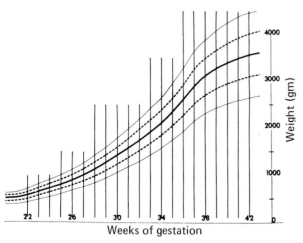

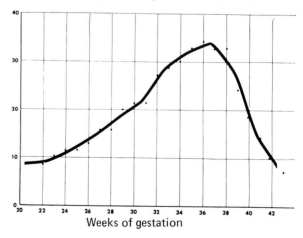

velopment. Each organ system has a definite time sequence for its appearance and differentiation and, as in the case of the urinary apparatus, for the disappearance of primitive early structures and their replacement by later definitive ones. In addition, the sequence of events in one system is related to the sequence of events in other systems. If deviations occur from these normal sequences and relationships, fetal abnormality results.

The sequential and predetermined nature of fetal development has two practical corollaries: a noxious event cannot influence the development of a structure if the event takes place prior to the appearance of the structure in the embryo, and if the noxious event occurs well after the structure has been differentiated and is undergoing growth only, deletion of the structure is exceedingly unlikely. Thus, rubella causes congenital cataracts only if the fetus is infected at the precise time when the lens is developing; infection earlier or later does not produce the defect. Table 17-2 indicates the period of gestation during which certain common malformations may occur.

Development Subsequent to Differentiation

When differentiation is completed (11th week), the infant should no longer be referred to as an embryo; it should be called a fetus. Its growth continues in terms of increasing development of organ systems to a degree of maturity that will permit extrauterine survival.

Intrauterine circulation, respiratory gas exchange, and thermoregulation are discussed in Chapter 42 in connection with the changes in these mechanisms associated with birth. Intrauterine development of the other organs and systems is discussed in the following sections.

Heart

The function of the myocardium is the same in the fetus as in the infant or adult. Of all the characteristics that can be observed before birth, the fetal heart rate is the most susceptible to quantitation.

The heartbeat can be detected by ultrasound devices, which use the Doppler principle, as early as the ninth menstrual week of pregnancy. Then and for the remainder of pregnancy, the heart rate is between 120 and 160 beats/minute. There is no trend in rate with time for an individual fetus or for fetuses as a group, and a fetal heart rate may fluctuate a great deal from week to week. Contrary to persistent superstition, the rate is not related to the sex of the fetus.

The fetal electrocardiogram is essentially indistinguishable from that of the newborn, except that multiple leads cannot be studied. An occasional instance of complete fetal heart block is observed, manifest by a steady heart rate of 60 or below, when there has been no obstetric accident and persisting for days and weeks. This continues during labor and into the newborn period

Table 17-2
Period of Gestation During Which Certain Fetal Malformations Occur

Week After Ovulation	Potential Malformation
3	Ectopia cordis
	Omphalocele
	Ectromelia
	Sympodia
4	Omphalocele
	Ectromelia
	Tracheoesophageal fistula
	Hemivertebra
5	Tracheoesophageal fistula
	Hemivertebra
	Nuclear cataract
	Microphthalmia
	Facial clefts
	Carpal or pedal ablation
6	Microphthalmia
	Carpal or pedal ablation
	Harelip, agnathia
	Lenticular cataract
	Congenital heart disease
	Gross septal and aortic anomalies
7	Congenital heart disease
	Interventricular septal defects
	Pulmonary stenosis
	Digital ablation
	Cleft palate, micrognathia
	Epicanthus, brachycephaly
8	Congenital heart disease
	Epicanthus, brachycephaly
	Persistent ostium primum
	Nasal bone ablation
	Digital stunting

and may be associated with anatomic defects. Even rarer instances of *in utero* atrial tachycardia with rates up to 220 beats/minute have been seen. This can result in intrauterine cardiac failure. However, the rate may revert to normal after birth, with complete recovery. Rarer still are irregularities of rate, sometimes due to a wandering pacemaker. These also ordinarily vanish shortly after birth.

Abnormalities of fetal heart rate associated with the acute changes of labor or cord obstruction are described in Chapter 41.

Fetal Blood Analysis

It is possible, once labor has begun, to obtain small samples of fetal blood directly from the fetal scalp or buttock. Use of an analysis of this blood as an early warning of fetal distress, especially in correlation with changes in fetal heart rate, has been intensely investigated. In these studies it is important to determine that the mother's acid–base balance is normal, because maternal acidosis is rapidly reflected in the fetus.

In normal early labor, the pH of fetal capillary blood is about 7.3; the lower limit is about 7.2. The carbon dioxide pressure is approximately 40 mm Hg, and the base deficit 6.5 mEq. The oxygen pressure is 22 mm Hg. As labor progresses, the fetal pH tends to decrease.

Lungs

Although they are present quite early in fetal life, the lungs are lined at first by columnar epithelium in the upper reaches of the respiratory tree and by transitional cuboidal epithelium in its lower portions. Gradually, the alveolar ducts differentiate from the terminal bronchioles, and the epithelium thins out. At the same time, capillaries proliferate toward the surfaces of the air sacs. Eventually, rudimentary alveolar sacs appear, but these are not present in large numbers prior to the 32nd week (Fig. 17-27).

FIG. 17-27. (A) Section of lung of 18-week stillborn infant. Air space is lined with cuboidal epithelium. (B) Section of lung of 38-week stillborn infant. Lumen of air space is much greater, but lining cells are so dispersed that they are not visible. (Both ×541, reduced) (Valdes-Dapena MA: Atlas of Fetal and Neonatal Histology. Philadelphia, JB Lippincott, 1957)

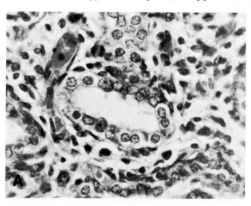

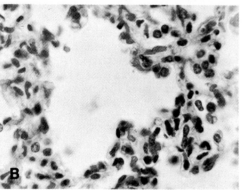

Anatomic maturity is, of course, essential for extrauterine survival, but the lungs must also be functionally prepared. Functional maturity depends largely on the formation of *surfactant,* a surface-active material that lines the pulmonary alveoli and reduces surface tension at the tissue–air interface. The alveolar epithelium consists of squamous lining cells (type I) and septal cells (type II). The main characteristic of the type-II cells is the presence of osmiophilic lamellar inclusion bodies (Fig. 17-28), which are responsible for the synthesis of surfactant. The type-I and type-II cells differentiate between 20 and 24 weeks' gestation, and the lamellar bodies appear shortly thereafter. The number of type-II cells rapidly increases, and increasing numbers of inclusion bodies are discharged into the alveoli and then into the amniotic fluid, correlating with the increasing alveolar surfactant and the increased amounts of surface-active lecithin in the amniotic fluid.

Gluck and Kulovich noted a rapid late gestational surge of total amniotic fluid phospholipids and observed that the ratio of amniotic fluid lecithin to sphingomyelin (L/S ratio) correlates directly with pulmonary maturity and, hence, with the likelihood that the preterm newborn would develop respiratory distress syndrome (RDS). In this syndrome, surfactant deficiency leads to incomplete postnatal lung expansion, expiratory atelectasis, and impaired gas exchange. The following L/S ratios are found in normal, uncomplicated pregnancy: at 12 weeks, 0.5:1, at 31 weeks, 1:1; at 31 to 33 weeks, 1:1; at 35 weeks, 2:1, and at term, 4:1. RDS does not occur in the newborn if the L/S ratio is 2:1 or higher. The L/S ratio and cortisol levels in amniotic fluid show high correlation, and the evidence suggests that fetal cortisol is probably the important physiologic regulator of surfactant production. Hence, preterm infants suffer a serious anatomic disadvantage in effecting gas exchange across the lung.

It is likely that vigorous respiratory activity conditioned by effective central nervous system stimulation and an adequate circulation may facilitate the expansion of alveoli and the progressive thinning of the epithelial lining. Thus, there is a fine interdependence among the general condition of the baby at birth, the anatomic and functional maturity of the lungs, and the infant's chances for survival. The maturity of the epithelial lining of the lung probably establishes the lower limit for viability of the human newborn, because this structure's prompt function for gaseous exchange is absolutely essential to the maintenance of homeostasis once the placental circulation has been interrupted. Recent studies of fetal breathing suggest that the respiratory movements of the human fetus can be a valuable aid in determining fetal well-being (see Chap. 41).

Kidneys

Although the preterm kidney is not efficient, it suffices for the limited needs of a normal fetus, assuming that acid–base regulation can be achieved by gas exchange in the lung. The kidney excretory system is fully

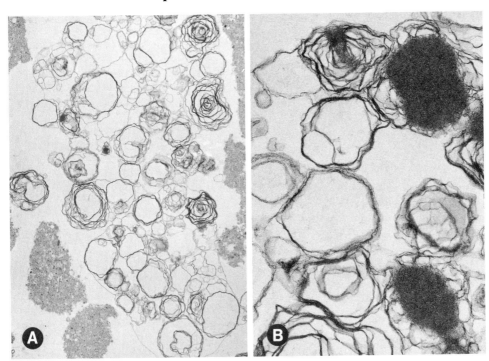

FIG. 17-28. (*A*) Large cluster of lamellar bodies from a term infant. Peripheral lamellae of adjacent lamellar bodies are closely associated with each other in this complex. Amorphous flocculent debris is also present. (×5250) (*B*) Laminar strands formed by "unwinding" of peripheral portions of lamellar bodies. Two lamellar bodies exhibit conspicuous electron-opaque cores that are also continuous with laminar strands. Same specimen as shown in *A*. (×20800) (Lee W, Bell M, Novy MJ: Pulmonary lamellar bodies in human amniotic fluid: Their relationship to fetal age and the lecithin/sphingomyelin ratio. Am J Obstet Gynecol 136:60, 1980)

differentiated quite early in fetal life, but the renal cortex is by no means fully formed even at the time of birth. On gross examination irregularities in the surface, which are referred to as *fetal lobulations* (Fig. 17-29), persist. At the time of birth and for several weeks thereafter, glomeruli continue to differentiate from the area immediately under the renal cortex. This provides a microscopic appearance that is characteristic of the newborn kidney and distinguishes it from that of the adult. Remarkably enough, these anatomic chnges are not accompanied by striking alterations of function. Obviously, there are sufficient numbers of glomeruli to produce a large glomerular filtrate, and the tubules are sufficiently differentiated to perform efficiently in the reabsorption of essential materials. There may be minor limitations in the ability of the fetal and newborn kidney to retain electrolytes, but it is certainly able to dilute and concentrate urine immediately after birth even in the pre-term infant; failure to survive is never attributable to renal immaturity.

Adrenals

The adrenals of the human fetus in the third trimester and at delivery are remarkable structures; they are very nearly the same size as the kidneys. Almost all of this bulk is made up of the fetal, or X, zone, which is part of the adrenal cortex. The adrenal medulla is unremarkable, and all of the normal infant and adult layers of the adrenal cortex are present. In addition, there is a wide zone of cells that do not differ in microscopic appearance from those of the zona glomerulosa. Involution of this zone begins shortly after birth and is completed within the first few weeks of life, reducing the adrenals to their normal size proportionate to the kidneys.

This zone is absent only from the grossly abnormal adrenals associated with major defects of the central nervous system, such as anencephaly. At the present time, however, nothing certain is known about the function of this fetal adrenal zone. It is not observed in most other mammalian fetuses. There are no unique adrenal steroids excreted by the human fetus or newborn that conceivably could be produced in this zone, nor does there seem to be any unique function associated with intrauterine life that is suddenly lost at the time of birth, when this zone begins to undergo regression. The normal human newborn, furthermore, does not exhibit signs of adrenal insufficiency, so necrosis of the adrenal

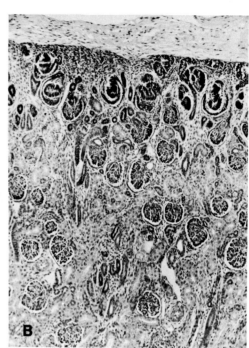

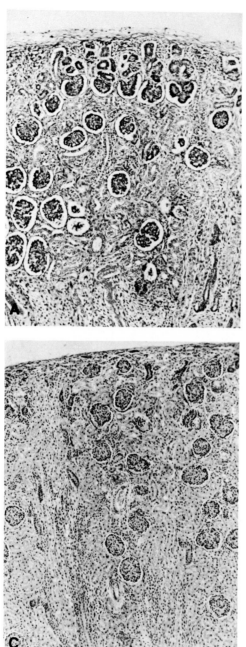

FIG. 17-29. (*A*) Section of kidney of 16-week stillborn infant. Many glomeruli are incompletely differentiated and tubules are not developed. (*B*) Section of kidney of 24-week infant who lived 4 hours. Glomeruli are still forming from cortex and are much more developed than at 16 weeks (*A*). Tubules occupy more space in parenchyma. (*C*) Section of 40-week infant who lived 2.5 days. Glomerular formation from cortex is still in progress, but cortex has achieved almost adult appearance. (All ×68, reduced) (Valdes-Dapena MA: Atlas of Fetal and Neonatal Histology. Philadelphia, JB Lippincott, 1957)

cortex in the newborn is apparently a selective process. The nature of the stimulus for this regression is unknown; it has never been observed prior to birth and always occurs after birth.

As outlined in Chapter 19, the fetal adrenals, in conjunction with the fetal liver and the placenta, play a key role in the production of estrogens in pregnancy. As pregnancy advances, they are also a potent and increasing source of cortisol, much of which is transferred to the amniotic fluid. The increasing cortisol concentration in amniotic fluid correlates well with the L/S ratios, and it has been theorized that the demonstrated increase in cortisol production by the fetal adrenals may be responsible for inducing fetal lung maturation. Specifically, the evidence supports the hypothesis that one function of the fetal adrenal cortex is to control the differentiation of the alveolar epithelium and, hence, the synthesis of phospholipid surfactant.

The possible role of the fetal adrenals in precipitating the onset of labor is considered in Chapter 31.

Central Nervous System

The central nervous system of the fetus is functional well before birth. The strongest evidence of this is that electroencephalograms have been obtained from the fetus *in utero*. The low amplitude and random nature of the waves suggest that there is little sensory input to the central nervous system. However, the diencephalon is not essential for fetal growth and development; infants who are born with cerebral agenesis may appear almost entirely normal in the neonatal state and may exhibit no external anomalies. It is unlikely that function of the midbrain is necessary for normal fetal development, although this is difficult to decide because anomalies of midbrain development are often associated with other congenital defects.

Gastrointestinal Tract

The gastrointestinal tract, which is almost completely developed rather early in fetal life, is also func-tional well before term. This has been demonstrated by the injection of radiopaque material into the amniotic fluid (Fig. 17-30). The opaque medium can be observed as it enters the fetal stomach and passes through the fetal gastrointestinal tract.

The solid material in amniotic fluid that may be swallowed by the fetus consists primarily of the des-quamated surface epithelium of the fetus, fetal hairs, and particles of vernix caseosa. The remaining material in amniotic fluid is in solution or suspension but, in either event, is available for absorption through the small intestine. Since under ordinary circumstances defecation does not take place *in utero*, the large intestine becomes packed with the partially digested or undigested remnants of the solid material of the amniotic fluid mixed with bile pigment and unaltered by bacterial decomposition. This viscid greenish black material is known as *meconium*. A certain portion of the material reabsorbed from the gastrointestinal tract is excreted by the fetal kidney into the excretory apparatus and then into the amniotic fluid, from which it is reabsorbed. The same material also enters the fetal circulation and may be exchanged with the mother directly through the intervil-

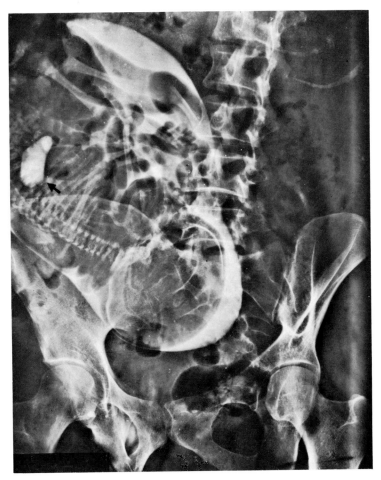

FIG. 17-30. Roentgenographic demonstration of radiopaque medium in amniotic fluid and stomach of fetus at 35 to 36 weeks' gestation. Hypaque was injected into amniotic fluid by transabdominal amniocentesis 1 hour earlier. Head can be seen in contrast; *arrow* indicates stomach. (McLain CR: Amniography studies of the gastrointestinal mobility of the human fetus. Am J Obstet Gynecol 86:1079, 1963)

lous space. The material in the amniotic fluid may be directly transferred to the maternal circulation across the membranes.

Water and electrolytes are absorbed from the amniotic fluid by the bronchioles and bronchi as well as by the gastrointestinal tract. The secretions from these viscera and from the upper respiratory tract add to the contents of the amniotic fluid. The importance of these mechanisms in the normal turnover of amniotic fluid can be appreciated from the impact of anomalies on that system. Atresia high in the gastrointestinal tract, for example, in the esophagus, stomach, or duodenum, which interferes with the swallowing of amniotic fluid and its passage into the small intestine, is frequently associated with marked hydramnios. Obstruction lower down in the gastrointestinal tract, the most striking example of which is imperforate anus, has no such result. On the other hand, agenesis of the kidneys or marked obstruction in the excretory system from the kidney is ordinarily associated with severe oligohydramnios. It has been demonstrated by the artificial production of oligohydramnios in the primate fetus by *in utero* bilateral nephrectomy that the unusual quantities of amniotic fluid are a direct result of the organ defect and not associated anomalies.

Musculoskeletal System

Normal differentiation of the musculoskeletal system is essential for the fundamental framework for fetal growth. The skull forms mostly from membranous bone, whereas the spinal column and the extremities form primarily from cartilaginous bone. For this reason, the ossification centers of the spinal column can be identified roentgenographically far earlier than the skull itself. This evidence of the existence of the fetus can sometimes be seen as early as the 14th week of pregnancy and almost always by the 18th week.

Capacity for Antibody Formation

The fetus synthesizes its own proteins, and there is little evidence of placental transfer of intact proteins from the mother. The concentration of albumin and globulins other than the γ-immunoglobulins of the fetus is about equal to the mother's throughout the last trimester, while that of the γ-globulins is much lower.

Transfer of maternal immunoglobulins, specifically IgG, is accomplished by a splitting of the parent molecule into an Fab fragment, which contains the antigen-binding activity, and an Fc fragment, which contains the biologic activity in an inactive form. The Fc then crosses the placenta and presumably unites with Fab of fetal origin to reconstitute IgG. Such proteins as albumin and human growth hormone, which are smaller than IgG, do not cross the placenta.

The molecular weight of IgG is 144,000, and its half-life is 23 to 30 days. There is a rising curve of transfer

(as Fc) as term approaches, and the IgG level in newborns is 700 mg to 1300 mg/dl. The IgG level is about 90 mg/dl in colostrum. The IgG falls after birth, depending principally on breast-feeding and minimally on infant production. By six months of age, levels vary from 200 mg to 1200 mg/dl. IgG has marked activity against bacterial toxins.

IgM has a molecular weight of 880,000 and does not cross the placenta in any form. It has a half-life of 5 days. The response of IgM production is very rapid, and mole for mole it is much more potent than IgG. The latter gradually replaces IgM in the antibody response to a given antigen.

IgM manifests marked activity against gram-negative bacilli and minimal antitoxin potency. In the newborn, IgM levels range from 0 mg to 30 mg/dl in contrast to 10 mg to 90 mg/dl at six months of age. Curiously, perhaps as a reflection of the short half-life, IgM levels may not be elevated with proved but mild infections, so a low level does not rule out infection. The IgM level in colostrum is 40 mg to 50 mg/dl.

The normal fetus and newborn can synthesize IgG, but the rate by body weight is less than 1% of that of an adult. The extent of newborn protection, with an IgG half-life of 30 days, is directly proportional to maternal plasma concentrations. Furthermore, to achieve proper active immunization of infants, it is necessary to wait until the IgG level has fallen below threshold after birth.

The maternal antibody responsible for isoimmunization and erythroblastosis fetalis is an IgG and consequently transfers readily to the fetus.

Alpha-Fetoprotein

α-Fetoprotein (AFP) is formed by the yolk sac and fetal liver, beginning as early as the fourth week of pregnancy. It increases rapidly in the fetal serum and makes its appearance in the amniotic fluid shortly thereafter. AFP can be detected in the serum of nonpregnant women at levels up to 10 ng/ml, but the higher levels in pregnancy are due specifically to production of this protein by the fetus. The first elevation of the AFP level in maternal serum is detected after ten weeks; at 12 weeks, the level is approximately 25 ng/ml. Serum levels may vary from one laboratory to another, but serial tests show that they rise rapidly in the second trimester and more slowly thereafter, reach a maximum at about 32 weeks, and then decline toward term (Fig. 17-31). The serum levels of AFP are elevated in certain circumstances (*e.g.,* recent transplacental amniocentesis, endothelial changes in the placental vessels as in Rh disease or preeclampsia, fetal death, neural tube defects, twins) and may have diagnostic usefulness (see p. 370). Serum levels of AFP are also elevated in the presence of ovarian tumors that contain a significant vitelline component, as in, for example, an endodermal sinus tumor. In contrast, AFP levels may be significantly lowered when the fetus is trisomic.

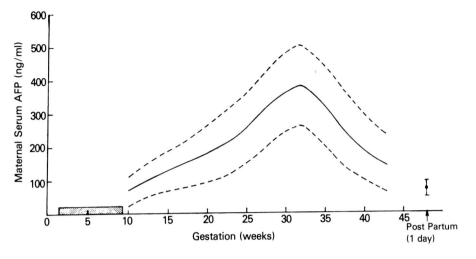

FIG. 17-31. Normal range for maternal serum α-fetoprotein according to gestation. (Hay DM, Forrester PI, Hancock RL et al: Maternal serum alpha-fetoprotein in normal pregnancy. Br J Obstet Gynaecol 83:534, 1976)

Enzyme Systems

There is considerable evidence that not all enzyme systems are functioning at maximum efficiency at the time of birth. Perhaps the most important of these is the glucuronyl transferase system in the liver. In many newborns this system functions quite efficiently, but the less mature the infant, the less effective is the glucuronyl transferase system. As a consequence, substances in the blood that pass through the glomeruli and become available for renal excretion only when they are conjugated as glucuronides are not efficiently conjugated and tend to accumulate in the circulation. They may then be able to pass through capillary membranes and into the tissues in high concentrations. The classic example of such a substance is bilirubin, which, under ordinary circumstances, is conjugated to a diglucuronide and readily excreted in the urine. If the glucuronyl transferase system is inefficient, either because it is immature or because other substances are competing with bilirubin for its activity, the bilirubin may accumulate in the blood. The adaptive importance of this can be appreciated in light of the fact that conjugated bilirubin is highly polar and hence, when excreted into the intestines, is not readily reabsorbed. The unconjugated form, being lipid soluble, crosses the placenta easily, and the mother disposes of fetal unconjugated bilirubin efficiently. This system is limited not by enzymatic immaturity, but by the availability of transport protein in the fetus.

Relation of Fetal Maturity to Survival

The physiological maturity of the fetus is directly related to its ability to survive in an extrauterine environment. However, the curve describing the relation of fetal age to survival is asymptotic. There is a striking increase in survival from the 33rd to the 37th week, but changes occurring beyond that time are trivial.

REFERENCES AND RECOMMENDED READING

Adamson YR, Bowden DH: Reaction of cultured adult and fetal lung to prednisolone and thyroxine. Arch Pathol 99:80, 1975

Adamsons K (ed): Diagnosis and Treatment of Fetal Disorders. New York, Springer-Verlag, 1968

Assali NS (ed): Biology of Gestation, Vols I, II. New York, Academic Press, 1968

An assessment of the hazards of amniocentesis. Report to the Medical Research Council by their working party on amniocentesis. Br J Obstet Gynaecol 85, Suppl 2, 1978

Benirschke K, Driscoll SG: Handbuch der speziellen pathologischen Anatomie und Histologie, Vol 7, Part 5, pp 98–616. Berlin, Springer, 1967

Boddy K: Fetal breathing: Its physiologic and clinical implications. Hosp Prac 89, 1979

Bourne G: Human Amnion and Chorion. London, Lloyd–Luke, 1962

Cowchock FS: Use of maternal blood protein levels in identification and management of high risk obstetric patients. Clin Obstet Gynecol 21:341, 1978

Danforth DN, Hull RW: Microscopic anatomy of the fetal membranes with particular reference to the detailed structure of the amnion. Am J Obstet Gynecol 75:536, 1958

Fencl M deM, Tulchinsky D: Total cortisol in amniotic fluid and fetal lung maturation. N Engl J Med 292:113, 1975

Fox H: Pathology of the Placenta. Philadelphia, WB Saunders, 1978

Freese UE, Maciolek JJ: Plastoid injection studies of the uteroplacental vascular relationship in the human. Obstet Gynecol 33:160, 1969

Gluck L, Kulovich M: Lecithin sphingomyelin ratios in amniotic fluid in normal and abnormal pregnancy. Am J Obstet Gynecol 115:539, 1973

Golbus MS, Louchman WD, Epstein CS et al.: Prenatal genetic diagnosis in 3000 amniocenteses. N Engl J Med 300:157, 1979

Grudzinskas JG, Evans DG, Gordon YB et al.: Pregnancy-specific beta₁ glycoprotein in fetal and maternal compartments. Obstet Gynecol 52:43, 1978

Hay DM, Forrester PI, Hancock RL et al.: Maternal serum alpha-fetoprotein in normal pregnancy. Br J Obstet Gynaecol 8:534, 1976

Hendricks CH: Patterns of fetal and placental growth: The second half of pregnancy. Obstet Gynecol 24:357, 1964

Horne CHW, Towler CM: Pregnancy-specific beta₁ glycoprotein: A review. Obstet Gynecol Surv 33:761, 1978

Hutchinson DL, Gray MJ, Plentl AA et al.: The role of the fetus in the water exchange of the amniotic fluid of normal and hydramniotic patients. J Clin Invest 38:971, 1959

Hytten FE, Leitch I: Physiology of Human Pregnancy, 2nd ed. Oxford, Blackwell, 1971

Lee W, Bell M, Novy MJ: Pulmonary lamellar bodies in human amniotic fluid: Their relationship to fetal age and the lecithin/sphingomyelin ratio. Am J Obstet Gynecol 136:60, 1980

McLain CR: Amniography studies of the gastrointestinal mobility of the human fetus. Am J Obstet Gynecol 86:1079, 1963

Merkatz IR, Nitowsky HM, Macri JN et al: An association between low maternal serum α-fetoprotein and fetal chromosomal abnormalities. Am J Obstet Gynecol 148:886, 1984

Moghissi KS, Hafez ESE: Biology of Mammalian Fertilization and Implantation. Springfield, IL, Thomas, 1972

Moskalewski S, Pitak W, Czarnik Z: Demonstration of cells with IgG receptor in human placenta. Biol Neonate 26:268, 1975

Page EW: Transfer of materials across the human placenta. Am J Obstet Gynecol 74:705, 1957

Queenan JT, Thompson W, Whitfield CR et al.: Amniotic fluid volumes in normal pregnancies. Am J Obstet Gynecol 114:35, 1972

Ramsey EM, Houston ML, Harris JWS: Interactions of the trophoblast and maternal tissues in three closely related primate species. Am J Obstet Gynecol 124:647, 1976

Ramsey EM, Martin CB Jr., Donner MW: Fetal and maternal placental circulations. Am J Obstet Gynecol 98:419, 1967

Report of UK Collaborative Study on alpha-fetoprotein in relation to neural-tube defects. Lancet 1:1323, 1977

Reynolds SRM: The care and feeding of embryos. Int J Gynaecol Obstet 7:43, 109, 1969

Reynolds SRM: Mechanisms of placentofetal blood flow. Obstet Gynecol 51:245, 1978

Shields JR, Resnick R: Fetal lung maturation and the antenatal use of glucocorticoids to prevent the respiratory distress syndrome. Obstet Gynecol Surv 34:343, 1979

Streeter GL: Developmental horizons in human embryos: Age Groups XI to XXIII. Contrib Embryol, Vol II. Washington, DC, Carnegie Institution, 1951

Thorsson AV, Hintz RL: Insulin receptors in the newborn. N Engl J Med 297:908 1977

Valdes–Dapena MA: Atlas of Fetal and Neonatal Histology. Philadelphia, JB Lippincott, 1957

Van Herendael BJ, Oberti C, Brosens I: Microanatomy of the human amniotic membranes. Am J Obstet Gynecol 131:872, 1978

Warkany J, Monroe BB, Sutherland BS: Intrauterine growth retardation. Am J Dis Child 102:294, 1961

Wilkin P: Pathologie du placenta. Paris, Masson, 1965

Maternal Changes in Pregnancy

Thomas C. Key
Robert Resnik

18

The physiologic alterations that occur in all organ systems in the pregnant woman are among the most remarkable events in normal biology. These changes result in symptoms and physical findings that mimic innumerable pathologic states. Consequently, the physician caring for the pregnant woman must develop a thorough understanding of these changes to clearly delineate and separate normal from abnormal physiology.

It has been assumed that these maternal alterations represent natural adaptive efforts to provide metabolic fuels and an optimum environment for the growing fetus, while at the same time maintaining maternal health. As the scientific foundations of reproductive biology have expanded, it has become increasingly apparent that this assumption is correct. Furthermore, the mechanisms involved frequently have their origins in the steroid and protein hormones of the fetoplacental unit.

Although this chapter discusses each organ system separately, the systems are integrated by a series of complex interactions that serve to enhance maternal well-being and fetal development.

CARDIOVASCULAR CHANGES

Because of the expanding uterus, the diaphragm is elevated, pushing the heart upward and rotating it forward. This lateral displacement results in the radiologic appearance of cardiomegaly, although the actual increase in cardiac volume is only 10% to 12%.

Cardiac output has been extensively studied during pregnancy, and the results have been markedly divergent. Although all studies have demonstrated a progressive increase in cardiac output that is present as early as the end of the first trimester of pregnancy, the exact time and magnitude of these changes have been subjects of continuing controversy, largely owing to differences in techniques of evaluation and maternal positioning during measurement. Invasive techniques to measure cardiac output involve central arterial and venous catheterization and the use of indicators such as indocyanine green dye and chilled saline (thermodilution). Echocardiography is the primary noninvasive technique. It was originally believed that cardiac output increases slowly, reaching a maximum between 28 and 32 weeks of gestation, and either remaining at that level or decreasing toward term. However, dye dilution studies performed on women serially throughout pregnancy with the patients in the lateral recumbent position have demonstrated that cardiac output peaks by the end of the first trimester, rising to approximately 1.5 liters per minute above the nonpregnant value (Fig. 18-1). Data obtained with echocardiographic techniques have helped clarify many of these issues (Table 18-1). These observations emphasize the importance of maternal positioning during measurement. When the patient is in the supine position, the pregnant uterus impinges on the inferior vena cava, decreasing venous return to the right side of the heart and thereby causing a decrease in stroke volume and cardiac output. These findings have led to clinical policies that encourage women to labor on their sides rather than in the supine position.

Stroke volume also increases during pregnancy by approximately 30%. Various studies have shown that stroke volume peaks by the end of the first half of gestation and either remains the same or decreases as term approaches. Differences found in stroke volume, like those found in cardiac output, may be traced to differences in maternal position while the studies are performed. Measurements performed with patients in the lateral recumbent position reveal no decrease in stroke volume after the 20th week of gestation.

Heart rate increases during pregnancy by 10% to 15%, and it should be considered normal to have a pulse of 85 to 90 beats per minute at term. Systolic and diastolic arterial pressures are among the most important

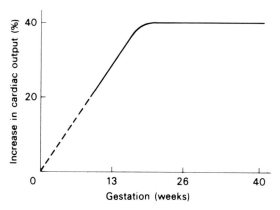

FIG. 18-1. Percentage increase in cardiac output during the course of pregnancy. Note the substantial increase by the end of the first trimester. (Hytten F, Chamberlain G: Clinical Physiology and Obstetrics. Oxford, Blackwell Scientific Publications, 1980)

parameters measured clinically during pregnancy. When the measurements are obtained with the patient sitting or standing, minimal changes are observed in systolic pressure; however, diastolic pressure decreases progressively, reaching a low point at 28 weeks' gestation, approximately 10 mm Hg below nonpregnant values. As term approaches, diastolic pressure returns closer to nonpregnant levels. Systolic and diastolic arterial pressures measured with the patient in the supine and left lateral positions both decrease substantially starting toward the end of the first trimester, and they reach a low

point between 28 and 32 weeks' gestation. Thereafter, both values begin to return to nonpregnant levels. These changes are summarized in Table 18-1.

As a result of these normal physiologic cardiovascular changes, as well as of a dramatic increase in blood volume, results of a cardiac examination are also altered. Phonocardiography is a highly accurate technique for describing changes in *heart sounds* during pregnancy. One of the most frequent findings is an early systolic to midsystolic ejection murmur heard along the left sternal border; this should be considered a flow murmur of no clinical significance. In some women a third sound may be heard, representing an insignificant diastolic flow murmur across the tricuspid valve. However, this is usually detectable only by phonocardiography, and it is generally agreed that only diastolic murmurs detected by routine auscultation should be considered abnormal and warrant more extensive evaluation.

Electrocardiographic changes are the result of the positional change of the heart. The most common finding is a modest degree of left axis deviation. Other less common changes include inverted or flattened T waves in lead III, deep Q waves, and S–T segment depression.

Although *venous pressure* in the upper extremities does not change during pregnancy, femoral venous pressure increases dramatically (Fig. 18-2) owing to the obstruction of blood flow by the large uterus on the iliac veins and interior vena cava. As a consequence of these pressure alterations, the rate of blood flow in the lower extremities decreases, and pregnant women are predisposed to edema in the lower extremities, to varicosities, and in some cases to thrombophlebitis. Centrally, no pressure changes are noted in the right atrium, and the

Table 18-1
Hemodynamic Parameters Throughout Pregnancy

Parameter	Patient Position	1st Trimester	2nd Trimester	3rd Trimester	Postpartum
Heart rate	L	77 ± 2	85 ± 2	88 ± 2	69 ± 2
(beats/min)	S	76 ± 2	84 ± 2	92 ± 2	70 ± 2
Stroke volume	L	75 ± 2	86 ± 4	97 ± 5	79 ± 3
(ml/min)	S	82 ± 5	85 ± 4	87 ± 5	79 ± 3
Cardiac output	L	3.53 ± 0.21	4.32 ± 0.22	4.85 ± 0.27	3.30 ± 0.17
$1/min/m^2$	S	3.76 ± 0.24	4.19 ± 0.21	4.54 ± 0.28	3.33 ± 0.21
Left ventricular ejection time	L	302 ± 2	290 ± 5	281 ± 4	310 ± 5
(msec)	S	301 ± 3	286 ± 4	260 ± 4	307 ± 5
Systolic blood pressure	L	98 ± 2	91 ± 2	95 ± 2	97 ± 2
(mm Hg)	S	106 ± 2	102 ± 2	106 ± 2	110 ± 2
Diastolic blood pressure	L	53 ± 2	49 ± 2	50 ± 2	57 ± 2
(mm Hg)	S	57 ± 2	60 ± 1	65 ± 2	65 ± 1

L, lateral; *S*, supine.

(After Katz R, Karliner JS, Resnik R: Effects of natural volume overload state (pregnancy) on left ventricular performance in human subjects. Circulation 58: 434, 1978)

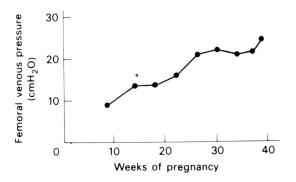

FIG. 18-2. Femoral venous pressure in normal pregnancy. (Hytten F, Chamberlain G: Clinical Physiology and Obstetrics. Oxford, Blackwell Scientific Publications, 1980)

central venous pressure remains between 2 cm and 5 cm of water.

Right ventricular and pulmonary artery pressures are unchanged during pregnancy, consistent with the high degree of compliance of the pulmonary vasculature. As cardiac output expands, pulmonary blood flow increases accordingly. The physiological importance of this characteristic of the pulmonary vasculature becomes readily apparent when one considers the risks of pulmonary hypertension during pregnancy. When this pathologic condition exists, the pulmonary circuit can not accommodate the increase in cardiac output; this results either in right ventricular failure or in the infusion of poorly oxygenated blood into the left side of the circulation through an atrial or ventricular septal defect.

CHANGES IN UTERINE BLOOD FLOW

Uterine blood flow in the nonpregnant state, as extrapolated from studies in large laboratory animals, is approximately 30 ml to 50 ml per minute. As term approaches, uterine blood flow increases dramatically to between 500 ml and 1000 ml per minute. The mechanism of this striking increase in flow is not well understood. However, it is known that 17β-estradiol, estriol, and to a lesser extent estrone all initiate marked increases in uterine blood flow in the nonpregnant and pregnant uterus. Indeed, as little as 1 μg 17β-estradiol injected directly into the uterine artery of a nonpregnant sheep results in a uterine blood flow approximating midpregnancy levels within 90 to 120 minutes of injection (Fig. 18-3). Evidence also suggests that the uterine neurovasculature undergoes a progressive depletion of adrenergic tone during gestation, while maintaining the ability to respond to norepinephrine by vasoconstriction. The combination of decreased uterine vascular adrenergic tone and exquisite sensitivity to estrogens of placental origin may be responsible for the increase in uterine blood flow. The 10- to 20-fold increase in flow above nonpregnant levels provides metabolic fuels and

oxygen for fetal development. Approximately 85% of the increase in uterine blood flow is directed toward placental tissues; the remainder is distributed to the endometrium and myometrium.

RESPIRATORY SYSTEM CHANGES

During the course of pregnancy, oxygen consumption increases by 30 ml to 60 ml per minute. This is a result of the increased demands of the mother as well as of the needs of the fetus and placenta (Fig. 18-4). The partial pressure of oxygen (PaO_2) does not rise during pregnancy, and the arteriovenous oxygen content decreases in association with the increase in oxygen consumption; therefore, *ventilation* must increase to meet these increased oxygen needs. Since the respiratory rate is unchanged, this increase in ventilation is accomplished by a rise in *tidal volume* (the volume of gas inspired or expired with each respiration) from about 500 ml to 700 ml; minute ventilation (tidal volume × respiratory rate) thus rises from 7.5 liters to 10.5 liters per minute. Furthermore, *residual volume* (the volume of gas remaining in the lungs at the end of maximal expiration, not including the anatomic dead space) decreases by 20%, as does *expiratory reserve volume* (the maximum amount of air that can be expired at the end of normal expiration). The *functional residual capacity* (residual volume + expiratory reserve volume) is thus diminished, which reduces the amount by which tidal volume is diluted during each breath. These combined changes serve to increase effective alveolar ventilation.

The timed vital capacity and *maximum breathing capacity* (the maximum amount of ventilation accomplished by forced voluntary breathing) is slightly increased during pregnancy (Fig. 18-5). This is a valuable parameter to monitor in patients with cardiac or respiratory disorders.

FIG. 18-3. The effects of 17β-estradiol and estriol on uterine blood flow in nonpregnant sheep following direct injection into the uterine artery. (Resnik R, Killam AP, Battaglia FC et al: The effect of various vasoactive compounds upon the uterine vascular bed. Am J Obstet Gynecol 125:201, 1976)

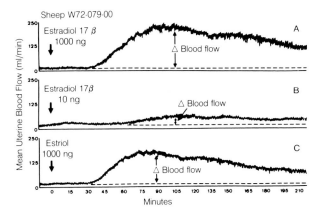

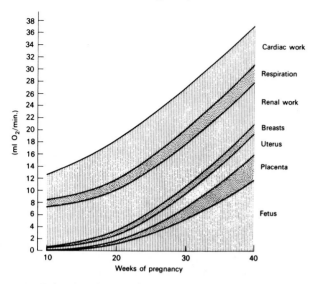

FIG. 18-4. Distribution of the increased oxygen consumption during pregnancy among organs. (Hytten F, Chamberlain G: Clinical Physiology and Obstetrics. Oxford, Blackwell Scientific Publications, 1980)

The increase in respiratory tidal volume, associated with no change in the respiratory rate, leads to an increase in the respiratory minute volume known as *hyperventilation of pregnancy.* Characterized by frequent sighing, this leads to a slight decrease in alveolar carbon dioxide and a lower partial pressure of carbon dioxide ($PaCO_2$) from 38 mm Hg to 31 mm Hg at term. This decrease is accompanied by a slight fall in plasma bicarbonate concentration, leading to a partially compensated respiratory alkalosis and an elevation of the *p*H from 7.35 to 7.4 as term approaches. The increase in ventilation and fall in $PaCO_2$ are believed to be due to increasing plasma concentration of progesterone. This hormone is thought to directly stimulate the respiratory center or lower its threshold of response to $PaCO_2$.

Dyspnea is common during pregnancy; about half of all pregnant women experience breathlessness by 20 weeks' gestation, and this number increases as term approaches. No physiological basis is known to explain this symptom, although its time course appears to be related to the fall in $PaCO_2$. It has been suggested that dyspnea occurs when the ventilatory response is inappropriate to the demand. Tests of respiratory function are usually normal in dyspneic pregnant women.

BLOOD CHANGES

There is a rapid expansion of *blood volume* during pregnancy, with sharp increases noted in both plasma and red cell components. The increase is approximately 45% over nonpregnant levels and reaches its peak by the middle of the third trimester. The rise in blood vol-

ume is slow and progressive, and the increase in plasma volume precedes that of red blood cell mass. This results in a *physiologic anemia of pregnancy,* in which the packed cell volume is decreased despite an increase in red cell mass. The total red blood cell mass reaches levels of 250 ml to 450 ml over nonpregnant values, an increase of 20% to 30%. This increase requires approximately 500 mg of additional iron during pregnancy. Another 300 mg is required within the fetal compartment. The pregnant woman should therefore receive iron supplementation so that she will not deplete her iron stores following delivery and nursing.

The mechanism controlling the increase in blood volume is unclear. Pregnancy is accompanied by increases in aldosterone production as well as by marked increases in total body water, most of which is extracellular. Increases in erythropoietin activity are presumably responsible for the expansion of the red blood cell mass.

Pregnancy is also characterized by an increase in *white blood cell* count. The change, which is limited to neutrophils, begins as early as the second month. By the end of the second trimester, total counts range between 9 and 15×10^9 cells per liter. Twenty percent of pregnant women have total counts greater than 10×10^9 cells per liter. About 20% of women also have more immature white blood cells in the peripheral smear.

Platelet counts have been reported to remain the same, rise, or fall during pregnancy. The consensus is that all changes are insignificant. Accordingly, the acceptable normal platelet count range for nonpregnant normal persons ($140–440 \times 10^9$ platelets per liter) should be applied to pregnant women as well.

Significant increases during pregnancy are observed in levels of several of the factors required for blood

FIG. 18-5. Components of lung volume in the nonpregnant and late pregnant female. (Hytten F, Chamberlain G: Clinical Physiology and Obstetrics. Oxford, Blackwell Scientific Publications, 1980)

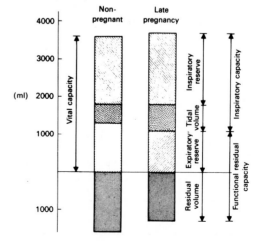

coagulation. Among the most striking are levels of fibrinogen and factor VIII. Changes in coagulant levels during pregnancy are summarized in Table 18-2.

CHANGES IN THE KIDNEYS AND LOWER URINARY TRACT

Changes in kidney function begin in the first trimester and parallel changes in blood volume and cardiac output. The *glomerular filtration rate* (GFR) is determined for experimental purposes by estimates of inulin clearance and clinically by estimates of creatinine clearance. GFR begins to increase early in the first trimester and by the 20th week of gestation is 40% above nonpregnant levels. From that point on, GFR increases at most by only an additional 10%. Whether GFR remains at that level or decreases slightly during the remainder of pregnancy is controversial. However, among women in whom clearances have been measured while they were in the lateral recumbent position following volume expansion, it appears that GFR tends to decrease towards term. Normal values during the second half of pregnancy range from 110 ml to 150 ml per minute. *Renal plasma flow* also increases during pregnancy in a pattern similar to that of GFR, reaching values 35% above the nonpregnant mean.

Renal tubular function demonstrates some clinically significant alterations during pregnancy. *Renal glycosuria* frequently develops even when blood glucose is normal. This may be due to the increased GFR's presenting a glucose load that overwhelms the tubular reabsorption mechanism; there is no evidence for an increase in tubular reabsorption (T max) capability during pregnancy. The finding at prenatal examinations of glucose in the urine dictates further evaluation to determine whether hyperglycemia also exists.

Aminoaciduria also increases during pregnancy and may reach 2 g per 24 hours. Glycine, hystidine, threonine, serine, and alanine are all excreted in large amounts early in pregnancy, and their excretion increases progressively toward term. Lysine, cystine, taurine, phenylalanine, valine, leucine, and tyrosine are also excreted in large quantities in early pregnancy, but their excretion decreases late in gestation. The significance of these observations is unknown.

Serum *uric acid* levels decrease significantly during the first and second trimesters, only to return to nonpregnant values during the third trimester. Renal excretion of uric acid is extremely sensitive to changes in extracellular volume and decreases with volume contraction. This may be a significant factor in the increases in serum uric acid concentration observed among women with pregnancy-induced hypertension, inasmuch as that entity is associated with plasma volume contraction.

The manner in which the renal tubules handle *electrolytes* is also altered during pregnancy. Potassium is normally secreted in the distal nephron, and during the course of gestation a net positive potassium balance is observed amounting to 300 mEq to 350 mEq. Also observed is an increase in the tubular reabsorption of *sodium*. The mechanisms regulating the handling of sodium by the kidneys are complex, being integrated with changes in GFR, increases in antidiuretic hormone and aldosterone, decreases in vascular resistance, and increases in plasma volume. Thus, it is likely that a combination of physiological and hormonal factors, rather than one isolated physiological event, is responsible for the retention of sodium during pregnancy. Ironically, there is a slight decrease in plasma sodium during gestation owing to the fact that water retention is slightly in excess of solute retention.

Coincidental with the functional changes in the urinary tract are anatomic changes of great significance, including dilatation of the calyces, renal pelvis, and ure-

Table 18-2
Changes in Procoagulant Levels or Activity During Pregnancy

Factor	Level in Nonpregnant Normal Subjects	Level During Second and Third Trimesters
I (Fibrinogen)	150–300 mg/100 ml	250–600 mg/100 ml
II (Prothrombin)	50–200%	No change
V	50–200%	No change
VII	50–200%	120–200%
VIII (Antihemophilic factor)	50–200%	100–300%
IX (Christmas factor)	50–200%	Slight increase
X	50–200%	120–200%
XI	50–200%	Slight decrease
XIII	50–200%	Slight decrease

(Anderson H: Maternal hematologic disorders. In Creasy RK, Resnik R (eds): Maternal–Fetal Medicine: Principles and Practice. Philadelphia, WB Saunders, 1984)

ters (Fig. 18-6). These changes occur to a greater extent, and earlier in gestation, in the right collecting system. The cause of hydronephrosis and hydroureter during pregnancy is ureteral compression by the expanding uterus plus the effects of progesterone on the ureter. The preponderance of findings on the right side has been attributed to dextrorotation of the uterus, the striking enlargement of the right ovarian vein, and the fact that the left ureter is protected by its anatomic position within the sigmoid colon mesentery.

This generalized dilatation and decreased peristalsis combine to increase the capacity of the urinary tract during pregnancy; it has been estimated that the volume within the system may reach 200 ml late in gestation. Ureteral reflux is also common. This increase in volume and decrease in urinary flow rates predispose pregnant women to urinary tract infections.

METABOLIC CHANGES

Dramatic changes occur in metabolic homeostasis during pregnancy to allow the fetus to undergo appropriate growth and development. Early in pregnancy there are

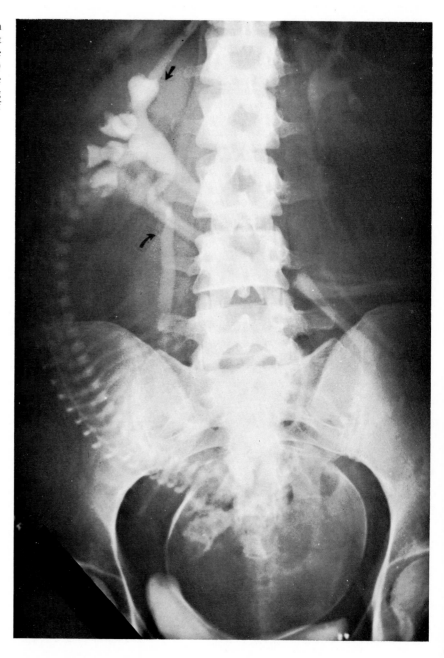

FIG. 18-6. Intravenous pyelogram showing normal urinary tract changes at 7.5 months of pregnancy. Note excessive dilatation of renal pelvis (*upper arrow*) and ureter (*lower arrow*) on right. Note also ureteral kink (asymptomatic) owing to ureteral lengthening and distortion of bladder by fetal head.

increases in plasma concentrations of estrogen and pro-gesterone. Later in pregnancy there are increases in plasma concentrations of human chorionic somato-mammotrophin (hCS), human placental lactogen (hPL), prolactin (probably of pituitary and decidual origin), and cortisol. In addition, pancreatic β-cell hyperplasia and increased insulin secretion lead to an increase in tissue glycogen storage and peripheral glucose utiliza-tion, together with a decrease in maternal fasting glucose levels. As this process continues, there is a shift toward increased production of free fatty acids and ketones. These changes have been described as "accelerated starvation" when food is unavailable and "facilitated anabolism" when food is ingested. The changes are summarized in Table 18-3.

During normal pregnancy, women experience in-sulin resistance, which is characterized by a decrease in the hypoglycemic action of insulin. In all likelihood, this is due to the combined effects of steroid and poly-peptide hormones of placental and decidual origin, which act in concert at various levels of insulin–glucose modulation.

All aspects of lipid metabolism are altered during pregnancy. *Free fatty acid* (FFA) levels decrease at midpregnancy and then increase toward term. There is also marked hypertriglyceridemia, which is due in large part to an increase in very low-density lipoprotein. *Cho-lesterol* and *phospholipid* levels increase as well.

THYROID CHANGES

During pregnancy maternal thyroid function is un-changed, but tests of function change dramatically as a result of alterations in the levels of various binding pro-teins. Although free thyroxine levels remain unchanged, an increase in serum total thyroxine (T_4) occurs early in the first trimester as a result of an increase in *thyroid-binding globulin* (TBG). This augmented production is a consequence of progressively increasing plasma es-trogen levels. As a result, the upper limits of normal during pregnancy are 2 μg to 4 μg per 100 ml higher than in nonpregnancy. There is a slight elevation in free triiodothyronine (FT_3), but this does not achieve levels higher than those found in normal nonpregnant con-trols.

Maternal thyroid-stimulating hormone (TSH) has been reported to remain at nonpregnant levels or to decrease slightly in early pregnancy. However, other thyroid stimulators of placental origin are present in increased amounts. Of particular interest is the fact that the α-subunit of human chorionic gonadotropin (hCG) has marked structural similarity to the α subunit of TSH and has been demonstrated to have maternal thyrotropic activity. Very low levels of placental TSH have been measured, but they do not appear to have any regulatory effect on the maternal thyroid. Finally, thyrotropin-re-leasing hormone (TRH) has been identified in human

---

Table 18-3
Carbohydrate Metabolism in Early and Late Pregnancy Demonstrating the Relationship Between Hormonal Changes and Their Metabolic Effects

Hormonal Change	Effect	Metabolic Change
Carbohydrate Metabolism in Early Pregnancy (to 20 Weeks)		
↑ Estrogen *and* ↑ Progesterone ↓	↑ Tissue glycogen storage ↓ Hepatic glucose production	Anabolic
Beta cell hyperplasia *and* ↑ Insulin secretion	↑ Peripheral glucose utilization ↓ Fasting plasma glucose	↑ Due to sex steroids *plus* Hyperinsulinemia
Carbohydrate Metabolism in Late Pregnancy (20 to 40 Weeks)		
↑hCS	"Diabetogenic" ↓ Glucose tolerance	Facilitated anabolism during feeding *and*
↑ Prolactin	Insulin resistance	Accelerated starvation during fasting ↓
↑ Bound and free cortisol	↓ Hepatic glycogen stores ↑ Hepatic glucose production	Ensures glucose and amino acids to fetus

(Hollingsworth DR, Cousins L: Endocrine and metabolic disorders. In Creasy RK, Resnik R (eds): Maternal–Fetal Medicine: Principles and Practice. Philadelphia, WB Saunders, 1984)

placental extracts. What, if any, effect this substance has on maternal or fetal thyroid activity is not known.

PARATHYROID CHANGES

During growth and development the fetus accumulates up to 30 g calcium, normally without there being a decrease in maternal bone calcification. For this appropriate transfer of calcium to the fetal compartment to occur, there are several changes in calcium homeostasis.

Although maternal serum calcium falls during pregnancy, this decrease represents a decrease only in serum albumin; the metabolically active ionized calcium is unchanged. *Parathyroid hormone* (PTH) acts under normal conditions at two sites. In bone it causes a shift of calcium from the osteocyte into the plasma. In the kidney it causes reabsorption of calcium and magnesium. PTH concentrations rise slightly during pregnancy, although remaining in the normal range. Levels of *calcitonin,* a calcium-lowering hormone produced in the thyroid, increase during pregnancy, although it is not known why.

Vitamin D is produced in the skin and to a lesser extent absorbed into the maternal gastrointestinal tract. It is converted in the liver to 25-hydroxyvitamin D (25[OH]D) and then in the renal proximal tubule to the biologically active forms, $1\alpha,25(OH)_2D_2$ and $1\alpha,25(OH)_2D_3$. This conversion is catalyzed by the enzyme 1α-hydroxylase, the synthesis of which is stimulated by PTH. Thus, the maternal concentration of calcium at any given time is the result of a complex interrelationship among PTH, calcitonin, and metabolites of vitamin D acting on the maternal kidney, bone, and intestinal tract. The placenta may hydroxylate vitamin D and is permeable to some of the vitamin's metabolites. Calcium transfer from mother to fetus is facilitated by a placental ATPase pump.

ADRENAL CHANGES

In longitudinal studies *adrenocorticotropic hormone* (ACTH) levels have been observed to increase during gestation, but the ranges are lower than those seen in normally ovulating women. This increase may be due to the secretion of placental ACTH. Plasma *cortisol* concentrations increase in parallel with ACTH, although most of this increase is due to the binding of cortisol to cortisol-binding globulin (CBG), the level of which doubles during pregnancy owing to estrogen stimulation. Additionally, there is a rise in unbound cortisol as well as a loss of diurnal variation. Consequently, in all likelihood, there is a slight increase in exposure of tissues to unbound cortisol during pregnancy.

WEIGHT GAIN

Few subjects in the physiology of pregnancy have received as much attention as what represents an appropriate weight gain. There have been numerous reports on average weight gain during normal pregnancy. Ranges of increase depend on variations in maternal age, size, ethnic origin, nutritional status, and various life-style factors, as well as fetal weight. Under what might be considered "normal" nutritional conditions, the average weight gain during pregnancy in the normal primigravid woman is approximately 22 lb to 27 lb. However, wide ranges may be associated with a normal outcome.

The weight gained is distributed among the fetus, placenta, amniotic fluid, uterus, mammary glands, blood, and extravascular fluids (Table 18-4). The normal pregnant woman needs to ingest about 300 kcal per day more than normal for adequate fetal nutrition.

GASTROINTESTINAL TRACT CHANGES

The gastrointestinal tract is altered anatomically and physiologically during pregnancy. As a result, as many as 90% of pregnant women experience bothersome gastrointestinal symptoms at some time during pregnancy.

The hormonal changes of pregnancy influence the soft tissues, smooth muscle, and epithelial surfaces of the *oral cavity.* Estrogen increases keratinization and subsequent desquamation of oral cavity epithelium. The net result is that epithelial turnover is increased. The ground substance becomes less dense, and blood flow to the oropharynx increases. Gingival hyperplasia results from increased mitotic activity. Thus, the tissues of the oral cavity bleed easily; as many as 75% of women bleed from the gums or oral pharynx during pregnancy.

Although it has been said that *salivation* increases during pregnancy, cannulation of salivary gland ducts does not reveal an increase in secretion rates. However, salivary composition is altered during pregnancy. Calcium and sodium concentrations are reduced in submandibular saliva, and potassium concentration is increased. In the parotid gland sodium concentration is decreased and potassium concentration increased; calcium concentration remains unchanged. The *p*H of saliva is also slightly increased during pregnancy. *Ptyalism* is a pathologic condition that occurs infrequently during pregnancy and is almost always associated with nausea. A result of glandular hypersecretion, the condition is characterized by excessive salivation. It is not unusual for individuals with ptyalism to salivate in excess of 2 liters per day. Ptyalism usually develops early during pregnancy and always remits postpartum. The factors responsible for the disorder are obscure.

Nausea and vomiting during pregnancy are common and are probably due to elevated hCG levels. Because they are so common, nausea and vomiting during early pregnancy have been accepted as presumptive evidence of pregnancy. They characteristically appear early in gestation (4–6 weeks), are usually mild, and remit during the late first or early second trimester. The physiologic basis for *hyperemesis gravidarum* is not well understood. In the nonpregnant individual, nausea and

Table 18-4
Distribution of Maternal Weight Gain

Tissues and Fluids Accounted for and Weight Gained	Approximate Increase in Weight (g) Up To			
	10 Weeks	20 Weeks	30 Weeks	40 Weeks
Fetus	5	300	1500	3400
Placenta	20	170	430	650
Amniotic fluid	30	350	750	800
Uterus	140	320	600	970
Mammary gland	45	180	360	405
Blood	100	600	1300	1250
Extracellular extravascular fluid				
Minimal or no edema	0	30	80	1680
Generalized edema	0	500	1526	4897
Total				
Minimal or no edema	340	1950	5020	9155
Generalized edema	340	2420	6466	12,372
Total weight gained*				
Minimal or no edema	650	4000	8500	12,500
Generalized edema	650	4500	10,000	14,500

* Note that the total weight gained is greater than can be accounted for by maternal stores alone.

(After Hytten F, Chamberlain G: Clinical Physiology in Obstetrics, p 221. Oxford, Blackwell Scientific Publications, 1980)

vomiting are regulated by the emetic center located in the reticular formation in the floor of the fourth ventricle. The center is near those controlling salivation and respiration. Stimuli from higher cortical centers have input on the emetic center, which in turn regulates the activities of medullary centers that produce the patterned activity known as vomiting. At least in part, hyperemesis gravidarum appears to be related to psychic and emotional factors. It has been noted that as many as 80% of patients with severe hyperemesis during pregnancy have identifiable contributing psychologic disturbances. However, neural and endocrine alterations that occur during pregnancy may also alter the threshold of resistance to nausea and vomiting. The appearance of nausea and vomiting parallels the rise in serum chorionic gonadotropin. Further, in pregnancies in which hCG levels are elevated, such as multiple gestations and pregnancies associated with gestational trophoblastic disease, nausea and vomiting are more common than usual. Although most women with hyperemesis note complete relief of their symptoms following termination of the pregnancy, the relationship of this condition to the presence of increased concentrations of circulating pregnancy hormones is not clear.

Appetite changes are also noted during the course of gestation. A modest degree of anorexia is common during the first trimester, particularly in women with hyperemesis. This is followed by an increase in appetite during the second trimester. More striking are qualitative differences in appetite, including cravings for and aversions to certain foods without apparent reason. The threshold for all forms of taste (salt, sour, sweet, and bitter) is raised. Pregnant women frequently have an increased desire for savory and flavored foods and may feel an aversion to coffee, alcohol, fried foods, red meat, and certain spices, as well as to tobacco products. Occasionally, pathologic cravings for bizarre foods, known as *pica,* may develop. Women with pica have bizarre cravings for starch, clay, paper, and ice; they should be evaluated for nutritional and hematologic disturbances.

Several alterations are observed in *esophageal* function during pregnancy. The esophagus is bounded by two cavities, the oropharynx and stomach, which have positive pressures in the resting state. In contrast, the esophagus has a negative intraluminal pressure in the resting state. The movement of food from the mouth to the stomach requires coordinated contractions of smooth muscle within the wall of the esophagus as well as the physiologic actions of sphincters located at the proximal and distal boundaries of the esophagus. During pregnancy the tone of the lower esophagus is decreased. This reduction in sphincter tone is at its peak at 36 weeks but can be demonstrated throughout the second half of pregnancy. As uterine enlargement causes increased intragastric pressure, the lower esophageal sphincter may become incompetent, allowing the reflux of gastric contents into the esophagus. Esophageal reflux produces inflammation of the lower esophageal mucosa, leading to symptoms of *heartburn.*

Pregnancy appears to produce a general protective effect against peptic ulcer disease. This effect is not due to control of gastric acid secretion by the polypeptide hormone gastrin, which is released from the antrum of the stomach during gastric distention. Gastrin levels in pregnant women are comparable to levels in nonpregnant women. Furthermore, gastric acid production varies widely. Nor is it due to changes in hormone levels; exogenously administered estrogen and progesterone have no effect on gastric acid secretion in nonpregnant women. However, radiologic studies in which contrast is ingested with a meal do demonstrate decreased *gastric motility* during pregnancy, and when serial radiologic studies are performed to follow movement through the gastrointestinal tract, significant delays in transit are noted. This decrease in motility, rather than changes in gastrin or gastric acid secretion, may play some role in the amelioration of ulcer symptoms frequently seen during pregnancy.

During labor and delivery there is a further prolongation of gastric emptying time and a decrease in gastric motility. It is not unusual for gastric retention to occur up to five hours following ingestion of a meal during labor. During the second stage of labor expulsive efforts increase intraabdominal and intragastric pressures, making esophageal reflux and the possibility of vomiting and aspiration more likely. These physiologic changes have important implications from the anesthetic standpoint; because the woman in labor is at greater risk than normal for vomiting and aspiration, meticulous attention must be paid to airway management.

Because of decreased gastrointestinal motility and increased transit times during pregnancy, water absorption from the large bowel is increased, and symptoms of *constipation* are intensified. Indeed, constipation is one of the most frequent and disturbing symptoms in pregnant women.

LIVER AND GALLBLADDER CHANGES

The *liver* does not increase its weight during pregnancy. Clinical estimation of liver size is difficult, since the gravid uterus enlarges and extends into the right upper quadrant beyond the second trimester. However, actual determinations of liver weight demonstrate no differences between pregnant and nonpregnant women. As a result, any demonstrable increase in liver size is likely to represent a pathologic rather than a pregnancy-specific change. Minor histologic changes are normally observed in the liver architecture, including variations in the size of the hepatocytes, irregularities in cell nuclei, and occasionally an increase in fat and glycogen deposition. Whereas cardiac output increases substantially during pregnancy, hepatic blood flow is unchanged. The net result could be construed as a relative decrease in blood flow, since this absence of net change occurs at the same time as an increase in cardiac output and blood volume. This observation may explain the decrease in hepatic clearance that occurs particularly during the last half of gestation.

Striking changes in protein synthesis during pregnancy are similar to changes noted in nonpregnant women following administration of exogenous estrogen.

Total serum protein concentration decreases by 20%, the major decline resulting from diminished concentrations of *albumin.* This decrease in serum albumin in part reflects dilutional changes that occur with an increase in circulating intravascular volume but is also partially due to an increase in catabolism without commensurate increases in synthesis. Slight increases are noted in the α- and β-globulin fractions, while γ-globulin concentrations decrease. The *procoagulant* factors like fibrinogen have been discussed earlier in this chapter. Other proteins the levels of which increase during pregnancy are transferrin, ceruloplasmin, TBG, sex-hormone-binding globulin, and various carrier proteins. These changes must be taken into consideration in the interpretation of laboratory profiles of pregnant women.

The clinical observation of normal or increased serum values of *enzymes* of hepatic origin determines the presence or absence of hepatocellular disease. Serum alkaline phosphatase concentrations increase during pregnancy. However, this increase is largely due to alkaline phosphatase production by the placenta, which is heat stable. The test is not useful clinically unless heat-stable and heat-labile forms of the enzyme are differentiated. In contrast, serum glutamic oxaloacetic transaminase (SGOT) and serum glutamic pyruvic transaminase (SGPT) are unchanged during pregnancy. Accordingly, any elevation of these serum enzymes should be considered an indication of intrinsic liver disease.

The *gallbladder* is also influenced by the hormonal and physiologic changes of pregnancy. Supersaturation of bile occurs whenever there is a high rate of cholesterol excretion or a diminished rate of bile salt secretion. Pregnancy may increase the secretion of cholesterol into bile. Moreover, women are known to have smaller bile salt pools than men, thus limiting the amount of cholesterol that can be retained in solution. Estrogen decreases the amount of chenodeoxycholic acid in the bile; this is of clinical significance because the amount of cholesterol soluble in bile is inversely related to the amount of chenodeoxycholic acid present in bile. Thus, an alteration in bile salt composition and an increase in the amount of cholesterol made available to the gallbladder may combine to increase the possibility of biliary cholesterol saturation and subsequent stone formation.

Progesterone appears to have a smooth muscle–relaxing effect by which it impairs gallbladder contractility. It does this by inhibiting the contractions produced by cholecystokinin, which is the major stimulus for gallbladder contraction following food ingestion. This leads the gallbladder to have increased capacity, increased residual volume, and impaired contractility. Sonographic studies of gallbladder function during pregnancy demonstrate significant increases in gallbladder volume during each trimester. These changes in gallbladder contractility, combined with the previously mentioned alterations in the bile salt pool, explain why pregnant women are predisposed to gallbladder disease.

PANCREATIC CHANGES

Pancreatic enzyme production is increased during late gestation. Serum amylase concentrations increase slightly, and the upper limit of normal during pregnancy may reach 200 units per 100 ml. Pregnant women are predisposed to pancreatitis because of increases in intra-abdominal pressure late in gestation and because of the gallbladder changes described in the last section.

SKIN CHANGES

The skin also responds to the physical and hormonal changes of pregnancy. An increase in *pigmentation* is common; it is highly variable but is present to some extent in virtually all women. Although generalized pigmentation can occur, it tends to be localized to areas of melanin hyperpigmentation. These areas include the areola and nipples, the vulvar and perianal regions, the axilla, and the linea alba. Under the influence of pregnancy, the linea alba may be transformed into what is known as the *linea nigra*. Approximately 70% of pregnant women experience hyperpigmentation of the forehead, cheeks, bridge of the nose, and chin. This hyperpigmentation is generally symmetric and begins as early as six to seven weeks of gestation. Characteristically, *chloasma,* or the "mask of pregnancy," has a blotchy appearance that results from irregular melanin deposi-

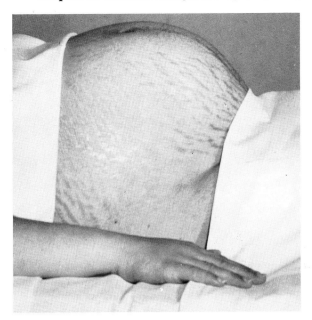

FIG. 18-8. Abdomen of patient at term, showing striae gravidarum and prominent linea nigra. (Bookmiller MM, Bowen GL: Textbook of Obstetrics and Obstetric Nursing. Philadelphia, WB Saunders, 1963)

tion (Fig. 18-7). Identical changes may be observed in women taking oral contraceptives. Following pregnancy the pigmentation changes remit. Experimental data suggest that these changes may reflect the activity of β-melanocyte-stimulating hormone, levels of which are increased throughout pregnancy and during lactation. Nevi, preexisting pigmented moles, and freckles also become darker during pregnancy. During pregnancy nevi may appear for the first time or old ones may enlarge. Melanocyte-stimulating hormone levels increase early in the second trimester and may be responsible for these changes.

Estrogens appear to have a significant effect on skin perfusion; vascular proliferation frequently results. Telangiectasis is caused by the dilatation of small arterioles. Such changes occur during the second trimester in approximately 70% of women, primarily in areas that are exposed to sunlight. *Palmar erythema* is also a common finding, with diffuse redness occurring over the entire palmar surface or on the thenar and hypothenar eminences.

The connective tissue is also affected by pregnancy. *Striae gravidarum* (Fig. 18-8) occur to some degree in most pregnant women; they are oriented perpendicular to the anatomic skin lines and are found predominantly over the lower abdomen, hips, and breasts. The initial pink to blue areas of discoloration gradually become depressed white bands of skin. The exact basis for striae formation is unknown. Histologic examination of striae demonstrates decreased collagen content and lack of elastic fibers.

FIG. 18-7. Chloasma, mask of pregnancy. Pigmentation is often most prominent on bridge of nose and forehead. (Bookmiller MM, Bowen GL: Textbook of Obstetrics and Obstetric Nursing. Philadelphia, WB Saunders, 1963)

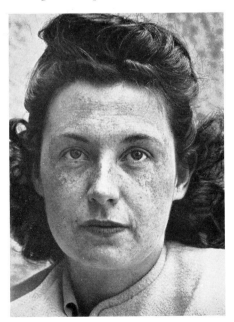

Hair growth is altered in a striking way during pregnancy and postpartum. The increased concentrations of circulating estrogen decrease the duration of anagen (follicle-growing phase) as well as the number of hair follicles in telogen (resting, or dormant, phase). In the postpartum period, the percentage of follicles in telogen increases sharply. This results in increased shedding of hair during the first three to four months postpartum. The loss of hair is uniform about the scalp, and virtually all the hair is replaced within six to nine months.

REFERENCES AND RECOMMENDED READING

General

Creasy RK, Resnik R (eds): Maternal–Fetal Medicine: Principles and Practice. Philadelphia, WB Saunders, 1984

Hytten F, Chamberlain G (eds): Clinical Physiology and Obstetrics. Oxford, Blackwell Scientific Publications, 1980

Cardiovascular Changes

Bader RA, Bader ME, Rose DJ et al: Hemodynamics at rest and during exercise in normal pregnancy as studied by cardiac catheterization. J Clin Invest 34:1524, 1955

Cutforth R, McDonald CD: Heart sounds and murmurs in pregnancy. Am Heart J 71:741, 1966

Katz R, Karliner JS, Resnik R: Effects of natural volume overload state (pregnancy) on left ventricular performance in human subjects. Circulation 58:434, 1978

Lees MM, Taylor SH, Scott DB et al: A study of cardiac output at rest throughout pregnancy. J Obstet Gynecol Br Commonw 74:319, 1967

Macgillivray I, Rose GA, Rowe B: Blood pressure survey in pregnancy. Clin Sci 37:395, 1969

Metcalfe J, Ueland K: Maternal cardiovascular adjustments to pregnancy. Prog Cardiovasc Dis 16:363, 1974

Changes in Uterine Blood Flow

Greiss FC Jr., Anderson SG: Uterine vascular changes during the menstrual cycle. Am J Obstet Gynecol 103:629, 1969

Makowski EL, Meschia G, Droegemuller W et al: Distribution of uterine blood flow in pregnant sheep. Am J Obstet Gynecol 101:409, 1968

Metcalfe J, Romney SL, Ramsey LH et al: Estimation of uterine blood flow to women at term. J Clin Invest 34:1632, 1955

Resnik R, Killam AP, Battaglia FC et al: The stimulation of uterine blood flow by various estrogens. Endocrinology 94:1192, 1974

Rosenfeld CR, Morriss FH Jr., Battaglia FC et al: Effect of estradiol-17β on blood flow to reproductive and nonreproductive tissues in pregnant ewes. Am J Obstet Gynecol 124:618, 1976

Respiratory System Changes

Alaily AB, Carrol KB: Pulmonary ventilation in pregnancy. Br J Obstet Gynecol 85:518, 1978

Anderson GJ, James GB, Mathers NP et al: The maternal oxygen tension and acid base status during pregnancy. Am J Obstet Gynecol 100:1, 1969

Campbell EJM, Howell JBL: The sensation of breathlessness. Br Med Bull 19:36, 1963

Comroe JH: Physiology of Respiration, 2nd ed. Chicago, Year Book Medical Publishers, 1974

Kelman GR, Templeton A: Maternal blood gases during human pregnancy. Physiology 244:66, 1975

Krumholz RA, Echt CR, Ross JC: Pulmonary diffusing capacity, capillary blood volume, lung volumes and mechanics of ventilation in early and late pregnancy. J Clin Med 63:648, 1964

Milne JA, Howie AD, Pack AI: Dyspnoea during normal pregnancy. Br J Obstet Gynecol 84:448, 1978

Ueland K, Novy MJ, Metcalfe J: Cardiorespiratory responses to pregnancy and exercise in normal women and patients with heart disease. Am J Obstet Gynecol 115:4, 1973

Blood Changes

Chesley LC: Plasma and red cell volumes during pregnancy. Am J Obstet Gynecol 123:440, 1972

Kuvin SF, Brecher G: Differential neutrophil counts in pregnancy. N Engl J Med 266:877, 1962

Lange RD, Dynesius R: Blood volume changes during normal pregnancy. Clin Haematol 2:433, 1973

Pritchard JA: Changes in blood volume during pregnancy and delivery. Anesthesiology 26:393, 1965

Changes in the Kidneys and Lower Urinary Tract

Chesley LC, Sloan CM: The effect of posture on renal function in late pregnancy. Am J Obstet Gynecol 89:754, 1964

Davison JM, Dunlop W, Ezimokhai M: Twenty-four hour creatinine clearance during the third trimester of normal pregnancy. Br J Obstet Gynecol 87:107, 1980

Lindheimer M, Katz AI: Renal function in pregnancy. Obstet Gynecol Annu 1:139, 1972

Sims EAH, Krantz KE: Serial studies of renal function during pregnancy and the puerperium in normal women. J Clin Invest 37:1764, 1958

Metabolic Changes

Cousins L, Rigg L, Hollingsworth D et al: The twenty-four hour excursion and diurnal rhythm of glucose, insulin, and C-peptide in normal pregnancy. Am J Obstet Gynecol 136:483, 1980

Freinkel N, Metzger BE, Nitzan M et al: Facilitated anabolism in later pregnancy: Some novel maternal compensations for accelerated starvation. In Malaise WJ, Pirart J (ed): Proceedings of the Eighth Congress of the Diabetes Federation. Amsterdam, Excerpta Medica, 1974

Hollingsworth DR: Alterations of maternal metabolism in normal and diabetic pregnancies. Differences in insulin dependent, non-insulin dependent and gestational diabetes. Am J Obstet Gynecol 146:417, 1983

Kitzmiller JL: The endocrine pancreas in maternal metabolism.

In Tulchinsky D, Ryan KJ (ed): Maternal–fetal endocrinology. Philadelphia, WB Saunders, 1980

Thyroid Changes

Burrow GN: Hyperthyroidism during pregnancy. N Engl J Med 298:150, 1978

Harada A, Hershman JM, Reed W et al: Comparison of thyroid stimulators in thyroid hormone concentrations in the sera of pregnant women. J Clin Endocrinol Metab 48:793, 1979

Hershman JM: Placental thyroid stimulators and thyroid function in pregnancy. In Novy MJ, Resco JA (ed): Fetal Endocrinology. New York, Academic Press, 1981

Parathyroid Changes

Cohn DV, MacGregor RR: Biosynthesis, intracellular processing and secretion of parathormone. Endocr Rev 2:1, 1981

Cole DEC, Kremer R, Goltzman D: The parathyroids in calcium homeostasis. In Collu R, Ducharme JR, Guyda HG (eds): Pediatric Endocrinology. New York, Raven Press, 1981

Pitkin RM, Reynolds WA, Williams GA et al: Calcium metabolism in normal pregnancy: A longitudinal study. Am J Obstet Gynecol 133:781, 1979

Gastrointestinal Tract Changes

Arafat A: Periodontal status during pregnancy. J Periodont 45: 741, 1974

Bernstine RL, Friedman MHF: Salivation in pregnant and non-pregnant woman. Obstet Gynecol 10:184, 1957

Braverman DZ, Johnson ML, Kern F: Effects of pregnancy and contraceptive steroids on gallbladder function. N Engl J Med 302:363, 1980

Clark DH, Tankel HI: Gastric acid in plasma histaminase during pregnancy. Lancet 2:886, 1954

Corlett RC, Mishell DR: Pancreatitis in pregnancy. Am J Obstet Gynecol 113:281, 1972

Davison JS, Davison MC, Hay DM: Gastric emptying time in late pregnancy and labor. J Obstet Gynecol Br Commonw 77:37, 1970

Fairweather DVI: Nausea and vomiting in pregnancy. Am J Obstet Gynecol 102:135, 1968

Fisher RS, Roberts GS, Grabowski CJ et al: Altered lower esophageal sphincter function during early pregnancy. Gastroenterology 74:1233, 1978

Mendelson CL: The aspiration of stomach contents into the lungs during obstetric anesthesia. Am J Obstet Gynecol 52:191, 1946

Ulmsten U, Sundstrom G: Esophogeal manomatry in pregnant and non-pregnant women. Am J Obstet Gynecol 132:260, 1978

Van Thiel DH, Galvaler JS, Joshi SN et al: Heartburn of pregnancy. Gastroenterology 63:1066, 1977

Endocrine Physiology of Pregnancy

Samuel S. C. Yen

19

Alterations of neuroendocrine functions during pregnancy represent a most remarkable adaptive phenomenon in biologic systems. Within the pregnant uterus, the fetal–placental–decidual units produce extraordinary amounts of steroid and protein hormones and neuropeptides. They appear to interact and function in a fashion similar to that of the hypothalamic–hypophyseal–ovarian system. It seems logical that the fetus determines its own destiny and that these newly added endocrine units conduct the unidirectional flow of nutrients from the mother to the fetus, provide a favorable environment within the uterus for cellular growth and maturation, and convey signals when the fetus is ready for extrauterine existence.

Thus, the initiation, maintenance, and termination of pregnancy are dependent largely on the interaction of hormonal and neural factors. Proper timing of these neuroendocrine events within and between compartments (*i.e.,* maternal compartment, fetal–placental compartment, amniotic fluid) is critical to appropriate fetal maturation, parturition, and lactation.

FORMATION AND SECRETION OF STEROID HORMONES

Corpus Luteum of Pregnancy

Within hours following implantation, the primitive trophoblast of the blastocyst secretes a luteotropic hormone, human chorionic gonadotropin (hCG). This appears in the maternal circulation almost immediately and "rescues" corpus luteum function, which otherwise would regress. A rise in circulating progesterone, 17-hydroxyprogesterone, and estradiol reflects continued and augmented corpus luteum activity in response to hCG stimulation (Fig. 19-1).

Relaxin, a peptide hormone, is detectable in serum eight to ten days after conception. Human corpus luteum extract contains biologic active relaxin, and hCG can induce biosynthesis and secretion of relaxin by the mature corpus luteum (Fig. 19-2). Ovarian relaxin may function in conjunction with progesterone to reduce spontaneous uterine activity and thus play a major role in early pregnancy maintenance.

The corpus luteum remains the major source of progestational steroids through approximately the ninth week of gestation; thereafter the placental trophoblast and decidua assume this role, which continues until the time of parturition (Fig. 19-3). Ovariectomy or corpus luteum removal before the eighth week of gestation invariably results in abortion but after the ninth week of gestation has no influence on the course of gestation. Thus, the integrity of early pregnancy is dependent on the corpus luteum. Relaxin appears to be secreted by the corpus luteum throughout pregnancy. However, the relative contribution of decidual relaxin during late pregnancy remains to be determined.

Maternal–Placental and Fetoplacental Units as Endocrine Organs

The human placenta achieves its mature architecture by the end of the first trimester of pregnancy. The functional unit is the chorionic villus, which consists of a central core of loose connective tissue with abundant capillaries connected with the fetal circulation. Around this core are two layers of trophoblast, an outer syncytium (syncytiotrophoblast) and an inner layer of discrete cells (cytotrophoblast), the latter becoming discontinuous as the placenta matures.

The developing fetus and its placenta form an interdependent partnership in regulating the normal

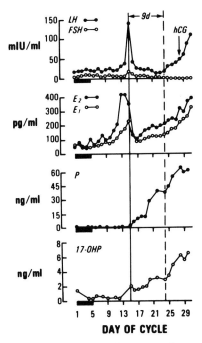

FIG. 19-1. Hormonal patterns of a conception cycle in which hCG may be detectable in blood 9 days after luteinizing hormone peak. Note the rise of steroid hormones by the corpus luteum of early pregnancy. *LH,* luteinizing hormone; *FSH,* follicle-stimulating hormone; E_2, estradiol; E_1, estrone; *P,* progesterone; *17-OHP,* 17-hydroxyprogesterone.

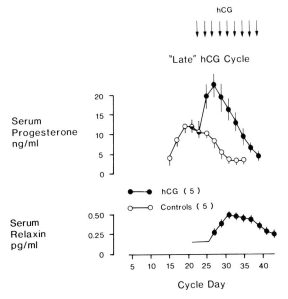

FIG. 19-2. Circulating concentrations (mean ± standard error) of progesterone and relaxin during the luteal phase of the cycle. Treatment with hCG (2500 IU intramuscularly every 2 days), as indicated by *arrows,* resulted in an augmented and prolonged progesterone elevation and a concomitant rise in relaxin levels. (After Quagliarello J, Goldsmith L, Steinetz B et al: Induction of relaxin secretion in nonpregnant women by human chorionic gonadotropin. J Clin Endocrinol Metab 51:74, 1980)

course of pregnancy. This functional relationship, commonly known as the fetoplacental unit, is a unique endocrine system that produces a substantial number of hormones, including peptide, neuropeptides, and steroid hormones. Many of these hormones are identical to or at least mimic those produced by the hypothalamic–hypophyseal–gonadal system.

Estrogens, androgens, and progestins are involved in pregnancy from the time of implantation to parturition. They are produced and metabolized in a complex pattern involving the fetus and placenta as well as the mother.

Formation of Progesterone

The classic experiments by Bloch and by Hellig and associates demonstrated that progesterone is synthesized by the placenta through hydroxylation from maternal cholesterol. This process is independent of fetal precursor or steroidogenesis, as evidenced by unchanged plasma progesterone and urinary pregnanediol levels following fetal death *in utero.* Thus, the formation of progesterone by the placenta, with an almost unlimited amount of maternal substrate, represents an endocrine process exclusively of maternal–placental interaction (Fig. 19-4).

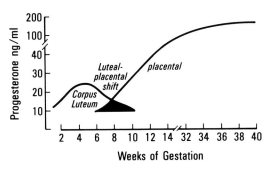

FIG. 19-3. A shift of progesterone production from the corpus luteum to the placenta occurs around the eighth or ninth week of gestation. The *black area* represents the estimated duration of this functional transition.

Cholesterol is carried in maternal circulation by lipoproteins, which consist of particles coated by proteins and packaged within its triglycerides and cholesteryl esters. Specific high-affinity receptors for low density lipoprotein (LDL) but not high density lipoprotein (HDL) are present on the cell membranes of the trophoblasts. Following binding of LDL to surface receptors, internalization through the process of active endocytosis takes place (Fig. 19-5). Within the trophoblast

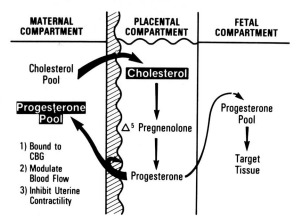

FIG. 19-4. The placental biosynthetic pathway for progesterone. *CBG,* cortical binding globulin.

from 40 ng/ml to 160 ng/ml from the first to the third trimester of pregnancy. The placenta at term produces approximately 250 mg of progesterone per day, secreting 90% to the maternal compartment and 10% to the fetal circulation. Because of the relative sizes of the compartments, fetal plasma concentration is sevenfold higher than maternal plasma concentration. In plasma progesterone is bound to corticosteroid-binding globulin (CBG) and albumin, with approximately 10% to 15% remaining in free form.

The myometrium contains receptors for progesterone. As noted in Chapter 30, progesterone decreases uterine sensitivity to oxytocin and appears to act synergistically with relaxin to reduce uterine motility and to inhibit propagation of uterine contractions.

In contrast to serum progesterone levels, 17-hydroxyprogesterone concentrations at midpregnancy are low, comparable to those observed during the luteal phase of the menstrual cycle. This is due to a lack of 17-hydroxylase activity in the placenta. The substantial rise of 17-hydroxyprogesterone levels after the 32nd week of gestation is largely due to activity of the fetal adrenal gland, which produces both 17-hydroxyprogesterone and 17-hydroxypregnenolone, the latter of which can be converted by the placenta to 17-hydroxyprogesterone. Thus, circulating levels of 17-hydroxyprogesterone in late pregnancy reflect functional activity of the fetal adrenal gland and the placenta (Fig. 19-6).

Formation of Deoxycorticosterone from Progesterone

Plasma concentrations of deoxycorticosterone (DOC), a potent mineralocorticosteroid, are elevated during pregnancy. Quantitative time course studies have revealed a two- to fivefold increase in circulating DOC during the first trimester over nonpregnancy levels. This

these LDL particles fuse with lysosomes, after which hydrolysis by lysosome enzyme occurs; the protein cast gives rise to amino acids, while hydrolysis of cholesteryl esters gives rise to fatty acids and cholesterol. The possibility that these amino acids and fatty acids may serve as intracellular substrate is attractive but has yet to be shown to be true. The liberated cholesterol is then available to serve as a precursor for formation of pregnanolone. Pregnanolone is readily converted to progesterone in a reaction catalyzed by 3β-hydroxysteroid dehydrogenase and Δ^5-Δ^4 isomerase enzymes. Regulation of progesterone formation appears to be autonomous. Because of the abundance of lipoprotein substrate in the maternal circulation, the magnitude of progesterone formation by the placenta is likely determined by placental size and perfusion.

Maternal plasma progesterone concentration rises

FIG. 19-5. Diagrammatic illustration of pathways of lipoprotein–cholesterol metabolism and biosynthesis of progesterone. (Courtesy of J Schreiber)

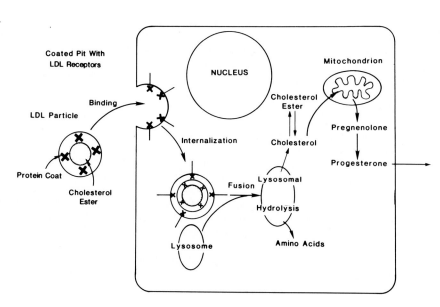

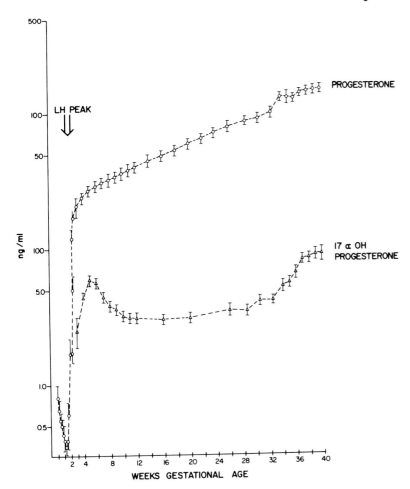

FIG. 19-6. Relative circulating concentrations (mean ± standard error) of progesterone and 17α-hydroxyprogesterone during the course of human pregnancy. (Courtesy of J R Marshall)

is followed by a progressive rise to levels at term of more than tenfold the nonpregnant value (Fig. 19-7). Winkel and collaborators have demonstrated unequivocally the extra-adrenal biosynthesis of DOC. The presence of steroid 21-hydroxylase activity in the human kidney is evidence of this conversion of plasma progesterone to DOC. Production of extra-adrenal 21-hydroxylase appears to be stimulated by estrogen. The rate of formation of DOC from plasma progesterone is proportional to the concentration of circulating progesterone in normal and adrenalectomized subjects. This finding is consistent with the poor response of DOC to adrenocorticotropic hormone (ACTH) stimulation and dexamethasone suppression in late pregnancy. Of course, there is marked individual variation in the conversion of progesterone to DOC.

Since DOC is a salt-retaining and hypertensive agent, it may play a role in the genesis of pregnancy-induced hypertension. Although DOC levels are not significantly different from normal in women with pregnancy-induced hypertension, it is possible that DOC concentrations are increased at the site of production and action (*i.e.,* the kidney) in these women and are thus a pathogenetic factor in the development of pregnancy-induced hypertension.

Placenta As an Androgen Sink

The placenta lacks 17-hydroxylase and 17,20-desmolase activity and hence cannot convert C_{21} to C_{19} steroids. The sources of placental androgens are the maternal and fetal adrenals. The placenta extracts dehydroepiandrosterone sulfate (DHAS) from the maternal and fetal circulations and, by hydrolyzing the sulfate (via sulfatase), converts it to free dehydroepiandrosterone (DHA). The placenta is capable of converting DHA to androstenedione (A) and testosterone (T), which are readily aromatized to form estrone (E_1) and estradiol (E_2) and released, mainly into the maternal circulation (Fig. 19-8). Maternal serum T and A levels rise two- or threefold during pregnancy, and most of serum T is bound to sex hormone–binding globulin (SHBG), which is markedly elevated in the maternal compartment but very low in the fetal compartment, independent of the sex of the fetus (Fig. 19-9).

In contrast to A and T concentrations, maternal cir-

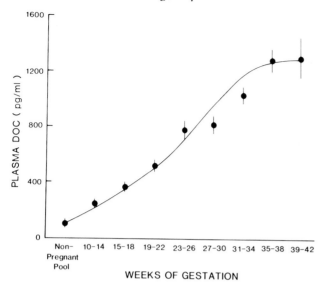

FIG. 19-7. The progressive increase in plasma deoxycorticosterone (*DOC*) concentrations (mean ± standard error) during the course of normal pregnancy. (After Parker CR Jr., Everett RB, Whalley PJ: Hormone production during pregnancy in the primigravid patient. II. Plasma levels of deoxycorticosterone throughout pregnancy of normal women and women who developed pregnancy-induced hypertension. Am J Obstet Gynecol 138:626, 1980)

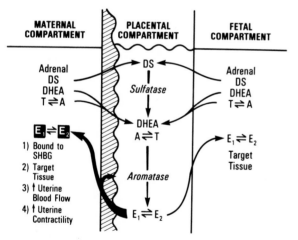

FIG. 19-8. Diagrammatic illustration of the placental formation of estradiol (E_2) and estrone (E_1) from maternal and fetal androgen precursors: dehydroepiandrosterone (*DHEA*) and its sulfate (*DS*), testosterone (*T*), and androstenedione (*A*). *SHBG*, sex steroid–binding globulin.

culating levels of DHAS and DHA do not change significantly during pregnancy. Placental extraction of DHAS and DHA from the maternal circulation accounts for the eightfold increase in the metabolic clearance rate of DHAS, which parallels placental growth. The metabolic clearance rate of DHA is 2.5-fold higher and its loss from the circulation is thus 2 times faster in late

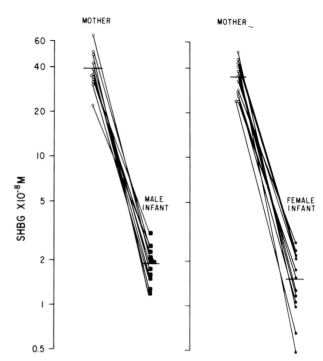

FIG. 19-9. Sex steroid–binding globulin (*SHBG*) concentrations in the paired sample from maternal and infant (cord blood) circulation. Note that there is no difference between male and female infants. (Courtesy of D Anderson)

pregnancy than in the nonpregnant state. Thus, the placenta functions to dispose of androgens, which are irreversibly aromatized to estrogens, a process of fundamental importance in pregnancy. The fetal adrenals produce DHAS in both the definitive and the fetal zones, and this production is stimulated by both hCG and ACTH in the first part of pregnancy with a shift to ACTH only after midgestation.

Formation of Estrogens

ESTRONE (E_1) AND ESTRADIOL (E_2).   The conversion by the placenta of Δ^4-C_{19} steroids A and T to E_1 and E_2 provides an essential barrier against androgen action that might otherwise cause virilization of the female fetus (see Fig. 19-8). The placenta is not capable of "aromatizing" 19-nor steroids, which are known to effect virilization *in utero,* causing female pseudohermaphroditism. The circulating DHAS used to form E_1 and E_2 is provided equally by the fetal and maternal adrenals. Therefore, placental E_1 and E_2 production depends only partially on the availability of a fetal precursor.

Because of a lack of 16-hydroxylase, the placenta cannot form estriol (E_3) from E_1 or E_2. The placenta secretes E_1 and E_2 into both the maternal and fetal circulations, and the fetus rapidly inactivates biologically active E_2 by the processes of hydroxylation and sulfurylation.

Maternal serum E_2 levels rise throughout pregnancy until term, reaching levels of 20 ng/ml to 30 ng/ml.

Because SHBG has a particularly high affinity for E_2, total maternal serum E_2 levels are higher than levels of E_1 and E_3 (Fig. 19-10), despite the fact that E_1 and E_3 production exceeds E_2 production, as evidenced by the urinary excretion rate of these three estrogens. Maternal urinary E_1 and E_2 excretion rates increase 100-fold from their preovulatory values to term. In contrast, urinary E_3 excretion increases 1000-fold over the same time period. The maternal liver metabolizes and conjugates E_1 and E_2, but only a small portion of these substances is converted to E_3.

ESTRIOL (E_3) AND ESTETROL (E_4). The demonstration by Ryan in 1959 that the placenta contains an unlimited amount of aromatase enzyme has permitted a rapid advance in the understanding of estrogen formation by the placenta. DHAS from the fetal adrenal is converted by the fetal liver to 16-hydroxydehydroepiandrosterone sulfate (16OH-DS); this is the principal fetal contribution to E_3 biosynthesis. In the placenta 16OH-DS is cleaved by sulfatase to 16OH-DHA. The placenta converts 16OH-DHA initially to 16OH-androstenedione and 16OH-testosterone and then aromatizes these compounds to E_3 (Fig. 19-11). Thus, the fetus and placenta play a joint and obligatory role in E_3 biosynthesis.

Without fetal ACTH stimulation, there is little or no DHAS production by the fetal adrenal. This situation is found in cases of congenital absence of the pituitary gland and anencephaly, as well as when corticosteroids given to the mother cross the placenta and suppress fetal ACTH secretion. Rarely, a fetus may lack 16-hydroxylase activity. In these instances there is relatively normal E_1 and E_2 but very little E_3 formation.

The placenta secretes E_3 into the maternal as well as into the fetal circulation; in the fetus E_3 is predominantly sulfurylated but is also converted into glucosiduronates. Unconjugated E_3 crosses the placenta most readily. In the mother E_3 metabolism consists almost entirely of conjugation, after which E_3 is excreted in the urine as glucosiduronates. Urinary E_3 excretion at term averages 30 mg per 24 hours. The binding affinity of E_3 to estrogen receptors is similar to that of E_1 and E_2. However, because of the short retention time of E_3 in the cytoplasmic estrogen receptors, manifestations of biologic activity require sustained and large amounts of E_3 delivered to the target cells. Because it is produced in such large quantity, E_3 is considered biologically important in estrogen-mediated events of pregnancy, such as the increase in uterine blood flow.

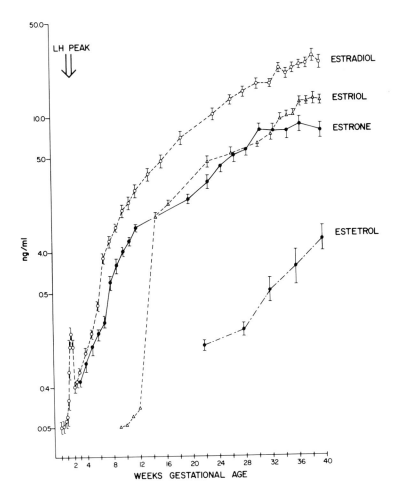

FIG. 19-10. The relative concentrations (mean ± standard error) and the incremental patterns of the four major estrogens plotted in the log scale during the course of pregnancy. (Courtesy of J Marshall)

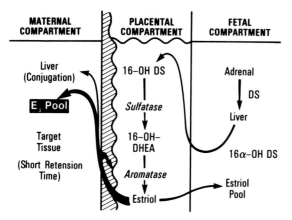

FIG. 19-11. Diagrammatic illustration of placental formation of estriol (E_3) exclusively from the fetal precursor 16α-hydroxydehydroepiandrosterone sulfate (*16αOH DS*). *16-OH-DHEA,* 16-hydroxydehydroepiandrosterone.

Estetrol, E_4, is 15-hydroxyestriol, distinguished from E_3 by a fourth hydroxyl group on carbon atom 15. This fourth hydroxyl group is introduced predominantly in the fetal liver by the action of 15-hydroxylase. The secretion of E_4 increases progressively after midgestation (see Fig. 19-10). This uniquely fetal estrogen is capable of binding to estradiol receptors but is devoid of estrogenic activity and has therefore been considered an endogenous antiestrogen. E_4 may have a "neutralizing" effect in pregnancy.

Placental Sulfatase Deficiency

France and Liggins first reported a case of very low urinary estrogen excretion and prolonged gestation in two consecutive pregnancies. Subsequent studies have con-

firmed their findings of placental sulfatase deficiency and inability to cleave steroid sulfates both *in vitro* and *in vivo* (Fig. 19-12*A*). However, the aromatization of free DHEA to estrogens by the placenta remains intact (Fig. 19-12*B*). Thus, E_1 and E_2 levels in maternal circulation may be in the low normal range, whereas E_3 and E_4 levels are strongly affected. This relative lack of estrogens appears to cause a delay in the onset of labor, which may lead to postmaturity and intrauterine death unless a cesarean section is performed. Patients with placental sulfatase deficiency are resistant to induction of labor by oxytocin. These observations, together with the prolongation of pregnancy in the case of an anencephalic fetus, support the concept that estrogens play an important role in determining the onset of labor. Placental sulfatase deficiency occurs in families as an X-linked genetic somatic inherited disease. The affected offspring are male. Thus, a careful family history may provide clues for prospective diagnostic exclusion (*e.g.,* measurement of urinary E_3 in suspected cases).

HUMAN CHORIONIC PEPTIDE AND NEUROPEPTIDE HORMONES

The intimate association between cells yielding neuropeptides (cytotrophoblast) and those producing protein hormones (hCG, human placental lactogen [hPL], syncytiotrophoblast) suggests the possibility of a trophoblastic control system resembling a compressed hypothalamic–pituitary complex. This idea is supported by the function of the decidua, a specialized endocrine compartment that borders the fetal membranes and the myometrium, that produces prolactin, relaxin, and prostaglandins, and that contains oxytocin receptors; these substances may perform local functions as well as act as links between the fetus and its environment.

FIG. 19-12. (*A*) Demonstration of the inability of placenta from a patient with placental sulfatase deficiency to cleave-labeled ^{3}H-dehydroepiandrosterone sulfate ([^3H]*DS*) to ^{3}H-dehydroepiandrosterone ([^3H]*D*), in contrast to normal placenta (*control*). (*B*) Although the placental conversion of DHAS to free DHA is impaired in patients with sulfatase deficiency (as shown in *A*), the formation of E_1 and E_2 from free DHA (*D*) is functionally intact. (Osathanondh R, Canick J, Ryan KJ et al: Placental sulfatase deficiency: A case study. J Clin Endocrinol Metab 43:208, 1976. Copyright © 1976, The Endocrine Society)

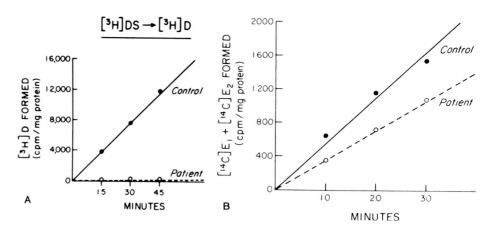

Human Chorionic Gonadotropin

Human chorionic gonadotropin (hCG) is a double-chained glycoprotein (molecular weight, 39,000), the α chain of which is biochemically and immunologically similar to the α chain of the three pituitary glycoprotein hormones: luteinizing hormone (LH), follicle-stimulating hormone (FSH), and thyroid-stimulating hormone (TSH). The β-chain is immunologically distinct, a unique feature that has been used in the development of radioimmunoassays; β-chains are both hormone and species specific. The separated subunits of hCG are virtually devoid of biologic activity. Each subunit contains 30% carbohydrate by weight. Dahl and associates have shown that asialo hCG is almost as potent as hCG but has much shorter half-life than the 5 to 10 hours reported for hCG. A major function of the carbohydrate residue of hCG may be prolongation of its half-life.

hCG is produced by the syncytiotrophoblast and secreted into the intervillous space; it is first detectable in maternal serum 9 days following a conceptual ovulation (see Fig. 19-1). This corresponds closely to the time of penetration of the trophoblast-covered blastocyst into the endometrial stroma and its consequent direct apposition to the maternal circulation. Serum hCG levels

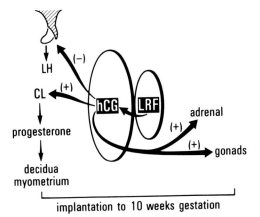

FIG. 19-14. Diagrammatic representation of the functional role of hCG in the maternal and fetal compartment during the first ten weeks of gestation. Note the potential control of synthesis and secretion (syncytiotrophoblast) by GnRH (cytotrophoblast). *LH,* luteinizing hormone; *CL,* corpus luteum; *LRF,* luteinizing hormone–releasing factor.

rise rapidly over the 10 days following implantation with a doubling time of 1.7 days. This exponential rise reaches a peak of about 100 IU/ml at the ninth week of gestation (Fig. 19-13) and is followed by a fall to a plateau of 10 IU/ml for the remainder of pregnancy. In women with twin pregnancies, hCG levels at four to five weeks after the last menstrual period are more than twofold higher than in women carrying singletons. During the last two thirds of pregnancy, increasing amounts of subunits of hCG are produced with relatively little intact hCG. This may account for the rather wide discrepancy between a higher immunoassayable and a lower bioassayable hCG in middle and late pregnancy. The renal clearance rate of hCG remains unchanged throughout pregnancy. The matabolic clearance rate is about 5 liters per day, and the initial half-life is about 5 to 10 hours. Relatively small but significant amounts of hCG appear in the fetal circulation.

The functional role of hCG in pregnancy is depicted in Figure 19-14. As already indicated, hCG provides the stimulus for the continued production of progesterone and relaxin by the corpus luteum that is essential for the maintenance of early pregnancy. Circulating hCG may also function to inhibit maternal gonadotropin secretion by the hypothalamic–pituitary axis through an autoregulatory mechanism. In fact, during pregnancy LH virtually disappears from the maternal pituitary gland (Fig. 19-15). In addition to its luteotropic function, hCG also provides gonadotropic and adrenotropic input to the fetus during the first trimester of pregnancy. The regulation of hCG secretion and synthesis is unclear. Recent evidence supports the idea that chorionic GnRH is a controlling factor; this is discussed in further detail below.

A remarkable characteristic of hCG (or hCG-like material) is its broad distribution. It is found in most,

FIG. 19-13. The exponential rise of circulating hCG following implantation and during first trimester of pregnancy. *BBT,* basal body temperature. (Braunstein GD, Karow WG, Gentry WC et al: First-trimester chorionic gonadotropin measurements as an aid in the diagnosis of early pregnancy disorders. Am J Obstet Gynecol 131:25, 1978)

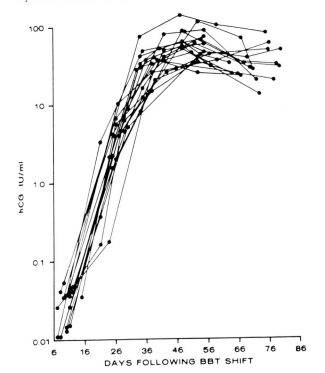

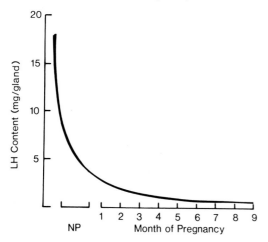

FIG. 19-15. The disappearance of luteinizing hormone (*LH*) in the human pituitary gland during pregnancy. *NP,* not pregnant. (After de la Mastra M, Llados C: Luteinizing hormone content of the pituitary gland in pregnant and non-pregnant women. J Clin Endocrinol Metab 44:921, 1977)

if not all, normal human tissues, in the urine and serum of normal men and women, and in many types of cancerous tissue. The hCG molecule has also been found in the human pituitary gland. The production of hCG-like material may represent incomplete suppression or depression in adult tissues of the fetal genome responsible for hCG biosynthesis. Alternatively, hCG-like material may be produced by relatively undifferentiated stem cells, which are responsible for cell renewal and which may not have differentiated to the stage of repression of the hCG genome.

Human Placental Lactogen

Human placental lactogen (hPL), a single-chain 191–amino acid polypeptide hormone (molecular weight, 23,000) produced by the syncytiotrophoblast, is also known as *chorionic growth hormone prolactin* and *human chorionic somatomammotropin.* Within the 191–amino acid sequence, there are remarkable similarities between human pituitary growth hormone and prolactin, suggesting a common ancestral gene. Unlike hCG levels, serum hPL levels rise concomitantly with placental growth (Fig. 19-16); daily hPL production at term averages 1 g to 2 g. The metabolic clearance rate of hPL is 175 liters per day, and hPL disappears rapidly from the blood following delivery of the placenta (half-life, 10–12 minutes). The functional role of hPL is shown in Figure 19-17. Although hPL has lactogenic properties and may participate in the mammotropic effect of pregnancy, it apparently is not involved in milk production in humans. Very little hPL is found in the fetal compartment; most is secreted into the maternal circulation, where it may function to inhibit maternal pituitary growth hormone secretion, which is markedly attenuated during pregnancy. Importantly, hPL may function to invoke some of the metabolic changes characteristic of pregnancy. Most noteworthy are its glucose-sparing and lipolytic effects, which can be attributed to its anti-insulin action.

FIG. 19-16. Circulating concentrations of hCG and hPL during the course of pregnancy. Note the contrasting patterns and the shift in the secretory activity of the two hormones by the syncytiotrophoblast at midgestation. Data expressed as μg/ml; 1 μg = 20 IU of hCG. *LMP,* last menstrual period.

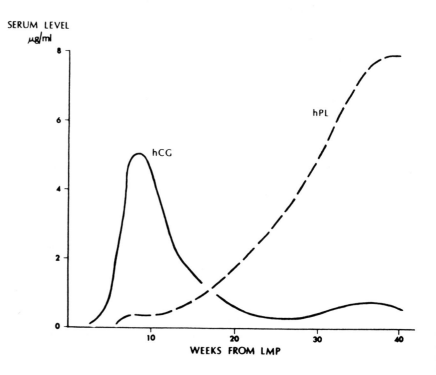

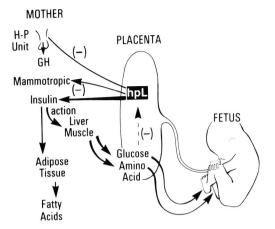

FIG. 19-17. The assumed and documented functional role of hPL in the readjustment of maternal metabolic homeostasis with preferential transfer of amino acid and glucose to the fetus. (−) indicates inhibitory effect. *H-P*, hypothalamus-pituitary; *GH*, growth hormone.

In this manner, the placenta directs maternal nutrients to the fetus, ensuring an uninterrupted supply of glucose and amino acids. The transplacental flux of free fatty acids, abundantly available through the lipolytic action of hPL in the maternal compartment, is limited, and free fatty acids are thus preserved as metabolic fuel for the mother. The active transport of amino acids by the placenta from the maternal circulation to the fetus results in maternal hypoaminoacidemia and limitation of the substrates (especially alanine) required for gluconeogenesis. This, together with hPL-induced lipolysis, accounts for the rapid development of hypoglycemia and ketonemia during fasting in pregnant women.

Human Chorionic Thyrotropin

The demonstration in 1955 by Akasu and colleagues that the human placenta contains a thyrotropic substance was followed by the isolation of a glycoprotein with a molecular weight of 28,000. The amino acid composition of this glycoprotein is distinct from that of hCG, and its carbohydrate content is only about one tenth that of hCG (3.5% versus 30%). This substance was named *human chorionic thyrotropin* (hCT). Unlike pituitary TSH, it does not cross-react with antiserum to hCG. Unexpectedly, it cross-reacts with antisera to TSH of bovine and porcine origin but not of human origin. It does not respond to hypothalamic thyrotropin-releasing factor (TRF). While pituitary TSH levels remain unchanged, hCT levels rise from about 7 μg/ml in early pregnancy to 30 μg/ml near term. Much greater amounts of hCT are found in neoplastic trophoblastic tissue. In some cases of hydatidiform mole and choriocarcinoma, serum thyroxine levels are elevated, and there may be clinical manifestations of hyperthyroidism. These

changes are attributed to hCT, since the intrinsic TSH-like activity is not sufficient to account for them. The true function of hCT is unknown.

Neuropeptides of Chorionic Origin

During the past few years, several neuropeptides, originally discovered in the brain, have been found in the placental villi, decidua, and chorionic membranes. These include gonadotropin-releasing hormone (GnRH), thyrotropin-releasing factor (TRF), somatostatin (SS), corticotropin-releasing factor (CRF), and ACTH–endorphin. In contrast to hCG and hPL, which are of syncytiotrophoblastic origin, these neuropeptides are exclusively located in the cytotrophoblast of the placental villi. This intimate association between the cells yielding neuropeptides and those producing protein hormones suggests the possibility of a trophoblastic control system, analogous to the neuroendocrine control of the hypothalamic–pituitary complex.

Human Chorionic Gonadotropin-Releasing Hormone

Gonadotropin-releasing hormone (GnRH), principally recognized as the hypothalamic decapeptide acting on the adenohypophysis to stimulate the synthesis and release of LH and FSH, has also been found in amniotic fluid and placenta. Gibbons and associates first reported the presence of a GnRH-like substance in the human placenta. *In vitro* incubation of homogenates of human term placenta with tritium-labeled amino acids results in the incorporation of radioactivities into a peptide with an elution profile similar to that of tritium-labeled GnRH as seen in ion-exchange chromatography. This GnRH-like substance is biologically active in stimulating the release of LH *in vivo*. The results of this study were confirmed by Khodr and Siler-Khodr, who also found that placental tissues cultured *in vitro* exhibit a fivefold to 40-fold net increase in immunoreactive GnRH content. The identity of this placental factor as GnRH decapeptide was later confirmed with use of a high-pressure liquid chromatographic system.

Immunofluorescence and immunohistochemical studies have demonstrated that the human chorionic GnRH-like substance is located mainly in the cytotrophoblasts of the placental villi, whereas hCG and hPL are of syncytiotrophoblastic origin. Studies on human placental tissue have yielded evidence suggesting that GnRH has the ability to stimulate the release of bioactive hCG. Measurement of the subunits of hCG indicates that GnRH stimulates the production of both α- and β-subunits of hCG in placental explants *in vitro*. These studies are consistent with the reported GnRH stimulation of hCG release by human choriocarcinoma cells *in vitro* and by the observed GnRH stimulation of monkey chorionic gonadotropin *in vivo*. Recently, Currie and co-workers demonstrated the presence of GnRH binding sites in human placenta, providing evidence that GnRH has a direct stimulatory effect on the biosynthesis and secretion of hCG by the syncytiotrophoblast (Fig. 19-18). Thus, it is proposed that placental GnRH plays paraendocrine role and that the human placenta resembles a ''compressed'' hypothalamic–pituitary unit that operates through intraplacental regulatory mechanisms.

Human Chorionic Thyrotropin-Releasing Factor

TRF-like material has been found in amniotic fluid, and the biosynthesis of TRF by the placenta has been demonstrated. Further information about TRF is not available.

Human Chorionic Somatostatin

Radioimmunoassayable amounts of SS-like substance are found in the chorionic villi and decidua of pregnant women. The presence of SS in the cytotrophoblast but not in the syncytiotrophoblast has been demonstrated by immunoperoxidase and indirect immunofluorescence techniques. Furthermore, there appears to be a progressive reduction in immunostaining SS but an increase in hPL as pregnancy advances. This decrease in cytotrophoblastic SS with maturation of the

FIG. 19-18. Intraplacental control system for the secretion of hCG and hPL; GnRH or luteinizing hormone–releasing factor (*LRF*) produced by the cytotrophoblast may play a regulatory role in the synthesis and secretion of hCG by the syncytiotrophoblast. hCG is synthesized on membrane-bound ribosomes, and its α- and β-subunits are translated from separate mRNAs rather than synthesized in tandem from one mRNA. Synthesis of the β-subunit constitutes a rate-limiting step in the production of intact hCG. First-trimester mRNA directs the synthesis of sixfold more α- than β-subunit, whereas term placental mRNA directs the synthesis of eightfold less α-subunit than does early placental mRNA and no β-subunit. The relationship between hPL synthesis and secretion is similar but reversed, and in this case the inhibitory action of somatostatin (*SS*) may be operational.

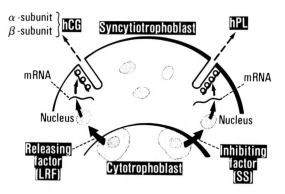

placenta may be involved in the progressive increase in hPL secretion by the adjacent syntiotrophoblast (see Fig. 19-18). The role of SS in control of the elaboration of hPL by the placenta merits further study.

Human Chorionic Corticotropin-Releasing Factor, ACTH, and β-Endorphin

It has been suggested that during pregnancy the placenta produces ACTH and is responsible for the relative resistance of glucocorticoids to negative feedback suppression of ACTH levels. Several investigators have reported the presence of both bioactive and immunoreactive ACTH in placental extracts.

Recent studies have established the existence of a family of peptides originating from a common precursor, a glycosylated molecule with a molecular weight of 31,000. This large peptide, referred to as *31K ACTH-endorphin,* or *pro-opiocortin,* is broken down into several smaller component peptides, including β-lipotropic hormone (β-LPH), ACTH, α-melanocyte–stimulating hormone (α-MSH), and β-endorphin (Fig. 19-19). It has been unequivocally established that ACTH, α-MSH, and β-endorphin, and β-LPH are present in the brain as well as in the pituitary gland of several species, including humans. However, the concentration of these peptides in humans is many times higher in the pituitary than in the brain. ACTH and β-endorphin have been found in the same hypophysial cells in humans. The presence of β-LPH, ACTH, and β-endorphin in human placental extract has been described in several reports. Furthermore, the fact of placental biosynthesis of this family of pro-opiocortin peptides has now been convincingly demonstrated. The recent demonstration of biologic active CRF-like peptide in the human placenta reinforces the concept of local neuroendocrine control of peptide hormone synthesis and release by the trophoblast.

Plasma levels of β-endorphin remain relatively low (mean, 15 pg/ml) throughout pregnancy. With the onset of labor, there is a several-fold increase in β-endorphin levels, with a further rise at delivery (Fig. 19-20). However, the molar ratio of β-endorphin to β-LPH does not change during pregnancy and labor, suggesting that pituitary processing of the precursor molecule is the same in the pregnant and in the nonpregnant state, as well as during the stress of delivery. High levels of β-endorphin (mean, 105 pg/ml) have been found in the cord plasma of term infants; these levels are parallel to those of ACTH, suggesting that both peptides are actively secreted either by the fetal pituitary or by the placenta (Fig. 19-21). There is evidence to suggest that hypoxia and acidosis may be major stimuli in the release of β-endorphin, β-LPH, and ACTH. Thus, β-endorphin elevation during labor and delivery and in fetal hypoxia-acidosis may reflect expression of the stress response. β-endorphin administered intrathecally (dose, 1 mg) has been shown to induce rapid and relatively lasting analgesia in labor patients.

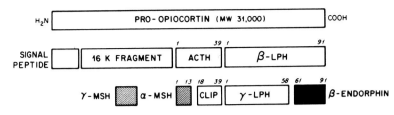

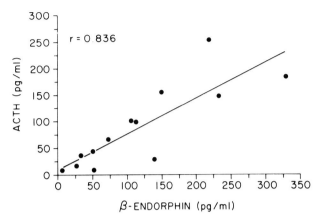

FIG. 19-19. Proteolytic processing of pro-opiocortin to form a family of peptides. *ACTH,* adrenocorticotropic hormone; *β-LPH, β*-lipotropic hormone; *α-MSH, α*-melanocyte–stimulating hormone.

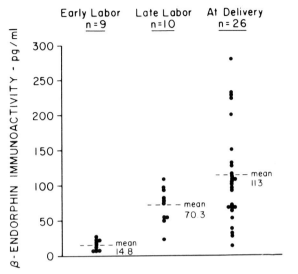

FIG. 19-20. Concentrations of *β*-endorphin in the plasma of women during early labor, during late labor, and at delivery. (Goland RS, Wardlaw SL, Stark RI et al: Human plasma *β*-endorphin during pregnancy, labor, and delivery. J Clin Endocrinol Metab 52:74, 1981. Copyright © 1981, The Endocrine Society)

FIG. 19-21. Correlation of *β*-endorphin and ACTH immunoreactivity in the umbilical cord plasma of a term fetus. (Goland RS, Wardlaw SL, Stark RI et al: Human plasma *β*-endorphin during pregnancy, labor, and delivery. J Clin Endocrinol Metab 52:74, 1981. Copyright © 1981, The Endocrine Society)

PROLACTIN IN PREGNANCY

Prolactin in the Mother

In pregnancy, serum prolactin begins to rise in the first trimester and increases progressively by term to 10 times the concentration found in nonpregnant women. When serum prolactin concentrations are determined serially at weekly intervals in the same individual throughout pregnancy, an approximately linear pattern of increase is seen (Fig. 19-22). This increase in prolactin concentration is probably due to supramaximal estrogen stimulation and reflects hypertrophy and hyperplasia of pituitary lactotropes.

The pulsatile nature of prolactin release observed in nonpregnant women appears to be maintained during pregnancy. Sleep-induced prolactin release also persists, but with pulses of higher magnitude. In pregnant women, as in nonpregnant women, an acute release of prolactin and cortisol occurs in synchrony with food ingestion. Thus, the food-associated release of prolactin by the hypothalamic–pituitary system is also functionally unaltered during pregnancy (Fig. 19-23). The physiological role of food-entrained prolactin and cortisol during pregnancy is unclear. Prolactin infusion in humans induces glucose intolerance and an increase in plasma free fatty acids. In hyperprolactinemic women, Gustafson and co-workers have observed a reduction in glucose tolerance associated with an exaggerated insulin response, as well as greater than normal suppression of glucagon by glucose, metabolic findings resembling those in normal pregnant women. Thus, food-entrained prolactin release may be subservient to endocrine–metabolic homeostasis in pregnancy.

Prolactin in the Fetus

The pituitary gland of the human fetus is able to synthesize, store, and secrete prolactin early in gestation; during the last few weeks of intrauterine life, there is an accelerated increase in these functions. At term the mean umbilical vein concentration of prolactin is higher than the mean maternal plasma levels (see Fig. 19-22). This high prolactin level declines progressively to the normal children's range by the end of the first week of postnatal life. Serum prolactin levels in anencephalic infants are essentially the same as those in normal infants (see Fig. 19-22). Since lactotropes are anatomically iso-

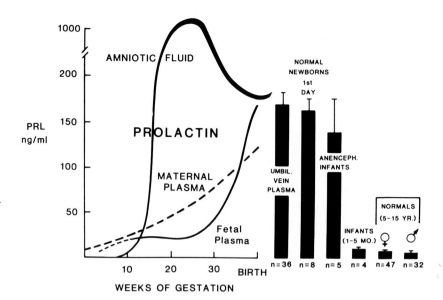

FIG. 19-22. Comparison of patterns of maternal, fetal, and amniotic fluid prolactin (*PRL*) levels during the course of human pregnancy. On the *right,* plasma levels of prolactin in normal and anencephalic newborns are compared with those of normal infants and adults.

lated from the hypothalamus in the anencephalic fetus, this observation provides confirming evidence that the principal hypothalamic control of prolactin secretion by the fetal, as by the adult, pituitary is through inhibitory mechanisms. The increase in fetal prolactin secretion is probably due to direct estrogenic stimulation of the fetal lactotropes. Although estriol production is markedly lower than normal in anencephalic infants, estrogen precursors of maternal adrenal origin are present, and 17β-estradiol and estrone cord blood values are in the low normal range. The physiologic role of fetal prolactin is unknown. However, experimental evidence indicates that prolactin in the fetal compartment may participate in fetal lung maturation. Administration of prolactin in pharmacologic amounts (1 mg) to the rabbit fetus leads to an increase in pulmonary lecithin levels; most notable is a rise in dipalmitoyl–lecithin, an active component of lung surfactants.

FIG. 19-23. Mean (±standard error) percent change (Δ) in serum prolactin levels (*PRL*) in seven pregnant women during fasting and after food ingestion at 1200 hours. (Quigley ME, Ishizuka B, Ropert JF et al: The food-entrained prolactin and cortisol release in late pregnancy and prolactinoma patients. J Clin Endocrinol Metab 54:1109, 1982. Copyright © 1982, The Endocrine Society)

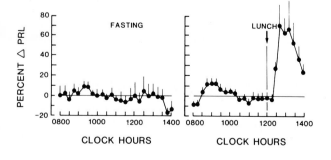

Prolactin in the Amniotic Fluid

The highest prolactin concentration is found in amniotic fluid, where it is five- to tenfold greater than in maternal serum. This high concentration is present as early as the first trimester of pregnancy, when both fetal and maternal prolactin levels are still relatively low (see Fig. 19-22). The human chorion decidua (but not the placenta) is capable of *de novo* biosynthesis of prolactin, and this prolactin is immunologically and chemically identical to prolactin derived from the pituitary. The secretion of prolactin by human decidual tissue *in vitro* is not influenced by dopamine or dopamine agonists, which are known to modify pituitary prolactin release. Prolactin binding has been demonstrated in the amnion, lung, adrenal, and liver of the fetal rhesus monkey. Furthermore, a 50% decrease in amniotic fluid volume can be induced in rhesus monkeys by an intra-amniotic injection of ovine prolactin; the effect persists for about 24 hours. Thus, it appears that prolactin produced locally may participate in the regulation of osmotic exchange in the amniotic fluid compartment. Additionally, decidua prolactin may serve in concert with decidua relaxin to modulate uterine contractility (see below).

Prolactin During Parturition

Prolactin secretion during and after labor follows a remarkable multiphasic pattern not found in patients who have undergone elective cesarean section. Serum prolactin concentration, which rises continuously throughout pregnancy, declines precipitously during active labor, reaching a nadir approximately two hours before delivery. Just before and immediately after delivery is a surge of prolactin release, which reaches a peak within two hours postpartum. Although the neuroendocrine mechanism behind this pattern of prolactin release is unknown, it is postulated that a transient increase in tubero-infundibular dopaminergic activity during active labor is responsible.

Lactogenesis and Lactation

Prolactin is the key hormone controlling milk production. The entire process of lactogenesis, however, requires a number of hormonal interactions. Growth of the duct system is dependent on estrogen synergized by the presence of growth hormone, prolactin, and cortisol. Development of the lobuloalveolar system requires both estrogen and progesterone in conjunction with prolactin. The synthesis of milk protein (casein and α-lactalbumin) and fat is regulated principally by prolactin and is facilitated by insulin and cortisol.

Neuroendocrinology of the Suckling Reflex

The maintenance of lactation in the puerperium is dependent on mechanical stimulation of the nipple by suckling. Sensory signals originating in the nipple during suckling are conveyed in an afferent pathway through the spinal cord, ultimately reaching the hypothalamus and inducing an acute response of the neuronal systems that control the release of oxytocin and prolactin. Denervation of the nipple or lesions of the spinal cord and brain stem abolish the normal response to the suckling reflex.

Three interrelated neuroendocrine events result from suckling: First, oxytocin release is induced by afferent signals to both paraventricular and supraoptic nuclei without concomitant release of vasopressin. The myopepithelial cells in the mammary alveoli and ducts are targets for oxytocin, which brings about contraction of these cells to induce the ejection of milk. An increase in episodic oxytocin release occurs when the mother plays with the infant or anticipates feeding. Milk "letdown" can then be observed; this phenomenon clearly illustrates the involvement of "psychic centers" in the neuroendocrine control of oxytocin secretion.

Second, when nursing is initiated, there is a prompt and large release of prolactin that is temporally associated with but independent of episodic oxytocin release. This transient increase in prolactin secretion is sufficient to maintain lactogenesis and an adequate milk supply for the next feeding.

Third, gonadotropin secretion is inhibited during pregnancy and lactation. Evidence suggests that hypothalamic β-endorphin may function as an inhibitor of hypothalamic GnRH secretion. The inhibitory effect of endogenous opioids appears to be increased during the postpartum period and to diminish progressively once lactation stops; at the same time, gonadotropin secretion increases, as does gonadotrope responsiveness to exogenous GnRH. This set of conditions may account for

the transient hypogonadotropinism of the puerperium. Prolongation of postpartum hypogonadotropinism during lactation is probably due to episodic hyperprolactinemia induced by suckling.

THE DECIDUA AS AN ENDOCRINE COMPARTMENT

The decidua is considered to be a specialized and complex endocrine structure as well as endocrine target tissue. To date the following endocrine features of the decidua have been described:

De novo biosynthesis of prolactin
De novo biosynthesis of relaxin
Prostaglandin synthesis
Presence of oxytocin receptors
Presence of $1,25(OH)_2D_3$ receptors
1α-Hydroxylase activity

The decidua is a membrane-like structure that is cast off after the termination of pregnancy. The decidual cell is a plump, glycogen-rich cell of stromal origin that appears during the late luteal phase of the endometrium and proliferates in early gestation. Anatomically, three portions of decidua can be recognized: d. basalis, which is present at the site of implantation and constitutes the maternal portion of the placenta; d. capsularis, which covers the gestational sac and disappears late in pregnancy; and d. parietalis, which lines the rest of uterine cavity and becomes laminated to the chorion. Thus, decidua can communicate directly with the fetus by way of the amniotic fluid and with the adjacent myometrium by simple diffusion.

Endocrine Characteristics of Decidua Prolactin and Relaxin

Explants of human decidua synthesize and release prolactin *in vitro*. When placenta and fetal membranes free of decidua are incubated under similar conditions, no prolactin release is found. Thus, it appears that trophoblast or amnion does not produce prolactin and that high amniotic fluid concentrations could be due to decidual prolactin synthesis. This idea is supported by the fact that decidual prolactin would be strategically placed to mediate local functions such as osmoregulation and myometrial activity. Furthermore, human prolactin and sera from hyperprolactinemic patients produce a prompt increase in the frequency and amplitude of myometrial contractility.

It has been clearly established that relaxin, an insulin-like peptide, is produced by the decidua and basal plate of the placenta. The long-held view that relaxin inhibits contractions of the uterine myometrium, promotes an increase in the distensibility of the cervix, and induces interpubic ligament formation has been confirmed in experimental conditions. Although the physiological role of relaxin in the normal progression of human gestation and parturition has yet to be established, it is possible that relaxin and prolactin play a role in the modulation of spontaneous uterine activity.

Oxytocin Receptors and Prostaglandin Production

Fuchs and colleagues have demonstrated that the number of oxytocin receptors in human myometrium and decidua increases progressively and in parallel fashion during gestation, reaching a maximum at the time of parturition. Furthermore, *in vitro* oxytocin induces prostaglandin production by the decidua but not by the myometrium. It stimulates uterine contractions by acting both directly on the myometrium and indirectly on decidual prostaglandin production. A fivefold increase in oxytocin receptors may be the first step in the initiation of labor, despite the absence of an increase in maternal oxytocin concentration even during the active phase of labor. Oxytocin from the fetus has the most direct route for delivery to its target cells. Such an oxytocin-initiated increase in uterine contractility might stimulate decidual prostaglandin synthesis, and these prostaglandins could then be conveniently diffused into adjacent myometrium to amplify uterine contractions. Thus, the combination of oxytocin receptor activation and prostaglandin synthetase activity in the decidua may be a decisive step in initiating human parturition. Other factors bearing on the initiation of labor are considered in Chapter 31.

Decidual Enzymes

As already indicated, the decidua has the unique capacity to produce 1α-hydroxylase, which is required to transform 25-OHD$_3$ to $1,25(OH)_2D_3$ (D$_3$). The implications are obvious. First, biologically active D$_3$ may participate in local calcium regulation, which is necessary to appropriate myometrial activity. Second, D$_3$ in the amniotic fluid may be ingested by the fetus.

Thus, the decidua is an endocrine structure as well as an endocrine target and may ultimately be shown to play an important role in the onset of labor, the regulation of amniotic fluid volume, and the control of calcium homeostasis and metabolism in the myometrium and in the fetus.

REFERENCES AND RECOMMENDED READING

Akasu R, Kawahara S, Ohki H et al: Thyroid stimulating hormone extracted from human placenta. Endocrinol Jpn 1: 297, 1955

Aubert ML, Grumbach MM, Kaplan SL: The ontogenesis of human fetal hormones. III. Prolactin. J Clin Endocrinol Metab 56:155, 1975

Ayala AR, Nisula BC, Chen C-C et al: Highly sensitive radioimmunoassay for chorionic gonadotropin in human urine. J Clin Endocrinol Metab 47:767, 1978

Bahl OP: Human chorionic gonadotropin. I. Purification and physicochemical properties. J Biol Chem 2244:567, 1969

Bahl OP: Human chorionic gonadotropin. II. Nature of the carbohydrate units. J Biol Chem 244:575, 1969

Bahl OP, Carlsen RB, Bellisario R, Swaminathan L: Human chorionic gonadotropin: Amino acid sequence of the α and β subunits. Biochem Biophys Res Commun 48:416, 1972

Bahl OP, Channing CP, Kammerman S: Effects of hCG, asialo hCG, and the subunits of the hCG upon luteinization of monkey granulosa cell cultures. Endocrinology 93:1035, 1973

Baulieu EE, Dray F: Conversion of ${}^3H$-dehydroisoandrosterone (3β-hydroxy-Δ^5-androsten-17-one) sulfate to ${}^3H$-estrogens in normal pregnant women. J Clin Endocrinol Metab 23: 1298, 1963

Belisle G, Guevin J-F, Bellabarba D, Lehoux J-G: Luteinizing hormone-releasing hormone binds to enriched human placental membranes and stimulates *in vitro* the synthesis of bioactive human chorionic gonadotropin. J Clin Endocrinol Metab 59:119, 1984

Belisle G, Schiff I, Tulchinsky D: The use of constant infusion of unlabeled dehydroepiandrosterone for the assessment of its metabolic clearance rate, its half-life, and its conversion into estrogens. J Clin Endocrinol Metab 50:117, 1980

Bigazzi M, Nardi E: Prolactin and relaxin: Antagonism on the spontaneous motility of the uterus. J Clin Endocrinol Metab 53:665, 1981

Bigazzi M, Pollicino G, Nardi E: Is human decidua a specialized endocrine organ? J Clin Endocrinol Metab 49:847, 1979

Bigazzi M, Ronga R, Lancranjan I et al: A pregnancy in an acromegalic woman during bromocriptine treatment: Effects on GH and PRL in the maternal, fetal and amniotic compartments. J Clin Endocrinol Metab 48:9, 1979

Bloch K: Biological conversion of cholesterol to pregnanediol. J Biol Chem 157:661, 1945

Bolté E, Mancuso S, Eriksson G: Studies on the aromatization of neutral steroids in pregnant women. I. Aromatization of C-19 steroids by placentas perfused *in situ*. Acta Endocrinol 45:535, 1964

Boyar RM, Finkelstein JW, Kapen S, Hellman L: Twenty-four hour prolactin secretory pattern during pregnancy. J Clin Endocrinol Metab 40:1117, 1975

Braunstein GD, Kamdar V, Rasor J et al: A chorionic gonadotropin-like substance in normal human tissues. J Clin Endocrinol Metab 49:917, 1979

Braunstein GD, Karow WG, Gentry WC et al: First-trimester chorionic gonadotropin measurements as an aid in the diagnosis of early pregnancy disorders. Am J Obstet Gynecol 131:25, 1978

Braunstein GD, Vaitukaitis JL, Carbone PO, Ross GT: Ectopic production of human chorionic gonadotropin by neoplasms. Ann Intern Med 78:39, 1973

Brown JB: Urinary excretion of oestrogen during pregnancy, lactation and the re-establishment of menstruation. Lancet 1:704, 1956

Brown RD, Strott CA, Liddle GW: Plasma deoxycorticosterone in normal and abnormal human pregnancy. J Clin Endocrinol Metab 35:736, 1972

Bryant-Greenwood GD: Relaxin as a new hormone. Endocr Rev 3:62, 1982

Cassmer O: Hormone production of the isolated human placenta. Acta Endocrinol (Suppl) 45:9, 1959

Catt KJ, Dufau ML, Vaitukaitis JL: Appearance of HCG in pregnancy plasma following the initiation of implantation of the blastocyst. J Clin Endocrinol Metab 40:537, 1975

Chatterjee M, Munro HN: Changing ratio of human chorionic gonadotropin subunits synthesized by the early and full-term placental polyribosomes. Biochem Biophys Res Commun 77:426, 1977

Csapo AI, Pulkkinen MO, Wiest WG: Effects of luteectomy and progesterone replacement in early pregnant patients. Am J Obstet Gynecol 115:759, 1973

Csontos K, Rust M, Höllt C et al: Elevated plasma β-endorphin levels in pregnant women and their neonates. Life Sci 25:835, 1979

Cummings SW, Hatley W, Simpson ER, Ohashi M: The binding of high and low density lipoproteins to human placental membrane fractions. J Clin Endocrinol Metab 54:903, 1982

Currie AJ, Fraser HM, Sharpe RM: Human placental receptors for luteinizing hormone releasing hormone. Biochem Biophys Res Commun 99:332, 1981

Diczfalusy E: Endocrine functions of the human fetoplacental unit. Fed Proc 23:791, 1964

Felig P: Body fuel metabolism and diabetes mellitus in pregnancy. Med Clin North Am 61:43, 1977

Fliegner JRH, Schindler I, Brown JB: Low urinary oestriol excretion during pregnancy associated with placental sulphatase deficiency or congenital adrenal hypoplasia. J Obstet Gynaecol Br Comm 79:810, 1972

France JT, Liggins GC: Placental sulfatase deficiency. J Clin Endocrinol Metab 29:138, 1969

France JT, Seddon RJ, Liggins GC: A study of a pregnancy with low estrogen production due to placental sulfatase deficiency. J Clin Endocrinol Metab 36:1, 1973

Frandsen VA, Stakeman G: The site of production of oestrogenic hormones in human pregnancy. I. Acta Endocrinol (Kbh) 38:383, 1961

Freinkel N, Metzger BE, Nitzan M et al: Facilitated anabolism in late pregnancy: Some novel maternal compensations for accelerated starvation. In Malaisse WJ, Pirart J (eds): Diabetes, International Series No. 312, p 474. Amsterdam, Excerpta Medica, 1973

Fuchs AR, Fuchs F, Husslein P: Oxytocin receptors and human parturition: A dual role for oxytocin in the initiation of labor. Science 215:1396, 1982

Gant NF, Hutchinson HT, Siiteri PK, MacDonald PC: Study of the metabolic clearance rate of dehydroepiandrosterone sulfate in pregnancy. Am Obstet Gynecol 111:555, 1971

Genazzani AR, Bennuzzi-Baldoni M, Felber JP: Human chorionic somatomammotropin (hCSM): Lipolytic action of a pure preparation on isolated fat cells. Metab Clin Exp 18:593, 1969

Genazzani AR, Fraioli F, Hurlimann J et al: Immunoreactive ACTH and cortisol plasma levels during pregnancy. Detection and partial purification of corticotrophin-like placental hormone: The human chorionic corticotrophin (hCG). Clin Endocrinol (Oxf) 4:1, 1975

Gibbons JM, Mitnick M, Chieffo V: *In vitro* biosynthesis of TSH- and LH-releasing factors by the human placenta. Am J Obstet Gynecol 121:127, 1975

Goland RS, Wardlaw SL, Stark RI, Frantz AG: Human plasma β-endorphin during pregnancy, labor, and delivery. J Clin Endocrinol Metab 52:74, 1981

Golander A, Hurley T, Barrett J et al: Prolactin synthesis by human chorion-decidual tissue: A possible source of prolactin in the amniotic fluid. Science 202:311, 1978

Gray TK, Lowe W, Lester GE: Vitamin D and pregnancy: The maternal-fetal metabolism of vitamin D. Endocr Rev 2:264, 1981

Grumbach MM, Kaplan SL, Sciarra JJ, Burr IM: Chorionic growth hormone-protein (CGP): Secretion, disposition, biologic activity in man, and postulated function as the "growth hormone" of the second half of pregnancy. Ann NY Acad Sci 148:501, 1968

Gurpide E et al: Fetal and maternal metabolism of estradiol during pregnancy. J Clin Endocrinol Metab 26:1355, 1966

Gustafson AB, Banasiak MF, Kalkhoff RK et al: Correlation of hyperprolactinemia with altered plasma insulin and glucagon: Similarity to effects of late human pregnancy. J Clin Endocrinol Metab 51:242, 1980

Hamosh M, Hamosh P: The effect of prolactin on the lecithin content of fetal rabbit lung. J Clin Invest 59:1002, 1977

Hellig H, Gattereau D, Lefebvre Y, Bolte E: Steroid production from plasma cholesterol. I. Conversion of plasma cholesterol to placental progesterone in humans. J Clin Endocrinol 30:624, 1970

Hennen G, Pierce JG, Freychet P: Human chorionic thyrotropin: Further characterization and study of its secretion during pregnancy. J Clin Endocrinol Metab 29:581, 1969

Hershman JM, Kojima A, Friesen HG: Effect of thyrotrophin-releasing hormone on human pituitary thyrotropin, prolactin, placental lactogen, and chorionic thyrotrophin. J Clin Endocrinol Metab 36:497, 1973

Hussa RO: Biosynthesis of human chorionic gonadotropin. Endocr Rev 3:268, 1980

Hwang P, Guyda H, Frieson H: A radioimmunoassay for human prolactin. Proc Natl Acad Sci 68:1902, 1971

Ishizka B, Quigley ME, Yen SSC: Postpartum hypogonadotropinism: Evidence for increased opioid inhibition. Clin Endocrinol 20:573, 1984

Jailer JW, Knowlton J: Stimulated adrenocortical activity during pregnancy in an addisonian patient. J Clin Invest 19:1430, 1950

Johansson EDB: Plasma levels of progesterone in pregnancy measured by a rapid competitive protein binding technique. Acta Endocrinol 61:607, 1969

Josimovich JB: Placental protein hormones in pregnancy. Clin Obstet Gynecol 16:46, 1973

Josimovich JB, Merisko K, Boccella L: Amniotic prolactin control over amniotic and fetal extracellular fluid water and electrolytes in the rhesus monkey. Endocrinology 100:564, 1977

Josimovich JB, Merisko K, Boccella L, Tobon H: Binding of prolactin by fetal rhesus cell membrane fractions. Endocrinology 100:557, 1977

Jovanovic L, Landesman R, Saxena BB: Screening for twin pregnancy. Science 198:738, 1977

Kanazawa S, Nakamura A, Saida K, Tojo S: Placento-thyroidal relationship in normal pregnancy. Acta Obstet Gynecol Scand 55:201, 1976

Kenny FM, Angsusingha K, Stinson D, Hotchkiss J: Unconjugated estrogens in the perinatal period. Pediatr Res 7:826, 1973

Khodr GS, Siler-Khodr TM: Localization of luteinizing hormone–releasing factor in the human placenta. Fertil Steril 29:523, 1978

Khodr GS, Siler-Khodr TM: The effect of luteinizing hormone-releasing factor on human chorionic gonadotropin secretion. Fertil Steril 30:301, 1978

Khodr GS, Siler-Khodr TM: Placental luteinizing hormone–releasing factor and its synthesis. Science 207:315, 1980

Konner M, Worthman C: Nursing frequency, gonadal function,

and birth spacing among !Kung hunter-gathers. Science 207:788, 1980

Krieger DT, Liotta AS: Pituitary hormones in brain: Where, how, and why? Science 205:366, 1979

Kumasaka T, Nishi N, Jai Y et al: Demonstration of immuno-reactive somatostatin-like substance in villi and decidua in early pregnancy. Am J Obstet Gynecol 134:39, 1979

Leake RD, Weitzman RE, Glatz TH, Fisher DA: Plasma oxytocin concentrations in men, nonpregnant women, and pregnant women before and during spontaneous labor. J Clin Endocrinol Metab 53:730, 1981

Lee J-N, Seppälä M, Chard T: Characterization of placental luteinizing hormone–releasing factor-like material. Acta Endocrinol (Copenh) 96:394, 1981

Levitz M, Young BK: Estrogens in pregnancy. Vitam Horm 35:109, 1977

Li CH, Dixon JS, Chung D: Primary structure of the human chorionic somatomammotropin (hCS) molecule. Science 173:56, 1971

Liotta AS, Houghten R, Krieger DT: Identification of a β-endorphin-like peptide in cultured human placental cells. Nature 295:593, 1982

Liotta A, Osathanondh R, Ryan KJ, Krieger DT: Presence of corticotropin in human placenta: Demonstration of *in vitro* synthesis. Endocrinology 101:1552, 1977

Lyons WR: Hormonal synergism in mammary growth. Proc R Soc Lond 149:303, 1958

MacDonald PC, Cutrer S, MacDonald SC et al: Regulation of extra-adrenal steroid 21-hydroxylase activity: Increased conversion of plasma progesterone to deoxycorticosterone during estrogen treatment of women pregnant with a dead fetus. J Clin Invest 69:469, 1982

Madden JD et al: The pattern and rates of metabolism of maternal plasma dehydroisoandrosterone sulfate in human pregnancy. Am J Obstet Gynecol 125:915, 1976

Magendantz HG, Ryan KJ: Isolation of an estriol precursor, 16α-hydroxydehydroepiandrosterone from human umbilical sera. J Clin Endocrinol Metab 24:1155, 1964

Marshall JR, Hammond CB, Ross GT: Plasma and urinary chorionic gonadotropin during early human pregnancy. Obstet Gynecol 32:760, 1968

Martucci C, Fishman J: Direction of estrogen metabolism as a control of its hormonal action–uterotropic activity of estradiol metabolites. Endocrinology 101:1709, 1977

McCoshen JA, Tomita K, Fernandez C, Tyson JE: Specific cells of human amnion selectively localize prolactin. J Clin Endocrinol Metab 55:166, 1982

McGarry EE, Beck JC: Some metabolic effects of ovine prolactin in man. Lancet 2:915, 1962

McNeilly AS, Robinson CAF, Houston MJ, Howie PW: Release of oxytocin and PRL in response to suckling. Br Med J 286:257, 1983

Mishell DR, Nakamura RM, Barberia JM: Initial detection of human chorionic gonadotropin in serum in normal gestation. Am J Obstet Gynecol 118:990, 1974

Morgan FJ, Canfield RE, Vaitukaits JL, Ross GT: Properties of the subunits of human chorionic gonadotropin. Endocrinology 94:1601, 1974

Nakai Y, Nakao K, Oki S, Imura H: Presence of immunoreactive β-lipoprotein and β-endorphin in human placenta. Life Sci 23:2013, 1978

Nisula BC, Morgan FJ, Canfield RE: Evidence that chorionic gonadotropin has intrinsic thyrotropic activity. Biochem Biophys Res Commun 59:86, 1974

Noel GL, Suh HK, Frantz AG: Prolactin release during nursing and breast stimulation in postpartum and nonpostpartum subjects. J Clin Endocrinol Metab 38:413, 1974

Nolten WE, Lindheimer MD, Oparil S, Ehrlich EN: Deoxycorticosterone in normal pregnancy. I. Sequential studies of the secretory patterns of desoxycorticosterone, aldosterone, and cortisol. Am J Obstet Gynecol 132:414, 1978

Oakey RE, Cawood ML, MacDonald RR: Biochemical and clinical observations in a pregnancy with placental sulphatase and other enzyme deficiencies. Clin Endocrinol 3:131, 1974

Odagiri E, Sherrell BJ, Mount CD et al: Human placental immunoreactive corticotropin, lipotropin, and β-endorphin: Evidence for a common precursor. Proc Natl Acad Sci 76:2027, 1979

Osathanondh R, Canick J, Ryan KJ, Tulchinsky D: Placental sulfatase deficiency: A case study. J Clin Endocrinol Metab 43:208, 1976

Oyama T, Matsuki A, Taneichi T et al: β-Endorphin in obstetric analgesia. Am J Obstet Gynecol 137:613, 1980

Parker CR Jr., Everett RB, Whalley PJ et al: Hormone production during pregnancy in the primigravid patient. II. Plasma levels of deoxycorticosterone throughout pregnancy of normal women and women who developed pregnancy-induced hypertension. Am J Obstet Gynecol 138:626, 1980

Parker CR Jr., Winkel CA, Rush AJ Jr. et al: Plasma concentrations of 11-deoxycorticosterone in women during the menstrual cycle. Obstet Gynecol 58:26, 1981

Pelletier G, Leclerc R, Labrie F et al: Immunohistochemical localization of β-lipotropic hormone in the pituitary gland. Endocrinology 100:770, 1977

Quagliarello J, Goldsmith L, Steinetz B et al: Induction of relaxin secretion in nonpregnant women by human chorionic gonadotropin. J Clin Endocrinol Metab 51:74, 1980

Quagliarello J, Szlachter N, Steinetz BG et al: Serial relaxin concentrations in human pregnancy. Am J Obstet Gynecol 135:43, 1979

Quigley ME, Ishizuka B, Ropert JF, Yen SSC: The food-entrained prolactin and cortisol release in late pregnancy and prolactinoma patients. J Clin Endocrinol Metab 54:1109, 1982

Quigley ME, Yen SSC: A mid-day surge in cortisol levels. J Clin Endocrinol Metab 49:945, 1979

Rees LH, Burke CW, Chard T et al: Possible placental origin of ACTH in normal human pregnancy. Nature 154:620, 1975

Resnik R, Killam AP, Battaglia FC et al: Stimulation of uterine blood flow by various estrogens. Endocrinology 94:1192, 1974

Riddick DH, Kusmik WF: Decidua: A possible source of amniotic fluid PRL. Am J Obstet Gynecol 127:187, 1977

Riddick DH, Luciano AA, Kusnik WF, Maslar IA: *De novo* synthesis of prolactin by human decidua. Life Sci 23:1913, 1978

Rigg LA, Lein A, Yen SSC: The pattern of increase in circulating prolactin levels during human gestation. Am J Obstet Gynecol 129:454, 1977

Rigg LA, Yen SSC: Multiphasic prolactin (PRL) secretion during parturition in humans. Am J Obstet Gynecol 128:215, 1977

Ryan KJ: Biological aromatization of steroids. J Biol Chem 234:268, 1959

Samaan NA, Yen SSC, Gonzalez D, Pearson OH: Metabolic effects of placental lactogen (HPL) in man. J Clin Endocrinol Metab 28:485, 1968

Schindler AE, Siiteri PK: Isolation and quantitation of steroids from normal human amniotic fluid. J Clin Endocrinol Metab 28:1189, 1968

Serón-Ferré M, Lawrence CC, Jaffe RB: Role of hCG in regulation of the fetal zone of the human fetal adrenal gland. J Clin Endocrinol Metab 46:834, 1978

Shibasaki T, Odagiri E, Shizume K, Ling N: Corticotropin-releasing factor–like activity in human placental extracts. J Clin Endocrinol Metab 55:384, 1982

Shiu RPC, Friesen HG: Mechanism of action of prolactin in the control of mammary gland function. Ann Rev Physiol 42:83, 1980

Siiteri PK, MacDonald PC: The utilization of circulating dehydroisoandrosterone sulfate for estrogen synthesis during human pregnancy. Steroids 2:713, 1963

Siler-Khodr TM, Khodr GS: Luteinizing hormone–releasing factor content of the human placenta. Am J Obstet Gynecol 130:216, 1978

Siler-Khodr TM, Khodr GS: Dose response analysis of GnRH stimulation of hCG release from human term placenta. Biol Reprod 25:353, 1981

Simpson ER, MacDonald PC: Endocrine physiology of the placenta. Ann Rev Physiol 43:163, 1981

Simpson ER, Porter JC, Milewich L et al: Regulation by plasma lipoproteins of progesterone biosynthesis and 3-hydroxy-3-methyl glutaryl coenzyme A reductase activity in cultured human choriocarcinoma cells. J Clin Endocrinol Metab 47:1099, 1978

Szlachter N, O'Byrne EM, Goldsmith L et al: Myometrial inhibiting activity of relaxin containing extracts of human corpora lutea of pregnancy. Am J Obstet Gynecol 136:584, 1980

Teodorczyk-Injevan J, Jewett MAS, Kellen JA, Malkin A: Gonadoliberin (LHRH) mediated release of choriogonadotropin in experimental human and animal tumors *in vitro.* Endocr Res Commun 8:19, 1981

Tojo S, Kanazawa S, Nakamura A et al: Human chorionic TSH (hCTSH, hCT) during normal or molar pregnancy. Endocrinol Jpn 20:505, 1973

Tulchinsky D, Hobel CJ: Plasma human chorionic gonadotropin, estrone, estradiol, estriol, progesterone and 17α-hydroxyprogesterone in human pregnancy. III. Early normal pregnancy. Am J Obstet Gynecol 117:884, 1973

Tulchinsky D, Hobel CJ, Yeager E, Marshall JR: Plasma estrone, estradiol, estriol, progesterone and 17-hydroxyprogesterone in human pregnancy. I. Normal pregnancy. Am J Obstet Gynecol 112:1095, 1972

Tulchinsky D, Okada DM: Hormones in human pregnancy. IV. Plasma progesterone. Am J Obstet Gynecol 121:293, 1975

Tyson JE, Hwang P, Guyda H, Friesen HG: Studies of prolactin secretion in human pregnancy. Am J Obstet Gynecol 113:14, 1972

Vaitukaitis JL: Changing placental concentrations of human chorionic gonadotropin and its subunits during gestation. J Clin Endocrinol Metab 38:755, 1974

Vaitukaitis JL, Boss GT, Braunstein GD, Rayford PL: Gonadotropins and their subunits: Basic and clinical studies. Recent Prog Horm Res 32:289, 1976

Vaitukaitis J, Braunstein GD, Ross GT: A radioimmunoassay which specifically measures human chorionic gonadotropin in the presence of human luteinizing hormone. Am J Obstet Gynecol 113:751, 1972

Voloschin LM, Dottaviano EJ: The channeling of natural stimuli that evoke the ejection of milk in the rat. Effect of transections in the midbrain and hypothalamus. Endocrinology 99:49, 1976

Wardlaw SL, Stark RI, Baxi L, Frantz AG: Plasma β-endorphin and β-lipotropin in the human fetus at delivery: Correlation with arterial pH and pO$_2$. J Clin Endocrinol Metab 79:888, 1979

Watkins WB, Yen SSC: Somatostatin in cytotrophoblast of the immature human placenta: Localization by immunoperoxidase cytochemistry. J Clin Endocrinol Metab 50:969, 1980

Weiss G, O'Byrne EM, Steinetz BG: Relaxin: A Product of the human corpus luteum of pregnancy. Science 194:948, 1976

Wide L: Early diagnosis of pregnancy. Lancet 2:863, 1969

Wilkes MM, Watkins WB, Stewart RD, Yen SSC: Localization and quantitation of β-endorphin in human brain and pituitary. Neuroendocrinology 30:113, 1980

Winkel CA, Milewich L, Parker CR Jr. et al: Conversion of plasma progesterone to deoxycorticosterone in men, nonpregnant and pregnant women, and adrenalectomized subjects: Evidence for steroid 21-hydroxylase activity in non-adrenal tissue. J Clin Invest 66:803, 1980

Winkel CA, Simpson ER, Milewich L, MacDonald PC: Deoxycorticosterone (DOC) biosynthesis in human kidney tissue: The potential for the formation of a potent mineralocorticosteroid in its site of action. Proc Natl Acad Sci 77:7069, 1980

Winkel CA, Snyder JM, MacDonald PC, Simpson ER: Regulation of cholesterol and progesterone synthesis in human placental cells in culture by serum lipoproteins. Endocrinology 106:1054, 1980

Yen SSC: Endocrine regulation of metabolic homeostasis during pregnancy. Clin Obstet Gynecol 16:130, 1973

Yen SSC, Llerena O, Little B, Pearson OH: Disappearance rate of endogenous luteinizing hormone and chorionic gonadotropin in man. J Clin Endocrinol Metab 28:1763, 1968

Yen SSC, Vela P, Tsai CC: Impairment of growth hormone secretion in response to hypoglycemia during early and late pregnancy. J Clin Endocrinol Metab 31:29, 1970

Yoshimoto Y, Wolfsen AR, Hirose F, Odell WD: Human chorionic gonadotropin–like material: Presence in normal human tissues. Am J Obstet Gynecol 134:729, 1979

Course and Conduct of Normal Pregnancy

Neil K. Kochenour

20

Early in this century pregnant women in the United States received no prenatal care, and the physician or midwife was involved only with labor and delivery. The subsequent development of widespread, systematic prenatal care has contributed significantly to the decrease in maternal and perinatal mortality seen in this country in the past three-quarters of a century. Today the concept of prenatal care encompasses risk assessment, medical care, social services, nutritional counseling, patient education, and psychological support; for many patients it actually begins before conception.

Major goals of prenatal care are as follows:

1. To define the health status of the mother and fetus.
2. To determine the gestational age of the fetus and to monitor fetal development.
3. To identify the patient at risk for complications and to minimize that risk whenever possible.
4. To anticipate and prevent problems before they occur.
5. To educate the patient.

To accomplish this, a systematic, comprehensive healthcare plan is required. In this chapter a framework is presented for providing good prenatal care.

PRECONCEPTUAL COUNSELING

Various factors have combined in the last several decades to improve perinatal outcome dramatically. With aggressive perinatal care, survival rates of 45% in infants born at 26 weeks of gestation and greater than 90% in infants born at 28 weeks have been reported. It has become apparent that if optimal care is to be provided to the mother, the fetus, and the newborn, the perinatal interval should be extended to the preconceptual period. There are a number of ways in which the outcome

of pregnancy can be improved by preconceptual intervention; for example, preconceptual metabolic control in the diabetic patient may decrease the incidence of congenital abnormalities. Additionally, in those instances where a pregnancy may have an adverse effect on maternal health or where a maternal condition may have an adverse effect on a pregnancy or on the fetus, preconceptual counseling allows couples to make an informed decision concerning pregnancy. All physicians providing care to women during their reproductive years should be aware of the effects of medical conditions and medications on pregnancy, as well as the consequences of a pregnancy on a woman's health. These issues should be discussed with women prior to conception.

Maternal Disease That May Be Adversely Affected by Pregnancy

The effects that the normal adaptations to pregnancy have on maternal medical conditions must be considered. For example, most women with heart disease can tolerate pregnancy successfully; however, there are some conditions in which the maternal risk presented by pregnancy is excessive. Maternal mortality for women with primary pulmonary hypertension has been reported to be as high as 50% and for patients with Eisenmenger's complex, to be as high as 25%. It has been estimated that patients who have had thromboembolic disease have a 10% to 15% risk of a recurrence of the condition during pregnancy. Another medical condition that may place the mother at increased risk is Marfan's syndrome. The maternal mortality for this condition has been reported to be very high; however, recent data indicate that the risk is related to dilation of the aortic root. If the aortic root is not dilated, the risk to these patients is not increased. When pregnancy will pose an increased risk to patients, they should be advised of that risk before undertaking pregnancy.

History of Poor Pregnancy Outcome

Patients with a history of recurrent pregnancy loss may benefit from preconceptual evaluation and therapy. The lupus anticoagulant, an autoantibody directed against phospholipid, has been associated with recurrent spontaneous abortions and midtrimester fetal demise. Recent evidence indicates that treatment with corticosteroids and low-dose aspirin improves pregnancy outcome in these patients. Women with a history of preterm deliveries are at risk of recurrent preterm labor. Preconceptual evaluation of these women may reveal the problem to have a treatable cause, such as a uterine anomaly.

Maternal Medications That May Adversely Affect Pregnancy

Epilepsy complicates approximately 0.15% of pregnancies. The teratogenicity of some anticonvulsants has recently been recognized. For patients with seizure disorders who are contemplating pregnancy, it is essential that an effective medication with the least risk to the fetus is prescribed. Many women have been on anticonvulsant medication for a long time without adequate follow-up. The time to evaluate the need for continued medication is before conception, not during pregnancy. Although the teratogenicity of all anticonvulsant medications is not completely known, it appears that some are more dangerous than others. Phenobarbital is probably one of the safest anticonvulsants and trimethadione, one of the more dangerous. When a fetus is exposed *in utero* to diphenylhydantoin (Dilantin), the risk of the fetus developing the fetal hydantoin syndrome may be as high as 10%, with an additional one-third of fetuses displaying some characteristics of this condition.

A number of medical conditions require the use of anticoagulants. The most commonly prescribed anticoagulants are heparin and warfarin (Coumadin). Warfarin is commonly used for long-term anticoagulation. It crosses the placenta and has been shown to be a teratogen when used early in pregnancy. It has been implicated in central nervous system damage to the fetus when used later in pregnancy. Heparin does not cross the placenta in appreciable amounts and is recommended by many for use throughout pregnancy when anticoagulant therapy is indicated.

Isotretinoin (Accutane), a medication used for severe acne, is a human teratogen and its use should be discontinued before a planned pregnancy is begun. It is now clear that isotretinoin use during the early part of pregnancy is associated with a high rate of spontaneous abortions and congenital malformations. Anomalies reported singly and in combination include very small, malformed, or absent ears, atretic ear canals, cleft palate, cortical blindness, severe congenital heart defects particularly involving the great vessels and interrupted aortic arch, and central nervous system malformations (hydrocephaly, decreased cerebral tissue, and posterior fossa cysts). The exact timing and dosage needed to produce these abnormalities has not been established. Women who are placed on medications that are potentially deleterious to a developing fetus should be cautioned to use adequate contraceptive measures. Both prescribed and over-the-counter medications should be reviewed whenever a couple is planning a pregnancy.

The principles of teratology are discussed in detail in Chapter 30.

Immunizations

The rubella virus was first recognized as a teratogen in 1941 by an Australian ophthalmologist named Gregg. More than 20,000 cases of congenital rubella occurred during the 1964 epidemic in the United States. Attempts to prevent the congenital rubella syndrome in this country have focused mainly on the immunization of young children. Since the widespread use of vaccines began in this country, only 25 to 90 cases of congenital rubella have been reported each year. Approximately 10% to 15% of the adult population in the United States has no detectable rubella antibody titer and is at risk for infection. A strong case can be made for the assessment of rubella antibody titers preconceptually. Several states require an assessment of rubella antibody titer as part of their premarital screening.

Social Habits That May Adversely Affect Pregnancy

The fetal alcohol syndrome (FAS) was rediscovered in the early 1970s. Neither the amount of alcohol required to produce the stigmata of FAS nor the amount of alcohol that can safely be consumed is known. However, it appears that the greater the exposure, the greater the risk. In one prospective study of 685 women, 32% of the infants born to heavy drinkers had congenital anomalies, whereas only 9% of infants born to those abstaining from alcohol or drinking only rarely showed anomalies; 14% of infants born to moderate drinkers had birth defects. It appears that when less than one ounce of alcohol is consumed per day, the risk for obvious abnormalities is low; however, if animal studies are an indication, it is not zero. For those who drink between 1 oz and 2 oz per day, the risk may approach 10%, whereas for those who drink 2 oz or more per day, the risk approaches 20%. The stigmata of FAS have been found both in chronic alcoholics and in binge drinkers. Preconceptual counseling on the adverse effects of alcohol in pregnancy allows patients to abstain if they desire and can prevent months of guilt and uncertainty in patients who drink heavily either before they are aware of a pregnancy or before they have been apprised of the dangers of alcohol consumption during pregnancy.

That smoking has harmful effects was recognized as early as the 16th century, but it was not until the mid-1930s that concern was first expressed about the adverse effects of smoking during pregnancy. In 1936, Sonntag and Wallace investigated the effects of cigarette smoking in pregnancy. They concluded that there "are definite and real effects of smoking on the rate of the fetal heart." Subsequently, numerous investigators have examined the question, "What are the effects of maternal smoking on reproductive performance?" Although most reports are not well controlled for potential compounding factors that may affect fetal growth, the overwhelming consensus from both prospective and retrospective studies is that women who smoke during pregnancy will have smaller babies. The decrease in birth weight averages about 200 g and appears to be dose-dependent. There is also evidence to suggest that preterm labor is more common in women who smoke.

Genetic Risks

The risk of delivering an infant with a chromosomal abnormality increases with advancing maternal age. Although the most common abnormality is Down's syndrome, the incidence of other chromosomal abnormalities is also increased. These risks are discussed in detail in Chapter 2.

DIAGNOSIS OF PREGNANCY

The possibility of pregnancy must always be considered when medical care is being provided for women of reproductive age. Women with symptoms of pregnancy are not infrequently evaluated for some gastrointestinal disturbance; x-rays are occasionally ordered when it is not known that the patient is in the early stages of pregnancy; medications that are potentially teratogenic are ordered without counseling the patient; and patients with medical conditions that may be adversely affected by pregnancy are frequently not told of potential problems until after conception.

Although women frequently suspect that they are pregnant, this is not always the case. The diagnosis of pregnancy can occasionally be crucial. There are a number of methods for establishing the presence of a pregnancy, depending upon the stage of gestation. Physical examination, biochemical tests, and imaging methods can all be used. In general, the signs and symptoms that aid in the diagnosis of pregnancy can be divided into three groups: positive, probable, and presumptive evidence of pregnancy.

Positive evidence of pregnancy
    Demonstration of the fetal heart
    Appreciation of fetal movement
    Visualization of the fetus
Probable evidence of pregnancy
    Enlargement of the abdomen
    Uterine changes (size, shape, and consistency)
    Cervical changes
    Palpation of the fetus
    Braxton Hicks' contractions
    Endocrine tests
Presumptive evidence of pregnancy
    Cessation of menses
    Breast changes
    Congestion of the vagina
    Skin changes
    Nausea
    Bladder irritability
    Fatigue
    Perception of fetal movement

Positive Evidence of Pregnancy

The positive signs of pregnancy are (1) demonstration of a fetal heart distinct from that of the mother, (2) appreciation of fetal movement by someone other than the mother, and (3) visualization of the fetus with a technique such as ultrasound or x-rays.

Demonstration of the Fetal Heart

The identification of the fetal heart rate distinct from the maternal heart rate establishes a diagnosis of pregnancy. Fetal heart activity can be detected as early as five weeks after conception with the use of echocardiography. If real-time ultrasound imaging is used, fetal heart motion can be visualized by the seventh week of pregnancy. Any of a number of instruments that use the Doppler effect to detect the movement of the fetal heart or blood can be used to detect fetal cardiac activity between the 10th and 12th weeks of pregnancy. The fetal heart can usually be auscultated with a fetoscope by 17 weeks and almost always by 19 weeks of gestation (Fig. 20-1).

Appreciation of Fetal Movement

From about 20 weeks of gestation on, fetal movements can intermittently be felt through the maternal abdominal wall. Although these movements can be recognized by the mother weeks earlier, unequivocal evidence of pregnancy is provided only when someone else verifies these movements.

Visualization of the Fetus

As discussed in Chapter 15, the normal intrauterine pregnancy can be visualized ultrasonically by five to six weeks of amenorrhea and appears as a ring or circular

1. Enlargement of the abdomen
2. Uterine changes
3. Cervical changes
4. Palpation of the fetus
5. Braxton Hicks' contractions
6. Results of hormone tests

Enlargement of the Abdomen

The uterus is a pelvic organ until about the 12th week, at which time it can usually be palpated abdominally. However, prior to this, the patient may experience a sensation of fullness in the pelvis or a feeling that her abdomen is swelling. The uterus gradually enlarges throughout the course of pregnancy; this enlargement may seem more pronounced in multiparous women than in nulliparas because of loss of abdominal muscle tone in the former. This difference is frequently noticed by the patient, who feels that she may either have twins or be further along than her last menstrual period would indicate.

Uterine Changes (Size, Shape, and Consistency)

A few weeks after implantation, the distinct enlargement of the uterus can be felt on bimanual examination. Progressive enlargement noted during successive examinations several weeks apart is especially helpful as a diagnostic sign. The uterus changes during pregnancy from a pear-shaped configuration to a globular contour. When implantation has occurred near one of the cornua, the uterus is felt as an asymmetric organ (Piskacek's sign) with a well-defined soft prominence of the cornu on the side of the implantation. In later months, the uterus is elongated as the fundus grows upward. Hegar's sign is a palpable softening of the lowest part of the corpus that appears at about the sixth week of gestation. To elicit this sign, the examiner places two fingers of one hand behind the cervix in the posterior vaginal fornix, then compresses the lower part of the corpus anteriorly by retropubic pressure of the other hand. In pregnant patients a distinct area of uterine softening can be noted between two firmer structures—the fundus above and the cervix below. An experienced examiner can place great reliance on Hegar's sign, since very few conditions other than pregnancy cause it. The inexperienced examiner, on the other hand, may mistake the cervix for a small uterus, and the softer uterine fundus may either not be appreciated or may be thought to be a tumor of the adnexa. McDonald's sign, which is positive when the uterine body and cervix can easily be flexed against one another, depends on the localized softening responsible for Hegar's sign.

Cervical Changes

Softening of the cervix (Goodell's sign) can be detected by the beginning of the second month. The fibrous cervix of the nonpregnant woman normally feels

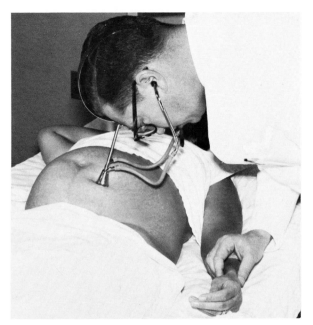

FIG. 20-1. Auscultation of fetal heartbeat with DeLee–Hillis fetoscope. Maternal pulse is checked simultaneously.

structure within the uterus. This echo pattern is known as a gestational sac and confirms the presence of an intrauterine gestation. By the eighth week of amenorrhea, fetal echoes can be seen within the sac, and a measurement of the crown-rump length (CRL) can be used to estimate the gestational age of the pregnancy accurately. A loss of definition of the gestational sac or the absence of a fetus by seven to eight weeks of amenorrhea is consistent with the diagnosis of a blighted ovum. By 11 weeks of amenorrhea, the gestational sac is not usually distinctly visible; however, fetal cardiac activity can usually be identified by this stage of gestation. By the 14th week, the fetal head and thorax can be visualized, and subsequently, the placenta can be localized. As pregnancy progresses, ultrasound visualization allows numerous fetal measurements and organ imaging. Assessments of fetal gestational age and growth and of the presence or absence of various fetal anomalies are all possible with the use of ultrasound.

After about 16 weeks of gestation, the fetus can usually be visualized on x-ray; nevertheless, because of the wide availability of ultrasound and the potential hazards of x-ray exposure, this technique is rarely, if ever, justified to diagnose a pregnancy.

Probable Evidence of Pregnancy

Probable evidence that a pregnancy exists includes the following:

like the tip of the nose. The effects of pregnancy alter its consistency to approximate that of the lips. Between the sixth and eighth weeks, the mucous membranes of the vulva, vagina, and cervix become congested and take on a bluish-violet hue (Chadwick's sign); it is especially well defined in the tissues around the vaginal opening and in the anterior vaginal wall, but it is also present to some extent throughout the vagina and on the cervix. Estrogen-progesterone contraceptives can also cause some softening and discoloration of the cervix.

Palpation of the Fetus

Early in the second half of pregnancy, the volume of the fetus is small in relation to the volume of the amniotic fluid. Sudden pressure exerted on the uterus may cause the fetus to sink in the amniotic fluid, and its rebound to the original position can be detected by the examiner (ballottement). As the fetus grows, it may be palpated through the abdominal wall. The fetus can usually be palpated earlier and more easily in multiparous patients because of their more relaxed abdominal musculature.

Braxton Hicks' Contractions

Beginning near the end of the first trimester, the uterus contracts intermittently. These contractions are usually irregular and painless. As pregnancy advances they become more frequent and are occasionally painful but, in general, remain irregular in timing and intensity.

Endocrine Tests

Pregnancy tests are laboratory determinations designed to detect the presence of human chorionic gonadotropin (hCG), a glycoprotein produced by the placental trophoblastic cells as early as the 23rd day after the first day of the last menstrual period. hCG has an α unit nearly identical to the α subunits of LH, FSH, and TSH. The β subunit of hCG is distinct from the other hormones. A first-voided morning urine specimen contains levels of hCG approximately the same as those in the serum; however, random urine samples usually have lower levels. Serum hCG levels increase exponentially between 21 and 70 days after the first day of the last menstrual period. After peaking at about 70 days, the serum level gradually falls until about 120 days, after which it remains at 5 to 20 IU/ml. These changes are discussed in Chapter 19.

Before the 1960s, a number of bioassays were used to reveal the presence of hCG in the urine. Pregnancy was indicated by the presence of various physiological effects of hCG in the bioassay animal following the injection of patient urine. For example, the Asheim-Zondek assay, developed in the late 1920s, relied on the formation of corpora hemorrhagica in the mouse to diagnose pregnancy. During the 1960s, many slide and

test tube tests for detecting urinary hCG by hemagglutination inhibition, latex particle agglutination inhibition, and latex particle agglutination were marketed. The slide tests, which were designed to detect urinary hCG levels of 0.5 to 4.0 IU/ml, could be performed in one to two minutes. One to two hours are required to perform the test tube tests, which are capable of detecting urinary hCG levels of 0.2 IU/ml to 2.1 IU/ml. The ability to recognize the β subunit of hCG is the most recent innovation in the evolution of endocrine tests for pregnancy.

With the hemagglutination inhibition method, anti-hCG is added to a sample of the patient's urine and then hCG-coated erythrocytes are added. If there is hCG in the patient's urine, it binds the anti-hCG and prevents the agglutination of the hCG-coated erythrocytes. Thus, a positive result is indicated by the failure of the erythrocytes to agglutinate. Examples of this type of test include Gravindex tube, Neocept tube, Pregnosticon tube, UCG tube, and UCG Beta tube. The principle of the latex agglutination inhibition test is the same except that latex particles rather than erythrocytes are coated with the hCG. Examples of this type of test are Gravindex slide, Pregnosis slide, Pregnosticon slide, Gest-State slide, UCG slide, UCG Beta slide, Placentex tube, and Sensi-Tex tube tests. In the latex particle agglutination test, anti-hCG-coated latex particles are agglutinated by hCG in the patient's urine. The DAP slide test is an example of this type of test.

In the middle 1970s, a radioreceptor assay for serum hCG was developed. This test is based on the principle that hCG in the test serum prevents the binding to pregnant bovine corpus luteum membranes of subsequently added hCG ^{125}I. Biocept G is an example of this type of test.

Currently, the most widely used technique for detecting low levels of serum hCG is the qualitative β subunit radioimmunoassay. This test is performed by adding β-hCG antibody to the patient's serum. If hCG is present, subsequently added hCG ^{125}I is unable to bind to the reagent β-hCG antibody, and the separated hCG:β-hCG antibody complexes will have low radioactivity. With the specificity of the β subunit antibody and the sensitivity of the radioimmunoassay technique, objective evidence of pregnancy can be obtained as early as the 23rd day after the first day of the last menstrual period.

Although with sensitive laboratory techniques, pregnancy can be diagnosed as early as the ninth day after the first day of the last menstrual period, this level of sensitivity is rarely necessary. The results obtained with urine pregnancy tests are inferior to those with serum tests; nevertheless, the sensitivity of urine tests is sufficient for the diagnosis of pregnancy in the vast majority of cases. A number of urinary tests are sensitive enough to detect urinary levels of 150 to 250 mIU/liter of hCG. These tests will record negative results in 90% to 100% of nonpregnant patients and positive results in 60% to 90% of patients with 200 to 1000 mIU β-hCG/liter. Recently, a number of pregnancy tests have claimed sensitivity of 1250 mIU/liter. The test will be negative in about 98% of nonpregnant patients but will only identify about 80% of pregnant patients who have a serum β-hCG level of 1000 to 10,000 mIU/liter. The range of serum hCG from 49 to 56 days after the first day of the last menstrual period is 17,000 to 20,000 mIU/liter.

Presumptive Evidence of Pregnancy

Presumptive evidence of pregnancy are signs and symptoms that can be recognized by the patient. The signs include:

1. Cessation of menses
2. Breast changes
3. Congestion of the vaginal mucosa
4. Increased skin pigmentation and the appearance of abdominal striae

The symptoms include:

1. Nausea
2. Frequency of urination
3. Fatigue
4. Perception of fetal movement

Cessation of Menses

Pregnancy should be suspected whenever a woman who has had regular menstrual cycles notices the abrupt cessation of menses. By the time the second menstrual period is missed, the probability of pregnancy is high. Although the cessation of menses is usually a reliable sign of pregnancy, pregnancy can occur without prior menstruation. Pregnancy has occurred prior to menarche; during lactation, when most women do not menstruate; and in women who believe they have passed the menopause. Additionally, about 8% of pregnant women will have a small amount of bleeding on or before the 40th day. This bleeding is thought to be related to implantation. This sign is difficult to evaluate in a patient with an irregular bleeding pattern. When oral contraception is stopped, pregnancy sometimes intervenes before the occurrence of spontaneous menstruation.

Breast Changes

Shortly after the first missed menstrual period, the pregnant woman notices a heavy sensation in the breasts, accompanied by tingling and soreness. The changes in the breasts that accompany pregnancy are caused by hormonal stimulation of the ducts and alveoli of the breast parenchyma and may also occur just before a menstrual period. If there is accessory breast tissue in the axilla, it may show marked enlargement during pregnancy or on the second or third postpartum day

(Fig. 20-2). Occasionally, changes in the breasts similar to those of pregnancy are seen in women with high levels of prolactin, as seen with prolactin-secreting pituitary tumors and as a consequence of use of certain tranquilizers.

Vaginal Mucosa Congestion

As noted previously, the mucosa of the vulva and vagina become congested and take on a bluish-violet hue.

Skin Changes

Increased pigmentation and the appearance of abdominal striae are common in pregnancy and can also be seen in women taking combined estrogen-progesterone contraceptives.

Nausea

About one-half of pregnant women develop nausea with or without vomiting early in pregnancy. This symptom usually appears between the 2nd and 12th weeks of pregnancy and subsides six to eight weeks later. Occasionally, it persists throughout pregnancy, and only rarely does it first appear after the first trimester. The nausea is commonly most severe on awakening in the morning and tends to lessen as the day progresses. Sim-

FIG. 20-2. Pregnancy hypertrophy of axillary breast tissue.

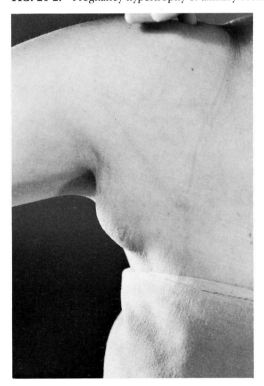

ple treatments, such as crackers before rising, frequent snacks, and avoidance of foods that promote nausea, are usually adequate therapy; however, medication is occasionally required.

Bladder Irritability

Early in pregnancy, the enlarging uterus exerts pressure on the bladder. The consequent bladder irritability and reduced capacity frequently result in urinary frequency. This symptom usually resolves by the second trimester, only to return late in pregnancy when the fetal head descends into the pelvis.

Fatigue

Fatigue is a common, sometimes severe, symptom of early pregnancy. This fatigue is often out of proportion with what would be expected, and its cause is unclear. It usually, but not always, resolves by the 20th week.

Perception of Fetal Movement

Between the 16th and 18th weeks of pregnancy in a multipara and usually several weeks later in a primipara, the patient becomes aware of a peculiar sensation in the abdomen, often described as a fluttering. This is caused by fetal movement, and the time it is first recognized is referred to as "quickening." Multiparas tend to notice quickening somewhat earlier, presumably because the symptom is remembered from a previous pregnancy.

Differential Diagnosis of Pregnancy

Although the progressive changes that occur during pregnancy are characteristic, it may be difficult to differentiate early pregnancy from other conditions.

Leiomyomas

Uterine enlargement secondary to leiomyomas can simulate the enlargement of pregnancy. In the patient with leiomyomas, however, breast changes do not occur, the uterus is usually firmer and more irregular in contour than in pregnancy, amenorrhea occurs only coincidentally, and the pregnancy test results are negative.

Ovarian Cysts

The soft consistency of an ovarian cyst can closely resemble that of the pregnant uterus; however, neither the softening of the cervix nor the discoloration of the vagina is present. When the mass is large, the differentiation between an ovarian cyst and a pregnancy can be made by ultrasonography.

Hematometra

An imperforate hymen or vaginal or cervical stenosis may result in an enlarged, intermittently contractile uterus in association with amenorrhea. Breast, vaginal, and cervical changes do not occur, and the pregnancy test results are negative. Ultrasound scanning will fail to reveal a fetus or placenta.

Pseudocyesis

Although most often found in women nearing menopause, pseudocyesis (imaginary pregnancy) occurs also in young women who have a strong, unfulfilled desire for pregnancy. It is associated with all the subjective symptoms of true pregnancy. The abdomen may appear enlarged and the patient interprets gas in the intestines or other abdominal sensations as fetal movement. On examination, the uterus is not enlarged, and there are no pelvic signs of pregnancy. Results of pregnancy testing are negative, and there is no objective evidence of a fetus. The physician may encounter difficulty in convincing the patient with pseudocyesis that she is not pregnant. In such cases, the patient should be referred to a psychiatrist.

DIAGNOSIS OF FETAL LIFE OR DEATH

Signs of Fetal Life

The widespread availability of Doppler and real-time ultrasound devices has greatly simplified the diagnosis of fetal life. Proof of fetal life is provided by hearing the fetal heart with either a stethoscope or a Doppler instrument, visualizing the fetal heart with a real-time ultrasound device, or palpating fetal movements. As noted previously, fetal cardiac activity can usually be discerned as early as the seventh week of pregnancy with real-time ultrasound and by the 10th to 12th week with Doppler techniques.

Diagnosis of Fetal Death

Early in pregnancy, fetal death is accompanied initially by a failure of uterine growth and by the regression of many of the signs of pregnancy. Repeated examinations that indicate a failure of the uterus to grow or even a decrease in size are strongly suggestive of embryonic or fetal death. Because the placenta may continue to produce hCG for several weeks after embryonic or fetal death, positive endocrine tests do not necessarily indicate a continuing viable pregnancy. Real-time ultrasound scanning is the primary method for establishing the diagnosis of fetal death. Very early in pregnancy, however, a single ultrasound examination may be inadequate to diagnose embryonic death beyond question. A gestational sac without a fetus, for instance, may be the result of a blighted ovum or may be a normal pregnancy that is earlier than anticipated. In this instance, reexamination after an interval of one to two weeks should enable the physician to differentiate between these possibilities.

Later in pregnancy, the failure to feel fetal movement may alert the mother to the possibility of a fetal death. If the fetal heart cannot be auscultated or detected with a Doppler device, fetal death is likely; however, the diagnosis must be established beyond a doubt before measures to terminate the pregnancy are initiated. Real-time ultrasound is the best method for confirming the diagnosis of fetal demise. Preferably, two independent observers should document the lack of fetal cardiac activity before this diagnosis is made. Caution must also be exercised, especially by an inexperienced observer, before the diagnosis of fetal demise is ruled out because transmitted maternal pulsations can produce heart motion resembling fetal bradycardia in a dead fetus. When the fetus dies, maternal weight gain usually ceases and breast changes regress.

If ultrasound is not available, the fetus has been dead for at least a few days, and the pregnancy has progressed to a point where the fetus is visible on radiography, x-rays can be used to establish the diagnosis definitively. There are three principal radiographic signs of fetal death:

1. Overlapping of the fetal cranium (Spalding's sign), which follows liquefaction of the fetal brain. Similar overlapping can occasionally be seen in a living fetus when the head is compressed in the maternal pelvis.
2. Exaggerated curvature of the fetal spine because of deterioration of the spinous ligaments.
3. Presence of gas in the fetal abdomen (Robert's sign).

When a fetus has been dead for several days, the amniotic fluid becomes a dark brown; however, this sign is not diagnostic, since hemorrhage into the amniotic cavity can cause a similar discoloration.

ESTIMATION OF THE DURATION OF PREGNANCY

Pregnancy begins with the fertilization of the ovum. Since the exact time of this event is not usually accurately known, the exact duration of a pregnancy generally is unknown. Nevertheless, because duration is one of the most important parameters to be considered when clinical judgments are being made, an accurate determination of gestational length is one of the important functions of prenatal care. Several methods can be used to estimate the duration of a pregnancy with reasonable accuracy.

Nägele's Rule

The mean duration of pregnancy is approximately 266 days from conception. Since the date of conception is rarely known, it is clinically more useful to measure the length of gestation from the first day of the last menstrual period. Several large studies have found the average duration of pregnancy from the first day of the last menstrual period to range between 279 and 282 days. A convenient method of estimating the date of confinement is Nägele's rule: to the last day of the last normal menstruation, add seven days, subtract three months, and add one year to obtain the estimated date of confinement (EDC). For example, if the first day of the last normal menstrual period began on May 5, 1986, the EDC would be February 12, 1987. Obviously, this method is based on the premise that most women ovulate about day 14 of a 28-day cycle. When the time of conception is known or when a woman has a cycle that varies significantly from 28 days, a more accurate estimation of the EDC can be made by using the 266-day average length of gestation.

Timing from Quickening

Maternal perception of fetal movement can furnish a rough estimate of the duration of a pregnancy. Movement is usually perceived initially between the 16th and 18th weeks in a multipara and several weeks later in a primipara. This method is useful more as a confirmation of the other parameters than as a primary method of assessing gestational age.

Height of the Fundus

The progressive enlargement of the uterus can be followed during pregnancy and the height of the fundus used to estimate gestational age (Fig. 20-3). The fundus can usually be felt above the pubic symphysis 12 weeks after the last menstrual period. At 16 weeks it rises to approximately halfway between the symphysis and the umbilicus, and it is at the umbilicus by 20 weeks. By the 36th week, the fundus is just below the ensiform cartilage, where it may remain until the onset of labor in the multipara. In most primigravidas, the fundal height drops slightly at the time of lightening.

Several methods have been devised in an attempt to relate the height of the uterine fundus to the gestational age. Spiegelberg compiled a table relating the distance from the symphysis to the fundus to the duration of pregnancy (Table 20-1). A modified form of this method is incorporated in *McDonald's rule,* which states that the fundus-to-symphysis arc in centimeters divided by 3.5 gives an approximation of the lunar month of pregnancy after the sixth month (Fig. 20-4). A number of investigators have reported that the height of the fundus, measured from the symphysis in centimeters when the bladder is empty, is approximately equal to the weeks of gestation between 20 and 31 weeks. Although these methods are not accurate enough to calculate gestational age precisely, when measurements are taken at each prenatal visit, they do corroborate other clinical

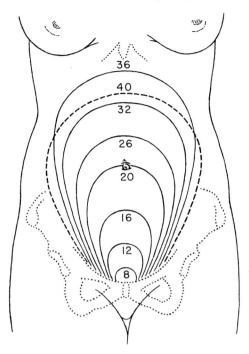

FIG. 20-3. Height of fundus at comparable gestational dates varies greatly from patient to patient. Those shown are most common. Convenient rule of thumb is that at five months' gestation, fundus is usually at or slightly above umbilicus.

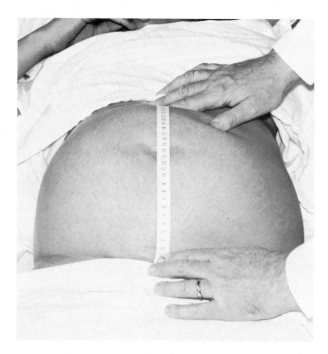

FIG. 20-4. Measuring fundus-to-symphysis distance by McDonald's method.

Table 20-1
Spiegelberg's Table of Relations Between Linear Distance from Symphysis to Fundus and Length of Gestation

Linear Distance Symphysis to Fundus (cm)	Estimated Fetal Age (weeks)
26.7	28
30.0	32
32.0	36
37.7	40

estimations of gestational age or may alert the physician to a discrepancy between the estimated gestational age and the height of the fundus. If the fundus is smaller than expected, the possibility of an earlier gestation or oligohydramnios should be considered. If the height of the fundus is larger than expected, a later gestation, polyhydramnios, or twins should be considered. If the uterus fails to grow as anticipated, the possibility of intrauterine growth retardation (IUGR) should be considered.

Since deviations from the expected rate of growth can alert the clinician to abnormalities of pregnancy, some measurement of fundal height should be recorded at each prenatal visit.

Ultrasound

Although clinical estimates of gestational age are useful and reasonably accurate in women who have regular menstrual cycles and who remember the first day of their last menstrual period, the obstetrical care provider frequently must estimate gestational age in the face of inadequate clinical information. For example, women can become pregnant following discontinuance of oral contraceptives or while lactating, can have irregular menstrual cycles, or may not remember their last menstrual period or may first be seen late in gestation. Recent advances in ultrasound imaging have made fetal age and growth assessment possible with a reasonable degree of accuracy. This subject is discussed in Chapter 15.

The accurate determination of gestational age is one of the most important goals of prenatal care. It is reasonable for the obstetrical care provider to ask at about 20 weeks, "Am I confident of this patient's gestational age?" If not, ultrasound should be used to determine the gestational age prior to the third trimester.

PRENATAL CARE: THE FIRST VISIT

The Record

An important contribution of modern obstetrics to the reduction in maternal and perinatal morbidity and mortality has been the systematization of prenatal care. Implicit in this emphasis on systematization is the assumption that all data that are gathered will be clearly recorded and available to all members of the health-care team when needed. To this end a number of standardized prenatal, intrapartum, and postpartum forms have been developed, many of which have the advantage of providing a built-in risk assessment system. (The details of risk assessment are discussed in Chapter 41.) It is certainly not necessary to use one of these forms to provide optimal prenatal care; nevertheless, it is the responsibility of the care provider to guarantee that all requisite historical, physical examination, and laboratory data are appropriately recorded and accessible when required.

Initial History and First Physical Examination

The first step in evaluation of the obstetric patient is the taking and recording of a general history and making a detailed physical examination. These must be sufficiently penetrating to uncover any current abnormalities and any prior ones that could have a bearing on the course of pregnancy. The details of the history and physical examination are outlined in Chapter 9.

Outline of Prenatal Care for the
Normal Obstetric Patient

First Prenatal Visit
Confirm pregnancy
Take history
Perform physical examination
    Pap smear
    Clinical pelvimetry
Order laboratory tests
    CBC, blood type and Rh, antibody screen, serologic test for
        syphilis, rubella antibody titer, urinalysis, screen for
        bacteriuria
Perform risk assessment
    Additional testing as indicated by risk factors
Facilitate patient education
    Instruct about danger signs, give handouts, answer
        questions

Subsequent Prenatal Visits
12 weeks
    Review prenatal laboratory tests, assess fetal heart tones
        with Doppler device
14 to 16 weeks
    Assess growth, order indicated genetic tests: amniocentesis
        or maternal serum α-fetoprotein
20 weeks
    Auscultate fetal heart with fetoscope
    Reassess gestational age if clinical dates not confirmed
    Consider ultrasound examination
24 weeks
    Begin education for birthing
28 weeks
    Administer Rh immune globulin when indicated
    Perform glucose screen for women over 25 years of age
    Repeat hematocrit determination
    Repeat risk assessment

30 to 40 weeks
    Observe for complications
    Initiate fetal surveillance when indicated
41 weeks
    Plan for postdate pregnancy

Every Visit
    Subjective: assess for vaginal discharge, bladder function,
        fetal activity, contractions
    Objective: assess blood pressure, weight, FHTs, fundal
        height, urine for protein/sugar; perform Leopold's
        maneuvers
    Answer questions
    Further patient education

Initial Laboratory Studies

Several basic laboratory tests should be performed early in pregnancy.

COMPLETE BLOOD COUNT. The hematocrit, hemoglobin, red cell indices, white blood cell count, and platelet count should be determined.

BLOOD GROUP STUDIES. Blood type and Rh positivity or negativity should be determined. All patients should be screened for the presence of antibodies. Although irregular antibodies occur in only about 1% of the population, several of them can cause erythroblastosis fetalis if present.

OTHER BLOOD TESTS. A serologic test for syphilis should be done on all patients and a test for the presence of rubella antibodies should be done if not previously performed.

URINE. A clean-voided specimen of urine should be tested for the presence of glucose and protein. If the patient has significant nausea and vomiting, the urine should also be tested for the presence of ketones. All patients should have either a quantitative urine culture or one of the several available screening tests to detect the presence of significant bacteriuria.

Patient Education

The initial prenatal visit provides the ideal time for the physician to begin what is a very important function of prenatal care: patient education. Usually it is possible to reassure the patient that she can anticipate an uneventful pregnancy and an uncomplicated delivery. If, however, risk factors have been identified during the initial visit, they should be discussed with the patient. She should also be instructed about the danger signs of pregnancy:

1. Vaginal bleeding of any amount
2. Persistent vomiting
3. Chills or fever

4. Dysuria
5. Abdominal pain or uterine cramping
6. Swelling of the face or fingers
7. Cerebral or visual disturbances: dizziness, mental confusion, or spots before the eyes are signs of severe preeclampsia
8. Oliguria: a marked reduction in the amount of urine can be a sign of severe preeclampsia
9. Headaches: any headache that does not respond to simple household remedies
10. Leakage of fluid from the vagina
11. Marked decrease in intensity or frequency of fetal movements

The expectant mother should be given information about many subjects, including diet, exercise, sleep, bowel habits, smoking, alcohol ingestion, medication usage, and sexual relations. It is impossible to impart at one visit all of the information the woman should have at the time her pregnancy is diagnosed. It is recommended that she be given printed information at this time, either in the form of notes that are prepared by the obstetrician to fit his or her particular needs, or as one of the paperback books that have been written for lay persons. If the latter, the obstetrician should have read the book carefully to be certain it supplies the kind of information that is desired. It is also extremely important to allow the patient the opportunity to ask questions and express any anxieties or fears she may have.

PRENATAL CARE: SUBSEQUENT VISITS

The routine examination of obstetric patients on subsequent visits is less detailed than the initial evaluation but has the same basic components. Certain measurements should be made at each prenatal visit, a history since the last visit should be elicited, a limited physical examination should be performed, the opportunity should be used for patient education, and the patient should be given ample time to ask questions and to discuss matters of concern to her.

Weight

The patient's weight should be recorded at each prenatal visit. A brief dietary history will elicit any major nutritional deficiencies or excesses.

Blood Pressure

Normally, both the diastolic and systolic blood pressures fall slightly during the second trimester of pregnancy and then return to prepregnant and early pregnancy levels during the third trimester. Patients with underlying hypertensive disease have an increased incidence of

preeclampsia, and the first sign of developing preeclampsia is usually the development of hypertension above prepregnant levels. A blood pressure reading in the third trimester of 140/90 or greater or an increase of 30 mm Hg in the systolic or 15 mm Hg in the diastolic pressure is cause for concern and requires further evaluation.

Urinalysis

Trace amounts of protein can appear in the urine as a result of contamination with vaginal discharge. As a general rule, proteinuria requires evaluation, and in the presence of hypertension it suggests preeclampsia; proteinuria in excess of 5 g per day in the absence of hypertension usually indicates nephrotic syndrome. Vaginal or urinary tract infection should be considered when small amounts of protein are present in the urine in the absence of hypertension. Glucosuria is seen in approximately 15% of pregnant women and is not necessarily abnormal. It is usually a consequence of the increase in glomerular filtration rate together with impaired tubular reabsorption of filtered glucose. Nevertheless, the possibility of diabetes cannot be ignored, and pregnant women with persistent glucosuria should be evaluated for glucose intolerance.

Systematic Examination of the Abdomen

By midpregnancy the fetus can usually be palpated through the anterior abdominal and uterine walls. After the fetal body becomes palpable, its position within the uterus is determined and recorded at each prenatal visit. The fetal position is determined by a systematic series of maneuvers, the *maneuvers of Leopold*. The first three maneuvers are accomplished with the examiner facing the patient's head and standing to one side of her as she lies supine on the examining table; the final maneuver is done with the examiner facing the patient's feet. Each maneuver is designed to answer by palpation a specific question regarding the relation of the fetal body to that of the mother.

FIRST MANEUVER. The first maneuver (Fig. 20-5) answers the question, "What fetal part occupies the fundus?" The examiner palpates the fundal area and distinguishes between the irregular, nodular breech and the round, mobile, and ballotable head.

SECOND MANEUVER. The second maneuver (Fig. 20-6) answers the question, "On which side is the fetal back?" The palms of the hands are placed on either side of the abdomen. On the one side a linear, bony ridge—the back—is felt, whereas on the other side are numerous nodular parts. This maneuver also enables the fetal

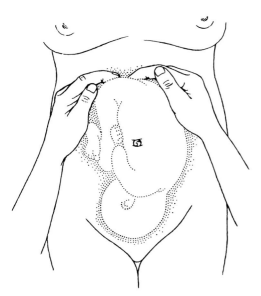

FIG. 20-5. Leopold's first maneuver. Answers question: What fetal part occupies fundus?

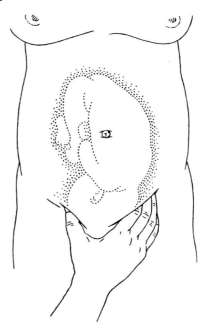

FIG. 20-7. Leopold's third maneuver. Answers question: What fetal part lies over pelvic inlet?

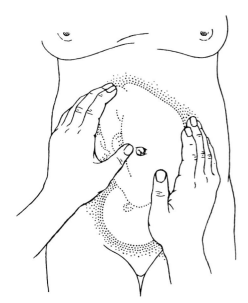

FIG. 20-6. Leopold's second maneuver. Answers question: On which side is fetal back?

position to be determined by disclosing whether the back is in an anterior, transverse, or posterior orientation.

THIRD MANEUVER. The third maneuver (Fig. 20-7) answers the question, "What fetal part lies over the pelvic inlet?" A single examining hand is placed just above the symphysis so as to grasp between the thumb and third finger the fetal part that overrides the symphysis. If the head is unengaged, it will be readily recognized

as a round, ballotable object that can be easily displaced upward. After engagement, a shoulder is felt as a relatively fixed, knoblike part. In breech presentations, the irregular, nodular breech is felt in direct continuity with the vertebral column in the dorsoanterior position. In frank and complete breech presentations, a knee or a foot may be felt in the dorsoposterior position.

FOURTH MANEUVER. The fourth maneuver (Figs. 20-8 and 20-9) answers the question, "On which side is the cephalic prominence?" The maneuver can be performed only when the head is engaged; if the head is floating the maneuver is inapplicable. The examiner faces the patient's feet and places a hand on either side of the lower pole of the uterus just above the inlet. When pressure is exerted in the direction of the inlet, one hand can descend further than the other. The part of the fetus that prevents the deep descent of one hand is called the *cephalic prominence*. In flexion attitudes, it is on the same side as the small parts, while in extension attitudes, it is on the same side as the back.

If the foregoing maneuvers disclose a significant abnormality (*e.g.,* transverse or oblique lie, breech presentation), further management depends upon the imminence of labor, as judged by both the duration of pregnancy and the condition of the cervix. If labor is considered not imminent, the abnormality should be noted in the patient's record but nothing further should be done, since the problem may correct itself before the onset of labor. If the cervix is soft and partly dilated and there is reason to believe labor is imminent, then

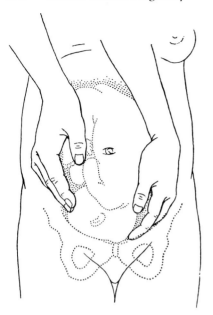

FIG. 20-8. Leopold's fourth maneuver. Answers question: On which side is cephalic prominence? In flexion attitude, cephalic prominence is on same side as small parts.

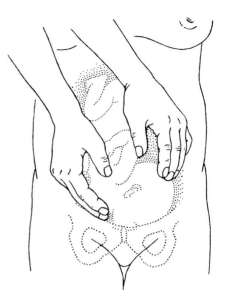

FIG. 20-9. Leopold's fourth maneuver. Answers question: On which side is cephalic prominence? In extension attitude, cephalic prominence is on same side as back.

specific evaluation and management should be undertaken.

External Cephalic Version

If the Leopold maneuvers disclose a breech presentation, the question of external version arises, a subject that has been a matter of debate for many decades. By the late 1970s, cesarean section was being utilized for the majority of breech deliveries at many institutions. Although improved outcomes have been reported for preterm and macrosomic infants, there is little evidence that abdominal delivery improves outcome for the breech fetus between 2500 g and 4000 g. Responses to the widespread use of cesarean section for breech presentation include protocols for vaginal delivery in selected cases, (*i.e.,* the frank breech between 2500 g and 4000 g), and a renewed interest in external cephalic version. Several large series have been reported in which an overall success rate of about 70% without morbidity or mortality has been achieved with external version in the late third trimester in carefully selected patients. Most investigators recommend that the procedure should be performed only after 37 weeks of gestation and only in a place where facilities for immediate cesarean section are available. The presenting part should be unengaged and a nonstress test should be reactive before version is attempted. The procedure is accomplished under tocolysis and continuous fetal monitoring. Real-time ultrasound is used to monitor the fetal position. The occurrence of fetal and maternal hemorrhage during this procedure has been reported; therefore, Rh immune globulin should be given to all Rh-negative women with Rh-positive partners. Contraindications to external version include marked oligohydramnios, placenta previa, rupture of the membranes, previous third-trimester bleeding, and previous myomectomy or metroplasty. It appears that external cephalic version in selected patients is a safe alternative for management of the patient with a breech presentation near term.

Other Obstetric Examinations

AUSCULTATION. At each prenatal visit, the fetal heart rate should be auscultated for rate and regularity.

VAGINAL EXAMINATION. A vaginal examination may be performed at any time during pregnancy if the information gained is necessary for the management of the pregnancy. However, routine pelvic examination, especially before term, should be discouraged, since it can lead to premature rupture of the membranes.

Other Tests During Pregnancy

In addition to routine laboratory baseline studies that are performed at the time of the first visit, various other tests may be indicated during the course of a pregnancy.

α-FETOPROTEIN. The advisability of routine screening of maternal serum for α-fetoprotein by immunoassay to detect fetal open neural tube defects is still under debate because of its cost and uncertainty as to what use is to be made of the information. Milunsky found the frequency of neural tube defects in the offspring of diabetic patients (19.5 per 1000) to be more than ten times higher than normal and recommended that pregnant diabetic women (optimally between 16 and 18 weeks) be routinely screened for elevated levels of serum α-fetoprotein. He also observed that the serum α-fetoprotein values were lower in diabetic patients than in nondiabetic patients. Screening is appropriate for pregnant women with family history of neural tube defects or a prior pregnancy that was so complicated.

GLUCOSE TOLERANCE TESTING. Glucose intolerance during pregnancy has been shown to be associated with an increase in perinatal morbidity and mortality, especially in women who are over 25 years of age or are overweight. In 1972, O'Sullivan showed that clinical history was an inadequate method for selecting patients at risk for gestational diabetes. He showed that a sensitive (88%) and specific (82%) screening test for the detection of glucose intolerance in pregnancy is a 50-g glucose load followed by a one-hour blood glucose determination. If the blood glucose level at one hour is greater than 130 mg/100 ml (150 mg/100 ml serum glucose), a full three-hour glucose tolerance test is indicated. Subsequent studies by Carpenter have shown that if the plasma glucose is less than 135 mg/100 ml, the chance of diabetes is less than 1%. If the plasma glucose at one hour is greater than 185 mg/100 ml, the probability of diabetes is greater than 95%. He suggested that the threshold for screening be lowered to 135 mg/100 ml plasma glucose. Lavin has estimated that the cost of screening per patient is less than $5.00 and the cost per case of gestational diabetes identified is approximately $330.00. Consideration should be given to screening all patients over the age of 25 at about 28 weeks of gestation.

SERIAL ULTRASOUND EXAMINATION. Although routine ultrasound screening of all pregnant patients is not recommended, serial sonographic examinations should be considered in a number of high-risk circumstances in which fetal growth may be in jeopardy or if gestational dates are uncertain. In patients at risk for intrauterine growth retardation (IUGR) or multiple gestation, for example, management may be aided by serial ultrasound determinations of fetal growth (see Chapter 15).

ANTEPARTUM Rh IMMUNE GLOBULIN. The widespread use of Rh immune globulin has significantly reduced the incidence of Rh isoimmunization. Unfortunately, 1% to 2% of Rh-negative women bearing Rh-positive infants will be sensitized before delivery. The postpartum use of Rh immune globulin will not prevent sensitization. The idea of antepartum prophylaxis was suggested in the late 1960s. Clinical trials were begun in Canada in 1968 and found that a 300-μg dose of Rh immune globulin given at 28 weeks of gestation reduced the incidence of sensitization from the expected 1.6% to 0.11% in the treated population. Subsequent trials have demonstrated both the efficacy and the safety of this regimen. This subject is considered in Chapter 24.

Weight Gain

During a normal singleton pregnancy, the pregnancy itself accounts directly for approximately 22 lb (10 kg) of weight gain. About 13.5 lb (6.1 kg) are accounted for by the uterus and its contents: 7.5 lb (3.4 kg) for the fetus, 1.5 lb (680 g) for the placenta, 2 lb (907 g) for the amniotic fluid, and 2.5 lb (1.1 kg) for the increase in uterine muscle mass. The normal maternal physiological adjustments to pregnancy account for another 7 lb to 9 lb (3.4 kg to 4 kg), of which 3.5 lb (1.6 kg) is for the increase in blood volume, 2 lb (907 g) for the increased breast tissue, and 2 lb to 3 lb (1 kg to 1.4 kg) for the increase in interstitial fluid.

The ideal weight gain for a woman during pregnancy has been a source of debate for decades. It is, in fact, impossible at this time to assign a specific "ideal" weight gain for a specific patient. There are, however, several generalizations that can serve as guidelines when counseling the pregnant patient about weight gain. For women who are of normal weight at the beginning of pregnancy, a weight gain of 20 lb to 27 lb (9 kg to 12 kg) is associated with the lowest rate of complications and incidence of low birth-weight babies. Both a low prepregnancy weight and a low weight gain during pregnancy are associated with an increased incidence of low birth-weight infants who have a higher perinatal morbidity and mortality. Women with a low prepregnancy weight should be encouraged to gain more than the average of 20 lb to 27 lb (9 kg to 12 kg). Women who are overweight at the onset of pregnancy should be encouraged to gain at least 20 lb (9 kg) during pregnancy. Failure to gain weight or weight loss during pregnancy are ominous signs. If a patient has not gained 10 lb by the 20th week of pregnancy, her dietary intake should be carefully reviewed.

Nutrition

A comprehensive discussion of nutrition in pregnancy can be found in Chapter 11.

Exercise

As more women engage in strenuous physical activity, the question of the influence of exercise on pregnancy outcome is more frequently asked. Concerns about the interaction of exercise and pregnancy include the potential effects of reductions in uterine blood flow as a consequence of the redistribution of blood during exercise, of increased maternal oxygen consumption during exercise, and of increased body temperature.

Data from which to answer these questions come primarily from two sources: animal studies, which in general address the issue of the effects of acute exercise on the physiological parameters of pregnancy, and human studies, which tend to address the effect of chronic exercise on pregnancy-outcome variables. There are several difficulties with this approach. Physiological parameters in animals may not directly relate to human responses. Human studies have tended to study healthy women who had trained before pregnancy and continued to exercise during pregnancy. The human studies have frequently been retrospective. In spite of these limitations, several generalizations can be drawn. Animal studies have shown that physical activity during pregnancy results in marked cardiovascular adjustments in the mother, including a reduction in uterine blood flow; however, because of simultaneous hemoconcentration and increased oxygen extraction, uterine oxygen consumption remains constant. In spite of marked changes in maternal physiology, fetal changes are small. The fetal arterial oxygen tension and oxygen content decrease slightly, but the other fetal variables remain essentially constant. This suggests that acute exercise does not represent a major hypoxic stress to the fetus. The most likely effect of chronic exercise appears to be fetal growth retardation, but the reports in humans are contradictory. Some investigators found no adverse consequences in women who regularly engaged in moderately heavy exercise; others reported a higher incidence of premature labor and small-for-gestational-age (SGA) infants. Because many factors influence fetal growth, large prospective studies are needed to answer these questions adequately. The effect of exercise on women with preexisting disease is also not known. A Bulletin published by the American College of Obstetricians and Gynecologists in May 1985 presents a program of home exercises and makes recommendations for exercise during pregnancy and the postnatal period.

It can be stated with reasonable certainty that women who have enjoyed good physical health before pregnancy will carry themselves and their fetuses safely through pregnancy while continuing established exercise patterns. Conversely, it would seem prudent to limit the activity of women with certain high-risk conditions such as multiple gestations, hypertension, previous premature delivery, and previous SGA infants.

Employment

As more women enter the work force, questions about the influence of work on pregnancy and the influence of pregnancy on work become more important. Categorical statements about the wisdom of continued work during pregnancy cannot be made from the available information. There is some evidence to suggest that working during pregnancy is associated with a decrease in infant birth weight. Other studies have failed to confirm this finding. Obviously, the range of activity and stress varies widely from occupation to occupation.

Recommendations should be individualized and take into account the type of job and the risk factors of the pregnant woman.

Immunization During Pregnancy

This subject is considered in the section on Viral and Protozoan Infections in Pregnancy in Chapter 30, and is summarized in Table 30-16.

Travel

Travel by the usual means does not directly jeopardize pregnancy. Any disadvantages to travel are indirect ones, involving such drawbacks as changes in dietary and sleep patterns and the possibility of not having competent obstetric care immediately available, should an emergency arise.

Prolonged periods of sitting, which entail the possibility of increased venous stasis, should be avoided during pregnancy. Long automobile trips should be broken up with frequent stops to allow the pregnant woman periods of walking. Pregnant women should also avoid prolonged sitting in aircraft by occasionally walking in the aisle. Travel in pressurized aircraft does not pose an additional risk to the pregnant woman.

Nausea and Vomiting

Nausea and vomiting are common complaints of early pregnancy. Typically, the symptoms begin early in pregnancy and continue until about the fourth month. Occasionally, the symptoms may continue throughout gestation. The etiology of this condition is unclear. Although some have postulated that it is caused by high levels of hCG because it seems to be more common and more severe in patients with conditions that lead to high levels of hCG, such as multiple gestations and hydatidiform mole, objective data have failed to confirm this association. Emotional factors appear to play a role in this condition but are probably only a contributing factor. Eating small frequent meals usually alleviates but rarely totally relieves the symptoms. Antinausea medications are occasionally required, but none predictably cure the condition. When ketonuria is present, the administration of fluids intravenously on an outpatient basis may provide relief. Infrequently, patients with severe vomiting must be hospitalized to correct fluid and electrolyte imbalances. Severe persistent nausea and vomiting of pregnancy is referred to as *hyperemesis gravidarum*.

Heartburn

A burning sensation in the epigastrium accompanied by a feeling of fullness is a common complaint especially toward the latter part of pregnancy. It is usually caused by the reflux of acid gastric contents into the lower esophagus. The upward displacement of the stomach by the uterus and the progesterone-mediated relaxation of the esophageal sphincter both probably contribute to this symptom. Relief is usually provided by the ingestion of liquid antacids such as aluminum hydroxide, magnesium trisilicate, or magnesium hydroxide and the avoidance of excessively large meals. It has been suggested that bile regurgitation may cause heartburn in some patients, and Atlay has suggested that patients who do not respond to alkali therapy should be treated with an acid mixture. The symptoms are often aggravated by lying flat. Late evening is a common time for the pain to appear, and elevation of the head of the bed may help alleviate the symptoms.

Varicosities

The increased venous pressure in the lower extremities that accompanies advancing pregnancy aggravates varicosities of the lower extremities and occasionally the vulva. The treatment of this condition consists of rest with elevation of the feet and the use of elastic support stockings. Support stockings should be the full-length, pantyhose type rather than calf or thigh length. Vulvar varicosities usually respond to support given by the wearing of several perineal pads.

Sexual Relations and Vaginal Hygiene

Until very recently it was generally accepted that sexual intercourse had no adverse effect on pregnancy outcome. Many practitioners advised against coitus in the last month of pregnancy, but even this admonition was not based on reliable data. In fact, until very recently, the question had not been studied. Several recent studies have suggested that sexual intercourse during pregnancy may be detrimental to some patients. Naeye has suggested that intercourse during pregnancy may be associated with amniotic fluid infections leading to premature rupture of the membranes with subsequent preterm delivery, neonatal respiratory distress, and perinatal death. Goodlin has suggested that orgasm after 32 weeks' gestational age may predispose to premature labor. Others have failed to confirm their findings. Nevertheless, until well-designed studies answer the question of the effect of coitus on pregnancy outcome, it would seen prudent to counsel high-risk patients about the possible adverse effects. Patients at risk may include those with a previous history of premature rupture of the membranes or premature labor and those who experience strong uterine contractions following coitus. At this point it does not appear that the data justify a dogmatic stance either for or against.

Douching is rarely indicated during pregnancy. If, however, it is required, the following guidelines should be adhered to.

1. Use only a douche bag and never a bulb syringe.
2. Do not place the douche bag higher than two feet above the level of the hips.
3. Insert the nozzle no more than three inches through the vulva.

Tub baths may be taken at will throughout pregnancy, since water does not enter the vagina under usual circumstances.

Bowel Habits

Constipation is a common complaint during pregnancy, presumably because of the steroid-induced suppression of bowel motility and the compression of the intestines by the enlarging uterus. Constipation aggravates hemorrhoids, which are another common complaint during pregnancy. Women who had normal bowel habits before pregnancy can usually maintain reasonably normal bowel function during pregnancy by drinking water liberally and having generous amounts of fruits, vegetables, and salads in the diet. Mild laxatives, such as milk of magnesia, bulk-producing substances, or stool-softening agents, may be used to maintain regular bowel habits. The use of strong cathartics or enemas should be avoided.

Alcohol

As noted previously, the fetal alcohol syndrome (FAS) is a distinct, dysmorphic condition characterized by prenatal and postnatal growth deficiency, facial abnormalities, cardiac defects, joint malformations, and mental deficiency. Alcohol intake should be sharply reduced—or, preferably, eliminated—during pregnancy.

Smoking

There is considerable evidence that women who smoke during pregnancy have infants who are an average of 200 g lighter than infants of women who do not smoke. In addition, smoking during pregnancy has been associated with a number of other complications, including premature labor, placental abruption, pregnancy bleeding, and premature rupture of the membranes.

Caffeine

Caffeine, a naturally occurring substance similar in structure to the DNA-base pair adenine and guanine, is probably the most widely used psychoactive drug in the United States. It is a central nervous system stimulant ingested by a large segment of the population in natural sources such as coffee, tea, chocolate, and as a food additive in many cola beverages. Although this drug has been generally recognized as safe, there has been some concern, centered primarily on caffeine as a mutagen and a teratogen and about its effects on catecholamine metabolism. Most of the incriminating evidence is based on animal studies in which the dosage levels and method of administration are often not comparable to the human experience.

One retrospective study suggested that reproductive loss is increased in women who ingest more than 600 mg of caffeine per day. This study did not control for confounding factors and does not prove any cause-and-effect relationship. Several recent, large studies in humans failed to show that caffeine has any deleterious effects when ingested in customary amounts.

Childbirth Education

Over the years a number of programs for preparation for childbirth have been developed. Their primary goal is to educate couples and thus reduce the fear and anxiety frequently associated with the birth process. These courses are designed to provide information about pregnancy, labor and delivery, and breathing and relaxation techniques. Care of the newborn is also usually discussed. Their ultimate objective is to decrease the need for analgesia and to minimize the need for intervention during labor. Classes are frequently designed for a specific group of patients. For example, the following classes are offered at the University of Utah.

1. *Preparation for Childbirth.* Six weekly classes emphasizing the birth process, breathing techniques, and care of the newborn.
2. *Single Mom Series.* Six weekly classes discussing aspects of pregnancy, preparation for labor and delivery, and single parenting.
3. *Refresher Course.* Three weekly classes intended as a review for persons who have previously taken a full six-week course in childbirth preparation.
4. *Early Pregnancy.* Three weekly classes to promote optimal health for mother and baby throughout pregnancy.
5. *Early Discharge.* One class for parents planning on a short (less than 24-hour) hospital stay.
6. *High-Risk/Cesarean Birth Series.* A two-class series to assist patients at high obstetric risk and those anticipating a cesarean birth.
7. *Early Parenting Series.* A two-class series addressing such concerns of new parents as feeding, safety, illnesses, and behavior in infants ages two weeks to three months.
8. *Diabetic Mother Series.* A series of classes especially designed to address the needs of the couple when the mother is diabetic.
9. *Breastfeeding Class.* A one-session class to prepare expectant mothers for the experience of breastfeeding.
10. *Sibling Preparation for Birth Class.* A class devoted to preparing older brothers and sisters for the actual birth of the new baby and adjusting to life with a new family member.
11. *Exercise Classes.* A twice-weekly activity class offering a good but not too strenuous nonaerobic workout.

Childbirth educators can be certified by several groups including the American Society for Psychoprophylaxis in Obstetrics (ASPO), the International Childbirth Educators Association (ICEA), and the Bradley group.

The widespread availability of childbirth education with its concomitant increase in patient knowledge has undoubtedly affected obstetric practice in this country. For the most part, this influence has been a positive one. Some have suggested, however, that the emphasis on "natural" childbirth and nonintervention has occasionally resulted in unrealistic expectations on the part of the patient and her partner. Obviously, the approach taken by individual instructors is extremely important in establishing the expectations of couples.

REFERENCES AND RECOMMENDED READING

Preconceptual Counseling

Badaracco MA, Vessey M: Recurrence of venous thromboembolic disease and use of oral contraceptives. Br Med J 1: 215, 1974

Clarren SK, Smith DW: The fetal alcohol syndrome. N Engl J Med 298:1063, 1978

Feldman GL, Weaver DD, Lovrien EW: The fetal trimethadione syndrome. Report of an additional family and further delineation of this syndrome. Am J Dis Child 131:1378, 1977

Hall JG: Vitamin A: A newly recognized human teratogen. Harbinger of things to come? J Pediatr 105:583, 1984

Hanson JW, Smith DW: The fetal hydantoin syndrome. J Pediatr 87:285, 1975

Harrod MJE, Sherrod PS: Warfarin embryopathy in siblings. Obstet Gynecol 57:673, 1981

Herschel M, et al: Survival of infants born at 24 to 28 weeks gestation. Obstet Gynecol 60:154, 1982

Hollingsworth DR, Jones OW, Resnik R: Expanded care in obstetrics for the 1980s: Preconception and early postconception counseling. Am J Obstet Gynecol 149:811, 1984

Jones AM, Howitt G: Eisenmenger syndrome in pregnancy. Br Med J 1:1627, 1965

Jones KL, Smith DW: Recognition of the fetal alcohol syndrome in early infancy. Lancet 2:999, 1973

Levy HL, Waibren SE: Effects of untreated maternal phenylketonuria and hyperphenylalaninemia on the fetus. N Engl J Med 309:1269, 1983

Lieberman E, Faich GA, Simon PR et al: Premarital rubella screening in Rhode Island. JAMA 25:1333, 1981

Longo LD: Environmental pollution and pregnancy: Risks and uncertainty for the fetus and infant. Am J Obstet Gynecol 137:162, 1980

Lott IT, Bocian M, Pribram H et al: Fetal hydrocephalus and ear anomalies associated with maternal use of isotretinoin. J Pediatr 105:597, 1984

Miller E, Hare J, Clohery J et al: Elevated maternal hemoglobin A_{1c} in early pregnancy and major congenital anomalies in infants of diabetic mothers. N Engl J Med 304:1331, 1981

Ouellette EM, Rosett H, Rosman NP et al: Adverse effects on offspring of maternal alcohol abuse during pregnancy. N Engl J Med 297:528, 1977

Pedersen J: The Pregnant Diabetic and Her Newborn: Problems

and Management, 2nd ed, p 191. Baltimore, Williams & Wilkins, 1977

Pirani BBK: Smoking during pregnancy. Obstet Gynecol Surv 33:1, 1978

Schoenbaum SC, Hyde JN, Bartsohesky L et al: Benefit-cost analysis of rubella vaccination policy. N Engl J Med 294:306, 1976

Smith DW: Teratogenicity of anticonvulsive medications. Am J Dis Child 131:1337, 1977

Sontag LW, Wallace RF: The effect of cigarette smoking during pregnancy upon the fetal heart rate. Am J Obstet Gynecol 23:405, 1963

Streissguth AP, Herman CS, Smith DW: Intelligence, behavior, and dysmorphogenesis in the fetal alcohol syndrome: A report on 20 patients. J Pediatr 92:363, 1978

Swiet MD: Management of thromboembolism in pregnancy. Practical Ther 18:478, 1979

Diagnosis of Pregnancy

Campbell S: The assessment of fetal development by diagnostic ultrasound. Clin Perinatol 1:2, 507, 1979

Chilcote WS, Asokan S: Evaluation of first trimester pregnancy by ultrasound. Clin Obstet Gynecol 20:253, 1977

Rasor JL, Farber S, Braunstein GD: An evaluation of ten kits for determination of human choriogonadotropin in serum. Clin Chem 29:1828, 1983

Rippey JH: Pregnancy tests: Evaluation and current status. CRC Crit Rev Clin Lab Sci 19:353, 1984

Ryder KW, Munsick RA, Oei TO et al: An evaluation of four serum tests for pregnancy. Clin Chem 29:561, 1983

Ryder KW, Munsick RA, Tjien OO et al: Five recent urinary tests for early pregnancy evaluated. Clin Chem 29:1812, 1983

Subir R, Klein TA, Scott JZ et al: Diagnosis of pregnancy with a radioreceptor assay for hCG. Obstet Gynecol 50:401, 1977

Duration of Pregnancy

Hohler CW, Quetel TA: Comparison of ultrasound femur length and biparietal diameter in late pregnancy. Am J Obstet Gynecol 14:759, 1981

Jimenez JM, Tyson JE, Reisch JS: Clinical measures of gestational age in normal pregnancies. Obstet Gynecol 61:436, 1983

Kopta MM, May RR, Crane JP: A comparison of the reliability of the estimated date of confinement predicted by crown–rump length and biparietal diameter. Am J Obstet Gynecol 145:562, 1983

Sabbagha RE, Barton EA, Barton FB et al: Sonar biparietal diameter. II. Predictive of three fetal growth patterns leading to a closer assessment of gestational age and neonatal weight. Am J Obstet Gynecol 126:485, 1976

Sabbagha RE, Barton FB, Barton EA: Sonar biparietal diameter. I. Analysis of percentile growth differences in two normal populations using same methodology. Am J Obstet Gynecol 126:479, 1976

Sabbagha RE, Hughey M, Depp R: Growth adjusted sonographic age (GASA): A simplified method. Obstet Gynecol 51:383, 1978

Worthen N, Bustillo M: Effect of urinary bladder fullness on fundal height measurements. Am J Obstet Gynecol 138:759, 1980

Prenatal Care

Bowman JM: Suppression of Rh isoimmunization. Obstet Gynecol 52:385, 1978

Carpenter MS, Coustan DR: Criteria for screening tests for gestational diabetes. Am J Obstet Gynecol 144:768, 1982

Macri JN, Haddow JE, Weiss RR: Screening for neural tube defects in the United States. Am J Obstet Gynecol 133:119, 1979

Maternal serum alpha-fetoprotein screening for neural tube defects. Results of a Consensus Meeting. Prenat Diagn 5:77, 1985

Milunsky A: Prenatal detection of neural tube defects. JAMA 244:2731, 1980

Milunsky A, Alpert E, Kitzmiller JL et al: Prenatal diagnosis of neural tube defects. Am J Obstet Gynecol 142:1030, 1982

Milunsky A, Elliot A, Neff RK et al: Prenatal diagnosis of neural tube defects. Obstet Gynecol 55:58, 1980

Naeye RL: Weight gain and the outcome of pregnancy. Am J Obstet Gynecol 135:3, 1979

O'Sullivan JB, Mahan CM, Charles D et al: Screening criteria for high-risk gestational diabetic patients. Am J Obstet Gynecol 116:895, 1973

Proceedings: McMaster conference on prevention of Rh immunization. Vox Sang 36:50, 1979

Zipursky A, Israels IG: The pathogenesis and prevention of Rh immunization. Can Med Assoc J 97:1245, 1967

General Problems and Questions

Atlay RD, Weekes ARL, Entwistle GD et al: Treating heartburn in pregnancy: Comparison of acid and alkali mixtures. Br Med J 2:919, 1978

Council on Scientific Affairs: Effects of pregnancy on work performance. JAMA 251:1995, 1984

Jimenez MH, Newton N: Activity and work during pregnancy and the postpartum period: A cross-cultural study of 202 societies. Am J Obstet Gynecol 135:171, 1979

Lenihan JP, Jr: Relationship of antepartum pelvic examinations to premature rupture of the membranes. Obstet Gynecol 83:33, 1984

Linn S, Schoenbaum SC, Monson RR et al: No association between coffee consumption and adverse outcomes of pregnancy. N Engl J Med 306:141, 1982

Lotgering FK, Gilbert RD, Longo LD: The interactions of exercise and pregnancy: A review. Am J Obstet Gynecol 149:560, 1984

Mills JL, Harlap S, Harley EE: Should coitus late in pregnancy be discouraged? Lancet 2:136, 1981

Naeye RL: Factors that predispose to premature rupture of the fetal membranes. Obstet Gynecol 60:93, 1982

Naeye RL: Coitus and associated amniotic-fluid infections. N Engl J Med 301:1198, 1979

Rayburn WF, Wilson RA: Coital activity and premature delivery. Am J Obstet Gynecol 137:972, 1980

PART III

Abnormal Pregnancy

Spontaneous Abortion   *James R. Scott*

21

Spontaneous abortion (also called miscarriage) is the natural termination of pregnancy before the fetus is capable of extrauterine life. The criteria for viability are generally considered to be gestation of at least 20 weeks and fetal weight of at least 500 g.

INCIDENCE

It is now appreciated that the incidence of natural embryo loss is higher than the previously estimated and often quoted figure of 15% of pregnancies ending in a first-trimester spontaneous abortion. The relatively high incidence of blighted ova (Fig. 21-1) found in hysterectomy specimens in Hertig's classic study,[1] recent data on very early pregnancies detected only with sensitive β-hCG assays during the luteal phase of the cycle,[2-4] and experience with *in vitro* fertilization indicate that the loss rate in early pregnancy is closer to 40% to 50%. The frequency of occult or subclinical abortions is undoubtedly even higher in women with irregular or late menses and those with infertility of undetermined etiology.

ETIOLOGY

In view of the complicated hormonal, immunologic, and cellular events that require precise integration for fertilization and nidation, it is remarkable that successful pregnancy occurs as often as it does. An abortion is an unfortunate event for the couple involved, but a high proportion of aborted conceptuses are abnormal. This selective process appears to eliminate about 95% of morphologic and cytogenetic errors.

Embryonic Factors

The vast majority of single sporadic abortions are due to nonrepetitive intrinsic defects in the developing conceptus, which can be caused by such conditions as abnormal germ cells, defective implantation of normal trophoblast, accidental injury to the developing embryo, and perhaps other causes as yet unrecognized.

The frequency of chromosome abnormalities in spontaneously aborted embryos decreases from 60% in the first trimester to 7% by the end of the 24th week (Fig. 21-2). If very early aborted conceptuses from unrecognized pregnancies were included, the incidence would probably be even higher. Autosomal trisomy is the most common chromosomal anomaly, making up 51.9% of the total. However, the relative frequency of different types of trisomy differs considerably. Trisomy 16, which accounts for about one third of all trisomic abortions, has not been reported in liveborn infants and is therefore considered highly lethal. Trisomy 22 and 21 are the next most frequent types in abortions, and trisomy 21 is also frequent in liveborn infants. The principal mechanism leading to trisomy is meiotic nondisjunction: that is, failure of homologous chromosomes to separate. In families with a child with trisomy 21, the extra chromosome has been traced to the mother in 81% of the informative families, and to the father in the remaining 19%.[10] These data suggest that the relative frequency of nondisjunction leading to trisomic offspring is higher in oocytes than in spermatocytes. The second most frequent type of chromosome anomaly in spontaneously aborted fetuses is monosomy X (45,XO), which accounts for 18.9% of the total (Fig. 21-3). Triploidy accounts for 15.5%, tetraploidy for 5.6%, translocations for 3.8% and mosaicism for 1.5%. The mutagenic factors that cause monosomy X, triploidy, and tetraploidy

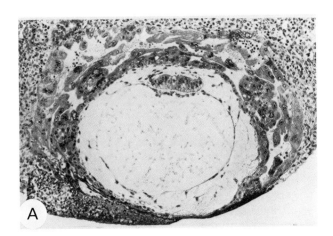

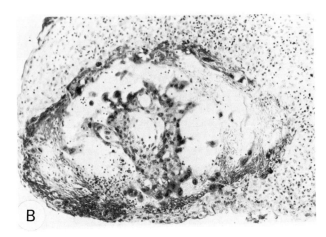

FIG. 21-1. Histologic comparison of (*A*) a morphologically normally implanted human ovum estimated as being about 11 to 12 days of age with (*B*) a "blighted" ovum showing defective trophoblast with pathologically large lacunae and an empty chorionic sac that is destined to abort. (From Hertig AT, Rock J, Adams EC: A description of 34 human ova within 17 days of development. Am J Anat 98:435, 1956)

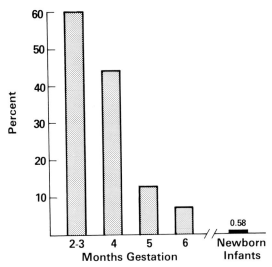

FIG. 21-2. The frequency of chromosome anomalies among 3040 spontaneously aborted fetuses related to the duration of pregnancy.[5-8] For comparison, the frequency of chromosome anomalies among 54,749 newborn infants is also shown.[9]

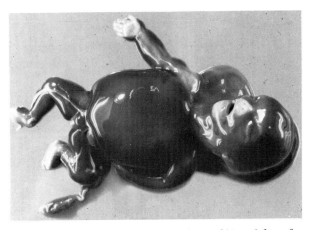

FIG. 21-3. Fetus with Turner's syndrome (45,XO) from first-trimester spontaneous abortion. Note the characteristic edema of the posterior neck, which could be missed without careful inspection.

are at present unknown, but none of them are dependent on maternal age. Chromosome marker studies of triploidy indicate that the supernumery haploid chromosome set originates from the father in 83% of cases and from the mother in only 17%.[11]

Parental Factors

Two situations exist among the parents of chromosomally abnormal abortuses. In most instances the couple is chromosomally normal and the abortuses' abnormalities occur in random and sporadic fashion. In a small percentage of cases, one member of the couple is a

carrier of a balanced translocation; offspring of these parents may be repeatedly aborted. Treatable maternal or paternal factors, which are discussed in the section on recurrent abortion, account for relatively few cases of first-trimester spontaneous abortions. However, new causes continue to be discovered. For example, isotretinoin (Accutane, Roche Laboratories), which is a recently marketed drug for acne and other skin conditions, has been associated with spontaneous abortions and fetal abnormalities and should not be used by women who are pregnant or who have immediate plans to become pregnant.[12,13]

PATHOLOGY

Most spontaneous abortions occur one to three weeks after the death of the embryo or rudimentary anlage. Initially, there is hemorrhage into the decidua basalis and necrosis and inflammation in the region of implantation. The conceptus becomes partially or entirely detached and is essentially a foreign body in the uterus. Uterine contractions and dilatation of the cervix usually result in expulsion of most or all of the products of conception. When the sac is opened, fluid is commonly found surrounding a small macerated fetus, or, alternatively, there may be no visible fetus in the sac: the so-called blighted ovum. Hydropic degeneration of the placental villi, caused by retention of tissue fluid, is commonly seen on histologic examination (Fig. 21-4).

There are distinct patterns of spontaneous abortion. The amniotic sac and contents may be evacuated with the chorion and decidua; the embryo may be expelled, with rupture of the amniotic sac and passage of the fetus alone; or the entire pregnancy and the decidua may be passed intact.

When expulsion of the conceptus is delayed for a prolonged period after embryonic death (missed abortion), hemorrhage around the ovum may result in the formation of a firm, nodular, fleshy mass. This is called a *carneous* or *blood* (*Breus*) *mole.*

CLINICAL ASPECTS AND TREATMENT

The possibility of an unrecognized pregnancy episode must always be kept in mind in any woman in the reproductive age range who presents with abnormal bleeding or pain. Moreover, each pregnant patient should be instructed at the first antepartum visit to immediately notify her physician should vaginal bleeding occur. It is convenient to consider the clinical aspects of spontaneous abortion under the following subgroups: threatened, inevitable, incomplete, complete, missed, septic, and habitual abortion.

Threatened Abortion

Any uterine bleeding that occurs during the first half of pregnancy is classified as *threatened abortion*. Since 20% to 25% of pregnant women have some spotting or

FIG. 21-4. Curettings from incomplete abortion, showing cellular debris, blood, and chorionic villi in varying stages of degeneration. (*A*) Hyaline (*left*) and hydropic (*right*) degeneration. (×250) (*B*) Villi, showing hyaline degeneration and necrosis. (×90)

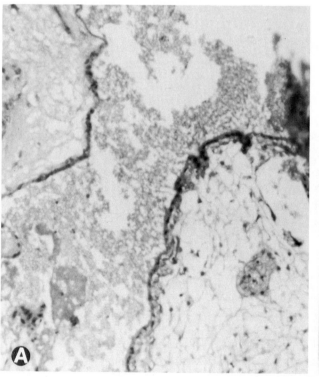
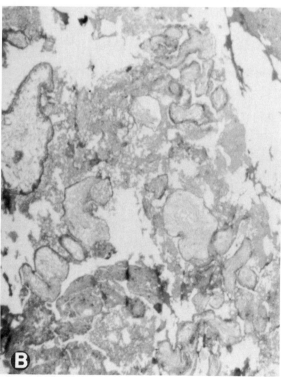

bleeding during the early months of gestation, it is a very common diagnosis. Of those women, only about one-half actually abort. The bleeding associated with threatened abortion is usually scanty, varies from a brownish discharge to bright-red bleeding, and may occur repeatedly in the course of many days. It usually precedes any mild pain that may occur in the form of cramping or low backache. There is no tissue loss and pelvic examination reveals that the cervix is closed and uneffaced. The differential diagnosis includes ectopic pregnancy, trophoblastic disease, vaginal ulcerations, cervical erosions, polyps, or carcinoma. Although there is no convincing evidence that any treatment regimen favorably influences the course of threatened abortion, a sympathetic attitude on the part of the physician as well as continuing support and follow-up are extremely important to the patient. Management includes a tactful explanation of the pathologic process and the prognosis. Over 90% of pregnancies with first-trimester bleeding will continue if fetal life has been demonstrated ultrasonically, and the perinatal mortality and frequency of congenital anomalies are no higher in these pregnancies than in normal pregnancies.[14] Initially, it is wise to advise the patient to restrict activity and coitus and to remain at home near a telephone until it can be determined whether the symptoms will persist or stop. Continued observation is indicated as long as the bleeding and cramping are mild, the cervix remains closed, and the uterus is growing in size. If the bleeding and cramping continue or increase, the prognosis becomes worse. Other findings associated with an unfavorable outcome are two consecutive analyses of blood or urine that are negative for human chorionic gonadotropin (hCG), sonographic evidence of a gestational sac with no central echoes from the embryo (Fig. 21-5), serial sonograms indicating that the gestational sac is decreasing in size

and is smaller than appropriate for gestational age, and a uterus that, on pelvic examination, is not increasing in size or is becoming smaller. When careful clinical evaluation indicates that the conceptus is no longer viable, the uterus should be evacuated.

Inevitable and Incomplete Abortions

Although usually classified as different entities, inevitable and incomplete abortions present a similar clinical problem and are treated in the same way. An abortion is considered *inevitable* when bleeding or rupture of the membranes is accompanied by pain and dilatation of the internal os of the cervix. The abortion is *incomplete* when the products of conception have partially passed from the uterine cavity, are protruding from the external os or are found in the vagina, and bleeding and cramping persists. A gentle vaginal examination under aseptic conditions is usually enough to establish the diagnosis. Occasionally, however, one conceptus will be aborted and a normal twin will be retained and proceed to delivery at term.[15] This unusual situation can be diagnosed by ultrasonography at the time of bleeding during the first trimester. There is otherwise no fetal survival in inevitable or incomplete abortions, so attempts at preservation of the pregnancy are futile, and the aim of therapy is evacuation of the uterus to prevent complications from further hemorrhage or infection.

In most cases, a vacuum or suction curettage can be carried out promptly and safely in an outpatient setting with analgesia and a paracervical block after beginning an intravenous infusion of 1000 ml normal saline containing 10 to 20 units of oxytocin. A plastic suction curette of appropriate size is inserted into the uterine cavity after being attached to the tubing on the suction

FIG. 21-5. Ultrasonic comparison of (*A*) a blighted ovum with no fetal tissue that is destined to abort with (*B*) a normal gestational sac with a transonic area, echogenic rim, and fetal pole.

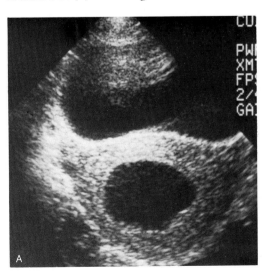
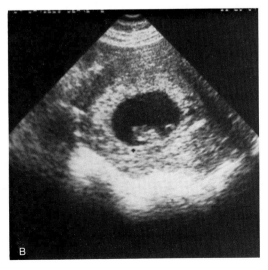

machine. As curettage proceeds, tissue will be seen flowing into the curette and tubing. The curette is rotated 360 degrees clockwise as it is withdrawn, and the procedure is repeated in a counterclockwise direction. When a grating sensation is noted and no more tissue is obtained, the endometrial cavity is usually curetted gently with a sharp curette, and this is followed by one brief suction curettage.

Appropriate backup and preparation must be available since adverse reactions can occur, such as allergic reactions to medication, uterine atony, uterine perforation, seizure, or cardiac arrest. A hemoglobin level should be obtained, and if the hemorrhage has been severe, blood replacement may be necessary. At the initial pelvic examination, placental fragments can often be removed from the cervical canal and lower uterine segment with ring forceps to facilitate uterine contraction and hemostasis. If measures taken in the emergency room fail to control the bleeding promptly, the patient should be taken directly to the operating room for an examination under anesthesia and evacuation of the uterus. After a curettage, the patient is observed for 4 to 6 hours and, if stable, can then be discharged to be followed as an outpatient. Each Rh-negative woman should receive either 50 μg or the standard 300-μg dose of Rh immune globulin to prevent Rh immunization. Oral methylergonovine maleate tablets cause persistent uterine cramping and are unnecessary if evacuation of the uterus is complete. All tissue obtained should be carefully studied to confirm the presence of products of conception, to rule out the possibility of ectopic pregnancy, and to try to ascertain whether the abortion is related to defective germ plasm or to some factor that has caused the uterus to empty itself of a normal ovum.

Complete Abortion

The physician following a patient with a threatened abortion should instruct her to save all tissue passed so it can be inspected. Complete abortion is identified by the cessation of pain and bleeding after the entire conceptus has been passed. If the diagnosis is certain, further therapy may not be necessary. If there is any question about whether the uterus has been completely evacuated, a suction curettage can be performed. Curettage removes any remaining necrotic decidua, decreases the incidence of postabortion bleeding, and shortens the recovery time.

Missed Abortion

The term *missed abortion* is applied when the conceptus dies but is not passed. The reason that some nonviable embryos do not proceed to spontaneous abortion is not clear, but it has been shown that a threatened abortion can be converted to a missed abortion by treatment with potent progestational agents. Typically, the patient reports that pregnancy symptoms have regressed, pregnancy tests become negative as chorionic function ceases, no fetal heart beat can be detected on Doppler ultrasound, and real-time ultrasound examinations reveal no fetal activity. Most patients with a missed abortion eventually abort spontaneously, and coagulation defects due to the dead fetus syndrome are rare in the first half of pregnancy. However, expectant management is emotionally trying, and many women with a missed abortion prefer to have the pregnancy terminated. During the first trimester, this is done by suction curettage. The procedure is best performed in a hospital setting with intravenous fluids and blood available, since profuse bleeding can occasionally occur in this situation. In the second trimester, the uterus is emptied by dilatation and evacuation (D&E) or induction of labor with intravaginal prostaglandin E$_2$ (PGE$_2$) suppositories. The D&E is a procedure that is an extension of both the traditional D&C and the vacuum curettage. It is especially appropriate in pregnancies of 13 to 16 weeks of gestation, although many proponents use this method up through 20 weeks. First, laminaria are used to accomplish a gradual and relatively atraumatic mechanical dilation of the cervix. The quantity of amniotic fluid is often markedly decreased following fetal death, limiting the usefulness of intra-amniotic techniques of induction. PGE$_2$ suppositories are very useful in induction labor in second-trimester missed abortions. One 20-mg suppository is placed high in the posterior vaginal vault every 3 to 4 hours until the fetus and placenta are expelled. Diphenoxylate hydrochloride (Lomotil), 2.5 mg to 5 mg given orally, and prochlorperazine (Compazine), 10 mg intramuscularly, are usually given at the onset and during the procedure as needed to control diarrhea and nausea respectively. Both medications can potentiate the effects of narcotics used to relieve the pain of uterine contractions. The duration of vaginal PGE$_2$ procedures averages about 14 hours.

Septic Abortion

Septic abortion, once a leading cause of maternal mortality, has become less frequent as liberalized abortion laws have made physician-induced abortions available to women with unwanted pregnancies. However, any threatened, inevitable, or incomplete abortion can be complicated by infection. The infection is most commonly metritis, parametritis, or peritonitis, as evidenced by fever, abdominal pain, and uterine tenderness, but it may progress to septicemia and septic shock. The polymicrobial infection usually mirrors the endogenous vaginal flora such as *Escherichia coli* and other aerobic enteric gram-negative rods, group B β-hemolytic streptococci, anaerobic streptococci, *Bacteroides* species, staphylococci, and microaerophilic bacteria.

Initial evaluation and management should include:

1. Physical and pelvic examination
2. Determination of CBC, electrolytes, BUN, creatinine levels
3. Typing and crossmatching of blood
4. Taking of smears from cervix for gram stain
5. Aerobic and anaerobic cultures of endocervix, blood, and any products of conception available
6. Installation of indwelling Foley catheter
7. Urinalysis and urine culture
8. Administration of intravenous fluids (saline or Ringer's lactate) through a large-bore angiocath
9. Administration of tetanus toxoid 0.5 ml subcutaneously for immunized patients or 250 U tetanus immune globulin deep intramuscularly
10. Taking of supine and upright films of the abdomen for free air or foreign bodies

Optimal therapy has two key components: (1) evacuation of the uterus and (2) aggressive use of parenteral antibiotics before, during, and after removal of any necrotic tissue by curettage. Prompt removal of infected necrotic tissue is an important therapeutic procedure and should be performed within a few hours after antibiotic therapy is begun. Numerous antibiotic regimens have been recommended, but high-dose, broad-spectrum coverage is essential.

Although most patients with septic abortions respond favorably to treatment, there is a danger of septic shock syndrome, which is a serious complication and can eventually lead to acute renal failure, coagulopathy, adult respiratory distress syndrome, and death. The pathophysiologic events in spetic shock are very complex, but the pattern is one of initially decreased peripheral vascular resistance, increased cardiac output, and low central venous pressure (early phase), followed by a fall in cardiac output, compensatory peripheral arterial vasoconstriction, and, in the absence of concomitant blood loss, a rising central venous pressure. The details for the management of septic shock are presented in Chapter 38.

However, it is essential to realize that the most common cause of death in cases of septic shock is the development of shock lung, or the adult respiratory distress syndrome. All patients with overwhelming septicemia are hypoxic and acidotic; therefore, oxygen therapy should be started immediately and arterial blood gases monitored carefully. Most important, the physician must initiate mechanical ventilatory support with a volume-cycled respirator at the earliest sign of decreased pulmonary compliance.

Recurrent (Habitual) Abortion

The commonly accepted definition of habitual abortion is the occurrence of three or more consecutive first-trimester spontaneous abortions. The condition occurs in approximately one in 200 couples, and in many cases is a chance phenomenon. Since at least 60% of embryonic tissues derived from first-trimester abortions are chromosomally abnormal, it is apparent that treatable maternal causes are present in the minority of cases. The problem is further complicated by the fact that the efficacy of some common diagnostic and therapeutic regimens is not well substantiated.

There is little scientific evidence that poor nutrition, thyroid disorders, undetected diabetes mellitus, or ABO incompatibility cause spontaneous abortion.[16] Various infections have been suspected, but although *Listeria monocytogenes* and *Toxoplasma gondii* may be responsible for a few cases, such organisms as *Mycoplasma hominis* and *Ureaplasma urealyticum* remain to be proven as clinically important etiologic agents. Moreover, chronic medical diseases are rarely implicated unless the patient is extremely debilitated, and psychological factors are most likely the result rather than the cause of this frustrating experience.

A decreased maternal immune response to HLA or cross-reactive trophoblast/lymphocyte antigens with inadequate production of the blocking factors necessary for fetoplacental allograft survival has recently been suggested as an immunologic cause of some cases of recurrent abortion, but this hypothesis remains controversial.[17-20] Some of these patients have been treated with injections of third party donor leukocytes or paternal lymphocytes, but it is not yet known whether this treatment is safe and effective.

The following generally accepted causes of recurrent abortion are worthy of clinical investigation, but it should be pointed out that few of the treatment regimens recommended have been subjected to prospective randomized trials to establish their efficacy.

Anatomic Uterine Defects

Hysterosalpingography or hysteroscopy can rule out the presence of a septate uterus (Fig. 21-6) or other müllerian anomaly, of intrauterine synechiae, or of submucous leiomyomas, which are thought to produce an inhospitable implantation site by interfering with vascularization and distorting or reducing the size of the uterine cavity. All other causes of recurrent abortion should be eliminated by a careful clinical investigation before surgical correction is considered. Following appropriate surgery, successful pregnancy rates are in the range of 70% to 90%.

Endocrine Factors

Inadequacy of the corpus luteum, a controversial entity defined as abnormal ovarian function with inadequate progesterone production, is most often diagnosed on the basis of low postovulatory serum progesterone levels and the histologic appearance of endometrial biopsies taken on the 26th to 28th day of the cycle. However, inadequate progesterone production

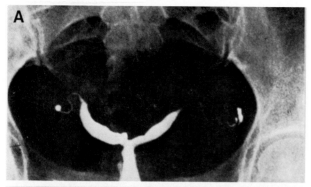

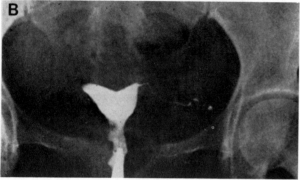

FIG. 21-6. (*A*) Preoperative hysterosalpingogram of uterus with a large septum in a patient with recurrent abortion. (*B*) Same uterus after surgical repair with metroplasty.

by the ovary or placenta is probably rarely responsible for recurrent abortion, and the demonstration of a progesterone deficiency does not categorically mean that abortion is inevitable. It has been shown that abnormally low levels of urinary pregnanediol excretion spontaneously revert to normal in 80% of patients and that pregnancy proceeds to term.[21,22] Furthermore, progesterone secretion may be low in a pregnancy doomed to abort because of defective germ tissue, a condition that is obviously not amenable to hormone treatment. The ratonale for progesterone replacement was derived from observations that spontaneous abortion occurred when the corpus luteum was surgically removed before 6 to 8 weeks of gestation. In carefully selected patients, supplemental progesterone beginning after ovulation and continued throughout pregnancy has been reported to reduce the incidence of spontaneous abortion.[23] The progesterone is most often given in the form of vaginal suppositories 25 mg twice daily. However, enthusiasm for this regimen should be tempered by consideration of the possibility of producing a missed abortion and by double blind studies that show no difference in aborton rates in treated and placebo groups.[21,22,24] Clomiphene and other ovulatory agents have also been tried in an attempt to improve follicular development, which in turn might improve corpus luteum function, but the results are variable.[25]

Chromosome Abnormalities

Although parental chromosome anomalies are not a frequent cause of repeated abortions, they occur more commonly in couples affected by the problem than in the general population. In approximately 5% to 10% of couples with repetitive abortions, one parent will have a translocation or inversion. Therefore, cytogenetic examinations of both partners may be helpful in predicting recurrence as well as in forming a basis for genetic counseling. Depending on the abnormality found, therapeutic possibilities include amniocentesis if a subsequent pregnancy progresses past 14 weeks of gestation, artificial donor insemination, or counseling about adoption.

Lupus Anticoagulant

Lupus anticoagulant is an acquired immunoglobulin first described in patients with systemic lupus erythematosus (SLE). Its presence is revealed by a prolonged activated partial thromboplastin time (APTT) and a positive tissue thromboplastin inhibition test (TTI). Many patients with this inhibitor have no evidence of SLE but have a false positive test for syphilis or other autoantibodies. The lupus anticoagulant rarely causes clinical bleeding and is more often associated with a tendency toward thrombotic episodes. An association with recurrent spontaneous abortion and midtrimester fetal deaths has also been reported.[26] The decidua and placenta in affected pregnancies show progressive thrombosis and infarction, but delivery of live infants has been achieved by treatment throughout pregnancy with immunosuppressive doses of prednisone (40–60 mg/day) and aspirin 75 mg/day. Corticosteroids theoretically suppress autoantibody synthesis and inhibit antigen-antibody interaction, and low-dose aspirin is used to attempt to restore a normal prostacyclin-thromboxane balance in these patients. Even with this regimen, careful surveillance is necessary, since severe fetal growth retardation, thrombocytopenia, and pregnancy induced hypertension are common. In addition, the incidence of positive antinuclear antibody tests is higher in women with repetitive abortions than in the normal population.[27] Even though the lupus anticoagulant and subclinical autoimmune diseases are rare causes of recurrent abortion, they are worthy of consideration when the patient presents with suggestive signs and symptoms or when the rest of the evaluation has been unrewarding.

It should be emphasized that in most patients with habitual abortion, none of the previously discussed abnormalities will be found. However, this information can be used in a positive way to reassure the couple, since at least 70% of these patients eventually deliver healthy offspring. In fact, supportive care alone resulted in successful pregnancies in 86% of patients in one study,[28] which emphasizes that caution is necessary in attributing success to any one treatment regimen. There is no evidence that the woman who has habitually aborted spontaneously is at greatly increased risk of having an abnormal child when she finally carries her pregnancy to term.

Cervical Incompetence

The term *incompetent cervix* is applied to a rather discrete obstetric entity characterized by painless dilatation of the cervix during the midtrimester of pregnancy followed by rupture of the membranes and subsequent expulsion of a fetus that is so immature that it almost never survives. Abortion from incompetence of the cervix is believed to be an entirely different and distinct entity from spontaneous abortion in the first trimester and premature labor in the third trimester; it results from different factors, presents a different clinical picture, and requires different management. Whereas spontaneous abortion in the first trimester and premature labor in the third trimester are common complications of pregnancy, incompetence of the cervix is relatively rare.

The cervix is fundamentally a connective tissue structure, in contrast to the corpus, which is basically muscular. The cause of cervical incompetence is obscure, and a variety of etiologic factors have been proposed.[29] Previous trauma to the cervix, especially in the course of a dilatation and curettage, amputation, conization, cauterization, or traumatic delivery, appears to be a factor in some cases. In other instances, congenital structural defects, such as infiltration of the connective tissue with smooth muscle, uterine anomalies, or abnormal cervical development associated with *in utero* exposure to diethylstilbestrol, appear to play a role.

There is little agreement regarding the diagnosis of cervical incompetence except that it is one of exclusion that requires careful evaluation to rule out other potential causes of midtrimester abortion. The abosolute diagnosis can only be made by actual visualization of the fetal membranes bulging through the partially dilated cervix of a patient in the midtrimester of pregnancy who

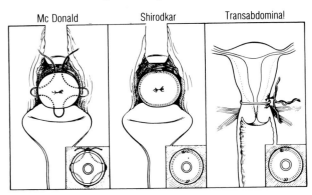

FIG. 21-8. Treatment of incompetent cervix (*A*) McDonald cerclage procedure—A multiple bite suture of large monofilament nylon is placed around the cervix and tied securely to reduce the diameter of the cervical canal to a few mm. (*B*) Shirodkar procedure—Mersiline tape encircling the cervix is passed under the mucosa and anchored to the cervix anteriorly and posteriorly with silk ligatures. (*C*) Transabdominal cervicoisthmic cerclage—Mersiline band is placed in an avascular space medially to the uterine vessels at the level of the cervicouterine junction.

is not in labor (Fig. 21-7). A presumptive diagnosis is perhaps most reliably made from the characteristic history of repeated silent dilatation of the cervix followed by rupture of the membranes and a relatively painless, rapid labor with delivery of an immature infant. On inspection in the nonpregnant state, the cervix may be shortened with a patulous os or may be deformed with lacerations that sometimes extend to the vaginal fornix. It has been suggested that the condition can be diagnosed in early pregnancy or during the nonpregnant state by sonographic methods designed to calibrate the diameter of the endocervical canal, but more information is needed. Moreover, the accurate prediction of whether or not a given cervix will be incompetent in a subsequent pregnancy is difficult.

Other causes of second-trimester abortions are abruptio placentae, chorioamnionitis, and uterine anomalies, but these usually present clinical pictures different from that of cervical incompetence. If these conditions have been ruled out, the generally accepted treatment of incompetent cervix is surgical. A variety of methods have been described, but the McDonald or Shirodkar procedures (Fig. 21-8) are the ones most commonly employed.[30,31] These are pursestring techniques performed vaginally, usually under regional anesthesia, that are designed to reinforce the cervix at the level of the internal os. If there is insufficient cervical tissue to allow placement of a cerclage, an abdominal approach is sometimes used.[32] The reinforcement suture is placed at approximately 12 to 14 weeks of gestation: after the risk of spontaneous abortion from chromosome anomalies has passed and before the cervix starts to dilate. The procedure should not be used if the diagnosis is in doubt, if membranes are ruptured,

FIG. 21-7. Cervical incompetence with bulging membranes at 20 weeks of gestation. (Barter R, Dusbabek JA, Riva HL et al: Am J Obstet Gynecol 75:511, 1958)

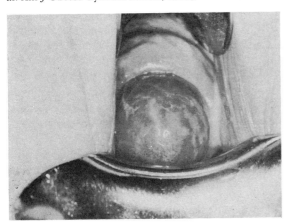

or if vaginal bleeding and cramping are part of the clinical picture. There is no evidence that postoperative antibiotics, progesterone, or tocolytic agents are useful adjuvants. If membranes rupture or labor ensues at any time, the cerclage should be removed to prevent chorioamnionitis, sepsis, cervical laceration, and rupture of the uterus. Otherwise the suture is removed when fetal maturity is achieved (usually after 37 weeks of gestation). Removal is often followed by the onset of labor and a relatively rapid delivery. If the patient desires further pregnancies, some physicians leave the cerclage in place and deliver the patient by cesarean section.

When patients are carefully selected, this type of management is 80% to 90% successful in preventing delivery of an immature fetus. There is little difference in the fetal survival rates between the McDonald and Shirodkar technique.[33] Gradually the idea has grown that the procedure might be used much more often prophylactically even for patients with previous preterm deliveries with less convincing evidence for cervical incompetence.[34] However, two recent prospective randomized studies have found no difference in perinatal outcome between treated and untreated groups when cerclage was used in this manner.[35,36]

REFERENCES

1. Hertig AT, Rock J, Adams EC: A description of 34 human ova within 17 days of development. Am J Anat 98:435, 1956
2. Miller JF, Williamson E, Glue J et al: Fetal loss after implantation. Lancet 2:554, 1980
3. Edmonds DK, Linsay KS, Miller JF et al: Early embryonic mortality in women. Fertil Steril 38:447, 1982
4. Whittaker PG, Taylor A, Lind T: Unsuspected pregnancy loss in healthy women. Lancet 1:1126, 1983
5. Boue J, Boue A, Lazar P: Retrospective and prospective epidemiological studies of 1500 karyotyped spontaneous human abortions. Teratology 12:11, 1975
6. Lauritsen JG: Aetiology of spontaneous abortion. A cytogenetic and epidemiological study of 288 abortuses and their parents. Acta Obstet Gynecol Scand (Suppl) 52:1, 1976
7. Creasy MR, Crolla JA, Alberman ED: A cytogenetic study of human spontaneous abortions using banding techniques. Hum Genet 31:177, 1976
8. Kajii T, Ferrier A, Niikawa N et al: Anatomic and chromosomal anomalies in 639 spontaneous abortions. Hum Genet 55:87, 1980
9. Nielsen J, Sillsen I: Incidence of chromosome aberrations among 11,148 newborn children. Humangenetik 30:1, 1975
10. Mikkelsen M, Poulsen H, Grindsted J et al: Nondisjunction in trisomy 21: Study of chromosome heteromorphisms in 110 families. Ann Hum Genet 44:17, 1980
11. Lauritsen JG, Bolund L, Friedrich U et al: Origin of triploidy in spontaneous abortuses. Ann Hum Genet 43:1, 1979
12. Rosa FW: Teratogenicity of isotretinoin. Lancet 2:513, 1983
13. Benke PJ: The isotretinoin teratogen syndrome. JAMA 251:3267, 1984
14. Jouppila P, Koivisto M: The prognosis in pregnancy after threatened abortion. Ann Chir Gynaecol [Fenn] 63:439, 1974
15. Finberg HJ, Birnholz JC: Ultrasound in multiple gestation with first trimester bleeding: The blighted twin. Radiology 132:137, 1979
16. Glass RH, Golbus MS: Habitual abortion. Fertil Steril 29:257, 1978
17. Taylor C, Faulk WP: Prevention of recurrent abortion with leucocyte transfusions. Lancet 2:68, 1981
18. Beer AE, Quebbeman JF, Ayuers JWT et al: Major histocompatibility complex antigens, maternal and paternal responses, and chronic habitual abortions in humans. Am J Obstet Gynecol 141:987, 1981
19. Caudle MR, Rote NS, Scott JR et al: Histocompatibility and recurrent spontaneous abortion and normal fertility. Fertil Steril 39:793, 1983
20. Oksenberg JR, Peritz E, Amar A et al: Maternal-paternal histocompatibility: Lack of association with habitual abortions. Fertil Steril 42:389, 1984
21. Goldzier JW: Double-blind trial of progestin in habitual abortion. JAMA 188:561, 1964
22. Shearman RP, Garreth WJ: Double-blind study of effect of 17-hydroxy-progesterone caproate on abortion rate. Br Med J 1:292, 1963
23. Jones GS: Luteal phase defects. In Behrman SJ, Kistner RW (eds): Progress in Infertility, 2nd ed, p 299. Boston, Little, Brown & Co, 1976
24. Klopper A, MacNaughton MD: Hormones in recurrent abortion. J Obstet Gynaecol Br Commonw 72:1022, 1965
25. Cook CL, Schroeder JA, Yussman MA et al: Induction of luteal phase defect with clomiphene citrate. Am J Obstet Gynecol 149:613, 1984
26. Lubbe WF, Butler WS, Palmer SJ et al: Fetal survival after prednisone suppression of maternal lupus-anticoagulant. Lancet 1:1361, 1983
27. Harger JH, Archer DF, Marchese SG et al: Etiology of recurrent pregnancy losses and outcomes of subsequent pregnancies. Obstet Gynecol 62:574, 1983
28. Stray-Pedersen B, Stray-Pedersen S: Etiologic factors and subsequent reproductive performance in 195 couples with a prior history of habitual abortion. Am J Obstet Gynecol 148:140, 1984
29. Danforth DN, Buckingham, JC: Cervical incompetence: A reevaluation. Postgrad Med 32:345, 1962
30. McDonald IA: Incompetent cervix as a cause of recurrent abortion. J Obstet Gynaecol Br Commonw 70:105, 1963
31. Shirodkar VN: A new method of operative treatment for habitual abortions in the second trimester of pregnancy. Antiseptic 52:299, 1955
32. Novy MJ: Transabdominal cervicoisthmic cerclage for the management of repetitive abortion and preterm delivery. Am J Obstet Gynecol 143:44, 1982
33. Harger JH: Comparison of success and morbidity in cervical cerclage procedures. Obstet Gynecol 56:543, 1980
34. Crombleholme WR, Minkoff HL, Delke I et al: Cervical cerclage: An aggressive approach to threatened or recurrent pregnancy wastage. Am J Obstet Gynecol 146:168, 1983
35. Rush RW, Isaacs S, McPherson K et al: A randomized trial of cervical cerclage in women at risk of spontaneous preterm delivery. Br J Obstet Gynaecol 91:724, 1984
36. Lazar P, Gueguen S, Dreyfus J et al: Multicentered controlled trial of cervical cerclage in women at moderate risk of preterm delivery. Br J Obstet Gynaecol 91:731, 1984

Gestational Trophoblastic Neoplasms

Robert D. Hilgers
John L. Lewis Jr.

22

Trophoblastic neoplasms are by tradition divided into three groups: (1) hydatidiform mole, (2) invasive mole (chorioadenoma destruens), and (3) choriocarcinoma. (A more recently described entity, partial hydatidiform mole, represents a subset that is not part of the original trilogy.) Before the advent of chemotherapy, approximately 90% of women with metastatic trophoblastic neoplasms died of their disease. The discovery by Li, Hertz, and Spencer in 1956 that methotrexate may cure patients with metastases not only provided the first dramatic evidence of the efficacy of chemotherapy in malignant disease, but it is also the basis for the present understanding of trophoblastic neoplasia. In 1961, Hertz and his co-workers reported the first five-year study of the effect of methotrexate in metastatic choriocarcinoma and presented evidence of the interrelationship of the three pathologic entities as they were then defined. They concluded that strict segregation of the three entities obscured the important fact that these tumors comprise a continuing spectrum, each merging imperceptibly with the other (Fig. 22-1). This dynamic process became known as "gestational trophoblastic disease," and the concept of "gestational trophoblastic neoplasia" was introduced to emphasize a developmental relationship between the benign and the malignant processes. The qualifying term *gestational* is needed because trophoblastic disease is not always associated with pregnancy; it may occur in the testicle or the ovary. Because these tumors produce human chorionic gonadotropin (hCG) and respond predictably to therapy, it has been possible to develop a new classification that includes the entire pathologic spectrum and also permits categorization according to both prognosis and selection of treatment. At present, complete remission can be achieved in 75% to 90% of the cases of metastatic gestational trophoblastic disease, depending on the distribution of patients in the high-risk category.

PATHOLOGY

The histopathologic features of gestational trophoblastic neoplasms are characterized by hyperplasia of the trophoblast and changes in the stroma of the chorionic villi. In choriocarcinoma, chorionic villi are absent and there is an overgrowth of anaplastic trophoblastic cells. The generic term *gestational trophoblastic neoplasia* is especially useful when histology is unknown or is suspected to have changed. The degree or kind of histologic change does not necessarily bear any relationship to the biologic behavior of the lesion and is not useful in making decisions relating to management or to surveillance during the follow-up period.

Hydatidiform Mole

In the past, all hydatidiform moles were lumped together in a single category. Utilizing newer cytogenetic techniques, Vassilakos, and later Szulman and Surti, demonstrated that there are two separate and distinct kinds of moles: *complete moles,* which conform to the familiar, classic hydatidiform mole and are a part of the continuing spectrum of trophoblastic neoplasia; and *partial moles,* which, despite the features they have in common with the classic mole, are different indeed and may or may not be part of the accepted continuum of trophoblastic neoplasia.

Complete Mole

Grossly, the complete mole resembles a bunch of white grapes (Fig. 22-2). It is characterized by smooth, translucent, avascular pale pink or gray hydropic vesicles that vary in size from microscopic to more than 2 cm in

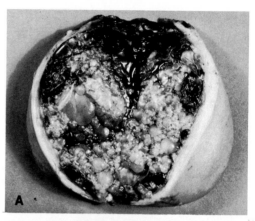

HYDATIDIFORM MOLE	CHORIOADENOMA DESTRUENS	CHORIO-CARCINOMA

METASTATIC

FIG. 22-1. The continuing spectrum of gestational trophoblastic neoplasms.

diameter and are held together by tenuous stems of connective tissue. The hydropic vesicles grow rapidly, and they quickly fill and distend the uterine cavity, often causing the uterus to be larger than one would expect from the menstrual dates. The embryo or fetus is usually absent and there is no definitive placenta, amniotic sac, or fluid, and the intervillous space is typically abnormal. The maternal blood arriving from the spiral arterioles is not transferred through the placental site, giving rise to hemorrhage into the uterine cavity and subsequent vaginal bleeding.

The histologic features are highlighted by proliferation of the trophoblastic cells overlying the chorionic villi (Fig. 22-3). Trophoblastic proliferation is extremely variable and is analogous to the trophoblastic proliferation found in the previllous stages of implantation (see Fig. 17-7C); in isolated high-power fields the distinction between the two may be impossible. One or both layers of trophoblast may be involved in the proliferation. Proliferating syncytiotrophoblast appears as sheets of vacuolated pink-staining cytoplasmic masses spotted with numerous hyperchromatic nuclei without mitoses. The Langhans cells appear as closely packed cuboidal or polyhedral cells with deeply staining nuclei. Although such changes are much more common and more marked in trophoblastic neoplasia, they are also found in normal pregnancy. Large or hydropic villi may appear with a transitional mole, blighted ovum, or normal first-trimester pregnancy and require differentiation from a hydatidiform mole, although as a rule hyperplasia and more disordered growth patterns (*i.e.,* anaplasia) are observed. Trophoblastic hyperplasia of greater or lesser degree occurs in almost all chorionic villi; the more extensive its occurrence, the higher the risk of developing choriocarcinoma following a complete hydatidiform mole. Although a general correlation exists between the morphologic and clinical malignancy of any given mole, histologic grading of trophoblastic proliferation cannot be used to predict accurately the possibility of malignant sequelae. Physical, roentgenologic, and laboratory (hCG) monitoring is needed.

Complete hydatidiform moles associated with twin fetuses are rare. The fetus usually aborts; however, on occasion it may reach term. It is important to distinguish the presence of complete hydatidiform moles in these patients, since there is a potential for malignant sequelae.

Complete hydatidiform moles are known to result from fertilization of an egg the nucleus of which is lost

or inactivated (Fig. 22-4). Androgenesis results when a haploid sperm (23X) duplicates, reconstituting the diploid number (46XX) but rendering the complete mole homozygous. The conceptus is genetically female, but it is also a paternally derived parthenogenone and a total allograft to the mother. In approximately 90% of hydatidiform moles, 46XX diploid and chromatin-positive cellular patterns are found. As progression toward choriocarcinoma occurs, the percentage of aneuploid cells increases.

FIG. 22-2. (*A*) Uterine cavity filled with hydatidiform mole. *Dark areas* denote hemorrhage. (*B*) Vesicular appearance of hydropic villi.

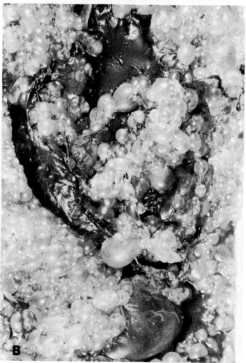

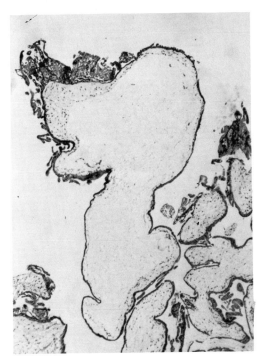

FIG. 22-3. Hydatidiform mole. Chorionic villus demonstrates marked interstitial fluid accumulation, and there are fetal vessels. Area of trophoblastic proliferation is seen at one margin of villus. (H&E, ×40)

Partial Hydatidiform Mole

A different etiology appears to exist for a partial hydatidiform mole. There is evidence of an embryo or fetus, and embryonic membranes are present. The histologic pattern is often a mosaic of nonhydropic villi intermixed with hydropic villi of the kind seen in the complete mole. Because of this mosaic-like pattern, extensive placental sampling is required; the one or two paraffin blocks taken routinely for pathologic examination are inadequate in this situation. Fetal vessels are present and, not uncommonly, fetal erythroblasts can be seen. Proliferation of the trophoblast is often inconspicuous, and it is uncommon to detect marked hyperplasia as is seen in complete hydatidiform moles. Usually the hyperplasia is confined to the syncytiotrophoblast, and only a few cases show cytotrophoblastic proliferation. As a consequence, the potential for malignant transformation is much less than that associated with the complete hydatidiform mole. In some cases, vesicles may be identified grossly; for the most part, the diagnosis is made by the pathologist at microscopic examination of aborted tissue.

The karyotype of partial hydatidiform mole is normal diploid, trisomic, or triploid (Fig. 22-5). Maternal genes do exist, and where the origin of the triploid has been determined, dispermy has been found to be the

most likely explanation. Both diandry (one maternal and two paternal sets of chromosomes) and digyny (two maternal and one paternal sets of chromosomes) can occur. The differences between complete and partial hydatidiform mole are summarized in Table 22-1. Karyotyping is needed for definitive diagnosis.

Invasive Mole (Chorioadenoma Destruens)

An invasive mole is a complete hydatidiform mole that has invaded the myometrium. The majority of cases are recognized within the six-month period following evacuation of a hydatidiform mole. The reason for penetration may lie in an immunologic alteration of host resistance to the developing trophoblast (see Chap. 12). Regardless of the cause, plaques and columns of molar tissue penetrate the myometrium and invade the blood vessels, resulting in local hemorrhage and, in some cases, metastatic transport of fragments to other parts of the body. The advancing mole may penetrate the entire thickness of the myometrium, causing uterine rupture with intra-abdominal hemorrhage and secondary involvement of adjacent pelvic structures.

The histologic characteristics of an invasive mole are identical to those of a complete hydatidiform mole that is confined to the uterine cavity. The villous pattern is well preserved. Abnormal mitotic figures do not accompany either hydatidiform mole or invasive mole. Curettings are helpful in making the diagnosis only if they include a sample of myometrium that is large enough to demonstrate actual invasion (Fig. 22-6).

FIG. 22-4. Chromosomal origin of a complete mole. A single sperm fertilizes an "empty egg." Reduplication of its 23,X set gives a completely homozygous diploid genome of 46,XX. A similar process follows fertilization of an empty egg by two sperms with two independently drawn sets of 23,X or 23,Y; note that both karyotypes 46,XX and 46,XY can ensue. (Szulman AE: Syndromes of hydatidiform moles. J Reprod Med 29: 788, 1984)

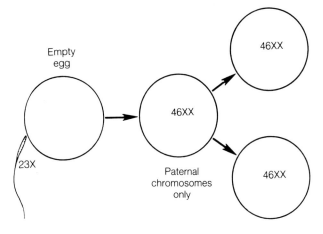

FIG. 22-5. Chromosomal origin of the triploid, partial mole. A normal egg with a 23,X haploid set is fertilized by two sperms that can carry either sex chromosome, to give a total of 69 chromosomes with a sex configuration of XXY, XXX, and XYY. A similar result can be obtained by fertilization with a sperm carrying the unreduced paternal genome 46,XY (resulting sex complement, XXY only). (Szulman AE: Syndromes of hydatidiform moles. J Reprod Med 29:788, 1984)

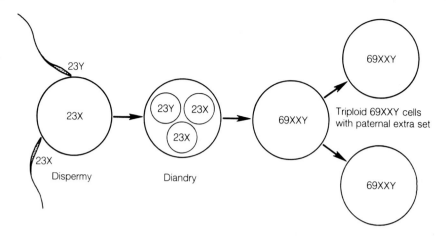

Table 22-1
Complete and Partial Hydatidiform Moles

Feature	Complete Mole	Partial Mole
Karyotype	46XX	Triploid
Embryo/fetus	Absent	Present
Trophoblast proliferation	Often marked	Focal, mild
Stromal edema	Pronounced	Variable
Fetal vessels	Absent	Present
Malignant potential	Expected	Remote

Choriocarcinoma

Choriocarcinoma is a highly malignant, pure epithelial tumor derived from uncontrolled proliferation of trophoblastic cells. There are no chorionic villi; there are only sheets of anaplastic trophoblastic tissue intermixed with areas of necrosis, hemorrhage, and vacuolation that form the plexiform cellular pattern that characterizes this tumor (Fig. 22-7). Abnormal mitoses, multinucleated cells, hyperchromatism, and anisonucleosis are characteristic. Grossly, the cut surfaces of the lesions have a red granular appearance (Fig. 22-8). The malignant tissue invades the myometrium and blood vessels, and metastases quickly follow. The most common sites are the lungs and vagina, although the brain, kidney, liver, and vulva are other possible sites of metastatic lesions. The malignant transformation of the chorionic tissue may occur either in the uterus (or fallopian tube) or, when benign trophoblast reaches the maternal circulation, in the bloodstream or in target tissues.

Although the microscopic findings of choriocarcinoma are characteristic, it may be difficult to diagnose from curettings unless the entire specimen is carefully processed. The lack of chorionic villi is a striking and diagnostic feature, but curettage may have dislodged the foci of trophoblastic cells from underlying villi that would have been evident if the entire uterine specimen had been available for study. When curettage is done

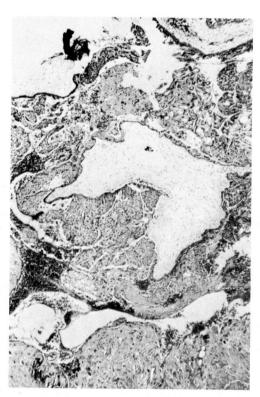

FIG. 22-6. Invasive mole (chorioadenoma destruens) invading myometrium. Villous architecture is preserved. (H&E, ×30)

for postpregnancy bleeding, it is important to process the entire material histologically, since small isolated areas of choriocarcinoma may be found. The similarity of the trophoblastic cells of an implanting blastocyst to the proliferation of trophoblastic disease has been mentioned earlier, but this should not cause confusion in diagnosis.

Unlike invasive mole, choriocarcinoma can follow any kind of pregnancy; hydatidiform mole, tubal pregnancy, blighted ovum, spontaneous or induced abortion,

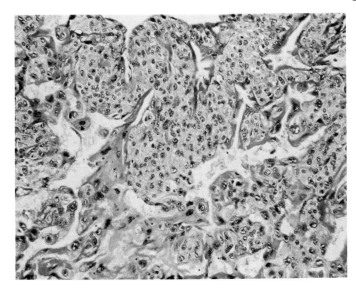

FIG. 22-7. Choriocarcinoma. Cords of cytotrophoblasts are surrounded by syncytiotrophoblasts, with intervening vascular spaces. (H&E, ×120)

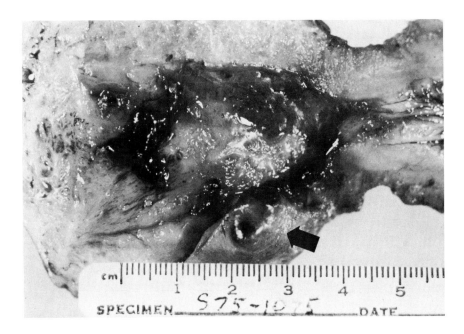

FIG. 22-8. Surgical specimen. After evacuation of hydatidiform mole, hCG titers dropped progressively for four weeks, then increased. Hysterectomy specimen showed no trophoblastic tissue in uterine cavity; intramural nodule (*arrow*) proved microscopically to be choriocarcinoma. Titers are shown in Figure 22-10.

or term pregnancy. Latent choriocarcinoma has been observed several years after the last known pregnancy. Spontaneous regression has also been known to occur, and some metastases have disappeared after removal of the primary tumor, which accounts for the occasional cures that were achieved before the advent of chemotherapy.

INCIDENCE

Complete hydatidiform moles occur in approximately 1 in 1500 pregnancies in the United States; a coexistent fetus occurs in approximately 1 in 20,000 pregnancies. The risk of developing a second mole is 4 to 5 times higher than the risk of the first. The possibility of three independent moles in the same patient is 1500^3 (1 in 3,375,000,000). There is marked geographic variation in the incidence of hydatidiform mole in relation to the known number of pregnancies. The incidence is 5 to 15 times higher in the Far East and Southeast Asia than it is in the Western world; as a consequence, the incidence of all types of malignant trophoblastic neoplasia is similarly increased. Approximately 80% of hydatidiform moles regress spontaneously; 15% continue as nonmetastatic gestational trophoblastic disease, and 5% become metastatic gestational trophoblastic disease. Of patients with metastatic trophoblastic disease, 50% develop the tumors as sequelae of a molar pregnancy.

The incidence of *partial hydatidiform mole* is difficult to estimate. Many escape unnoticed because of inadequate sampling of tissue from aborted or term pregnancy; there is inconsistency in the pathologic criteria needed for diagnosis; and karyotyping is seldom done. In the series of Szulman and colleagues, partial moles constituted 9.4% of all moles studied.

Invasive mole occurs in approximately 1 in 15,000 pregnancies, or one tenth as frequently as noninvasive mole.

It has been estimated that in the United States 1 in 40 moles, 1 in 5000 ectopic pregnancies, 1 in 15,000 abortions, and 1 in 150,000 normal pregnancies result in *choriocarcinoma*. Choriocarcinoma is preceded by hydatidiform mole in 50%, by abortion in 25%, by normal pregnancy in 22.5%, and by ectopic pregnancy in 2.5%.

Approximately 3000 new cases of hydatidiform mole and 500 to 750 new cases of malignant gestational trophoblastic neoplasia are expected to occur in the United States each year.

According to incidence figures for all pregnancies, 67 cases of gestational trophoblastic neoplasia should be encountered among every 100,000 induced abortions. This number is small, but it indicates the need for gross and microscopic examination of every induced abortion specimen.

PATHOPHYSIOLOGY

Since the three major trophoblastic neoplasms are part of a continuing spectrum of trophoblastic proliferation, it follows that the systemic responses to the three neoplasms are similar.

Human Chorionic Gonadotropin

There is no documented exception to the observation that human trophoblastic cells produce hCG when they grow. The formation, function, and detection of hCG in normal pregnancy are discussed in Chapter 18. The amount of hCG produced correlates directly with the amount of viable trophoblastic tissue present (Table 22-2). In trophoblastic neoplasia, the hCG production greatly exceeds that of normal pregnancy, providing the single most important measure for evaluating the response to therapy.

In normal pregnancy, hCG is produced in minimal but detectable amounts as early as 1 day after implantation, increases rapidly to peak levels of about 50,000 mIU/ml serum about 65 days after implantation, and declines for the remainder of pregnancy to levels that vary from 15,000 mIU to 30,000 mIU/ml. It disappears from the maternal bloodstream and urine 10 to 14 days after delivery or after the successful treatment of trophoblastic neoplasia.

Early in the course of trophoblastic disease, hCG levels are not helpful in diagnosis unless they exceed

Table 22-2
*Tumor hCG Production**

Volume	No. of Cells	hCG (IU)
1 mg	10^6	10^2
1 g	10^9	10^5
1 kg	10^{12}	10^8

* Based on exponential growth of tumor cells.

100,000 mIU/ml serum, since such levels are sometimes found in normal pregnancy. However, if a hydatidiform mole has been evacuated, if choriocarcinoma is suspected after a normal pregnancy, or if there is a possibility of metastasis from an invasive mole, hCG levels assume preeminent importance. The available tests and their range of sensitivity are discussed in Chapter 20. Since in the aforementioned cases the amounts of hCG may vary widely at either high or low levels, it is apparent that a sensitive and specific test is needed and that ordinary tests for the diagnosis of pregnancy are not appropriate. When hCG levels are extremely high, as in the early stages of trophoblastic neoplasia, rapid radioreceptorassay tests (RRA) or immunologic agglutination assays can be used. However, when hCG levels below 1000 mIU/ml are encountered, it is preferable to employ radioimmunoassay (RIA) for the beta subunit of hCG in order to avoid confusion with human luteinizing hormone (hLH). For practical purposes, the RIA β-hCG test is specific, and it can detect hCG concentrations of less than 2 mIU/ml serum. Immediate availability of these tests is an essential part of the armamentarium for management and follow-up of trophoblastic neoplasia.

Preliminary studies suggest that as the assays for pregnancy-specific β_1-glycoprotein become more specific, tests for this protein may serve as a useful adjunct to hCG for the evaluation and monitoring of trophoblastic disease.

Theca Lutein Ovarian Cysts

Because of the intense stimulation of the theca interna by very high levels of hCG, theca lutein cysts are a common finding in gestational trophoblastic neoplasia. They occur in at least 30% of cases. The cysts are multilocular, bilateral, red gray to purple gray, and measure up to 10 cm to 12 cm in diameter. The locules are lined by plump theca interna or granulosa cells, and the cyst contents often test positively for gonadotropins. Such cysts sometimes become refractory to hCG and may subside during the course of the disease. They invariably regress spontaneously after resolution of trophoblastic activity and are to be left in place without surgical intervention (see Fig. 59-7).

Thyroid-Stimulating Activity

Thyroid-stimulating activity has been observed in patients with extensive trophoblastic neoplasia, and approximately 5% of patients with metastatic disease suffer from thyrotoxicosis. The evidence suggests that the thyroid-stimulating hormone (TSH) of trophoblastic disease is chemically different from the similarly acting hormone secreted by the placenta (see page 349) and the pituitary, and that it is hCG *per se* that has this quality. Compared with pituitary TSH, its activity is estimated to be approximately 1:4000. The condition clears dramatically after eradication of all trophoblastic tissue.

Estrogens

The estrogens (notably estriol) that require fetal participation in synthesis are decreased in patients with hydatidiform mole. Total estrogen level is low normal for early pregnancy, and estradiol is somewhat increased, especially in the presence of theca lutein cysts. This leads to a reversal of the pregnancy ratio of estriol:estradiol + estrone.

Serum Progesterone

Significant increases in serum progesterone levels occur with both hydatidiform mole and choriocarcinoma. Both molar trophoblast and theca lutein cysts contribute to the elevated progesterone levels. In choriocarcinoma, the ovaries are the major source of progesterone. Since progesterone levels are invariably elevated in trophoblastic disease, they have been used to monitor the course of the disease; however, they are far less reliable than hCG determinations.

Preeclampsia

Preeclampsia occurs in about 15% of women with hydatidiform mole, the only circumstance in which this complication occurs before 20 weeks' gestation. Its cause is unknown. Factors that may be involved are uterine distention, excessive levels of hCG, and immunobiologic phenomena.

STAGING AND CLASSIFICATION

As noted above, the course of gestational trophoblastic disease is so variable and so unpredictable that the pathologist's classification in three major categories (hydatidiform mole, invasive mole, and choriocarcinoma) is not adequate either for evaluating an individual case or for outlining or monitoring therapy. Clinical findings are of major importance in categorizing patients for treatment, and a classification must take these findings into account to be clinically useful.

In 1982, the Fédération Internationale de Gynécologie et Obstétrique (FIGO) adopted a staging system for trophoblastic disease that is based on anatomic criteria and conforms to the FIGO staging systems for other gynecologic malignancies, as follows:

Stage I: Disease confined to the corpus uteri
Stage II: Metastases to pelvis and vagina
Stage III: Metastases to lung
Stage IV: Metastases to brain, liver, spleen, or gastrointestinal tract

This staging system is useful in assigning risk and prognosis in stage-I disease (where usually the risk is low and the outlook is good) and in stage-IV disease (where the risk is high and the outlook is much less favorable); it is less helpful in stages II and III, since patients who are at both low risk and high risk may fall into either group.

The clinical classification that has been used in the United States (Table 22-3) takes into account factors that alter the risk for certain groups of patients and has been valuable as a guide to therapy. The factors considered to be of special importance in assigning risk are the duration of disease, the magnitude of the hCG value, and the sites of metastases.

More recently, prognostic scoring systems have been introduced in an effort to achieve greater precision in the assignment of risk and, hence, in selection of therapy. The World Health Organization (WHO) prognostic scoring system is shown in Table 22-4. The additional risk factors that the prognostic scoring systems take into account are the patient's age, the nature of the prior pregnancy (*i.e.,* whether mole, abortion, or term

---

Table 22-3
Clinical Classification

I. Nonmetastatic trophoblastic disease
   A. Hydatidiform mole
      1. Undelivered
      2. Delivered (<8 weeks)
   B. Persistent mole (>8 weeks)
   C. Invasive mole or choriocarcinoma confined to the uterus
II. Metastatic trophoblastic disease
   A. Low-risk metastatic
      1. Short duration (<4 months)
      2. Low hCG titer (<100,000 IU/24 hrs)
      3. Lung or vaginal metastasis
   B. Intermediate-risk metastatic
      1. Long duration (>4 months)
      2. High hCG titer (>100,000 IU/24 hrs)
      3. Metastasis other than central nervous system or liver
   C. High-risk metastatic
      1. Central nervous system metastasis
      2. Liver metastasis

(Modified from Lewis JL Jr: Ann Clin Lab Sci 9:387, 1979)

Table 22-4
WHO Prognostic Scoring System for Trophoblastic Disease

	Score*			
Prognostic Factors	*0*	*1*	*2*	*4*
Age (years)	≤39	>39		
Antecedent pregnancy	HM	Abortion	Term	
Interval†	4	4–6	7–12	12
hCG (IU/liter)	<10^3	10^3–10^4	10^4–10^5	>10^5
ABO groups (female × male)		O × A	B	
		A × O	AB	
Largest tumor, including uterine tumor		3–5 cm	5 cm	
Site of metastases		Spleen	Gastrointestinal tract	Brain
		Kidney	Liver	
Number of metastases identified		1–4	4–8	8
Prior chemotherapy			Single-drug	2 or more drugs

* Total score ≤4, low risk; 5–7, intermediate risk; ≥8, high risk.

† Interval: time (months) between end of antecedent pregnancy and start of chemotherapy.

WHO, World Health Organization; *HM,* hydatidiform mole.

pregnancy), the interval since the last pregnancy, the ABO blood groups, the size of the largest tumor, the site and number of metastases, and the nature of any prior chemotherapy. The weight given to these factors is shown in the table. A total score of 4 or less assigns the patient to the low-risk group; a score of 5 to 7 indicates intermediate risk; a score of 8 or higher indicates high risk.

NONMETASTATIC GESTATIONAL TROPHOBLASTIC DISEASE

Nonmetastatic trophoblastic disease refers to gestational trophoblastic neoplasms that are confined to the uterus. They include hydatidiform mole (either preevacuation or postevacuation), invasive mole (chorioadenoma destruens), and choriocarcinoma confined to the uterus.

Hydatidiform Mole

Signs and Symptoms

In the early stages, hydatidiform mole cannot be distinguished from a normal pregnancy. Ultimately, vaginal bleeding occurs in almost every case. It may be dark brown ("prune juice") in appearance, or bright red, scant or profuse, and may continue for only a few days or intermittently for weeks. Scant bleeding occurs in approximately 10% of all early pregnancies; therefore, most patients with bleeding during early pregnancy do not have a hydatidiform mole. Prolonged bleeding, however, should suggest this possibility.

At first examination, only half of the patients have a uterus significantly larger than one would expect from the menstrual dates. The percentage of patients with an excessively enlarged uterus increases as the length of time from the last menstrual period increases. Approximately 25% of patients will have a uterus smaller than would be expected from the menstrual dates.

Anemia from blood loss, nausea and vomiting, and abdominal cramps due to uterine distention are relatively common. Anemia results from intrauterine bleeding and in some patients may be disproportionate to the amount of visible blood loss. Preeclampsia occurs in about 15% of cases, usually between 9 and 12 gestational weeks. Hyperthyroidism and pulmonary embolization of trophoblastic elements occur less frequently but are serious complications of hydatidiform mole. Ovarian enlargement due to theca lutein cysts is detected in approximately 10% of women at the time of uterine evacuation; in 20% of cases, ovarian enlargement is detected one to four weeks after a mole has been evacuated.

Many moles abort spontaneously. When hydropic vesicles are passed vaginally and the patient has the wit to save the specimen, the diagnosis can be established with certainty.

Diagnosis

The finding of one or more grapelike hydropic vesicles in the vagina, or passed vaginally, is diagnostic of hydatidiform mole. Unfortunately, no clinical sign or symptom permits a diagnosis before tissue is passed. The problem of diagnosis prior to uterine evacuation may be difficult and often requires additional means of detection.

The most reliable means of detecting a mole prior to uterine evacuation are ultrasonography and amniography. Ultrasonography (see page 278) is noninvasive, safe, and reasonably reliable for early diagnosis. The sonographic pattern of a molar pregnancy is characterized by diffuse sonodense echoes distributed in a "snowstorm" pattern (see Fig. 15-16). Uncommonly, this picture may be mimicked by uterine fibroids, intrauterine fetal death, and, rarely, a normal uterine pregnancy. Few diagnostic errors occur when the sonogram is evaluated by a qualified examiner. Any uncertainty is usually clarified by an accurate clinical history, an accurate hCG titer, and, if necessary, a repeat sonogram in two weeks. *Amniography* is an invasive procedure in which radiopaque material is instilled into the uterus transabdominally. A moth-eaten or honeycomb pattern establishes the diagnosis of hydatidiform mole. A 3% failure rate has been reported for this procedure, but for practical purposes it is almost invariably diagnostic. The latter technique is rarely needed if ultrasonography is available.

A baseline serum hCG level is required prior to evacuation of the uterus. This is not considered diagnostic, since the required information is usually provided by the clinical history, physical examination, and ultrasound study. If ultrasonography and the clinical picture are equivocal, hCG concentrations significantly higher then those of normal early pregnancy can be suggestive. The customary hCG level in hydatidiform mole of six to eight weeks' duration is 200,000 mIU to 300,000 mIU/ml, but in occasional cases much higher values may be found, especially if the mole is very large. Following the baseline hCG determination, follow-up hCG levels at weekly intervals will determine the natural behavior of the disease and will monitor the response to chemotherapy.

Treatment

In the past, dilatation and curettage (D&C) was recommended if the uterus was 12 weeks' gestational size or less, and abdominal hysterotomy was recommended if the size of the uterus was larger than 12 weeks' gestational size. More recently, suction curettage has been found to be safe and effective for most hydatidiform moles, regardless of size. When the uterus is larger than 12 weeks' gestational size, a laparotomy set-up should be immediately available; the larger the uterus, the greater the possibility of perforation and uncontrolled hemorrhage. An oxytocin infusion (30 U/liter 5% DW, 40–60 drops/minute) should be started when the uterus has been approximately 50% evacuated or if disturbing bleeding occurs. After the uterus is thoroughly emptied by suction curettage, gentle sharp curettage is performed. The curettings are submitted for separate study, since there may be different degrees of trophoblastic proliferation in each of the specimens. When a hydatidiform mole regresses spontaneously, serum hCG levels drop rapidly and should return to nonpregnant levels within 8 to 12 weeks.

Although suction curettage is usually appropriate, hysterectomy may be considered for patients of high parity, those 40 years of age or older, and those who have completed their desired families. The malignancy rate in women over age 40 reaches 35%, and in those of high parity it approximates 15%. Women over age 40 are not only more likely to develop malignant sequelae after a molar pregnancy but are also likely to have more problems with chemotherapy, which may be avoided by surgery. It is emphasized that surgical removal of the uterus does not dismiss the physician from the responsibility for meticulous follow-up.

Chemotherapy is not recommended for prophylaxis or therapy of uncomplicated hydatidiform mole. In 80% of cases, retained molar tissue regresses spontaneously; of those who do develop malignant sequelae, all can be cured by presently available techniques.

Subsequent Clinical Course

Eighty percent of complete hydatidiform moles undergo spontaneous regression following uterine evacuation, with a prompt fall-off in serum hCG levels, resumption of cyclic menses, and no subsequent development of malignant disease. The rate and constancy of hCG production by any remaining viable tumor cells predict the outcome. If the hCG level remains elevated eight weeks after uterine evacuation of a hydatidiform mole and there is no evidence of extrauterine disease, a persistent mole, invasive mole, or nonmetastatic gestational choriocarcinoma may be present. The clinical features of patients at greatest risk for the development of malignant sequelae are those with a large uterus and bilateral ovarian enlargement. In two reviews of hydatidiform mole, 57% and 62% of patients with these characteristics required chemotherapy for persistent trophoblastic disease. Approximately 30% of patients with nonmetastatic and 25% of patients with metastatic disease have an enlarged uterus and theca lutein cysts.

The malignant potential of partial moles is unsettled. A few cases have been reported in which chemotherapy was required, but these cases may be suspect. Szulman observed that no case of transformation of partial mole to choriocarcinoma has yet been reported, and Dodson pointed out that no case of partial mole that required treatment has both fulfilled the histologic criteria of a partial mole *and* been demonstrated to have a karyotype (*e.g.*, triploidy) that is inconsistent with a complete mole. The consensus appears to be that partial mole may have malignant potential, but the question remains open.

Follow-Up

The principal objective of follow-up is to detect persistent uterine or metastatic disease as early as possible. Approximately 20% of patients with hydatidiform mole have an elevated serum hCG titer eight weeks after uterine evacuation. Of these, 50% develop clinical or histologic malignancy, that is, invasive mole or chorio-carcinoma. The initial pathologic diagnosis is of little value in predicting whether an individual patient will develop subsequent trophoblastic malignancy. Clinical findings such as prompt uterine involution, regression of enlarged ovarian cysts, and cessation of bleeding are all optimistic clinical signs, but definitive follow-up after molar pregnancy requires determination of serial hCG levels. Figure 22-9 illustrates a normal β-hCG regression curve in a patient with a hydatidiform mole treated by suction curettage.

The following protocol should be rigidly adhered to in the follow-up of all patients with complete hydatidiform mole:

1. *Weekly hCG assay until complete remission* (weekly normal hCG titers for three consecutive weeks). RRA is suitable if hCG levels exceed 1000 mIU/ml serum; RIA should be used for levels of β-hCG below 1000 mIU/ml. *After complete remission,* β-hCG should be measured by RIA every month for six months and then every two months for the next six months. In patients who require chemotherapy or who develop malignant disease, β-hCG should be measured by RIA every six months for five years after complete remission.

FIG. 22-9. β-hCG levels in 27-year-old gravida 2 para 0 after evacuation of hydatidiform mole by suction curettage. Values returned to within normal range (below 10 mIU/ml serum) in about seven weeks.

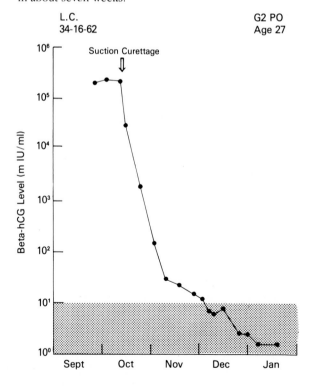

2. *Physical and pelvic examination at two-week intervals* until complete remission has occurred, the uterus and ovaries have returned to normal size, and uterine bleeding has ceased.
3. *Chest x-ray film at the time of evacuation of mole.* Further chest films are not needed if hCG levels continue to fall spontaneously and complete remission follows. When chemotherapy is required, chest films are necessary for staging purposes and for determining prognostic factors.
4. *Avoidance of pregnancy* for one year after evacuation of a hydatidiform mole. If there are no contrary indications, oral contraception may be prescribed. There is no confirmation for the suggestion that trophoblastic disease may regress more slowly if oral contraception is started before serum hCG levels return to normal.
5. Prompt institution of *chemotherapy* if hCG levels plateau or rise, or if metastases appear.

A *cure* is defined as complete absence of all clinical and hormonal evidence of disease for five years.

Just as the malignant potential of partial hydatidiform mole is unsettled, there is also no agreement as to the depth of follow-up that is appropriate. Until more information is available, some consider it prudent to make the same follow-up as for complete mole, as outlined above. Others consider it reasonable to relax the protocol and to follow hCG levels only until they return to normal.

Persistent Hydatidiform Mole

Retention of molar tissue and continued elevation of serum hCG levels eight weeks after evacuation of a hydatidiform mole is referred to as a *persistent hydatidiform mole.* Clinically, the uterus remains soft and enlarged and uterine bleeding is often present. Persistent theca lutein cysts may be palpable. Under these circumstances it is essential to rule out extrauterine disease by a metastatic survey. This includes physical examination, chest film, intravenous pyelogram, liver and brain scan, liver and kidney function tests, ultrasound, and selected computed tomography (CT) scan of the abdomen and pelvis. If the results of these tests are negative, it can be presumed that the disease is limited to the uterus. Persistent hydatidiform mole is one of the three conditions that may produce this picture. The other two possibilities include invasive mole and choriocarcinoma limited to the uterus. Regardless of the diagnosis, the initial clinical and therapeutic approach is the same.

Treatment

CHEMOTHERAPY. It is emphasized that chemotherapy, like surgery and radiation therapy, is a major therapeutic modality and should be used only by those who are properly schooled in its administration and its side-effects, who are knowledgeable in the nuances of trophoblastic disease, and who have at hand the supporting services required. A major risk factor that has emerged in recent years in regional trophoblastic disease centers is that of late death resulting from drug resistance. The risk of developing drug resistance is related both to the relative degree of prognostic factors present and the manner in which the patient is managed at the time of initial treatment and before referral to a regional trophoblastic disease center. The risks that a patient faces therefore are a function of both the disease status and the clinical management. When the risk of developing drug resistance is low, simple and safe chemotherapy can be given. Where the risk of drug resistance is increased, more complex and hazardous methods are required. Brewer and co-workers have shown a significant difference in remission rates between those originally treated at the Northwestern Trophoblastic Disease Center and those who were referred after treatment failure. Of those who died, 34% were in the latter group and 21% were in the former.

Single-agent chemotherapy is used as first-line treatment for persistent hydatidiform mole as well as for invasive mole and choriocarcinoma limited to the uterus. Single-agent chemotherapy may also be appropriate for some patients with low-risk prognostic scores whose disease is stage II or III. Once a diagnosis has been made, chemotherapy should be started immediately. Historically the two agents that have been shown to be most effective in treating early, or low-risk, disease are methotrexate and dactinomycin (actinomycin-D). Either methotrexate or actinomycin-D may be used initially if renal and hepatic functions are normal. If these are impaired, the use of methotrexate is generally avoided. The two drugs have similar response rates and there is no crossover in drug resistance. Therefore, if resistance appears under therapy with one drug, the other drug may be used.

Toxicity is a major problem associated with chemotherapy. Chemotherapy must be given in maximally tolerated doses at frequent intervals if drug resistance is to be avoided. Maximally tolerated doses are designed to produce intentional toxicity without producing irreversible toxicity. Inadequate doses of chemotherapy or prolonged delays between courses may lead to drug resistance and, in some, a fatal issue. Appropriate surveillance is essential before and during each course of chemotherapy if irreversible toxicity is to be avoided. Predictable, but usually not dose-limiting, side-effects include alopecia, stomatitis, dermatitis, nausea and vomiting, severe gastroenteritis, and bone marrow suppression. The decision to prevent irreversible toxicity is made during the time that the drug is being administered, not later. Overwhelming toxicity, which may prove to be fatal, does not usually occur until five to ten days after the termination of the course of treatment. Therefore, careful judgments need to be made on the basis of rather subtle changes in hematopoietic, renal, or hepatic tests in order to avoid unnecessary complications.

The following tests are ordered before administration of the first dose of chemotherapy: leukocyte count (WBC), granulocyte count, platelet count, hematocrit, serum glutamic-oxaloacetic transaminase (SGOT), serum blood urea nitrogen (BUN), and serum creatinine. The usual nadir following single-agent chemotherapy with methotrexate and actinomycin-D occurs 7 to 12 days following chemotherapy. The drug should be withheld until the results return to the following values: hematocrit above 30%, WBC above $3000/\mu l$, granulocyte count above $1500/\mu l$, platelet count above $100,000/\mu l$, SGOT below 50 units, and serum BUN and creatinine stable and not rising.

The usual five-day schedule for administering methotrexate or actinomycin-D has been replaced by Bagshawe's eight-day schedule of intermediate-dose methotrexate given on alternate days, followed on the intervening days with citrovorum factor. This method allows good clinical response as well as virtual elimination of morbidity. Toxicity with the five-day schedule of methotrexate or actinomycin-D is often cumulative, and after several courses it may become prohibitive. More than 80% of patients treated with one course of 8-day methotrexate and citrovorum factor require only one course of chemotherapy. The course may be repeated every 8 days, and should resistance be identified, crossover to the conventional 5-day course of actinomycin-D is suggested. The criteria for changing chemotherapeutic agents in this instance are (1) a rising or plateau hCG titer; (2) evidence of metastases; and (3) excessive drug toxicity using the 5-day course of chemotherapy. Serum hCG levels are measured each week. When they are within normal range in each of three consecutive weeks, chemotherapy is stopped and routine follow-up is started as for a complete hydatidiform mole.

DILATATION AND CURETTAGE. When the uterus remains subinvoluted and there is evidence of uterine bleeding with suspicion of a retained mole, a D&C may be performed on the third day of chemotherapy. Uterine curettage may be therapeutic in this instance, but chemotherapy must be resumed later and continued until complete remission occurs.

HYSTERECTOMY. Hysterectomy is appropriate treatment in the patient with the clinical diagnosis of persistent hydatidiform mole if the patient is 40 years of age or older, if she is of high parity, or if she desires no further pregnancies. The hysterectomy specimen provides an intact uterus that may be examined microscopically for diagnosis as well as for extent of myometrial disease. It should be warned, however, that hysterectomy does not eliminate the need for rigid follow-up according to the protocol outlined for hydatidiform mole. If hysterectomy is indicated, it is performed on the third day of a 5-day course of chemotherapy or on the fifth day of an 8-day course of chemotherapy. Hysterectomy may also be performed when drug failure occurs.

Invasive Mole

When an invasive mole is confined to the uterus, there are no symptoms to distinguish it from a hydatidiform mole except that bleeding may be very heavy as a result of involvement of the myometrial vasculature. Large intramural nodules may occasionally be palpated on pelvic examination; at the time of surgery, the uterus may be irregular with a nodular swelling arising from its wall. Pelvic arteriography and ultrasonography are essential if the uterus is to be conserved. In the patient in whom preservation of childbearing function is important, single-agent chemotherapy, as described above, is indicated. In some instances, uterine perforation may occur, and intraperitoneal bleeding requires an immediate hysterectomy to control the hemorrhage. When single-agent chemotherapy fails, drug-resistant choriocarcinoma may be present and a hysterectomy is recommended during the first course of second-line chemotherapy. The diagnosis of invasive mole (chorioadenoma destruens) is made when locally invasive trophoblastic disease is identified histologically. Regardless of whether the lesion is treated by hysterectomy or chemotherapy, the same follow-up is required as for uncomplicated hydatidiform mole.

Nonmetastatic Choriocarcinoma

The woman with a choriocarcinoma limited to the uterus presents a somewhat more difficult problem. In 2% to 5% of patients with persistent hydatidiform mole, the tumor undergoes transition to gestational choriocarcinoma. Of more concern therapeutically is the problem of choriocarcinoma that develops after a term delivery or a spontaneous abortion. Choriocarcinoma following term delivery or nonmolar abortion tends to be diagnosed at a more advanced stage because the index of suspicion is not as acute. When the tumor is confined to the uterus, uterine subinvolution and bleeding may be present. The diagnosis is based on an elevated hCG titer, histologic diagnosis of choriocarcinoma (when possible), and lack of extrauterine metastases. Establishing the diagnosis of intrauterine choriocarcinoma by curettage may be difficult.

Treatment of nonmetastatic gestational choriocarcinoma depends on the desire of the patient to retain her ability to have children. If she desires more children, it is reasonable to start treatment with chemotherapy. However, it may not be safe to wait until the patient's disease has failed to respond to chemotherapy before turning to hysterectomy, since metastases have been reported to occur during chemotherapy. If no more children are desired, the wise policy is to perform a hysterectomy on the third day of the first course of chemotherapy. Figure 22-10 illustrates a β-hCG curve with an initial rise in titer. Because the patient desired no more children, a hysterectomy was performed on the third day of chemotherapy. The surgical specimen (see Fig. 22-8) showed a solitary intramural nodule of choriocarcinoma. When retention of childbearing ability is important, chemotherapy is recommended until the disease clears or until it becomes evident that the patient is not responding to the drugs selected, in which case hysterectomy should be performed during the first course of subsequent treatment selected.

Response

Complete remission occurs in 100% of patients with nonmetastatic gestational trophoblastic disease who are treated with single-agent chemotherapy. In 5% to 10% of cases, a hysterectomy is required. Thus, reproductive function is preserved in more than 90% of patients. The cure rate of 100% by chemotherapy alone and chemotherapy plus surgery amply exceeds the reported cure rate of approximately 40% for uterine choriocarcinoma treated by hysterectomy alone.

The patient's ability to become pregnant and the subsequent outcome of the pregnancy are matters of concern for both the patient and her physician. Prior chemotherapy does not seem to cause an adverse effect on future pregnancies with regard to congenital malformations or other serious obstetric problems. Nor does the incidence of second malignancies appear to be increased. Patients who received chemotherapy are reported to experience a slightly higher incidence of spontaneous abortion and focal placenta accreta, although this has not been confirmed. There is still concern that chemotherapy may cause mutagenic effects in first or later generations. At present there is no information to settle this question.

METASTATIC GESTATIONAL TROPHOBLASTIC DISEASE

Metastatic gestational trophoblastic disease is defined as trophoblastic disease that extends beyond the limits of the uterus. The diagnosis of metastatic disease is simplified when there is a prior history of hydatidiform mole; these patients are observed more closely because of the known risk of malignant sequelae. Symptoms of metastatic disease may be the first evidence of choriocarcinoma following a full-term delivery or abortion. The tumor commonly metastasizes to the lungs and, less frequently, to the vagina, brain, or liver. Metastases may occur in multiple sites and have been observed in unusual areas such as the breast, bone, lymph nodes, or a branch of the coronary artery. Their growth pattern often leads to unexpected manifestations of disease if the first symptoms are due to metastases in organs distant from the reproductive tract.

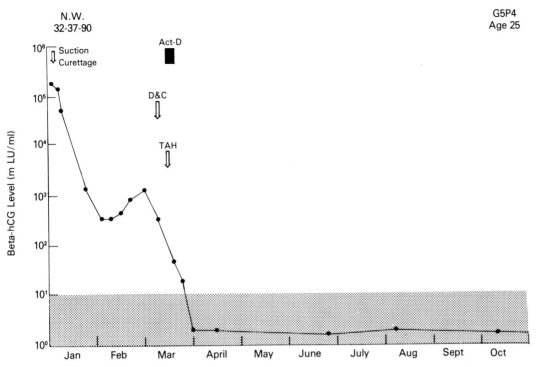

FIG. 22-10. β-hCG regression curve. Following suction curettage of molar pregnancy, serial β-hCG values declined as expected but four weeks later began to rise. Studies revealed no evidence of extrauterine disease. There was no trophoblastic tissue on uterine curettage. Hysterectomy specimen (Fig. 22-8) showed intramural choriocarcinoma.

While symptoms of trophoblastic neoplasms usually develop soon after delivery, long asymptomatic intervals may occur; in the interim, normal menstruation may resume and pregnancy tests may remain negative. It is in cases of this kind that diagnostic errors are especially common. Unfortunately, in these cases the diagnosis is often not made until after the patient has undergone a craniotomy, thoracotomy, resection of a segment of the small bowel, or nephrectomy. One third of patients with metastatic gestational trophoblastic disease seek medical care because of symptoms due to metastases; thus, it is especially critical to recognize the nongynecologic manifestations of this disease (Table 22-5). *Any woman with bleeding or a tumor in any organ who has had a recent or even remote history of molar pregnancy, abortion, or term delivery should have at least one hCG assay to be sure that metastatic gestational trophoblastic disease is not the cause of her problem.*

When metastatic gestational trophoblastic neoplasia is suspected, the following are used to determine the extent of metastatic disease: clinical history and physical examination, chest x-ray film, intravenous pyelogram, liver and brain scans, liver and kidney function tests, ultrasound, and selected CT examinations of the pelvis and abdomen. Brain metastases are usually absent if the chest film is normal. If pulmonary metastases are found, however, a CT scan of the brain and determination of

cerebrospinal fluid levels of hCG may be needed to rule out cerebral metastases. It must be cautioned that metastases detected on full lung tomograms of the chest may not be seen on a plain roentgenogram of the chest. The prognosis depends on the variables noted in the prognostic scoring system (see Table 22-4). It is emphasized again that if patients are treated with inadequate doses or improper chemotherapeutic agents, the response will be seriously jeopardized.

Patients with metastatic gestational trophoblastic neoplasia are divided into low-, intermediate-, and high-

Table 22-5
Extrauterine Manifestations of Metastatic Trophoblastic Disease

I. Pulmonary: coin lesion, progressive dyspnea or hemoptysis, plain-film appearance of pneumonia, unexplained pulmonary hypertension

II. Central nervous system: signs of an expanding lesion, hemorrhage (intracerebral, subarachnoid, or subdural)

III. Gastrointestinal: hemorrhage (lesions of small or large bowel)

IV. Genitourinary: hemorrhage (renal or bladder), ureteral obstruction

risk groups according to the probability of cure in response to chemotherapy. In low-risk and intermediate-risk cases, the rate of cure approaches 100%. In the high-risk group, the outlook is less favorable.

Low-Risk Metastatic Disease

Patients with metastases to either the lung or vagina associated with other optimal risk factors invariably respond to single-agent chemotherapy. These patients are treated initially with either methotrexate or actinomycin-D daily for 5 days, and the course is repeated every 10 to 14 days. Some patients fail to respond to one drug and require treatment with the other. Although the 8-day method of alternating methotrexate with citrovorum factor has been shown to be effective in some patients, the response rate is not yet sufficiently predictable for its use to be recommended. Serum β-hCG levels and the number and size of metastatic lesions are measured serially to evaluate response. Single-agent chemotherapy results in a complete remission rate of 100% when treatment is given in the appropriate manner.

Intermediate-Risk Metastatic Disease

Data affecting the choice of chemotherapy in patients with intermediate-risk metastatic gestational trophoblastic disease are more limited. Chemotherapy is more effective when administered early in the course of the disease, and single-agent chemotherapy is associated with poor response rates when treatment is delayed. Accordingly, combination chemotherapy appears to be the more appropriate choice when initial treatment is delayed more than four months from the antecedent pregnancy and when serum hCG levels are above 100,000 mIU/ml. MAC (methotrexate, actinomycin-D, chlorambucil) and MAC III (methotrexate, citrovorum factor, actinomycin-D, cyclophosphamide) are examples of multiagent chemotherapy that is used in the intermediate-risk group. Although the toxicity and morbidity may be marked, particularly with the former regimen, this form of therapy ordinarily yields a prognosis equivalent to that of the low-risk group. Once the toxic response to the first course of chemotherapy has subsided, the next course is begun.

High-Risk Metastatic Disease

The presence of metastatic choriocarcinoma in the brain and liver significantly increases the severity of the disease but does not preclude cure. Cerebral choriocarcinoma should be considered in any woman of reproductive age with a brain tumor, increased intracranial pressure, or intracranial bleeding. Brain metastases are diagnosed in approximately 10% to 20% of patients with metastatic gestational trophoblastic disease and must be confirmed or excluded in all patients at the start of chemotherapy. CT is a major advance in the detection of cerebral metastases, but serum/spinal fluid ratios for hCG are also sensitive indicators. Hemorrhage into a metastatic brain lesion is a common fatal event that some prefer to avoid by removal of such lesions when they are diagnosed. Others reserve craniotomy for life-threatening hemorrhage.

Liver metastases are insidious in onset, and they may be extensive before symptoms appear. A palpable abdominal mass or evidence of intra-abdominal hemorrhage may be the first sign. Abnormal liver function values are seldom observed in early disease, and transient abnormalities may follow chemotherapy; if they persist, the possibility of extensive liver metastases should be considered. When asymptomatic metastases are suspected, a liver scan or CT scan of the upper abdomen may be helpful in detecting the disease. Pain and intra-abdominal bleeding following acute distention and rupture of Glisson's capsule may indicate extensive liver metastases. Ordinarily, such bleeding can be controlled with primary suture of the lesion or hepatic artery ligation and packing.

The chemotherapy of high-risk trophoblastic disease involves the use of multiple agents, and an effort is made to utilize all, or nearly all, of the potent drugs at an early stage of treatment. Examples of currently used drug combinations are CHAMOCA (hydroxyurea, methotrexate, vincristine, cyclophosphamide, actinomycin-D, adriamycin) and EMA-CO (using etoposide with methotrexate, dactinomycin, vincristine, and cyclophosphamide). The regimens call for rotation of the drugs, with brief rest periods that should not be extended without good cause. Bagshawe has reviewed the details of the regimens that are in current use.

High-dose methotrexate is critically important both in prevention of cerebral metastases and in management when they do occur. In the presence of brain lesions, doses of methotrexate in the range of 1 g to 3 g/m² allow the drug to reach effective concentrations in the central nervous system; when lesser doses are used, intrathecal methotrexate should be given at regular intervals between courses of chemotherapy.

REFERENCES AND RECOMMENDED READING

Athanassiou A, Begent RHJ, Newlands ES et al: Central nervous system metastases of choriocarcinoma: 28 years experience at Charing Cross Hospital. Cancer 52:1728, 1983

Baggish MS, Woodruff JD, Tow SH et al: Sex chromatin pattern in hydatidiform mole. Am J Obstet Gynecol 102:362, 1968

Bagshawe KD: Trophoblastic tumors: Chemotherapy and developments. Br Med J 2:1303, 1963

Bagshawe KD: Choriocarcinoma. In Bagshawe KD: The Clinical Biology of the Trophoblast and Its Tumors. Baltimore, Williams & Wilkins, 1969

Bagshawe KD: Risk and prognostic factors in trophoblastic neoplasia. Cancer 38:1373, 1976

Bagshawe KD: Treatment of high-risk choriocarcinoma. J Reprod Med 29:813, 1984

Bagshawe KD, Harland S: Immunodiagnosis and monitoring of gonadotropin-producing metastases in the central nervous system. Cancer 38:112, 1976

Bandy LC, Clarke–Pearson DL, Hammond CB: Malignant potential of gestational trophoblastic disease at the extreme ages of reproductive life. Obstet Gynecol 64:395, 1984

Berkowitz RS, Goldstein DP, Marean AR et al: Oral contraceptives and postmolar trophoblastic disease. Obstet Gynecol 58:474, 1981

Brewer JI, Rinehart JJ, Dunbar R: Choriocarcinoma. Am J Obstet Gynecol 81:574, 1961

Brewer JI, Smith RT, Pratt GB: Choriocarcinoma: Absolute five year survival rates of 122 patients treated by hysterectomy. Am J Obstet Gynecol 85:841, 1963

Cohen BA, Burkman RT, Rosenshein NB et al: Gestational trophoblastic disease within an elective abortion population. Am J Obstet Gynecol 135:452, 1979

Cotton DB, Bernstein SG, Read JA et al: Hemodynamic observations in evacuation of molar pregnancy. Am J Obstet Gynecol 138:6, 1980

Curry SL, Hammond CB, Tyrey L et al: Hydatidiform mole: Diagnosis, management, and long term follow-up of 347 patients. Obstet Gynecol 45:1, 1975

Delfs E: Quantitative chorionic gonadotropin: Prognostic value in hydatidiform mole and chorionepithelioma. Obstet Gynecol 9:1, 1957

Dodson MG: New concepts and questions in gestational trophoblastic disease. J Reprod Med 28:741, 1983

Fisher RA, Sheppard DM, Lawler SD: Twin pregnancy with complete hydatidiform mole (46XX) and fetus (46XY): Genetic origin proved by analysis of chromosome polymorphisms. Br Med J 1:1218, 1982

Gestational Trophoblastic Diseases: World Health Organization Technical Report Series 692. Geneva, World Health Organization, 1983

Hammond CB, Borchert LG, Tyrey L et al: Treatment of metastatic trophoblastic disease: Good and poor prognosis. Am J Obstet Gynecol 115:451, 1973

Hertig AT, Mansell H: Tumors of the female sex organs: Part 1. Hydatidiform mole and choriocarcinoma. In Hertig AT, Mansell H: Atlas of Tumor Pathology, pp 1-63. Washington, DC, Armed Forces Institute of Pathology, 1956

Hertig AT, Sheldon WH: Hydatidiform mole: A pathologico-clinical correlation of 200 cases. Am J Obstet Gynecol 53:1, 1947

Hertz R, Lewis JL Jr., Lipsett MB: Five years' experience with the chemotherapy of metastatic choriocarcinoma and related trophoblastic tumors in women. Am J Obstet Gynecol 82:631, 1961

Hilgers RD, Lewis JL Jr.: Gestational trophoblastic neoplasms. Gynecol Oncol 2:460, 1974

Hilgers RD, Standefer JC, Rutledge JM et al: Trophoblastic cell sensitivity to 8 day chemotherapy in nonmetastatic gestational trophoblastic neoplasia. Gynecol Oncol 17:386, 1984

Jacobs PA, Hunt PA, Matsura JS et al: Complete and partial hydatidiform mole in Hawaii: Cytogenetics, morphology and epidemiology. Br J Obstet Gynaecol 89:258, 1982

Jacobs PA, Szulman AE, Funkhouser J et al: Human triploidy: Relationship between the parental origin of chromosomes and the development of partial mole in the placenta. Ann Hum Genet 46:223, 1982

Javey H, Borazjani G, Behmard S et al: Discrepancies in the histological diagnosis of hydatidiform mole. Br J Obstet Gynaecol 86:480, 1979

Jones WB, Lewis JL Jr., Lehr M: Monitor of chemotherapy in gestational trophoblastic neoplasm by radioimmunoassay of the beta subunit of human chorionic gonadotropin. Am J Obstet Gynecol 121:669, 1975

Kajii T, Ohama K: Androgenetic origin of hydatidiform mole. Nature 268:633, 1977

Kato M, Tanaka K, Takeuchi S: The nature of trophoblastic disease initiated by transplantation into immunosuppressed animals. Am J Obstet Gynecol 142:497, 1982

Kenimer JG, Herschmen JM, Higgins HP: The thyrotropin in hydatidiform moles in human chorionic gonadotropin. J Clin Endocrinol Metab 40:482, 1975

Lawler SD, Fisher RA, Pickthall VJ et al: Genetic studies on hydatidiform moles: I. The origin of partial moles. Cancer Genet Cytogenet 5:309, 1982

Lawler SD, Povey S, Fisher RA et al: Genetic studies on hydatidiform moles: II. The origin of complete moles. Ann Hum Genet 46:209, 1982

Lewis JL Jr.: Human leukocyte antigens and ABO blood groups in gestational trophoblastic neoplasms. In Seventh National Cancer Conference Proceedings, pp 205–211. New York, American Cancer Society, 1973

Lewis JL Jr.: Current status of treatment of gestational trophoblastic disease. Cancer 38:620, 1976

Lewis JL Jr.: Treatment of gestational trophoblastic neoplasms: A brief review of development in the years 1968 to 1978. Am J Obstet Gynecol 136:163, 1980

Lewis JL Jr., Gore H, Hertig AT et al: Treatment of trophoblastic disease with rationale for use of adjunctive chemotherapy at the time of indicated operation. Am J Obstet Gynecol 96:710, 1966

Li MC, Hertz R, Spencer DB: Effect of methotrexate therapy upon choriocarcinoma and chorioadenoma. Proc Soc Exp Biol Med 93:361, 1956

Lurain JR, Brewer JI: Invasive mole. Semin Oncol 9:174, 1982

Lurain JR, Brewer JI, Torok EE et al: Gestational trophoblastic disease: The effect of duration of disease and hCG titer on response to therapy. J Reprod Med 27:401, 1982

Maroulis GB, Hammond CB, Johnsrude IS et al: Arteriography and infusional chemotherapy in localized trophoblastic disease. Obstet Gynecol 45:397, 1975

Marshall JR, Hammond CB, Ross GT et al: Plasma and urinary chorionic gonadotropin during human pregnancy. Obstet Gynecol 32:760, 1968

Miller JM, Surwit EA, Hammond CB: Choriocarcinoma following term pregnancy. Obstet Gynecol 53:207, 1979

Morrow CP, Kletzky OK, DiSaia PJ et al: Clinical and laboratory correlates of molar pregnancy and trophoblastic disease. Am J Obstet Gynecol 128:424, 1977

Nisula BC, Morgan FJ, Canfield RE: Evidence that chorionic gonadotropin has instrinsic thyrotropic activity. Biochem Biophys Res Commun 59:86, 1974

Nisula BC, Taliadouros GS: Thyroid function in gestational trophoblastic neoplasia: Evidence that the thyrotropic activity of chorionic gonadotropin mediates the thyrotoxicosis of choriocarcinoma. Am J Obstet Gynecol 138:77, 1980

Novak E, Seah CS: Choriocarcinoma of the uterus. Am J Obstet Gynecol 67:933, 1954

Osathanondh R, Goldstein DP, Pastorfide GB: Actinomycin D as the primary agent for gestational trophoblastic disease. Cancer 36:863, 1975

Park WW: Choriocarcinoma: A general review, with analysis of 516 cases. Arch Pathol 49:73, 1951

Pastorfide GB, Goldstein DP: Pregnancy after hydatidiform mole. Obstet Gynecol 42:67, 1973

Patillo RA, Gey GO, Delfs E et al: Human hormone production in vitro. Science 159:1467, 1968

Ross GT: Congenital anomalies among children born of mothers receiving chemotherapy for gestational trophoblastic neoplasms. Cancer 37:1043, 1976

Ross GT, Goldstein DP, Hertz R et al: Sequential use of methotrexate and actinomycin D in the treatment of metastatic choriocarcinoma and related trophoblastic diseases in women. Am J Obstet Gynecol 93:223, 1965

Ross GT, Hammond CB, Hertz R et al: Chemotherapy of metastatic and nonmetastatic gestational trophoblastic neoplasms. Tex Rep Biol Med 24:326, 1966

Sasaki M, Fukuschima T, Makino S: Some aspects of the chromosome constitution of hydatidiform moles and normal chorionic villi. Gann 53:101, 1962

Smith JP: Chemotherapy in gynecologic cancer. Clin Obstet Gynecol 18:109, 1975

Soules MR, Tyrey L, Hammond CB: The utility of a rapid assay for human chorionic gonadotropin in the management of trophoblastic disease. Am J Obstet Gynecol 135:384, 1979

Stone M, Bagshawe KD: An analysis of the influences of maternal age, gestational age, contraceptive method, and the primary mode of treatment of patients with hydatidiform moles on the incidence of subsequent chemotherapy. Br J Obstet Gynaecol 86:782, 1979

Stone M, Dent J, Kardana A et al: Relationship of oral contraception to development of trophoblastic tumor after evacuation of a hydatidiform mole. Br J Obstet Gynaecol 83:913, 1976

Surwit EA, Hammond CB: Treatment of metastatic trophoblastic disease with poor prognosis. Obstet Gynecol 55:565, 1980

Szulman AE: Syndromes of hydatidiform mole: Partial vs. complete. J Reprod Med 29:788, 1984

Szulman AE, Ho-Kei MA, Wong LC et al: Residual trophoblastic disease in association with partial hydatidiform mole. Obstet Gynecol 57:392, 1981

Szulman AE, Surti U: Syndromes of hydatidiform mole: I. Cytogenetic and morphologic correlations. Am J Obstet Gynecol 131:665, 1978

Szulman AE, Surti U: The syndromes of hydatidiform mole: II. Morphologic evolution of the complete and partial mole. Am J Obstet Gynecol 132:20, 1978

Tsuji K, Yagi S, Nakano R: Increased risk of malignant transformation of hydatidiform moles in older gravidas: A cytogenetic study. Obstet Gynecol 58:351, 1981

Twiggs LB, Marrow CP, Schlaerth JB: Acute pulmonary complications of molar pregnancy. Am J Obstet Gynecol 135: 189, 1979

Van Thiel DH, Grodin JM, Ross GT et al: Partial placenta accreta in pregnancies following chemotherapy for gestational trophoblastic neoplasms. Am J Obstet Gynecol 112:54, 1972

Vassilakos P, Riotton G, Kajii T: Hydatidiform mole: Two entities. A morphologic and cytogenic study with some clinical considerations. Am J Obstet Gynecol 127:167, 1977

Vaughn IC, Surwit EA, Hammond CB: Late recurrences of gestational trophoblastic neoplasia. Am J Obstet Gynecol 138: 73, 1980

Walden PAM, Bagshawe KD: Reproductive performance of women successfully treated for trophoblastic tumors. Am J Obstet Gynecol 125:1108, 1976

Weed JC, Hammond CB: Cerebral metastatic choriocarcinoma: Intensive therapy and prognosis. Obstet Gynecol 55:89, 1980

Ectopic Pregnancy

William Droegemueller

23

Ectopic pregnancy is a pregnancy that is implanted outside the uterine cavity, that is, at a site that is not designed either to receive the conceptus or to permit it to develop. The most common site for ectopic pregnancy is the fallopian tube (Fig. 23-1). Most cases culminate in disaster of one kind or another; the conceptus is almost invariably lost, and the condition may also be fatal to the mother. With modern care, the death rate from ectopic pregnancy is about 1 in 1000 cases. From 8% to 12% of all maternal deaths and about 16% of deaths from hemorrhage during pregnancy are due to ectopic pregnancy. There has been a slight decrease in mortality from this cause, but even so, in a recent series of cases, 75% of the deaths were considered preventable. The major sources of disease and death are patient delay in reporting early symptoms and physician delay in making the diagnosis and instituting appropriate treatment.

The true incidence of ectopic pregnancy is difficult to determine. It varies from one population to another, and some of the cases, notably tubal abortion, may resolve spontaneously without diagnosis. In recent years, the incidence of diagnosed cases has been increasing. Although there are many causes, the increasing incidence is believed to be related primarily to the greater frequency of pelvic inflammatory disease.

Between 52,500 and 57,500 ectopic pregnancies occur in the United States each year. The reported incidence ranges from 1 in 80 to 1 in 200 live births. Ectopic pregnancy is more common among the poor than among the affluent. Jamaica has one of the highest incidences of ectopic pregnancies in the world—1 in 28 live births.

Almost 100 years have passed since the publication of Tait's classic paper on the *Modern Management of Ectopic Pregnancy*. He discussed the difficulty of making the diagnosis but emphasized the importance of early surgery. "If an operation is to be done, it must be done without delay," according to Tait. He was the first to establish the importance of exploratory laparotomy if ruptured tubal pregnancy is a reasonable diagnosis. Before his paper, most women died of either hemorrhage or infection.

Ectopic pregnancy, "the great masquerader," can mimic many other abdominal and pelvic problems. If patients report symptoms early, if the physician has a high index of suspicion, and if modern methods of diagnosis are used, the diagnosis is missed in only a few cases. Early diagnosis depends on the clinical caveat "think ectopic." In all women between menarche and menopause who complain of lower abdominal pain, the possibility of ectopic pregnancy should be considered, and discarded only if it is untenable.

TUBAL PREGNANCY

Etiology

The common denominator in most theories of etiology is delay in ovum transport, but several other factors have been associated or implicated in women who develop ectopic pregnancy. There is no suitable animal model, as ectopic pregnancy is unknown in lower animals and rarely occurs in subhuman primates. Only 3 tubal pregnancies have been reported among 3000 pregnancies observed in monkeys in captivity.

Tubal Abnormalities

Chronic pelvic inflammatory disease is a common cause of tubal pregnancy. The adherent mucosal folds may either trap the fertilized ovum or alter its transport. Cases of acute pelvic inflammatory disease are reaching epidemic numbers in the United States, and many epidemiologists relate this disease directly to the increase in the incidence of ectopic pregnancy. A history of prior

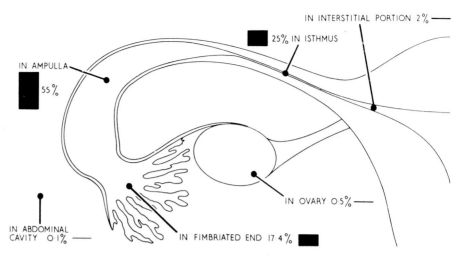

FIG. 23-1. Sites of ectopic gestation implantation with relative frequency of occurrence. (Llewellyn-Jones D: Fundamentals of Obstetrics and Gynaecology, Vol 1, Obstetrics. London, Faber & Faber, 1969)

salpingitis is obtained from 30% to 50% of women operated on for ectopic pregnancy. In tubes excised for ectopic pregnancy, histologic evidence of chronic salpingitis is found in approximately half the cases. Before the advent of antibiotic therapy, gonorrheal infections usually resulted in total occlusion of the tube. Of the women now treated with antibiotics for acute pelvic inflammatory disease, complete tubal occlusion occurs in only about 15%. In the remainder, some escape with no tubal lesion, but others may be left with lesions that interfere with the function of the epithelium and agglutination of adjacent mucosal folds, with the formation of blind pockets. Pregnancies following tuberculous salpingitis are at an even higher risk of ectopic location, approximately one pregnancy of every three being located in the tube.

Peritubal adhesions can distort tubal anatomy and function. The initial insult may have resulted from pelvic inflammatory disease, especially postpartum or postabortion, previous ruptured appendix, or sterile inflammation produced by endometriosis.

Other anatomic abnormalities that may lead to ectopic pregnancy include accessory tubal ostia, convolutions, and diverticula. Tubal diverticula can be congenital or acquired as a result of infection. Extrinsic masses, such as uterine or tubal myomas, and adnexal masses (see Fig. 23-2) may cause kinking or displacement of the tube.

Other often mentioned but less popular theories on the etiology of ectopic pregnancy include the mechanical effect of retrograde menstrual bleeding and endometriosis. There is speculation about the exact pathophysiology that relates endometriosis to ectopic pregnancy. Possibly the chemotaxis of the aberrant endometrium attracts the conceptus to the ectopic location.

Abnormalities of the Zygote

Various developmental abnormalities of the zygote, including an abnormal zona pellucida, have been implicated in tubal pregnancy. Chromosomal analysis of material from such a pregnancy reveals an abnormal karyotype in approximately one third of the cases. Detailed morphologic studies of the embryos have revealed grossly disorganized growth and a high incidence of neural tube defects in many cases. Whether or not the defects result from the poor vascular supply of the ectopic implantation is unknown.

A male factor has been implicated in some cases. The incidence of ectopic pregnancy is reported to be highest if the male has an abnormal sperm count and especially if he has a high percentage of abnormal spermatozoa.

Endocrine Disorders

Some investigators have related ectopic pregnancy to an inadequacy of the corpus luteum or to delayed ovulation, which, because of altered estrogen–progesterone relationships, may affect tubal and cilial motility and ovum transport. An increased incidence has been reported following ovulation induction with human pituitary and chorionic gonadotropin. Prostaglandins, catecholamines, and other substances can also affect tubal motility and function so that transport of the fertilized ovum is delayed in the tube. It has been estimated that hormonal factors may be responsible for about 50% of those cases in which no recognizable mechanical or structural abnormality can be found.

Prior Tubal Pregnancy

Regardless of the cause, a history of prior ectopic pregnancy is an important etiologic factor. A woman who has had one ectopic pregnancy has a 10% to 20% chance that her subsequent pregnancies will be ectopic.

Contraceptive Failure

INTRAUTERINE DEVICE. Of pregnancies that occur in women using intrauterine devices, 4% to 9% are ectopic; one of eight is a primary ovarian pregnancy. Ap-

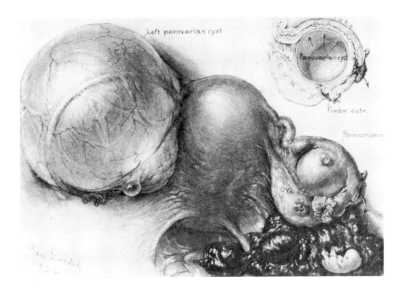

FIG. 23-2. Ruptured tubal pregnancy (*right*), possibly caused by a parovarian cyst. The pelvic organs are viewed from behind. The pregnancy was situated in the ampulla of the right tube, which has ruptured at a point 2 cm from the fimbriated end (*arrow*). The blood, fetus, and products of conception are collected behind the right broad ligament. The right tube is drawn over the parovarian cyst and compressed proximal to the point of nidation (*insert*). The corpus luteum of pregnancy is located in the right ovary near the fimbria. On the *left* side is a larger parovarian cyst, with the fallopian tube drawn out over its surface and the ovary beneath it. This case illustrates the relation of tubal constriction to tubal pregnancy. (Brady L: Report of a case of tubal pregnancy probably caused by a par-ovarian cyst. Bull Johns Hopkins Hosp 33:442, 1933. Drawing by Max Brödel)

proximately 2 ectopic pregnancies occur per 1000 intrauterine device users per year. Although the incidence of pregnancy diminishes with long-term use of the intrauterine device, among those who do become pregnant the likelihood of ectopic pregnancy increases. The cause of ectopic pregnancy among users of intrauterine devices is unsettled. Some have suggested that the effect of the intrauterine device on tubal motility delays ovum transport or that tubal infection may be the cause.

There is little difference in the incidence of ectopic pregnancy according to the type of intrauterine device, except in the case of the progesterone-bearing Progestasert; in one series, 16% of the pregnancies that occurred were extrauterine.

PROGESTIN-ONLY ORAL CONTRACEPTION. The minipill, or progestin-only oral contraceptive, has been associated with an incidence of ectopic pregnancy about five times as high as the customary incidence. In women taking the minipill, 4% to 6% of pregnancies are ectopic. There is no increased incidence of ectopic pregnancy with combination oral contraceptives.

TUBAL LIGATION. Sterilization by tubal ligation may fail because of fistula formation and recanalization. Approximately 15% of pregnancies following tubal ligation or application of spring-loaded clips are ectopic. When silastic rings fail, more than 50% of the resulting pregnancies are ectopic.

TUBAL SURGERY. With the recent advances in microsurgery and changes in our society, many more women are requesting reversal of a previous sterilization operation. Approximately 5% of women who conceive following a tuboplasty operation have an ectopic implantation.

"MORNING-AFTER PILL." Pregnancy is rare after the postcoital administration of large doses of estrogen.

However, when this contraceptive method fails, there is a tenfold increase in the incidence of ectopic pregnancy.

Elective Abortion

Studies differ as to whether elective abortion increases or does not significantly change the incidence of ectopic pregnancy. One study suggested an increased relative risk of ectopic pregnancy after elective abortion. However, this report comes from Greece, a country in which elective abortion is illegal, and therefore its conclusion may be related to an increase in postabortal infection. In countries where early abortion is legal and is usually performed by suction curettage, no increase in later ectopic pregnancy has been reported.

Pathology

As the trophoblast penetrates the wall of the tube, hemorrhage is an inevitable consequence of either erosion of capillaries or blood vessels, or rupture of the viscus containing the conceptus. The stroma adjacent to the conceptus may show a feeble decidual response that is insufficient to nurture or to limit advancement of the conceptus, leading to its early death and also to the erosion of its blood supply. There is some evidence to suggest that even after the death of the embryo, the trophoblast may remain viable for a time and continue its erosive activity in the retroperitoneal space.

At first, the tube enlarges locally at the point of implantation, but there is little discoloration; later, the whole tube is usually distended, has a dark red to purple-gray color, and contains both clotted and fresh blood. A gestational sac is sometimes seen, but an embryo may not be evident. If the tube is ruptured or if a significant amount of blood has escaped from the ostium, the tube may be surrounded by clot. If chorionic villi cannot be found in the tubal lumen, the surrounding debris must be searched for evidence of the pregnancy. The presence of an embryo is, of course, proof of pregnancy. If none can be found, the mere presence of hematosalpinx is not sufficient for diagnosis, because at least one chorionic villus, either within the tube or the retroperitoneal space, or among the extruded clots, is needed for diagnosis.

The course and outcome of tubal pregnancy, and consequently the clinical picture, vary according to the site of implantation.

Ampullar Implantation

Ampullar pregnancy is by far the most common type of ectopic pregnancy, but its true incidence is unknown because in many cases the manifestations are so trivial that they are not observed by the patient. As noted in Figure 23-3, a very early conceptus may die and be absorbed without producing any notable symptoms; another conceptus, also quite early, may be extruded into the abdominal cavity and be absorbed without incident (complete tubal abortion). If there is extensive erosion of capillaries or if a major tubal vessel is opened, free blood may collect at the fimbriated end of the tube. Some of this leaks into the cul-de-sac, and some of it collects around the conceptus, which may be partially

extruded through the ostium (incomplete tubal abortion). In some cases, repeated choriodecidual hemorrhages occur around the dead conceptus, giving rise to a tubal blood mole or carneous mole (Fig. 23-4). The amount of blood reaching the cul-de-sac varies in amount, being least in cases of complete tubal abortion and greater (pelvic hematocele) in incomplete tubal abortion.

Isthmic Implantation

The lumen of the isthmic portion of the tube is quite narrow and is much less distensible than the ampullary portion. Implantation in this area predisposes to early and dramatic tubal rupture (Fig. 23-5) as a result of either erosion of the trophoblast through the tubal wall or distention by the conceptus and rapidly collecting blood. (According to Munro Kerr's clinical grouping, it is usually in isthmic pregnancy that "the woman is struck down suddenly with abdominal pain and becomes collapsed.") The site of the rupture is ordinarily toward the peritoneal cavity (Figs. 23-6 and 23-7), but in some cases rupture occurs between the leaves of the broad ligaments. In either case, bleeding is usually heavy and may be fatal if it is not dealt with promptly. Intraligamentous bleeding may diminish as the pressure builds in the broad ligament, but the anterior or posterior leaf

FIG. 23-3. Sequelae of tubal abortion. (Llewellyn-Jones D: Fundamentals of Obstetrics and Gynaecology, Vol 1, Obstetrics. London, Faber & Faber, 1969)

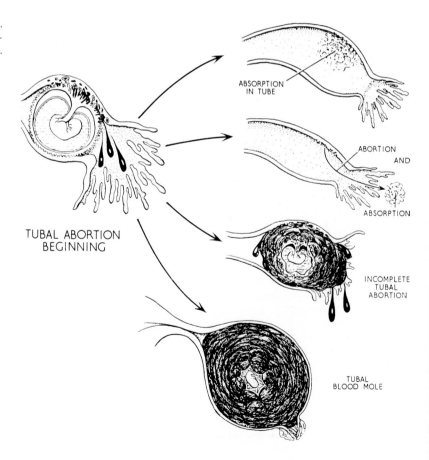

TUBAL ABORTION BEGINNING

ABSORPTION IN TUBE

ABORTION AND ABSORPTION

INCOMPLETE TUBAL ABORTION

TUBAL BLOOD MOLE

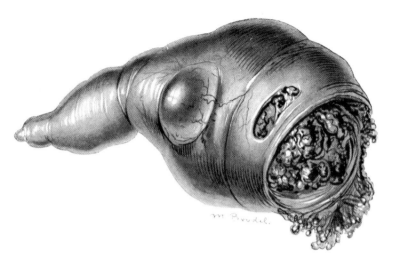

FIG. 23-4. Tubal blood mole. The bleeding is checked by a large coagulum distending and thinning out the tube; the fimbriated opening is greatly distended, but the greater diameter of the clot in the ampulla prevents its escape. Wall of tube averages 1 mm in thickness. Operation. Recovery, July 7, 1896. Natural size. (Kelly HA: Operative Gynecology. New York, D Appleton, 1898. Drawing by Max Brödel)

may ultimately give way in response to recurrent hemorrhage.

Interstitial Implantation

In interstitial pregnancy, the implantation site is partially surrounded by myometrium, which can hypertrophy as needed to accommodate the enlarging conceptus. Rupture therefore occurs after implantation occurs in the isthmus, being delayed usually until 12 to 14 weeks. When the disaster occurs, it is no less dramatic, however; indeed, rupture of the rich blood supply of the cornual area leads quickly to intra-abdominal hemorrhage that can be massive, and must be dealt with at once if the patient is to survive.

Changes in the Uterus

The response of the myometrium to the hormones of early tubal pregnancy is identical to its response to the hormones of intrauterine pregnancy. The uterus first becomes softened and then enlarges as a result of both hypertrophy and hyperplasia of the myometrial cells. If the tubal pregnancy is apparent at a very early stage, the uterine enlargement may not be clinically detectable (Table 23-1), just as it may be difficult to discern uterine enlargement before 6 weeks in a normal intrauterine pregnancy. If a tubal pregnancy extends beyond 6 weeks, the uterus is usually found to be slightly enlarged. (In an interstitial pregnancy of six to eight weeks' duration, an irregularity may be found at one side of the fundus. This gradually enlarges and becomes tender, making it difficult to determine whether there is a combination of degenerating fibroid and intrauterine pregnancy, or an interstitial pregnancy.)

The endometrium also responds to a tubal pregnancy as it does to an intrauterine pregnancy: the stroma is transformed to decidua, and the endometrial glands assume the feathery pattern commonly found in early pregnancy. The atypical glandular patterns that characterize the Arias–Stella reaction (see p. 87) may also be found. However, in tubal pregnancy, the gestational changes usually last for only a short time, because the early death of the embryo and trophoblast results in the

FIG. 23-5. Ruptured tubal pregnancy, seven weeks' gestation. Note contraction of tubal musculature opposite rupture. (×3) (DN Danforth)

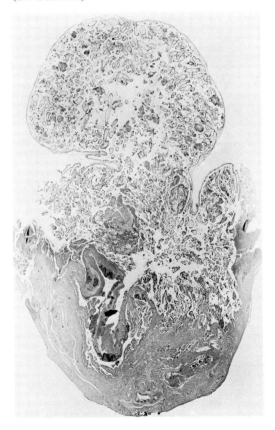

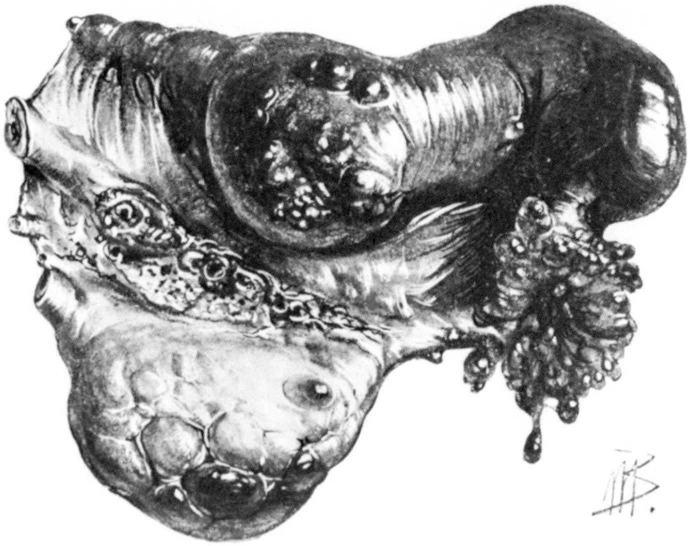

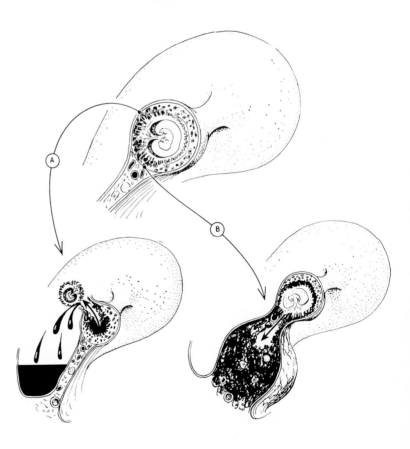

FIG. 23-6. Ruptured left extrauterine pregnancy with large, free intraperitoneal hemorrhage. The rupture is at the junction of the ampulla and the isthmus; the rest of the ampulla is dilated and infiltrated down to a narrow neck just behind the fimbriated end. Enucleation; saline infusion. Recovery. February 25, 1895. Natural size. (Kelly HA: Operative Gynecology. New York, D Appleton, 1898. Drawing by Max Brödel)

FIG. 23-7. Sequelae of tubal rupture in cases of ectopic gestation. (*A*) Intraperitoneal hemorrhage and pelvic hematocele. (*B*) Broad ligament hematoma. (Llewellyn-Jones D: Fundamentals of Obstetrics and Gynaecology, Vol 1, Obstetrics. London, Faber & Faber, 1969)

withdrawal of the hormones responsible for the endometrial changes. In one series of cases in which curettage was performed before laparotomy for tubal pregnancy, no decidua was found in more than 80% of the cases. Usually, the decidua breaks down gradually over the course of days or weeks, giving rise to the intermittent, occasionally heavy vaginal bleeding that commonly occurs in ectopic pregnancy. In some cases, the decidua may be shed abruptly in the form of a flat, triangular, reddish brown, shaggy decidual cast of the uterine cavity. It consists of two layers of tissue each made up of decidual cells, sparse endometrial glands in varying stages of collapse, thin-walled blood vessels that are either thrombosed or filled with red cells, and scattered areas of lymphocytes, plasma cells, and neu-trophils. Passage of a decidual cast should alert the physician to the possibility of ectopic pregnancy, but it should not be considered diagnostic since endometrial casts may also be passed at the time of normal menstruation.

Symptoms and Signs

Like appendicitis, the myriad of clinical pictures presented by tubal pregnancy can be divided into two major groups: those that follow the classic "textbook" picture or a recognizable variation thereof, and those that are entirely bizarre and cannot be solved by logic alone. Wharton recalled that the preeminent Howard A. Kelly once remarked in the course of one of his clinics that a physician who is confronted with a pelvic problem that follows no rules and conforms to no standards should think first of ectopic pregnancy and second of pelvic tuberculosis. Classically, the first symptoms of tubal pregnancy are the first symptoms of any early pregnancy (nausea, breast tenderness, overdue menstruation). They are followed, in order, by lower quadrant discomfort, spotting, faintness, and, finally, sharp exacerbation of pain as rupture occurs or is imminent, and syncope with shoulder pain as the abdomen fills with blood that finds its way between the liver and diaphragm. In such cases, the diagnosis can be made over the telephone; but usually, the picture is less tidy. The variations are due principally to the unpredictable character of vaginal bleeding and abdominal pain, the differences in the anatomic location of the tubal implantation, the abruptness of tubal rupture or distention, and the magnitude and speed of hemorrhage.

The admission symptoms and signs in 300 consecutive surgically treated cases of ectopic pregnancy are listed in Table 23-1. It should be noted that abdominal pain was more commonly diffuse than localized; that abnormal uterine bleeding and amenorrhea of at least two weeks' duration occurred in most of the cases; that adnexal tenderness occurred in almost all cases, but an adnexal mass could be felt in only half; that in two thirds of the cases the uterus was thought to be of normal size; that leukocytosis appeared in only half the cases; and that fever was extremely unusual.

Diagnosis

Although the diagnosis is obvious in occasional cases, in most cases it is not. A sufficiently penetrating history usually leads to at least a suspicion of tubal pregnancy that makes it mandatory to proceed at once to more definitive diagnostic measures.

Physical Examination

Depending on the rate and amount of bleeding, the patient's general status may vary from only slight pallor to hemorrhagic shock. Since bleeding tends to be re-

Table 23-1

Admitting Signs and Symptoms in 300 Consecutive Cases of Ectopic Pregnancy

Sign or Symptom	Cases (%)
Abdominal Pain	99.3
Generalized abdominal	44.3
Unilateral abdominal	32.7
Radiating to shoulder	22.3
Abnormal Uterine Bleeding	74.3
Amenorrhea ≤ 2 Weeks	68.3
Syncopal Symptoms	37
Adnexal Tenderness	96.3
Unilateral Adnexal Mass	53.7
Uterus	
Normal size	70.7
6–8 weeks' size	25.7
9–12 weeks' size	3.3
Uterine Cast Passed Vaginally	6.7
Admission Temperature > 37°C	2.3

(After Brenner PF, Roy S, Mishell DR Jr.: Ectopic pregnancy: A study of 300 consecutive surgically treated cases. JAMA 243:673, 1980)

current as successive clots are dislodged, serial determinations of pulse and blood pressure should be made while the patient is being prepared for surgery. Progressive loss of fluid from the circulatory compartment may become evident by first noting the pulse and blood pressure in the reclining posture, then in the sitting posture.

The abdominal signs vary. Deep lower quadrant tenderness is usually present; occasionally, guarding and rebound tenderness are also seen. Cullen's sign (bluish discoloration of the skin around the umbilicus), if it appears, is striking evidence of extensive intra-abdominal hemorrhage; but it is found so rarely, even when the hemorrhage is massive, that its absence by no means rules out extensive bleeding.

On pelvic examination, the findings vary from the presence of a large mass to completely negative findings. As noted in Table 23-1, tenderness is present in most of the cases, and a mass is found in about half. In many cases, the mass is vague and ill defined; it may consist of not only the tubal pregnancy, but also of adherent omentum, blood clots, and small bowel. A tender, boggy mass in the cul-de-sac, when present, is due to the collection of blood in this area, a pelvic hematocele.

When an adnexal mass is suspected, it is not uncommon for the physician to repeat the examination with the patient under anesthesia in order to avoid laparotomy if nothing is found. This practice is extremely dangerous if there is a reasonable possibility of tubal pregnancy. A tube about to rupture may indeed rupture if the slightest pressure is exerted on it; no mass is felt, and, since the patient cannot react or protest, the rupture is unnoticed until shock ensues. Ian Donald records two fatal cases of this kind, and Jeffcoate refers to three cases in which the patient died within 30 minutes of being moved from the operating room. In suspected tubal pregnancy, pelvic examination should be done under anesthesia only if laparotomy is to be done immediately, regardless of the findings.

Culdocentesis

The value of culdocentesis is emphasized in Table 23-2, because it shows that blood appeared in the fluid obtained by this method in 95% of 300 proven cases. The procedure is simple and rapid, and it can be diagnostic of intraperitoneal bleeding. When blood escapes into the abdominal cavity, it undergoes the clotting process and subsequent fibrinolysis, after which it fails to clot. With the patient's legs in stirrups and her hips slightly lower than her thorax so that any blood will pool in the cul-de-sac, a tenaculum is placed on the cervix and, with slight traction, an 18-gauge needle is introduced through the posterior vaginal vault without anesthesia. If the aspirated blood clots, its probable source is a vessel that was punctured en route to the

Table 23-2
Admitting Laboratory and Other Data in 300 Consecutive Cases of Ectopic Pregnancy

Laboratory or Other Data	Cases (%)
Pregnancy Test (HI, urine, sensitive to 700 mIU hCG/ml)	
Positive	82.5
Negative	17.5
Not done (surgical emergency)	16.3
Hematocrit	
>30%	72.3
Between 21% and 30%	23.0
<21%	4.7
White Blood Cell Count	
<10,000/mm^3	49
Between 10,000 and 15,000/mm^3	35.7
Between 15,000 and 20,000/mm^3	10.7
>20,000/mm^3	4.7
Culdocentesis	
Nonclotting blood obtained	95
Hematocrit value on blood > 15%	97.5
Hematocrit value on blood < 15%	2.5
No blood or fluid obtained	5

HI, hemagglutination inhibition test; *hCG*, human chorionic gonadotropin.

(After Brenner PF, Roy S, Mishell DR Jr.: Ectopic pregnancy: A study of 300 consecutive surgically treated cases. JAMA 243:673, 1980)

cul-de-sac. Failure to obtain any fluid may suggest that the culd-de-sac was not entered. Culdocentesis is a valuable diagnostic aid, especially when unclotted blood with an hematocrit value of 15% or higher is obtained. The purpose of the procedure is to determine whether there is any free blood in the abdomen. Of course, no blood will be present if a tubal pregnancy is unruptured or has not leaked from the ostium. If result of culdocentesis is negative, further diagnostic tests should be made; if it is positive; laparotomy should be performed at once.

Laparoscopy

Laparoscopy is not needed if culdocentesis reveals free blood in the abdominal cavity or if the clinical picture of tubal rupture is classic. It is invaluable if unruptured tubal pregnancy is suspected or is even considered as part of the differential diagnosis of some other pelvic problem. Before the advent of laparoscopy, most suspected cases were managed by observation and repeated pelvic examination; at present, such problems can be solved quickly by laparoscopy, permitting early laparotomy and, in some of the cases, preservation of the affected tube.

Pregnancy Tests

A positive result to the test for human chorionic gonadotropin (hCG) confirms pregnancy, but gives no indication whether the pregnancy is intra- or extrauterine. In tubal pregnancy, the need for diagnosis usually arises at six or seven weeks' gestation when hCG levels are relatively low either because it is so early in the pregnancy or because the trophoblast had undergone abruption or degeneration. Such low levels of hCG are readily detectable by radioimmunoassay (RIA) and also by radioreceptorassay (see Chapter 20). If a urine slide or tube agglutination test yields positive results, they can be relied on, but negative results do not rule out the presence of hCG in amounts below the sensitivity level of the test. Consequently, it is important to select a test with a sensitivity of 35 mIU βhCG/ml serum or less. Even at a sensitivity of 35 mIU/ml, the test is negative in 2% of ectopic pregnancies.

Ultrasound

The place of ultrasound in the diagnosis of tubal pregnancy is discussed on page 278. Occasionally, the procedure can be definitive, but more frequently, its value is in demonstrating the presence of an intrauterine pregnancy, which would make the possibility of a simultaneous tubal pregnancy extremely unlikely.

Dilatation and Curettage

In cases in which the leading symptom is abnormal bleeding, dilatation and curettage (D and C) may be performed with a presumptive diagnosis of dysfunctional uterine bleeding or incomplete abortion. In the presence of an unsuspected tubal pregnancy, the returns are usually scant, consisting only of decidua in which the Arias–Stella reaction (see page 87) may be noted. If no chorionic villi are found in such a case, it may be prudent to request that the pathologist make deeper cuts in the paraffin block, because finding even one chorionic villus in the curettings establishes the diagnosis of intrauterine pregnancy. If none is found in the presence of decidua with or without the Arias–Stella reaction, the possibility of ectopic pregnancy must be considered and steps taken to establish or rule out the diagnosis.

Posterior Colpotomy

Before the introduction of laparoscopy, posterior colpotomy was an excellent method of directly visualizing the pelvic organs. Occasionally, definite surgery for tubal pregnancy is accomplished through the posterior cul-de-sac. Obviously, it should be used with caution if there is frank hemorrhage.

Differential Diagnosis

A careful and painstaking history is of more value than physical findings in raising the question of tubal pregnancy and ruling out other conditions that may be confused with it. The following conditions are among those most frequently confused with tubal pregnancy.

CORPUS LUTEUM CYST. Amenorrhea, spotting, and unilateral pelvic pain are common. The patient does not have the symptoms and signs of early pregnancy, the pain is less severe than that in tubal pregnancy, there is no history of faintness, and RIA or RRA tests for hCG are negative. The uterus is firm and not enlarged, and the adnexal mass of a corpus luteum cyst is usually well defined, smooth, cystic in consistency, and freely movable. A ruptured corpus luteum cyst with intra-abdominal hemorrhage is usually a surgical emergency unless bleeding stops spontaneously, as it does occasionally. Laparotomy is usually performed with a presumptive diagnosis of ruptured tubal pregnancy. The corpus luteum of pregnancy may attain a size of 3 cm to 6 cm and is usually an incidental finding on first pelvic examination in early pregnancy. There is no pain, and the structure is round, usually nontender, freely movable, and cystic in consistency. Ultrasound usually discloses the nature of the contents and also permits diagnosis of an early intrauterine pregnancy.

THREATENED OR INCOMPLETE ABORTION. The period of amenorrhea in threatened or incomplete abortion is usually longer than that in tubal pregnancy. The pain, if any, is midline and crampy, and it is less severe; bleeding is usually heavier and is not accompanied by fainting. There is no vaginal or adnexal tenderness, and no adnexal mass unless a corpus luteum of pregnancy should be palpated. The uterus is usually larger and softer than in tubal pregnancy.

PELVIC INFLAMMATORY DISEASE. Salpingitis is usually bilateral, movement of the cervix produces equal bilateral adnexal pain, and both adnexa are extremely tender. There is usually no history of amenorrhea or fainting, the breasts are soft and not tender, and the results of the hCG test are negative. The traditional case of gonorrheal salpingitis is accompanied by fever, leukocytosis, and dysuria. Other organisms that cause salpingitis and some gonorrheal strains may produce a lesser systemic reaction; in one series of cases, 50% of proven cases had no fever or leukocytosis. Although the manifestations of salpingitis and tubal pregnancy may seem to be so different that there should be no difficulty in distinguishing them, this is not true. In emergency rooms, this can be one of the most puzzling diagnostic problems.

ACUTE APPENDICITIS. In some cases, appendicitis may be confused with tubal pregnancy, because appendicitis may produce bizarre clinical pictures. Typical cases of appendicitis differ from cases of tubal pregnancy in that vomiting is more likely, fainting and amenorrhea do not occur, low-grade fever and leukocytosis are much more common, the breasts are soft and nontender, and right lower quadrant rigidity and rebound tenderness are usually more pronounced.

DEGENERATING FIBROID. Fibroids tend to become painful and to enlarge in pregnancy. If such a tumor is small in early pregnancy and is located in the cornual area of the uterus, it may be impossible to distinguish it from an interstitial pregnancy. Ultrasound should be helpful in determining the nature of the enlarging mass. If the matter is not solved by ten weeks' gestation, the diagnosis should be made by laparotomy (not laparoscopy).

NORMAL INTRAUTERINE PREGNANCY AND AN ASSOCIATED ABDOMINAL OR PELVIC PROBLEM. As Osler emphasized, the physician should avoid assigning two simultaneous causes for a single group of symptoms. However, in considering the differential diagnosis of tubal pregnancy, it is important to consider such possibilities as a normal intrauterine pregnancy with tortion of the tube and ovary, tortion of an ovarian cyst, or a pedunculated fibroid. Finally, a normal intrauterine pregnancy *and* a tubal pregnancy may coexist, a rare combination but by no means a medical curiosity.

INTRAUTERINE DEVICE. Spotting, pelvic pain, and unilateral pelvic infections are complications that can result from the use of an intrauterine device (IUD). Tubal pregnancy is also more common in women using an IUD. The distinction between IUD complications and tubal pregnancy is extremely important and may be difficult. When the patient does not have amenorrhea or any other signs of early pregnancy and the results of a sensitive test for β-hCG are negative, she is unlikely to have a tubal pregnancy.

Treatment

Routine Procedure

Laparotomy is urgently indicated as soon as the diagnosis of tubal pregnancy is made. In the past, the presence of massive intra-abdominal bleeding and shock led to debate over whether the first step should be to stop the bleeding, or whether surgery should be deferred until the circulation is restored. Before blood and blood substitutes were readily available, a prompt clinical diagnosis and rapid, skillful surgery were usually rewarded by a healthy patient. In one series of 174 ectopic pregnancies reported in 1947, most of the operations were done in 20 minutes or less, and 17 patients were transfused. Four women died. Of these, it is reasonable to presume that two, and possibly three, would have survived if modern methods of circulatory support and monitoring had been available. At present it is usually possible for medical and surgical therapy to be started simultaneously.

If the woman's condition is at all precarious, the simplest procedure that will control the bleeding should be selected. A midline incision can usually be made more rapidly than a transverse one. Sufficient blood is cleared away so that *both* adnexa can be readily visualized. The operation of choice is a total salpingectomy. The tube is removed from the mesosalpinx by clamping with successive Kelly clamps and placing transfixation sutures of 4-0 Dexon or Vicryl (Fig. 23-8).

It is preferable to perform a modified cornual resection. This should be superficial in order to avoid a myometrial defect that could rupture in a subsequent pregnancy. Following the cornual resection, it is important to peritonealize this area; the adjacent round ligament can be used for this purpose. (Fig. 23-8*C*). All old blood and clots are removed from the peritoneal cavity, and the pelvis is irrigated with warm saline. This step is important for future fertility because it reduces the possibility of damage as a result of pelvic adhesions. The ipsilateral ovary is not removed unless there is an extensive hematoma of the infundibulopelvic or broad ligaments. The contralateral tube and ovary should be inspected. Hematosalpinx of the contralateral tube is a frequent finding in acute tubal pregnancy, but it requires no treatment. Several years ago, some physicians recommended that the ovary on the side of the ectopic pregnancy be routinely removed so that all future ovulations would occur from the ovary with the remaining tube, thus preventing loss of ova from the opposite side and improving fertility. This theory is interesting, but there is as yet no proof of its efficacy.

FIG. 23-8. Salpingectomy. (*A*) Removal of tube, including wedge of uterine cornu that contains interstitial part of tube. Dissection hugs fallopian tube to avoid ovarian blood supply. (*B*) Cornu closed by figure-of-eight suture, mesosalpinx ligated by transfixation. (*C*) Modified Coffey suspension of uterus; knuckle of round ligament anchored to posterior aspect of uterus to peritonealize area and suspend ovary. Anterior and posterior leaves of broad ligament attached to round ligament may now be tacked to uterus if needed to cover raw surfaces. (Wharton LR: Gynecology with a Section on Female Urology. Philadelphia, WB Saunders, 1943)

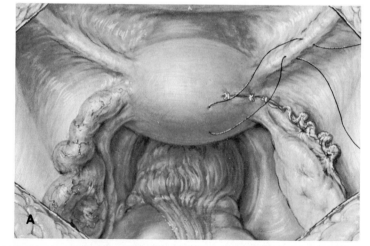

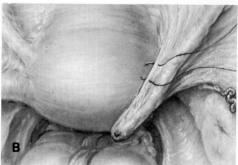

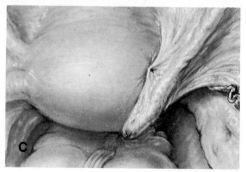

Rh-negative women who are unsensitized should receive an injection of anti-D γ-globulin after surgery.

Alternative Procedures

The most pressing problem is control of active bleeding. If the woman has been in shock, no matter how stable her condition seems at the moment, it is wise to complete the necessary procedure (salpingectomy) as quickly as possible and close the abdomen. If the tube is unruptured or if bleeding has been minimal, certain alternative or additional procedures can be considered.

EXPRESSION OF A TUBAL BLOOD MOLE. In some cases of tubal blood mole, the contents of the tube can be easily expressed from the fimbriated end.

SALPINGOSTOMY. In unruptured, and in some ruptured, tubal pregnancies, salpingostomy with removal of the pregnancy and conservation of the tube is feasible. The past five years have seen a dramatic improvement in the early diagnosis of unruptured ectopic pregnancy. This has fostered an interest in conservative surgery for ectopic pregnancies and in adaptations in microsurgical techniques to improve future fertility. Many groups gradually have increased their indications for conservative surgery and now perform salpingostomy even with a normal contralateral tube.

A linear incision is made on the antimesenteric aspect of the tube. The products of conception are gently removed from the tube, usually by washing of the area with warm saline. Hemostasis is achieved by bipolar cauterization or with individual sutures of 6-0 Dexon or Vicryl. The majority of gynecologists leave the surgical incision in the fallopian tube open and let it close by secondary intention.

If the pregnancy is in the narrow isthmus, it is best to do a segmental resection of the tube. If this is the last remaining tube, an end-to-end tuboplasty is performed in a subsequent operation.

In one large series of cases, 80% of the patients experienced an intrauterine pregnancy following conservative surgery for ectopic pregnancy. The recurrence rate for tubal pregnancy was 12%. It is hoped that future series will have the same optimistic results. Throughout the literature, conservative surgery is not shown to increase the incidence of repeat ectopic pregnancy. Therefore, there is no negative side to the consideration of performing conservative surgery.

APPENDECTOMY. In uncomplicated gynecologic operations, appendectomy is often performed as in incidental procedure. In connection with operations for tubal pregnancy, there is no evidence to suggest that it is hazardous. Although complications from elective appendectomy are extremely unusual, many consider it to be contraindicated if the woman desires further preg-

nancies because of the theoretic possibility of contamination and subsequent formation of adhesions in the region of the tube.

HYSTERECTOMY. Hysterectomy may be appropriate if the woman desires no further pregnancies, if the uterus is diseased, and if she clearly desires this to be done at the time the tubal pregnancy is dealt with (provided the physician considers the additional operation to be reasonable under the circumstances). Hysterectomy is usually the procedure of choice in ruptured interstitial pregnancy, since the cornu may be so damaged that repair is time-consuming, unsatisfactory, and accompanied by considerable blood loss.

RARE FORMS OF ECTOPIC PREGNANCY

Ectopic pregnancies located at sites other than the fallopian tube are extremely rare, but they are encountered from time to time.

Abdominal Pregnancy

There are two types of abdominal pregnancy: primary peritoneal implantation, which has occurred, but is so rare as to be almost a medical curiosity; and implantation secondary to tubal rupture, in which the fetus escapes cleanly from the tube through a rupture or through the fimbriated end, leaving the chorion, and usually the amnion, attached to the tube. The chorion continues to develop, attaching itself to surrounding structures and forming a placenta which, although insecure, may be sufficient to permit subsequent development of the fetus. After the tubal rupture, the pregnancy progresses normally from the patient's viewpoint, except for the considerable discomfort that results from the adhesions and peritoneal irritation and is accompanied by flatulence, abdominal discomfort, nausea, occasional vomiting, and diarrhea and constipation. Fetal movements may be painful. As the pregnancy advances, the presenting part is found to be high; the fetus is usually felt in a transverse position lying superior to the uterus, which can often be felt lower in the abdomen. Maternal mortality is 5% to 10%, and fetal mortality is more than 90%. Congenital malformations are common. Ultrasound provides an unequivocal diagnosis.

The treatment for abdominal pregnancy is laparotomy as soon as the diagnosis is made. This is not to be undertaken lightly; although some of the operations are quite simple, others may be extremely difficult because of adhesions and because of inadvertent dislodgement of the placenta. The objective is to remove the fetus, cutting the umbilical cord close to the placenta without disturbing it. The placenta is allowed to be absorbed; if left alone, it rarely presents problems of bleeding or infection. The placenta should be removed only if it is attached to the posterior part of the tube, ovary, broad ligament, and the uterus, and its blood supply can be readily ligated. Attempts to remove the placenta from other intra-abdominal organs have resulted in massive hemorrhage because of the invasive properties of the trophoblast and the lack of cleavage planes. The abdomen is closed without drainage.

Some abdominal pregnancies escape notice because the patient misinterprets the episode of tubal rupture as a miscarriage or some other minor accident. Or, as in the Clark case (Fig. 23-9), operation may have been refused when the problem was originally diagnosed. In patients who refuse treatment for this length of time, the fetus is converted to a lithopedion, and its removal may be a very hazardous procedure.

Cornual Pregnancy

In cornual pregnancy, a variant of interstitial pregnancy, implantation takes place in the cornual area at the uterine end of the interstitial portion of the tube. As it is when implantation takes place in the tube, the decidual reaction is imperfect. The implications are much the same as those of interstitial pregnancy, except that the greater mass of myometrium permits the pregnancy to advance to a somewhat later date, as late as 16 weeks in some of the cases, before rupture occurs. As noted

earlier, an asymmetric pregnant uterus with a tender, enlarging mass in the cornual area may be the first sign, and the physician may first suspect an enlarging fibroid. However, it is vitally important that an exact diagnosis be made, preferably by 10 weeks and no later than 12 weeks; when rupture occurs, the collapse that follows is so rapid and so profound that it may be fatal.

Pregnancy in a Rudimentary Uterine Horn

The cavity of a rudimentary uterine horn usually is not connected with the cavity of the horn that communicates with the cervix (see Fig. 5-17). In such cases, conception results from external migration of the spermatozoa or the fertilized ovum. The myometrium of the rudimentary horn is usually poorly developed, and the time of rupture depends on the degree to which the myometrium can grow in response to the pregnancy (Fig. 23-10). In early pregnancy, bimanual examination may disclose what appears to be an adnexal mass lateral to the uterus. An ultrasound scan should disclose the pregnancy, and the rudimentary horn should be removed promptly when this condition is diagnosed. If no bimanual examination is made in early pregnancy, the first sign may be intense abdominal pain and massive intra-abdominal hemorrhage. Laparotomy is performed with a presumptive diagnosis of ruptured interstitial pregnancy.

FIG. 23-9. Lithopedion lying undisturbed in the abdominal cavity. The strong adhesions holding it in place and its position are well shown. The patient was a 45-year-old woman who had had her last child at age 38. Four years before entering the clinic she became pregnant, with all the usual signs, and was taken with perfectly normal labor pains at the expected time. Dr. Barnum, who saw her two months later, recognized an abdominal pregnancy. The mind of the patient was unbalanced, and she would not allow any interference until after four years had passed. Operation by Dr. Clark. Recovery. B.H., August 14, 1896. (Kelly HA: Operative Gynecology. New York, D Appleton, 1898. Drawing by Max Brödel)

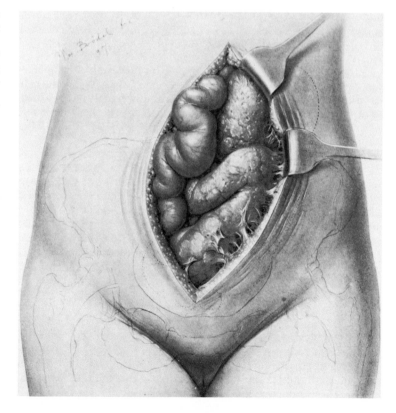

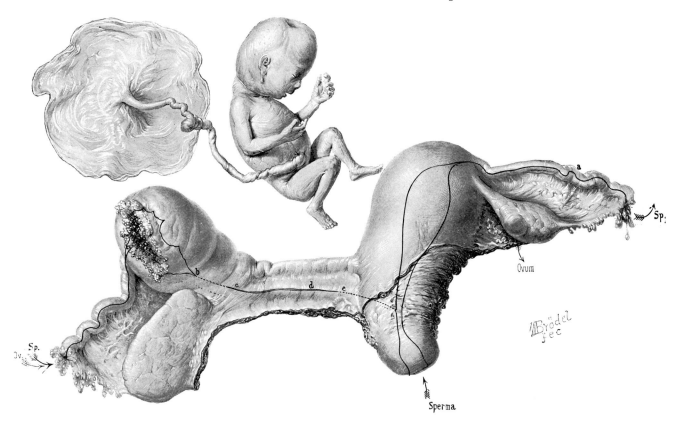

FIG. 23-10.   Pregnancy in rudimentary left uterine horn: rupture and death. Viewed from behind. To *right,* a well-developed uterus. Attached to cornu is normal right tube. Ovary of usual size, and at its inner and lower portion corpus luteum of pregnancy. Springing from left side of uterus at internal os is muscular band that merges into rudimentary uterine horn, on posterior surface of which is point of rupture. Placental remains protrude through rent. Left tube passes off from outer side of rudimentary horn. Left ovary flattened. Line on well-developed uterus indicates size of uterine cavity. Lines *b, c, d, e* indicate course of left Müller's duct between *c* and *d* containing a lumen; *dotted lines* indicate solid muscular cord. Above the specimen are the placenta and fetus drawn in normal size. (Kelly HA: Gynecology. New York, D Appleton, 1928. Drawing by Max Brödel)

Cervical Pregnancy

An extremely rare form of ectopic pregnancy, cervical pregnancy produces profuse vaginal bleeding without associated cramping pain. The differential diagnosis is difficult because the physician initially is apt to suspect a cervical carcinoma or either an incomplete or septic abortion. The combination of necrotic tissue, marked vascularity, and, occasionally, secondary infection adds to the problem of differential diagnosis. Initial attempts can be made to stop the hemorrhage by local removal of the products of conception; if hemostasis is obtained, this is adequate treatment. Because of the depth of trophoblastic invasion, however, major blood vessels are often involved, and hysterectomy may be necessary. Bilateral internal iliac artery ligation has been recommended as a possible substitute, because this procedure preserves reproductive function.

The above discussion applies to pregnancies that are implanted in the cervix itself. David has recently described a variant, shown to have been implanted in the upper cervix, in which growth of the conceptus extended upward into the isthmic area, such that the surrounding myometrium was able to enlarge sufficiently to retain the conceptus until delivery at term by cesarean section–hysterectomy. This report reviews 11 similar cases previously reported and suggests a new classification for the variants of cervical pregnancy.

Ovarian Pregnancy

The signs and symptoms of ovarian pregnancy are similar to those of tubal pregnancy. Usually, the diagnosis is not made until a laparatomy is done. The incidence of ovarian pregnancy is increasing because of the increased

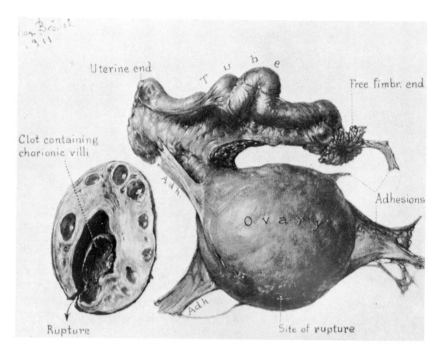

FIG. 23-11. (*Right*) Posterior view of the ovary and uterine tube before it was cut open. *Adh* = adhesions. (*Left*) Transverse section through the ovary at the point of follicle rupture, which resulted in an extensive hemorrhage. The clot is covered with an inverted chorion and contains villi. (Mall FP, Cullen EK: An ovarian pregnancy located in the graafian follicle. Surg Gynecol Obstet 17: 698, 1913. Drawing by Max Brödel)

use of the IUD. The classic criteria of Spiegelberg that are used to diagnose an ovarian pregnancy include the following: the fetal sac must occupy a portion of the ovary, the fallopian tube must be normal and intact on the affected side of the pelvis, the ovary and sac must be connected to the uterus by the ovarian ligament, and ovarian tissue must be identified in the sac (Fig. 23-11).

Many early ovarian pregnancies grossly resemble a bleeding corpus luteum, and the diagnosis is rarely established except by histologic examination of the specimen. Treatment consists of resection of the trophoblast from the ovary, preserving as much ovarian tissue as possible. Salpingo-oophorectomy is rarely necessary.

Ectopic Pregnancy Coexisting with Unrelated Pelvic Problems

Different types of ectopic pregnancy have been reported in the same patient. Ectopic pregnancy may also coexist with a normal intrauterine pregnancy, a condition known as *heterotopic pregnancy*. The incidence of heterotopic pregnancy is approximately one per 17,000 to 30,000 pregnancies. Rarely, an ectopic pregnancy may be the factor that unmasks some other pelvic abnormality. The prize for such an event must go to the case, which is probably unique, of a tubal pregnancy that abutted, cell to cell, against one of the rarest of pelvic cancers, adenocarcinoma of the fallopian tube.

REFERENCES AND RECOMMENDED READING

Arias–Stella J: Atypical endometrial changes associated with the presence of chorionic tissue. Arch Pathol 58:112, 1954

Barnes AB, Wennberg CN, Barnes BA: Ectopic pregnancy: Incidence and review of determinant factors. Obstet Gynecol Surv 38:345, 1983

Beacham WD, Collins CG, Thomas EP et al: Ectopic pregnancy. JAMA 136:365, 1948

Beral V: An epidemiological study of recent trends in ectopic pregnancy. Br J Obstet Gynaecol 82:775, 1975

Beswick IP, Gregory MM: The Arias–Stella phenomenon and the diagnosis of pregnancy. J Obstet Gynaecol Br Commonw 78:143, 1971

Brady L: Report of a case of tubal pregnancy probably caused by a par-ovarian cyst. Bull Johns Hopkins Hosp 33:442, 1922

Breen JL: A 21-year survey of 654 ectopic pregnancies. Am J Obstet Gynecol 106:1004, 1970

Brenner PF, Roy S, Mishell DR Jr.: Ectopic pregnancy: A study of 300 consecutive surgically treated cases. JAMA 243:673, 1980

Bronson RA: Tubal pregnancy and infertility. Fertil Steril 28:221, 1977

Brown TW, Filly RA, Laing FC et al: Analysis of ultrasonographic criteria in the evaluation for ectopic pregnancy. Am J Roentgenol 131:967, 1978

Bryson SC: β-Subunit of human chorionic gonadotropin, ultrasound, and ectopic pregnancy: A prospective study. Am J Obstet Gynecol 146:163, 1983

Bukovsky I, Langer R, Herman A et al: Conservative surgery for tubal pregnancy. Obstet Gynecol 53:709, 1979

Burrows S, Moors W, Pekala B: Missed tubal abortion. Am J Obstet Gynecol 136:691, 1980

Capraro VJ, Chuang JT, Randall CL: Cul-de-sac aspiration and other diagnostic aids for ectopic pregnancy: A 22-year analysis. Int Surg 53:245, 1970

Carapeto R, Nogales FF Jr., Matilla A: Ectopic pregnancy coexisting with a primary carcinoma of the fallopian tube: A case report. Int J Gynaecol Obstet 16:263, 1978

Cartwright PS, DiPietro DL: Ectopic pregnancy: Changes in serum human chorionic gonadotropin concentration. Obstet Gynecol 63:76, 1984

Carty MJ, Barr RD, Ouna N: The coagulation and fibrinolytic properties of peritoneal and venous blood in patients with ruptured ectopic pregnancy. J Obstet Gynaecol Br Commonw 80:701, 1973

Danforth WC: Referred pain in the shoulder in ruptured tubal pregnancy. Am J Obstet Gynecol 12:883, 1926

Danforth WC: Ectopic pregnancy: A study of 174 cases. J Mt Sinai Hosp (NY) 14:269, 1947

David MKP, Bergman A, Delighdish L: Cervico-isthmic pregnancy carried to term. Obstet Gynecol 56:247, 1980

DeCherney AH, Maheaux R, Naftolin F: Salpingostomy for ectopic pregnancy in the sole patent oviduct: Reproductive outcome. Fertil Steril 37:619, 1982

DeCherney AH, Kase N: The conservative management of unruptured ectopic pregnancy. Obstet Gynecol 54:451, 1979

Donald I: Practical Obstetric Problems, p 39. London, Lloyd–Luke, 1979

Dorfman SF: Deaths from ectopic pregnancy, United States, 1979 to 1980. Obstet Gynecol 62:334, 1983

Dotters D, Davis JR, Christian CD: Sex ratio in ectopic gestations. Fertil Steril 41:778, 1984

Fienberg R, Lloyd HED: The Arias–Stella reaction in early normal pregnancy—An involutional phenomenon. Hum Pathol 5:183, 1974

Freakley G, Norman WJ, Ennis JT et al: Diverticulosis of the fallopian tubes. Clin Radiol 25:535, 1974

Gabbe SG, Kitzmiller JL, Kosasa TS et al: Cervical pregnancy presenting as septic abortion. Am J Obstet Gynecol 123:212, 1975

Gitstein S, Ballas S, Schujman E at al: Early cervical pregnancy: Ultrasonic diagnosis and conservative treatment. Obstet Gynecol 54:758, 1979

Gray CL, Ruffolo EH: Ovarian pregnancy associated with intrauterine contraceptive devices. Am J Obstet Gynecol 132:134, 1978

Halbrecht I: Healed genital tuberculosis: A new etiological factor in ectopic pregnancy. Obstet Gynecol 10:73, 1957

Hallatt JG: Repeat ectopic pregnancy: A study of 123 consecutive cases. Am J Obstet Gynecol 122:520, 1975

Hallatt JG: Ectopic pregnancy associated with the intrauterine device: A study of seventy cases. Am J Obstet Gynecol 125:754, 1976

Halpin TF: Ectopic pregnancy: The problem of diagnosis. Am J Obstet Gynecol 106:227, 1970

Harralson JD, van Nagell JR Jr., Roddick JW Jr.: Operative management of ruptured tubal pregnancy. Am J Obstet Gynecol 115:995, 1973

Helvacioglu A, Long M Jr., Yang S: Ectopic pregnancy—an eight-year review. J Reprod Med 22:87, 1979

Hochberg CJ: Tubal amylase. Obstet Gynecol 43:129, 1974.

Honoré LH, O'Hara KE: Failed tubal sterilization as an etiologic factor in ectopic tubal pregnancy. Fertil Steril 29:509, 1978

Jarvinen PA, Nummi S, Pietila K: Conservative operative treatment of tubal pregnancy with postoperative daily hydrotubations. Acta Obstet Gynecol Scand 51:169, 1972

Jeffcoate N: Principles of Gynaecology, 4th ed, p 214. London, Butterworths, 1975

Kamrava MM, Taymor ML, Berger MJ et al: Disappearance of human chorionic gonadotropin following removal of ectopic pregnancy. Obstet Gynecol 62:486, 1983

Kallenberger DA, Ronk DA, Jimerson GK: Ectopic pregnancy: A 15-year review of 160 cases. South Med J 71:758, 1978

Katz J, Marcus RG: The risk of Rh isoimmunization in ruptured tubal pregnancy. Br Med J 3:667, 1972

Kauppila A, Rantakyla P, Huhtaniemi I et al: Trophoblastic

markers in the differential diagnosis of ectopic pregnancy. Obstet Gynecol 55:560, 1980

Kelly MT, Santos–Ramos R, Duenhoelter JH: The value of sonography in suspected ectopic pregnancy. Obstet Gynecol 53:703, 1979

Kersztúry S: Examination of curettage material for the diagnosis of ectopic pregnancy. Acta Morphol Acad Sci Hung 24:359, 1976

Kumar S, Oxorn H: Ectopic pregnancy following tubal sterilization. Can Med Assoc J 22:156, 1978

Lancet M, Bin–Nun I, Kessler I: Angular and interstitial pregnancy. Int Surg 62:107, 1977

Langer R, Bukovsky I, Herman A et al: Conservative surgery for tubal pregnancy. Fertil Steril 38:427, 1982

Liukko P, Erkkola R, Laakso L: Ectopic pregnancies during use of low-dose progestogens for oral contraception. Contraception 16:575, 1977

McCausland A: High rate of ectopic pregnancy following laparoscopic tubal coagulation failures. Am J Obstet Gynecol 136:97, 1980

McElin TW: Discussion of intraligamentous pregnancy. Am J Obstet Gynecol 70:182, 1955

McElin TW, Iffy L: Ectopic gestation: A consideration of new and controversial issues relating to pathogenesis and management. Obstet Gynecol 5:241, 1976

McElin TW, LaPata RE: Angular pregnancy: Report of a case. Obstet Gynecol 31:849, 1968

Mall FP, Cullen EK: An ovarian pregnancy located in the graafian follicle. Surg Gynecol Obstet 17:698, 1913

May WJ, Miller JB, Greiss FC Jr.: Maternal deaths from ectopic pregnancy in the South Atlantic region, 1960 through 1976. Am J Obstet Gynecol 132:140, 1978

Meirik O, Nygren KG: Ectopic pregnancy and IUDs: Incidence, Risk Rate and Predisposing Factors. Acta Obstet Gynecol Scand 59:425, 1980

Milwidsky A, Adoni A, Miodovnik M et al: Human chorionic gonadotropin (β-subunit) in the early diagnosis of ectopic pregnancy. Obstet Gynecol 51:725, 1978

Myerscough PR: Monro Kerr's Operative Obstetrics, 9th ed, p 662. Baltimore, Williams & Wilkins, 1977

Nelson RM: Bilateral internal iliac artery ligation in cervical pregnancy: Conservation of reproductive function. Am J Obstet Gynecol 134:145, 1979

Niebyl JR: Pregnancy following total hysterectomy. Am J Obstet Gynecol 119:512, 1974

Nyberg DA, Laing FC, Filly RA et al: Ultrasonographic differentiation of the gestational sac of early intrauterine pregnancy from the pseudogestational sac of ectopic pregnancy. Radiology 146:755, 1983

Olson CM, Holt JA, Alenghat E et al: Limitations of qualitative serum beta-hCG assays in the diagnosis of ectopic pregnancy. J Repro Med 28:838, 1983

Panayotou PP, Kaskarelis DB, Miettinen OS et al: Induced abortion and ectopic pregnancy. Am J Obstet Gynecol 114:507, 1972

Pauerstein CJ: From fallopius to fantasy. Fertil Steril 30:133, 1978

Pent D, Loffer FD: The natural history of an hematosalpinx. Obstet Gynecol 47:2s, 1976

Poland BJ, Dill FJ, Styblo C: Embryonic development in ectopic human pregnancy. Teratology 14:315, 1976

Pugh WE, Vogt RF, Gibson RA: Primary ovarian pregnancy and the intrauterine device. Obstet Gynecol 42:218, 1973

Pusey J, Taylor PJ, Leader A et al: Outcome and effect of medical intervention in women experiencing infertility following removal of ectopic pregnancy. Am J Obstet Gynecol 148:524, 1984

Rasor JL, Barunstein GD: A rapid modification of the Beta-hCG radioimmunoassay: Use as an aid in the diagnosis of ectopic pregnancy. Obstet Gynecol 50:553, 1977

Rothe DJ, Birnbaum SJ: Cervical pregnancy: Diagnosis and management. Obstet Gynecol 42:675, 1973

Rubin GL, Peterson HB, Dorfman SF et al: Ectopic Pregnancy in the United States. JAMA 249:1725, 1983

Saito M, Koyama T, Yaoi Y et al: Site of ovulation and ectopic pregnancy. Acta Obstet Gynecol Scand 54:227, 1975

Sanders EP: Subacute ectopic pregnancy. NZ Med J 87:41, 1978

Saxena BB, Landesman R: Diagnosis and management of pregnancy by the radioreceptorassay of human chorionic gonadotropin. Am J Obstet Gynecol 131:97, 1978

Schenker JG, Evron S: New concepts in the surgical management of tubal pregnancy and the consequent postoperative results. Fertil Steril 40:709, 1983

Schenker JG, Eyal F, Polishuk WZ: Fertility after tubal pregnancy. Surg Gynecol Obstet 135:74, 1972

Schinfeld JS, Reedy G: Mesosalpingeal vessel ligation for conservative treatment of ectopic pregnancy. J Repro Med 28:823, 1983

Schneider J, Berger CJ, Cattell C: Maternal mortality due to ectopic pregnancy: A review of 102 deaths. Obstet Gynecol 49:557, 1977

Schoen JA, Nowak RJ: Repeat ectopic pregnancy: A 16-year clinical survey. Obstet Gynecol 45:542, 1975

Seppala M, Venesmaa P, Rutanen EM: Pregnancy-specific β-1 glycoprotein in ectopic pregnancy. Am J Obstet Gynecol 136:189, 1980

Sherman D, Langer R, Sadovsky G et al: Improved fertility following ectopic pregnancy. Fertil Steril 37:497, 1982

Spiegelberg O: Zur Casuistik der Ovarialschwangerschaft. Arch Gynaekol 13:73, 1878

Strafford JC, Ragan WD: Abdominal pregnancy: Review of current management. Obstet Gynecol 50:548, 1977

Stromme WB: Conservative surgery for ectopic pregnancy: A twenty-year review. Obstet Gynecol 41:215, 1973

Tait RL: Five cases of extra-uterine pregnancy operated upon at the time of rupture. Br Med J 1:1250, 1884

Tatum HJ, Schmidt FH: Contraceptive and sterilization practices and extrauterine pregnancy: A realistic perspective. Fertil Steril 28:407, 1977

Wharton LR: Gynecology with a Section on Female Urology, p 693. Philadelphia, WB Saunders, 1943

Wolf GC, Kritzer L, DeBold C: Heterotopic pregnancy: Mid-trimester management. Obstet Gynecol 54:756, 1979

Wolfman W, Holtz G: Update on ectopic pregnancy. Can Med Assoc J 129:1265, 1983

Isoimmunization in Pregnancy

James R. Scott

24

Erythroblastosis fetalis is a disease of the fetus and newborn caused by an incompatibility of fetal and maternal blood; the Rh-negative mother becomes immunized by exposure to Rh-positive fetal erythrocytes during pregnancy or delivery (or occasionally as the result of an incompatible blood transfusion). The antibodies formed by the mother pass through the placenta to the fetal circulation where they react with the Rh-positive fetal erythrocytes, causing hemolytic anemia.

Although the first description of hemolytic disease of the newborn dates back to 1609, no rational treatment was possible until the 20th century, when the ABO blood groups and Rh factor were discovered. In the ensuing years, advances in therapy dramatically reduced perinatal mortality, and Rh immune globulin (RhIgG) was developed to prevent the condition. Figure 24-1 shows that the incidence of hemolytic disease of the newborn has gradually decreased but not disappeared since the introduction of RhIgG. Paradoxically, as the disorder becomes less frequent, it is increasingly difficult to keep abreast of the new and sometimes controversial recommendations for prophylaxis as well as sophisticated advances in treatment. The purpose of this chapter is to present a practical and up-to-date approach to the management of the pregnant Rh-negative woman.

PATHOPHYSIOLOGY

Nomenclature

The Rh blood group was originally given its name because rabbits immunized with rhesus monkey erythrocytes produced an antibody that agglutinated red blood cells from 85% of Caucasians. Subsequently, the human blood group system has been found to be extremely complex.[1] The genetic locus for Rh antigens is located on the short arm of chromosome 1, but there is no consensus as to the number of genes controlling their synthesis. Nevertheless, the final gene product on the human erythrocyte is a small protein of 7000 daltons to 10,000 daltons that has multiple antigenic determinants. Rh antigens associated with membrane phospholipid are distributed in nonrandom clusters on the red cell surface, and the number of antigenic sites for a specific erythrocyte is dependent on the genotype.

Although several systems of terminology have been proposed, the Fischer–Race nomenclature is the most widely used in obstetrics and has been recommended by the World Health Organization (WHO) Expert Committee on Biological Standardization in the interest of simplicity and uniformity. This system assumes the presence of three genetic loci, each with two possible alleles. Antigens produced by these alleles are identified by specific antisera and have been lettered C, c, D, E, and e. No antiserum specific for d has been found, and therefore *d* signifies the absence of a discernible allelic product. The following gene complexes have been identified: CDe, cDE, cde, cDe, cdE, Cde, and CDE. Genotypes are indicated as pairs of gene complexes such as CDe/cde. Although the alleles are always written in this order, the actual chromosome order is D(d), C(c), E(e). For most clinical purposes it is sufficient to divide human beings into Rh positive and Rh negative, and the distinction is made by testing their red cells with anti-D antiserum.

There are several variations of D antigen expression that make up a heterogeneous group called *Du variants* (Fig. 24-2). Du phenotypes (those antigens expressed on the erythrocyte surface) that strongly express D antigen may react with sera containing anti-D; other Du phenotypes are distinguished from d phenotypes only by very sensitive assays. Du variant patients are usually considered to be Rh positive, since their erythrocytes

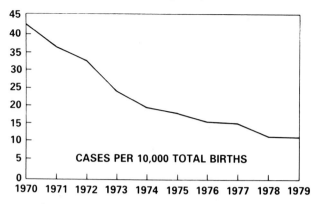

FIG. 24-1. Incidence of Rh hemolytic disease of the newborn by year in the United States, 1970–1979. (Centers for Disease Control: Rh hemolytic disease—Connecticut, United States, 1970–1979. MMNR 30(2):13, 1981)

can stimulate the production of anti-D antibodies, and these persons rarely produce anti-D antibodies themselves.

Fetomaternal Hemorrhage

Fetal blood often gains entry to the maternal circulation during pregnancy and in the immediate postpartum period. Fetal red cells have been detected in 6.7% of pregnant women during the first trimester, 15.9% during the second trimester, and 28.9% during the third trimester.[2] Although the minimum number of Rh-positive fetal red cells necessary to cause immunization in the pregnant Rh-negative woman is still a subject of controversy, as little as 0.1 ml of Rh-positive blood has been shown to sensitize Rh-negative volunteers. A fetomaternal hemorrhage sufficient to cause immunization is most common at the time of delivery, but in more than half the cases, the amount of fetal blood found in the maternal circulation is 0.1 ml or less.[2] The obstetric factors that increase the risk of transplacental transfer of fetal red cells are listed below:

Amniocentesis
Threatened abortion, placenta previa, placental abruption
Abdominal trauma
External version
Fetal death
Sinusoidal fetal heart tracing
Multiple pregnancy
Cesarean section
Anemic infant

Factors influencing Rh immunization are the following:

Incidence and size of fetomaternal hemorrhage
ABO compatibility between mother and fetus
Rh phenotype of fetal red cells

Sex of the baby
Genetic predisposition (responder)

Even though the quantity of fetal red cells in the maternal circulation is usually small, larger transplacental bleeds sometimes occur, often in an unpredictable manner.

The *Kleihauer–Betke test* was the first method described to detect fetal red cells.[3] Adult hemoglobin (HbA) in the maternal erythrocyte is eluted through the cell membrane in the presence of an acidic buffer, but fetal hemoglobin (HbF) in the fetal red cell is resistant to removal. When a film of blood is fixed on a slide and prepared in this fashion, it is stained with erythrosin and the fetal cells containing stained HbF can be distinguished microscopically from the adult erythrocyte ghost cells (Fig. 24-3). A count is made of fetal and adult cells on the smear, and the size of the fetomaternal bleed is determined according to the following formula:

$$\frac{\text{number of fetal red cells}}{\text{number of maternal red cells}}$$

$$= \frac{X \text{ (ml of fetomaternal bleed)}}{\text{estimated maternal blood volume}}$$

A number of modifications of the original acid elution technique have been introduced, and rapid, simplified commercial tests are now available in kit form (Fetaldex, Ortho Diagnostics; BMC Reagent Set, Boehringer Mannheim Corp.). An erythrocyte rosetting test (Fetalscreen, Ortho Diagnostics) that specifically detects Rh-positive red cells can also be used. However, because

FIG. 24-2. Mechanism for the determination of D and Du positivity. One theory suggests that the density of the D antigen on the surface of the red cell determines the results of red cell typing. Patients with no antigen are typed Rh−, patients with low densities of the antigen will be typed Du+, and patients with high density of the antigen will be typed Rh+. (Kochenour NK, Scott JR: Rh isoimmunization in pregnancy. In Scott JR, Rote NS (eds): Immunology in Obstetrics and Gynecology, p 143. Norwalk, CT, Appleton–Century–Crofts, 1984)

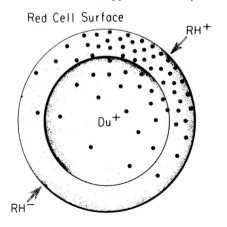

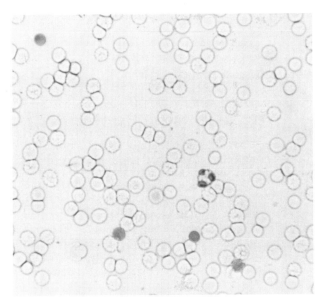

FIG. 24-3. Peripheral smear showing dark fetal red cells in contrast to light-colored maternal cells. The larger dark-staining cell near the middle is a maternal neutrophil. (Scott JR, Warenski JC: Tests to detect and quantitate fetomaternal bleeding. Clin Obstet Gynecol 25:277, 1982)

this test is qualitative, positive results must be followed by a quantitative acid elution test.

Immunology

Unlike the ABO system in which persons produce antibodies against similar or identical antigens on bacteria or other substances, Rh-negative patients develop circulating titers of anti-D only when exposed to Rh-positive red cells. Moreover, about 30% of Rh-negative persons are never sensitized (nonresponders) even when challenged with large volumes of Rh-positive blood.[4] Other factors that influence whether a particular mother will become immunized are listed above. The maternal humoral immune system responds relatively slowly to Rh antigens, first by synthesizing low levels of IgM antibodies, and later by producing IgG antibodies, which are usually detectable within six weeks to six months. These antibodies, which are 7S immunoglobulins, are capable of crossing the placenta and can destroy fetal Rh-positive red cells. However, the heterogeneity of the IgG subclasses produced and the differences in transplacental transfer may be partially responsible for the variability of fetal involvement among patients.

The reaction of anti-D antibody with D antigens results in the eventual destruction of Rh-positive cells, but the exact mechanism is unclear. It is not a complement-fixing reaction, and most IgG-coated red cells are hemolyzed extravascularly in the splenic reticuloendothelial system. Antibody-dependent cellular cytotox-

icity mechanisms may also contribute. Mononuclear phagocytes and some lymphoid cells have receptors that can interact with a portion of the antibody on the red cell surface to lyse the target cells (as has been shown *in vitro* with anti-D–coated erythrocytes).

Clinical Manifestations

In the fetus, red cell destruction leads to hyperbilirubinemia, anemia, and ultimately to erythroblastosis fetalis, characterized by heart failure, edema, ascites, pericardial effusion, and extramedullary hematopoiesis. The severe anemia is associated with tissue hypoxia and acidosis, and extensive liver erythropoiesis results in replacement of normal hepatic parenchyma and architectural distortion. The consequences include a decrease in protein production, portal hypertension, ascites, and generalized anasarca.

In the neonate, the primary clinical problem is hyperbilirubinemia, but bleeding problems and heart failure can also occur. Although hemoglobin breakdown products (primarily bilirubin) are found in increased levels in amniotic fluid and cord blood, excessive amounts are readily cleared by the placenta and metabolized by the mother. However, low levels of glucuronyltransferase in the newborn preclude the conjugation of large amounts of bilirubin and result in high levels of serum bilirubin, which lead to kernicterus by the deposition of the bilirubin complexes in the basal ganglia of the central nervous system.

PREVENTION

Mechanisms

Immunization to the D antigen can be prevented by the administration of RhIgG either before or shortly after exposure to Rh-positive cells. There are three potential mechanisms of action from an immunologic standpoint:[5]

Antigen blocking–competitive inhibition. This classic explanation assumes that passively administered antibodies produce suppression by attaching or "covering" antigenic sites on the Rh-positive red cells, rendering them unavailable to the receptors on the maternal lymphoid cells, which are necessary to initiate the immune response. Evidence against this theory is the fact that a ratio of 20 μg of exogenous antibody per milliliter of red cells prevents the synthesis of endogenous anti-D antibody even though only a small percentage of the antigenic sites is bound.

Clearance and antigen deviation. This theory is based on the concept that the antigen is directed away from the reticuloendothelial system, preventing the formation of antibodies. Presumably, ABO incompatibility protects against Rh immunization in this manner. Since other antigens such as C and E, which are present on the carrier molecule, are also directed away from the immune system, the use of RhIgG should prevent the formation of antibodies to C and E in addition to antibodies to D. Some evidence for this type of nonspecificity suggests that antigen deviation may in some way be involved in antigen-mediated immune suppression for the Rh system.

Central inhibition. Immune responses are modulated much like a thermostat by effector lymphocytes, which are responsible for augmenting (helping) or abrogating (suppressing) the response. Suppressor cells have membrane receptors for the altered Fc portion of IgG and can be stimulated by IgG-containing immune complexes. This suggests that the immune response to the D antigen can be prevented by the generation of antigen-specific suppressor cells near the time of exposure to Rh-positive erythrocytes. RhIgG, in the presence of fetal Rh-positive erythrocytes, may generate the immune complexes responsible for the induction of these cells (Fig. 24-4). This hypothesis is consistent with the observation that antibody-mediated immune suppression appears to prevent only a primary response and has no effect on the secondary response in Rh-sensitized patients.

Clinical Use of RhIgG

RhIgG, first released for general use in 1968, has proved to be remarkably successful in the prevention of sensitization to the Rh antigen. One vial of RhIgG (300 μg of anti-D) can suppress immunity to approximately 30 ml of whole Rh-positive blood or 15 ml of packed Rh-positive red cells. Unfortunately, failure to utilize this protection remains a significant public health problem and contributes to the persistence of Rh hemolytic disease. In order to reduce the morbidity and mortality of Rh erythroblastosis fetalis to the minimum, it is imperative that all women at risk be identified and treated. RhIgG is 100% effective immunologically if given before sensitization, but reasons for postabortal and postpartum clinical failures include the following:

Failure to type the patient's blood at the first prenatal visit or to order RhIgG when indicated
Error in transmitting the proper blood type to the mother's chart and to the physician
Error in typing the mother's, father's, or baby's blood
Failure to administer RhIgG when ordered
Unrecognized fetomaternal hemorrhage during pregnancy
Inadequate RhIgG dosage for the volume of fetomaternal hemorrhage
Patient choice

In each pregnancy, a woman should have her blood and Rh type determined and an antibody screen performed as early as practical so that she can be managed appropriately (Table 24-1). If the father is homozygous for D, then all his offspring will be D positive. On the other hand, if he is heterozygous, there is a 50% chance that any given child of his will be Rh negative and unaffected by Rh hemolytic disease due to D.

First-Trimester Abortion

The D antigen has been identified on the fetal red cell as early as the 38th day of gestation, and the risk of sensitization in both induced and spontaneous abortions is 3% to 5.5% but varies with length of gestation.[6-8] The embryo has a circulation by four weeks postconception, and transplacental passage of erythrocytes can occur theoretically by six to eight weeks' gestation. How early and often this actually happens has not been well documented, and the necessity for prophylaxis following menstrual extractions or spontaneous abortions with blighted ova before six weeks has never been resolved satisfactorily. Nevertheless, until the minimum amount of Rh-positive blood necessary to immunize is more firmly established, and because the fetal blood type is not usually known, all Rh-negative women with any type

FIG. 24-4. The theoretic mechanism that best explains the known facts about Rh prophylaxis is central inhibition of antibody production. The immune response to the Rh antigen is modulated by effector lymphocytes that augment (helper cells; *Th*) or suppress (suppressor cells; *Ts*). Suppressor cells can be stimulated by the Fc portion of IgG in immune complexes with Rh antigen to produce soluble substances that suppress the stimulating effect of helper lymphocytes. This blocks the production of endogenous antibody against the Rh antigen. (Kochenour NK, Scott JR: Rh isoimmunization in pregnancy. In Scott JR, Rote NS (eds): Immunology in Obstetrics and Gynecology, p 143. New York, Appleton–Century–Crofts, 1984)

Central Inhibition of Antibody Production

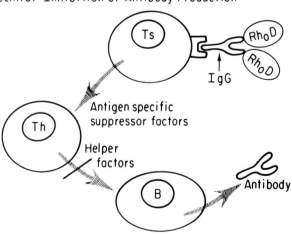

Table 24-1
Evaluation and Management of an Unsensitized Rh-Negative, Du-Negative Pregnant Patient

Time in Gestation	Management
First prenatal visit	Determine ABO blood group and Rh, including Du Antibody screen (indirect Coombs' test)
28 weeks	Antibody screen negative: administer 300 μg RhIgG Antibody screen positive: check Rh of baby's father and manage as Rh-sensitized
35 weeks	Antibody screen negative (<1:4): observe Antibody screen positive: manage as Rh-sensitized
Postpartum	Antibody screen negative: administer 300 μg RhIgG if infant is Rh-positive or Du-positive Antibody screen positive: manage next pregnancy as Rh-sensitized

of abortive episode should be protected with RhIgG when the pregnancy is terminated. Unfortunately, this source of sensitization has not been attacked vigorously enough, and the RhIgG utilization rate is far below that of term pregnancies. Commercially available 50-μg RhIgG preparations (Mini-Gamulin Rh, Armour Pharmaceutical Co.; MICRhoGAM, Ortho Diagnostics) protect against 5 ml of whole fetal blood (or 2.5 ml of packed red cells) and are sufficient prophylaxis against all fetomaternal hemorrhages occurring during the first trimester.[9]

A similar potential for sensitization exists with ectopic pregnancy, but whether RhIgG is necessary after a hydatidiform mole is more conjectural. Histologic analysis of hydatidiform moles reveals no nucleated fetal red cells or fetal vessels in the villi, and most investigators have found that trophoblastic cells do not contain Rh antigens.[10,11] In the only reported case of Rh immunization associated with a hydatidiform mole, it is likely that antepartum sensitization during the next pregnancy was actually the cause.[12]

Amniocentesis

Amniocentesis for intrauterine diagnosis of genetic disease carries a risk of fetomaternal hemorrhage and sensitization in Rh-negative patients, even when performed under ultrasound direction.[13] Therefore, until further data show a more selective protocol to be safe, it is recommended that all Rh-negative patients undergoing second-trimester amniocentesis receive 300 μg of RhIgG. One theoretical risk of RhIgG used in this way is the phenomenon of "enhancement." This term refers to facilitation of an immune response in the presence of a very low antibody level at the time of antigen exposure.[14] Because the half-life of RhIgG is about 25 days, augmentation could take place in the third trimester as fetal red cells gain access to the maternal circulation. Although immunologic enhancement has not been clearly proved in this situation, it is one reason to avoid the 50-μg dose of RhIgG with amniocentesis and to make sure that the patient receives an additional 300-μg dose at 28 weeks' gestation.

Even in the third trimester, the use of ultrasound for amniocentesis and the absence of macroscopic blood in the amniotic fluid are not adequate guarantees against the appearance of fetal red cells in the maternal circulation.[15] However, if delivery is to be accomplished within 72 hours, it is reasonable to withhold RhIgG at the time of amniocentesis and to administer it immediately after delivery if the infant is found to be Rh positive.

Antepartum Bleeding

Although the risk of sensitization with threatened abortion is not known, fetomaternal bleeding may be more common in this setting. One way to manage the situation is to test for fetal red cells in maternal blood and to administer RhIgG if they are present. If this course is followed, RhIgG should be given and repeated again at 28 weeks' gestation if the pregnancy continues. If the pregnancy proceeds to abortion, it is unlikely that more RhIgG is necessary.

It may also be worthwhile to look for fetal red cells in the maternal circulation during certain other obstetric complications known to increase the risk of fetomaternal hemorrhage. These include cases of antepartum bleeding from placenta previa or abruptio placentae, abdominal trauma, fetal hydrops, sinusoidal fetal heart rate patterns, and unexplained fetal demise.[16]

Antepartum Prophylaxis

It has become apparent that the standard postpartum RhIgG regimen fails to protect 1% to 2% of Rh-negative women who deliver an Rh-positive infant. Most often this failure is due to occult transplacental transfer of a sufficient number of fetal red cells during the pregnancy.[17] Antepartum prophylaxis was first suggested in 1967,[18] and trials of antepartum administration of RhIgG were started in Canada in 1968.[19] Sensitization occurred in only two of 1799 Rh-negative women who delivered Rh-positive infants, representing a failure rate of 0.11% compared with the expected failure rate of 1.6%. The beginning of the third trimester and a 300-μg dose were chosen because the majority of sensitizations occur after this time, and with this dose adequate levels of RhIgG are still present at the end of pregnancy.

Despite its demonstrated efficacy by clinical trials, the

use of antepartum prophylaxis has not been universal. Some have expressed concern that it may not be immunologically safe for the fetus, but there is no clinical or laboratory evidence of any harm in tens of thousands of infants delivered after their mothers received antenatal Rh prophylaxis. The main controversy in the United States has centered around the cost/benefit ratio, despite analysis by a variety of statistical approaches.[16,20–24] However, the cross-match has now been eliminated, fewer indirect Coombs' tests are necessary, and the price of RhIgG is half that of when it was introduced. Consequently, the present cost to the patient of the combined antepartum–postpartum regimen compares favorably with the previously recommended postpartum regimen.

A protocol for the antepartum administration of RhIgG is shown in Figure 24-5. Whether an anti-D titer is necessary at 35 weeks' gestation to detect the rare patient who might become sensitized despite antepartum RhIgG is unresolved at this time. This never occurred in 1357 pregnancies when the indirect Coombs' test at 28 weeks' gestation was negative prior to administration of RhIgG,[25] and it would be extremely unlikely that such a case would require active intervention before delivery.

Problems encountered in instituting such a program are primarily logistical or involve education of the patients, physicians, and laboratory personnel. For example, it is important to realize that the patient has recently received RhIgG if blood is cross-matched at delivery and to remember that the infant may have a weakly positive direct Coombs' test. Each patient should be thoroughly informed and given a card showing that she has received antepartum RhIgG in case she is seen later by a different physician or delivers at another hospital. Otherwise, postpartum RhIgG might be withheld because of a mistaken diagnosis of Rh immunization based on a positive indirect Coombs' test from the circulating anti-D antibody.

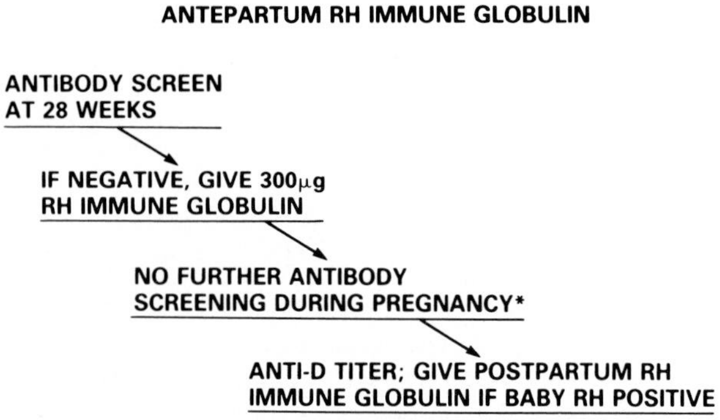

ANTEPARTUM RH IMMUNE GLOBULIN

**ANTIBODY SCREEN
AT 28 WEEKS**

**IF NEGATIVE, GIVE 300µg
RH IMMUNE GLOBULIN**

**NO FURTHER ANTIBODY
SCREENING DURING PREGNANCY***

**ANTI-D TITER; GIVE POSTPARTUM RH
IMMUNE GLOBULIN IF BABY RH POSITIVE**

FIG. 24-5. Two-dose (antepartum–postpartum) regimen for unimmunized Rh-negative patients. (*, Some authorities recommend obtaining an anti-D antibody titer at 35 weeks' gestation because a titer of 1:4 or higher represents active immunization [lower levels of antibody can be detected because of the circulating RhIgG].)

Postpartum Use

The most common cause of Rh immunization is delivery of an Rh-positive or Du-positive child by an Rh-negative woman. Ordinarily, 300 µg of RhIgG injected intramuscularly within 72 hours of delivery will prevent sensitization. Moreover, there is evidence that it is effective even when given later than this arbitrarily chosen time limit. Therefore, RhIgG should be administered as soon as possible after delivery, but it is still indicated after 72 hours if an error is recognized. Postpartum administration of RhIgG protects the mother only against sensitization by the just completed pregnancy. It is necessary to test and treat the mother as needed after delivery of each subsequent Rh-positive or Du-positive child.

Even when appropriately timed, approximately 0.4% of patients will have a fetomaternal hemorrhage so large that 300 µg of RhIgG will not be sufficient prophylaxis.[26] Ideally, the volume of the fetomaternal bleed can be determined by use of one of the acid elution tests, but since the incidence of patients not protected by 300 µg is so low, it is probably not cost effective to screen every Rh-negative woman for fetal red cells at the time of delivery. However, if a large fetomaternal hemorrhage is found either on routine screening or because clinical suspicion has led to the test, additional RhIgG at a dose of 300 µg for each 15 ml of fetal red cells is indicated.

One confusing scenario is the pregnant woman who is reported to be Rh negative, Du positive late in pregnancy or after delivery. This can mean either that the patient is actually Du positive (and does not require RhIgG) or that she is Rh negative but has a large number of Rh-positive fetal cells in her circulation (and therefore is a candidate for RhIgG). In this case, it is helpful to have prior information about the patient's blood type either when she was not pregnant or early in pregnancy. If there is any question, it is best to check for the presence of Rh-positive fetal cells in the maternal circulation before deciding against giving RhIgG.

MANAGEMENT

Once a pregnant patient is identified as being Rh immunized, the goal is to time the delivery so that morbidity and mortality risks to the infant are minimized. With this in mind, patients are grouped into one of three categories:

1. Fetuses that are mildly affected can be allowed to remain *in utero* until they have achieved pulmonary maturation.
2. Moderately affected fetuses may need to be delivered before pulmonary maturity but without active intrauterine fetal treatment of the condition.
3. The most severely affected fetuses will require active intervention to reach a gestational age at which the risks of delivery and neonatal intensive care are less than the risks of *in utero* therapy.

Maternal Antibody Titers

Anti-D antibody titers are used primarily to diagnose Rh immunization or to alert the physician to perform the first amniocentesis earlier in pregnancy if the titer is higher than expected. Serial titers have commonly been advocated as a guide for determining the need for amniocentesis in the first sensitized pregnancy. This advice has been based on the experience at a given hospital where severely affected infants were not seen below a "critical" titer. However, anti-D titers differ among laboratories, and the decreasing frequency of this condition has made it more difficult for each institution to reliably determine which values are safe to follow. It is apparent that a fetus can become severely involved with titers as low as 1:16 or 1:32. Therefore, it is much safer to rely on amniotic fluid ΔOD450 values to evaluate the severity of fetal involvement in any questionable situation.

Fetal Assessment

In general, the status of a particular infant can be predicted by review of the mother's previous obstetric history, since the condition tends to worsen with each subsequent pregnancy. Nevertheless, for accurate clinical judgments to be made in a given patient, more specific information is required.

Amniocentesis and Amniotic Fluid Analysis

Although not excreted in large amounts by the fetal kidneys, bilirubin diffuses into the amniotic fluid across such fetal membranes as the skin and umbilical cord. Spectrophotometric analysis of amniotic fluid bilirubin concentration remains the single most reliable method for evaluating the fetal status.[27]

Timing of the initial amniocentesis is a matter of judgment as to when the risk of intrauterine morbidity becomes appreciable. Factors involved in the decision include antibody titers and maternal history of severity of infant involvement in previous pregnancies. The amniocentesis is done under ultrasound guidance, and the aspirated amniotic fluid is placed in a brown bottle to protect it from sunlight, which can cause a falsely low bilirubin determination. For analysis, a beam of light is passed through the standardized sample of amniotic fluid, and the absorption of light is measured at various known wavelengths (Fig. 24-6). Using the Liley graph, the optical density at 450 μ (ΔOD450) is then plotted on a semilogarithmic scale versus gestational age (Fig. 24-7). To understand the Liley curve, it is important to remember that the concentration of bilirubin pigments in the amniotic fluid gradually declines during a normal pregnancy. A significant hemolytic process will result in a higher ΔOD450 level that is constant or rising. The absolute value as well as the trend plotted against gestational age determines the plan of management for an

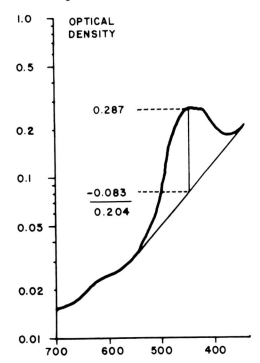

FIG. 24-6. Spectrophotometric scan of amniotic fluid containing bilirubin. Arbitrary line (*heavy line*) has been drawn to show where scan would have been traced if there had been no increase in bilirubin. The peak absorption of bilirubin occurs at 450 μ. The difference between the peak and the arbitrary line equals 0.204. (Liley AW: Amniocentesis and amniography in hemolytic disease. In Greenhill JP (ed): Yearbook of Obstetrics and Gynecology, 1965–65 series, p 256. Copyright © 1964 by Year Book Medical Publishers, Inc., Chicago)

individual pregnancy. When the bilirubin concentration is in the lower zone (zone I), the baby is Rh negative or is only mildly affected. In zone II the majority of fetuses are moderately affected, and values in zone III indicate that the infant is severely affected with erythroblastosis fetalis and in danger of dying *in utero*. Figure 24-8 illustrates how the Liley graph can be used as a guideline for the management of Rh-sensitized patients.

Ultrasound

Serial ultrasound examinations are also helpful to evaluate fetal status in Rh immunization. Since there is not complete correlation between amniotic fluid ΔOD450 values and ultrasound findings, the two should be used together (Fig. 24-9). Ascites and soft tissue edema are definite signs of severe fetal involvement with erythroblastosis fetalis. Several other parameters such as pericardial effusion, hepatic and splenic size, and umbilical blood flow have also been suggested as useful in assessing fetal status, but their value is yet to be determined.

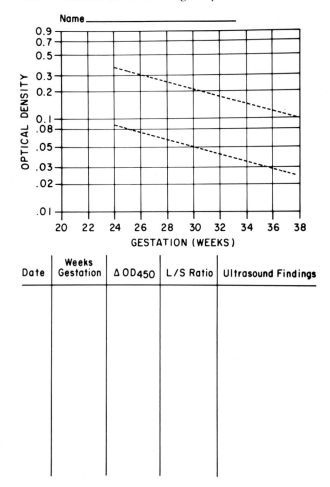

FIG. 24-7. Form used to record serial data on each Rh-immunized patient. The modified Liley graph is divided into three zones to predict the outcome of the pregnancy in terms of umbilical cord blood hemoglobin, intrauterine deaths, or unaffected fetuses.

FIG. 24-8. Modified Liley graph outlining management guidelines currently in use at the University of Utah Medical Center. (Kochenour NK, Scott JR: Rh isoimmunization in pregnancy. In Scott JR, Rote NS (eds): Immunology in Obstetrics and Gynecology, p 152. Norwalk, CT, Appleton–Century–Crofts, 1984)

Fetal Monitoring

Although antepartum fetal monitoring has been reported to be helpful,[28] its exact role in Rh immunization is unclear at this time. This is in part because important management decisions are often made during the late second and early third trimesters of pregnancy, when these tests are of little value. It has been observed that the severely compromised fetus moves less frequently than a normal infant.[29] The lack of fetal movement, either as visualized by ultrasound or as perceived by the mother, has been used as a sign of worsening fetal condition. The appearance of a sinusoidal pattern also suggests a significant worsening of the fetal anemia.[30] However, there are no published data to evaluate the usefulness of the nonstress test in a large number of sensitized pregnancies, and contraction stress tests have not always been reliable in following these fetuses. As with any high-risk pregnancy, intrapartum electronic monitoring is recommended.

Fetal Management

The Mildly to Moderately Involved Fetus

Ultrasound determination of gestational age is obtained at 14 to 16 weeks to avoid errors in dating. Unless the maternal antibody titer is very low, amniotic fluid analysis will be used to follow the status of the infant. If the current pregnancy is the first sensitized pregnancy or if the last infant was only mildly involved, the first amniocentesis should be performed at about 26 to 28 weeks' gestation. The timing of each subsequent amniocentesis as well as the optimal time of delivery will depend on the results of the previous amniotic fluid analyses as outlined in Figure 24-8.

The amniotic fluid lecithin:sphingomyelin ratio is extremely helpful in making management decisions regarding these patients. If the $\Delta OD450$ value is in zone II and falling, delivery should be accomplished as soon

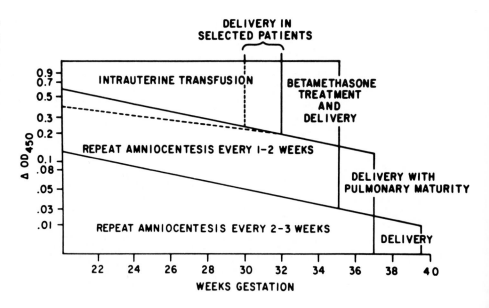

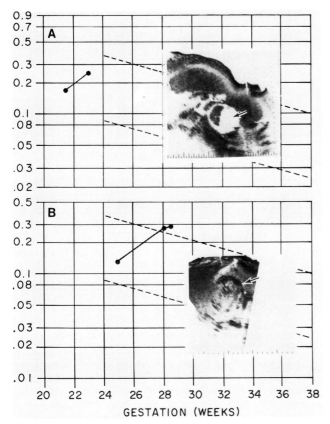

FIG. 24-9. Ultrasound findings in two patients with severe Rh immunization. (*A*) Marked fetal ascites (*broken line*) is already demonstrated by sonogram at 23 weeks' gestation, even though the amniotic fluid ΔOD450 value has not yet reached the upper zone on the Liley graph. (*B*) The amniotic fluid ΔOD450 value is in the upper zone by 30 weeks' gestation with no ultrasound evidence of fetal hydrops (*broken line*). (Kochenour NK, Scott JR: Rh isoimmunization in pregnancy. In Scott JR, Rote NS (eds): Immunology in Obstetrics and Gynecology, p 153. Norwalk, CT, Appleton–Century–Crofts, 1984)

The Severely Involved Fetus

The initial ultrasound examination is performed at 14 to 16 weeks' gestation and repeated between 20 and 22 weeks' gestation to look for fetal ascites and edema and to direct the first amniocentesis. Subsequent amnioceteses and management are determined by ultrasound findings and amniotic fluid ΔOD450 values. When amniotic fluid analysis indicates that the fetus is endangered by Rh hemolytic disease, induction of labor is not always the treatment of choice because the hazard of preterm delivery may be too great. In general, it is preferable to delay delivery until 32 weeks' gestation. However, this figure is being lowered each year as survival rates for low-birth-weight infants continually improve in neonatal intensive care units.

INTRAUTERINE TRANSFUSION. Recent technical advances in the performance of intrauterine transfusions have resulted in perinatal survival rates of 80% to 92%.[31,32] Intrauterine transfusions are indicated in severely Rh-immunized patients when rising amniotic ΔOD450 values reach high zone II or zone III on the Liley graph between 22 and 32 weeks' gestation. The transfused red cells are absorbed from the fetal peritoneal cavity by way of the subdiaphragmatic lymphatics, thoracic duct, and venous circulation to correct the anemia.

Under sedation and with sterile technique, the patient is first scanned with either static or real-time ultrasound to assess fetal position, placental location, and the presence of fetal ascites or peripheral edema. The orientation of the fetal spine to the side or posterior facilitates the transfusion. The transfusion site and the necessary depth of the needle insertion are then calculated. With the patient under local anesthesia and the bladder used as a landmark, a 15-gauge Touhy needle is guided into the fetal abdominal cavity with real-time ultrasound (Fig. 24-10). A small air bubble is introduced

as the fetus is mature. If the ΔOD450 level is in zone II and level or rising, it may be appropriate to deliver the baby before maturity. If so, 12 mg of betamethasone is given 48 and 24 hours before delivery. However, in many instances, the ΔOD450 value will be in zone I, and delivery should be undertaken between 38 and 40 weeks' gestation, as soon as the cervix is favorable for induction.

One of the most common errors in the management of the Rh-sensitized patient is underestimation of the severity of the condition. When a fetus has attained pulmonary maturity, there is little reason not to deliver, since the condition will continue to worsen *in utero.* Even when the ΔOD450 is very low, indicating that the infant may be Rh negative, the patient should be delivered by 40 weeks' gestation in an institution with the personnel and facilities to treat the baby with unexpected hyperbilirubinemia with exchange transfusions.

FIG. 24-10. Real-time ultrasound image shows transfusion needle (*arrow*) advancing into fetal abdomen. (Larkin RM, Knochel JQ, Lee TG: Intrauterine transfusions: New techniques and results. Clin Obstet Gynecol 25:303, 1982)

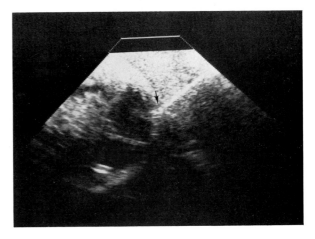

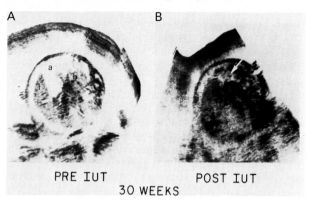

PRE IUT   POST IUT
30 WEEKS

FIG. 24-11. (*A*) Sagittal scan of fetus shows marked ascites (*a*). Fetal liver (*l*) and fetal bowel (*b*) are also seen. (*B*) Sagittal scan following removal of ascitic fluid and performance of intrauterine transfusion shows blood (*arrow*) in fetal peritoneal cavity. *IUT,* intrauterine transfusion.

to verify the intra-abdominal placement of the needle. Type O-negative, leukocyte-poor, high-hematocrit, packed red cells that have been maternally cross-matched and deglycerized are then infused at a rate of 5 ml to 10 ml per minute through the needle or a polyethylene catheter. The formula for the amount of blood transfused is as follows:

$$(\text{number of weeks' gestation} - 20) \times 10 \text{ ml}$$

If fetal ascites is present, some of the fluid should be removed prior to the transfusion in order to avoid excessive intra-abdominal pressure (Fig. 24-11). Depending on fetal position, the infused blood is almost always visualized in the peritoneal cavity of the fetus by real-time ultrasound. During the transfusion, it is important to monitor the fetal heart rate. This can be done either with real-time ultrasound or the hand-held Doppler. An increase in fetal heart rate usually is associated with a good outcome, whereas bradycardia is ominous.

Fetal heart tones are again monitored carefully after completion of the procedure. If the fetus is less than 26 weeks' gestation, the heart tones are checked every 4 hours and the mother is discharged in 12 to 24 hours. If the fetus is more than 26 weeks' gestation, the patient is transferred to the labor and delivery suite where continuous electronic fetal monitoring is performed. If signs of fetal distress such as persistent bradycardia occur, delivery is accomplished.

Once the infant has been transfused, frequent ultrasound examinations are extremely useful for timing the next intrauterine transfusion. Specifically, ultrasound evidence of increasing or decreasing fetal peritoneal fluid accumulation can be used to determine whether transfusion intervals should be decreased or increased.[31,32] If transfusion is unsuccessful or if severe fetal hydrops does not improve with transfusion, delivery is considered as early as the 30th gestational week. When it is determined that a preterm fetus with immature lungs must be delivered, the mother is given a course of corticosteroids to decrease the incidence of respiratory distress syndrome (RDS). Because the cervix is usually unfavorable for vaginal delivery at this stage of pregnancy, cesarean section is often necessary. Studies of long-term follow-up indicate that children who have required intrauterine transfusions for severe erythroblastosis fetalis do very well (Table 24-2).

EXPERIMENTAL METHODS OF TREATMENT. Aggressive and early use of new diagnostic techniques and

Table 24-2
Long-Term Follow-Up Studies of Infants Who Received Intrauterine Transfusions

Author	No. of Infants	Type of Handicap	Normal (%)	Minor Handicap (%)	Major Handicap (%)
Ellis[33]	48	Neurologic	84	7	9
		Physical	88	12	0
Bock[34]	17	Neurologic	94	6	0
		Physical	59	35	6
White[35]	15	Neurologic	100	0	0
		Physical	57	53	0
Hardyment[36]	21	Neurologic	61	29	10
		Physical	86	14	0
Knobbe[37]	15	Psychological	100	0	0
Bowman[38]	89	Neurologic	83	12	4

(After Kochenour NK, Scott JR: Rh isoimmunization in pregnancy. In Scott JR, Rote NS (eds): Immunology in Obstetrics and Gynecology, p 160. Norwalk, CT, Appleton–Century–Crofts, 1984)

advances in fetal therapy, proper timing of delivery, and modern changes in neonatal care have all contributed to the improved perinatal outcome for severely Rh-immunized patients. Therefore, it is doubtful that some of the measures advocated in the past are justified today except in the otherwise hopeless situation in which fetal hydrops is already present before an intrauterine transfusion can be performed at about 22 weeks' gestation. Second-trimester intrauterine transfusion under direct vision with fetoscopy and ultrasound-fetoscopy–directed transfusions into the umbilical vein show promise in these cases.[39,40] There is little convincing evidence that plasmapheresis, treatment with immunosuppressive agents such as promethazine, corticosteroids, or azathioprine, or oral desensitization regimens significantly improve the outcome in severely Rh-sensitized patients, and each poses some risk to the mother and infant.[41]

NEONATAL CARE. One of the most important facets of the overall management of the Rh-affected baby is the close cooperation necessary among the obstetric and pediatric teams and the blood bank. The successful management of markedly premature erythroblastotic infants requires all the resources of a tertiary intensive care nursery including respiratory assistance, correction of acidosis, and exchange transfusion.

Table 24-3
Hemolytic Disease Resulting from Irregular Antibodies

Blood Group System	Antigen	Severity of Hemolytic Disease	Proposed Management	Blood Group System	Antigen	Severity of Hemolytic Disease	Proposed Management
Rh subtype	C	+ to +++	AF ΔOD450	Lutheran	Lua	+	Expectant
	Cw	+ to +++	AF ΔOD450		Lub	+	Expectant
	c	+ to +++	AF ΔOD450	Diego	Dia	+ to +++	AF ΔOD450
	E	+ to +++	AF ΔOD450		Dib	+ to +++	AF ΔOD450
	e	+ to +++	AF ΔOD450	P	P	−	None
Lewis	Lea	−	None		PP1Pk (Tja)	+ to +++	AF ΔOD450
	Leb	−	None	Xg	Xga	+	Expectant
I	I	−	None	Public antigens	Yta	+ to +++	AF ΔOD450
Kell	K	+ to +++	AF ΔOD450		Ytb	+	Expectant
	k	+	Expectant		Lap	+	Expectant
	Ko	+	Expectant		Ena	+ to ++	AF ΔOD450
	Kpa	+	Expectant		Ge	+	Expectant
	Kpb	+	Expectant		Jra	+	Expectant
	Jsa	+	Expectant		Coa	+ to +++	AF ΔOD450
	Jsb	+	Expectant		Coab	+	Expectant
Duffy	Fya	+ to +++	AF ΔOD450	Private antigens	Batty	+	Expectant
	Fyb	−	None		Becker	+	Expectant
	Fy3	+	Expectant		Berrens	+	Expectant
Kidd	Jka	+ to +++	AF ΔOD450		Biles	+ to ++	AF ΔOD450
	Jkb	+ to +++	AF ΔOD450		Evans	+	Expectant
	Jk3	+	Expectant		Gonzales	+	Expectant
MNSs	M	+ to +++	AF ΔOD450		Good	+ to +++	AF ΔOD450
	N	−	None		Heibel	+ to ++	AF ΔOD450
	S	+ to +++	AF ΔOD450		Hunt	+	Expectant
	s	+ to +++	AF ΔOD450		Jobbins	+	Expectant
	U	+ to +++	AF ΔOD450		Radin	+ to ++	AF ΔOD450
	Mia	++	AF ΔOD450		Rm	+	Expectant
	Mta	++	AF ΔOD450		Ven	+	Expectant
	Vw	+	Expectant		Wrighta	+ to +++	AF ΔOD450
	Mur	+	Expectant		Wrightb	+	Expectant
	Hil	+	Expectant		Zd	+ to ++	AF ΔOD450
	Hut	+	Expectant				

−, not a proven cause of hemolytic disease of the newborn; +, mild; ++, moderate; +++, severe; expectant, no further diagnostic testing or intervention is necessary until delivery; AF ΔOD450, amniocentesis with amniotic bilirubin studies may be necessary.

(After Weinstein L: Irregular antibodies causing hemolytic disease of the newborn: A continuing problem. Clin Obstet Gynecol 25:321, 1982)

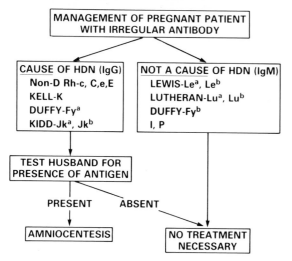

FIG. 24-12. Flow sheet for the management of a pregnant patient with irregular antibodies. It is important to determine that the husband is the father of the baby before deciding against amniocentesis.

ATYPICAL ANTIBODIES

Coinciding with the decrease in hemolytic disease of the newborn secondary to antibodies to the D antigen has been a relative increase in antibodies directed against minor or unusual antigens on the red cell. Many can produce severe hemolytic disease of the newborn, and the pathogenesis is similar to Rh immunization. The differences in the frequencies of irregular antibodies and resultant hemolytic disease of the newborn depend on the following variables: (1) size and frequency of the antigenic stimulus, (2) relative potency of the antigen, (3) capacity of the patient to respond to the antigenic stimulus, (4) alteration of the antigen when it combines with Rh-positive cells, (5) the type of antibody response (IgG or IgM), and (6) the development of fetal red cell antigens. In order to cause erythroblastosis, the antigen must be present on the fetal red cell and absent in the mother. The most frequent clinically important irregular antibodies are anti-c, anti-E, anti-K, and anti-Fy[a]; a complete list is presented on Table 24-3. It is important to remember that both Rh-positive and Rh-

Table 24-4
Comparison of Rh and ABO Incompatibility

	Rh	**ABO**
Blood Group Set-Up		
Mother	Negative	O
Infant	Positive	A or B
Type of Antibody	IgG	IgM and IgG
Clinical Aspects		
Occurrence in firstborn	1%–2%	40%–50%
Stillbirth or hydrops	Frequent	None
Severe anemia	Frequent	Rare
Degree of jaundice	+++	+
Hepatosplenomegaly	+++	+
Laboratory Findings		
Direct Coombs' test (infant)	+	+ or −
Maternal antibodies	Always present	Not clear-cut
Treatment		
Need for antenatal measures	Yes	No
Exchange transfusion		
Frequency	Approximately 2/3	Approximately 1/100
Donor blood type	Group-specific when possible	Rh same as infant; group O only
Incidence of late anemia	Common	Rare

(After Oski FA, Naiman JL: Hematologic problems in the newborn. In Oski FA, Naiman JL: Major Problems in Clinical Pediatrics, vol 6, 2nd ed, p 232. Philadelphia, WB Saunders, 1972)

negative mothers can produce these antibodies. Therefore, all pregnant women (or all who have received blood products previously or who are multiparous) should have an antibody screen as part of their initial prenatal blood work. If the antibody screen is positive, it should be serially titrated, and the patient is managed as shown in Figure 24-12.

ABO Hemolytic Disease

A comparison of Rh and ABO incompatibility is important, since these are the two most frequent causes of immune hemolytic disease in the neonatal period (Table 24-4). In approximately 20% to 25% of all pregnancies there is ABO incompatibility between mother and infant, but a clinically recognizable hemolytic process in the baby occurs in only 10%. ABO hemolytic disease affects the firstborn child in approximately 50% of cases, and it is not uncommon for multiple siblings to be affected with comparable severity.

The pathophysiology involves the transplacental passage of maternal antibody and its interaction with fetal or neonatal red cell antigens, yielding erythrocyte destruction, variable anemia, and hyperbilirubinemia. Clinically, ABO hemolytic problems are confined almost exclusively to the A (specifically A1 rather than A2) or B infants of group O mothers. Anti-A and anti-B "natural" antibodies produced early in life by group A or B persons are predominantly IgM. In contrast, group O persons produce anti-A or anti-B that is predominantly IgG and capable of crossing the placenta. However, for reasons not completely understood, it is extremely rare that these antibodies cause harm during pregnancy. There is no relationship between the antibody titer and the severity of hemolytic disease. The discordance between the high frequency of ABO-incompatible pregnancies and the low frequency of hemolytic disease, as well as the broad spectrum of the severity, has been attributed to such factors as (1) immature, weak, nonspecific or altered antigens on the fetal red cell, (2) absorption of the antibodies by ABO antigens present in all body tissues, and (3) presence of soluble blood group substances in fetal plasma and tissue fluids that can neutralize maternal antibody (secretor status).[42] There is no single test that will forewarn the physician of impending ABO hemolytic disease. However, since this does not occur until after birth, there is no justification for performing amniocentesis or preterm induction of labor. The most common manifestations of ABO incompatibility in the neonate are early-onset (24 hours) jaundice and a variable elevation of the indirect bilirubin fraction. In contrast to Rh disease, kernicterus and anemia are rare. The cornerstones of management of ABO incompatibility are bilirubin surveillance, phototherapy (required in approximately 10% of infants), and occasionally exchange transfusion.

REFERENCES

1. Rote NS: Pathophysiology of Rh isoimmunization. Clin Obstet Gynecol 25:243, 1982
2. Cohen F, Gustafson C, Evans MM: Mechanisms of isoimmunization: The transplacental passage of foetal erythrocytes in homospecific pregnancies. Blood 23:621, 1964
3. Kleihauer E, Braun H, Betke K: Demonstration von fetalem hamoglobin in den erythrocyten eines blutausstrichs. Klin Wochenschr 35:637, 1957
4. Pollack W, Ascari WQ, Crispen JF et al: Studies on Rh prophylaxis after transfusion with Rh positive blood. Transfusion 11:340, 1971
5. Pollack W, Gorman JG, Freda VJ: Rh immune suppression: Past, present and future. In Frigoletto FD, Jewett JF, Konugres AA (eds): Rh Hemolytic Disease: New Strategy for Eradication, p 37. Boston, GK Hall, 1982
6. Katz J, Marcus RG: Incidence of Rh immunization following abortion: Possible detection of lymphocyte priming to Rh antigen. Am J Obstet Gynecol 117:261, 1973
7. Freda VJ, Gorman JG, Galen RS et al: The threat of Rh immunization from abortion. Lancet 2:147, 1969
8. Leong M, Duby S, Kinch RAH: Fetal-maternal transfusions following early abortion. Obstet Gynecol 54:425, 1979
9. Louis K, Nager B: Small dose anti-Rh therapy after first trimester abortion. Int J Gynaecol Obstet 15:235, 1977
10. McCormick JN, Faulk WP, Fox H et al: Immunohistological and elution studies of the human placenta. J Exp Med 133: 1, 1971
11. Goto S, Nishi H, Tomodo Y: Blood group Rh-D factor in human trophoblast determined by immunofluorescent method. Am J Obstet Gynecol 137:707, 1980
12. Price JR: Rh sensitization by hydatidiform mole. N Engl J Med 278:1021, 1968
13. Dubin CF, Staisch KJ: Amniocentesis and fetal-maternal blood transfusion: A review of the literature. Obstet Gynecol Surv 37:272, 1982
14. Mollison PL: Can primary Rh immunization be augmented by passively administered antibody? In Frigoletto FD, Jewett JF, Konugres AA (eds): Rh Hemolytic Disease: New Strategy for Eradication, p 161. Boston, GK Hall, 1982
15. Harrison R, Campbell S, Craft I: Risks of fetomaternal hemorrhage resulting from amniocentesis with and without ultrasound placental localization. Obstet Gynecol 46: 389, 1975
16. Scott JR: Antenatal prophylaxis: Experience at Utah. In Frigoletto FD, Jewett JF, Konugres AA (eds): Rh Hemolytic Disease: New Strategy for Eradication, p 191. Boston, GK Hall, 1982
17. Scott JR, Beer AE, Guy LR: Pathogenesis of Rh immunization in primigravidas: Fetomaternal versus maternafetal bleeding. Obstet Gynecol 49:9, 1977
18. Zipursky A, Israels LG: The pathogenesis and prevention of Rh immunization. Can Med Assoc J 97:1245, 1967
19. Bowman JM: Suppression of Rh isoimmunization. Obstet Gynecol 52:385, 1978
20. Lim OW, Fleisher AA, Zeil HK: Reduction of Rho(D) sensitization: A cost-effective analysis. Obstet Gynecol 59:477, 1982
21. Kochenour NK, Beeson JH: The use of Rh-immune globulin. Clin Obstet Gynecol 25:283, 1982
22. Adams MM, Marks JS, Kaplan JP: Cost implications of routine antenatal administration of Rh immune globulin. Am J Obstet Gynecol 149:633, 1984

23. Hensleigh PA: Reduction of Rh(D) sensitization: A cost-effective analysis. Obstet Gynecol 61:537, 1983

24. Torrance GW, Zipursky A: Cost-effectiveness of antepartum prevention of Rh immunization. Clin Perinatol 11:267, 1984

25. Bowman JM: Efficacy of antenatal prophylaxis. In Frigoletto FD, Jewett JF, Konugres AA (eds): Rh Hemolytic Disease: New Strategy for Eradication, p 143. Boston, GK Hall, 1982

26. Lloyd LK, Miya F, Hebertson RM et al: Intrapartum feto-maternal bleeding in Rh negative women. Obstet Gynecol 56:285, 1980

27. Liley AW: Liquor amnii analysis in management of pregnancy complicated by rhesus sensitization. Am J Obstet Gynecol 82:1359, 1961

28. Rochard F, Schifrin B, Goupil F et al: Non-stressed fetal heart rate monitoring in the antepartum period. Am J Obstet Gynecol 126:699, 1976

29. Sadovsky E, Laufer N, Beyth Y: The role of fetal movements assessment in cases of severe Rh immunized patients. Acta Obstet Gynaecol Scand 58:313, 1979

30. Elliot JP, Monanlou HD, O'Keefe DF et al: Significance of fetal and neonatal sinusoidal heart rate pattern: Further clinical observations in Rh incompatibility. Am J Obstet Gynecol 138:227, 1980

31. Scott JR, Kochenour NK, Larkin RM et al: Changes in the management of severely Rh immunized patients. Am J Obstet Gynecol 149:336, 1984

32. Bowman JM, Manning FA: Intrauterine transfusions: Winnipeg 1982. Obstet Gynecol 61:203, 1983

33. Ellis MI: Follow-up study of survivors after intrauterine transfusion. Dev Med Child Neurol 22:48, 1980

34. Bock JE, Winkel S: A follow-up study on infants who received intra-uterine transfusions because of severe rhesus hemolytic disease. Acta Obstet Gynecol Scand Suppl 53:37, 1976

35. White CA, Goplerud CP, Kisker CT et al: Intrauterine transfusion, 1965–1976, with an assessment of the surviving children. Am J Obstet Gynecol 130:933, 1978

36. Hardyment AF, Salvador HS, Towell ME et al: Follow-up of intrauterine transfused surviving children. Am J Obstet Gynecol 133:235, 1979

37. Knobbe T, Meier P, Wenar C et al: Psychological development of children who received intrauterine transfusions. Am J Obstet Gynecol 133:877, 1979

38. Bowman JM: The management of Rh-isoimmunization. Obstet Gynecol 52:1, 1978

39. Rodeck CH, Holman CA, Karnicki J et al: Direct intravascular fetal blood transfusion by fetoscopy in severe rhesus isoimmunization. Lancet 1:625, 1981

40. Bang J, Bock JE, Trolle D: Ultrasound-guided fetal intravenous transfusion for severe rhesus haemolytic disease. Br Med J 284:373, 1982

41. Caudle MR, Scott JR: The potential role of immunosuppression, plasmapheresis, and desensitization as treatment modalities for Rh immunization. Clin Obstet Gynecol 25:313, 1982

42. Cook LN: ABO hemolytic disease. Clin Obstet Gynecol 25:333, 1982

Bleeding in Late Pregnancy

Clifford P. Goplerud

25

Third-trimester bleeding occurs in 2% to 3% of patients. It may be due to a trivial cause (cervical polyp or "bloody show") or to a far more serious condition of the uterus (invasive carcinoma of the cervix or rupture of the uterus). The most common source of significant bleeding in late pregnancy is the placental site, as in placenta previa and premature separation of the normally implanted placenta. These two complications are potentially fatal to mother, fetus, or both. Hence, it is an obstetric maxim that all patients with third-trimester bleeding be admitted to the hospital immediately and that no rectal or vaginal examination be done until preparations to deal with any abnormality that may be found or any hemorrhage that the examination may provoke have been made.

PLACENTA PREVIA

The term *placenta previa* is used to describe the condition in which the placenta is implanted in the lower pole of the uterus; usually, a portion of the placenta precedes the presenting part of the fetus. Since the relation of the placenta to the internal os of the cervix is important in the management and outcome of pregnancy, certain descriptive terms are necessary. The commonly used terminology is illustrated in Figure 25-1. In total placenta previa the entire internal cervical os is covered by placenta (Figs. 25-2 and 25-3). In partial placenta previa, only a portion of the os is covered; this is expressed as the percentage of the os covered at the time the definitive diagnosis is made. If the placenta is implanted near the internal os but does not extend beyond its edge, it is referred to as a low-lying placenta or a low implantation.

Incidence

Placenta previa occurs in approximately 1 in 200 deliveries and is more common among women who have had more than one prior delivery. At the University of Iowa Hospitals, the incidence among 90,000 deliveries was 0.49%. The total incidence is decreasing, apparently as the result of the decline in the number of women of high parity and an increase in the number of primigravidas (Table 25-1). This alteration of patient population results from several factors. Among the most important are better and more readily available means of contraception and more liberal attitudes toward surgical sterilization.

Etiology

The specific cause of placenta previa is unknown. A number of factors may affect the place of implantation in any pregnancy. Early or late fertilization, variability in the implantation potential of the blastocyst, and the receptivity and adequacy of the endometrium, which vary from cycle to cycle, may all play a role. However, it is probable that more than chance controls the site of nidation. Multiple pregnancy may predispose to placenta previa because of the increased surface area of placenta or placentas. In patients who have scar from a uterine incision after such operations as cesarean section, hysterotomy, myomectomy, or metroplasty, it is quite common to find that subsequent placental sites include the area of the scar. There is an increased incidence of placenta previa in patients previously delivered by low cervical cesarean section, regardless of whether the uterine incision was vertical or transverse. This may result from alteration in blood supply to the area, from change in

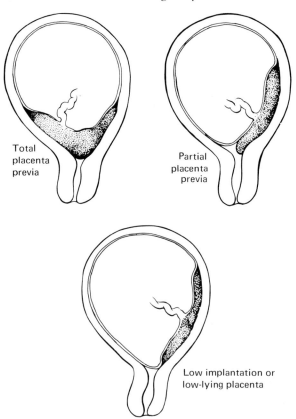

Total
placenta
previa

Partial
placenta
previa

Low implantation or
low-lying placenta

FIG. 25-1.   Variations of placenta previa.

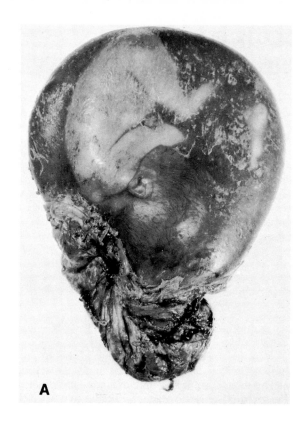

A

the quality and depth of the endometrium, or from change in the shape and contour of the uterine cavity. The change in size and contour of the uterine cavity after any pregnancy may account for the fact that placenta previa is more common in multiparas. Not only does the incidence increase with parity, but the higher the pregnancy order, the more marked the rate of increase. The vessels at the previous placental sites undergo changes that may decrease the blood supply to those regions of the endometrium. In subsequent pregnancies, therefore, more surface area may be required for placental attachment to provide adequate maternal blood flow to the intervillous space, which would in-

→

FIG. 25-2.   Total placenta previa. (*A*) Intact conceptus. Previable fetus can be seen in its amniotic sac; placenta covers entire lower uterine segment. (*B*) Amniotic sac opened to show relation of fetal head to placenta. Patient (gravida 4, para 3) was admitted to delivery room in shock due to heavy vaginal bleeding and promptly expelled 6-month conceptus intact. This is unusual outcome for patients with placenta previa; without definitive treatment, exsanguination usually occurs before cervix is sufficiently dilated to permit delivery and consequent closing of uterine sinusoids by retraction of myometrium.

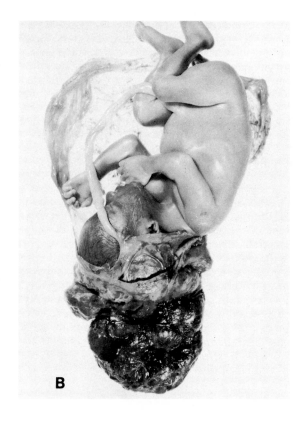

B

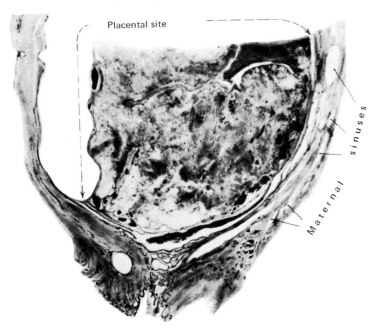

FIG. 25-3. Section through lower uterine segment and cervix in case of total placenta previa. Note pathologic lower uterine segment. Extensive vascularization and increased thickness of uterine wall are results of this abnormal placental location.

crease the possibility of encroachment on the internal cervical os. The placenta from a patient with placenta previa is thinner and the maternal surface area is greater than in the normally implanted placenta.

Clinical Course

Painless bleeding is the hallmark of placenta previa. It is usually limited to the third trimester, but it can occur as early as 20 weeks.

During late pregnancy, the lower pole of the uterus becomes somewhat thinner, and the softening cervix begins to efface and dilate; if the placenta is implanted in the lower pole, the size and margins of the implantation site are altered by these uterine changes. Some separation at the placental margin results, and maternal bleeding occurs from the intervillous space. To a greater or lesser degree, this occurs in all types of placenta previa. The earlier in pregnancy the lower segment begins to form, and the lower the placenta, the earlier the first episode of bleeding. Unless the initial bleeding episode coincides with the onset of labor, the patient ex-

periences no pain and the uterus remains soft. Blood loss associated with the first bleeding ranges from slight to heavy. Unless major uterine sinuses have been opened, the initial bleeding tends to stop as clots form, but may recur with renewed violence as further adjustments occur.

The bleeding may occur while the patient is resting in bed or during any type of activity. The blood is bright, like the fresh bleeding from an incision or laceration, rather than dark, like menstrual blood or that usually associated with premature separation of the normally implanted placenta.

About one fourth of patients experience the first bleeding episode before the end of the 30th week of gestation. In slightly more than half, the initial bleeding occurs between the 34th and 40th weeks. The baby is not affected unless placental exchange is compromised by major placental detachment or maternal hypovolemia due to blood loss. Preterm delivery is the greatest threat to the infant, and the stage of pregnancy during which the first bleeding occurs may be the most important factor in fetal salvage. Rarely, asymptomatic placenta previa is found at the time of repeat cesarean section, or the

Table 25-1
Occurrence of Placenta Previa at University of Iowa Hospitals, 1926 to 1963 and 1964 to 1982

	Number of Deliveries	Number of Cases of Placenta Previa	Frequency of Placenta Previa	Incidence (%)
1926 to 1963	42,896	224	1:192	0.52
1964 to 1982	47,146	220	1:214	0.46

patient may bleed for the first time after labor is well established.

Painless bleeding in the third trimester of pregnancy, regardless of whether it is heavy or minimal, must be considered to be due to placenta previa until this complication is ruled out.

Diagnosis

History

Painless vaginal bleeding is the classic and cardinal sign of placenta previa. Its occurrence in the second half of pregnancy should instantly suggest the possibility of this complication.

Indirect Methods of Diagnosis

The indirect methods of diagnosis are applicable only if the initial hemorrhage has stopped and if there is a clear advantage in deferring delivery until the baby is more mature. Since less than half the patients who experience painless vaginal bleeding have placenta previa, it may be of major importance either to confirm or to rule out placenta previa so that prolonged observation in the hospital will not be needed.

The most commonly used method of placental localization is ultrasound, a procedure whose accuracy is confirmed by many reports in the literature. It must be emphasized that this procedure is not indicated in cases in which hemorrhage is extreme and immediate delivery by cesarean section is indicated. If the bleeding has stopped or diminished and the mother's cardiovascular status is stable, ultrasound is indicated. If placenta previa is ruled out, bleeding is considered to be due to minor separation of the normally implanted placenta or to a local genital lesion. If placenta previa is diagnosed, a plan of management can be formulated. However, if this complication cannot be confirmed or excluded, the patient must be treated as though the diagnosis had been confirmed.

Definitive Diagnosis

The definitive antepartum diagnosis of placenta previa is made by palpation of the placenta on vaginal examination. Regardless of the amount of prior bleeding, this examination can provoke violent hemorrhage, sufficient enough to endanger the mother's life. Hence, it is to be performed only if preparations for immediate cesarean section, should it prove necessary, have been made and if expectant management is not appropriate. The need for this type of examination diminishes with the increased experience of the sonographer.

Management

General Evaluation of the Patient

On admission to the hospital, the patient should be placed at bed rest in an area of high-intensity care, such as the labor–delivery suite. Unless the bleeding has stopped or is minimal, an intravenous catheter should be inserted; blood drawn for typing, crossmatching, and hemogram; and fluids started. The systemic manifestations of hemorrhage depend on the amount of blood lost. The bleeding episodes usually occur during the phase of pregnancy when the circulating blood volume is increased by 20% to 40%; thus, the medical staff may be lulled into a false sense of security if there are no major changes in pulse and blood pressure. Evidence of hypovolemia suggests that the hemorrhage has been severe unless there is some unrelated factor (*e.g.,* preeclampsia, previous hemorrhage, recent use of diuretics) that has caused a decrease in blood volume.

The exact details of the episode, the history of previous bleeding, and the past obstetric and medical history should be obtained. How detailed this history must be depends on the patient's clinical and hemodynamic status. Physical examination should be complete except for vaginal and rectal examinations, which are omitted at this time. Any or all of the manifestations of hypovolemic shock may be present. Observation of the lower extremities and perineum usually reveals blood. On examination of the abdomen, the uterus is usually found to be soft, normal in tone, and not tender. With a longitudinal presentation, the fundus is usually higher than expected, since the presenting part is held high by the placenta. Breech, oblique, and transverse lies are common. Antepartum fetal death is unusual, and the fetal heart tones are usually found easily. As a rule, fetal distress or fetal death occurs only if a significant portion of the placenta is detached from the uterus or if the mother suffers hemorrhagic shock.

Concepts of Therapy

The philosophy of treatment of placenta previa has changed. Before blood was readily available and before potent antibacterial drugs were developed, immediate treatment was usually necessary to prevent the mother's death. This treatment was designed to tamponade the placenta, control bleeding, and induce delivery, usually vaginally. The result was a maternal mortality that in some series of cases was more than 10% and a fetal mortality that exceeded 50%. In the 1940s, it became evident that many of the maternal deaths could be prevented by immediate cesarean section, and this means of therapy was quickly accepted. The results for the baby were less salutary, however; many of these preterm infants died.

Expectant Treatment

In 1945 Johnson and Macafee, in separate papers, introduced the current expectant treatment of selected cases of placenta previa (notably, those in which the baby is preterm and in which immediate delivery is not mandatory to stop hemorrhage). In large series of cases, they demonstrated that the first vaginal hemorrhage from placenta previa is rarely, if ever, fatal as long as vaginal or rectal examinations are not performed. The purpose of expectant treatment is to extend the period of gestation and, hence, to increase the probability of fetal survival. It is of no value in the presence of persistent or recurrent heavy bleeding, and it is not appropriate if the pregnancy is near term. Two recent reports, one by Cotton and colleagues and one by Silver and colleagues, suggest that selected patients with placenta previa and premature contractions may be treated with tocolytic agents, but they stress the importance of maternal hemodynamic stability before these drugs are used. Blood replacement should be utilized to keep the maternal hemoglobin at 10 g/dl to 11 g/dl or the hematocrit at 30% or higher.

Expectant treatment involves a period of observation in the hospital until persistent or recurring hemorrhage or the onset of labor, which is nearly always accompanied by bleeding, demands intervention. If bleeding is not sufficient to terminate expectant treatment, amniocentesis studies to determine fetal pulmonary maturity should be done at about 37 weeks. If the fetal lungs are mature, delivery should be undertaken with or without double setup examination, depending on the sonographic findings and the accrued local data confirming their accuracy. To wait longer is to invite another episode of hemorrhage that could unnecessarily endanger the mother and the fetus.

Definitive Treatment

Before the advent of blood replacement, modern anesthesia, and antibiotics, the metreurynter (intrauterine bag), traction on a fetal foot after internal podalic version, or traction on the fetal scalp or buttocks with Willett forceps was used in efforts to tamponade the placenta. With the rarest exceptions, these practices have no place in the modern management of placenta previa. Current treatment is limited almost entirely to amniotomy for the lesser degrees of placenta previa, and cesarean section for the remainder. The decision about which of these is applicable may be made by the sonographic findings if the evidence of total placenta previa is unquestionable. Otherwise the decision is made by the digital findings at double setup examination. The following requirements for double setup examination should be observed stringently:

1. The examination should be conducted in an operating room or a delivery room in which major surgery can be performed.
2. The nursery and pediatric staff should be notified to expect a high-risk infant.
3. Personnel must include a scrub nurse, a circulating nurse, the physician who will perform the examination and treatment, at least one physician assistant, an anesthetist or anesthesiologist, and someone to provide immediate care for the baby.
4. Instruments must be ready for either vaginal or abdominal delivery, since vaginal examination may precipitate instant and massive bleeding.
5. A vein must be kept open with a large-bore catheter,

and fluids should be running. If not already being administered, whole blood must be available in the room.

When all of these conditions have been met and the patient has been prepared for either vaginal or abdominal delivery, the aseptic vaginal examination is begun by visualization of the cervix. At this point, one finger should be carefully passed into the cervical canal. If placental tissue covers the os, there is a gritty feel to the tissue palpated. When only a portion of the internal os is covered, the placental edge can be felt. The examination should be stopped immediately in either case, because even a gentle examination may precipitate severe hemorrhage. If no placental tissue is palpated over the os or at its margins, the membranes should be stripped away from the uterine wall and the finger inserted along the surface of the lower uterine segment. This area should be palpated as far as the examining finger can reach. Low-lying placenta is diagnosed if placental tissue is palpated during this maneuver. Because this examination may cause heavy bleeding, it must not be undertaken unless immediate diagnosis is essential or prompt delivery is planned.

The following considerations are important in the use of a double setup examination in patients with a history of recent bleeding unless placenta previa has been ruled out definitely by ultrasound:

1. Any patient pregnant 37 weeks or more, as determined by accurate data from early in pregnancy (dates, first examination, quickening, auscultation of fetal heart, or early ultrasound) or amniotic fluid data, should have a double setup examination as soon as the maturity of the baby can be ascertained definitely. If placenta previa is found, treatment should be instituted at that time.
2. Any patient who has persistent or heavy bleeding or is in labor, regardless of the duration of pregnancy, should have an immediate double setup examination. If placenta previa is found, appropriate treatment should be carried out at that time.
3. Any patient who has a preterm fetus, is not bleeding heavily, and is not in labor should be carefully observed at bed rest for 48 hours. No vaginal or rectal examination should be performed during that time. When the bleeding has stopped, a careful speculum examination should be performed to rule out traumatic, infectious, or neoplastic lesions of the vagina and cervix. If none are found, the patient may be allowed out of bed gradually unless there is a recurrence of bleeding. If placenta previa cannot be ruled out by the indirect methods, the patient should remain under close observation until the fetus has matured. At that time an elective double setup examination is indicated. Therapy appropriate for the diagnosis made at this examination should be instituted. If labor begins or if persistent or heavy bleeding recurs prior to the attainment of adequate fetal maturity, conservative or expectant management

must be abandoned and double setup examination and appropriate therapy instituted.

AMNIOTOMY. If at the time of double setup examination the cervix is found to be dilated 3 cm or more and the placenta covers not more than 10% of the internal os, rupture of the membranes permits the presenting part to advance against the placenta and hence to tamponade it against the bleeding maternal sinuses. If this does not control the bleeding and labor does not ensue and progress, cesarean section is indicated unless the baby is dead, in which case the presenting part may be grasped with Willett forceps and pressure maintained against the placenta by a weight attached to the handle; if the bleeding is controlled, progression of labor and vaginal delivery may be awaited.

CESAREAN SECTION. When the placenta completely covers the internal os, the bleeding is usually violent and rarely stops until the infant is delivered. Hence, the treatment of total placenta previa is abdominal delivery in all cases, regardless of the stage of gestation or the condition of the baby. The same is true of partial but major degrees of placenta previa.

Cesarean section without prior double setup examination is a proper procedure for the classic case in which there is bleeding of shock-producing proportions, a soft uterus, and a viable baby in good condition. With such signs, the likelihood that bleeding is due to something other than placenta previa is minuscule; vaginal examination to confirm what is already a virtual certainty only increases the bleeding, regardless of its source, and delays delivery. If placenta previa is not confirmed at cesarean section, scrupulous examination must be made for cervical or vaginal lesions that could produce this kind of bleeding. (Invasive carcinoma of the cervix is sometimes mentioned as such a lesion, but most obstetricians never encounter major hemorrhage from this source in pregnancy.)

If there are other indications for cesarean section, such as a scarred uterus or abnormal presentation, the double setup examination is unnecessary. Similarly, if both the history of bleeding and unquestionable sonographic evidence confirm the presence of total placenta previa, the double setup examination may be omitted.

Opinions differ regarding the type of cesarean section that should be performed in patients with placenta previa (*i.e.,* classic or lower segment with vertical or transverse incision). The location of the placenta and the fetal presentation should be revealed by the sonogram. With this knowledge a logical choice can be made. If the placenta, although completely covering the cervical os, extends upward along the posterior uterine wall, either a transverse or vertical incision in the lower segment will avoid the placental tissue and permit easy delivery with a polar lie. However, if the placenta extends upward along the anterior wall for any distance or if there is a transverse lie, a vertical incision is the best choice. If the placenta is encountered, a path around to the edge should be found, the membranes ruptured,

and the baby delivered with dispatch. It is possible to incise the placenta and deliver the baby promptly, but this may involve additional fetal blood loss. In either case, the cord should be clamped quickly and the pediatrician should be advised to check the infant's hemoglobin level or hematocrit.

Complications

Maternal disease and death may result from the placenta previa itself, from the treatment, or from a combination of both. Antepartum hemorrhage may be fatal or nearly so, and prolonged hypotension short of death may produce cerebral or renal damage. In most instances the latter can be reversed with proper therapy. Sheehan's syndrome may occur, but it is far more likely to be associated with abruptio placentae. Clotting defects have been reported with placenta previa, but they are far less common than with abruption. Severe postpartum hemorrhage in patients with placenta previa may occur in the presence of a well-contracted or atonic uterus. At the site of implantation, the lower uterine segment, the muscle content is diminished, and the natural mechanism to control bleeding—interlacing muscle bundles contracting around open vessels—may be less effective. In this event, bimanual compression of the uterus and the administration of oxytocic drugs are of little or no value. Uterine packing, a procedure that has been abandoned in most institutions, rarely has a place in the treatment of postpartum hemorrhage from placenta previa. The other means used for control of postpartum hemorrhage are bilateral hypogastric artery ligation and hysterectomy.

The anatomy and physiologic capabilities of the endometrium of the lower uterine segment may contribute to a type of complication that may manifest antepartum but is not usually apparent until after delivery. The thinness of the endometrium, its inability to control the invasive qualities of the trophoblast, or both allow for an increase in the reported incidence of placentae accreta, increta, and percreta, which usually require hysterectomy for control of postpartum hemorrhage.

Complications associated with treatment include sepsis, operative trauma to structures adjacent to the uterus, severe hemorrhage from examination or labor, blood transfusion reactions, serum hepatitis, and problems related to anesthesia. During the treatment of hemorrhage, hypovolemia must be reversed without overtransfusion or overinfusion. Continuous monitoring of central venous or pulmonary wedge pressure by intravenous catheter permits precise control of blood and fluid replacement. The maternal mortality from placenta previa in most institutions is less than 1%.

Perinatal Mortality

Perinatal deaths resulting from placenta previa have decreased progressively because of the combination of better pediatric care, the use of expectant management, and the increasing use of cesarean section for delivery. The major problem is preterm delivery. Most reports indicate a slightly higher than usual incidence of serious congenital anomalies. Perinatal mortality has been reduced from over 40% before 1950 to less than 5% at present.

PREMATURE SEPARATION OF PLACENTA (ABRUPTIO PLACENTAE)

Abruptio placentae is the term used to describe the partial or complete detachment of the placenta from a site of normal implantation in the corpus uteri at any time before delivery of the infant. It commonly occurs in the third trimester, but may occur at any time after 20 weeks' gestation. It occurs in varying degrees in about 1% of pregnancies. The detachment may be complete or partial, or only the placental margin may be involved. The latter is sometimes referred to as *marginal sinus rupture* or *marginal sinus bleeding* (Fig. 25-4), but for practical purposes, it is considered a variant of abruption. Bleeding from the placental site may dissect beneath the

FIG. 25-4. Various degrees of separation of normally implanted placenta.

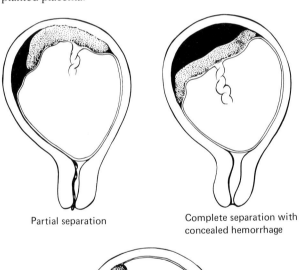

Partial separation

Complete separation with concealed hemorrhage

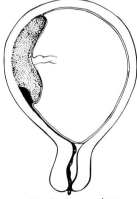

Marginal separation

membranes and find its way to the outside (external, or revealed, bleeding); it may remain trapped (concealed bleeding); or it may do both, the external bleeding representing only a portion of the blood loss from the maternal circulation. As a rule, the clinical signs vary according to the degree of detachment. In the marginal type they are usually trivial, but complete detachment may be quickly fatal if it cannot be dealt with at once; hence the clinical designations of mild, moderate, or severe abruptio placentae.

Cause

The cause of spontaneous premature separation of the placenta is obscure. It occurs far more frequently in multipara than in primigravid patients, and it is more common in patients over the age of 35. Preeclampsia clearly predisposes a patient to this complication, especially when there is underlying renovascular disease.

Trauma is the cause in some cases. A direct blow to the uterus, forceful external version, or placental site bleeding resulting from needle puncture at amniocentesis have produced abruptio placentae, but they are rare causes. The rapid reduction of uterine size after rupture of the membranes in hydramnios has been cited as a possible cause. Several cases of separation have been reported apparently as the result of spinal anesthesia when it is used as terminal anesthesia in the midst of an explosive second stage of labor; the precipitating factor appears to be the added uterine tone in a uterus that is already excessively irritable.

Folic acid deficiency has been suggested as a causal factor, but recent studies have failed to support this hypothesis.

Pathology

In patients who are predisposed to this complication, spontaneous rupture of blood vessels at the placental bed may result from lack of resiliency or other changes in the uterine vasculature. The problem is compounded by hypertension and by the fact that the uterus, being distended, cannot contract sufficiently to close off the torn vessels. Hypovolemia from the loss of a significant amount of blood from the maternal circulation results in shock. The blood may flow beneath the placenta, shearing it off completely or in part, and may eventually separate the membranes from the uterine wall and appear in the vagina. If there is no easy egress for the blood, its force may cause rupture through the fetal membranes into the amniotic sac, or it may extravasate between the muscle fibers of the myometrium, or both. This increases uterine tone and irritability, and uterine relaxation is incomplete. Areas of ecchymosis are common; if the extravasation is severe enough to render the uterus almost entirely blue or purple, or to prevent it from contracting normally after delivery, the condition is referred to as *uteroplacental apoplexy* or *Couvelaire uterus.* In such cases, the uterus is boardlike and tender before delivery.

Large quantities of thromboplastin are released into the maternal circulation as a result of myometrial damage and retroplacental clotting; in severe cases, this produces disseminated intravascular clotting. Much of this clotting is reduced by the circulating fibrinolysin, but the laying down of fibrin both within the blood vessels and especially in the retroplacental clot may be sufficient to deplete fibrinogen more rapidly than it can be restored. The consumption coagulopathy that results may cause increased bleeding from the uterus, as well as from other organs.

Renal disturbance is a predictable consequence of the foregoing chain of events. Renal perfusion may be impaired by vascular spasm resulting from shock or by intravascular clotting. Oliguria and proteinuria may be ominous signs of either acute tubular necrosis, which may be reversible, or acute cortical necrosis, which is irreversible.

Time seems to be an important factor in the development of both clotting defects and renal lesions. The longer the interval before delivery, the more likely and more serious these complications are.

The effects on the fetus depend mainly on the degree to which the uteroplacental interface is disrupted. Marginal separation may have no apparent effect. Intermediate degrees of separation may produce fetal embarrassment, which varies according to the extent to which placental exchange is lost and the degree to which uterine blood flow is impaired by continuous partial contraction of the uterine musculature. In severe cases, with complete or almost complete abruption, total anoxia and fetal death are virtually certain to occur.

Signs and Symptoms

Mild Abruptio Placentae

In marginal and other minor degrees of premature separation of the placenta, there is usually no evident effect on the fetus; the heart tones remain strong and regular, and there is no excessive fetal movement. The maternal vital signs are unchanged because there is only minimal blood loss from the maternal circulation. Scant to moderate dark vaginal bleeding may occur (unless the bleeding is entirely concealed), and the uterus may fail to relax completely between contractions. Vague lower abdominal discomfort and tenderness may be present. Leopold's maneuvers may be unsatisfactory because a firm uterine contraction may result from each effort to outline the fetus. Although these signs rarely demand immediate action, uterine irritability must be given serious consideration because it may herald a grave degree of separation.

In some cases external, usually dark, bleeding is the only sign, and the major diagnostic differentiation is from placenta previa.

Moderate Abruptio Placentae

The separation of more than one fourth but less than two thirds of the placental surface from the uterine wall is considered moderate abruptio placentae. The onset of symptoms may be gradual, beginning with the symptoms of a mild separation, or it may be abrupt, with the sudden appearance of continuous abdominal (uterine) pain that is followed promptly by dark vaginal bleeding. Although external bleeding is usually moderate in amount, the total blood loss from the circulation may be up to 1000 ml by the time the patient is seen. There may be evidence of shock (cold clammy skin, tachycardia, hypotension, oliguria), and the fetus may show evidence of embarrassment. The uterus is clearly tender and, of major diagnostic importance, manifests a sustained firm or partial contraction. Regardless of any prior or accompanying signs, failure of the uterus to relax between contractions inevitably suggests the possibility of premature separation of the placenta.

Because the uterine contraction is sustained, the fetal heart may be difficult to hear with certainty. An ultrasonic fetal pulse detector may be needed to determine the condition of the fetus. Labor, if not already in progress, usually ensues within two hours. Clotting defects and renal sequelae occur in both mild and moderate forms of abruption, but they occur most frequently in the severe form.

Severe Abruptio Placentae

In severe abruptio placentae, more than two thirds of the placenta is separated from the uterus. The onset is usually abrupt, with no or very brief premonitory signs. The clinical picture is classic. Uterine pain is agonizing and is described as tearing, knifelike, and unremitting. The uterus is continuously boardlike and tender. External bleeding is usually moderate, or there may be no external bleeding at all. The fetus is almost invariably stillborn. Shock ensues with astonishing speed, and unless the condition is promptly brought under control, oliguria and consumption coagulopathy should be expected.

Treatment

Mild Abruptio Placentae

When there is slight to moderate external bleeding, the uterus appears to relax well, and there is no fetal distress, abruption must be distinguished from placenta previa. If the gestation period is less than 37 weeks and external bleeding is less than moderate, a sonogram should be performed. If placenta previa definitely can be ruled out, if external bleeding stops, and if no new signs of separation occur after a period of ambulation and observation, the patient may be sent home. However, she must be given complete and unequivocal directions regarding the exact circumstances under which she must return to the hospital. If placenta previa is ruled out but moderate bleeding continues, a speculum and vaginal examination should be performed. If no cervical or vaginal lesion can be found to account for the bleeding and blood loss is minimal, the physician may await the onset of labor or the appearance of new signs to suggest the need for intervention. If the patient is already in labor, the membranes should be ruptured, which usually accelerates labor and minimizes bleeding because of uterine adjustment to smaller contents. An oxytocin infusion may help if labor is desultory or incoordinate.

If the gestation period is more than 37 weeks, a double setup examination should be made after admission of the patient to the hospital. If placenta previa is ruled out, the membranes should be ruptured and an oxytocin infusion started if labor does not begin immediately. Electronic monitoring of the fetus is essential. Continued bleeding, failure of the uterus to relax between contractions, and fetal distress are indications for cesarean section.

Moderate Abruptio Placentae

The immediate objectives of treatment for moderate abruptio placentae are to restore blood loss and to initiate delivery. Other objectives are to maintain constant surveillance of the condition of the fetus and to anticipate and deal with clotting defects.

When moderate abruption with actual or impending shock is diagnosed, the following should be done at once and almost simultaneously:

1. At least 3 units of blood should be matched, and, pending their administration according to need, a vein should be kept open with a large-bore catheter and infusion of Ringer's lactate solution or a plasma expander other than dextran should be started.
2. A vaginal examination should be carried out and the membranes ruptured, regardless of whether the patient is in shock and regardless of whether abdominal or vaginal delivery is anticipated. Standard management dictates that if labor does not ensue promptly, an oxytocin infusion should be started at a rate of 2 mU/minute and increased at appropriate intervals until effective labor occurs. Cesarean section should be performed under the following conditions: if fetal distress occurs, as evidenced by change in fetal heart rate and pattern obtained by electronic monitor or by evidence of fetal acidemia; if effective labor is not established within six hours; or if delivery cannot be anticipated within eight hours. Before operation, the exact clotting status should be determined and defects corrected.
3. If shock is present or appears imminent, central venous or pulmonary wedge pressure monitoring should be started at once, provided the clotting mechanism is intact, and a Foley catheter should be inserted for accurate appraisal of urinary output. In all cases of moderate placental abruption, the fetus is at high risk. Continuous electronic monitoring of the fetus is essential if abnormalities are to be noted in time for the obstetrician to deal with them.
4. Clotting defects are common even in the mild degrees of abruptio placentae. Tests for fibrinogen and circulating fibrinolysin must be set up immediately and repeated at frequent intervals until the patient is out of danger. The tests and correction of defects are outlined in Chapter 30.

Recently cesarean section has been used much more liberally in the treatment of both mild and moderate abruptio placentae than in the past. In Knab's study of 388 cases, 75% of the fetal deaths occurred more than 90 minutes after the patients' admission to the hospital, and almost 70% of all perinatal deaths involved infants who had been delivered more than two hours from the time of diagnosis. In these cases, early abdominal delivery might have prevented at least some of these fatalities.

Severe Abruptio Placentae

The procedures outlined for the treatment of moderate abruptio placentae are applicable for severe separation except that blood replacement is needed in a much greater amount, the clotting defect is far more profound and needs much closer vigilance, and with the rarest exceptions, consideration does not need to be given to the fetus because it almost surely will be stillborn. Also, renal complications are more common.

The membranes should be ruptured at once, regardless of shock, and blood should be replaced as quickly as possible (two to four liters are usually needed). The clotting status must be determined promptly and corrected as necessary. Most patients deliver vaginally and with reasonable dispatch. Cesarean section is used only if there is a chance that the infant may still be liveborn, if effective labor does not follow promptly, or if there is little likelihood that vaginal delivery will follow within four to six hours. If delivery is delayed longer, the probability of serious maternal renal complications increases.

Complications

Maternal complications associated with moderate and severe placental separation may result either from the disease itself or from the treatment.

Postpartum hemorrhage should be anticipated, especially in severe separation. Although the uterus may feel firm, its contractile efficiency (and hence its ability to close off bleeding sinuses) may be greatly impaired by extravasation of blood between the muscle fibers throughout the myometrium, as in the Couvelaire uterus. The problem may be compounded by the persistence of a clotting defect (see Chap. 30). If conservative measures fail (correction of clotting defect, bimanual compression of the uterus, administration of oxytocic drugs), the ultimate means of controlling the bleeding is by ligation of the hypogastric arteries (see p. 732 and Fig. 38-3) or by hysterectomy.

Renal failure may result from ischemia, which may be caused by shock, vascular spasm, intravascular clotting, or a combination of these factors. Incompatible emergency blood transfusion may produce renal shutdown; the frequency of this complication is directly proportional to the number of units of blood transfused either because of the severity of a condition that requires massive amounts of blood or because of the increasing statistical possibility of a mismatch. Prevention of this rare but potentially fatal complication consists mainly of the early detection and treatment of shock, the meticulous replacement of blood loss, and the proper treatment of any infection that may be present or anticipated. Monitoring the response of the central venous or pulmonary wedge pressure and urinary output to a provocative test may allow early detection of renal difficulty and prevent renal failure.

Pituitary necrosis (Sheehan's syndrome), which may follow ischemia, results from the same changes that precipitate renal failure. This condition is discussed in Chapter 46. Lactation at the proper time in the puerperium suggests that the pituitary gland has escaped serious damage. Thyrotropic, adrenotropic, and gonadotropic pituitary function may be destroyed singly or in combination. Return of menses is adequate evidence of gonadotropic activity. Tests of thyroid and adrenal function four to six months after delivery are part of the proper follow-up of patients who have suffered severe abruptio placentae.

CIRCUMVALLATE PLACENTA

Another cause of bleeding in late pregnancy is circumvallate placenta, although this is less common than placenta previa (see Fig. 43-3). The bleeding is bright red in color and moderate in amount and nearly always occurs without pain. When bleeding occurs before fetal maturity, the patient may be treated expectantly. Placental localization usually rules out placenta previa. If bleeding is persistent or heavy, if the patient is in labor, if the fetus is known to be mature, and if placenta previa cannot be completely ruled out, double setup examination is indicated.

In most cases the treatment is induction of labor, unless there is another indication for cesarean section. At times this complication is responsible for the spontaneous onset of preterm labor; as a result, there is an increased perinatal mortality. The diagnosis is made by inspection of the placenta following delivery.

PLACENTA ACCRETA

Normally, the placenta spontaneously separates from the uterine wall a few minutes after delivery of the infant. The most common causes of delayed delivery of the placenta are inadequate uterine contraction and retraction or failure of a portion of the normally attached placenta to separate from the implantation site. In placenta accreta, the placenta is abnormally adherent, the decidua is underdeveloped, and the physiologic cleavage plane through the spongy layer of the decidua is not present. When the villi extend through the myometrium, the condition is called *placenta increta;* when they reach or even penetrate the uterine serosa, it is termed *placenta percreta.*

Abnormal adherence of the placenta is most often associated with conditions that adversely affect decidual formation. These include placenta previa, previous cesarean section or curettage, intrauterine synechiae, and multiparity. Although antepartum bleeding and even uterine rupture can occur, the pregnancy and labor are usually normal until after delivery of the infant. Then the problems associated with the delivery of the placenta depend on the degree of adherence. With extensive involvement, no plane of cleavage can be found on manual exploration, and severe bleeding or uterine inversion may result from an attempt to remove the placenta.

When only a small part of the placenta is adherent, that portion can sometimes be removed by additional manipulation and the bleeding controlled with massage and intravenous administration of oxytocin. If efforts to detach the placenta are unsuccessful and bleeding continues, the safest treatment is to institute prompt blood replacement and proceed with hysterectomy. Attempts at curettage, suturing of the bleeding site, or packing of the uterus have been advocated for young women who would like to remain fertile, but these conservative measures present definite risks and should be abandoned if bleeding persists.

INVERSION OF THE UTERUS

Although acute puerperal inversion of the uterus is a rare complication, it is one that demands immediate diagnosis and rapid treatment to avoid a catastrophic result. The majority of cases are associated with umbilical cord traction and fundal pressure. The uterus is partially or completely inverted so that the top of the endometrial cavity protrudes through the cervix into the vagina and even outside the introitus.

Diagnosis

The beefy red mass at the introitus may be erroneously diagnosed as a prolapsed submucous myoma. If the placenta is still attached, it can be felt in the lower vagina with the inverted uterus above it. In addition pain, bleeding, and shock rapidly develop.

Management

The keystone of successful treatment is rapid reinversion of the uterus, because delay in treatment appreciably increases the possibility of disease and death. An anesthesiologist and other personnel should be summoned immediately, and an intravenous infusion of lactated Ringer's solution and blood through a large-bore catheter should be started.

The exact time at which the placenta should be removed is controversial and depends on the situation, but general anesthesia is induced as soon as possible, and the fundus is grasped in the palm of the hand with the fingers directed toward the posterior fornix. The uterus is lifted out of the pelvis and forcefully held in the abdominal cavity while pressure is applied to push the fundus upward through the cervix. After the uterus is restored to its normal configuration, the anesthesia used to provide relaxation is discontinued and oxytocin is started while the obstetrician maintains the position. The inverted uterus can usually be restored by this maneuver; but if vaginal attempts are unsuccessful, laparotomy should be performed. The round ligaments are grasped with instruments used for traction while an assistant elevates the fundus by inserting a hand into the vagina. When a constriction ring prevents reposition, it is incised posteriorly to allow ample room to reinvert the uterus. If the placenta is still attached, it is removed manually, the incision is closed, and the patient is given oxytocin and prophylactic antibiotics.

RUPTURE OF THE UTERUS

Either spontaneous or traumatic rupture of the uterus may occur before or during labor. It is a serious hazard to the mother, and the fetus usually dies if it is extruded into the peritoneal cavity or if the maternal hypovolemia is so profound that fetal oxygenation is inadequate. The major causes of rupture of the uterus are weakness of the uterine wall because of incision (previous cesarean section, hysterotomy, myomectomy, metroplasty) and difficult operative delivery (breech extraction, difficult forceps delivery, especially version and extraction). Injuries, such as those resulting from automobile accidents or gunshot wounds, account for a small percentage of cases. Improperly monitored or inappropriate use of oxytocic agents has been associated with a significant number of cases. Lower uterine segment rupture because of neglected obstructed labor should never occur in developed countries.

As in any ruptured viscus, pain usually, but not always, precedes the definitive tear. Severe pain and shock follow as rupture occurs, after which the pain is apt to subside. In uterine rupture, local bleeding, which may be scant or heavy, usually ensues; depending on the location of the tear, some of the blood may escape vaginally.

Rupture of a cesarean section scar is the most common type of uterine rupture. Classic vertical scars clearly predispose a patient to uterine rupture; lower segment transverse scars are least apt to give way. In rupture of the classic scar, the clinical picture includes fleeting pain, often for several days before rupture; this is followed by severe pain, shock, and cessation of fetal heart tones. The pain abates after rupture, but the collapse

continues and may be compounded if it is accompanied by intra-abdominal hemorrhage. Immediate laparotomy is lifesaving for the mother but of little help to the fetus, which may have already escaped into the abdominal cavity. In rupture of the lower segment scar, the picture is apt to be less dramatic, but the condition is potentially as serious. The therapeutic procedure must be tailored to the problem. If the tear is clean and amenable to repair, the edges may be freshened and the defect sutured. If repair is not reasonable, the uterus should be removed. If the patient's condition is compromised, a supravaginal hysterectomy solves the immediate emergency more quickly and easily, and as definitely, as a total hysterectomy.

Version and extraction, except for delivery of a second or later born infant in a multiple birth, breech extraction, and difficult midforceps deliveries are decreasing in use and should be eliminated. In addition to the possible injury to the fetus, the potential danger of traumatic uterine rupture is ever present. Currently, delivery by cesarean section is safer than vaginal delivery for both the mother and the infant. The diagnosis of uterine rupture in these cases is made by manual exploration of the uterus. If uterine rupture is diagnosed, laparotomy should be undertaken immediately with due attention to vigorous appropriate management of hemorrhage and collapse. In this situation, a total hysterectomy should be done because the tears often involve the lower uterine segment and extend into the cervix and vaginal fornix.

The protean lesions produced by injury cannot be categorized. Rupture has resulted from a seatbelt injury, for example. (This is not to suggest that pregnant women should abandon seatbelts; uterine rupture is less serious than possible death if this protection is not used.) The major signs of the lesions are intra-abdominal hemorrhage, pain, and collapse. The procedure at laparotomy depends on the problem presented; it may be necessary to empty the uterus by hysterotomy if its bulk interferes with exposure and control of bleeding.

Oxytocin infusions can cause uterine rupture and must be used with meticulous care, especially in parous women. The use of constant infusion pumps allows for safer administration, and the continuous monitoring of the frequency, duration, and strength of uterine contractions by either machine or an experienced attendant is mandatory. Uterine tetany must be avoided.

Lower uterine segment rupture is a predictable consequence of neglected obstructed labor.

RUPTURED VASA PREVIA

Ruptured vasa previa is a rare complication of late pregnancy or labor that can sometimes be confused with abruptio placentae or placenta previa. If a major fetal vessel is the source of the vaginal bleeding, fetal death is virtually certain—delivery can rarely be completed quickly enough to prevent fetal exsanguination. The presence of scant vaginal bleeding may suggest bleeding from a small vessel, if the uterus is soft and there is

Table 25-2
Differential Diagnosis of Bleeding in Late Pregnancy

	Placenta Previa	*Marginal Separation*	*Moderate Abruption*	*Severe Abruption*	*Antepartum Rupture of Scarred Uterus*
External bleeding	Mild to catastrophic	Minimal to mild	None to moderate	None to moderate	None to mild
Color of blood	Bright	Dark	None, dark	None, dark	None, bright
Back pain	None	None	None to moderate	None to moderate	None
Myometrial tone	Normal	Normal	Hypertonicity, localized or diffuse	Hypertonicity, diffuse	Normal if infant is in uterus; contracted if infant extruded
Uterine tenderness	None	Nearly always none; localized if present	Marked, usually diffuse	Marked and diffuse	None to moderate; localized if present; abdomen generally tender
Fetal status at first examination	Nearly always alive; occasionally in jeopardy	Nearly always alive; rarely in jeopardy	Frequently alive but in jeopardy	Usually dead; if alive, in jeopardy	Usually dead; if alive, in jeopardy
Presentation	High incidence of breech, oblique, transverse	Normal distribution	Normal distribution	Normal distribution	Normal distribution if not extruded
Station of presenting part	High	High to engaged	High to engaged	High to engaged	High
Shock	Uncommon	None	Frequent	Very common	Frequent
Coagulopathy	Very rare	Very rare	Occasional	Frequent	Rare
Association with hypertensive states	Normal distribution	Normal distribution	Increased	Increased	Normal distribution

evidence of fetal distress. The presence of nucleated red cells in a sample of expelled blood confirms the diagnosis, and the infant should be delivered by the most expeditious means.

In some cases, depending on the clinical picture, the physician may proceed at once to cesarean section without awaiting confirmation by a stained blood smear or chemical test for fetal hemoglobin. In a recent case, the membranes ruptured spontaneously when the cervix was dilated 3 cm. The amniotic fluid was port-wine colored, which may be an important sign. Decelerative fetal heart rate patterns followed, and the infant was delivered by cesarean section within 10 minutes. Ruptured vasa previa involving a small vessel was confirmed. The infant's condition was good, except for a hemoglobin of 12 g/dl, and the subsequent course was uneventful.

OTHER CAUSES OF LATE PREGNANCY BLEEDING

Traumatic lesions of the vagina and cervix rarely cause bleeding late in pregnancy. Lacerations of vaginal septa can occur during labor and delivery. A friable condyloma acuminatum may bleed from minor trauma and must be differentiated from other sources of bleeding. Cervical erosions and polyps rarely produce bleeding in late pregnancy. Invasive cervical carcinoma as a cause of painless vaginal bleeding in late pregnancy must be considered, although proper early prenatal care, including cervical cytology, should enable diagnosis of this entity before the second half of pregnancy.

The differential diagnosis of bleeding in late pregnancy is summarized in Table 25-2.

REFERENCES AND RECOMMENDED READING

Brenner WE, Edelman DA, Hendricks CH: Characteristics of patients with placenta previa and results of "expectant management." Am J Obstet Gynecol 132:180, 1978

Carter B: Premature separation of the normally implanted placenta: Six deaths due to gross bilateral cortical necrosis of kidneys. Obstet Gynecol 29:30, 1967

Cotton DB, Read JA, Paul RH et al: The conservative aggressive management of placenta previa. Am J Obstet Gynecol 137: 687, 1980

Crenshaw C, Jones DED, Parker RT: Placenta previa: A survey

of twenty years experience with improved perinatal survival by expectant therapy and cesarean delivery. Obstet Gynecol Surv 28:461, 1973

Golan A, Sandbank O, Rubin A: Rupture of the pregnant uterus. Obstet Gynecol 56:549, 1980

Hobbins JC, Winsberg F: Ultrasonography in Obstetrics and Gynecology, pp 49–58. Baltimore, Williams & Wilkins, 1977

Johnson HA: The conservative management of some varieties of placenta previa. Am J Obstet Gynecol 50:248, 1945

Knab DR: Abruptio placentae: An assessment of the time and method of delivery. Obstet Gynecol 52:625, 1978

Macafee CHG: Placenta previa. J Obstet Gynaecol Brit Emp 52:313, 1945

Macafee CHG, Millar WG, Harley G: Maternal and fetal mortality in placenta previa. J Obstet Gynaecol Br Commonw 69:203, 1962

Pent D: Vasa previa. Am J Obstet Gynecol 134:151, 1979

Pritchard JA, Mason R, Carley M et al: Genesis of severe placental abruption. Am J Obstet Gynecol 108:22, 1970

Sheehan HL, Murdoch R: Postpartum necrosis of anterior pituitary: Pathological and clinical aspects. J Obstet Gynaecol Br Emp 45:456, 1938

Silver R, Depp R, Sabbagha RE et al: Placenta previa: Aggressive expectant management. Am J Obstet Gynecol 150:15, 1984

Spaulding LB, Gallup DG: Current concepts of management of rupture of the gravid uterus. Obstet Gynecol 54:437, 1979

Pregnancy-Induced Hypertension

Richard J. Worley

26

Pregnancy-induced hypertension (PIH) complicates about 5% to 7% of pregnancies in otherwise normal primigravid women, and as many as 20% to 40% of pregnancies in women with chronic renal disease or vascular disorders such as essential hypertension, diabetes mellitus, and lupus erythematosus. In some areas of the world, including many regions of the United States, hypertension complicating pregnancy is the most prominent cause of maternal and infant illness and death. The hazard of PIH to the fetus results mainly from the decreased placental perfusion typical of this vasospastic disorder. The major maternal hazard is that of eclampsia, or *grand mal* seizures, resulting from profound cerebral effects of the disease. Fortunately, with proper management PIH can often be ameliorated and eclampsia largely if not entirely prevented. To these ends, however, two admonitions bear repeated emphasis:

Do not underestimate the importance of even a mild degree of hypertension complicating pregnancy.
Acknowledge that no one can predict accurately which patients with PIH will develop eclampsia.

Failure to heed these principles is a factor in most instances of preventable poor outcome in pregnancies complicted by hypertension. It is especially crucial to acquire at the outset lasting respect for the clinical implications and potential consequences of PIH. Even minimal PIH can lead rapidly to catastrophic complications such as eclampsia or abruptio placentae that have no parallel in the nonpregnant individual with a comparably mild form of hypertension. Timely recognition of the disease is of no value, however, if the physician does not heed the diagnosis by taking proper measures to arrest progression of the disorder (if possible), prevent eclampsia, and provide safe delivery of the infant.

CLASSIFICATION AND DEFINITION OF PREGNANCY-INDUCED HYPERTENSION

The classification of hypertensive disorders of pregnancy used in this chapter is as follows:

1. PIH
    a. Without proteinuria
    b. With proteinuria (preeclampsia)
    c. Eclampsia
2. Chronic hypertension preceding pregnancy (any etiology)
3. Chronic hypertension (any etiology) with superimposed PIH
    a. Without proteinuria
    b. With proteinuria (superimposed preeclampsia)
    c. Superimposed eclampsia
4. Late or transient hypertension

PIH is defined as a blood pressure of 140/90 mm Hg during the second half of pregnancy in a previously normotensive woman. A rise in systolic blood pressure of 30 mm Hg or in diastolic pressure of 15 mm Hg over baseline values also defines the condition. The diagnosis is established by the finding of these blood pressure changes on at least two occasions six or more hours apart. The addition of proteinuria to PIH signifies a more advanced stage of the disorder, called *preeclampsia.*

Preeclampsia has for many years been defined as the development of PIH plus proteinuria and/or generalized edema. Because the edema characteristic of preeclampsia is typically difficult to distinguish from the edema prevalent in normal pregnant women, and because edema per se is far more commonly correlated with maternal and fetal well-being than with hypertension,[1] many authorities restrict use of the term *pre-*

eclampsia to women with PIH who have proteinuria, defined as 500 mg protein or more in a 24-hour urine specimen or a semiquantitative reaction of 2+ or more in a random urine specimen. The term *preeclampsia* of course signifies a stage in the evolution of PIH at which a seizure, or eclampsia, has yet to occur. The term also implies that it is from preeclampsia rather than simple PIH that eclampsia is most likely to ensue. The concept is accurate, but it can dangerously mislead the clinician for two reasons: first, the rise in perinatal mortality rate associated with PIH begins with the appearance of hypertension alone, before proteinuria occurs;[2] second, eclampsia can nevertheless occur in women with PIH who do not have proteinuria. These important observations justify heeding the disease clinically as soon as it can be recognized, that is, with the appearance of hypertension, regardless of whether there is associated proteinuria.

It is useful to envision PIH as existing in two different forms. One, a so-called pure form, has a peculiar predilection for occurring only in first pregnancies. The other form seems to be incited by chronic hypertension, renal disease, diabetes mellitus, collagen vascular diseases, and the like. This form, known as *superimposed PIH* when it complicates chronic hypertension, tends to recur in subsequent pregnancies, often in increasingly virulent form. Although the pathophysiologies of the two different forms of PIH seem to be similar, if not identical, the form associated with chronic vascular disease often occurs earlier in pregnancy and in more severe fashion than the pure type. Moreover, its propensity to recur may contraindicate a subsequent pregnancy for some women with chronic disease, whereas the otherwise normal primigravida who has the pure form of PIH can expect not to develop the disorder in subsequent pregnancies.

Chronic hypertension complicating pregnancy is easily distinguished from PIH when there is a history of hypertension antedating pregnancy, hypertension appears before the 20th week of gestation, or hypertension persists indefinitely following delivery. The occasional case of PIH associated with a hydatidiform mole is the only recognized exception to the generalization that hypertension during the first half of pregnancy is not gestational in origin. Additional historical factors suggestive of chronic hypertension are multiparity or the occurrence of hypertension in a previous pregnancy. When the patient is not seen for obstetric care until after the 20th week of gestation, however, chronic hypertension may be difficult to distinguish from PIH. Both normal women and many with chronic hypertension exhibit a decrease in blood pressure during the middle and early third trimesters of pregnancy. Thus, a patient with unrecognized chronic hypertension who is seen for the first time at the 24th week of pregnancy may appear normal, but early in the third trimester her blood pressure may rise to the unrecognized hypertensive level

that preceded the pregnancy and was doubtless present during its early months. Sometimes it is impossible to distinguish PIH from chronic hypertension in such a case, but the following clinical findings suggest that the disorder is chronic in nature:

Retinal hemorrhages and exudates
Plasma urea nitrogen concentration above 20 mg/dl
Plasma creatinine concentration above 1 mg/dl
The presence of diabetes mellitus, renal disease, collagen vascular disease, or other disorders that predispose to chronic hypertension

Ability to distinguish between PIH and chronic hypertension is of both clinical and investigative importance. The threat to the pregnancy of PIH, either alone or superimposed on chronic hypertension, is greater than that of otherwise uncomplicated mild chronic hypertension. A great effort, often entailing hospitalization, may be in order to treat PIH remote from term, but the woman with simple mild chronic hypertension can usually be managed in the office and at home. Inability to distinguish between chronic hypertension and PIH also frustrates the scientific investigator, for pathophysiologies of the two disorders are decidedly different. The student of scientific publication regarding PIH should be alert to this problem.

Unlike uncomplicated mild chronic hypertension, which often has a benign obstetric impact, severe chronic hypertension and PIH superimposed on chronic hypertension are commonly harsh on the pregnancy. Superimposed PIH consists of acute aggravation of preexisting hypertension and often rapid development of proteinuria and edema (superimposed preeclampsia). Eclampsia may ensue quickly. Diagnostic criteria for superimposed PIH are as follows:

1. Documented evidence that the patient has chronic hypertension
2. Evidence of a superimposed, acute process as demonstrated by
   a. Elevation of systolic blood pressure 30 mm Hg or of diastolic blood pressure 15 mm Hg above baseline on two occasions at least six hours apart
   b. Development of proteinuria or edema (superimposed preeclampsia)

The diagnosis of superimposed PIH may be difficult to establish precisely in some cases, especially when the woman has a labile form of chronic hypertension.

Late or transient hypertension describes the brief, often nonrecurrent elevations in blood pressure that some pregnant women exhibit only during labor or in the early puerperium. The nature of the disorder may range from mild PIH to latent or early chronic hypertension.

ETIOLOGY

In 1916 the German physician Zweifel called pre-eclampsia the disease of theories. Seventy years later this characterization is still accurate. Chesley's contemporary words (written in 1970) are testimony to the continuing bewilderment about the etiology of PIH:

> Everyone from allergist to zoologist has proposed hypotheses and suggested rational therapies based upon them, such as mastectomy, oophorectomy, renal decapsulation, trephination, alignment of the patient with the earth's magnetic field with her head pointing to the North Pole, and all sorts of medical regimens.[3]

Three major concepts are prominent in current thinking about the etiology of PIH: increased vasoconstrictor tone, abnormal prostaglandin action, and immunologic factors.

Increased Vasoconstrictor Tone

A central point on which all observers agree is that PIH is characterized by widespread (but seemingly not ubiquitous) vasospasm. The dominant view is that the vasospasm results mainly, or wholly, from an abnormal sensitivity of vascular smooth muscle to the vasoconstrictive effects of pressor substances. Nearly 50 years ago Dieckmann and Michel showed that vascular reactivity to the pressor effects of a vasoactive agent, in this case crude vasopressin, is greater in preeclamptic than in normotensive pregnant women.[4] It was not recognized until 25 years later, however, that normal pregnant women are far less responsive than nonpregnant women to infused vasoactive agents; that is, they are relatively refractory to the pressor effects of agents such as angiotensin II (A-II).[5]

To investigate patterns of pressor substance refractoriness during pregnancy, Gant and colleagues in the early 1970s conducted a prospective analysis of vascular responsiveness to A-II throughout pregnancy in 192 primigravidas.[6] The subjects were recruited from an adolescent population at high risk for PIH, and 72 of the 192 subjects developed the disorder. The investigators were thus able to contrast the pattern of vascular responsiveness during pregnancy in normal women with that in women who developed PIH.

In this and other studies like it, a vascular response was defined as a rise in diastolic blood pressure of 20 mm Hg or more after infusion of a given amount of A-II, expressed in nanograms of angiotensin per kilogram of body weight per minute of infusion. This amount of A-II, referred to as the *effective pressor dose* (EPD A-II), in nonpregnant subjects averages about 7.5 ng/kg/minute.

The results of Gant's study are depicted in Figure 26-1. As the figure shows, both normal and subsequently hypertensive pregnant women were already relatively refractory to infused A-II by the 18th week of pregnancy. This state of refractoriness persisted throughout the remainder of pregnancy in the 120 who remained normal; in contrast, after midpregnancy the mean EPD A-II in the 72 who developed PIH fell, such that after about the 34th week these women exhibited a mean EPD A-II lower than nonpregnant subjects. Remarkably, the women who developed PIH were clinically normal most of the time they were losing pregnancy-acquired refractoriness to A-II; hypertension was typically detected only during the last few weeks of pregnancy.

This observation, probably more than any other, constitutes the basis for recognizing that PIH, a kind of acute hypertension of pregnancy, is nevertheless the result of a surprisingly protracted disease process, confined by definition to pregnancy but often occurring throughout the entire second half of gestation. The concept that PIH becomes clinically evident only after a

FIG. 26-1. The amount of angiotensin II required to evoke a pressor response during pregnancy in 120 primigravidas who remained normal (*black dots*) and in 72 who developed pregnancy-induced hypertension (*open circles*). Vertical bars represent the standard error of the mean. Differences between the two groups were highly significant after the 22nd week of gestation. (Gant NF, Daley GL, Chand S et al: A study of angiotensin II pressor responsiveness throughout primigravid pregnancy. Reproduced from *The Journal of Clinical Investigation*, 1973, 52: 2682, by copyright permission of The American Society for Clinical Investigation.

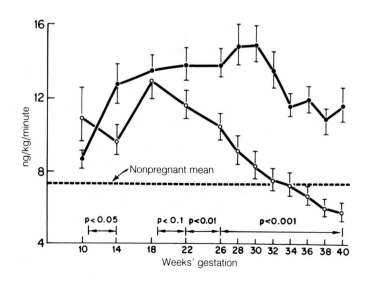

relatively long, clinically inapparent pathophysiologic prelude has two important clinical implications. First, the clinician must recognize that by the time even mild cases of PIH are detected, intervillous perfusion is already compromised and other organ systems may also be affected (see the section on Pathophysiology below). Second, the existence of a lengthy and silent prelude to PIH allows for the possibility that a means of recognizing the disorder at a preclinical stage and forestalling it might be devised. Although an ideal means of recognizing PIH in its preclinical state has yet to be developed, some potentially useful maneuvers have been described (see the section on Prophylaxis of Pregnancy-Induced Hypertension below).

Although there is little argument that women with PIH exhibit much greater sensitivity to infused vasoactive agents than normal pregnant women, there is considerable uncertainty about the exact mechanism of the hypertension in PIH. In general, subjects who are most sensitive to infused A-II have low plasma renin activity, and conversely, those who are least sensitive have high renin activity.[7] Consistent with this relationship, nonpregnant subjects exhibit a positive correlation between plasma A-II concentration and EPD A-II,[8] as often do pregnant women. However, pregnancy alters the relationship between angiotensin concentration and vascular responsiveness to pressor agents. Whereas in nonpregnant subjects pressor responsiveness to A-II depends principally on plasma A-II concentration, in pregnant women it depends principally on degree of vascular smooth muscle responsiveness or refractoriness to vasoactive agents and is largely independent of circulating A-II concentration.[9] Thus, although different investigators report widely varying circulating concentrations of vasoactive agents in women with PIH, the blood vessels invariably exhibit abnormal sensitivity to infused angiotensin.

Although vascular sensitization to vasoactive agents appears to play a central role in the pathophysiology of PIH, it is not clear what role any of the pressor agents plays in the genesis of PIH. With regard to antiotensin, for instance, administration of the converting enzyme inhibitor SQ 20881, which inhibits A-II generation, does not relieve PIH, at least when given postpartum.[10] In fact, administration of a converting enzyme inhibitor may have catastrophic consequences for the fetus. When Symonds and colleagues administered captopril to pregnant rabbits and ewes, 40% of the fetal rabbits and 80% of the fetal lambs succumbed.[11]

It seems probable that A-II is no more a specific cause of PIH than are any of the other pressor agents. There is limited evidence, for instance, that catecholamines may circulate in higher concentrations in preeclamptic than in normal women.[12] In addition, serum deoxycorticosterone (DOC) concentration averages 1200 times higher in normal pregnant women at term than in nonpregnant women. The increased generation of this potent mineralocorticoid during pregnancy is mainly due to extra-adrenal 21-hydroxylation of pro-gesterone and thus is largely independent of adrenal function or electrolyte distribution. Nevertheless, mean concentrations of DOC in women with PIH do not differ significantly from those in normal pregnant women.[13]

It is possible that an anomaly of cation distribution or availability may contribute to the increased vasomotor responsiveness of women with PIH. Sodium has long been recognized as a sensitizer of vascular smooth muscle to the action of vasoactive agents. Infusion of hypertonic (but not isotonic) sodium is one of the few methods whereby vascular refractoriness to A-II can be temporarily abolished in normal pregnant women.[14] Dietary sodium restriction has of course been a mainstay of antihypertensive regimens in nonpregnant patients for some time. Some of the alterations in sodium homeostasis that occur during pregnancy might seem at first glance to be capable of promoting hypertension. Normal pregnant women accumulate about 750 mEq of sodium during gestation. Women with preeclampsia accumulate even more, and in contrast with normal pregnant women, excrete a sodium load poorly. At least one group of investigators found sodium–potassium ATPase in cord blood erythrocytes to be lower in women with PIH than in normal pregnant women.[15] Another electrolyte distribution system, sodium–sodium countertransport, is reportedly elevated in nonpregnant subjects with essential hypertension.[16] This cation flux, usually measured as sodium–lithium countertransport, is also sizably elevated during pregnancy, but there do not appear to be discernible differences in measurements between normal and hypertensive pregnant women.[17]

However, there is little reason to believe that altered sodium homeostatsis is central to the pathogenesis of PIH. The serum concentration of sodium in both normal and preeclamptic pregnant women averages about 5 mEq/liter lower than in nonpregnant subjects, reflecting the relatively greater retention of water than of sodium. During pregnancy there is both an increase in glomerular filtration rate and a marked elevation in circulating concentration of progesterone (acting as an aldosterone antagonist). To overcome these powerful natriuretic influences, pregnant women undergo more than a tenfold increase in the rate of secretion of aldosterone in order to maintain osmotic homeostasis, an effort that amounts to a physiological struggle to conserve sodium. Furthermore, neither restricting sodium intake nor promoting its excretion reduces the incidence or severity of PIH.[18] In fact, judging from the physiological effort necessary to conserve sodium during pregnancy, it is no surprise that dangerous hyponatremia has occasionally resulted from sodium restriction; thiazide diuretic therapy in particular may pose critical hazards to the fetus.[19] Given that sodium restriction and diuretic therapy are not efficacious and are even potentially hazardous, all contemporary authorities concur that both regimens are contraindicated in the management of PIH.

Calcium is another prominent cation that is linked to blood pressure control, and there is a growing body of evidence that hypertension is generally associated with increased intracellular calcium accumulation sensitizing vascular smooth muscle to constrictor stimuli. Mendlowitz hypothesized that PIH may result from the defective generation of intracellular calcium–transporting protein.[20] However, there are also contrasting views. Belizan and associates proposed that the problem is dietary calcium deficiency, and they provided evidence that women who received calcium supplementation had a lower mean blood pressure during the last trimester of pregnancy than did nonsupplemented controls.[21] McCarron and colleagues concluded from a large dietary survey that nonpregnant individuals with chronic hypertension generally consume significantly less calcium than do normotensive subjects.[22] McCarron also reported that the mean serum ionized calcium concentration is lower in subjects with essential hypertension than in normal individuals.[23] Nevertheless, Richards and associates were unable to find a difference in circulating ionized calcium concentration between normal and hypertensive pregnant women,[24] and Belizan and colleagues did not find that calcium supplementation alters the incidence of PIH.[21]

Abnormal Prostaglandin Action

The data depicted in Figure 26-1 give rise to two obvious questions: By what mechanism do normal pregnant women acquire refractoriness to vasoactive agents? What disturbance in this mechanism leads to the loss of refractoriness that precedes and characterizes PIH? Altered prostaglandin or prostanoid generation or action increasingly appears to be central to the answers to both questions.

Prostaglandins are potent mediators of vascular reactivity to vasoactive agents in both pregnant and nonpregnant women. Numerous observations support the contention that during pregnancy prostaglandin generation in blood vessel walls blunts the response to pressor substances. As depicted in Figure 26-2, inhibition of prostaglandin synthesis by administration of indomethacin abolishes A-II refractoriness in normal pregnant women.[25] Aspirin, in a dosage of 600 mg every 6 hours, produces a comparable effect. However, the relationship between prostaglandin synthetase inhibition and PIH is not straightforward. Many women take aspirin in unsupervised fashion during pregnancy, and even when the effect of the aspirin is sufficient to delay labor slightly, hypertension does not occur with unusual frequency. Zuckerman and colleagues gave enough indomethacin to 50 women in premature labor to interrupt their contractions entirely, yet none of these women became hypertensive.[26]

If vasodilating prostaglandin generation is requisite to pregnancy-acquired refractoriness to pressor agents, one reason that acute prostaglandin synthetase inhibition does not lead to PIH is undoubtedly because the development of hypertension involves more than mere loss of refractoriness. As shown in Figure 26-1, women

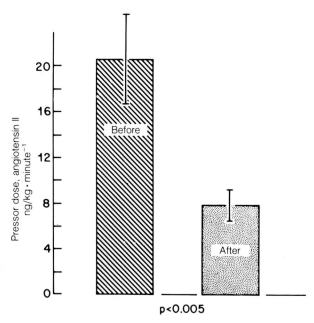

FIG. 26-2. The mean effective pressor dose of angiotension II before and during indomethacin treatment in 11 normotensive women studied late in pregnancy. (Gant NF, Worley RJ: Hypertension in Pregnancy, p 29. Norwalk, CT, Appleton-Century-Crofts, 1980)

who developed PIH in that study became hypertensive only at the end of a period of as long as 20 weeks, during which they relentlessly lost refractoriness to A-II. Between the 28th and 32nd weeks of gestation, many of these women already exhibited an EPD A-II less than the nonpregnant mean, even though they were clinically normal; over 90% of them later developed PIH.

Moreover, prostaglandins are not the only substances that influence vascular responsiveness to vasoactive agents. Steroid hormones may also have an effect. When infused intravenously, the progesterone metabolite 5α-dihydroprogesterone restores angiotensin refractoriness to A-II–sensitive women with mild PIH.[27] In normal pregnant women this steroid can also reverse the A-II sensitivity that results from administration of indomethacin, implying that its action either overcomes the prostaglandin block or, more likely, is independent of the prostaglandin effect. What role, if any, 5α-dihydroprogesterone may play in the genesis of PIH is unclear. The circulating concentration of 5α-dihydroprogesterone is the same during pregnancy in women who remain normotensive as in those who develop PIH.[28]

Another factor that influences vascular responsiveness to pressor agents is the cyclic nucleotide apparatus. Administration of theophylline to A-II–sensitive women with mild PIH restores vascular refractoriness,[29] which effect may be interpreted to mean that the agent, acting as a phosphodiesterase inhibitor, promotes accumulation of vasorelaxing cyclic nucleotides in vascular smooth muscle. There are probably other modifiers of vascular responsiveness to vasoactive agents that would confound the issue, but it seems clear that prostaglandin or prostanoid generation is a key modulator during pregnancy.

If PIH is a kind of prostaglandin deficiency syndrome, the problem could be deficiency of a prostaglandin precursor, reduced prostaglandin synthetase activity, or defective prostaglandin action. Several groups of investigators have pondered whether dietary deficiency of essential fatty acids might be a factor in the genesis of PIH. In pregnant rabbits such dietary restriction leads to increased sensitivity to infused A-II;[30] however, such a dietary factor has yet to be identified in humans. Gant and associates found no difference in incidence of PIH between pregnant women who received large daily supplements of the prostaglandin precursor homo-γ-linoleic acid and placebo-treated controls.[31]

The evidence is better that PIH is due to reduced prostaglandin generation. Prostaglandin E2, but not F2a, production is reduced in preeclamptic women, and infusion of the agent into pregnant women blunts their response to infused A-II.[32,33] There are also data, derived mainly from *in vitro* and acute surgical studies, that A-II stimulation during pregnancy leads to prostaglandin E2 generation in the uteroplacental bed and other tissues.[34] Such a mechanism might augment uterine perfusion during pregnancy and protect selected vascular beds, that of the uterus included, from undesirable vasoconstriction.

The prostanoid compounds thromboxane (TXA2) and prostacyclin (PGI2) may exert even more direct effects than the major prostaglandins on vasomotor tone during both normal and hypertensive pregnancy. These compounds are synthesized in the manner depicted in Figure 26-3. The cyclo-oxygenase enzyme system rapidly converts free arachidonic acid to the ephemeral intermediates known as endoperoxides. These agents can be metabolized in one of two ways: they may be converted either to the familiar prostaglandins of the series E, F, A, and so on, or to one of the prostanoids, PGI2 or TXA2, the most potent vasoactive agents known. TXA2 is a more powerful vasoconstrictor than A-II, and PGI2 is a more potent vasodilator than prostaglandin E2. In addition to having opposing effects on vascular smooth muscle, these agents exert opposing effects on platelet aggregation and adherence, TXA2 promoting them and PGI2 inhibiting them.

The prostanoid compounds have short half-lives (TXA2, 30 seconds; PGI2, 2–3 minutes). As a result, it is necessary to measure stable metabolites of the compounds as an indication of their respective production rates. The stable hydration product of TXA2 is thromboxane B2 (TXB2); the stable metabolite of PGI2 is 6-keto-prostaglandin F1a (6-keto-PGF1a). The prostanoids exert action at their respective sites of formation. They are virtually unmeasureable in circulation, so to assay them one must measure the capacity of specific tissues to generate them. The predominant assay systems involve estimation of PGI2 generation by vascular endothelium and TXA2 generation by platelets.

Because of the opposing effects of the prostanoids, it is useful to envision the consequences of their actions as a balance of their respective rates of generation. During normal pregnancy both prostanoids are produced in increased amounts, in many ways the action of one balancing that of the other. Many investigators, however, have found evidence of reduced PGI2 generation in women with PIH.[35–40] Selectively reduced PGI2 production in association with substantial TXA2 action is a plausible mechanism for the widespread vasospasm, and perhaps the A-II sensitivity, of women with PIH. The impairment may be even worse in the fetus than in the mother. Remuzzi and co-workers found that the decrement in PGI2 generation was considerably greater in umbilical than in maternal vasculature,[36] implying that fetal–placental blood flow is impaired more than maternal–placental flow during PIH. Dadak and colleagues also found considerably reduced umbilical artery PGI2 generation in preeclamptic women, as well as marked disruption of the umbilical vascular endothelium in affected pregnancies.[39]

It is thus possible that a pivotal defect in PGI2 synthesis is of major importance in the pathophysiology of PIH. If so, one would expect that a selective stimulus to PGI2 generation, or selective inhibition of TXA2 production, would resolve the syndrome. The search for

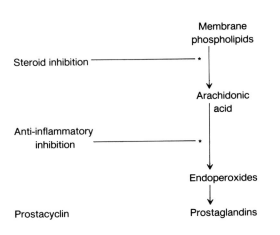

Membrane phospholipids

Steroid inhibition

Arachidonic acid

Anti-inflammatory inhibition

Endoperoxides

Prostacyclin   Prostaglandins

Phospholipase A2

Cyclo-oxygenase

Thromboxane

FIG. 26-3. Basic scheme of endoperoxide and prostaglandin formation. The phospholipase A2 and cyclo-oxygenase reactions are indicated, as are known inhibitors of each enzyme.

agents that can accomplish either of these tasks has yielded a couple of possibilities. Aspirin, given in small doses, may be one of them. Masotti and associates suggest that 3.5 mg per kg of body weight, or about half an aspirin tablet every 3 days, increases the ratio of PGI2 to TXA2 generated in tissues;[40] Hanley and associates claim that 40 mg to 50 mg daily, about half a baby aspirin, is effective.[41]

It is perplexing that, on the one hand, administration of prostaglandin synthetase inhibitors, aspirin among them, abolishes pregnancy-acquired refractoriness to vasoactive agents, and in so doing reproduces one of the key events in the pathophysiology of PIH, while on the other hand, it is alleged that low-dose aspirin therapy may be salutary. Keys to the dichotomy are likely the dosage of aspirin involved and the ratio of PGI2 to TXA2 generation at the time of treatment. Although both PGI2 and TXA2 production are augmented during normal pregnancy, it is natural to speculate that the vasorelaxing effects of PGI2 predominate and perhaps play a role in promoting refractoriness to vasoactive agents. It is conceivable that relatively intense prostaglandin synthetase inhibition, which indomethacin or standard-dose aspirin treatment provides, might in this circumstance reduce both PGI2 and TXA2 production to levels characteristic of the nonpregnant state, and in this manner altogether abolish refractoriness to A-II, as has been shown.[25] However, if low-dose aspirin treatment selectively inhibits TXA2 generation to a degree, thereby increasing the ratio of PGI2 to TXA2,[40,41] it could conceivably benefit women who have or are likely to develop PIH. In fact, at least one group of investigators has suggested that the incidence of preeclampsia is lower in women who consume aspirin during pregnancy than in those who do not.[42] The hypothesis, however, is otherwise largely untested, and evidence in support of the concept is not yet sufficient to warrant use of low-dose aspirin to prevent or treat PIH in clinical practice.

Another agent studied for its ability to alter prostanoid generation is dazoxiben, a relatively selective inhibitor of TXA2 synthesis and promoter of PGI2 generation. Van Assche and colleagues gave dazoxiben to four women with severe PIH for periods of between three and ten weeks and found that the drug appeared to produce clinical improvement in most of the patients.[43] Two of the four infants died, however, one *in utero* in the 27th week and the other after cesarean section for fetal distress in the 29th week. The two infants who survived were delivered in the 33rd and 37th weeks of pregnancy.

More evidence is required before we can judge whether selective promotion of PGI2 generation or inhibition of TXA2 synthesis could be effective in reducing the incidence of PIH or in treating it once it is established. Direct infusion of PGI2 into women with PIH has had catastrophic effects on the babies and unpleasant effects on the mothers. Three women with severe preeclampsia who received PGI2 infusions suffered weakness, nausea, headache, hypotension, and bradycardia;

two of their infants died, and the third was delivered by emergency cesarean section for severe fetal bradycardia.[44,45]

In addition to being a critical factor in the development of PIH, defective PGI2 production could also account for the thrombocytopenia and microangiopathy that are sometimes prominent in women with PIH (see the section on Pathophysiology of Severe Pregnancy-Induced Hypertension below). In several ways PIH is strikingly similar to at least three syndromes seen in nonpregnant individuals: hemolytic uremic syndrome, thrombotic thrombocytopenic purpura, and the lupus anticoagulant syndrome. In all four conditions hypertension, renal impairment, thrombocytopenia, and microangiopathy are variously present, and all entail a defect in PGI2 generation.[46-48]

It is possible that many of the features of PIH result directly from a central underlying defect, such as altered prostanoid formation, and are neither proportionate to nor consequent upon the hypertension. Such a view does not in any way lessen the clinical importance of hypertension to the syndrome, but it does provide a basis for understanding the protean nature of PIH. The concept would account, for instance, for the frequent instances in which features of the PIH syndrome such as thrombocytopenia, microangiopathy, impaired regional perfusion, and convulsions are prominent while hypertension is only moderate or mild in severity.

Immunologic Factors

Several characteristics of PIH provide grounds for the belief that the disorder may have an immunologic basis. Principal among these characteristics is the tendency of PIH to occur only in first pregnancies; pure PIH (not superimposed on chronic hypertension) is 10 times more common in first pregnancies than in subsequent pregnancies.[49]

It is difficult to explain this first-pregnancy preponderance of PIH without invoking the idea of an immune mechanism whereby exposure to fetal antigens somehow protects the mother from acquiring PIH in subsequent pregnancies. Strictly speaking, exposure to fetal antigens is not necessary to the development of PIH, since the disorder is a well-known, occasional complication of hydatidiform mole. Trophoblastic tissue is fetal in nature, but it is a remarkably bland antigen, and trophoblastic membranes contain neither major transplantation nor histocompatibility antigens.[50] Nevertheless, pregnant women do form antibodies against fetal HLA antigens, although the mechanisms behind this antibody formation are undefined. The incidence of such antigen formation increases with parity, so one might anticipate an inverse relationship between antifetal HLA antigen formation and occurrence of PIH. Indeed, women with PIH exhibit reduced HLA antibody formation and increased HLA compatibility with their sexual partners.[51] Although there is no particular relationship between maternal HLA typing and the occurrence of PIH, Redman and associates found that women with PIH are more likely to be homozygous for HLA-B than are normal women.[52] They proposed that, when associated with HLA-B homozygosity, the defect could lie in a recessive immune response gene linked to HLA.

Other researchers have wondered whether PIH is associated with an increase in circulating immune complexes. If maternal antibody response to fetal antigen were deficient, or the antigen burden excessive, pathologic immune complexes formed as a consequence could produce vasculitis, glomerular changes, and alterations in the coagulation system like those seen in PIH. However, most investigators have been unable to identify circulating immune complexes in women with PIH.[53,54]

In addition to there being evidence of a possible histocompatibility basis, and hence a genetic basis, for PIH, it has long been observed that a familial factor can contribute to the incidence of the disorder. Sutherland and associates proposed that the maternal genotype is even more important than fetal antigens to immunologic processes that could contribute to severe PIH.[55] Other investigators have found that a paternal factor, presumably immunologic in nature, occasionally appears to exert a potent influence.[56] Other features of PIH also lend themselves to immunologic analysis. Occasionally, offspring of preeclamptic women exhibit features of their mothers' syndrome; in the case of thrombocytopenia, for instance, it may be that the preeclamptic mother's platelet consumption may have an immunologic basis and that the infant who also suffers from thrombocytopenia may be a victim of the same immunologic attack.[57]

PATHOPHYSIOLOGY

Mild Pregnancy-Induced Hypertension

The precise sequence in which PIH evolves is not well established, but a reasonable surmise is that the process begins with vasospasm, which then leads to reduced blood flow to the uterus and other organs, reduced intravascular volume, and ultimately, hypertension.

Vasospasm

All observers concur that vasospasm is invariably present in women with PIH. The circumstantial evidence is probably sufficient to warrant the conclusion. As is discussed below, women with PIH are routinely found to have reduced perfusion of the uterus, kidneys, and other organs. It is difficult to conceive of a mechanism other than vasospasm by which compromise in organ perfusion occurs in hypertensive persons who have normal cardiac output. Numerous observers have directly observed arteriolar constriction in the retinas, conjunctiva, and nailbeds of women with PIH. Retinal examination is an especially helpful way to differentiate

between PIH and chronic hypertension. Vascular tortuosity, angiosclerosis (*e.g.*, copper or silver wire effect and arteriovenous nicking), hemorrhage, and exudates may be seen in subjects with long-standing chronic disease; in contrast, arteriolar constriction is the sole retinal finding in more than 80% of women with PIH. Retinal edema is far less common, and hemorrhages and exudates are found in under 2% of women with PIH.

Retinal vasospasm, the most commonly cited direct evidence of arteriolar constriction in women with PIH, is a late development in the evolution of PIH. Retinal changes are often undetectable until the blood pressure exceeds 150/100 mm Hg or so, and the degree of arteriolar constriction generally parallels the clinical severity of the syndrome. Nevertheless, the reasons for postulating that vasospasm is an early and progressive feature of PIH are that (1) it clearly appears at some point in the development of the disease, (2) it is a logical early consequence of increasing vascular sensitivity (loss of refractoriness) to A-II (see Fig. 26-1), and (3) evidence of reduced organ perfusion precedes the appearance of hypertension.

Reduced Uterine and Renal Blood Flow

Intervillous perfusion is reduced in women with PIH, not only owing to vasospasm. Over 30 years ago Zeek and Assali described in the decidual spiral arterioles of women with preeclampsia a morphologic alteration that markedly narrows the arteriolar lumen (Fig. 26-4).[58] The combination of vasospasm and intimal atherosis in women with PIH leads to a reduction in intervillous perfusion to about 35% to 50% of normal, a decrement that is typically found regardless of the severity of the PIH.[59]

One technique of assessing intervillous perfusion involves measuring the volume of blood cleared of dehydroepiandrosterone sulfate (DHAS) in the placenta for estradiol (E_2) synthesis. Measurements of the placental clearance of DHAS by this route (PC DS-E2) provide evidence that during the first half of two thirds of pregnancy, women who develop PIH have normal, or even greater than normal, intervillous perfusion, but that as sensitivity to A-II becomes more intense, intervillous perfusion declines to 35% to 50% of normal about two to four weeks before hypertension is detectable. Unfortunately, clinical improvement, such as may result from bed rest, is accompanied neither by improved intervillous perfusion as reflected in the PC DS-E2,[59] nor by an increase in refractoriness to A-II.[60] There must be relatively enormous placental reserve for fetuses of women with PIH to tolerate an insult of this magnitude as well as they commonly do. However, further reductions in intervillous blood flow—as produced by diuretic therapy, antihypertensive treatment, or conduction anesthesia—could well cause serious fetal jeopardy. Impaired intervillous perfusion is certainly the main cause of perinatal illness and death associated with hypertension complicating pregnancy.[61]

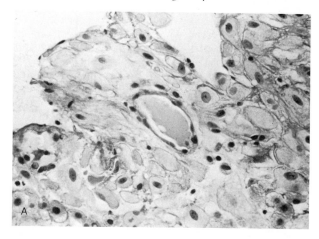

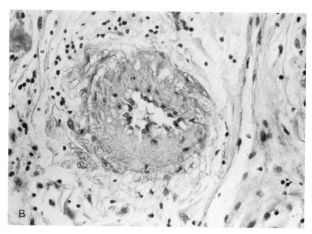

FIG. 26-4. The impact of PIH on decidual spiral arterioles. (*A*) Photomicrograph of a spiral arteriole in the decidua of a normotensive primigravida who underwent cesarean section at term because of dystocia. (*B*) Photomicrograph of a spiral arteriole in the decidua of a primigravida with PIH who underwent cesarean section in the 37th week of pregnancy because of fetal distress. Note the considerable compromise in vascular lumen caused by prominent atherosis.

Blood flow through the kidneys is also often reduced in women with PIH, as reflected in measurements of endogenous creatinine clearance. More specific and sensitive measurements provide evidence that renal plasma flow is typically reduced about 20% (para-aminohippurate clearance) and glomerular filtration about 30% (inulin clearance). As shown in Figure 26-5, however, the compromise can be severe.

Proteinura, defined as the excretion of 500 mg or more protein per 24 hours, is another reflection of renal involvement in PIH. Proteinuria is widely accepted as a late development in the evolution of PIH. There is no useful selectivity to the distribution of the proteins that escape the compromised kidney, making detailed analysis of the excreted proteins of no help in differentiating PIH from other potential causes of proteinuria. The amount of protein in the urine, when present, generally reflects the severity of the PIH. The perinatal mortality rate is higher in cases of PIH with proteinuria than in cases of PIH without proteinuria. Urinary excretion of more than 5 g protein per day in a patient with PIH is a sign of severe preeclampsia.

Reduced Intravascular Volume

Women with PIH are commonly found to have reduced blood volume, especially late in the progression of the disease. The development is expressed clinically as hemoconcentration and is identified by a rising hematocrit level. In cases of severe PIH, it is not uncommon for the blood volume to be 10% to 20% less than nonpregnant values. It is not entirely clear whether the decrease in blood volume precedes, coincides with, or follows the onset of hypertension, but it seems probable that it precedes the hypertension. If PIH occurs as a consequence of relentless loss of vascular refractoriness to vasoconstrictive agents (see Fig. 26-1), it is plausible that in a late phase of the vasoconstriction that results, blood pressure control could still be maintained, at least transiently, by a reduction in intravascular volume. Indeed, the hematocrit commonly rises during the days before overt PIH appears, reflecting passage of crystalloid from intravascular to extravascular spaces, and as a consequence, the edema characteristic of preeclampsia makes its appearance. Another correlate of this flux is rapid weight gain, a phenomenon that is commonly observed shortly before the appearance of PIH. The weight gain presumably results from the combination of already compromised glomerular perfusion and the passage of a substantial volume of fluid into extravascular spaces, from which it cannot readily circulate to the kidneys for excretion.

Hypertension

After an often long-standing, progressive increase in sensitivity to vasoactive agents, the consequent vasospasm, and ultimately a decrease in intravascular volume, hypertension ensues. The clinical challenge is great. Although the intravascular compartment of the woman with PIH is typically diminished in volume, the presence of hypertension argues persuasively that the compartment is not underfilled. Regimens of intravascular volume expansion for PIH have not been shown to provide lasting therapeutic benefit, and they increase the risk of pulmonary edema. Nor is pharmacologic reduction of blood pressure appropriate unless the degree of acute hypertension threatens the mother's health. The clinician is confronted by a pregnancy in which the mother has acute hypertension and the fetus is jeopardized by reduced intervillous perfusion. The evidence is abundant that most methods lowering the blood pressure also further lower intervillous perfusion and do not reverse the pathophysiology of PIH. Given that by definition the hypertension of mild PIH (<160/110 mm

Hg) does not normally constitute an acute threat to the mother, authorities concur that antihypertensive and diuretic therapy are contraindicated for mild PIH (see the section on Management below).

Placental Complications

PIH predisposes to certain placental problems. First, the placenta may fail to grow properly and remain abnormally small. Second, there may be reduced function in a normally developed placenta owing to decreased blood flow. Abruptio placentae occurs in 2% to 10% of cases, depending on the severity of the disease.

Severe Pregnancy-Induced Hypertension

PIH is regarded as severe when one or more of the following is found:

Blood pressure of at least 160 mm Hg systolic or 110 mm Hg diastolic on two occasions at least six hours apart while the patient is on bed rest
Proteinuria of at least 5 g per 24 hours, or 3+ to 4+ by semiquantitative assay
Oliguria (24-hour urinary output less than 400 ml)
Cerebral or visual disturbances, such as altered consciousness, headache, scotomata, or blurred vision
Pulmonary edema or cyanosis
Thrombocytopenia or markedly deranged liver function

Understandably, the threat of severe PIH to both the fetus and the mother is greater than that of mild PIH. The threat to the mother is so much increased, however, as to become an overriding factor in management (see below). The risk of eclampsia rises, as do the hazards of cardiac, pulmonary, cerebral, hepatic, and coagulation disorders. In some ways severe PIH constitutes simply a worse form of mild PIH; the hypertension is more severe, the renal involvement more profound, and intervillous perfusion more compromised. In other respects, however, the features of severe PIH often differ entirely from those seen in the milder syndrome.

Hypertension

Blood pressure elevation in severe PIH constitutes an acute threat to the mother. Pressures higher than 200/140 mm Hg are occasionally encountered. Cerebral hemorrhage and cardiac decompensation are potential complications of such blood pressure elevations. Anesthesia becomes difficult to provide safely.

Cardiac and Pulmonary Complications

Heart failure, one of the most common causes of maternal death due to PIH, is rarely encountered in young, otherwise healthy women despite the severity of PIH. In the older gravida, however, heart failure can

be a devastating complication, especially if the hypertension is difficult to bring under control. Elderly multiparas who have experienced repeated hypertensive pregnancies also occasionally fall prey to a condition described as circulatory collapse, which consists of an abrupt decrease in systolic blood pressure by 70 mm Hg or more and clinical evidence of shock. Circulatory collapse may occur either before or during labor, but it most often has been reported a few hours after delivery. Many cases of a few decades ago were associated with profound electrolyte depletion resulting from injudicious restriction of sodium intake and prescription of saliuretic drugs. As many as 10% of women with severe preeclampsia who develop circulatory collapse die as a result.

Pulmonary edema is another serious complication of severe PIH. Fortunately, it is rare, probably less common among preeclamptic women than seizures. The cause of pulmonary edema in untreated patients is unknown, but it is reasonable to presume that the generalized edema of advanced PIH may also occur in the pulmonary interstitium. Differentiation of pulmonary edema due to PIH from pulmonary edema associated with organic heart disease can be difficult. Typically, however, women with pulmonary edema due to PIH have severe generalized edema, whereas those with edema due to heart disease do not. Electrocardiographic tracings are typically normal in women with PIH who have the syndrome but show characteristic abnormalities in patients with heart disease. Pulmonary edema is a far more common complication of the treatment provided for severe PIH than it is of the hypertensive syndrome itself. Protracted oxytocin administration, fluid administration to compensate for sympathetic blockade resulting from conduction anesthesia, or overreplacement of fluid losses at cesarean section are typical causes of iatrogenic intravenous fluid overload. Pulmonary edema and congestive heart failure are virtually the only accepted indications for diuretic therapy during pregnancy.

Cerebral Involvement

Vascular resistance in the brain is unaltered during normal pregnancy but is increased by about 50% in patients with PIH. Given that there is little evidence that cerebral blood flow is substantially reduced in either preeclamptic or eclamptic women, it appears that for most patients the hypertension is sufficient to overcome the increased cerebrovascular resistance. However, for some women the hypertension is too much, and in these cases cerebral hemorrhage ensues. One of the most common causes of maternal death due to PIH, cerebral hemorrhage is best avoided by adequate control of severe hypertension.

Some patients with severe PIH may experience cerebral edema, which perhaps occurs by the same mechanism as pulmonary or generalized edema. Headache, altered consciousness, scotomata, and blurred vision are

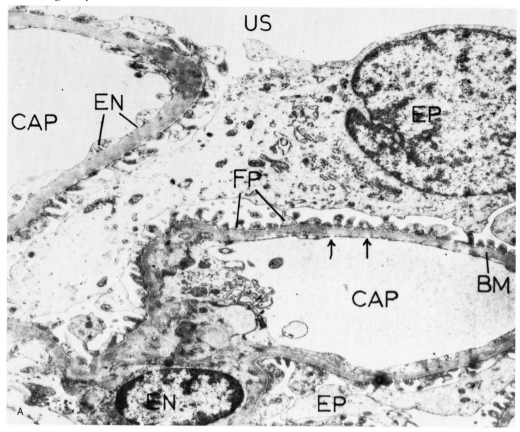

FIG. 26-5. (*A*) Normal glomerular capillary from 25-year-old man demonstrating capillary lumen (*CAP*), endothelium (*EN*), basement membrane (*BM*), foot processes (*FP*), epithelium (*EP*), and urinary space (*US*). (×10,000) (*B*) Glomerular loop from a patient with preeclampsia. Pronounced swelling has greatly restricted capillary lumen (*CAP*). Fibrinoid (*fib*) is present between endothelium (*END*) and basement membrane (*BM*) (subendothelial location) and to some extent between endothelial cells (interendothelial location). Epithelial foot processes (*fp*) and basement membrane appear essentially normal. *EP*, epithelium; *RBC*, red blood cell. (×11,500) (Hopper J, Farquhar MG, Yamauchi H et al: Obstet Gynecol 17:271, 1961)

typical symptoms of cerebral edema. They also typically presage eclampsia.

Impaired Liver Function

Liver function is impaired in women with PIH more commonly than is often thought. The degree to which the liver is affected is proportional to the severity of the disease. Chesley collated the data from numerous reports (Table 26-1) and computed that half of women with severe PIH have an increased serum glutamic oxaloacetic transaminase (SGOT) concentration.[62] A variety of liver function tests and circulating enzyme concentrations may be deranged in women with severe PIH. I have seen a mother's serum bilirubin concentration as high as 14 mg/dl due to severe preeclampsia. As ominous as these findings may seem, the figures revert to normal rapidly once the severe preeclampsia is treated by delivering of the fetus.

Coagulopathy

For almost a century, students of PIH have debated whether the condition is a result of or results in disseminated intravascular coagulation (DIC). One rarely sees DIC in women with PIH, and there is no good evidence that the coagulopathy causes the hypertensive syndrome. Pritchard and co-workers studied indices of DIC in nearly 100 eclamptic women and rarely found hypofibrinogenemia or fibrin products (Table 26-2).[63] Thrombocytopenia was the most common coagulation abnormality they found; the platelet count was lower than 150,000 in 25% of the patients. Other researchers have confirmed this general pattern of altered coagulation factors in PIH,[64] which is most typically one of a selective reduction in platelet count without a significant alteration of other factors. The findings suggest that microangiopathy, not DIC, is involved in PIH. Microangiopathic thrombocytopenia is the consequence of abnormal in-

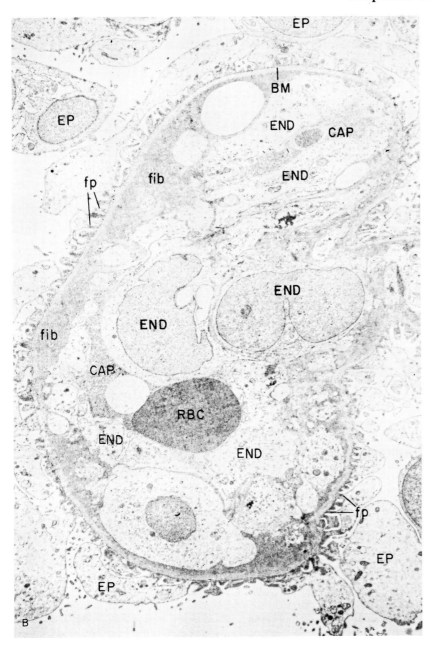

Fig. 26-5. (*Continued*)

Table 26-1
Serum Glutamic Oxaloacetic Transaminase Concentration Late in Pregnancy in Normal and Hypertensive Subjects

	Normal Pregnancy	Mild Preeclampsia	Severe Preeclampsia	Eclampsia
Cases	269	148	131	50
Number elevated	9	35	66	42
Percentage	3.3	23.6	50.3	84

(After Chesley LC: Hypertensive Disorders in Pregnancy, p 268. Norwalk, CT, Appleton-Century-Crofts, 1978)

Table 26-2
*Measurements of Coagulation Factors That Imply
Intravascular Coagulation in Women with Eclampsia*

Factor	Number	Percentage of Total
Plasma fibrinogen		
< 250 mg/dl	7/92	7.6
Fibrin degradation products		
> 16 μg/ml	2/65	3
Fibrin monomer	1/20	5
Platelet count < 150,000	28/95	29.5

(After Pritchard JA, Cunningham FG, Mason RA: Coagulation changes in eclampsia: Their frequency and pathogenesis. Am J Obstet Gynecol 124: 855, 1976)

teraction between platelets and vascular endothelium,[65] an interaction that could be produced by defective PGI2 generation.

Whether as the consequence of disrupted vascular endothelium or of deficient PGI2 formation or of both, platelet consumption is becoming widely recognized as a more common feature of severe PIH than many clinicians have suspected. It is difficult to propose a figure for the incidence of this phenomenon, but it is fair to say that it occurs in a substantial minority of women with severe preeclampsia. When present, thrombocytopenia must be recognized as a sign of severe PIH, regardless of the degree of hypertension, and treated accordingly. Thrombocytopenia in preeclamptic women is often accompanied by hemolysis and deranged liver function, reflecting the trauma that microangiopathy inflicts on erythrocytes and the compromise in organ function (in this case, of the liver) that impaired perfusion produces.[66]

Eclampsia

The pathophysiology of eclampsia is almost as unclear as the etiology of PIH in general. Women who develop eclampsia may have any or many of the possible signs of severe preeclampsia. In addition, they may have one or more major motor seizures. Most likely, eclampsia ultimately results from cerebral vasospasm or cerebral edema.

Sheehan and Lynch attribute eclampsia principally to cerebral vasospasm.[67] It is plausible that vasospasm in a variety of tissues is more intense in women with severe than in women with mild forms of PIH, and the brain could be one of those tissues. The heart could be another; coronary artery spasm may also be an important cause of maternal death from eclampsia.[68] Arterial spasm sufficient to cause death when it occurs in the heart should also be sufficient to produce a seizure when it occurs in the brain. Although, as noted above, cerebral

blood flow in eclamptic women is not markedly lower (only about 5%) than in normal or preeclamptic gravidas, cerebral oxygen consumption is about 20% lower. It is not clear, however, whether this decrement in cerebral oxygen utilization leads to or results from the convulsions.

Over seventy years ago Zangemeister concluded that cerebral edema is the cause of eclampsia.[69] He opened the skulls of three living eclamptic women (!) and found the dura to be tense and hard. When he opened the dura, large amounts of fluid escaped and the convulsions subsided. Indeed, with the modern technique of computed tomographic (CT) scanning, substantial cerebral edema has been identified in some eclamptic women.[70,71] The characteristic picture is one of symmetrically reduced density of the intracranial capsules coupled with marked, symmetric compression of the ventricles. Cerebral edema is the likely cause of the infrequent, profound central nervous system dysfunction that may persist for several days after eclamptic seizures, then resolves rapidly, and often completely.[71] An extension of this central process of edema is thought to produce the occasional case of transient blindness that is associated with eclampsia.[70]

MANAGEMENT

The management of PIH is based on severity of the hypertensive syndrome and duration of the pregnancy in question. The guidelines are presented in Table 26-3.

Pregnancy-Induced or Chronic Hypertension at Term

The management of PIH or chronic hypertension when the fetus is mature is straightforward, especially when the patient presents in labor. When the condition is found in the office and the patient is not in labor, one should typically hospitalize the woman and prepare to deliver the fetus. This injunction applies to any woman with PIH who has a mature fetus. In that circumstance there is no further advantage to prolonging the pregnancy, and to do so only incurs the risk that the PIH will worsen, perhaps to the point of eclampsia.

The condition can be frustrating to manage, however, when the patient's cervix is not favorable for induction of labor and the severity of disease does not warrant prompt delivery at all costs. Such a patient with truly mild disease who nevertheless continues to be hypertensive in the hospital is best managed by continued surveillance and reappraisal in the hospital until labor can be induced successfully. The woman whose PIH becomes normotensive in the hospital may, as the next best alternative, be managed with bed rest at home until the cervix ripens, providing that a family member or friend is available to record her blood pressure at least twice daily and return her to the office if hypertension recurs.

Table 26-3
Management of Hypertension Complicating Pregnancy

Clinical Condition	Therapy
PIH (or chronic hypertension) when the fetus is mature	Definitive 1. Prevent convulsions 2. Control blood pressure 3. Deliver fetus
PIH (or chronic hypertension) when the fetus is premature but there is 1. Severe preeclampsia (or superimposed preeclampsia) 2. Fetal growth retardation 3. Fetal jeopardy	Definitive 1. Prevent convulsions 2. Control blood pressure 3. Deliver fetus
Eclampsia, whether the fetus is mature or premature	Definitive 1. Treat convulsions 2. Control blood pressure 3. Stabilize mother 4. Deliver fetus
PIH or chronic hypertension when the fetus is premature	Expectant 1. Ambulatory treatment 2. Hospitalization
Hypertension in the first 20 weeks	Dependent on severity

In the absence of superimposed PIH, the patient with mild chronic hypertension whose cervix is not ripe for induction can usually be followed successfully as an outpatient until labor is inducible. It is anticipated that in the near future the problem of the unripe cervix can be remedied by the application of prostaglandin E2 suppositories or gels, which are presently undergoing clinical trials.

Sometimes a clear decision to deliver the fetus is frustrated by uncertainty about the length of gestation. As indicated in the following section, if the syndrome is severe one should most always deliver the fetus promptly regardless of the duration of the pregnancy. If the disease is mild, however, and the dates are uncertain, one may choose to manage the patient with carefully supervised bed rest until spontaneous labor occurs, try to ascertain the duration of gestation sonographically, or base the decision for delivery on analysis of amniotic fluid indices of fetal lung maturity. Often the best plan is careful surveillance until labor ensues. Ultrasonic estimation of pregnancy duration is notoriously less accurate late in pregnancy than earlier, and it may be difficult to differentiate between a premature fetus and one afflicted with intrauterine growth retardation. Sometimes the results of amniotic fluid analysis are of great help in reaching a clinical decision, but only in selected circumstances. Amniocentesis is never the first order of business in developing a plan of management for PIH.

In preparing the patient for delivery it is imperative to perform a thorough physical examination, even when the physician has cared for the woman throughout her entire course. All too often the mistake is made of equating the degree of hypertension with the extent of systemic pathophysiology. This is a dangerous and erroneous assumption. No matter how mild the hypertension is, intervillous perfusion is already compromised, and any women with PIH, no matter how mild, can develop eclampsia. The lungs should be auscultated for evidence of pulmonary edema. The right upper quadrant of the abdomen should be palpated to detect liver tenderness. The biophysical indicators of fetal well-being should be studied by application of an external monitor, and the status of the cervix should be verified. Examination of the ankle and patellar reflexes rarely provides a clue to impending eclampsia. Many pregnant women exhibit hyperactive reflexes during labor even though they have no evidence of PIH. Nevertheless, any woman with PIH who has sustained ankle clonus, or any patient who is obviously tremulous or obtunded, should be treated promptly for imminent eclampsia.

Laboratory studies to be obtained for the laboring woman who has PIH include a hematocrit, a urinalysis, a chemistry profile, and a platelet count. It is advisable at least to have the patient's ABO and Rh blood types verified, her blood screened for antibodies, and type-specific blood made available in the blood bank should it be needed. A serum fibrinogen assay is unnecessary unless abruptio placentae is suspected. The hematocrit is an important means of identifying evidence of hemoconcentration, which must be considered in any decision about fluid replacement during the puerperium. The urinalysis will of course reveal proteinuria, if present. It may also provide evidence of unsuspected conditions such as hemoglobinuria, almost surely a reflection of microangiopathic hemolysis and hence of advanced PIH. If the count is below about 50,000/mm³, the wisdom of platelet transfusion should be considered in light of the anticipated route of delivery.

Magnesium Sulfate Therapy

Labor is the most likely time for eclampsia to occur. Hence, all laboring women with PIH should receive prophylaxis against eclamptic convulsions. Magnesium sulfate is the preferred agent for this purpose. It typically prevents or controls the seizures of eclampsia without sedating the mother, which barbiturates, tranquilizers, and narcotics do; as a result, it makes airway problems and aspiration of stomach contents less likely than do these other agents. Moreover, magnesium sulfate does not further compromise the already jeopardized fetus, in contrast to barbiturates or diazepam, which in anticonvulsant doses may have depressant fetal effects. Diphenylhydantoin, the major anticonvulsant used for prophylaxis of epileptic seizures, has too slow an onset of action to be of use in preventing or treating eclampsia.

Magnesium sulfate must be given parenterally. One may elect either an intramuscular or an intravenous regimen. The intramuscular regimen is probably safer, requiring less attention by the nursing staff and less experience on the part of the physician. The intramuscular regimen used for prophylaxis consists of 10 ml of 50% magnesium sulfate (5 g) injected deeply into the upper outer quadrant of each buttock through a 3-inch, 20-gauge needle; this provides a 10-g loading dose. The patient who complains of headache, scotomata, or other visual disturbances or who has ankle clonus also receives a 4-g loading dose intravenously (see the section on Eclampsia below). The patient is evaluated for maintenance treatment every 4 hours after administration of the loading dose. If her respiratory rate is not depressed (12/minute or greater), the patellar reflex is present, and urinary output during the preceding four hours has been at least 100 ml, 10 ml of 50% magnesium sulfate (5 g) is given intramuscularly in alternating buttocks. To reduce the local discomfort of injection, 1 ml of 2% lidocaine may be drawn into the syringe after it is loaded with the 50% magnesium sulfate solution. If six or more hours lapse between maintenance doses, anticonvulsant therapy should be reinstituted with the full 10-g loading dose.

The normal concentration of magnesium in serum is 1.5 mEq/liter to 2 mEq/liter. When 10 g of magnesium sulfate is administered intramuscularly, the plasma concentration rises progressively during the first one to two hours to a concentration of about 3.5 mEq/liter to 6 mEq/liter and, in the absence of further injections, declines to the preinjection level over about six hours. The intramuscular injection of 10 g of magnesium sulfate followed by 5 g every four hours usually stabilizes the serum magnesium concentration at about 4 mEq/liter to 7 mEq/liter. In the experiences of both Chesley[72]

and Pritchard,[73] this regimen is safe for all hypertensive pregnant women, even those with impaired renal function, provided that the aforementioned precautions are taken before the administration of each maintenance dose every 4 hours. Because of the discomfort of the intramuscular injections, many institutions prefer to use the continuous intravenous route of administration; nevertheless, the intramuscular regimen is both safer and efficacious.

If magnesium sulfate is given by continuous intravenous infusion, one should administer the agent in 5% dextrose in water through an infusion pump. At our institution we begin with an infusion rate of 2 g/hour. If the solution is prepared by the addition of 10 g magnesium sulfate (20 ml of 50% solution) to 500 ml dextrose in water, the appropriate initial infusion rate is 100 ml/hour. Slower rates of fluid administration can be achieved, if necessary, by the preparation of more concentrated solutions of magnesium sulfate. A therapeutic level of magnesium can be achieved more rapidly if a 4-g loading dose is given before the intravenous infusion is started. This amount is contained in 20 ml of 20% magnesium sulfate, or in 8 ml of 50% solution. If the latter is used, it should be diluted with sterile water to a volume of 20 ml for intravenous administration. The loading dose should be injected over about a 3-minute period. For reasons that are not entirely clear, women who receive magnesium sulfate intravenously sometimes seem to require more of the agent per unit of time than women who receive it intramuscularly.[74] For this reason, beginning about two hours after the infusion is started, the serum magnesium concentration should be measured periodically during intravenous therapy to ensure that the level is appropriate. The therapeutic range of serum magnesium concentration for anticonvulsant purposes is between 4 mEq/liter and 7 mEq/liter, more than twice the normal concentration (1.5–2 mEq/liter). If the measured concentration falls outside the therapeutic range, appropriate adjustments in the infusion rate must be made.

Excessive accumulation of magnesium can be fatal. As the concentration rises above 7 mEq/liter, signs of toxicity appear. The patellar reflex disappears at magnesium concentrations of 7 mEq/liter to 10 mEq/liter. Respiratory depression, and later respiratory arrest, occur at levels of 10 mEq/liter to 15 mEq/liter. Finally, cardiac arrest ensues if the magnesium concentration reaches approximately 30 mEq/liter. The antidote for magnesium toxicity is calcium gluconate, 1 g given intravenously over 3 minutes. Administration of this antidote in combination with respiratory support nearly always leads to an uneventful recovery unless the magnesium concentration is high enough to cause cardiac arrest.

The importance of neither overtreating nor undertreating with magnesium sulfate cannot be overemphasized. It is mandatory to monitor the respiratory rate, urinary output, and patellar reflexes of every woman receiving the agent, regardless of the route employed, at least every four hours. It is always appropriate to monitor the serum magnesium concentration during intravenous therapy, and in cases of concern during intramuscular treatment as well. In typical circumstances magnesium administration can be safely discontinued 24 hours after delivery. If the patient remains severely preeclamptic, however, it is appropriate to continue the prophylaxis accordingly.

Antihypertensive Therapy

The antihypertensive effect of magnesium sulfate is at best transient, and in truth practically negligible. Thus, even when magnesium treatment is provided, one must monitor the patient's blood pressure carefully throughout labor to be sure that the hypertension has not become severe. As pointed out earlier in this chapter, because of the danger of further reducing intervillous perfusion, antihypertensive therapy is not given for PIH unless the hypertension constitutes an acute threat to the mother, and diuretics are never used except for pulmonary edema or congestive heart failure. The goal of antihypertensive therapy in the management of PIH at term is only to protect the mother's heart and brain long enough to get the baby delivered.

Antihypertensive therapy is indicated when the mother's blood pressure nears or exceeds 160/110 mm Hg. The goal is to lower the blood pressure to a mildly hypertensive level, such as a diastolic pressure between 90 mm Hg and 100 mm Hg. Hydralazine is the preferred agent. The initial dose should be 5 mg, given slowly by intravenous injection. The blood pressure should be recorded every 5 minutes after administration of the hydralazine. If suitable lowering does not occur within 20 minutes, 10 mg hydralazine should be given. The dose should be increased by 5 mg to 10 mg every 20 minutes until suitable control of blood pressure is achieved. A desirable blood pressure is usually reached after a total dose of 5 mg to 50 mg hydralazine has been given. A suitable dose is repeated whenever the diastolic blood pressure rises to 110 mm Hg or higher. Because hydralazine has a duration of action of several hours, adequate control of severe hypertension can often be achieved from one or two intravenous treatments. Also because of the long duration of action of the agent, continuous intravenous infusion can easily produce dangerous overlowering of blood pressure after a while.

Delivery

Labor, whether spontaneous or induced because of PIH, is commonly uneventful despite the compromise in intervillous perfusion. Because of possible fetal jeopardy, however, electronic fetal monitoring should be employed throughout the labor. Cesarean section is generally carried out according to standard obstetric indications. If labor cannot be successfully induced, the decision whether to deliver the fetus by cesarean section or attempt to induce labor at a later date is based on severity of the PIH.

Relief of pain during labor may be accomplished in either of two ways. The simplest approach is to give doses of meperidine or fentanyl intravenously every two to four hours as needed, then to administer a pudendal block for delivery. Alternatively, epidural analgesia may be provided. The epidural technique provides excellent relief of discomfort during labor and, especially when both lumbar and caudal catheters are inserted, highly satisfactory anesthesia for delivery and perineal repair. The block should be given and maintained by an anesthesiologist, however, especially one who is knowledgeable about PIH and experienced in giving conduction anesthesia to hypertensive patients.

The feared complication of conduction anesthesia in a woman with PIH is that the induced sympathetic blockade and consequent pooling of blood in the capacitance vasculature will lead to profound hypotension because of the already contracted blood volume. Severe fetal bradycardia commonly ensues in such instances. This complication can often be forestalled by infusion of crystalloid solution to expand intravascular volume before sympathetic blockade occurs. However, rapid expansion of blood volume in a woman with severe hypertension is not recommended; antepartum volume expansion is one of the most common preludes to pulmonary edema in preeclamptic women. Often the acute blood pressure drop from epidural analgesia can be avoided by unusually gradual induction of the block. When given by a knowledgeable, attentive anesthesiologist, epidural anesthesia can be an acceptable means of providing pain relief for the laboring woman with mild PIH.

Severe Pregnancy-Induced Hypertension Remote from Term

As reflected in Table 26-3, management of severe PIH remote from term does not differ from management of PIH at term, but the situation is decidedly different in that the fetus must be delivered for maternal reasons even though it is probably not mature. In general, the indication for early delivery is persistence of any of the features of severe preeclampsia, as defined earlier. There is some room for judgement, however. Pulmonary edema, cerebral symptoms, or worsening thrombocytopenia certainly forces the issue, but persistence only of substantial proteinuria without ominous hypertension or other features of severe preeclampsia does not always mandate early delivery. If fetal growth and development are appropriate as judged by an experienced ultrasonographer, results of the nonstress or other fetal heart rate tests are normal, and the mother is stable despite abundant proteinuria, one may elect not to deliver the fetus as long as the indices of fetal well-being are encouraging and the mother's clinical and laboratory findings do not worsen.

Oral antihypertensive therapy should not be instituted to prolong the pregnancy. Such therapy only serves to reduce intervillous perfusion further in women who have PIH. Antihypertensive medication should be given for severe PIH and only then to produce a modest reduction in blood pressure for the time necessary to deliver the fetus. Oral antihypertensive treatment during pregnancy is reserved for women with chronic hypertension (see below).

When PIH is particularly severe, especially in the absence of proteinuria, consideration should be given to the possibility that the disorder may be due to a cause other than pregnancy. Renal artery stenosis, pheochromocytoma, or heretofore occult lupus erythematosus is an unlikely diagnosis, but it is simple to auscultate over the kidneys for an arterial bruit, obtain urinary catecholamine assays, and search for antinuclear antibody. Most often, of course, one is dealing with PIH.

Even when severe preeclampsia necessitates early delivery, the infant's condition is often good. Offspring of hypertensive women commonly undergo accelerated lung maturation, so it is unusual for them to experience severe respiratory distress syndrome (RDS) even when they are delivered as early as the 32nd week. The earlier the delivery, of course, the greater is the risk of RDS. The most anguishing dilemma comes when one is confronted with severe PIH before the 28th week of gestation. Management must always be individualized, but delivery of the fetus is usually warranted.

In most ways, appropriate induction of labor and delivery for severe PIH remote from term is the same as that described for PIH at term. However, a few aspects of management of severe PIH, either at term or short of it, deserve additional emphasis. Because severe PIH is a more urgent indication for delivery than is mild PIH, the delivery should usually be carried out within 24 to 48 hours of the decision to end the pregnancy. Hence, a vigorous approach to induction of labor is appropriate. Insertion of laminaria should be considered if the cervix is not ripe, and early amniotomy is often appropriate. The hypertension may be hard to bring under control, but one should make every reasonable effort to succeed with the hydralazine regimen recommended earlier. Hydralazine is the only agent suitable for lowering the blood pressure acutely that has been shown not to further lower intervillous perfusion; in fact, the drug may even produce an increase in placental blood flow.[75] Ultimately it may be necessary to give 20 mg or more per injection to control severe PIH, but the alternatives are clearly less attractive. Diazoxide produces often catastrophic fetal compromise,[76,77] and nitroprusside can theoretically cause cyanide toxicity in the fetus.[78]

Used judiciously, however, a nitroprusside drip may be the next best choice when hydralazine is inadequate to control a hypertensive crisis.[79] At many institutions, women with severe preeclampsia are usually not given epidural block analgesia, so if cesarean section is performed, general anesthesia is required. Women with severe PIH commonly exhibit frightening increases in blood pressure during the process of endotracheal intubation. To guard against a hypertensive catastrophe in this situation, some practitioners begin a nitroprusside infusion just before intubation in order to control the anticipated surge in blood pressure. Since the infant is usually delivered with a short time of intubation, toxic levels of nitroprusside do not occur.

Because blood volume may be markedly contracted in severely preeclamptic women, crystalloid replacement and blood transfusion, when indicated, may be difficult to manage safely. Placement of a Swan–Ganz catheter is often helpful[80] but not always required. In fact, subclavian catheterization may be contraindicated by thrombocytopenia, as may be placement of an epidural catheter. In this circumstance central blood pressure monitoring, if incorporated, must be accomplished by antecubital insertion. Platelet transfusion is of course indicated if thrombocytopenia is severe.

Eclampsia

Most of the principles of treating eclampsia are contained in the two previous sections. The first orders of business are to turn the patient on her side, administer 4 g magnesium sulfate intravenously over about a 3-minute period, establish an airway after the seizure ceases, and then institute maintenance magnesium therapy. If convulsions recur within about 20 minutes of initial treatment, the patient should receive an additional 2 g magnesium sulfate intravenously if she is small or of average size, 4 g if she is large. In the exceptional circumstance in which convulsions still persist, a slow intravenous injection of up to 250 mg sodium amobarbital should control the seizures. In this case the obstetrician must warn the pediatrician who is to care for the infant that the barbiturate was given so proper care can be provided for the neonate, who may suffer from central or respiratory depression.

One should neither deliver the fetus immediately following an eclamptic seizure, by cesarean section, for instance, nor delay in taking appropriate steps to terminate the pregnancy in a timely fashion. Eclamptic seizures produce a marked metabolic insult to both the mother and the fetus. Induction of anesthesia and performance of major surgery during this time can be disastrous for both patients. Instead it is best to allow a period of roughly three to six hours to pass before taking steps to deliver the infant. In general, once the mother becomes responsive and oriented after her seizure, it is reasonable to presume sufficient recovery has taken place that one can proceed safely.

During this period of stabilization, intense clinical observation is necessary. Pulmonary edema, prolonged coma, hyperthermia, and marked oliguria worsen the prognosis. A weak, rapid pulse, lowered blood pressure, and pulmonary rales suggest circulatory failure, for which rapid digitalization and probably diuresis with furosemide are indicated. If unilateral neurologic signs or prolonged coma ensues, neurologic consultation and contrast-enhanced CT scanning of the brain are warranted.[70,71,81] Fluids should be infused intravenously at a rate sufficient to replace the sum of measured and insensible loss, usually between 60 and 120 mg/hour. We typically use 5% dextrose in water and lactated Ringer's solution in alternating fashion.

Mild Hypertension Remote from Term

After Midpregnancy

Mild PIH or chronic hypertension occurring during the latter half of pregnancy but before the fetus is mature is best managed by at least brief hospitalization of the mother, then surveillance and reduced physical activity either until the fetus is mature or until the PIH worsens and mandates delivery. The reason for hospitalizing most such patients is to ensure that the hypertension abates with bed rest and to have the patient under close scrutiny long enough to conclude that she is not in the throes of fulminating PIH that could progress rapidly to eclampsia. Sometimes overnight hospitalization is all that is required. About 80% of such patients become normotensive in response to bed rest, and in a similar percentage of cases delivery can be deferred safely until the fetus is mature.[82]

Once the physician is satisfied that the disease is mild and responsive to bed rest, the patient can usually be discharged safely to rest at home. There should be no special dietary restrictions. A family member, friend, or visiting nurse should record the patient's blood pressure once or twice daily and notify the physician if it rises significantly, such as to 140/90 mm Hg or more. Each day the patient should record her weight and urinary protein reaction according to a paper strip indicator. Her activity should largely be limited to bed rest and lounging around the house; someone else should do the housework and shopping. The physician should usually see the patient in the office each week, but in selected instances perhaps even less often if he is comfortable with periodic telephone reports. Indications for delivery in patients managed this way are fetal maturity, fetal distress, or progression to severe PIH, however far along the pregnancy.

In the First Half of Pregnancy

As pointed out in the introduction to this chapter, mild chronic hypertension sometimes has no discernible adverse effects on pregnancy, but when superimposed PIH ensues, the consequences are often severe. Unfortunately, there is no good evidence that the manner in which mild chronic hypertension is managed early in pregnancy affects the incidence, time of appearance, or intensity of superimposed PIH. In particular, there is no evidence that prophylactic antihypertensive therapy forestalls superimposed PIH, but it is conventional wisdom to recommend the regimen of rest at home described in the previous section throughout

at least the second half of pregnancy for women with mild chronic hypertension.

Prophylaxis of Pregnancy-Induced Hypertension

Prevention is the best treatment of any disease. It is not presently possible to prevent or deter PIH with great reliability, but some advances have been made. The reader is referred elsewhere for an analysis of this subject.[83] An accurate, clinically practicable means of identifying women who are likely to develop PIH later in pregnancy, and a useful method of deterring or ameliorating the disease, would be of enormous benefit.

POSTPARTUM MATERNAL MANAGEMENT AND PROGNOSIS

PIH typically resolves promptly after the infant and placenta are delivered. Even when the disease is severe, mother and child often are able to leave the hospital two or three days after vaginal delivery or at the customary time after cesarean section. As stated earlier, magnesium sulfate prophylaxis usually should be provided for 24 hours postpartum. One exception is the patient with mild disease who rapidly becomes normotensive after delivery and remains so for eight consecutive hours; for such a patient it is probably safe to discontinue the prophylaxis. Another exception is the patient whose PIH remains severe or worsens during the first 24 hours postpartum; in this case it is wise to continue the prophylaxis even longer. The likelihood of a seizure in such a patient is remote but not unheard of.

Occasionally hypertension remains severe and difficult to control after delivery. Now that the infant is no longer *in utero,* a wider array of therapies may be used to treat the mother. If necessary, for instance, diazoxide could be given without fear for its effects on the fetus. Instead, at our institution, severe hypertension that either does not respond to hydralazine or continues to require its administration after 18 to 24 hours postpartum is often treated with clonidine. One can administer 0.1 mg to 0.2 mg of the agent orally every hour until the blood pressure is controlled, then prescribe roughly the total amount required in divided doses on subsequent days. If suitable control is achieved with a total dose of 0.4 mg, for instance, the expected maintenance dose would be about 0.2 mg every 12 hours. It is our practice to discharge without antihypertensive treatment women whose blood pressure remains elevated but is less than about 160/110 mm Hg after delivery. The blood pressure should be monitored every week or two for about a month. If hypertension persists, further evaluation and care are in order.

The occurrence of PIH raises two important questions about contraception and prognosis: Does the disorder contraindicate oral contraception? Is the patient predisposed to recurrence of hypertension in a subsequent pregnancy?

PIH does not contraindicate oral contraception as long as the patient has become normotensive by the time the pill is prescribed, typically between the fourth and sixth weeks postpartum. Freedom to use oral contraceptives extends even to women who suffer eclampsia if they meet the above criteria. Women who develop pill-induced hypertension after experiencing PIH do so with about the same frequency as never-hypertensive women of comparable age. Pill-induced hypertension following PIH is often a reflection of underlying chronic vascular disease or essential hypertension.[84]

In general, the patient is not predisposed to recurrence of hypertension in a subsequent pregnancy if she has experienced the so-called pure form of PIH, which typically occurs only in first pregnancies and does not coexist with other forms of hypertension or vasculorenal disease. However, the risk of recurrent hypertension during pregnancy is substantially increased in women who were normotensive in the first pregnancy but in whom PIH occurred in one or more subsequent pregnancies and in women who developed PIH both in their first pregnancies and in one or more subsequent pregnancies.[85]

Increased risk of hypertension complicating pregnancy does not necessarily mean that a patient should not undertake another pregnancy. As indicated earlier, some women with recurrent, mild forms of PIH negotiate pregnancy with little difficulty. However, in the following circumstances it is reasonable to counsel against another pregnancy and for sterilization:[86]

Severe PIH superimposed on chronic hypertension. The chance of repetition is about 70%, and the disorder tends to recur earlier and in more virulent fashion.

Chronically impaired renal function. The perinatal mortality rate can be as high as 40% to 80%, depending on the degree of impairment.

Severe chronic hypertension (diastolic blood pressure above 120 mmHg)

Old retinal exudates or fresh hemorrhages

Intrinsic cardiac disease characterized by cardiac enlargement or electrocardiographic indications of ischemia or heart strain, or a history of previous cardiac failure

Presence of a chronic, irreversible hypertensive disease severe enough to warrant pregnancy termination before fetal viability.

REFERENCES

1. Robertson EG: The natural history of oedema during pregnancy. J Obstet Gynaecol Br Commonw 78:520, 1971
2. Friedman EA, Neff RK: Pregnancy outcome as related to hypertension, edema, and proteinuria. In Lindheimer MD, Katz AI, Zuspan FP (eds): Hypertension in Pregnancy, p 13. New York, John Wiley & Sons, 1976
3. Chesley LC: Hypertensive disorders in pregnancy. In Hellman LM, Pritchard JA: Williams' Obstetrics, 14th ed, p 716. New York, Appleton-Century-Crofts, 1971
4. Dieckmann WJ, Michel HL: Vascular–renal effects of posterior pituitary extracts in pregnant women. Am J Obstet Gynecol 33:131, 1937
5. Abdul-Karim R, Assali NS: Pressor response to angiotensin in pregnant and nonpregnant women. Am J Obstet Gynecol 82:246, 1961
6. Gant NF, Daley GL, Chand S et al: A study of angiotensin II pressor responsiveness throughout primigravid pregnancy. J Clin Invest 52:2682, 1973
7. Kaplan NM, Silah JF: The effect of angiotensin II on the blood pressure in humans with hypertensive disease. J Clin Invest 43:659, 1964
8. Chinn RH, Düsterdieck G: The response of blood pressure to infusion of angiotensin II: Relation to plasma concentrations of renin and angiotensin II. Clin Sci 42:489, 1972
9. Gant NF, Worley RJ: Hypertension in Pregnancy. Concepts and Management, pp 16–25. New York, Appleton-Century-Crofts, 1980
10. Sullivan JM, Palmer EJ, Schoeneberger AA et al: SQ20881: Effect on eclamptic–preeclamptic women with postpartum hypertension. Am J Obstet Gynecol 131:707, 1978
11. Broughton Pipkin F, Turner SR, Symonds EM: Possible risk with captopril in pregnancy: Some animal data. Lancet 1:1256, 1980
12. Lindheimer MD, Katz AI: Kidney Function and Disease in Pregnancy, pp 188–221. Philadelphia, Lea & Febiger, 1977
13. Parker CR, Everett RB, Whalley PF et al: Hormone production during pregnancy in the primigravid patient: II. Plasma levels of deoxycorticosterone throughout pregnancy of normal women and women who developed pregnancy-induced hypertension. Am J Obstet Gynecol 138:626, 1980
14. Gant NF, Chand S, Whalley PJ, MacDonald PC: The nature of pressor responsiveness to angiotensin II in human pregnancy. Obstet Gynecol 43:854, 1974
15. Kuhnert BR, Kuhnert PM, Murray BA, Sokol RJ: Na/K and Mg-ATPase activity in the placenta and in maternal and cord erythrocytes of preeclamptic patients. Am J Obstet Gynecol 127:56, 1977
16. Canessa M, Adragna N, Solomon HS et al: Increased sodium–lithium countertransport in red cells of patients with essential hypertension. N Engl J Med 302:772, 1980
17. Worley RJ, Hentschell WM, Cormier C et al: Increased sodium–lithium countertransport in erythrocytes of pregnant women. N Engl J Med 307:412, 1982
18. Chesley LC: Hypertensive Disorders in Pregnancy, pp 302–306. New York, Appleton-Century-Crofts, 1978
19. Gant NF, Worley RJ: Hypertension in Pregnancy. Concepts and Management, pp 95–96. New York, Appleton-Century-Crofts, 1980
20. Mendlowitz M: Toxemia of pregnancy and eclampsia. Obstet Gynecol Surv 35:327, 1980
21. Belizan JM, Villar J, Zalazar A et al: Preliminary evidence of the effect of calcium supplementation on blood pressure in normal pregnant women. Am J Obstet Gynecol 146:175, 1983
22. McCarron DA, Morris CD, Cole C: Dietary calcium in human hypertension. Science 217:267, 1982
23. McCarron DA: Low serum concentrations of ionized calcium in patients with hypertension. N Engl J Med 307:226, 1982
24. Richards SR, Nelson DM, Zuspan FP: Calcium levels in normal and hypertensive pregnant patients. Am J Obstet Gynecol 149:168, 1984

25. Everett RB, Worley RJ, MacDonald PC, Gant NF: Effect of prostaglandin synthetase inhibitors on pressor response to angiotensin II in human pregnancy. J Clin Endocrinol Metab 46:1007, 1978

26. Zuckerman H, Reiss U, Rubinstein I: Inhibition of human premature labor by indomethacin. Obstet Gynecol 44:787, 1974

27. Everett RB, Worley RJ, MacDonald PC, Gant NF: Modification of vascular responsiveness to angiotensin II in pregnant women by intravenously infused 5α-dihydroprogesterone. Am J Obstet Gynecol 131:352, 1978

28. Parker CR, Everett RB, Quirk JG et al: Hormone production during pregnancy in the primigravid patient. I. Plasma levels of progesterone and 5a-pregnane-3,20-dione throughout pregnancy of normal women and women who developed pregnancy-induced hypertension. Am J Obstet Gynecol 135:778, 1979

29. Everett RB, Worley RJ, MacDonald PC, Gant NF: Oral administration of theophylline to modify pressor responsiveness to angiotensin II in women with pregnancy-induced hypertension. Am J Obstet Gynecol 132:359, 1978

30. O'Brien PMS, Pipkin FB: The effects of deprivation of prostaglandin precursors on vascular sensitivity to angiotensin II and on the kidney in the pregnant rabbit. Br J Pharmacol 65:29, 1979

31. Gant NF: Personal communication

32. Pedersen EB, Christensen NF, Christensen P et al: Preeclampsia—A state of prostaglandin deficiency? Hypertension 5:105, 1983

33. Symonds EM: Hormonal influences on blood pressure during pregnancy. In Proceedings of the Eighth International Congress on Nephrology, pp 429–439. Basel, Karger, 1981

34. Chesley LC: Hypertensive Disorders in Pregnancy, pp 229–246. New York, Appleton-Century-Crofts, 1978

35. Downing I, Shepherd GL, Lewis PJ: Reduced prostacyclin production in pre-eclampsia. Lancet 2:650, 1980

36. Remuzzi G, Marchesi D, Zoja C et al: Reduced umbilical and placental vascular prostacyclin in severe pre-eclampsia. Prostaglandins 20:105, 1980

37. Ylikorkala O, Makila UM, Viinikka L: Amniotic fluid prostacyclin and thromboxane in normal, pre-eclamptic, and some other complicated pregnancies. Am J Obstet Gynecol 141:487, 1981

38. Goodman RP, Killam AP, Brash AR, Branch RA: Prostacyclin production during pregnancy: Comparison of production during normal pregnancy and pregnancy complicated by hypertension. Am J Obstet Gynecol 142:817, 1982

39. Dadak C, Kefalides A, Sinzinger H, Weber G: Reduced umbilical artery prostacyclin formation in complicated pregnancies. Am J Obstet Gynecol 144:792, 1982

40. Masotti G, Poggesi L, Galanti G et al: Differential inhibition of prostacyclin production and platelet aggregation by aspirin. Lancet 2:1213, 1979

41. Hanley SP, Bevan J, Cockbill SR, Heptinstall S: Differential inhibition by low-dose aspirin of human venous prostacyclin synthesis and platelet thromboxane synthesis. Lancet 1:969, 1981

42. Crandon AJ, Isherwood DM: Effect of aspirin on incidence of preeclampsia. Lancet 1:1356, 1979

43. Van Assche FA, Spitz B, Vermylen J, Deckmijn H: Preliminary observations on treatment of pregnancy-induced hypertension with a thromboxane synthetase inhibitor. Am J Obstet Gynecol 148:216, 1984

44. Lewis PJ, O'Grady JP: Clinical Pharmacology of Prostacyclin, pp 141–143. New York, Raven Press, 1981

45. Lewis PJ, Shepherd GL, Ritter J: Prostacyclin and pre-eclampsia. Lancet 1:559, 1981

46. Jorgensen KA, Pedersen RS: Familial deficiency of prostacyclin production stimulating factor in the hemolytic uremic syndrome of childhood. Thromb Res 21:311, 1981

47. Remuzzi G, Imperti L, DeGaetano G: Prostacyclin deficiency in thrombotic microangiopathy. Lancet 2:122, 1981

48. Carreras LO, Defreyn G, Machini SJ et al: Arterial thrombosis, intrauterine death and "lupus" anti-coagulant: Detection of immunoglobulin interfering with prostacyclin formation. Lancet 1:244, 1981

49. McGillivray I: Some observations on the incidence of preeclampsia. Br J Obstet Gynaecol 65:536, 1958

50. Redman CWG: Immunological factors in the pathogenesis of preeclampsia. Contr Nephrol 25:120, 1981

51. Jenkins DM, Need J, Rajah SM: Deficiency of specific HLA antibodies in severe pregnancy pre-eclampsia/eclampsia. Clin Exp Immunol 27:485, 1977

52. Redman CWG, Bodmer JG, Bodmer WF et al: HLA antigens in severe pre-eclampsia. Lancet 2:397, 1978

53. Balasch J, Mirapeix E, Borche L et al: Further evidence against preeclampsia as an immune complex disease. Obstet Gynecol 58:435, 1981

54. Rote NS, Caudle MR: Circulating immune complexes in pregnancy, preeclampsia, and autoimmune diseases: Evaluation of Raji cell enzyme–linked immunosorbent assay and polyethylene glycol precipitation methods. Am J Obstet Gynecol 147:267, 1983

55. Sutherland A, Cooper DW, Howie PW et al: The incidence of severe pre-eclampsia amongst mothers and mothers-in-law of pre-eclamptics and controls. Br J Obstet Gynaecol 88:785, 1981

56. Astin M, Scott JR, Worley RJ: Pre-eclampsia/eclampsia: A fatal father factor. Lancet 2:533, 1981

57. Mirro R, Brown DR: Edema, proteinuria, thrombocytopenia, and leukopenia in infants of preeclamptic mothers. Am J Obstet Gynecol 144:851, 1982

58. Zeek PM, Assali NS: Vascular changes in the decidua associated with eclamptogenic toxemia. Am J Clin Pathol 20:1099, 1950

59. Worley RJ, Everett RB, Madden JD et al: Fetal considerations: Metabolic clearance rate of maternal dehydroisoandrostenone sulfate. Semin Perinatol 2:15, 1978

60. Whalley PJ, Everett RB, Gant NF et al: Pressor responsiveness to angiotensin II in hospitalized primigravid women with pregnancy-induced hypertension. Am J Obstet Gynecol 145:481, 1983

61. Lin CC, Lindheimer MD, River P, Moawad A: Fetal outcome in hypertensive disorders of pregnancy. Am J Obstet Gynecol 142:255, 1982

62. Chesley LC: Hypertensive Disorders in Pregnancy, p 268. New York, Appleton-Century-Crofts, 1978

63. Pritchard JA, Cunningham FG, Mason RA: Coagulation changes in eclampsia: Their frequency and pathogenesis. Am J Obstet Gynecol 124:855, 1976

64. Gibson B, Hunter D, Neame PB, Kelton JG: Thrombocytopenia in preeclampsia and eclampsia. Thromb Haemost 8:234, 1982

65. Bern MM, Driscoll SG, Levitt T: Thrombocytopenia complicating preeclampsia. Obstet Gynecol 57:289, 1981

66. Weinstein L: Syndrome of hemolysis, elevated liver enzymes, and low platelet count: A severe consequence of hypertension in pregnancy. Am J Obstet Gynecol 142:159, 1982

67. Sheehan HL, Lynch JB: Pathology of Toxaemia of Pregnancy. London, Churchill Livingstone, 1973

68. Bauer TW, Moore GW, Hutchins GM: Morphologic evidence for coronary artery spasm in eclampsia. Circulation 65:255, 1982
69. Chesley LC: Hypertensive Disorders in Pregnancy, p 80. New York, Appleton-Century-Crofts, 1978
70. Beeson JH, Duda EE: Computed axial tomography scan demonstration of cerebral edema in eclampsia preceded by blindness. Obstet Gynecol 60:529, 1982
71. Gaitz JP, Bamford CR: Unusual computed tomographic scan in eclampsia. Arch Neurol 39:66, 1982
72. Chesley LC: Parenteral magnesium sulfate and the distribution, plasma levels, and excretion of magnesium. Am J Obstet Gynecol 133:1, 1979
73. Pritchard JA: Standardized treatment of 154 consecutive cases of eclampsia. Am J Obstet Gynecol 123:543, 1975
74. Sibai BM, Lipshitz J, Anderson GD, Dilts PV: Reassessment of intravenous MgSO4 therapy in preeclampsia–eclampsia. Obstet Gynecol 57:199, 1981
75. Gant NF, Worley RJ: Hypertension in Pregnancy. Concepts and Management, pp 93–94. New York, Appleton-Century-Crofts, 1980
76. Morris JA, Arce JJ, Hamilton CJ et al: The management of severe preeclampsia and eclampsia with intravenous diazoxide. Obstet Gynecol 49:675, 1977
77. Neuman J, Weiss B, Rabello Y et al: Diazoxide for the acute control of severe hypertension complicating pregnancy: A pilot study. Obstet Gynecol (Suppl) 53:50, 1979
78. Lieb SM, Zugaib M, Nuwayhid KB et al: Nitroprusside-induced hemodynamic alterations in normotensive and hypertensive pregnant sheep. Am J Obstet Gynecol 139:925, 1981
79. Shoemaker CT, Meyers M: Sodium nitroprusside for control of severe hypertensive disease of pregnancy: A case report and discussion of potential toxicity. Am J Obstet Gynecol 149:171, 1984
80. Henderson DW, Vilos GA, Milne KJ, Nichol PM: The role of Swan–Ganz catheterization in severe pregnancy-induced hypertension. Am J Obstet Gynecol 148:570, 1984
81. Beck DW, Menezes AH: Intracerebral hemorrhage in a patient with eclampsia. JAMA 246:1442, 1981
82. Gilstrap LC, Cunningham FG, Whalley PJ: Management of pregnancy-induced hypertension in the nulliparous patient remote from term. Semin Perinatol 2:73, 1978
83. Worley RJ: Early identification of the pregnant woman at high risk of developing pregnancy-induced hypertension. In Di Renzo GC, Hawkins DF (eds): Perinatal Medicine: Problems and Controversies. New York, Raven Press, 1984
84. Pritchard JA, Pritchard SA: Blood pressure response to estrogen progestin oral contraceptive after pregnancy-induced hypertension. Am J Obstet Gynecol 129:733, 1977
85. Chesley LC: Hypertensive Disorders in Pregnancy, pp 445–476. New York, Appleton-Century-Crofts, 1978
86. Gant NF, Worley RJ: Hypertension in Pregnancy. Concepts and Management, pp 194–195. New York, Appleton-Century-Crofts, 1980

Fetal Growth Retardation

William N. Spellacy

27

Discrepancies in fetal growth patterns have always occurred, yet only in the last two decades have perinatologists paid any considerable attention to this important problem. A major difficulty with the clinical management of abnormal intrauterine growth is that neither of the two pieces of information required to establish the diagnosis—gestational age and fetal weight—is precisely or easily obtained in the perinatal period. Largeness for gestational age, or macrosomia, is generally defined as a birth weight of more than 4500 g. The major problem associated with macrosomia is trauma during the delivery process. *Small-for-gestational age* (SGA) infants, those suffering from intrauterine growth retardation (IUGR), are infants whose weight for age falls in the tenth percentile in standard weight-for-age tables (Fig. 27-1).[1] There are about 3.5 million births per year in the United States, meaning that more than 350,000 cases of IUGR occur per year.[2] SGA infants are at high risk for fetal and neonatal problems, including death. As the management of other high-risk conditions has improved, the management of the growth-retarded fetus has become a major perinatal problem and now commands the prime attention of researchers and clinicians alike.[3] This chapter reviews current information about the control of normal fetal growth, the etiology of IUGR, the tests that can be used to detect abnormal fetal growth, and the clinical importance and management of the pregnancy with this high-risk complication.

CONTROL OF FETAL GROWTH

In normal pregnancy the fetus and placenta grow at different rates. The placenta expands early and develops into a large and tertiary villous structure whose maximum surface area for exchange, about 11 m², is normally reached at about 37 weeks of gestation.[4] At that point the placenta weighs about 500 g.[5] This placental development seems to be in response to the environment of oxygenated maternal blood bathing the cotyledons from open uterine spiral arteries. Many other parameters of pregnancy also peak at 37 weeks, including amniotic fluid volume and maternal blood human placental lactogen levels, which suggests that placental function also peaks at that point. From 37 weeks until delivery there is a slight decline in placental surface area as senescence sets in.

Fetal growth continues throughout pregnancy. In the last few weeks, beginning at about the 36th to 37th week, the rate of weight increase per week begins to decrease.[6] The fetus is then normally depositing fat in the form of C-16 palmitate derived from the two carbon acetate segments resulting from glucose metabolism. Since fat has a high caloric content, in normal pregnancy the fetus continues to accumulate calories rapidly until term, despite a slowed absolute rate of weight gain in the last 3 to 4 weeks.

The requirements for normal fetal growth are as follows:

1. Large placental membrane (11 m²)
2. Adequate uterine and umbilical blood flow
3. Substrate (especially glucose, amino acids, oxygen)
4. Fetal "growth factors"

As noted in this list, the fetus requires three major forms of substrate for its growth. First, it receives glucose freely across the placenta from the maternal blood by facilitated diffusion.[4] In a steady state, the maternal and fetal blood glucose levels are similar, the fetal level being about 80% that of the mother. Since this form of transfer requires a coupling mechanism at the placental membrane border, any elevation of the maternal level above fasting results in a widening of the maternal-fetal gradient. Second, the maternal amino acids are all actively transported to the fetus and thus are in higher concen-

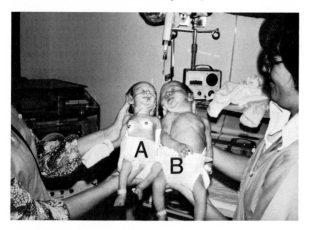

FIG. 27-1. IUGR in a twin pregnancy. It is readily apparent that twin A is much smaller than twin B, though both are the same age.

tration in fetal than in maternal blood. This active transport process for amino acids seems to be controlled by the concentration of cyclic-AMP in the placental syncytiotrophoblast.[8] Finally, oxygen freely diffuses from the maternal blood to the fetal blood, and the degree of transfer depends on the blood flow rates through the uterus and placenta and on the concentration gradients, as noted in the Fick principle. Although many other minor ingredients are necessary for fetal metabolism, these three are key. *In utero* the glucose is burned with oxygen to produce energy in the form of ATP. The energy is utilized to convert the amino acids into protein, and the result is a growing intrauterine infant. Regulation of this growth rate is dependent on not only the placental transfer of these three substrates, but also on fetal hormones, such as insulin and somatomedins, which act as "growth factors."[9] Fetal pituitary growth hormone does not seem to be needed since congenitally growth-hormone–deficient infants (ateliotic sexual dwarfs) are of normal size at birth. Excess or deficiency of substrate and growth factors leads to overgrowth (macrosomia) or undergrowth (IUGR).

ETIOLOGY

Although there are many causes of fetal growth retardation, they can be conveniently grouped into three broad categories relating to the substrate, namely:

1. *Maternal*—Substrate availability
2. *Placental*—Substrate transfer
3. *Fetal*—Substrate utilization

In each category there are important subgroups. For example, the *maternal causes* center on the requirements for the critical substrate—namely glucose, amino acids, and oxygen—in the blood. Maternal nutrition before and during pregnancy is very important for fetal growth.[10] Although the average weight gain in pregnancy is about 22 lb to 27 lb, good fetal outcome requires larger weight gains from thin than from obese women.[11] Thus, malnourished women who become pregnant tend to deliver smaller than normal infants. Abnormalities can also occur if there is poor nutrition during pregnancy, or if the mother has diseases such as cyanotic heart disease (low blood oxygen) or malabsorption syndromes (following gastrointestinal bypass procedures, for example, or abnormal bowel syndromes manifest by low, flat glucose tolerance curves). Those suffering from malabsorption do not have an adequate substrate level in the blood despite having a good diet. Some mothers consume little food because they use their resources for other things—drug addicts, for example, will often buy drugs rather than food.[12] Alcohol, especially beer, can also adversely affect fetal growth.[13]

The *placental causes* of IUGR include poor uterine blood flow or a small placental surface area. If there is maternal vascular disease, such as hypertension with constricted decidual spiral arteries, the growth phase of the placenta may stop even earlier, resulting in a smaller placenta that not only weighs less but also has a reduced surface area for exchange. The uterine blood flow can be reduced by diseased blood vessels or vessels that are in spasm.[14] Smoking also can affect uterine blood flow, since it causes the release of both epinephrine and norepinephrine, which can induce uterine blood vessel spasm and reduced uterine blood flow. In addition, in the mother who smokes, the fetal vessel endothelial layer produces less prostacyclin, and blood flow is reduced. Many studies have shown that the infants of smokers weigh 150 g to 300 g less than nonsmokers. Controlled studies of smokers who stop during pregnancy have shown that their infants are larger than those of mothers who continue to smoke.[16] The most common clinical symptom of constricted uterine blood vessels is maternal hypertension, which is also the most common maternal factor associated with IUGR. A rarer problem is a deficiency in the cyclic-AMP content of the placental syncytiotrophoblast.[8]

The *fetal causes* of IUGR include those cases in which even though substrate is in the mother's blood and indeed crosses the placenta, it is not utilized normally by the fetus. There are two general conditions responsible for this inability to utilize the substrate. The first is the presence of major congenital anomalies. Cardiovascular anomalies are the most common, but extreme inability to utilize substrate is often associated with even more serious problems, such as trisomy 13 or 18. The second fetal problem group is accelerated fetal metabolism due to an infection with any of the TORCH agents. These include toxoplasmosis, rubella, cytomegalovirus, herpes simplex, and others like β-streptococcus. About half of these TORCH–affected infants are growth retarded. If infection is a possibility, a complete blood screen is needed.

DIAGNOSIS

The diagnosis of IUGR depends on a simple inexpensive clinical screen and then on more expensive laboratory tests to confirm or refute the diagnosis. Several risk-scoring systems have been developed that can define a population to be concerned about.[17] These systems usually include uterine fundal height measurements. Clinical palpation for fetal size is known to be inaccurate.[18] However, the serial tape measurement of uterine fundal height, from the symphysis over the uterus to the top of the fundus, has been shown to be a useful index of fetal growth. Many factors can affect that result, including the placement of the tape and changes in fetal engagement and position, urine bladder volume, amniotic fluid volume, and fetal weight. Several studies have shown an accuracy of about 75% in diagnosing IUGR with this test, however, and the cost for the test is minimal. The routine measurement of uterine fundal height at each prenatal visit, as well as the plotting of this measurement on a graphic chart, is one key to early diagnosis. An example of a chart to do this that can become part of the prenatal record is shown in Fig. 27-2.

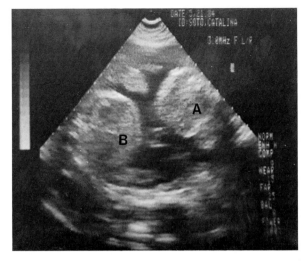

FIG. 27-3. Ultrasound studies of the fetal abdomen at the level of the umbilical vein in a twin pregnancy. Note that twin A is much smaller than twin B, suggesting IUGR.

FIG. 27-2. Uterine fundal weight chart that can be placed in the prenatal record. If the measurement from the symphysis over the uterus to its top falls below the tenth percentile line at any week, the pregnancy becomes at risk for IUGR, and other diagnostic tests can be done.

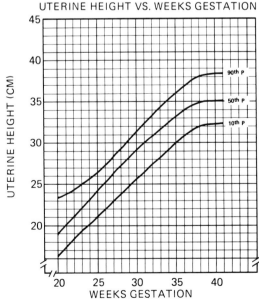

The clinical suspicion of IUGR can be confirmed by more sophisticated and expensive tests.[19] The first tests are biophysical in type. The ultrasonographic visualization of the intrauterine cavity has greatly assisted in the diagnosis. The first studies were of fetal head size, but their accuracy was only about 50%. This is not too surprising, since nature allows the brain to continue to grow in the most adverse circumstances as a natural protection for CNS function.[5] Thus, since the brain is the last organ affected, there is a "brain sparing effect" in IUGR. The growth pattern of the storage organs like the liver is affected very early and is therefore a much better index of fetal nutrition. More precise ultrasound measurements include abdominal or chest circumference studies in which the scan is taken across the umbilical vein as it enters the fetal liver (Fig. 27-3). Ultrasound measurements of fetal bone growth (femur length) and amniotic fluid volume are also helpful. Other studies that can be useful are measurements of placental and fetal biochemical factors that are present in the maternal circulation and are related to fetal or placental weight. These factors include estriol, human placental lactogen (HPL), and SP$_1$ protein.[21,22] Amniotic fluid levels of the C-peptide fragment of proinsulin and of glucose levels are also of assistance in the diagnosis.[3,23] With IUGR, levels of all of these biochemical markers tend to be low. Several studies of maternal serum α-fetoprotein levels in early pregnancy (16 weeks) have shown that high levels are often associated with the later development of IUGR. The high levels in such cases may reflect early placental disruption and resultant leakage of fetal α-fetoprotein into the maternal blood. Placental breaks of this kind also inhibit the subsequent development of the placenta, which in turn affects fetal growth.

COMPLICATIONS

The complications of IUGR principally affect the infant.[24,25] By definition it is small for its gestational age.[1] If the condition has been present for a relatively short period, the central nervous system has continued to grow, yet other systems, and especially storage organs like the liver and fat depots, are small. This gives the clinical picture of "asymmetrical" IUGR. If, however, the process has been going on for a long time, then even brain growth will be adversely affected and IUGR is "symmetrical," meaning that body and head are both small for gestational age. Symmetrical IUGR is generally more severe because it usually has been present for a longer time, and it often is a consequence of congenital anomalies, including the trisomies, or the congenital TORCH infection. Since the placenta of fetuses whose growth retardation has a placental cause is often small, these fetuses have only marginal respiratory reserves. They do not tolerate uterine contractions well: about 30% of IUGR cases have a positive oxytocin contraction stress (OCT) test, while about 50% develop fetal hypoxia or acidosis during labor,[26] conditions that may be accompanied by the passage and aspiration of meconium, leading to respiratory difficulties in the nursery. In addition, probably because of their marginal oxygenation *in utero* and the low amniotic fluid volume, these fetuses often develop variable heart rate decelerations in nonstress tests that are similar to those seen in umbilical cord compression.[27] The fetus may have attempted to compensate for the poor placental transfer of oxygen by developing a marked polycythemia (hyperviscosity syndrome) with hematocrits of greater than 65%. After birth these fetuses can have problems of multiple organ thrombosis, cardiac failure and hyperbilirubinemia.[3] Since there is generally very little fat deposited on these fetuses, they tend to develop hypoglycemia in early neonatal life if they are not fed, for they cannot mobilize free fatty acids for metabolism and instead utilize their glucose for neonatal fuel. Depending on the etiology of the IUGR, there may be other problems too—for example, like anomalies or intrauterine infections, such as with rubella, cytomegalovirus or herpes simplex or drug withdrawal.

It is not surprising then that both fetal and neonatal death rates are significantly increased in the presence of IUGR; the extent of the increase depends on the severity of the problem. In general, the overall perinatal mortality for the IUGR infant is about six to eight times higher than that observed in normal pregnancies. The management of IUGR, therefore, is one of the most serious problems facing the physician dealing with high-risk pregnancies.

Another major concern is the subsequent development of the infants that do survive. Many longitudinal studies have been done to investigate this aspect of the problem. In the first year after birth, IUGR infants remain smaller than matched controls. They are lighter, shorter, and have reduced circumferences of organs like the head and chest.[28] There are also significantly reduced neurologic evaluation indices suggesting lower intelligence levels.[28] The brain has a tremendous reserve, however, and in the children over five years of age, detectable differences in neurologic development or function are uncommon.[29]

MANAGEMENT

Because of the many serious problems that can occur in the fetus and neonate that is growth retarded, pregnancies with IUGR generally need to be managed by an experienced perinatal team in a tertiary referral center. The management of these pregnancies depends upon several general principles:

1. Early detection (*e.g.,* by screening of high-risk groups, testing)
2. Elimination of contributing factors (*e.g.,* poor diet, smoking, drugs)
3. Increasing uterine blood flow (*e.g.,* by instituting bed rest)
4. Serial fetal surveillance (*e.g.,* by weekly oxytocin stress testing)
5. Early delivery in perinatal center

In order to introduce a management program one first needs to detect the cases. Early diagnosis is best because it provides time for intervention before fetal damage occurs. Clinicians must therefore be aware of the problem and test for it, especially in pregnancies at risk, such as those in women who have hypertension, are smokers, demonstrate poor nutrition, or show little weight gain. Second, the contributing factors must be eliminated. These include inadequate dietary intake, smoking, and drug abuse. The details of diet in pregnancy are discussed in Chapter 11, and the rules that are outlined are of special importance in prevention of IUGR. Pregnant women require about 300 extra calories per day and therefore all pregnant women should be instructed that their calorie intake should be about 2100-2300 calories/day. The composition of the diet has been shown to be less important than the number of calories.[30,31] Nonetheless a protein content of 1.3 g to 1.5 g is recommended. Women on this diet will gain weight differently depending on their prepregnancy weights. The normal–weight woman will gain about 22 lb to 27 lb, whereas the thin woman will gain more and the obese woman will gain less.[11] No studies have shown a clear need for prenatal vitamin supplementation if the diet is adequate, although additional exogenous iron is clearly needed. All women should also be encouraged to stop smoking and to stop drinking alcohol during pregnancy. If the patient is a substance abuser she should seek rehabilitation, (a methadone program is an example). Other identifiable causes of IUGR should also be eliminated if possible. For example, strenuous work and physical activity should be avoided by women whose vascular system is poor, as evidenced by hypertension. Intrauterine feeding of the fetus and hyperalimentation of the mother have been tried but still are experimental, although further studies in these areas may prove rewarding.[32,33]

The third principle of IUGR management is to increase uterine blood flow as much as possible. In general this means that blood pressure is not lowered in pregnant hypertensive women unless it presents a serious risk to the mother's health, since uterine blood flow is directly related to maternal blood pressure. The other very important point is to have the woman remain at bedrest, preferably on her left side, where uterine blood flow will be maximal. Although exercise and physical activity do not seem to threaten the infant in normal pregnancy, they are considered to be contraindicated in high-risk pregnancies.[34] The question of the advisability of continuing to work during pregnancy arises here. If the pregnancy is normal and the work is not strenuous, then a "six-week window" of leave is usual, with two weeks being taken before delivery and four weeks after. If the pregnancy is complicated by, for example, hypertension or IUGR, bed rest for extended periods of time may be necessary.

The fourth principle of IUGR management is to put the fetus into an intensive surveillance program. This should be started as soon as there is a chance to do something about an abnormal result. Since most perinatal centers now have normal survivors at about 26 weeks of gestation, this is about the time to start these studies if the diagnosis of IUGR has been made. Usually, however, the diagnosis is not made until much later in the pregnancy. Evaluation tests must be done serially until the pregnancy is terminated. The most practical test seems to be the weekly oxytocin uterine contraction test (OCT) which seems to be more sensitive than the nonstress test.[35,36] Other parameters of fetal and placental health can also be monitored, such as estriol, human placental lactogen, and amniotic fluid volume levels, and fetal weight and growth can be estimated by ultrasound studies.

Since intrauterine monitoring is not perfect, and since IUGR can result in injury or death, early delivery of infants with IUGR seems reasonable. When all surveillance test results are normal, the optimal time for delivery, appears to be about the 38th week of pregnancy. If the surveillance test results become abnormal before that time, an assessment of fetal maturity needs to be made. This often involves the use of amniocentesis with measurements of the fetal lung surfactant content, usually using a test like the lecithin/sphingomyelin (L/S) ratio. Depending on the outcome of these tests, delivery before 38 weeks may be necessary. Delivery prior to 38 weeks is also indicated if the serial ultrasound studies of biparietal diameter show that head (brain) growth is also becoming affected. When brain growth is affected, the infant has a high risk of developing CNS dysfunction.

During labor the continuous assessment of fetal well-being is also important because many infants with IUGR develop hypoxia. Assessment is most easily done by continuous electronic measurements of fetal heart rates, using an internal fetal electrode when technically feasible. Any alteration in basal rate, pattern, or short-term variability that suggests fetal hypoxia and acidosis should be confirmed by fetal scalp blood sampling. If acidosis is confirmed, (*i.e.,* if fetal scalp blood pH is <7.20) intrauterine resuscitation and rapid delivery, usually by cesarean section, are needed. Fetal resuscitation can be done by instituting maternal hydration, positioning the mother on her left side, administering oxygen, and stopping uterine activity with uterine tocolytics, such as the β-mimetics (*e.g.,* terbutaline 0.25 mg SC). After delivery the umbilical cord should be clamped quickly so that the infant, who may have polycythemic hyperviscosity syndrome, will not receive a further transfusion of red blood cells.

The care of the growth-retarded neonate is equally important. If meconium has been passed, immediate intubation is necessary to remove the meconium from the airway before it is pulled down into the lungs. If the infant is hypoxic and depressed it needs rapid resuscitation with such measures as intubation, artificial breathing assistance, oxygen, cardiac massage, hydration, and occasionally drugs. Such etiologic factors as congenital anomalies and intrauterine infections must be rapidly assessed for and appropriately managed if detected. Hematocrit level will indicate whether the hyperviscosity syndrome is present. If it is, therapy may include phlebotomy or plasma exchange. Blood glucose levels should be monitored in the early hours of life so that hypoglycemia can be detected and treated. If blood glucose level falls below 30 mg/dl, parenteral glucose is needed. Maintaining body temperature at about 35°C will minimize the metabolic rate and therefore oxygen consumption. Finally, long-term follow-up of these children is important in order to assess the success of the treatment program.

SUMMARY

Infants with intrauterine growth retardation are those whose weight is in the tenth percentile for gestational age. About 350,000 such infants are born in the United States each year. The condition may be due to maternal, placental or fetal factors. Early diagnosis is important, and clinical suspicion induced by slow growth patterns in the uterine fundal height can be confirmed by ultrasound and biochemical testing. Since IUGR significantly increases infant morbidity and mortality, pregnancies in which IUGR is present need special care. Therapy includes good nutrition; avoidance of confounding factors, such as smoking and drug use; and bedrest to improve uterine blood flow. Fetal health must be serially monitored with such tests as weekly contraction stress tests. Carefully timed and monitored early delivery in a tertiary center with appropriate neonatal care is of great importance. The long-term development of survivors seems to be adequate.

REFERENCES AND RECOMMENDED READING

1. Battaglia FC, Lubchenco LO: A practical classification of newborn infants by weight and gestational age. J Pediatr 71:159, 1967
2. Reed MS, Catz C, Grave G et al: Introduction. Intrauterine growth retardation: Identification of research needs and goals. Semin Perinatol 8:2, 1984
3. Lin CC, Evans MI: Intrauterine Growth Retardation: Pathophysiology and Clinical Management. New York, McGraw-Hill, 1984
4. Page EW: Human fetal nutrition and growth. Am J Obstet Gynecol 104:378, 1969
5. Gruenwald P: Chronic fetal distress and placental insufficiency. Biol Neonate 5:215, 1963
6. Hendricks CH: Patterns of fetal and placental growth: The second half of normal pregnancy. Obstet Gynecol 24:357, 1964
7. Bonds DR, Mwape B, Kumar S et al: Human fetal weight and placental weight growth curves: A mathematical analysis from a population at sea level. Biol Neonte 45:261, 1984
8. Matsuda T, Nakano Y, Nishikawa Y et al: Fetomaternal amino acid patterns and cyclic AMP in the human placenta with abnormal pregnancies, particularly with SFD. Tohoka. J Exp Med 121:253, 1977
9. Susa JB, Widness JA, Hintz R et al: Somatomedins and insulin in diabetic pregnancies: Effects on fetal macrosomia in the human and Rhesus monkey. J Clin Endocrinol Metab 58:1099, 1984
10. Eastman NJ, Jackson E: Weight relationships in pregnancy I. The bearing of maternal weight gain and pre-pregnancy weight on birth weight in full term pregnancies. Obstet Gynecol Surv 23:1003, 1968
11. Naeye RL: Weight gain and the outcome of pregnancy. Am J Obstet Gynecol 135:3, 1979
12. Kandall SR, Albin S, Lowinson J et al: Differential effects of maternal heroin and methadone use on birth weight. Pediatrics 58:681, 1976
13. Bottoms SF, Judge NE, Kuhnert PM et al: Thiocyanate and drinking during pregnancy. Alcoholism 6:391, 1982
14. Lunell ND, Sarby B, Lewander R et al: Comparison of uteroplacental blood flow in normal and in intrauterine growth-retarded pregnancy measurements with indium-113 M and a computer-linked gammacamera. Gynecol Obstet Invest 10:106, 1979
15. Busacca M, Balconi G, Pietra A et al: Maternal smoking and prostacyclin production by cultured endothelial cells from umbilical arteries. Am J Obstet Gynecol 148:1127, 1984
16. Sexton M, Hebel JR: A clinical trial of change in maternal smoking and its effect on birth weight. JAMA 251:911, 1984
17. Wennergren M, Karlsson K, Olsson T: A scoring system for antenatal identification of fetal growth retardation. Br J Obstet Gynecol 89:520, 1982
18. Bossak WS, Spellacy WN: Accuracy of estimating fetal weight by abdominal palpation. J Reprod Med 9:58, 1972
19. Rosso P, Winick M: Intrauterine growth retardation. A new systematic approach based on the clinical and biochemical characteristics of this condition. J Perinat Med 2:147, 1974
20. Manning FA, Hill LM, Platt LD: Qualitative amniotic fluid volume determination by ultrasound: Antepartum detection of intrauterine growth retardation. Am J Obstet Gynecol 139:254, 1981
21. Low JA, Galbraith RS, Boston RW: Maternal urinary estrogen patterns in intrauterine growth retardation. Obstet Gynecol 42:325, 1973
22. Spellacy WN, Buhi WC, Birk SA: Human placental lactogen and intrauterine growth retardation. Obstet Gynecol 47:446, 1976
23. Marin RD, Hood W: Significance of amniotic fluid glucose in late pregnancy. Aust NZ J Obstet Gynaecol 19:91, 1979
24. Bard H: Intrauterine growth retardation. Clin Obstet Gynecol 13:511, 1970
25. Jones MD Jr, Battaglia FC: Intrauterine growth retardation. Am J Obstet Gynecol 127:540, 1977
26. Low JA, Boston RW, Pancham SR: Fetal asphyxia during the intrapartum period in intrauterine growth-related infants. Am J Obstet Gynecol 113:351, 1972
27. Pazos R, Vuolo K, Aladjem S et al: Association of spontaneous fetal heart rate decelerations during antepartum nonstress testing and intrauterine growth retardation. Am J Obstet Gynecol 144:574, 1982
28. Low JA, Galbraith RS, Muir D et al: Intrauterine growth retardation: A preliminary report of long-term morbidity. Am J Obstet Gynecol 130:534, 1978
29. Low JA, Galbraith RS, Muir D et al: Intrauterine growth retardation: A study of long-term morbidity. Am J Obstet Gynecol 142:670, 1982
30. Lechtig A, Habicht JP, Delgado H et al: Effect of food supplementation during pregnancy on birth weight. Pediatrics 56:508,1975
31. Stein Z, Susser M, Rush D: Prenatal nutrition and birth weight: Experiments and quasi-experiments in the past decade. J Reprod Med 21:287, 1978
32. Mesaki N, Kubo T, Iwasaki H: A study of the treatment for intrauterine growth retardation. Nippon Sanka Fujinka Gakkai Zasshi 32:879, 1980
33. Charlton V, Johengen M: Amelioration of intrauterine growth retardation by fetal intragastric nutritional supplementation. Clin Res 30:140A, 1982
34. Jarrett JC II, Spellacy WN: Jogging during pregnancy: An improved outcome? Obstet Gynecol 61:705, 1983
35. Freeman RK, Anderson G, Dorchester W: A prospective multi-institutional study of antepartum fetal heart rate monitoring. II. Contraction stress test versus nonstress test for primary surveillance. Am J Obstet Gynecol 143:778, 1982
36. Barrett JM, Salyer SL, Boehm FH: The nonstress test: An evaluation of 1,000 patients. Am J Obstet Gynecol 141:153, 1981

Multiple Pregnancy

Allan Killam
Kenneth F. Trofatter

28

Multiple pregnancies occur in only about 1% of gestations carried beyond 20 weeks but account for 10% of all perinatal mortality. The fear and, occasionally, reverence afforded multiple pregnancies since antiquity have been replaced by a healthy respect for the challenges they present to the safety of the mother and the fetuses. Although controversy still exists about the best methods of managing such pregnancies, such diagnostic tools as ultrasound and antepartum fetal monitoring now aid in critical decision-making and contribute to improved outcomes.

DIAGNOSIS

Early diagnosis, allowing well-planned antepartum, intrapartum, and neonatal care, is a critical aspect of the management of multiple gestations. Unfortunately, in the past the diagnosis was often made late or remained unsuspected until the time of delivery. Multiple pregnancies in which the diagnosis is not made until delivery contribute a significant percentage to the total morbidity and mortality associated with multiple pregnancies because in such pregnancies there is an increased chance that intrapartum decisions will be inappropriate, neonatologists, will be unprepared, and facilities will be inadequate for managing preterm or compromised infants.

Pertinent history, physical examination, and a high index of suspicion go a long way toward establishing an early diagnosis of multiple pregnancy. The frequency of twinning increases with both maternal age and parity. It is more likely to occur following the use of drugs for ovulation-induction, in the months after discontinuation of oral contraceptives, and as a result of *in vitro* fertilization. Twins are also more common among blacks and among patients with a strong family history or previous obstetric history of dizygous multiple gestation.

On physical examination, twins should be suspected whenever uterine size is greater than expected for gestational age as predicted by date of last menstrual period. Uterine size with twins exceeds that expected for singletons early in the second trimester and the discrepancy can be detected by 16 to 18 weeks. Auscultation of more than one distinct fetal heartbeat helps to verify the diagnosis, but failure to detect more than one is not useful in ruling it out. Confirmation of multiple gestation is best done with real-time ultrasonography. This can be used to determine the number of fetuses as early as 6 to 7 weeks of gestation.

Many biochemical tests have been proposed to aid in the diagnosis and management of multiple gestations, but currently, none will differentiate definitively between one and more than one fetus. For example, maternal serum α-fetoprotein measurement, aside from its use in detection of neural tube defects, has been advocated as a screening method for multiple gestation, and elevated levels may lead to this diagnosis. However, when the test is used for this purpose alone, both specificity and sensitivity are low, and even if multiple gestation is detected, one cannot exclude the possibility of associated congenital abnormalities or pregnancy at risk for preeclampsia or early delivery.

MATERNAL AND FETAL RISKS

Prematurity

Premature labor and delivery is the single most important cause of morbidity and mortality related to multiple gestations. It occurs in 25% to 40% of all twin pregnancies and is seen most commonly with nulliparous patients, monozygotic and, especially, monoamnionic twins, and male fetuses. Proposed reasons for premature labor include physical factors, such as expansion of intrauterine volume at a rate exceeding myometrial accommodation, the effects of mass on cervical integrity, abnormal placentation, and congenital anomalies. In addition, hydramnios associated with congenital abnormalities, diabetes, growth discordancy, and twin-to-twin transfusion syndromes occurs in a high percentage of multiple pregnancies and further increase the risk of premature delivery.

The perinatal mortality among twins is three to four times that among singletons and is mainly related to complications of prematurity and low birth weight, such as traumatic delivery, respiratory distress syndrome, intracerebral hemorrhage, necrotizing enterocolitis, and sepsis. As an added factor, the risk of intrauterine growth retardation among twins is also at least four times that among singletons.

Fetal Wastage

Fetal wastage, as manifested by spontaneous abortion, delivery prior to fetal viability, and intrauterine fetal demise, is also high in multiple gestations. A unique aspect of this problem is the so-called vanishing twin phenomenon. Reports of serial ultrasound examiners beginning in early pregnancy have shown that only about 30% to 50% of multiple gestations actually result in all the fetuses being carried to viability. Fetal demise with complete resorption or even miscarriage, manifested only by slight vaginal bleeding, may occur, with survival of the remaining fetuses and continuation of the pregnancy.

Death of a fetus at later gestational ages can affect the surviving fetus and mother in various ways. Consequences can range from death of the surviving fetus (usually within 48–72 hours) and premature labor to uncomplicated continuation of the pregnancy. Occasionally the only indication that a twin pregnancy occurred is the finding of a fetus compressus or papyraceous at delivery. Disseminated intravascular coagulopathy can occur in the mother if one twin dies and remains *in utero* for a prolonged period (generally 4 weeks or longer) but is most common if both fetuses have been dead for an extended period.

Congenital Abnormalities

Multiple gestations are at increased risk for congenital abnormalities. The rates for both major and minor malformations are two to four times as high as those for singletons and are highest among monozygotic/monoamnionic twins. Malformations can range from being identical or similar to being extensive in one fetus and absent in the other. As an extreme example, conjoined twins may result if the twinning process is begun after the embryonic disc and rudimentary amniotic sac have been formed and the division of the embryonic disc is incomplete. Such twins can be joined along their anterior (thoracopagus), posterior (pyopagus), cephalic

(craniopagus), or caudal (ischiopagus) aspects. Thoracopagus twins are the most common type of conjoined twins.

Maternal Complications

Mothers with multiple gestations have a three to five times higher risk of pregnancy-induced hypertension, which is estimated to occur in 20% to 40% of all twin pregnancies. Multiple gestations probably also increase the risk that gestational diabetes will develop in predisposed women.

In the course of singleton pregnancies, blood volume increases by about 30% to 40%. Generally there is a disproportionate increase of plasma volume over red cell volume, resulting in a relative hemodilution or "pregnancy anemia"; this effect may be more pronounced in multiple gestations, where blood volume increases 50% or more. In addition, in multiple gestations the pregnancy anemia is more likely to be a real anemia because of the increased fetal and maternal demands. It is estimated that the risk of anemia related to iron or folate deficiency with twins is two to three times that with singletons. Furthermore, women with multiple gestations are at higher risk for hemorrhage antepartum, intrapartum, and postpartum due to the increased chance of placenta previa, abruptio placentae, and uterine atony and as a result of complications related to operative deliveries.

Complications of Labor

Labor in multiple pregnancy is often complicated by dysfunctional patterns that are commonly attributed to uterine overdistention. Fetuses are at risk antepartum and intrapartum for cord accidents, such as prolapse, entanglement, and vasa previa. In addition it is often difficult to monitor fetal heart rate patterns accurately. Fetal malpresentation and the increased necessity of operative and manipulative deliveries pose hazards to mother and fetuses during the delivery process itself. Hemorrhagic complications of such deliveries have been already mentioned.

ANTEPARTUM ASSESSMENT AND CARE

General Measures

Once the diagnosis of multiple gestation is suspected, it should be confirmed by ultrasonography and a best estimated gestational age determined. Such a pregnancy should immediately be considered high risk and managed by a fully qualified obstetrician with access to a hospital equipped and staffed to handle preterm or compromised infants.

In general the management of multiple gestations should be directed toward assessment of congenital abnormalities, detection of coincident maternal disease, prevention of preterm delivery, ensuring of adequate maternal nutrition, assessment of fetal growth and well-being, preparation for delivery, and intervention when a maximum benefit of intrauterine existence has been achieved. Regular clinic visits should be scheduled at one- to two-week intervals from 16 weeks on. Evaluation at each visit should include determinations of maternal weight, blood pressure, hemoglobin, urine analysis, fundal height, and fetal heart rates.

Today, ultrasonography forms the cornerstone for management of multiple pregnancy. Not only does it help to confirm the number of fetuses and the gestational age, but it is essential for assessment of congenital anomalies, number of separate sacs, location of placentas, fetal positions, interval fetal growth, and late complications of pregnancy. An ultrasound study should be done early in pregnancy, and as part of antepartum fetal assessment as the pregnancy progresses.

Maternal nutritional needs with multiple pregnancy exceed those of singletons. With twins, caloric requirements increase by 300 kcal to 600 kcal and, as in any pregnancy, should be made up of a balanced intake of protein, carbohydrate, vitamins, minerals, and essential fatty acids. Prenatal vitamins, including 60 mg to 100 mg iron in simple salt, is recommended each day. Supplementation with folic acid (1 mg/day) has been suggested to ensure that fetal and maternal needs are met.

Prevention of Premature Labor

Prevention of premature labor and delivery in otherwise uncomplicated multiple pregnancies remains a controversial area of management. Unresolved are the relative benefits of simple bed rest, restricted activity, and the prophylactic use of tocolytic agents.

Although various studies have supported, and others refuted, the benefits of bed rest in delaying preterm delivery of multiple gestations, no study has demonstrated a contraindication to its use. Furthermore, even if bed rest does not result in pregnancy prolongation, it is generally correlated with higher fetal weights for gestational age, probably because uterine perfusion is increased and maternal nutritional demands are minimized. For these reasons we advocate staged bed rest to our patients from 20 weeks on. Although no ideal bed rest schedule has been defined, it is not unreasonable to suggest two to three rest periods of one to two hours per day in addition to an eight- to ten-hour period of sleep at night. The patient should be advised to rest on her side, preferably in the left lateral decubitus position. If not begun sooner, bed rest should be encouraged between 26 and 32 weeks, when neonatal survival rates rise from less than 10% to greater than 90%. Arguments can also be made for discontinuing work, heavy lifting, and even intercourse during this period.

Other measures for prolonging the multiple pregnancy are open to considerable debate. Prophylactic placement of a cerclage has been suggested but has not been found to be effective in either prolonging gestation or improving fetal outcome. Prophylactic use of tocolytic β-mimetic agents, such as terbutaline or ritodrine, has not been shown unequivocally to reduce prematurity rates in twins. Prolonged use of these drugs is not without risk and requires careful surveillance of fetal growth, maternal electrolytes, and glucose tolerance. In addition, women with twins on β-mimetics have been found to be at greater risk for developing pulmonary edema. At this point we cannot advocate the use of these drugs on a routine basis in multiple gestations except for appropriate clinical indications. Similarly, administration of progestational agents, such as 17-hydroxyprogesterone caproate (Delalutin) has been ineffective in the prevention of prematurity in twin pregnancy.

Antepartum Testing

One factor that appears to be having a beneficial effect on the management of multiple gestation is the use of antepartum fetal testing. Currently we advocate the use of nonstress testing weekly starting at 30 to 32 weeks, and sooner for fetal or maternal indications. The nonstress test is particularly valuable when combined with a brief ultrasound examination and assessment of the fetal biophysical profiles: fetal movement, tone, and "breathing" activities, with particular attention to differences in amniotic fluid volumes or fetal ascites. When any abnormality is suggested, the frequency of nonstress testing is increased to at least semiweekly.

A nonstress test to which even one fetus does not react has been correlated with an increased incidence of perinatal morbidity, fetal distress, asphyxia, and intrauterine growth retardation, and a perinatal death rate six times as high as that of reactive twins. When a nonreactive nonstress test result is obtained, an oxytocin challenge test is generally performed if not contraindicated. A positive result in one or both fetuses in an oxytocin challenge test has been associated with a very high risk of fetal death within 24 to 48 hours and is an indication for delivery. Obvious pitfalls of these procedures relate to technical difficulties, including the interpretive skills of the examiner and the inadvertent detection of a single fetal heart rate in more than one location. Success rates can be improved by using ultrasound to confirm the best locations for monitoring the different fetal hearts.

Amniocentesis

On occasion it will be necessary to perform amniocentesis in a multiple pregnancy for reasons such as genetic counseling, Rh isoimmunization, or assessment of pulmonary maturity. Several points should be kept in mind when this procedure is being considered. Genetic amniocentesis should be performed for usual maternal or fetal indications, such as advanced maternal age, elevated α-fetoprotein levels, congenital anomaly, and previous personal or family history of a genetic abnormality for which diagnostic tools are available. When more than one fetus is present, it is necessary to attempt to obtain fluid from each sac. Ultrasound guidance of needle placement has proved invaluable in this regard. A dye such as indigo carmine can be instilled in each sac following removal of fluid to avoid the possibility of acquiring fluid from a sac more than once. When amniocentesis is performed for assessment of Rh and other isoimmunization it is again necessary to sample each sac separately because fetuses can be discordant for blood types and severity of hemolysis.

Under ideal circumstances, when amniocentesis is used to assess pulmonary maturity, each sac should again be sampled, although recent findings have suggested that L/S ratios will usually be similar in the absence of labor, irrespective of sex, zygosity, and discordancy. Amniotic fluid should be coincidentally analyzed for the presence of phosphatidylglycerol and for foam stability. The foam stability index is particularly valuable as a means of assessing the actual functional ability of the surfactant that is present. If the patient is in labor, the presenting twin usually has a pulmonary maturity profile more advanced than subsequent babies, and, if one is anticipating interruption of labor, sampling of amniotic fluid is advisable.

It has generally been found that multiple-gestation fetuses achieve pulmonary maturity several weeks earlier than singletons. However, in anticipation of premature delivery, particularly when more than two fetuses are present, it has been suggested that one consider the weekly prophylactic administration of β-methasone or other corticosteroid capable of accelerating pulmonary maturity, starting at 26 weeks. Certainly, there appear to be few contraindications to this except in patients who are diabetic, in whom an aberration of blood sugar control usually will be found following administration of these drugs.

Discordancy

Discordancy of twin growth can be found with congenital abnormalities, with differences in sex (or even race), with unequalities in nutrition and intrauterine growth retardation resulting from different sites of placentation and unequal placental perfusion, and in "twin-to-twin transfusion" syndromes. When discordant growth is suspected, efforts should be made to determine its etiology and to confirm fetal well-being. Ultrasonography, antepartum testing, and, occasionally, amniocentesis for genetic and other reasons are helpful in this regard. If intrauterine growth retardation is suspected as the cause of discordancy, a reactive nonstress test, presence of normal amounts of amniotic fluid in each gestational sac, and a negative oxytocin challenge test, are reassuring. Increased fetal surveillance is in order under these circumstances, with serial nonstress tests

and ultrasound studies being done at least semiweekly until labor ensues or delivery is necessitated. A suspicious nonstress test result or sudden change in amniotic fluid volume is an ominous sign, and delivery should be expedited—usually it should take place within 24 to 48 hours.

Because fetuses can be discordant for fetal anomalies, chromosomal abnormalities, and inborn errors of metabolism, one may have to address a situation in which one normal fetus is coexistent with one or more abnormal fetuses. Approaches to this problem in the past have included either termination of the pregnancy or expectant management. It has been advocated recently that "selective feticide," usually accomplished by cardiac puncture, be considered under these circumstances. However, this is not without risk: death of the remaining fetuses and disseminated intravascular coagulation in the mother have been described following selective feticide. Also, the procedure carries heavy moral, ethical, and psychologic implications that must be addressed.

Intrauterine Fetal Demise

It is not unusual to have to contend with a multiple pregnancy that has been complicated by intrauterine demise of one fetus. When such a condition is detected, hospitalization for proper evaluation is often indicated. The well-being of remaining fetuses should be confirmed using nonstress testing, ultrasound, and if necessary, oxytocin challenge testing. Coincident maternal disease, such as preeclampsia and disseminated intravascular coagulation, should be ruled out. In pregnancies confirmed to be beyond 34 weeks or in the presence of fetal distress, it is best to consider delivery.

If the pregnancy is less than 34 weeks, and there is no evidence of fetal distress or maternal disease, expectant management can be considered. This should include daily nonstress tests for at least 72 hours after fetal demise and at least semiweekly thereafter. If the surviving fetuses are clearly premature or have immature amniotic fluid pulmonary profiles, the use of β-methasone or other corticosteroid should be considered. The mother should be screened at least weekly for evidence of disseminated intravascular coagulation. Platelet count, fibrinogen, fibrin split products, prothrombin time and activated partial thromboplastin time can be assessed simultaneously for this purpose. A sudden decrease in fibrinogen associated with an increase in fibrin split products is usually the first aberration detected. The occurrence of transient hypofibrinogenemia shortly after the death of one twin has been described; this has been successfully managed with heparin infusions.

Twin-to-Twin Transfusion

A problem unique to the multiple gestation, and presenting an unusual challenge to the practicing obstetrician, is that of twin-to-twin transfusion syndrome (see

Chapter 44). Twin-to-twin transfusion results from vascular anastomoses between monochorionic or fused placentas. Often fetuses suffering from twin-to-twin transfusion syndromes present with discordancy of growth, hydramnios, or evidence of acute heart failure in one or both twins. Once begun, the process generally follows an unrelenting course resulting in the intrauterine death of one or both fetuses or premature labor. Regardless of gestational age, timely delivery is the only reasonable course of action if survival of both infants is sought. Even with timely delivery, it is not unusual to lose at least one of the infants, usually the polycythemic/plethoric one, in the neonatal period. If twin-to-twin transfusion is suspected before the gestational age of viability, expectant management can be considered in the hope that at least one infant will survive.

MANAGEMENT OF LABOR AND DELIVERY

Timing of Delivery

Perhaps the most controversial aspects of caring for patients with multiple gestation relate to management of labor and delivery. The first question to be considered in this regard is, when is the best time for delivery? Several indications for expediting delivery have been addressed in the previous section; however, proper timing of delivery in the uncomplicated pregnancy may also be critical to maternal and fetal outcome.

In many instances, the question of intervention never arises because labor begins early. Most twin gestations will spontaneously go into labor by 37 to 38 weeks of gestation, and the mean length of gestation for triplets and quadruplets is even shorter (35 and 34 weeks, respectively). Indeed, more than 50% of twins will be less than 37 weeks at delivery and weigh less than 2500 g. Perinatal mortality in uncomplicated twin pregnancies appears to be lowest at 37 to 38 weeks.

The question then arises, should all twins be delivered at 37 to 38 weeks? Although a flexible approach is always advocated in this situation, generally, with accurate dates and good prenatal care, including early ultrasound, and with difficulty assuring fetal well-being beyond 38 weeks, even with frequent follow-up, serious consideration should be given to induction of labor, or even cesarean section if indicated. However, when plans are made for expectant management, repeated nonstress tests with biophysical assessment of fetal well-being should be done. In general no twin gestation should be allowed to continue beyond 40 weeks, except in extraordinary circumstances.

Route of Delivery

Once labor has begun or has been determined to be necessary, the first issue one must address is the best route of delivery. Several factors must be taken into consideration when this decision is made: fetal presentations, gestational age, and weight, status of the membranes and cervix, parity, presence of coincident fetal complications (*e.g.*, congenital anomalies, discordancy, intrauterine growth retardation, twin-to-twin transfusion, fetal distress, and polyhydramnios), as well as maternal complications (*e.g.*, preeclampsia and diabetes).

Abnormal presentation is more likely with twins than with a single fetus. The first twin may be expected to present by the vertex in only about 80% of cases; the second twin in only about 50% of cases. Combinations of presentations (Fig. 28-1) occur with the following approximate frequency:

Cephalic-cephalic	39%
Cephalic-breech	37%

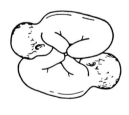
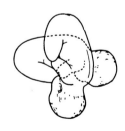
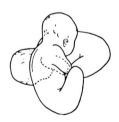
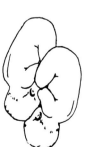
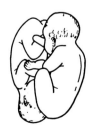
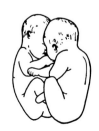

FIG. 28-1. Combinations of presentations of twins (Beck AC, Rosenthal AH: Obstetrical Practice. Baltimore, Williams & Wilkins, 1955)

Breech-breech	10%
Cephalic-transverse	8%
Breech-transverse	5%
Transverse-transverse	1%

A rare complication of labor and delivery in twin pregnancy is fetal entanglement, or locking. This has been reported to occur once in 817 twin deliveries and once in 87 twin deliveries with breech–vertex combinations. The most common type can be termed "interlocking" (Fig. 28-2). This occurs at or below the pelvic inlet, characteristically when the first twin presents by the breech. In this condition, the neck of the baby is elongated and its head is locked above the head of the second twin, which has descended into the pelvis. Other types of entanglement may occur above the pelvic brim and can be termed "collisions." For example, the two heads may descend simultaneously so that neither one can enter the pelvis, or the arm of one twin may be around the neck of the other. Conjoined twins may present a similar difficulty in labor and delivery.

As a general recommendation for multiple gestations, cesarean section is preferred over vaginal delivery whenever the first fetus is in a malpresentation, especially in nulliparas, or when delivery of the first fetus is complicated by conditions such as deflexion of the head, transverse arrest, or a contracted pelvis. Cesarean section is also indicated whenever conjoined twins or collision is diagnosed with reasonable certainty, and when congenital abnormality compatible with life, such as myelomeningocele, is suspected and where minimizing birth trauma and infectious morbidity might improve postpartum outcome. As a general rule, any pregnancy with three or more fetuses is best handled primarily by cesarean section.

In the absence of the complications discussed above, cephalic-cephalic twins of any gestational age can often be safely delivered vaginally. When the first fetus is cephalic and the second is in a malpresentation, the route of delivery depends to a large degree on the experience of the attending obstetrician. Some have advocated routine cesarean section under these circumstances, but, if the gestation is beyond 34 weeks, estimated fetal weight exceeds 1500 g, discordancy is minimal, and there is no evidence of fetal distress, outcomes from cesarean and vaginal births are similar. When a vaginal delivery is anticipated, an operator skilled in the art of internal and external podalic version must be present in the delivery room. Indeed, such a precaution is necessary even with cephalic-cephalic twins because the presentation of the second twin can change with delivery of the first and at least 40% of second twins will require a manipulative delivery.

There has been a growing reluctance to perform vaginal delivery even on healthy fetuses, regardless of presentation, if low birthweight (<1500 g) is suspected. Low birthweight, prematurity, and intrauterine growth retardation, place the malpositioned fetus at higher risk for head entrapment and complications of traumatic delivery because of the increased likelihood that head circumference will exceed abdominal circumference. In addition, these infants have a greater tendency intrapartum to develop acidosis and asphyxia, which can potentiate both respiratory distress syndrome and intracerebral hemorrhage. It is suggested, therefore, that liberal, though not invariable, use of cesarean section is indicated for the delivery of the low birthweight twin pregnancy, particularly when either fetus is malpresenting. Ideally, if cesarean section is selected as the route of delivery, it should be performed expeditiously, before labor is prolonged, since the labor process itself may contribute to perinatal asphyxia and intracerebral bleeding in the premature infant.

Care in Labor

Once labor has been established, or induction deemed necessary, in the patient with multiple pregnancy, the following steps are taken to minimize maternal and fetal complications:

1. The senior obstetricians, neonatologists, and anesthesiologists are notified of the patient's presence and any pregnancy complications.
2. An intravenous infusion of lactated Ringer's solution is begun using a large bore (18 gauge or lower) indwelling catheter.
3. Routine laboratory preparation is begun, including complete blood count, urine analysis, and cross match for two units of compatible blood.
4. The patient is positioned on her side, preferably in the left lateral decubitus position.
5. Fetal presentations are determined and, ideally, confirmed with ultrasound.
6. Fetal heart rates are monitored continuously using

FIG. 28-2. Fetal interlocking. (Clyne DGW: Textbook of Gynaecology and Obstetrics. London, Longmans, 1963)

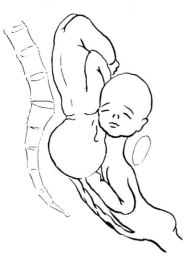

either two external monitors or a combination of one internal and one external monitor. (Inability to follow fetal heart rates due to an unavailability of monitors or maternal obesity may be another indication for cesarean section).

7. A delivery area is prepared in which a general anesthetic can be administered and a cesarean section can be performed.

8. If oxytocin is used for induction or augmentation of labor, it is administered in a dilute solution, starting at 1–2 mU per minute, and increased cautiously at intervals of no less than 15 minutes.

9. Pain in labor can be managed with judicious administration of narcotics, intravenously, during contractions, or with a continuous epidural anesthetic. If the continuous epidural anesthesia is anticipated, adequate fluid load is necessary to prevent hypotension resulting from sympathetic blockade.

10. If labor progresses well, the patient is taken to the delivery room in time to enable attending obstetricians, neonatologists, and anesthesiologists to prepare adequately.

Delivery of the Second Twin

Once the first baby is delivered and the cord singly clamped, the position of the next baby must be quickly ascertained, using as necessary internal, external, and even ultrasound examination. At this point, adequate anesthesia, assuring maternal cooperation and uterine relaxation, becomes one of the most crucial aspects of delivery care; general anesthesia may be necessary even if an epidural anesthetic is functional. Monitoring of the second fetus continues during and after delivery of the first. If the fetal head can be guided into the pelvis, membranes are ruptured, and oxytocin augmentation is begun if needed. Once adequate descent has been achieved, the second stage of labor can be shortened by the use of forceps or vacuum extraction. When the infant is delivered, the placental side of the umbilical cord is doubly clamped to indicate birth order.

If the presenting part is not the fetal head, several options are available. Traditionally, breech extraction has been performed promptly prior to contraction of the lower uterine segment. To do this, both feet are identified and firmly grasped through the membranes and drawn into the pelvis. The membranes are then ruptured and the baby delivered using a careful and patient technique. During this process, gentle suprapubic pressure or use of Piper forceps can help to maintain the head in flexion, facilitating delivery and minimizing trauma.

Alternatively, external version can be attempted before rupture of membranes, using ultrasound, if available, for guidance. When an undeliverable presentation exists and external version cannot be accomplished safely, when fetal distress develops, or when the malpresenting fetus appears to be significantly larger than the first, as 40% will be, cesarean section should be performed expeditiously. One is not committed to delivering both babies vaginally, and if adequate preparations have been made, extraordinary heroics should be avoided.

Classical teaching has encouraged delivery of the second twin between 5 and 20 minutes after delivery of the first. Undue haste can result in an unnecessarily traumatic delivery, and a prolonged interval places the fetus in danger of placental insufficiency or premature separation, cervical retraction, and cord accidents. Generally, we prefer to adhere to delivery within this time frame, but with careful monitoring and a well-prepared operative team, delay in delivery of the second infant can be safely managed.

Once the babies are delivered, and while the cervix is dilated and anesthesia is available, the placenta can be manually removed. It should be inspected carefully, as an aid in determining zygosity and as a means of diagnosing any pathologic conditions, such as vascular communications between fetuses, which existed during the pregnancy. Following delivery of the placenta, oxytocin infusion is begun and the uterus is manually explored for rupture, which might have occurred secondary to forceps or manipulative delivery. At this point hemorrhage may ensue from poor myometrial contractility resulting from overdistention, anesthesia, retained placental fragments, or uterine perforation. If uterine contraction and control of hemorrhage cannot be achieved with oxytocin and fundal massage, then methergine (0.1–0.2 mg. IV or IM) or prostaglandin (PGE_2 or 15-methyl-$PGF_2\alpha$) can be administered. Both physician and patient should embark on any delivery of a multiple gestation aware that hysterectomy may be necessary if hemorrhagic complications cannot be controlled by conservative measures.

POSTPARTUM CARE

When the delivery room is left behind, the obstetrician must remain aware of the special needs of mothers with multiple pregnancies. Aside from medical complications, the patient is at high risk for prolonged fatigue and depression because of both the stress of the pregnancy itself and the extra efforts involved in caring for more than one baby. If the infants are compromised or in the intensive care nursery, bonding may be difficult. Mothers who have made plans to breastfeed their babies may find that this is impractical, further potentiating feelings of inadequacy. Discharge of such a patient should be delayed until she has dealt with the acute phase of these problems and recovered from her delivery.

Before discharge careful plans should be made for contraceptive management. The patient should be encouraged to maintain in close contact with her obstetrician and pediatrician about questions and complications that may arise. In some areas local support groups for "parents with twins" have been formed to help in dealing with the special difficulties of having more than one baby. This is particularly important because products of multiple gestations have been found to be at high risk for neglect and child abuse, especially when they are born prematurely. If a patient is known to come from an environment where the babies will be at higher risk for abuse, social services should be contacted and follow-up arranged even before she is discharged from the hospital.

REFERENCES AND RECOMMENDED READING

Berkowitz R: Twin gestation. Perinat Care 2:28, 1978

Chervenak FA, Johnson RE, Berkowitz RL et al: Intrapartum external version of the second twin. Obstet Gynecol 62:160, 1983

Chervenak FA, Johnson RE, Berkowitz RL et al: Is routine cesarean section necessary for vertex-breech and vertex-transverse twin gestations? Obstet Gynecol 148:1, 1984

Chervenak FA, Johnson RE, Youcha S et al: Intrapartum management of twin gestation. Obstet Gynecol 65:119, 1985

Galea P, Scott JM, Goel KM: Feto-fetal transfusion syndrome. Arch Dis Child 57:781, 1982

Hanna JH, Hill JM: Single intrauterine fetal demise in multiple gestation. Obstet Gynecol 63:126, 1984

Hartikainen-Sorri A, Kauppila A, Tuimala R: Inefficacy of 17α-hydroxyprogesterone caproate in the prevention of prematurity in twin pregnancy. Obstet Gynecol 56:692, 1980

Hartikainen-Sorri A, Kauppila A, Tuimala R et al: Factors related to improved outcome for twins. Acta Obstet Gynecol Scand 62:23, 1983

Hawrylyshyn PA, Barkin M, Bernstein A et al: Twin pregnancies: A continuing challenge. Obstet Gynecol 59:463, 1982

Holcberg G, Biale Y, Lewenthal H et al: Outcome of triplet gestations. Obstet Gynecol 59:472, 1982

Leveno KJ, Santos-Ramos R, Duenhoelter JH et al: Sonar cephalometry in twin pregnancy: Discordancy of the biparietal diameter after 28 weeks' gestation. Am J Obstet Gynecol 138:615, 1980

McCarthy BJ, Sachs BP, Layde PM et al: The epidemiology of neonatal death in twins. Am J Obstet Gynecol 141:252, 1981

Newton ER, Genest DR, Cetrulo CL: Management of a nonreactive nonstress test in a twin gestation. J Reprod Med 28:345, 1983

Romero R, Duffy TP, Berkowitz RL et al: Prolongation of a preterm pregnancy complicated by death of a single twin in utero and disseminated intravascular coagulation. N Engl J Med 310:772, 1984

Ron-El R, Caspi E, Schreyer P et al: Triplet and quadruplet pregnancies and management. Obstet Gynecol 57:458, 1981

Tabshe KM, Crandall B, Lebherz TB et al: Genetic amniocentesis in twin pregnancy. Obstet Gynecol 65:843, 1985

Vaughn TC, Powell C: The obstetrical management of conjoined twins. Obstet Gynecol 52:67S, 1979

Weekes ARL, Menzies DN, de Boer CH: The relative efficacy of bed rest, cervical suture, and no treatment in the management of twin pregnancy. Br J Obstet Gynaecol 84:161, 1977

Other Complications Due to Pregnancy

David N. Danforth

29

PREMATURE RUPTURE OF THE MEMBRANES

Premature rupture of the membranes is defined as the leakage of amniotic fluid prior to the onset of labor. The implications are less serious when rupture occurs at term than when the membranes rupture earlier in pregnancy.

Premature rupture of the membranes occurs in 10% of patients at term, whereas the incidence among women who deliver before term is more than 15%. About 30% of infants delivered after premature rupture of the membranes are of low birth weight.

At term, spontaneous rupture of the membranes is usually followed by the onset of labor in 24 to 48 hours; earlier in pregnancy, however, the latent period is usually much longer, and the leakage sometimes persists without labor for several weeks.

Cause

The cause of premature rupture of the membranes is unknown, and rupture usually occurs without warning in a woman whose pregnancy appears to be progressing normally.

The strength of the fetal membranes is imparted almost entirely by the connective tissue layer to which the epithelial cells of the amnion are attached (see Fig. 17-21). Premature rupture may result if this supporting layer is either inherently weak or damaged by substances released from the cervix or some other source.

Several studies have suggested that there is no difference in the tensile strength of the membranes regardless of whether they rupture prematurely or remain intact throughout labor. However, Skinner and colleagues have found that the collagen content of the amnion declines as term approaches and that it is present in significantly lower amounts in membranes that rupture prematurely. They have suggested that these

changes in the collagen layer may be related to the softening and increasing compliance of the cervix in late pregnancy and may be caused by similar factors. Although Al-Zaid and colleagues could not confirm these findings, perhaps because of differences in sampling or methodology, the question remains an important one and should be pursued.

Lenihan suggests that the practice of weekly vaginal examination during the month before term may lead to an increased incidence of premature rupture of the membranes, possibly by introducing bacteria into the cervix. More information is needed because this conclusion is at variance with the clinical opinion of those who routinely follow this practice. More recently, Minkoff and colleagues have found a positive correlation between the earlier presence of vaginal pathogens (*Trichomonas vaginalis, Bacteroides,* and *Ureaplasma urealyticum*) and premature rupture of the membranes, suggesting the possibility that patients at risk may be identified early in pregnancy.

Fortunately, the question of lunar and barometric influences appears to be solved—Marks and colleagues found no correlation.

Complications

The major complications of premature rupture of the membranes are the precipitation of labor and ascending intrauterine infection.

The major cause of perinatal disease and death because of premature rupture of the membranes is preterm delivery. When the membranes have ruptured, ascending intrauterine infection also is a constant threat to fetal survival. Amnionitis, omphalitis, congenital pneumonia, and, occasionally, fetal septicemia have ominous implications; maternal septicemia and fatal septic shock have often occurred as the result of ruptured membranes. In the low-birth-weight infant, the primary risks of preterm delivery are respiratory distress syndrome (RDS), hyaline membrane disease, and intraventricular hemorrhage. In the term infant, the major risk is neonatal sepsis.

Diagnosis

The diagnosis is obvious if the membranes rupture with a gush that is followed by continued and copious leakage of watery fluid from the vagina. A diagnostic problem may arise if the watery leakage is slight and intermittent, as occurs in many women because of urinary incontinence. If it continues immediately after voiding, the membranes are probably ruptured, but the following tests can be helpful if there is doubt:

1. Examination with a vaginal speculum in place may show amniotic fluid draining from the cervical canal. If there is doubt, the discharge can be tested with nitrazine paper (amniotic fluid is alkaline; vaginal secretions are acidic). This test is often inconclusive, however.
2. A drop of the liquid can be mixed with 0.1% nile blue sulfate and permitted to dry on a glass slide for five minutes. The presence of *any* orange-staining fetal squames confirms that the liquid is amniotic fluid.
3. The presence of anucleate fetal squames, lanugo, and the frond crystallization pattern of dried amniotic fluid that is not contaminated by blood or meconium identifies the liquid as amniotic fluid.
4. Gahl and colleagues have reported that the presence of diamine oxidase in the vaginal pool suggests that the membranes have ruptured. Maternal blood, seminal fluid, and iodine antiseptics interfere with the accuracy of the test, which can be performed in about one hour. A scintillation counter is required, and the value of the test appears to be for cases in which conventional tests are equivocal.
5. Rochelson and co-workers have described a rapid, sensitive latex-agglutination test for α-fetoprotein (AFP). The AFP concentration in amniotic fluid declines after 35 weeks' gestation; therefore, the test's value is for pregnancies of 35 weeks' gestation or less. No equivocal or negative tests were found before 35 weeks; most of the false-negative results occurred at term.

Management

The management of premature rupture of the membranes is determined chiefly by the time in pregnancy at which it occurs. The major considerations are the potential for serious maternal or perinatal complications at the various stages of pregnancy. With regard to fetal outlook, a liveborn infant's chance of survival is excel-

lent after 36 weeks' gestation and is good between 34 and 36 weeks' gestation. At 28 to 34 weeks the prognosis must be considered fair to poor, depending upon the size and condition of the infant upon arrival in the nursery, the skill of the medical team that provides the neonatal care, and the physical facilities available in the nursery. In approaching the problem of premature rupture of the membranes, the physician should be aware that under the most optimal circumstances, a liveborn infant weighing 2001 g to 2500 g has a 97% chance of surviving, a liveborn weighing 1501 g to 2000 g has at least a 90% chance of surviving, and a liveborn weighing 1001 g to 1500 g has a 65% to 80% chance of surviving. Special perinatal centers are reporting survivorship of newborns weighing 750 g to 1000 g. With these figures in mind, the obstetrician can make a reasonable judgment of perinatal risks versus benefits of intervention in a given case.

In all cases of premature rupture of the membranes, the patient should be admitted to the hospital. At admission a sterile speculum examination is made to determine whether a pool of amniotic fluid may be present. The question of whether sterile vaginal examination should be done at admission is unsettled. Most obstetricians consider it essential in ruling out cord prolapse and determining the status of the cervix. Some avoid vaginal examination until labor is established or the decision to deliver the infant within 24 hours has been made. Reasons for avoiding vaginal examination include the possibility of introducing pathogenic organisms and the possibility of causing prostaglandin release by manipulation of the cervix, thus contributing to the precipitation of labor. If the examination is conducted gently and with dispatch, the information to be gained appears to outweigh the hazards. No other vaginal examinations should be done until the patient is committed to delivery.

In most cases, an ultrasound examination is done to determine cephalometry and placental localization. The lecithin/sphingomyelin (L/S) ratio or equivalent test should be done if fetal maturity is in doubt; the vaginal pool may be an appropriate source of the fluid, but, if it is not, amniocentesis should be done. If the latter is needed, the fluid should be cultured. Cotton suggests the following guidelines for amniocentesis:

Before 32 weeks' gestation it is not needed. Even if the lungs are shown to be mature, neonatal morbidity is sufficiently probable that expectant treatment is advisable unless contraindicated.

Between 32 and 34 weeks' gestation amniocentesis for L/S ratio or equivalent test, Gram stain, and aerobic and anaerobic cultures are helpful in deciding whether delivery should be initiated.

After 34 weeks' gestation amniocentesis is of questionable value unless there are risk factors for RDS, as there are in cases of diabetes mellitus. The lungs are usually mature at this stage, and even if RDS does occur, it is usually mild or moderate and responsive to treatment.

The risks of amniocentesis in this situation have been debated, but in the experience of Yeast and colleagues, the procedure is quite safe and is without demonstrable maternal or fetal risk.

After 37 Weeks

Spontaneous rupture of the membranes after 37 weeks is usually followed by the onset of labor within 48 hours, but in these patients, the risk of ascending infection is significant, and an oxytocin induction is usually started if labor has not begun within 24 hours. Because of both theoretic and documented risks of prolonged oxytocin administration, the attempt should be abandoned if labor has not started within five hours of the initiation of the infusion, and cesarean section delivery should be seriously considered.

Before 34 Weeks

Premature rupture of the membranes before 34 weeks may be managed either conservatively (*i.e.*, observation either until the infant is mature enough to survive without intensive care, or until infection or labor intervenes) or aggressively (*i.e.*, prompt delivery by induction of labor or cesarean section).

CONSERVATIVE MANAGEMENT. The purpose of conservative management is to prolong the *in utero* existence of the fetus in an effort to minimize the serious complications of preterm delivery. It is important to remember that during the last two months of pregnancy the baby grows at a rate of about a half pound per week. Also, a latent period of more than 16 hours between rupture of the membranes and preterm delivery may enhance fetal lung maturation and, hence, reduce the incidence of RDS. In the large series reported by Kappy and co-workers, the latent period from rupture of membranes to spontaneous onset of labor exceeded seven days in 19% of women whose pregnancies were of less than 37 weeks' duration and in only 4% of those beyond 37 weeks' duration. The longest latent period was 58 days.

Bed rest is an essential feature of conservative management, and it is advisable for the patient to remain in the hospital as long as there is active leakage. A complete blood count and urinalysis at admission, continuous external electronic record of the fetal heart rate at admission to exclude occult cord or fetal tachycardia, daily white blood count, and a four times daily record of fetal heart rate (auscultation for 30 seconds), temperature, pulse, and respiration are required.

If prolonged hospitalization is not feasible, the patient may be discharged after five days with a full explanation that this is less than optimal treatment. Home care should include bed rest with bathroom privileges; avoidance of intercourse, douches, and tampons; recording of oral temperature in the morning, afternoon, and evening; and white blood cell count at least once

every other day. The physician should be notified of fever, a change in the character or odor of the vaginal discharge, onset of contractions, or any change in fetal movements. If the leakage stops during the hospital stay, the patient may also be discharged, with the same instructions except that bed rest is not required. If the leakage resumes or if fever develops, she should be readmitted immediately.

PROPHYLACTIC ANTIBIOTICS. Prophylactic antibiotics are not recommended in cases of uncomplicated premature rupture of the membranes. Their use does not influence the incidence of amnionitis or neonatal sepsis, and the growth of resistant organisms is a major threat. Moreover, such treatment will interfere with proper bacterial studies of the newborn.

EFFORTS TO STOP LABOR. The clinical use of tocolytic agents is discussed in Chapter 35. With few exceptions, they are generally contraindicated in the presence of ruptured membranes.

PREVENTION OF RESPIRATORY DISTRESS SYNDROME. The events in the normal maturation of the fetal lung are considered on page 320. The question of whether a latent period of 16 to 24 hours between premature rupture of the membranes and preterm delivery per se leads to accelerated pulmonary maturation and, hence, to a reduced incidence of RDS is still unsettled. Current evidence suggests that such a latent period is indeed beneficial. The ability of glucocorticoids to accelerate lung maturation, as first suggested by Liggins, has been confirmed by numerous clinical trials. In women whose pregnancies are of 24 to 34 weeks' duration and in whom delivery can be delayed for at least 24 hours, the administration of betamethasone (10 mg to 12 mg/24 hours in divided intramuscular doses, continued, if possible, for 48 to 72 hours) is reported to significantly reduce the incidence of RDS, as well as the incidence of death from hyaline membrane disease and intraventricular hemorrhage. The most favorable cases are those of 30 to 32 weeks' gestation; no benefits accrue if pregnancy is of more than 34 weeks' duration or if delivery occurs before 24 hours or after seven days from the time of the first injection. For those who are to be managed conservatively, treatment must be repeated weekly until examination of the amniotic fluid indicates pulmonary maturity (see p. 798).

Although most reports are favorable, Iams and colleagues found that injection of hydrocortisone, with delivery occurring 48 to 82 hours later, has no advantage over simple observation without intervention or use of steroids.

To date, no short-term adverse effects of preterm glucocorticoids on the infant have been demonstrated, and preliminary psychometric studies at four or more years of age suggest no long-term detrimental effects. As Shields and Resnik note, however, extensive well-controlled clinical trials with long-term follow-up are needed to answer the question of possible long-term sequelae.

Severe preeclampsia is a specific contraindication to glucocorticoids. Possible maternal complications include increased susceptibility to, or masking of, intra-uterine or other infection and, when glucocorticoids are used in conjunction with β-mimetic tocolytic agents, postpartum pulmonary edema and shock. The latter complication responds quickly to oxygen and diuretics.

AGGRESSIVE MANAGEMENT. In the event of am-nionitis, the infant should be delivered within eight hours, by induction of labor if it is feasible and by ce-sarean section if it is not. Cervical and blood cultures are taken at once. If delivery is imminent, antibiotics are withheld until after delivery in order to facilitate bacterial studies of the newborn; if delivery will be de-layed for several hours, intravenous antibiotics are started at once.

The onset of amnionitis may be difficult to pinpoint. Warning signs may include a morning temperature of 99°F, a single white blood cell count above 18,000/μL and fetal tachycardia above 160 beats/minute. The di-agnosis is made without hesitancy in the presence of maternal fever, white blood cells counts above 18,000/μL, a tender uterus, and persistent fetal tachycardia. In some cases, a fetid vaginal discharge is present.

Quantitative estimation of C-reactive protein (CRP) appears to be valuable when used in conjunction with other tests in the surveillance of patients who are at risk for amnionitis. The organisms that usually cause am-nionitis are those that are indigenous to the lower female genital tract, such as groups B and D streptococci and vaginal anaerobes. Gravett and co-workers have recov-ered bacterial metabolites in amniotic fluid by gas–liquid chromatography (GLC) before the appearance of clinical signs or other evidence of amnionitis. The test is rapid and relatively specific. A culture is needed to identify the organism, but a positive GLC may permit the phy-sician to act before amnionitis significantly threatens the condition of the mother and the fetus.

Between 34 and 37 Weeks

Unless there are other complications, the decision regarding management is based on tests for pulmonary maturity. If the tests suggest immaturity of the fetal lungs, conservative management is indicated unless there are compelling reasons to terminate the preg-nancy. Glucocorticoids are not helpful at this stage of pregnancy. The L/S ratio or its equivalent is determined once a week; when a mature ratio is obtained, the infant is delivered by induction of labor with oxytocin, or by cesarean section if there is a malpresentation or other reason for abdominal delivery.

At the time of amniocentesis, Gram stain and aerobic and anaerobic cultures are made. The presence of bac-teria in the Gram stain or positive culture is an indication for prompt delivery.

POSTTERM PREGNANCY

Postterm pregnancy is defined differently by different authors. For practical purposes, delivery before 42 weeks' gestation can be considered within normal limits. If the infant is still undelivered at the end of 42 weeks (two weeks after the projected date of labor as estimated by Nägele's rule), the possibility of postterm pregnancy should be considered and, if possible, verified. Most of the cases are accounted for by an error in menstrual dates; in others, pregnancy is actually longer than the accepted limits of normal. The data vary, but it is esti-mated that about 12% of women are undelivered at the end of 42 weeks' gestation. In one series, 7.3% of women delivered after 43 weeks.

Etiology

Failure to begin labor within a normal time range results from a defect in one or more of the myriad of factors that are concerned in the normal onset of labor at term, as discussed in Chapter 30. It is usually futile to attempt to identify the particular cause of a given case of post-term pregnancy. One exception is the postterm preg-nancy that occurs with an anencephalic fetus; the fetus has no hypothalamus, the pituitary is consequently hy-poplastic, and the adrenals are also hypoplastic because of a lack of adrenocorticotrophic hormone (ACTH). The fetal pituitary gland produces no fetal oxytocin, which some investigators have implicated in the normal onset of labor, and the secretion of cortisol by the fetal ad-renals is also impaired. The latter substance is clearly concerned in the onset of labor in the sheep, and it may also play some role in humans. A second exception is placental sulfatase deficiency, which interferes with es-triol formation and is accompanied by prolonged preg-nancy. The diagnosis can be made when estriol excre-tion fails to increase after intra-amniotic instillation of dehydroepiandrosterone sulfate (see also p. 346).

Hazards

The risks to the mother are largely those of delivering an infant that has grown beyond its optimal size. They include such problems as dysfunctional labor, midpelvic arrest, and cephalopelvic disproportion.

Although many infants are unaffected, several re-ports provide evidence that the postterm fetus is at added risk of serious perinatal illness and perinatal death, as occurred, for example, in 13% of the postterm babies in the series of cases reported by Knox and colleagues. The fetal insults appear to be threefold. The first is im-posed by delivery of an excessively large fetus; even if the head does come through without incident, the like-lihood of shoulder dystocia exists, which sometimes re-sults in neonatal illness and death. The second is im-posed by entrapment of the umbilical cord by the uterine wall and fetal parts as a result of oligohydramnios, a common finding in the "postmaturity syndrome." The third insult is imposed by an aging postterm placenta with failing transport mechanisms. The normal life span of the placenta is about 40 weeks; after this time, its capacity and reserve are progressively reduced in the face of increasing demands by the growing fetus. If delivery is delayed too long, intrauterine death must ultimately result. In Zwerdling's huge series, the perinatal mortality of infants born at 37 to 42 weeks' gestation was 1.2%; for those born after 43 weeks, it was 2.4%. Nakano's findings were similar: a perinatal mortality of 0.7% for babies born at term compared with a rate of 2.2% for those born after 42 weeks' gestation.

Diagnosis

If labor has not started at the end of the 42nd week of pregnancy, all of the pertinent data bearing on the duration of pregnancy should be reassessed.

Menstrual Dates

Complete information should have been obtained at the first visit, but, too frequently, the blank space on the record is filled in with the response to the single query: "When was your last period?" The obstetrician must also know if the period was normal, whether it began on time, and whether the customary periodicity is every 28 to 30 days or every one to two months (in the latter case, the projected date of labor may be highly unreliable). Since amenorrhea may occur after oral contraceptives have been used, it is important to know whether oral contraception was used prior to the pregnancy; if used within three months of the last normal menstrual period, the dates may be spurious. The obstetrician should know also whether the basal body temperature (BBT) was monitored prior to the pregnancy: a persistently elevated BBT can provide a reliable indication of when the pregnancy began. Coupled with an exact date of the last menstrual period, it can be used without hesitancy to calculate the duration of pregnancy.

PREGNANCY TESTS. The date of the first positive human chorionic gonadotropin (hCG) test can be helpful in the timing of some pregnancies. However, it is important to know the sensitivity of the test used. As noted in Chapter 20, the most sensitive tests can diagnose pregnancy 24 hours after implantation, but others do not indicate positive results until much later.

Pelvic Examination

The timing of pregnancy by estimation of uterine size is much more accurate at six or seven weeks than it is after three months. Accordingly, a pelvic examination in early pregnancy is more reliable as an index of pregnancy duration than an examination after three months.

Auscultation of the Fetal Heart

When fetal heart tones can be heard with the stethoscope (not Doppler instrument) for the first time, the pregnancy is of at least 20 weeks' duration. This date may be useful in extrapolating the estimated date of labor.

Quickening

It is believed that fetal movements are first felt at about 16 weeks' gestation, but this is highly unreliable and should not be used as a means to date pregnancy.

Ultrasonic Cephalometry

At some time between 20 and 26 weeks' gestation, ultrasonic cephalometry should be done if the menstrual dates are suspect, and a second scan should be done at 31 to 33 weeks. As noted in Chapter 15, these two measurements can predict gestational age within a five-day range. They are also useful if there is a risk of fetal growth retardation or if it seems essential to establish a term date with some accuracy.

The aforementioned factors are all used in the timing of pregnancy. In the Knox series, a diagnosis of postterm pregnancy (beyond 42 weeks) was made according to the following criteria. If the menstrual dates were considered to be accurate and reliable and oral contraceptives had not been used within three months of the last period, then at least one of the following clinical confirmations was needed: pelvic examination prior to 12 weeks, auscultation of unamplified fetal heart tones for at least 22 weeks, or ultrasonic cephalometry between 20 and 30 weeks' gestation. If the menstrual history was unreliable, at least two of these clinical confirmations were required.

Evaluation and Treatment

Beginning after 42 weeks' gestation, it is essential that fetal welfare be determined and monitored until delivery. As noted before, in many cases, perhaps 50%, labor will intervene before any evidence of fetal distress appears (in the Cario series, 50% of the patients went into spontaneous labor within the first three days of monitoring). Unfortunately, all of the applicable tests are indirect, and many have not been validated by noting the results of nonintervention when the tests are abnormal.

Nonstress Testing (NST) of Fetal Heart Rate

Beginning at the end of the 42nd week, nonstressed testing of the fetal heart rate should be done two or three times weekly. Gradually decreasing reactivity, as manifested by either a changing baseline or less frequent or smaller accelerations, should be followed promptly by a contraction stress test (CST) or by an oxytocin challenge test (OCT). Use of these tests is considered in Chapter 41. If the contraction stress test is positive, the infant should be delivered.

Real-Time Ultrasound for Amniotic Fluid Volume

The finding of oligohydramnios in a postterm pregnancy is an ominous sign that calls for prompt delivery. Using real-time ultrasound, the volume of amniotic fluid can be estimated as adequate, as appearing only in pockets, or as less than 300 ml, which indicates oligohydramnios (Fig. 29-1). The scans may be scheduled two or three times weekly, to follow the NST tests.

Fetal Movements

There is evidence that the mother's estimate of fetal activity may have prognostic value. Her impression of reduced fetal motion may constitute evidence of fetal jeopardy.

Estriol Studies

Views of estriol testing as a means of surveillance are changing, and it is now used more frequently than in the recent past. Twenty-four-hour urinary excretion or plasma determinations may be used, or, as recommended by Rayburn and colleagues, a single-voiding urine specimen may be collected at any time of the day to determine the estrogen:creatinine (E:C) ratio. Laboratory norms must be established; for the latter test, the mean ratio for all postterm pregnancies was 28 ± 5. The subnormal ratio was less than 19, providing strong evidence that the baby was indeed postmature and therefore at special risk. The tests were taken on the days of NST testing.

If the estimate of gestation is accurate *and* if the conditions for induction of labor are favorable (see p. 747), labor is induced at the end of the 43rd week. If the conditions for induction are not favorable, it is advisable to continue meticulous surveillance until the end of the 44th week. However, the patient should be

delivered when 44 weeks have been completed, regardless of the normal findings of the various tests. In those for whom induction of labor is considered appropriate, the membranes should be ruptured as the initial step in the procedure. If the amniotic fluid is meconium-stained, a more expeditious delivery than usual is needed; if the induction is to proceed, the application of a scalp electrode is of special importance.

Management

The mere fact of postterm pregnancy imposes a sense of urgency. There is general agreement that if the conditions for induction are favorable, labor should be induced at the end of 42 weeks; if the conditions are clearly unfavorable for induction, it is permissible to defer delivery until the end of the 43rd week, unless *any* evidence of fetal jeopardy should appear, in which case the baby should be delivered promptly. When the gestational dates are definite, it is recommended that the baby be delivered at the end of the 43rd week, by induction of labor if this is feasible and appropriate, or by cesarean section if it is not.

If labor is to be induced, the membranes should be ruptured as the initial step in the procedure. The presence of meconium requires special vigilance and special precautions at the time of delivery (see p. 658). If the conditions for induction of labor are extremely favorable (cervix soft, thin, anterior, and 3 or more cm dilated; vertex presenting at station +2 to +3), most women will start labor within one hour after the membranes are ruptured; if not, an oxytocin infusion should be started at a rate of 0.5 mU/minute and increased by increments of 0.5 mU/minute every 15 minutes until either satisfactory laborlike contractions occur or the maximum rate (in postterm patients) of 4 mU/minute is reached. If labor is not established within six hours of the start of the infusion or if the continuous monitoring of fetal heart rate (an essential part of any induction) suggests fetal distress, then cesarean section should be selected.

Cesarean section should also be selected if prior contraction stress tests were positive or if delivery is

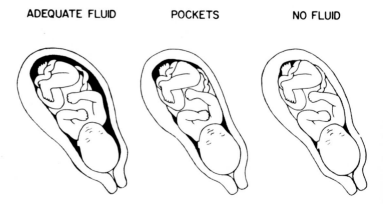

FIG. 29-1. Classification of amniotic fluid volume as visualized by real-time ultrasonography. A lack of amniotic fluid results in oligohydramnios. (Rayburn WF, Motley ME, Stempel LE, Gendreau M: Antepartum prediction of postmature infant. Obstet Gynecol 60:148, 1982. Reprinted with permission from The American College of Obstetricians and Gynecologists)

ADEQUATE FLUID   POCKETS   NO FLUID

indicated and the conditions for induction are not favorable.

MISSED LABOR (DEAD FETUS SYNDROME)

Missed labor refers to intrauterine death after 20 weeks' gestation, with retention of the dead fetus within the uterus. The term *missed abortion* is used when the fetal death occurs before the end of the 20th week of pregnancy. Although rare, the fetus occasionally remains in the uterus for many months, or even years, and becomes calcified.

The fetal death may be due to such factors as a knot in the umbilical cord, Rh isoimmunization, diabetes, or placental insufficiency. In many cases, there is no apparent cause. Failure of labor to start results from failure of some combination of factors normally responsible for the onset of labor at term (see Chap. 30); in missed labor, the most striking defects are lack of increasing uterine stretch, loss of fetal oxytocin and fetal cortisol, and disruption of the fetal contribution to estrogen synthesis, any of which might delay labor.

The diagnosis of missed labor is usually not difficult. As a rule, pregnancy progresses normally until suddenly, usually at some time after 28 weeks, the patient fails to perceive fetal movements. The uterus is silent, and no fetal heartbeat can be detected by real-time or time-motion ultrasonography. Missed labor is diagnosed if labor fails to ensue within 48 hours of fetal death. The differential diagnosis includes abdominal pregnancy and pregnancy in a rudimentary horn.

Most women carrying a dead fetus ultimately go into labor, but the emotional impact of waiting indefinitely for this to occur is significant. In addition, fibrinogen levels generally begin a linear descent approximately three to four weeks after the fetus dies, and severe coagulation problems, especially disseminated intravascular coagulation (see p. 540), can develop in women who remain undelivered for a month or more. Current policy is to await spontaneous labor for a period not exceeding two weeks, unless the membranes rupture before this time, in which case induction is started promptly. Oxytocin may be used.

The use of prostaglandin E_2 in viscous gel, either intravaginally or intracervically, seems especially appropriate if the condition of the cervix is not favorable for the induction of labor. Intra-amniotic saline is not recommended, because the reduced amount of amniotic fluid increases the probability of hypernatremia, coagulation disorders, infection, and cardiovascular collapse.

Induction of labor is contraindicated in certain circumstances, regardless of whether the fetus is living or dead; cesarean section should be used for delivery in the presence of cephalopelvic disproportion, abnormal presentation (transverse lie is common in this syndrome), previous uterine incision, advanced maternal age, grand multiparity, and any maternal condition in which labor is contraindicated.

HYDRAMNIOS

Hydramnios refers to the accumulation of excessive amounts (2000 ml or more) of amniotic fluid. The term *polyhydramnios* is sometimes used to refer to this condition. In the series reported by Queenan and colleagues, the conditions commonly associated with hydramnios were diabetes mellitus (25%), Rh incompatibility (11%), multiple pregnancy (8%), and congenital malformations.

The factors responsible for the normal formation and exchange of amniotic fluid are discussed on page 316. Under ordinary circumstances, the sources of amniotic fluid appear to be secretion by the amnion itself, transudation from maternal serum, and fetal urine, each of which is an ongoing process that provides, at 38 weeks, a production estimated at about 500 ml/hour. This is normally balanced by the hourly removal of an equivalent volume of amniotic fluid by absorption across the fetal membranes and fetal swallowing.

The cause of hydramnios has not been explained. An imbalance between fetal swallowing and voiding could be responsible, but it has been shown that the normal ranges of swallowing (87 ml to 287 ml/day) and voiding (mean average of 23.6 ml/hour) are unchanged in cases of hydramnios. We therefore conclude that the basic derangement is in other water transport mechanisms. Among these, the complex and highly developed amnion cells overlying the placenta seem to be the most likely source of this dysfunction, but there are no published data regarding the possibility that these cells may be concerned.

The fact that hydramnios has always been associated with a high incidence of fetal abnormalities is not helpful in defining its etiology, because no specific etiologic factors are found in any case. The diverse abnormalities that occurred in 100 consecutive cases of hydramnios are shown in Table 29-1. It should be noted that there were no fetal abnormalities in 61 of the cases. In other large series of cases, the incidence of fetal anomalies was less: 18% in the series by Alexander and colleagues, and 21% in the series by Queenan and colleagues.

Diagnosis and Treatment

Hydramnios is usually first suspected after seven months' gestation when the uterus is found to be somewhat tense and larger than it should be for the gestational dates, when fetal parts are difficult to palpate but are readily ballotable, and when the fetal heartbeat is not easily heard with the stethoscope. The diagnosis is confirmed by stage-I ultrasound scanning (see p. 263). Because of the frequent association with diabetes mellitus and Rh incompatibility, a three-hour oral glucose tolerance test and Coombs' test are ordered. Regardless of the outcome of the stage-I scan, a stage-II scan is performed at this time to permit detailed study of the fetus. Magnetic resonance scanning is reported to be especially

Table 29-1
Conditions Found with 100 Consecutive Cases of Clinical Hydramnios

Condition	Number of Cases
Fetal Abnormality	39
Anencephaly	23
Esophageal atresia	3
Duodenal atresia	1
Hydrops fetalis	3
Tumor of chest causing pressure on esophagus	1
Occipitocervical meningocele	1
Hydrocephalus	3
Achondroplasia	2
Skin disease	1
Spina bifida	1
Multiple Pregnancy	9
Diabetes Mellitus	7
Normal Fetus, Normal Mother	45

(From Gadd RL: The liquor amnii. In Philipp EE, Barnes J, Newton M [eds]: Scientific Foundations of Obstetrics and Gynaecology, 2nd ed. London, William Heinemann, 1977)

helpful in the diagnosis of fetal anomalies (see p. 1190). If a major abnormality is found, the mother should be informed, and if she approves, steps should be taken to terminate the pregnancy. If no abnormality is found, the pediatrician should be alerted, at the time of delivery, to the presence of hydramnios during pregnancy and to the possibility of some surgical emergency, such as duodenal or esophageal atresia.

The collection of amniotic fluid can be enormous, amounting to upwards of five liters. In such cases, abdominal discomfort and dyspnea can be severe, often accompanied by difficulty in moving about and edema of the abdominal wall and extremities. Bed rest, salt restriction, and diuretics have been recommended but are rarely beneficial. Minor degrees of hydramnios are usually tolerated without difficulty, but, in the more severe cases, withdrawal of amniotic fluid by amniocentesis can be extremely helpful. An intravenous catheter such as the Angiocath is inserted into the uterus (after sonography to localize the placenta so that it will not be punctured) and is connected to an intravenous infusion set, the tubing of which is threaded through the infusion–withdrawal pump mechanism. The negative pressure helps to prevent clogging by particulate matter and permits even withdrawal at a rate of about 500 ml/hour. Depending on the magnitude of the hydramnios, removal of 1500 ml to 2000 ml usually suffices to relieve the symptoms. The fluid sometimes collects again rather rapidly, and the procedure may be repeated as needed. Sometimes labor intervenes. As the uterus

contracts after removal of significant amounts of fluid, the obstetrician should be alert to the possibility, although rare, that the diminished intrauterine surface may result in premature separation of the placenta. Like other conditions in which the uterus is overly distended, hydramnios predisposes the woman to postpartum hemorrhage; it is prudent to have an oxytocin infusion running after delivery.

Acute Hydramnios

The term *acute hydramnios* refers to the very rapid accumulation of huge amounts of amniotic fluid over the course of a few days to two weeks. The condition, which appears to be associated invariably with monoamniotic twin pregnancy, is characterized by varying degrees of upper abdominal discomfort, dyspnea, and marked abdominal, vulval, and dependent edema. The condition usually occurs between 21 and 28 weeks' gestation and may terminate by premature rupture of the membranes or preterm labor. In the series of cases studied by Weir and co-workers, 14 of 16 infants were normally formed, but none survived. Transabdominal amniocentesis was not tried; since hydramnios occurs in early gestation, however, it is doubtful that amniocentesis would be of more than temporary benefit. The important differential diagnosis is placental abruption, which would be quickly clarified by an ultrasound scan.

UMBILICAL CORD ACCIDENTS

The serious umbilical cord accidents that are encountered most frequently are prolapse and entrapment. Such problems as true knots, stricture, umbilical thrombosis, and the like are discussed in Chapter 43. They are less common, and they are also less amenable to early diagnosis and effective treatment.

Prolapse of the Cord

Cord prolapse occurs when the umbilical cord descends in advance of the presenting fetal part. The prolapse may be overt, protruding through the cervix into, and sometimes escaping from, the vagina, or it may be occult, lying beside the presenting part. The term *cord* or *funic presentation* is used when the membranes are intact and the cord can be felt in the bag of waters.

Causes

When the presenting part does not fit evenly into the pelvic inlet, a loop of cord may advance beside it and become caught between the bony pelvis and the presenting part. Predisposing factors are a floating presenting part, a small presenting part (as in the preterm fetus), abnormal presentations (*e.g.,* a transverse or oblique lie), breech presentation (especially footling breech), and some cases of multiple pregnancy, multiparity, and hydramnios. Cord prolapse may occur when the membranes rupture, either immediately or as the uterus adjusts to its smaller volume. It is most likely to occur in the presence of one of the predisposing factors mentioned above, but it can also occur unexpectedly. This is an important reason for performing a vaginal examination promptly after spontaneous rupture of the membranes; it also underscores the need for special vigilance whenever the membranes are ruptured artificially.

Frequency

Cord prolapse occurs in ratio of about 1:200 deliveries. In the Berkus series, the incidence among 63,769 deliveries was 1:190.

Diagnosis

The diagnosis of cord prolapse is obvious if a loop of cord protrudes through the introitus or is palpated on vaginal examination. If the cord is pulsating, the baby is alive. If it is not pulsating, the baby is either dead or dying. If the diagnosis is not obvious, indirect means of diagnosis may indicate cord prolapse before the baby is seriously jeopardized.

ELECTRONIC FETAL MONITORING (EFM). Variable decelerations in heart rate are classically associated with cord compression (see Chap. 41). If the abnormal patterns are not eliminated by changing the mother's position, it should be inferred that they are due to cord prolapse.

ULTRASOUND SCAN. The position of the cord can be determined by ultrasound scan. The technique is useful if occult cord prolapse or cord presentation is suspected. If the problem is not confirmed and labor is imminent, the scan is recommended for patients in whom any of the predisposing factors mentioned earlier is present.

Treatment

If the baby is dead, labor is allowed to proceed and terminate naturally, unless there are complicating factors (e.g., cephalopelvic disproportion, transverse lie) that should be dealt with by cesarean section.

If the baby is alive and instant delivery by fundal pressure or outlet forceps (not midforceps) is feasible, delivery should be initiated. If not, a successful outcome depends on protection of the baby while preparations are being made for delivery.

MEASURES TO PROTECT THE BABY. The woman is placed in the knee-chest position immediately, oxygen is administered, and the presenting part is elevated by insertion of two fingers into the vagina and exertion of pressure against it. If any delay in delivery is anticipated, ritodrine tocolysis may be started, and the device recommended by Katz may be used: 500 ml to 700 ml of saline may be introduced into the bladder by a catheter in an effort to relieve cord compression.

Delivery

Many of the methods that were formerly used for delivery in cases of cord prolapse (e.g., Dührssen's incisions, version and extraction, midforceps delivery) are no longer acceptable. At present, vaginal delivery is appropriate only if it can be accomplished at once and with less trauma to the infant than would be imposed in delivery by cesarean section. This includes cases in which the head is low and the infant can be delivered easily by slight or moderate fundal pressure, or outlet forceps, and some cases of breech presentation in which the second stage is sufficiently advanced that assisted breech delivery would be safest. Cesarean section is appropriate for all other cases of cord prolapse, with the possible exception of cases in which the fetus is very small. In these cases cesarean section is usually selected only if the fetus is not seriously compromised and is believed to be large enough to survive. (However, in the experience of Robertson, infants delivered both by cesarean section and vaginally at gestations of less than 31 weeks have a low survival rate; at 32 to 37 weeks Robertson found a slightly increased risk of respiratory distress syndrome with cesarean section, but this was rarely fatal and was not sufficient evidence to rule out cesarean section if labor would present appreciable hazard to the fetus.)

Cesarean section for cord prolapse is an emergency procedure that is done in the interests of a fetus who is in serious jeopardy. Rapid intravenous anesthesia should be used. A midline abdominal incision is preferable to the transverse incision, which many prefer when time is not a factor. At term, the low cervical incision can usually be made with as much dispatch as the classic incision and with less threat to the mother.

ENTRAPMENT OF THE UMBILICAL CORD

Entrapment of the umbilical cord occurs when the circulation through the cord is compromised because of pressure between a firm fetal part and the uterine wall. It is sometimes suspected in the course of routine fetal monitoring because of the appearance of variable decelerations in the fetal heart rate, which are usually eliminated by changes in the mother's position and administration of oxygen. If the variable decelerations persist or become severe (repetitive, lasting one minute or more, with rates of 70 beats/minute or less), the patient should be delivered.

Entrapment often occurs in the presence of oligohydramnios, which is considered by Leveno and colleagues to be the most frequent cause of fetal distress in postterm pregnancy. The presence of oligohydramnios, as diagnosed by ultrasound scan, is a serious complication and requires immediate electronic fetal monitoring. If the tracings are normal, labor should be induced by amniotomy, which can be augmented by oxytocin if necessary. Amniotic fluid that is more than slightly stained with meconium and severe decelerative heart rate patterns are ominous signs that indicate the need for prompt cesarean section. Scalp sampling can be used to verify the indications for cesarean section in cases of cord entrapment with oligohydramnios: a pH of 7.25 or less is an indication for cesarean section.

REFERENCES AND RECOMMENDED READING

Premature Rupture of Membranes

Al-Zaid NS, Bou-Resli MN, Goldspink G: Bursting pressure and collagen content of fetal membranes and their relation to premature rupture of the membranes. Br J Obstet Gynaecol 87:227, 1980

Artal R, Burgeson RE, Hobel CJ et al: An in vitro model for the study of enzymatically mediated biochemical changes in the chorioamniotic membranes. Am J Obstet Gynecol 133:656, 1979

Artal R, Sokol RJ, Neunam N et al: The mechanical properties of prematurely and non-prematurely ruptured membranes. Methods and preliminary results. Am J Obstet Gynecol 125:655, 1976

Berkowitz RL: Premature rupture of the membranes: A review and treatment plan. Contemp Ob/Gyn 10:35, 1977

Cotton DB, Hill LM, Strassner HT et al: Use of amniocentesis in preterm gestation with ruptured membranes. Obstet Gynecol 63:38, 1984

Danforth DN, Hull RW: Microscopic anatomy of the fetal membranes with particular reference to the detailed structure of the amnion. Am J Obstet Gynecol 75:536, 1958

Danforth DN, McElin TW, States MN: Studies on the fetal membranes: I. Bursting tension. Am J Obstet Gynecol 65:480, 1953

Farb HF, Arnesen M, Geistler P et al: C-reactive protein with premature rupture of membranes and premature labor. Obstet Gynecol 62:49, 1983

Gahl WA, Kozina TJ, Fuhrmann DD et al: Diamine oxidase in the diagnosis of ruptured fetal membranes. Obstet Gynecol 60:297, 1982

Garite TJ, Freeman RK, Linzey EM et al: The use of amniocentesis in patients with premature rupture of the membranes. Obstet Gynecol 54:226, 1979

Gibbs RS, Castillo MS, Rodgers PJ: Management of chorioamnionitis. Am J Obstet Gynecol 136:709, 1980

Gravett MG, Eschenbach DA, Spiegel–Brown CA et al: Rapid diagnosis of amniotic-fluid infection by gas-liquid chromatography. N Engl J Med 306:725, 1982

Iams JD, Talbert ML, Barrows H et al: Management of preterm prematurely ruptured membranes: A prospective randomized comparison of observation versus use of steroids and timed delivery. Am J Obstet Gynecol 151:32, 1985

Kappy KA, Cetrulo CL, Knuppel RA et al: Premature rupture of the membranes: A conservative approach. Am J Obstet Gynecol 134:655, 1979

Lenihan JP Jr.: Relationship of antepartum pelvic examinations to premature rupture of the membranes. Obstet Gynecol 63:33, 1984

Liggins GC, Howie RN: A controlled trial of antepartum glucocorticoid treatment for prevention of respiratory distress syndrome in premature infants. Pediatrics 50:515, 1972

Marks J, Church CK, Benrubi G: Effects of barometric pressure and lunar phases on premature rupture of the membranes. J Reprod Med 28:335, 1983

Minikoff H, Grunebaum AN, Schwarz RH et al: Risk factors for prematurity and premature rupture of the membranes: A prospective study of the vaginal flora in pregnancy. Am J Obstet Gynecol 150:965, 1984

Pagageorgiou AN, Desgranges MF, Masson M et al: The antenatal use of betamethasone in the prevention of respiratory distress syndrome: A controlled double-blind study. Pediatrics 63:73, 1979

Rochelson BL, Richardson DA, Macri JN: Rapid assay for alpha-fetoprotein—Possible application in diagnosis of premature rupture of the membranes. Obstet Gynecol 62:414, 1983

Schreiber J, Benedetti T: Conservative management of preterm premature rupture of the fetal membranes in a low socio-economic population. Am J Obstet Gynecol 136:92, 1980

Selle J, Harris TR: Association of premature rupture of membranes with idiopathic respiratory distress syndrome. Obstet Gynecol 49:167, 1977

Shields JR, Resnik R: Fetal lung maturation and the antenatal use of glucocorticoids to prevent the respiratory distress syndrome. Obstet Gynecol Surv 34:343, 1979

Skinner SJM, Campos GA, Liggins GC: The collagen content of human amniotic membranes: Effect of gestation length and premature rupture. Obstet Gynecol 57:487, 1981

Tinga DJ, Aarnoudse JG, Rogge P et al: Letter to the Editor (regarding adverse maternal effects of combined use of terbutaline and corticosteroids). Lancet 1:1026, 1979

Yeast JD, Garite TJ, Dorchester W: The risks of amniocentesis in the management of premature rupture of the membranes. Am J Obstet Gynecol 149:505, 1984

Young BK, Klein SA, Katz M et al: Intravenous dexamethasone for prevention of neonatal respiratory distress: A prospective controlled study. Am J Obstet Gynecol 138:203, 1980

Postterm Pregnancy

Anderson GG: Postmaturity: A review. Obstet Gynecol Surv 27:65, 1972

Callenbach JC, Hall RT: Morbidity and mortality of advanced gestational age: Postterm or postmature. Obstet Gynecol 53:721, 1979

Cario GM: Conservative management of prolonged pregnancy using fetal heart rate monitoring only: A prospective study. Brit J Obstet Gynaecol 91:23, 1984

Cohen AW: Movement as a yardstick for fetal well-being. Contemp OB/GYN 26(2):61, 1985

Crowley P, O'Herlihy C, Boylan P: The value of ultrasound measurement of amniotic fluid volume in the management of prolonged pregnancies. Brit J Obstet Gynaecol 91:444, 1984

Eden RD, Gergely RZ, Schifrin BS et al: Comparison of antepartum testing schemes for the management of postdate pregnancy. Am J Obstet Gynecol 144:683, 1982

Grandos JL: Survey of the management of postterm pregnancy. Obstet Gynecol 63:651, 1984

Klapholz H, Friedman EA: The incidence of intrapartum fetal distress with advancing gestational age. Am J Obstet Gynecol 127:405, 1977

Knox GE, Huddleston JF, Flowers CE Jr.: Management of prolonged pregnancy: Results of a prospective randomized trial. Am J Obstet Gynecol 134:376, 1979

Leveno KJ, Quirk JG Jr., Cunningham FG et al: Prolonged pregnancy. I. Observations concerning the causes of fetal distress. Am J Obstet Gynecol 150:465, 1984

Liggins GC: Fetal influences on myometrial contractility. Clin Obstet Gynecol 16, No. 3:148, 1973

Nakano R: Postterm pregnancy: Five-year review from Osaka National Hospital. Acta Obstet Gynecol Scand 51:217, 1972

Park GL: Duration of pregnancy. Lancet 2:1388, 1968

Phelan JP, Platt LD, Sze-Ya Yeh et al: Continuing role of the nonstress test in the management of postdate pregnancy. Obstet Gynecol 64:624, 1984

Rayburn WF, Motley ME, Stempel LE et al: Antepartum prediction of the postmature infant. Obstet Gynecol 60:148, 1982

Shime J, Gare DJ, Andrews J et al: Prolonged pregnancy: Surveillance of the fetus and the neonate and the course of labor and delivery. Am J Obstet Gynecol 148:547, 1984

Tabei T, Heinrichs WL: Diagnosis of placental sulfatase deficiency. Am J Obstet Gynecol 124:409, 1976

Yeh S-Y, Read JA: Management of post-term pregnancy in a large obstetric population. Obstet Gynecol 60:282, 1982

Zwerdling MA: Factors pertaining to prolonged pregnancy and its outcome. Pediatrics 42:202, 1967

Missed Labor

Aoskan S, Portela L, Nijenson E et al: Fetal demise, an accurate diagnosis. IMJ 155:153, 1979

Mackenzie IZ, Davies AJ, Embrey MP: Fetal death in utero managed with vaginal prostaglandin E_2 gel. Br Med J 1:1764, 1979

Wingerup L, Anderson KE, Ulmsten U: Ripening of the uterine cervix and induction of labour at term with prostaglandin E_2 in viscous gel. Acta Scand Obstet Gynecol 57:403, 1978

Hydramnios

Abramovich DR, Garden A, Jandial L et al: Fetal swallowing and voiding in relation to hydramnios. Obstet Gynecol 54:15, 1979

Alexander ES, Spitz HB, Clark RA: Sonography of polyhydramnios. Am J Roentgenol 138:343, 1982

Danforth DN, Hull RW: The microscopic anatomy of the fetal membranes with particular reference to the detailed structure of the amnion. Am J Obstet Gynecol 75:536, 1958

Flowers WK III: Hydramnios and gastrointestinal atresias: A review. Obstet Gynecol Surv 38:685, 1983

Gadd RL: The liquor amnii. In Philipp EE, Barnes J, Newton M (eds): Scientific Foundations of Obstetrics and Gynaecology, 2nd ed. London, William Heinemann, 1977

Queenan JT: Managing polyhydramnios. Contemp Ob/Gyn, August 1983, p. 17

Queenan JT: Recurrent acute polyhydramnios. Am J Obstet Gynecol 106:652, 1970

Queenan JT, Gadow EC: Polyhydramnios: Chronic versus acute. Am J Obstet Gynecol 108:349, 1970

Quinlan RW, Cruz AC, Martin M: Hydramnios: Ultrasound diagnosis and its impact on perinatal management and pregnancy outcome. Am J Obstet Gynecol 145:306, 1983

Weir PE, Ratten GJ, Beischer NA: Acute polyhydramnios—A complication of monozygous twin pregnancy. Br J Obstet Gynaecol 86:849, 1979

Cord Accidents

Berkus M: Coping successfully with cord prolapse. Contemporary Ob/Gyn, July 1983, p. 199

Katz Z, Lancet M, Borenstein R: Management of labor with umbilical cord prolapse. Am J Obstet Gynecol 142:239, 1982

Levy H, Meier PR, Makowski EL: Umbilical cord prolapse. Obstet Gynecol 64:499, 1984

Robertson NRC: Caesarean section—paediatric outcome. In Beard RW, Paintin DB: Outcomes of Obstetric Intervention in Britain, p. 126. London, Royal College of Obstetricians and Gynaecologists, 1980

Wolfman WW, Purohit DM, Self SE: Umbilical cord thrombosis at 32 weeks' gestation with delivery of a living infant. Am J Obstet 146:468, 1983

Medical and Surgical Complications of Pregnancy

30

Cardiovascular Disease

Dwight P. Cruikshank

Maternal cardiac disease complicates 0.5% to 1% of pregnancies. In the past, the vast majority of these patients suffered from rheumatic disease, but with the declining incidence of rheumatic fever coupled with better surgical treatment of congenital heart lesions in early childhood, rheumatic lesions are now responsible for only about half the cases of heart disease complicating pregnancy. The other half of cases is due to congenital lesions.

CONGENITAL HEART DISEASE

Left-to-Right Shunts

Atrial Septal Defect

The atrial septal defect (ASD) is the most common congenital lesion seen in pregnancy. With an ASD there is shunting of blood from the left to the right atrium, which leads to an increased load on the right ventricle and increased pulmonary blood flow. This is usually well tolerated by the pulmonary vasculature, and there may be no rise in pulmonary pressure for many years. Most patients demonstrate right ventricular hypertrophy or right bundle branch block on electrocardiogram, but heart failure is uncommon in persons under 30 years of age. Atrial arrhythmias (fibrillation, flutter, paroxysmal atrial tachycardia) are also more commonly associated with ASD than with any other congenital lesion, but they too are usually not seen in young persons.

The great majority of patients with uncorrected ASD tolerate pregnancy well. Careful antepartum care and prophylaxis against endocarditis at the time of labor and delivery are indicated (see the section on General Principles of Management). In the unlikely event that congestive failure refractory to medical management develops during pregnancy, surgical closure of the defect is indicated.

Shunt reversal is the major risk during pregnancy for the patient with an uncomplicated ASD. If systemic blood pressure falls abruptly, such that the pulmonary pressure exceeds the systemic pressure, the shunt will reverse, blood will move from the right to the left atrium, and there will be underperfusion of the lungs, cyanosis, and circulatory collapse. This is most likely to occur in one of two circumstances: (1) hypovolemia secondary to obstetric hemorrhage of any cause and (2) injudicious use of epidural or spinal anesthesia with systemic hypotension from sympathetic blockade. Thus, it is important to have cross-matched blood readily available during labor, delivery, and the puerperium for patients with an ASD, and efforts should be made to minimize blood loss. Conduction anesthesia should be administered by an experienced anesthesiologist after volume expansion has been performed with 500 ml to 1000 ml crystalloid solution, and the supine position must be avoided.

The uncommon patient who has developed pulmonary hypertension secondary to an ASD and who has a bidirectional or right-to-left shunt in effect has Eisenmenger's syndrome; for such a patient pregnancy is a grave risk (see below).

Ventricular Septal Defect

A small ventricular septal defect (VSD) is usually hemodynamically insignificant, and a patient with such a VSD usually tolerates pregnancy well. In fact, most patients with a VSD who reach childbearing age without corrective surgery are symptom free. With larger defects there is shunting of blood from the left to the right ventricle, with increased pulmonary blood flow. As with an ASD, pulmonary resistance usually remains normal for many years, so even patients with a large VSD tolerate pregnancy well, although congestive failure can occur.

The great majority of patients with an uncorrected VSD do quite well in pregnancy. There is a significant risk of bacterial endocarditis, and prophylaxis is indicated in the peripartum period. As with an ASD, the major risk is shunt reversal leading to circulatory collapse and cyanosis. Thus, blood loss must be minimized and systemic hypotension avoided. In Mendelson's series of 110 pregnant patients with uncorrected VSDs, congestive failure developed in nine (8%), and six (5.5%) died. Three of the deaths were due to shunt reversal following delivery; the others were due to one case each of congestive heart failure, endocarditis, and parodoxical embolism.

If they develop pulmonary hypertension, patients with VSDs have all the pregnancy risks associated with Eisenmenger's syndrome.

Patent Ductus Arteriosus

Formerly the second most common congenital lesion encountered during pregnancy, patent ductus arteriosus (PDA) is now a rare complication, almost all cases being surgically corrected in childhood. Most patients with PDA tolerate pregnancy well, but occasionally a patient develops congestive heart failure. If this condition does not respond promptly to medical management, surgical correction during pregnancy is indicated, provided the patient does not have pulmonary hypertension. Once pulmonary pressure equals or exceeds systemic pressure, closure of the ductus is inadvisable. These patients with pulmonary hypertension have Eisenmenger's syndrome and must be managed accordingly.

All patients with uncorrected PDA need peripartum subacute bacterial endocarditis (SBE) prophylaxis. As with other left-to-right shunts, shunt reversal is the major pregnancy-associated risk.

Totally Corrected Shunts

Patients who have had complete surgical correction of an ASD, VSD, or PDA are at no increased risk during pregnancy and need only good obstetric care. SBE prophylaxis is not necessary at delivery. However, patients whose defects have been only partially corrected should be managed as outlined above.

Cyanotic Heart Disease (Right-to-Left Shunts)

Tetralogy of Fallot

Tetralogy of Fallot, the most common form of cyanotic congenital heart disease, consists of (1) pulmonic stenosis, often both valvular and infundibular, (2) a ventricular septal defect, (3) dextroposition of the aorta, so that it overrides the septal defect, and (4) right ventricular hypertrophy. The pulmonic stenosis leads to increased right ventricular pressure, which causes the right ventricular hypertrophy and leads blood to be shunted from right to left through the ventricular septal defect and overriding aorta. Because the septal defect can be large or small and the degree of pulmonic stenosis may vary, there is a wide spectrum of signs and symptoms. However, symmetric cyanosis, clubbing of the fingers and toes, and dyspnea on exertion are common findings.

Without surgical treatment, most patients do not survive childhood, and 95% are dead by age 25. Most patients now have total surgical correction in childhood and later tolerate pregnancy well. It is not uncommon to see women with partial or palliative surgical corrections, however. These include anastomoses of the subclavian artery to pulmonary artery (Blalock-Taussig), descending aorta to left pulmonary artery (Potts), and ascending aorta to right pulmonary artery (Waterston-Cooley). Patients with such partial corrections are at increased risk during pregnancy, and patients who have had no surgical treatment are at greatly increased risk.

Pregnancy tends to increase the degree of right-to-left shunting, because the progesterone-induced fall in systemic resistance lowers the left-sided pressure, while the right-sided pressure remains high because of the pulmonic stenosis and right ventricular hypertrophy. Serious complications such as bacterial endocarditis, brain abscess, and cerebral thrombosis are more common during pregnancy than in the nonpregnant state. Congestive failure is rare in tetralogy of Fallot, but the incidence is increased somewhat in pregnancy. Overall maternal mortality is 5% to 10%. Especially poor prognostic signs are syncope, hematocrit greater than 60%, peripheral arterial oxygen saturation below 80%, and right ventricular pressure of 120 mm Hg or more. Patients with these findings should be advised against pregnancy, and those who are already pregnant should consider first-trimester abortion.

Systemic hypotension is even more dangerous in pregnant patients with tetralogy of Fallot than in those with left-to-right shunts because of the increased right ventricular systolic pressure. Excessive blood loss, sympathetic blockade, and supine hypotension can lead to essentially all blood being shunted away from the lungs, with severe hypoxia, circulatory collapse, and death resulting. Thus, at delivery every effort must be made to minimize blood loss, blood must be immediately available for transfusion, and the supine position must be avoided. Spinal and epidural anesthesia should be avoided unless meticulously done by an anesthesiologist experienced in both obstetric and cardiac anesthesia.

The perinatal mortality associated with tetralogy of Fallot is reported to be 30% to 40%. As with other states of severe maternal hypoxia, intrauterine growth retardation is common. Patients without total correction who elect to continue their pregnancies should have an obstetric ultrasound exam at 18 to 24 weeks of amenorrhea to document the duration of gestation, and after 28 weeks they should have serial ultrasound exams every three to four weeks to detect aberrations of fetal growth. Chronic oxygen treatment may be necessary.

Eisenmenger's Syndrome

Eisenmenger's syndrome is any right-to-left shunt accompanied by pulmonary hypertension. The shunt can be at any level (PDA, VSD, ASD, transposition of the great vessels with VSD). Patients begin life with left-to-right shunts, but when chronically elevated pulmonary flow leads to increased pulmonary resistance, pulmonary pressure exceeds systemic, the shunt becomes right to left, and cyanosis ensues.

Pregnancy is exceedingly hazardous for patients with Eisenmenger's syndrome. With the possible exception of primary pulmonary hypertension, no other maternal heart disease carries a more grave prognosis. In a review of 44 well-documented cases of Eisenmenger's syndrome in pregnancy in the literature, Gleicher and co-workers found that 52% of these women died during or immediately following pregnancy. Some women did not die until the second or third pregnancy, so the maternal mortality for any given pregnancy was 30.3%.

Pregnancy worsens the right-to-left shunting and hypoxia, because systemic resistance falls owing to the influence of progesterone but pulmonary vascular resistance is fixed and cannot fall. Labor and delivery are the most critical times, because blood loss may lower left-sided pressure and straining increases right-sided pressure, and these hemodynamic changes can cause profound hypoxia and fatal arrhythmias.

Women with Eisenmenger's syndrome should be offered sterilization. If pregnancy occurs, early abortion should be recommended. Suction abortions seem safe in the first trimester provided systemic hypotension is avoided. The same cannot be said for later abortions. The review of Gleicher and colleagues revealed only three midtrimester abortions: two successful intra-amniotic instillations (it is not stated what drug was used), and one hysterotomy, which resulted in maternal death. I have observed two maternal deaths associated with midtrimester abortion in Eisenmenger's syndrome patients: one associated with saline infusion and one associated with prostaglandins. Most observers believe that the hazards of late abortion are no less than those of term delivery in these patients.

If sterilization or early abortion is not acceptable to the pregnant patient with Eisenmenger's syndrome, she needs intensive antepartum and peripartum care. She probably should be hospitalized when the diagnosis of pregnancy is made, and certainly no later than at 20 weeks' gestation, and remain hospitalized until about two weeks after delivery. Bed rest is essential. Some data indicate that oxygen administered by nasal cannula will reduce pulmonary vascular resistance, and this should be used continuously, with frequent monitoring

of arterial blood gases. If congestive failure develops, it should be treated with digitalis and diuretics, as it would be in a nonpregnant patient. An early ultrasound examination for dating of the gestation is often helpful. Fetal surveillance should be intensive as well, with serial ultrasound studies every three to four weeks after 28 weeks' gestation and weekly fetal heart rate testing beginning at 32 weeks' gestation. Spontaneous labor is preferable to induced labor in that it is associated with a lower risk of cesarean delivery, but induction has the advantage of allowing delivery to occur under controlled circumstances, when all the necessary team members—obstetricians, cardiologists, anesthesiologists, neonatologists, and intensive care nurses—are present. Therefore, induction of labor after 37 weeks is acceptable if the condition of the cervix is favorable and fetal maturity is assured.

In labor, monitoring with a Swan–Ganz catheter and a maternal cardiac monitor is essential, and an arterial line may be helpful as well. Administration of high concentrations of oxygen is recommended, with frequent monitoring of arterial blood gases. Epidural anesthesia is indicated if it can be expertly done without producing systemic hypotension. The patient should not be in the supine position, blood should be available for transfusion, and systemic hypotension should be treated pharmacologically if necessary (intravenous ephedrine offers some advantages over other agents). The Valsalva maneuver should be avoided; uterine contractions alone should be allowed to bring the fetal head to the perineum, and delivery should then be effected by use of low forceps. SBE prophylaxis is of course mandatory.

The standard wisdom is that cesarean delivery should be avoided if possible. Gleicher's review found 75% maternal mortality with cesarean delivery, but this was in a group of only four women, too small a number to permit a definitive statement to be made. Spinnato and associates have stated that elective cesarean with epidural anesthesia is an acceptable delivery alternative in these patients, but the results of their one case need to be confirmed by others.

Other Congenital Lesions

Coarctation of the Aorta

Coarctation of the aorta is usually corrected in childhood, and pregnancy in women with a corrected coarctation is without undue risk. In persons with uncorrected coarctation, systolic blood pressure in the head and right arm is much higher than in the legs. Whether the left arm blood pressure is high depends on whether the coarctation is proximal or distal to the left subclavian artery.

The risks of coarctation are those of hypertension, as well as those of aortic rupture or dissection. In addition, some patients with coarctation have associated congenital cerebral aneurysms, and up to 50% of patients have a bicuspid aortic valve that is predisposed to bacterial endocarditis. Mortality in pregnant women with coarctation is about 3.5%; death may be due to aortic rupture or dissection, cerebrovascular accident, congestive failure, or bacterial endocarditis. Management during pregnancy consists of limitation of activity and control of blood pressure with antihypertensives. Coarctations have been successfully repaired during pregnancy, but surgery should be delayed until after pregnancy unless dissection, congestive failure unresponsive to medical therapy, or uncontrollable hypertension occurs. The literature suggests that coarctation per se is not an indication for cesarean delivery, since most aortic ruptures in pregnancy occur before labor. Epidural anesthesia and avoidance of the Valsalva maneuver are essential during labor.

Perinatal mortality as high as 25% has been reported with coarctation, many of the deaths probably due to reduced uterine blood flow. Patients should be monitored with serial ultrasound exams for fetal growth, and weekly fetal heart testing after 32 weeks' gestation seems prudent.

Isolated Pulmonic Stenosis

Most patients with isolated pulmonic stenosis tolerate pregnancy well. The major risk associated with this lesion is right-sided heart failure, which may occur in 5% to 10% of patients and which usually responds to medical therapy. If failure unresponsive to medical therapy occurs during pregnancy, pulmonary valvotomy is indicated.

Congenital Aortic Stenosis

Congenital aortic stenosis is a rare complication of pregnancy. Most patients with this disorder tolerate pregnancy well, but they are at risk for left ventricular failure and for sudden death from asystole or ventricular fibrillation. Reduced physical activity and extra bed rest are important throughout pregnancy. The reported maternal mortality rate is about 17%, but the number of cases involved is small.

RHEUMATIC HEART DISEASE

Mitral Stenosis

Rheumatic heart disease in women usually involves the mitral valve, and mitral stenosis accounts for 90% of rheumatic heart disease seen in pregnancy. Pregnancy worsens the hemodynamic problem of mitral stenosis, and the overall mortality of these patients is 1% during pregnancy. In more severe cases (New York Heart Association functional classes III and IV), mortality is 4% to 5%, and in cases associated with atrial fibrillation, mortality rates as high as 15% have been reported. Because pregnancy aggravates mitral stenosis, one must not be lulled into a false sense of security because the patient is asymptomatic at the onset of pregnancy.

The basic problem in mitral stenosis is obstruction to left ventricular filling. This leads to increased left atrial pressure, left atrial enlargement, and increased pulmonary venous and capillary pressures. The enlarged left atrium is predisposed to thrombus formation and to arrhythmias, especially atrial fibrillation. Pregnancy aggravates mitral stenosis for a variety of reasons: (1) the physiologic tachycardia of pregnancy, which shortens diastole and thus reduces the time available for blood flow across the mitral valve; (2) the increased blood volume of pregnancy, including increased pulmonary capillary blood volume; (3) the need for increased cardiac output during pregnancy, which necessitates further increases in left atrial and pulmonary capillary pressures; (4) the decreased serum albumin concentration of pregnancy, which allows the development of pulmonary edema at lower pulmonary capillary pressures; and (5) the increased incidence of atrial arrhythmias during pregnancy. Therefore, the woman with mitral stenosis is closer to pulmonary edema when pregnant than when not pregnant, and the risk of this complication rises progressively to term. Properly managed labor does not seem to increase the risk of pulmonary edema over that present in late pregnancy, unless atrial fibrillation occurs. The early puerperium is a dangerous time, since venous return to the heart is promoted by the relief of uterine obstruction of the vena cava and by the mobilization of extracellular fluid into the vascular compartment. Congestive failure complicates about 8% of pregnancies in women with mitral stenosis. Other major complications of pregnancy include atrial arrhythmias (6%) and embolic phenomena (1–2%).

Management of the pregnant patient with mitral stenosis includes reduced activity and extra bed rest. Many authors recommend rheumatic fever prophylaxis, such as a monthly intramuscular injection of 1.2 million units of benzathine penicillin, in addition to SBE prophylaxis at delivery. The onset of atrial fibrillation calls for anticoagulation and digitalis therapy, and if pulmonary congestion occurs, cardioversion should be performed promptly. Congestive failure unresponsive to medical therapy during pregnancy is an indication for mitral valvotomy.

Chesley has shown that single or even repeated pregnancies do not accelerate the course of rheumatic heart disease. Although women with the disorder are at increased risk during pregnancy, if they survive the gestation itself their life expectancy is not shortened.

Patients with severe mitral stenosis of long duration may develop pulmonary hypertension. Pregnancy is a grave risk in these patients, with maternal mortality approaching 25%. These patients should have first-trimester abortions and should have sterilization recommended to them. In a patient with severe mitral stenosis, it is crucial to learn early in pregnancy whether pulmonary hypertension is also present. All previous cardiac catheterization data should be reviewed. If recent data are not available, and if signs or symptoms suggest the possibility of pulmonary hypertension, use of a Swan–Ganz catheter to measure pulmonary pressures may be justified early in pregnancy.

Mitral Insufficiency

Mitral insufficiency accounts for about 6% of cases of rheumatic heart disease in pregnancy. Women with the condition generally tolerate pregnancy well, but women with severe mitral regurgitation are at risk for atrial fibrillation, and some authors recommend that they receive prophylactic digitalis therapy. Antibiotic prophylaxis against endocarditis is indicated during labor and delivery.

Aortic Stenosis

Rheumatic aortic stenosis is rarely encountered during pregnancy, accounting for only about 1% of cases of rheumatic heart disease seen. Patients with mild aortic stenosis tolerate pregnancy well, but severe aortic stenosis, manifested by syncope or angina, can be a serious threat to maternal life. Overall maternal mortalities as high as 17% have been reported. In patients with severe aortic stenosis, any fall in cardiac output may cause fatal cerebral or cardiac ischemia. Thus, venous return to the heart must be maintained by avoidance of the supine position, of excessive blood loss at the time of delivery, and of injudicious conduction anesthesia. Antibiotic prophylaxis during labor is recommended.

Aortic Insufficiency

Aortic insufficiency accounts for 2% to 3% of cases of rheumatic heart disease encountered during pregnancy. Although the pregnancy-induced increase in blood volume theoretically should induce an increased load on the left ventricle, in reality the increased heart rate leads to shorter diastole and reduces the amount of blood regurgitating from the aorta into the left ventricle. In the rare circumstance in which pulmonary edema develops, restriction of activity, digitalis, and diuretics are indicated. All patients with aortic insufficiency should receive SBE prophylaxis during labor.

CARDIOMYOPATHIES

Peripartum Cardiomyopathy

Peripartum cardiomyopathy (PPCM) has many synonyms, including *postpartum cardiomyopathy, cardiomyopathy of pregnancy,* and *postpartum heart disease.* The disease is rare, complicating between 1 in 1500 and

1 in 4000 pregnancies. Three criteria must be met to establish the diagnosis: (1) development of congestive heart failure in the last month of pregnancy or the first five months of the puerperium, (2) lack of any determinable cause of heart failure, and (3) lack of any demonstrable evidence of heart disease before the last month of pregnancy.

The cause of PPCM is unknown. In the past there has been controversy as to whether the disease is caused by viral infection, alcohol intake, hypertension, or coronary artery disease, but the bulk of data refutes all of these. The disease is most common among black multiparas. Furthermore, 7% of cases follow twin pregnancy, and 15% to 30% of affected patients have preeclampsia. The time of onset of the disease is variable, with 7% of cases beginning in the last month of pregnancy, 82% in the first three months after delivery, and 11% in the fourth or fifth month postpartum. Patients exhibit all the symptoms, clinical signs, and radiographic, electrocardiographic, and echocardiographic features of biventricular congestive failure. Systemic and pulmonary embolism complicates 25% to 30% of cases and should be considered an integral part of the disease. Arrhythmias are also common, with 40% of patients demonstrating ventricular ectopic beats and 20% atrial fibrillation. Medical management of the disease should include digitalis, diuretics, and anticoagulation. The mainstay of treatment is prolonged, complete bed rest. Most authors recommend bed rest until three months after heart size has returned to normal. If cardiac enlargement persists, bed rest should be continued for 6 to 12 months.

The prognosis in PPCM depends on whether the heart returns to normal size with bed rest. Demakis and colleagues found that the hearts of 50% of patients returned to normal size within six months, and none of these patients died of heart disease during an 11-year follow-up period. However, approximately 50% of patients had persistent cardiomegaly after six months of bed rest, and 85% of these women died of cardiac failure within five years.

PPCM tends to recur in subsequent pregnancies, especially in women whose hearts have not returned to normal size. All patients who have had PPCM should be urged to consider sterilization. Oral contraceptives are contraindicated because of the risk of thromboembolism.

Hypertrophic Cardiomyopathy

This disease is also known as *obstructive cardiomyopathy* and *idiopathic hypertrophic subaortic stenosis.* It is an autosomal dominant disorder characterized by obstruction of the outflow tract of the left ventricle due to muscular hypertrophy, often asymmetric with greater hypertrophy of the ventricular septum. Many of these patients also have mitral regurgitation because the mitral valve is pulled open during systole. The basic problem is obstruction to left ventricular outflow, which is made worse by tachycardia and by anything that reduces diastolic ventricular filling, such as peripheral vasodilitation, hypotension, blood loss, epidural anesthesia, and the Valsalva maneuver. Patients are prone to sudden death, usually due to ventricular arrhythmias, and unfortunately there is no clinical, electrocariographic, echocardiographic, or hemodynamic feature by which to identify those at risk. Most patients are treated with β-blocking agents such as propranolol. These should be continued during pregnancy, with careful attention to fetal growth by serial ultrasound examination, since such therapy may cause intrauterine growth retardation. Unfortunately, propranolol does not prevent the serious ventricular arrhythmias that may cause death. Therefore, investigation during pregnancy should include exercise testing and ambulatory Holter monitoring, and patients with subclinical ventricular arrhythmias should be treated with more specific antiarrhythmic agents.

In hypertrophic cardiomyopathy as in most cardiac diseases, cesarean delivery is indicated only for obstetric reasons. Many authors regard epidural anesthesia as contraindicated because of the risk of hypotension and reduced venous return to the heart, although there are studies that demonstrate no increased risk from carefully administered epidural anesthesia.

Primary Pulmonary Hypertension

Although a rare disorder, primary pulmonary hypertension (PPH) is associated with an exceedingly high mortality rate (>50%) during pregnancy.

The basic processes in PPH are progressive constriction, muscularization, and fibrosis of the pulmonary arterioles. Pulmonary artery pressure is quite high, but because the obstruction is proximal to the capillary bed, pulmonary wedge pressure is normal, and pulmonary edema does not occur. There is progressive right ventricular hypertrophy. Death is usually due to right ventricular failure or ventricular arrhythmia. Patients usually have decreased arterial oxygen partial pressure and oxygen saturation. Pulmonary function studies are usually normal, although carbon dioxide diffusing capacity may be low. Electrocardiograms and echocardiograms show right ventricular hypertrophy, and chest x-ray films demonstrate an enlarged right atrium and right ventricle and dilatation of the pulmonary trunk. Symptoms such as dyspnea, fatigue, syncope, and chest pain usually occur late in the course of the disease. Unfortunately, the presence or absence of symptoms before pregnancy does not seem to be an indication of who will die during gestation. Death can occur any time during pregnancy, but the last months of pregnancy and the early puerperium are especially dangerous. The mechanism of death in pregnancy is not clear but seems to be the increased blood volume and cardiac output of pregnancy leading to right ventricular failure and fatal arrhythmias.

Patients with PPH should be counseled against pregnancy. If pregnancy occurs, first-trimester abortion is indicated. Patients who refuse abortion should be hospitalized at bed rest from the 20th week of gestation until two weeks after delivery. Right ventricular failure should be treated with digitalis and diuretics. Anticoagulation is of questionable value.

MITRAL VALVE PROLAPSE

Also called the *click–murmur syndrome* and *floppy mitral valve,* mitral valve prolapse is a common condition found in 6% to 10% of reproductive-aged women. The chordae tendinae are long and thin, and the mitral valve leaflets prolapse into the left atrium during ventricular systole. This may lead to some degree of mitral regurgitation. The anatomic defects lead to the auscultatory hallmarks of the syndrome, the midsystolic click and late systolic murmur. Most patients are asymptomatic, but a few have chest pain or palpitations secondary to arrhythmias, which usually respond to propranolol therapy. Although sudden death is a much feared complication in these patients, it has not been reported in pregnancy. In fact, patients with this disorder tolerate pregnancy well; the auscultatory signs may even diminish owing to increased left ventricular end diastolic volume. Patients who require propranolol therapy when they are not pregnant should continue with it during pregnancy if they have persistent chest pain or arrhythmias. Whether these patients need antibiotic prophylaxis during labor and delivery is controversial, but the majority opinion seems to favor it at this time.

MARFAN'S SYNDROME

An autosomal dominant disease, Marfan's syndrome is characterized by connective tissue weakness leading to ocular lens dislocation, joint deformities, and weakness of the aortic root and aortic wall. Up to 90% of patients have mitral valve prolapse, and 25% have aortic insufficiency. There is an increased risk of aortic dissection and rupture during pregnancy, and maternal mortality is reported at 25% to 50%. If the aortic root is found on echocardiography to be dilated to more than 4 cm, pregnancy is contraindicated. Other patients should be managed by restricted activity, and propranolol should be given to decrease the force of myocardial contractions.

GENERAL PRINCIPLES OF MANAGEMENT OF HEART DISEASE

Antepartum

The general goal of prenatal care in cardiac patients is the prevention or early detection of the major complications of congestive failure, arrhythmias, and embolism. Cardiac patients should be seen more frequently than other patients, approximately every two weeks during the first half of pregnancy and weekly during the second half. Bed rest reduces cardiac work, so an extra two to four hours per day of bed rest is indicated for asymptomatic patients and more for those with symptoms. Diuretics and sodium restriction are indicated if they have been part of the patient's prepregnancy regimen or if the patient shows signs of congestive failure. Because anemia increases cardiac work, it should be diagnosed and corrected if present; all anemic patients need appropriate iron and folate supplementation. Infection also increases cardiac work, so early signs should be sought and even seemingly trivial infections treated vigorously. Monthly screening for asymptomatic bacteriuria, accompanied by appropriate therapy, should reduce the risk of pyelonephritis. Preeclampsia is the third condition that can increase cardiac work and precipitate heart failure—hospitalization and bed rest are indicated at the earliest sign of increasing blood pressure or proteinuria. All patients except those with totally corrected congenital lesions should be hospitalized near term to ensure that labor begins under optimal conditions and in the absence of congestive failure.

Intrapartum and Postpartum

Excellent pain relief during labor reduces cardiac work by about 20%. Epidural is the anesthetic of choice for most cardiac patients. However, it may be contraindicated in patients with hypertrophic cardiomyopathy. Furthermore, patients with shunts at any level are at risk for pulmonary hypoperfusion if they develop systemic hypotension and should therefore receive epidurals only from experienced obstetric anesthetists. The Valsalva maneuver is to be avoided in most cardiac patients—the presenting part should be allowed to descend to the perineum by the force of uterine contractions alone, after which a low forceps delivery should be performed. Blood should be immediately available for transfusion should excessive blood loss occur, so that hypotension can be avoided.

The role of antibiotic prophylaxis against SBE is controversial. Because bacteremia complicates under 5% of vaginal deliveries, some physicians no longer use routine prophylaxis. However, 10% of all cases of SBE follow obstetric delivery, and most obstetricians continue to treat all cardiac patients except those with totally corrected congenital lesions. Three acceptable regimens of SBE prophylaxis are presented below. The first dose should be given as early as possible during labor.

Prophylaxis Against Subacute Bacterial Endocarditis

Penicillin G, 2 million units IM or IV
Gentamicin, 1.5 mg/kg body weight IM or IV
} every 8 hours for 3 doses

or

Ampicillin, 1 g IM
Streptomycin, 1 g IM
} every 12 hours for 3 doses

For penicillin-allergic patients

Vancomycin, 1 g IV
Streptomycin 1 g IM
} every 12 hours for 3 doses

There is no cardiac condition that in and of itself is an indication for cesarean delivery; this operation should be reserved for usual obstetric indications.

Patients with significant heart disease should be intensively monitored during labor and delivery with maternal cardiac monitors and arterial lines. Most should also have a Swan–Ganz catheter inserted, although this is contraindicated in patients with VSD and tetralogy of Fallot, in whom passage of the catheter through the septal defect into the left ventricle may precipitate a fatal arrhythmia.

The immediate puerperium is an especially dangerous time for patients with heart disease. Venous return to the heart increases, owing to mobilization of extracellular fluid and reduced obstruction of the inferior vena cava, and can lead to congestive failure. Therefore, intensive monitoring must be continued for several days after delivery. Cardiac output returns to nonpregnant levels by two weeks after delivery.

CHRONIC HYPERTENSION

For purposes of this discussion, chronic hypertension is assumed to be essential hypertension. Although the management of the hypertensive gravida with chronic renal disease, coarctation of the aorta, collagen vascular disease, or diabetes is in some respects similar to that to be described here, the specifics of management of those diseases during pregnancy are discussed elsewhere.

A pregnant woman is assumed to have chronic hypertension if she has a history anteceding pregnancy of a blood pressure of 140/90 mm Hg or greater, or if she has a persistent blood pressure of 140/90 mm Hg or greater during the first 20 weeks of gestation. In a parous woman who was normotensive during her first pregnancy, the development of preeclampsia is highly suggestive of underlying chronic hypertension.

Many patients with mild chronic hypertension experience a fall in both systolic and diastolic blood pressure during the second trimester, as do normal women. Therefore, the diagnosis of chronic hypertension may not be readily apparent in the patient who first presents for care in the second trimester. An even more difficult problem is presented by the patient who first presents for care in the third trimester, is found to be hypertensive, and has not had her blood pressure checked for years. It is difficult to know whether such a patient has preeclampsia (pregnancy-induced hypertension) or chronic hypertension. The absence of proteinuria and a serum uric acid level in the normal pregnancy range support the diagnosis of chronic hypertension in such circumstances. Examination of the optic fundi may also aid in the differential diagnosis.

The perinatal problems associated with chronic maternal hypertension include intrauterine growth retardation, stillbirth (especially term stillbirth), abruptio placentae, and fetal distress during labor. The development of superimposed preeclampsia further increases the risk of these perinatal problems. Intrauterine fetal growth retardation occurs in at least 15% of fetuses of chronic hypertensives.

The perinatal mortality of fetuses of treated chronic hypertensives has been reported as 16 to 32 per 1000 births. That of fetuses of untreated patients has been reported as 5 per 1000, but that result was obtained in mildly hypertensive women who had intensive surveillance during pregnancy; the outcome in most untreated cases would undoubtedly be worse. In fact, in Virginia in 1983 nearly half of the antepartum deaths of fetuses that were not malformed and that weighed more than 2500 g were due to untreated or undertreated maternal hypertension.

The association between maternal hypertension and abruptio placentae is striking. Eleven percent of patients who have abruptio placentae are chronic hypertensives, and abruptions complicate up to 10% of pregnancies among chronic hypertensives.

Superimposed preeclampsia is strictly defined as a rise in systolic and diastolic blood pressure of 30 mm Hg and 15 mm Hg, respectively, accompanied by sustained and significant proteinuria and generalized edema in a patient with chronic hypertension. The incidence according to this definition has been reported at between 14% and 23%. If the condition is more loosely defined, by blood pressure criteria alone, the incidence probably approaches 50%; in other words, 50% of untreated hypertensives will eventually demonstrate a significant rise in blood pressure during pregnancy.

Antepartum management of patients with chronic hypertension should include an ultrasound examination between 16 and 26 weeks for pregnancy dating, with subsequent studies at 30 to 32 weeks and again at 35 to 37 weeks to document fetal growth. The patient should be seen every two weeks during the first two trimesters and weekly during the third. Baseline renal function studies (creatinine clearance, 24-hour urinary protein excretion) should be performed early in pregnancy and repeated every six to eight weeks thereafter. Urine cultures should be performed monthly for the detection of asymptomatic bacteriuria, since some patients might have compromised renal function, which would be worsened by pyelonephritis. Fetal surveillance with weekly nonstress testing should be instituted at 32 to 34 weeks' gestation.

Regardless of whether they were treated before pregnancy, most chronic hypertensives should be treated with antihypertensive agents during pregnancy. The drug of choice is α-methyldopa (Aldomet) in divided doses two or three times a day up to a maximum dose of 2 g per day. Long-term follow-up has demonstrated no adverse effects from this drug on children exposed *in utero*. For patients who do not respond satisfactorily to α-methyldopa, hydralazine may be added to the regimen in divided doses of up to 200 mg per day.

The use of β-blocking agents in the management of chronic hypertension in pregnancy is controversial. In the past, all sorts of fetal/neonatal complications, including preterm labor, fetal bradycardia, neonatal hypoglycemia, and respiratory depression were ascribed to maternal treatment with propranolol. However, this theory has not withstood the test of time; only intrauterine growth retardation remains a concern. In theory propranolol may reduce umbilical blood flow. However, when Eliahou treated a large group of seriously hypertensive gravidas with propranolol throughout pregnancy, he noted only a 10% incidence of intrauterine growth retardation, hardly a surprising result if growth retardation is defined as birthweight below the tenth percentile. In addition, propranolol therapy reduced fetal mortality from 48% in previous pregnancies to 15% in the treated pregnancies.

The new β1-blockers such as metoprolol theoretically should have less effect than propranolol on umbilical blood flow. After more data become available, these agents may become the drugs of choice for treating hypertension during pregnancy. At present, however, the drug of choice remains α-methyldopa.

Certain antihypertensives should be avoided during pregnancy. Captopril, the angiotensin-converting enzyme inhibitor, has been associated with reduced uteroplacental perfusion and fetal death in experimental animals. Clonidine has not been studied enough in pregnancy to be considered safe. The calcium channel blockers (nifedipine and others) have been reported to reduce uterine blood flow in animals and therefore should be avoided, at least until more data are available. Diuretics should not be started during pregnancy as treatment for hypertension, since their use is associated with reduced plasma volume expansion and therefore probably reduced uteroplacental perfusion. Although this risk probably does not exist in the patient who is taking thiazide diuretics chronically before pregnancy, it is our practice to switch women to another drug once pregnancy is diagnosed.

The timing of delivery is crucial in the management of chronically hypertensive patients. Waiting for the cervix to become favorable once the fetus is mature unnecessarily increases the risk of fetal death. Even if all the surveillance techniques indicate fetal well-being, there is no test to predict the occurrence of abruptio placentae. Therefore, our practice is to perform an amniocentesis at 37 to 38 weeks and to effect delivery if the fetus's lungs are mature. Superimposed preeclampsia, intrauterine growth retardation, or abnormal fetal heart rate testing of course mandates even earlier delivery.

VASCULAR DISEASE

The causes of venous thrombosis and pulmonary embolism are Virchow's classic triad of changes in blood clotting factors, vessel wall damage, and stasis. Although pregnancy is often referred to as a hypercoagulable state because of increased blood levels of fibrinogen, factor VIII, and factor XII, there is little evidence that these increases lead to an increased incidence of thromboembolic disease in pregnancy. In fact, some clotting factors, especially factors XI and XIII, are usually decreased in pregnancy. However, levels of antithrombin III, an inhibitor of activated blood coagulation factors, are decreased during pregnancy, and therefore inherited deficiencies of antithrombin III may become manifest as pulmonary embolism during pregnancy.

Vessel wall damage does not occur during normal pregnancy but can occur during delivery. Most often pelvic vessel wall damage occurs during cesarean delivery, but improper or prolonged use of stirrups for vaginal delivery may lead to vessel wall damage in the legs.

Stasis of blood in the lower extremities is common in pregnancy. Venous distensibility increases in the first trimester, and by 28 weeks' gestation venous pressure in the legs is twice nonpregnant levels. Furthermore, the enlarging uterus interferes with venous return from the legs, so that by term the velocity of venous flow in the legs is reduced by half.

Contrary to popular belief, there is only a slightly increased incidence of thromboembolic disease during pregnancy. The incidence increases as pregnancy progresses, so that by term it is about 50% above nonpregnant values. The time of the most significant risk, however, is the early puerperium, when the incidence is 5 to 6 times higher than it is in nonpregnant women. It is thus evident that endothelial damage is the most important etiologic factor in thromboembolic disease.

Deep Vein Thrombosis

The clinical diagnosis of deep vein thrombosis (DVT) is not reliable. Up to 50% of patients with clinical signs of the disorder (pain, tenderness, swelling, Homan's sign) have entirely normal veins on venography; conversely, 30% to 50% of patients with DVT demonstrable on venography are asymptomatic.

The tests used to diagnose DVT are compromised by pregnancy. Venography, the definitive test, ideally requires irradiation of the pelvis. In pregnancy it can be done with shielding of the uterus, but this makes

visualization of the external and common iliac veins impossible. Impedance plethysmography (IPG) and Doppler ultrasound examinations are insensitive to calf vein thrombosis even in nonpregnant patients. However, they are useful in the diagnosis of proximal thrombosis during the first and second trimesters. By the third trimester the compression caused by the enlarged uterus may yield a false-positive result.

Therefore, the diagnosis of DVT during pregnancy is best made by a combination of impedance plethysmography or Doppler ultrasound and limited venography with pelvic shielding. During the first two trimesters the initial test in a patient in whom one suspects DVT should be IPG or Doppler ultrasound. A positive result establishes the diagnosis. If the result is negative, limited venography should be performed to evaluate the vessels of the calf and thigh; if this is also negative, DVT has been ruled out. In the third trimester there seems to be little point in doing IPG or Doppler ultrasound, because a negative test would require venography to rule out calf disease, and a positive test would require venography to rule out compression by the uterus. One should not hesitate to perform venography as indicated, since it may spare the patient the hazards of unnecessary anticoagulation.

The mainstay of therapy for DVT is anticoagulation (to be discussed later in this chapter). Another important measure is bed rest with the leg elevated about 8 inches until pain and edema subside. The leg is better elevated by bed blocks than by pillows, which flex the hip and may impede femoral flow. Moist heat should be continuously applied to involved areas. As soon as symptoms subside, the patient should be fitted with elastic support panty hose with a decreasing pressure gradient from ankle to thigh, and ambulation should be encouraged. Prolonged bed rest does not prevent thrombus detachment and enhances venous stasis. Sitting with the legs dependent must be avoided, as must wrapping the legs with elastic bandages.

Pulmonary Embolism

Nearly all patients with pulmonary embolism demonstrate tachycardia, tachypnea, and dyspnea. Many patients show only clinical manifestations, but some present with pulmonary infarction with pleuritic pain, hemoptysis, and pleural effusion; acute right-heart failure; or cardiovascular collapse with shock or arrhythmias.

If a pulmonary embolism is suspected during pregnancy, the most important diagnostic test is a perfusion lung scan using technetium 99 coupled to human albumin, which does not cross the placenta. A normal perfusion scan rules out pulmonary embolism. If the perfusion scan is not normal, it should be coupled with a xenon 133 ventilation scan. Perfusion deficits without ventilation abnormalities are generally due to pulmonary emboli, whereas matched perfusion and ventilation deficits are usually due to some other disease process.

Chest x-ray films are helpful only in the proper interpretation of the perfusion scan. Alone they are not useful in diagnosing pulmonary embolism, since they are often normal or show only nonspecific abnormalities.

Pulmonary angiography is the most definitive method of diagnosis but should be performed only if surgical intervention is contemplated.

Arterial blood gas determinations are of limited value. Although an arterial oxygen partial pressure of more than 80 torr during breathing of room air makes the diagnosis unlikely, overall the test is nonspecific and insensitive. The electrocardiogram is also often normal; only 40% of patients with pulmonary embolism show nonspecific ST-T wave changes, and the classic picture of right-axis deviation with strain is only seen after extensive embolization has occurred.

In summary, if pulmonary embolism is suspected in pregnancy, a perfusion lung scan should be performed, coupled with a ventilation scan if the perfusion scan is abnormal.

The mainstay of therapy is anticoagulation (discussed below). Bed rest is indicated for five to seven days, and if the embolus can be attributed to DVT in the lower extremities, measures similar to those described for DVT should be undertaken. Oxygen therapy should be used as necessary to maintain a normal maternal arterial oxygen partial pressure.

Anticoagulation in Pregnancy

Contrary to what used to be taught, the use of oral anticoagulants is contraindicated throughout pregnancy. These agents cross the placenta readily, and anatomic and physiologic deficits due to intrafetal bleeding have been associated with their use in any trimester. Heparin is the anticoagulant of choice throughout pregnancy; critical analysis of the literature does not reveal conclusive evidence of increased perinatal loss due to its use. There is a report of a 14% prematurity rate and a 13% stillbirth rate associated with heparin use, but most of these losses occurred in women being treated with heparin for preeclampsia, and it is probable that the adverse perinatal outcomes reported were due to the underlying disease rather than to the treatment.

Pregnant patients who develop DVT or pulmonary embolism should be fully anticoagulated with a continuous intravenous infusion of heparin for 10 to 14 days. The dosage should be adjusted to keep the activated partial thromboplastin time (aPTT) at 1.5 to 2 times the pretreatment level. Because of elevated factor VIII levels during pregnancy, many patients have a shortened aPTT before the institution of heparin therapy. This may give the appearance of heparin resistance, but to raise the aPTT to twice the nonpregnant control level may require very large doses of heparin and may cause serious hemorrhage. Therefore, it is preferable to use the patient's own pretreatment aPTT level as her control value.

The dosage and duration of heparin therapy after the acute episode are controversial, but the regimen of Kelton and Hirsh seems reasonable (Table 30-1). In women who develop DVT or a pulmonary embolus during the first half of pregnancy, 10 to 14 days of full intravenous therapy should be followed by 10,000 units SC twice a day for three months, and then 5000 units SC twice a day for the duration of pregnancy. Heparin therapy should be stopped at the onset of labor and resumed 24 hours after delivery at a dosage of 10,000 units SC twice a day for one to two weeks. The patient who experiences an acute event in the second half of pregnancy should be maintained on 10,000 units SC twice a day for the duration of pregnancy and the first one to two weeks of the puerperium, with discontinuation of therapy during labor and the first 24 hours after delivery. Women who have experienced DVT or pulmonary embolism in previous pregnancies or in the nonpregnant state should be maintained on low-dose heparin (5000 units SC twice a day) throughout pregnancy and the early puerperium, except during labor and the 24 hours after delivery.

Table 30-1
Anticoagulation with Heparin During Pregnancy

Diagnosis	Acute Event	Duration of Pregnancy	Puerperium
DVT or PE (first 20 weeks)	Full dose × 10–14 days	Moderate dose × 3 months Low dose for duration of pregnancy	Moderate dose × 1–2 weeks
DVT or PE (second 20 weeks)	Full dose × 10–15 days	Moderate dose for duration of pregnancy	Moderate dose × 1–2 weeks
Past history of DVT or PE		Low dose throughout pregnancy	Low dose × 1–2 weeks

Full dose = heparin IV to keep aPTT at control level × 2; *moderate dose* = 10,000 units SC b.i.d.; *low dose* = 5000 units SC b.i.d.
DVT, deep vein thrombosis; PE, pulmonary embolism.

Superficial Thrombophlebitis

Superficial thrombophlebitis occurs in approximately 1 in 600 women during pregnancy and 1 in 100 women in the puerperium. The diagnosis is usually apparent from physical examination, which reveals a painful, tender, red superficial vein. Edema may also be present. If there is any question of DVT, Doppler ultrasoud or IPG and venography should be performed. Therapy involves bed rest, elevation of the limbs, moist heat, and the use of aspirin or acetaminophen for analgesia. Anticoagulation is not indicated. Symptoms should resolve in one to two weeks, although the course may be more protracted in women with severe varicose veins.

Varicose Veins

In most persons there is one valve in the external iliac or common femoral vein; because the inferior vena cava and common iliac veins are without valves, this one valve must support all the hydrostatic venous pressure from the heart to the groin. However, in 8% of persons there is bilateral absence of this valve, and in 29% there is unilateral absence. In these persons the valves of the saphenous veins must support any increase in hydrostatic pressure. The hormonal effects of pregnancy cause a reduction in venous tone, and the resultant venous dilitation may render previously competent saphenous valves incompetent. Increased venous pressure due to uterine compression of the inferior vena cava and common iliac veins compounds this problem, causing the development of varicose veins.

Varicose veins usually improve or disappear after delivery and therefore rarely require surgical therapy during pregnancy. Daily bed rest for 1 hour every 4 hours should be prescribed for patients with varicose veins. During this time the legs should be elevated about 8 inches. This is better accomplished by placement of blocks under the foot of the bed than by use of pillows, which flex the hips and may impede blood flow through the femoral veins. The patient should be advised to avoid standing motionless or sitting with the legs dependent; sitting with the legs crossed must be studiously avoided. Custom-fitted support panty hose with a pressure gradient from ankle to thigh are quite beneficial in two ways: they reduce the amount of blood in the legs, and probably also cause some venous valve cusps to reapproximate, thereby restoring the function of the muscle pump mechanism.

REFERENCES AND RECOMMENDED READING

Abdella TN, Sibai BM, Hays JM, Anderson GD: Relationship of hypertensive disease to abruptio placentae. Obstet Gynecol 63:365, 1984

Baston GA: Cyanotic congenital heart disease and pregnancy. J Obstet Gynaecol Br Cmwlth 81:549, 1974

Chesley LC: The remote prognosis for pregnant women with rheumatic cardiac disease. Am J Obstet Gynecol 100:732, 1968

Chesley LC: Superimposed preeclampsia or eclampsia. In Chesley LC: Hypertensive Disorders in Pregnancy. New York, Appleton-Century-Crofts, 1978

Chesley LC: Severe rheumatic cardiac disease and pregnancy: The ultimate prognosis. Am J Obstet Gynecol 136:552, 1980

Conradsson TB, Werko L: Management of heart disease in pregnancy. Prog Cardiovasc Dis 16:407, 1974

Demakis JG, Ramimtoola SH, Sulton GC et al: Natural course of peripartum cardiomyopathy. Circulation 44:1053, 1971

Eliahou HE, Silverberg DS, Reisin E et al: Propranolol for the treatment of hypertension in pregnancy. Br J Obstet Gynaecol 85:431, 1978

Elkayam U, Gleicher N: Cardiac Problems in Pregnancy. Diagnosis and Management of Maternal and Fetal Disease. New York, Alan R Liss, 1982

Ferris TF: Toxemia and hypertension. In Burrow GN, Ferris TF (eds): Medical Complications During Pregnancy, 2nd ed. Philadelphia, WB Saunders, 1982

Gleicher N, Midwall J, Hochberger D, Jaffin H: Eisenmenger's syndrome and pregnancy. Obstet Gynecol Surv 34:721, 1979

Gunsted M, Cockburn J, Moar VA, Redman CW: Maternal hypertension with superimposed pre-eclampsia: Effects on child development at 7 plus years. Br J Obstet Gynaecol 90:644, 1983

Kelton JG, Hirsh J: Venous thromboembolic disorders. In Burrow GN, Ferris TF (eds): Medical Complications During Pregnancy, 2nd ed. Philadelphia, WB Saunders, 1982

Mendelson CL: Cardiac Disease in Pregnancy. Philadelphia, FA Davis, 1960

Pritchard JA, Pritchard SA: Standardized treatment of 154 cases of eclampsia. Am J Obstet Gynecol 123:543, 1975

Redman CWG: Treatment of hypertension in pregnancy. Kidney Int 18:267, 1980

Sibai BM, Abdella TN, Anderson GD: Pregnancy outcome in 211 patients with mild chronic hypertension. Obstet Gynecol 61:571, 1983

Spinnato JA, Kraynack BJ, Cooper MW: Eisenmenger's syndrome in pregnancy. Epidural anesthesia for elective cesarean section. N Engl J Med 304:1215, 1981

Szekely P, Snaith L: Heart Disease and Pregnancy. London, Churchill Livingstone, 1974

Whittemore R, Hobbins JC, Engle MA: Pregnancy and its outcome in women with and without surgical treatment of congenital heart disease. Am J Cardiol 50:641, 1982

Pulmonary Disease

Dwight P. Cruikshank

ASTHMA

Asthma, the only chronic obstructive lung disease encountered with significant frequency during pregnancy, occurs in 0.4% to 1.3% of gestations.

The effect of pregnancy on asthma is quite variable.

Patients with mild disease have little problem with pregnancy, but women with severe disease have about an 80% exacerbation rate during pregnancy. Patients tend to repeat the same pattern of response in each pregnancy; a patient who experiences worsening of asthma in one pregnancy is likely to do so in subsequent pregnancies as well.

Asthma does not appear to cause any maternal pregnancy complications. Most series demonstrate increased neonatal mortality among the offspring of asthmatics, all deaths apparently being due to an increased frequency of premature labor and low birth weight. Bahna and Bjerkedal reported an incidence of delivery at less than 37 weeks' gestation of 7.4% among asthmatics, as compared with 5% among controls (p < 0.01). The incidence of birth weight under 2500 g was 7.1% for infants of asthmatics and 3.7% for infants of control subjects (p < 0.001).

The chronic medical management of asthma is the same during pregnancy and in the nonpregnant state. The drug regimen that is most successful in keeping the patient's disease under control when she is not pregnant should usually be continued. Xanthine bronchodilators, the mainstay of therapy, do not appear to be harmful to the fetus. The dosage of theophylline should be adjusted to maintain serum levels of 10 μg/ml to 20 μg/ml, the usual dosage being 100 mg to 200 mg every 6 hours. Catecholamine bronchodilators may also be useful. The drug with the longest track record is the β-agonist terbutaline; although it has not been approved for the treatment of asthma in pregnancy, it is not associated with any teratogenicity, and it preserves or even enhances uterine blood flow, unlike drugs that have both α- and β-agonist activity. An oral dose of terbutaline between 2.5 mg twice a day and 5 mg 3 times a day is usually effective; the major side-effect is tremor. Theoretically, oral terbutaline may inhibit uterine contractions, and thus at term the dosage should be reduced or the drug discontinued if possible.

Corticosteroids are usually reserved for short courses of therapy in patients with refractory symptoms. In these patients, 60 mg to 100 mg prednisone orally per day for three to four days should be followed by rapid tapering over a five to ten-day period. If steroids cannot be discontinued, an alternate day regimen is preferable. There are no human data to suggest that corticosteroids are teratogenic. Furthermore, fetal adrenal suppression does not occur following maternal therapy with cortisol or prednisone, although estriol excretion is reduced. Women being treated with steroids need an increased dose during labor, delivery, and the puerperium, however, because of maternal adrenal suppression. An effective regimen is 100 mg of hydrocortisone intramuscularly or intravenously every 8 hours during labor and the first 24 to 48 hours postpartum.

The safety of beclomethasone inhalation in pregnancy has not been clearly established, but since there are many fewer maternal systemic side-effects with beclomethasone treatment than with systemic steroid therapy, one would expect few if any adverse effects on the fetus. The usual dosage is 100 mg (2 inhalations) 3 or 4 times per day.

The data about inhaled cromolyn sodium in pregnancy are insufficient to ensure this agent's safety, and the manufacturer does not recommend its use during pregnancy; however, to date no evidence suggests increased fetal risk associated with cromolyn use, and animal studies suggest that the drug is safe.

Expectorants are not generally useful in the management of asthma, and those containing iodides must be scrupulously avoided, because their chronic use is associated with a significant risk of fetal goiter.

The pregnant patient with an acute asthma attack should be evaluated with arterial blood gas determinations, complete blood count, serum electrolytes, spirometry, and, if she is febrile, a chest radiograph. Initial drug therapy is subcutaneous epinephrine, 0.3 ml to 0.5 ml of 1:1000 solution every 15 to 20 minutes. If there is no response after the second injection, intravenous theophylline, 6 mg per kg of body weight in 1 dl should be infused over 20 to 30 minutes (if the patient has taken oral theophylline in the past 18 hours, the loading dose should be reduced to 4.5 mg/kg), followed by a maintenance dose of 0.9 mg/kg/hour. If the patient has been seriously ill for more than six hours and does not respond promptly to therapy with epinephrine and theophylline, she should be hospitalized and steroid therapy begun using 4.5 mg/kg intravenous hydrocortisone every 4 to 12 hours. Careful attention to arterial blood gas determinations is important. In a pregnant patient, a carbon dioxide partial pressure (pCO_2) of greater than 35 mm Hg, a pH of less than 7.35, or an oxygen partial pressure (pO_2) of less than 60 mm Hg signifies impending respiratory failure, and the patient should be transferred to an intensive care unit for possible assisted ventilation. More typical blood gas findings during an acute asthma attack are those of respiratory alkalosis due to hyperventilation, with a reduced pCO_2 and elevated arterial pH. Maternal alkalosis causes a marked reduction in uterine blood flow, and the fetus may become quite hypoxic even though the mother's pO_2 is normal. Therefore, if significant maternal respiratory alkalosis is present (pH $\geq$ 7.60, $pCO_2 \leq$ 17 mm Hg), it is important to maintain the mother's pO_2 at high levels with supplemental oxygen and to remove the stimulus to hyperventilation by relieving the airway obstruction as quickly as possible.

TUBERCULOSIS

There is no evidence that the natural history of tuberculosis is altered in any way by pregnancy, nor do recent data suggest that tuberculosis increases the risk of any pregnancy complications, including spontaneous abortion, congenital anomalies, premature labor, or stillbirth. However, it is important that tuberculosis be detected and aggressively treated during pregnancy, because a newborn exposed to undiagnosed, active pulmonary tuberculosis has a 50% chance of developing tuberculosis in the first year of life and a significant risk of death.

All pregnant women should be screened at their first prenatal visit with an intradermal test of intermediate-strength purified protein derivative (PPD). Pregnancy does not depress reactivity to PPD, and tuberculin skin testing is valid throughout pregnancy. Chest radiographs are not indicated except for the following patients: patients with positive skin tests known to be negative in the past, patients with positive skin tests and unknown prior status, and patients whose histories or examinations suggest tuberculosis, even if their skin tests are negative.

The pregnant patient with a positive skin test and a positive or suspicious x-ray film should be hospitalized, and at least three early morning sputum specimens should be obtained from her for culture. If the patient is bacteriologically positive, or presumptively positive on the basis of history, physical examination, and chest x-ray film, chemotherapy should be begun. The drugs recommended for use in pregnancy are isoniazid (INH) and ethambutol. In most studies INH has not been shown to be teratogenic, even when given in the first trimester, and most of its toxic effects can be prevented by simultaneous administration of pyridoxine. Nor has teratogenicity been reported with first-trimester ethambutol use. Therefore, therapy should be begun with INH, 300 mg per day; pyridoxine, 100 mg per day; and ethambutol, 25 mg/kg per day for 6 weeks followed by 15 mg/kg per day thereafter. This regimen must be maintained for 12 to 18 months. Consultation with a pulmonary disease specialist is essential.

There is some controversy over whether recent PPD convertors should be treated during pregnancy. I believe that the pregnant patient who is known to have converted her skin test within the past 12 months should be treated with INH, 300 mg per day, and pyridoxine, 100 mg per day, for one year beginning at the end of the first trimester.

The mother with active tuberculosis must be separated from her newborn until she is bacteriologically negative and appropriate prophylaxis for the infant has been undertaken. Whether neonatal prophylaxis should be daily INH for one year or vaccination with BCG is beyond the scope of this chapter—both methods have supporters among pediatric infectious disease specialists. All other members of a tuberculous mother's household must be screened and appropriately treated before the newborn is permitted to enter that environment.

SARCOIDOSIS

There is no evidence that sarcoidosis has any adverse effect on pregnancy, unless maternal pulmonary or cardiac disease is severe enough to endanger the mother's life. Many authors report that pregnancy has an amelio-

rating effect on sarcoidosis, and this is often ascribed to the elevation in free plasma cortisol levels that occurs in pregnancy. Scadding summarized the effects of pregnancy on sarcoidosis, noting that patients with normal chest x-ray films tend to remain normal, patients with resolving radiographs continue to show resolution, and patients with active disease tend to show partial or complete resolution of their x-ray findings during pregnancy. Most patients in the latter group tend to have an exacerbation of their disease three to six months after delivery, however.

Patients with sarcoidosis should be evaluated with chest x-ray films and pulmonary function tests early in pregnancy. These should be repeated every three months in patients who show evidence of active disease or in whom symptoms appear. Treatment with steroids is indicated if there is rapid progression of symptoms, deterioration seen on chest x-ray films (an unlikely event), central nervous system or eye involvement, or development of hypercalcemia.

VIRAL PNEUMONIAS

During the influenza epidemics of 1918 to 1919 and 1957 to 1958, there was high mortality associated with pregnancy, with half of the deaths of women of reproductive age occurring during pregnancy. The cause of death in these cases was influenzal pneumonia rather than secondary bacterial infection. Because of this apparently increased risk during pregnancy, many physicians recommend that pregnant women be vaccinated against influenza when an epidemic threatens. The vaccines are made from killed virus, and there are no data to suggest that they are teratogenic.

Varicella is not a common infection during pregnancy, most persons having been immune since childhood. Nonetheless, there seems to be an increased risk of life-threatening varicella pneumonia in pregnant women who contract chickenpox. About 10% of all reported cases of varicella pneumonia have occurred in pregnant women, and although the number of cases is small (approximately 20), the mortality is 45% among pregnant women, compared with 15% to 20% among nonpregnant individuals. The profound maternal hypoxia that occurs in this disease is associated with a greater than normal risk of spontaneous abortion, premature labor, and stillbirth.

CYSTIC FIBROSIS

More than 140 pregnancies have been reported in patients with cystic fibrosis (CF). Women with CF who conceive generally were much older when their disease was diagnosed (mean age, 11 years) than were all CF patients (mean age, 3.7 years), suggesting that the disease of the former group is less severe than that of the latter group. A survey of CF centers in the United States revealed 129 pregnancies in 100 patients. Maternal mortality was quite high (12% within six months of delivery, 18% within two years), but the observed death rates were not greater in this group than in nonpregnant CF patients of the same age. This suggests that pregnancy itself does not lead to increased mortality. Among CF patients, perinatal mortality is 11%, about 4 times higher than normal, and the incidence of premature labor is about 27%, also a fourfold increase. Cyanosis and dyspnea are poor prognostic signs, as is a vital capacity of less than 50% the predicted value. Some patients show transient acceleration of deterioration in pulmonary function, but in general pregnancy does not appear to change the general trend of deterioration over several years. Corkey and associates reported a subgroup of CF patients with no pancreatic insufficiency who did not deteriorate during pregnancy and whose maternal and perinatal mortality rates were much lower than those of CF patients with pancreatic insufficiency.

Cor pulmonale and pulmonary hypertension are absolute contraindications to pregnancy in CF patients; pregnancy termination and sterilization should be recommended to CF patients with these additional disorders. Other patients should be managed on an individual basis, with frequent measurements of arterial blood gases and pulmonary function. A rapid decline in these parameters during pregnancy is an indication for pregnancy termination, whereas a gradual decline probably is not. Pulmonary infection is a serious threat to CF patients, and antibiotics should be used as indicated bacteriologically, without regard to pregnancy, although tetracycline should be avoided if possible. Penicillin analogs such as carbenicillin exert less fetal toxicity than do the aminoglycosides.

REFERENCES AND RECOMMENDED READING

Bahna SL, Bjerkedal T: The course and outcome of pregnancy in women with bronchial asthma. Acta Allergol (Kbh) 27: 397, 1972

Brown Z: Tuberculosis and pregnancy. In Sciarra JJ (ed): Gynecology and Obstetrics, Vol. 3. Philadelphia, Harper & Row, 1984

Cohen LF, Di Sant'Agnese PA, Friedlander J: Cystic fibrosis and pregnancy. A national survey. Lancet 2:842, 1980

Corkey CWB, Newth CJL, Corey M, Levison H: Pregnancy in cystic fibrosis: A better prognosis in patients with pancreatic function. Am J Obstet Gynecol 140:737, 1981

Giesler CF, Webster JR: Pulmonary disease in pregnancy. In Sciarra JJ (ed): Gynecology and Obstetrics, Vol. 3. Philadelphia, Harper & Row, 1984

Good JT, Iseman MD, Davidson PT et al: Tuberculosis in association with pregnancy. Am J Obstet Gynecol 140:492, 1981

Scadding JG: Sarcoidosis. London, Eyre & Spottiswoode, 1967

Turner ES, Greenberger PA, Patterson R: Management of the pregnant asthmatic patient. Ann Intern Med 6:905, 1980

Weinberger SE, Weiss ST, Cohen WR et al: Pregnancy and the lung. Am Rev Resp Dis 121:559, 1980

Weinstein AM, Dubin BD, Podleski WK et al: Asthma and pregnancy. JAMA 241:1161, 1979

Urinary Tract Disease

Dwight P. Cruikshank

INFECTION

Urinary tract infections are a common medical complication of pregnancy, occurring in 10% to 15% of women, and acute pyelonephritis is a frequent indication for hospitalization during pregnancy. The organisms most commonly responsible for these infections are *Escherichia coli* (75–90% of cases), *Klebsiella* (10–15%), and *Proteus* (5%). Other responsible organisms include *Pseudomonas, Staphylococcus,* and group-D and group-B *Streptococcus.* Group-B *Streptococcus* is a potent, albeit uncommon, urinary tract pathogen. When urine cultures from pregnant women show the presence of this organism, cervical cultures should also be obtained; neonatal infection with group-B *Streptococcus* is associated with high morbidity and mortality.

Asymptomatic Bacteriuria

Asymptomatic bacteriuria is found in 4% to 10% of all sexually active women; the incidence is the same in pregnant women. Women with sickle trait have about twice the normal incidence of this condition.

The usual definition of asymptomatic bacteriuria is the finding of over 100,000 organisms per milliliter in the urine of a woman without fever, chills, dysuria, frequency, or flank pain. However, Lenke and associates have shown that pure cultures of gram-negative bacteria with colony counts of over 1000 organisms per milliliter are significant, as are counts of over 10,000 gram-negative bacteria per milliliter with concomitant growth of only one other organism. Contaminated cultures usually demonstrate over 1000 gram-negative organisms per milliliter with concomitant growth of at least two other organisms, often including gram-positive ones. Colony counts below 100,000 organisms per milliliter may also be significant in partially treated patients and in patients who have voluntarily increased their fluid intake.

The effect of asymptomatic bacteriuria on pregnancy is controversial, but the bulk of evidence supports the view that bacteriuria does not in and of itself lead to an increased incidence of low birth weight or prematurity. However, there is no doubt that women with asymptomatic bacteriuria are at increased risk for acute pyelonephritis during pregnancy. In fact, of women with asymptomatic bacteriuria who are not treated, 25% to 30% will develop pyelonephritis later in pregnancy. At least two thirds of these cases can be prevented by eradication of bacteriuria early in pregnancy.

All pregnant women should be screened periodically for asymptomatic bacteriuria. One simple and inexpensive way is with the nitrite test, a dip-stick method, which should be performed at each prenatal visit. Patients with a positive nitrite test should provide a clean-catch urine sample for culture. Patients at high risk for urinary tract infection should have a culture of clean-catch urine, rather than the nitrite test, as the screening test. These include patients at increased risk for bacteriuria (those with a past history of urinary infections, with sickle trait, or with nephrolithiasis) and for serious sequelae of urinary infection (those with chronic renal disease, hypertension, or diabetes). These patients should have their urine cultured at their first prenatal visit, and every four to six weeks thereafter. Although urine specimens obtained by catheterization yield more accurate results (95%) than clean-voided specimens (80%), the 4% to 5% incidence of infection caused by catheterization is unacceptably high. Furthermore, the accuracy of the clean-void technique is 90% in cases in which two specimens reveal the same organisms. When providing a voided specimen for culture, the patient should separate the labia and swab the vulva with distilled water or a plain soap solution. Antiseptics should be avoided; they may result in a false-negative culture.

Patients with asymptomatic bacteriuria should be treated with therapeutic doses of sulfonamide, ampicillin, nitrofurantoin, or sulfamethoxazole–trimethoprim (co-trimoxazole). Sulfonamide and co-trimoxazole should be avoided near term, and because it has not been proved that trimethoprim is free of teratogenicity, co-trimoxazole is best avoided in the first trimester. Nitrofurantoin (Macrodantin) has the distinct advantage of being associated with a very low incidence of bacterial resistance even with prolonged or repeated use, but it does cause nausea and vomiting in 10% to 15% of patients. A repeat urine culture should be obtained one week after completion of therapy, and every four to six weeks thereafter, unless nitrite testing indicates the need for more frequent cultures.

Cystitis

Acute cystitis is defined as bacteriuria accompanied by symptoms of urinary urgency, frequency, dysuria, and pyuria. Fever and flank pain are absent. A clean-void urine culture should be obtained before the initiation of therapy, and follow-up cultures should be performed as outlined for patients with asymptomatic bacteriuria.

It is inadvisable to make the diagnosis of urinary tract infection solely on the basis of pyuria. The presence of more than 50 leukocytes per high-power field on a spun specimen is evidence of urinary infection. Lesser amounts of pyuria found in voided samples are probably not significant unless accompanied by other unequivocal signs or symptoms.

Acute Pyelonephritis

Infection of the renal parenchyma complicates 1% to 2.5% of pregnancies. The diagnosis is based on the findings of fever, costovertebral angle tenderness, pyuria, and bacteriuria. Symptoms may include chills, urgency, frequency, dysuria, and nausea and vomiting. Acute pyelonephritis frequently is associated with premature labor. Furthermore, Whalley and co-workers have shown transient but significant reductions of creatinine clearance during episodes of acute pyelonephritis.

When the diagnosis of acute pyelonephritis is made, the patient should be hospitalized. After a urine culture is obtained, intravenous antibiotic therapy should be started. A dosage of ampicillin of 1 g to 2 g every 4 hours is a good initial regimen, although comparable doses of a cephalosporin are acceptable. It is important to maintain adequate hydration, and febrile patients should receive at least 200 ml/hour of intravenous fluid. Once the patient has been afebrile for 24 hours, she may be switched to oral antibiotics. If she remains afebrile for another 24 hours on oral antibiotics, she may be discharged from the hospital to complete a 10-day course of antibiotics.

If the patient remains symptomatic after 48 hours of single-drug intravenous therapy, consideration should be given to adding or switching antibiotics. If antibiotic sensitivity tests are available, switching to a better drug is ideal; if they are not available, intravenous gentamicin should be added to the antibiotic regimen. If flank pain and fever persist beyond four to five days of appropriate antibiotic therapy, the diagnosis of calculus or perinephric abscess should be considered. Renal ultrasound may be helpful in diagnosing the latter condition, but intravenous pyelography may be necessary to rule out stone disease. This can usually be accomplished with two x-ray films: a scout film and a 20-minute film.

Whether to maintain the patient on chronic suppressive antimicrobial therapy for the duration of pregnancy after one bout of pyelonephritis is controversial. The incidence of recurrence of pyelonephritis during the same gestation is 10% to 18%. Harris and Gilstrap found a 2.7% incidence of recurrence in patients maintained on suppressive therapy for the remainder of pregnancy. However, Lenke and colleagues found almost identical recurrence rates in patients given suppressive therapy (7%) and in patients who received no therapy but were closely monitored with frequent urine cultures (8%). They did find that suppressive therapy reduced the incidence of asymptomatic bacteriuria, however.

It is our practice to use suppressive therapy after the first episode of acute pyelonephritis only in patients with underlying renal disease, urinary calculi, or a history of recurrent urinary infections in previous pregnancies. All other patients are followed with monthly urine cultures and are begun on suppressive therapy if they develop a second urinary tract infection. Adequate suppressive therapy consists of 100 mg nitrofurantoin or one double-strength tablet of co-trimoxazole taken at bedtime after emptying of the bladder. The practice of acidifying the urine with high doses of ascorbic acid should be avoided during pregnancy, because the fetus may become conditioned to a high–vitamin C environment and develop scurvy in the neonatal period. If the patient had persistent or recurrent disease, it is important to evaluate the renal anatomy 12 or more weeks postpartum with an intravenous pyelogram and voiding cystogram.

URINARY CALCULI

The reported incidence of urinary calculi complicating pregnancy is 0.05% to 0.35%. It appears that pregnancy does not increase the risk of stone formation or the severity of stone disease. Coe and co-workers studied 78 women with established nephrolithiasis during 148 pregnancies and concluded that the incidence of stone formation or passage was not higher than the nonpregnant rate.

Furthermore, the only adverse effect of stones on pregnancy is an increased frequency of urinary tract infection. The incidence of urinary infection in pregnant patients with calculi is 20% to 45%. The incidence of spontaneous abortion, premature labor, and hypertensive complications is not higher than usual.

Patients known to have nephrolithiasis should be followed with monthly urine cultures. Chronic antibacterial suppression with nitrofurantoin or co-trimoxazole is recommended by most authors, and aggressive treatment of all urinary infections is necessary.

Patients who should be investigated for possible stone disease during pregnancy include those with painful hematuria, colicky flank and loin pain, and unusually severe or unresponsive pyelonephritis. An intravenous pyelogram consisting of two x-ray films may be necessary.

Management of pregnant patients with urinary tract stones must be individualized. Most stones pass spontaneously, so most patients need only be treated with analgesics (often in substantial doses), hydration, and, if infection is present, antibiotics. Unrelenting pain, complete ureteral obstruction, or persistent infection may require surgical intervention.

Approximately 85% to 90% of stones seen in pregnant women contain calcium (oxalate or phosphate) and are radiopaque. Uric acid stones, which are radiolucent, constitute 10%; minimally radiopaque cystine stones are rare. Interestingly, 10% of the patients in the series of Coe and associates had hyperparathyroidism, a condition that should be ruled out because it has deleterious effects during pregnancy.

CHRONIC RENAL DISEASE

It used to be taught that pregnancy in women with renal disease led to progression of renal lesions and permanent worsening of renal function. However, recent studies do not support this view.

Leppert and colleagues evaluated the subsequent pregnancies of 133 women hospitalized during childhood for acute glomerulonephritis, the nephrotic syndrome, or acute pyelonephritis. When compared with two control groups—their female siblings and another group of women hospitalized during childhood for respiratory diseases—these women were no different in terms of incidences of live births, spontaneous abortions, stillbirths, or pregnancy-induced hypertension. Interestingly, the incidences of low-birth-weight offspring in the group with previous kidney disease (13.6%) and the group with respiratory disease (18.3%) were much higher than in the group of siblings (3.5%). The authors concluded that childhood kidney disease that heals without significant impairment in renal function has no adverse effect on pregnancy outcome other than causing birth weight to be low.

Katz and associates reported on 121 pregnancies in 89 women with proved renal disease. Before pregnancy 16% of these patients had been hypertensive ($\geq$140/90); of these, 4% had been severely hypertensive (>170/110). In addition, 34% had proteinuria of more than 1 g/24 hours, including 6% with severe proteinuria (>3 g/24 hours). As summarized in Table 30-2, 23% of the 121 patients developed significant hypertension during pregnancy, the condition being most pronounced in patients with diffuse or membranous glomerulonephritis and arteriolar nephrosclerosis. Half of these women had been hypertensive before they became pregnant. Serum urea and creatinine levels rose during pregnancy in 16% of cases, most frequently in patients with diffuse glomerulonephritis. Increased proteinuria was the most common finding, occurring in nearly half of cases, and in two thirds of these patients proteinuria exceeded 3 g/24 hours. The incidence of all three complications was low in patients with interstitial nephritis (chronic pyelonephritis).

Eighty women were also studied 3 months to 23 years after delivery. At follow-up, five women had progressed to end-stage renal disease; however, in four there clearly was no connection between pregnancy and ultimate outcome, and in the fifth it was not clear whether there was an association.

These authors also found that patients with chronic renal disease showed a mean increase in glomerular filtration rate of 50% during pregnancy, although the absolute levels achieved were below those seen in normal women. These data suggest that, in the words of Katz and co-workers, "although renal disease may become clinically manifest or worsen during pregnancy, its natural course is probably not affected by gestation."

Table 30-2
Effect of Pregnancy on Maternal Renal Disease

Diagnosis	Number	Increased Blood Pressure (%)*	Decreased Renal Function (%)†	Increased Proteinuria (%)‡
Diffuse glomerulonephritis	33	33	33	73
Focal glomerulonephritis	26	23	8	35
Interstitial nephritis (chronic pyelonephritis)	26	12	4	8
Membraneous nephropathy	10	0	0	80
Arteriolar nephrosclerosis	8	63	25	38
Lipoid nephrosis	6	0	0	33
Membranoproliferative glomerulonephritis	4	0	25	75
Other renal disease	8	38	25	75
Overall		23	16	47

* Blood pressure of ≥160/110 mm Hg, or an increase of ≥30/20 mm Hg above prepregnancy levels.

† Blood urea nitrogen of ≥25 mg/dl or serum creatinine of ≥1.5 mg/dl, or an increase in either of ≥50% over prepregnancy levels.

‡ 24-hour protein excretion of ≥3 g or an increase of 100% over prepregnancy levels.

(After Katz AI et al: Contrib Nephrol 25:53, 1981)

Although Katz and associates avoided use of the term, superimposed preeclampsia is usually diagnosed in the case of worsening blood pressure and proteinuria during pregnancy in association with renal disease. In a summary of 424 pregnancies in 365 women with chronic renal disease, Ferris found an incidence of superimposed toxemia of 16% in women who had been normotensive before pregnancy and of 50% in women who had been hypertensive before pregnancy.

In all series of pregnant women with renal disease, fetal mortality is increased. Katz and colleagues reported fetal mortality of 4.1%, whereas Ferris reported fetal mortality of 7% in normotensive women and 45% in hypertensive women.

All patients with chronic renal disease should have baseline renal function studies (creatinine clearance, protein excretion) performed early in pregnancy and an ultrasound examination carried out between 16 and 24 weeks to document the duration of gestation. Because renal infection is a threat to these patients, monthly urine cultures and vigorous treatment of asymptomatic bacteriuria are indicated. Ultrasound examinations at 32 and 36 weeks to document appropriate fetal growth seem prudent. Hypertensive patients should have antepartum fetal surveillance with electronic heart-rate testing and delivery when fetal pulmonary maturity is established. The development of superimposed preeclampsia may mandate preterm delivery.

ACUTE RENAL FAILURE

The incidence of acute renal failure in pregnant women has fallen dramatically in recent years, probably owing to a dramatic reduction in the number of septic criminal abortions performed as well as to better and more ag-

gressive management of obstetric complications such as severe preeclampsia and eclampsia. In France the percentage of cases of acute renal failure in pregnancy fell from 40% in 1966 to 4.5% in 1978. The Pritchards reported 154 consecutive cases of eclampsia with only 1 case of acute renal failure. Nonetheless, acute renal failure occurs in pregnancy, and although the majority of cases involve acute tubular necrosis, up to 21% of cases lead to bilateral cortical necrosis and chronic renal failure. This is especially common in cases of acute renal failure following abruptio placentae, and this diagnosis should be suspected in any patient in whom the anuric or oliguric phase of acute renal failure lasts more than ten days. Grunfeld and associates reported cortical necrosis in 54% of 13 patients who developed acute renal failure following placental abruption but in only 8% of patients who developed acute renal failure secondary to toxemia. They also found abruption to be the leading cause of acute renal failure in pregnancy (13 of 57 cases), followed by severe preeclampsia or eclampsia (12 cases) and prolonged intrauterine fetal death associated with coagulopathy (6 cases). Acute renal failure also occurred secondary to postpartum hemorrhage, amniotic fluid embolism, acute pyelonephritis, dehydration caused by hyperemesis gravidarum, and acute fatty liver of pregnancy.

In many cases the precipitating cause of acute renal failure in pregnancy (*e.g.,* abruptio placentae, eclampsia) will necessitate delivery, and in most other cases delivery should be effected if the fetus is beyond 34 weeks' gestation.

Hemodialysis during pregnancy has been reported in patients with acute renal failure and more commonly in patients with chronic renal failure. The incidence of premature labor in these women is extraordinarily high, approaching 75% in some series. It has been postulated that this might be due to the removal of progesterone by dialysis; it is therefore our practice to treat these women with 100 mg intramuscular progesterone in oil during each episode of dialysis. Because of reduced peripheral resistance, systemic hypotension is more common than usual during hemodialysis of pregnant women and must be scrupulously guarded against. Avoidance of the supine position is important in this regard.

There have been reports of at least four cases of acute renal failure secondary to ureteral obstruction by an overdistended uterus in otherwise normal patients. Three of these patients had twin gestations, and all had polyhydramnios. All presented with oliguria, azotemia (blood urea nitrogen, 42–77 mg/dl), and elevated serum levels of creatinine (3.8–7.6 mg/dl) and uric acid (10.6–11.1 mg/dl). In all cases, delivery was followed promptly by diuresis and a return of renal function to normal.

REFERENCES AND RECOMMENDED READING

Coe FL, Parks JH, Lindheimer MD: Nephrolithiasis during pregnancy. N Engl J Med 298:324, 1978

Ferris TF: Renal diseases. In Burrow GN, Ferris FT: Medical Complications During Pregnancy, 2nd ed. Philadelphia, WB Saunders, 1982

Grunfeld JP, Ganeval D, Bournerais F: Acute renal failure in pregnancy. Kidney Int 18:179, 1980

Harris RE, Gilstrap LC: Prevention of recurrent pyelonephritis during pregnancy. Obstet Gynecol 44:637, 1974

Katz AI, Davison JM, Hayslett JP et al: Pregnancy in women with kidney disease. Kidney Int 18:192, 1980

Kleinknecht D, Grunfeld JP, Cia Gomez P et al: Diagnostic procedures and long-term prognosis in bilateral renal cortical necrosis. Kidney Int 4:390, 1973

Lenke RR, Van Dorsten JP, Schifrin BS: Pyelonephritis in pregnancy. A prospective randomized trial to prevent recurrent disease evaluating suppressive therapy with nitrofurantoin and close surveillance. Am J Obstet Gynecol 146:953, 1983

Leppert P, Tisher CC, Cheng SS, Harlan WR: Antecedent renal disease and the outcome of pregnancy. Ann Intern Med 90:747, 1979

Pritchard JA, Pritchard SA: Standardized treatment of 154 cases of eclampsia. Am J Obstet Gynecol 123:543, 1975

Surian M, Imbasciati E, Cosci P et al: Glomerular disease in pregnancy: A study of 123 pregnancies in patients with primary and secondary glomerular diseases. Nephron 36:101, 1984

Whalley PJ, Cunningham FG, Martin FG: Transient renal dysfunction associated with acute pyelonephritis of pregnancy. Obstet Gynecol 46:174, 1975

Neurologic Disease

Dwight P. Cruikshank

CENTRAL NERVOUS SYSTEM

Cerebrovascular Disease

Hemorrhagic Stroke

Hemorrhagic strokes are an uncommon but catastrophic complication of pregnancy. The most common cause is rupture of an intracranial aneurysm, usually in the angle of bifurcation of vessels in the circle of Willis or the proximal regions of their branches. The second most common cause is arteriovenous malformation (AVM) or angioma, most commonly located in the parietal, frontoparietal, or temporoparietal region. In some series, AVM has been reported to be nearly as common as aneurysm. Other much less common causes are subacute bacterial endocarditis and cerebral metastases from choriocarcinoma.

Most commonly, the initial symptom of a hemorrhagic stroke is a headache of sudden onset, often described as bursting or "the worst headache of my life" (Table 30-3). Other prominent early symptoms are nuchal rigidity and nausea and vomiting. Hemiplegia and seizures are not dominant signs. The patient may have an elevated temperature, mild proteinuria, and fluctuating blood pressure elevations.

The workup of pregnant patients with hemorrhagic stroke is decided on neurosurgical grounds and should proceed as in nonpregnant patients. Almost always a lumbar puncture is indicated and reveals grossly bloody cerebrospinal fluid (CSF). If more than 6 hours have elapsed since the stroke, the CSF supernatant will be xanthochromic. Computed tomography (CT) will demonstrate intracerebral hemorrhage and may suggest the site of bleeding, but all authorities agree that angiography of all four major intracranial arteries is necessary. Again, the timing of angiography is decided solely on a neurosurgical basis.

The occurrence of a ruptured aneurysm is not related to increased parity, 50% to 65% occurring in primigravidas. The first bleeding episode usually occurs in the third trimester or late second trimester (23–36 weeks' gestation), and the risk appears to increase as term approaches. Labor appears to play a small role, if any, in the initiation of bleeding. None of the 21 patients reported by Amias bled during labor, although two bled in the early puerperium. However, six patients with marked pathology (severe hypertension, multiple aneurysms) did not bleed until several weeks after delivery. In fact, a review of the entire literature regarding

Table 30-3
Cerebrovascular Disease in Pregnancy

	Hemorrhagic		Occlusive	
	Aneurysm	*Arteriovenous Malformation*	*Arterial*	*Venous*
Principal Initial Symptom	Headache	Headache	Sensory and motor deficits	Seizures
Other Symptoms	Nausea and vomiting, nuchal rigidity	Nausea and vomiting, nuchal rigidity	Headache, seizures, coma	Headache, coma, paralysis
Time of Occurrence	16–20 weeks' gestation	23–36 weeks' gestation	Throughout pregnancy, first week of puerperium	1–4 weeks postpartum
Usual Treatment	Surgical	Surgical	Medical	Medical

104 ruptured aneurysms in pregnancy revealed only 11 cases occurring during labor. A possible explanation for this is that, with contractions, blood pressure and CSF pressure increase in parallel while the intracranial transvessel pressure gradient does not change.

The association between ruptured intracranial aneurysms and systemic hypertension is well known; chronic hypertensives are at increased risk for intracranial aneurysms, and up to 60% of patients with ruptured aneurysms are hypertensive. Antihypertensive therapy is indicated for persons with severe preeclampsia who have blood pressure of 160/110 or more, since up to 5% of such patients may have undiagnosed aneurysms. It may be hard to differentiate between a ruptured aneurysm and eclampsia (Table 30-4); the presence of grossly bloody CSF suggests an aneurysm, whereas proteinuria greater than 1+ suggests eclampsia.

Bleeding from AVMs, unlike bleeding from aneurysms, is more common in multiparas than in primigravidas, suggesting that a malformation is unlikely to bleed in a first pregnancy. However, AVMs tend to bleed earlier in pregnancy than aneurysms, in the first or early second trimester. Donaldson states that the most common time for the first bleed is at 16 to 20 weeks' gestation, but in 21% of cases bleeding occurs in the first trimester. Bleeding during labor is more common with AVMs than with aneurysms, occurring in 11% of cases.

The immediate management of pregnant patients with intracranial hemorrhage is supportive, consisting of prevention of seizures, control of hypertension, and high-dose steroid therapy to combat cerebral edema. The use of hyperosmolar mannitol to prevent tentorial herniation may be necessary, but this drug has profound effects on the fetus, including dehydration, marked reduction in blood volume, hypoxia, and bradycardia, and should therefore be avoided if possible. Unless the lesion is inoperable, surgical treatment of both aneurysms and AVMs is associated with the best prognosis for the mother, and it eliminates the risk of rebleeding during pregnancy or labor. The type and timing of surgical intervention should be decided strictly on the basis of neurosurgical principles, as if the patient were not

Table 30-4
Ruptured Intracranial Aneurysm Versus Eclampsia

Signs and Symptoms	*Aneurysm*	*Eclampsia*
Headache	Sudden, severe, constant, generalized	Gradual onset; throbbing, frontal
Seizures	25%	100%
Lumbar puncture	Grossly bloody	Usually clear; may be slightly bloody
Proteinuria	50%; mild	99–100%; usually marked

pregnant. Surgery under hypothermia is without apparent adverse effect on the fetus. Similarly, neurosurgery using controlled hypotension has been followed by normal pregnancy outcome, although fetal bradycardia of 60 beats to 80 beats/minute may occur during the hypotensive period.

Obstetric management of the patient who has bled from an aneurysm or AVM has been likened to that for patients with heart disease. Abortion is not indicated if the patient bleeds early in pregnancy. Amias states the opinion of all authorities but one when he says, "termination does not alter the prognosis and has virtually no place in present day management of cerebral vascular lesions." In the case of the patient who bleeds later in pregnancy, the question of vaginal or cesarean delivery must be considered. In Amias' series of 38 patients with aneurysms or AVMs that bled before delivery, 5 mothers died undelivered at under 29 weeks' gestation, 15 delivered vaginally, and 18 delivered by cesarean section. Maternal outcome in terms of death or severe neurologic disability was identical in the vaginal and cesarean groups, as was neonatal outcome. In a retrospective analysis of the 18 delivered by cesarean section, the author concluded that "in only two cases did there appear to have been a genuine indication for this form of delivery."

Since cesarean delivery has the potential for more rapid hemodynamic changes and more coughing, vomiting, and straining in the postoperative period, it probably is much more stressful than a well-conducted vaginal delivery. The Valsalva maneuver should be avoided in patients with an aneurysm or AVM, for although the intracranial transvessel pressure gradient is unchanged during straining, when the strain is released there is a sudden increase in cardiac output, arterial pressure, and blood flow, which could cause intracranial hemorrhage. Low forceps delivery is indicated in these patients. For the most part, cesarean delivery should be reserved for cases with the usual obstetric indications. Even patients who are stabilized but not yet surgically treated can be safely delivered vaginally. However, for the rare patient who suffers a hemorrhagic stroke during labor, cesarean delivery may be life saving for the baby.

Occlusive Stroke

It has long been taught that most occlusive strokes associated with pregnancy are venous (sagittal sinus, cortical veins), but more recent series demonstrate that arterial occlusions are more common. Most venous occlusions do occur in association with pregnancy, the puerperium, or use of oral contraceptives, but arterial occlusive strokes are more common in pregnancy than are venous occlusions.

Cerebral arterial occlusions may be the result of thrombosis, embolism, or vasculitis. The differential diagnosis is listed below:

Thrombosis
Idiopathic (atheromatous)
Thrombotic thrombocytopenic purpura
Sickle hemoglobinopathy

Embolism
Atrial fibrillation
Mitral stenosis
Peripartum cardiomyopathy
Mitral valve prolapse (?)
Subacute bacterial endocarditis
Parodoxical embolus
Choriocarcinoma

Vasculitis
Systemic lupus erythematosus

Atheromatous plaques are most commonly found in patients experiencing cerebral arterial occlusions during pregnancy. The vessels most commonly involved are the middle cerebral artery (35%) and the internal carotid (20%). Vertebrobasilar occlusions are rare during pregnancy. The most characteristic presenting symptom of an arterial occlusive stroke is the sudden onset of motor and sensory deficit (see Table 30-3). Headaches, seizures, and vomiting may occur but are not typical. The occurrence of arterial occlusions seems evenly distributed throughout pregnancy and the first week of the puerperium.

The workup and management is decided on neurologic grounds and usually begins with a lumbar puncture, which should reveal no red cells in the CSF. CT scans and arteriography are usually indicated as well. Although surgical intervention (thrombectomy) or anticoagulation may be indicated in highly selected cases, the usual course is conservative management. This consists of supportive care, anticonvulsants, and high-dose steroids to combat cerebral edema. Maternal mortality is about 30%; another third of patients survive with severe disability, and the last third recover completely.

Cerebral vein thrombosis in pregnancy may involve either the cortical veins (this is most common) or the sagittal sinus. Although headache is a common prodrome, the onset of seizures, which may be focal or generalized, is usually the first sign. Coma and paralysis usually ensue. Recurrence of seizures implies spreading of the thrombus. Fever is a common finding and in the absence of other signs does not indicate infection. There may be blood in the CSF because of the rupture of numerous small vessels draining into the obstructed vein. Therefore, cerebral vein thrombosis is often confused with subarachnoid hemorrhage, and CT and arteriography are necessary to establish the diagnosis.

Cerebral vein thrombosis is rare during pregnancy; it most often occurs one to four weeks after delivery. Treatment consists of supportive care and administration of anticonvulsants and agents to combat cerebral edema. The use of anticoagulants is generally contraindicated, since these agents may promote hemorrhage from areas of infarcted brain. The use of antihypertensive drugs is also generally inadvisable, since the rise in systemic blood pressure seen after venous thrombosis is probably a compensatory mechanism to maintain cerebral blood flow.

Maternal mortality with cerebral vein thrombosis is higher than with arterial occlusion, being reported as 30% to 50%. However, patients who survive usually have less residual disability than patients with arterial stroke. In Amias' series 55% of patients recovered without residual damage and 45% died.

Brain Tumors (Excluding Pituitary Tumors)

The coexistence of brain tumors and pregnancy seems to be coincidental. Every category of tumor has been reported in pregnancy, but none with greater frequency than in the general population. There is evidence that all brain tumors enlarge during pregnancy, especially in the last half of gestation. This is probably due to fluid retention in the tumor. Any tumor may demonstrate remission after delivery, and small acoustic neuromas and meningiomas may be symptomatic only during late pregnancy. Therefore, signs and symptoms that appear during pregnancy warrant immediate neurologic evaluation. The most common symptoms are unilateral scotomata and oculomotor defects.

Benign Intracranial Hypertension (Pseudotumor Cerebri)

Patients with pseudotumor cerebri universally have headaches as an initial symptom, and about 10% of patients also have blurred vision or diplopia. Such complaints are common in pregnant women but should be investigated by an ophthalmoscopic exam. Papilledema, which suggests pseudotumor, is an indication for performance of a CT scan to rule out the presence of space-occupying lesions; a lumbar puncture should also be performed. If the opening pressure is elevated and the CSF composition normal, the diagnosis is established.

Eighty percent of patients with pseudotumor cerebri are women of reproductive age, and 90% are obese. When it complicates pregnancy, pseudotumor usually has its onset between 12 and 20 weeks' gestation. Symptoms may abate in one to two months, although intracranial pressure remains elevated. Remission usually occurs after delivery, but the disease recurs in subsequent pregnancies in 5% to 10% of patients.

Although pseudotumor cerebri is usually self limited, treatment is necessary to prevent permanent visual damage. In pregnancy the best therapy is repeated lumbar punctures to reduce intracranial pressure combined with glucocorticoid therapy if necessary. Weight reduction and diuretic therapy are often helpful in nonpreg-

nant persons but should be avoided during pregnancy because of adverse fetal consequences.

There are no special recommendations for the management of labor and delivery in patients with this condition, although shortening of the second stage with low forceps seems reasonable.

Headache

Muscle contraction or tension headaches occur with the same frequency during pregnancy as in the nonpregnant state. Many pregnant women suffer unnecessarily from headaches because of an unwarranted fear of simple analgesics. Aspirin in usual doses is clearly not teratogenic in humans and can safely be taken for relief of headaches up until 36 weeks' gestation (earlier if the patient has a past history of premature labor or threatened premature labor). However, because maternal aspirin intake does alter coagulation indices in the newborn, it should be avoided when there is the possibility of labor within one week. Acetaminophen has not been shown to be more or less safe than aspirin in terms of teratogenicity; however, it does not have aspirin's problem of being associated with neonatal coagulation alterations.

Classic migraine is mainly a disease of women of reproductive age, but most patients experience relief during pregnancy. Up to 30% of migraine victims are completely asymptomatic during pregnancy, and another 50% have fewer and less severe attacks. Unfortunately, about 20% of patients fail to improve, worsen, or have the onset of migraine headaches during pregnancy.

The usual treatment of migraine, ergot alkaloids, should be avoided during pregnancy because some of them cause intense uterine contractions. Orally administered ergotamine tartrate has no oxytocic effect. Ergonovine maleate, also known as ergometrine maleate and sold under the brand name Ergotrate, does have considerable oxytocic activity. Since ergotamine and Ergotrate can easily be confused because of the similarity of their names, the safest course during pregnancy is simply to avoid this class of drugs. Migraine headaches that occur during pregnancy should be managed with analgesics and sedatives. Avoidance of precipitating factors in the diet, such as red wine, strong cheese, chicken livers, and monosodium glutamate, is recommended.

Multiple Sclerosis

Multiple sclerosis has no apparent effect on pregnancy. The incidence of all pregnancy complications and the duration of labor are the same in patients with multiple sclerosis as in the general population. No changes in the management of labor and delivery are necessary, although most anesthesiologists are reluctant to use conduction anesthesia in these patients for medicolegal reasons.

If pregnancy has an effect on multiple sclerosis, it is small. Some studies demonstrate no increase in the relapse rate during pregnancy and the puerperium, but others report it at 50% to 100%. Interestingly, most relapses occur in the first three months of the puerperium, and it has been postulated that fatigue from caring for a new baby may be the most important inciting factor.

Seizure Disorders

The incidence of seizure disorders among pregnant women is 0.3% to 0.5%. During pregnancy, 45% to 50% of patients experience an increase in seizure frequency, perhaps owing to decreased plasma anticonvulsant levels resulting from expanding plasma volume, enhanced hepatic metabolism, and increased renal clearance. Such an increase in seizure frequency usually begins by the end of the first trimester. Interestingly, 45% to 50% of epileptic women experience no change in seizure frequency during pregnancy, and approximately 5% have a decrease in frequency. Knight and Rhind reported that increased seizure frequency during pregnancy is seen in most women who before pregnancy experienced one or more seizures a month but in only about one fourth of women whose prepregnancy seizure frequency was less than one in nine months.

Maternal seizure disorders do not increase the risk of spontaneous abortion, premature delivery, intrauterine growth retardation, or multiple gestation. The incidence of toxemia is the same among epileptics as among control subjects, but seizures during the last weeks of pregnancy or during labor are a special problem in epileptic patients, for one must decide whether they are due to epilepsy or eclampsia. As a rule, diastolic blood pressure is rarely above 95 mm Hg after an epileptic seizure, whereas it is often much higher in eclampsia. Therapy with parenteral magnesium sulfate seems prudent until the diagnosis is clear.

Of major concern is the effect of maternal epilepsy and its treatment on the fetus and newborn. Epileptic women often ask about the risk of their offspring's having seizure disorders. There appears empirically to be a fourfold increase in risk to about 2%. The risk of congenital malformations in the offspring of treated epileptics (6–10%) is two- to threefold higher than in the offspring of normal subjects (3%). The most frequently encountered anomalies are those of midline closure–orofacial clefts (1.5% risk) and cardiac septal defects (2% risk). There does not appear to be an increased risk among the offspring of untreated epileptics, a fact that would seem to implicate anticonvulsant drugs. However, there are very few untreated epileptics, and women who are so classified probably have had no seizures for a long period of time. Therefore, whether the risk is en-

tirely due to drugs, or whether it is also related to seizure frequency and severity of disease, is not entirely clear.

A fetal hydantoin syndrome has been described that is characterized by hypoplasia of the distal phalanges, rudimentary nails, growth deficiency, mental retardation, and characteristic facies. The incidence of this syndrome is about 5% to 10% among the offspring of hydantoin-treated women. A second disorder associated with maternal anticonvulsant therapy is the fetal trimethadione (Tridione) syndrome, a constellation of developmental delay, growth retardation, V-shaped eyebrows, low-set ears, irregular teeth, speech disturbances, ocular defects, and microcephaly; it has been firmly established that this syndrome is caused by maternal trimethadione intake, so this drug should be avoided during pregnancy. No specific malformation syndromes have been associated with the use of primidone (Mysoline) or carbamazepine (Tegretol) during pregnancy. There are some reports that maternal therapy with valproic acid may increase the risk of orofacial cleft more than therapy with other drugs, but this observation remains to be confirmed.

The neonates of women treated with hydantoin or phenobarbital may be deficient in vitamin K–dependent clotting factors despite normal maternal levels. This is prevented by the routine administration of 1 mg phytonadione (vitamin K) to the newborn shortly after birth. Prophylactic administration of vitamin K to the mother in late pregnancy is neither necessary nor helpful.

The anticonvulsant management of the pregnant epileptic consists of administration of the fewest drugs at the lowest effective dose. A patient who has never been tried on phenobarbital and whose disease theoretically should be controlled with it should be switched to that agent with the consent of her neurologist. Patients who need hydantoin for control of their seizures should be treated with the lowest effective dose. Measurement of serum hydantoin levels is helpful in the management of patients who are experiencing an increase in seizure frequency; serum levels may fall during pregnancy in women on a constant hydantoin dose. However, lowered serum levels should not be taken as an indication to increase the hydantoin dosage in a patient who is free of seizures. In women who are taking hydantoin for trivial or nonexistent indications, the drug should be stopped during pregnancy after consultation with a neurologist. Use of anticonvulsants by pregnant epileptics should not be routinely discontinued, however, because the hypoxia associated with repeated maternal seizures may damage the fetus at any stage of gestation.

Hydantoin therapy causes malabsorption of folate from the gut, so women treated with this agent often have low serum folate levels. Interestingly, during pregnancy, if hydantoin levels drop, serum folate levels may rise. Pregnant women taking hydantoin should usually receive folic acid supplementation of 1 mg per day. Larger supplements do not reduce the risk of fetal malformation and may make seizure control more difficult. In fact, increasing seizure frequency despite larger doses of hydantoin may be a reason to discontinue folate supplementation.

PERIPHERAL NERVOUS SYSTEM

Bell's Palsy

The incidence of idiopathic facial paralysis due to compression of the facial nerve in the temporal bone may be increased during pregnancy. Adour reported a threefold increase in the incidence of Bell's palsy from 0.017% in nonpregnant women of reproductive age to 0.057% in pregnant women and women in the early puerperium. The increased incidence did not seem to be related to parity or to the presence of preeclampsia.

If treatment is begun within a week of the onset of symptoms, a 10-day course of prednisone, 40 mg to 60 mg per day, increases the chance of complete recovery. This regimen is also acceptable during pregnancy. Surgical decompression of the facial nerve is not helpful.

Carpal Tunnel Syndrome

Compression of the median nerve by the flexor retinaculum in the wrist is more common in pregnant than in nonpregnant women, probably because of fluid retention in the involved tissues. The principal symptoms are numbness, tingling, and especially pain in the lateral two thirds of the hand (thumb, index and middle fingers, and lateral aspect of the ring finger). Percussion over the wrist may cause pain (Tinel's sign). Nerve conduction velocity across the wrist is slowed. Often only the dominant hand is involved.

Initial treatment consists of splinting of the wrists at night, with a plastic splint on the dorsum of the wrist holding the hand in a neutral or slightly flexed position. If symptoms persist, the patient should be advised to discontinue activities that involve heavy use of the wrist and hand, such as typing. If symptoms remain, injection of glucocorticoids into the carpal tunnel usually provides relief. Injection may need to be repeated weekly for three to four weeks. Surgical division of the carpal tunnel is curative but rarely necessary in pregnancy, since nearly all patients recover completely after delivery.

Meralgia Paresthetica

Meralgia paresthetica consists of pain, numbness, and tingling in the middle third of the lateral thigh. It is caused by compression of the lateral femoral cutaneous nerve by the inguinal ligament. It may appear in the third trimester owing to increased lumbar lordosis, which stretches the nerve and makes it more vulnerable to compression. The symptoms may be bilateral or uni-

lateral and disappear after delivery. Usually reassurance is the only therapy necessary.

NEUROMUSCULAR DISEASE

Myasthenia Gravis

Myasthenia gravis is an autoimmune disease characterized by the presence of high titers of IgG antibodies against acetylcholine receptors in striated muscle (anti-AChR). There may be an alteration of cell mediated immunity as well. In any event, there is a reduction of over 70% in available ACh receptor sites in striated muscle, leading to weakness. The most prominent symptoms often are due to weakness of muscles innervated by the cranial nerves, and visual symptoms and difficulty with speech and swallowing are common. There may also be weakness of the limbs and the muscles of respiration; repetitive actions lead to progressive weakness. Women account for 55% to 70% of cases, and the peak incidence in women occurs between 21 and 30 years of age, so it is a disease of reproductive-age women.

Accepted therapeutic modalities include anticholinesterase drugs, glucocorticoids, and thymectomy. Less well proven treatments include immunosuppressive drugs (*e.g.* azathioprine) and plasmapheresis. Thymectomy, immunosuppressives, and plasmapheresis should be avoided in pregnancy. The choice between anticholinesterase drugs and glucocorticoids should be made by the patient's neurologist, according to what has been most effective for her in the nonpregnant state. Steroids are not contraindicated; there is no evidence that they cause malformations in humans.

The most frequently used anticholinesterase drugs are pyridostigmine (Mestinon) and neostigmine (Prostigmin). Both are quaternary ammonium compounds that delay the degradation of acetylcholine at the motor end plate; because they are quaternary ions they cross the placenta minimally. Equivalent oral doses are pyridostigmine 60 mg and neostigmine 15 mg. Both drugs are available in parenteral forms, and for each the intramuscular dose is one tenth the oral dose and the intravenous dose one thirtieth the oral. Excessive doses of either may cause cholinergic crises, with muscle weakness that is difficult to differentiate from myasthenic crises due to inadequate doses.

The effect of pregnancy on myasthenia is variable. Plauché (1979) reviewed 292 pregnancies in 202 myasthenic women and reported that remission occurred in 30% of pregnancies, exacerbation in 40%, and no change in 35%. Unfortunately, outcome in individual cases cannot be predicted by past pregnancy history, since the course of myasthenia may vary greatly in different pregnancies in the same patient. About 30% to 40% of patients will have an exacerbation of some degree in the puerperium. Among Plauché's 202 cases there were 9 maternal deaths (4.4%), at least 8 of which were attributed to myasthenia gravis. Aspiration is the leading cause of death.

The effect of myasthenia on pregnancy is small. There is no increased risk of abortion or premature labor, nor is there an increase in uterine inertia or dysfunctional labor, since the smooth muscle of the myometrium is unaffected by the disease. The response to oxytocin is normal. Cesarean delivery is indicated only for the usual obstetric reasons.

The most important aspects of the antepartum care of these patients are extra bed rest, early recognition and treatment of infections of all types, and alertness for exacerbation. The drug regimen should be determined in consultation with a neurologist.

During labor, the patient's drug regimen should be continued by a parenteral route. If she has been on steroids, increased doses will be necessary during labor, because of maternal adrenal suppression. An increase in the dose of anticholinesterase drugs may or may not be necessary. Low forceps should be used to shorten the second stage of labor. Regional anesthesia is preferred, although only amide agents such as lidocaine or bupivacaine (Marcaine) should be used if the patient is being treated with anticholinesterases. Local anesthetics that are esters, such as tetracaine (Pontocaine), procaine (Novocain), and chloroprocaine (Nesacain) are metabolized by cholinesterase, and toxic reactions have been reported in patients taking anticholinesterase drugs. Other drugs to be avoided include curare and other nondepolarizing muscle relaxants, ether, chloroform, Fluothane, aminoglycoside antibiotics, quinine, and quinidine. Special mention must be made of magnesium sulfate, since it diminishes the action and the amount of acetylcholine at the motor end plate and thus may precipitate a myasthenic crisis. Such crises will not respond to calcium therapy, but should respond to edrophonium (Tensilon). Thus, myasthenia gravis represents the one circumstance in which use of magnesium sulfate should be avoided in the management of preeclampsia.

The IgG anti-AChR crosses the placenta, and 12% to 20% of the offspring of myasthenic mothers will develop neonatal myasthenia gravis, a transient condition characterized by mild to severe muscle weakness. Of those neonates destined to be involved, 80% become symptomatic in the first 24 hours of life, and all will have symptoms by 4 days. These symptoms may persist for 2 to 4 weeks and usually require therapy with anticholinesterase drugs.

Myotonic Dystrophy

Myotonic dystrophy is an autosomal dominant disease characterized by weakness and wasting of the muscles of the face, neck, and distal limbs, and myotonia of the hands and tongue. There is marked variation in the age of onset and clinical severity, and many times the diagnosis is not recognized in the mother until the birth of an affected child prompts a more thorough search. There is no effective treatment for the muscle weakness (dystrophy), although the myotonia may be treated with diphenylhydantoin, quinine, or procainamide.

Pregnancy may cause increased weakness or myotonia, especially after 28 weeks of gestation, although in some patients these symptoms remain constant rather than increase. Prolonged bed rest will cause further muscle weakness and should be avoided if possible.

There appears to be an increased risk of spontaneous abortion associated with this disease. The incidence of premature labor is certainly increased, probably due to the associated polyhydramnios (see below). The first stage of labor is usually normal in length, and in these patients the uterus responds normally to oxytocin. Due to voluntary muscle weakness the second stage may be prolonged, and outlet forceps delivery is recommended. Regional anesthesia is recommended. If general anesthesia is required, depolarizing muscle relaxants (e.g., succinylcholine) should be avoided, since they may cause severe muscle spasms and hyperthermia. Nondepolarizing agents (e.g., d-tubocurarine, gallamine, pancuronium) may be used safely, although the dose may need to be reduced.

From an obstetric perspective, the most important aspect of the disease is congenital myotonic dystrophy. Affected infants lack myotonia but have marked muscle weakness, feed poorly, have respiratory difficulty, and often have arthrogryposis. The condition begins *in utero* and since these fetuses do not swallow properly, polyhydramnios often results. Neonatal myotonic dystrophy apparently is due to the interaction of the myotonic dystrophy gene carried by the fetus with some humoral factor transported across the placenta from an affected mother, for it only occurs in infants who inherit the gene from an affected mother. Infants who inherit the gene from an affected father (a less common event because testicular atrophy is part of the disease) are at risk for the disease later in life, but do not exhibit polyhydramnios *in utero* or weakness in the early neonatal period.

There is close linkage between the myotonic dystrophy and secretor genes. Therefore, by testing parents, siblings, and children, matings can be identified where prenatal diagnosis by amniocentesis is possible. This is only true in 20% to 35% of matings, however, and these couples should therefore be evaluated by competent genetic counselors.

REFERENCES AND RECOMMENDED READING

Adour KK, Wingerd J: Idiopathic facial paralysis (Bell's palsy): Factors affecting severity and outcome in 446 patients. Neurology 24:1112, 1974

Amias AG: Cerebral vascular disease in pregnancy. I. Haemorrhage. J Obstet Gynaecol Br Cmwlth 77:100, 1970

Amias AG: Cerebral vascular disease in pregnancy. II. Occlusion. J Obstet Gynaecol Br Cmwlth 77:312, 1970

Copelan EL, Mabon RF: Spontaneous intracranial bleeding in pregnancy. Obstet Gynecol 20:373, 1962

Donaldson JO: Neurology of Pregnancy. Philadelphia, WB Saunders, 1978

Knight AH, Rhind EG: Epilepsy and pregnancy: A study of 153 pregnancies in 59 patients. Epilepsia 16:99, 1975

Nazir MA, Dillon WP, McPherson EW: Myotonic dystrophy in pregnancy. J Reprod Med 29:168, 1984

Plauché WC: Myasthenia gravis in pregnancy: An update. Am J Obstet Gynecol 135:691, 1979

Young DC, Leveno KJ, Whalley PJ: Induced delivery prior to surgery for ruptured cerebral aneurysm. Obstet Gynecol 61:749, 1983

Endocrine and Metabolic Diseases

Dwight P. Cruikshank

THYROID DISEASE

Hyperthyroidism

Hyperthyroidism complicates approximately 1 in 500 pregnancies, an incidence of 0.2%. The vast majority of cases are caused by Grave's disease (toxic diffuse goiter), although cases due to toxic nodular goiter, solitary adenoma, Hashimoto's thyroiditis, and hydatidiform mole have been reported.

Many of the usual signs and symptoms of hyperthyroidism occur in normal pregnancy, including palpitations, heat intolerance, fatigue, skin warmth, and tachycardia. Nonetheless, a resting heart rate of greater than 100 beats per minute, especially if it does not slow during a Valsalva maneuver, is a suggestive sign, as are tremor and failure to gain weight despite increased appetite. The eye signs frequently associated with Grave's disease (exophthalmos, lid lag, globe lag) and pretibial myxedema (infiltrative dermopathy) may or may not be present, and may be present in the absence of hyperthyroidism. The best readily available laboratory evidence of hyperthyroidism during pregnancy is a serum total thyroxine (TT_4) level above the usual pregnancy level. Values above 15 $\mu g/dl$ are suggestive, although exact values vary according to the assay used. The radioactive triiodothyronine (T_3) uptake (RT_3U), usually reduced in normal pregnancy, will be in the euthyroid range in hyperthyroid pregnant women, but because of the pregnancy-associated rise in thyroxine binding globulin (TBG), the free thyroxine index calculated from the TT_4 and RT_3U values is inaccurate during pregnancy. Furthermore, high levels of TBG interfere with all the methods for directly measuring free thyroxine

(FT_4) except the equilibrium dialysis technique, so even direct measurement of FT_4 is inaccurate in diagnosing or following the progress of hyperthyroidism during pregnancy. Thus one is left with the TT_4 level as the best diagnostic test, keeping in mind that normal TT_4 values are higher in pregnancy than in the nonpregnant state. In the rare instance of the patient who is clinically thyrotoxic but has levels of TT_4 that are normal for pregnancy, the possibility of T_3 thyrotoxicosis should be considered.

There are some data to suggest that preexisting hyperthyroidism may be somewhat ameliorated by pregnancy, with recrudescence after delivery. This is thought to be due to alterations in both humoral and cell-mediated immunity during pregnancy; indeed some patients with Grave's disease have been shown to have lower thyroid antibody levels during pregnancy. Nonetheless, many cases of hyperthyroidism appear or are first diagnosed during pregnancy.

The literature is full of conflicting statements about the effect of hyperthyroidism on fertility and pregnancy. It appears that mild to moderate hyperthyroidism does not interfere with fertility. The principal adverse effect of hyperthyroidism on pregnancy is the possibility that labor or delivery will precipitate a life-threatening thyroid storm. Although women with untreated hyperthyroidism may show a slight increase in perinatal mortality and in the incidence of low-birth-weight babies, no increase is seen in treated subjects. The previously reported association between thyrotoxicosis and an increased incidence of preeclampsia is doubtful.

The mainstay of therapy during pregnancy is the thioamide group of drugs, propylthiouracil and methimazole (Tapazol). Because methimazole may be associated with an increased incidence of the scalp lesion aplasia cutis in the offspring, and because propylthiouracil blocks peripheral conversion of T_4 to T_3 in addition to blocking synthesis in the gland, propylthiouracil is the drug of choice. However, patients with intolerable side effects from propylthiouracil may tolerate methimazole quite well, and it should be tried in those circumstances. One milligram of methimazole is equivalent to 10 mg propylthiouracil in terms of thyroid suppression. The pregnant woman diagnosed as hyperthyroid should be started on 300 mg to 450 mg propylthiouracil daily, depending on the severity of the disease. In a few patients, doses of 600 mg per day may be necessary. The drug should be given in doses of 100 mg to 150 mg every 8 hours, and this dose should be maintained for two to three weeks. TT_4 measurements should be obtained every two weeks. Because of the speed at which propylthiouracil has its effect, more frequent laboratory testing is superfluous. If, at the end of two to three weeks, the patient is clinically improved in terms of heart rate, tremor, and weight gain, and if her TT_4 level is falling, the dose should be halved, to 150 mg to 200 mg per day in divided doses. This dose is maintained for two weeks or until the TT_4 level is in the normal pregnancy range, at which time the dose is reduced by 50 mg per day every two weeks to the lowest dose that maintains her in the euthyroid range, usually 50 mg to 100 mg per day. Some have recommended stopping propylthiouracil entirely after the patient has been euthyroid for 4 to 8 weeks, but Mestman (1980) reports that about 70% of patients will relapse when the drug is completely stopped, and recommends this course of action only in those patients with mild symptoms, small goiters, and short duration of disease. If relapse does occur, it is necessary to resume treatment at 300 mg per day and then taper the drug as before. For this reason, I prefer not to stop the drug during pregnancy, but to keep all patients on the lowest dose that maintains clinical and laboratory euthyroidism. It is important to continue measuring TT$_4$ every two weeks, because hypothyroidism must be avoided. Between 1% and 5% of patients taking propylthiouracil will develop a skin rash, pruritus, or nausea. If these symptoms are severe, the patient should be switched to methimazole, since there is little cross-reactivity. Agranulocytosis occurs in 0.3% of patients treated with thioamides and causes death in 1 of 10,000 treated patients. It usually occurs four to eight weeks after initiation of therapy, and the initial symptoms are fever and sore throat. Patients should be advised to stop the drug immediately should these symptoms occur. Periodic white cell counts are not helpful, since agranulocytosis may develop in 24 hours or less. If it does occur, the patient must be isolated and treated with antibiotics and glucocorticoids.

Propranolol is often used in the treatment of nonpregnant patients with hyperthyroidism but should be used sparingly during pregnancy. The patient who is quite toxic may be given propranolol 40 mg every 6 hours for two to three weeks, until her disease is brought under control with thioamides. Iodide therapy is contraindicated except during thyroid storm, because of its propensity for causing fetal hypothyroidism and goiter. Likewise, therapy with radioactive iodine is absolutely contraindicated, because it will cause destruction of the fetal thyroid.

Surgical therapy (subtotal thyroidectomy) is rarely indicated during pregnancy—I have not yet seen a case in which it was necessary. It is indicated only in patients with hypersensitivity to both propylthiouracil and methimazole or in the rare instance when neither drug is effective. If thyroidectomy becomes necessary it should be performed in the second trimester.

Thyroid storm may be triggered by labor, vaginal or cesarean delivery, or infection. It is a life-threatening state marked by fever as high as 41°C (105.8°F), tachycardia, nausea and vomiting, dehydration, prostration and mental confusion. The maternal mortality is 20% to 25%. Therapy of thyroid storm is as follows:

1. Hydration: 5 to 6 liters of intravenous fluid per day
2. Hyperthermia control:
   Cooling blanket
   Alcohol baths
   Aspirin suppositories
3. Propranolol:
   IV, 1.0 mg per minute to maximum of 10 mg
   PO, 40 mg every 6 hours
4. Propylthiouracil:
   PO, 300 mg every 4 to 6 hours for 3 to 5 days, then 150 mg every 6 hours
5. Sodium iodide:
   IV, 1.0 g,
   then PO, SSKI, 5 drops every 8 hours
6. Glucocorticoids:
   IV dexamethasone, 12 mg every 24 hours,
   or
   IV hydrocortisone sodium succinate (Solu-Cortef), 300 mg every 24 hours,
   or
   IV methylprednisolone sodium succinate (Solumedrol), 60 mg every 24 hours

Because of the threat to maternal life, these drugs should be used without regard to possible adverse fetal effects.

About 1% to 5% of fetuses exposed to propylthiouracil develop a goiter and transient neonatal hypothyroidism. This is not strictly dose dependent. Furthermore, the goiters are small and not life threatening, unlike those seen after prolonged maternal iodide therapy. The addition of thyroid hormone to the mother's treatment regimen does not prevent this problem, since the amount of thyroid hormone that crosses the placenta is insignificant. The only effect of giving thyroid hormone to the mother is to increase her requirement for propylthiouracil, and thus the practice has largely been abandoned.

Another possible complication in the offspring of women with Grave's disease is neonatal thyrotoxicosis, which occurs in 1% to 2% of such infants. It is probably due to transfer of thyroid-stimulating immunoglobulins (LATS, LATS-protector) across the placenta. The disease may not become apparent for five to ten days after birth in infants exposed to thioamides *in utero*. It is not a benign condition (mortality rates up to 15% have been reported), and thus these children need careful observation. Although the use of radioactive iodine (^{131}I) in pregnancy is absolutely contraindicated, mention should be made of the management of the patient to whom the drug is given inadvertently. This most commonly occurs when a woman is given a diagnostic dose of ^{131}I for a thyroid uptake and scan before she is found to be pregnant. The patient should be reassured and nothing further need be done, since the amount of ^{131}I administered is too small to be of concern. A greater problem is when a woman is inadvertently given a therapeutic dose of ^{131}I during pregnancy. If the dose is given before eight weeks of gestation, the risk of fetal damage is small, since the fetal thyroid does not begin to trap iodine until the tenth week and most of the drug is cleared from the maternal circulation within two weeks after administration. The offspring of women treated with ^{131}I after eight weeks of gestation, however, will have thyroid ablation with its attendant risks of congenital hypothyroidism and cretinism, and most likely an increased risk of malignancy later in life. These patients should be offered pregnancy termination, but if this is impossible or unacceptable to the patient, consideration should be given to *in utero* treatment of the fetus with thyroid hormone to prevent the stigmata of cretinism. Therapy should be started at 32 weeks of gestation, and the calculated intrafetal dose necessary is 500 μg every two weeks thereafter. This dose requires injections of large volumes of drugs into the fetus, which may be technically difficult. Since the fetus swallows amniotic fluid, a simpler therapeutic approach may be injection of 500 μg of thyroxine into the amniotic fluid weekly after 32 weeks.

Hypothyroidism

Myxedema is a rare complication of pregnancy, only about 50 cases having been reported. Older studies that suggest increased rates of spontaneous abortion, stillbirth, congenital anomalies, and neonatal developmental delay secondary to maternal hypothyroidism suffer from serious methodologic shortcomings. Most recent reports suggest that maternal hypothyroidism is associated with minimal perinatal morbidity and no increase in perinatal mortality.

Since most cases of hypothyroidism are primary, due either to ablation of the gland by previous therapy or to an intrinsic defect of thyroid hormone production, the most accurate diagnostic indicator is an elevated maternal serum TSH level. In normal pregnancy, TSH levels are the same as in the nonpregnant state.

Patients with hypothyroidism diagnosed during pregnancy should be treated with oral L-thyroxine, beginning with an initial dose of 0.15 mg daily. After three weeks, the TT_4 level should be checked, and the replacement dose adjusted upward until the TT_4 value is in the normal pregnancy range. Adequate replacement can also be judged by finding that the TSH level has fallen into the normal range, although this may not occur until after six to eight weeks of adequate replacement therapy. In most hypothyroid pregnant women, a replacement dose of 0.15 mg to 0.20 mg daily is sufficient, although some patients may require 0.25–0.30 mg.

A more commonly encountered problem concerns pregnant patients who have been taking thyroid hormone replacement for some time prior to pregnancy, often for obscure reasons. Although many of these patients are not hypothyroid, discontinuation of the medication during pregnancy could result in five to six weeks of transient hypothyroidism until their thyroid resumes unsuppressed functioning. The most prudent course in these women is to continue the replacement, increasing the dose if necessary to keep their TT_4 in the normal pregnant range, and then to stop the drug after the puerperium.

Thyroid Nodules

Thyroid nodules are no more common during pregnancy than in the nonpregnant state, but the medical attention received by pregnant women may increase the chances of discovery at that time. Likewise, thyroid carcinoma is no more or less common during pregnancy, and pregnancy does not influence the course of thyroid cancer.

The solitary thyroid nodule discovered during pregnancy should be evaluated by ultrasound. If it is cystic, the cyst should be aspirated and the fluid sent for cytologic examination. If solid, fine-needle biopsy should be performed. In either case, if the microscopic examination suggests malignancy, surgery is indicated despite the pregnancy. Thyroid cancer is not an indication for pregnancy termination. If the microscopic examination of the aspirate or fine-needle biopsy is benign, the patient's thyroid function should be suppressed with 0.2 mg L-thyroxine daily until after delivery, when further evaluation, including radioactive iodine scanning and uptake, can be performed.

Goiter

The thyroid gland normally enlarges by 30% to 50% during pregnancy. The patient with a greater degree of diffuse thyroid enlargement (simple goiter), or with a multinodular goiter, should be evaluated with thyroid function tests, including an assessment of TSH level, to rule out primary hypothyroidism.

The patients with a euthyroid goiter should be treated with suppressive doses of L-thyroxine, 0.15 mg to 0.20 mg daily, to prevent further growth of the goiter. Only 30% to 50% will regress in size. The patient with a goiter due to primary hypothyroidism should be treated as outlined above.

PARATHYROID DISEASE

Hyperparathyroidism

Hyperparathyroidism is more common in women than in men. Approximately 60% to 80% of cases diagnosed during pregnancy are caused by a solitary parathyroid adenoma, most of the remainder being due to diffuse hyperplasia of all four parathyroids.

Many patients with hyperparathyroidism are asymptomatic, although fatigue, muscle weakness, and a variety of nonspecific aches and pains are common symptoms. Patients with longstanding disease may have polydipsia and polyuria secondary to hypercalcemia, as well as signs and symptoms secondary to nephrocalcinosis or ureterolithiasis. In addition, nausea and vomiting may be more pronounced in pregnant women with hyperparathyroidism. Hypertension is present in 5% to 10% of patients.

The diagnosis of hyperparathyroidism rests on the finding of hypercalcemia. While 90% of pregnant patients with the disease will have a serum total calcium concentration of greater than 12.0 mg/dl, the reported range varies from 9.5 mg/dl to 20.6 mg/dl. It is important to remember that the normal pregnant woman has a serum total calcium concentration lower than a nonpregnant subject because of reduced serum albumin concentration, and serum total calcium levels persistently above 10 mg/dl are suggestive of hypercalcemia and should lead to further work-up. Serum ionized calcium levels in normal pregnancy are identical to nonpregnant values. Therefore, in patients with persistently elevated total calcium levels, an ionized calcium should be obtained; an elevated value is very suggestive of hyperparathyroidism, although other causes of hypercalcemia must be considered.

The causes of hypercalcemia, in order of frequency are as follows

Primary hyperparathyroidism
Malignancy with bone metastases
Use of thiazide diuretics
Thyrotoxicosis
Sarcoidosis
Multiple myeloma
Vitamin D intoxication
Milk-alkali syndrome
Prolonged immobilization
Familial hypocalcuric hypercalcemia

Radiographic examination of the hands may reveal subperiosteal bone resorption in patients with hyperparathyroidism. Serum parathyroid hormone (PTH) levels will be elevated, but it must be remembered that PTH levels rise in normal pregnancy beginning at about 20 weeks, and by term are 33% to 50% higher than in the nonpregnant state.

Hyperparathyroidism has a very deleterious effect on pregnancy. In most series, the perinatal mortality rate is 25% to 30%, with half the losses being stillbirths. The incidence of premature labor is as high as 20%. Between 15% and 50% of the offspring of these women develop neonatal tetany due to fetal parathyroid suppression secondary to *in utero* hypercalcemia.

Because of the poor perinatal outcome when disease is left untreated, surgical treatment is indicated during pregnancy. In the immediate postoperative period, severe maternal hypocalcemia may occur, which may require therapy with intravenous calcium gluconate.

The patient with preeclampsia and undiagnosed hyperparathyroidism may present a special problem. This author has treated one woman with severe preeclampsia who developed seizures despite treatment with intravenous magnesium sulfate in doses of 4 g to 5 g per hour. In retrospect it appeared that her greatly elevated serum calcium levels were effectively neutralizing the therapeutic effect of magnesium.

Hypoparathyroidism

Hypoparathyroidism usually is iatrogenic, due to intentional or inadvertent removal of the parathyroids. Patients demonstrate hypocalcemia and its associated signs and symptoms, such as numbness and tingling, weakness, tetany, carpopedal spasm, and mental aberrations.

Untreated hypoparathyroidism in pregnancy leads to fetal and neonatal hyperparathyroidism, but treated patients appear to have no increase in incidence of ad-

verse pregnancy outcome. Therapy is much the same as in nonpregnant subjects, consisting of daily supplementation with 50,000 IU to 150,000 IU of vitamin D, and 2.0 g elemental calcium (equivalent to 24 g calcium gluconate or 8.0 g calcium lactate). Salle and co-workers have reported successful treatment during pregnancy with daily doses of calcitriol (1,25-dihydroxy-vitamin D_3) 0.5–2.0 mcg and calcium 1.0 g.

ADRENAL DISEASE

Cushing's Syndrome

The association of Cushing's syndrome and pregnancy is rare, since most patients with the syndrome are anovulatory. Of those cases that do occur during pregnancy, however, a disproportionate number are due to adrenal adenomas or carcinomas. In the nonpregnant population, 70% of cases are caused by adrenal hyperplasia secondary to excessive pituitary ACTH production (Cushing's disease), 20% are due to adrenal neoplasms, and 10% to ectopic ACTH production. However, Kreines and DuVaux reported adrenal adenomas in seven of ten pregnant patients with Cushing's syndrome.

The diagnosis of Cushing's syndrome in pregnancy is difficult, since many of the usual signs and symptoms including weight gain, edema, striae, weakness, hypertension, and glucose intolerance may be caused by pregnancy or its common complications. Easy bruisability, acne, and increasing hirsutism do not usually accompany normal pregnancy, but are common in Cushing's syndrome. Furthermore, many of the usual laboratory tests for Cushing's syndrome are invalidated by pregnancy. Normal pregnancy is associated with elevated total and free cortisol levels, diminished diurnal variation in plasma cortisol levels, failure of cortisol levels to suppress with the overnight 1.0 mg dexamethasone suppression test, and elevated urinary free cortisol levels. In fact, the diagnosis of Cushing's syndrome in pregnancy can only be made with a full dexamethasone suppression test. In this test, plasma cortisol is measured after administration of dexamethasone 0.5 mg every 6 hours for 48 hours ("low-dose test") and again after administration of 2.0 mg every 6 hours for 48 hours ("high-dose test"). The cortisol levels of normal pregnant women will be suppressed with the low-dose test, whereas high cortisol levels due to pituitary-dependent adrenal hyperplasia will be suppressed only with the high-dose test and high cortisol levels that are due to adrenal neoplasms will not be suppressed with either test.

Cushing's syndrome in pregnancy is associated with high perinatal morbidity and mortality. In the small series of Kreines and DeVaux, 25% of pregnancies ended in spontaneous abortion, 25% in stillbirth, and 50% in premature live birth. The associated maternal hypertension and carbohydrate intolerance both impart added risks to the fetus and neonate. For this reason, Burrow states that all cases of Cushing's syndrome diagnosed during pregnancy should be treated surgically, those due to adrenal hyperplasia with transsphenoidal hypophysectomy and those due to adrenal neoplasms with adrenalectomy. On the other hand, Mestman recommends surgical treatment in pregnancy only for primary adrenal disease. If one adopts this philosophy, untreated patients will need intensive treatment to control maternal blood pressure and blood sugar levels, as well as antepartum fetal surveillance with serial ultrasound examinations and heart rate testing, coupled with delivery as soon as fetal pulmonary maturity can be documented.

The only pregnant patient with Cushing's syndrome managed by this author died in the antepartum period from hemorrhage during attempted resection of an adrenal carcinoma.

Addison's Disease

Chronic adrenocortical insufficiency is characterized by weakness, fatigue, weight loss, low blood pressure (especially postural hypotension), nausea, vomiting, anorexia, diarrhea, fasting hypoglycemia, and increased skin pigmentation. Since many of these are present in normal pregnant women, making the diagnosis during pregnancy can be difficult. Weight loss and persistent nausea and vomiting should alert the physician, but the diagnosis can only be definitively made by demonstrating a failure of cortisol levels to rise after ACTH infusion. In fact, some patients with undiagnosed Addison's disease tolerate pregnancy remarkably well without therapy, only to develop Addisonian crises due to the stress of labor or the effect of the diuresis that occurs in the puerperium.

Patients with previously diagnosed Addison's disease usually can be maintained on the same dose of glucocorticoid replacement during pregnancy as they required in the nonpregnant state. In most cases a daily dose of 37.5 mg cortisone acetate or 7.5 mg prednisone is sufficient, with two thirds of the dose being given in the morning and one third in the evening. During labor and the immediate puerperium, these patients should receive supplemental glucocorticoids, such as hydrocortisone sodium succinate (Solu-Cortef) 100 mg intravenously every 6 hours. These patients also require mineralocorticoid replacement in the form of fludrocortisone 0.05 mg to 0.10 mg daily. The dose of mineralocorticoid may need to be increased during pregnancy to compensate for the sodium-losing effects of progesterone.

Pregnancy in patients with treated Addison's disease usually has a normal perinatal outcome. There does not appear to be an increased incidence of spontaneous abortion, stillbirth, or preterm labor. The offspring of these women rarely demonstrate any transient adrenal insufficiency, but it seems reasonable to monitor their blood sugar closely during the first hours of life.

Pheochromocytoma

Pheochromocytoma is a rare complication of pregnancy—fewer than 100 cases have been reported in the English-language literature—but its consequences for both mother and fetus can be disastrous. Schenker and Chowers reviewed 89 cases and found a maternal mortality of 48% and a perinatal mortality of 54%.

Ninety percent of these tumors arise in the adrenals; 10% to 15% are bilateral, and 10% are malignant. Hypertension is the most common symptom, occurring in 80% to 90% of patients. It may be sustained or paroxysmal. In Schenker and Chower's series, 67 of 89 cases were misdiagnosed during pregnancy and of these, 43% were diagnosed as preeclampsia/eclampsia and 16% as chronic hypertension. Other signs and symptoms include headaches, palpitations, sweating, nervousness, weakness, tremor, weight loss, and glycosuria. Therefore, marked or paroxysmal hypertension in a patient whose other symptoms suggest hyperthyroidism should alert one to the possibility of pheochromocytoma. The differential diagnosis between this disease and preeclampsia can be quite difficult, especially in those 16% of patients with pheochromocytoma who also have proteinuria. Most disconcerting, in 17 reported cases, there was remission of symptoms and signs between pregnancies, with the manifestations of the disease becoming progressively more severe in each pregnancy. Facts such as these have led Schenker and Chowers to state that "laboratory tests for pheochromocytoma should be performed in every case of hypertension during pregnancy." Although one need not agree with such a universal approach, their recommendation should clearly be heeded in every case of paroxysmal or atypical hypertension in pregnancy, and in all hypermetabolic states unless the thyroid function studies make the diagnosis of hyperthyroidism obvious.

The diagnosis is best made by measurement of 24-hour urinary catecholamines. The normal values for these assays do not change during pregnancy, and are 0–20 μg/24 hr for epinephrine and 10–70 μg/24 hr for norepinephrine. Once the diagnosis has been made, tumor localization is important. The first step in this investigation is abdominal CT scan, which should be done despite the pregnancy. To quote Ferris, "concern about the danger of using x-ray to localize the tumor is inappropriate with this potentially lethal condition." If the tumor cannot be seen by CT scan, vena cava catheterization, venography, and differential adrenal venous sampling for catecholamine levels are indicated. The critical importance of making the diagnosis during pregnancy is emphasized by the fact that maternal mortality is 58% in undiagnosed cases and 17% in diagnosed cases. The perinatal mortality is about 55% in both circumstances. Maternal death is usually due to cerebrovascular accident, cardiac arrhythmia, acute pulmonary edema, or shock.

Once the diagnosis is made, surgical removal of the tumor is indicated, after pretreatment for one to two weeks with α- and β-adrenergic blockers (phenoxybenzamine and propranolol). If the pregnancy is advanced beyond 32 weeks, or if the enlarged uterus precludes surgical approach to the tumor, cesarean delivery should be performed. Vaginal delivery should be avoided in all untreated patients, because of the potential for sudden discharge of catecholamines into the circulation, probably as a result of mechanical compression of the tumor. Among all patients, both diagnosed and undiagnosed, the maternal mortality is 39% following vaginal delivery and 19% following cesarean.

PITUITARY DISEASES

Tumors

Pituitary adenomas are common, being found in 8% to 22% of asymptomatic individuals at autopsy. The chromophobe adenoma is most common, accounting for 80% to 85% of tumors, and commonly secretes prolactin. Eosinophilic adenomas, which may secrete prolactin or growth hormone, account for another 10% to 15% of tumors. These tumors are defined as microadenomas if they are less than 10 mm in diameter and are confined to the sella turcica; all others are considered macroadenomas.

Pituitary adenomas can enlarge rapidly during pregnancy, although the exact incidence of this complication is unknown. Jewelewicz and Van de Wiele followed 25 patients with untreated microadenomas through pregnancy, and none developed neurologic or visual symptoms. Randall and associates followed 34 pregnancies in 25 patients with untreated microadenomas, 6 pregnancies in 5 patients with untreated macroadenomas, and 10 pregnancies in 7 patients with previously treated macroadenomas; in none was there evidence of tumor growth during pregnancy. On the other hand, Magyar and Marshall reported headaches in 23% and visual symptoms in 25% of 73 previously untreated patients with pituitary tumors, and headaches in 4% and visual disturbances in 5% of 73 previously treated women. Of the previously untreated patients, 22 required surgery or radiation therapy during pregnancy or the puerperium because of severe symptoms. In their series, the rates of spontaneous abortion and perinatal mortality were the same as for normal subjects in all groups of patients, whether untreated or treated before or during pregnancy. There is agreement that macroadenomas should be treated before pregnancy is attempted; no such consensus exists regarding microadenomas.

All patients with pituitary tumors, whether treated or untreated, regardless of tumor size, should be seen frequently during gestation and questioned closely about headaches and visual symptoms. Those with untreated microadenomas or previously treated tumors of any size should have formal visual field examinations three times during pregnancy, once in each trimester. Those with untreated macroadenomas should have such examinations monthly. Blood prolactin levels stay elevated and are therefore of no help in managing the pregnancy. Management options for patients who develop visual field defects during pregnancy include hypophysectomy or medical therapy with corticosteroids or bromocriptine. Bromocriptine appears to be the best alternative; although not conclusively proven safe in pregnancy, its use has been evaluated in over 1500 pregnancies and no deleterious effects have been found. Maeda and associates reported successful management of an enlarging macroadenoma in pregnancy with 7.5 mg bromocriptine per day. If bromocriptine therapy becomes necessary, induction of labor as soon as fetal pulmonary maturity can be demonstrated seems prudent, since many of these tumors regress after delivery.

Diabetes Insipidus

The reported incidence of diabetes insipidus in pregnancy ranges between 1 in 16,000 and 1 in 80,000 deliveries. The patient presents with polydipsia and polyuria and a very low urine specific gravity. The diagnosis is made by the water deprivation test, showing low urine osmolality despite increasing serum osmolality and correction of the abnormalities by vasopressin. This test should be performed very cautiously during pregnancy.

Hime and Richardson (1978) reviewed 67 patients and concluded that diabetes insipidus worsened during pregnancy in 58%, perhaps because of increased requirement for antidiuretic hormone (ADH) as a result of the increased glomerular filtration rate, or because of the antagonistic effect of progesterone on ADH. However, 20% of patients improved during pregnancy and 15% were unchanged.

Pregnancy is not adversely affected by the disease, the incidence of spontaneous abortion, premature labor, and stillbirth being the same as in control subjects. The course of labor is usually normal.

Treatment is with intranasal L-deamino-8-d-arginine vasopressin (DDAVP) in doses of 0.1 ml three to four times daily.

METABOLIC DISEASE

Maternal Phenylketonuria (PKU)

Phenylketonuria is an autosomal recessive error of amino acid metabolism. Individuals homozygous for the gene are unable to convert phenylalanine to tyrosine at a normal rate. They therefore have elevated serum phenylalanine levels, which, if untreated, result in mental retardation and seizure disorders. Treatment with a phenylalanine-restricted diet in childhood, however, leads to normal development, and after mental developmental maturity has been achieved, the restricted diet can be abandoned without deleterious effect. Once the diet is abandoned, these patients develop elevated serum phenylalanine levels, and fall into one of three groups: those with phenylalanine levels of 20 mg/dl or more (classic PKU), those with phenylalanine levels between 9 mg/dl and 20 mg/dl (atypical PKU), and those with phenylalanine levels of less than 9 mg/dl (mild hyperphenylalaninemia). If such women become pregnant, their elevated phenylalanine levels cause elevated phenylalanine levels in the fetus and lead to mental retardation, microcephaly, and congenital heart disease, even though the fetus has not inherited the PKU gene.

Two controversies exist regarding pregnancy in such patients. The first concerns the level of phenylalanine in maternal serum that is deleterious to the fetus, and the second is whether maternal dietary phenylalanine restriction during pregnancy can result in the birth of normal offspring.

In a national survey of 490 pregnancies in women with PKU on unrestricted diets, Lenke and Levy found significantly increased frequencies of mental retardation and microcephaly among the offspring of all such women, even those with serum phenylalanine levels of 3 to 10 mg/dl (Table 30-5). The risk correlated with maternal phenylalanine levels, such that among offspring of women with serum phenylalanine of 20 mg/dl or more, the incidence of mental retardation was 92% and of microcephaly 73%. The incidence of congenital heart disease was increased in offspring of women with serum phenylalanine levels greater than 11 mg/dl. However, the authors felt that ascertainment bias may have altered their findings, and therefore Levy and Waisbreu studied 53 offspring of 22 untreated mothers identified by routine cord blood screening. They found that all offspring born to women with serum phenylalanine levels of 20 mg/dl or more were microcephalic and mentally retarded. The offspring of mothers with serum phenylalanine levels of between 9 mg/dl and 20 mg/dl had a mean IQ of 95.2 ± 13.4, but only 1 of 13 was seriously retarded. Of the offspring in this group, 23% were microcephalic at birth, but only one child remained so at long-term follow-up. There were no cases of mental retardation or microcephaly among the offspring of women with serum phenylalanine levels below 9.0 mg/dl, and the mean IQ of these 10 children was 116.6 ± 13.6.

Dietary restriction of phenylalanine during pregnancy has been tried with some success. All such reports must be viewed with some scepticism, since compliance with the unpalatable diet must be quite difficult once one has grown accustomed to regular food. Lenke and

Levy (1980) reported 34 pregnancies managed with a low-phenylalanine diet, in which maternal serum phenylalanine levels were "generally maintained at 4–12 mg/dl, with some values below 1.90 mg/dl and some above 16 mg/dl." There did seem to be improvement in IQ and head circumference when treatment was begun early in gestation, but 4 of 11 infants whose mothers began phenylalanine restriction in the first trimester died of congenital heart disease. In two of three pregnancies in which phenylalanine restriction was begun before conception, the offspring were normal, but in the third, the child had a reduced IQ and head circumference. Michels and Justice reported a case in which maternal dietary restriction was begun at 6 weeks of gestation and serum levels were maintained between 1.7 mg/dl and 10.7 mg/dl; the infant had a congenital heart defect but was otherwise normal. Tenbrinck and Stroud reported a case in which dietary restriction was begun at 9 weeks of gestation; the patient's serum phenylalanine levels were kept between 1.1 mg/dl and 9.1 mg/dl and she delivered a normal infant.

A woman with PKU should be intensively counseled about the risks of abnormal offspring. If she decides to conceive, a phenylalanine-restricted diet should be begun preconceptually or as soon as possible after conception, with a goal of maintaining her serum phenylalanine level below 9.0 mg/dl.

REFERENCES AND RECOMMENDED READING

Burrow GN: Pituitary, adrenal and parathyroid disorders. In Burrow GN, Ferris TF (eds): Medical Complications During Pregnancy, 2nd ed. Philadelphia, WB Saunders, 1982

Hime MC, Richardson JA: Diabetes insipidus and pregnancy. Obstet Gynecol Surv 33:375, 1978

Jewelewicz R, Van de Wiele RL: Clinical course and outcome of pregnancy in twenty-five patients with pituitary microadenomas. Am J Obstet Gynecol 136:339, 1980

Kreines K, DeVaux WD: Neonatal adrenal insufficiency associated with maternal Cushing's syndrome. Pediatrics 47:516, 1971

Lenke RR, Levy HL: Maternal phenylketonuria and hyperphenylalaninemia: An international survey of the outcome of untreated and treated pregnancies. N Engl J Med 303:1202, 1980

Levy HL, Waisbren SE: Effects of untreated maternal phenylketonuria and hyperphenylalaninemia on the fetus. N Engl J Med 309:1269, 1983

Maeda T, Vshiroyama T, Okuda K et al: Effective bromocriptine treatment of a pituitary macroadenoma during pregnancy. Obstet Gynecol 61:117, 1983

Magyar D, Marshall J: Pituitary tumors and pregnancy. Am J Obstet Gynecol 132:739, 1978

Mestman JH: Endocrine disease in pregnancy. In Sciarra JJ (ed): Gynecology and Obstetrics, vol 3. Philadelphia, Harper & Row, 1984

Mestman JH: Management of thyroid diseases in pregnancy. Clin Perinatol 7:371, 1980

Michels VV, Justice CL: Treatment of phenylketonuria during pregnancy. Clin Genet 21:141, 1982

Randall S, Laing I, Chapman AJ et al: Pregnancies in women

Table 30-5
Frequency of Abnormalities in Offspring of Women with Untreated Phenylketonuria

Maternal Phenylalanine Level (mg/dl)	Mental Retardation (Percent)	Microcephaly (Percent)	Congenital Heart Disease (Percent)
≥20	92	73	12
16–19	73	68	15
11–15	22	35	6
3–10	21	24	0

(Adapted from Lenke RR, Levy HL: Maternal phenylketonuria and hyperphenylalaninemia: An international survey of the outcome of untreated and treated pregnancies. N Engl J Med 303:1202, 1980)

with hyperprolactinemia: Obstetric and endocrinologic management of 50 pregnancies in 37 women. Br J Obstet Gynaecol 89:20, 1982

Salle BL, Berthezene F, Glorieux FH et al: Hypoparathyroidism during pregnancy. Treatment with calcitrol. J Clin Endocrinol Metab 52:810, 1981

Schenker JG, Chowers I: Pheochromocytoma and pregnancy: Review of 89 cases. Obstet Gynecol Surv 26:739, 1971

Schenker JG, Granat M: Phaeochromocytoma and pregnancy— an updated appraisal. Aust NZ J Obstet Gynaecol 22:1, 1982

Schreyer P, Caspi E, El-Hindi JM et al: Ceirbosis-pregnancy and delivery: A review. Obstet Gynecol Surv 37:304, 1982

Shangold MM, Dor N, Welt SI et al: Hyperparathyroidism and pregnancy: A review. Obstet Gynecol Surv 37:217, 1982

Tenbrinck MS, Stroud HW: Normal infant born to a mother with phenylketonuria. JAMA 247:2139, 1982

Diseases of the Alimentary Tract

Dwight P. Cruikshank

GASTROINTESTINAL DISEASES

Nausea and Vomiting of Pregnancy

Nausea and vomiting, or "morning sickness," complicate up to 70% of pregnancies. It typically has its onset between 4 and 8 weeks' gestation and continues to about 14 to 16 weeks. Although the symptoms often are quite distressing, the condition seldom leads to evidence of disturbed nutritional status such as weight loss, ketonemia, or electrolyte disturbances. The cause is not well understood, although relaxation of the smooth muscle of the stomach probably plays a role. There is some evidence that elevated levels of steroid hormones and human chorionic gonadotropin (hCG) may be involved. However, there does not appear to be a good correlation between maternal serum hCG levels and degree of nausea and vomiting, either in patients with normal pregnancies or in patients with hydatidiform moles. Interestingly, nonmolar pregnancies complicated by nausea and vomiting often have a more favorable outcome than those without nausea and vomiting.

Treatment is largely supportive, consisting of reassurance and psychologic support. The patient should be counseled to avoid foods that trigger nausea and to eat frequent, small meals. Until June of 1983, the best pharmacologic treatment of "morning sickness" was a combination of doxylamine succinate, 10 mg, and pyridoxine, 10 mg (Bendectin, Merrell Dow). The drug was proven effective, and there was no evidence that it was associated with teratogenicity. Two tablets at bedtime, and one each midmorning and midafternoon, usually provided marked relief. However, owing to legal pressures and the economic burden of product liability insurance, the manufacturer withdrew the drug from the market. In March of 1985, a U.S. District Court jury in Cincinnati, Ohio, found that "Bendectin did not cause the birth defects of children whose mothers took the drug during pregnancy." Now that legal opinion is being reconciled with scientific information, perhaps the drug will again become available. In the meantime, the two components of Bendectin, doxylamine succinate and pyridoxine, both remain available as over-the-counter preparations.

Hyperemesis gravidarum, a more pernicious form of nausea and vomiting associated with weight loss, ketonemia, electrolyte imbalance, dehydration, and possible hepatic and renal damage, often persists throughout pregnancy. In patients with this condition one must rule out underlying diseases such as pyelonephritis, pancreatitis, cholecystitis, and hepatitis. Hospitalization with parenteral replacement of fluids, electrolytes, and calories is often necessary. A continuous low-dose infusion of promethazine (Phenergan) is helpful in this situation. To each liter of intravenous fluid, up to 6 liters a day, 10 mg to 25 mg promethazine is added. Nothing is permitted by mouth, and parenteral therapy is continued for at least 48 hours after all vomiting has ceased to prevent rapid reappearance of symptoms.

Reflux Esophagitis

Reflux esophagitis, or heartburn, complicates up to 25% of pregnancies. The typical symptom is substernal burning, worsened after eating and upon lying down, bending over, or lifting heavy objects. It typically appears at the end of the second month of gestation and is most common and most severe at about 32 weeks.

Reflux esophagitis probably occurs because progesterone reduces lower esophageal sphincter pressure, and when intra-abdominal pressure rises as the uterus enlarges, acid from the stomach refluxes into the lower esophagus.

Therapy consists of use of a bed the head of which is elevated 4 inches, avoidance of food at bedtime, and use of antacids. It may be necessary to use antacids in doses of 30 ml 7 times a day (1 and 3 hours after each meal and at bedtime). Magnesium- and aluminum-containing antacids are all acceptable, but those containing large amounts of sodium (*e.g.,* Alka-Seltzer, Rolaids) probably should be avoided. Although calcium-containing antacids are generally not advised for nonpregnant patients because calcium stimulates acid secretion, they may be useful during pregnancy as a source of calcium supplementation as well as as an antacid. Cimetidine, ranitidine, and metoclopramide are not approved for use in pregnancy and should be avoided until further data about them are available.

Peptic Ulcer Disease

Pregnancy protects against the development of peptic ulcer disease, both gastric and duodenal. Furthermore, women with preexisting peptic ulcer disease usually show marked improvement of the condition when pregnant. Clark reported that 45% of such patients were symtpom free in pregnancy, 43% were much improved, and only 12% were no better or worse. The mechanism of this pregnancy-induced improvement is not clear, since the data on gastric acid secretion in pregnancy are conflicting, but most authors suggest that gastric acid secretion is unchanged from the nonpregnant state. It is known that the delayed gastric emptying characteristic of pregnancy protects against the development of duodenal ulcers. Prostaglandins exert an ill-defined protective effect on the gastric mucosa; the relationship between prostaglandin levels and ulcer disease in pregnancy needs to be studied further.

The treatment of peptic ulcer disease during pregnancy, much the same as that described for reflux esophagitis, centers around antacid therapy and dietary manipulation. Cimetidine and other H2 blockers should be used only as a last resort.

In pregnant patients with intractable symptoms, especially those with upper gastrointestinal bleeding, the diagnostic procedure of choice is panendoscopy. Any visualized ulcer should be biopsied, since there have been several reports of ulcers in pregnancy caused by gastric carcinoma or lymphoma. Radiologic procedures should be avoided, if possible; tests such as gastric analysis and measurement of serum pepsinogen levels should also be avoided, since they have not proven reliable in pregnancy.

Inflammatory Bowel Disease

Ulcerative colitis and Crohn's disease (regional enteritis, granulomatous enterocolitis) frequently affect young adults, so their association with pregnancy is not uncommon.

There are pathologic differences between the two diseases, with ulcerative colitis consisting of ulcer formation in the mucosa and submucosa of the colon and Crohn's disease consisting of transmural ulceration and granuloma formation in any portion of the gastrointestinal tract from mouth to anus. However, many authors consider both entities to be part of the spectrum of a single disease, and since the medical therapies and courses of pregnancy are similar for the two, they will be considered together as inflammatory bowel disease (IBD).

Many widely held views regarding IBD in pregnancy are based on old data and simply are not true. These include the notions that IBD usually worsens during pregnancy, that it poses a serious threat to maternal and fetal life, and that therapeutic abortion should be recommended to patients with the disorder.

There is little evidence that IBD, either quiescent or active, adversely effects the course of pregnancy. Willoughby and Truelove found that live births occurred in 87% of pregnancies in women with quiescent ulcerative colitis, 82% of pregnancies in women with active disease, and 88% of pregnancies in women whose first attacks occurred during pregnancy. The incidences of spontaneous abortion, stillbirth, neonatal death, and congenital anomalies were no different among women with ulcerative colitis than in the general population. Data for Crohn's disease are similar.

Similarly, pregnancy does not seem to have an adverse effect on the course of IBD. The disease is one of relapses and remissions, and although relapses are common in pregnant women and women in the puerperium, they are not more frequent in this group than in nonpregnant female patients of similar age. Willoughby and Truelove found that 30% of patients with quiescent ulcerative colitis had relapses during pregnancy. Among patients with active disease at the time of conception, in 40% the condition improved during pregnancy, in 27% it was unchanged, and in 33% it worsened, either during pregnancy or in the puerperium. According to Sorokin and Levine, the same is true regarding Crohn's disease.

Medical therapy of IBD centers around diet, glucocorticoids, and sulfasalazine (Azulfidine). Glucocorticoids (usually prednisone) should be used for the same indications and in the same doses for pregnant and nonpregnant patients. As previously discussed, fear about adverse effects of prednisone in human pregnancy seems unfounded. Sulfasalazine is split in the gut into 5-aminosalicylic acid and sulfapyridine. Because sulfapyridine crosses the placenta, theoretically it could displace bilirubin from albumin and thereby increase the risk of kernicterus. However, data from Scandinavia and the United States demonstrate that the concentrations of sulfapyridine in the blood of fetuses whose mothers have received usual maternal doses of sulfasalazine are too low to cause significant bilirubin displacement; thus, sulfasalazine can be given without undue risk until delivery.

Complications of IBD are no more common than usual during pregnancy but are more difficult to diagnose and treat. Ultrasound may have some value, but if the physician suspects obstruction or perforation, radiologic examinations are indicated despite pregnancy. Close consultation among obstetrician, gastroenterologist, and surgeon is essential.

Management of labor and delivery in patients with IBD is usually not different from ordinary. However, the patient with Crohn's disease who has perirectal abscesses or fistulas may be a candidate for cesarean section, unless it is obvious that vaginal delivery can be accomplished without lacerations or an episiotomy.

Appendicitis

Appendicitis occurs with the same frequency during pregnancy as in the nonpregnant state, and cases tend to be distributed equally among all three trimesters. The incidence of appendicitis is approximately 1 in 1500 deliveries. Nevertheless, until recently mortality in pregnant women was about 2% overall and 7% in the third trimester, whereas mortality in the general population is 0.1% if no rupture has occurred and 2% to 3% with rupture. Several recent series report no maternal deaths, but the incidence of appendiceal rupture remains significantly higher during pregnancy than in the nonpregnant state.

Appendicitis is not a more rapidly progressive disease during pregnancy; the increase in maternal mortality is due to delay in diagnosis and treatment because pregnancy blunts the signs and symptoms of the disease. This effect is more marked later in pregnancy. Thus, Cunningham and McCubbin found no apparent delay in diagnosis and surgery in patients in the first trimester but an obvious delay in 18% of patients in the second trimester and 75% of patients in the third. As pregnancy progresses, the appendix is usually dislocated from the right lower quadrant. The appendix may be above the iliac crest by 16 weeks' gestation, and by 32 weeks it is above the iliac crest in 90% to 95% of subjects. Therefore, the location of abdominal pain associated with appendicitis in pregnancy is quite variable. As noted in Table 30-6, right lower quadrant pain is felt by all patients with appendicitis in the first trimester but in only 71% of second-trimester patients and 27% of third-trimester patients. The right upper quadrant may be the main site of pain in the second trimester and is the site of greatest pain in the third trimester in nearly half of patients.

As pregnancy advances, the abdominal wall is lifted away from the appendix, so that peritoneal signs such as rebound tenderness, guarding, and rigidity become less frequent; in the third trimester these are present in fewer than half of patients. As the appendix rises in the abdomen, it may come to overlie the ureter, resulting in sterile pyuria and hematuria in 15% to 20% of pregnant women with appendicitis. Anorexia occurs in about 67% of pregnant patients with appendicitis and fever in about 50%. Nausea, with or without vomiting, occurs in most patients; however, since it accompanies many pregnancy-related problems, especially in the first trimester,

Table 30-7
Appendicitis in Pregnancy—Differential Diagnosis According to Trimester

First	*Second*	*Third*
Ectopic pregnancy	Abortion/labor	Labor
Ruptured corpus luteum cyst	Chorioamnionitis	Chorioamnionitis
Round ligament syndrome	Round ligament syndrome	Abruptio placentae
Adnexal torsion	Degenerating myoma	Degenerating myoma
Pyelonephritis	Pyelonephritis	Pyelonephritis

it is not indicative of any particular problem. Leukocytosis with white blood counts of over 10,000 and a leftward shift on the differential are usually present but may also occur in the last two trimesters of normal pregnancies.

The differential diagnosis of appendicitis in pregnancy is given in Table 30-7. It is necessary to maintain a high index of suspicion in all patients with right-sided or generalized abdominal pain, especially those with nausea or anorexia. Laparotomy is indicated if appendicitis is suspected. In pregnant as in nonpregnant patients, however, the appendix will be found to be normal at laparotomy in 33% to 50% of cases. Given that in many cases of erroneous diagnosis the source of the problem is the uterus or its adnexa, most authors agree that the procedure of choice should always begin with a midline incision.

Even if the appendix is grossly normal at laparotomy, it should be removed; microscopic examination of the appendix may reveal inflammation, and its removal will eliminate confusion if the patient's original symptoms recur.

Occasionally the question arises as to whether to perform a cesarean section at the time of laparotomy if the appendicitis occurs near term. Although this does not appear to increase maternal morbidity if appendiceal rupture has not occurred, in general cesarean sections should be done for obstetric reasons only. If the appendix has ruptured, every effort should be made to avoid a cesarean section, since serious uterine infection may result. If cesarean delivery is absolutely necessary under such circumstances, consideration should be given to cesarean hysterectomy. Retention sutures are advised if the woman is undelivered, since labor and pushing could disrupt the wound.

PANCREATITIS

Acute pancreatitis is a rare complication of pregnancy, the reported incidence varying between 1 in 4000 and 1 in 12,000 deliveries. In more than two thirds of cases,

Table 30-6
Pregnancy and Appendicitis—Physical Findings

	Percentage per Trimester		
Finding	*First*	*Second*	*Third*
Direct tenderness			
Right lower quadrant	100	71	27
Right upper quadrant	0	7	47
Generalized	0	10	7
Flank	0	10	7
Rebound tenderness	100	70	47

(After Cunningham FG, McCubbin JH: Appendicitis complication pregnancy. Obstet Gynecol 45:415, 1975; Weingold AB: Appendicitis in pregnancy. Clin Obstet Gynecol 26:801, 1983)

pancreatitis in pregnancy is related to gallstones. This usually consists of a short-lived (24–48 hours) attack resulting from temporary impaction of a stone at the ampulla of Vater. Most other cases of pancreatitis result from ingestion of drugs, the most well known being alcohol. Thiazide diuretics have also been reported to cause pancreatitis and should be avoided during pregnancy.

The diagnosis of pancreatitis should be considered in any patient with right upper quadrant abdominal pain or right flank pain, especially when the pain is associated with nausea and vomiting. The differential diagnosis includes appendicitis, pyelonephritis, and cholecystitis. The diagnosis is established by the finding of elevated serum levels of amylase and lipase, both of which are unchanged in normal pregnancy. However, because both ptyalism and preeclampsia have been associated with elevated serum amylase levels, a high serum level should be corroborated by an elevated 24-hour urinary amylase excretion before the diagnosis is secure. Ultrasound examination may reveal a pancreatic pseudocyst. Since acute hemorrhagic pancreatitis may cause hypocalcemia, serum calcium levels should also be measured.

The mainstays of therapy are fluid replacement, suppression of pancreatic secretion, and pain relief. Since many liters of fluid may be sequestered in the abdomen of a patient with pancreatitis, careful attention to fluid and electrolyte balance is essential. A central venous pressure line or Swan–Ganz catheter may be helpful in this regard. Pancreatic suppression is best obtained by allowing the patient nothing by mouth and using nasogastric suction until she has been pain free for 24 hours. Pain relief is best accomplished with appropriate doses of meperidine (100–125 mg, intramuscularly, every 3–4 hours). Although it has been stated that this drug causes spasm of the sphincter of Oddi, the problem seems more theoretical than real. Antibiotics are reserved for patients with sepsis. Steroid therapy is not useful.

Wilkinson reviewed the literature on pancreatitis complicating pregnancy between 1950 and 1973 and found an overall maternal mortality of 37%. However, the reviewed series included at least 22 patients with "acute fatty liver of pregnancy," the exclusion of which cases reduced maternal mortality to 20%. Pancreatitis is a serious problem at any time, but it is especially so in pregnancy.

CHOLECYSTITIS

The effects of pregnancy on the incidence of gallstone disease is controversial. Clearly, exogenous estrogen administration increases the risk of cholesterol stone formation by decreasing the size of the bile acid pool and increasing the saturation of bile with cholesterol. Whether pregnancy also leads to these changes is controversial, but it is known that pregnancy alters gall-

bladder function. During pregnancy, fasting and residual gallbladder volumes are twice nonpregnant values, and the rate of emptying is markedly reduced. Whether these functional changes increase the risk of cholecystitis is disputed. It can be argued that the sluggish gallbladder serves a protective function by sequestering bile acids in the gallbladder, which leads to less feedback inhibition, increased bile acid synthesis, and large bile acid pool size, which in turn decreases cholesterol saturation of bile acids and makes stone formation less likely. Nonetheless, during pregnancy 3% to 4% of asymptomatic women have been found to have stones.

In any event, symptomatic cholecystitis is not common during pregnancy, cholecystectomy being required in only 1 in 2000 to 1 in 10,000 pregnancies. The usual signs of cholecystitis are intense constant or colicky pain in the midepigastrum, right upper quadrant, or right scapula and shoulder, and nausea and vomiting. Vomiting does not relieve the pain. Jaundice may be present, but only about 5% of jaundice in pregnancy is due to gallbladder disease, most being caused by hepatitis or intrahepatic cholestasis. In gallbladder disease there may also be elevated hepatic enzyme levels and mild leukocytosis.

The differential diagnosis for cholecystitis includes appendicitis, pyelonephritis, hepatitis, peptic ulcer disease (rare), and acute pancreatitis (in pregnancy the latter is usually caused by gallstones in the ampulla of Vater).

Ultrasound of the gallbladder is a useful diagnostic tool. At least in nonpregnant subjects it is accurate in the diagnosis of gallstones in 90% of cases.

The treatment for gallstones in pregnancy is very similar to that described for pancreatitis: ingestion of nothing by mouth, nasogastric suction, intravenous hydration, and narcotic analgesics until the pain subsides, which it should in 24 to 48 hours. Antibiotics should be used only in patients with sepsis for whom surgery is intended.

Indications for surgical treatment of gallstones during pregnancy include failure to respond to medical therapy within four days, ascending cholangitis, persistent pancreatitis, significant obstructive jaundice, suspected perforation, and inability to rule out other conditions such as appendicitis or perforated ulcer.

REFERENCES AND RECOMMENDED READING

Clark DH: Peptic ulcer in women. Br Med J 1:1254, 1953

Cordero JF, Oakley GP, Greenberg F, James LM: Is Bendectin a teratogen? JAMA 245:2307, 1981

Cunningham FG, McCubbin JH: Appendicitis complicating pregnancy. Obstet Gynecol 45:415, 1975

DeDombal MD, Watts JH, Watkinson G et al: Ulcerative colitis and pregnancy. Lancet 2:599, 1965

Geiger CJ, Fahrenbach DM, Healey FJ: Bendectin in the treatment of nausea and vomiting in pregnancy. Obstet Gynecol 14:688, 1959

Jarnerot G, Into-Malinberg MD, Esbjorner E: Placental transfer of sulfasalazine and sulfapyridine and some of its metabolites. Scand J Gastroenterol 16:693, 1981

Jarnfelt-Samsioe A, Samsioe G, Velinder G-M: Nausea and vomiting in pregnancy—A contribution to its epidemiology. Gynecol Obstet Invest 16:221, 1983

Kolata GB: How safe is Bendectin? Science 20:518, 1980

Medalie JH: Relationship between nausea and/or vomiting in early pregnancy and abortion. Lancet 2:117, 1957

Mogadam M, Dobbins WO, Korelitz BI: Pregnancy in inflammatory bowel disease: Effect of sulfasalazine and corticosteroids on fetal outcome. Gastroenterology 80:72, 1981

Shapiro S, Heinonen OP, Siskind V et al: Antenatal exposure to Bendectin in relation to congenital malformations, perinatal mortality rate, birth weight, and intelligence quotient score. Am J Obstet Gynecol 128:480, 1977

Sorokin JJ, Levine SM: Pregnancy and inflammatory bowel disease. A review of the literature. Obstet Gynecol 62:247, 1983

Soules MR, Hughes CL, Garcia JA et al: Nausea and vomiting of pregnancy. Role of human chorionic gonadotropin and 17-hydroxyprogesterone. Obstet Gynecol 55:696, 1980

U.S. Department of Health and Human Services: Indications for Bendectin narrowed. FDA Drug Bull 11:1, 1981

Wilkinson EJ: Acute pancreatitis in pregnancy. A review of 98 cases and a report of 8 new cases. Obstet Gynecol Survey 28:281, 1973

Willoughby CP, Truelove SC: Ulcerative colitis and pregnancy. Gut 21:469, 1980

Yerushalmy J, Milkovich L: Evaluation of the teratogenic effect of meclizine in man. Am J Obstet Gynecol 93:553, 1965

Liver Disease

Stuart C. Gordon
Eugene R. Schiff

The reticence of most obstetricians and internists in their approach to the pregnant women with liver disease may be attributed to the presumed rarity of these conditions. But it is increasingly evident that such situations may be neither as obscure nor as rare as previously thought, necessitating a better understanding of the clinical spectrum and accepted management of liver disease in pregnancy.

During most pregnancies, a certain deviation from "normal" may be observed in liver function tests, but this is usually of a minor degree. In up to 6% of uncomplicated pregnancies, the serum bilirubin may be elevated to 2 mg/dl. Elevations in alkaline phosphatase, up to double the nonpregnant value, are not related to the biliary tract, but rather reflect production of a heat-stable fraction by the placenta. A progressive decrease in total serum protein and albumin is related to positive water balance with a resultant increase in total body water. Finally, in normal pregnancies there is no change in serum transaminases, γ glutamyl transpeptidase,

5'-nucleotidase, or prothrombin time; these measurements, therefore, serve as the most sensitive indicators of liver disease in pregnancy.

It has become traditional to consider both the jaundice *of* pregnancy and the jaundice *in* pregnancy. Thus, for the purpose of this discussion, these disease entities will be classifed according to whether the disease is (1) peculiar to pregnancy, and presenting with acute fatty liver, intrahepatic cholestasis, and toxemia; or (2) not peculiar to pregnancy, and presenting with gallstones, intercurrent liver disease, viral hepatitis, chronic hepatitis and cirrhosis, tumors, and the Budd-Chiari syndrome.

ACUTE FATTY LIVER OF PREGNANCY

Recent reports have emphasized that acute fatty liver of pregnancy, formerly believed to be rare and almost invariably fatal for both mother and child, consists of a broad clinical spectrum that includes mild illnesses and that earlier reported cases represented only the tip of the iceberg. Although the disease is still the most catastrophic hepatic disease that can occur in the pregnant woman, it is now recognized that early detection, early cesarean section, and aggressive supportive care may significantly improve survival rates.

Acute fatty liver of pregnancy occurs between the 30th and 38th weeks of pregnancy, and may be more common with twin and male births and in primigravidas. The condition is characterized by nausea, repeated vomiting, and abdominal pain. Jaundice follows about a week later; in severe cases, this is associated with hepatic encephalopathy, renal failure, and hemorrhage, but numerous well-documented nonfatal cases in recent years have demonstrated that milder forms of the disease may exist. Routine biochemical profiles that have uncovered clinically occult cases of acute fatty liver of pregnancy in women without coagulopathy or encephalopathy have enabled earlier intervention.

Laboratory indications include raised serum transaminase levels, but rarely greater than 550 IU/liter, a feature helpful in ruling out acute hepatitis. Serum bilirubin levels tend to peak early in the clinical course, usually at less than 15 mg/dl. Hyperbilirubinemia is found without demonstrable hemolysis, unlike preeclampsia or eclampsia, where jaundice is rare except with hemolysis (as discussed later in this chapter). Mild leukocytosis with neutrophilia is common. High uric acid levels may be noted, perhaps as a result of tissue destruction and lactic acidosis. In severe cases, progressive liver failure leads to hyperammonemia, hypoglycemia, and coagulopathy that is unresponsive to parenteral vitamin K. Death is usually secondary to disseminated intravascular coagulation, gastrointestinal hemorrhage, or renal failure.

Acute fatty liver of pregnancy must be included in the differential diagnosis of all cases of hepatic dysfunction in the third trimester of pregnancy. Types A and B viral hepatitis can usually be excluded with the use of appropriate serologic markers. The patient's history should be examined for epidemiologic evidence for viral hepatitis, such as intravenous drug abuse. The patient should also be questioned about alcohol abuse and exposure to hepatotoxic drugs so that other forms of hepatocellular injury can be uncovered. Acute cholecystitis can generally be detected by ultrasonography and clinical history. Cholestasis of pregnancy presents with pruritus and a cholestatic chemical profile. The hemolytic uremic syndrome, with hepatic dysfunction, occasionally complicates pregnancy but is associated with oliguria and hemolytic anemia. The preeclampsia syndrome may feature mild and often subclinical liver disease, although jaundice may on occasion be deep. Proteinuria and edema, however, are rare in fatty liver of pregnancy. Although the differential diagnosis may be difficult, the treatment for toxemia and acute fatty liver is similar.

Despite the reluctance to perform a liver biopsy in a pregnant women—often, one with coagulopathy—this option should be considered before induced delivery or cesarean section. If clotting studies are normal, liver biopsy may be safely performed, preferably under ultrasound guidance because of the displacement of the liver in pregnancy. When coagulopathy is present, the transjugular approach can be used. Staining to detect microvesicular fat (oil red-0) must be done before formalin tissue fixing; plans to perform this stain should be made with the pathologist before the biopsy procedure is done. Alternatively, CT scans of the liver may be useful, since fat accumulation may be reflected in low attenuation ratios.

Treatment consists of supportive care. Early recognition of coagulopathy and treatment with fresh frozen plasma may decrease mortality from hemorrhage and postpartum bleeding. Lactulose therapy, protein restriction, avoidance of all central nervous system depressants, and prevention of hypoglycemia with continued dextrose infusions should lessen the likelihood of encephalopathy and thus improve survival. Finally, since early delivery appears to lower both infant and maternal mortality when acute fatty liver of pregnancy is present, prompt termination of pregnancy (without general anesthesia) should be performed if the disorder is strongly suspected. Acute fatty liver usually does not recur in subsequent pregnancies.

VIRAL HEPATITIS

Acute Hepatitis

Although acute viral hepatitis is probably the most common cause of jaundice during pregnancy, most of the literature dealing with it predates the advent of serologic markers for types A and B hepatitis. In general, uncomplicated viral hepatitis poses no significant threat to either mother or child. Following recovery, though, ele-

vated bilirubin levels may persist in the amniotic fluid, mistakenly suggesting an Rh-immunized fetus; elevated bilirubin levels, therefore, must be interpreted cautiously. Voluntary termination of pregnancy does not ameliorate the course of the disease. Indeed, surgery and anesthesia can be deleterious during acute hepatitis.

All available evidence suggests that acute type A hepatitis in pregnancy causes neither obstetric complications nor congenital malformations. There are no reports of perinatal transmission. The prophylactic administration of immune serum globulin (0.16 ml/kg) for newborns is indicated only when the mother is acutely infected during the perinatal period.

Similarly, the course of hepatitis B infection appears to be unaltered by pregnancy. Of far greater significance is the vertical transmission of hepatitis B, discussed below.

During an epidemic of presumed non-A, non-B hepatitis in India, severe disease was more common among pregnant than among nonpregnant women, and perinatal mortality was increased. Since viral markers were not then available, however, the data remain inconclusive. The diagnosis of acute non-A, non-B hepatitis is one of exclusion and, depending on the clinical setting, the differential diagnosis must include fatty liver of pregnancy and hepatic toxemia. When non-A, non-B viral disease is suspected, the newborn should be given immune serum globulin 0.5 ml intramuscularly at birth and probably again at one month.

Perinatal Transmission of Hepatitis B

Vertical transmission from mother to neonate is the most common mode of transmission of the hepatitis B virus. If, at the time of delivery, the mother is positive for both HBsAg and HBeAg, whether in an acute stage or in an asymptomatic "chronic carrier" state, the neonate will become infected in up to 90% of cases. Exposure is primarily perinatal but may occur by transplacental infection in 5% of cases. Approximately 90% of infected neonates will become chronic carriers of hepatitis B virus. The fact that these chronic carriers will eventually become infectious themselves and that 25% of them will die of cirrhosis or primary hepatocellular carcinoma underlies the need for rigorous surveillance and immunoprophylaxis against this worldwide health menace.

The identification of pregnant HBsAg carriers, regardless of HBeAg status, is crucial. Prenatal HBsAg screening is recommended for women of Asian, Mediterranean, Pacific Island, or Alaskan Eskimo descent, whether immigrant or US-born, as well as women born in Haiti or sub-Saharan Africa. Women with the following histories should also be screened:

Acute or chronic liver disease
Work or treatment in a hemodialysis unit
Work or residence in an institution for the mentally retarded

Rejection as a blood donor

Repeated blood transfusions

Frequent occupational exposure to blood in medical or dental settings

Household contact with a hepatitis B carrier or hemodialysis patient

Repeated episodes of venereal disease or history of multiple sex partners

Percutaneous use of illicit drugs

If not obtained prenatally, such screening should be done at the time of delivery, or soon after.

In an attempt to prevent the hepatitis B carrier state, and the rare occurrence of neonatal fulminant B hepatitis, both passive and active immunization is begun immediately postpartum in infants born of HBsAg carriers. Both hepatitis B immune globulin (HBIG, 0.5 ml) and hepatitis B vaccine (Heptavax-B, 0.5 ml) should be administered intramuscularly within 12 hours of birth, at separate sites. In addition, hepatitis B vaccine (0.5 ml) should be readministered at one month and six months after the first dose. This immunization program has proven to be quite effective; however, antigen and antibody testing should be performed following this vaccine sequence. Anti-HBs should then be detected; if instead, HBsAg is positive at six months, therapeutic failure has occurred.

CHRONIC LIVER DISEASE

The effect of pregnancy on preexisting chronic inflammatory liver disease (*chronic active hepatitis*) is uncertain. Although it is recognized that the disease is associated with an increase in fetal morbidity and mortality, it has been reported that pregnancy *per se* probably does not affect maternal survival or the number of recurrences of the hepatitis. Although pregnancy is not specifically contraindicated in women with chronic active hepatitis, it should be recognized that the disease itself has an ominous prognosis, with progression to cirrhosis even with corticosteroid therapy, so that the long-term outlook remains guarded. Prednisone and azathioprine, often used in the treatment of these disorders, have not been associated with teratogenicity or short-term complications in the children born to mothers on these medications. The more benign *chronic persistent hepatitis* has not been associated with problems during pregnancy. If the chronic hepatitis is of viral etiology, immunization of the neonate should be planned as outlined above in cases of chronic viral B disease.

Cirrhosis in pregnancy is rare and presents a unique set of problems. The rarity of the condition probably stems from the fact that disturbances in estrogen metabolism in cirrhosis often result in infertility. Furthermore, cirrhotic women tend to be in an older age range. But because most cirrhotics are clinically latent and have an adequate hepatic reserve, the reported incidence of cirrhosis in pregnancy may understate the true incidence.

The increased blood volume in pregnancy results in increased portal pressure, especially in the third trimester; the added pressure of the gravid uterus on the vena cava leads to transient esophageal varices in up to two thirds of healthy pregnant women. The added burden of cirrhosis, with baseline portal hypertension, may predispose to severe or even fatal hemorrhage. It has been suggested that prophylactic decompressive shunting may reduce the incidence of serious variceal hemorrhages in the pregnant woman with cirrhosis, but clearly this procedure remains controversial, and perhaps prophylactic endoscopic variceal sclerotherapy may be considered as a less invasive alternative.

INTRAHEPATIC CHOLESTASIS OF PREGNANCY

In contrast to the recent optimism about the prognosis of acute fatty liver of pregnancy, recent reports have challenged the long-accepted doctrine that the so-called benign cholestasis of pregnancy is, in fact, entirely benign for both mother and child. The recurrent nature of the disease, the intensity of the often unrelieved pruritus, and the occasional steatorrhea secondary to prolonged cholestasis and intestinal malabsorption can create profound anxiety and depression for the mother. It is now well recognized that the incidence of prematurity and perinatal mortality is markedly increased.

The exact pathogenesis and mode of inheritance of benign cholestasis of pregnancy is unclear, although its occurrence in family members and the apparent clustering of cases in Chile and Scandinavia have suggested a genetic incidence. It is of interest that among normal pregnant women, about 25% will have subclinical laboratory evidence of mild cholestasis attributable to elevated estrogen levels. It is felt that the clinical disorder is caused by an exaggerated response to the cholestatic effects of estrogen among genetically predisposed women. Furthermore, women with previous cholestasis of pregnancy will develop, without exception, the same syndrome with subsequent pregnancies and will also develop cholestasis when taking estrogen-containing oral contraceptives. Conversely, up to 50% of women who develop jaundice related to contraceptive steroids will have a history of jaundice during pregnancy.

The clinical spectrum of this disease is highly variable. Although usually presenting in late pregnancy, a prodrome of pruritus may begin as early as the sixth week of gestation and the entity should be easily recognizable. Itching is widespread and may be intense, often involving the palmar and plantar surfaces. Serum bile acids are increased 10 to 100 times and, indeed, may be raised before the onset of pruritus. In the condition known as *pruritus gravidarum* no further symptoms or laboratory abnormalities (specifically, hyperbilirubinemia) ensue.

In most cases, a cholestatic form of jaundice follows the pruritus by about two weeks. The serum bilirubin level rarely exceeds 6 mg/dl and bilirubin is primarily the conjugated form. Alkaline phosphatase is similarly raised. Serum transaminase may be slightly increased. In cases of prolonged jaundice, the prothrombin time may be prolonged. Pruritus and jaundice continue throughout the pregnancy.

The entities most likely to be confused with intrahepatic cholestasis of pregnancy are extrahepatic obstructive disease and viral hepatitis. The absence of typical biliary pain and the demonstration by ultrasonography of nondilated bile ducts should clearly rule out obstruction, although women with intrahepatic cholestasis have an increased risk of subsequent cholelithiasis and gall bladder disease. While the clinical setting of hepatitis is generally recognizable, a cholestatic form of viral hepatitis has been described in association with acute hepatitis A, and both type A and type B hepatitis should be serologically excluded. Non-A, non-B hepatitis can only be excluded on clinical and epidemiologic grounds since no serologic parameters are as yet available.

Cholestyramine binds bile acids in the gut and removes them from the enterohepatic circulation, thus lowering serum bile acid levels and providing the most physiologic means for the amelioration of symptoms. This agent may also have an estrogen-binding effect. Although cholestyramine is not always effective, a full therapeutic regimen should be attempted, since results may not be seen until after two weeks of treatment. The usual dose is 12 g/day; packets should be given 30 minutes before breakfast, 30 minutes after breakfast, and at bedtime. After one or two weeks, the dosage can usually be reduced to 9 g per day, but may have to be increased to 16 g per day if symptoms do not abate. Antihistamines and phenobarbital have been used with varying success, the antipruritic effects probably being related to central nervous system depression. A recent report noted that plasmapheresis resulted in clinical and biochemical improvement in two refractory patients in late pregnancy.

The risk to the fetus of a woman with cholestasis of pregnancy is substantial. As noted earlier, overall perinatal mortality is four times that of controls (6.4% in one series), and premature delivery may occur in 30% to 60% of cases. Furthermore, signs of fetal distress may be present in 40% of the pregnancies, perhaps because of altered steroid metabolism in the fetus following transplacental passage of maternal bile salts or other unknown substances. Clearly, intensive perinatal monitoring is essential; more important, because of this increased risk, some have suggested that induction of labor be commenced as soon as fetal lung maturity is established, usually before the onset of the 38th week of pregnancy. Monitoring the short-term variability of fetal heart rate has been found useful in selecting the time for induction of labor. Following delivery, all signs and symptoms abate; whereas the level of alkaline phosphatase may continue to increase for two weeks, serum bilirubin and transaminase levels start to decrease immediately. Pruritus ceases within one to two weeks. Should cholestasis persist following delivery, an underlying cholestatic disorder, such as primary biliary cirrhosis, should be considered, since occasionally this condition may become clinically manifest during pregnancy as a result of the superimposed estrogenic impact. As in any cholestatic condition of prolonged duration, fat malabsorption occurs; in addition, cholestyramine will further bind fat-soluble vitamins. Prothrombin times should be tested at term, but even in the absence of coagulopathy, vitamin K deficiency may develop, resulting in postpartum hemorrhage. Prophylactic treatment with intramuscular vitamin K is recommended in all patients with cholestasis of pregnancy.

TOXEMIA OF PREGNANCY AND RUPTURE OF THE LIVER

Subclinical liver dysfunction may be seen in cases of preeclampsia/toxemia, and the diagnosis of *hepatic toxemia* remains one of exclusion. Riely observed that some patients with acute fatty liver of pregnancy were found to be hypertensive and suggested that acute fatty liver may be part of a spectrum of toxemia, although conventionally these entities are regarded as different diseases.

Hepatic toxemia also presents in the third trimester, typically with nausea and epigastric or right upper quadrant pain in a patient with other signs of toxemia, including varying degrees of hypertension, edema, proteinuria, and hyperreflexia. There are few clinical hallmarks, and the diagnosis remains one of exclusion. Viral hepatitis and biliary tract disease have to be ruled out. The differentiation from acute fatty liver may be difficult. The biochemical abnormalities include elevations, sometimes marked, in transaminase levels and bilirubin elevation that is usually mild and related to an associated microangiopathic hemolytic anemia. Clinical jaundice is unusual and is a grave prognostic sign. Laboratory evidence of toxemia or of disseminated intravascular coagulation (elevated uric acid, BUN, fibrin split products, and thrombocytopenia) may be seen.

Because of the potentially ominous association of preeclampsia and liver dysfunction in late pregnancy, close observation is warranted. If the fetus is mature, delivery should be performed. If hepatic toxemia occurs earlier in gestation or is mild, supportive care may suffice. Although no specific therapy is available, the condition responds to the treatment of toxemia itself; chronic liver disease and liver failure do not develop.

A rare association, and perhaps complication, of hepatic toxemia is the spontaneous rupture of the capsule of the liver after development of a subcapsular hematoma. The pathogenesis of the hematoma is unknown, and the trigger of the rupture may be related to the trauma of parturition, vomiting, or the convulsions of toxemia. Typically occurring in a multiparous, hypertensive woman in the third trimester, progressive epigastric pain should lead to the suspicion of impending rupture, prompting ultrasonic examination searching for subcapsular hematoma. Early diagnosis and cesarean section may obviate the surgical catastrophe associated with the actual rupture of Glisson's capsule.

GALLSTONES

Despite recent evidence showing that gallbladder volume is increased and rate of gallbladder emptying is reduced during pregnancy, the incidence of obstructive jaundice due to gallstones in pregnancy is surprisingly low. When the condition is encountered, however, the diagnostic modalities and management do not differ from those used in nonpregnant patients. In cases of documented common bile duct obstruction, surgical intervention or endoscopic papillotomy should be attempted. Krejs recommends that surgery for common bile duct obstruction may be performed up to the 36th weeks of gestation, after which it should be delayed until after delivery. But in clinically obvious acute attacks of cholecystitis, management remains the same as in the nonpregnant patient. Pregnancy is not a contraindication to cholecystectomy.

BUDD-CHIARI SYNDROME

The increased incidence of *hepatic vein thrombosis* in both pregnant women and users of contraceptive steroids suggests that estrogen-related hypercoagulability is responsible for the predisposition to this dramatic clinical event.

Hepatic vein thrombosis generally presents as an acute illness, with abdominal pain, ascites, hepatosplenomegaly and variable laboratory abnormalities, and fatal hepatic failure usually follows. Attempts at clot lysis have been ineffective, although side-to-side portacaval shunt surgery may improve intractable ascites in chronic cases.

HEPATIC TUMORS IN PREGNANCY

Adenomas are the most common liver tumors in pregnancy and are frequently associated with a history of prior contraceptive steroid use. These highly vascular tumors enlarge in response to estrogen, often with resultant rupture and potentially fatal hemorrhage. Although successful pregnancy without recurrence of the neoplasm has been reported in a patient with a previously resected adenoma, pregnancy is contraindicated in patients with an unresected adenoma.

REFERENCES AND RECOMMENDED READING

Centers for Disease Control: Recommendation of the immunization practices advisory committee: Postexposure prophylaxis of hepatitis B. MMWR 33:285, 1984

Douvas SG, Meeks GR, Phillips O et al: Liver disease in pregnancy. Obstet Gynecol Surv 38:531, 1983

Gordon SC, Reddy KR, Schiff L et al: Prolonged intrahepatic cholestasis secondary to acute hepatitis A. Ann Intern Med 101:635, 1984

Henny CP, Lim AE, Brummelkamp WH et al: A review of the importance of acute multidisciplinary treatment following rupture of the liver capsule during pregnancy. Surg Gynecol Obstet 156:593, 1983

Krejs GJ: Jaundice during pregnancy. Sem Liver Dis 3:73, 1982

Pockros PJ, Peters RL, Reynolds TB: Idiopathic fatty liver of pregnancy: Findings in ten cases. Medicine 63:1, 1984

Reyes H: The enigma of intrahepatic cholestasis of pregnancy: Lessons from Chile. Hepatology 2:87, 1982

Riely CA: Acute fatty liver of pregnancy—1984. Dig Dis Sci 29:456, 1984

Riely CA, Romero R, Duffy TF: Hepatic dysfunction with disseminated intravascular coagulation in toxemia of pregnancy: A distinct clinical syndrome. Gastroenterology 80:1364, 1981

Schiff L, Schiff ER (eds): Diseases of the Liver, 5th ed. Philadelphia, J. B. Lippincott Co, 1982

Sherlock S: Acute fatty liver of pregnancy and the microvesicular fat diseases. Gut 24:265, 1983

Shreyer P, Caspi E, el-Hindi JM et al: Cirrhosis: Pregnancy and delivery: A review. Obstet Gynecol Surv 37:304, 1982

Steven MM: Pregnancy and liver disease. Gut 22:592, 1981

Wong VCW, Ip HMH, Reesink HW et al: Prevention of the HBsAg carrier state in newborn infants of mothers who are chronic carriers of HBsAg and HBeAg by administration of hepatitis-B vaccine and hepatitis-B immunoglobulin. Lancet 1:921, 1984

Diseases of the Blood

Sue M. Palmer
Janna Sherrill
John C. Morrison

Anemia is a very common disorder during pregnancy. It occurs in over 50% of gestations in the United States and may range from being an insignificant laboratory finding to being a serious disorder with consequences for both the mother and fetus.[1] Anemia by definition is a reduction in the oxygen-carrying capacity of the blood as reflected by a decrease in the hemoglobin content to less than 10 g/dl. Normally during pregnancy hormonal influences lead to a physiologic increase in plasma volume, and a "relative" anemia, or reduction in the ratio of hemoglobin to plasma volume, is noted. Absolute anemias, which involve a true decrease in red cell mass,

Supported in part by the Vicksburg Hospital Medical Foundation.

are characterized either by diminished red cell production (hypoproliferative anemia), increased blood cell loss, or an increase in erythrocyte destruction (proliferative anemia) as shown in Figure 30-1. The effect of red blood cell abnormalities (absolute anemias) on the mother/fetus/neonate is determined by the severity of the anemic process and its direct effect on oxygenation. These abnormalities, however, may affect normal hemostasis and indirectly damage the progeny.

DISORDERS OF HEMOGLOBIN STRUCTURE, FUNCTION AND SYNTHESIS

Hemoglobin is a complex protein composed of four heme groups each bound to one member of two dissimilar pairs of polypeptide chains. Human red blood cells contain a pair of α chains and a pair of β (hemoglobin A_1), γ (hemoglobin F), or δ (hemoglobin A_2) chains.[2] These protein chains are differentiated by their unique sequence of amino acids. Disorders of hemoglobin integrity most commonly involve globin structure in the erythrocyte. There are more than 300 types of abnormal hemoglobin and most of these involve single amino acid substitutions in one or more of the protein chains. Most commonly, these structural abnormalities involve the β chains, but at times both protein moieties can be unaffected and there is simply diminished production of structurally normal globin chains, as in thalassemia. The various hemoglobinopathies include sickle hemoglobins, unstable variant forms of hemoglobin, those with altered oxygen affinity, the M or cyanotic varieties, as well as disorders of production, such as thalassemia.

Sickle Hemoglobin

The most common hemoglobinopathy with clinically significant maternal and fetal effects involves sickle hemoglobin, or hemoglobin S.[3] This variety differs from normal hemoglobin by a single substitution of the amino acid valine for glutamic acid in both β chains. During deoxygenation, hemoglobin S molecules form hydrophobic bonds. These long strands of repetitive tetramers coalesce into microcables that cause sickling. *In vivo*, the sickling of red blood cells causes a sickle cell crisis.[4] These vaso-occlusive crises can cause infarction in many organs and adversely affect the mother or fetus. In the United States, the incidence of sickle cell anemia (HbS-S) is highest among blacks, where it reaches 1 in 500. Its clinically significant variants, such as hemoglobin SC disease (HbS-C) and hemoglobin S thalassemia (HbS-thal), which may cause increased morbidity and mortality in the mother and fetus/neonate, are also fairly common among blacks (1/800 and 1/1250 respectively).[1]

The manifestation of sickle hemoglobin may range from serious disease (it is responsible for some 80,000 deaths annually throughout the world) to absolutely no symptomatology, as is found in sickle cell trait (HbA-S). Sickle cell disease (SS, SC, or S-Thal) appears to entail significant maternal morbidity and patients with

FIG. 30-1. Classification of anemia.

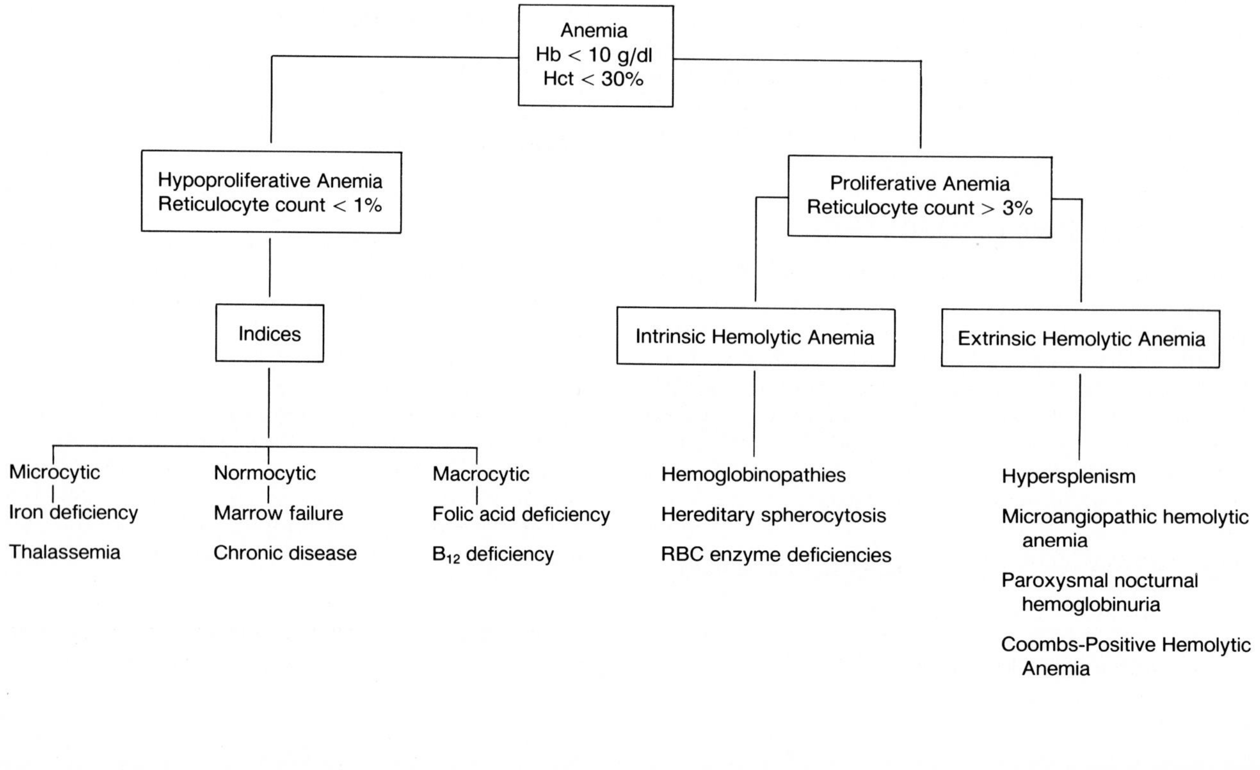

the disease should have intensive antepartal risk assessment, with particular emphasis on the detection of crises or infections.[5] The perinatal effects of maternal sickle cell disease include abortion, low birthweight, and stillbirth—outcome usually depends on the number of crises and other significant maternal morbidity. On the other hand, the patient with HbA-S is thought to be at no significant disadvantage amd may be managed in much the same way as patients with normal (AA) hemoglobin. The same can be said for patients with the "benign" hemoglobinopathies, such as homozygous C disease and hemoglobin SD and SE disorders. However, patients with HbA-S do have a twofold increase in urinary tract infections during pregnancy. They should therefore be screened with urine cultures at the first prenatal visit, and again at 32 weeks.

The diagnosis of sickle hemoglobinopathies may be made by a screening assessment, such as the Sickledex test.* Screening should be offered to all black patients during their antepartum care. If the test is positive, a hemoglobin electrophoresis using cellulose acetate is employed to identify the abnormal hemoglobin. After the diagnosis has been established, biweekly visits to the physician during the antepartum period are advocated.[1] Assessment for evidence of sickling crisis by blood film and clinical history is recommended. An intense search for and early treatment of infections is essential, since patients with sickle hemoglobin are immunocompromised by defective opsonization and complement fixation.[4] Some clinicians recommend the use of prophylactic partial exchange transfusions during the antepartum period to increase the concentration of hemoglobin A and decrease the concentration of hemoglobin S-containing cells, thus making the likelihood of sickling remote.[6,7] Others prefer to rely on intense antenatal surveillance and reserve transfusions for crises, infections, and other forms of maternal morbidity.[5,8] For those using prophylactic exchange transfusions, erythrocytapheresis is not only more rapid and accurate but it is also less costly than traditional transfusion techniques, since it does not involve hospitalization. Research in the treatment of patients with sickle cell disease is being directed toward the use of desickling agents, such as polypeptides and imidate compounds, and toward genetic induction of hemoglobin A or F by marrow transplantation.[9]

The treatment of patients with sickle cell disease during labor is usually no different from that of patients with other medical complications.[4] Intensive maternal and fetal monitoring is employed. Cesarean birth is used only for the usual obstetric indications. The care of the neonate is no different from that of the infant of a mother with normal hemoglobin, since there is enough hemoglobin F to prevent sickling even if the infant has homozygous disease. The protective benefit of hemoglobin F usually lasts for about four to six months after birth. Nevertheless, in these patients cord blood should be assessed to delineate the type of hemoglobinopathy.

Other Hemoglobinopathies

Other types of hemoglobin disorders involve the unstable hemoglobins, which are inherited by the autosomal dominant mechanism and are characterized by a hemolytic anemia (see Fig. 30-1). The hematologic picture is normocytic with Heinz body inclusions in the red cells. Electrophoresis is the method of diagnosis and the disorders usually have no effect on the parturient or the fetus unless the mother is exposed to certain drugs, such as sulfas and furantoin derivatives.[10] The mainstay of therapy involves removing offending agents as well as transfusion and splenectomy, the latter is usually not necessary during pregnancy.

Methemoglobin is formed when iron is oxidized to its ferric form and becomes unable to combine with oxygen. Although methemoglobinemia may result from treatment with various drugs, exposure to chemicals, or a deficiency in the enzyme hemoglobin reductase, it is usually associated with hemoglobin M and with structural abnormalities in the α or β chain.[10] Methemoglobinemia is autosomal dominant and is always heterozygous. It is diagnosed by its absorption spectral characteristics, but electrophoresis using electrofocusing techniques may be helpful. Methylene blue and ascorbic acid are useful in the treatment of the enzyme-deficient form of the disease but not in the forms associated with structural hemoglobin M disorders. Fortunately, methemoglobinemia is totally unaffected by pregnancy and never has an adverse effect on the mother or the fetus or newborn. Reassurance and proper diagnosis are the only therapy necessary.

There are nearly 50 hemoglobin disorders in which oxygen affinity is altered. About two thirds are associated with a high oxygen affinity and demonstrate polycythemia as well as an increased red cell mass without leukocytosis.[10] Usually, no symptomatology is noted although the patient may tire easily. Hemoglobinopathies associated with low oxygen affinity usually induce cyanosis. It is important, however, that more severe blood disorders associated with cyanosis or polycythemia be ruled out. Most variant forms of hemoglobin can be identified on electrophoresis using starch or agar gel. For both high-affinity and low-affinity varieties, no treatment is usually necessary. Although there is a theoretic increase in risk of thrombosis in patients with polycythemia, no cases have been reported in pregnancy.

The most common types of thalassemia are the heterozygous α or β varieties, for which no treatment is usually necessary.[11] Cooley's anemia, or homozygous β thalassemia, is rarely associated with pregnancy because the disorder is so devastating that the patient usually does not survive childhood. Homozygous α thalassemia, because of the way in which it alters the oxygen-carrying capacity of the blood, is usually incompatible with life,

---

* Ortho Pharmaceutical Corporation, Raritan, New Jersey.

with most fetuses being stillborn or succumbing shortly after birth. The laboratory diagnosis of heterozygous thalassemia is difficult because the hemoglobin is normal. Hemoglobin A_2 and F levels may be slightly elevated with heterozygous β thalassemia, but in α thalassemia frequently the diagnosis can only be made on the basis of family pedigree.

It is evident that the parturient with abnormal hemoglobin, as well as her fetus/newborn, is usually unaffected by most of these disorders. Only the severe sickling disorders and homozygous thalassemia have a consistent adverse effect on the mother and fetus/neonate. Nevertheless, it is imperative that proper diagnosis be confirmed so that more severe hemotalogic disorders may be discounted and the patient given reassurance.

HYPOPROLIFERATIVE ANEMIA

Iron Deficiency

Iron is essential for oxygen transport and is incorporated into hemoglobin. Requirements for this metal are increased during pregnancy. Iron deficiency anemia is the most common type of anemia seen during pregnancy, representing causation in 75% to 85% of those with low hemoglobin concentrations (<11 g/dl).[1] Indeed, some degree of iron depletion (which is the initial state of iron deficiency anemia) is present in all parturients, since the increase in requirements during pregnancy is not supplied by the diet. For example, the average North American diet supplies only 11 mg to 14 mg iron, which compensates only for basal losses. The additional maternal requirements and expanded blood volume during pregnancy, as well as the fetal and placental require-

ments, result in iron depletion in all pregnant women unless they receive supplementation. This is particularly true in the latter half of pregnancy, when the iron demand increases fivefold.

The symptomatology of iron deficiency is protean, but fatigue, irritability, and malaise usually precede hematologic laboratory evidence of anemia. As the iron depletion progresses to iron deficiency anemia, other systemic signs, such as pica and, finally, shortness of breath may be encountered as the hemoglobin drops below 10 g/dl and finally below 5 g/dl.[12]

Peripheral blood smears usually show some poikilocytosis and basophilic stippling although hypochromic microcytic erythrocytes are the rule (see Fig. 30-1). The mean corpuscular hemoglobin concentration (MCHC) is the most reliable index of iron deficiency anemia, and usually values of less than 30% indicate anemia. The diagnostic value of mean corpuscular volume (MCV) and mean corpuscular hemoglobin (MCH) is negated because of the changes that occur during pregnancy. Serum iron level normally decreases with advancing gestational age; however, a level below 30 μg/dl is diagnostic of iron deficiency.[13] The unsaturated iron binding capacity also increases during pregnancy but a value of more than 400 μg/dl strongly suggests iron deficiency anemia (Table 30-8). In addition, a transferrin saturation of less than 15% is virtually diagnostic of the disorder. Serum ferritin reflects iron stores; levels of 55–70 μg/dl during pregnancy are normal, values of less than 10 μg/dl are diagnostic of iron deficiency anemia. Serum ferritin is also helpful in assessing iron depletion in the absence of frank anemia. The serum free erythrocyte protoporphyrin (FEP) levels may also be helpful in diagnosis.

Treatment of iron deficiency anemia revolves around iron supplementation. Because all pregnancies

Table 30-8
Normal Laboratory Values for Anemia

Assessment	Pregnant	Nonpregnant
General		
Mean corpuscular volume	79–90 μ^3/cell	80–100 μ^3/cell
Mean corpuscular hemoglobin	23–31 pg/cell	27–34 pg/cell
Mean corpuscular concentration	Unchanged	32–35 g/dl/RBC
Hemoglobin	10–13 g/dl	12–16 g/dl
Packed cell volume	30–39%	37–45%
Red blood cell count	3.8–4.4 million/mm^3	4.2–5.4 million/mm^3
Reticulocyte count	1.0–2.0%	0.5–1.0%
Specific		
Serum iron	30–100 g/dl	50–110 g/dl
Unsaturated iron binding capacity	280–400 g/dl	250–300 g/dl
Transferrin saturation	15–30%	25–35%
Serum folate	4–10 ng/ml	4–16 ng/ml
Serum B_{12}	70–500 ng/dl	70–85 ng/dl

need some supplementation, prophylactic iron administration and proper diet counseling are considered the mainstay of iron depletion prevention during pregnancy.[14] Simple elemental iron as ferrous sulfate is usually adequate to prevent this problem but nausea, vomiting, and abdominal complaints during pregnancy often make iron replacement difficult (Table 30-9). Iron absorption can be enhanced and gastrointestinal symptoms reduced by taking this mineral with meals. Gastrointestinal side effects can be avoided by using ferrous sulfate syrup, slow release preparation, or enteric-coated iron capsules.[15] For those few parturients who cannot or will not take iron or who have intestinal problems limiting absorption, elemental iron complexed with carbohydrates may be given intramuscularly or intravenously.

Occasionally, patients who undergo operation during pregnancy or who have severe iron deficiency anemia may need red blood cell infusions. Usually this is not necessary in the postpartum period unless the parturient's packed cell volume is less than 25%, or she is symptomatic or is postoperative. Treatment with oral iron preparation should be continued during the postpartum period, particularly if the woman is lactating. The fetal effects of iron deficiency anemia are usually in proportion to the maternal deficiency state. No detrimental effects of mild iron depletion have been documented; however, hemoglobin concentrations of less than 6.5 g/dl have been associated with fetal growth retardation and stillbirth. Prophylactic iron supplementation in the mother appears to be safe for the fetus, and supplementation in the puerperium does not appear to have any effect on the breastfeeding neonate.

Megaloblastic Anemias During Pregnancy

Megaloblastic anemia during pregnancy is usually due to a deficiency of folic acid. Vitamin B_{12} deficiency, although it causes a similar hematologic picture, is rare in young women. Like iron deficiency anemia, folic acid deficiency is one of the hypoproliferative disorders (see Fig. 30-1), but it is characterized by megaloblastic cellular changes. Nuclear maturation and mitotic activity are delayed but cytoplasmic development progresses normally. Therefore the cells are much larger than normal. The deficiency of folic acid during pregnancy is usually attributed to the increasing demand for this vitamin by the trophoblast, the rapidly developing fetus (the condition is commoner in multiple pregnancy), and the expanding maternal red cell mass.[16] This increase in demand is usually coupled with inadequate nutrition. Prophylactic folic acid supplementation in the form of a vitamin supplement is usually recommended. Folate is present in a number of foods but extensive cooking, which is a western practice, destroys up to 90% of the element. Furthermore, storage capacity for folate is limited: the stores contained in the liver are usually sufficient for only 4 to 6 weeks.[17] The normal nonpregnant daily requirement of 50 μg folate is increased six- or sevenfold during pregnancy. In addition, the use of drugs during pregnancy, particularly anticonvulsant drugs such as diphenylhydantoin as well as certain antibiotics, impairs the absorption and utilization of folate.

Clinically folate deficiency is the second most frequent cause of anemia during pregnancy. This condition is noted in about 15% to 20% of patients with anemia

Table 30-9
Iron Preparations

Product	Manufacturers	Elemental Iron Content	Cost per 100 Tablets or Capsules	Retail Cost for Nine Months†
Ferrous sulfate† 300 mg	Generic	60 mg	$2.00	$15.10
Fer-In-Sol Caps	Mead Johnson	60 mg	$6.25	$47.25
Feosol Tablets	Menley-James (SKF)	65 mg	$5.05	$38.18
Ferrous Gluconate† (Fergon)	Breon	37 mg	$3.70	$46.62*
Ferro-Sequels	Lederle	50 mg	$10.56	$75.00
Feasol elixir	Menley-James (SKF)	44 mg/5 ml	$5.65/12 oz	$79.10
Ferrous sulfate elixir	Generic	60 mg/5 ml	$3.45/16 oz	$27.17
Imferon (parenteral)	Merrell	100 mg/2 ml	$7.38	$86.30 (avg)
Transfusion (packed cells)		250 cc	one unit	$104.00

* Based on 60 mg elemental iron three times per day.
† Ferrous sulfate = 20% elemental iron; ferrous gluconate = 12% elemental iron.

during pregnancy.[17] About half of these are diagnosed during the antepartum period, and the other half are found after delivery. Frank megaloblastic anemia occurs 1 in 70 to 1 in 250 pregnancies. Folate depletion is much more common and has been estimated to occur in 30% to 60% of pregnancies among socioeconomically deprived groups in the United States. The primary direct consequences of severe folic acid deficiency are the possibility that the mother will need transfusion therapy and that there is an increased risk of hemorrhage secondary to thrombocytopenia. Folic acid deficiency has been associated with abortion and abruptio placentae but other studies have been unable to establish a connection.[16]

The diagnosis of folate deficiency is usually made by findings of reduced levels of serum fasting folate (<3 ng/ml by radioassay) and the presence of leukocyte nuclear hypersegmentation.[13] Serum folate values in the pregnant woman usually decrease, and during pregnancy hypersegmentation of neutrophils is an accurate delineator of folic acid deficiency. In pregnancy, an erythrocyte folate level of less than 20 ng/dl has been suggested as the best biochemical index of folic acid deficiency.[18] Usually in these disorders of a macrocytic pattern, elevated serum iron concentrations, and elevated transferrin saturations are noted, along with increased LDH-1 and LDH-2 isoenzyme fractions.[13] Generally the diagnosis can be made without bone marrow aspiration.

Treatment of folic acid deficiency is given as 0.5 mg folic acid.[17] For prophylactic therapy, folic acid contained in multiple vitamins is usually sufficient. Dietary counseling is also important. A distinct elevation of the reticulocyte count and a decrease in hypersegmentation of the neutrophils are the earliest signs of remission and usually occur two to four days after folate therapy has begun. The hematocrit and hemoglobin concentration usually respond within a few weeks of the initiation of therapy.

If therapy does not seem to ameliorate the condition, B$_{12}$ deficiency must be considered. Because pernicious anemia usually affects older men and usually involves infertility in women, B$_{12}$ deficiency as a cause for megaloblastic anemia is rarely encountered during pregnancy, averaging 1 in 6000 to 1 in 8000 deliveries. It is most commonly associated with a strict vegetarian diet or tropical sprue. A vitamin B$_{12}$ level of less than 50 pg/ml is strongly suggestive of pernicious anemia. Six weekly injections of 1000 μg of hydroxycobalamine are recommended as standard treatment. The traditional histamine and Schilling tests for the disorder should be deferred until after the postpartum period so that their results will be valid. Breastfed neonates whose mothers are suffering from B$_{12}$ deficiency may themselves develop severe deficiency syndrome at about 4 to 12 months of age. The purported association between B$_{12}$ deficiency and anencephaly requires further study.[19]

Intrinsic Hemolytic Disorders

Occasionally, increased hemoglobin loss can result from increased destruction of the red blood cells. In these cases anemia usually results from an erythrocyte destruction that is in excess of the bone marrow erythropoietic capacity. In some cases, known as the intrinsic hemolytic processes, the destruction is due to a defect in the red blood cells. The intrinsic hemolytic processes involve hereditary spherocytosis and deficiencies in red blood cell enzymes. In spherocytosis which is inherited as an autosomal trait, the erythrocyte membrane is abnormally permeable to sodium, which leads to premature demise of the red blood cells. The diagnosis of hereditary spherocytosis is confirmed by an abnormal osmotic fragility test. Splenectomy is used to treat the disorder.[20]

Enzyme defects can also shorten the survival time of red blood cells. The two most common disorders of this kind are G6PD deficiency and pyruvate kinase deficiency. G6PD deficiency is an X-linked disorder with partial expression in the heterozygous female. It occurs most commonly in blacks, and about a quarter of black women are affected. If these patients are exposed to such drugs as nitrofurantoin or primaquin, acute hemolysis and accompanying hemoglobinuria follow. Also, acute infection with high fever can precipitate a hemolytic episode. The methemoglobin reduction test is the best assessment of G6PD deficiency.[13] Pyruvate kinase deficiency is an autosomal recessive disorder and most commonly is noted in people with northern European origin. It is usually diagnosed during childhood by the fluorescent spot test because the patient has a persistent anemia and jaundice. The maternal and fetal outcome are dependent on the severity of the disorder.

Extrinsic Hemolytic Disorders

The red blood cells may be normal but external or environmental factors may cause them to be destroyed earlier than usual thus leading to anemia.[21] Hypersplenism due to excessive red cell destruction is rare and reticulocyte counts usually remain less than 6%. Extrinsic hemolytic disorders may also be precipitated by collagen vascular diseases, treatment with the antihypertensive agent alpha methyldopa, and other drug reactions. There are also some Coombs'-positive hemolytic anemias in which an IgG antibody is fixed to the red cell membrane.[21] This type of hemolytic anemia is usually associated with a warm or cold antibody that causes premature lysis of the red blood cells. The cold autoantibodies are usually of the IgM class but may develop after infections by a virus or mycoplasma. IgM antibody does not become fixed to the red blood cell membrane but stimulates the production of complement that will bind to and cause lysis of the red cell.

In microangiopathic hemolytic anemias, histiocytes or red cell fragments are usually seen in large numbers in the peripheral blood smear. These disorders are usually due to changes in coagulation profiles or to small-vessel damage in the microcirculation that causes fragmentation and lysis of erythrocytes. Coombs'-positive hemolytic anemias are usually best treated by therapy directed toward the disorder that led to the anemia. After the offending agent has been removed, hemolysis usually will cease in two to three weeks, although the Coombs' test may remain positive for several months. Transfusion should be used only in emergencies, and corticosteroids are frequently of benefit only in patients with warm antibody hemolytic anemia. If corticosteroids fail, splenectomy is sometimes of value. The effect of these disorders on the mother, fetus, and neonate is usually dependent on the severity of the underlying disorder.

Anemia of Chronic Disease

Anemia that accompanies chronic disease may be mild and is usually nonprogressive. It can be caused by increased erythrocyte destruction but more usually is the result of insufficient compensatory erythropoeisis (see Fig. 30-1). This hypoproliferative anemia is usually normochromic and normocytic but may become hyperchromic if it is severe. Pregnancy appears to have no effect on the disorder, although there may be maternal or fetal morbidity as a consequence of the underlying disease process. The clinical presentation usually involves a slow decline in the hematocrit and hemoglobin associated with a chronic inflammatory process or illness. The degree of anemia is usually not correlated with the severity or duration of the underlying disorder. For example, solid tumors and lymphomas may produce this disorder, as may collagen vascular diseases, such as lupus erythematosis and rheumatoid arthritis. Due to improvements in antibiotics, anemia associated with chronic infectious processes is now uncommon, but tuberculosis, bacterial endocarditis, chronic renal disease, and chronic neurologic infections are still associated with anemia.

The laboratory findings in these patients reveal a hypoproliferative anemia that involves a depressed erythrocyte count.[13] There may be normal erythropoietin production, but iron and other constituents cannot be effectively utilized although they are present in adequate amounts. This underutilization appears to be not only a local effect in the bone marrow but also a systemic component affecting iron stores. The red blood cell indices usually reflect a normocytic, normochromic anemia and there is usually a reduction in the serum iron and unsaturated iron binding capacity but a normal to increased level of serum ferritin. Marrow iron stores are usually plentiful, in contrast to iron deficiency anemia.

The mainstay of treatment for these disorders, of course, is the elimination of the underlying defect. The prognosis in these disorders as well as their effect on the mother and fetus/neonate depends upon the ability to treat these disorders effectively.

Marrow Failure

Diagnosis of bone marrow failure or red cell aplasia usually requires a bone marrow analysis. Etiologies include myelophthisic, refractory, and aplastic anemias. In myelophthisic anemia, the marrow is replaced by myelofibrosis or malignant cells, and the peripheral smear is characterized by marked poikilocytosis, anisocytosis, nucleated red blood cells, and some myeloblasts.[22] A constant physical finding in this disorder is splenomegaly. Usually, bone marrow analysis can differentiate this from chronic myelocytic leukemia that has similar laboratory and clinical features. Metastatic carcinoma also needs to be ruled out, since the peripheral smear in such cases can be similar to that of myelofibrosis.

Refractory anemia is thought to be due to maturation failure of cells within the marrow and is associated with the intramedullary death of cells. Bone marrow analysis reveals the marrow not to be hypoplastic, a finding that differentiates the condition from aplastic anemia. Refractory anemia is usually caused by exposure to chemicals or drugs. Occasionally, a preleukemic state may also present and must be diagnosed.

The peripheral smear in aplastic anemia usually shows marked pancytopenia and severe anemia.[23] In spite of the severe anemia, nucleated red cells are not noted on the peripheral smear. Bone marrow analysis usually reveals hypoplasia. Aplastic anemia is also usually caused by exposure to drugs or chemicals.

Other Anemia Processes

Paroxysmal nocturnal hemoglobinuria (PNH) is a type of hemolytic anemia with no familial tendencies. There is intravascular hemolysis and hemoglobinuria, particularly during sleep.[24] It rarely accompanies pregnancy and, except in severe cases, does not appear to have an adverse effect on pregnancy. The mechanism for hemolysis appears to be an acquired membrane defect in the red blood cell, and it may be linked to aplastic anemia since 25% of patients have both disorders. At least in patients who also have aplastic anemia, PNH may be caused by a mutation that gives rise to increased membrane sensitivity. The diagnosis is confirmed with the sugar water test, which is highly specific for PNH.[13] The treatment is supportive and largely unsatisfactory.[24] Iron therapy sometimes leads to increased hemolysis. High-dose corticosteroids have been helpful as therapy in these patients due to their effect on complement deactivation.

In summary, anemia during pregnancy is a common event. Fortunately, the most frequent causes of anemia, iron deficiency and folic acid deficiency, are responsive to therapy and usually do not adversely affect pregnancy. However, the more severe hematologic disorders must be ruled out and consultation is recommended in all unresponsive or complicated cases. In general, the effect of all but the most severe anemias on the mother and fetus/neonate is minimal. Nevertheless, the provider must maintain a high index of suspicion.

REFERENCES AND RECOMMENDED READING

1. Morrison JC, Gookin KS: Anemia associated with pregnancy. In Depp R, Eschenbach DA (eds): Gynecology and Obstetrics: Maternal and Fetal Medicine, vol 3, p 1. New York, Harper & Row, 1984
2. Kaplan BH, Hunt T, London IM: The synthesis of heme and protein (globin). In Williams WJ, Buetler AJ, Ersler RW (eds): Hematology, p 149. New York, McGraw-Hill, 1977
3. Adachi I, Kelleher JF: Human hemoglobin variants. In Schwartz E (ed): Hemoglobinopathies in Children, p 25. Littleton, MA, PSG Inc, 1980
4. Martin JN, Morrison JC: Sickle cell crisis: recognizing it and treating it. Contemp OB/GYN 20:171, 1982
5. Carache S, Scott J, Neibyl J et al: Management of sickle cell disease in pregnant patients. Obstet Gynecol 55:407, 1980
6. Cunningham FG, Pritchard JA: Prophylactic transfusion of normal red blood cells during pregnancies complicated by sickle cell hemoglobinopathies. Am J Obstet Gynecol 135:994, 1979
7. Morrison JC, Schneider JM, Whybrew WD et al: Prophylactic transfusion in pregnant patients with sickle hemoglobinopathies: Benefit versus risk. Obstet Gynecol 46:274, 1980
8. Milner PF, Jones BR, Dobler J: Outcome of pregnancy in sickel cell anemia—hemoglobin C–disease. Am J Obstet Gynecol 138:239, 1980
9. Klotz IM, Haney DN, King LC: Rational approaches to chemotherapy: Antisickling agents. Science 213:724, 1981
10. Lehmann H, Huntsman RG: Man's Hemoglobins, p 156. Philadelphia, JB Lippincott, 1974
11. Weatherall DJ, Clegg JB: The Thalassemia Syndromes, 2nd ed, p 372. Oxford, Blackwell Scientific Publications, 1972
12. Garn SM, Ridella SA, Petzola AS et al: Maternal hematologic levels and pregnancy outcomes. Semin Perinatol 5:155, 1981
13. Roberts WE, Blake PG, Morrison JC: Evaluation of anemia in pregnancy. In Kitay DZ (ed): Hematologic Problems in Pregnancy. Boston, GK Hall, 1984
14. Pritchard JA, Mason RA: Iron stores of normal adults and replenishment with oral iron therapy. JAMA 190:897, 1964
15. Dallman PR, Simes MA, Stekel A: Iron deficiency in infancy and childhood. Am J Clin Nutr 33:86, 1980
16. Pritchard JA, MacDonald PC: Megaloblastic anemia. Williams Obstetrics, 16th ed, p 717. New York, Appleton-Century-Crofts, 1980
17. Kitay DE: Folic acid and reproduction. Clin Obstet Gynecol 22:809, 1979
18. Johan E, Magnus EM: Plasma and red blood cell folate during normal pregnancy. Acta Obstet Gynecol Scand 60:247, 1981
19. Schorah CJ, Smithells RW, Scott J: Vitamin B_{12} and anencephaly. Lancet 1:880, 1980
20. Eicher ER: Splenic function: Normal, too much and too little. Am J Med 66:311, 1979
21. Dalie JV: Autoimmune hemolytic anemia. Arch Intern Med 135:1293, 1975
22. Rappaport JM, Bunn HF: Bone marrow failure: Aplastic anemia and other disorders of the bone marrow. In Isselbacher KJ, Adams RD, Braunvald E et al (eds): Principles of Internal Medicine, 9th ed. New York, McGraw-Hill, 1980
23. Suda T, Omine M, Tsuchija J et al: Prognostic aspects of aplastic anemia in pregnancy. Blut 36:285, 1978
24. Hurd W, Meodovnik M, Step S: Pregnancy associated with paroxysmal nocturnal hemoglobinuria. Obstet Gynecol 60:742, 1982

Clotting Disorders

Edgar O. Horger III

Major changes occur in the blood coagulation system during pregnancy. These changes are designed teleologically to increase the coagulability of blood, but either genetic abnormality or systemic illness may prevent this normal adaptation. Pregnancy may occur in patients with congenital or acquired platelet disorders and defects in blood coagulation factors. Some complications of pregnancy may be responsible for clotting disorders.

This section discusses briefly the maintenance of hemostasis and the effects of pregnancy on this physiology, presents a simple evaluation of abnormal hemostasis during pregnancy, and discusses several of the disorders of coagulation and their associations with pregnancy.

HEMOSTASIS

Hemostasis is the term applied to the arrest of blood flow. It is dependent on a complex interrelationship of vascular integrity, platelet function, and plasma clotting factors. The initial response to vascular injury is contraction of the damaged blood vessel. Platelets adhere to the collagen fibrils exposed by endothelial damage in an effort to seal the vessel injury with a hemostatic plug. Platelet degranulation releases compounds that promote further platelet aggregation, and a self-perpetuating phenomenon is established. A lipoprotein component of the platelet membrane, platelet factor 3 (PF3), initiates generation of a fibrin clot from the plasma clotting factors.

The basic principle of coagulation involves the conversion of circulating plasma fibrinogen into a stable fibrin clot. This conversion involves a linked sequence of activation of inert clotting factors into enzymes, which then convert the clotting factors next in line into active enzymatic forms by a "cascade mechanism" (Fig. 30-2). The end result of this cascade may be reached by either of two pathways, which are termed *extrinsic* or *intrinsic* according to whether the changes are initiated outside or inside the vasculature. The extrinsic pathway is activated by tissue thromboplastin liberated from injured or necrotic tissue. Thromboplastin and calcium activate factor VII, which then activates factor X. Activated factor X enters the common pathway to convert prothrombin into thrombin. The intrinsic pathway is so named because tissue thromboplastin is not required; coagulation results entirely from plasma factors. The intrinsic pathway appears to begin with platelet aggregation and activation of PF3. Activation of factor XII then starts the complex cascade that ultimately activates factor X for entry into the common pathway and production of thrombin.

Thrombin enzymatically splits fibrinogen into soluble monomers that link to form insoluble but fragile fibrin polymers. The final step of stabilization is mediated by factor XIII and forms the stable fibrin clot.

FIBRINOLYSIS

The onset of coagulation also activates a system of clot lysis. Fibrin strands adsorb circulating plasminogen, which is hydrolyzed to produce plasmin, the enzymatic principle of the fibrinolytic system. Plasmin then digests the fibrin clot from within.

Clot lysis liberates fibrin degradation products (FDP), which have antihemostatic effects on platelets, thrombin, and fibrin polymerization. Other checks and balances on coagulation and fibrinolysis include the ability of plasmin to hydrolyze factors V and VIIIC and plasmin inactivators such as α_2-antiplasmin, α_2-macro-globulin, and antithrombin. The dynamic equilibrium produced allows appropriate fibrin clot formation along with rapid dissolution of microthrombi and removal of major clots in a manner that returns circulation to ischemic tissues.

EFFECTS OF PREGNANCY ON COAGULATION

Pregnancy causes significant changes in many coagulation factors (Table 30-10). There is no significant change in platelet counts during pregnancy, but some slight decrease may occur in the third trimester secondary to hemodilution and placental trapping. A marked increase in the platelet count of more than 100,000/mm^3 usually is noted by the third to fifth postpartum day.[1] All plasma coagulation factors except II, IV, XI, and XIII increase during pregnancy.[2] These changes lead to an increased ability to produce fibrin and a decreased ability to remove it—in summary, a hypercoagulable state.

EVALUATION OF ABNORMAL HEMOSTASIS

Screening for clotting disorders begins with a thorough medical history and careful physical examination. Easy bruising and bleeding problems beginning in infancy or early childhood suggest a congenital hemostatic defect, whereas symptoms beginning in adulthood indicate an acquired disorder. Many medications can cause bleeding problems, and a careful history of drug ingestion must be obtained.

No single test can screen patients for all bleeding disorders. However, a combination of three readily available laboratory tests can be very useful: platelet count, prothrombin time, and partial thromboplastin time (PTT).[3] Platelets may be counted directly or estimated with sufficient accuracy for screening from ex-

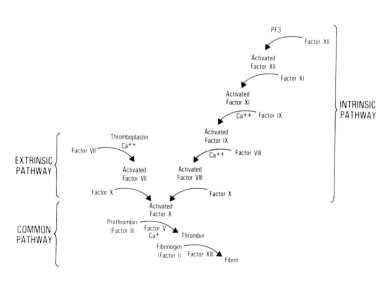

FIG. 30-2. Cascade mechanism of blood coagulation, showing activation of blood coagulation factors leading to production of fibrin. (Miller JM Jr., Horger EO III: Obstetric Hematology. In Wilds PL and Burdenell M [eds]: Medical and Surgical Problems in Pregnancy. Bristol, John Wright & Sons, 1984)

Table 30-10
Coagulation Factors and Changes During Pregnancy

Factor	Nonpregnant	Late Pregnancy
I Fibrinogen	200 mg/dl–400 mg/dl	350 mg/dl–650 mg/dl
II Prothrombin	75%–125%	100%–125%
III Thromboplastin	Unable to measure	Unable to measure
IV Calcium ions	4.7 mg/dl–5.5 mg/dl	4.7 mg/dl–5.5 mg/dl
V Proaccelerin	75%–125%	100%–150%
VII Proconvertin	75%–125%	150%–250%
VIII Antihemophilic globulin	75%–125%	200%–500%
IX Plasma thromboplastin component	75%–125%	100%–150%
X Stuart–Prower factor	75%–125%	150%–250%
XI Plasma thromboplastin antecedent	75%–125%	50%–100%
XII Hageman factor	75%–125%	100%–200%
XIII Fibrin-stabilizing factor	75%–125%	35%–75%

(Horger EO III: Disorders of hemostasis. In Sciarra JJ (ed): Gynecology and Obstetrics. Hagerstown, Harper & Row, 1981)

amination of a peripheral blood smear; each platelet seen per oil immersion field suggests a count of about 20,000/mm.[3,4] The mean platelet count in the healthy adult is about 250,000/mm.[3]

The prothrombin time averages 11 to 12 seconds in healthy persons. It is used to evaluate the extrinsic coagulation pathway and is prolonged if one or more of the factors in this pathway or in the common pathway (Fig. 30-2) fall below 30% of normal. The PTT normally averages 21 to 30 seconds and becomes prolonged if the plasma concentration of any coagulation factor other than factor VII falls below 30% of normal.[5]

Definitive assays can be performed for the various coagulation factors listed in Table 30-10. The most useful method for determining the presence and degree of fibrinolysis is measurement of fibrin breakdown products.

DISSEMINATED INTRAVASCULAR COAGULATION

Disseminated intravascular coagulation (DIC) is a clinical syndrome that implies widespread clotting within the blood vessels. In truth, widespread blood clots have been demonstrated only rarely. Clinical manifestations of DIC are variable and may include localized or generalized bleeding, petechiae and purpura, thrombotic and embolic phenomena, or complete absence of symptoms and only laboratory evidence of the coagulopathy.

DIC may develop as a complication of a vast array of disease processes and a variety of obstetric conditions. Activation of the coagulation mechanism may result from one or more of the following events: endothelial cell injury, exposure of plasma to collagen, and activation of the intrinsic pathway; release of thromboplastin from injured or necrotic tissue with activation of the extrinsic pathway; erythrocyte or platelet injury, with phospholipid release and activation of both intrinsic and extrinsic pathways. The clinical syndrome ultimately results from excess production of activated factor X and thrombin and concomitant decrease in circulating antithrombin III (AT III).[6] This uncontrolled activation of coagulation and accompanying fibrinolysis leads to depletion of platelets and clotting factors, with subsequent bleeding and further depletion.

The diagnosis of DIC is usually obvious. In acute and severe cases, however, shock or sepsis related to the underlying condition may be so pronounced that DIC is unsuspected and unrecognized. Simple laboratory tests will confirm DIC (Table 30-11). The most useful of these tests are the platelet count, fibrinogen concentration, and assessment of fibrinolysis by measurement of FDP.

DIC may be precipitated by many complications of pregnancy, including abruptio placentae, amniotic fluid embolism, preeclampsia–eclampsia, sepsis, saline-in-

Table 30-11
Laboratory Tests in DIC

Diagnostic Test	Abnormality
Platelets	Decreased
Fibrinogen	Decreased
Fibrin degradation products	Increased
Prothrombin time	Prolonged
Partial thromboplastin time	Prolonged
Thrombin clotting time	Prolonged
Factors V, VIII, X, XII, XIII	Decreased
Peripheral blood smear	Microangiopathic change

duced abortion, retained dead fetus, and hydatidiform mole. Each of these conditions involves liberation of thromboplastin or vascular endothelial damage. The initial retroplacental hemorrhage in abruptio placentae results in local tissue injury and thromboplastin release. DIC that accompanies retention of a dead fetus develops slowly and is caused by escape of thromboplastic substances from the degenerating conceptus. Endothelial damage may result from circulating endotoxin in septic shock or from intense segmental vasospasm in severe preeclampsia.

Since the primary management of all cases of DIC involves correction of the underlying cause, the pregnancy must be terminated as quickly as possible. In mild DIC, treatment other than delivery may not be needed. Severe DIC, however, may require cryoprecipitate or fresh-frozen plasma for replacement of the depleted clotting factors and AT III.[6] If the fibrinogen concentration is below 50 mg/dl, replacement therapy should be used to elevate the level above 100 mg/dl. One bag of cryoprecipitate is expected to increase plasma fibrinogen concentration by 2 mg to 5 mg/dl.[7]

Platelet transfusions are administered only when the patient has continued bleeding and significantly depressed platelet counts ($<20,000/mm^3$). Each unit of platelet concentrate will raise the platelet count by 7000 to $10,000/mm^3$,[8] and a level of $50,000/mm^3$ should be sought. Packed red blood cells may be transfused to correct anemia.

Heparin therapy has been recommended to inhibit coagulation activated by thromboplastin release. However, heparin anticoagulation is not recommended for the obstetric patient with DIC because the problem of DIC is short-lived and the depleted coagulants can be replaced, it may cause bleeding even if the DIC is corrected, and it may worsen bleeding in the presence of a disrupted vascular system.[7] DIC secondary to retained dead fetus may be an exception to this generalization. Significant depletion of clotting factors may develop over a period of weeks while the maternal vascular system remains intact, and no bleeding occurs. Heparin administration will halt this coagulopathy and allow clotting factors to rise prior to induction of labor or operative uterine evacuation.

Obstetric DIC usually improves promptly after delivery. If DIC worsens or does not improve within several hours, retained products of conception, sepsis, and liver disease must be considered.

PLATELET DISORDERS

Platelet counts below $100,000/mm^3$ represent thrombocytopenia. Spontaneous purpura seldom occurs with platelet counts greater than $30,000/mm^3$, and profuse bleeding is rare with counts above $50,000/mm^3$. Although pregnancy per se does not affect either platelet number of platelet function adversely, patients with congenital platelet abnormalities can become pregnant,

and acquired platelet disorders may appear before, during, or after pregnancy.

Immunologic thrombocytopenic purpura (ITP) is the most common form of thrombocytopenia diagnosed during pregnancy. The subject is discussed in Chapter 12.

Thrombotic Thrombocytopenic Purpura

The clinical syndrome of thrombotic thrombocytopenic purpura (TTP) is characterized by thrombocytopenia, microangiopathic hemolytic anemia, fluctuating neurologic manifestations, renal disease, and fever. The cause remains unknown and management is uncertain. When left untreated, TTP is almost invariably fatal; the long-term survival rate is only about 10%.[9] TTP during pregnancy has been reported only infrequently. Both maternal and perinatal mortality rates have been extremely high.[10]

Although thrombocytopenia is found in all cases of TTP and both hypofibrinogenemia and fibrin breakdown products have been found in some, other coagulation parameters are normal. The pathognomonic histologic feature is the widespread hyaline thrombi that occlude terminal arterioles and capillaries and occur most frequently in the heart, brain, kidneys, and pancreas. However, these characteristic thrombi are found in only about 50% of cases of TTP diagnosed clinically.[11] The basic defect appears to be platelet aggregation on injured vascular endothelium. Microangiopathic hemolytic anemia results from erythrocyte damage caused by collision with intraluminal thrombi in partially occluded smaller vessels. More complete vascular occlusion leads to ischemia and the characteristic neurologic and renal abnormalities.

Clinical similarities between TTP and severe preeclampsia suggest that many cases previously reported to be severe preeclampsia leading to maternal death actually may have been TTP.[12,13] Both TTP and the syndrome of hemolysis, elevated liver enzymes, and low platelet count (HELLP)[14] may represent extension of the pathophysiology operative in severe preeclampsia.

Management of TTP has included corticosteroids, heparin, urokinase, dextran, antiplatelet drugs, hemodialysis, and splenectomy, with only occasional remissions. Recent successes have been reported following whole blood exchange transfusions, exchange plasmapheresis, and plasma infusions.[11,15,16] A combination of plasma infusion or plasmapheresis and administration of antiplatelet agents such as dipyridamole and aspirin offers the most effective therapy.[11]

Management of TTP is not altered during pregnancy. The fetus has normal platelets and no evidence of coagulopathy, and delivery has no effect on the disorder. Nonetheless, because of the difficulty encountered in differentiating TTP from severe preeclampsia, when albuminuria and hypertension accompany thrombocytopenia in late pregnancy, prompt delivery seems advisable.

Preeclampsia

Thrombocytopenia is reported in 2.6% to 15.4% of patients with preeclampsia and in 9.1% to 29.5% of those with eclampsia.[17-19] Additional coagulation abnormalities have been reported inconsistently by various investigators. Preeclampsia is a microangiopathic disorder very similar to that described in TTP. Segmental vasospasm causes vascular endothelial damage, with subsequent platelet adhesion. A decrease in platelet number may be the first detectable abnormality in women who later develop preeclampsia.[20] The degree of thrombocytopenia correlates directly with the severity of preeclampsia. Some reports have emphasized that thrombocytopenia indicates a need for delivery despite the clinical appearance of control of the preeclampsia.[21-23]

Drug-Induced Platelet Disorders

Maternal drug administration may affect platelets both quantitatively and qualitatively. A partial listing of drugs that induce platelet disorders appears in Table 30-12. Fetal and neonatal platelets often are more susceptible to these agents than are those of the mother.

Thrombocytopenia may be induced by toxic suppression of bone marrow megakaryocytes, immunologic destruction of platelets, or a combination of these mechanisms. Acetylsalicylic acid (aspirin) is the most widely used drug that affects platelet function.

Table 30-12
Drug-Induced Platelet Disorders

Drug	Thrombo-cytopenia	Thrombo-pathia
Acetylsalicylic acid		+
Antibacterial agents		
Penicillin, carbenicillin	+	+
Cephalothin, cefamandole	+	
Sulfonamides	+	
Isoniazid	+	
Antihistamines		+
Anti-inflammatory nonsteroids	+	+
Barbiturates	+	
Diazepam		+
Digitalis	+	
Ethanol	+	+
Glyceryl guaiacolate		+
Heparin	+	+
Methyldopa	+	
Morphine, heroin	+	
Phenothiazine	+	+
Propranolol		+
Thiazide	+	

+, present.

Since aspirin combines irreversibly with platelets, a single 300-mg dose can impair platelet aggregation in both mother and fetus for seven to ten days.[24] Under normal circumstances, the effect of aspirin and similar thrombopathic agents is of minimal clinical significance. However, drug-induced platelet dysfunction may become clinically important to the obstetrician called upon to manage patients with other coagulation defects, those undergoing therapeutic or prophylactic anticoagulation therapy for phlebitis or valvular heart disease, and those experiencing difficult or traumatic deliveries.

Drug-induced platelet disorders logically require discontinuation of the offending agent. Glucocorticoid administration may be helpful in correcting thrombocytopenia after drug withdrawal but will have little effect on platelet dysfunction.[5] Since the thrombopathic effect of aspirin and similar agents is permanent and irreversible, correction of a prolonged bleeding time requires production of new platelets by the bone marrow.

HEREDITARY COAGULATION DEFECTS

Congenital disorders of coagulation characteristically involve a single coagulation factor that may be decreased quantitatively or altered functionally. Although more than 30 hereditary coagulopathies have been described, they are found infrequently. The absolute incidence in the general population is no greater than 1 in 10,000, and these disorders are seen even less frequently in obstetric patients. Pregnancy causes minimal or no alteration in the manifestations or management of these inherited defects. However, the more common of these disorders warrant some consideration.

Hemophilia A

Classic hemophilia (hemophilia A) is inherited as an X-linked recessive trait and is found almost exclusively in males. Although the affected male cannot transmit the disorder to his sons, each of his daughters will receive his X chromosome and be a carrier of hemophilia A. The carrier female then will transmit hemophilia to half of her sons and the carrier state to half of her daughters.

Hemophilia A has been reported in females only rarely.[25,26] Half of the daughters of a hemophilic male and a carrier female will be expected to have overt hemophilia. In addition, inactivation of the unaffected X chromosome in a carrier may result in dominance of the hemophilia gene on the intact X chromosome. Pregnancy has not been documented in a hemophiliac.

Plasma levels of factor-VIII coagulant activity (factor VIIIC) vary in hemophiliacs from 0% to 25% of normal.[27] Although the level of factor VIIIC cannot identify carriers of hemophilia A, the ratio between factor-VIIIC and factor-VIII–related antigen (factor VIII-RAg) may be very helpful.[28] Carrier identification allows selection of pregnancies for prenatal diagnostic studies.

Many hemophilia carriers have undergone amniocentesis for fetal sex determination. This technique can identify the male fetuses who have a 50% risk of hemophilia. More recently, pregnant carriers have undergone fetoscopy and aspiration of fetal blood. Assay for factor-VIII coagulant antigen (factor VIIIC Ag) has permitted successful identification of affected fetuses.[29]

Hemophilia B

Christmas disease (hemophilia B) is clinically indistinguishable from hemophilia A. It also is inherited as an X-linked recessive trait that causes extremely low or absent plasma levels of factor IX. Although pregnancy has not been reported in a patient with Christmas disease, carrier identification and counseling are important.

Von Willebrand's Disease

Von Willebrand's disease is inherited as an autosomal dominant trait. The disorder apparently involves several associated genetic defects, and gene penetrance and expressivity are highly variable. Decrease in the level of factor VIII-RAg parallels that of factor VIIIC in von Willebrand's disease, and both are undetectable in severe cases.[27]

Factor-VIIIC levels normally rise slowly during the first trimester of pregnancy, reach a plateau in the second trimester, and increase sharply near term.[27] Consequently, the hemorrhagic tendency in von Willebrand's disease usually improves during pregnancy. Perhaps the greatest pregnancy-associated risk is abortion or premature delivery before factor VIIIC has risen to a safe level.[30]

Replacement of factor VIIIC may be required in patients with von Willebrand's disease because of active bleeding, spontaneous or elective abortion, anticipation of cesarean section or other surgery, or failure of factor VIIIC to reach a satisfactory level prior to labor. In general, a factor-VIIIC plasma level of 60% or greater is associated with safe vaginal delivery. However, if cesarean section is necessary, a factor-VIIIC level of 100% should be achieved by replacement therapy.[30]

Cryoprecipitate contains most of the factor VIII of plasma and is recommended in the treatment of von Willebrand's disease. Since the liver cells of patients with von Willebrand's disease can synthesize factor VIIIC, infusion of small amounts of cryoprecipitate (1 bag/10 kg/day) will mobilize factor VIIIC from the liver and lead to much higher plasma levels than would be expected from the quantity infused.[5] Factor-VIIIC levels should be monitored for about seven days in postoperative and postpartum patients, and cryoprecipitate should be used to maintain a level of 25% or more.[31]

Acquired Factor-VIII Inhibitors

Severe coagulopathy secondary to an antibody that inhibits factor VIIIC has been reported in postpartum patients and patients with immunologic disorders such as systemic lupus erythematosus. Spontaneous remission usually occurs within a few months to several years, but deaths due to postpartum hemorrhage have been reported. While corticosteroids and immunosuppressives have been used in the management of this disorder, cryoprecipitate offers the most effective treatment. Subsequent pregnancies in those patients in remission have not caused reappearance of the inhibitor.

REFERENCES AND RECOMMENDED READING

1. Ygge I: Changes in blood coagulation and fibrinolysis during the puerperium. Am J Obstet Gynecol 104:2, 1969
2. Laros RK Jr., Alger LS: Thromboembolism and pregnancy. Clin Obstet Gynecol 22:871, 1979
3. Horger EO III, Keane MWD: Platelet disorders in pregnancy. Clin Obstet Gynecol 22:843, 1979
4. Kitay DZ: Purpura: Significance and management of the ITP and TTP syndromes. Contemp Obstet Gynecol 2:65, 1973
5. Moake JL, Funicella T: Common bleeding problems. Clinical Symposia 35:1, 1983
6. Rosenberg RD: The function of heparin. In Kalshar UU, Thomas DP (ed): Heparin: Chemistry and Clinical Usage, p 101. London, Academic Press, 1976
7. Talbert LM, Blatt PM: Disseminated intravascular coagulation in obstetrics. Clin Obstet Gynecol 22:889, 1979
8. Angiulo JP, Temple JT, Corrigan JJ et al: Management of cesarean section in a patient with idiopathic thrombocytopenic purpura. Anesthesiology 46:145, 1977
9. Cuttner J: Splenectomy, steroids, and Dextran-70 in thrombotic thrombocytopenic purpura. JAMA 227:397, 1974
10. May HV Jr., Harbert GM Jr., Thornton WN Jr.: Thrombotic thrombocytopenic purpura associated with pregnancy. Am J Obstet Gynecol 126:452, 1976
11. Myers TJ, Waken CJ, Ball ED et al: Thrombotic thrombocytopenic purpura: Combined treatment with plasmapheresis and antiplatelet agents. Ann Intern Med 92:149, 1980
12. Schwartz ML, Brenner WE: The obfuscation of eclampsia by thrombotic thrombocytopenic purpura. Am J Obstet Gynecol 131:18, 1978
13. Thiagarajah S, Harbert GM Jr., Caudle MR et al: Thrombotic thrombocytopenic purpura in pregnancy: A reappraisal. Am J Obstet Gynecol 141:20, 1981
14. Weinstein L: Syndrome of hemolysis, elevated liver enzymes, and low platelet count: A severe consequence of hypertension in pregnancy. Am J Obstet Gynecol 142:159, 1982
15. Bukowski RM, King JW, Hewlett JS: Plasmapheresis in the treatment of thrombotic thrombocytopenic purpura. Blood 50:413, 1977
16. Byrnes JJ, Khurana M: Treatment of thrombotic thrombocytopenic purpura with plasma. N Engl J Med 297:1386, 1977
17. Giles C: Intravascular coagulation in gestational hyperten-

sion and pre-eclampsia: The value of haematological screening tests. Clin Lab Haematol 4:351, 1982

18. Pritchard JA, Cunningham FG, Mason RA: Coagulation changes in eclampsia: Their frequency and pathogenesis. Am J Obstet Gynecol 124:855, 1976
19. Roberts JM, May WJ: Consumptive coagulopathy in severe pre-eclampsia. Obstet Gynecol 48:163, 1976
20. Redman CWG, Bonnar J, Beilin LJ: Early platelet consumption in pre-eclampsia. Br Med J 1:467, 1978
21. Goodlin R: Severe pre-eclampsia: Another great imitator. Am J Obstet Gynecol 125:747, 1976
22. Schwartz ML, Brenner WE: Pregnancy-induced hypertension presenting with life-threatening hemorrhage. Am J Obstet Gynecol 146:756, 1983
23. Trudinger BJ: Platelets and intrauterine growth retardation in pre-eclampsia. Br J Obstet Gynaecol 83:284, 1976
24. Weiss H, Aledort L: Impaired platelet/connective tissue reaction in man after aspirin ingestion. Lancet 2:495, 1967
25. Gilchrist GS, Hammond D, Melnyk J: Hemophilia A in a phenotypically normal female with XX/XO mosaicism. N Engl J Med 273:1402, 1965
26. Whissell DY, Hoag MS, Aggeler PM et al: Hemophilia A in a woman. Am J Med 38:119, 1965
27. Bloom AL, Peake IR: Molecular genetics of factor VIII and its disorders. Semin Hematol 14:319, 1977
28. Telfer MC, Chediak J: Factor VIII-related disorders and their relationship to pregnancy. J Reprod Med 19:211, 1977
29. Firschein SI, Hoyer LW, Lazarchick J et al: Prenatal diagnosis of classic hemophilia. N Engl J Med 300:937, 1979
30. Gorosky J, Klatsky A, Nobert GF et al: Von Willebrand's disease complicating second trimester abortion. Obstet Gynecol 55:253, 1980
31. Noller KL, Bowie EJW, Kempere RD et al: Von Willebrand's disease in pregnancy. Obstet Gynecol 41:865, 1973

Dermatologic Disorders

David N. Danforth
Stanley E. Huff

The normal integumentary response to pregnancy, mentioned in Chapter 18, includes the pigmentary changes (chloasma, linea nigra, and the increased pigmentation of normally pigmented areas) and the striae gravidarum (most pronounced over the abdomen, breasts, and hips). A third pregnancy response, palmar erythema, is also extremely common, asymptomatic, and of unknown cause; it usually clears after delivery. Vascular spiders and other cutaneous vascular reactions to pregnancy have been mentioned previously. In addition to these common and more or less trivial problems, certain other diseases of the skin, which are relatively rare and in some cases extremely serious, can result directly from pregnancy.

HAIR

During pregnancy there is a lengthening of the normal anagen (growing) hair phase. After delivery, the telogen follicles are converted to club (shedding) hairs; this may result in hair loss, especially in the frontal area, that is maximal two to four months after delivery; by six months postpartum the density of scalp hair should return to normal. Prolonged hair loss calls for an endocrine investigation or a search for a causative drug (*e.g.,* oral contraceptive).

GENERALIZED PRURITUS

Generalized pruritus is an uncommon disorder of the skin in pregnancy. Although it can be agonizing at times, it abates after delivery. There are no objective findings, except for the excoriations that may result from scratching. Speculation about its cause has not been rewarding, with the possible exception of the finding that many of the patients suffering from generalized pruritus have elevated serum bile acid values, and urobilin, urobilinogen, and bilirubin in the urine. These findings suggest that the pruritus is related to some hepatic disorder of pregnancy. Some suggest that this represents a mild form of intrahepatic cholestasis. A diet that is low in fat and high in protein and vitamins is believed to be helpful, along with antihistamines and added calcium. Sedatives, antipruritic lotions and sprays, and general supportive measures are needed in severe cases.

CUTANEOUS TAGS (MOLLUSCUM FIBROSUM GRAVIDARUM)

Skin tags, either pedunculated or sessile, are quite common in pregnancy and are most frequently found on the neck and upper chest. They are not inflammatory and evidently result from epithelial hyperplasia. The tags are removed by cautery or by excision.

PRURIGO GESTATIONIS

Prurigo gestationis is a skin eruption peculiar to pregnancy. It is characterized by small, highly pruritic papules, which are usually covered by bloody crusts that result from scratching. The papules are located especially on the extensor surfaces of the extremities, on the abdomen, and on the thorax. The condition clears spontaneously after delivery, leaving small areas of hyperpigmentation. Antipruritic sprays; oatmeal baths; oral antihistamines; ointments, creams and lotions; sedatives; and general supportive measures may all be helpful. The fetus is not affected.

PAPULAR DERMATITIS OF PREGNANCY

Papular dermatitis of pregnancy is not only incapacitating, but also has most serious implications for the fetus. It is a generalized eruption of intensely pruritic papules, usually covered by bloody crusts. Its generalized distribution and the extremely high levels of urinary hCG distinguish it from prurigo gestationis. The stillbirth rate in cases of papular dermatitis is high. The eruption clears after delivery and recurs in subsequent pregnancies. Corticosteroids may be helpful in treating this disease.

AUTOIMMUNE PROGESTERONE DERMATITIS OF PREGNANCY

Autoimmune progesterone dermatitis of pregnancy was described by Bierman in 1973. It is characterized by a severe acneiform eruption consisting of comedones, papules, pustules, and erosions with residual hyperpigmentation. Biopsies show histologic evidence of eosinophilic dermatitis and panniculitis. The disease is accompanied by profound peripheral eosinophilia (50%), hyperglobulinemia, and transient arthritis. It is reported to occur in the first trimester of pregnancy and to be associated with spontaneous abortion. Bierman suggests that the cause of this unusual disorder is related to hormone-dependent mechanisms, probaby because of cell-mediated immunity against endogenous progesterone produced during pregnancy. There is some evidence to support the thesis that progesterone hypersensitivity causes this disease, but several important questions remain unanswered.

HERPES GESTATIONIS (PEMPHIGOID GESTATIONIS)

This serious and debilitating autoimmune dermatitis is unique to pregnancy. It is characterized by generalized pruritus, followed shortly by the appearance of erythematous papules, plaques, and vesicobullous lesions about the umbilicus, which spread gradually over the entire body. Confluence of the vesicles leads to the formation of bullae, which may contain clear fluid, pus, or blood. Severe local burning, a febrile constitutional response, and eosinophilia up to 50% are characteristic. The outlook for the mother is good, except for the areas of pigmentation that may remain after the disease terminates. The symptoms may clear within a few days of delivery or, in unusual cases, may continue for extended periods. Exacerbation within three days of delivery may be an important characteristic, since it is reported to occur in a majority of cases. The disease can now be verified by immunofluorescent demonstration of complement and occasionally immunoglobulin G (IgG) in a linear deposition along the basement membranes of involved areas of the skin. Herpes gestationis recurs in subsequent pregnancies.

Management consists of supportive measures and local antibiotics to prevent infection. Systemic corticosteroids usually suppress the systemic manifestations, but Carruthers suggests that they may prolong the disease and hence should be used with "some reluctance." Termination of pregnancy may be considered in severe cases.

There is no agreement on the outlook for the fetus. Among 41 cases reported in two series, there was no increase in the rate of abortion, stillbirth, or fetal anomaly; the only fetal casualty was due to a therapeutic abortion. In other series of cases, the fetus has been shown to be at substantial risk of stillbirth, preterm delivery, and congenital disease. In the series of 28 cases by Shornick and colleagues, less than 5% of infants had cutaneous lesions, and no other unfavorable fetal complications were apparent. These researchers suggest that the high fetal morbidity in some series may result from the tendency to report "worst cases."

IMPETIGO HERPETIFORMIS

Impetigo herpetiformis is a rare, extremely serious inflammatory dermatitis of pregnancy that in some respects resembles pemphigus vulgaris. The disease can occur at any stage of pregnancy or the puerperium. Early reports suggested a mortality of 70% to 80%, but maternal death from this cause is now unusual. The primary lesion is a pustule from which no organisms can be cultured. The pustules, which are surrounded by a zone of erythema, coalesce to form large, oozing, crusted lesions of generalized distribution. Usually the genitocrural areas are most seriously affected. Itching is not a prominent symptom, but the systemic reaction is profound, including prostration, fever, leukocytosis, tachycardia, vomiting, and electrolyte imbalance. No organisms can be cultured from blood samples. The cause is unknown, and there is no specific therapy. Its special severity in pregnancy suggests that the conceptus may impose an added insult or, indeed, may precipitate the disease. Some studies suggest that the outlook for the fetus is poor, but, in any case, meticulous fetal surveillance is necessary. Delivery is advised as soon as there is evidence of pulmonary maturity. Topical and systemic corticosteroids have been used with benefit in some cases. Antibiotics may prevent secondary infection of the open lesions. The disease recurs with greater fury in subsequent pregnancies, and positive steps (e.g., sterilization) should be taken to prevent further pregnancy in those who have had the disease.

PRURITIC URTICARIAL PAPULES AND PLAQUES OF PREGNANCY (PUPPP)

This disease, which appears to be specific to pregnancy, was described by Lawley in 1979. Evidently, it is the same disease that was described by Spangler in 1962 and by Rahbari in 1978, and it probably occurs more frequently than the few reports suggest. The disease appears in the last trimester of pregnancy and is characterized by the eruption of red papules that change to small urticarial plaques. The eruptions begin on the abdomen and often spread to the thighs. In some cases the buttocks and arms are affected; facial lesions have not been reported, and the trunk is rarely affected above the umbilicus. No maternal or fetal mortality has been reported, but the question of nonlethal fetal effects is unsettled. However, the probable frequency of the disease suggests that if a cause-and-effect relationship exists, it would be noted in the literature. The disease responds promptly to topical corticosteroids and clears after delivery.

TELANGIECTASIA

Areas of capillary dilation about the ankles and less commonly on the thighs are common in pregnancy. They are related to varices and are sometimes confluent, producing raised, often disfiguring but rarely painful lesions for which there is no effective treatment except pressure bandages in extreme cases. They usually subside to an extent, but not completely, after delivery. Vascular spiders are extremely common in pregnancy. They are characterized by a bright red, punctate central point with branching hair-thin radials 1 to 2 mm in length. They are commonly found on the face, neck, arms, and upper part of the chest; usually, but not always, they clear after delivery.

The cause of telangiectasia and its variants is unknown, except as part of the general vascular response to pregnancy. There is nothing tangible to support the repeated allegation that high estrogen levels are responsible.

REFERENCES AND RECOMMENDED READING

Bierman SM: Autoimmune progesterone dermatitis of pregnancy. Arch Dermatol 107:896, 1973

Carruthers JA: Herpes gestationis: Clinical features of immunologically proved cases. Am J Obstet Gynecol 131:865, 1978

Heikkinen J, Mäentausta O, Ylöstalo P et al: Changes in serum bile acid concentrations during pregnancy, in patients with intrahepatic cholestasis of pregnancy and in pregnant women with itching. Brit J Obstet Gynaecol 88:240, 1981

Holmes RC, Black MM: The fetal prognosis in pemphigoid gestationis (Herpes gestationis). Br J Dermatol 110:67, 1984

Lawley TJ, Hertz KC, Wade TR et al: Pruritic urticarial papules and plaques of pregnancy. JAMA 241:1695, 1979

Lookingbill DP, Chez RA: Herpes gestationis. Clin Obstet Gynecol 26:605, 1983

Noguera J, Morena A, Moragas JM: Pruritic urticarial papules and plaques of pregnancy (PUPPP). Acta Derm Venereol 63:35, 1983

Rahbari H: Pruritic papules of pregnancy. J Cutan Pathol 5:347, 1978

Rogers PE, Katz S, Jordan W et al: Dermatoses and pregnancy. Hospital Med, January 1972

Ross MG, Tucker DC, Hayashi RH: Impetigo herpetiformis as a cause of postpartum fever. Obstet Gynecol 64:49S, 1984

Shornick JK, Bangert JL, Freeman RG et al: Herpes gestationis: Clinical and histologic features of twenty-eight cases. J Am Acad Dermatol 8:214, 1983

Spangler AS, Reddy W, Bardawill WC et al: Papular dermatitis of pregnancy. JAMA 181:577, 1962

Wade TR, Wade SL, Jones HE: Skin changes and diseases associated with pregnancy. Obstet Gynecol 52:233, 1978

Diabetes Mellitus

Steven G. Gabbe

The prognosis for the 2% to 3% of pregnancies that are complicated by diabetes mellitus has improved remarkably. This success may be attributed, in part, to a better understanding of the changes in maternal metabolism that alter fetal growth and development. Several maternal adaptations are made to provide the fetus with an uninterrupted supply of fuel. Pregnancy is characterized by maternal hyperinsulinemia associated with insulin resistance, changes that are most marked late in gestation (Table 30-13). Estrogen and progesterone directly alter maternal islet cell function, producing β-cell hyperplasia and hyperinsulinemia. Placental syncytiotrophoblast is the source of human placental lactogen (hPL), a growth hormone–like glycoprotein that produces insulin resistance and augments maternal lipolysis. Therefore, there is an accelerated progression of maternal ketosis. With increased maternal utilization of fats for energy, glucose is spared for fetal consumption. Levels of hPL are directly related to placental mass, increasing the "diabetogenic stress" as pregnancy pro-

Table 30-13
Metabolism in Pregnancy

	Early	*Late*
Fasting glucose	↓	↓
Free fatty acids	Normal	↑
Triglycerides	↑	↑↑↑
Fasting insulin	↑	↑↑
Postprandial insulin	↑	↑↑↑

↓, decreased; ↑, increased; ↑↑, moderately increased; ↑↑↑, greatly increased.

(Adapted from Kalkhoff RK et al: Semin Perinatol 2:291, 1978)

gresses. Other hormones that also produce this state of insulin resistance include free cortisol and possibly prolactin.

PERINATAL MORBIDITY AND MORTALITY

Maternal glucose crosses the placenta by carrier-mediated facilitated diffusion. In normal pregnancies, maternal plasma glucose levels rarely exceed 100 mg/dl with excursions between fasting levels of 60 mg/dl and postprandial levels of 120 mg/dl. Mean plasma glucose concentration during the third trimester is 86 mg/dl. Insulin does not cross the placenta, however, and although the fetus receives a continuous supply of maternal glucose, it is not affected by maternal insulin. In the pregnancy complicated by diabetes, periods of maternal hyperglycemia produce fetal hyperglycemia. Elevated levels of glucose then stimulate the fetal pancreas, resulting in fetal β-cell hyperplasia and hyperinsulinemia. This combination of fetal hyperglycemia and hyperinsulinemia contributes to much of the morbidity and mortality observed in the infant of the diabetic mother (Fig. 30-3).

Insulin is an important fetal growth hormone. Cord blood and amniotic fluid levels of C-peptide reflect endogenous insulin secretion and correlate well with birth weight. The combination of fetal hyperglycemia and hyperinsulinemia results in excessive fetal growth. Fetal macrosomatia has been associated with a significant incidence of traumatic complications during vaginal delivery, including perinatal asphyxia and injuries to the brachial plexus.

After 36 weeks' gestation, the frequency of fetal deaths in pregnancies complicated by diabetes is increased tenfold. Although the cause of these intrauterine deaths remains unknown, fetal hyperglycemia and hyperinsulinemia probably play important roles. Insulin infusions in fetal sheep increase the oxidative metabolism of glucose and reduce fetal arterial oxygen content. Patients who are poorly controlled, who have suffered a prior stillbirth, and who have pregnancy-induced hypertension and/or vasculopathy are also at greater than normal risk of intrauterine death.

In the past, obstetricians terminated the pregnancies of diabetic patients between 35 and 38 weeks' gestation to prevent these fetal losses. However, premature delivery may result in increased morbidity and mortality from the respiratory distress syndrome. Robert and co-workers demonstrated that at any gestational age, the infant of the diabetic is 5 to 6 times more likely to develop respiratory distress syndrome. Smith has found that fetal hyperinsulinemia impairs cortisol-stimulated lung surfactant synthesis *in vitro*.

Improved understanding of maternal metabolism and of the need to carefully regulate maternal glycemia as well as reliable techniques for fetal surveillance and improved neonatal care have markedly reduced perinatal mortality arising from intrauterine deaths, trauma, and respiratory distress syndrome. At present, the most important cause of perinatal loss in pregnancies complicated by insulin-dependent diabetes is a fatal congenital malformation. The frequency of major malformations reported in offspring of insulin-dependent diabetic patients is 6% to 8%, a rate 2 to 3 times higher than that observed in normal pregnancies. The caudal regression syndrome and cardiac, renal, and central nervous system anomalies are most common. Such malformations develop during the first seven weeks of embryogenesis, long before most diabetic patients seek prenatal care.

There is increasing evidence that these anomalies, which today account for 30% to 50% of all deaths in infants of diabetic mothers, may be attributed to inadequate control of maternal diabetes during the early weeks of pregnancy. Levels of hemoglobin A_{1C}, a glycosylated hemoglobin, reflect glycemic control in previous weeks and months. The incidence of major anomalies is significantly higher in pregnancies of diabetic mothers who have elevated hemoglobin A_{1C} concentrations during the first trimester. Fuhrmann and colleagues have reported that the incidence of major anomalies in offspring of insulin-dependent diabetic women who achieve physiologic glucose control during the early weeks of pregnancy is reduced to that observed in normal pregnancies.

After delivery, considerable neonatal morbidity has been reported in the offspring of diabetic women. The characteristic triad of hypoglycemia, hypocalcemia, and hyperbilirubinemia may be seen in as many as 25% of these babies. Infants of diabetic mothers may exhibit a cardiomyopathy associated with septal hypertrophy, polycythemia with hyperviscosity, and the small left colon syndrome. The incidence of subsequent insulin-dependent diabetes in the infants of those women who themselves have insulin-dependent diabetes is approximately 1.5%.

MATERNAL MORBIDITY AND MORTALITY

Patients with vasculopathy or unstable diabetes are at greatest risk of complications and death during pregnancy. Pregnancy does not shorten the life expectancy

FIG. 30-3. Possible fetal consequences of maternal hypoglycemia.

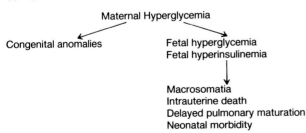

of women with diabetes. While maternal deaths are rare, women with diabetes who have coronary artery disease are at increased risk of dying. Pregnancy does not produce a permanent deterioration of renal function in women with diabetic nephropathy. However, there remains uncertainty concerning the course of diabetic retinopathy during gestation. Benign retinopathy may worsen as pregnancy advances but usually regresses after delivery. Women with proliferative retinopathy that has not been treated with laser therapy before pregnancy appear to be at greater risk for deterioration of vision.

The majority of maternal disorders observed in pregnancies complicated by diabetes can be attributed to the changes in maternal metabolism that cause deterioration of glycemic control. Before the use of home glucose monitoring techniques, severe hypoglycemic reactions requiring hospitalization occurred in approximately 10% of insulin-dependent patients. Early in gestation, nausea and vomiting may necessitate a reduction in insulin dosage. After delivery, the contrainsulin effects of hPL are lost, and hypoglycemia may again result. Ketoacidosis usually occurs during the second and third trimesters, when the "diabetogenic stress" of pregnancy is greatest. A viral illness or urinary tract infection is often the precipitating cause. The recently diagnosed diabetic is most likely to develop ketoacidosis in pregnancy because she fails to recognize its symptoms.

DETECTION OF DIABETES IN PREGNANCY

Gestational diabetes has been characterized as a state restricted to pregnant women in whom diabetes or impaired glucose tolerance begins or is first recognized during pregnancy. It constitutes 90% of all diabetes in pregnancy, occurring in approximately 30,000 to 90,000 women in the United States each year. Patients with gestational diabetes exhibit postprandial hyperglycemia and may demonstrate insulin resistance or abnormalities in the timing or amount of insulin secreted.

The diagnosis of gestational diabetes is made using a 100-g oral glucose tolerance test (oral GTT). A well-organized screening program should be established to detect carbohydrate intolerance in pregnancy (Table 30-14). In the past, screening was based on recognized historical or clinical clues, including a family history of diabetes; delivery of a macrosomatic infant, an infant with a malformation, or an unexplained stillborn; obesity; hypertension; or glycosuria. However, screening patients by such means is inadequate, since up to 50% of women who go on to develop gestational diabetes fail to manifest these clues. It is now recommended that all pregnant patients be screened for gestational diabetes at 24 to 28 weeks' gestation. The patient may be given a 50-g oral glucose load followed by a glucose determination 1 hour later (Table 30-14). This screening test has a sensitivity of 79% and a specificity of 87% when compared with subsequent glucose tolerance test results.

Table 30-14
Detection of Diabetes in Pregnancy (Upper Limits of Normal)

	Whole Blood (mg/dl)	Plasma (mg/dl)
Screening Test*		
50 g, 1 hr	130	140
Oral GTT†		
Fasting	90	105
1 hr	165	190
2 hr	145	165
3 hr	125	145

* Patients are not required to be in a fasting state to take the screening test. An abnormal screening test is followed by an oral GTT.

† The diagnosis of gestational diabetes is made when any two values are exceeded.

Approximately 10% to 15% of all gestational diabetics demonstrate significant fasting (>105 mg/dl plasma) or postprandial (>120 mg/dl plasma) hyperglycemia and require a program of care identical to that utilized for the pregestational diabetic. Patients who have been diagnosed as gestational diabetics should not subsequently receive oral contraceptive agents, since the hormones contained in these agents may produce the derangements in carbohydrate metabolism observed during pregnancy. Sterilization should be offered when the desired family size is achieved. As many as 35% to 50% of patients who exhibit gestational diabetes will show further deterioration of carbohydrate metabolism during the next 15 years of life.

RISK ASSESSMENT

A program of patient care may be best developed when the risks to the patient and her infant are first considered. The most widely applied risk assessment system has been that of Dr. Priscilla White. She observed that age at onset of diabetes, duration of the disorder, and the presence of maternal vascular disease—factors that could be determined before pregnancy—all have an important impact on pregnancy outcome (Table 30-15). In general, the earlier the onset of diabetes, the longer its duration, and the greater the degree of vasculopathy, the worse the prognosis in pregnancy. Maternal nephropathy has been associated with an increased risk of perinatal death, premature delivery, and fetal growth retardation. Of course, the quality of maternal glucose control must also be considered in assessing perinatal risk. Class-A diabetics, women who have gestational diabetes but maintain a normal fasting glucose, rarely experience an intrauterine death.

Pedersen noted that prognostically unfavorable signs of pregnancy, specifically ketoacidosis, pyelone-

Table 30-15
White's Classification of Diabetes in Pregnancy

Class	Age at Onset (yr)		Duration (yr)	Vascular Disease	Insulin
A	Any		Any	None	Diet only
B	>20		<10	None	+
C	10–19	or	10–19	None	+
D	<10	or	>20	Benign retinopathy	+
F	Any		Any	Nephropathy	+
R	Any		Any	Proliferative retinopathy	+
H	Any		Any	Heart disease	+

+, insulin required.

phritis, pregnancy-induced hypertension, and poor clinic attendance or neglect, are associated with an unfavorable outcome.

MANAGEMENT OF THE INSULIN-DEPENDENT PATIENT

Care of the insulin-dependent patient must begin before gestation. The patient should be assessed as to her suitability for pregnancy. Does she have proliferative retinopathy, nephropathy, or hypertension? The patient and her family should be advised of the financial demands of pregnancy and a program of contraception established.

Maternal glucose levels that duplicate those seen in normal pregnancies should be the therapeutic objective in pregnancies complicated by diabetes mellitus. Perinatal mortality rates of 30 to 50:1000 have been observed when maternal fasting plasma glucose levels are maintained between 100 mg and 150 mg/dl. However, the incidence of neonatal macrosomatia and hypoglycemia observed with this degree of control is unacceptably high. If physiologic glucose levels are achieved, the occurrence of macrosomia and neonatal morbidity can be reduced significantly. With increasing evidence that congenital malformations are related to poor control during early embryogenesis, insulin-dependent patients should be in optimum control at the time of conception and throughout the first trimester of pregnancy.

Maintenance of physiologic glucose levels in the pregnant insulin-dependent diabetic usually requires two to three injections of insulin daily as well as careful adjustment of dietary intake. Most patients require a mixture of intermediate-acting (NPH) and rapid-acting (regular) insulin in the morning. As a general guideline, the amount of NPH exceeds that of regular by 2:1. In the evening, equal amounts of NPH and regular insulin are injected. Patients usually receive two thirds of their total insulin dose at breakfast and the remainder at dinner. In the past, control was assessed primarily by review of the results of double-voided urine specimens tested for glucose and acetone and by weekly surveys of a 24-hour glucose profile. The physiologic glycosuria of pregnancy limited the value of tests. Today, patients can accurately monitor their control by using glucose oxidase–impregnated strips with a color chart or a glucose reflectance meter. This outpatient approach enables patients to assess their control following their usual pattern of diet and exercise. Initially a profile of glucose levels in the fasting state, before lunch, dinner, and bedtime should be monitored each day. If these levels remain elevated, the corresponding insulin dose should be increased by 20%. Glycosylated hemoglobin determinations may be made at the patient's first visit to provide a rapid assessment of her prior diabetic regulation and repeated subsequently in each trimester.

Early in gestation, hospitalization may be required to assess diabetic control and educate the patient. The initial hospitalization also provides an opportunity to evaluate the patient's vascular status with an ophthalmologic consultation, determination of baseline creatinine clearance and protein excretion, and an electrocardiogram. An initial urine culture is also obtained and repeated every four to six weeks.

Caloric intake must be carefully coordinated with the patient's insulin regimen and exercise. The average diet for a pregnant insulin-dependent diabetic patient derives 20% of its calories from protein, 35% from fats, and 45% from carbohydrates. The average daily caloric intake will range from 2000 kcal to 2400 kcal. Twenty-five percent of the calories are provided with breakfast, 30% with lunch, 30% with dinner, and 15% with a bedtime snack. Some patients may require snacks in the midmorning or midafternoon as well. A total weight gain of 22 lb to 25 lb is desired.

The stable and compliant patient with diabetes mellitus may be followed as an outpatient with visits every one or two weeks. Deterioration of control or hypertension may necessitate hospitalization. If benign retinopathy has been detected early in gestation, repeat ophthalmologic examinations should be obtained in the second and third trimesters. Proliferative retinopathy requires more intensive follow-up. Renal function should be assessed with a determination of creatinine clearance and protein excretion in each trimester.

During the third trimester, when sudden intrauterine deaths are most likely to occur, a program of fetal surveillance is initiated. Insulin-dependent patients who maintain glucose levels within the physiologic range will exhibit a low incidence of antepartum fetal distress. In these cases, antepartum fetal testing enables the obstetrician to delay delivery safely and gain further fetal maturity. The contraction stress test (CST) has proven to be an extremely valuable tool for fetal evaluation. Many studies have demonstrated that in a metabolically stable diabetic patient, a negative CST predicts fetal survival for one week. Positive CSTs have been observed in approximately 10% of insulin-dependent diabetic patients and are more frequently associated with perinatal death, fetal distress during labor, and neonatal depression. However, the CST has a significant false-positive rate of up to 60%. Most recently, the nonstress test (NST) performed twice weekly has been used as a screening test in the assessment of the diabetic pregnancy. If the initial NST is nonreactive, a CST must then be undertaken. A simple and practical additional approach to the evaluation of fetal condition has been the mother's daily assessment of fetal activity. Ultrasonography has permitted the assessment of fetal growth as well as the detection of hydramnios. A baseline scan may be obtained at 16 to 18 weeks' gestation and repeated at four- to six-week intervals. Although daily estriol analyses were once widely applied to monitor fetal well-being, biophysical tests are performed more easily, are less expensive, and have proven more reliable.

If the patient has been maintained in excellent glycemic control and all parameters of antepartum surveillance remain normal, delivery should be delayed until fetal pulmonary maturation has been achieved. For the highest risk patients, those who have been in poor control, who have had a previous stillbirth, or who have not been compliant, delivery at 38 weeks' gestation should be undertaken if fetal pulmonary maturation can be confirmed with a lecithin/sphingomyelin (L/S) ratio of 2 or greater and the presence of the acidic phospholipid phosphatidylglycerol (PG). Elective cesarean section may be required if the cervix is not favorable for induction. For patients without vasculopathy who remain in excellent control, the obstetrician may await the onset of spontaneous labor. If the pregnant diabetic patient develops pregnancy-induced hypertension, progressive proliferative retinopathy, hydramnios, or evidence of fetal distress on antepartum fetal testing, delivery prior to 38 weeks' gestation may be indicated. The timing of any delivery must be coordinated with the neonatologists who are to be present. If adequate neonatal care cannot be provided, the pregnant diabetic should be transferred to a hospital with an appropriately equipped nursery.

During labor, electronic fetal heart rate monitoring is mandatory. Labor should be allowed to progress as long as cervical dilatation and descent follow the estab-

lished normal labor curve. Any evidence of an arrest pattern should alert the physician to the possibility of cephalopelvic disproportion and fetal macrosomatia.

The incidence of neonatal hypoglycemia can be related to the level of maternal glycemia maintained during labor as well as to the degree of antepartum control. A continuous intravenous infusion of both insulin and glucose has proven effective in controlling maternal glucose levels during labor and delivery. Ten units of regular insulin may be added to 1000 ml of 5% dextrose. For most patients, regardless of antepartum insulin requirements, this combination infused at 100 ml per hour (1 unit of insulin/hour) usually results in good glycemic control. Glucose levels should be monitored hourly using glucose oxidase–impregnated strips. If an elective cesarean section is planned, the patient is maintained NPO the night before delivery and her morning insulin dose withheld. After the operation has been completed, glucose levels should be monitored every two to four hours and an intravenous solution containing 5% dextrose continued. No insulin may be required for the remainder of the operative day.

MANAGEMENT OF THE PATIENT WITH GESTATIONAL DIABETES

Women with gestational diabetes are usually identified late in pregnancy. Once the diagnosis has been established by glucose tolerance testing, these patients are started on a dietary program of approximately 2000 kcal per day with the exclusion of simple sugars. Their fasting and postprandial glucose levels should be evaluated at 2-week intervals until delivery. If fasting plasma glucose levels reach 105 mg/dl and postprandial glucose values exceed 120 mg/dl, insulin treatment should be initiated.

Gestational diabetic patients may be safely followed until 40 weeks as long as fasting glucose levels remain normal. If labor cannot be induced at 40 weeks, fetal surveillance should be initiated with twice weekly NSTs. The risk of intrauterine death is greater in the gestational diabetic who has had a prior stillbirth or who develops pregnancy-induced hypertension. In such a patient, therefore, a program of fetal surveillance using twice weekly NSTs should be initiated at 34 weeks' gestation.

REFERENCES AND RECOMMENDED READING

Fuhrmann K, Reiher H, Semmler K et al: Prevention of congenital malformations in infants of insulin-dependent diabetic mothers. Diabetes Care 6:219, 1983

Gabbe SG: Management of diabetes in pregnancy: Six decades of experience. In Pitkin RM (ed): 1980 Yearbook of Obstetrics and Gynecology, pp 37–49. Chicago, Year Book Medical Publishers, 1980

Gabbe SG, Mestman JH, Freeman RK et al: Management and outcome of diabetes mellitus, Classes B-R. Am J Obstet Gynecol 129:723, 1977

Gabbe SG, Mestman JH, Freeman RK et al: Management and

outcome of Class A diabetes mellitus. Am J Obstet Gynecol 127:465, 1977

Golde SH, Montoro M, Good–Anderson B et al: The role of non-stress tests, fetal biophysical profile, and contraction stress tests in the out-patient management of insulin-requiring diabetic pregnancies. Am J Obstet Gynecol 148: 269, 1984

Jorge CS, Artal R, Paul RH et al: Antepartum fetal surveillance in diabetic patients. Am J Obstet Gynecol 141:641, 1981

Jovanovic L, Druzin M, Peterson CM: Effect of euglycemia on the outcome of pregnancy in insulin-dependent diabetic women as compared with normal control subjects. Am J Med 71:921, 1981

Kitzmiller JL, Brown ER, Phillippe M et al: Diabetic nephropathy and perinatal outcome. Am J Obstet Gynecol 141: 741, 1981

Kitzmiller JL, Cloherty JP, Younger MD et al: Diabetic pregnancy and perinatal morbidity. Am J Obstet Gynecol 131: 560, 1978

Lavin JP Jr, Lovelace DR, Miodovnik M et al: Clinical experience with one hundred seven diabetic pregnancies. Am J Obstet Gynecol 147:742, 1983

Miller E, Hare JW, Cloherty JP et al: Elevated maternal hemoglobin A_1 in early pregnancy and major congenital anomalies in infants of diabetic mothers. N Engl J Med 304:1331, 1981

Mills JL: Malformations in infants of diabetic mothers. Teratology 25:385, 1982

O'Sullivan JB, Mahan CM, Charles D et al: Screening criteria for high-risk gestational diabetic patients. Am J Obstet Gynecol 116:895, 1973

Robert MF, Neff RK, Hubbell JP et al: Maternal diabetes and the respiratory distress syndrome. N Engl J Med 294:357, 1976

Smith BT, Giroud CJP, Robert M et al: Insulin antagonism of cortisol action on lecithin synthesis by cultured fetal lung cells. J Pediatr 87:953, 1975

Steel JM, Johnstone FD, Smith AF et al: Five years' experience of a ''prepregnancy'' clinic for insulin-dependent diabetics. Br Med J 285:353, 1982

Varner MW: Efficacy of home glucose monitoring in diabetic pregnancy. Am J Med 75:592, 1983

Workshop: Conference on Gestational Diabetes. Diabetes. Diabetes Care 3:501, 1980

Viral and Protozoan Diseases

Mary Ann South
John L. Sever

Women are susceptible to the same infectious diseases during pregnancy as in the nonpregnant state. The specific adaptive immune response is intact during pregnancy, and cellular immunity and antibody production can be demonstrated for newly acquired as well as previously experienced antigens. In contrast, the inflammatory response is depressed, probably because of changes in the prostaglandin system. This depression creates an increased likelihood of clinically apparent and prolonged infection.

The pregnant woman who becomes infected with certain viral and protozoan agents may transmit the agent to her fetus. Regardless of the severity of maternal symptoms, the fetus can be seriously or even fatally damaged. Because of immaturity of the fetal defense systems, such agents are poorly limited and may produce a chronic active infectious state as well as teratogenic effects on the developing organ systems. Therefore, these viral and protozoan infections assume great importance in the daily practice of obstetrics.

Diagnosis of viral and protozoan infections has been aided by the development of laboratory techniques for the measurement of antibody titers. The so-called TORCHES titers, for *t*oxoplasma, *r*ubella, *c*ytomegalovirus, *h*erpes, and *s*yphilis, have become popular as a screening method for the newborn who has symptoms of a congenital infection. Comparison of these immunoglobulin G (IgG) antibody levels in the mother and newborn infant may be helpful, at least in ruling out the infections for which the antibody is absent. Definitive diagnosis can be made only by other means, such as measurement of specific antibody in the IgM class. In interpreting these tests, the clinician should be aware that in indirect and capture techniques a false-positive IgM antibody can be caused by the presence of rheumatoid factor, and a false-negative result can be produced by the concurrent presence of IgG antibody, which blocks the reaction. The laboratory performing the test must properly absorb the serum to give reliable results in these crucial obstetric situations.

VIRAL INFECTIONS

Rubella

Rubella is a common childhood disease that is almost always mild in the pregnant woman, but it is important because of the devastating effects of *in utero* infection, the congenital rubella syndrome (CRS). The last pandemic of rubella, in 1964, produced CRS in 20,000 to 30,000 infants in the United States and many more in other areas of the world.

Epidemiology

In the United States rubella has been controlled to a great degree by use of rubella vaccine. The vaccine has been widely distributed, and there has not been a problem with waning of immunity in the vaccinees in over 15 years of follow-up. In 1984, only four cases of congenital rubella were reported. However, 15% to 20% of women of childbearing age are still seronegative. They were already through their childhood immunization programs when rubella vaccine became available in 1969 or failed to become immune from the vaccine (rubella vaccine is effective in 95% to 98% of normal vaccinees) or are from areas in which there is no effective vaccine program (many of the developing nations).

Clinical Presentation and Diagnosis

The incubation period for rubella is 14 to 21 days. Asymptomatic rubella infection is common. When symptomatic, it produces an erythematous maculopapular rash with lymphadenopathy. Arthralgia and arthritis are common in adults. Diagnosis of rubella requires serologic confirmation, since several other viral infections mimic rubella closely. A fourfold or greater rise in IgG or the presence of IgM antirubella antibody indicates recent infection. The IgM remains positive for about a month after the rash appears. Reinfection in seropositive persons has been documented but has never produced either clinical illness in the mother or CRS in the offspring.

Effect on the Fetus

Incidence of fetal damage from rubella is dependent on the gestational age of the fetus when infection occurs. Shortly before conception and during the first eight weeks of gestation, there is a 70% incidence of transplacental transmission of rubella virus. Virtually every fetus infected at this stage will be defective, and there is an increased rate of spontaneous abortion. Between 9 and 20 weeks, the transplacental transmission rate decreases steadily to 20% to 30%. Since the period of organogenesis is over, the incidence and severity of fetal malformation among those infected fetuses also decrease. In the last half of pregnancy, very few defects occur. Deafness, the cardiac defect of peripheral pulmonary artery stenosis, and mental retardation can result from fetal infection at 20 to 30 weeks' gestation, but the incidence of this damage decreases progressively. No fetal damage has been reported from maternal rubella during the last ten weeks of gestation.

In addition to having teratogenic effects on the heart, eyes, hearing, and mental capabilities, CRS may cause hepatosplenomegaly, lymphadenopathy, thrombocytopenia, anemia, encephalitis, pneumonitis, and osteitis. These symptoms of active viral infection are often observed immediately at birth and can produce difficulty in resuscitation. All infants with CRS are infectious and should be treated as such while diagnostic procedures are carried out. The placenta and amniotic fluid also are infectious.

Delayed effects may appear in the survivors of CRS many years after the acute stage is over. The most common of these is insulin-dependent diabetes mellitus. As many as 40% of persons with CRS have clinical or latent diabetes by the time they reach their 20s. Abnormalities in thyroid function occur in about 5% of CRS survivors; both hypothyroid and hyperthyroid states may follow an autoimmune (Hashimoto's) thyroiditis. Arterial stenosis can occur with delayed onset and produce hypertension. Other late effects are sudden hearing loss, glaucoma, and the very rare "slow-virus" form of encephalitis known as *progressive rubella panencephalitis.*

Treatment and Prevention

There is no antiviral agent that is effective in treatment of rubella infection, and prevention of fetal infection is the only intervention. Each pregnant woman should have verifiable serologic evidence of immunity to rubella. If she is seronegative, she should receive rubella vaccine postpartum. Women who have received rubella vaccine after a past pregnancy should have a rubella titer repeated to check the effectiveness of the vaccine. Even women who were themselves victims of CRS need to have a rubella titer performed, since among these persons, 5% lose their antibody and again become susceptible to rubella infection.

Immunoglobulin prophylaxis will not prevent rubella viremia, nor will it prevent transplacental transmission of the virus. However, the severity of symptoms in the fetus is reduced somewhat by the early presence of antibody. If a seronegative pregnant woman is exposed to rubella and interruption of the pregnancy is contemplated, she should not be given γ-globulin prophylaxis, since the presence of the passive antibody will cloud the serologic diagnosis of rubella (Table 30-16). If interruption of pregnancy is not to be considered, she should be given γ-globulin in a dose of 20 ml intramuscularly as soon as possible after the exposure. She should not be given vaccine during the pregnancy, since the rubella vaccine strain can be transmitted transplacentally. However, an inadvertent rubella vaccination during pregnancy is not an indication for termination of the pregnancy, since the vaccine strain has never been associated with teratogenicity.

The Herpes Group of Viruses

Human herpesviruses include herpes simplex types 1 ("oral") and 2 ("genital"), cytomegalovirus (CMV), varicella–zoster virus (VZV), and Epstein–Barr virus (EBV). These viruses can cause disease in the pregnant woman and can be acquired transplacentally or perinatally by the fetus.

All the members of the herpes group have a unique capacity for persistence in a latent phase throughout the lifetime of the infected person. All induce antibody, but the antibody does not alter the viral persistence, as shown by the fact that reactivation can occur even in the presence of great quantities of circulating antibody. Compromise of cellular immunity seems to be the crucial factor for reactivation as well as for dissemination of herpes infection. Cellular immunity is crucial for control of all viral agents, however, so that such a compromise does not explain the peculiar propensity for

Table 30-16
Immunization Against Viruses During Pregnancy

Virus	Active Immunizing Agent	Passive Immunizing Agent	Indications for Use During Pregnancy and in Newborns	Immunization Schedule
Hepatitis A	None	Pooled immunoglobulin	Postexposure prophylaxis; infant or mother ill at delivery	Adult: 0.02 ml/kg IM Newborn: 0.5 ml
Hepatitis B	Inactivated component vaccine	Hepatitis B immune globulin (HBIG)	Postexposure prophylaxis	See Table 30-17
Influenza	Inactivated vaccines, types A and B	None	Only for pregnant patients who have serious underlying disease, as in general population	Consult with public health authorities for current year's recommendations
Measles	Live attenuated virus vaccine	Pooled immune globulins	Postexposure prophylaxis with Ig only; vaccine contraindicated until postpartum	0.25 ml/kg, up to 15 ml, IM; must be given within 6 days of exposure
Mumps	Live attenuated virus vaccine	None	Contraindicated	
Poliomyelitis	Live attenuated virus (OPV) and inactivated virus (IPV) vaccine	Pooled immune globulin	IPV: series for preparation of susceptible traveler to endemic area OPV: epidemic situation when immediate protection necessary, or as part of mass immunization program	IPV: 3 doses at 4- to 8-week intervals, fourth dose in 6–12 months OPV: one dose, immunize with IPV postpartum
Rabies	Killed virus vaccine (human diploid)	Rabies immune globulin (RIG)	Postexposure prophylaxis not altered by pregnancy; consult public health authorities	RIG 20 IU, ½ in site of bite, ½ IM plus five doses rabies vaccine, 1 ml IM, days 0, 3, 7, 14, 28
Rubella	Live attenuated virus vaccine	Pooled immune globulin does not prevent infection but may decrease severity of fetal damage	Vaccine contraindicated; immune globulin for exposed susceptible woman if interruption of pregnancy not considered	Immune globulin 20 ml IM; vaccine is part of postpartum care
Vaccinia (smallpox vaccine)	Live attenuated vaccinia may be acquired from vaccinated contact	Vaccinia immune globulin (VIG)	VIG for complications in mother or baby: disseminated vaccinia, keratitis, eczema vaccinatum	Contact International Health Program Office*
Varicella	None	Varicella–zoster immune globulin (VZIG)	Probably indicated for postexposure prophylaxis of known susceptible woman; definitely indicated for newborn of woman with onset of chickenpox 5 days before to 2 days after delivery	Consult Massachusetts Public Health Service, Biologic Laboratories†, or regional offices of American Red Cross
Yellow fever	Live attenuated virus vaccine	None	Contraindicated except if exposure unavoidable	Single dose

* Centers for Disease Control, Atlanta, GA 30333.
† 617-522-3700.

persistence and reactivation displayed by the herpes group. An explanation may be furnished by further studies of direct effects of herpes viruses on T-cell function during primary infection.

Herpes Simplex Types 1 and 2

EPIDEMIOLOGY AND CLINICAL PRESENTATION. Herpes lesions are produced by two distinct but closely related viruses, the herpes simplex viruses (HSV). Type 1 is the agent causing common cold sores and thus is often called *oral herpes*. Type 2, because it is commonly transmitted venereally and produces genital blisters, is known as *genital herpes*. Each can produce disease in the other locale, and each can result in the serious complications of herpes encephalitis, herpes keratitis, eczema herpeticum, and herpetic whitlow. Both can be associated with disseminated visceral herpetic infection occurring in the immunocompromised host. Pregnancy is not in itself associated with disseminated herpes infection, and obstetric problems are presented most often by localized genital herpes. Between 5 and 20 million Americans have genital herpes, and at least 300,000 new cases occur annually.

EFFECT ON THE FETUS. Neonatal herpetic infection occurs in 150 to 300 infants per year in the United States. It can be produced by both herpes types but is more commonly due to type 2, which can be contracted by the infant during passage through an infected lower genital tract. Ascending infection is unusual, and transplacental transmission is rare. Thus, most cases of neonatal herpes can be prevented by cesarean section.

In the newborn, herpetic infection produces a spectrum of illness ranging from localized skin lesions to generalized systemic infection. Encephalitis can occur with or without other manifestations and is likely to produce severe residual brain damage in survivors. Symptoms can appear in the newborn immediately or up to four weeks after delivery. The average date of onset is day 6 for generalized disease and day 11 for localized central nervous system disease.

DIAGNOSIS. Definitive diagnosis is by culture of the virus. Both types of herpes will grow in tissue culture within three days or less. Several methods are being explored for making the diagnosis more rapidly.

TREATMENT AND PREVENTION. Pregnant women who develop genital herpes, who have a history of genital lesions, or who have a sexual partner with genital herpes should be monitored weekly during the last eight weeks of pregnancy. Women with HSV infection are likely to experience premature labor (50% of affected infants are born before 38 weeks' gestation), and this should be considered in planning monitoring. A cervical culture should be done at each weekly interval regardless of whether genital lesions are visible. A woman with clinical disease or with a positive culture within

two weeks of term should have cesarean section before the onset of labor and rupture of membranes. If membranes rupture spontaneously, cesarean section should still be performed if it can be accomplished in less than 24 hours. Breastfeeding may be allowed if the mother has no lesions on the breast and any other active lesions can be covered. She should observe careful handwashing technique. Mothers (and hospital personnel) with active or recurrent cold sores should be warned not to kiss infants.

There is no vaccine or prophylactic antiviral agent for herpes. Several antiviral agents can affect herpes simplex, including iododeoxyuridine (IDU), trifluridine, vidarabine (adenine arabinoside or Ara-A), and acyclovir. IDU and trifluridine are used topically, especially for herpes keratitis. Vidarabine has been used systemically to treat serious herpetic infection. It is too toxic for general use and will decrease viral excretion but will not cure the infection. Acyclovir is less toxic and may be used parenterally or orally. It, too, is ineffective in curing herpetic infection but has been shown to decrease symptoms and viral excretion. As of this writing, use during pregnancy has not been studied. Readers are advised to consult the most recent medical literature for update of this rapidly developing field.

Cytomegalovirus

EPIDEMIOLOGY. The CMVs are highly species specific; thus, human CMV grows only in human cells. CMV is ubiquitous, with no seasonal or epidemic occurrence. In the United States about 50% of adults are seropositive, with higher rates in the lower socioeconomic groups. The seropositivity rate approaches 100% in adults of some developing countries.

Among humans CMV can be transmitted venereally, by mucous membrane contact with infected secretions (including milk), and through blood transfusions. Because CMV is not an air-borne disease, careful handwashing techniques should be adequate to prevent spread of infection. The major epidemiologic problem exists in homes and day care centers in which there is congregation of large numbers of infants and children who may be asymptomatically excreting CMV. Immunocompromised persons (including neonates) and pregnant women who are seronegative or of unknown serologic status should be protected from patients known to be excreting CMV.

CLINICAL PRESENTATION. Most commonly, CMV infections are asymptomatic in normal children and adults. Upper respiratory symptoms, a flulike disease, or, rarely, infectious mononucleosis syndrome may result from primary infection. In contrast to the normal host, the immunocompromised host can experience fatal infection. Pneumonia and retinitis are the usual manifestations of either primary or reactivated CMV infection in these persons.

EFFECT ON THE FETUS. CMV is the viral agent most frequently acquired *in utero*. At least 1% of all newborns are excreting this virus at birth. Only 5% of these infected infants are symptomatic at birth with disseminated viral disease; another 5% may have milder symptoms. Almost all of these infants are offspring of women who experienced primary CMV infection during pregnancy. An additional 10% have some later effect attributable to the CMV infection, such as hearing loss, mental retardation, or neurologic abnormality. The remaining 80% of infected infants remain normal as they grow up but are long-term virus excreters and serve as a reservoir of infection.

DIAGNOSIS. Definitive diagnosis is by viral isolation. CMV can be recovered most easily from urine but also is present in most mucous membrane secretions during active infection. Serologic testing is valuable for describing experience with the virus but does not define whether the experience is primary or reactivated infection, since CMV-IgM can be present in both. The neonate's CMV-IgM level is of value if properly obtained to eliminate rheumatoid factor. In fact, rheumatoid factor is so frequently found in cord blood of infants with congenital CMV that it can serve as a nonspecific clue to congenital CMV infections.

TREATMENT AND PREVENTION. None of the antiviral agents has yet been proven to be beneficial against CMV. In severely immunocompromised patients, a combination of an antiviral agent and immunotherapy, such as CMV hyperimmune globulin, has been helpful in controlling symptoms but does not "cure" the virus infection. A CMV vaccine is being developed, but because of the ubiquitous nature of CMV and the problem of latency, there is at present no hope of containing the maternal–fetal CMV problem by means of vaccine. Attention should be given to the CMV serologic status of milk bank donors, as well as that of donors of blood transfusions given to pregnant women and newborns.

Varicella–Zoster Virus

EPIDEMIOLOGY. VZV produces chickenpox after primary infection and herpes zoster (shingles) upon recurrence. Since chickenpox is a highly contagious disease, with about 80% of cases occurring in children under nine years of age, only about 5% of American women of childbearing age are susceptible to primary VZV infections. Zoster also produces infective skin lesions, but the virus is not air borne as it is in chickenpox and thus has a lower degree of contagion.

CLINICAL PRESENTATION. Primary VZV infection is more severe in the adult than in the child and therefore is among the most serious infections in the pregnant woman. Interstitial pneumonitis is a frequent complication. Rare complications include central nervous system involvement (acute cerebellar ataxia, encephalitis, aseptic meningitis, myelitis), hepatitis, nephrosis, nephritis, arthritis, and myocarditis.

VZV has a predilection for neural tissue and persists in its latent phase in the peripheral ganglia. Herpes zoster is the manifestation of local reactivation of this latent virus. Cases of zoster during pregnancy have been reported, but they have not been especially frequent, considering that at least 95% of pregnant women have already experienced VZV infection. When zoster does occur, the severity and the occurrence of dissemination do not seem to be affected by the pregnancy, and transplacental transmission of the virus to the fetus has not been documented.

EFFECT ON THE FETUS. Fetal infection with VZV during the early part of pregnancy can result in congenital defects. The defects produced by VZV are clearly related to the neurotropism of the virus, generally occurring in a neural distribution. Some combination of limb deformity, cicatricial skin lesions, cortical atrophy, and ocular abnormalities can be produced. Since gestational chickenpox is unusual, it has not been possible to estimate frequencies of these defects.

Late gestational VZV can be manifest in the newborn by the characteristic skin lesions distributed like typical chickenpox or in the dermatomal manner typical of zoster. The most severe manifestations are in infants whose mothers had chickenpox so late in gestation that no antibody was transmitted transplacentally. In such infants, generalized varicella with pneumonia is the rule, and the mortality rate is approximately 30%.

TREATMENT AND PREVENTION. A vaccine against VZV is being developed, but the only prophylaxis presently available is passive immunization with varicella–zoster immune globulin (VZIG) (see Table 30-16). VZIG is not routinely indicated in healthy women exposed to varicella during pregnancy, since 95% of adult women are immune. In women who are known to be seronegative, VZIG may be indicated to prevent complications of varicella in the mother, but it is unknown whether this treatment will prevent fetal infection. VZIG is definitely indicated in the newborn infant of a woman who has had onset of varicella within five days before or two days following delivery. It is manufactured by the Massachusetts Public Health Biologic Laboratories* and is distributed by the regional offices of the American Red Cross Blood Services and other regional blood banking centers.

The antiviral agents vidarabine and acyclovir may be used in treatment of severe VZV infection in the pregnant woman. These agents are toxic to both mother and fetus, and expert help must be sought in their use during pregnancy.

---

* 24-hour phone: 617-552-3700.

Epstein–Barr Virus

EBV does not present a unique problem to the pregnant woman and is not known to produce any defects or disease in the fetus, although it can be transmitted transplacentally. Infectious mononucleosis syndrome in the pregnant woman does present a diagnostic problem, since it is important to mother and fetus to differentiate among the three known causes: EBV, cytomegalovirus, and *Toxoplasma gondii*. If the syndrome proves to be due to EBV, the mother can be reassured that the infant will probably not be affected adversely by her infection. The diagnosis is established by serologic means. The mono spot test, although not definitive, is often helpful, since the results are negative in infectious mononucleosis syndrome due to CMV or toxoplasmosis. In all cases of EBV infection during pregnancy, consultation should be sought with a large virologic center, since definitive serology is technically difficult. The exact extent of disease caused by this virus during pregnancy needs much more study.

Smallpox (Variola) and Vaccinia

In May 1980, the World Health Organization declared the world free of smallpox. Distribution of smallpox vaccine for civilian use was discontinued in the United States in 1983. Since there are no requirements for smallpox vaccination for international travelers, there is now no indication for smallpox vaccination except for persons in highly unusual circumstances such as certain laboratory workers. The U.S. Department of Defense maintains smallpox immune status for all active-duty personnel (including National Guard), and several hundred thousand of the military are vaccinated every year. Although the vaccinated population does not normally include pregnant women, the vaccine may still produce complications in pregnant contacts of a vaccinee. Complications include disseminated vaccinia, keratitis, and eczema vaccinatum. For advice on vaccine administration and contraindications and the use of vaccinia immune globulin, one can contact the International Health Program Office, Centers for Disease Control.*

Measles (Rubeola)

Epidemiology

Measles is a highly contagious infection due to a paramyxovirus. The virus is found in respiratory tract secretions, blood, and urine of infected persons. It can be transmitted by direct or indirect contact with infected secretions; it also can be air borne. Measles incidence has declined to very low levels since the introduction of killed measles vaccine in 1957 and live vaccine in

* Atlanta, GA 30333.

1967. Most cases of measles now occur in unimmunized adults, and as a result the percentage of cases occurring in pregnant women has increased.

Clinical Presentation

The incubation period ranges from 10 to 12 days. The regular course of rash, fever, and toxicity can be severe. Encephalitis follows measles in approximately 1 case per 1000, and the risk is greatest in adults. In addition, persons who were immunized in childhood with killed vaccine (1957–1967) can experience atypical measles, with a severe course that commonly includes pneumonia, on exposure to wild or even vaccine measles virus. Thus, measles infection is a hazard to women of childbearing age.

Effects on the Fetus

In early gestational measles, there have been reports of a small increase in numbers of congenital malformations. However, these malformations are so varied in type that no specific syndrome can be ascribed to measles virus. The abortion rate is probably higher than normal, and infant deaths before two years of age are more frequent.

Late gestational measles can result in infection of the fetus such that the infant is born with measles or acquires it in the first 12 days of life. These infants can experience severe respiratory disease with a rash. The infant of a woman who has measles at or shortly after the time of delivery should receive immune globulin prophylaxis.

Treatment and Prevention

Treatment of the susceptible pregnant woman who is exposed to measles is with pooled immunoglobulin, 0.25 ml/kg up to 15 ml (see Table 30-16). To be effective, the immune globulin must be given within six days of exposure. Live measles vaccine is contraindicated during pregnancy, and immunization of susceptible women is part of postpartum care. If immune globulin prophylaxis or blood transfusion has been used, vaccine administration should be deferred for at least three months.

Mumps

Mumps is caused by a pseudomyxovirus. Its most common manifestation is a generalized infection with parotitis. Other manifestations may include aseptic meningitis, meningoencephalitis, orchitis, pancreatitis, and sublingual or submaxillary gland involvement. These manifestations may precede, accompany, or follow the parotitis or occur without it. About one third of mumps infections are asymptomatic. The infection is transmitted by direct contact or droplet spread from saliva of infected persons. The incubation period is from 14 to 21 days. The diagnosis can be confirmed by serologic tests; elevation of serum amylase levels is a useful presumptive diagnostic finding.

Maternal mumps probably is associated with an increased abortion rate in the first trimester. There is highly questionable evidence of teratogenic potential of mumps virus. It has been associated with the occurrence of endocardial fibroelastosis in the infant, but a causal relationship has not been confirmed in this or any other congenital defect. Chronic mumps virus infection of the fetus has never been observed.

The incidence of mumps infection has declined 98% since the introduction of live mumps vaccine in 1967, but there is still a group of nonimmune women of childbearing age who could contract mumps during pregnancy. The vaccine is contraindicated in pregnant women because it is a live vaccine. Mumps immunization can be a part of postpartum care for women known to be seronegative.

Acquired Immune Deficiency Syndrome

Acquired immune deficiency syndrome (AIDS) is produced by a retrovirus that may render the infected person susceptible to serious opportunistic infection with a wide range of bacteria, viruses, protozoa, and fungi, and to development of lymphoreticular malignancy.

Epidemiology

The infectious virus is found in and can be transmitted by blood. It may also be transmitted transplacentally, even when the mother does not have any symptoms of AIDS. Of the 64 cases of infant AIDS reported through 1984, only a few were associated with blood transfusions, and the great majority occurred in infants of women with AIDS or with one of the risk factors for the disease. None of the infants was sick at birth, but in some symptoms developed within the first month after birth, suggesting transplacental rather than perinatal exposure of the infant. High-risk women include those who are sexual partners of bisexual men, intravenous drug users, Caribbeans, especially Haitians, and intimate contacts of AIDS patients.

Clinical Presentation

The incubation period of AIDS is varied, and symptoms may develop many years after infection occurs. The symptoms of opportunistic infections and malignancy may be preceded by the AIDS-related complex of lymphadenopathy, hepatosplenomegaly, weight loss, diarrhea, and hypergammaglobulinemia.

A test for antibody to HTLV-III, the causative agent of AIDS, has been developed and is useful for screening of blood products. It is not helpful diagnostically, since healthy persons may have antibody and AIDS patients may be antibody negative (probably because of the immune deficiency associated with the disease). At this writing, a test for the presence of HTLV-III antigen has not been approved.

Treatment and Prevention

There is no specific therapy or vaccine available. Treatment consists of care of the infections and malignancies that may develop during the course of the disease.

Influenza

Epidemiology

Influenza is produced by orthomyxoviruses, which fall into three antigenic types: A, B, and C. Types A and B cause epidemic disease. Influenza-A strains are subclassified by their hemagglutinin type (H1, H2, and H3) and their neuraminidase type (N1 and N2). These types undergo minor changes (antigenic drift) almost yearly, and major antigenic shifts occur at intervals of years, usually five to ten. These antigenic changes can render the "immune" person susceptible to the new A strain, and the major antigenic shifts usually result in epidemics or pandemics.

Clinical Presentation

Influenza is highly contagious, being spread by direct and indirect contact with infected nasopharyngeal secretions. After a short incubation period of one to three days, a syndrome of fever, chills, malaise, headache, diffuse myalgia, cough, and sore throat may develop. Some infected persons may have simple upper respiratory tract symptoms or be asymptomatic, but they are still infectious to others. Mortality among high-risk persons is high owing mainly to pulmonary complications.

Effects on the Fetus

Pregnancy has not constituted a high-risk factor except during the largest pandemics of 1918 to 1919 and 1957 to 1958. During these two periods there was also an increase in the abortion rate, but no fetal malformations have been associated with maternal influenza.

Treatment and Prevention

A new influenza vaccine is formulated yearly and should be given yearly to high-risk persons (see Table 30-15). The vaccine is indicated for the pregnant woman only if she has another risk factor such as a chronic cardiovascular or pulmonary disorder. Women with chronic metabolic disease (including diabetes mellitus), renal dysfunction, anemia, or immunosuppression are also at moderately increased risk and may receive vaccine. Finally, health professionals who have extensive contact with high-risk patients should be immunized to avoid exposing their patients to influenza. Although influenza vaccine is an inactivated vaccine and no teratogenicity has been demonstrated, it is prudent to avoid the vaccine in the first trimester of pregnancy whenever practical.

Amantadine is an effective prophylactic for influenza A and also may be of some benefit in the treatment of established infection. It is not effective for influenza B or for any other of the respiratory viruses, and it is not a substitute for immunization. It is indicated for interim prophylaxis of high-risk persons. Amantadine teratogenicity has not been observed, but it has not been studied adequately in humans; the agent is embryotoxic in rats at about 12 times the recommended human dose. Thus, amantadine should not be used freely during pregnancy.

The major cause of death in influenza is superinfection with bacteria, especially *Staphylococcus aureus*. In the pregnant woman as in all other influenza patients, bacterial superinfection must be promptly diagnosed and treated.

Arboviruses

The term *arbovirus* refers to an arthropod-borne virus. Only a few of this large group of viruses cause human disease in the Western hemisphere. The usual clinical manifestations are encephalitis (California, eastern equine, Powassan, St. Louis, Venezuelan equine, and western equine) and hemorrhagic fevers (dengue, Colorado tick fever, Mayaro, and yellow fever). All of these infections can follow a severe course with significant mortality but are not made more severe by pregnancy. Among the arboviruses, western equine encephalitis, Venezuelan equine encephalitis, and dengue are known to be transmitted transplacentally. Only Venezuelan equine encephalitis virus is known to produce fetal malformations: abortion, stillbirth, and neurologic malformations (cerebral, cerebellar, and medullary hypoplasia) have been reported.

A vaccine is available for yellow fever; it is a live vaccine and therefore should not be given during pregnancy unless exposure is unavoidable (see Table 30-16). Infection with the other arboviruses can be prevented only by control of the arthropod vector, use of protective clothing and insecticides, and avoidance of travel to epidemic and endemic areas. No specific antiviral therapy is available.

Rabies

Rabies virus infection causes a neurologic disease that is nearly 100% fatal. The virus is found in the saliva of infected animals and can be present as long as five days before the appearance of recognizable illness. The incubation period ranges from nine days to several months. There is no treatment for the established disease, but it is preventable by passive and active immunization. Any animal bite should be treated seriously, and prompt consultation should be sought with local or state public health officials for advice about the necessity for prophylaxis. The treatment consists of rabies immune globulin (RIG), 20 IU, half in the site of the bite and half intramuscularly (IM), plus 5 doses of rabies vaccine, 1 ml IM, on days 0, 3, 7, 14, and 28 (see Table 30-16).

The rabies vaccine now used is an inactivated form of the virus grown in human diploid cells. The number of serious reactions to this vaccine is much lower than the number produced by the old vaccine. Although the safety of rabies vaccine during pregnancy has not been established, pregnancy does not alter the necessity or the method of postexposure prophylaxis.

Enteroviruses: Polio, Coxsackie, and Echo

The enterovirus group contains a large number of virus strains. In the past they were classified as poliovirus, coxsackievirus, and echovirus. However, they are so closely related that newly defined members of this group are designated simply as enteroviruses.

Poliomyelitis is caused by one of the three types of poliovirus. Most poliovirus infections in normal persons are subclinical or cause only a minor illness, and in only a small percentage of infections does lower motor neuron paralytic disease result. The course tends to be more severe during pregnancy, however, and infection of the fetus or newborn is highly fatal, frequently producing paralysis in survivors. Thus, the polio immune status of the pregnant woman assumes great importance, even though in the United States effective vaccine programs have made paralytic polio rare. Two trivalent polio vaccines are available, the inactivated (IPV) and the live attenuated oral (OPV) (see Table 30-16). The administration of OPV has been associated with paralytic poliomyelitis in immunocompromised patients. Vaccine-induced paralysis also occurs in normal persons, in 1 person per 9 million doses of OPV distributed. Although this is an extremely small risk, it indicates that an adult of uncertain immune status who is not facing an epidemic situation should be immunized with IPV. However, immunization takes longer to achieve with IPV, so that in a high-risk or epidemic situation OPV is necessary. During pregnancy both vaccines should be avoided, although no adverse effects have been reported in either the pregnant woman or the developing fetus. IPV is indicated for the susceptible pregnant woman preparing to travel in endemic areas. If immediate protection against polio is needed, OPV, not IPV, is recommended for the pregnant woman.

Coxsackieviruses and echoviruses are the other large groups of enteroviruses that can cause serious disease, especially in newborn infants. These viruses usually cause minor respiratory symptoms in the pregnant woman, although rarely an influenza-like illness, pleurodynia, pericarditis, or aseptic meningitis may result. Regardless of the mother's symptoms, the newborn can develop fulminating encephalomyocarditis due to coxsackievirus group B, or hepatic necrosis from echovirus 11 infection. There are no specific preventive or therapeutic measures available. These infections are most common in young children, in late summer and early fall, with an incubation period of two to five days. Transmission is usually by the fecal–oral route, so that attention to handwashing and personal hygiene can help contain the infection.

Hepatitis

Primary hepatitis is caused by at least three different agents, which are classified according to their usual mode of transmission. *Hepatitis A* refers to infectious hepatitis, and *hepatitis B* and *non-A non-B* to serum hepatitis. Hepatitis B is caused by hepatitis-B virus (HBV), a member of a newly defined virus group. Any hepatitis having the clinical and epidemiologic characteristics of serum hepatitis but not due to HBV is called *non-A non-B hepatitis.* There are probably several causal agents.

Hepatitis A

Hepatitis A is usually transmitted by the fecal–oral route and has an incubation period of 15 to 40 days. It spreads easily in families and in day care centers. Children are likely to have anicteric hepatitis A and can then transmit the virus to their families. Adults, especially pregnant women, tend to have much more serious disease from hepatitis A than do children. There is an increased rate of abortion and prematurity, but transplacental or perinatal transmission is unusual. Fortunately this type of hepatitis does not produce chronic sequelae or a carrier state. Prophylactic immunoglobulin, in a dose of 0.02 ml/kg IM, is indicated as soon as possible after exposure (see Table 30-16). Infants of mothers with hepatitis A should receive γ-globulin, 0.5 ml IM, as soon as possible after birth. Strict enteric isolation procedures are necessary in care of a patient with acute hepatitis A.

Hepatitis B

HBV can be transmitted perinatally and by sexual contact as well as percutaneously in blood. HBV characteristically produces subacute illness; asymptomatic infection is common, and fulminant hepatitis is unusual. The incubation period is 40 to 180 days. Chronic liver disease or a chronic carrier state may follow HBV infection regardless of the symptoms produced initially. Between 6% and 10% of adults with HBV infection become carriers, and 25% of these carriers will have chronic active hepatitis. Newborn infants of carrier mothers positive for both surface and "e" antigen have

an 80% to 90% probability of becoming infected. Although the infection is rarely symptomatic, 90% of these infants become HBV carriers. It has been estimated that 25% of the chronic carriers of perinatally acquired HBV eventually die of cirrhosis or primary hepatocellular carcinoma. In addition, these infants are infectious, and eventually they may participate in another cycle of perinatal transmission, thus perpetuating the virus pool in the human population. The pregnant woman who contracts HBV may display more severe symptoms, especially during the third trimester, and may have an increased probability of abortion or prematurity. Any person who has a documented HBV contact, either percutaneous or mucous membrane, should be treated as outlined in Table 30-17.

HBV is transmitted transplacentally in about 5% of perinatally acquired cases. Thus, 95% are theoretically preventable by treatment of the infant at birth. A combination of hepatitis-B immune globulin (HBIG) and hepatitis-B vaccine is nearly 90% efficacious in preventing chronic infection of the infant. The recommended schedule is provided in Table 30-17. It is the responsibility of the obstetrician to inform the personnel caring for the infant of the mother's carrier status so that proper prophylaxis can be carried out in a timely manner. Therefore, screening for hepatitis-B surface antigen (HBsAg) is recommended during pregnancy for the high-risk groups listed below:*

Women of Asian, Pacific Island, or Alaskan Eskimo descent, whether immigrant or U.S.-born
Women born in Haiti or Sub-Saharan Africa
Women with histories of:

  Acute or chronic liver disease
  Work or treatment in a hemodialysis unit
  Work or residence in an institution for the mentally retarded
  Rejection as a blood donor
  Blood transfusion on repeated occasions
  Frequent occupational exposure to blood in medico-dental settings
  Household contact with an HBV carrier or hemodialysis patient
  Multiple episodes of venereal disease
  Percutaneous use of illicit drugs

PROTOZOAN INFECTIONS

Toxoplasmosis

Epidemiology

Toxoplasma gondii is a ubiquitous sporozoan organism that infects a variety of warm-blooded animals. Members of the cat family are definitive hosts. Infected

* (Immunization Practices Advisory Committee: MMWR 33: 285, 1984.)

Table 30-17
Hepatitis-B Virus Postexposure Recommendations

| Exposure | HBIG | | Vaccine | |
	Dose	Recommended Timing	Dose	Recommended Timing
Perinatal	0.5 ml IM	Within 12 hr of birth	0.5 ml (10 μg) IM	Within 7 days* repeat at 1 and 6 mo
Percutaneous	0.06 ml/kg IM or 5 ml for adults	Single dose within 24 hr	1.0 ml (20 μg) IM†	Within 7 days* repeat at 1 and 6 mo
		or‡		
	0.06 ml/kg IM or 5 ml for adults	Within 24 h, repeat at 1 month		
Sexual	0.06 ml/kg IM or 5 ml for adults	Within 14 days of sexual contact	§	

* The first dose can be given at the same time as the HBIG dose but at a separate site.
† For persons younger than age 10, use 0.5 ml (10 μg).
‡ For those who choose not to receive HB vaccine.
§ Vaccine is recommended for homosexually active males and for regular sexual contacts of chronic HBV carriers.
(Immunization Practices Advisory Committee: MMWR 33:285, 1984)

cats excrete oocysts in their stools, which become infective 48 hours after excretion and can persist in soil in the infective state for weeks. Other infected animals carry encysted organisms in muscle and various organs but do not excrete infectious forms. Humans become infected by ingesting poorly cooked infected meat or the sporulated oocysts from cat feces. Transfusion-related transmission has occurred only rarely.

Clinical Presentation

Infection in the pregnant woman is usually asymptomatic, although a range of symptoms from malaise and myalgia through infectious mononucleosis syndrome may occur. Serious manifestations can include encephalopathy, pneumonia, myocarditis, and acute or chronic chorioretinitis. The immunosuppressed woman is prone to widely disseminated disease.

Effect on the Fetus

Congenital infection can be asymptomatic or can cause severe symptoms. The infant may be born prematurely, may be small for gestational age, may have manifestations of active infection at birth (hepatosplenomegaly, lymphadenopathy, jaundice, thrombocytopenia), or may have meningitis and encephalitis. Central nervous system infection can result in hydrocephalus, microcephaly, chorioretinitis, and convulsions. The severely affected infant may die soon after birth; survivors may be profoundly mentally retarded, blind, and deaf. Such an outcome is rare; however, because this cause of fetal infection is now preventable by timely treatment of the pregnant woman, investigation of maternal exposures and even minor illness is warranted.

Prevention

Transmission of toxoplasmosis from pet cats can be limited by disposal of cat litter daily before oocysts become infective and by limitation of the cats' intake of food to prepared cat food only. Seronegative pregnant women should avoid cats altogether and should not garden in areas to which cats have access. All lamb, beef, and pork they eat should first be cooked thoroughly.

Diagnosis

Diagnosis of acute toxoplasmosis is by serologic means. IgM-specific antibodies can usually be detected by immunofluorescence by the end of the second week; they peak at one month and may persist for more than a year. Thus, a high titer of IgM antibody must be found in order to diagnose acute infection. IgG antibody may be detected by the Sabin–Feldman dye test, immunofluorescence, or enzyme-linked immunosorbent assay (ELISA). Seroconversion or a fourfold rise in IgG antibody in specimens analyzed concurrently suggests recent infection. In diagnosis of the newborn infant, maternal and cord serum specimens must be analyzed together. IgM-specific antibodies are detectable in the cord blood of only 20% of infected infants by methods used in studies to date; therefore, maternal serologic findings are of great importance.

Treatment

Pyrimethamine and sulfadiazine act synergistically against toxoplasma and are the drugs of choice for treatment of toxoplasmosis. Although these drugs are potentially embryotoxic, their use during pregnancy is warranted by the grave danger to the fetus posed by acute maternal toxoplasmosis. Folinic acid must be administered concurrently. Expert consultation should be sought for drug dosages and specific management techniques in each case of maternal toxoplasmosis.

Malaria

Malaria is transmitted by the *Anopheles* mosquito in many tropical and subtropical countries. Although this mosquito is not found in the United States, American travelers to endemic areas may become infected. Active and chronic cases are imported, especially in South American and Asian immigrants. Parasitemia may persist intermittently for as long as 40 years. The infection can be acquired from blood transfusions, and occasionally the pregnant woman transmits the infection to her fetus. Relapse of malaria is more likely during pregnancy and the puerperium. There is an increased incidence of abortion and premature labor during these relapses.

Chloroquine phosphate (Aralen) is the drug of choice for treatment and prophylaxis of malaria. It is given in a dose of 500 mg orally, once weekly. In some areas of the world, chloroquine-resistant strains of *Plasmodium falciparum* are found; the drug of choice for treatment of these infections is pyrimethamine–sulfadoxine (Fansidar). This drug is no longer recommended for prophylaxis because of its potential for producing severe cutaneous reactions. The pregnant woman is in double jeopardy, because pyrimethamine has a teratogenic potential as a folic acid antagonist and sulfadoxine may produce kernicterus in the newborn if used at term. The pregnant woman who must travel in an area endemic for chloroquine-resistant malaria should be instructed on measures to reduce contact with the night-feeding mosquitoes. She should take routine chloroquine prophylaxis and should be given a single-treatment dose of Fansidar along with folic acid supplementation to take promptly in event of a febrile illness if professional medical care is not available. In these cases, practitioners are urged to seek advice from state or local health officials, the Centers for Disease Control, or the U.S. Health Service annual publication, *Health Information for International Travel.*

REFERENCES AND RECOMMENDED READING

American College of Obstetricians and Gynecologists: Technical Bulletin No. 64, 1982

Amstey MS (ed): Virus Infection in Pregnancy. Orlando, FL, Grune & Stratton, 1984

Hanshaw JB, Dudgeon JA, Marshall WC: Viral Diseases of the Fetus and Newborn. Philadelphia, WB Saunders, 1985

Centers for Disease Control: Postexposure prophylaxis of hepatitis B: Recommendation of the Immunization Practices Advisory Committee. MMWR 33:285, 1984

Centers for Disease Control: Adult immunizations: Recommendation of the Immunization Practices Advisory Committee. MMWR 33 (Suppl 1):1, 1984

Centers for Disease Control: Revised recommendations for preventing malaria in travelers to areas with chloroquine-resistant *Plasmodium falciparum.* MMWR 34:185, 1985

Krugman S, Gershon AA (eds): Infections of the Fetus and the Newborn Infant. New York, Alan R. Liss, 1975

Remington JS, Klein JO (eds): Infectious Diseases of the Fetus and Newborn Infant. Philadelphia, WB Saunders, 1983

Report of the Committee on Infectious Diseases of the American Academy of Pediatrics, 19th edition, 1982

Sever JL, Larsen JW Jr, Grossman JH III: Handbook of Perinatal Infections. Boston, Little, Brown & Co, 1979

Reproductive Tract Disorders[*]

Howard C. Sharp

VAGINITIS IN PREGNANCY

Vaginitis is considered in Chapter 52, but its treatment may differ in pregnancy because of the teratogenicity of certain drugs. In general, the penicillins, cephalosporins, and erythromycin are among the drugs that may be safely used during pregnancy. The estolate salt of erythromycin has been observed to induce hepatotoxicity in pregnant women. While sulfonamides are teratogenic in some species of animals, they do not appear to pose a significant risk of malformation in humans. Their main danger is manifested when they are administered near term; in such circumstances, jaundice, hemolytic anemia, and, rarely, kernicterus may be observed in the newborn. Tetracycline is contraindicated in pregnancy because of adverse effects on fetal teeth and bones, maternal liver toxicity, and an increased incidence of minor fetal malformations, especially inguinal hernia. The use of metronidazole in pregnancy is still controversial despite reports of its safe use in over 800 pregnancies, including more than 300 in the first trimester. Two reports of midline facial defects with the drug's use in the first trimester and its carcinogenicity in rodents and mutagenicity in bacteria have given rise to concern. It has not been shown to be oncogenic in humans.

With the above considerations in mind, the following recommendations are given for treatment of specific vaginitis during pregnancy.

CANDIDIASIS. Clotrimazole or miconazole suppositories or cream should be inserted intravaginally twice daily for 3.5 days or nightly for one week. The cream is better than suppositories for local application when a vulvitis occurs concomitantly or a balanitis is

---

[*] This section is a revision of the material prepared by Robert E. L. Nesbitt for previous editions of this book.

present in the male partner. Boric acid capsules are also effective, and nystatin is somewhat less so.

TRICHOMONIASIS. Metronidazole is not appreciably absorbed from the vagina, and thus a 500-mg tablet may be used intravaginally daily during the first trimester (or later) to control symptoms. In most cases it will not clear the condition because of urethral and other involvement. After the first trimester it is probably best to treat the patient and her sexual partner with oral metronidazole, 250 mg 3 times per day for 7 days, or a single 2-g dose for each, since *Trichomonas* vaginitis has been known to be a risk factor for premature rupture of the membranes (30% risk).

GARDNERELLA VAGINALIS VAGINITIS. Ampicillin, 500 mg 4 times a day, can be expected to clear between 60% and 90% of cases. For those in whom the condition persists despite this therapy, metronidazole may be considered after the first trimester in a dose of 250 mg 3 times daily for 1 week. This regimen has been significantly more successful for this organism than the single 2-g dose. Sulfa vaginal cream and erythromycin have not proven clinically effective.

CHLAMYDIA TRACHOMATIS CERVICITIS AND URETHRITIS. Erythromycin, 500 mg, should be administered 4 times daily for 7 days.

NON–PENICILLINASE-PRODUCING NEISSERIA GONORRHOEAE CERVICITIS AND URETHRITIS. Recommended treatment includes the following: aqueous procaine penicillin G, 4.8 mu IM, with 1 g of probenecid orally; amoxicillin, 3 g, or ampicillin, 3.5 g, with probenecid.

PENICILLINASE-PRODUCING NEISSERIA GONORRHOEAE CERVICITIS AND URETHRITIS. Recommended treatment includes the following: cefotaxime, 1 g IM, with probenecid, 1 g PO; cefoxitin, 2 g IM, with probenecid; or spectinomycin, 2 g IM, for those who are allergic to penicillins or cephalosporins.

VULVAR VARICOSITIES

A 30-fold increase in circulation draining from the rapidly enlarging uterus into the tributaries of the iliac veins, compounded by pressure on these vessels at the end of the third trimester, is largely responsible for the development of vulvar varices in about one fifth of pregnant women. Normally these swollen, grapelike clusters of veins do not constitute a hazard to the patient, although an uncommon traumatic rupture of a varix may rapidly produce a sizable hematoma unless prompt pressure is applied. Women should be reassured that the varices will rapidly regress after delivery and most often become asymptomatic.

During pregnancy the aching and burning discomfort that may result can be controlled by a pad, piece of

foam rubber, or commercially available device held in place by a firm support around the pelvic girdle. A dramatic decrease in size of the varices is often apparent immediately with the delivery of the infant. Surgical therapy is not indicated during pregnancy. Usually, relief of pain is complete after and between pregnancies, although a significant number of women notice some discomfort with the onset of the menses. This is rarely severe enough to warrant surgery, which to be effective must eliminate a complex of veins drained by four or five drainage systems.

UTERINE PROLAPSE

Uterine prolapse during pregnancy is a rare occurrence; only 231 cases have been reported. It may present during any trimester as a bulging edematous mass protruding through the introitus, with or without previous history of prolapse. Most often the patient is multiparous, and the trauma of childbirth has contributed to laxity of the cardinal and uterosacral ligament support as well as herniation through the pelvic diaphragm. However, one fifth of patients are nulliparous.

Treatment consists of bed rest in slight Trendelenburg position until such time as the cervical edema subsides and replacement can be accomplished. In the first and second trimesters a Hodge or ring-type pessary precisely fitted without undue pressure may serve to elevate the cervix, enabling the patient to be ambulatory. As the later weeks approach, it may not be possible to prevent prolapse and massive cervical edema without bed rest. Cervical ulceration and fissuring are frequent and may be treated with saline packs and antibiotic ointments.

Premature labor and premature rupture of membranes often occur, and while vaginal delivery is to be expected, cesarean section may be necessary when the cervix is trapped and will not retract into the vagina. This is preferable to Dührssen's incisions and forceps extraction.

RETRODISPLACEMENT OF THE UTERUS

Retroflexion or retroversion of the uterus is observed frequently during the early months of pregnancy, but the normal position is usually assumed by the third month as the anterior wall undergoes hypertrophy and draws the organ up out of the pelvis (Fig. 30-4). Although retrodisplacement of the uterus has been implicated in spontaneous abortion, there is no clear evidence of a causal relationship, except in neglected cases of incarceration.

When the uterus is found to be retroverted at the ninth or tenth week, the cervix is usually seen to be high anteriorly, distorting and compressing the urethra and bladder neck. Patients with this condition are well advised to assume the knee-chest position before sleep-

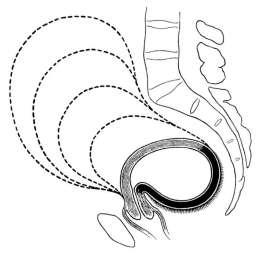

FIG. 30-4. Retrodisplacement of the uterus. (Bumm E: Grundriss zum Studium der Geburtshilfe. Munich, Bergmann, 1922)

ing and to unlock the vaginal vacuum digitally, thereby allowing the gravid uterus to fall from the hollow of the sacrum. After continuing this position for a minute or two, sleeping on the abdomen or side should maintain the uterus forward. If at any time she has difficulty voiding, the patient should be examined and catheterized if there is urinary retention. Replacement is usually successful when attempted in the knee-chest position but may require traction on the posterior lip of the cervix with a tenaculum (Fig. 30-5). Occasionally, anesthesia will be necessary to release the fundus; rarely, laparotomy may be required, possibly with release of adhesions.

Once the uterus is anteverted, it may be maintained in position with the use of a Hodge pessary until such time as it is large enough to rest well above the pelvic brim, usually an additional two weeks.

SACCULATION OF THE UTERUS

An extremely rare disorder of the uterus is the presence of a pouch or sac in the wall made up of very thin myometrium. A sacculation may occur at any point in the myometrium, and fetal parts can be readily palpated through it. In Danforth's case, the cranial sutures were readily palpable through the abdominal wall. Such sacculations are of unknown cause and do not necessarily recur in a subsequent pregnancy. When the condition is diagnosed, it is prudent to deliver by cesarean section.

INVERSION OF THE UTERUS

Puerperal inversion of the uterus is a rare complication that can lead to profuse hemorrhage, shock, and even death. The uterus is turned inside out so that the top of the endometrial cavity protrudes through the cervix into the vagina and even outside the introitus (Fig. 30-6). Inversion may be acute, subacute, or chronic, depending on when it is recognized, and occasionally it is partial rather than complete.

Multiparity with a lax uterus, fundal pressure following delivery, and excessive umbilical cord traction are the usual conditions associated with this complication. However, uterine inversion has occurred in primigravidas and with minimal manipulation of the uterus in the third stage of labor. Consequently, the exact cause is sometimes difficult to determine.

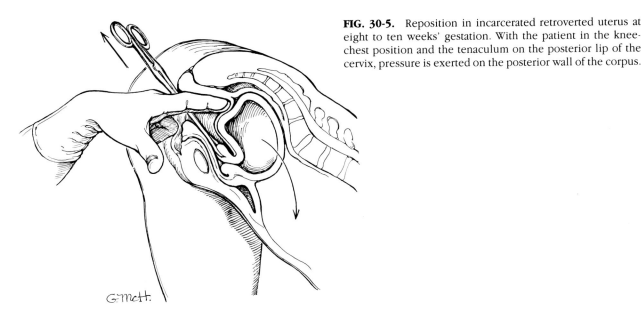

FIG. 30-5. Reposition in incarcerated retroverted uterus at eight to ten weeks' gestation. With the patient in the knee-chest position and the tenaculum on the posterior lip of the cervix, pressure is exerted on the posterior wall of the corpus.

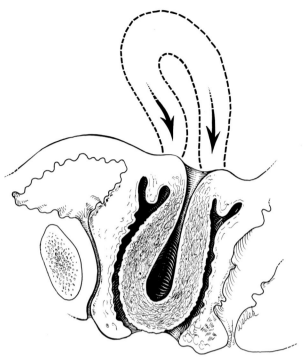

FIG. 30-6. Inversion of the uterus.

Diagnosis

The most important point to be made in the management of inversion is the necessity of early recognition. The diagnosis depends upon feeling an unusual hard mass filling the vagina or seeing a mass protruding from the introitus following delivery of the infant or placenta. Bimanual examination confirms that the fundus is not felt suprapubically. The uterus can usually be replaced vaginally in most early cases, since a contracted cervical ring does not usually form for 15 to 30 minutes.

Management

Immediate replacement of the uterus is the procedure of choice as soon as the diagnosis is made. Preferably with the patient under general anesthesia, the fundus is grasped in the palm of the hand with the fingers directed toward the posterior fornix. The uterus is lifted out of the pelvis and forcefully held in the abdominal cavity so the pull of the uterine ligaments will help the entire fundus snap back into its normal position. If this is done almost immediately, the bleeding is minimal, and the widely discussed syndrome of shock out of proportion to blood loss can often be avoided. If the placenta is still attached, it should be removed under direct vision to make replacement easier. If there is a placenta accreta, the fundus is replaced with the placenta *in situ.* Once the fundus is replaced, a hand should be kept in

the uterine cavity until the uterus contracts strongly under the influence of intravenous oxytocin infusion.

If the prolapsed mass cannot be replaced at once or there has been a delay in the diagnosis, expert anesthesiology, obstetric, and nursing assistance should be summoned, fluid started in two veins with large-bore catheters, blood made ready, and intravenous antibiotics begun. If further vaginal attempts at replacement of the fundus are unsuccessful, prompt performance of an abdominal operation in the delivery room is indicated. The abdomen is entered through a midline incision with the patient in the Trendelenburg position, and large Allis clamps are placed within the inversion tunnel (Huntington's procedure). As the fundus comes upward, traction is applied and more clamps are placed below the first group; this process repeated until the entire fundus is delivered.

In some cases a tight cervical ring makes reduction of the inversion possible only by Haultaim's operation. In this procedure the lower segment of the uterus is incised at the posterior end of the funnel so the inversion can be reduced, and the uterine incision is then closed with absorbable suture. If the inversion was due to a placenta accreta and bleeding continues, hysterectomy may be necessary.

TORSION OF THE UTERUS

Pathologic torsion of the pregnant uterus is diagnosed when a rotation of the uterus on its radial axis of 45 degrees or greater is discovered, usually in the presence of pain, thus ruling out the slight dextrorotation of the uterus that occurs in about 80% of all pregnancies. About two thirds of reported cases have been associated with intrinsic pelvic pathology such as myomas, uterine anomalies, ovarian cysts, or adhesions. Abdominal pain unassociated with uterine contractions occurs in about 95% of patients, and about 30% have circulatory shock, urinary or intestinal symptoms, and minor vaginal bleeding, thus mimicking abruptio placentae. Abnormal presentation, especially transverse lie, is often present, and when labor ensues, obstruction can be expected.

Torsion of the pregnant uterus has rarely been diagnosed before surgery. The finding of a broad ligament stretched obliquely across the lower abdomen, torsion of the upper vagina and/or cervix, and malposition of the urethra in the presence of pain should arouse suspicion. Successful detorsion by external manipulation has been reported, but immediate laparotomy in symptomatic patients is usually necessary to accomplish this. At the same time it may be possible to correct the condition leading to the torsion. Late in pregnancy cesarean section is usually advisable. It is most important to recognize the uterine landmarks and avoid incision into the broad ligament and its vasculature. Detorsion should precede the uterine incision, if possible, to permit hysterotomy at the normal site. At times this is not possible, and in extreme cases it may be necessary to incise the posterior wall of the uterus to effect delivery. Hysterectomy may be indicated when laparotomy has been long delayed, a situation that increases both maternal and fetal morbidity.

MÜLLERIAN ANOMALIES

The incidence of müllerian anomalies has been estimated to be as frequent as 1 in 250 and as uncommon as 1 in 1000. The genesis of these defects is discussed in Chapter 5. Most women with communicating anomalies have little, if any, increased difficulty conceiving, but fetal wastage is high, depending on the degree and type of defect.

The rare patients with cervical, fundal, tubal, or combined types of uterine agenesis or hypoplasia are usually sterile, as are most patients with vaginal agenesis despite vaginal anastomosis. Early diagnosis and surgical treatment of transverse vaginal septa have been rewarded by pregnancy in several instances, although the uteri are often anomalous. Ultrasound may be of use preoperatively to measure uterine and cervical length and to establish the presence of a uterocervical cavity.

Sagittal vaginal septa are found with 75% of didelphic uteri, 5% of bicornuate uteri, and 25% of septate uteri. In addition to being a source of dyspareunia and hygiene problems, they commonly produce dystocia during labor and may be forcefully avulsed from their attachment to the bladder or rectum with resultant hemorrhage and difficult repair. They are best treated surgically before pregnancy, or during the midtrimester when encountered during a pregnancy.

Of the uterine anomalies most commonly encountered in obstetric practice, septate uteri are associated with approximately twice the pregnancy wastage (two thirds or greater) as occurs in didelphic, unicornuate, or bicornuate uteri. This is thought to be due to implantation on the relatively avascular septum, and its abortion potential is apparently proportional to the length of the septum.

In addition, uterine configuration in all of these anomalies predisposes to breech presentation, and in the case of bicornuate and septate uteri to transverse lie as well, increasing the cesarean section rate toward 50%. In the absence of malpresentation or other incidental contraindications, the expulsive force of the uterus is usually normal, and vaginal delivery can be expected. Manual exploration of the uterus immediately after delivery will not only permit an accurate diagnosis of the anomalous condition but will prevent retention of placental fragments, the chief cause of postpartum hemorrhage, which has frequently been observed in these patients.

Unless separate horns of a bicornuate uterus are palpable on bimanual examination, the distinction between this diagnosis and that of septate uterus must be made by laparoscopy or laparotomy before or after a pregnancy, since the hysterosalpingographic (HSG) images may be indistinguishable.

In women with septate uteri who have repeated abortion or premature labor, fetal salvage rates may be improved to 80% to 90% by the Jones wedge procedure or Tompkins metroplasty. Recently, successful resection of the septum has been accomplished hysteroscopically with the urologic resectoscope and the CO_2 laser. These innovative procedures save hospital time and cost, lessen blood loss, speed recovery, and allow the possibility of vaginal delivery. Bicornuate uteri are appropriately treated, when necessary, by the Strassmann unification metroplasty.

Special consideration should be given to pregnancy in the rudimentary horn of a bicornuate uterus, a rare but potentially lethal condition (Fig. 30-7). In about 85% of cases there may be a fibromuscular connection between the two horns but no endometrial communication, requiring transperitoneal migration of spermatozoa to fertilize the ipsilateral or occasionally the contralateral ovum. Of the more than 350 cases reported, only 7 have resulted in the salvage of both mother and infant, the vast majority rupturing in the second trimester when not discovered and resected early. Intra-abdominal hemorrhage is so massive that death results in most cases within 10 to 15 minutes. (See also Fig. 23-10 and p. 414.)

Suspicion of this condition should be aroused when a soft, rapidly growing, nontender mass is palpated adjacent to a slightly enlarged uterus, with or without bleeding. Ultrasound examination should be performed. The presence of an extrauterine gestational sac with well-localized and defined placenta helps differentiate this condition from an abdominal pregnancy, which is more common. Proper treatment is early excision of the rudimentary horn and its tube, with preservation of the ipsilateral ovary.

FIG. 30-7. Pregnancy in a noncommunicating rudimentary horn of a bicornuate uterus.

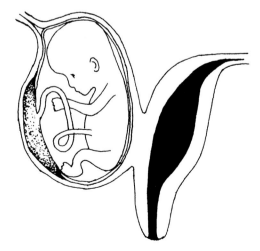

DIETHYLSTILBESTROL EXPOSURE *IN UTERO*

Between 1 million and 1.5 million women were exposed *in utero* to diethylstilbestrol (DES) administered to their mothers between the late 1940s and 1970, primarily for treatment of threatened abortion. These women are usually able to conceive, but many have poor pregnancy outcome. It has been found that 35% have vaginal epithelial changes (adenosis) and 24% have cervical structural changes. Such manifestations are associated with an increased incidence of abnormal HSG findings, which in turn imply increased risk of unfavorable pregnancy outcome. Forty-two percent of these women subjected to HSG have been found to have abnormal uterine cavity shape; the T shape and constriction defects are the most common and significant for prognosis. Thirty-five percent have had intrauterine defects; irregular margins, caused by myometrial thickening and consequent indentation, were most frequent and most significant (Fig. 30-8). Preterm delivery and ectopic pregnancy are experienced significantly more often than normal in women with HSG changes: preterm birth at some time in 22%, versus 7% of patients with a normal HSG, and ectopic pregnancy in 10%, versus fewer than 1%. Spontaneous abortion and stillbirth are not statistically different. Forty-six percent of women with abnormal HSGs have an unfavorable outcome at least once, and 31% never experience a favorable outcome. Comparable statistics for those with normal HSGs are 24% and 4%, respectively.

The 20-fold increase in ectopic pregnancy among women with DES stigmata on HSG should alert the clinician to take every precaution to make an early diagnosis of this complication. Frequent pelvic examinations may detect early effacement and dilatation of the cervix, although it remains to be seen whether cerclage will be effective in managing selected patients with a history of midtrimester abortion and preterm delivery. HSG for the woman who exhibits signs of DES exposure and who has had a poor obstetric outcome will allow a more accurate prognosis for that patient's childbearing future.

MYOMA UTERI

Although myomas are found in 40% to 50% of women at autopsy, less than a 1% incidence of myomas 3 cm or greater has been found in a large group of pregnant women subjected to ultrasound. While there may be dramatic enlargement of myomas in the first 12 weeks of pregnancy, relatively few increase in size beyond that time, and almost all regress to their original size in the puerperium.

Myomas may cause infertility, and when no other cause for infertility is found, myomectomy may be indicated. Spontaneous abortion may be caused by myomas, but the majority of implantation sites, as demonstrated by ultrasound, do not overlap the myoma; most pregnancies progress normally and terminate in vaginal delivery.

Large tumors may undergo secondary changes, notably carneous, hyaline, fatty, cystic, or calcific degeneration; infection and suppuration; and very rarely, sarcomatous transformation. These changes increase the probability of late abortion, preterm birth, and fetal death *in utero*. When extensive necrosis of the carneous type (red degeneration) occurs during pregnancy, the patient may complain of severe pain and marked tenderness over the uterus. This complication of myomas is characteristically associated with the gravid state, but it is observed occasionally in the nonpregnant uterus. Degeneration of blood vessels, local hemolysis, and resultant thrombotic processes account for low-grade fever, peritoneal irritation, and leukocytosis. Treatment of this condition is usually medical, with bed rest and analgesics. Ice packs may be helpful intermittently.

Torsion with subsequent gangrene of a subserous, pedunculated myoma is an indication for myomectomy, which usually can be performed safely without interrupting the pregnancy.

Pain in the right lower quadrant is less apt to be confused with appendicitis when an eary diagnosis of right-sided myoma is made during pregnancy.

Whenever myoma is suspected during pregnancy, an ultrasound scan should be performed to confirm the diagnosis, to measure the tumor, and especially to note the relationship between the myoma and the implantation site. The latter is much more important than tumor size in predicting risk during the pregnancy, since there is a 75% complication rate when the tumor and placenta overlap. Premature rupture of membranes and antenatal and postpartum hemorrhage commonly result.

While poor placentation may be caused by myomas, resulting in intrauterine fetal demise, a near-term living infant has been delivered by cesarean hysterectomy along with a 14-lb tumor.

FIG. 30-8. Composite illustration of the three most significant HSG DES stigmata: T shape, narrow cavity, irregular margins. External configuration is normal.

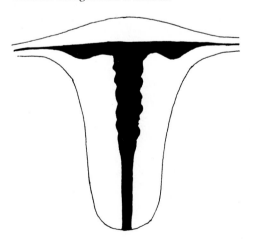

When a fetal death has been associated with a myoma, a myomectomy should be performed four to six months postpartum before the patient becomes pregnant again. The decision as to whether a subsequent infant is delivered vaginally or abdominally depends somewhat on the size of the myoma and the resulting defect requiring closure, but particularly on whether entrance into the endometrial cavity occurred. The latter indicates the need for cesarean section. The surgeon should dictate into the operative notes his impression as to the best management of future delivery.

A twofold increase in limb-defect anomalies has been reported in women having myomatous uteri, placing these patients at additional risk. At the onset of labor, it may be apparent that the myoma displaces the presenting fetal part or obstructs the birth canal. Moreover, the tumor may so interfere with the character and effectiveness of the uterine contraction pattern that labor is inert, dyskinetic, and prolonged. Any patient known to have a uterine myoma should have a sterile vaginal examination during the early part of the first stage of labor to determine fetal presentation and station and to rule out pelvic obstruction. Any patient who exhibits dystocia from an unknown cause should be examined carefully for the presence of a uterine tumor. If the myoma remains impacted in the pelvis and prevents descent of the presenting part, cesarean section is the preferred method of delivery. Multiple myomectomy is usually ill advised at this time, although large tumors that are likely to undergo marked degeneration and sepsis during the puerperium may necessitate hysterectomy. It is important to reserve judgment concerning the method of delivery until the onset of labor because myomas often rise out of the pelvis at term or in early parturition, especially when they arise from the anterior uterine wall.

If the birth canal is unobstructed, even though there are large tumors throughout the upper fundus, and fetal presentation is normal, vaginal delivery is usually possible. The principal hazard in delivery by this route is uterine bleeding due to a faulty third-stage mechanism and retention of part of the placenta. Inexpert attempts to remove the placenta manually may disrupt the tumor or even sever its uterine attachments. These accidents are associated with profuse hemorrhage and shock requiring repeated transfusions to maintain blood volume and prompt hysterectomy to control heavy bleeding.

Even if serious problems do not supervene during labor and delivery, not all danger has passed; uterine tumors may undergo extensive necrosis, infection, and suppurative degeneration during the puerperium. Moreover, vigorous manipulation of the uterus, as in manual removal of the placenta or in compression and massage to maintain muscle tone and minimize blood loss, may disrupt omental or peritoneal adhesions in the region of the tumor, giving rise to subsequent intra-abdominal hemorrhage. Thus, intensive supervision and care during this critical period should be routine for all patients.

OVARIAN TUMORS

Although any type of ovarian tumor may complicate pregnancy, the most common are the benign cysts, notably dermoids and serous or pseudomucinous cystadenomas. The corpus luteum of pregnancy may reach a diameter of 5 cm to 6 cm during the first trimester, but after that it gradually regresses. The possibility of its being confused with a true ovarian neoplasm is greatest when the structure is of maximum size, although repeated examination usually discloses reduction of its dimensions as gestation advances. During early pregnancy, the changes in size and consistency of ovarian cysts are easily discernible, once both the tumor and the uterus can be outlined as separate masses even though their relations may be variable. Later, the ovarian mass may come to lie in the abdomen or in a lateral gutter of the flank and may be exceedingly difficult to feel, even when it is large.

A true cystic ovarian neoplasm discovered during early pregnancy is best removed between the 16th and 18th weeks of gestation, a time when fewer than 2% of women will subsequently abort. During the first trimester, as many as 35% will abort; after 18 weeks preterm labor is much more common. Immediate operation is required, regardless of the duration of pregnancy, when acute symptoms develop or when the tumor is solid. Ultrasound may be helpful in assessing whether a tumor is solid or cystic.

The decision to remove any asymptomatic ovarian tumor is based on the seriousness of potential complications; these include the increased probability of abortion and the fourfold likelihood of torsion, necrosis, septic degeneration, hemorrhage into the capsule, rupture followed by peritonitis, preterm birth and neonatal death, and obstruction of the birth canal preventing normal delivery in 25% of cases. Even after normal delivery, torsion, necrosis, and eventual sepsis of an ovarian tumor constitute serious risks in the puerperium. Thus, an ovarian cyst diagnosed late in pregnancy or after delivery is best removed in the immediate postpartum period if the patient's general condition is satisfactory. An additional reason for removing an ovarian tumor is that its benign or malignant nature cannot be determined by pelvic examination alone. Most tumors under 5 cm do not produce symptoms, whereas most over 10 cm are symptomatic.

Hormone-producing tumors may affect the fetus, but it is thought that the placenta's ability to aromatize androgens to estrogens may prevent some virilization effect. Large quantities of estrogen produced by some granulosa cell tumors are apparently masked by the pregnancy.

Rarely an ovarian mass wedged below the promontory rises out of the pelvis spontaneously at term or in early labor and may interfere with descent of the presenting part. In obstructed labor, cesarean section is the preferred method of delivery; otherwise vaginal delivery should be accomplished and the tumor removed shortly thereafter. If the mass is found to be a dermoid cyst, the tumor can often be resected with preservation of normal ovarian tissue. The contralateral ovary should be bisected and inspected for the presence of an early tumor. If the mass is found to be a cystoma or a sex cord tumor, the entire ovary should be sacrificed and the opposite ovary examined thoroughly. If the cyst is multiloculated or papillary or if it contains areas of induration, a frozen section of suspicious tissue should be studied.

Malignant tumors of the ovary are exceedingly rare complications of pregnancy, and are dealt with according to the principles outlined in Chapter 59.

REFERENCES AND RECOMMENDED READING

Buttram VC Jr.: Müllerian anomalies and their management. Fertil Steril 40:159, 1983

Crona N, Bachrach I: Pathologic torsion of the pregnant uterus. Acta Obstet Gynecol Scand 63, No. 4:375, 1984

Danforth DN: Discussion of paper by Fields C, Pildes RB: Sacculation of the uterus. Am J Obstet Gynecol 87:507, 1963

Hill PS: Uterine prolapse complicating pregnancy: A case report. J Reprod Med 29, No. 8:631, 1984

Holden R, Hart P: First trimester rudimentary horn pregnancy: Prerupture ultrasound diagnosis. Obstet Gynecol 61, No. 35:565, 1983

Kaufmann RH, Noller K, Adam E et al: Upper genital tract anomalies and pregnancy outcome in diethylstilbestrol-exposed progeny. Am J Obstet Gynecol 148:973, 1984

Minkoff H, Grunebaum AN, Schwarz RH et al: Risk factors for prematurity and premature rupture of membranes: A prospective study of the vaginal flora in pregnancy. Am J Obstet Gynecol 150, No. 8:965, 1984

Sumner DS: Venous dynamics: Varicosities. Clin Obstet Gynecol 24, No. 3:743, 1981

Washington AE: Preventing complications of sexually transmitted disease: New treatment guidelines for expanded spectrum of problems. Drugs 28, No. 4:355, 1984

Winer–Muram HT, Muram D, Gillieson MS et al: Uterine myomas in pregnancy. Can Med Assoc J 128:949, 1983

Worthen NJ, Gonzales F: Septate uterus: Sonographic diagnosis and obstetric complications. Obstet Gynecol 64, No. 3S: 34S, 1984

Young RH, Dudley AG, Scully RE: Granulosa cell, Sertoli–Leydig cell, and unclassified sex cord-stromal tumors associated with pregnancy: A clinicopathological analysis of 36 cases. Gynecol Oncol 18, No. 2:181, 1984

Cancer

William L. Donegan

Cancer accompanies one of every 1008 pregnancies.[1] With 3.5 million live births in the United States each year, one can expect about 3571 cases of cancer. This represents 0.8% of the 422,000 women who develop cancers annually and 2.2% of the fertile women who do so, that is, those between the ages of 15 and 44 years.[2] One of every 118 women newly diagnosed with cancer will be pregnant.

Of all cancers of women, 12.8% occur during reproductive life. Those most likely to do so are thryoid, uterine cervix, melanoma of the skin, bones, and joints, and lymphomas. Almost half (49.8%) of all thyroid cancers and more than one third of all uterine cervix cancers occur in women 15 to 44 years of age. However, because of their numeric frequency, the cancers most likely to be seen in pregnant women are, in declining order, those of the breast, uterine cervix, ovary, lymphomas, and colorectum.

Pregnancy is generally considered to have an adverse effect on the course of cancer. One reason for suspecting this is the immunologic tolerance that characterizes pregnancy. The manifestations of tolerance include the depression of cellular immunity; the presence of circulating serologic blocking factors, probably an IgG immunoglobulin; the immunosuppressive effect of estrogen, progesterone, and human chorionic gonadotropin (hCG); the presence of suppressor T cells, the presence of a leukocyte migration enhancement factor; and decreased red blood cell immune adherence.[3,4] These mechanisms, which ensure the survival of the fetus, presumably also favor the progress of neoplasia.

The physician's objectives are to cure the patient of her cancer and to deliver a healthy, viable infant. Important concerns are whether pregnancy adversely influences the prospects for cure of cancers, what risk maternal cancer or its treatment poses to the fetus, and whether pregnancy following treatment of a malignant neoplasm is advisable.

CANCER OF THE BREAST

Cancer of the breast is the most frequent cancer of women, as well as the cause of most neoplastic deaths, now numbering 37,000 per year in the United States. After age 15 and until age 75, a woman is more likely to die of breast cancer than of any other type of cancer.[5] About 15% of the cases occur in women under 41 years of age, and about 3% of the cases occur during pregnancy, complicating approximately 1 in every 3000 pregnancies.

Opinions about diagnosis and management when breast cancer occurs coincident with pregnancy have undergone substantial change in recent years.[6–14] The high frequency of metastases to axillary lymph nodes and the poor survival of women with breast cancer during pregnancy have been offered as evidence that pregnancy has an adverse effect on the growth and spread of this cancer. Contributing influences include the increased vascularity of the breasts and stimulation by sex steroids of this often hormonally dependent tumor. However, delay in diagnosis and hesitant treatment may have contributed substantially to the poor results of earlier years. The histologic types of tumors that occur in pregnant women are not different from those seen in nonpregnant women. While a disproportionately high number of patients present with axillary node involvement, delayed diagnosis averages two to seven months longer for pregnant patients than for the nonpregnant.

Emphasis at present is upon prompt diagnosis of any mass in the breast of a pregnant or lactating woman and prompt treatment of the cancer, essentially ignoring the pregnancy and accepting a small risk of abortion. Needle aspiration of masses to distinguish cystic from solid lesions and biopsy of the latter under local anesthesia entail negligible risk to the fetus. Mammograms in the pregnant patient are compromised by the density of the breast tissues during pregnancy and do not influence the need for biopsy if a mass exists. Stage for stage, the outlook for the pregnant patient is almost as good as is that for the nonpregnant patient; the patient's best hope for successful treatment lies in the treatment of small tumors that have not yet spread to axillary lymph nodes. Masses in the breast of a pregnant woman prove to be cancer as often as in the nongravid female. In deference to the fetus, staging of the patient with proven cancer should not include radioisotopic scans.

Treatment is not different from that of the nonpregnant patient. Experience with treatment during pregnancy has virtually all been with radical mastectomy, but modified radical mastectomy, that is, removal of the breast and the axillary lymph nodes, is now the standard treatment for cancer of the breast in early clinical stages and is appropriate for the pregnant patient. The risk of spontaneous abortion after mastectomy is 1% depending on the duration of gestation, and this must be discussed with the patient in advance.[15] Treatment with primary irradiation to the breast is unwise in a pregnant patient. Intrauterine exposure during the first six weeks of pregnancy is likely to result in fetal death or congenital anomalies (Fig. 30-9).[16] A fetus located 25 cm below the base of the irradiation field to which 7500 rad is delivered would receive approximately 30 rad of irradiation.[17] Although the risk of teratogenesis is less during the second half of pregnancy, the fetus is higher in the abdomen and would be exposed to additional irradiation with the hazards of long-term carcinogenesis. The same risks apply to postoperative irradiation. The risk of teratogenic or mutagenic effects upon the fetus approximates 1:1000 per cGy (rad).[18]

Women with nodal metastases, still 75% of treated cases, are candidates for systemic chemotherapy because of their poor prognosis. As it happens, premenopausal women have benefited most from adjuvant chemotherapy, but since most chemotherapeutic drugs are teratogenic, therapeutic abortion is desirable in early pregnancy. If the patient is near term, chemotherapy might be delayed briefly until after early delivery. Normal infants have been delivered when systemic chemotherapy was given during pregnancy, but the reports are too few to clarify the long-term risks. Similar decisions must be made when postoperative irradiation is considered in patients with a high risk of local recurrence.

Diagnosis during the third trimester of pregnancy deserves no special considerations. There seems to be little justification for delay to achieve fetal viability in view of the small risk of premature delivery and the potentially adverse consequences for the patient.[12]

Unless indicated to permit adjuvant therapy, abortion has no therapeutic advantage for the patient. Nor is prophylactic castration of proven benefit; randomized trials have produced conflicting results.[19-21]

Although relatively advanced stage and frequent nodal involvement usually characterize patients treated during pregnancy or lactation, their prognosis is only slightly inferior to that of nonpregnant women with similar stages of the disease. Ribeiro and Palmer reported five-year survivals of 90%, 37%, 15%, and 0% for patients with clinical stages I, II, III, and IV, respectively. In contrast to the earlier reports of Peters, they found that the results for each stage were similar in each trimester of pregnancy and postpartum.[22] Overall, survival was 70% at five years.

Effective palliative therapy of advanced and disseminated breast cancer in the first or second trimester ordinarily requires termination of pregnancy. Chemotherapy or irradiation would entail considerable risk to the fetus, and endocrine therapy would also require its termination. In the third trimester a temporary delay of treatment for three or four weeks to permit fetal growth to 1500 g to 1800 g, at which survival is assured, might be considered if the patient's condition permits. Any such delay should be discussed and mutually agreed upon by the patient and physician.

Advice concerning pregnancies after potentially curative treatment for breast cancer has changed in recent years.[23] Up to 7% of fertile women have subsequent pregnancies, most often within five years of treatment. Opinion has traditionally been against further childbearing, but it has become increasingly apparent that pregnancies are not associated with excessive risk of

FIG. 30-9. Deaths and abnormalities at term after radiation exposure. Figures are estimated for humans based on animal data. (Brill AB, Forgotson EH: Radiation and congenital malformations. Am J Obstet Gynecol 90:1149, 1964)

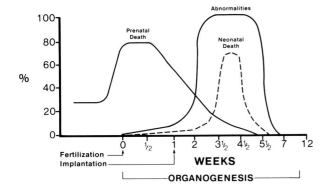

recurrence. Five-year survival rates of 58% to 77% are common. This is not a matter of patient selection in that only women without an early recurrence and with a good prognosis from the outset live to become pregnant. On the contrary, when patients are matched for clinical stage, age, status of axillary involvement, and length of survival to the time of the subsequent pregnancy, those who become pregnant survive as well as others who do not.[9,24] There is little ground, therefore, for advising against subsequent pregnancies for those who desire them and are free of recurrence. Whether the estrogen-receptor content of the tumor should have an influence on this decision is uncertain. Negativity in general would suggest no influence on the tumor but implies a poor prognosis for the patient. The patient's prospects for recurrence based on nodal status might influence this decision. Chances for recurrence are highest in the first three years after mastectomy (Fig. 30-10). Should a pregnancy occur, a decision for abortion is based upon the patient's overall prognosis and her desires; it has no therapeutic value.

GENITAL CANCER

A gynecologic malignancy accompanies 1 in every 407 pregnancies.[25] Most are carcinomas of the cervix (1:664 pregnancies), but others include vulvar cancer (1:8000), vaginal cancer (1:37,000), and ovarian cancer (1:9000). Ages range from 25 to 35 years. Proper prenatal care should result in early diagnosis of these cancers. A vaginal examination and Papanicolaou (Pap) smear should be routine, and during pregnancy an abnormal vaginal discharge, especially bloody, deserves investigation. Genital cancers are not known to be influenced by pregnancy.

FIG. 30-10. Annual risk of recurrence after mastectomy in 134 patients under 45 years of age.

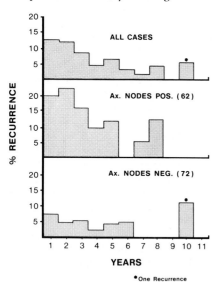

% RECURRENCE

YEARS

•One Recurrence

Cervical Cancer

From 2.7% to 3.5% of all cervical carcinomas occur during pregnancy, and management is the subject of many reports.[26-29] Diagnosis is similar to that in the nonpregnant state. The physician should be aware that pathophysiologic alterations of the cervical epithelium during pregnancy cannot be attributed to increased estrogen and progesterone levels. Vaginal bleeding due to cervical carcinoma is infrequent in the gravid female; most cases are discovered by vaginal examination and Pap smear.

Treatment is determined by the state of the cancer and the trimester of pregnancy. If a colposcopically directed biopsy shows carcinoma *in situ,* conization of the cervix is rarely necessary. The important distinction between carcinoma *in situ* and invasive carcinoma can often be made with colposcopically directed biopsies. The ultimate diagnosis can be made in 92% or more of such cases.[30] If conization is necessary, the complication rate is appreciable; spontaneous abortion, premature labor, and hemorrhage vary in frequency from 20% to 33%.

Carcinoma *in situ* may be managed safely with repeated colposcopic examinations and Pap smears and the patient allowed to deliver vaginally. Conization during pregnancy is not adequate therapy; as many as 50% of patients will demonstrate residual carcinoma *in situ* in postpartum hysterectomy specimens. Six to eight weeks after delivery, complete diagnostic studies, including Pap smear, colposcopy, and therapeutic conization, should be performed. In most cases conservative treatment of carcinoma *in situ* with conization, cryocautery, or CO_2 laser evaporation will be adequate therapy if margins are tumor free by colposcopic examination. Hysterectomy is reserved for the rare patient with persistent disease manifested by positive cytology or residual tumor at the margins of the cone.

Invasive carcinomas of the cervix discovered during the first two trimesters of pregnancy are managed as if the pregnancy did not exist. Early stages are commonly treated surgically; that is, stage 1A is treated with total abdominal hysterectomy, including a wide vaginal cuff, and stage 1B by radical hysterectomy with bilateral pelvic lymph node dissection. The ovaries are retained in young women. More advanced stages are treated with irradiation. External irradiation almost invariably induces a spontaneous abortion; if not, a hysterotomy is performed prior to radium insertion. In the third trimester a viable fetus is delivered by cesarean section followed by surgical treatment or irradiation. A brief delay is acceptable if necessary for the fetus to reach viability, after which the same procedure is followed. Vaginal delivery is deemed unwise on the grounds that cancer cells may be spread by the trauma of cervical dilation, but verification of this hazard is difficult to obtain.[29,31]

The prognosis of patients treated for carcinoma *in situ* is uniformly good, with recurrences in no more than 1.5%. Opinion is not uniform concerning the prognosis of women with invasive carcinoma. The opinion of some is that pregnancy has a negative effect on results; others have found the results superior for each stage.[29] Current thought suggests that stage for stage, the outlook is the same regardless of pregnancy. Sablinska and colleagues found that advanced stages became more frequent as pregnancy progressed, accounting for the superior results obtained in patients treated during the first trimester (73.2% survivors) compared with those in patients treated after delivery (36.5% survivors).[28] Young women (under 30 years of age) were diagnosed late in pregnancy, had a high frequency of advanced stages, and fared less well in each stage of disease than patients of similar age who were not pregnant.

Endometrial Cancer

Cases of endometrial carcinoma occurring with pregnancy are too few to permit reliable evaluation; only eight have been reported since 1900.[14] The rarity of this cancer reflects the fact that only 8% of all cases of endometrial carcinoma occur in women under 40 years of age.[32] Furthermore, premalignant or carcinomatous changes in the endometrium usually discourage successful implantation. Age at diagnosis has been between 21 and 43 years, and four of seven cases summarized by Sandstrom have been diagnosed as adenoacanthoma, usually a well-differentiated cancer.[32] Vaginal bleeding is a prominent symptom. Three patients have lived at least five years after treatment, which in two cases consisted of hysterectomy. One patient refused treatment after her diagnosis, became pregnant, and delivered a normal infant. She was well ten years later, raising some question about the diagnosis. Most of these tumors are small and well differentiated. The only patient known to have died had deep myometrial invasion. Total abdominal hysterectomy with bilateral salpingo-oophorectomy is indicated without delay if endometrial cancer is diagnosed in the first trimester of pregnancy or after abortion. Abdominal and pelvic lymphadenectomy is performed if the lesion warrants this approach (see Chap. 56).

Vulvar Cancer

Vulvar cancer is a disease of the aged, and only 2% are associated with pregnancy.[25] Nineteen cases were reported through 1977, the majority of which were squamous cell carcinomas. Three cases of sarcoma, two of adenocarcinoma of Bartholin's gland, one carcinoma *in situ,* and one melanoma completed the total. Invasive vulvar carcinoma associated with pregnancy has a poor prognosis. Only the patient with carcinoma *in situ* was cured in Lutz's series, although two others survived 10 and 18 years prior to death from recurrence.[25] Invasive vulvar cancer is treated with radical vulvectomy and inguinal–femoral node dissection performed at any time during pregnancy. Deep pelvic nodes are rarely involved

if inguinal–femoral nodes are histologically normal. Since deep pelvic lymph node dissection is so often attended by morbid lymphedema, most surgeons believe that it is not necessary unless superficial nodes are involved. Surgical treatment does not preclude vaginal delivery or a later pregnancy.

Vaginal Cancer

The genital cancer least frequently associated with pregnancy is vaginal carcinoma. The estimate is that only 1 of 77 cases of vaginal cancer will be associated with pregnancy. With only 11 cases reported, information regarding treatment is limited. Customarily, squamous cell carcinoma of the vagina is treated with radiation therapy if low in the vagina and either irradiation or radical surgery if in the upper vagina. Opinions are that vaginal delivery should be avoided and that optimum treatment should be administered without regard to the pregnancy. If the fetus has reached viability, treatment should be preceded by a cesarean section. A speculum examination for vaginal bleeding at any stage of pregnancy is the key to early diagnosis.

Ovarian Cancer

The frequency of ovarian malignancy has been placed at 1 in every 9000 to 25,000 deliveries.[33,34] Because ovarian cancer is rare in populations that do not practice birth control, some have suggested that pregnancy may protect against its development.[35] Diagnosis is difficult because ovarian cancers are obscured by an enlarged uterus, but ultrasound is valuable. Masses greater than 5 cm in the second trimester require diagnostic evaluation. Fortunately, only 5% of ovarian neoplasms found during gestation are malignant, compared with approximately 15% to 20% of those found in nonpregnant women. Furthermore, unusual types of tumors of a low malignant potential account for a high proportion of the total, and many are found at an early stage. If the tumor is unilateral, well encapsulated, associated with negative peritoneal cytology, and of a low histologic grade, unilateral oophorectomy may be considered, allowing the pregnancy to proceed to term. After 6 weeks' gestation or more, the placenta alone is capable of supporting pregnancy. Agreement is not uniform, however; some would limit unilateral oophorectomy to mucinous cystadenocarcinomas, dysgerminomas, or granulosa cell tumors, while others would exclude dysgerminomas.[33] Intraoperative decisions are facilitated by frozen sections. If excrescences are found on the surface of the tumor, omentum, or peritoneum, if the tumor is poorly differentiated or of an aggressive cell type, or if the disease is found in an advanced stage, aggressive surgery is indicated, followed by adjuvant therapy.

In 1980 Cunanan and associates reported the 25th case of choriocarcinoma of the ovary coexisting with pregnancy, only the third instance in which both the mother and infant survived.[36] Treatment was delayed until a term infant was delivered by cesarean section, following which the patient was treated with chemotherapy with actinomycin D, methotrexate, and chlorambucil. hCG levels returned to normal, and the patient was well three and one half years later. These authors emphasized the value of ultrasound in detecting ovarian tumors during gestation.

CANCER OF THE GASTROINTESTINAL TRACT

Cancer of the gastrointestinal tract complicates approximately 1 in 100,000 pregnancies;[37] most are cancers of the colon and rectum. The 19th case of carcinoma of the colon was reported in 1980. In one survey 7 cases of rectal cancer were found during 350,000 pregnancies, an incidence of 0.002%.[38,39] The total number of rectal carcinomas in the literature before 1967 was only 155.[40] The preponderance of rectal over colon cancers may be due to the attention given to the pelvis during pregnancy.

Pregnancy has no apparent influence on the growth of these cancers. Delayed diagnosis is the major problem, particularly when the tumor is situated above the level that can be easily reached on a digital rectal examination. The symptoms of abdominal pain, distention, nausea, vomiting, constipation, and rectal bleeding are often dismissed as the side-effects of pregnancy until intussusception, obstruction, or perforation of the colon discloses the error. Neoplasms have been discovered during all trimesters and during labor, and some patients have clearly had predisposing factors such as ulcerative colitis, familial polyposis, Gardner's syndrome, and villous tumors. In the interest of early diagnosis, symptoms related to the colon and rectum during pregnancy cannot be dismissed lightly. Digital rectal examination, a test of the stool for occult blood, and proctosigmoidoscopic examination can be performed safely during pregnancy and will detect more than 75% of carcinomas in the rectosigmoid region. A strong suspicion that colorectal cancer is present justifies further investigation, including a barium enema. To avoid irritation risk to the fetus, however, colonoscopy may be preferable to barium enema in the pregnant patient.

Appropriate treatment during the first two trimesters of pregnancy is surgical resection without delay. After the 33rd week of gestation, a cesarean section obtains a viable infant and permits the tumor to be resected at the same time. If the pregnancy is near term and the tumor is not in a position to cause dystocia, a vaginal delivery can be performed before the tumor is resected. The plan is similar for rectal tumors, although their location is more likely to complicate delivery.

Anterior resection or abdominal perineal resection is used as appropriate. Normal vaginal deliveries have followed both of these procedures.[41] Near term, either induced labor or cesarean section is appropriate, but if labor has begun, a vaginal delivery is preferred, followed after a short interval by surgical resection of the cancer. Large low-lying tumors or those that involve the anterior rectal wall may hemorrhage during labor or cause obstruction of labor, so in these cases a cesarean section is preferable to a vaginal delivery. It is not usually necessary to remove the uterus in order to resect the rectum during early pregnancy or after a cesarean section, since the uterus can be sufficiently displaced. Unless the uterus is involved by the tumor or must be removed for adequate margin around the tumor, it may be left intact. Abortion per se is not therapeutic and is not indicated. Curative resections were attended by a 15% fetal loss and a 10% operative mortality rate before 1947; presumably results have improved in recent years.[42]

If the rectal cancer is not curable, a viable fetus can be obtained, if the patient chooses, by withholding treatment until the fetus matures. Cesarean section can then be followed by palliative resection of the colon and supplemented with chemotherapy or irradiation as appropriate. Hemorrhage, obstruction, or perforation of the colon requires early intervention.

The prognosis of pregnant women with colon cancer has been poor, with no five-year survivors. By contrast, 10 of 16 women treated for rectal carcinoma at the Mayo Clinic (62%) survived for at least five years,[40] comparable to the overall survival rate of nonpregnant women with rectal cancer. Six were treated early in their pregnancy with abdominoperineal resection or anterior resection without disturbing the pregnancy. One died postoperatively of sepsis, another died subsequently during her pregnancy, and the remaining four had normal vaginal deliveries. Five had cesarean sections, with the loss of one infant.

Reports have been made of cancers at other sites in the gastrointestinal tract, including reticulum cell sarcoma of the duodenum and of the appendix, hepatocellular carcinoma, and cancer of the stomach, pointing out their infrequency and difficulty of diagnosis.[43,44] Wide excision without delay is advocated without interference with the pregnancy unless it is necessitated by involvement of the uterus, tubes, or ovaries. It is of interest that metastatic tumors to the ovaries (*i.e.,* Krukenberg tumors) can stimulate androgen production and cause masculinization of a female fetus.[45]

MALIGNANT MELANOMA

Melanoma is concentrated in the third and fourth decades of life, consequently among women in their reproductive years, and circumstantial evidence suggests that endocrine changes may influence its behavior.[46] A rapidly fatal course is sometimes observed in the pregnant female; pregnancy stimulates melanocytes, and estrogen-receptor proteins are found in melanomas. Conclusive evidence for either a beneficial or a deleterious effect of pregnancy, however, has not been forthcoming.[47-49]

Most authors have reported no significant difference in the five-year survival rates of pregnant and nonpregnant women and no influence of endocrine ablation or of therapeutic abortion on the course of the disease.[50] Nor have differences in local development or metastatic spread of implantable hamster melanomas been observed when both pregnant and nonpregnant hamsters were inoculated.[51] Clinical reviews have failed to be conclusive. In one, 115 patients up to 43 years of age who were pregnant at presentation or had a pregnancy after treatment had more advanced stages at the time of treatment than 141 patients of similar age who were not pregnant. Nevertheless, the clinical courses of the two groups were indistinguishable, with ten-year survivals of 42% and 45%. In a subsequent report, patients with involved nodes who were treated during pregnancy or who reported activation of a melanoma during a pregnancy had reduced survival compared with others. The suggestion was that pregnancy may adversely influence some melanomas, most evident among those with a high risk of residual disease. In a study of 101 patients compared with controls matched for important variables, Reintgen and co-workers found disease-free survival reduced in patients diagnosed during pregnancy, but subsequent pregnancies had no effect on recurrence or survival.[52]

Any suspicious change in a pigmented cutaneous lesion during pregnancy warrants a prompt biopsy, and a diagnosis of melanoma should be treated promptly in a manner that does not compromise the patient's chances for cure. The pregnancy is a secondary consideration in patients who are potentially curable. Standard treatment is wide resection of the primary along with dissection of clinically involved regional lymph nodes, en bloc with the primary if feasible. Prophylactic regional lymph node dissection is presently a subject of controversy, and practice varies with the convictions of individual surgeons. Data are available for and against prophylactic nodal dissections when melanoma arises in the extremities, but none that is specific for the pregnant patient.[53,54]

Some advise against future pregnancies for patients who had nodal metastases or who experienced activation of the lesion during gestation.[50] Others recommend that all women avoid pregnancy for three to five years after treatment.[49] In view of the possibly adverse effect of estrogenic substances, nonhormonal methods of contraception seem wise.

LYMPHOMA AND LEUKEMIA

Successful management of Hodgkin's disease depends on careful staging and comprehensive treatment, objectives that are difficult to achieve during pregnancy without risk to the fetus. Evaluation of the abdomen is the obvious handicap. Isotopic scans are contraindicated because of the radiation hazard, and staging laparotomy is avoided. Lymphangiography is of undisputed value,

but a modified technique, in which the contrast material is injected as usual but is followed by only a single abdominal film 24 hours after the injection,[55] is recommended.

Pregnancy has been found to have no influence on the pattern of curability of Hodgkin's disease, and it is important not to compromise treatment.[55] Stage-I and stage-II disease above the diaphragm, frequently nodular sclerosing in this youthful age group, can be treated with irradiation to an upper mantle with reasonably effective shielding of the abdomen, but fetal exposure increases with the stage of pregnancy as the uterus rises in the abdomen. Fundal dose has been calculated at approximately 10.4 rad at 16 weeks of pregnancy, with an increase to 100 rad at 30 weeks. If involvement of abdominal nodes is unequivocally present and the pregnancy is in its early months, the pregnancy must be terminated so that adequate treatment can be given. In advanced stages consideration should be given to therapeutic abortion because of the teratogenic effects of chemotherapy, a risk most critical in the first ten weeks of pregnancy. Chemotherapy later in pregnancy has been followed by delivery of normal infants.[56-58] Cesarean section or induced labor can be used before treatment is started if the fetus has reached viability.

Pregnancy is not advised for two years after treatment; 80% of recurrences appear within this period. After treatment for Hodgkin's disease, only 57% of pregnancies result in normal live births.[59] Thirty percent of fetuses are either premature or die, and 7.5% of live births have major malformations. In some reports, however, patients fared no worse than sibling controls. Whereas irradiation alone does not appear to increase these hazards, the combination of irradiation and chemotherapy does.[60] The risk extends to males treated with both irradiation and chemotherapy, whose wives are more likely to have spontaneous abortions than the wives of male controls.

Burkitt's lymphoma during pregnancy and lactation has a predilection for the breasts and runs a rapidly fatal course.[61] Dramatic swelling of the breasts occurs and has been mistaken for mastitis. This unusual presentation has been attributed to a favorable hormonal milieu or to lowered immunologic competence.

Leukemia accompanies fewer than 1 in 75,000 pregnancies; 300 cases were reported through 1976.[57] Pregnancy has no deleterious effect upon leukemia. On the other hand, leukemia poses a significant threat to the pregnancy with increased risk of infection, spontaneous abortion, and hemorrhage. A healthy live infant can be expected in fewer than 50% of patients if acute myelogenous leukemia develops in the first half of pregnancy.[62] The prospects are somewhat more favorable with acute lymphocytic leukemia. Patients require aggressive combination chemotherapy and diligent supportive care. If treatment is started in the first trimester, fetal abnormalities are high and termination of the pregnancy should be considered after remission is achieved. Initiation of treatment in the second or third trimester is less likely to be teratogenic. A number of reports have emphasized that treatment of leukemia does not preclude a successful pregnancy,[57,63-65] but the long-term effects upon infants exposed *in utero* are not completely known. Because the prognosis for women with acute leukemia is poor, the prospect for a newborn is that it will soon be motherless. The maternal mortality rate approaches 100% by the sixth month postpartum for patients with acute meylogenous leukemia.[62] Chronic leukemias generally have an indolent course with little threat to successful pregnancy.

THYROID

Thyroid cancer has an affinity for young women, but it is still an infrequent cancer and has no clear relationship to pregnancy. Pregnancy subsequent to the treatment of thyroid carcinoma is not believed to invite recurrence nor to accelerate growth.[66] Cunningham and Slaughter operated on 71 women who developed disease of the thyroid during pregnancy or shortly afterward and found 8 with carcinoma, a frequency of 11.2%.[67] These eight cases represented 13% of all thyroid carcinomas seen during a 12-year period. Five had operations during pregnancy, and three of the five were followed by spontaneous abortion; all three had required neck dissections. Thus, fetal loss was considerable after extensive surgery. Rosvoll and Winship studied the effect of pregnancy on 60 women who had been treated previously for thyroid carcinoma[68] and concluded that pregnancy did not stimulate the growth of thyroid carcinoma and that the presence of the latter was not sufficient cause for prevention of pregnancy or for therapeutic abortion. Hill and associates reached similar conclusions.[69]

Recently, ultrasonography to differentiate between solid and cystic nodules and fine-needle aspiration of thyroid nodules to obtain cytologic material have found increased use and are of particular value for evaluating the pregnant patient, reducing the number of negative explorations and the attendant hazard of spontaneous abortion. Management of thyroid carcinoma can be based on the trimester of pregnancy.[67] If the clinical situation strongly suggests carcinoma during the first or second trimester, the thyroid gland is promptly explored. In the third trimester exploration might be delayed until after delivery, since this cancer is relatively indolent and pregnancy does not seem to stimulate its growth. The high probability of spontaneous abortion, particularly if a neck dissection is required, is also a factor. Neck dissection is obligatory for patients with histologically proven cervical lymph node metastases. Radioactive iodine for diagnostic purposes, for ablation of residual thyroid tissue, or for treatment of distant metastases is inappropriate during pregnancy and should be delayed until after delivery.

SARCOMAS

Any specific influence of pregnancy upon the behavior of soft tissue sarcomas is obscured by diverse clinical presentations and varied treatments. Some reports suggest an adverse effect, with disproportionate numbers of advanced cases or recurrences coincident with pregnancy,[70,71] but convincing evidence is lacking.[70,72] In one review, 57 women pregnant during, or subsequent to, the treatment of a variety of soft tissue sarcomas had ten-year cancer-free survivals comparable to those of nonpregnant patients of reproductive age (55% and 75%, respectively).[70] Cantin and McNeer recommended that pregnant women be managed without regard for the pregnancy during the first two trimesters of gestation, but in the third trimester suggested that the pregnancy be completed before initiation of treatment. They found no medical basis for recommending the interruption of subsequent pregnancies in women who had been effectively treated. Jafari and associates recommended that the fetus be given primary consideration in the presence of widespread maternal sarcoma.[72]

Radical pelvic surgery, when it is indicated, is not always a deterrent to childbearing. Two cases have been reported in which hemipelvectomy for sarcoma was followed by pregnancy and normal vaginal delivery.[73] In a review of 33 collected bone sarcomas treated during pregnancy, giant cell tumors and osteosarcomas were the most frequent, followed by Ewing's sarcomas, lymphomas, malignant fibrous histiocytomas, and one fibrosarcoma.[74] No effect on the pregnancy could be appreciated, and recommendations for treatment were based on the trimester of pregnancy, the location of the tumor, and the tumor's type and grade. General guidelines were as shown in Table 30-18. If radiation to the femur, pelvis, or thoracolumbar spine is indicated, elective abortion or early delivery is indicated.

Table 30-18
Recommended Treatment of Sarcoma by Trimester of Pregnancy

Sarcoma	First Trimester	Second Trimester	Third Trimester
High-grade sarcoma	Surgery, with abortion if chemotherapy planned		Early induced delivery
Low-grade sarcoma	Surgery only and continue pregnancy	Surgery only and continue pregnancy	Spontaneous or early induced delivery

CARCINOMA OF THE PANCREAS

Carcinoma of the pancreas during pregnancy is rare, difficult to diagnose, and uniformly fatal. An association with the pancreatitis of pregnancy has been reported, another unusual event that is frequently fatal, usually idiopathic, and most often found in the third trimester or early puerperium.[75] The subject of the report, a 37-year-old woman, developed nausea, vomiting, and epigastric discomfort with meals during the seventh month of her pregnancy and had developed mild icterus by the time she delivered. Her symptoms and jaundice progressed, were associated with elevated levels of urine amylase, and at laparotomy six weeks postpartum a needle biopsy was consistent with pancreatitis. A pseudocyst was also found in the tail of the pancreas. Cholecystectomy and choledochoduodenostomy were performed without relief, and two months later a pancreatic cystogastrostomy was performed. The patient developed sepsis and had three additional laparotomies for abscesses but died 13 months after the onset of her illness. An adenocarcinoma of the pancreas was found at autopsy with metastases to regional lymph nodes, the liver, and spleen.

Carcinoma is notoriously difficult to detect in the presence of pancreatitis, being made premortem in only 62% of the patients in a recent series.[76] Endoscopic retrograde pancreatography with cytologic examination of pancreatic secretions may be the best method of making this diagnosis.

Gastrinomas during pregnancy are limited to two cases.[77,78] Both patients developed the Zollinger–Ellison syndrome immediately after delivery, suggesting that pregnancy somehow protected against the ulcer diathesis. Symptoms included heartburn, which after delivery became severe epigastric pain, nausea, vomiting, and diarrhea. Peptic ulceration was associated with increased gastric acid secretion and elevated levels of serum gastrin. In one patient, a 4-cm to 5-cm tumor was found in the pancreas associated with a hepatic metastasis, and the patient was treated with total gastrectomy.[77] The patient developed weakness and weight loss and subsequently was found to have bilateral adrenal cortical hyperplasia. Following an adrenalectomy 14 months after delivery, the patient died of sepsis and pulmonary embolism. Despite its rarity, the Zollinger–Ellison syndrome should be suspected when severe ulcer symptoms follow delivery.

Insulinoma has also been reported. The symptoms are characteristic: dizziness, periodic loss of balance, diplopia, bizarre behavior, and convulsions associated with hypoglycemia. Relief of symptoms with intravenous glucose administration fulfills Whipple's diagnostic triad. A high serum insulin to glucose ratio is characteristic. Although selective splenic angiography exposes the fetus to irradiation, it is justified for localizing the tumor and detecting multiple insulinomas. Because repeated episodes of hypoglycemia are a threat to both the patient and the fetus, early operation is desirable. Two reports exist of successful surgical removal of insulinomas during the first trimester of pregnancy without fetal loss.[79,80]

METASTASES TO THE FETUS

Metastasis of maternal cancers to the fetus occurs but is unusual. Between 1866 and 1981 only 44 cases were reported in which a malignancy of the mother metastasized to the placenta or fetus[81] (Table 30-19). Both carcinomas and sarcomas have done so, but malignant melanoma is the most frequent offender; leukemias or lymphomas and breast cancers follow in frequency. The patient always had disseminated cancer at the time of her pregnancy. In 35 of the 44 cases the placenta was involved by tumor, and in 12 the fetus contained metastases. In only three were both the placenta and the fetus involved, although the placenta was not always examined. An involved placenta free of villous invasion generally indicates that the fetus is intact. An exception was an infant whose mother had disseminated melanoma; the infant also died of melanoma at one month of age. In six cases with known villous invasion, one child died of melanoma at ten months of age. It is evident that villous invasion does not invariably result in fetal metastases. Almost all cases of fetal involvement were by leukemias, lymphomas, or malignant melanomas, and the placenta was involved by the tumor in all cases in which it was examined.

Villous invasion is probably the means by which tumor cells traverse the placenta and reach the fetus. Whether biologic protective mechanisms exist for the

Table 30-19

Placental and Fetal Metastases from Maternal Malignancies, 1866–1981

Tumor Type	Total Cases	Placenta	Fetus
Malignant melanoma	15	11	6
Leukemia/lymphoma	8	5	4
Breast carcinoma	6	6	
Bronchogenic carcinoma	4	4	
Gastric carcinoma	2	2	
Myxosarcoma	1	1	
Adrenal carcinoma	1	1	
Ethmoid carcinoma	1	0	1
Ovarian carcinoma	1	1	
Hepatic carcinoma	1	0	1
Colorectal carcinoma	1	1	
Pancreatic carcinoma	1	1	
Undifferentiated carcinoma	1	1	
Angioblastic sarcoma	1	1	
Total	44	35	12

(Read EJ Jr, Platzer PB: Placental metastasis from maternal carcinoma of the ovary. Obstet Gynecol 58, No. 3:387, 1981)

placenta and fetus is uncertain.[1] The fetus may be able to resist a maternal tumor that is not genetically identical to its own tissues. This may explain cases of spontaneous regression of melanoma in children born to mothers with disseminated melanoma.

The placenta resists neoplastic transmission in both directions. Five cases of primary fetal malignancy (three neuroblastomas, one melanoma, and one leukemia) have been reported without metastasis to the mother.[1]

The risk of fetal involvement from maternal cancer, particularly if the cancer is not disseminated, is too small to recommend therapeutic abortion for this reason. Nevertheless, careful examination of the placenta and observation of the infant are recommended, particularly if the tumor was a melanoma or of the leukemia/lymphoma group.

REFERENCES AND RECOMMENDED READING

1. Potter JF, Schoeneman XM: Metastasis of maternal cancer to the placenta and fetus. Cancer 25:380, 1970
2. U.S. Department of Health and Human Services: Vital Statistics Report: Annual Summary for the United States, 1979. 28, No. 13:1, 1980
3. Gleicher N, Siegel I: Common denominators of pregnancy and malignancy. In Gleicher N (ed): Reproductive Immunology, pp 339–353. New York, Alan R Liss, 1981
4. Gleicher N, Deppe G, Cohen CJ: Common aspects of immunologic tolerance in pregnancy and malignancy. Obstet Gynecol 549, No. 3:335, 1979
5. Silverberg E: Cancer Statistics, 1984. CA 34:7, 1984
6. Anderson JM: Mammary cancers and pregnancy. Br Med J, April 28, 1979, 1124
7. Clark RM, Reid J: Carcinoma of the breast in pregnancy and lactation. Int J Radiat Oncol Biol Phys 4:693, 1978
8. Sahni K, Sanyal B, Agrawal MS et al: Carcinoma of breast associated with pregnancy and lactation. J Surg Oncol 16:167, 1981
9. Harvery JC, Rosen PP, Ashikari R et al: The effect of pregnancy on the prognosis of carcinoma of the breast following radical mastectomy. Surg Gynecol Obstet 153:723, 1981
10. Zinns JS: The association of pregnancy and breast cancer. J Reprod Med 22, No. 6:297, 1979
11. Hubay CA, Barry FM, Marr CC: Pregnancy and breast cancer. Surg Clin North Am 58, No. 4:819, 1978
12. Ribeiro GG, Palmer MK: Breast carcinoma associated with pregnancy: A clinician's dilemma. Br Med J 2(6101):1524, 1977
13. Donegan WL: Breast cancer and pregnancy. Obstet Gynecol 50, No. 2:244, 1977
14. Orr JW Jr., Shingleton HM: Cancer in pregnancy. Curr Probl Cancer 8, No. 1:27, 1983
15. Byrd BF Jr., Bayer DS, Robertson JC et al: Treatment of breast tumors associated with pregnancy and lactation. Ann Surg 155:940, 1962
16. Brill AB, Forgotson EH: Radiation and congenital malformations. Am J Obstet Gynecol 90:1149, 1964
17. Denoix P: Treatment of malignant breast tumors: Indications and results. Recent Results Cancer Res 31:80, 1970
18. Mossman KL, Hill LT: Radiation risks in pregnancy. Obstet Gynecol 60, No. 2:237, 1982
19. Ravdin RG, Lewison EF, Slack NH et al: Results of a clinical trial concerning the worth of prophylactic oophorectomy for breast carcinoma. Surg Gynecol Obstet 131:1055, 1970
20. Bryant AJS, Weir JA: Prophylactic oophorectomy in operable instances of carcinoma of the breast. Surg Gynecol Obstet 153, No. 5:660, 1982
21. Meakin JW, Allt WEC, Beale FA et al: Ovarian irradiation and prednisone following surgery for carcinoma of the breast. In Salmon SE, Jones SE (eds): Adjuvant Therapy of Cancer. Amsterdam, Elsevier/North-Holland Biomedical Press, 1977
22. Peters MV: The effect of pregnancy in breast cancer. In Forrest APM, Kunkler PB (eds): Prognostic Factors in Breast Cancer, pp 65–80. Baltimore, Williams & Wilkins, 1968
23. Harvey JC, Rosen PP, Ashikari R et al: The effect of pregnancy on the prognosis of carcinoma of the breast following radical mastectomy. Surg Gynecol Obstet 153:723, 1981
24. Cooper DR, Butterfield J: Pregnancy subsequent to mastectomy for cancer of the breast. Ann Surg 171, No. 3:429, 1970
25. Lutz MH, Underwood PB Jr., Rozier JC et al: Genital malignancy in pregnancy. Am J Obstet Gynecol 129, No. 5: 536, 1977
26. Gilotra PM, Lee FYL, Krupp PJ et al: Carcinoma in situ of the cervix uteri in pregnancy. Surg Gynecol Obstet 142:396, 1976
27. Barclay DL, Frueh DM, Hawks BL: Carcinoma in situ of the cervix in pregnancy: Treatment with primary cesarean hysterectomy. Gynecol Oncol 5:357, 1977
28. Sablinska R, Tarlowska L, Stelmachow J: Invasive carcinoma of the cervix associated with pregnancy: Correlation between patient age, advancement of cancer and gestation, and result of treatment. Gynecol Oncol 5:363, 1977
29. Subrahmaniyam K, Pant GC, Sanyal B: Pregnancy complicated by cancer of the cervix: A study of 90 cases. Ind J Cancer 14:340, 1977
30. Stafl A, Mattingly RF: Colposcopic diagnosis of cervix neoplasia. Obstet Gynecol 41:168, 1973
31. Hacker NF, Berek JS, Lagasse LK et al: Carcinoma of the cervix associated with pregnancy. Obstet Gynecol 59, No. 6:735, 1982
32. Sandstrom RE, Welch WR, Green TH Jr.: Adenocarcinoma of the endometrium in pregnancy. Obstet Gynecol 53, No. 3(suppl):73S, 1979
33. Karlen JR, Akbari A, Cook WA: Dysgerminoma associated with pregnancy. Obstet Gynecol 53, No. 3:330, 1979
34. Novak ER, Lambrou CD, Woodruff JD: Ovarian tumors in pregnancy. Obstet Gynecol 46:401, 1975
35. Beral V, Fraser P, Chilvers C: Does pregnancy protect against ovarian cancer? Lancet 1(8073):1083, 1978
36. Cunanan RG Jr., Lipes J, Tancinco PA: Choriocarcinoma of the ovary with coexisting normal pregnancy. Obstet Gynecol 55, No. 5:669, 1980
37. Woolf RB: Gastrointestinal complications of pregnancy. In Gynecology-Obstetrics Guide, vol 1. Chicago, Commerce Clearing House, 1965
38. Girard RM, Lamarche J, Baillot R: Carcinoma of the colon associated with pregnancy: Report of a case. Dis Col Rect 24, No. 60:473, 1981
39. McLean DW, Arminski TC, Bardley GT: Management of primary carcinoma of the rectum diagnosed during pregnancy. Am J Surg 90:816, 1955
40. O'Leary JA, Pratt JH, Symmonds RE: Rectal carcinoma and pregnancy: A review of 17 cases. Obstet Gynecol 30:862, 1967

41. McGownan L: Cancer and pregnancy. Obstet Gynecol Surv 19:285, 1964

42. Bacon HE, Rowe RJ: Abdominoperineal proctosigmoidectomy for rectal cancer complicating pregnancy: Report of four cases. South Med J 40:471, 1947

43. Griffin WO Jr., Dilts PV Jr., Roddick JW Jr.: Non-obstetric surgery during pregnancy. Curr Probl Surg, Nov 1969, p 30

44. Egwuatu VE: Primary hepato carcinoma in pregnancy. Trans R Soc Trop Med 74:793, 1980

45. Vicens E, Martinez–Mora J, Potau N et al: Masculinzation of a female fetus by Krukenberg tumor during pregnancy. J Pediatr Surg 15:188, 1980

46. George PA, Fortner JG, Pack GT: Melanoma with pregnancy: A report of 115 cases. Cancer 13, No. 4:854, 1960

47. Hersey P, Stone DE, Morgan G et al: Previous pregnancy as a protective factor against death from melanoma. Lancet 1(8009):451, 1977

48. Elwood JM: Previous pregnancy and melanoma prognosis. Lancet 2(8097):100, 1978

49. Riberti C, Marola G, Bertani A: Malignant melanoma: The adverse effect of pregnancy. Br J Plas Surg 34:338, 1981

50. Shiu MH, Schottenfeld D, MacLean B et al: Adverse effect of pregnancy on melanoma: A reappraisal. Cancer 37:181, 1976

51. Shockert EC, Fortner JT: Melanoma and pregnancy: An experimental evaluation of a clinical impression. Surg Forum 9:671, 1958

52. Reintgen DS, McCarty KS Jr., Vallmer R et al: Malignant melanoma and pregnancy. Abstract for the Society of Surgical Oncology, 37th Annual Cancer Symposium, New York, NY, May 13–17, 1984

53. Veronesi U, Adamus J, Bandiera DC et al: Delayed regional lymph node dissection in stage I melanoma of the skin of the lower extremities. Cancer 49:2420, 1982

54. Balch MC, Murrad T, Soong S et al: Tumor thickness as a guide to surgical management of clinical stage I melanoma patients. Cancer 43:883, 1979

55. Thomas PRM, Peckham JMJ: The investigation and management of Hodgkin's disease in the pregnant patient. Cancer 38:1443, 1976

56. Durodola JI: Administration of Cyclophosphamide during late pregnancy and early lactation: A case report. J Natl Med Assoc 71, No. 2:165, 1979

57. Gokal R, Durrant J, Baum JD et al: Successful pregnancy in acute monocytic leukaemia. Br J Cancer 34:299, 1976

58. Newcomb M, Balducii L, Thigpen T et al: Acute leukemia in pregnancy: Successful delivery after Cytarabine and Doxorubicin. JAMA 239, No. 25:2691, 1978

59. McKeen EA, Mulvihill JJ, Rosner F et al: Pregnancy outcome in Hodgkin's disease. Lancet 2:590, 1979

60. Holmes GE, Holmes FF: Pregnancy outcome of patients treated for Hodgkin's disease: A controlled study. Cancer 41:1317, 1978

61. Durodola JI: Burkitt's lymphoma presenting during lactation. Int J Gynaecol Obstet 14:225, 1976

62. Lilliman JS, Hill AS, Anderson KJ: Consequences of acute myelogenous leukemia in early pregnancy. Cancer 40:1300, 1977

63. Estiu M: Successful pregnancy in leukaemia. Lancet 1(8008):433, 1977

64. Okun DB, Groncy PK, Sieger L et al: Acute leukemia in pregnancy: Transient neonatal myelosuppression after combination chemotherapy in the mother. Med Pediatr Oncol 7:315, 1979

65. Raich PC, Curet LB: Treatment of acute leukemia during pregnancy. Cancer 36:861, 1975

66. Burrow GN: The thyroid in pregnancy. Med Clin North Am 59, No. 5:1089, 1975

67. Cunningham MP, Slaughter DP: Surgical treatment of disease of the thyroid gland in pregnancy. Surg Gynecol Obstet 126:486, 1970

68. Rosvoll RV, Winship T: Thyroid carcinoma and pregnancy. Surg Gynecol Obstet 121:1039, 1965

69. Hill GS Jr., Clark RL, Wolf M: Effect of subsequent pregnancy on patients with thyroid carcinoma. Surg Gynecol Obstet 122:1219, 1966

70. Cantin J, McNeer GP: The effect of pregnancy on the clinical course of sarcoma of the soft somatic tissues. Surg Gynecol Obstet 125:28, 1967

71. Lysyj A, Bergquist JR: Pregnancy complicated by sarcoma: Report of two cases. Obstet Gynecol 21:506, 1963

72. Jafari K, Lash AF, Webster A: Pregnancy and sarcoma. Acta Obstet Gynecol Scand 57:265, 1978

73. Holzaepfel JH: Pregnancy and delivery post radical hemipelvectomy. Obstet Gynecol 42, No. 3:455, 1978

74. Simon MA, Phillips WA, Bonfidio M: Pregnancy and aggressive or malignant primary bone tumors. Cancer 53:2564, 1984

75. Boyle JM, McLeod ME: Pancreatic cancer presenting as pancreatitis of pregnancy. Am J Gastroenterol 70, No. 40:371, 1979

76. Gambrell EE: Pancreatitis associated with pancreatic carcinoma: A study of 26 cases. Mayo Clin Proc 46:174, 1971

77. Mentgen CN, Moeller DD, Klotz AP: Protection by pregnancy. J Kans Med Soc 75, No. 2:37, 1974

78. Waddell WR, Leonsins AS, Zuidema GD: Gastric secretory and other laboratory studies on two patients with Zollinger–Ellison syndrome. N Engl J Med 260:56, 1959

79. Rubens R, Carlier A, Thiery M et al: Pregnancy complicated by insulinoma: Case report. Br J Obstet Gynecol 84:543, 1977

80. Serrano–Rios M, Cifuentes I, Prieto JC et al: Insulinoma in a pregnant woman. Obstet Gynecol 47:361, 1976

81. Read EJ Jr., Platzer PB: Placental metastasis from maternal carcinoma of the ovary. Obstet Gynecol 58, No. 3:387, 1981

Principles of Teratology

Neil K. Kochenour

Until relatively recently it was thought that the uterus provided a protected environment and that external factors did not significantly affect the development of the mammalian fetus. In the early 1940s, however, Warkany and Nelson reported skeletal abnormalities in the offspring of rats reared on a deficient diet, and Gregg recognized the association between maternal rubella infection during pregnancy and neonatal cataracts. These two observations introduced the age of experimental teratology. Numerous reports documenting the effects of environmental manipulation on embryogenesis accumulated during the subsequent two decades. However, it was not until the early 1960s that an epidemic of limb-reduction malformations in newborns, due to maternal ingestion early in pregnancy of the sedative thalidomide, brought worldwide attention to the potential adverse effects of environmental factors on developing offspring.

Teratology can be defined as the study of causes, mechanisms, and manifestations of developmental deviations initiated between gametogenesis and functional or structural maturation in an otherwise normally developing embryo. A number of environmental factors have been shown to be capable of influencing the development of an embryo. Infectious agents, such as the rubella virus and cytomegalovirus; drugs, such as thalidomide and warfarin; chemicals, such as mercury; and radiation with x-rays are all known to be teratogenic. An excess or deficiency of substances that are required for normal development—vitamin A, for example—can cause abnormal development in animals. Hyperthermia and hypoxia have both been shown to be teratogenic in animals. Teratogens can cause a malformation by inducing chromosomal abnormalities, gene mutations, or mechanical or vascular disruption. Most commonly the mechanism is not known.

Although teratogenic agents vary markedly, certain general principles appear to be valid for all of them.

SPECIFICITY OF THE AGENT

It is possible that among very similar agents, some are teratogenic and others are not. For example, the rubella virus is extremely teratogenic when exposure occurs early in pregnancy. Approximately 50% of the fetuses exposed during the first month of development will be abnormal and between one-third and one-half of infants born with the congenital rubella syndrome will die within the first year of life. In contrast, the measles virus (rubeola) is rarely, if ever, teratogenic.

DOSAGE

At any given time, an embryo can respond to a teratogen in one of three ways: (1) a low dose may have no effect, (2) an intermediate dose may cause a malformation, and (3) a high dose may cause death. The route and the timing of the administration may also affect the consequences of a teratogen. Small doses administered over a period may have a different effect than the same total dose administered at one time.

STAGES OF DEVELOPMENT

Three stages of susceptibility can be identified. In the first few weeks of life the blastocyst appears to be relatively resistant to teratogenic insult. During this period teratogens tend either to be lethal or to have no effect on the embryo's development. Organ differentiation occurs between approximately the third and the eighth week, which is the period of maximum susceptibility. These four weeks constitute the most critical period of development. When organogenesis is complete, embryonic growth is characterized primarily by organ growth. Teratogenic agents can still affect the embryo but rarely produce visible malformations. There are, however, several exceptions to this generalization. The external genitalia are susceptible to hormonal influences throughout gestation, and androgenic hormones can masculinize a female fetus even late in pregnancy. The central nervous system also continues to develop and can be adversely affected by environmental influences throughout gestation (Fig. 30-11). The effects of ionizing radiation on the developing fetus illustrate the importance of the stage of development at the time of exposure. Permanent effects of radiation exposure on the mammalian embryo include growth retardation, death, and structural malformations. The organ system most consistently affected by exposure to radiation is the central nervous system. In the preimplantation embryo radiation can cause death but does not usually cause malformation. Survivors of preimplantation radiation exposure usually develop and grow normally. Gross malformations occur when the fetus is irradiated during the early organogenic period. Growth retardation can occur as a result of radiation exposure at any time after implantation. The importance of the timing of exposure to teratogens is clearly illustrated in the case of thalidomide (Table 30-20).

GENOTYPE OF THE MOTHER AND FETUS

The genotypes of the mother and fetus are important determinants of fetal response to teratogenic exposure. For example, the prevalence of corticosteroid-induced cleft palate varies markedly between different strains of mice: 10 mg of cortisol given between days 11 and 44 will produce cleft defects in almost all mice of one strain and in very few mice of another strain. The incidence of diaphragmatic hernias induced by vitamin-A deficiency is approximately 10% in one strain of rats and twice that in another strain. Thalidomide, a potent teratogen in humans, exerts essentially no effect on developing mice. The genotypic specificity of teratogenic agents is one of the factors that makes investigation of the teratogenic effects of new drugs so difficult.

DRUG INTERACTIONS

Agents administered in combination have different consequences than the same agents administered separately: the combination may enhance teratogenic potential or reduce it.

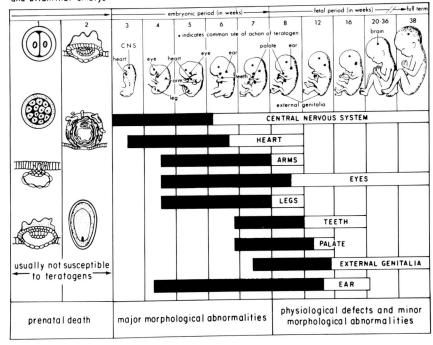

FIG. 30-11. Susceptibility to teratogens according to stage of fetal development.

VARIATION IN RESPONSE

Maternal exposure to identical doses of teratogen at the same time in gestation may lead to different effects in two fetuses of the same species. Variations in maternal absorption or metabolism may lead to different exposure at the fetal level. Genetic differences among fetuses may also contribute to differences in outcome.

Table 30-20
Sensitive Period for External Malformations Caused by Maternal Ingestion of Thalidomide

Malformation	Day After Last Menstrual Period
Anotia	34th–38th
Aplasia of thumb	38th–40th
Amelia of arms	38th–43rd
Dislocation of hips	38th–48th
Phocomelia of arms	38th–47th
Deformity of ears	39th–43rd
Amelia of legs	41st–45th
Phocomelia of legs	42nd–47th
Ectromelia of legs	45th–47th
Triphalangism of thumbs	46th–59th

ADVERSE EFFECTS ON PREGNANCY OUTCOME

A wide variety of agents have been shown to be capable of influencing the developing fetus. These agents can be responsible for such diverse consequences as death, growth retardation, mental retardation, structural deformities, functional impairment, and the subsequent development of cancer. These effects may occur immediately, or they may be delayed for many years. It is important for all professionals responsible for the care of pregnant women to keep these facts in mind when they prescribe medications or x-rays, or counsel pregnant women regarding environmental or work-related exposures.

Embryo Lethality

If administered at the appropriate time in the appropriate dose, a teratogen may cause the death of an embryo. At high doses, x-ray radiation administered before implantation is frequently lethal to an embryo.

Growth Retardation

One of the common consequences of teratogenic influence is interference with normal growth potential. Examples are seen in the fetal alcohol syndrome, congenital rubella, fetal hydantoin syndrome, and numerous others.

Mental Retardation

A number of teratogens, including hydantoin, alcohol, aminopterin, among others, lead to a reduction in the intelligence quotient of affected individuals.

Behavioral Effects

Although the area has been inadequately investigated, there is some evidence that teratogens may affect future behavior.

Structural Defects

One of the obvious consequences of teratogenic action is the development of structural abnormalities. The effect of thalidomide on the developing fetus illustrates this adverse effect.

Functional Impairment

Although it is frequently difficult to separate structural defects from functional impairment, there are instances where, in the absence of apparent structural abnormalities, agents can cause functional damage. An example of this is the effect on reproduction of *in utero* exposure to the drug diethylstilbestrol (DES). A number of studies have found the reproductive performance of women exposed *in utero* to DES to be much worse than that of control groups of women not exposed to this medication. This poor reproductive capability is sometimes, but not always, accompanied by demonstrable anatomic alterations. It has also been suggested that *in utero* ex-

posure to DES has led to alterations in male reproductive capability.

Carcinogenesis

Although not strictly a teratogenic consequence, the subsequent development of a malignancy because of *in utero* exposure to a particular agent must be included in a discussion of adverse outcomes related to drug exposure. Epidemiologic studies have shown that women who were exposed to DES *in utero* have an increased risk for the development of clear cell carcinoma of the vagina. There is also evidence that *in utero* exposure to diphenylhydantoin may lead to an increased incidence of neural crest tumors.

REFERENCES AND RECOMMENDED READING

Cousins L, Karp W, Lacey C et al: Reproductive outcome of women exposed to diethylstilbestrol in utero. Obstet Gynecol 56:70, 1980

Golbus MS: Teratology for the obstetrician: Current status. Obstet Gynecol 55:269, 1980

Gregg N: Congenital cataracts following German measles in the mother. Trans Ophthalmol Soc Aust 3:3536, 1941

Herbst AL, Cole P, Colton T et al: Age-incidence and risk of diethylstilbestrol-related clear cell adenocarcinoma of the vagina and cervix. Am J Obstet Gynecol 128:43–50, 1977

Herbst AL, Hubby MM, Blough RR et al: A comparison of pregnancy experience in DES-exposed and DES-unexposed daughters. J Reprod Med 24:62, 1980

Lenz W: Kindliche Missbildungen nach Medikament-Einnahgme wahrend der Graviditat. Dtsch Med Wochenschr 86:2555, 1961

McBride WG: Thalidomide and congenital abnormalities. Lancet 2:1358, 1961

Smith DW, Clarren SK, Harvey MAS: Hyperthermia as a possible teratogenic agent. J Pediatr 92:878, 1978

Warkany J, Nelson RC: Appearance of skeletal abnormalities in the offspring of rats reared on a deficient diet. Science 92:383, 1940

PART IV

Normal Labor

Physiology of Uterine Action

David N. Danforth
Kent Ueland

31

The sole function of the uterus is childbearing, and its structural features, its position, its supports, and its physiological reactions are designed to accomplish and to facilitate this single purpose. An understanding of the means by which this function is carried out requires a knowledge of the actions and reactions of the myometrium, and of the dynamics and structural changes in the uterus in pregnancy and labor.

THE CAUSE OF THE ONSET OF LABOR

Since the time of Hippocrates, simple causes or mechanisms have been sought to explain the onset of labor. As knowledge has increased, it has become evident that there is no simple explanation of why previously sporadic, haphazard, and wholly uncoordinated uterine contractions should suddenly, over the course of hours or days, increase in coordination and strength so that ultimately and inexorably the uterus is evacuated. In recent years, a resurgence of interest in this question has resulted in a prodigious literature that examines the many factors that are concerned in the regulation of uterine activity. As new data become available, it is apparent that the onset of labor results from the convergence of a number of factors, each of which, like the instruments in a symphony orchestra, must bear an optimal relationship to all of the others. Unfortunately, some investigators focus upon a single factor and declare it to be of preeminent importance as *the* cause of the onset of labor; however, all of the factors related to the physiology of the myometrium affect the onset of labor. Some of these are needed to set the stage for labor, after which others can act as direct or indirect precipitating factors.

The Physiology of the Myometrium

The uterus possesses no intrinsic nervous mechanism similar to the Purkinje system of the heart. Hence, in the uterus the propagation of the contraction wave resembles that of a syncytium, in which the contraction of one muscle cell triggers the contraction of the adjacent one. The resulting wave spreads for variable distances over the myometrium. The ability of one muscle cell to "fire" when the adjacent one contracts and the distance the wave advances depend on many factors, including estrogen, progesterone, and prostaglandin (PG) influences; electrochemical phenomena at the cell surfaces; actomyosin and adenosine triphosphate (ATP) concentrations; electrolyte environment; stretch; and, apparently, the density of the postganglionic nerve axons and gap junctions, which varies according to the physiological state of the uterus.

These factors are also responsible for the increasing reactivity of the uterus as pregnancy progresses. Oxytocin is one of the most effective drugs used for stimulation of the uterus and for testing its reactivity. In early pregnancy, the uterus is exceptionally refractory to oxytocin; large doses are required to produce contractions even vaguely resembling those seen in early labor (Fig. 31-1). In the final weeks of pregnancy, the uterus becomes increasingly responsive to oxytocin, and by the time labor begins, it is acutely sensitive (Figs. 31-1 and 31-2). Doses of oxytocin that in early pregnancy have little effect can, at term, produce the most violent and sustained tetany.

Much has been learned of myometrial physiology by noting the effects of administered agents and by testing the circulating blood for levels of critical constituents. In interpreting such studies, it must be remem-

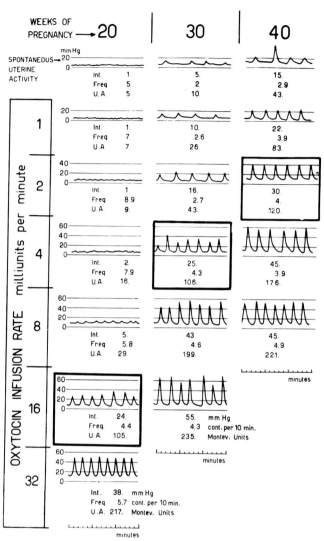

FIG. 31-1. Response to increasing doses of oxytocin administered by constant pump infusion at 20, 30, and 40 weeks' gestation. Contraction pattern in heavy squares is within range usually observed in normal labor that begins spontaneously. Hypercontractility and increased tonus result from administration at excessive rate; this abnormally high activity may interfere with fetal oxygen supply and occasionally may even cause rupture of uterus. (Caldeyro–Barcía RC, Sica–Blanco Y, Poseiro JJ et al: A quantitative study of the action of synthetic oxytocin on the pregnant human uterus. J Pharmacol Exp Ther 121:128. Copyright © 1957, Williams & Wilkins, Baltimore)

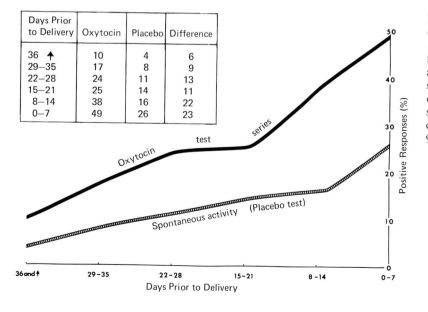

Days Prior to Delivery	Oxytocin	Placebo	Difference
36 ↑	10	4	6
29–35	17	8	9
22–28	24	11	13
15–21	25	14	11
8–14	38	16	22
0–7	49	26	23

FIG. 31-2. During final weeks before onset of labor, spontaneous uterine activity (*dotted line*) increases steadily, reaching peak in last few days before onset of labor. Response to a given dose of oxytocin (*solid line*) increases somewhat between 35th and 38th weeks; during 39th and 40th weeks, oxytocin response increases much more rapidly. (Hendricks CH, Brenner WE: Am J Obstet Gynecol 90:485, 1964)

bered that the observed effects of administered agents, even if they are also produced *in vivo,* give no significant information about the physiological effects of the same agents as they are normally produced and secreted endogenously, and that blood levels of specific constituents cannot be used as a measure of endogenous production or release unless the rates of clearance and degradation are also known.

Properties of Uterine Muscle

The major properties of uterine muscle are the same as those of smooth muscle in general: contraction, relaxation, coordination, and changes in length without changes in tension.

CONTRACTION AND RELAXATION. Autonomous, spontaneous, rhythmic contraction and relaxation are inherent properties of smooth muscle that clearly distinguish it from skeletal muscle. Such activity is of myogenic origin, and it occurs in completely denervated preparations and in preparations under the influence of ganglion- and nerve-blocking agents. Uterine muscle strips that have been refrigerated for two weeks in saline or Locke's solution quickly resume spontaneous activity when they are warmed.

COORDINATION. During pregnancy, prior to the onset of labor, the uterus contracts intermittently, sometimes very forcefully. These contractions, known as Braxton Hicks contractions, are totally irregular in duration, intensity, and frequency. Although they do not significantly affect the evacuation of the uterus, Braxton Hicks contractions do partially empty the uterus of blood and hence provide for the frequent movement of blood in the uterine sinuses and intervillous space. They also may help to move the fetus about in the uterus and cause the fetus to move its muscles.

Braxton Hicks contractions are triggered from various parts of the uterus, most commonly in one of the cornual areas, and spread for variable distances over the myometrium. Some ultimately involve the entire uterus and may be just as intense as labor "pains," but most are propagated only for short distances.

As labor approaches, the intermittent contractions gradually become more regular in frequency, duration, and intensity, and they are propagated for increasing distances over the myometrium. In normal labor, an impressive coordination is achieved: the contractions spread inferiorly from the fundus to involve the entire uterus, and as labor progresses, their frequency, duration, and intensity increase. Thus, at the onset of labor the uterus is converted from an uncoordinated, protective domicile for the infant to a powerfully active and precisely coordinated unit whose contractions are designed to expel the conceptus. When labor is fully es-

tablished, the process is inexorable: it does not stop, and it cannot be permanently stopped until the uterus is empty. Some drugs appear to arrest labor for variable periods, but they are unpredictable and much less effective if labor has advanced to the point at which the cervix is dilated 4 cm or more.

CHANGES IN LENGTH WITHOUT CHANGES IN TENSION. Adjustments in length without changes in tension are essential for the orderly development of the uterus in pregnancy, as well as for the development of the lower uterine segment and ultimate evacuation of the uterus (see p. 604). Such changes are by no means unique to the uterus. The stomach adjusts to accommodate a full meal without significant changes in intragastric pressure, and the urinary bladder can be partially emptied without significant change in intravesical pressure. These essential properties of smooth muscle are termed brachystasis and mecystasis. *Brachystasis* is a state manifested by a muscle fiber after it has assumed a relatively fixed decrease in length. At this shorter length it resists stretch, contracts and relaxes, and manifests the same tension as before shortening. Brachystasis is the process whereby the longitudinal component of the myometrium shortens in labor, or "retracts," and allows evacuation of the conceptus (Fig. 31-3). *Mecystasis* is a state manifested by a muscle fiber after it has assumed a relatively fixed increase in length. At this longer length it resists stretch, contracts and relaxes, and manifests the same tension as before lengthening. Mecystasis occurs in the lower circular component of the myometrium to permit the unfolding of the lower pole of the uterus in early pregnancy and the formation of the lower uterine segment in late pregnancy and labor.

Effects of Distention and Stretch

Gillespies' classic diagram (Fig. 31-4) emphasizes the inevitability of the onset of labor. The fetus grows at a rapidly accelerating rate, more than doubling its weight in the last two months of pregnancy; uterine growth at this time is trivial, and the consequent stretching of the uterine wall reduces its thickness. The importance of this relation has not been enunciated, although it is certain that many of the uterine phenomena of advancing pregnancy are the direct result of myometrial stretch.

Most of the studies regarding the effects of distention have been done in the rabbit, and with a few exceptions, they are considered to be applicable to humans. The important work of Reynolds on the effects of uterine distention can hardly be summarized in a few sentences, but some of his conclusions can be cited. Even in the castrated rabbit, uterine distention (by cylindrical paraffin pellets of known sizes) was found to constitute a specific stimulus to uterine growth. The

Mecystasis   Brachystasis

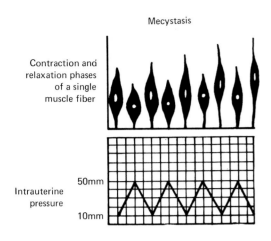

Contraction and
relaxation phases
of a single
muscle fiber

Intrauterine
pressure

50mm

10mm

FIG. 31-3. Mecystasis and brachystasis. In mecystasis, as muscle fiber contracts, intrauterine pressure increases; with relaxation, intrauterine pressure returns to resting tone and fiber assumes longer length than before contraction. Reverse effect occurs in brachystasis.

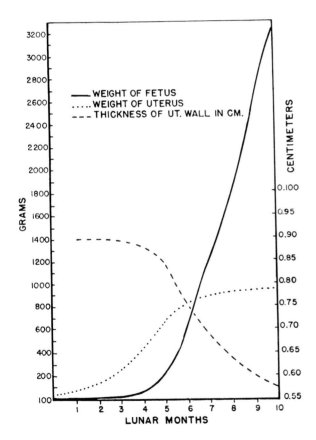

FIG. 31-4. Fetouterine relation. Note reduced uterine growth and progressive thinning of uterine wall as fetus develops most rapidly after fourth month. (Gillespie CG: Am J Obstet Gynecol 59:949, 1950)

number of cells in the myometrium increased appreciably, the cells were larger, and as many as 50 mitotic figures in metaphase were counted in the circular muscle of a single cross-section of the myometrium (Fig. 31-5). When the distention–growth response was studied in animals treated with estrogens, it was clear that this hormone limited the capacity of the uterus to grow when distended. Hence, when estrogen is acting, distention is incapable of acting as a stimulus to uterine growth. Conversely, in progesterone-treated animals, the general effect was equivalent to that in the castrated animals; but apparently because of uterine relaxation, much greater distention was required to produce equivalent effects. In sum, it seems possible to conclude, in general terms, that estrogen inhibits the growth response to distention, while progesterone enhances it. These observations have important implications when Gillespie's curves (Fig. 31-4) are considered in light of estrogen and progesterone levels in normal pregnancy.

In addition to causing uterine growth, distention per se directly stimulates the mechanical activity of the uterus, causing an increase in the electrical activity and orderly propagation of the impulse (Fig. 31-6). This response has been shown to be enhanced by estrogen and depressed by progesterone, providing additional evidence for the importance of progesterone in accommodation of the fetus.

In humans, distention per se appears to influence the duration of pregnancy. Preterm labor is the rule in multiple pregnancy. The influence of distention is also important in the rabbit, where there is a direct relation between the degree of uterine stretch and the onset of labor. In this animal, a measure of uterine distention is obtained by comparing the total weight of the conceptus

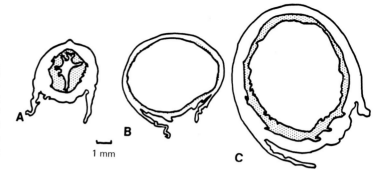

FIG. 31-5. Extent of uterine growth in untreated ovariectomized rabbit resulting from simple distention of uterus. (*A*) Cross-section of undistended part of uterus. (*B*) Section of uterus taken immediately after distention. (*C*) Section taken two weeks after distention. *C* is 161% greater in area than *A,* as measured with planimeter. (Reynolds SRM, Kaminester S: Am J Physiol 116:510, 1936)

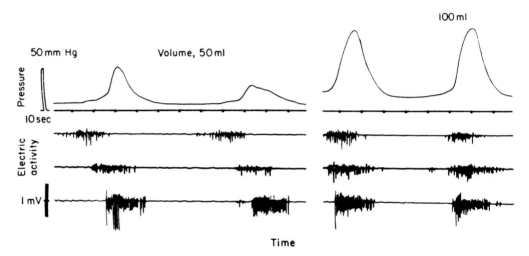

FIG. 31-6. Effect of volume changes on electric and mechanical activity of uterus. Note that when uterine volume is 50 ml, propagation of electric activity from ovarian to cervical end is slow (~20 sec). Slow propagation results in relative asynchrony. Pressure is moderate and its development irregular. Volume increase to 100 ml facilitates propagation; uterine horn becomes active at its whole length within short period (~2 sec), resulting in synchrony. Synchrony in electric activity results in increase in pressure and regularity in shape of pressure curves. Rate of pressure rise also increases. (Csapo AI, Takeda H, Wood C: Am J Obstet Gynecol 85:813, 1963)

with the weight of the uterus. When this ratio reaches 1:1.5, labor begins (Fig. 31-7).

There is now convincing evidence that, in the estrogen-dominated uterus, the availability of prostaglandin $F_{2\alpha}$ ($PGF_{2\alpha}$) is determined by the degree of stretch. With increasing stretch, the synthesis, myometrial concentration, and release of $PGF_{2\alpha}$ are all proportionately increased. Csapo and colleagues found that the instillation of as little as 150 ml isotonic solution into the uterine cavity at term consistently produced increased uterine activity. The mechanism is presumed to be increased prostaglandin (PG) production and release as the result of stretch.

These observations indicate that uterine distention is *one* of the important forces that influence the myometrial changes of normal pregnancy and labor, although it does not appear to be crucial. For example, in both the monkey and the rat removal of the fetus(es) leaving the placenta(s) *in situ* does not influence the normal length of pregnancy; the placentas are delivered at term. Also, in extrauterine abdominal pregnancy, the empty uterus contracts at term. Perhaps, as in the case

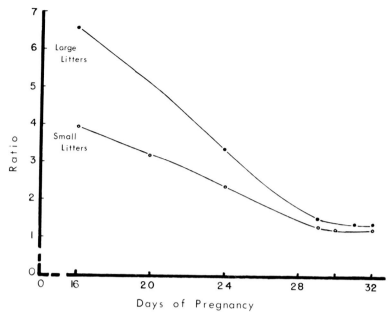

FIG. 31-7. Relation of uterine distention to onset of labor in rabbit. With six fetuses (large litters), uterus weighs 480 g at term; with three fetuses (small litters), it weighs 280 g. Ratio of uterine weight to total conceptus weight gives measure of uterine distention. After ratio becomes 1.5:1, labor occurs. In human uterus simplex, ratio is 3:1. (Reynolds SRM: Symposium on Fertility and Sterility, East Lansing, MI, Michigan State University, 1956)

of distention and consequent stretch, some of the other factors that seem important, since they are operative in normal pregnancy, are not necessarily essential to the orderly structural and functional development of the uterus.

Effects of Estrogens and Progesterone

Estrogens have many myometrial effects, a few of which are mentioned here.

Estrogens are essential for the coordinated activity and reactivity of the uterus. After castration, the uterus becomes increasingly inactive, the organized pattern of myometrial motility disappears, the uterus becomes increasingly unresponsive to oxytocic agents, and atrophic changes begin. All of these regressive changes are quickly reversed by estrogens. In achieving these effects, each of three classic estrogens is uniformly effective, but estradiol is most potent, estriol is least potent, and estrone is intermediate.

Estrogens restrict the growth response of the uterus to distention, and they affect the myometrial concentrations of the contractile protein actomyosin, its enzyme adenosine triphosphatase, and the energy source for contraction. These relations are discussed below.

The resting membrane potential, which is a measure of the level of membrane polarization and, hence, of the excitability and conductive ability of the myometrial cells, is elevated by estrogens.

The innervation density (*i.e.,* the density of the terminal nerve axons, each of which makes contact with several myometrial cells) is increased by estrogens. Similarly, the concentrations of neurotransmitter substance (norepinephrine) are also increased.

Estrogens, notably estradiol, appear to cause the synthesis as well as release of $PGF_{2\alpha}$ from the uterus, and it has been suggested that the myometrial effects of estrogens are mediated through the action of $PGF_{2\alpha}$.

Under the influence of estrogens, the contraction wave is propagated in an orderly manner from one part of the uterus to the next. This is believed to result from the electrical coupling of the myometrial cells, forming a physiological syncytium. The morphologic sites for the coupling (Fig. 31-8) may be the "gap junctions" or "nexuses" where the sarcolemma of one cell is closely applied to that of the next cell, thus providing low-resistance pathways between cells. In the species studied, gap junctions are either lacking or sparse throughout pregnancy until term, at which time their frequency increases sharply. They attain their highest frequency and size during labor and revert to prelabor frequency after delivery. Garfield and others consider the gap junctions to be essential to the coordinated contractions of labor and attribute their formation to the hormonal changes that precede labor.

The primary myometrial effect of progesterone is its interference with conduction from one cell or group of cells to another; it therefore prevents the orderly

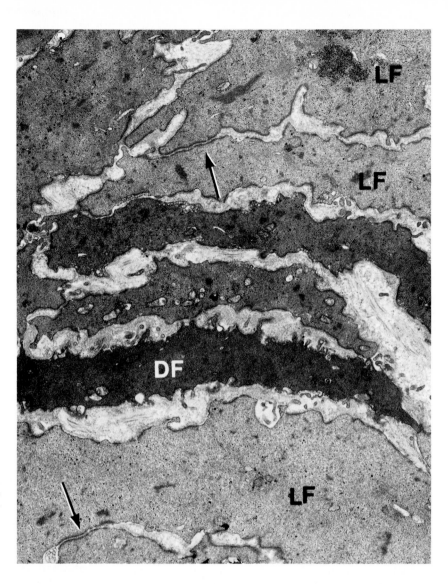

FIG. 31-8. Electron micrograph of human myometrium. *DF,* contracted fibril, *LF,* relaxed fibril. Thinned areas (*arrows*) probably represent nexuses or junctional gaps that provide low-resistance pathways between myometrial fibrils (×8000). (Dessouky DA: Am J Obstet Gynecol 125:1099, 1976)

propagation of the contraction wave from one part of the uterus to the next, and tends to prevent contraction of the entire organ at the same time. This effect, termed the *progesterone block* by Csapo, probably results from the sequestration of calcium in the sarcoplasmic reticulum, which suppresses both conduction and excitability. By this means, in addition to enhancing the growth response to distention, progesterone counters the stimulatory effects of both estrogens and stretch in pregnancy.

In 1956 Csapo proposed the progesterone block thesis, which was based on the evidence to date and also on his own elegant studies in the rabbit. This theory proposed that progesterone dominance ensures the

continuation of pregnancy by preventing coordinated uterine contractions; when the block is lifted, labor ensues. Some have criticized the thesis because progesterone levels do not decrease before labor. However, as noted earlier, progesterone dominance may be lost without significant changes in progesterone production or level if the impact of opposing factors is increased. Another consideration cited in opposition to the theory is the failure of progesterone to stop labor that is in progress. This point is probably not pertinent because although small amounts of placental progesterone reach the peripheral circulation in humans, the myometrial inhibitory effect is largely achieved by direct suffusion of progesterone into the myometrium. When labor has started, systemically administered progesterone may not reach the myometrium in sufficient concentration to be effective.

A theory that was popular for many years was that the normal onset of labor at term results from an increase in the production of estrogen and a decline in that of progesterone. Until recently, studies to clarify this relationship produced conflicting results. At present, it is generally accepted that there is no decline in serum progesterone before the onset of labor and that, although estrogen rises steadily throughout pregnancy, there is no abrupt increase in estrogen before labor. However, ultimately the point at which the estrogen:progesterone balance is upset by the increasing estrogen levels is reached.

Preterm labor has been effectively prevented by prior administration of progesterone. Also, in increasing dosages, progesterone is reported to be effective in preventing late abortion and preterm labor in cases of abnormal ("muscular") cervix, congenital absence of the cervix, and septate uterus, in which there was a history of late abortion or preterm labor.

Effects of Prostaglandins

Prostaglandins are synthesized in the microsomes of virtually all tissues from unsaturated fatty acids. When administered vaginally, orally, or by injection, PGs cause a variety of effects, but there is no agreement or real knowledge about whether these observed effects exactly represent the physiological functions of normally synthesized endogenous PGs. They are widely distributed throughout the body, but are not stored to any extent, and have an extremely short half-life of only a few min-

utes. They are almost completely degraded by one circulation through the lung. They appear to act directly in the sites where they are synthesized. (One exception to this rule is luteolysis in the nonpregnant, and probably also the pregnant, animal, which results from $PGF_{2\alpha}$ that is formed in the uterus.) The release of PGs from cells has been shown to be enhanced by nervous, humoral, chemical, and physical stimuli. Indeed, mere handling of tissues can cause their release, as can the trauma of venesection or the clotting of blood, which must account for the spurious conclusions of some earlier investigations.

Administered PGs (notably of the E and F series) have been shown to enhance uterine activity and coordination, to lower the uterine threshold to oxytocin, and to produce uterine contractions that are virtually indistinguishable from spontaneous contractions. In general, administered PGs of the E series have approximately ten times the potency of those in the F series. Uterine sensitivity to these substances is much greater during pregnancy, and they have been used to evacuate the uterus at all stages of pregnancy. They are also of great value in treating postpartum hemorrhage caused by uterine atony (15-methyl $PGF_{2\alpha}$ appears to have special value for this purpose).

Arachidonic acid, which is the obligatory precursor of PGs, has been used successfully to terminate pregnancy by intra-amniotic instillation in the middle trimester, and it has been proposed that the release of this acid by the action of lysosomal enzymes may result in increased $PGF_{2\alpha}$ synthesis as a part of the normal sequence of events leading to labor (see Fig. 31-9).

The physiological contributions of PGs to normal pregnancy and labor have been determined chiefly by

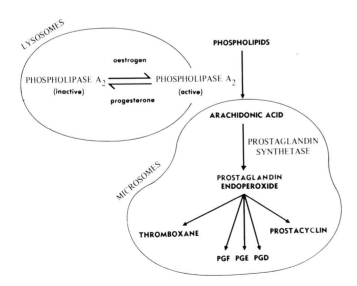

FIG. 31-9. Pathway for biosynthesis of primary prostaglandins, thromboxanes, and prostacyclins. Arachidonic acid "cascade" is shown in bold capital letters and bold arrows. Main rate-limiting step is activation of phospholipase A_2 (*top left*). (Liggins GC: Initiation of parturition. Br Med Bull 35:145, 1979)

measuring their metabolites. In the case of PGE_2 the results have been conflicting because of methodological problems and the instability of the principal metabolite 13,14-dihydro-15-keto PGE_2. Discovery of a stable degradation product (bicyclo PGEM) has identified a compound suitable for assay. In the series by Brennecke and co-workers, this metabolite did not change significantly during the second or third trimester or during labor.

Although increases in plasma $PGF_{2\alpha}$ have not been found before labor, significant elevations have been reported during labor, with significant declines two hours after delivery. The maximum $PGF_{2\alpha}$ concentrations occur between 100 and 120 seconds after the peak of a uterine contraction and between 40 and 60 seconds before the peak of the next contraction. The evidence therefore suggests that $PGF_{2\alpha}$ has a more important physiological role in labor than PGE_2.

In vitro studies in animals have shown that the highest concentration of $PGF_{2\alpha}$ is found in uterine epithelium. The myometrium produces predominantly PGI_2, but it also produces substantial amounts of $PGF_{2\alpha}$. For the most part, PGE_2 synthesis is confined to the cervix, although relatively high concentrations of PGI_2 are found also. The latter compounds are present in higher concentrations during pregnancy, and in animals, the concentrations increase sharply when spontaneous cervical effacement occurs.

The mode of action of PGs in stimulating myometrial activity and coordination has been the subject of intense investigation. As noted later in this chapter, calcium ion transport is essential for uterine contraction, and there is evidence that PGs cause the release of some of the calcium that is bound in the sarcoplasmic reticulum. Indeed, the ability of PGs to alter calcium trans-

port in smooth muscle as well as across other biologic membranes is probably the universal mechanism of PG action. It is known that stretch of the myometrial fibers causes an increased endogenous production of PGs, and it is likely that not only PG synthesis but also its cellular concentration and local release are functions of stretch.

Other aspects of the physiology of prostaglandins are considered in Chapter 7.

Contractile System of the Myometrium

The basic elements of the contractile system are actin, myosin, the high-energy phosphate compound adenosine triphosphate (ATP), and the enzyme adenosine triphosphatase (ATPase). The myofilaments of the structural unit contain threadlike proteins; the thin filaments contain actin, and the thick filaments contain myosin. During relaxation, the actin filaments are separated from the myosin filaments; during contraction, however, the actin-containing filaments slide past and combine with the myosin-containing filaments, producing actomyosin (AM). AM is the contractile protein of smooth, cardiac, and skeletal muscle. ATP supplies the energy for contraction. ATPase is the enzyme that splits ATP so that the required energy is released.

The working capacity of the uterus is determined by the concentration of AM, ATP, and ATPase. Uniquely among all smooth muscle, the myometrial concentration of these elements is influenced by the ovarian hormones. The concentrations are lowest in postmenopausal women and in animals after castration, but they are quickly restored to or even above their former levels by the administration of estrogens (Figs. 31-10 and 31-11). The concentrations of these substances are also increased by stretch; thus, for pregnancy, estrogens and

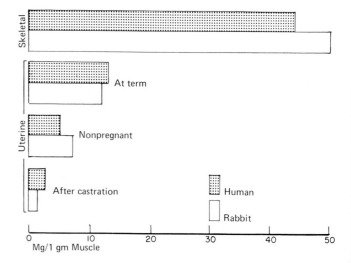

FIG. 31-10. Concentration of actomyosin in human and rabbit skeletal muscle and uterus. Note decreased quantities in nonpregnant and postcastration states. (Csapo A: Am J Physiol 162:405, 1950)

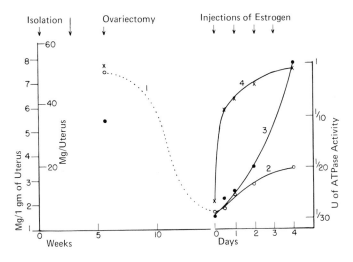

FIG. 31-11. Effect of castration and subsequent estrogen administration on contractile system of rabbit uterus. (*Curve 1*) Loss of system by two weeks after castration. (*Curve 2*) Concentration of actomyosin after estrogen administration. (*Curve 3*) Actomyosin content after estrogen administration. (*Curve 4*) ATPase activity after estrogen administration. Note beginning recovery in 12 hours; before this, estrogen causes hyperemia (in 30 min) and increase in water content (in six hours). (Csapo A: Am J Physiol 162:406, 1950)

stretch have a dual influence on the working capacity of the uterus. Through these actions, the myometrium is maintained in a "functional readiness" for contraction that increases as pregnancy advances.

As noted later in this chapter, the contraction event is calcium-dependent because the interaction of actin and myosin occurs only in the presence of available calcium ions.

Effects of Mineral Ions

Much is known of the complex interactions of the mineral ions in the contraction and relaxation of smooth muscle. The movements of ions (notably Ca^{2+}, K^+, Na^{2+}, and Mg^{2+}) are fundamentally involved in the regulation of membrane permeability, resting membrane potential, and membrane polarization, each of which is involved in muscle contraction and excitability. Movements of these ions have been shown to be influenced and, in the case of the uterus, controlled by estrogen and progesterone.

CALCIUM. The oxytocic effect of calcium was first noted by W. Blair Bell* and Hick in 1909. At that time, these researchers stated that "we admit that we have been unable in our experiments to show definitely that

---

* In later years, William Blair Bell's name was hyphenated (Blair–Bell); his earlier articles are to be found under the name Bell and later ones, Blair–Bell. Blair Bell, the name that is now used, was cofounder, with Sir William Fletcher Shaw, of the Royal College of Obstetricians and Gynaecologists. Sir John Peel described him as a restless, ruthless, intolerant but dynamic torchbearer. He was preeminent among the obstetrician–gynecologists of the early 1900s.

labour *is* produced by the action of calcium salts in the blood, . . . [but] so far as we have gone we incline to the belief that calcium salts . . . play the most important role in this connexion." Like many of Blair Bell's prophetic observations, this statement is astonishing when considered in light of present knowledge of the role of calcium in uterine contractility. Note, for example, a 1979 statement by Liggins, one of the leading modern students of the physiology of parturition: "Human labour is undoubtedly initiated by increased intracellular Ca^{2+} in myometrial smooth muscle, but there is less certainty of the factors causing the changes in Ca^{2+}." It has been demonstrated that available calcium is specifically necessary for uterine contraction both *in vivo* and *in vitro,* and that, without it, the uterus is not only quiescent but fails to respond to oxytocin or PGs; spontaneous activity and reactivity are restored by the presence of available calcium.

It is now well documented that calcium can be mobilized from intracellular binding sites for purposes of contraction. Chief among the binding sites is the sarcoplasmic reticulum surrounding the individual myofibrils; mitochondria and the plasma membrane and its surface vesicles are involved to a lesser extent. The binding sites are considered intracellular compartments that alternately sequester and release Ca^{2+} to inhibit and to activate the contractile apparatus (Fig. 31-12). Calcium uptake by the sarcoplasmic reticulum is dependent on an energy source, ATP, and is mediated by an enzyme, ATPase (which is different from the actomyosin ATPase of the myofibril); as calcium accumulates, relaxation results. Fluctuations in cyclic adenosine monophosphate (cAMP) are also part of this process. Carsten suggests that cAMP may diminish the size of the calcium pool, leaving less calcium available for contraction and promoting relaxation.

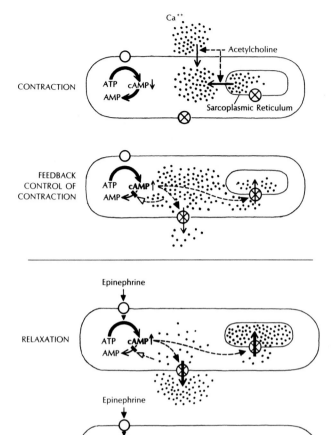

FIG. 31-12. Acetylcholine produces contraction of smooth muscle by triggering calcium influx into cytoplasm from medium and sarcoplasmic reticulum (SR). Calcium also serves as feedback control, blocking breakdown of cAMP by phosphodiesterase; increased cAMP levels then produce reaccumulation of calcium in SR. Epinephrine acts in opposite way, triggering rise in cAMP that causes calcium reaccumulation in SR; drop in cytoplasmic calcium produces feedback control by unblocking breakdown of cAMP. (Rasmussen H: Ions as "second messengers." Hosp Pract 9:99, 1974)

Watterson and colleagues suggest that in principle, relaxation of the uterus can be brought about in two ways. The first is to facilitate production of cAMP, a response that follows stimulation of β-2-adrenergic receptors and relaxin receptors. The other is to reduce Ca^{2+} influx into the cell by using calcium-entry blockers such as verapamil or nifedipine. Indeed, Huszar has suggested that calcium channel blocking agents, or calcium antagonists, are likely to be the most powerful agent in tocolytic therapy in the future.

The contraction–relaxation event in the myometrium, like virtually all other calcium-dependent intracellular processes, appears to be modulated by calmodulin, the preeminent member of a group of proteins that reversibly bind to calcium ions when the Ca^{2+} concentration increases in response to a stimulus. This induces a change in the shape of the calmodulin molecule, which enables the calmodulin–calcium complex to bind to any of several enzymes, thus activating the enzyme and setting in motion the biochemical changes that produce the response to the stimulus. Marx observes that "calmodulin is hardly a household word, but in the world of cell biology it is one of the most exciting discoveries since recombinant DNA."

Progesterone enhances calcium binding in the storage depots, and this action may constitute the basis for the progesterone block. It is now apparent that oxytocin and PGs inhibit calcium binding in the sarcoplasmic reticulum. They also promote the release of previously bound calcium, and their actions as uterine stimulants are mediated through this device.

As would be expected, calcium antagonists severely depress uterine activity (Fig. 31-13). Although each of the several calcium antagonists seems to affect the calcium-dependent activation mechanism differently, it seems clear that they all selectively inhibit the influx of calcium into the myofibril.

Effects of Nervous Mechanisms

The role of nervous influences in the control of uterine activity is poorly understood. For a time, this mechanism was entirely dismissed as unimportant because placentation, pregnancy, and labor can all proceed unhindered after transection of the spinal cord, after lumbar sympathectomy, and after section of all the extrinsic uterine nerves and removal of the uterovaginal ganglion. Theobald refers to the report of Kurdinowsky, which describes the onset of labor and coordinated activity that resulted in delivery of all pups by the totally isolated and perfused uterus of a bitch at term.

Although these observations are dramatic, there are important reasons why they cannot be interpreted to mean that nervous mechanisms play no role in the normal function of the myometrium. The first reason is the mass of clinical evidence in which the motor activity of the uterus is clearly altered by neural or reflex stimuli. For example, labor may temporarily stop when the husband or the physician first appears. Labor is rarely effective when the presenting part does not fit evenly into the lower uterine segment (*e.g.,* in transverse lie, occiput

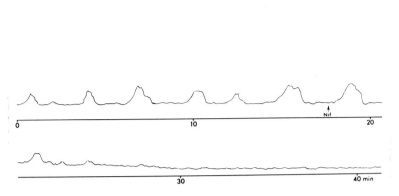

FIG. 31-13. External recording of uterine activity in a woman in 34th week of gestation. Cervix was effaced and dilated 3 cm. Nifedipine (*Nif*) was given orally in a dose of 30 mg. A transient flushing was observed after about 10 minutes, and there was an increase in pulse rate from 90 to 105 beats/minute. Systolic blood pressure was not affected. Fetal heart rate was unchanged. Inhibiting effect on uterine activity lasted for more than six hours. (Andersson K-E: Inhibition of uterine activity by the calcium agonist nifedipine. In Anderson A, Beard R, Brudenell JM et al [eds]: Pre-term Labour, p 101. London, Proceedings of the 5th Study Group of the Royal College of Obstetricians and Gynaecologists, 1977)

posterior position, or a severely asymmetric pelvis) or when the head is held up by inlet disproportion. Labor may start after administration of an enema, especially if it is large and somewhat irritating to the bowel. Stripping the membranes from their loose adhesion to the lower uterine segment can initiate labor (Fig. 31-14). The most efficient means of initiating labor is rupture of the membranes, but, since the withdrawal of 5% to 10% of the amniotic fluid by transabdominal amniocentesis is not followed by labor, it is clear that much more is involved than simple adjustments of the muscle fibers and stretch responses. (It has been shown in both sheep and humans that manipulation of the cervix causes release of PGs, and that the augmentation of uterine activity as a result of such procedures as rupture or stripping of the membranes is more likely due to PG release than to the stimulation of nerve endings. Perhaps both mechanisms are concerned.)

The second reason to presume that nervous mechanisms may be important in myometrial function is that the short uterine postganglionic nerve fibers do not degenerate when the spinal cord is transected or when the preganglionic nerves are cut. Hence, intrinsic neural activity within the myometrium is retained despite section of the extrinsic nerves. Moreover, the density of this intrinsic adrenergic innervation and of the transmitter (norepinephrine) content of the individual nerves (each of which makes contact with many muscle cells) is altered by pregnancy and by the administration of estrogens and progesterone. The predominant transmitter substance is norepinephrine; little, if any, epinephrine is present. In essence, estrogens have been thought to increase both the innervation density and the norepinephrine content of the myometrium. The changes induced by estrogen can be reversed by progesterone. Both α- and β-adrenergic receptors are present in the myometrium, and the dominance of one over the other was conveniently thought to be determined in large measure by the hormonal status of the uterus,

with estrogen causing the α-receptors and progesterone the β-receptors to function predominantly. More recent work has shown that at term all fluorescent adrenergic nerves in the myometrium have disappeared and the norepinephrine concentration is reduced to almost zero. By contrast, the acetylcholine-synthesizing enzyme, choline acetyl-transferase, is unchanged, suggesting both the presence of cholinergic nerves in the uterus and some possible function for them in the control of uterine activity.

There is much confusion about the uterine effects of stimulation of the hypogastric nerves and the action of adrenergic agents. The conflicting reports are partly due to species differences, which in this case are very real, and to differences in methodology. In general, the response to these stimuli appears to vary according to whether the α- or the β-receptors are predominantly concerned. In the case of the human uterus, it is generally agreed that a contractile response is initiated through the α-receptors, while a relaxation effect is mediated through the β-receptors.

Acupuncture is reported to be useful for either the induction or inhibition of labor, depending on the sites used for stimulation. If this should be confirmed, it is presumed that the nervous system must somehow be concerned.

Although the exact role of the autonomic nervous system in the uterus is unknown, it is unreasonable to presume that this or any other organ would possess such a system if it did not have a real function in the control of its physiological activity. What this role is remains to be seen.

Effects of Catecholamines

Investigators have been interested in the effects of catecholamines on the uterus for many years. In recent years, increasing efforts to control the activity of the human uterus during labor have led to clinical trials of the

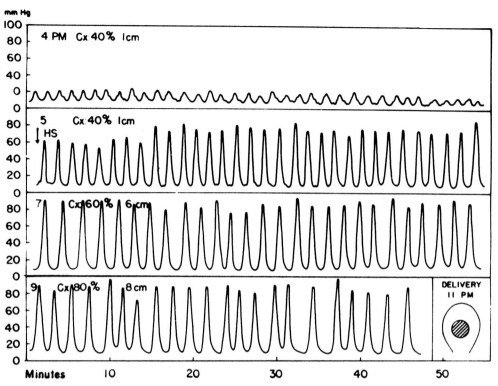

FIG. 31-14. Effect of "high sweeping" (*HS*), with rubber finger, on amniotic pressure. Original record taken from series of 50. All pressure tracings obtained through extraovular technique. Cervical progress is established by repeated vaginal examination. Placental implantation site is determined by manual exploration immediately postpartum. (*Row 1*) Amniotic pressure before high sweeping. (*Rows 2 to 4*) Amniotic pressure after high sweeping. Note increase in active pressure induced by high sweeping (in this case "active pressure area," increased by 11.6 sq cm/30 min). Labor was induced effectively by high sweeping alone, that is, without rupturing membranes and without oxytocin stimulation. (Csapo AI: Effects of the placenta on uterine contractility. In Marshall JM, Burnett WM (eds): Initiation of Labor, p 135. Public Health Service Publication No 1390. Bethesda, MD, US Department of Health, Education, and Welfare, 1963)

uterine response to many catecholamines and catecholamine derivatives. In general, the human uterus responds according to whether the agents are α- or β-mimetic; as noted earlier, α-mimetic agents (*e.g.,* norepinephrine) tend to stimulate (and are sufficiently unpredictable to have no place in clinical obstetrics), while β-mimetic agents depress. Epinephrine activates both α- and β-receptors, with the β-receptors predominating. The result is a depression of uterine activity; however, the uterus recovers after (and even during) the infusion, suggesting later α-receptor activation. Also, a severe rebound effect occurs when the infusion is stopped. This fact, plus the profound cardiovascular stimulation, makes epinephrine impractical for clinical use as a uterine depressant.

The role of endogenous catecholamines in the physiological control of uterine motility is not clear.

The only direct observation has to do with the effects of stress; the blood level of epinephrine is elevated in the presence of marked anxiety, a circumstance that is reported to be associated with longer and less efficient labor.

The clinical use of β-mimetic catecholamine derivatives in the management of preterm labor is considered in Chapter 35. The β-agonists appear to act by stimulating adenyl cyclase and increasing cAMP levels, which leads to calcium binding in the sarcoplasmic reticulum, interference with propagation of the contractile impulse, and myometrial relaxation.

Effects of the Fetus

In normal pregnancy, the fetus exerts at least two influences on myometrial activity. The first of these is due to its bulk, which increases at an accelerating rate and provides the stimulus of stretch. As noted elsewhere, the factor of distention is not introduced until 12 to 14 weeks' gestation; after 16 to 18 weeks, the uterine wall becomes progressively thinner, and increasing stretch is an important factor in all of the subsequent myometrial reactions to pregnancy.

The second fetal influence results from endocrine factors, with the fetal hypothalamus, pituitary, and adrenal cortex being the organs most concerned. It is known that pregnancy is likely to be prolonged in the presence of anencephaly, a fetal anomaly in which there is usually no hypothalamus. The fetal pituitary is hypoplastic for lack of stimulation by the releasing hormones, as are the adrenals for the lack of adrenocorticotropic hormone (ACTH). The degree to which pregnancy is prolonged correlates with the degree of pituitary and adrenal hypoplasia. It is a reasonable conclusion that fetal cortisol is concerned in the onset of labor, and there are considerable experimental data to support this hypothesis: infusing ACTH into fetal lambs provokes enlargement of the adrenals, marked elevation of fetal cortisol levels, and the onset of preterm labor within a few days; in the fetal lamb, hypophysectomy, destruction of the fetal pituitary or hypothalamus, or section of the pituitary or hypothalamus, or section of the pituitary stalk causes atrophic adrenal changes, and pregnancy is prolonged indefinitely; pregnancy is prolonged in the sheep and goat after bilateral fetal adrenalectomy. Based on these studies, as well as other data, Liggins has concluded that "the hormonal changes preceding parturition in the sheep consist of an increase of fetal cortisol, which acts on placental enzymes to cause a fall in the production of progesterone, and an increase in the production of unconjugated estrone and estradiol. This reversal of the ratio of progesterone–estrogen stimulates the formation of $PGE_{2\alpha}$ in the maternal placenta and myometrium." The myometrial consequences of the latter changes are outlined elsewhere in this chapter.

It seems likely that in women, as well as in sheep, cattle, and goats, cortisol is indeed related to the myometrial events surrounding the onset of labor, as exemplified by the clinical syndrome of prolonged pregnancy as the result of fetal anencephaly. The counterpart of this syndrome occurs in adrenal hyperplasia, and Turnbull has found that the weight of the fetal adrenal is greatly increased in cases of spontaneous, "unexplained" preterm labor compared with adrenal weights of infants born early as a result of antepartum hemorrhage, preeclampsia, or some equivalent pregnancy complication. In untreated Cushing's syndrome caused either by pituitary or adrenal neoplasms or by ACTH-secreting bronchial carcinoma, spontaneous labor occurs before the 34th week. In human labor at term, increased levels of cortisol are found in both the maternal

and fetal circulation. The amniotic fluid cortisol also increases with advancing pregnancy; the steepest rise occurs after 40 weeks, suggesting that this value could be used as part of the evaluation of postterm pregnancy.

However, large doses of corticosteroids injected at or before term into pregnant women, into the amniotic cavity, or into the human fetus have consistently failed to initiate labor. Although the fetal adrenal appears to be concerned in the myometrial changes of labor in the sheep, its role in human labor is still not clear. If cortisol is concerned, its influence appears to be mediated through its effects on progesterone secretion, with all the attendant consequences mentioned earlier.

Catecholamines, presumably of fetal origin, have been demonstrated in the amniotic fluid. The concentrations of epinephrine, norepinephrine, and especially dopamine are significantly elevated near term. It is not clear whether these changes have physiological significance, or if they merely reflect the increasing contribution of fetal urine to the amniotic fluid volume as term approaches.

A question has also been raised as to the possible role of the fetal pineal gland in labor. Melatonin is present in amniotic fluid in increased amounts at term, and the melatonin content of the fetal pineal gland is significantly greater during the five days before birth than earlier in pregnancy.

Effects of Fetal Membranes and Decidua

As already noted, arachidonic acid is the obligate precursor of PGs. Gustavii has proposed that the breakdown of lysosomes releases active phospholipase A_2, thus freeing arachidonic acid from the phospholipid stores and making it available for PG synthesis. It is also proposed that progesterone stabilizes the lysosomes of fetal membranes and decidua during most of pregnancy and that, upon breakdown, these lysosomes serve as a substantial source of arachidonic acid for PG synthesis. Liggins has suggested that this membrane mechanism may constitute a sort of "biological clock," genetically motivated, that may be part of the system determining the time of labor in different species. He also suggests that Gustavii's hypothesis may explain preterm labor in such circumstances as intrauterine infection, hemorrhage, overdistention of the uterus by hydramnios or multiple pregnancy, or rupture of the membranes, all of which could result in lysosomal disruption in the fetal membranes and decidua. Such a breakdown of decidual lysosomes could also explain the delivery of the placenta(s) at the correct time for labor after prior removal of the fetus(es).

Effects of Oxytocin

Oxytocin is a cyclic polypeptide containing eight amino acids and having a molecular weight of about

1000. It is produced in the hypothalamus and is stored in and released from the posterior pituitary.

Oxytocin is the agent *par excellence* for stimulating the uterus and for testing its reactivity. Synthetic preparations are used extensively for the induction and stimulation of labor, and the uterus becomes increasingly responsive as pregnancy advances. As noted elsewhere, oxytocin acts by causing the release of previously bound calcium from the sarcoplasmic reticulum, thus activating the contractile system. The clinical use of oxytocin in the induction and stimulation of labor is considered in Chapter 39.

MATERNAL OXYTOCIN. The hypothesis that labor is initiated as the direct result of oxytocin release from the maternal pituitary is no longer tenable. Concentrations of oxytocin in the maternal blood increase slightly as pregnancy advances, but there is no significant change at the time of the onset of labor. However, it will be recalled that the sensitivity of the uterus to oxytocin increases as pregnancy advances; increasing uterine responsiveness to unchanging oxytocin levels could have the same effect as an increase in oxytocin concentration. In humans, Fuchs and colleagues have found that the concentration of myometrial *oxytocin receptors* parallels the increasing oxytocin sensitivity of the uterus, which reaches a maximum level in early labor. It is likely that the increased number of receptors plays a role in the increasing uterine sensitivity. However, as in the case of other receptors, it will be interesting to note how many of the new receptors are occupied, and whether all occupied receptors are capable of initiating a subsequent response.

Late in labor, significant elevations do occur in blood oxytocin, which lends credence to the old concept of the *Ferguson reflex* (a spurt release of oxytocin in response to the stimulus of the presenting part on the cervix and upper vagina) and suggests a neurohumoral reflex that is still undefined. Further support is offered by the finding that such elevations are suppressed by spinal or pelvic regional anesthesia. *Nipple stimulation* also produces an elevation in plasma oxytocin level, which then provokes uterine contractions.

With regard to the role of the posterior pituitary in normal labor, it has been noted repeatedly that neither the onset nor the maintenance of labor is abnormally affected in patients with diabetes insipidus. In one case of idiopathic diabetes insipidus, a surge in plasma oxytocin similar to that of normal pregnancy was found during labor and the puerperium. In the interpretation of such data, it should be recalled that the defect causing diabetes insipidus may not involve the entire posterior lobe, or that it may be "nephrogenic" in origin, resulting from a tubular defect that interferes with water reabsorption. In cases in which the entire posterior lobe is involved, ocytocin in the peripheral blood must be assumed to be either of fetal origin or to have reached the bloodstream directly from the hypothalamus. Among patients who have had total hypophysectomy, sponta-

neous labor is the rule, but no oxytocin studies of such patients have been reported.

FETAL OXYTOCIN. The role of fetal oxytocin in the normal course of labor is not clear. Khan–Dawood and colleagues have found that the oxytocin concentration in the human fetal pituitary gland is greatly increased with advancing pregnancy. During spontaneous labor, umbilical cord blood contains far higher concentrations of oxytocin than does maternal blood, and the concentration in umbilical artery blood is about twice that of umbilical venous blood. It was noted earlier that in anencephaly and after fetal hypophysectomy, labor is usually delayed or may be prevented. However, in anencephaly and after fetal decapitation in the rat, the amniotic fluid does contain considerable amounts of oxytocin, suggesting that it may arise from a source other than the fetal pituitary.

The placenta is an important source of enzymes that destroy oxytocin. Accordingly, fetal oxytocin would probably be suffused into the myometrium across the fetal membranes, rather than introduced into the maternal circulation through the placenta. One of these enzymes, oxytocinase, appears in the plasma of pregnant women. It is produced only in the placenta of the primate, with plasma levels rising throughout pregnancy to term. It rapidly inactivates oxytocin; this fact has led many workers to the belief that oxytocinase serves to protect pregnancy through prompt inactivation of any oxytocin suddenly released to the bloodstream and, consequently, to prevent excessive uterine activity. The presence of abnormally large or abnormally small amounts of the enzyme has been postulated as a possible explanation for a wide spectrum of clinical problems, such as preterm labor, inefficient labor, and failure of the uterus to respond within normal limits to exogenous oxytocin.

However, the metabolism of oxytocin is very rapid in males and in nonpregnant females, as well as in pregnant females. Oxytocin is excreted in the maternal urine and also appears to be inactivated in kidney tissues. Therefore, while oxytocinase is undeniably present in the plasma of pregnant women, its clinical importance remains undemonstrated, especially since the high concentrations of oxytocin in amniotic fluid suggest that the most direct route by which fetal oxytocin could reach the myometrium is suffusion through the fetal membranes. High concentrations of biologically active oxytocin have now been demonstrated in the human placenta, but the significance of this finding is unclear. Perhaps oxytocin that reaches the placenta from fetal and maternal circulations and by suffusion from amniotic fluid is deactivated more slowly than was formerly thought.

The Onset of Labor

When the Gillespie curves (Fig. 31-4) are examined, it is obvious that the continuation of pregnancy beyond a given point is impossible, for the uterus must either empty or rupture. Moreover, it seems clear that nature's design for the duration of pregnancy must be unique for each species; in the evolutionary scale, as brain and head size increased, the pelvis became smaller. This, as Page has pointed out, posed a serious problem for the higher phyla, for delivery must occur before the fetal head becomes so large it cannot traverse the pelvis. In the case of *Homo sapiens,* the solution was delivery at a time when, compared with most other mammals, the fetus is approximately one year preterm—judged by such parameters as the development of enzyme systems; neuromuscular coordination; ability to stand, communicate, and forage for food; and other attainments not achieved by the human until about one year of age. These observations lend credence to the probability that the timing of the changes leading to labor is set by a "genetic clock" that is unique for each species.

As new data become available, it is apparent that the onset of labor results from the gradual convergence of a number of factors, each of which must bear an optimal relation to all the others. According to the classic theory of Csapo, the gradually accelerating factors that tend to stimulate coordinated uterine activity are effectively counterbalanced during pregnancy by the similarly increasing production of progesterone (Fig. 31-15). The stimulatory factors include the consequences of increasing estrogens and stretch, the development of the contractile system, the increasing availability of PGs, and the continuing availability of oxytocin. The ability of progesterone to counterbalance these factors and to "block" the development of coordinated contractions appears to be twofold. Progesterone stabilizes the pools of calcium in the sarcoplasmic reticulum, making them unavailable for activation of the contractile system; also, progesterone may change the membrane potentials such that the threshold to the stimulating effects of oxytocin and PGs is raised. Oxytocin and PGs have effects that are opposite to those of progesterone, causing calcium mobilization and lowering of membrane potentials. Key words are *progesterone dominance:* as long as progesterone is dominant

uterine activity in pregnancy is limited to the sporadic and incoordinated Braxton Hicks contractions; when the balance shifts so that the simulatory factors are dominant, labor starts.

Evidence is accumulating to support the hypothesis that the lysosomes of the fetal membranes and decidua serve as a primary source of arachidonic acid for PG synthesis. It has been proposed that progesterone receptors appear in the fetal membranes, competing with the lysosomes for progesterone. As a consequence, the lysosomes become more fragile, their contents spill, PGs are produced in quantity, and the progesterone dominance gives way. As noted before, this thesis is attractive, since rupture of membranes and decidual lysosomes could explain the onset of labor after such insults as rupture or stripping of the membranes, intrauterine infection, the instillation of hypertonic saline for late abortion, or the trauma and hypoxia associated with preterm separation of the placenta. It therefore follows that multiple factors are concerned and that the "trigger" for labor, as Chard proposes, may be a random series of events. He suggests that the factors that may be involved in the onset of labor can be divided into the following three types:

Type 1 includes factors that might constitute a primary stimulus to labor, such as oxytocin, ACTH, and related peptides.
Type 2 factors are fairly specific to labor but are dependent on a primary stimulus. Some examples are estrogen, progesterone, cortisol, oxytocin receptors, and relaxin.
Type 3 factors are nonspecific and are involved in the activation of smooth muscle at any site. Some examples are prostaglandins, autonomic mediators, calcium, gap junctions, and cyclic nucleotides.

According to this thesis, the weight of the several factors may vary not only from one species to another according to special needs, but also from one person to another.

The determination of the cause of the onset of labor is not merely an academic exercise, for it is through this

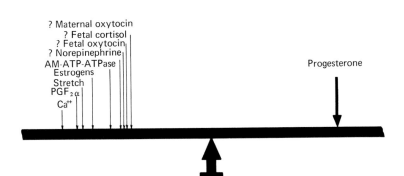

? Maternal oxytocin
? Fetal cortisol
? Fetal oxytocin
? Norepinephrine
AM-ATP-ATPase
Estrogens
Stretch
$PGF_{2\alpha}$
Ca^{++}

Progesterone

FIG. 31-15. Oversimplified summary of regulatory mechanism of pregnant uterus, illustrating balance between stimulants and suppressor. As pregnancy advances, gradual increase in progesterone balances (and effectively negates) influence of gradually increasing stimulants. At term, progesterone dominance gives way and stimulatory factors are unopposed. (AI Csapo)

knowledge that the most pressing clinical problem in obstetrics will be answered—the absolute control of uterine contractility, that is, the ability to start or to stop coordinated contractions at will. The first may have been solved already, because oxytocin and PGs may be the ultimate agents for producing coordinated uterine contractions. The second, the ability to arrest coordinated contractions with equal precision and predictability, remains a problem for the future. As more is learned about the factors that normally converge to produce labor, it will be possible to intervene with precision at some point in the cascade of events, and so to terminate labor that is established or to prevent it among those who are predisposed to preterm labor.

UTERINE RESPONSES TO PREGNANCY AND LABOR

The two parts of the uterus, the corpus and the cervix, react differently to pregnancy. It is important to remember that the corpus is composed basically of muscle, the cervix of connective tissue; and that the corpus undergoes growth and is subject to distention, while the cervix, although slightly softened, maintains its continuity as a relatively firm, more or less closed, fibrous ring until late in pregnancy. The corpus thus functions to *contain* the products of conception, the cervix to *retain* them.

Structural Changes in Pregnancy

The nonpregnant uterus weighs 60 g to 80 g; the term uterus, 900 g to 1200 g. This enormous increase is due almost entirely to proliferation of the myometrium. In early pregnancy (but not past the third month), there is hyperplasia of the muscle cells, and mitotic figures are common. In the second and third trimesters, uterine growth is due almost entirely to hypertrophy, the individual muscle cells increasing 10 to 12 times in length and 2 to 7 times in width.

Uterine growth in pregnancy results from two major factors: hormonal effects, which alone are operative until 12 to 14 weeks' gestation; and distention and consequent stretching, which begins at about the fourth month of pregnancy. The proliferation of new muscle bundles is accounted for by the influence of estrogens. The proliferation of new fibers comes to an end as the progesterone level increases. Further growth is primarily a hypertrophic response to distention and is enhanced by progesterone.

Architecture and Development of the Myometrium

Goerttler has clarified the architectural arrangement of the myometrium. In the unfused uterus (*e.g.,* rabbit)

the muscle bundles in each uterus take a spiral course from outside in and from above downward. Similar systems are present in the fused (primate) uterus, one arising in each uterine cornu, proceeding caudad, and interdigitating as they approach the midportion of the corpus (Fig. 31-16). In the middle and upper portions of the corpus the two systems are at right angles to one another; in the lower corpus they are almost parallel. These relations are accentuated as pregnancy advances, and it seems clear that in labor a uterine contraction in the middle or upper portion of the corpus would tend to pull upward on the more transversely arranged bundles of the lower pole of the uterus. It is therefore convenient to refer to the *upper longitudinal component* of the myometrium, which pulls cephalad on the *lower circular* or *transverse component.*

In early pregnancy, the fundus becomes increasingly convex because of the upward pushing of the proliferating muscle. Consequently, the tubes and round ligaments insert at an increasingly lower point in the corpus as pregnancy advances. In addition, the corpus becomes globular, rather than flattened as before pregnancy, and the uterine cavity enlarges. In the first trimester and in part of the second, these changes occur almost precisely symmetrically so that the uterine appendages insert at the same level in the exact midfrontal plane of the corpus. A uterine abnormality or a uterine tumor (fibroid) in pregnancy is suggested by asymmetry of the uterus or irregularity in the attachment of its appendages.

In the first 12 to 14 weeks of pregnancy, the myometrium grows at a faster rate than the conceptus. On

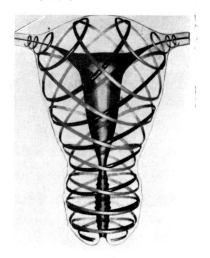

FIG. 31-16. Architecture of nonpregnant uterus. Note spiral course and bilateral symmetric arrangement of muscle fibers in planes of different inclination. Fibers cross each other at right angles in upper segment, but at obtuse angles in lower segment. (Goerttler K: Gegenbaurs Morphologisches Jahrbuch 65:45, 1930)

bimanual examination the corpus is felt to be softened and enlarged. These changes in the corpus are termed *Hegar's sign* (see p. 361) and can usually be elicited between 5 and 10 weeks. At about 14 weeks, the conceptus begins to grow at a more rapid rate than the corpus. The reflected decidua comes in contact with the parietal decidua, and the isthmic segment unfolds (Fig. 31-17); because of the resulting distention, pressure is exerted upon the cervix. If the cervix is normal and is able to resist this pressure, the pregnancy continues; if it is structurally abnormal or sufficiently injured by a prior pregnancy, late abortion results.

The unfolding of the lower pole of the uterus to receive the enlarging conceptus involves mecystatic adjustments in length of the lower circular component of the myometrium that are similar to those that occur in the urinary bladder as it fills and in the stomach as a meal is eaten. As the fibers lengthen circumferentially, the thickness of the involved area is reduced, and for the remainder of pregnancy, the myometrium at the lower pole of the uterus is somewhat thinner than in the midportion and the fundus. The transition is extremely gradual and does not necessarily bear any relation to the site of the former anatomic internal os.

As a rule, the uterus can be readily palpated abdominally at three months' gestation, the fundus reaches the level of the umbilicus at five months' gestation, and the uterus reaches the level of the costal margins and the xiphoid at eight to nine months' gestation and drops slightly thereafter as the presenting part engages in the pelvis during the last week of pregnancy.

After five months' gestation, as the uterus grows, it gradually turns to the right. This dextrorotation is usually attributed to the presence of the sigmoid colon on the left and is of practical importance at the time of cesarean section, because immediately beneath a midline abdominal incision the blood vessels of the left broad ligament may be encountered.

Along with the changes in size and thickness of the myometrium, striking changes occur in the blood vessels of the corpus. The uterine arteries undergo considerable enlargement, and there is an enormous increase in the size and capacity of the ovarian vessels. Particularly in the region of the placental site, the radial arteries that traverse the myometrium enlarge considerably and form the large trunks that open into the intervillous space.

The uterus is traversed by large veins, which not only empty the placenta at its base and its margins but also carry the large blood supply afforded the uterine muscle. Although there is some information about the gross blood flow through the uterus at term, it has not yet been possible to sort out what proportion of this flows into the intervillous space and what proportion into the uterine muscle. It is not unusual to encounter large venous sinuses in the uterine wall opposite the location of the placenta; indeed, the blood loss from these sinuses may account for most of the bleeding at the time of cesarean section, which usually amounts to an average of 1000 ml.

At term, the venous blood from the uterus traverses the broad ligament in large blood vessels, many of them greater than 2 cm in diameter. Some vessels drain upward through the infundibulopelvic ligaments, but most proceed to the pelvic sidewall where they join the hypogastric vein. Although it is not improper to speak of the uterine artery, there is no such structure as the uterine vein; the veins are always multiple. These large veins are remarkably thin-walled and are often located directly

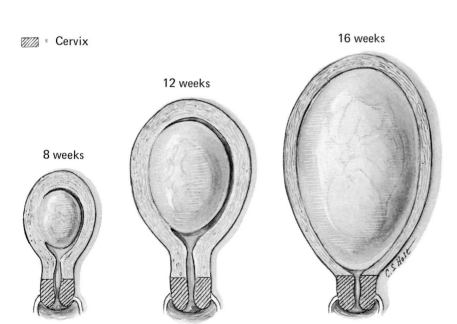

⬛ = Cervix

8 weeks
12 weeks
16 weeks

FIG. 31-17. Changes in corpus relative to cervix in early pregnancy. Cervix, crosshatched in diagram, is principally fibrous and exhibits little change in this period. Corpus, principally muscular, undergoes marked growth, and at 12 weeks, the fact that conceptus has not yet expanded to fill growing uterus results in lengthening isthmic segment. With accelerating fetal growth, this space is filled by 16th week. Unfolding normally stops at fibrous cervix, where adaptive relaxation is not possible. (Danforth DN: Fibrous nature of the human cervix and its relation to the isthmic segment in gravid and nongravid uteri. Am J Obstet Gynecol 53:541, 1947)

under the posterior peritoneum of the broad ligament. Although they are unusual, ruptures into the peritoneal cavity and fatal hemoperitoneum have been reported.

Structural Changes in Labor

The structural changes that occur in the uterus and allow its orderly evacuation at term have been the subject of much study and speculation. Unfortunately, it is not possible to watch the uterus directly as it undergoes these changes, or even to study it with contrast media and x-ray films as the stomach and other hollow viscera can be studied. The methods of studying uterine contractions have provided an excellent and probably a true picture of the contraction patterns and activities of the different parts of the uterus, but the structural changes produced are more difficult to determine. One means of determining such changes is by examination of intact uteri at the different stages of labor, but such specimens are (fortunately) unusual in humans; when they do occur, the manipulations needed for excising them distort not only the uterus but its relation to the pelvic landmarks. Frozen sagittal sections in humans are even more rare, but reports of 60 to 70 of them have been published (most near the turn of the century). The freezing techniques were slow, and the obstetric problems they portrayed were often horrendous. An example of such a specimen is shown in Figure 37-10. An alternative, which can probably be interpreted directly in terms of the structural changes in the human uterus, is the examination of frozen sagittal sections made during labor in *Macaca rhesus* or other primate having a fused uterus simplex like that of humans. Distortion of the uterus necessarily enters here, too, because the rapid freezing methods must cause significant contraction of the tissue. However, the results are informative and appear to give much insight into the structural changes of labor.

The monkey uterus is like the human uterus except for the presence of an inner lip, or colliculus, at the superior extremity of the cervix. This does not hamper the observations; rather it is helpful, because it can be used to mark on the intact specimen the exact upper end of the cervix. A second important feature of pregnancy in *Macaca rhesus* is that the placenta is bidiscoidal; the two disks are of about equal size, and one is attached to the anterior aspect of the corpus and one to the posterior. The two disks are connected by vessels that traverse one lateral aspect of the uterine cavity. A series of these frozen sections is shown in Figures 31-18 through 31-27. Although the concern here is with the uterus, these sections also show the relation of the bladder to the pelvis and uterus; the great length of the vagina in the second stage; the effectiveness of the forewaters as a dilating wedge when the membranes are intact (in Fig. 31-20 the membranes have "hourglassed" through and not only are of no use but may be hazardous if an edge of the placenta should be pulled off); and

the placental stage of labor (in Fig. 31-26 part of the placenta can be seen in the vagina immediately after delivery).

These sections show that, during the first stage of labor, the lower pole of the uterus is gradually pulled up over the presenting part and there is no appreciable advancement of the head until the cervix is fully dilated. They demonstrate that, beginning with the first stage and continuing through labor, there is progressive shortening of the uterus. The relative rate and extent of the shortening are shown by measurements of the internal circumference of the uterus in the sagittal plane (Fig. 31-28). This progressive, ratchetlike shortening of the uterus is referred to as *retraction* or *brachystasis* (see p. 584) and is one of the properties of uterine muscle. Although demonstration of brachystasis in a single fiber is not possible, this phenomenon provides the only reasonable explanation for the retractive changes that are known to occur and that result, over the course of the first stage of labor, in progressive shortening and thickening of the corporeal musculature and, in the second stage, in delivery.

Retraction of the myometrium is necessary not only for expelling the infant from the uterus but also for controlling bleeding after delivery. Under normal circumstances, the uterus contracts firmly and remains well contracted after the delivery of the placenta (Fig. 31-29). By this means, the vessels and sinusoids of the uterus are closed off, and bleeding from the placental site and the adjacent denuded areas of the uterus is controlled. If the uterus fails to remain well contracted after delivery, heavy bleeding invariably results. Although postpartum hemorrhage may result from lacerations and clotting defects, its usual cause is atony of the uterus. This is a leading cause of maternal death.

Role of the Uterine Supports

It has been noted that the work of the first stage of labor is devoted to preparation of the lower uterine segment, dilatation of the cervix, and retraction of the cervix over the presenting part. Although the head may advance as cervical resistance diminishes, the active advance of the fetus and delivery are second-stage events. It is when the cervix is fully dilated and has completed its upward excursion that the uterine supports (notably the cardinal ligaments, the pubocervical fascia, and the uterosacral ligaments) begin their important role in uterine evacuation, because these supports enable the uterus to expel the infant through the birth canal. In the monkey, the supports are relatively longer than in humans; consequently, the cervix rises to a higher level before the taut supports stop its upward excursion. In humans, x-ray films of metal clips on the cervix show clearly that the supports limit the upward excursion of the cervix to the plane of the inlet (Fig. 31-30). If the supports were elastic at this point in labor, a second-stage contraction, instead of advancing the baby, would merely

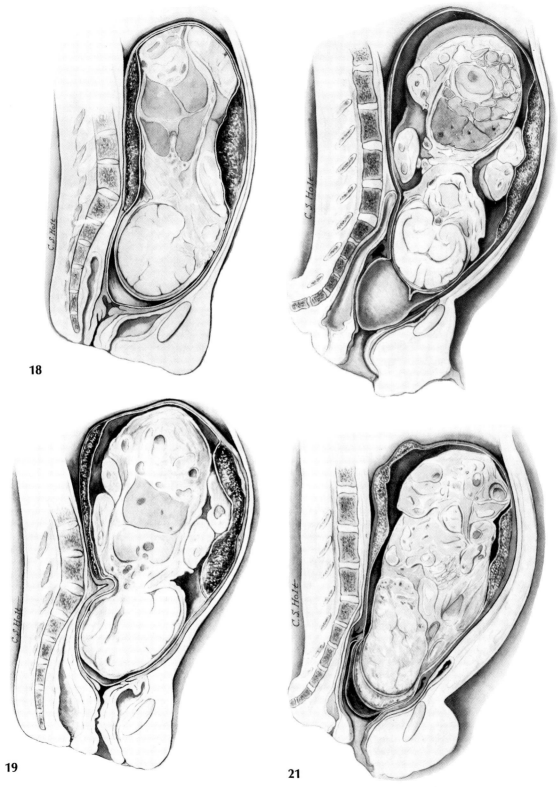

FIGS. 31-18 through 31-21.   Frozen sagittal sections of *Macaca rhesus,* first stage of labor. Nembutal anesthesia. Rapid freezing by immersion in alcohol chilled to −80°C. (Danforth DN, Graham RJ, Ivy AC: Functional anatomy of labor as revealed by frozen sagittal sections in the *Macaca rhesus* monkey. Surg Gynecol Obstet 74:188, 1942)

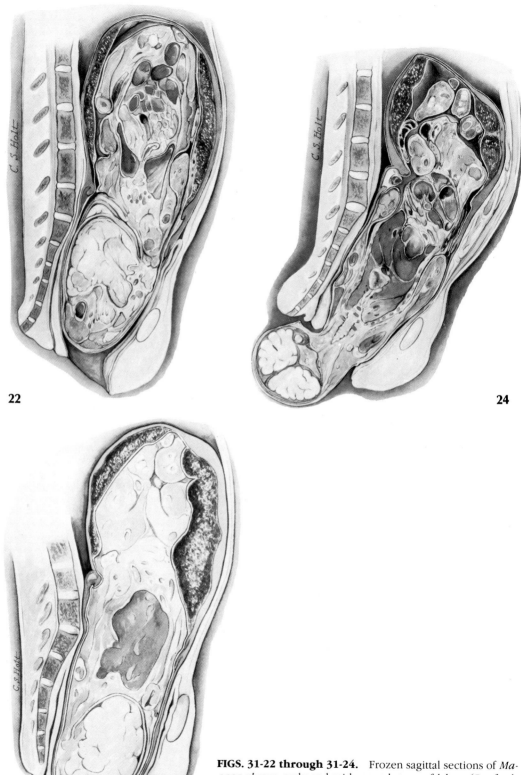

FIGS. 31-22 through 31-24. Frozen sagittal sections of *Macaca rhesus,* early and mid-second stage of labor. (Danforth DN, Graham RJ, Ivy AC: Functional anatomy of labor as revealed by frozen sagittal sections in the *Macaca rhesus* monkey. Surg Gynecol Obstet 74:188, 1942)

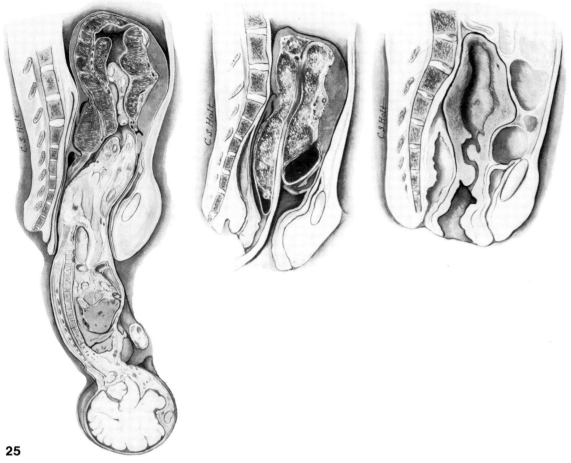

25

FIGS. 31-25 through 31-27. Frozen sagittal sections of *Macaca rhesus*, late second stage (Fig. 31-25), mid-third stage (Fig. 31-26), and 15 minutes after delivery (Fig. 31-27). (Danforth DN, Graham RJ, Ivy AC: Functional anatomy of labor as revealed by frozen sagittal sections in the *Macaca rhesus* monkey. Surg Gynecol Obstet 74:188, 1942)

pull the cervix higher. The supports act as stout, unyielding guy ropes against which the uterus works during the second stage of labor (Fig. 31-31). The stress or strain upon these ligaments is proportional to the resistance to delivery offered by the bony pelvis or by the soft parts. The longer or more violent the second stage, the higher the probability of injury and ecchymosis within the structure of the ligaments.

Historical Aspects

For many years controversy surrounded the concept of the lower uterine segment. The term was introduced by Bandl in 1875 and engendered a huge and at times vitriolic literature because of the violent dissension about its origin and physiological behavior. Some of the German papers are diatribes of monographic size. All agreed that, either during labor or just prior to labor, the corpus becomes divided into a thicker "upper segment" and a thinner "lower segment." The debate centered on the question of whether the lower segment is active or passive and whether the cervix is or is not a part of the lower uterine segment. Aschoff's definition of the isthmus in 1905, although now shown to be inaccurate, brought order to the chaos by the simple statement that the lower uterine segment is derived neither from the corpus nor from the cervix, but from the isthmus. In 1949, this comfortable concept was upset by data that showed that the isthmus is not a distinct and separate entity as Aschoff held, but rather is an integral part of the corpus with properties similar to those of the remainder of the corpus; and that the cervix is basically a connective-tissue structure and therefore has no contractile function.

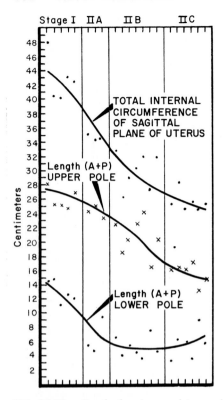

TOTAL INTERNAL
CIRCUMFERENCE
OF SAGITTAL
PLANE OF UTERUS

Length (A+P)
UPPER POLE

Length (A+P)
LOWER POLE

FIG. 31-28. Graph showing total internal circumference in sagittal plane of uterus during labor. Measurements made in 21 monkeys, of which 5 were sacrificed in first stage of labor (*I*), 3 in early second stage (*IIA*), 7 in mid-second stage (*IIB*), and 6 in late second stage (*IIC*). Lower edge of placenta was used in all specimens as arbitrary point for measuring length changes in lower pole of uterus and is contrasted in this graph with equivalent changes in upper part of uterus. Lines are fitted by inspection. In these specimens, first-stage shortening of uterus appears to be almost entirely due to retraction of lower pole of uterus as it pulls up over fetal head. Additional uterine shortening in second stage appears to be almost entirely due to retraction of upper pole of uterus. (Danforth DN, Graham RJ, Ivy AC: Functional anatomy of labor as revealed by frozen sagittal sections in the *Macaca rhesus* monkey. Surg Gynecol Obstet 74:188, 1942)

Formation of the Lower Uterine Segment

The lower uterine segment is first formed as a definitive entity during the uterine changes before labor or as the first stage of labor begins. It is well known that, as labor advances, the entire length of the uterus shortens, the midportion and fundal areas thicken, and the lower pole becomes thinner as it is pulled upward about the presenting part. As the lower circular component of the myometrium is pulled upward around the presenting part, the transverse fibers must elongate; as they do so, the myometrial thickness must diminish. This is a mecystatic adjustment (see p. 585) that is limited to the lower reaches of the myometrium, which must dilate in order to permit the fetus to pass. There

is a point on the uterine wall below which circumferential dilatation must occur as the myometrium is pulled upward and above which the diameter is already great enough so that no further dilatation need occur. The *physiologic retraction ring* necessarily appears at this point and marks the junction of the upper and the lower uterine segments. The physiologic retraction ring is evident as a ledge, thicker cephalad and thinner caudad, around the entire internal circumference of the uterus. The level at which this ring occurs in any given uterus is determined only by the relation between the size of the presenting part and its level in the uterine cavity. The *lower uterine segment* is therefore defined as the band of myometrium at the lower pole of the uterus that must undergo circumferential dilatation, and consequent thinning, as it is pulled upward around the presenting part (Fig. 31-32). It is marked superiorly by the physiologic retraction ring and inferiorly by the fibromuscular junction of the cervix and the corpus.

The progressive total shortening of the uterus, the gradual thickening of the upper segment, and the upward advancement of the lower segment are the result of brachystatic adjustments in the muscle fibers of the longitudinal component of the myometrium. Brachystasis and retraction of the upper segment are progressive and do not cease until the uterus is empty; indeed, such changes are essential to supply the force needed to advance the fetus and to maintain the advantage gained at each contraction.

FIG. 31-29. Schematic representation of blood vessels coursing through myometrium. (*A*) During pregnancy. (*B*) Postpartum, occluded by myometrial retraction. Changes in individual muscle fibers shown by *numbers*. (After Bumm E: Grundriss zum Studium der Geburtshilfe, 13th ed. Munich, Bergmann, 1921)

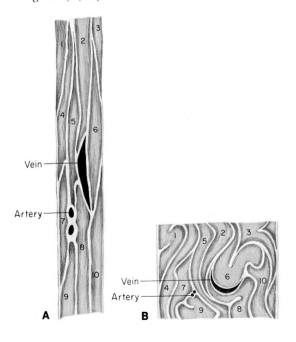

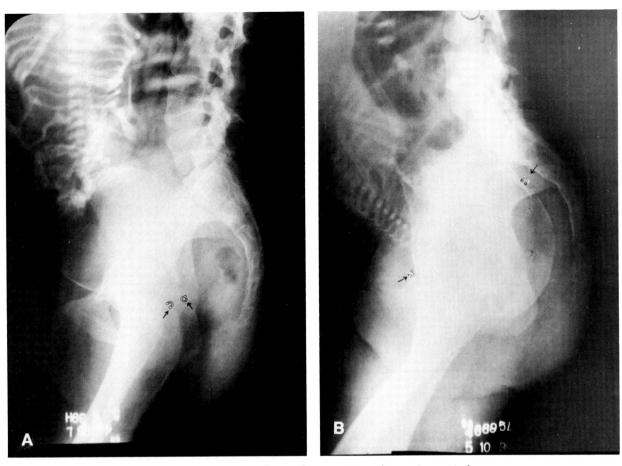

FIG. 31-30. Lateral x-ray films showing metal clips (*arrows*) on anterior and posterior cervical lips. (*A*) Early labor. Head not engaged, clips below spines. Clips retouched. (*B*) Full dilatation. Anterior clip superior to pubic ramus, posterior clip about 2 cm below pelvic brim, head deeply engaged; delivery occurred moments after film was taken. (Courtesy James Stillman)

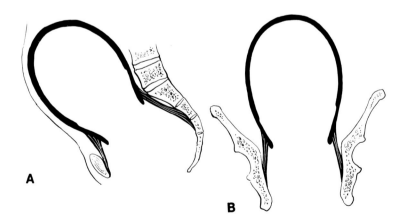

FIG. 31-31. (*A*) Lateral and (*B*) coronal diagrams showing functions of ligamentary supports of uterus in limiting upward excursion of cervix in labor. Undue tension at this time (due to obstruction to advancement of baby) may damage supports. (Danforth DN: Cervical incompetency. In Davis CH, Carter AB [eds]: Gynecology and Obstetrics. Hagerstown, WA Prior, 1962)

At full dilatation the cervix is pulled upward approximately to the level of the inlet and is prevented from going higher by the stout uterine supports that are now pulled taut. Further changes in the uterus are wholly dependent upon the amount of effort expended by the uterus in overcoming the obstruction offered by the soft parts and the bony pelvis. If there is no obstruction, as in the case of some multiparas, the uterus shortens as a whole and empties. Since the supports limit the upward excursion of the cervix, significant obstruction in the

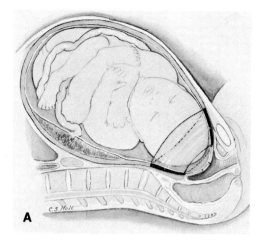

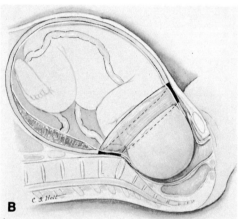

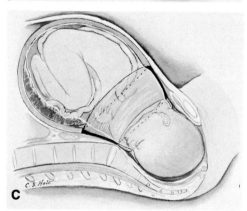

FIG. 31-32. Lower uterine segment. (*A*) At onset of labor. (*B*) Precisely at full dilatation. (*C*) After full dilatation in presence of significant obstruction to advancement of fetus. Bandl's ring beginning to form. (Danforth DN, Ivy AC: The lower uterine segment: Its derivation and physiologic behavior. Am J Obstet Gynecol 57:831, 1949)

face of progressive brachystatic shortening must inevitably result in damage to the uterus, and the weakest part will give way. The weakest portion of the musculature is the thinned lower uterine segment. If the obstruction is only slight or moderate, the lower segment is lengthened to a degree by the brachystatic contractions of the powerful upper uterine segment, but the fetus advances slightly with each contraction. If the obstruction is absolute, however, and the baby cannot advance, the upper segment continues to thicken and the lower segment becomes excessively thinned (Fig. 31-32). The physiologic retraction ring, formerly only a small ledge, now becomes pronounced and is known as *Bandl's ring* or *pathologic contraction ring*. The formation of Bandl's ring heralds the imminent rupture of the uterus. It is sometimes evident as an indentation or transverse groove on the abdomen at a point between the symphysis and the umbilicus and has the same general appearance as a full bladder. However, the ring rises as contractions continue, and uterine rupture through the greatly thinned lower uterine segment is inevitable unless the obstruction to delivery is immediately relieved (see discussion of rings in Chap. 37).

UTERINE CONTRACTIONS IN PREGNANCY AND LABOR

The year 1872 marked the opening of an important new era in clinical obstetrics. It was then that Dr. John Braxton Hicks presented a paper, "On the Contractions of the Uterus Throughout Pregnancy: Their Physiological Effects and Their Value in the Diagnosis of Pregnancy," before the Obstetrical Society of London. There Hicks gave evidence that the pregnant uterus contracts and relaxes from the third month of pregnancy. He noted that careful palpation of the gravid uterus would allow the examiner to feel contractions, usually occurring every 5 to 20 minutes, but occasionally coming only once every 30 minutes. He felt that such contractile activity "is a natural condition of pregnancy" and stated that the pregnant woman is not usually conscious of these contractions, but that they may be painful on some occasions. More than 100 years after these observations were published, it is agreed that Hicks was right on all counts. The frequently used term *Braxton Hicks contractions* is a fitting tribute to Hicks's clinical acumen.

About the same time Hicks was presenting his findings in London, Schatz, in Germany, published the first tracings of uterine contractility in labor. Using an intrauterine balloon for recording, Schatz demonstrated the pattern of uterine contractility throughout labor. Among other observations, he noted the effect of postural change upon uterine contractility and demonstrated the relatively large increase in intrauterine pressure brought about by bearing down in the second stage of labor.

These two brilliant clinicians laid the foundation for a significant portion of present-day understanding of the physiology of labor. Hicks provided part of the knowledge of prelabor and its relation to active labor. Schatz increased the understanding of the process of parturition. His pioneering technique was the all-important first step toward the now common practice of monitoring uterine activity during the course of labor.

Today the monitoring of uterine contractility has

been brought to a high degree of practical usefulness. Either external or internal measurements of uterine activity may be made. The latter provides a more accurate picture of the contractility pattern, because it permits direct documentation of changes in the intrauterine pressure. This method enables the attendant to note the general contour of the contraction, the intensity (in millimeters of mercury), the frequency of contractions, and the tonus (the "resting pressure" between contractions). The record of intrauterine pressure, properly interpreted, can help the physician identify and follow the course of normal labor. Moreover, the recording can help the clinician realize when abnormal types of uterine activity that might have a deleterious effect upon the woman or her fetus are developing.

To provide a graphic portrayal of uterine activity, Caldeyro–Barcía and Alvarez used the term *Montevideo unit.* This is the product obtained by multiplying the frequency of the contractions (the number occurring in 10 minutes) by the intensity of the contractions (the average intrauterine pressure peaks of all contractions occurring in the 10-minute span). The use of this device is illustrated in Figure 31-33.

Development of Uterine Activity During Pregnancy

The uterus remains relatively quiescent during the first half of pregnancy. Nevertheless, there is always some evidence of myometrial activity. There may be frequent localized (regional) contractions that may increase the intrauterine pressure only 1 mm Hg to 5 mm Hg above the resting pressure (Fig. 31-34). The resting pressure between contractions (tonus) is relatively constant throughout pregnancy and early labor, ranging from 5 mm Hg to 10 mm Hg. Even in early pregnancy, however, there may be bursts of greatly increased activity—much larger contractions that appear without evident cause, are not sensed by the patient, and usually subside spontaneously after a few minutes.

Toward the end of the second trimester, the regional activity persists, but it is occasionally interrupted by the appearance of isolated contractions that in form and intensity are quite typical of the contractions observed in normal labor (Fig. 31-35). These isolated, usually painless contractions (Braxton Hicks contractions) tend to become more frequent as pregnancy advances into the last trimester, and they appear to play an important role in prelabor changes.

The Contractions of Prelabor

Prelabor is that all-important period in late pregnancy when the uterus is undergoing preparatory changes that under normal conditions help to ensure efficient labor. For the last four weeks before the onset of labor, the pattern of uterine contractility evolves toward that of active labor. The regional activity tends to persist into advanced prelabor, but the laborlike contractions appear with increasing frequency and tend to become better

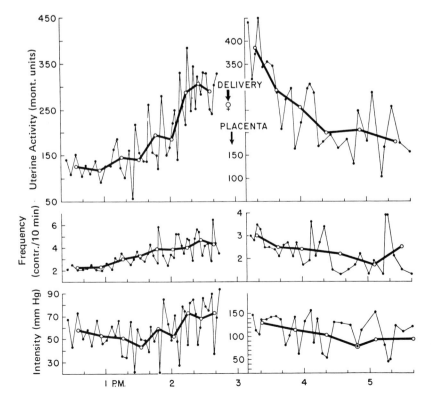

FIG. 31-33. Comparison of one subject's uterine activity in late labor (*left*) and in early puerperium (*right*). (Hendricks CH: Uterine contractility at delivery and in the puerperium. Am J Obstet Gynecol 83:890, 1962)

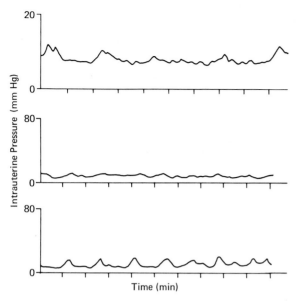

FIG. 31-34. Uterine activity in early pregnancy. (*Top*) At 11 weeks, spontaneous regional type contractions develop 1 to 5 mm Hg intrauterine pressure above resting pressure. (*Middle*) At 14 weeks, spontaneous activity is noted. (*Bottom*) At 14 weeks, same patient as in middle graph shows slight response to large dose of oxytocin (100 mU/min). (Hendricks)

coordinated as the time for labor approaches (Fig. 31-36). Although the exact cause of cervical effacement is unknown, there is some evidence that the agent responsible for the contractions of prelabor (probably PGs) may also be responsible for the effacement and slight dilatation that usually occur before the onset of true labor (Fig. 31-37).

Most Braxton Hicks contractions are painless and are noticed by the woman, if she perceives them at all, only as an intermittent tightening of the uterus. While the contractility pattern is substantially the same in women of all parities, the woman's perception of these contractions is altered considerably by previous childbearing experience. In the first pregnancy, Braxton Hicks contractions are generally painless until an hour or so before the onset of true labor; but, with each succeeding pregnancy, painful contractions are likely to precede the onset of true labor by an increasingly long period. A woman in her eighth or ninth pregnancy may find painful Braxton Hicks contractions extremely troublesome as early as the fifth or sixth month.

When these painful contractions come in bursts, the woman (and her physician) may form the mistaken impression that she is in labor. The fact that it is a false labor becomes apparent only in retrospect, when the bursts of contractility have subsided and it becomes evident that the contractions are not going to progress further toward active labor. It is clinically important not to confuse these bursts of contractions with active labor and not to treat such a woman for dystocia before there has been any real evidence of true active labor.

The Braxton Hicks contractions of late pregnancy gradually become more frequent, and their presence is announced by increasing discomfort. At the very end of pregnancy, these contractions merge by slow, imperceptible degrees into the progress of clinically recognizable active labor.

The Contractions of Labor

As a general rule, labor begins with uterine contractions occurring every 15 to 20 minutes. Before labor, the contractions often appear uncoordinated or of insufficient intensity to be recognized as effective labor contractions, although there are many exceptions.

As labor approaches, large areas of the myometrium become involved in coordinated contractile activity. The question of *pacemakers,* which are specialized areas from which the contractions of labor are triggered, is not entirely settled. Ivy, Hartman, and Koff observed the laboring monkey uterus directly and found that the contractions started simultaneously in the cornual areas, spreading to involve the entire uterus. In the human

FIG. 31-35. Uterine activity in midpregnancy. (*Top*) At 21 weeks, much spontaneous regional activity is present, with intermittent superimposition of poorly coordinated contractions developing 10 to 25 mm Hg pressure. (*Middle*) At 21 weeks, in same patient as in top graph, oxytocin infused at 80 mU/minute produces only minimal increment in activity. (*Bottom*) At 26 weeks, regional activity persists. During 10-minute period shown, one well-coordinated contraction appeared, developing 35 mm Hg intrauterine pressure. In form and intensity, this Braxton Hicks contraction is indistinguishable from those frequently recorded in active spontaneous labor. (Hendricks)

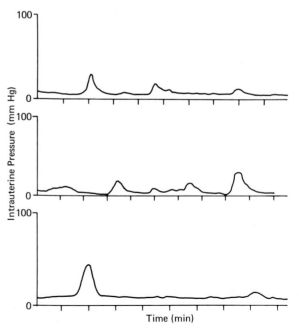

609 Physiology of Uterine Action

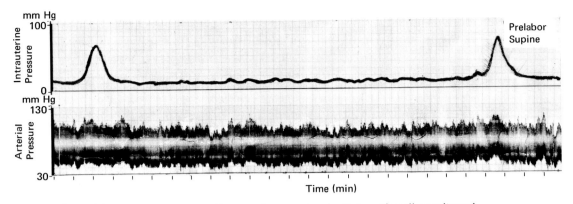

FIG. 31-36. Prelabor at term pregnancy. Note persistent regional activity with well-coordinated laborlike contractions developing more than 50 mm Hg pressure at about 20-minute intervals. (Hendricks CH: Symposium of Modern Obstetrical Practices. New York, Karger, 1970)

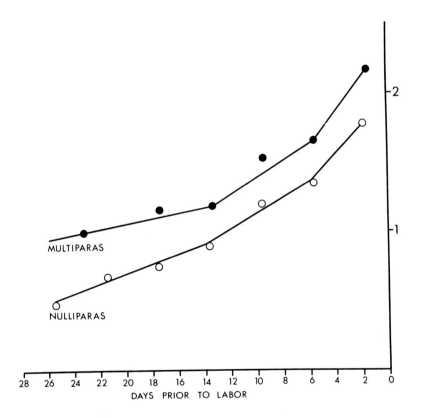

FIG. 31-37. Cervical dilatation before labor in multiparous and nulliparous women. In both, dilatation progresses steadily during last four weeks of gestation, but multipara's dilatation tends to exceed that of nullipara throughout this period. (Hendricks)

uterus, Caldeyro–Barcía found that the contractions began in one or the other cornu and only rarely on both sides simultaneously (Fig. 31-38). More recently, strain-gauge studies have demonstrated one dominant pacemaker area in the uterine fundus, the exact location of which may vary in the same patient in different labors. While the notion of a pacemaker is appropriate, it appears that, under proper conditions, each myometrial cell potentially should be capable of initiating an adequate contraction that involves the entire uterus. Fortunately the anatomic arrangement of the myometrium allows parturition to be carried out successfully whether or not there is a sharply delineated pacemaker site. Because the concentration of myometrial cells is greatest at the fundus, the probability is always greater that an effective contraction will be triggered from there rather than from the lower portion of the uterus, which is less well endowed with myometrial components. Furthermore, because of this concentration of muscular components in the fundus, the greatest contractile effort is applied at that point. Thus, as one contraction succeeds another, the lower portion of the myometrium is pulled

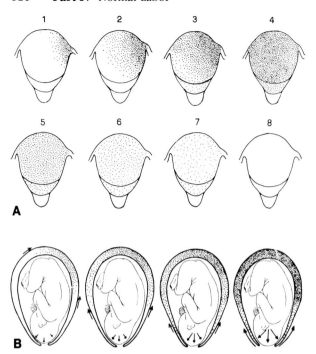

FIG. 31-38. Contractions of labor, often but not necessarily arising in one or the other cornual area, propagated evenly to involve entire musculature and, as a rule, painful. (*A*) Surface view. (*B*) Coronal section. (R Caldeyro–Barcía)

up by the overwhelmingly greater muscular component at the top of the fundus. As a result the lower portion is drawn thinner and thinner as labor progresses.

It is both desirable and inevitable that efficient contractions in normal labor exhibit fundal dominance, which implies that the contraction arises somewhere in the fundus of the uterus and spreads smoothly throughout the fundus and downward over the more caudal parts of the uterus, with the greatest force developing in the fundus. The number of these contractions required to finish labor is determined in large measure by the completeness of the prelabor changes in the lowermost portions of the uterus.

During the active phase of labor, the contractions occur at intervals of 3 to 5 minutes and the frequency may increase to as often as one contraction every two minutes during the last half of the first stage (Figs. 31-39 and 31-40). At the outset, the contractions usually average at least 300 mm Hg in intensity above the resting pressure. As labor advances, the average intensity rises to almost 50 mm Hg; in some, the intensity may reach 80 mm Hg to 100 mm Hg. The resting pressure remains within the range of 5 mm Hg to 10 mm Hg until very late in labor, when it may rise to 12 mm Hg to 14 mm Hg. Thus, as labor advances, both the frequency and the intensity of contractions increase. Even in the best labor, however, some contractions deviate significantly from the ideal frequency and intensity pattern. In abnormal labor, the pattern may be seriously disturbed in form, and the contractions can lose all ability to produce further cervical dilatation.

Various attempts have been made to express the work performed by the uterine contractions during first-stage labor. A somewhat arbitrary way of comparing the course of differing types of labors is to use the peak intensities of all contractions recorded during the first stage as a rough estimate of this work. In general, it may be observed that less uterine work is required to accomplish dilatation in multiparas than in nulliparas, and in anterior than in transverse positions (Fig. 31-41).

In order for the coordinated uterine contractions in labor to be effective, there must be even and uniform fitting of the presenting part to the lower uterine segment (possibly the nerve endings mentioned earlier are concerned). Optimal fitting occurs with the head in the occiput anterior or transverse position. When the head is in the posterior position, the fitting is less favorable, and this is one of the explanations frequently given for the clinical observation that labor with the fetal head in the posterior position may be longer than when the head is positioned anteriorly. In a transverse lie, cervical dilatation may proceed normally as long as the membranes fit neatly; when the membranes rupture, further dilatation of the cervix is likely to be impeded unless the shoulder or the breech moves down to replace the stimulus to the lower segment. In cases of disproportion at

FIG. 31-39. Intrauterine pressure changes in normal labor and in premature separation of placenta. (Caldeyro–Barcía R, Alvarez H: J Obstet Gynaecol Br Emp 59:646, 1952)

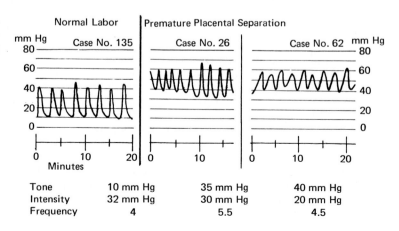

	Normal Labor	Premature Placental Separation	
	Case No. 135	Case No. 26	Case No. 62
Tone	10 mm Hg	35 mm Hg	40 mm Hg
Intensity	32 mm Hg	30 mm Hg	20 mm Hg
Frequency	4	5.5	4.5

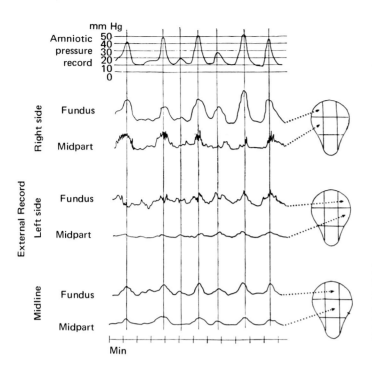

FIG. 31-40. Normal first stage of labor. Combined internal pressure recording and external recording. Note fundal dominance, especially on right side, and decreased activity toward left and middle parts of uterus. Note how external contraction patterns are reflected in internal pressure variations. (Caldeyro–Barcía R, Alvarez H: J Obstet Gynaecol Br Emp 59:646, 1952)

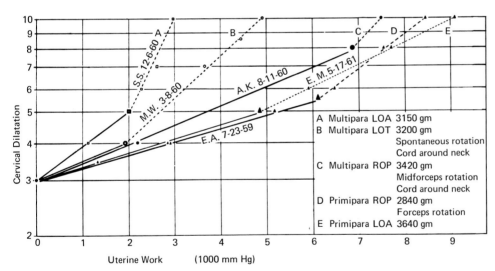

FIG. 31-41. Representation of uterine work during labor expressed as cumulative sum of intensities of contractions plotted against progress in cervical dilatation (semilog). Factors tending to reduce amount of work required to complete first stage of labor are multiparity, anterior position of fetal head, and small fetal size. Slopes of lines give good indication of relative efficiency of labor. Consistent steepening of slope of dilatation after amniotomy (*broken lines*) illustrates increased efficiency resulting from this procedure. (Cibils LA, Hendricks CH: Am J Obstet Gynecol 91:391, 1965)

the inlet, when the head is prevented from entering the pelvis and fitting properly, the stimulus also may be inadequate.

As the second stage of labor is reached, the contractions occur every 1.5 to 2 minutes and last 1 to 1.5 minutes. The intensity of second-stage contractions is about the same as that in the late first stage, but the intrauterine pressure may be raised substantially by the patient's voluntary bearing-down efforts (Fig. 31-42).

Immediately after delivery of the infant, the recorded intrauterine pressure increases dramatically, producing intrauterine and intramyometrial pressures of approximately 250 mm Hg. With delivery of the infant, the uterine content is reduced by approximately seven

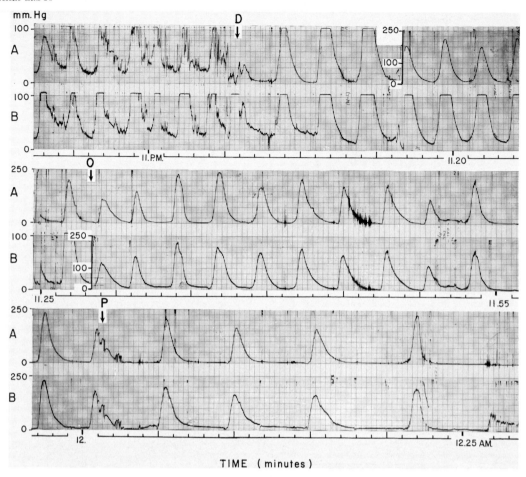

FIG. 31-42. Continuous record of uterine activity at delivery (*D*) and postpartum. (*Line A*) Intrauterine pressure. (*Line B*) Intramyometrial pressure. Record is characteristic of spontaneous uterine activity, but these particular contractions resulted from oxytocin infusion started two hours before delivery for induction of labor and stopped at point *O* on graph. Placenta, which had been visible at introitus, was delivered at point *P* by gentle traction on cord. (Hendricks CH: Uterine contractility at delivery and in the puerperium. Am J Obstet Gynecol 83:890, 1962)

eighths. The delivery of the placenta brings about another sharp reduction in intrauterine volume. Thus, the continuing activity of the same contractile mass that prior to delivery produces pressures of 70 mm Hg to 80 mm Hg, in contracting around the much smaller intrauterine volume, engenders pressures that have been recorded above 250 mm Hg. The tracings in Figures 31-33, 31-42, and 31-43 illustrate typical situations of labor, delivery, and puerperium.

EFFECTS OF DRUGS ON UTERINE CONTRACTILITY

In the discussion of the physiology of the myometrium earlier in this chapter, reference was made to several agents that affect uterine motility when they are administered. Some of these have been used clinically either to stimulate or to depress uterine activity. In addition to those used in a deliberate effort to control uterine action, there is a group of agents used for other purposes that may incidentally alter the motility of the uterus.

Oxytocics

Oxytocin

Over the years, oxytocin has produced almost as many disasters as benefits. However, if it is used properly, it is the safest and most effective pharmacologic agent for the stimulation of uterine activity. In 1909 W. Blair Bell, a pioneer in so many areas of obstetrics, was the first to employ extracts of whole posterior lobe for the clinical stimulation of uterine activity. A few years later B. P. Watson recommended its use for the induction

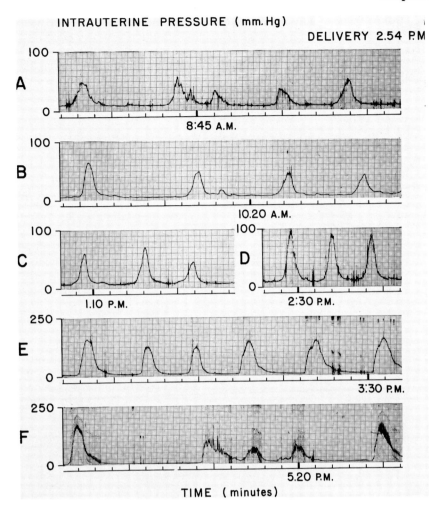

FIG. 31-43. Uterine activity as recorded through same single intrauterine catheter. (*A*) Late prelabor, 6 hours antepartum (cervix 2 cm dilated, effaced 50%, station −2). (*B*) Early labor, 5 hours antepartum. (*C*) Active labor, 2 hours antepartum (cervix 3 cm dilated, effaced 70%, station O). (*D*) Late labor, predelivery (cervix 9 cm dilated, station 0+). (*E*) Spontaneous activity 0.5 hour postpartum (note change in pressure scale). (*F*) Spontaneous activity 2.5 hours postpartum. (Hendricks CH: Uterine contractility at delivery and in the puerperium. Am J Obstet Gynecol 83:890, 1962)

of labor and in 1920 described a large series of cases in which there were no significant complications from the method. As the technique was adopted, others experienced an increasing number of uterine ruptures caused by overstimulation and, of almost equal importance, severe hypertensive responses because of the presence of vasopressin in the extracts. In 1928 Kamm and colleagues achieved the separation of oxytocin from the pressor–antidiuretic fraction of the posterior lobe. The next important advance was Theobald's recommendation that more precise control could be achieved by the intravenous administration of dilute solutions of oxytocin. Finally, in 1954, Du Vigneaud synthesized oxytocin; this was the first successful synthesis of a biologically active peptide.

The commercial preparations of oxytocin now available (Pitocin, Oxytocin, and Syntocinon) are synthetic preparations that are virtually identical, highly uniform, and standardized in similar manner. Dosage is expressed in international units (IU) or milliunits (mU). The 1-ml ampule contains 10 IU, or 10,000 mU. A single milligram of synthetic oxytocin contains approximately 435 IU.

Oxytocin is very rapidly metabolized, its biologic half-life being in the range of 3 to 4 minutes. Administered as a constant intravenous infusion, its effect on contractility becomes evident within 2 to 4 minutes and the peak effect is attained in 10 to 15 minutes. When given intramuscularly (as may be done after, but rarely before, delivery), increased contractility of the uterus is noted within 3 to 5 minutes, the peak response appears in 15 to 25 minutes, and most of the increased activity has subsided 30 to 40 minutes after the injection.

Nonpregnant and early pregnant uteri are relatively, but not absolutely, refractory to oxytocin, and large doses beyond the ordinary pharmacologic range are required to produce even a minimal response. The same relative refractoriness occurs also at midpregnancy (Figs. 31-34 and 31-35) and accounts for the ineffectiveness of oxytocin as an abortifacient. It is not useful for this purpose in the first trimester, and in the second trimester, some other agents (*e.g.,* PGs, intra-amniotic saline) are also required.

As pregnancy advances into the third trimester, the uterus becomes increasingly responsive to oxytocin (Figs. 31-1 and 31-2), and at term it is especially sensitive to extremely small doses. It is in this group of patients that oxytocin has its greatest usefulness as a uterine stimulant.

The objective of uterine stimulation at term is to produce contractions equivalent to those that occur in spontaneous labor (*i.e.,* contractions that occur every 2 to 3 minutes, last 40 to 50 seconds, and produce intrauterine pressures of 50 mm Hg to 60 mm Hg). Contractions of this kind can usually be achieved by the intravenous infusion, at a constant rate, of 1 mU to 10 mU oxytocin/minute. If this dose range is exceeded, or if the uterus is excessively responsive to lesser doses, the resting tone increases, the interval between contractions is reduced, and the contractions become much more forceful. Rupture of the uterus is the ultimate consequence. This is an obstetric disaster of the first order and causes oxytocin stimulation to be regarded as a major obstetric procedure to be used only by those who are fully informed of its action and who are willing to provide the constant observation that is essential. Accidents resulting from overstimulation caused the Food and Drug Administration (FDA) to interdict the use of oxytocin for the elective induction of labor. This action appears to be more an indictment of improper and inappropriate use than a condemnation of the drug itself. The clinical use of oxytocin for stimulation is described in Chapter 37.

Immediately postpartum, the uterus remains sensitive to oxytocin but to a somewhat lesser degree. Many physicians administer an ampule (10 IU) intramuscularly after delivery of the placenta to ensure adequate contraction of the uterus in the early puerperium. This is especially helpful in patients who receive general anesthesia for delivery, since general anesthesia tends to diminish uterine contractility and may be associated with excessive bleeding after delivery. The rapid intravenous injection of even 5 IU oxytocin postpartum is contraindicated because it may cause transient but profound hypotension.

Ergot

From an ergot alkaloid, originally obtained from a fungus growing on rye, several useful drugs have been isolated, and several have been synthesized. Ergonovine and ergometrine are identical substances synthesized almost simultaneously by American and British investigators and named by the individual workers. (Ergonovine is the American preparation.) Their use is limited to the puerperium, either immediately after delivery or for the later control of bleeding due to atony. The duration and intensity of their effects in pharmacologic doses are so great that they should never be given to an undelivered patient. In the past, impure products administered over a long period produced a serious vascular disorder called *ergotism;* this is unusual with modern preparations, however, and if it occurs at all it results from prolonged use at high dosages.

Ergonovine maleate (Ergotrate) may be given orally, intramuscularly, or if necessary, intravenously. The usual dose is 0.2 mg given orally, intramuscularly, or intravenously. This dose causes uterine contractions of high intensity; since the effect persists for hours (Fig. 31-44), this is a useful drug for maintaining good uterine contractility during the early pospartum period.

The extent of the uterine response is directly related to the dose and time of administration. This may be seen by comparing Figures 31-44 and 31-45. In the latter case, 0.015 mg (one thirteenth of the usual dose) er-

FIG. 31-44. Kymographic tracings of uterine activity following administration of ergonovine six to eight days after delivery (*A*) intravenously, (*B*) orally, and (*C*) intramuscularly. Note immediate response after intravenous administration. There is a 15- to 20-minute lag after both oral and intramuscular administration, but intramuscular response is more marked. (Davis ME, Rubin R [eds]: DeLee's Obstetrics for Nurses, 17th ed. Philadelphia, WB Saunders, 1962)

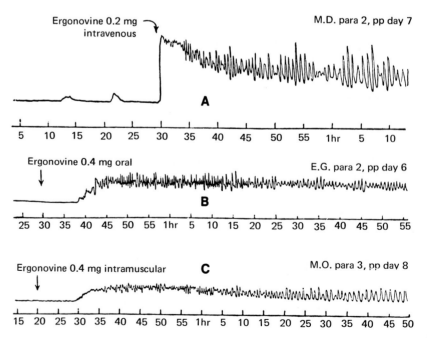

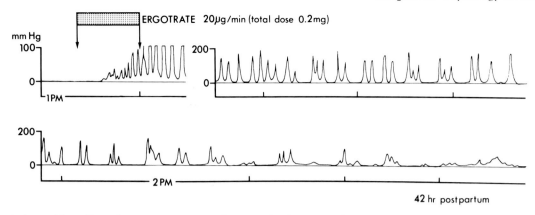

FIG. 31-45. Effect of 0.2 mg ergonovine (Ergotrate) administered intravenously by constant infusion pump over 10-minute period. Hypercontractility and transient hypertonus ensued, but no evidence of tetanic response. (Hendricks)

gonovine maleate given intravenously induces only a gentle increase in contractility in the early postpartum uterus. If the usual dose of 0.2 mg is given intravenously over a ten-minute period rather than as a bolus (Fig. 31-45), hypercontractility and mild hypertonus may be observed, but the dramatic tetanic response shown in Figure 31-44 is lacking.

Methylergonovine tartrate (Methergine) is also in wide current use as a powerful oxytocic and has similar effects on uterine contractions.

Both drugs, when administered intravenously, have been noted to induce hypertension in some patients, but methylergonovine tartrate is less likely to cause this undesirable side-effect. The likelihood that hypertension will occur with either drug is minimized by using either the intramuscular or the oral route of administration.

Prostaglandins

As noted earlier in this chapter, the effects of PGs on uterine contractility are like those of oxytocin, and their mode of action appears to be similar. Also, the uterus becomes increasingly responsive as pregnancy advances. However, the uterus is not refractory to PGs in early and middle stages of pregnancy, as it is to oxytocin, and PGs can produce evacuation of the uterus at any stage of pregnancy.

In the United States, use of these substances is limited by an edict of the FDA that limits the use of PGs to cases in which the fetus is dead or is not expected to survive; the three applicable conditions are missed abortion, induced abortion (Fig. 31-46), and intrauterine fetal death. Their use for induced abortion is discussed in Chapter 14. In countries other than the United States, PGs are widely used for the induction of labor at term and appear to have special usefulness if the cervix is "unripe." As noted elsewhere, PGs (notably the 15-methyl analog of $PGF_{2\alpha}$) are highly effective in dealing with postpartum hemorrhage caused by uterine atony. On many services they are used as second-line therapy instead of ergonovine if oxytocin fails.

Other Drugs with Oxytocic Properties

Several other drugs have oxytocic properties, but they are not indicated for purposes of stimulating uterine contractions and are best avoided in pregnancy. They

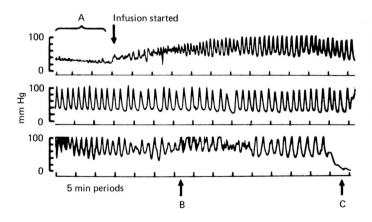

FIG. 31-46. Effect of continuous intravenous infusion of 50 μg/minute $PGF_{2\alpha}$ on pregnant uterus at 18 weeks' gestation. (A) Part of control period spontaneous activity. (B) Sitting up to pass urine. (C) Intact sac expelled. (Karim SMM, Hillier K: The role of prostaglandins in myometrial contractions. In Josimovich JB [ed]: Uterine Contraction: Side Effects of Steroidal Contraceptives. New York, John Wiley, 1973)

include dimenhydrinate (Dramamine), propanolol, norepinephrine (Levophed), and acetylcholine. Disopyramide (Norpace), a cardiac antiarrhythmic agent, appears to have special usefulness for treatment of cardiac arrhythmia in nonpregnant women. In pregnancy it may induce sustained uterine contractions, and another drug should be selected.

Drugs That Depress Uterine Contractility

The drugs that have been used clinically in an effort to terminate preterm labor are discussed in Chapter 35. They include β-mimetic catecholamines, ethanol, antiprostaglandins, calcium antagonists, and magnesium sulfate. Examples of the effects of ritodrine, ethanol, and magnesium sulfate are shown, respectively, in Figures 31-47, 31-48, and 31-49. The effect of a calcium antagonist, nifedipine, is illustrated in Figure 31-13.

Diazoxide (Hyperstat) is a nondiuretic thiazide that is used for the treatment of severe hypertensive crises. It causes immediate arteriolar dilatation and a drop in blood pressure. It also has a marked tocolytic effect, but it should not be selected as a uterine relaxant. If the drug is used in labor to treat a hypertensive crisis for which no other drug is appropriate, the uterine contractions may be expected to stop, but the other obstetric and fetal effects cannot be predicted.

Aminophylline has been reported to be an effective tocolytic agent; this effect evidently results from its ability to cause an accumulation of cAMP. The cardiovascular side-effects are sufficiently severe that its use for the deliberate arrest of uterine contractions is not acceptable.

FIG. 31-47. Effect of ritodrine in a case of preterm labor. Patient G6 P2, 32 weeks' gestation, cervix 3 cm dilated, presenting part floating. Contractions on admission characteristic of true labor, diminishing very rapidly after infusion of ritodrine (100 µg/min) started. Note slight decline in diastolic blood pressure, slight increase in pulse pressure, and definite increase in pulse rate. Patient was later discharged on oral medication and readmitted 32 days later; labor was allowed to continue, and she delivered a 2675-gram infant in good condition. (Cibils LA, Zuspan FP: Pharmacologic control of premature labor. Clin Obstet Gynecol 16:199, 1973)

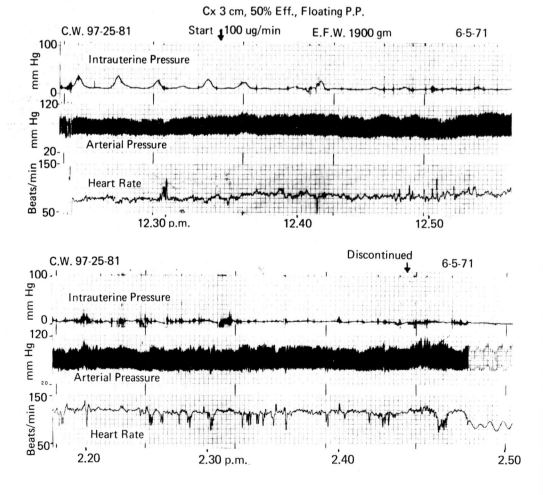

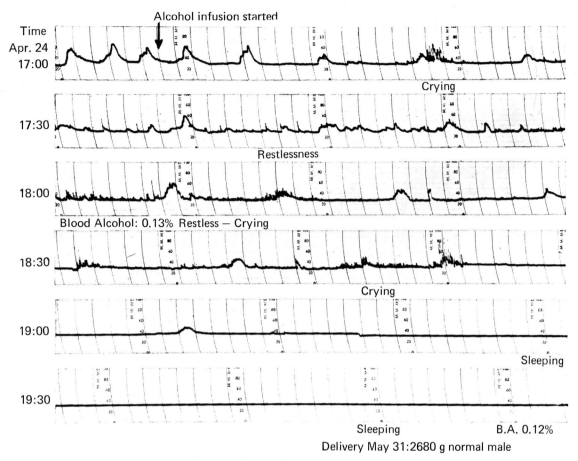

FIG. 31-48. Effect of alcohol in arresting preterm labor in patient 32 weeks' pregnant, with 2 cm cervical dilatation and intact membranes (Fuchs F: Effect of ethyl alcohol upon spontaneous uterine activity. J Obstet Gynaecol Br Commonw 72:1011, 1965)

FIG. 31-49. Effect of magnesium sulfate on uterine contractility. Oxytocin induction (5 mU/min, intravenously), membranes intact. Total of 3.9 g magnesium sulfate was given intravenously at rate of 0.5 g/minute. Note mild tachycardia (*top line*), transient depression of uterine contractility (*middle line*), moderate depression of arterial blood pressure (*bottom line*), and prompt recovery. (Hendricks CH: Clin Obstet Gynecol 9:535, 1966)

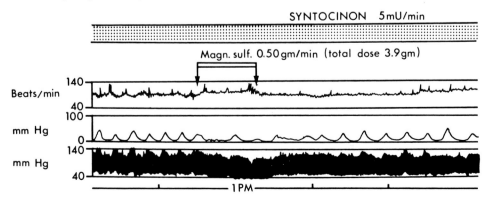

Analgesics, Sedatives, and Tranquilizers

From time to time other agents have been considered as possible suppressants of uterine activity. For many years, morphine was sometimes administered in an attempt to relax the uterus, but objective studies have demonstrated that even after large doses of morphine there is no diminution of uterine action (Fig. 31-50). Likewise, the administration of meperidine does not produce any measurable diminution in uterine contractility. To the contrary, work of Sica–Blanco and his colleagues indicates that, under certain conditions, a single intravenous dose of meperidine hydrochloride (Demerol) may initiate active labor.

As a general rule, the usual doses of analgesic, sedative, antispasmodic, and tranquilizing drugs employed in obstetric practice exert no demonstrable effect upon uterine contractility. The exceptions are aspirin and indomethacin, which are capable of blocking the synthesis of PGs. Lewis and Schulman found that a group of women who were taking large doses of acetylsalicylic acid for chronic disease tended to have longer labors and longer gestations than did control groups of women who were not taking the drug.

Anesthetics

General Anesthetics

Of the general anesthetic agents commonly used, nitrous oxide and thiopental (Pentothal) have little effect upon uterine action.

Ether and halothane (Fluothane) are capable of inducing complete uterine relaxation. Ether is a specific depressant of uterine activity; uterine activity can be rapidly abolished by halothane.

It is well to remember that in addition to complete uterine relaxation, these agents also induce a deep general anesthesia that abolishes the ability of the parturient to bear down. Likewise, deep suppression of uterine contractility may be followed by postpartum hemorrhage; this danger can be partially reduced by the appropriate use of oxytocic drugs.

FIG. 31-50. Effect on uterine activity of 8.3 mg morphine sulfate infused in 8.3 minutes. No effect is discernible on oxytocin-induced contractions characteristic of labor. (Eskes TK: Effect of morphine upon uterine contractility in late pregnancy. Am J Obstet Gynecol 84: 281, 1962)

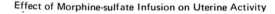
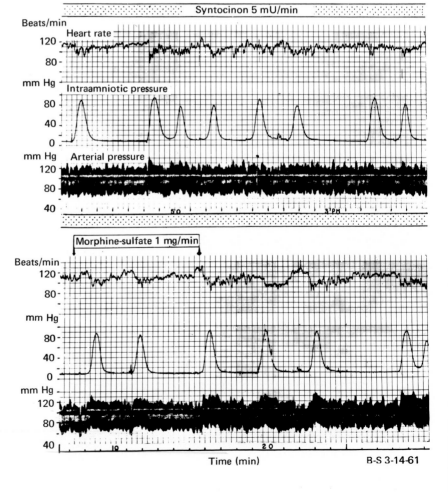

In modern obstetric practice, the need for inducing profound surgical planes of anesthesia to abolish uterine contractility occurs less often than it has in the past because practices that involve major intrauterine maneuvers are being replaced by less dramatic but safer alternative methods of management.

Regional Anesthetics

The major regional blocks commonly employed are caudal, lumbar epidural, and spinal anesthesia. Under optimal conditions, none of these is associated with a significant reduction in uterine contractility (Fig. 31-51). It has been noted that when anesthetic agents containing epinephrine are used, a mild transient depression may be observed in uterine contractility, usually lasting only about 10 minutes and not enduring beyond 30 minutes after injection. Vasicka and associates have found that spinal anesthesia is accompanied by a significant reduction in uterine contractility only when the patient is severely hypotensive.

Uterine contractility, as recorded by accurate methods of tokodynamometry, is not significantly affected by the induction of a major regional anesthetic block. Nevertheless, there is a widespread belief that the major blocks often slow the progress of labor. A number of possibilities have been suggested to explain the apparent discrepancy between the uterine contractility record and the impression that labor has slowed.

1. If the block was administered so early that the patient was not yet in active labor, the block is associated with (but not responsible for) lack of progress in cervical dilatation.
2. The contrast between the uncomfortable patient before the onset of regional anesthesia and the tranquil patient after her pain has been relieved may lead the attendants (physician or nurse–midwife) to believe that labor has been arrested.
3. In the second stage, progress may be slowed because the patient does not feel the need to push (as occurs in all major blocks) or cannot cooperate by pushing when directed to do so (as with spinal block).
4. Vaginal examination of the newly relaxed patient just after initiation of a block sometimes results in the head being pushed to a somewhat higher level. This may disturb the finely balanced adaptation between head and cervix, making the uterine contractions less

effective, even though the contractions recorded on the tracing continue and are not altered in appearance. The fetal head is particularly likely to rise to a higher position in the pelvis if the mother's legs are elevated to counteract a sudden drop in blood pressure.

5. Epinephrine administered with the blocking agent, or the release of epinephrine because of the stress of the procedure, may bring about mild reductions in uterine contractility. Such reductions may be too minor to be evident on examination of the tracing.
6. Severe hypotension, such as may occur in conduction anesthesia, actually does reduce uterine contractility.

THE PAIN OF LABOR

Pain is likely to be most intense during the latter part of the first stage of labor, less so during the second stage, and virtually absent during and after the third stage.

The pain associated with labor has never been well explained; but, since it is clearly related to the occurrence of the uterine contractions, the words *contraction* and *pain* have come to be synonymous. The sense of pain generally begins before the height of a contraction. Pain is usually perceived at an intrauterine pressure of about 25 mm Hg, but this is not always the case; painful contractions have been noted at much lower intensity and painless ones at much higher. In the beginning of the first stage, the contractions last 15 to 30 seconds. As they become more intense and longer, the pain increases. In most normal labors, the distress is felt in the suprapubic areas and laterally, both sides equally, for 6 cm to 8 cm from the midline. Backache occurs most commonly in labors in which dilatation of the cervix is not proportional to the strength of the contractions; the presence of backache with the contractions suggests faulty dilatation of the cervix or improper fitting of the presenting part to the lower pole of the uterus, as may occur in certain malpositions (*e.g.,* occiput posterior) or malpresentations (*e.g.,* in certain cases of breech). Pain referred from the back down the legs is explained by similar causes.

When the cervix becomes fully dilated, a reflex is produced that causes the parturient to make a voluntary effort to expel the baby by bearing down. A trained observer can often recognize the onset of the second stage by the grunting sound made by the patient at this junc-

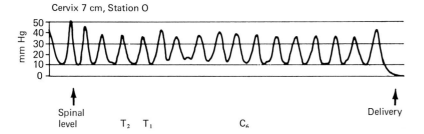

FIG. 31-51. Effect of administration of high spinal block in late labor on uterine contractility pattern. No significant effect is noted. (Bonica JJ: Principles and Practice of Obstetric Analgesia and Anesthesia. Philadelphia, FA Davis, 1972. After Vasicka A, Kretchmer H: Am J Obstet Gynecol 82:600, 1961)

ture in labor. (In the anesthetized postpartum dog, and probably other animals as well, the sudden distention of the cervix by a balloon causes the characteristic grunting, bearing-down effort.) It is reported that the more vigorous the bearing-down efforts, the less the discomfort of the contractions. Whether this is true or whether the patient is distracted by the fact that she may now actually participate is a moot question. As the presenting part approaches the pelvic floor, a new distress occurs as a result of the pressure and often the actual tearing of these tissues as they are increasingly distended.

In discussing the pain of labor, note must be made of the marked variation among patients. A patient's reaction to labor cannot be predicted from her evident emotional patterns before labor; the most stoic may disintegrate emotionally, and the most apprehensive may labor with equanimity. Psychologic factors (confidence in the attendants, attitude toward the baby, proximity of relatives) are clearly concerned.

It is curious that an adequate explanation of the mechanism that produces the uterine pain has not been offered. Uterine ischemia during contractions has been suggested; since the intrauterine pressure in certain painless Braxton Hicks contractions has been recorded as exceeding 100 mm Hg, however, this explanation leaves something to be desired. Moreover, contractions of the third stage and immediately after delivery may produce pressures of 250 mm Hg to 300 mm Hg, but they are not painful. Additional causes of pain in labor may be stretching of the cervix; traction upon the peritoneum, adnexa, and supporting ligaments; distention of the soft parts before the advancing head; and pressure upon the urethra and bladder. All may contribute, and it is emphasized that the uterus is not necessarily the only source of the pain of labor.

A multiplicity of nerve endings in the lower pole of the uterus just superior to the cervix has been described. They appear to be receptor structures. Since they are limited to this part of the uterus, it is possible that the stimulation of these nerve endings is responsible for the pain of labor as the lower pole of the uterus dilates before the presenting part. The fact that labor pain is often relieved by local anesthesia applied to the uterosacral ligaments, to the paracervical structures, or to the area of the pudendal nerve is not helpful in explaining its causation.

CHANGES IN THE CERVIX IN PREGNANCY AND LABOR

The function of the cervix is to retain the conceptus until the uterus is prepared to evacuate its contents. Figure 31-17 shows the manner in which this function is carried out, and emphasizes also that the cervix is not called upon to resist the stress of uterine distention until about the 16th week of pregnancy. Late abortion is a predictable consequence if the cervix is sufficiently

damaged, as by deep laceration or conization; if it is congenitally abnormal, as the so-called muscular cervix or the cervix sufficiently affected by intrauterine exposure to diethylstilbestrol (DES); or if it should soften sufficiently and dilate prematurely in the middle trimester.

Physical Changes

In the cervix, the physical changes caused by pregnancy are well known, since this structure has been a focal point for all who are concerned with the conduct of pregnancy and labor.

One of the early signs of pregnancy is softening of the cervix, *Goodell's sign,* which is evident first at about five to six weeks' gestation and remains without significant change until the beginning of preparations for labor a month or so before term. This sign is probably due largely to the vascular changes characteristic of pregnancy; edema may be concerned to an extent, but the actual accumulation of water is negligible and is not sufficient to account for Goodell's sign. In addition, duskiness (cyanosis) of the cervix can be noted very early in pregnancy (*Chadwick's sign*). It is due to the increased vascularity and becomes more marked as pregnancy advances; at term, the cervix is usually light to deep purple in color.

The endocervix reacts to pregnancy by marked proliferation of the endocervical glands, which produce a tenacious mucus that acts to seal the cervical canal by the so-called mucous plug of pregnancy. The mucous plug ordinarily remains in place, especially in a primigravida, until early labor, when it may be extruded from the vagina almost intact as a blob of mucus to which a few cells of the endocervix may adhere.

Although there are no changes in the squamous epithelium of the portio vaginalis that are diagnostic of pregnancy, certain findings are present more often in the pregnant than in the nonpregnant woman. They include a higher percentage of mitotic figures in the basilar zone, a higher percentage of large so-called active nuclei in the midzone, an increased submucosal infiltration with lymphocytes and plasma cells, and the occasional presence of atypical mitotic figures, especially near the squamocolumnar junction. If present in marked degree, the normal pregnancy changes may resemble carcinoma *in situ.* During pregnancy the squamocolumnar junction migrates toward and sometimes into the cervical canal, causing this area to be less accessible to colposcopic examination.

Cervical Effacement and Dilatation

Although the cervix is slightly softened to the touch, it remains thick, rigid, and closed until a few weeks before term, and the cervical canal maintains its nonpregnant length of 2 cm to 3 cm. Several weeks before the onset of labor, the cervix begins to unfold from above downward (Fig. 31-52) and to become perceptibly softer. This change is referred to as *effacement*. As effacement begins, the cervix also dilates slightly so that it becomes possible to introduce a finger into the cervical canal without resistance. When labor starts, the cervix is usually soft and mushy; about half of the canal has been taken up; and the external os is dilated to the extent of about 2 cm or more (Fig. 31-53).

As the contractions of labor become established, further shortening occurs and the cervix becomes thin-

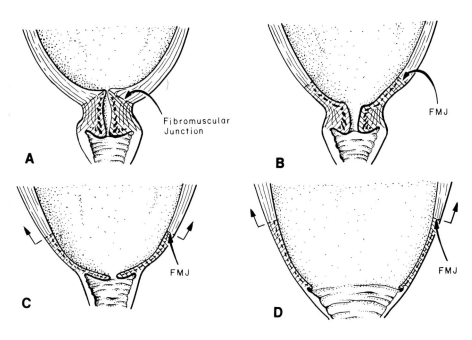

A Fibromuscular Junction

B FMJ

C FMJ

D FMJ

FIG. 31-52. Effacement and dilatation of cervix in primigravida. (*A, B*) Cervical shortening generally occurs first, and (*B, C*) is followed by progressive thinning and dilatation. In multipara, there is no consistent pattern, although dilatation is often well established before there is notable effacement.

FIG. 31-53. Mean cervical dilatation by parity in patients without signs of gross dysfunctional labor in prelabor and active labor. *Dashed lines* are extrapolation of best fitting line drawn back from means of active labor to point of intersection with extrapolation of best fitting line of known means of prelabor. Time zero is time of admittance to hospital. (Hendricks CH, Brenner WE, Kraus G: The normal cervical dilatation pattern in late pregnancy and labor. Am J Obstet Gynecol 106:1065, 1970)

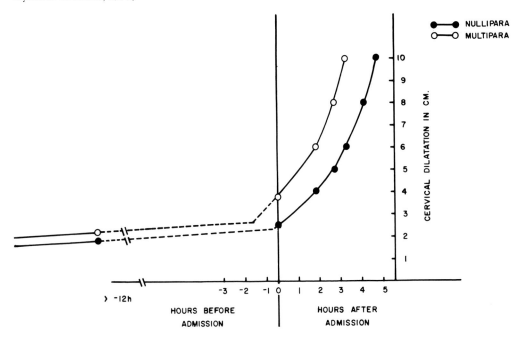

●——● NULLIPARA
○——○ MULTIPARA

CERVICAL DILATATION IN CM.

HOURS BEFORE ADMISSION   HOURS AFTER ADMISSION

⟩ -12h   -3 -2 -1 0   1   2   3   4   5

ner, but it cannot be forcibly dilated without injury. As a rule, when labor is well established, effacement proceeds rapidly, and at 6 cm to 7 cm dilatation the cervical thinning and softening are complete. When effacement is complete, the cervix is said to be "negotiable," that is, it can usually be dilated manually without significant injury. Within a month after delivery, the cervix is restored to its former rigid, undilatable state.

It is to be noted that the cervix is fundamentally a fibrous connective tissue structure. The myometrium ends at the cervix and inserts into it much as a skeletal muscle inserts into an aponeurosis. Hence, the brachystatic contractions of labor pull the cervix upward about the presenting part as labor advances. However, the mechanical traction of labor contractions can produce full dilatation of the cervix only when effacement is complete. Indeed, cases have been recorded in which the effacement mechanisms have failed, and the force of labor contractions has resulted in annular detachment of the undilated cervix. Also, in many induced late abortions, the cervix is not prepared to dilate, and posterior cervical ruptures result.

Contrast stains show that the nonpregnant cervix is composed predominantly of tight bundles of collagen fibers. A few muscle cells are irregularly scattered at random, and, at the periphery of the cervix, there is a thin layer of attenuated smooth muscle that is contin-uous with the smooth muscle of the vaginal vault. With these inconsequential exceptions, the cervix is fibrous connective tissue. Reticulum fibers are present in predictable quantity. Elastin has been found in the cervix, and elastic fibers are sparsely scattered. In the cervix at the time of full dilatation, the collagen bundles are seen to be loosely and widely scattered and very sparse (Fig. 31-54).

The question of whether upward traction on the cervix in labor may be necessary for cervical softening appears to have been settled by the study of Ledger and colleagues. In these studies in sheep, the cervix was physically separated from the corpus, and cervical softening during labor occurred in the absence of any direct mechanical or local vascular connection between cervix and corpus.

Biochemical Changes

There is ample evidence to support the theory that the physiological changes in cervical resistance and morphology are determined by the status of the connective tissue framework. The collagen concentration, as determined by hydroxyproline analysis, is about 85% in the nonpregnant cervix; in pregnancy at ten weeks this concentration is reduced to 70%, and at term the collagen content is only 30% (see Fig. 31-55). The collagen

FIG. 31-54. Photomicrograph of tissue from posterior lip of cervix, approximately 1 cm above plane of external os. (*A*) Nonpregnant. (*B*) Immediately postpartum. These changes were originally attributed to edema and dispersion of collagen fibers, but they are now known to be largely due to actual destruction of collagen and accumulation of glycosaminoglycans. (Milligan's trichrome stain for collagen, ×835) (Danforth DN, Buckingham JC, Roddick JW Jr.: Connective tissue changes incident to cervical effacement. Am J Obstet Gynecol 80:939, 1960)

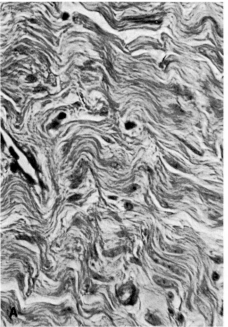
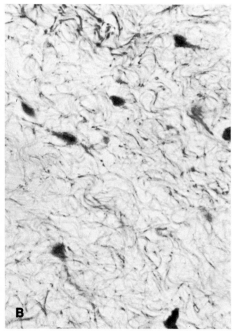

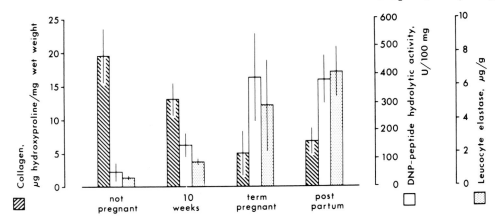

FIG. 31-55. Hydroxyproline (collagen), DNP peptide hydrolytic activity (collagenase), and leukocyte elastase concentration in the lower part of the human uterine cervix in nonpregnant women of fertile age, in pregnant women, and immediately postpartum. The *vertical bars* represent 1 SD limit. (Uldbjerg N, Ekman G, Malmström A et al: Am J Obstet Gynecol 147:662, 1983. Reproduced with permission of CV Mosby)

loss appears to result from the destruction of collagen by the increasing quantities of collagenase. Moreover, the degree of compliance appears to be a function of the collagen content. Uldbjerg and colleagues found that the time required for cervical dilatation was long in women with high concentrations of cervical collagen and short in women with low concentrations.

Huszar and Naftolin have reviewed the biochemical changes leading to ripening of the cervix and found that before pregnancy the collagen fibers are tightly bound by the glycosaminoglycans and dermatan and chondroitin sulfates, ensuring that the cervix remains securely closed. As one or more of the factors leading to the onset of labor appear, the cervix also responds by breaking down collagen and dermatan and chondroitin sulfates, and an increase in water and hyaluronic acid results. These changes lead to cervical softening and rapidly increasing compliance.

The Role of Prostaglandins

The mechanism by which PGs could cause the changes of effacement and dilatation is yet to be determined. The explanation will undoubtedly come through greater understanding of the connective-tissue degradation and remodeling processes that are responsible for the marked morphologic changes. It seems clear that collagenases and proteases will be involved, and preliminary data suggest that, like so many other phenomena of pregnancy, the effects of estrogens and progesterone will be shown to be part of the process.

The details of the remarkable phenomenon of cervical ripening are discussed in both the Liggins review and the Naftolin–Stubblefield symposium. The interested reader is referred to these sources.

Liggins has observed that no hypothesis for the initiation of human labor is complete unless it includes a satisfactory explanation of the structural changes in the cervix. He has reviewed the current status of this question; in addition, Naftolin and Stubblefield devoted a symposium to an exploration of the physiology of cervical dilatation. As noted earlier in this chapter, there is evidence that the arachidonic acid released from disturbed lysosomes in the fetal membranes is the source of substantial quantities of PGs, which are synthesized by the decidua. Although the evidence is indirect, PGs appear to play a key role in the initiation of labor. It is now apparent that these same substances can also cause effacement of the cervix (a process also known as *cervical ripening* or *compliance*). There is no direct evidence that endogenous PGs are physiologically responsible for cervical ripening, but the circumstantial evidence is impressive. PGs administered intravenously or applied locally in the form of a viscous vagnal gel suppository cause significant cervical softening. They have also been shown to be especially useful in producing cervical ripening prior to induced late abortion or induction of labor when the condition of the cervix is unfavorable. When applied *in vitro,* they greatly increase the stretch modulus of the cervix. Moreover, Ekman and colleagues have shown that in women with an "unfavorable," (noncompliant) cervix, the intracervical application of PGE_2 results in a significant decline in collagen concentration. This, plus other indirect evidence cited earlier in this chapter, suggests the possibility that the local release of PGs could be the trigger that leads to cervical effacement. Local release of PGs could also explain the efficacy of laminaria in producing effacement, and the severe uterine cramps and ultimate effacement, and dilatation of the cervix as a predunculated submucous fibroid moves through the lower pole of the uterus.

REFERENCES AND RECOMMENDED READING

Cause of the Onset of Labor

General

Bottari S, Thomas JP, Vokaer A et al (eds): Uterine Contractility. New York, Masson Publishing USA, Inc, 1984

Chard T: The human fetal hypothalamus-pituitary in the initiation of labour. In Bottari S, Thomas JP, Vokaer A et al (eds): Uterine Contractility. New York, Masson Publishing USA, Inc, 1984

Creasy RK, Liggins GC: Aetiology and management of preterm labour. In Stallworthy J, Bourne G (eds): Recent Advances in Obstetrics and Gynaecology, Vol 13, Chap 2. Edinburgh, Churchill Livingstone, 1979

Csapo AI: The regulatory interplay of progesterone and prostaglandin $F_{2\alpha}$ in the control of the pregnant uterus. In Josimovich JB (ed): Uterine Contraction—Side Effects of Steroidal Contraceptives, Chap 15, p 251. New York, John Wiley, 1973

Csapo AI: The "see–saw" theory of the regulatory mechanism of pregnancy. Am J Obstet Gynecol 121:578, 1975

Csapo AI: The uterus: Model experiments and clinical trials. In Bourne GH (ed): The Structure and Function of Muscle, 2nd ed, Vol II, p 17. New York, Academic Press, 1973

Fuchs AR, Fuchs F: Endocrinology of human parturition. Brit J Obstet Gynaecol 91:948, 1984

Liggins GC, Forster CS, Grieves SA et al: Control of parturition in man. Biol Reprod 16:39, 1977

Liggins GC: Initiation of parturition. Br Med Bull 35:145, 1979

Liggins GC: What factors initiate human labor? Contemp Ob/Gyn 13:147, 1979

Reynolds SRM: Physiology of the Uterus, 2nd ed. New York, Hoeber, 1949. Reprint: New York, Hafner, 1965

Ryan KJ: Maintenance of pregnancy and the initiation of labor. In Tulchinsky D, Ryan KJ (eds): Maternal–Fetal Endocrinology, Chap 16, Philadelphia, WB Saunders, 1980

Effects of Distention and Stretch

Csapo AI, Jaffin H, Kerenyi T et al: Volume and activity of the pregnant human uterus. Am J Obstet Gynecol 85:819, 1963

Effects of Estrogens and Progesterone

Boroditsky RS, Reyes FI, Winter JDS et al: Maternal serum estrogen and progesterone concentrations preceding labor. Obstet Gynecol 51:686, 1978

Csapo AI: Progesterone block. Am J Anat 98:273, 1956

Csapo AI, Pohanka O, Kaihola HL: Progeterone deficiency and premature labor. Br Med J 1:137, 1974

Csapo AI, Resch BA: Induction of preterm labor in the rat by antiprogesterone. Am J Obstet Gynecol 134:823, 1979

Danforth DN: Cervical incompetency. In Davis CH, Carter AB (eds): Obstetrics and Gynecology. Chap 10-A. Hagerstown, WA Prior, 1962

Danforth DN, Buckingham JC: Cervical incompetence—A reevaluation. Postgrad Med 32:4, 1962

Demianczuk N, Towell ME, Garfield RE: Myometrial electrophysiologic activity and gap junctions in the pregnant rabbit. Am J Obstet Gynecol 149:485, 1984

Garfield RE: Myometrial ultrastructure and uterine contractility. In Bottari S, Thomas JP, Vokaer A et al: Uterine Contractility. New York, Masson Publishing USA, Inc, 1984

Haning RV Jr., Barrett DA, Alberino SP et al: Interrelationships between maternal and cord prolactin, progesterone, estradiol, 13,14-dihydro-15-keto-prostaglandin $F_{2\alpha}$ and cord cortisol at delivery with respect to initiation of parturition. Am J Obstet Gynecol 130:204, 1978

Johnson JWC, Austin KL, Jones GS et al: Efficacy of 17 α-hydroxyprogesterone caproate in the prevention of premature labor. N Engl J Med 293:675, 1975

Johnson JWC, Lee PA, Zachary AS et al: High-risk prematurity—Progestin treatment and steroid studies. Obstet Gynecol 54:412, 1979

Kauppila A, Kivela A, Kontula K et al: Serum progesterone, estradiol, and estriol before and during induced labor. Am J Obstet Gynecol 137:462, 1980

Mathur RS, Landgrebe S, Williamson HO: Progesterone, 17α-hydroxyprogesterone, estradiol, and estriol in late pregnancy and labor. Am J Obstet Gynecol 136:25, 1980

Mitchell MD, Flint APF: Progesterone withdrawal: Effects on prostaglandins and parturition. Prostaglandins 14:611, 1977

Saito Y, Sakamoto H, MacLusky NJ et al: Gap junctions and myometrial steroid hormone receptors in pregnant and postpartum rats: A possible cellular basis for the progesterone withdrawal hypothesis. Am J Obstet Gynecol 151:805, 1985

Verhoeff A, Garfield RE, Ramondt J et al: Electrical and mechanical uterine activity and gap junctions in prepartal sheep. Am J Obstet Gynecol 153:447, 1985

Effects of Prostaglandins

Brenner WE, Hendricks CH, Braaksma JT et al: Intraamniotic administration of prostaglandin $F_{2\alpha}$ to induce therapeutic abortion. A. Efficacy and tolerance of two dosage schedules. Am J Obstet Gynecol 114:781, 1972

Brennecke SP, Castle BM, Demers LM et al: Maternal plasma prostaglandin E_2 levels during human pregnancy and parturition. Brit J Obstet Gynaecol 92:345, 1985

Bruce SL, Paul RH, Van Dorsten JP: Control of postpartum uterine atony by intramyometrial prostaglandin. Obstet Gynecol (Suppl)59:475, 1982

Challis JRG: Physiology and pharmacology of PGs in parturition. Prostaglandins, Series G, pp 47ff, 1974

Dubin NH, Johnson JWC, Calhoun S et al: Plasma prostaglandin in pregnant women with term and preterm deliveries. Obstet Gynecol 57:203, 1981

Keirse MJNC, Hicks BR, Mitchell MD et al: Increase of the prostaglandin precursor, arachidonic acid, in amniotic fluid during spontaneous labour. Br J Obstet Gynaecol 84:937, 1977

Kirton KT: Biochemical effects of prostaglandins as they might relate to uterine contraction. In Josimovich JB (ed): Uterine Contraction—Side Effects of Steroidal Contraceptives, Chap 12, p 193. New York, John Wiley, 1973

Kurzrok R, Lieb D: Biochemical studies of human semen: Action of semen on human uterus. Proc Soc Exp Biol Med 28:268, 1930

Lackritz R, Tulchinsky D, Ryan KJ et al: Plasma prostaglandin metabolites in human labor. Am J Obstet Gynecol 131:484, 1978

Liggins GC, Campos GA, Roberts CM: Production rates of prostaglandin F, 6-keto-$PGF_{1\alpha}$ and thromboxane B_2 by perfused human endometrium. Prostaglandins, 19:461, 1980

MacDonald PC, Schultz M, Duenhoelter J et al: Initiation of

human parturition: I. Mechanism of action of arachidonic acid. Obstet Gynecol 44:829, 1974

Mitchell MD, Flint AFP, Bibby J et al: Rapid increases in prostaglandin concentrations after vaginal examination and amniotomy. Br Med J 2:1183, 1977

Mitchell MD, Flint AFP, Turnbull AC: Increasing uterine response to vaginal distension in sheep. J Reprod Fertil 49: 35, 1977

Mitchell MD, Flint AFP, Turnbull AC: Stimulation by oxytocin of prostaglandin F levels in uterine venous affluent in pregnant and puerperal sheep. Prostaglandins 9:47, 1975

Novy MJ, Cook MJ, Manaugh L: Indomethacin block of normal onset of parturition in primates. Am J Obstet Gynecol 118:412, 1974

Novy MJ, Liggins CG: Role of prostaglandins, prostacyclin, and thromboxane in the physiologic control of the uterus in parturition. Semin Perinatol 4:45, 1980

Satoh K, Yasumizu T, Fukuoka H et al: Prostaglandin $F_{2\alpha}$ metabolite levels in plasma, amniotic fluid, and urine during pregnancy and labor. Am J Obstet Gynecol 133:886, 1979

Schulman H, Saldana L, Lin C-C et al: Mechanism of failed labor after fetal death and its treatment with prostaglandin E_2. Am J Obstet Gynecol 133:742, 1979

Toppozada M, El-Bossaty M, El-Rahmen HA et al: Control of intractable atonic postpartum hemorrhage by 15-methyl prostaglandin $F_{2\alpha}$. Obstet Gynecol 58:327, 1981

Zuckerman H, Reiss U, Atad J et al: Prostaglandin $F_{2\alpha}$ in human blood during labor. Obstet Gynecol 51:311, 1978

Contractile System of the Myometrium

Perry SV, Grand RJA: Mechanisms of contraction and the specialized protein components of smooth muscle. Br Med Bull 35:219, 1979

Effects of Mineral Ions

Anderson NC Jr.: Physiologic basis of myometrial function. Semin Perinatol 2:211, 1978

Andersson K-E: Inhibition of uterine activity by the calcium antagonist nifedipine. In Anderson A, Beard R, Brudenell JM et al (eds): Pre-term Labour. Proceedings of the 5th Study Group of the Royal College of Obstetricians and Gynaecologists, London, 1977

Andersson K-E, Ingemarsson I, Ulmsten U et al: Inhibition of prostaglandin-induced uterine activity by nifedipine. Br J Obstet Gynaecol 86:175, 1979

Bell WB, Hick P: Observations on the physiology of the female genital organs. Br Med J, March 27, 1909

Carsten ME: Calcium accumulation by human uterine microsomal preparation: Effects of progesterone and oxytocin. Am J Obstet Gynecol 133:598, 1978

Carsten ME: Hormonal regulation of myometrial calcium transport. Gynecol Invest 5:269, 1974

Carsten ME: How does calcium control uterine contraction? Contemp Ob/Gyn 8:61, 1976

Carsten ME: Prostaglandins and cellular calcium transport in the pregnant human uterus. Am J Obstet Gynecol 117: 824, 1973

Carsten ME: Prostaglandins and oxytocin: Their effects on uterine smooth muscle. Prostaglandins 5:33, 1974

Carsten ME: Regulation of myometrial composition, growth, and activity. In Assali NS (ed): Biology of Gestation, Vol I, p 393. New York, Academic Press, 1968

Carsten ME: Sarcoplasmic reticulum from pregnant bovine uterus: Calcium binding. Gynecol Invest 4:84, 1973

Carsten ME: Sarcoplasmic reticulum from pregnant bovine uterus: Prostaglandins and calcium. Gynecol Invest 4:95, 1973

Carsten ME, Miller JD: Involvement of cyclic AMP in calcium accumulation by uterine sarcoplasmic reticulum. Abstracts of the 1980 meeting of the Society for Gynecologic Investigation, p 86

Danforth DN, Ivy AC: A consideration of the cause of the onset of labor. Int Abstr Surg (Surg Gynecol Obstet) 69:351, 1939

Danforth DN, Ivy AC: Effect of calcium on uterine activity and reactivity. Proc Soc Exp Biol Med 38:550, 1938

Danforth DN, Ivy AC: Effect of calcium on uterine contractions and on uterine response to intravenously injected oxytocics. Am J Obstet Gynecol 37:184, 1939

Fleckenstein A: Specific pharmacology of calcium in myocardium, cardiac pacemakers, and vascular smooth muscle. Annu Rev Pharmacol Toxicol 17:149, 1977

Huszar G: Cellular basis for new approaches to tocolytic therapy. In Bottari S, Thomas JP, Vokaer A et al (eds): Uterine Contractility. New York, Masson Publishing USA, Inc, 1984

Liggins GC: Initiation of parturition. Br Med Bull 35:145, 1979

Liggins GC, Forster CS, Grieves SA et al: Control of parturition in man. Biol Reprod 16:39, 1977

Marx JL: Calmodulin: A protein for all seasons. Science 208: 274, 1980

Perry SV, Grand RJA: Mechanisms of contraction and the specialized protein components of smooth muscle. Br Med Bull 35:219, 1979

Rasmussen H: Cell communication: Calcium ion and cyclic adenosine monophosphate. Science 170:404, 1970

Rasmussen H: Ions as "second messengers." Hosp Pract 9:99, 1974

Rasmussen H, Goodman DBP, Tenehouse A: The role of cyclic AMP and calcium in cell activation. CRC Crit Rev Biochem 1:95, 1972

Ulmsten U, Andersson K-E, Forman A: Relaxing effects of nifedipine on the nonpregnant uterus in vitro and in vivo. Obstet Gynecol 52:436, 1978

Watterson JG, Schaub MC, Büchi K: Control of the contractile process in uterus smooth muscle. In Bottari S, Thomas JP, Vokaer A et al (eds): Uterine Contractility. New York, Masson Publishing USA, Inc, 1984

Effects of Nervous Mechanisms

Daniel EE, Lodge S: Electrophysiology of the myometrium. In Josimovich JB (ed): Uterine Contraction—Side Effects of Steroidal Contraceptives, p 19. New York, John Wiley, 1973

Moawad AH: The sympathetic nervous system and the uterus. In Josimovich JB (ed): Uterine Contraction—Side Effects of Steroidal Contraceptives, Chap 4, p 71. New York, John Wiley, 1973

Thorbert G, Alm P, Bjorklund AB et al: Adrenergic innervation of the human uterus: Disappearance of the transmitter and transmitter-forming enzymes during pregnancy. Am J Obstet Gynecol 135:223, 1979

Tsuei JJ, Lai Y-F, Sharma SD: The influence of acupuncture stimulation during pregnancy: The induction and inhibition of labor. Obstet Gynecol 50:479, 1977

Effects of Catecholamines

Cibils L, Pose S, Zuspan F: Effect of 1-norepinephrine infusion on uterine contractility and cardiovascular system. Am J Obstet Gynecol 84:307, 1962

Krall JF: Molecular basis of drug action on uterine smooth muscle. In Anderson A, Beard R, Brudenell JM et al (eds): Preterm Labour. Proceedings of the 5th Study Group of the Royal College of Obstetricians and Gynaecologists, London, 1977

Kroeger EA, Marshall JM: Beta-adrenergic effects on rat myometrium: Role of cAMP. Am J Physiol 226:1298, 1974

Lederman RP, Lederman E, Work BA Jr. et al: The relationship of maternal anxiety, plasma catecholamines, and plasma cortisol to progress in labor. Am J Obstet Gynecol 132:495, 1978

Phillippe M, Ryan KJ: Catecholamines in human amniotic fluid. Am J Obstet Gynecol 139:204, 1981

Pose SV, Cibils L, Zuspan F: Effect of 1-epinephrine infusion on uterine contractility and cardiovascular system. Am J Obstet Gynecol 84:297, 1962

Effects of Fetus and Fetal Membranes

Bjorkhem I, Lantto O, Lunell N-O: Total and free cortisol in amniotic fluid during late pregnancy. Br J Obstet Gynaecol 85:446, 1978

Cawson MJ, Anderson ABM, Turnbull AC et al: Cortisol, cortisone, and 11-deoxycortisol levels in human umbilical maternal plasma in relation to the onset of labor. J Obstet Gynaecol Br Commonw 81:737, 1974

Gustavii B: Release of lysosomal acid phosphatase into the cytoplasm of decidual cells before the onset of labor in humans. Br J Obstet Gynaecol 82:177, 1975

Gustavii B: Studies on the mode of action of intra-amniotically and extra-amniotically injected hypertonic saline in therapeutic abortion. Acta Obstet Gynecol Scan (Suppl)25:5, 1973

Haukkamaa M, Lahteenmaki P: Steroids of human myometrium and maternal and umbilical cord plasma before and during labor. Obstet Gynecol 53:617, 1979

Katz Z, Lancet M, Levavi E: The efficacy of intraamniotic steroids for induction of labor. Obstet Gynecol 54:31, 1979

Kauppila A, Koivisto M, Pukka M et al: Umbilical cord and neonatal cortisol levels: Effects of gestational and neonatal factors. Obstet Gynecol 52:666, 1978

Kennaway DJ, Matthews CD, Seamark RF et al: J Steroid Biochem 8:559, 1977

Liggins GC: Fetal influences on myometrial contractility. Clin Obstet Gynecol 16:148, 1973

Liggins GC: Fetal influences on uterine contractility. In Josimovich JB (ed): Uterine Contraction: Side Effects of Steroidal Contraceptives, Chap 13, p 208. New York, John Wiley, 1973

Mitchell MD, Sayers L, Heirse MJNC et al: Melatonin in amniotic fluid during human parturition. Br J Obstet Gynaecol 85:684, 1978

Okazaki T, Casey ML, MacDonald PC et al: Prostaglandin biosynthesis and degradation in human fetal membranes and uterine decidua vera. Abstracts of the 1980 meeting of the Society for Gynecologic Investigation, p 22

Page EW: The fetus as a factor in the initiation of labor. In Marshall JM (ed): Initiation of Labor, p 167. Public Health Publication 1390. Bethesda, MD, National Institue of Child Health and Human Development, Department of Health, Education and Welfare, 1963

Phillippe M, Ryan KJ: Catecholamines in human amniotic fluid. Am J Obstet Gynecol 139:204, 1981

Roopnarinesingh S, Alexis D, Lendore R et al: Fetal steroid levels at delivery. Obstet Gynecol 50:442, 1977

Schwarz BE, MacDonald PC, Johnston JM: Initiation of human parturition: XI. Lysosomal enzyme release in vitro from amnions obtained from laboring and nonlaboring women. Am J Obstet Gynecol 137:21, 1980

Effects of Oxytocin

Bell WB: Infundibulin in primary uterine inertia and in the induction of labour. Proc R Soc Med 8:71, 1915

Bell WB: The pituitary body: Therapeutic value of the infundibular extract in shock, uterine atony, and intestinal paresis. Br Med J 1609, 1909

Caldeyro–Barcía R, Heller H (eds): Oxytocin. New York, Pergamon Press, 1962

Caldeyro–Barcía R, Sica–Blanco Y, Poseiro JJ et al: A quantitative study of the action of synthetic oxytocin on the pregnant human uterus. J Pharmacol Exp Ther 121:128, 1957

Chard T, Boyd NRH, Fosling AS et al: The development of a radioimmunossay for oxytocin: The extraction of oxytocin from plasma and its measurement during parturition in human and goat blood. J Endocrinol 48:223, 1970

Dawood MY: Neurohypophyseal hormones. In Fuchs F, Klopper A (eds): Endocrinology of Pregnancy, 3rd ed. Philadelphia, JB Lippincott, 1983

Dawood MY, Pociask C, Raghaven KS et al: Oxytocin levels in mother and fetus during parturition. Gynecol Invest 7:29, 1976

Dawood MY, Raghaven KS, Pociask C et al: Oxytocin in human pregnancy and parturition. Obstet Gynecol 51:138, 1978

DuVigneaud V: Hormones of the posterior pituitary gland: Oxytocin and vasopressin. London, Harvey Lecture 50:1, 1954–1955

Fields PA, Eldridge RK, Fuchs A-R et al: Human placental and bovine luteal oxytocin. Endocrinol 112:1544, 1983

Fuchs A-R, Fuchs F, Husslein P et al: Oxytocin receptors and human parturition: A dual role for oxytocin in the initiation of labor. Science 215:1396, 1982

Hill WC, Moenning RK, Katz M et al: Characteristics of uterine activity during the breast stimulation stress test. Obstet Gynecol 64:489, 1984

Kamm O, Aldrich TB, Grote IW et al: The active principles of the posterior lobe of the pituitary gland. I. The demonstration of the presence of two active principles. II. The separation of the two principles and their concentration in the forms of potent solid preparations. J Am Chem Soc 50:573, 1928

Khan–Dawood FS, Dawood MY: Oxytocin content of human fetal pituitary glands. Am J Obstet Gynecol 148:420, 1984

Kumaresan P, Anandarangam PB, Dianzon W et al: Plasma oxytocin levels and labor as determined by radioimmunoassay. Am J Obstet Gynecol 119:215, 1974

Leake RD, Weitzman RE, Fisher DA: Pharmacokinetics of oxytocin in the human subject. Obstet Gynecol 56:701, 1980

Ray BS: Some inferences from hypophysectomy in 450 human patients. Arch Neurol 3:121, 1960

Swaab DF, Oosterbaan HP: Exclusion of fetal brain as the main source of rat and human amniotic fluid oxytocin. Brit J Obstet Gynaecol 90:1160, 1983

Takahashi K, Diamond F, Bieniarz J et al: Uterine contractility and oxytocin sensitivity in preterm, term, and postterm pregnancy. Am J Obstet Gynecol 136:774, 1980

Theobald GW, Graham A, Campbell J et al: The use of postpituitary extract in physiological amounts in obstetrics. Br Med J 2:123, 1948

Viegas OAC, Arulkumaran S, Gibb DMF et al: Nipple stimulation in late pregnancy causing uterine hyperstimulation and profound fetal bradycardia. Brit J Obstet Gynaecol 91:364, 1984

Watson BP: Induction of labor: Indications and methods, with special reference to the use of pituitary extract. Transactions of the American Gynecological Society, 45:31, 1920

Uterine Responses to Pregnancy and Labor

Structural Changes in Pregnancy and Labor

Danforth DN, Chapman JCF: Incorporation of the isthmus uteri. Am J Obstet Gynecol 59:979, 1950

Danforth DN, Graham RJ, Ivy AC: Functional anatomy of labor as revealed by frozen sagittal sections in the *Macaca rhesus* monkey. Surg Gynecol Obstet 74:188, 1942

Danforth DN, Ivy AC: The lower uterine segment: Its derivation and physiologic behavior. Am J Obstet Gynecol 57:831, 1949

Uterine Contractions

Alvarez H, Caldeyro-Barcía R: Contractility of the human uterus recorded by new methods. Surg Gynecol Obstet 91:1, 1950

Beard RW: Controlling and quantifying uterine activity. Contemp Ob/Gyn 13:75, 1979

Blair-Bell W, Datnow MM, Jeffcoate TNA: The mechanism of uterine action and its disorders. J Obstet Gynaecol Br Emp 40:541, 1933

Caldeyro-Barcía R, Poseiro JJ: Physiology of the uterine contraction. Clin Obstet Gynecol 3:386, 1960

Danforth DN, Graham RJ, Ivy AC: The physiology of the uterus in labor. Quart Bull Northwestern Univ Med Sch 15:1, 1941

Duey JA Jr., Miller FC: The evaluation of uterine activity: A comparative analysis. Am J Obstet Gynecol 135:252, 1979

Hendricks CH: Uterine contractility at delivery and in the puerperium. Am J Obstet Gynecol 83:890, 1962

Hicks JB: On the contractions of the uterus throughout pregnancy: Their physiological effects and their value in the diagnosis of pregnancy. Trans Obstet Soc Lond 13:216, 1872

Ivy AC, Hartman CG, Koff A: The contractions of the monkey uterus at term. Am J Obstet Gynecol 22:388, 1931

Jeffcoate TNA: Abnormalities of uterine action in labour. In Bowes K (ed): Modern Trends in Obstetrics and Gynaecology. New York, Hoeber, 1950

Lowenstein WR: Cellular communication by permeable membrane junctions. Hosp Pract 9:113, 1974

Marshall JM: Physiological principles of contraction in uterine muscle. In Marshall JM (ed): Initiation of Labor, pp 24, 25, 96. Public Health Publication 1390. Bethesda, MD, National Institute of Child Health and Human Development, Department of Health, Education, and Welfare, 1963

Marshall JM: Physiology of the myometrium. Norris HJ, Hertig AT, Abell MR (eds): The Uterus, p 89. Baltimore, Williams & Wilkins, 1973

Miller FC, Mueller E, Velick K: Quantitation of uterine activity: Clinical evaluation of a new method of data presentation. Obstet Gynecol 55:388, 1980

Mizrahi J, Karni Z, Polishuk WZ: Strain uterography in labour. Br J Obstet Gynaecol 84:930, 1977

Reynolds SRM: The uses of Braxton Hicks contractions. Obstet Gynecol 32:134, 1968

Richardson JA, Sutherland IA: Letter: A cervimeter for continuous measurement of cervical dilatation in labour—Preliminary results. Br J Obstet Gynaecol 85:975, 1978

Schatz P: Beitrage zur physiologischen Geburtskunde. Arch Gynaekol 3:58, 1872

Seitchik J, Chatkoff ML: Intrauterine pressure wave forms characteristic of successful and failed first stage labor. Gynecol Invest 8:246, 1977

Seitchik J, Chatkoff ML: Induced uterine hypercontractility pressure wave forms. Obstet Gynecol 48:436, 1977

Turnbull AC, Anderson ABM: Uterine function in human pregnancy and labour. In MacDonald RR (ed): Scientific Basis of Obstetrics and Gynaecology, 2nd ed. Edinburgh, Churchill Livingstone, 1978

Wolfs GMJA, Van Leeuwen M: Electromyographic observations on the human uterus during labour. Acta Obstet Gynecol Scand (Suppl)58:90, 1979

Drug Effects

Akamatsu TJ, Bonica JJ: Spinal and extradural analgesia-anesthesia for parturition. Clin Obstet Gynecol 17:183, 1974

Barden TP: The effect of drugs on uterine contractility. In Quilligan EJ, Kretchmer N (eds): Fetal and Maternal Medicine. New York, John Wiley, 1980

Caritis SN, Edelstone DI, Mueller-Heubach E: Pharmacologic inhibition of preterm labor. Am J Obstet Gynecol 133: 557, 1979

Cibils LA, Zuspan FP: Pharmacology of the uterus. Clin Obstet Gynecol 11:34, 1968

Datta S, Kitzmiller JL, Ostheimer GW et al: Propranolol and parturition. Obstet Gynecol 51:577, 1978

Eskes TK: Effect of morphine upon uterine contractility in late pregnancy. Am J Obstet Gynecol 84:281, 1962

Fuchs F: Effect of ethyl alcohol upon spontaneous uterine activity. J Obstet Gynaecol Br Commonw 72:1011, 1965

Hendricks CH, Brenner WE: Cardiovascular effects of oxytocic drugs used postpartum. Am J Obstet Gynecol 108:751, 1970

Lewis RB, Schulman JD: Influence of acetylsalicylic acid, an inhibitor of prostaglandin synthesis, on the duration of human gestation and labor. Lancet 2:1159, 1973

Lipshitz J: Uterine and cardiovascular effects of aminophylline. Am J Obstet Gynecol 131:716, 1978

Niebyl JR, Blake DA, Johnson JWC et al: The pharmacologic inhibition of premature labor. Obstet Gynecol Surv 33: 507, 1978

Pauerstein CJ: Use and abuse of oxytocic agents. Clin Obstet Gynecol 16:262, 1973

Sica-Blanco Y, Rozada H, Remedio M: Effect of meperidine on uterine contractility during pregnancy and prelabor. Am J Obstet Gynecol 97:1096, 1967

Tepperman HM, Beydoun SN, Abdul-Karim RW: Drugs affecting uterine contractility in pregnancy. Clin Obstet Gynecol 20:423, 1977

Vasicka A, Hutchinson HT, Eng MM et al: Spinal and epidural anesthesia, fetal and uterine response to acute hypo- and hypertension. Am J Obstet Gynecol 90:800, 1964

Zuckerman H, Reiss U, Rubinstein I: Inhibition of human premature labor by indomethacin. Obstet Gynecol 44:787, 1974

Changes in the Cervix in Pregnancy and Labor

Beier HM: Anatomy of cervical changes at the end of pregnancy. Z Geburts Perinatol 183:83, 1979

Buchanan D, Macer J, Yonekura ML: Cervical ripening with

prostaglandin E_2 vaginal suppositories. Obstet Gynecol 63:659, 1984

Buckingham JC, Selden R, Danforth DN: Connective tissue changes in the cervix during pregnancy and labor. Ann NY Acad Sci 97:733, 1962

Conrad JT, Ueland K: Reduction of stretch modules of human cervical tissue by prostaglandin E_2. Am J Obstet Gynecol 126:218, 1976

Conrad JT, Ueland K: The stretch modules of human cervical tissue in spontaneous, oxytocin-induced and prostaglandin E_2-induced labor. Am J Obstet Gynecol 133:11, 1979

Danforth DN: Distribution and functional significance of the cervical musculature. Am J Obstet Gynecol 68:1261, 1954

Danforth DN: Fibrous nature of the human cervix and its relation to the isthmic segment in gravid and nongravid uteri. Am J Obstet Gynecol 53:541, 1947

Danforth DN: The morphology of the human cervix. Clin Obstet Gynecol 26:7, 1983

Danforth DN: The squamous epithelium and squamocolumnar junction of the cervix during pregnancy. Am J Obstet Gynecol 60:985, 1950

Danforth DN, Buckingham JC: Connective tissue mechanisms and their relation to pregnancy. Obstet Gynecol Surv 19: 715, 1964

Danforth DN, Buckingham JC, Roddick JW Jr.: Connective tissue changes incident to cervical effacement. Am J Obstet Gynecol 80:939, 1960

Danforth DN, Veis A, Breen M et al: The effect of pregnancy on the human cervix: Changes in collagen, glycoproteins, and glycosaminoglycans. Am J Obstet Gynecol 120:641, 1974

Ekman G, Forman A, Marsal K et al: Intravaginal versus intracervical application of prostaglandin E_2 in viscous gel for cervical priming and induction of labor in patients with an unfavorable cervical state. Am J Obstet Gynecol 147: 657, 1983

Ekman G, Malmström A, Uldbjerg N et al: Cervical collagen—An important regulator of cervical function in term labor. Obstet Gynecol (in press)

Grunberger W, Husslein P: "Portio priming" in post date and low pelvic score. Geburtshilfe Frauenheilkd 39:793, 1979

Hendricks CH, Brenner WE, Kraus G: The normal cervical dilatation pattern in late pregnancy and labor. Am J Obstet Gynecol 106:1065, 1970

Herbst AL, Hubby MM, Blough RR et al: A comparison of pregnancy experience in DES-exposed and DES-unexposed daughters. J Reprod Med 24:62, 1980

Huszar G, Naftolin F: The myometrium and uterine cervix in normal and preterm labor. N Engl J Med 311:571, 1984

Junqueira LCU, Zugaib M, Montes GS et al: Morphologic and histochemical evidence for the occurrence of collagenolysis and for the role of neutrophilic polymorphonuclear leukocytes during cervical dilatation. Am J Obstet Gynecol 138:273, 1980

Kleissl HP, Van der Rest M, Naftolin F et al: Collagen changes in the human uterine cervix at parturition. Am J Obstet Gynecol 130:748, 1978

Ledger WL, Webster M, Harrison LP et al: Increase in cervical extensibility during labor induced after isolation of the cervix from the uterus of pregnant ewes. Am J Obstet Gynecol 151:397, 1985

Prins RP, Bolton RN, Markm Carl III et al: Cervical ripening with intravaginal prostaglandin E_2 gel. Obstet Gynecol 61:459, 1983

Roddick JW Jr., Buckingham JC, Danforth DN: The muscular cervix—A cause of incompetency in pregnancy. Obstet Gynecol 17:562, 1961

Rossavik IKR: Total uterine impulse and cervical resistance at parturition. Am J Obstet Gynecol 136:579, 1980

Sokamato S, Sokamato M, Goldhaber P: Collagenase activity and chemical bone resorption induced by prostaglandin E_2 in tissue culture. Proc Soc Exp Biol Med 161:99, 1979

Stys SJ, Clewell WH, Meschia G: Changes in cervical compliance at parturition independent of uterine activity. Am J Obstet Gynecol 130:414, 1978

Uldbjerg N, Ekman G, Malmström A et al: Ripening of the human uterine cervix related to changes in collagen, glycosaminoglycans, and collagenolytic activity. Am J Obstet Gynecol 147:662, 1983

Uldbjerg N, Ulmsten U, Ekman G: The ripening of the human uterine cervix in terms of connective tissue biochemistry. Clin Obstet Gynecol 26:L14, 1983

Ulmsten U, Wingerup L, Andersson K-E: Comparison of prostaglandin E_2 and intravenous oxytocin for induction of labor. Obstet Gynecol 54:581, 1979

Weiss G, O'Bryne FM, Hochman J et al: Distribution of relaxin in women during pregnancy. Obstet Gynecol 52:569, 1978

Wilson PD: A comparison of four methods of ripening the unfavorable cervix. Br J Obstet Gynaecol 85:941, 1978

General and Miscellaneous References

Daniel EE, Lodge S: Electrophysiology of the myometrium. In Josimovich JB (ed): In Uterine Contraction—Side Effects of Steroidal Contraceptives, Chap 3, p 19. New York, John Wiley, 1973

Garfield RE, Rabideau S, Challis JRG: Ultrastructural basis for maintenance and termination of pregnancy. Am J Obstet Gynecol 133:308, 1979

Garfield RE, Sims S, Daniel EE: Gap junctions: Their presence and necessity in myometrium during parturition. Science 198:958, 1977

Garfield RE, Sims SM, Kanna MS: Possible role of gap junctions in activation of myometrium during pregnancy. Am J Physiol 235:C168, 1978

Kirsch RE: Study on the length of gestation in the rat with notes on maintenance and termination of gestation. Am J Physiol 122:86, 1938

Peel J: The Royal College of Obstetricians and Gynaecologists, 1929 to 1979. Br J Obstet Gynaecol 86:673, 1979

Wynn RM (ed): Biology of the Uterus, 2nd ed. New York, Plenum, 1977

Leiman G, Harrison NA, Rubin A: Pregnancy following conization of the cervix: Complications related to cone size. Am J Obstet Gynecol 136:14, 1980

Liggins GC: Ripening of the cervix. Semin Perinatol 2:261, 1978

MacLennan AH, Green RC: A double blind dose trial of intravaginal prostaglandin $F_{2\alpha}$ for cervical ripening and the induction of labour. N Z J Obstet Gynecol 20:80, 1980

MacLennan AH, Green RC: Cervical ripening and induction of labour with intravaginal prostaglandin $F_{2\alpha}$. Lancet 1:117, 1979

Naftolin F, Stubblefield PG (eds): Dilatation of the Uterine Cervix: Connective Tissue Biology and Clinical Management. New York, Raven Press, 1980

Nimrod C, Currie J, Yee J et al: Cervical ripening with labor induction with intracervical triacetin base prostaglandin E_2 gel: A placebo-controlled study. Obstet Gynecol 64: 476, 1984

O'Herlihy C, MacDonald HN: Influence of preinduction prostaglandin E_2 vaginal gel on cervical ripening and labor. Obstet Gynecol 54:708, 1979

Mechanism of Normal Labor

David N. Danforth

32

The mechanism of labor refers to the sequence of attitudes and positions that must be assumed by the fetus as it passes through the birth canal. As a general rule, the changes in position are determined by the configuration of the mother's bony pelvis; for each configuration, there is a single optimum mechanism. The physician must be aware of the normal pelvic variations in order to appreciate the details of the normal mechanism of labor.

Modern concepts of the obstetric pelvis and its influence on the mechanism of labor are based on the classic work of Caldwell and Moloy. Prior to the publication of their work, certain grossly deformed pelves were recognized as variants, but there was no understanding of the variations commonly encountered in a normal population. Caldwell and Moloy studied the human pelves in the American Museum of Natural History in New York and the large collection of T. Wingate Todd at the Western Reserve University. On the basis of this analysis, they classified normal pelves into four major groups according to the general shape of the pelvic inlet. They pursued their investigations at the Sloane Hospital for Women, using an instrument known as the *precision stereoscope,* which was developed by Moloy. This instrument resembles a standard stereoscope except that it uses prisms instead of mirrors. By aligning the optical system, it is possible to place a rule on any part of the phantom image; this permits reasonably accurate direct measurement of the size of the pelvic inlet, the interspinous diameter, and the important diameters of the fetal head. Caldwell and Moloy used this technique in the study of many hundreds of labors, and their findings form the basis of the concept of pelvic classification and the mechanism of labor that has become an integral part of the discipline of obstetrics.

THE OBSTETRIC PELVIS

Anatomy

The bones and articulations comprising the pelvis are considered in Chapter 3. For practical purposes, the obstetrician is concerned only with the "true" pelvis, which includes the inlet, the midpelvis, and the outlet.

The *pelvic inlet* can be traced anteriorly from the iliopectineal lines along the pectineal eminence and the pubic crest to the symphysis (Fig. 32-1). Posteriorly, the inlet is bounded by the sacrum at the level of termination of the iliopectineal lines. (The sacral promontory is slightly superior to this and hence lies above the inlet.) The *plane of the inlet* is a flat surface that is bounded as noted and is generally inclined at an angle of 40° to 60° with the horizontal when the patient is standing. This angle is called the *pelvic inclination,* and it may have much practical significance. If the angle with the horizontal is wide, for example, such that the pelvis is inclined posteriorly, the axis of drive or force into the pelvis may be sufficiently faulty to interfere with the progress of labor.

For obstetric purposes, the plane of the pelvic inlet is considered in terms of four diameters: the anteroposterior diameter, the widest transverse diameter, and the oblique diameters. The anteroposterior diameter (superior strait, obstetric conjugate) extends from the posterosuperior border of the symphysis pubis to the sacrum at the level of the iliopectineal lines. For descriptive purposes, the anteroposterior diameter is divided into anterior and posterior sagittal diameters to designate the amount of space anterior and posterior to the widest transverse diameter. In the description of inlet x-ray films, the anterior and posterior sagittal

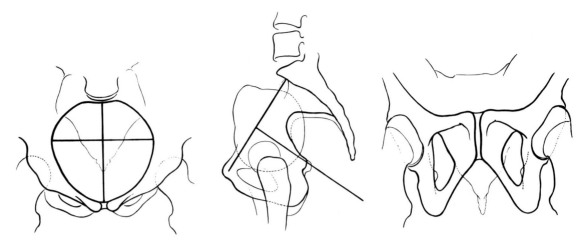

FIG. 32-1. Inlet, lateral, and front views of pelvis.

lengths, when considered together with the widest transverse diameter, provide instant knowledge of the general shape and capacity of the inlet. The widest transverse diameter is invariably located posterior to the center of the pelvis and, except in asymmetric pelves, transects the anteroposterior at right angles. The right oblique diameter extends from the right sacroiliac joint to the left iliopectineal eminence and takes its name from the posterior landmark. The left oblique diameter extends from the left sacroiliac joint to the right iliopectineal eminence (Fig. 32-2).

Two additional conjugates should be noted. The true conjugate (conjugata vera, CV) lies immediately superior to the obstetric conjugate and extends from the top of the pubis to the tip of the sacral promontory. It is a little longer than the obstetric conjugate, except in pelves in which the promontory hangs over the inlet. The diagonal conjugate (DC) extends from the undermargin of the symphysis to the sacral promontory. It is believed to be approximately 1.5 cm longer than the true conjugate and hence to be useful in assessing the

FIG. 32-2. Right and left oblique diameters of pelvic inlet and forepelvis.

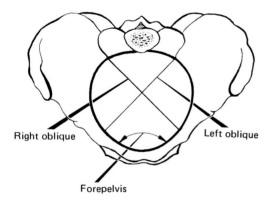

Right oblique

Left oblique

Forepelvis

anteroposterior diameter of the inlet. However, Eastman has shown that, although the correlation is good in some cases, in others it is sufficiently poor to give a spurious impression of the anteroposterior diameter. Therefore, this measurement is of questionable value.

The *forepelvis* is the angle described by the posterior aspects of the symphysis and the pubis (Fig. 32-2). Although it is illustrated in diagrams of the inlet, this angle also affects the capacity of the midpelvis.

The *midpelvis*, for obstetric purposes, is bounded anteriorly by the posterior aspect of the symphysis and pubis, posteriorly by the sacrum at the level of S3 or S4, and laterally by the sidewalls and ischial spines.

The *sidewalls* extend from the level of the inlet at the point of the widest transverse diameter inferiorly and forward to the lower portion of the ischial tuberosities. The sidewalls are more or less straight lines; when they converge from above downward, they may limit the transverse diameter of the pelvis in the same manner in which the transverse space can be limited by very prominent spines.

The *pelvic outlet* is bounded anteriorly by the inferior aspect of the symphysis (the subpubic arch), posteriorly by the tip of the sacrum (*not* the coccyx), and laterally by the ischial tuberosities.

The *axis of the pelvis* (the obstetric axis) is the general curve of the birth canal described by a line drawn through the center of each of the planes mentioned previously (Fig. 32-3). The line curves anteriorly as the outlet is approached.

Caldwell–Moloy Classification of Pelvic Types

Although the Caldwell–Moloy classification designates the four types of pelves in terms of the configuration of the inlet, certain features of the lower pelvis are also characteristic of each type. Thus the classification is based upon normal variations in the following pelvic features:

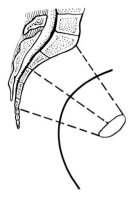

FIG. 32-3. Axis of pelvis (curve of Carus). Note that curve is more or less straight through inlet, curving anteriorly in mid-pelvis. *Dashed lines* indicate planes of inlet, midpelvis and outlet.

Shape of inlet (width of forepelvis, ratio of widest transverse to longest anteroposterior diameter, ratio of anterior sagittal to posterior sagittal diameter)
Splay of sidewalls

Prominence of spines
Height of symphysis
Transverse diameter of outlet (bituberous)
Width of subpubic arch
Curvature and inclination of sacrum

Four basic categories that identify all the possible normal variations in these individual features are recognized. It is emphasized that the basic types are virtually hypothetical, because it is extremely unusual to find any pelvis that conforms exactly—from front to back, from side to side, and from top to bottom—to any of them. Rather, most pelves are mixed types, showing not only combinations of the various characteristics but also much difference in size. To make an accurate assessment of the mechanism of labor, the physician must be aware both of the variations and of their influence on the posture and position of the fetus.

The four basic types of pelves are gynecoid, android, anthropoid, and platypelloid. The *gynecoid pelvis* (Fig. 32-4) is the so-called normal type of female pelvis. The inlet is rounded, with the anteroposterior diameter very slightly shorter than the widest transverse diameter. The posterior sagittal diameter at the inlet is only slightly

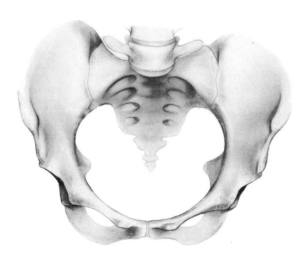

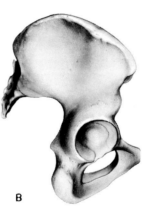

FIG. 32-4. Typical gynecoid pelvis. (*A*) Inlet view. Inlet is nearly round. (*B*) Lateral view. Sacrosciatic notch is of average size; sacrum has average inclination; descending rami of pubes pass straight down to tuberosities. (*C*) Subpubic arch view. Arch is spacious and well curved; sidewalls are straight. (Steer CM: Moloy's Evaluation of the Pelvis in Obstetrics, 2nd ed. Philadelphia, WB Saunders, 1959)

A

B

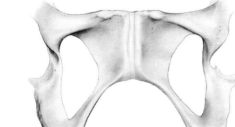

C

shorter than the anterior sagittal. The sidewalls of the pelvis are virtually straight, the spines are not prominent, the height of the symphysis is about 6 cm, the subpubic arch is wide, the transverse diameter of the outlet is about 10 cm, and the sacrum is inclined neither anteriorly nor posteriorly, but has a gentle concavity that is midway between these two extremes.

The *android pelvis* (Fig. 32-5) is the so-called male type of pelvis. The inlet is wedge-shaped; the forepelvis is narrowed; and, although the anteroposterior and widest transverse diameters of the inlet may be about the same, the posterior sagittal diameter at the inlet is much shorter than the anterior sagittal. The sidewalls are typically convergent, the ischial spines are prominent, the height of the symphysis is more than 6 cm, the transverse diameter of the outlet is less than 10 cm, and the subpubic arch is narrowed. In addition, the bone structure is characteristically heavy, and the sacrum is inclined forward, especially in its lower third.

The *anthropoid pelvis* (Fig. 32-6) is characteristic of the ape and monkey but also commonly occurs in humans. It differs from the gynecoid pelvis in shape of the inlet, splay of the sidewalls, and position of the sacrum. The inlet is elongated anteroposteriorly, with the widest transverse diameter being shorter than the anteroposterior diameter. The posterior sagittal diameter at the inlet is longer than that in the gynecoid pelvis, and the forepelvis is slightly narrowed. The sidewalls are characteristically divergent, and the sacrum is inclined posteriorly. The last two characteristics account for the term "blunderbuss" pelvis.

The *platypelloid (flat) pelvis* (Fig. 32-7) is similar to the gynecoid in all respects, except for anteroposterior narrowing at all levels. At the inlet, therefore, the anteroposterior diameter is significantly shorter than the widest transverse, and the sacrum is forward throughout.

Table 32-1 summarizes the features of the four basic pelvic types.

Clinical Evaluation

Pelvic characteristics can be determined by x-ray films (see p. 645) or, with less exact but nonetheless sufficient detail for most purposes, by clinical examination.

FIG. 32-5. Typical android pelvis. (*A*) Inlet view. Inlet is more triangular than round; iliopectineal lines are nearly straight, making forepelvis narrow; widest transverse diameter is close to sacrum. (*B*) Lateral view. Sacrosciatic notch is narrow; sacrum has forward inclination; descending rami of pubes incline backward to tuberosities. (*C*) Subpubic arch view. Descending rami arise from bottom of bodies of pubes and are straight rather than curved; sidewalls tend to converge. (Steer CM: Moloy's Evaluation of the Pelvis in Obstetrics, 2nd ed. Philadelphia, WB Saunders, 1959)

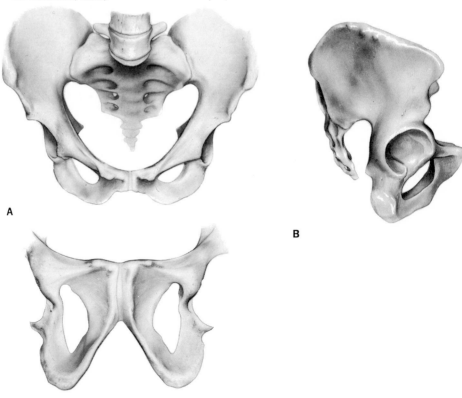

A

B

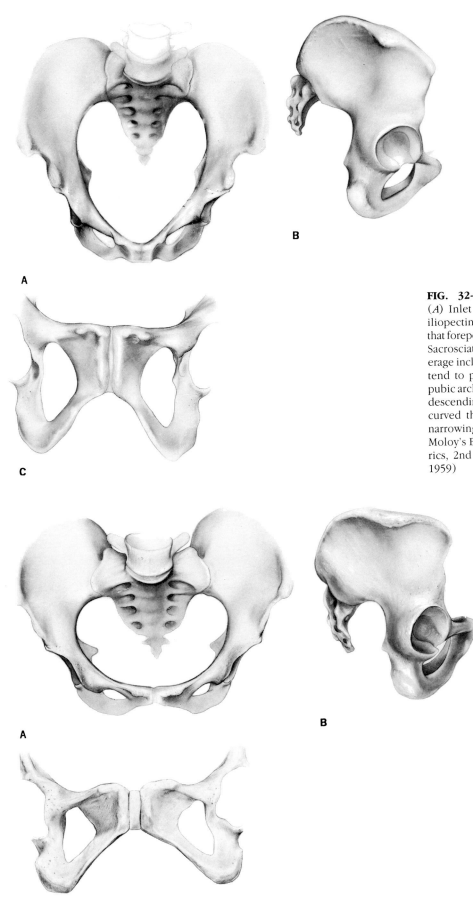

FIG. 32-6. Typical anthropoid pelvis. (*A*) Inlet view. Inlet is long and narrow; iliopectineal lines are not well curved, so that forepelvis is narrowed. (*B*) Lateral view. Sacrosciatic notch is wide; sacrum has average inclination; descending rami of pubes tend to pass backward slightly. (*C*) Subpubic arch view. Arch is rounded at top, but descending rami are apt to be less well curved than in gynecoid type and some narrowing of arch may occur. (Steer CM: Moloy's Evaluation of the Pelvis in Obstetrics, 2nd ed. Philadelphia, WB Saunders, 1959)

FIG. 32-7. Typical platypelloid pelvis. (*A*) Inlet view. Inlet is wide transverse oval. (*B*) Lateral view. Sacrosciatic notch appears narrow because it passes in more transverse direction, although it is actually wide; descending rami are straight. (*C*) Subpubic arch view. Arch is very wide throughout; spines are somewhat more prominent than is usually considered characteristic of simple flat pelvis. (Steer CM: Moloy's Evaluation of the Pelvis in Obstetrics, 2nd ed. Philadelphia, WB Saunders, 1959)

Table 32-1
Characteristics of Four Basic Types of Pelves of Average Size

Characteristic	Type of Pelvis			
	Gynecoid	Android	Anthropoid	Platypelloid
Anteroposterior diameter of inlet	11 cm	11 cm	12+ cm	10 cm
Widest transverse diameter of inlet	12 cm	12 cm	<12 cm	12 cm
Forepelvis	Wide	Narrow	Narrow	Wide
Sidewalls	Straight	Convergent	Divergent	Straight
Ischial spines	Not prominent	Prominent	Not prominent	Not prominent
Sacrosciatic notch	Medium	Narrow	Wide	Narrow
Inclination of sacrum	Medium	Forward (lower third)	Backward	Forward
Subpubic arch	Wide	Narrow	Medium	Wide
Transverse diameter of outlet	10 cm	<10 cm	10 cm	10 cm
Bone structure	Medium	Heavy	Medium	Medium

Definitive typing of a pelvis usually should not be attempted prior to the completion of 7.5 or 8 months' gestation. If delivery occurs before that time, the fetus will be so small that the bony architecture will have no bearing upon the course of labor. Moreover, clinical evaluaton of the pelvis is easier and causes far less discomfort to the patient if it is done after the soft parts have reached the maximum relaxation and softening that occurs about a month before term. Finally, when the examination is performed a month or two weeks before term, the presenting part has attained a considerable size, and a more accurate appraisal can be made of the capacity of the pelvis and its relation to the fetus. Early pelvic typing may be necessary, however, if the pelvis is grossly distorted by rickets or an old fracture, or if the fetus is clinically of eight months' size despite menstrual dates that suggest a pregnancy of lesser duration.

Typing the pelvis requires a thorough knowledge of the landmarks of the pelvis and their spatial relations. This should be obtained first by study and palpation of a pelvic model. The clinical evaluation of the pelvis is illustrated in Figures 32-8 through 32-11. With practice, a satisfactory clinical appraisal can be made of most pelves; if more precise information is needed, x-ray pelvimetry should be done (see p. 645). For the beginner, assessment of the ischial spines may be difficult. If the spines are prominent, they may project into the pelvis like spikes; if they are flush with the pelvic sidewalls, they may be difficult to locate except by first identifying the sacrospinous ligament and following it forward to its anterior termination.

External Pelvimetry

It was formerly believed that a reasonable appraisal of the obstetric adequacy of the pelvis could be obtained by measuring the distance between certain external pelvic landmarks. The diameters selected for measurement were the intercristal (between the iliac crests), the interspinous (between the anterosuperior iliac spines), the intertrochanteric (between the femoral trochanters), and the Baudelocque or external conjugate (from the most promient part of the pubic bone to the dimple under the last lumbar spine). The technique of external pelvimetry is of historic interest, but the comparison of such measurements with those obtained by x-ray pelvimetry has shown conclusively that external pelvimetry has no practicel value. The external pelvic measurements have the same kind of relation to the internal diameters of the pelvis as the biparietal and bitemporal diameters of the head have to the distance between the upper molar teeth.

FIG. 32-8. Evaluation of transverse diameter. Lateral motion of fingers is restricted in transversely narrowed pelvis. (Steer CM: Moloy's Evaluation of the Pelvis in Obstetrics, 2nd ed. Philadelphia, WB Saunders, 1959)

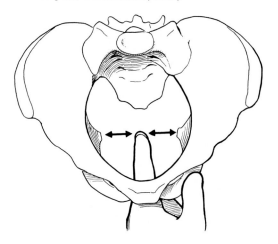

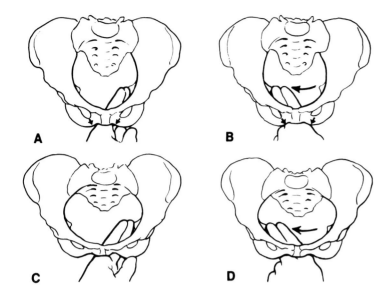

FIG. 32-9. Estimation of width of subpubic arch and interspinous diameter by act of pronation. (*A, B*) Transversely narrowed diameters in mid- and lower pelvis. (*C, D*) Wide transverse diameters in mid- and lower pelvis. (Steer CM: Moloy's Evaluation of the Pelvis in Obstetrics, 2nd ed. Philadelphia, WB Saunders, 1959)

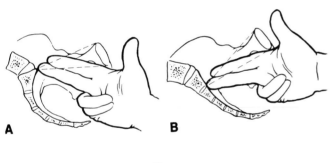

FIG. 32-10. Measurement of diagonal conjugate. When promontory is reached, index finger of opposite hand marks point of undersurface of symphysis. Distance from this point to tip of extended middle finger is length of diagonal conjugate; subtracting 1.5 cm is said to represent length of true conjugate. Promontory may be difficult to reach in early pregnancy before vagina and supports are relaxed, and in late pregnancy may be impossible to reach without disengaging presenting part. (If head is engaged, this information is not needed).

Even if accurately measured, there is great variation in its relation to the true conjugate. Since it is rarely useful and often impossible to determine, this measurement should be discarded from modern obstetric practice. (Steer CM: Moloy's Evaluation of the Pelvis in Obstetrics, 2nd ed. Philadelphia, WB Saunders, 1959)

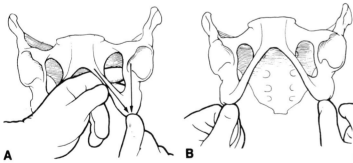

FIG. 32-11. Estimation of intertuberous diameter. (*A*) Identification of ischial tuberosity at point of convergence of pubic rami and pelvic sidewalls. (*B*) Measurement of intertuberous diameter. (Steer CM: Moloy's Evaluation of the Pelvis in Obstetrics, 2nd ed. Philadelphia, WB Saunders, 1959)

THE FETAL HEAD

The fetal skull is composed of three major parts: the roof or vault, the face, and the base. The face and base are more or less fixed because the bones are well fused. The vault, however, is composed of bones that are not fused; hence, this portion of the head can make the adjustments in shape that may be needed as the head passes through the narrower diameters of the pelvis. These changes in shape are referred to as *molding* (Fig. 32-12).

The bones that form the vault are the two frontal bones, the two parietal bones, and the occipital bone. They are separated from one another by sutures and by

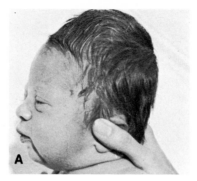
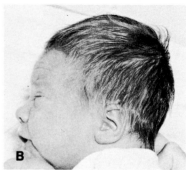

FIG. 32-12. (*A*) Well-molded head of newborn infant. (*B*) Same head three days later.

the two fontanels. The sutures and fontanels are arranged in a sufficiently distinctive way, and palpation of these landmarks prior to delivery permits instant determination of the position of the head. This information may be of fundamental importance in following the course of labor and predicting its outcome. The relations of the sutures, fontanels, and bones of the vault are shown in Figure 32-13.

The term *fetal attitude* refers to the relation of the fetal parts to one another. In the case of the head, the reference is to its relation to the thorax, that is, whether it is flexed anteroposteriorly or laterally, or extended. The atlanto-occipital articulation and the flexibility of the neck permit slight lateral mobility of the head and considerable anteroposterior mobility. The lateral mobility is occasionally important. For practical purposes, the lateral diameter of the head presented to the pelvis is the biparietal diameter (Fig. 32-13); in a baby weighing about 7 lb, this diameter is about 9 cm. The presenting biparietal diameter, of course, is not influenced by the amount of flexion or extension of the head. The head usually enters the pelvis with the sagittal suture lying in the transverse plane of the mother's pelvis; when this suture lies about midway between symphysis and sacrum, the situation is referred to as *synclitism* (Fig. 32-14). When the head flexes to the right or left, and the sagittal suture approaches the symphysis or the sacrum, the situation is referred to as *asynclitism*. Depending on the direction of flexion toward or away from the sacrum, the terms *anterior* or *posterior parietal bone presentation,* respectively, may be used (Fig. 32-15). Asynclitism may occur in normal labor as a result of a change in the axis of force (through changes in position of the uterus), or it may be a sign that the pelvis is too small to permit the head to advance into the inlet.

Although the lateral diameter that presents is not influenced by anteroposterior flexion or extension, such flexion or extension is important in determining the anteroposterior diameter of the head that will be presented to the pelvis and, hence, in determining the amount of space required for its advance through the pelvis. In about 95% of cases, the fetus is delivered headfirst; in most of these, full flexion automatically results because

the occipital condyles are located near the posterior aspect of the skull, with about two thirds of the head lying anterior to this articulation (Fig. 32-16). As the head is thrust into the inlet (and is confined by the lower pole of the uterus), the longer segment of the lever yields to the pressure and flexion results. When the head is fully flexed, with chin on the chest, the shortest anteroposterior diameter, the suboccipitobregmatic, is presented. Accordingly, the position of full flexion offers the smallest circumference of the head to the narrower planes of the pelvis. The suboccipitobregmatic diameter is slightly longer than the biparietal; it measures approximately 9.5 cm in a 7-lb infant (Fig. 32-13).

In some situations, full flexion does not occur, and the result is the presentation of an anteroposterior diameter that is longer than the suboccipitobregmatic. The important variations in flexion are shown in Figure 32-17 and are named for the portion of the skull that is presented. The major attitudes when the fetus presents headfirst are vertex, sincipital, brow, and face.

In the sincipital presentation (the so-called military attitude), the occipitofrontal plane of the head is presented, with an anteroposterior diameter of about 12 cm. In the case of brow presentation, which has the longest anteroposterior diameter of the head of the four attitudes, the occipitomental plane is presented. As further extension occurs, the anteroposterior diameter decreases until, in the extreme situation of face presentation, the anteroposterior diameter presented to the pelvis is only slightly longer than the suboccipitobregmatic that presents in the customary situation of full flexion.

Of the four attitudes noted, full flexion is the ideal circumstance. A military attitude gradually changes to one of flexion as the head advances into the pelvis unless mobility is impaired in the fetal neck or in the atlanto-occipital articulation. A face presentation, as explained in Chapter 36, permits advancement through the pelvis, but a brow presentation does not unless the head is extremely small or the pelvis huge. A brow presentation can sometimes be converted to face or to vertex presentation. If not, the fetus must be delivered by cesarean section unless the pelvis is enormous.

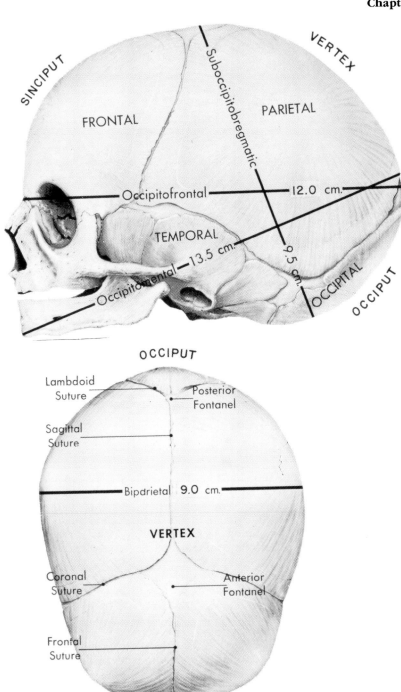

FIG. 32-13. Relation of bones, fontanels, sutures, and diameters of fetal head. (Phenomena of Normal Labor, Brochure 345, 20C. Columbus, Ohio, Ross Laboratories)

PRESENTATION, POSITION, AND LIE

Certain terms are used specifically to describe the fetopelvic relations. *Lie* refers to the relation of the long axis of the fetus to the long axis of the mother (Fig. 32-18). The two possibilities are longitudinal (which is common and normal) and transverse (which is uncommon and potentially serious). Oblique lie, a variant of the transverse lie, may also occur.

Presentation (or presenting part) refers to the part

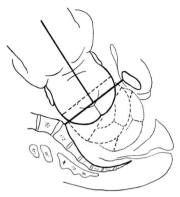

FIG. 32-14. Synclitism. Head entering pelvis with plane of biparietal diameter parallel (or synclitic) to plane of inlet. *Dotted lines* indicate changes in position as head advances. (Beck AC, Rosenthal AH: Obstetrical Practice, 6th ed. Copyright © 1955, Williams & Wilkins, Baltimore)

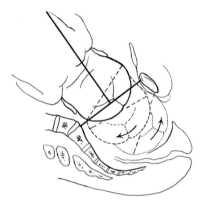

FIG. 32-15. Asynclitism. Prior to engagement, head is laterally flexed and is referred to as "anterior synclitism" or "posterior parietal bone presentation." Subsequent changes in attitude (*dotted lines*) are due both to adaptation of head to pelvis and to effect of lower uterine segment and cervix. (Beck AC, Rosenthal AH: Obstetrical Practice, 6th ed. Copyright © 1955, Baltimore, Williams & Wilkins)

of the fetus lying over the inlet. The three major possibilities are cephalic (which occurs in about 95% of cases), breech (which occurs in perhaps 5% of labors at term), and shoulder (which is extremely rare but is ominous for both mother and fetus). Cord presentation occurs when the umbilical cord advances into the inlet before the fetus.

Point of direction (denominator, point of reference) refers to an arbitrary, and usually the most dependent, portion of the presenting part. In cephalic presentation with a well-flexed head, the occiput is the point of direction. When the fetus is in the military attitude, the occiput is also the point of direction, despite the fact that the parietal bones may be in a dependent position. In brow presentation, the anterior fontanel (bregma) is the point of direction; in face presentation, it is the chin

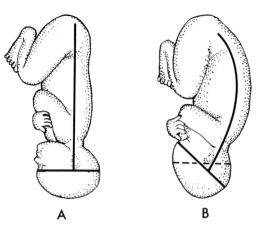

A   **B**

FIG. 32-16. (*A*) Relation of head to spinal column prior to flexion. (*B*) Relation of head to spinal column after flexion.

(mentum); and in breech presentation, the sacrum is the point of direction.

The head is engaged when the biparietal diameter has passed through the plane of the inlet.

Station refers to the level of the head (or presenting part) in the pelvis. When the most dependent part of the head is at the level of the ischial spines, the station is referred to as zero. Levels 1, 2, or 3 cm above or below the level of the spines are referred to as station −1, −2, −3, or +1, +2, +3, respectively (Fig. 32-19). Station 0 is generally considered exact engagement, indicating that the biparietal diameter is at the level of the inlet. However, with heavy molding of the head or caput succedaneum, the biparietal diameter may lie a significant distance above the inlet when the tip of the vertex reaches the interspinous diameter.

Position refers to the relation of the point of direction to one of the four quadrants or to the transverse diameter of the maternal pelvis. The point of direction may lie in either of the two posterior quadrants (right or left posterior), in either of the two anterior quadrants (right or left anterior), or in the direct transverse diameter (right or left transverse). It may also lie either directly to the front of the pelvis or directly to the back (direct anterior or direct posterior).

In defining position, the following abbreviations are used: O (occiput) in cephalic presentation, M (mentum or chin) in face presentation, and S (sacrum) in breech presentation. The abbreviations are further related to the appropriate part of the pelvis: ROA (right occiput anterior), LST (left sacrum transverse), LMA (left mentum anterior), and so forth. Several of the positions are illustrated in Figures 32-20 through 32-23.

THE MECHANISM OF LABOR

In considering the "normal" mechanism of labor, it is customary to list the following five steps by which the head traverses the pelvis: descent, flexion, internal ro-

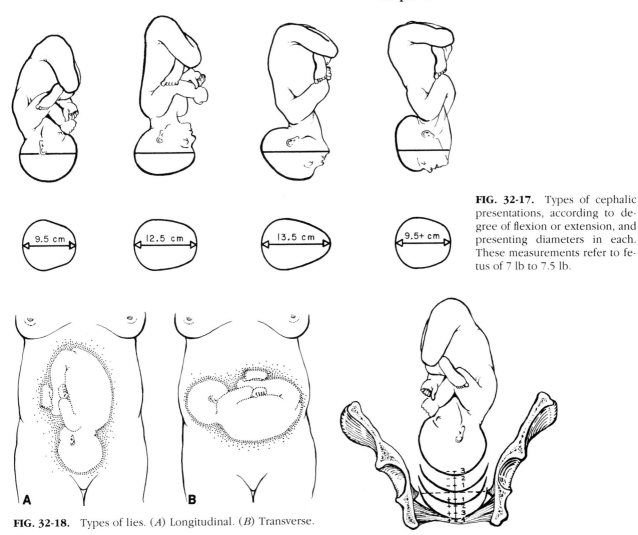

FIG. 32-17. Types of cephalic presentations, according to degree of flexion or extension, and presenting diameters in each. These measurements refer to fetus of 7 lb to 7.5 lb.

FIG. 32-18. Types of lies. (*A*) Longitudinal. (*B*) Transverse.

FIG. 32-19. Stations of fetal head.

FIG. 32-20. Cephalic presentation. (*A*) Right occiput anterior (ROA) position. (*B*) Left occiput anterior (LOA) position. (Bumm E: Grundriss zum Studium der Geburtshilfe. Munich, Bergmann, 1922)

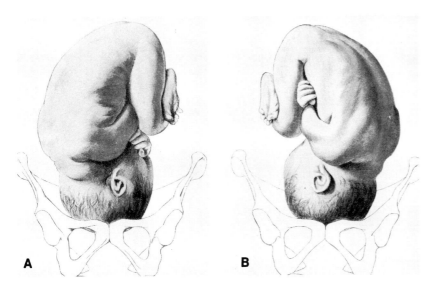

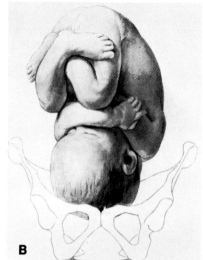

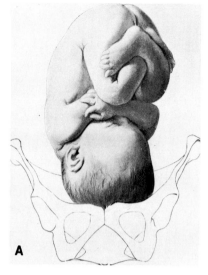

FIG. 32-21. Cephalic presentation. (*A*) Right occiput posterior (ROP) position. (*B*) Left occiput posterior (LOP) position. (Bumm E: Grundriss zum Studium der Geburtshilfe. Munich, Bergmann, 1922)

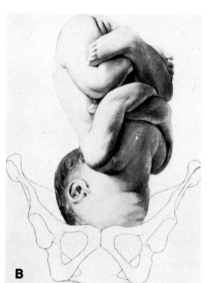

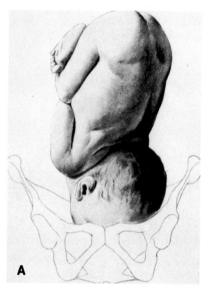

FIG. 32-22. Face presentation. (*A*) Right mentum posterior (RMP) position. (*B*) Left mentum anterior (LMA) position. (Bumm E: Grundriss zum Studium der Geburtshilfe. Munich, Bergmann, 1922)

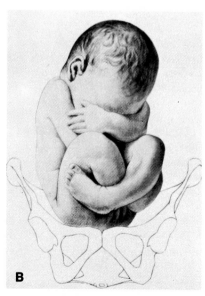

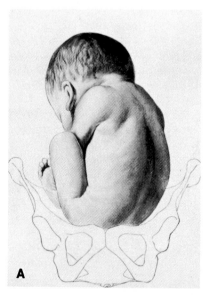

FIG. 32-23. Breech presentation. (*A*) Left sacrum anterior (LSA) position. (*B*) Right sacrum posterior (RSP) position. (Bumm E: Grundriss zum Studium der Geburtshilfe. Munich, Bergmann, 1922)

tation, extension, and external restitution. These steps are illustrated in Figure 32-24 and are entirely accurate and appropriate for an average-sized gynecoid pelvis and an average-sized infant with the occiput the point of direction. However, no two pelves are exactly the same, just as no two faces are the same. For each pelvis there is an optimum mechanism that may be wholly different from the so-called normal mechanism described in the figure.

In most labors, which are efficient and require no intervention, the details of mechanism are of only academic interest; but a precise knowledge of each mechanism may be of transcendent importance if the head arrests and must be delivered by forceps from a level above the outlet, because traction in the wrong pelvic diameter can be lethal to the fetus and highly damaging to the mother. It must be remembered that the bony pelvis may show great variation in individual features and that the birth canal is curved anteriorly (Fig. 32-3). The presenting part (for purposes of this discussion the head, with occiput the point of direction) must negotiate both the pelvic curve and any narrow areas that may be present in the pelvis.

Several other variables also influence the ease or difficulty with which the head traverses the pelvis. Among these are the quality of the uterine contractions and the ability of the head to mold; marked molding and extremely efficient uterine powers can often overcome rather high degrees of disproportion between the size of the head and the size of the pelvis. The importance of flexion of the head has already been mentioned. If the baby is small enough and the pelvis is large enough, the head can advance without being influenced in any way by the configuration of the pelvis. As the disparity in size is reduced, a point is reached at which the head must rotate one way or another to negotiate the narrow diameters and the pelvic curve. Efficient contractions, average molding, adequate flexion, and a fetus large enough to use the pelvic space that is available are all that are required in the normal mechanism of labor. If any of these conditions are not met, the anticipated mechanism may be altered.

Influence of Individual Pelvic Features

Two dicta are extremely important in determining the changes in position that the head undergoes as it passes through the pelvis:

The biparietal is the narrowest presenting diameter of the head, and it must therefore go through the narrowest diameter of the pelvis at any given level.
The occiput generally tends to rotate to the widest or most ample portion of the pelvis at any given level.

On the basis of these maxims, the mechanism of labor can be predicted by considering first the effect of each individual pelvic feature and then the relation of each of the features to one another.

Shape of the Inlet

When the available space is used, the position of engagement is largely determined by inlet shape (Fig. 32-25). Thus, in the flat inlet, with anteroposterior narrowing, the biparietal diameter must go through this narrowed area, and engagement occurs in the occiput transverse position. In the anthropoid inlet, with transverse narrowing, engagement occurs with the sagittal suture in the sagittal plane of the pelvis. In the anthropoid pelvis, however, the forepelvis is invariably narrowed and the posterior segment is deep; hence, engagement in the posterior position is the rule. In the android inlet, with a narrow forepelvis and a short posterior segment, the occiput rotates away from both these areas and engages in the transverse position. Transverse engagement also occurs in 70% of gynecoid pelves because the anteroposterior diameter is slightly shorter than the widest transverse diameter.

Shape of the Forepelvis

When the forepelvis is wide, the occiput tends to rotate anteriorly both at the inlet and in the midpelvis. When it is narrowed, the occiput tends to rotate away from the symphysis both at the inlet and in the midpelvis.

Prominence of the Ischial Spines and Splay of the Sidewalls

The presence of prominent spines, converging sidewalls, or both has the effect of transverse narrowing in the midpelvis, and the biparietal diameter tends to descend through this narrowed area. If the interspinous diameter is wide, the head may pass this level in the direct transverse position.

Position and Configuration of the Sacrum

If the sacrum is far posterior at all levels, providing ample posterior space throughout, the head may traverse the entire pelvis in the posterior position. If the sacrum is directed somewhat anteriorly in its lower portion, the occiput tends to rotate into the more ample anterior pelvis. If the sacrum is forward throughout, as in the flat pelvis, the head tends to descend through the midpelvis in the transverse position.

Width of the Subpubic Arch and Transverse Diameter of the Outlet

When the subpubic arch is wide, the occiput may stem closely under the symphysis, using all of the space (Fig. 32-26). If the arch is narrowed or if the transverse diameter of the outlet is shortened, the head is prevented from stemming under the symphysis and is forced to pass more posteriorly than it normally would. If the sacrum is far posterior, narrowing of the arch may have no practical significance except to require a wider episiotomy. If the sacrum is anterior, however, serious outlet disproportion may result.

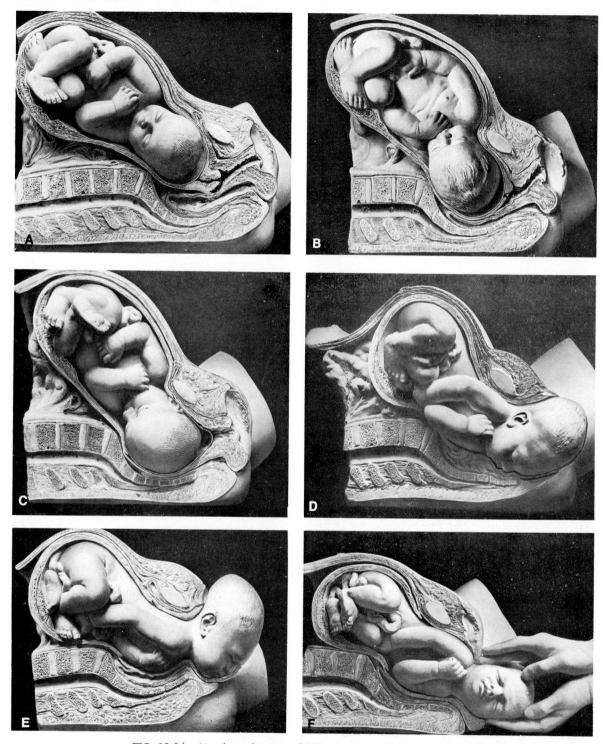

FIG. 32-24. Usual mechanism of labor in gynecoid pelvis. (*A*) Head engages in transverse position. (*B*) It flexes a bit more and descends into midpelvis, and (*C*) begins its internal rotation to occiput anterior position. (*D, E*) As head advances, it negotiates pelvic curve by extension. (*F*) Since shoulders traverse pelvis in oblique diameter without rotation, head undergoes external restitution toward its former transverse position immediately after it is delivered. (Reproduced with permission from Birth Atlas, 5th ed, 1960. Published by Maternity Center Association, New York)

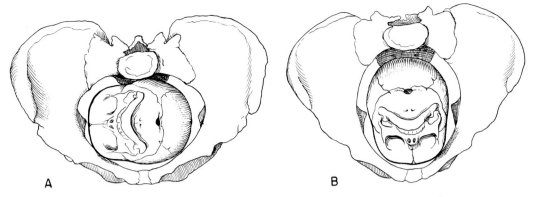

FIG. 32-25. Influence of inlet shape on engagement. Long axis of fetal head adjusts to longest inlet diameter. (*A*) Transverse positions occur in platypelloid type of pelvis. (*B*) Posterior or anterior oblique positions occur in anthropoid type. (Steer CM: Moloy's Evaluation of the Pelvis in Obstetrics, 2nd ed. Philadelphia, WB Saunders, 1959)

Figure 32-27 shows the mechanism of labor that characterizes each of the four pure pelvic types. Since most pelves are mixed types that do not conform exactly to any one of these, the mechanism of labor may differ from the classic mechanisms shown in the diagram, in accordance with the particular pelvic features that obtain at each level of the pelvis. It is emphasized that, no matter how badly formed the pelvis may be, the head can traverse it without incident if the pelvis is large enough and the fetus is small enough.

Among the most formidable conditions are those presented by the effort of an average-sized head to traverse an average-sized android, or "funnel," pelvis in which the spines are prominent, the sidewalls converge, the lower sacrum is forward, and the subpubic arch is narrow. If vaginal delivery is to be attempted, the physician must determine which pelvic diameter—the anteroposterior or the transverse—is the narrowest and try to bring the biparietal diameter through it. If traction in the occiput anterior position meets heavy resistance, the head may be rotated to the transverse position and traction attempted to test whether the anteroposterior diameter can accommodate the biparietal and whether the interspinous diameter is long enough to permit the head to pass this area in the transverse position. If this also offers heavy resistance, cesarean section is the

proper solution because injudicious traction either in the wrong diameter or against undue resistance may irretrievably damage the fetus and seriously injure the mother.

Influence of the Pelvic Axis

With a gynecoid pelvis and a cephalic presentation in the occiput transverse position, internal rotation occurs in the midpelvis, and the pelvic curve is negotiated by extension of the head (Fig. 32-24). In the case of a face presentation with mentum anterior, the pelvic curve can also be readily negotiated by flexion of the head, with the chin instead of the occiput stemming behind and under the symphysis. A different problem is presented when the head enters the pelvis with either the occiput or the chin in the posterior position (Figs. 32-28 and 32-29). In the occiput posterior position, the head is already flexed, with chin on chest, to the maximum extent. Hence, it can advance only if the sacrum is far posterior, as it is in the monkey (in which delivery with face to pubes is the rule); or if it can rotate to the anterior position. In the first instance, if the posterior segment of the pelvis is very wide at all levels, the head may reach the pelvic floor in the direct posterior positon

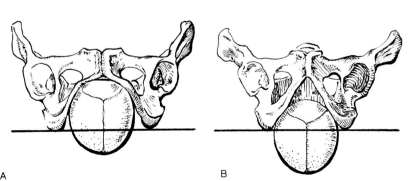

FIG. 32-26. Influence of shape of subpubic arch. (*A*) Wide (gynecoid) subpubic arch, head stemming closely under symphysis. (*B*) Narrow (android) arch, directing head posteriorly and requiring ample posterior segment at outlet and a wide episiotomy.

A   B

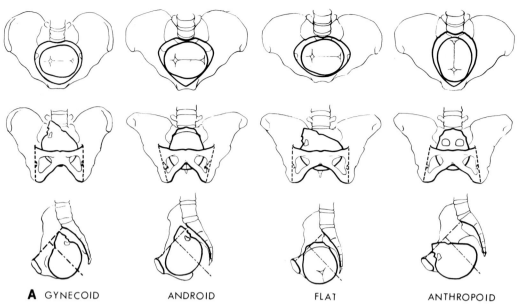

A GYNECOID   ANDROID   FLAT   ANTHROPOID

FIG. 32-27.   Influence of characteristic pelvic variations on labor mechanism. (Danforth DN, Ellis AH: Mid-forceps delivery: A vanishing art? Am J Obstet Gynecol 86:29, 1963)

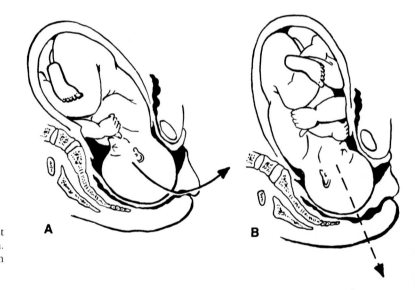

FIG. 32-28.   Cephalic presentation. (*A*) Occiput anterior position. (*B*) Occiput posterior position. Head cannot advance at posterior unless sacrum is far back.

and, in fact, may deliver face to pubes. If the posterior segment is shorter, spontaneous rotation may occur when the occiput strikes this narrowed area; this happens in about 70% of cases. If rotation fails to occur either because prominent spines mechanically prevent rotation or because the uterine contractions fail to supply the needed force, artificial rotation is required.

A mentum posterior presentation offers much more difficulty than an occiput posterior, because it is impossible for a normal-sized head to pass through a normal-sized pelvis in this position. In about one half of cases in which labor starts as mentum posterior, the head ro-

tates spontaneously to chin anterior and, as noted in Chapter 36, normal delivery usually follows. If spontaneous rotation to the anterior fails to occur, cesarean section is needed for delivery because attempts to rotate artificially are almost uniformly unsuccessful and highly damaging.

Breech Presentation

In breech presentation, the following three separate mechanisms are important: the mechanism of the breech, the mechanism of the shoulders, and the mech-

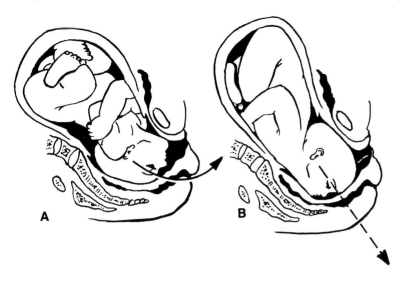

FIG. 32-29. Face presentation. (*A*) Mentum anterior position. (*B*) Mentum posterior position.

anism of the after-coming head. In each case, just as in vertex presentation, the shortest diameter of the fetus passes through the shortest diameter of the pelvis. At the level of the breech, the bitrochanteric diameter is the longer, and it usually (in gynecoid, android, and flat pelves) engages in the transverse position with the sacrum anterior. The breech descends in this position until the sacrum or pelvic floor is encountered and the pelvic curve must be negotiated. Since the anteroposterior mobility of the spine is very limited (especially if it is splinted by the legs), the pelvic curve must be negotiated by lateral flexion of the lumbar spine (Fig. 32-30). The anterior buttock then stems beneath the symphysis, with the fetal back lying either to one side or in an oblique diameter. As the shoulders approach the inlet, the longer bisacromial diameter adapts to the longer transverse diameter of the inlet, rotating to the oblique in the midpelvis, and the anterior shoulder later appears beneath the symphysis. After delivery of both shoulders, the back is usually directly anterior and consequently the head is in the direct occiput anterior position. In the anthropoid pelvis, the head can immediately enter the pelvis in the anterior position without rotation; for this reason an anthropoid pelvis of large size is considered most favorable for breech delivery. Pelves of the gynecoid, android, or flat type, in which cephalopelvic relations are such that all the space must be used, are unfavorable because the head must sometimes be rotated to the transverse position so that the narrow biparietal diameter can pass through the narrower anteroposterior diameter of the inlet. This is a maneuver that can be very awkward when the shoulders are already delivered. After engagement, the head negotiates the pelvic curve and is delivered by increasing flexion.

X-RAY PELVIMETRY

A suitable technique for x-ray pelvimetry is described by Steer in *Moloy's Evaluation of the Pelvis in Obstetrics.* The three basic films that are needed are a standing lateral film; an inlet film, to show the shape of the inlet;

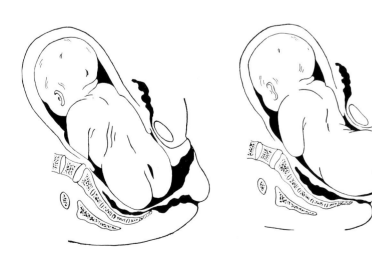

FIG. 32-30. Lateral flexion in breech presentation. (Beck AC, Rosenthal AH: Obstetrical Practice, 6th ed. Copyright © 1955, Williams & Wilkins, Baltimore)

and a subpubic arch film, to show the splay of the side-walls. Examples of the resulting views are shown in Figure 32-27. Techniques that give inadequate information are still commonly used; it is understandable that physicians who insist on using such techniques believe that x-ray pelvimetry is obsolete. When a correct technique is used and the films are interpreted by someone who understands the mechanism of labor, x-ray pelvimetry can be extremely helpful if vaginal delivery is contemplated and there is question about the pelvic diameters.

REFERENCES AND RECOMMENDED READING

Caldwell WE, Moloy HC, Swenson PC: Use of the roentgen ray in obstetrics. Am J Roentgenol Radium Ther Nucl Med 41:305, 505, 719, 1938. (These three articles are the classic summary reference to the work of Caldwell and Moloy. Dr. Caldwell was Professor of Obstetrics and Gynecology and Associate Director of the Sloane Hospital for Women, Columbia University. Dr. Moloy was Assistant Clinical Professor of Obstetrics and Gynecology in the same institution. Dr. Swenson was Assistant Attending Radiologist, Presbyterian Hospital and Vanderbilt Clinic, New York City, and was actively concerned in the development and clinical application of the Caldwell–Moloy thesis.)

Danforth DN: Clinical pelvimetry. In Sciarra JJ: Gynecology and Obstetrics, Vol 2, Chap 51. Hagerstown, Harper & Row, 1979

Danforth DN, Ellis AH: Mid-forceps delivery: A vanishing art? Am J Obstet Gynecol 86:29, 1963

Duff P: Diagnosis and management of face presentation. Obstet Gynecol 57:105, 1981

Eastman NJ: Pelvic mensuration: A study in the perpetuation of error. Obstet Gynecol Surv 3:301, 1948

Steer CM: Moloy's Evaluation of the Pelvis in Obstetrics, 3rd ed. New York, Plenum, 1975

Conduct of Normal Labor

David N. Danforth

33

DEFINITIONS

Certain terms that are used in this and succeeding chapters must be defined. The clinical designation of *weeks' gestation* refers to the number of weeks that have elapsed since the first day of the last normal menstrual period, *not* the number of weeks since the date of presumed ovulation or conception. *Labor* is defined as the sequence of events by which the uterus expels the products of conception into the vagina and into the outer world. The term is reserved for pregnancies of more than 20 weeks' duration. Miniature labor does occur in pregnancy terminated before that time, but if delivery occurs prior to the end of 20 weeks' gestation, the term *abortion* must be applied.

The time at which the fetus attains viability has been a point of some confusion. Historically, survival of an infant born before 28 weeks' gestation was so unusual that 28 weeks was usually considered the time of viability. Within the last decade, however, survival of infants born at 27 weeks, 26 weeks, and sometimes even earlier has become increasingly frequent. In a 1979 ruling, the U.S. Supreme Court considered the diagnosis of viability to be the individual physician's determination, one that is not necessarily based on weight, weeks' gestation, or any other parameter. The Court stated that "viability is reached when, in the judgment of the attending physician on the particular facts of the case before him, there is reasonable likelihood of the fetus's sustained survival outside the womb, with or without artificial support."

A *preterm labor* is one that occurs after the 20th but before the end of the 37th week of pregnancy. A *term birth* is one that occurs after the 37th week of pregnancy and before the 43rd week. Delivery occurring after the beginning of the 43rd week of pregnancy is referred to as *postterm birth;* it is quite rare. Some cases of alleged postmaturity are actually term births because confusion

about dates can arise if the patient's menstrual history is inaccurate or if conception was preceded by one to two months of amenorrhea. Similarly, some preterm births are actually term births, because the pregnancy was dated not from the last normal menstrual period but rather from an episode of vaginal bleeding during the first six weeks of pregnancy.

A *parturient* is a woman who is in labor. A woman is said to be *parous* if she has given birth (either vaginally or by cesarean section) to an infant after the 20th week of pregnancy, and her *parity* refers to the number of such deliveries she has had. A *nullipara* has had no deliveries at more than 20 weeks' gestation. A *primipara* has had one delivery at more than 20 weeks' gestation; a *multipara,* more than one. The term *gravida* followed by an arabic or Roman numeral refers to the total number of previous pregnancies (including ectopic pregnancy, hydatidiform mole, abortion, and normal intrauterine pregnancy); *para* followed by an arabic or Roman numeral refers to the number of deliveries after the 20th week of pregnancy (live birth or stillbirth, single or multiple, vaginal or cesarean section). In this context a woman who has had one spontaneous abortion, one ectopic pregnancy, and viable twins delivered by cesarean section is designated as gravida 3 para 1. A group of digits, for example, 0–3, 0–2, is sometimes used to define a woman's reproductive history. The first digit refers to the number of term infants she has delivered, the second to the number of preterm infants, the third to the number of abortions, and the fourth to the number of children currently living. Although this device is intended to be more precise than the traditional designation, it can be confusing. The series of digits given in the example could refer to a woman who has had three preterm births, of whom two children are now living; it could also refer to a woman who has had preterm triplets of whom two survived or to a woman who has had one preterm single labor and one preterm twin labor with two currently living children. The traditional designation of parity and gravidity is recommended and should be supplemented by additional information as needed.

A *precipitate labor* is one that lasts less than three hours. *Prolonged labor* was formerly defined as a labor lasting more than 24 hours. However, the Terminology Committee of the American College of Obstetricians and Gynecologists suggests that prolonged labor is active labor that continues more than 20 hours. Most obstetricians are satisfied that 18 hours is the upper limit for normal labor.

THE PRODROMES OF LABOR

There are three major prodromes of labor: lightening, Braxton Hicks contractions, and cervical effacement. In the primigravid patient, *lightening,* which refers to the settling of the presenting part into the pelvis, usually occurs two to four weeks before labor. If a primigravid patient goes into labor with the presenting part unengaged, there is a high probability of inlet disproportion. In the multiparous patient, however, lightening may not occur until after the beginning of labor. The disparity between primigravid and multiparous patients in this regard suggests that the phenomenon may result from differences in uterine tone (the multipara having the more relaxed uterus), but the muscular tone of the myometrium in the multipara does not differ significantly from that in the primigravida. Simple relaxation of the lower pole of the uterus as a passive phenomenon does not explain the disparity. It has been shown that before lightening the lower pole of the uterus is conical, whereas after lightening it is cup-shaped. Since intense myometrial activity is characteristic of pregnancy, the best explanation is that the changes result from the active pulling up of the lower pole of the uterus around the presenting part. It is reasonable also to presume that the presenting part does not merely fall into the pelvis, but rather is pushed there by myometrial activity pulling against the pericervical axis and supports. Lightening usually occurs gradually over the course of weeks. The patient is usually aware of it because of the added comfort and ease of breathing that result, but these advantages are balanced by increased distress from pelvic pressure, urinary frequency, and constipation.

The rhythmic tightening of the uterus, known as *Braxton Hicks contractions* (see p. 606), may be painful but is for the most part irregular in frequency, duration, and intensity. In the first pregnancy, Braxton Hicks contractions are generally painless until an hour or so before the onset of labor, but with each succeeding pregnancy such painful contractions are likely to precede the onset of true labor by an increasingly long period. A woman in her eighth or ninth pregnancy may find Braxton Hicks contractions extremely painful as early as the fifth or sixth month. Such contractions are often difficult to distinguish from true labor pains and may be referred to, usually in retrospect, as *false labor.* Despite their painful

nature, careful examination usually discloses the irregularity in frequency, duration, intensity, or all three.

The softening and thinning of the cervix, which are referred to as *cervical effacement* (see p. 620), generally become evident in both primigravida and multigravida about a month before term and are usually accompanied by slight dilatation of the cervix. *Bloody show,* a discharge of pink mucus, sometimes results from the cervical changes and may precede labor by periods varying from an hour to a week or more.

In addition to the three major prodromes, the following phenomena commonly occur in the days or weeks preceding labor:

Loss of 1 lb to 3 lb in weight because of water loss resulting from electrolyte shifts that in turn are produced by changes in estrogen and progesterone levels

Increase in frequency of urination because of reduction in bladder capacity by pressure of the presenting part

Increase in vaginal secretions due to the extreme congestion of the vaginal mucous membranes

Increasing backache and sacroiliac distress due to relaxation of the pelvic joints.

THE STAGES OF LABOR

Labor is divided into three stages. The first stage begins with the onset of regular uterine contractions accompanied by progressive dilatation of the cervix. It ends when the cervix is fully dilated. The first stage, then, is the stage of dilatation of the cervix. The exact moment of its onset may be difficult to record.

The second stage of labor begins when the cervix is completely dilated and ends when the fetus is completely delivered. Although there is slight advancement of the presenting part in the first stage, it is not until the second stage, when the uterus gains purchase on the ligamentary supports, that uterine evacuation actually begins (see Fig. 31-31). The second stage, then, is the stage of delivery.

The third stage of labor begins when delivery of the infant is complete and ends when the placenta and membranes are delivered. This is the placental stage.

Character of Contractions

As noted in Chapter 31, at the onset of the first stage, contractions usually occur every five to eight minutes, last 20 to 30 seconds, and achieve intrauterine pressures of 20 to 30 mm Hg. As the first stage advances, the contractions gradually improve in quality; by the end of the first stage, they occur every two to four minutes, last 30 to 50 seconds, and produce intrauterine pressures of about 50 mm Hg. Second-stage contractions normally occur every two to three minutes and last about 60 seconds, producing intrauterine pressures of about 100 mm Hg, but bearing-down efforts may cause these pressures to exceed 100 mm Hg. In the third stage, the contractions are rarely painful, although intramyometrial pressures of 250 mm Hg are common.

Length of Labor

During the days, and occasionally weeks, before the actual onset of labor, the cervix gradually begins to soften, to become thinner, and to dilate slightly. Hence, when labor starts, the cervix is already dilated 1 to 3 cm in both nulliparous and multiparous patients. As a rule, the first stage of labor is completed within eight hours in a first labor and within four to six hours in subsequent labors. If the first stage of labor lasts more than 12 hours, or if cervical dilatation arrests for more than two hours, labor is considered abnormal.

The duration of the second stage depends entirely on the amount of resistance to be overcome. In a multipara with a small baby, the second stage may be only momentary, and delivery may occur promptly when the cervix is fully dilated. In a primipara, or in a multipara with a large baby, considerable voluntary effort (bearing down) may be needed to advance the baby through the birth canal. The second stage of labor is considered prolonged, although not necessarily abnormal, if it lasts more than one hour. An active, vigorous second stage must be terminated (by vaginal delivery or cesarean section) after two hours because of the threat of uterine rupture, constriction ring dystocia, or fetal injury.

It is well known that succeeding labors tend to be shorter until the fifth or sixth pregnancy, after which labor is apt to lengthen. The shortening of labor is usually attributed to the somewhat more lax cervix and the progressively decreased resistance offered by the soft parts; the lengthening of labor after the fifth or sixth pregnancy is attributed to an increase in the connective tissue of the myometrium with consequent impairment of uterine coordination.

CONDUCT OF THE FIRST AND SECOND STAGES OF LABOR

In all fields of medicine new knowledge begets new procedures and new regimens whose purpose is to improve results. In obstetrics, the new methods and new approaches have produced a decline in both maternal mortality (from 37.1 per 100,000 live births in 1960 to 9.9 per 100,000 live births in 1977) and also in perinatal mortality (from 29.3 per 1000 live births in 1960 to 19.6 per 1000 in 1977). Both rates continue to decline, and perinatal mortality has dropped by 47% since 1965. These spectacular advancements are largely caused by an increase in the availability and quality of prenatal care, new developments in the conduct and monitoring of labor, and pediatric advances in the care of the newborn.

The new hospital routines that have made so important a contribution to reducing maternal and perinatal mortality have not been fully accepted. Many regard childbirth as an intensely personal experience to be shared by other members of the family, and specific criticism has been leveled at the restricted, sterile, and sometimes stark conditions of the labor and delivery rooms, the immense "gadgetry," and the increased cesarean section rate, which some allege to be the direct result of fetal monitoring. Many women with these attitudes seek delivery at home, a practice that major health organizations have determined to be accompanied by unacceptably greater risk to both mother and infant. Many hospitals have responded to the criticisms by providing what is referred to as "family-centered maternity care," which has the enthusiastic approval of the organizations comprising the Interprofessional Task Force on the Health Care of Women and Infants.* The recommended practices include allowing the husband or "supporting other" to be present as much as possible during and after labor; a flexible program that allows the mother to keep the newborn in her room; special visiting dispensations for children; optional early release from the hospital; breastfeeding and handling the baby immediately after delivery; childbirth preparation classes for expectant couples; and availability of a "birthing room," which is a combination labor and delivery room that has a homelike atmosphere and is adjacent to the delivery room in case of emergency, but has no external evidence of the standard monitoring and support systems.

The protocol for birthing rooms varies from one hospital to another; even the same hospital may offer different options. In some, indoctrinated children are permitted to remain throughout labor. Some hospitals accede to the request for no electronic monitoring; some recommend such monitoring for 15 minutes every hour; some require monitoring for the first 30 minutes after admission (to record baseline characteristics and possible decelerative patterns) and again continuously after the cervix reaches 8 cm dilatation. Usually, labor must be conducted in a standard labor room if electronic monitoring, either optional or indicated, is to be continuous. In some birthing rooms, patients must rely entirely on Lamaze training or its equivalent for analgesia, while a partial or full range of analgesia and anesthesia is available in others. Spontaneous delivery without episiotomy is an objective in most birthing rooms, and procedures such as episiotomy and outlet forceps require removal to a standard delivery room; in other facilities, these procedures may be performed in the birthing room.

---

* American Academy of Pediatrics, American College of Nurse–Midwives, American College of Obstetricians and Gynecologists, American Nurses' Association, Nurses Association of the American College of Obstetricians and Gynecologists.

Obstetricians must recognize these new challenges to traditional obstetric practice. Also, they must be aware of the emotional needs and societal forces that have generated the new attitudes, as well as the data that bear on the propriety of the requested protocols. Having evaluated all of these factors, physicians must select the range of options that they can conscientiously offer their patients and should deviate from this only if a new service or option will offer greater safety or an improved result. The desire to let nature take its course must never be carried so far that the basic principles of good obstetric practice are neglected.

Three fundamental concepts must be kept in mind. First, in the vast majority of cases, labor and delivery are physiologic processes and do not, in the true sense, require "management." Second, the functions of the medical attendant are to promote the successful termination of the process and to anticipate and deal with abnormal conditions. Third, precautions must be taken at all times to avoid endangering or injuring either the mother or the baby.

At the onset of labor most patients are confident and prepared for the task in store, but there is also an element of uncertainty and emotional stress, regardless of the patient's mien or her parity. This will be compounded if the medical attendant (physician or nurse–midwife) manifests hesitance, flippancy or thoughtlessness, or haste that is inconsistent with the needs of that particular patient. Reassurance and support, both emotional and physical, are keystones of the successful conduct of labor.

When to Come to the Hospital

The woman should be advised to come to the hospital when any of the following three circumstances occur:

1. Uterine contractions. It is reasonably certain that labor is starting when contractions have occurred every ten minutes for as long as an hour and have begun to be painful. If the pain is unremitting or severe, the patient should not wait for an hour to pass, but should come to the hospital at once.
2. Ruptured membranes. This may occur as a sudden uncontrollable gush of watery fluid or as continuous slow leakage of fluid from the vagina. The latter must be distinguished from urinary incontinence, which is not uncommon in the later months of pregnancy; if the leakage continues after voiding, the membranes are probably ruptured and the patient should be admitted to the hospital.
3. Bleeding. Active bleeding, equivalent to a normal menstrual period, is an indication for admission to the hospital even if it is not accompanied by discomfort. Bloody show, which results from the cervical changes of early labor or prelabor, usually consists of a pink, mucoid discharge; it suggests that labor may start within hours or days, but unaccompanied

by other signs, it is not an indication for admission to the hospital.

Admission to the Hospital

For all registered patients a detailed medical, surgical, and obstetric history (see p. 164), as well as the results of a complete physical examination, should be on file in the delivery room. If no information is available, it should be obtained before delivery if time permits; if not, it must be obtained after delivery.

General Evaluation and Preparation

While assisting the patient to bed, the nurse should obtain the following information and record it in the chart: the time of onset and frequency of the contractions; whether the membranes appear to be ruptured or intact; whether there has been any vaginal bleeding and, if so, its character; the time and content of the last meal; and whether the patient wears dentures or contact lenses. The nurse should also take and record the patient's temperature, pulse, and rate of respiration; collect a urine specimen for analysis; and either take or order an admission hematocrit.

The attendant should then evaluate the patient's obstetric status at once, before proceeding to other matters. In order to determine whether delivery is imminent or whether there is any major obstetric problem, the attendant should perform the following:

1. Take the patient's blood pressure.
2. Listen to the fetal heart between contractions and immediately after a contraction. The heart tones should be regular, and the rate should be 120 to 160 beats/minutes. Irregularity or rates outside these limits may suggest fetal hypoxia.
3. Feel a uterine contraction to note its duration, intensity, and whether the uterus relaxes well between contractions.
4. If there is no history of bleeding, make a sterile vaginal examination to determine the station and symmetry of the presenting part; the effacement, dilatation, and position of the cervix; and the adequacy of the pelvis.

A *sterile vaginal examination* includes an antiseptic wash or spray of the introitus and adjacent skin, use of sterile gloves, and separation of the labia by the index and middle fingers of the opposite hand before the examining fingers are introduced. A sterile lubricant is desirable unless there is discharge of blood or mucus, in which case it is not needed. The index finger is usually sufficient for this examination and is considerably less uncomfortable for the patient than an examination with index and middle fingers, especially in a primigravida.

The *station of the presenting part* and the method of recording it are discussed on page 638. *Symmetry,* in vertex presentation, means that the head should be found on vaginal examination to be symmetric, firm, and rounded. With persistence it is usually possible to feel some of the sutures in the fetal head and to determine its exact position, but the attempt at this stage only increases discomfort, prolongs the examination, and produces information that is rarely needed until labor is more advanced. Accordingly, the obstetrician should be content if the initial examination shows the head to be symmetric and well engaged (station +1 or lower) and if the head advances progressively. If the presenting part is found to be irregular (asymmetric), the possibilities of brow, face, or breech presentation, or a monstrosity, must be considered, and steps must be taken at once to make an exact diagnosis. Ultrasound scan may be helpful. An x-ray film of the abdomen is definitive.

Effacement of the cervix (see p. 620) is recorded as a percentage figure: an uneffaced (0%) cervix is firm and about 2.5 cm long; 50% effacement implies that the cervix is about 1 cm thick and somewhat softer; a completely effaced cervix (100%) is soft and only a few millimeters thick. Cervical dilatation is recorded in centimeters. It is important to know the *position of the cervix.* If it is far posterior in early labor and difficult to reach, the labor may be longer than usual because the first part of it, before significant dilatation occurs, is devoted to advancing the cervix anteriorly into the axis of the vagina. If the cervix is difficult to reach, it can often be made more accessible if the head is moved posteriorly by suprapubic pressure during the vaginal examination. There is no good explanation of why this maneuver may bring the cervix sufficiently anterior for the obstetrician to determine its dilatation more easily.

The method of *estimating pelvic capacity* is considered in Chapter 32, and such an estimation should be noted on the prenatal record. When the patient goes into labor, however, the question of whether her particular pelvis is large enough to accommodate her particular fetus must be answered. In a primigravid patient, the head should be engaged at the onset of labor (and usually a few weeks before); if it is unengaged in early labor, the possibility of inlet disproportion should be considered and kept in mind if the head fails to advance as labor progresses. If the head is already engaged, the possibility of inlet disproportion is eliminated, and attention should be directed to the ischial spines and the position of the sacrum. Excessively prominent spines may suggest transverse narrowing of the midpelvis, with the attendant problems that are considered in Chapter 32. If the head is engaged to station +2, there should be ample space to insert the index finger between the head and the sacrum; if this space is snug, it may suggest anteroposterior flattening, which may need to be taken into account at the time of delivery.

If delivery is not imminent, the prenatal record should be read carefully and specific questions asked to determine whether there is any current or recent sore throat or upper respiratory infection, whether there has

been any recent illness, whether any pregnancy problems have occurred that might not be entered on the prenatal record, whether the patient is taking any medications or drugs, and whether she is allergic to any medications. A complete history should be taken if no prenatal record is available.

The physical examination during labor is extremely important, but it need not be as detailed as the customary physical examination unless no prenatal information is available; in the latter event, a detailed examination should be made. The routine labor examination should include blood pressure, throat and teeth, heart, and lungs; the sacral and pretibial areas should be examined for edema. The relevant information to be gained on examination of the abdomen is supplied by the Leopold maneuvers (see Figs. 20-5 to 20-9) in the course of which the presentation and position can be determined and the size of the infant can be estimated. It is not possible to estimate the infant's weight within a pound with any regularity, and sometimes this estimate is even more incorrect. An effort should be made, however, to obtain an accurate estimate of whether the baby is large, small, or of average size.

The remainder of the admission procedure consists of a shower (if needed and feasible), the "prep," and, usually, an enema. It was formerly believed that asepsis required shaving the pubic, vulvar, and perineal hair, but it is now agreed that this is uncomfortable and unnecessary. Accordingly, the shave is limited to the area of the possible episiotomy, and long pubic and vulvar hair is clipped with scissors. There is some difference of opinion regarding the need for an enema. Most obstetricians prefer that one be given shortly after admission unless labor is extremely active, delivery is imminent, or there is a history of recent bleeding. If there is adequate time, the enema may reflexly stimulate and improve coordination of uterine contractions, and it also gives reasonable assurance that the lower bowel will be empty and the fecal column will not be expelled as the head advances, contaminating the delivery field. If the patient objects to an enema, it can usually be omitted.

Determination of the State of Membranes

The membranes may rupture before the onset of labor, at any time during labor, or when the head emerges. A damp area under the buttocks may suggest that the membranes have ruptured, but it may be caused by urine, which can be identified by odor. The management of labor depends in many cases on whether the membranes are ruptured. The usual methods of determining this are listed on page 482.

Labor

Diagnosis of Onset

The onset of labor is marked by the beginning of progressive cervical dilatation in response to regular, usually painful, uterine contractions. This point may be impossible to define precisely, especially if it is preceded by a prodromal period of fairly regular, forceful, painful contractions that have no influence on the cervix. Thus, the diagnosis of prodromes of labor and false labor is usually retrospective, because a period must pass before it can be determined whether the cervix has undergone change.

In some cases, labor starts abruptly; more frequently, and especially in nulliparous women, there is a prodromal period of one to eight more hours during which the contractions occur at intervals of 10 to 15 minutes, cause only slight discomfort, and are quite short. The interval between contractions then shortens progressively, and the contractions gradually lengthen and become more intense. As a rule, the patient is considered to be in labor when contractions of good quality have occurred at regular intervals of six minutes or less for at least one hour. The probability of labor is strengthened if there is also bleeding caused by the opening of small blood vessels in the cervix as effacement and dilatation begin, or if the membranes rupture. The physiology of the transition from prodromal to actual labor is described in Chapter 31.

False labor is defined as a period of fairly regular, painful contractions that are not accompanied by effacement or dilatation of the cervix and that may either stop completely or be followed, either promptly or ultimately, by the onset of true labor. False labor is a form of disordered uterine action and is discussed further in Chapter 37.

It is important that false labor be diagnosed. By using an external monitor for uterine contractions, it is usually possible to make the distinction between true and false labor without waiting several hours to note whether cervical dilatation has begun. It has been mentioned that the contractions of true labor are absolutely regular and are all of the same or gradually increasing intensity and duration. Although the contractions of false labor may be forceful at times, they do not exhibit the absolute regularity of actual labor. Two or three contractions, or more, of excellent quality may occur at intervals of two to three minutes, to be followed by an eight- or ten-minute interval of quiescence; or the regular intense contractions, after ten minutes or more, may be followed by a few fleeting contractions of low intensity. If false labor occurs, its nature should be explained to the patient and her family so they will be aware that delivery is not imminent. In some instances, anxiety and pain are severe, and sedatives and analgesics are required for their relief. These drugs must be used with caution. Morphine may be given in a single dose in an effort to terminate false labor; repeated doses should be avoided, however, because addiction is always a hazard.

Cervical dilatation is the fundamental clinical phenomenon of the first stage of labor. The cervix normally dilates just far enough to permit the passage of whatever fetal part is presented to the cervix. The diameter of the flexed head of an average-sized fetus is between 9 cm and 10 cm. Full or complete dilatation is considered to be about 10 cm. The body of the average fetus will easily pass through a cervix dilated enough to permit the passage of the head. Note, however, that if the largest diameter of the presenting fetal head is only 8 cm (because of prematurity or microcephaly), from a physiological point of view 8 cm is full dilatation.

For the first stage of labor to be considered normal, complete dilatation must be reached within 12 hours, but the average is much less than that. Multiparas usually reach full dilatation in about half the time that nulliparas do. After the fifth or sixth delivery, labor tends to get longer. Dilatation does not ordinarily proceed at a constant rate. Typically, dilatation is slow until a dilatation of 4 cm to 5 cm is reached, then rapid until dilatation is nearly complete, then slower until full diltation is achieved. If the cervix can be felt on vaginal examination, dilatation is not complete.

One of the duties of the professional attendant during labor is to determine the amount of cervical dilatation from time to time. It will then be known how labor is progressing. The curves of the normal rate of dilatation (Fig. 36-3) should be kept in mind. Significant deviations from the normal rate of progress should alert the physician to the presence of abnormality.

The First Stage of Labor

Several matters require consideration during the first stage of labor.

CHARTING. A chart note is required at least every hour during the first stage. This may be either a written note or an entry in the labor sheet; if progress is not rapid, only the character of the contractions and apparent progress as judged by abdominal examination may be noted. The partogram (see Fig. 37-1) is an extremely useful device that permits immediate and exact appraisal of the course and quality of labor. Normally the cervix dilates at a rate of approximately 1 cm/hour. Utilizing this observation, Philpott and Castle recommended that dilatation be plotted on a graph on which "alert" and "action" lines have been constructed (Fig. 37-3). In normal labor the dilatation curve remains in zone 1; if dilatation lags, the curve enters zone 2, which indicates dysfunctional labor and the need for special evaluation. If the curve enters zone 3, intervention is strongly indicated. To account for the differing cervical dilatation at the time of admission, Studd and Duignan constructed a series of curves to show mean progressive cervical dilatation of normal primigravidas according to admission dilatation. Using a stencil, the correct curve is affixed to the patient's chart; any deviations from the normal curve are immediately evident.

A narrative note should be written if any abnormalities occur or if intervention is contemplated. It should be emphasized that all notes in the chart must be legible, signed, timed, and dated. The labor may need to be reconstructed a year or so hence for medical or legal reasons and it can be immensely frustrating to try to decipher an untimed, scribbled note by one whose signature is illegible (Fig. 33-1).

Tromans and colleagues have reported a method for continuous feto–maternal surveillance in labor that uses a microcomputer. This is a technique that will probably be used increasingly in the future.

EXAMINATIONS. Careful evaluation of the patient's subjective and objective symptoms and accurate interpretation of the findings on abdominal examination are sufficient for following the progress of most of the labor. At least three vaginal examinations are needed: on admission, midway through the first stage when discomfort becomes more marked or medication is requested, and when the signs suggest that the cervix is fully dilated. Vaginal examination should also be done when the membranes rupture (to be sure a loop of cord has not prolapsed), and at other times as needed to determine progress or the lack of it. Arterial pulsations are sometimes felt either inside the cervix or peripheral to it. If they are synchronous with the maternal pulse, they are produced by an artery in the rectovaginal septum or cervix. If they are synchronous with the fetal heartbeat, they are due to cord prolapse or vasa previa and are invariably of ominous portent.

POSTURE IN LABOR. When in normal labor, the patient may sit in a chair or walk when the labor is not too active, the membranes are intact, and no analgesia has been administered. If she is in bed, the lateral recumbent posture, as opposed to the supine, is preferred because deviations in fetal pulse tracings occur less frequently in this position, and the possibility of the supine hypotensive syndrome (see p. 734) is eliminated.

NUTRIMENT AND FLUIDS. The emptying time of the stomach is greatly prolonged in labor; in some cases, vomitus may contain food ingested 24 hours earlier. Consequently, nothing is permitted by mouth after labor starts. Fluids are essential, however, and an infusion of 5% dextrose in water is usually started shortly after ad-

FIG. 33-1. Example of vexing narrative chart note: no date or time is recorded, and both note and author's signature are illegible.

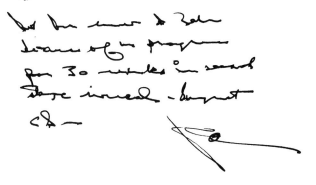

mission, to run at the rate of 1000 ml every eight hours. This may be omitted if labor is expected to be terminated by vaginal delivery within a few hours.

ANTACIDS. Aspiration of gastric contents is the most common cause of anesthetic death in obstetrics and is a serious threat if general anesthesia is suddenly required. Its effects can be minimized if the acidic gastric juice is neutralized, and some physicians have advocated administration of magnesium trisilicate or an equivalent every two hours during labor. Since the particulate matter of such antacids can cause severe and sometimes massive pneumonitis if aspirated, a clear antacid (*e.g.,* 15 ml of 0.3 M sodium citrate in 20% syrup) is preferred and is given as a single dose a few minutes before the induction of anesthesia. The preventive value of antacids is not improved by administering them at regular intervals throughout labor.

ANALGESIA. Obstetric analgesia is discussed in Chapter 34. In addition to its pain-relieving qualities, analgesia may also help to relax parturients who are tense and apprehensive.

BLADDER. A full bladder can reflexly impede the course of labor. The woman should be asked to void every several hours during labor; if she cannot void, the bladder should be emptied by catheter whenever it can be felt abdominally. In advanced labor, catheterization can often be avoided by inserting two fingers vaginally, one on either side of the urethra, and applying suprapubic pressure during the active phase of a contraction.

TEMPERATURE, PULSE, RESPIRATION, AND BLOOD PRESSURE. Measurements of temperature, pulse, respiratory rate, and blood pressure should be taken and recorded every four hours during labor. These measurements should be taken more often if any are abnormal.

FETAL MONITORING. There are differing opinions on whether normal women who are at low risk benefit from continuous electronic monitoring of fetal heart rate and uterine contractions (see Chap. 41), but there is no question that this practice is clearly indicated and may be lifesaving among those whose fetuses are at risk. Since unexpected fetal hypoxia can occur among low-risk women (*e.g.,* due to a low-lying cord), the burden of proof appears to be on those who deliberately ignore the information to be gained from the routine monitoring of all women in labor. If continuous electronic monitoring is not being used, auscultation of the fetal heart should be done every 15 minutes during the first stage of labor and every 5 minutes for periods of 30 seconds in the second stage.

PSYCHOLOGIC SUPPORT. Of all the devices for the psychologic support of the patient during labor, the most important is the physical presence of another person.

The person need not be qualified to provide medical assistance; for example, the husband can be invaluable for this duty. Other psychologic aids are pleasantness, optimism, patience, gentleness, and an ability to convince the patient that she is the chief concern at the moment. The attendant should never discuss unpleasant aspects of some other patient's labor with the patient or within her hearing.

Amniotomy

The membranes usually rupture spontaneously during the first or second stage of labor. If not, they may sometimes retard progress, and amniotomy (artificial rupture) may be done. Some form of clamp or sharp instrument should be used. The patient must be prepared for vaginal examination. Sterile gloves should be worn by the examiner. If the membranes bulge far in advance of the head, and especially if the presenting part is at or above station +1, the membranes should be punctured between uterine contractions. If they are broken during a contraction, the amniotic fluid may be expelled with such force that the cord prolapses. Descent and dilatation usually accelerate after amniotomy. When labor is especially active, the possibility of amniotic fluid embolism appears to be lessened if as much fluid as possible is drained by slightly elevating the presenting part when the first flow stops. Stewart and colleagues found that early amniotomy significantly shortens the length of labor and reduces the need for augmentation and instrumental delivery. They found no adverse effects on the fetus.

Summary of Danger Signs in Labor

One of the major functions of the professional attendants during labor is careful and continued observation for the detection of abnormalities. These should be suspected in every labor, because no labor can be called normal until it is completed. Some of the danger signs are listed in Table 33-1.

Signs of Full Dilatation of the Cervix

A subtle or abrupt change in the patient's mien often occurs when the cervix becomes fully dilated. Most commonly, involuntary bearing-down efforts are noted. An episode of vomiting late in the first stage may suggest full dilatation, as may a significant increase in the amount of bloody show. Sweat collects on the upper lip in many women at this time, and its sudden appearance should suggest the possibility of full dilatation. Certain evidence of full dilatation must be obtained by vaginal examination. Perineal bulging and gaping of the anus appear late in the second stage, when delivery is imminent.

The Second Stage of Labor

The second stage of labor should normally be completed, and the infant delivered, within one hour after the cervix becomes fully dilated.

Bearing-down efforts are usually reflexive and spontaneous. In some multiparas, and occasionally in primigravidas, two or three bearing-down efforts may suffice to advance the baby through the birth canal and to complete delivery. More frequently, and especially in the primigravida, significant voluntary effort is needed, and encouragement by the attendant can be extremely helpful. The knees should be hyperflexed toward the flanks so the force of uterine contractions (the axis of drive) is directly into the pelvic inlet. The woman should take a deep breath at the onset of the contraction and bear down exactly as though she were attempting to have a bowel movement. She should relax fully when the contraction is over. In some cases, the effectiveness of bearing down can be improved if two or three breaths of 50% nitrous oxide and 50% oxygen are taken at the beginning of the contraction. As a rule, the head advances slightly, but sometimes imperceptibly, with each contraction. When the perineum bulges and the scalp is visible, an episiotomy may permit spontaneous delivery; if it does not, the use of outlet forceps (a "lift-out delivery") is infinitely preferable to allowing prolonged pressure of the head against the pelvic floor in an effort to avoid forceps delivery.

Preparation for Delivery

Asepsis is a prime consideration in the delivery room. All personnel must wear freshly laundered clothing, cap, and mask. Clean shoe covers minimize the danger of tracking dirt from outside the labor and delivery areas. The basic purpose of antisepsis is to prevent the transfer of potentially virulent organisms from patient to patient or from personnel to patient. Prevention is at least as important as antibiotics in reducing the incidence and severity of puerperal infection.

In some hospitals there is a trend toward following the European custom of using the same bed for labor and delivery. If this is not followed, the patient should be transferred from the labor room to the delivery room in ample time to permit the usual preparations for delivery, but not so early that she will have to spend much time on the uncomfortable delivery table before she is ready to deliver. As a rule, the patient in her first labor should be moved to the delivery room when the head has advanced sufficiently to cause the perineum to bulge during contractions, or if in the second stage there is evidence of fetal distress, or if her bearing-down efforts would be assisted by inhalation analgesia (50% nitrous oxide, 50% oxygen) during the contractions. The multiparous patient, depending upon the speed of labor, should be moved to the delivery room when the cervix is dilated 6 cm to 8 cm.

When the patient has been moved to the delivery table, she must not be left unattended. If she has had medication for pain relief, the attendant must not turn away from her even for an instant.

For spontaneous delivery, a flat surface is usually preferred; if the woman is on a delivery table, the end should not be "broken," and she may assume whatever

Table 33-1
Summary of Danger Signs in Labor

Observation or Finding	Possible Significance
Fetal heart rate rapid, slow, or irregular	Fetal distress; prolapsed or occult cord
Presenting part	
Irregular	Breech, face, brow presentation; fetal monstrosity
Not palpable in pelvis	Transverse or oblique lie
Unengaged	Inlet disproportion; malpresentation (brow)
Failure to descend after cervix fully dilated	Midpelvic disproportion or error in estimate of cervical dilatation
Uterine contractions	
Decrease in frequency, intensity, or duration	Uterine inertia; too much medication
Tetany or failure to relax well between contractions	Premature separation of placenta
Failure of cervix to dilate progressively	False labor; cervical dystocia; abnormal uterine action; excessive medication; cephalopelvic disproportion; error in estimate of cervical dilatation
Vaginal discharge	
Active bleeding	Placenta previa; abruptio placentae; maternal laceration (cervix, uterus, vagina); clotting defect
Amniotic fluid	
Meconium-stained (vertex presentation)	Fetal distress
Port wine-colored	Ruptured vasa previa; abruptio placentae
Foul or "fruity" odor	Intrauterine infection (amnionitis)
Blood pressure	
Elevated	Preeclampsia
Low	Shock; supine hypotensive syndrome; reaction to drug; internal bleeding
Dyspnea, sense of suffocation	Amniotic fluid embolism (may be earliest sign)
Maternal tachycardia	Impending shock; maternal dehydration; atropine reaction
Continuous abdominal pain	Premature separation of placenta; ruptured uterus; extrauterine intra-abdominal surgical emergency
Fever	Infection, either intrauterine or elsewhere
Unconsciousness	Postconvulsive eclampsia or epilepsy; shock; heavy sedation; amniotic fluid embolism
Prolapsed umbilical cord	Without instant action by attendant, intrauterine fetal death

position is most comfortable. In England, the left lateral recumbent (Sims) position has been preferred for many years and is probably most physiologic because it avoids the pressure of the gravid uterus on the inferior vena cava. The supine posture is most commonly used in the United States.

For operative delivery, including delivery by outlet forceps, the lithotomy position is preferred because it improves exposure and provides easier access. The buttocks should project about 2 inches over the end of the table. The stirrups that are usually used are not without hazard, and the legs should not be put into them until delivery is immediately imminent; prolonged pressure from stirrups and straps may cause thrombosis in leg veins or damage to important nerves. A desirable alternative to the use of stirrups, if both a scrub nurse and an assistant are available, is to hold the legs in the manner shown in Figure 33-2. This avoids the stress of stirrups and permits the knees to be advanced as the head crowns, thus minimizing the chance of laceration or extension of the episiotomy.

The final preparations for delivery are now made. The vulva, inner thighs, and abdomen (at least up to the umbilicus) should be thoroughly scrubbed with soap

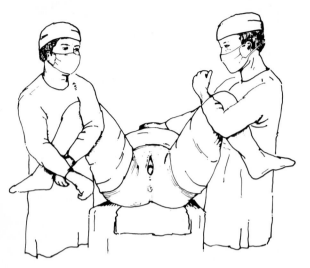

FIG. 33-2. Method of holding legs that avoids sciatic strain and pressure injury, and permits knees to be moved downward as head delivers, or, in breech delivery, as shoulders engage. (After Danforth WC: Forceps. In Curtis AH [ed]: Obstetrics and Gynecology. Philadelphia, WB Saunders, 1933)

and water and rinsed. An antiseptic solution may be applied. The vagina should not be entered during this procedure. Sterile drapes should then be used to cover the leg from toe to crotch, the abdomen, and at least as far up as the nipple line. The draping must be done by someone who has scrubbed and is wearing sterile gown and gloves. Breaks in technique are the joint responsibility of the attendant and all other personnel in the delivery room. Anyone whose sterile covering touches an unclean or unsterile area must drop out at once and change gloves, gown, or both.

Routine catheterization is often carried out, but there is a trend away from this procedure. The danger of introducing infection into the bladder may be greater than the danger of a full bladder.

A vaginal examination is now made to determine the presenting part, its position and station; whether the cervix is fully dilated; and whether the membranes are ruptured. If the membranes are still intact, they should be ruptured.

Delivery

As a general rule, if the head crowns (*i.e.,* distends the vulva, showing at the introitus a patch of scalp 3 cm to 4 cm in diameter), it can be readily delivered either spontaneously or by exerting slight pressure on the fundus (Kristeller expression). If anesthesia is used, the head may not reach the level of crowning or may recede; in this case outlet forceps should be used if the head does not readily advance with slight fundal pressure.

Spontaneous Delivery

Most patients deliver spontaneously if simply left undisturbed (Fig. 33-3). The physician's function is to protect the perineum from excessive damage by encouraging the slow emergence of the head; to prevent cord complications; to assist with delivery of the shoulders, if necessary; to clear the infant's air passages; to encourage the infant to breathe; to assess the condition of the infant; to clamp and cut the cord; to supervise procedures to minimize maternal blood loss; to supervise the delivery of the placenta; to investigate or inspect the uterus, cervix, and vagina; and to suture as needed.

The essence of assistance during spontaneous delivery is promotion of slow distention of the perineum and dilatation of the vaginal orifice and slow delivery of the head and shoulders (the shoulders may cause tearing even when the head did not). The urge to bear down is so violent in some patients that the head or shoulders cause almost complete disintegration of the perineum. Anyone assisting at delivery should try to counteract the violent expulsive efforts by repeated instruction to the patient and should make an episiotomy in ample time if it is needed. As noted earlier, moving the knees forward a few inches tends to relax the perineum and so reduces the possibility of laceration or extension of the episiotomy.

A special procedure to minimize perineal damage is *Ritgen's maneuver.* When the head has advanced far enough so that the chin has passed the mother's coccyx, the fetal head can be grasped by placing one hand on the scalp and the other on the chin through the postanal tissue (the fingers should be covered with several layers of sterile gauze or towel to prevent contamination of the glove). The patient should be cautioned not to bear

FIG. 33-3. Spontaneous delivery. (*A*) Episiotomy, if needed, is made as head begins to crown. (*B, C*) Pressure against perineum causes head to stem closely beneath symphysis, minimizing possibility of extension of episiotomy. (*C, D*) Soft parts may be pushed gently over head as it advances. (*E*) By depressing head slightly and exerting pressure upon fundus, posterior shoulder moves into hollow of sacrum, and anterior shoulder stems beneath symphysis. (*F, G*) Anterior arm is delivered by applying pressure in antecubital fossa. (*H*) Gentle elevation of head delivers posterior shoulder, and (*I*) posterior arm is then delivered. (*J, K*) Thorax, abdomen, and legs follow. (*L*) Immediately after delivery of legs, infant is held up by feet to encourage accumulated secretions to drain before infant takes first breath. (Evanston Hospital. Photos by D. Sherline)

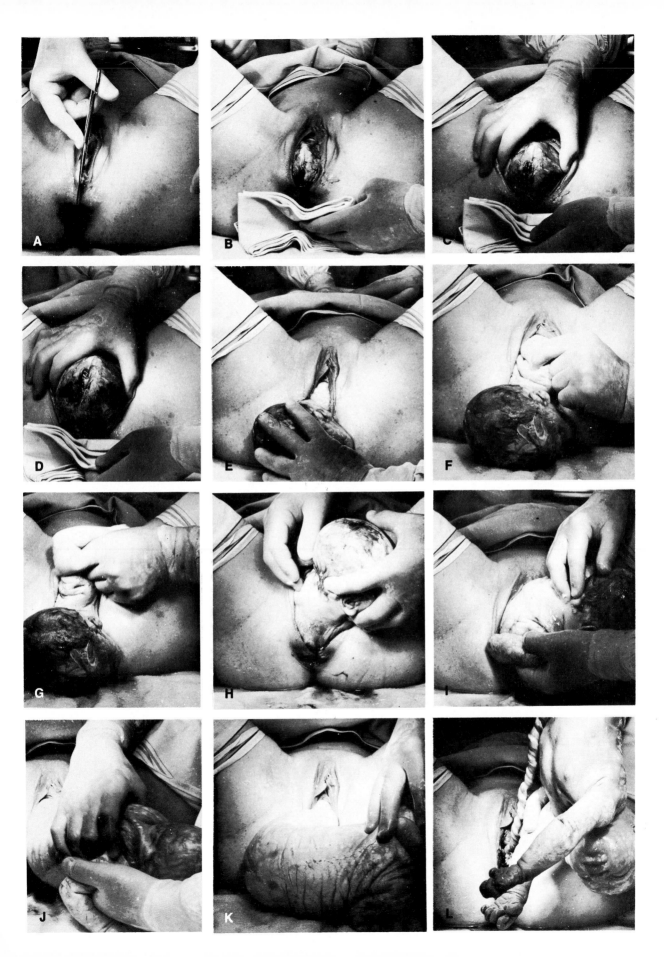

down any more, and the head can then be slowly maneuvered through the vaginal orifice, always under complete control of the operator.

As soon as the head emerges, the infant's neck region should be palpated. Usually, nothing abnormal is felt. In many cases, however, one to six loops of umbilical cord may be felt loosely or tightly wound around the infant's neck. If the loops are tight, circulation through the cord may already have ceased and the infant will probably try to breathe at once. Its airway should therefore be cleared promptly. Other possibilities are that the cord has ruptured; that the cord will rupture as the fetus descends further; that further descent will result in separation of the placenta; or that, as delivery proceeds, the traction on the cord will cause the uterus to turn inside out, an extremely rare but serious complication. If the loops are relatively loose, they can often be relaxed or enlarged so that the infant is delivered through the loops. If there are many loops or they are tight, two clamps should be placed close together on the most easily accessible bit of cord and the cord cut between the clamps. The cord can then be unwound. If either clamp slips off, that end of the cord must be reclamped at once, since it is impossible to know at that moment which end of the cord is attached to the baby and which to the placenta.

After the head emerges, in a completely unaided delivery there may be a pause. The head is no longer pressing on the perineum, and the shoulders have not descended far enough to press on it, so temporarily the patient has no urge to bear down. In addition, the amount of baby in the uterus has suddenly decreased, and it may take a few moments for the uterus to adjust to this decreased volume. Mucus, amniotic fluid, and perhaps a slight amount of blood (maternal) can be seen running out of the infant's mouth and nose (the infant's face is usually directed downward at this time). The infant may move its head, blink its eyes, grimace, gasp, and even cry. Shortly, as the uterus resumes effective contractions, the shoulders are forced into and down through the pelvis, at the same time rotating so that one shoulder is behind the pubis and the other in the hollow of the sacrum. This rotation of the shoulders into the anteroposterior diameter of the pelvis causes the infant's head to rotate, with the back of the head facing toward the side of the mother where the fetal back was positioned during labor. This is the external restitution phase of the mechanism of labor. The anterior shoulder stems or pivots beneath the symphysis, and the posterior shoulder is forced outward. If the delivery is assisted, both shoulders should not be permitted to deliver at once. Just as one would negotiate a porthole, the posterior shoulder should be pushed back slightly and the anterior arm delivered by exerting pressure in the antecubital fossa (Fig. 33-3 *F* and *G*). As the posterior shoulder emerges over the perineum, the rest of the infant follows without delay or particular mechanism.

Immediately after delivery, the infant is held with its head down for a few seconds to permit secretions to drain (Fig. 33-3 *L*) and is then placed supine, either on the end of the delivery table or, if the obstetrician is seated, on a tray placed across his knees. Clearing the airway involves removing foreign material from the infant's mouth and throat. A considerable amount can be removed simply by scooping it out with the finger. Squeezing the nose between the fingers may express small masses of thick mucus. Stroking the upper neck from the larynx toward the mandible (milking) seems to help. A soft rubber suction bulb can be used. Mechanical suction pumps (the tubing must be sterile) are sometimes employed. The gag reflex can be elicited by irritating the base of the tongue or the nasopharynx with the finger. This causes the infant to vomit, and a surprising amount of liquid may be ejected. This prophylactic procedure partially obviates the danger that the infant will vomit and aspirate gastric contents several minutes after delivery without being noticed by the attendant.

In vertex presentation, the presence of meconium in the amniotic fluid is not necessarily a cause for concern, but electronic fetal monitoring is indicated. If the meconium is thick, dark, and copious, and if it appears early in labor, special precautions should be taken to prevent the syndrome of *meconium aspiration*. As soon as the infant's head is delivered, before delivery of the shoulders, a DeLee suction catheter should be passed through the nares to the level of the nasopharynx and any mucus or meconium aspirated. The delivery is then completed routinely. The vocal cords should be visualized with an infant laryngoscope; the presence of meconium at the cords suggests the need for tracheal aspiration.

The official time of birth is the instant at which all of the infant is outside the mother's body. It has nothing to do with breathing, crying, cutting the cord, or any other factor. The second stage of labor terminates and the third stage starts at that moment.

The Apgar score (see p. 811) is taken at one minute and five minutes after birth. Both scores are recorded on the infant's chart.

TIME OF CUTTING THE UMBILICAL CORD.   After delivery, the umbilical cord continues to pulsate for about two minutes. During this time, the infant receives a significant quantity of blood through the cord. The amount varies according to the level, with respect to the introitus, at which the infant is held after delivery. If the infant is held at or below the introitus, the "placental transfusion" amounts to as much as 100 ml; if held above the introitus (for example, placed on the mother's abdomen), the amount of blood received is much less. The volume of the placental transfusion is also time-related; in infants delivered by cesarean section, Ogata and colleagues have shown that after 40 seconds, the direction of net blood flow reverses so that any benefits from the prior transfusion are lost. After vaginal delivery, it is therefore prudent to hold the baby at or below the level of the introitus and to delay clamping the cord for at least 20 seconds and not more than 40 seconds. This time can usually be well spent in making a preliminary evaluation of the infant's condition and thoroughly clearing the airway.

The cord should be cut promptly if the mother is receiving general anesthesia or if there is a maternal–fetal blood group incompatibility, an obvious cardiovascular anomaly, or severe asphyxia, in which case resuscitative measures should be taken at once. The mechanics of cutting the cord are simple. With sterile scissors (bacteria can readily enter the umbilical circulation by this route) the cord is cut between clamps placed about 3 cm from the umbilicus.

PREVENTION OF OPHTHALMIA NEONATORUM. The prevention of blindness due to ophthalmia neonatorum is usually the responsiblity of the obstetrician, and it is essential that it be carried out within one hour of delivery. The classic offending organisms is *Neisseria gonorrhoeae,* but other organisms may also cause the disease by infecting the eyes of the fetus as it passes through the birth canal. Prophylaxis is usually carried out immediately after cutting the cord. For many years the standard agent for this purpose was 1% silver nitrate: one drop instilled in each eye and followed by saline irrigation not less than one minute later. More recently this has given way to ophthalmic solutions of erythromycin, tetracycline, or penicillin, which are just as effective and do not produce the intense conjunctivitis that usually follows the use of silver nitrate.

Resuscitation, Apgar scoring, and physical examination of the infant are discussed in Chapter 42.

Use of Outlet (Prophylactic) Forceps

Perhaps especially in the United States, the use of prophylactic or outlet forceps has become so much a part of normal obstetrics that it can be considered a part of normal delivery. Its purpose is to supply the final force required to deliver the head through the vaginal orifice. It is considered prophylactic because the delivery is controlled by the operator, rather than being dependent upon the unpredictable voluntary effort of the patient; the head, by being lifted out over the perineum, is spared an unpredictable period of stress while it presses against the perineum; and injury to maternal soft parts is minimized if the procedure is combined with episiotomy.

These comments should not be construed to suggest that the use of outlet forceps is preferable to a spontaneous delivery that occurs promptly either without episiotomy or immediately after episiotomy is made, as occurred in the delivery shown in Figure 33-3. However, if the head does not emerge immediately after the skull reaches the pelvic floor, the use of outlet forceps can prevent the damage to the delicate structures of the fetal brain that may result from prolonged pressure of the head against the perineum while the mother attempts to expel it. Some women insist upon spontaneous de-

livery, but most obstetricians believe that this is not in the best interests of the infant except when the head is expelled promptly after the skull reaches the pelvic floor. If there is delay at this point in labor, use of outlet forceps is preferable.

For the use of outlet forceps, the following conditions must exist: the scalp must be or have been visible at the introitus without separating the labia, the skull must have reached the pelvic floor, the sagittal suture must be in the sagittal plane of the pelvis, the membranes must be ruptured. Episiotomy is usually a part of the procedure and anesthesia is usually required. Such methods as pudendal block, local infiltration of the perineum, saddle block, and epidural are satisfactory. These techniques of anesthesia are outlined in Chapter 34.

The *obstetric forceps* consists of two matched parts that articulate, or lock. Each part is composed of blade, shank, lock, and handle (Fig. 33-4). The blades possess two curves: the cephalic curve, which makes it possible to apply the instrument accurately to the curved lateral aspects of the fetal head, and the pelvic curve, which corresponds to the curved pelvic axis. The blades are referred to as left and right, according to the side of the mother's pelvis on which they lie after application. The *rule of the forceps* is "left blade, left hand, left side of the pelvis; and right blade, right hand, right side of the pelvis." According to this rule, the left blade is held in the operator's left hand and applied to the left side of the mother's pelvis (and, in occiput anterior position, to the left side of the fetal head); using the right hand, the right blade is then applied to the right side of the pelvis. When the blades are applied in this order, the right shank lies upon the left shank in such a manner that they immediately articulate, or lock.

The technique of their use in the operation of outlet forceps is illustrated in Figures 33-5 through 33-9. After

FIG. 33-4. DeLee's modification of Simpson forceps. Note smooth handles and wider crossbar for traction; lock, shank, and blade are essentially same as those of original Simpson instrument. Blades are loosely articulated to show characteristic features of English lock.

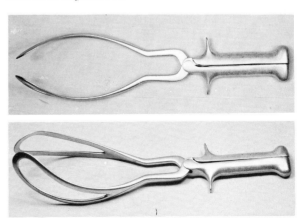

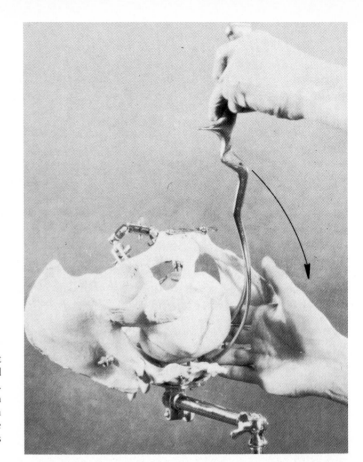

FIG. 33-5. Introduction of left blade (left blade, left hand, left side of pelvis). Handle is held with fingers and thumb, not clenched in hand. Handle is held vertically. Blade is guided with fingers of right hand. After application of blade to side of head, handle is swung downward in an arc (*arrow*) so that it protrudes as shown in Figure 33-7. (Danforth WC: Forceps. In Curtis AH [ed]: Obstetrics and Gynecology. Philadelphia, WB Saunders, 1933)

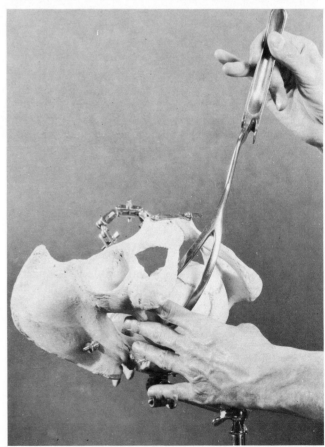

FIG. 33-6. Introduction of right blade (right blade, right hand, right side of pelvis). Left blade (already in place) not shown. Handle is grasped with fingers and thumb, not gripped in whole hand. Handle is held vertical for introduction, and swung downward as in Figure 33-5. (Danforth WC: Forceps. In Curtis AH [ed]: Obstetrics and Gynecology. Philadelphia, WB Saunders, 1933)

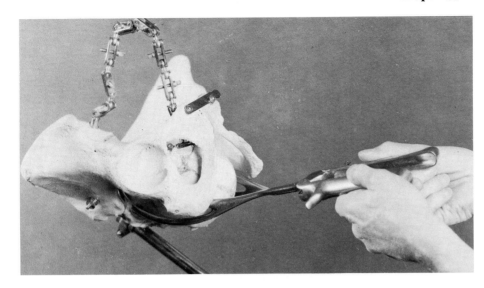

FIG. 33-7. Both blades introduced. The two blades are brought together, or locked. If application is correct, handles lock precisely, without force. (Danforth WC: Forceps. In Curtis AH [ed]: Obstetrics and Gynecology. Philadelphia, WB Saunders, 1933)

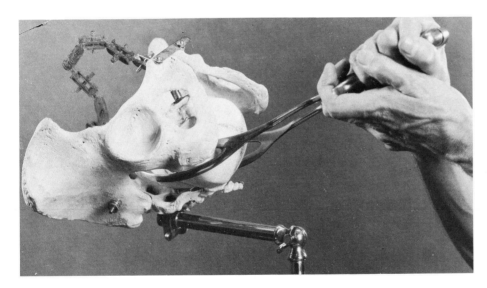

FIG. 33-8. Traction on forceps. Note grip of hands. Position of left hand as shown is used by most obstetricians. Some prefer to place fingers of right hand in crotch of instrument to facilitate traction. Either grip may be used. If heavier traction is needed, no more force should be used than can be exerted by flexed forearms. (Danforth WC: Forceps. In Curtis AH [ed]: Obstetrics and Gynecology. Philadelphia, WB Saunders, 1933)

delivery of the head, the remainder of the delivery is conducted as described for spontaneous delivery. The use of forceps for procedures other than outlet forceps is considered in Chapter 35.

Vacuum Extractor

The vacuum extractor is used with satisfaction instead of forceps in many parts of the world, but it has met with no enthusiasm in the United States. The instrument consists of a round metal or plastic cup that is 3 cm to 6 cm in diameter and to which are attached a rubber hose and a pump. The cup is pressed against the fetal scalp, and air is pumped out of the device. A partial vacuum is created, causing the cup to adhere to the scalp. Traction on the hose can then be applied with force sufficient to pull the head through the birth canal. There

is ample evidence of its safety when it is correctly used, and the instrument is a useful alternative for those who eschew all forceps deliveries except those by outlet forceps. Readers interested in information about the use and limitations of the vacuum extractor should consult the Chalmers and Baggish references.

Episiotomy

Episiotomy is the surgical incision of the perineum. It is made just prior to delivery, and its purposes are to provide sufficient space for delivery so that the pelvic floor will not be torn as the baby delivers, and to provide a clean, incised wound that can be accurately repaired, with restoration of normal relationships. Some women request that delivery be conducted with no episiotomy and "no stitches." It has been estimated, however, that

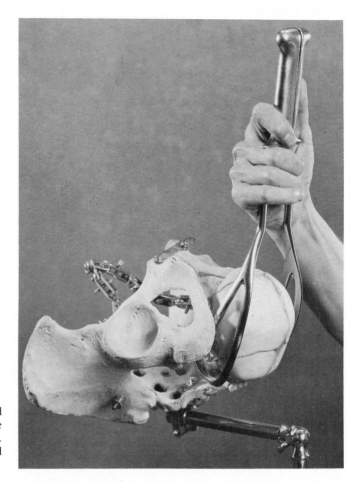

FIG. 33-9. Delivery. As head extends, handles are raised until they pass vertically over infant's head, but little force is needed. One hand suffices; other may support perineum. (Danforth WC: Forceps. In Curtis AH [ed]: Obstetrics and Gynecology. Philadelphia, WB Saunders, 1933)

without episiotomy at least one in four women will sustain serious and avoidable injury to the pelvic floor. Second- and third-degree lacerations can be repaired, but the result is less satisfactory than a well-repaired episiotomy. If such lacerations are not repaired, they ultimately heal, but usually leave some distortion, loss of function, or, occasionally, real disability. No disadvantages of episiotomy come to mind except for the occasional woman who does not need it.

The incision begins precisely in the midline. It may extend either directly posterior through the perineal body itself (median episiotomy), or it may extend in a mediolateral direction to the right or left. The median episiotomy is preferred if the perineum is of normal length, if the subpubic arch is of average width, and if no difficulty in delivery is anticipated. Extension to or through the anal sphincter occurs in 2% to 3% of median episiotomies, but loss of function is unusual if it is recognized at once and properly repaired. The incidence of extension is reduced by advancing the legs as the head crowns (compare position of legs in Figs. 33-3A and 33-3C).

The mediolateral episiotomy reduces the possibility of traumatic extension of the incision into the rectum if the perineum is short, if the subpubic arch is narrow, or if there should be difficulty in delivery. In either median or mediolateral episiotomy, the incision should be extended upward for 2 cm to 3 cm along the vaginal mucous membrane because this clearly reduces the possibility of extension. One method of episiotomy repair is shown in Figure 33-15.

Maternal–Infant Bonding

Maternal–infant bonding appears to be very important in eliminating many of the serious problems related to the psychologic development of the infant and the family unit. Indeed, Klaus and Kennell, who are largely responsible for the concept, asserted that "it is our hypothesis that the entire range of problems from mild maternal anxiety to child abuse may result largely from separation and other unusual circumstances which occur in the early newborn period as a consequence of present hospital care policies." The policies are better than they were when this was written; but the hypothesis is still relevant, and continued efforts are being made to improve family relationships from the moment of birth.

The essential components of bonding are touching,

eye-to-eye contact between mother and infant, parallel facial position (*en face*), and the immediate presence of the husband or supporting other. The newborn infant is suctioned, shown to the parents, dried, assessed briefly, loosely wrapped, and given to the mother for approximately 10 minutes. Breastfeeding may be attempted at this time if it is desired. The infant is then taken to the nursery for the necessary examinations and returned to the mother, preferably in a rooming-in atmosphere, as soon as it is appropriate.

Maternal–infant bonding has received the enthusiastic approval of the American Medical Association (AMA) and the Interprofessional Task Force on the Health Care of Women and Infants, and hospitals have responded by promoting both this and other aspects of family-centered maternal and infant care.

CONDUCT OF THE THIRD STAGE OF LABOR

From the standpoint of maternal risk, the third stage of labor is the most important phase of parturition. Although it occupies an insignificant period of time compared with the many hours devoted to labor, this short period involves many hazards for the mother. Postpartum hemorrhage contributes appreciably to maternal illness and is a leading cause of maternal death. Although the immediate blood loss is important, the manipulations necessary to control the bleeding increase the hazard of infection, which may also result in illness and death directly attributable to the third stage, although often not credited to this period.

Mechanism of Placental Delivery

The normal mechanism of the placental stage consists of two distinct phases: separation and expulsion. The physician should not initiate the latter until the former is completed. The first phase involves a slow, progressive separation of the placenta from the uterine wall and is brought about by physical changes that take place upon the evacuation of the fetus from the uterine cavity.

The placenta normally remains attached to the uterus until the expulsion of the fetus. The sudden diminution in size of the uterine cavity results in a reduction of the placenta site, which is the surface area of the uterine wall to which the placenta is attached. The semirigid, noncontractile placenta cannot alter its surface area, and thus it partially or completely separates from its attachment (Fig. 33-10). The speed with which the uterine surface area is reduced determines the completeness of the separation.

After separation, blood accumulates behind the placenta, and the uterus rises in the abdomen. A firm uterine contraction now begins, usually within two minutes of delivery, and the uterus changes from a flattened, soft, discoid organ to one that is firm and globular. If the Brandt maneuver (Fig. 33-11) is started at the

time of this first contraction (not before and not after), the placenta is usually delivered without incident. The Brandt maneuver consists of the following steps:

1. Firm downward pressure on the fundus (at the time of the first contraction), followed immediately by
2. Suprapubic pressure directly against the lower pole of the corpus, while, simultaneously, steady traction is made on the cord to advance the placenta into the lower uterine segment. This is followed promptly by
3. Suprapubic upward pressure on the corpus to move it toward the umbilicus. As the cord is held steady, the uterus moves away from the placenta, which now enters the vagina and can be readily delivered by gentle cord traction.

It is emphasized that the Brandt maneuver should be started when the first contraction occurs; if this is missed because of preoccupation with the fetus or for other reasons, the maneuver should not be attempted until the uterus again contracts firmly. It should be remembered that, whereas a rising hard uterus means that the placenta is separated and a contraction is occurring, a rising soft uterus may mean intrauterine bleeding. If the uterus is soft and enlarging or if fresh vaginal bleeding occurs, gentle massage of the fundus may provoke a contraction, which permits the Brandt maneuver to be attempted. If this should fail, manual removal of the placenta is indicated (Fig. 33-12).

The two major mechanisms for delivery of the placenta were described many years ago by Schultze and by Duncan (Fig. 33-13). In the Schultze mechanism, said to be the most common, the fetal surface of the placenta slips through the opening in the fetal membranes and appears at the introitus. The membranes then peel off the surface of the uterine cavity, usually uniformly and intact. In this case, the liquid blood and retroplacental clots are contained within the folded placenta and are not evident until the placenta is delivered and examined. In the Duncan method, one edge of the placenta first slips through the cervix and into the vagina. The remainder of the placenta follows, and the fetal membranes are peeled from the uterus as traction is exerted on the following edge of the placenta. The liquid blood and retroplacental clots escape from the uterus as the maternal surface of the placenta is delivered. The designations "shiny Schultze" and "dirty Duncan" have been a part of obstetric parlance for a long time. In addition to the fact that it is less tidy, the Duncan mechanism is more frequently followed by retained fragments of the fetal membranes.

Conduct of the Immediate Puerperium

The following steps are to be undertaken immediately after delivery of the placenta:

1. An oxytocic may be given, but there is not full agreement that oxytocics are routinely needed. The uterus

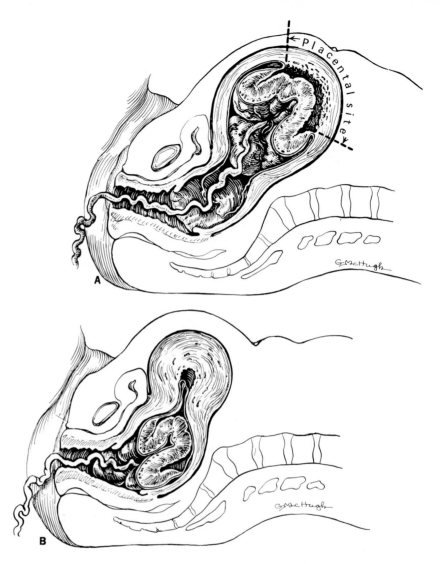

FIG. 33-10. Uteroplacental relations in third stage of labor. (*A*) Immediately after infant has been expelled from uterus and placenta has separated from its uterine attachment. Note great decrease in surface area of placental site, thickened uterine wall, and change in uterine contours. (*B*) After expulsion of placenta into lower uterine segment and vagina. Corpus uteri has become globular and has risen; lower uterine segment is distended by separated placenta. (Davis ME, Boynton MW: Am J Obstet Gynecol 43:775, 1942)

normally contracts firmly after delivery of the placenta, and this is usually sufficient to maintain closure of the uterine sinuses. Despite evidence of the competence of nature to prevent excessive bleeding, many obstetricians prefer to administer an oxytocic after delivery of the placenta. This appears to be especially prudent in women who are predisposed to postpartum hemorrhage (*i.e.*, previous twins, hydramnios, prolonged or dysfunctional labor; grand multiparity; over age 35; postpartum hemorrhage after a prior delivery; general anesthetic used for delivery).

The customary agent is oxytocin, and the preferable route is by infusion (40 units in 1000 ml 5% dextrose in water). For undelivered women, an infusion pump is essential for accurate administration of oxytocin; for use after delivery, precision is not needed and a drip is preferable. The speed of the infusion should be adjusted according to the amount of bleeding and the tone of the uterus. It must not be run too rapidly, because an intravenous bolus of as little as five units of oxytocin can cause a transient but profound drop in blood pressure.

In the past ergonovine was a standard agent for routine use after delivery; because of occasional hypertensive responses to this drug, it is now reserved, for the most part, for cases in which the uterus remains boggy despite an oxytocin infusion. In such a case,

FIG. 33-11.	Technique of delivery of placenta. (*A, B, C, D*) Brandt's maneuver, which is begun when uterus has assumed globular shape and has risen in abdomen. (*E, F, G*) Subsequent steps in delivery of placenta and membranes. (Willson JR: Atlas of Obstetric Technique. St. Louis, CV Mosby, 1961)

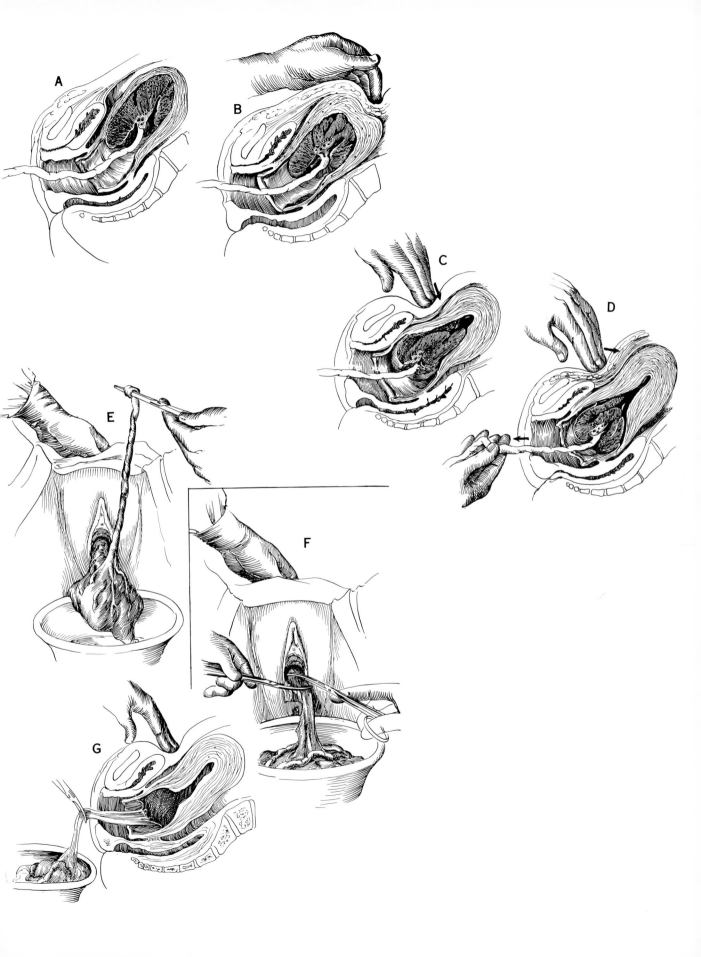

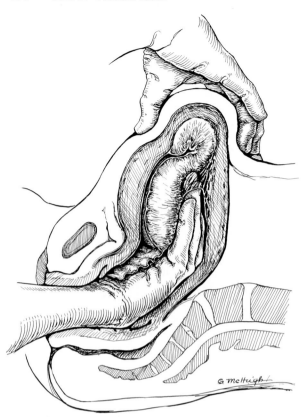

FIG. 33-12. Manual removal of placenta. Physician carefully separates attached placenta in proper plane before attempting its removal from uterus. (Davis ME, Rubin R [eds]: DeLee's Obstetrics for Nurses, 17th ed. Philadelphia, WB Saunders, 1962)

FIG. 33-13. Mechanism of delivery of placenta. (*A*) Schultze mechanism. (*B*) Duncan mechanism. (After Myles MF: Textbook for Midwives. London, Livingstone, 1956)

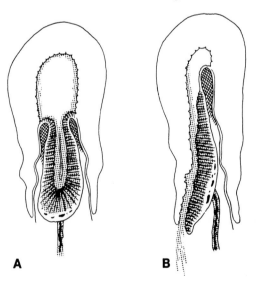

0.2 mg ergonovine is given intramuscularly. If bleeding and uterine atony continue, the administration of calcium gluconate (10 ml 10% solution intravenously) may have an instant and salutary oxytocic effect. If this fails, prostaglandins should be used.

2. The placenta and membranes should be inspected (Fig. 33-14). If there is an obvious placental defect, the uterus should be digitally explored and the frag-

FIG. 33-14. Examination of placenta. (*A*) Maternal surface is carefully sponged of clots; inspection will reveal whether it is complete or a fragment is missing. (*B*) Fetal surface is then examined and note is made whether blood vessels disappear at periphery of placenta. If a patent vessel continues to edge of membranes, retained succenturiate lobe is suggested.

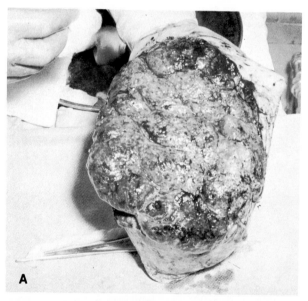

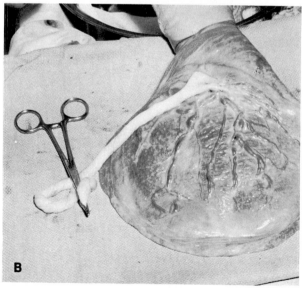

ment retrieved. Despite its popularity among some obstetricians of high competence, routine exploration is not recommended; it is probably not harmful, but there is nothing to suggest that it is of any real benefit in preventing postpartum hemorrhage caused by retained secundines. Exploration is recommended only if there is a missing placental fragment of sufficient size to be detected at the first inspection or if the labor or delivery was of such character that uterine rupture must be ruled out.

3. The vagina (especially in the vaginal sulci and over prominent ischial spines) and the cervix should be inspected, and lacerations immediately repaired.

4. The episiotomy (if one was made) should now be repaired. One technique of episiotomy repair is shown in Figure 33-15. Probably no two obstetricians repair an episiotomy in exactly the same way; but most repairs accomplish the same result. The obstetrician should use the simplest and most expeditious repair that will provide a firm pelvic floor.

5. The fundus should be palpated. It should now be positioned below the level of the umbilicus and should be firmly retracted. If the uterus is at or above the umbilicus, the bladder may be full or blood may have collected in the uterus. The distinction is important, and intrauterine blood should be expelled by Credé's maneuver (a technique designed to expel the placenta, no longer used for this purpose but valuable for emptying the uterus of clots) in which the uterus is grasped anteriorly and posteriorly and squeezed.

6. The patient should be moved to the obstetric recovery room.

The obstetrician should not leave the patient until satisfied that there is no active bleeding, the uterus is firm and well retracted, and the pulse and blood pressure are within normal limits. If general anesthesia was used for delivery, the obstetrician should not leave until the patient is fully reacted.

Recovery Room Care

A recovery room for obstetric patients is essential to modern obstetric care. The required equipment includes suction and oxygen from a wall source and a fixed sphygmomanometer. Fluids, plasma expanders, an immediate source of blood, a tray or kit containing the drugs ordinarily used for dealing with shock and preeclampsia, central venous pressure monitoring apparatus, laryngoscope, endotracheal catheters, and a good light should be immediately available. A cart equipped with side rails is generally preferable to a bed for the patient in the obstetric recovery room. Defibrillator and electronic monitoring devices for pulse and blood pressure should be part of the standard equipment.

As a rule, obstetric patients remain on the delivery table until vital signs are stable. Then they are moved to the recovery room, where they should remain under

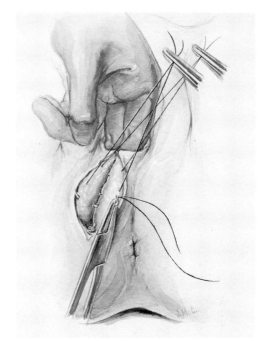

FIG. 33-15. One technique for episiotomy repair. (Right mediolateral episiotomy is shown, but same technique is applicable to median or to left mediolateral.) Vaginal mucosa has been approximated with running suture. Lifting sutures placed as shown cause perineal structures to stand out and facilitate their approximation. Fingers inserted into vagina push rectum away and bring vaginal sutures down so depth of incision can be closed readily. Skin is closed with interrupted sutures unless, as frequently occurs, edges fall together, in which case Allis clamps, allowed to remain in place for 10 minutes, suffice and usually produce less discomfort than sutures. Subcuticular sutures do not improve cosmetic result, prevent egress of any blood that may collect, and they prolong procedure unnecessarily.

constant surveillance for at least one hour. At intervals of at least every 15 minutes the following observations should be made and recorded on an appropriate chart: pulse, blood pressure, height and consistency of the fundus, and estimate of the amount of uterine bleeding (*i.e.,* whether slight, moderate, or heavy).

The complications for which special vigilance should be maintained in the first hour after delivery include excessive uterine bleeding (usually due to uterine atony, obstetric lacerations, retained placental fragments, or clotting defects); hematoma formation in the episiotomy site, vagina, or, rarely, in the lower portion of the broad ligament; shock (due to blood loss, sepsis, anesthesia, or aspiration); hypertension (due to postpartum preeclampsia or vasospasm precipitated by an oxytocic agent); and convulsions (occurring as a complication of regional anesthesia, eclampsia, epilepsy, or cerebral hemorrhage). The diagnosis and management of these complications are considered elsewhere.

When hemorrhagic shock occurs in the obstetric patient, it is usually instant and precipitous. The compensatory mechanisms to resist blood loss hold up much longer than in the nonobstetric patient, and the gradual decline in blood pressure and elevation of pulse, that are valuable in assessing blood loss in other surgical situations are rarely seen. In the obstetric patient, the best guide to the imminence of hemorrhagic shock is the clinical estimate of blood loss, *not* pulse and blood pressure, which may remain normal until moments before the collapse. When excessive bleeding occurs, measures against hemorrhagic shock should be taken at once.

REFERENCES AND RECOMMENDED READING

Abouleish E: Vomiting, regurgitation, and aspiration in obstetrics. In Abouleish E: Pain Control in Obstetrics, Chap 8, pp 138–159. Philadelphia, JB Lippincott, 1977

Annexton M: Parent–infant bonding. Birthing: A real family affair in California center. JAMA 240:823, 1978

Anonymous. A study of physicians' handwriting as a time waster. JAMA 242:2429, 1979

Baggish MS: Vacuum extraction. In Iffy L, Kaminetzky HA: Textbook of Obstetrics and Perinatology, Chap 87. New York, Wiley, 1981

Bruce SL, Paul RH, Van Dorsten JP: Control of postpartum uterine atony by intramyometrial prostaglandin. Obstet Gynecol (Suppl)59:475, 1982

Carson BS, Losey RW, Bowes WA Jr., Simmons MA: Combined obstetric and pediatric approach to prevent meconium aspiration syndrome. Am J Obstet Gynecol 126:172, 1976 (See also Letter to the Editor, ibid, 133:934, 1979)

Chalmers JA: The Ventouse: The Obstetric Vacuum Extractor. Chicago, Year Book, 1971

Danforth DN, Ivy AC: The effect of calcium upon uterine contractions and upon the uterine response to intravenously injected oxytocics. Am J Obstet Gynecol 37:194, 1939

Drouin P, Nasah BT, Nkounawa F: The value of the partogram in the management of labor. Obstet Gynecol 53:741, 1979

Executive Board, American College of Obstetricians and Gynecologists: Nonhospital deliveries should be discouraged. ACOG Newsletter 27:1, May 1983

Fliegner JRH: Third stage management: How important is it? Med J Aust 2:190, 1978

Goldenberg RL, Hale CB, Houde J et al: Neonatal deaths in Alabama. III. Out-of-hospital births, 1940–1980. Am J Obstet Gynecol 147:687, 1983

Hemminki E, Saaroski S: Ambulation and delayed amniotomy in the first stage of labor. Eur J Obstet Gynecol Reprod Biol 15:129, 1983

Jeffcoate N: Medicine versus nature: The James Y Simpson memorial lecture. J R Coll Surg Edinb 21:246, 1976

Klaus MH, Kennell JH: Maternal–Infant Bonding. St. Louis, CV Mosby, 1976

McClellen MS, Cabianca WA: Effects of early mother–infant contact following cesarean birth. Obstet Gynecol 56:52, 1980

Nichols DH, Randall CL: Vaginal Surgery, pp 39–40. Baltimore, Williams & Wilkins, 1976

Notelovitz M: The single-unit delivery system—A safe alternative to home deliveries. Am J Obstet Gynecol 132:889, 1978

Ogata ES, Kitterman JA, Kleinberg F et al: The effect of time of cord clamping and maternal blood pressure on placental transfusion with cesarean section. Am J Obstet Gynecol 128:197, 1977

Pearse WH: Home birth. JAMA 241:1039, 1979

Peltonen T: Placental transfusion: Advantage and disadvantage. Eur J Pediatr 137:141, 1981

Philpott RH: The management of labour. In Stallworthy J, Bourne G (eds): Recent Advances in Obstetrics and Gynaecology. Edinburgh, Churchill Livingstone, 1979

Shamsi HH, Petrie RH, Steer CM: Changing obstetric practices and amelioration of perinatal outcome in a university hospital. Am J Obstet Gynecol 133:855, 1979

Siegel E: Early and extended maternal–infant contact: A critical review. Am J Dis Child 136:251, 1982

Sosa R, Kennell J, Klaus M et al: The effect of a supportive companion on perinatal problems, length of labor, and mother–infant interaction. N Engl J Med 303:597, 1980

Stewart KS: The second stage. In Studd J (ed): Progress in Obstetrics and Gynaecology, Vol 4. Edinburgh, Churchill Livingstone, 1984

Stewart P, Kennedy JH, Calder AA: Spontaneous labour: When should the membranes be ruptured? Brit J Obstet Gynaecol 89:39, 1982

Studd J: Partograms and nomograms of cervical dilatation in management of primigravid labour. Br Med J 4:451, 1973

Studd JW, Cardozo LD, Gibb DMF: The management of spontaneous labour. In Studd J (ed): Progress in Obstetrics and Gynaecology, Vol 2. London, Churchill Livingstone, 1982

Taylor PM (ed): Parent–infant relationships. Semin Perinatol 3:1, 1979

Toppozada M, El-Bossaty M, El-Rahmen HA et al: Control of intractable atonic postpartum hemorrhage by 15-methyl prostaglandin $F_{2\alpha}$. Obstet Gynecol 58:327, 1981

Tromans PM, Sheen MA, Beazley JM: Feto–maternal surveillance in labour: A new approach with an on-line microcomputer. Brit J Obstet Gynaecol 89:1021, 1982

Yao AC, Lind J: Placental transfusion. Am J Dis Child 127:128, 1974

Obstetric Analgesia and Anesthesia

Ezzat Abouleish

34

Obstetric anesthesia is unique because it is the only branch of anesthesia in which two individuals, mother and fetus, are cared for simultaneously. The drugs and techniques must be chosen with due awareness that a drug or a technique that is desirable for one may be undesirable for the other. Therefore, the proper choice of obstetric anesthesia or analgesia requires a knowledge not only of the anatomy, physiology, and psychology of obstetric pain, but also of the transmission of drugs across the placenta and their effects on the fetus and neonate.

Obstetric anesthesia and analgesia includes techniques and drugs used for either vaginal delivery or cesarean section.

During the first stage of labor, uterine contractions may be associated with pain. These nociceptive impulses are carried from the uterus and cervix to the spinal cord by way of sympathetic afferent fibers. These fibers proceed from the uterus and cervix to the inferior hypogastric plexus (Fig. 34-1). A local anesthetic injected bilaterally on both sides of the cervix, a technique called paracervical block, induces pain relief by interrupting the nociceptive impulses at this site. The next station of the nociceptive fibers is at the nerve plexus between the bifurcation of the aorta, the superior hypogastric plexus. The fibers then proceed to the spinal cord to relay at the four spinal segments, T10 through L1 (Fig. 34-2). From there, the nociceptive impulses cross to the opposite side and proceed to the higher centers, where they are perceived as pain stimuli.

The pain of the first stage of labor is due to contraction of the uterine muscle, stretching and dilatation of the cervix, and pull on the attached ligaments. The pain is not felt in the pelvis, but is referred to the somatic areas that share segments (T10 to L1) with the pelvic organs initiating the pain (see Fig. 34-2). The areas of referred pain extend from the umbilical region (T10) to the inguinal region and upper part of the thigh (L1)

and to the sides and lower back, all of which share the same segments (T10 through L1). Therefore, when epidural analgesia is administered and relieves the pain of labor, associated analgesia is produced in these areas, as can be tested by pinprick.

During the second stage of labor, additional pain results from distension, stretching, and sometimes tearing of the perineal structures as the presenting fetal part advances. This latter pain is somatic in nature, and is carried by the sacral and coccygeal nerves. Therefore, in order to achieve pain relief at the second stage of labor, in addition to the segments T10 through L1, the sacral and coccygeal nerves should be blocked. This can be done by pudendal nerve block by extending the epidural analgesia caudad to involve these nerves; by caudal block, or by a subarachnoid block. Therefore, in the second stage of labor analgesia affects larger areas, the doses of the drug used are higher, and the expected complications are greater.

PAIN RELIEF IN THE FIRST STAGE OF LABOR

It is emphasized that there is great variation in the need for pain relief in the first stage of labor. It is the obstetrician's responsibility to determine the patient's needs and wishes, and to act in accordance with them. Large doses and major techniques should not be used if smaller doses and minor methods will suffice.

The methods most commonly used in the first stage are systemic analgesia, epidural analgesia, and paracervical block.

Systemic Analgesia

For systemic analgesia, the drugs of choice are a tranquilizer to relieve apprehension and anxiety, and a narcotic to relieve pain. All drugs that cross the blood-brain

669

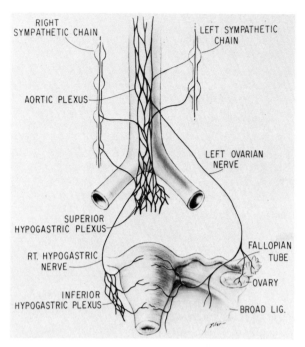

FIG. 34-1. Sympathetic nerve supply of the uterus (pelvic and abdominal distribution). Uterine nerves arise from (1) the upper part of the uterus (upper uterine segment), the contraction of which contributes to pain; (2) the lower part of the uterus (lower uterine segment), the distention of which contributes to labor pain; and (3) the cervix, the dilatation of which contributes to pain. The ovarian nerve supplies the ovary, fallopian tube, broad ligament, round ligament, and the side of the uterus, and communicates with the uterine plexus. Note that sympathetic efferent and afferent fibers are shown together. (Abouleish E: Pain Control in Obstetrics. Philadelphia, JB Lippincott, 1977)

barrier also cross the blood-placenta barrier. Accordingly, the dose of systemic agents should be limited, and the drugs should be given early enough that they will be largely metabolized and excreted before delivery.

Tranquilizers

Agents commonly used are phenothiazine 25 mg or hydroxyzine 50 mg intramuscularly. Hydroxyzine, in a dose not exceeding 1.5 mg/kg injected intramuscularly, has no depressant effect on the neonate despite an appreciable transmission across the placenta, as shown by the relative concentrations of the drug in the maternal and umbilical circulation, which are as follows: maternal venous blood, 1.0; umbilical venous blood, 0.71; umbilical arterial blood, 0.47. Diazepam in excess of 10 mg is inadvisable because of its long duration of action, particularly in the premature fetus and newborn, and because fetal blood levels of the drug may exceed maternal levels. Diazepam also causes hypotonia and difficulty with temperature regulation in the neonate.

Barbiturates and scopolamine have no analgesic properties and are even considered to have antianalgesic effects. This combination of drugs was popular some 50 years ago because it produced total amnesia for the events of labor. However, it also caused severe respiratory depression of the newborn, and the mothers became highly agitated and disoriented. It is no longer used in modern obstetrics.

Narcotics

Meperidine 25 mg is commonly administered intramuscularly early in labor. The total dose of meperidine should not exceed 100 mg during the course of labor because of the drug's depressant effect on neonates, especially those of low birth weight. The depressant effect is due not only to meperidine itself but also to its metabolites, particularly normeperidine, which easily cross the placenta. The maximum depressant effects of meperidine after intramuscular injection are manifested between one and four hours from delivery. Intravenous administration is superior to the intramuscular administration of narcotics because control of analgesia is better, onset of action is quicker, and du-

FIG. 34-2. Nerve supply of the uterus (segmental distribution). (Abouleish E: Pain Control in Obstetrics. Philadelphia, JB Lippincott, 1977)

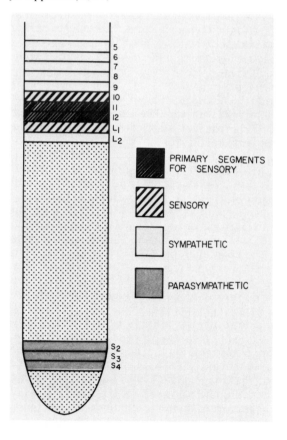

ration of action is shorter. With intramuscular injection or oral administration of a drug, the rate and extent of absorption into the blood stream are quite variable, and so are the subsequent pharmacologic effects.

A new group of narcotic agonist-antagonist drugs, such as, for example, butorphanol or nalbuphine, offers certain advantages, at least theoretically. Because of their inherent antinarcotic effect, these drugs cause less respiratory depression of the mother and fetus than do pure agonist narcotics. However, these drugs as well as pure agonist narcotics should be used cautiously in women delivering premature infants.

All central nervous system depressants cross the blood-placental barrier, as mentioned before, leading to fetal depression, which can present in the form of loss of beat-to-beat variability. Therefore, when beat-to-beat variability is essential in evaluating the condition of the fetus, central nervous system depressants should not be used until after the evaluation is made.

Intrathecal Morphine Analgesia

A more recent method of administering narcotic drugs is by the intrathecal route. This approach is based on the existence of narcotic receptors along the pain pathway in the spinal cord, in the brain stem, and in the thalamus. Since these receptors are specific for narcotics, a minute quantity (*e.g.,* 0.5 mg morphine) produces marked analgesia lasting 12 to 24 hours. The patient becomes comfortable in 20 to 30 minutes and the effect lasts for the whole course of labor, sometimes extending into the postpartum period. There is no associated sympathetic blockade; therefore, resultant maternal hypotension is not a problem. Also, the motor power remains intact, thus preserving the patient's ability to bear down during the second stage of labor. However, intrathecal injection of morphine has undesirable side effects. These are:

1. Respiratory depression: Cephalad extension of morphine to the fourth ventricle can depress the respiratory centers. Patients given an intrathecal injection of morphine require careful monitoring of respiration for up to 24 hours; equipment to support respiration should be readily available; and naloxone 0.4 mg should be drawn in a syringe and kept in the patient's room.
2. Nausea and vomiting: Cephalad spread of morphine to the fourth ventricle stimulates the chemoreceptor trigger zone (CTZ) and causes nausea and vomiting.
3. Pruritus: The mechanism of this side effect is unknown; however, it can be quite annoying.
4. Retention of urine: Postpartum bladder atony is common following intrathecal injection of narcotics.
5. Inadequate control of somatic pain: for forceps delivery and episiotomy repair, other methods of analgesia (e.g., epidural, caudal or pudendal nerve

block) are required to supplement intrathecal injection of the narcotic.
6. Somnolence: The patient is somnolent and sometimes difficult to arouse between contractions.

All these side effects are dose related: with 2 mg intrathecal morphine the patient is difficult to arouse, but with 0.5 mg morphine analgesia is usually satisfactory, but the woman is much more alert.

The side effects of intrathecal injection of morphine are considerable, and to most obstetricians the benefits of the technique are not sufficient to warrant its routine use. However, the intrathecal injection of morphine may lead to a more rational approach to pain control in which a drug is injected as close to the specific receptor as possible. Other narcotics, natural, synthetic, or agonist-antagonist, are under trial to maximize the beneficial effects and minimize the side effects of the intrathecal narcotic technique.

Epidural Analgesia

Epidural analgesia is an important means of controlling the pain of the first stage of labor. The principle of epidural analgesia is to inject a local anesthetic into the epidural space to block the spinal segments T10 through L2. The epidural space is located inside the vertebral column surrounding the dural sac (Figs. 34-3, 34-4). The ligamentum flavum constitutes the posterior border of the epidural space and the dural sac lies anteriorly to it (see Fig. 34-3). The spinal epidural space extends cephalad to the base of the skull and caudad to the sacral hiatus, where it is bordered by the posterior sacrococcygeal ligament. This space is quite narrow, the distance from ligamentum flavum to the dura being only 5 mm (see Fig. 34-4). The ligamentum flavum is a thick ligament that offers resistance to the advancing needle; the loss of resistance as the epidural needle traverses it and reaches the epidural space is the cardinal means of identifying the epidural space. If the needle is advanced too far, the dura will be punctured.

The best approach to the epidural space is in the midline, where the ligamentum flavum is thickest so that loss of resistance is most easily identified. Also, in the midline the epidural space is widest, so the risk of dural puncture is lessened, and blood vessels are scarce, so the possibility of intravascular injection of drug is minimized.

When the needle reaches the epidural space and no blood or cerebrospinal fluid has been seen to drip from its hub, a test dose of 2 ml of the local anesthetic is injected, and a soft long catheter is inserted through the needle. The needle is then withdrawn, leaving the catheter in the epidural space for further injections of the local anesthetic. The epidural catheter is taped to the patient's body and remains in place until delivery has been completed.

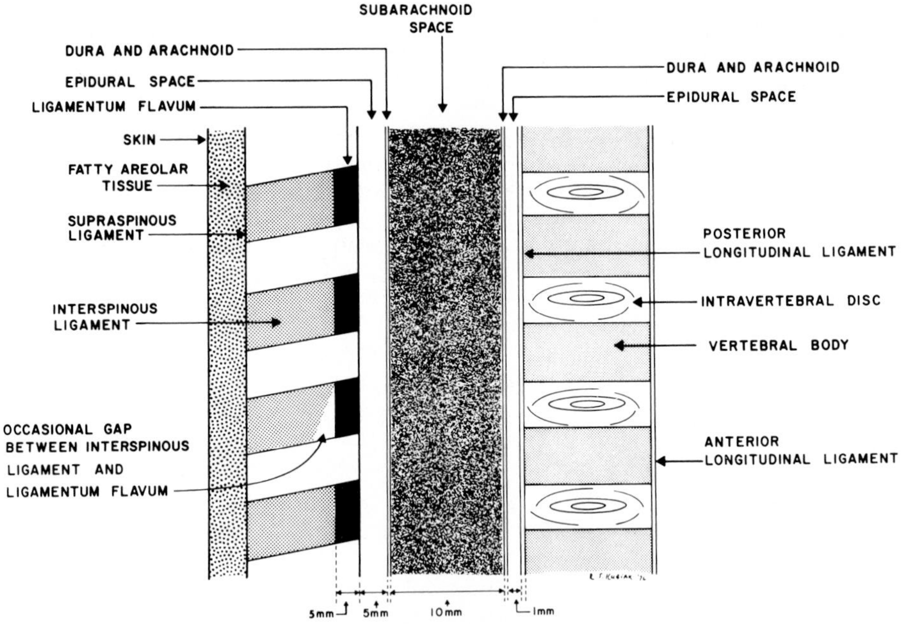

FIG. 34-3. Diagrammatic sagittal section of the back at the lumbar region. Note the structures traversed by the needle from skin to epidural space; the slightly caudad direction of the spinous processes; the thickness of the ligamentum flavum and the diameters of the epidural and subarachnoid spaces; and the occasional gap between the interspinous ligament and ligamentum flavum. (Abouleish E: Pain Control in Obstetrics. Philadelphia, JB Lippincott, 1977)

During labor, long-acting local anesthetics are preferred to reduce the frequency of injections. Bupivacaine is an amide-type local anesthetic that is metabolized in the liver. It has a two-hour duration of action, and no harmful effect on fetus or newborn. Moreover, its analgesic qualities are excellent, and the minimal muscular paralysis permits the patient to bear down effectively when the second stage is reached. When epidural anesthesia is being induced in active labor, a test dose of 2 ml of 0.5% bupivacaine is first administered through the epidural catheter to exclude subarachnoid injection. Two minutes later another test dose of 4 ml of 0.5% bupivacaine is injected to exclude intravascular injection. If no untoward reaction occurs in 30 seconds, another 4 ml of 0.5% bupivacaine is injected. In earlier labor, 0.25% bupivacaine is preferred. Continuous analgesia can be obtained by intermittent injections of similar doses, or by a continuous infusion of half the initial effective dose per hour. An alternative drug is lidocaine, which is also an amide-type local anesthetic.

It is usually administered in four times the concentration and in the same volume as bupivacaine. Its duration of action is about 60 to 75 minutes and it can also be administered by the intermittent or continuous epidural infusion technique. These two drugs differ from chloroprocaine, which is an ester-type local anesthetic metabolized by plasma cholinesterase. Chloroprocaine has a more rapid onset and a shorter duration (45 minutes). Because of its short duration, it is unsuitable for the first stage of labor unless the continuous infusion technique is used. It is also used in the same volume as bupivacaine at four times the concentration.

Advantages

The advantages of epidural analgesia are as follows:

1. The technique has been used extensively, it is effective and predictable, and the incidence of significant complications is very low.

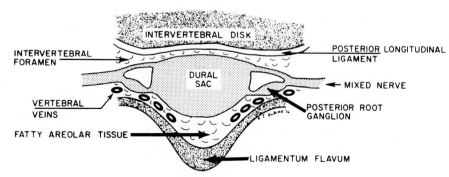

FIG. 34-4. Diagrammatic cross-section of the vertebral canal showing contents of the epidural space. Note that the ligamentum flavum is thickest in the midline, the epidural space is widest in the midline, and the nerves and blood vessels are in the anteriolateral part of the epidural space. (Abouleish E: Pain Control in Obstetrics. Philadelphia, JB Lippincott, 1977)

2. The patient is alert and cooperative.
3. It can be administered continuously through the epidural catheter. Thus, the patient remains comfortable throughout labor.
4. When the second stage is reached, the dose, volume, and type of local anesthetic drug can be modified to allow the mother to push, to produce perineal analgesia, and to permit forceps delivery if required.
5. If an indication for cesarean section arises, the epidural block can be extended to provide analgesia for this operation.

Disadvantages

There are certain disadvantages to epidural analgesia. These are as follows:

1. Although epidural analgesia usually does not adversely affect the course of labor, it may prolong labor if the block becomes too extensive. This problem can be managed by an oxytocin infusion. Since the patient perceives no pain, meticulous attention to the monitoring of uterine contractions and fetal heart rate is essential.
2. Maternal blood pressure may drop as a result of the sympathetic blockade that follows cephalad extension of the epidural anesthetic. The sympathetic nerve fibers for the body as a whole arise from T1 to L2. Therefore, if the block extends unintentionally above the T10 level, more sympathetic fibers are blocked, vasodilation occurs, and hypotension results. The following measures are helpful in avoiding this complication, and should be used routinely:
   a. Prehydration of the mother by administering 500 ml to 1000 ml lactated Ringer's solution not more than 20 minutes before epidural block is induced.
   b. Limiting the dose of local anesthetic so it does not exceed the patient's needs
   c. Keeping the mother in the lateral position as much of the time as possible to avoid vena caval compression.
   Since maternal hypotension can endanger the life of the mother or fetus, proper monitoring of the blood pressure is essential. The use of noninvasive electronic blood pressure monitoring is helpful in maintaining the necessary surveillance. If maternal hypotension occurs, 10 mg ephedrine is injected and the fluid infusion is accelerated. Other increments of 10 mg ephedrine can be used if required to maintain maternal blood pressure at or above 90% of the original level.
3. If the local anesthetic is accidentally injected intravascularly, manifestations of central nervous system toxicity may appear. The degree and magnitude of these manifestations depend on the dosage. A relatively small intravenous dose may cause ringing in the ears, a metallic taste in mouth, blurred vision, drowsiness, decrease in awareness, or delirium. These symptoms should be considered warning signs to stop further injection of the local anesthetic. They usually occur during the test dose, or when the therapeutic dose is fractionated at 5-ml increments. If the policy of a test dose and fractionization of the therapeutic dose is ignored and the full dose is administered to a sensitive patient, the central nervous system toxicity may result in grand mal seizures that cannot be stopped or prevented by thiopental or diazepam. As the patient convulses, she consumes oxygen and energy, while at the same time being unable to breathe. This leads to severe, rapidly progressive metabolic and respiratory acidosis. Acidosis, asphyxia, and the local anesthetic itself lead to marked cardiac depression that may culminate in cardiac arrest and death. The seizures terminate as the local anesthetic is distributed to other body tissues, such as muscle and fat. If respiration and circulation are maintained for a few minutes, convulsions end and are followed by postictal amnesia. Therefore, when using local anesthetic drugs for any purpose, one must keep in mind their central nervous system and cardiac toxicities. A test dose should always be used and the therapeutic dose fractionated at 30-second intervals to detect accidental intravascular injection. Capability for cardiopulmonary resuscitation must be immediately available.

   If convulsions occur, the first priorities are to stop the convulsions, to secure the airway, and to hyperventilate with 100% oxygen. The following steps are taken at once:
   a. An assistant applies cricoid pressure (to occlude the esophagus by compressing it between the cricoid ring and the sixth cervical vertebra).
   b. Succinylcholine is administered to induce generalized paralysis.
   c. An endotracheal tube is inserted and the cuff inflated.
   d. Hyperventilation with 100% oxygen is begun and is continued, using an Ambu bag or an anesthetic machine.
   e. An ECG monitor is applied, and continuous monitoring of pulse and blood pressure is started.
   f. Attention is now turned to the fetus, who will not be compromised if effective maternal ventilation can be established at once. Initially, fetal bradycardia may occur due to hypoxia, hypercarbia, and the direct effect of the transmitted local anesthetic. The bradycardia is quickly reversed as the mother's condition stabilizes and as the anesthetic is dispersed.
4. If the local anesthetic is accidentally injected into the subarachnoid space, spinal analgesia results. The dose used for epidural block is about six times that for spinal block to the same dermatomal level. Therefore, if the epidural dose is injected into the subarachnoid space by mistake, the level of the block becomes too extensive and a total spinal block results. This leads to complete respiratory paralysis. Maternal hypotension also occurs because the sym-

pathetic nerve fibers, from T1 to L2, are all blocked. Loss of consciousness follows and loss of airway reflexes predisposes to aspiration pneumonitis. If accidental intrathecal injection is to be avoided, attention must be given to the following:

a. The method is not to be approached casually. To be effective and safe, it requires the expertise and constant attendance of one who is properly trained in this technique.
b. Dural puncture should be excluded by ensuring that aspiration does not draw cerebrospinal fluid before the local anesthetic is injected.
c. A test dose should be injected to detect intrathecal injection of the local anesthetic drug (2 ml of 0.5% bupivacaine will cause pain relief in two minutes if injected intrathecally but has no effect if injected epidurally).

If a total spinal block occurs, cricoid pressure should be applied, respiration controlled, and hypotension corrected. Intubation is performed, the endotracheal cuff is inflated to seal the trachea, and respiration is maintained until anesthesia wears off (one to three hours, depending on the anesthetic used). The fetal heart rate is monitored and usually remains normal after the maternal condition has been stabilized. Total spinal block is not *per se* an indication for cesarean section.

5. Fetal heart rate decelerations may be associated with epidural analgesia. The possible mechanisms are:
a. Maternal hypotension.
b. Aortic compression by the gravid uterus, which reduces the uterine and intervillous blood flow. This can be prevented or alleviated if the mother remains on her side, preferably the left.
c. Local anesthetic drug toxicity. This only occurs with accidental intravascular injection, as explained above, and is usually temporary.
d. Maternal hypoxia (*e.g.,* from convulsions or total spinal block).
e. Uterine vasoconstriction as the block ascends. The local anesthetic is injected into the lumbar region and extends to the thoracic region. As it ascends, the sympathetic nerve fibers of the lower limbs are paralyzed before those of the uterus. To maintain the blood pressure and compensate for the vasodilation of the lower limbs, there is vasoconstriction of the blood vessels above the block, including the uterine blood vessels. The decrease in uterine blood flow may lead to fetal bradycardia. This complication can be minimized by prehydrating the mother before starting epidural block, thus reducing the vasoconstriction.

In summary, when epidural anesthesia is being used, an intravenous line must be set up and 500 ml of lactated Ringer's solution should be infused before the block is started; fetal heart rate should be monitored; the vital signs should be recorded; and facilities for cardiopulmonary resuscitation, including oxygen and suction, should be immediately available.

Contraindications to Conduction Analgesia

There are certain contraindications to epidural analgesia that apply equally to caudal and subarachnoid block:

1. *Antepartum hemorrhage.* Acute hypovolemia leads to increased sympathetic tone to maintain the blood pressure; any anesthetic technique that blocks the sympathetic fibers can lead to significant hypotension that can endanger the lives of the mother and baby.
2. *Anticoagulant therapy or bleeding disorder.* If a blood vessel is injured in a patient receiving anticoagulant therapy or with a bleeding disorder, the resulting hematoma may compress the cauda equina or the spinal cord, leading to serious central nervous system sequelae.
3. *Infection at the injection site.* Infection can be spread intravertebrally if the needle traverses an infected area. Amnionitis, on the other hand, is not a contraindication to intravertebral blocks.
4. *Tumor at the injection site.* A tumor at the injection site is an unusual but definite contraindication.

Relative Contraindications

Relative contraindications to intravertebral blocks include patient refusal, extensive back surgery, morbid obesity or anatomic abnormality in which landmarks cannot be identified, and current or prior disease of the central nervous system.

Caudal Analgesia

Caudal anesthesia is an epidural technique in which the local anesthetic is injected through the posterior sacrococcygeal ligament covering the sacral hiatus (Fig. 34-5). The nerves to be blocked are the coccygeal and sacral nerves first, followed by the lumbar and lower thoracic nerves. The risk of dural puncture is less with caudal analgesia than with lumbar epidural technique, since the dural sac ends at the second sacral bony segment, about 5 cm superior to the sacral hiatus.

During the first stage of labor, pain relief requires block of segments T10 through L1. With caudal analgesia, the sacral and lumbar nerves must be blocked before T10 can be reached. Consequently, a much higher dose of local anesthetic is required, early paralysis of the pelvic floor may interfere with internal rotation of the fetal head, and anesthesia of the pelvic floor prevents the patient from pushing reflexly. For these reasons caudal analgesia is rarely used for labor, but it is still used in a single dose for delivery. If lumbar epidural anesthesia is used for the first stage of labor, a

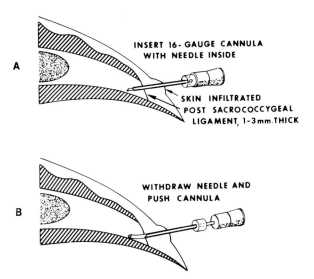

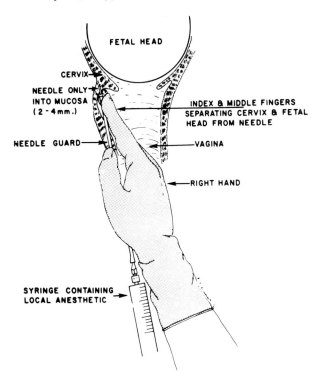

FIG. 34-5. Insertion of the needle and cannula in single-dose caudal analgesia. (*A*) The needle pierces the posterior sacrococcygeal ligament and enters the caudal canal at 45-degree angle with the patient's back. (*B*) The angle of entry is changed to 30 degrees and the needle is advanced in the canal for 1 cm to 2 cm. (Abouleish E: Pain Control in Obstetrics. Philadelphia, JB Lippincott, 1977)

caudal catheter may also be inserted when the epidural catheter is introduced, a technique called "double-catheter technique." When the patient is ready to deliver, a local anesthetic is injected through the caudal catheter to achieve perineal analgesia quickly and efficiently; the lumbar epidural catheter is utilized to control uterine pain by blocking T10 through L1. This technique is particularly appropriate when the block must be precise and excessive doses of the local anesthetic are to be avoided (as in, for example, preeclampsia, cardiac disease, or respiratory disease).

Paracervical Block

During active labor with the cervix 4 cm to 6 cm dilated, nociceptive impulses from the uterus and cervix can be blocked by injecting 5 ml of local anesthetic on either side of the cervix at the 4 o'clock and 8 o'clock positions (Fig. 34-6). This technique cannot be utilized if the cervix is fully effaced and dilated because of absence of landmarks. The drug used depends on the desired duration of effect: chloroprocaine is used for short duration and lidocaine for medium duration. Bupivacaine is no longer used for paracervical block because of possibility of prolonged fetal myocardial depression if the drug reaches the fetus in a sufficient concentration. Chloroprocaine (10 ml of 1% solution injected in two divided doses) is readily hydrolyzed by cholinesterase in maternal blood, placenta, and fetal blood, and is the safest drug for paracervical block.

Paracervical block is a simple technique that does not require the presence of an anesthesiologist, causes no sympathetic paralysis or hypotension, and produces rapid pain relief. Unfortunately, fetal bradycardia, occurring 2 to 10 minutes following the block and lasting between 5 and 30 minutes, develops in 33% of cases. Fetal acidosis, neonatal depression, and even perinatal death may follow in some cases.

Depression by the local anesthetic may occur because higher drug levels are achieved in the fetus than the mother. Because of the proximity of the fetus and placenta to the site of injection, the drug can be accidentally injected into the fetal head, the placenta, the lower uterine segment, or a blood vessel reaching the placenta. Decreased intervillous circulation may result from the uterine vasoconstriction and increased uterine tone caused by the local anesthetic. Therefore, paracervical block is contraindicated in a compromised fetus when a decrease in uterine blood flow could lead to fetal death. As a further precaution, the fetal heart rate should be continuously monitored for 10 minutes before and after this block is used in any patient. Repeated paracervical blocks should be avoided because of the

FIG. 34-6. Technique of paracervical block. Note the position of the hand and fingers in relation to the cervix and fetal head and the shallow depth of the needle insertion. Note also that no undue pressure is applied at the vaginal fornix by the fingers or needle guide. (Abouleish E: Pain Control in Obstetrics. Philadelphia, JB Lippincott, 1977)

increasing incidence and severity of fetal bradycardia with each injection. Because of the potential fetal morbidity and mortality, many obstetricians have abandoned the use of this technique in both compromised and normal fetuses.

PAIN RELIEF IN THE SECOND STAGE OF LABOR

The available options for pain relief during the second stage are epidural analgesia, subarachnoid block, pudendal block, and inhalation techniques.

Epidural Analgesia

When epidural anesthesia is used, the spinal segments to be blocked extend from T10 through the coccygeal nerve (a total of 14 segments). Therefore, 10 to 20 minutes before the expected time of delivery, the local anesthetic (15–20 ml) is injected to allow time for the agent to reach and block the sacral segments. If the double catheter technique has been used, 6 ml to 8 ml of chloroprocaine is injected through each catheter to anesthetize the required nerves, and the time to obtain analgesia is shortened to 10 minutes. Some obstetricians prefer to use epidural analgesia for labor, allow the patient to push and deliver spontaneously without analgesia, then do any perineal repair under local anesthesia. Recent studies have found that interruption of epidural analgesia does not shorten the course of labor.

Subarachnoid Block

If the patient has no epidural or caudal catheter in place, subarachnoid block is an excellent technique for vaginal delivery. If spontaneous delivery is anticipated, lumbar puncture is performed with the patient in a sitting position and the dose is 30 mg of 5% lidocaine in 7.5% dextrose, a solution whose specific gravity is greater than

that of cerebrospinal fluid. This dose produces adequate perineal analgesia for episiotomy and repair. The anesthesia is comparable to that of a pudendal nerve block, but onset is much faster (2 minutes for saddle block, 10 minutes for pudendal block). The area blocked is identical to the area in contact with the saddle when riding a horse, hence the name "saddle block." If a forceps delivery is required, a block to T10 is needed, so the dose of lidocaine is increased to 40 mg to 50 mg. The details of the technique, precautions, and contraindications of subarachnoid block are described below, under the heading Anesthesia for Cesarean Section.

Pudendal Nerve Block

Pudendal nerve block is performed 10 to 20 minutes before perineal analgesia is needed. The block is obtained by injecting the local anesthetic, for example, 10 ml of 1.5% lidocaine, on each side. Each pudendal nerve arises from the sacral plexus, S2 through S4, and leaves the pelvis through the greater sciatic foramen to pass behind the junction of the ischial spine with the sacrospinous ligament. Lateral and posterior to it lie the posterior cutaneous nerve of the thigh then the sciatic nerve. The pudendal nerve reenters the pelvis through the lesser sciatic foramen. It then accompanies the pudendal vessels in the pudendal canal, which lies along the lateral wall of the ischiorectal fossa. It divides into three branches, as shown in Figure 34-7. The *inferior hemorrhoidal nerve* carries motor fibers to the external anal sphincter muscle and sensory nerve fibers to the perineum in the anal region. It usually arises from the pudendal nerve just before the latter enters the pudendal canal. However, sometimes it arises higher up or even separately from the sacral plexus. Variations in the nerve's course are common, and may explain some of the failures to obtain analgesia following pudendal nerve block. The *perineal nerve* carries motor fibers to the muscles of the pelvic floor and sensory fibers to the perineum and the corresponding labia majus and minus. The *dorsal nerve of the clitoris* supplies the clitoris and corresponding corpus cavernosum.

FIG. 34-7. The pudendal nerve and its branches. The inferior hemorrhoidal nerve can arise higher up from the pudendal nerve or separately from the sacral plexus. (Abouleish E: Pain Control in Obstetrics. Philadelphia, JB Lippincott, 1977)

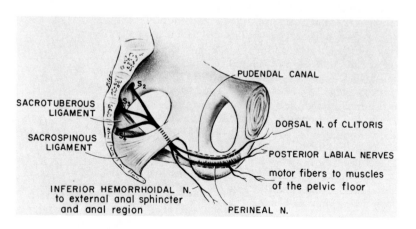

Although the pudendal nerve is the main nerve supply of the perineum, it is not the only one. Other nerves participate, namely the posterior cutaneous nerve of the thigh (S1, S2, and S3), the ilioinguinal nerve (L1), the genital branch of the genitofemoral nerve (L1 and L2), and the sacrococcygeal nerve (S4, S5, and coccygeal nerve) (Fig. 34-8). Therefore, to obtain adequate perineal analgesia, local infiltration of the line of incision is required as well as transvaginal block of the pudendal nerve, the inferior hemorrhoidal nerve, and the posterior cutaneous nerve of the thigh.

The block is performed by locating the ischial spine, and depositing the local anesthetic at the expected site of the pudendal nerve behind the sacrospinous ligament just distal to the ischial spine. The needle is advanced a further 1 cm and the local anesthetic is injected to block the inferior hemorrhoidal nerve in case it arises separately. Then it is advanced 1 cm more to block the posterior cutaneous nerve of the thigh, which supplies the skin of the labia and adjacent part of the thigh. A total of 10 ml of 1.5% lidocaine is injected on each side.

The combination of pudendal nerve block and inhalation analgesia is suitable for vaginal delivery in high-risk patients, since the block neither changes the hemodynamic or respiratory functions of the parturient nor adversely affects the fetus. However, it entails the same risk of toxicity as all regional anesthesia blocks. Therefore, to avoid intravascular injection, aspiration should be performed before the local anesthetic is injected, one minute should elapse before the other pudendal nerve is blocked, facilities for cardiopulmonary resuscitation should be readily available, and the person performing the block should be capable of resuscitating the mother if an accident should occur. The main disadvantages of pudendal nerve block are that it does not relieve the pain of uterine contractions, it does not permit instrumental vaginal delivery except low forceps,

and it does not allow uterine exploration or manual removal of the placenta.

Local Infiltration of the Perineum

Local infiltration of the perineum is a suitable technique for a patient who has had an easy labor and delivery. It is safe and simple. The local anesthetic used is usually 1% lidocaine in a volume of 10 ml to 20 ml.

Inhalation Analgesia

Inhalation analgesia is achieved when sufficient anesthetic is administered to provide pain relief without loss of consciousness. All inhalation anesthetics can be used for this purpose provided they are administered in half-MAC (minimal alveolar concentration needed to produce anesthesia) amounts. Inhalation analgesia is widely used in the United Kingdom and is administered by midwives who use a premixed combination of 50% nitrous oxide in oxygen. It is sometimes self-administered during contractions.

The advantages of this technique are safety and hemodynamic and respiratory stability. The disadvantage is that it is much less effective than epidural or caudal techniques. If it is used for prolonged periods, air pollution may result, making it desirable to have a scavenging system to collect the exhaled anesthetic.

Inhalation Anesthesia

If full inhalation anesthesia is to be used for delivery, the same precautions as noted for cesarean section must also be observed.

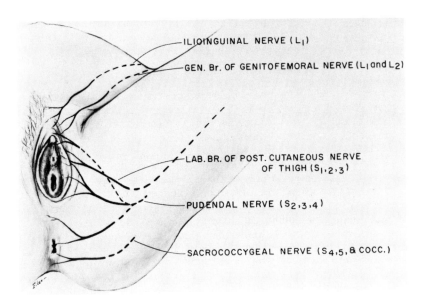

FIG. 34-8. Nerve supply of the perineum. (Abouleish E: Pain Control in Obstetrics. Philadelphia, JB Lippincott, 1977)

ILIOINGUINAL NERVE (L₁)

GEN. Br. OF GENITOFEMORAL NERVE (L₁ and L₂)

LAB. BR. OF POST. CUTANEOUS NERVE OF THIGH (S₁,₂,₃)

PUDENDAL NERVE (S₂,₃,₄)

SACROCOCCYGEAL NERVE (S₄,₅,& COCC.)

PSYCHOLOGIC METHODS OF PAIN RELIEF

Prepared childbirth, hypnosis, and acupuncture are techniques designed to deal with psychophysiologic aspects of pain. Pain perception in an individual patient is dependent on a variety of interrelated and complicated factors, including physical condition, expectations, distraction, motivation, and education. Pain during labor appears to be accentuated by fear of the unknown, insecurity, anger, apprehension, and previous unpleasant experiences. On the other hand, it seems to be lessened or better tolerated if the patient has confidence, understanding of the birth process, realistic expectations, and uses breathing exercises, conditioned reflexes, emotional support, and other techniques of distraction. Proper selection of patients is important for the success of all psychologic methods. Among the factors associated with the best results are enthusiasm of the patient and her coach or support person for the technique, higher socioeconomic and educational levels, previous good experiences, and a normal labor and delivery.

Prepared Childbirth

Prepared childbirth usually consists of a series of weekly meetings which the father of the child is encouraged to attend (see Chapter 20). Lectures, audiovisual aids, and group discussions are used to educate the parents about pregnancy, labor, and the puerperium. The mother is taught how to relax and how to exercise to strengthen the back and abdominal muscles, improve body tone, and to loosen such joints as the hips and pelvis. She is coached on how to use certain breathing patterns with uterine contractions during the first and second stages of labor and at the actual delivery of the fetal head.

Although prepared childbirth reduces the reaction to pain, the need for pain relief is approximately the same as in control groups. However, the time of request for analgesia is usually later in the course of labor. These facts make it wise to discuss this situation during antenatal classes and avoid the implication that medications will not be required or are harmful to the fetus. If this is not done, the result may be a sense of frustration and failure when medications are needed for pain relief. Most recent studies indicate that epidural anesthesia and other accepted analgesic techniques, if properly administered, have no long-term harmful effects on the infant.

Hypnosis

Hypnosis is a state of altered consciousness; it is not a state of sleep. Awareness becomes restricted, and concentration is deep. A typical hypnosis course consists of weekly sessions for 5 or 6 weeks during which the patient learns how to relax and how to enter a hypnotic trance easily and effectively. With the onset of labor, the patient can initiate the trance and continue until delivery has been accomplished. The mechanism of hypnosis is multifactorial, as are other methods of psychologic pain relief through suggestion, motivation, conditioned reflex, and education. Although all body systems remain stable, patient selection is essential since the technique is not successful in every case.

Acupuncture

Acupuncture is an art and a philosophy; it is not yet a science. According to Chinese culture, each organ has a certain amount of energy. A proportion of this energy is used locally by the organ, and the remainder travels in a circular pathway away from and then back to the same organ. These pathways are called "meridians" and are located beneath the skin. When an organ either is diseased or is a source of pain, the energy produced by that particular organ is abnormal—either too much or too little. The insertion of needles at points along the corresponding meridian can relieve pain by restoring energy to a normal level. An added element specific to acupuncture involves the "gate theory of pain." Vibration of the needles closes these gates in the central nervous system or liberates endorphins that interfere with transmission of the nociceptive impulses. It is likely that the mechanism of action also involves suggestion, expectation, motivation, and conditioning. Theoretically, acupuncture should be ideal for pain relief in childbirth. However, pain relief is usually only partial and most patients need other analgesia or anesthesia for the second stage of labor. The method is of interest, but there is no reason to believe that it will ever assume importance as a method of obstetric analgesia or anesthesia.

ANESTHESIA FOR CESAREAN SECTION

Three methods are in common use for cesarean section: subarachnoid block, epidural block, and general anesthesia.

Subarachnoid Block

Subarachnoid block is an excellent method for elective cesarean section, and for cases in which there is no fetal distress or other urgency. A local anesthetic is injected into the subarachnoid space to achieve a dermatomal block up to the T5 segment. Anesthesia of the pelvic and abdominal organs is thus produced, since all the nerves supplying the pelvis and abdomen, including the splanchnic nerves, are blocked with the exception of the vagus and phrenic nerves. The local anesthetic used is usually lidocaine 5% in 7.5% dextrose. Its specific gravity is higher than that of CSF, hence it is called hyperbaric lidocaine. Other local anesthetics are 1% tetracaine and more recently 0.75% bupivacaine, which has proven to be an excellent anesthetic for cesarean section.

It is essential that certain rules be followed if spinal analgesia is to be used safely for cesarean section:

1. The dose of local anesthetic must be one-third less than the amount used to achieve the same dermatomal level for nonpregnant patients (mainly because of the reduced amount of cerebrospinal fluid during pregnancy). The dose is 8.25 mg bupivacaine for a 150-cm woman (5 feet) with the addition of 0.75 mg bupivacaine for each 7.5 cm (3 inches). For example, if the patient is 165 cm tall (5'6"), the dose is 9.75 mg bupivacaine.
2. Hypotension, which is the principal problem associated with spinal analgesia in pregnant women, can be avoided by
   a. Displacing the uterus to the left to ensure adequate venous return to the heart
   b. Infusing lactated Ringer's solution 15 ml/g body weight within 20 minutes of the block in anticipation of vasodilation
   c. Injecting intravenously ephedrine in 10-mg increments to maintain the blood pressure between 90% and 100% of the original level
   d. Monitoring of the blood pressure closely, preferably by use of the modern noninvasive, automatic device
   e. Administering oxygen by plastic face mask. Oxygen does not prevent hypotension but counteracts some of its effects.
3. Respiration should be closely monitored during spinal analgesia; if there is any doubt about respiratory adequacy, respiration should be assisted or controlled.

Spinal analgesia has many advantages. The mother is awake and her reflexes are intact, which lowers the risk of aspiration pneumonitis. With spinal anesthesia the support person can attend the operation and be at the mother's side. Spinal analgesia is a simple technique with a clear end point that is evidenced by the appearance of cerebrospinal fluid before the anesthetic is injected. It takes effect quickly, and within a few minutes analgesia is usually complete. Spinal analgesia carries a lower risk of cardiovascular or central nervous system toxicity than epidural analgesia because the dose of local anesthetic injected is small. Finally, spinal analgesia is not costly.

The main disadvantage of spinal analgesia is that it can cause hypotension. This can be avoided or reduced to a minimum if appropriate precautions are taken. If hypotension does occur, it can be easily treated by rapid infusion of fluid and injection of ephedrine. Many obstetricians and anesthesiologists avoid spinal analgesia if the fetus is compromised, since any degree of hypotension could be dangerous. Nevertheless spinal analgesia can be used safely for some high-risk pregnancies when proper precautions are taken. Spinal anesthesia is a one-dose technique, which limits the duration of its effect. Severe post-lumbar-puncture cephalgia is

much less common than in former years. Use of the smaller 26-gauge spinal needle and more experience with the technique have reduced the incidence of this complication to about 1%, a frequency similar to that following epidural anesthesia and accidental dural puncture.

Epidural Analgesia

Epidural analgesia is better than spinal anesthesia in the following respects: the rapidity and magnitude of hypotension are less, encroachment on respiratory function with a high segmental block is less, and by using the continuous technique, the duration of the block can be prolonged as needed for the surgery or for postoperative analgesia. However, if used for cesarean section, epidural anesthesia can be dangerous because of the higher possibility of cardiovascular and central nervous system toxicity.

For a patient who is 150 cm (5 ft) tall, the dose is 20 ml of 0.5% bupivacaine or equivalent dose of other agent. An additional 1.5 ml is given for each 2.5 cm (one inch) of extra height. The dose is fractionated into 4 ml to 5 ml every 30 seconds to avoid toxicity.

Epidural analgesia is a superior method of analgesia for women in labor, and it is valuable for cesarean section in conditions where sudden and marked fluctuations in the blood pressure may impose excessive risk. However, it is a more complicated technique than spinal block and its success rate is lower.

General Anesthesia

The principal use of general anesthesia for cesarean section is in the case in which there is a need for rapid delivery or there are contraindications to conduction anesthesia. Some obstetricians prefer general anesthesia because they believe uterine relaxation is greater than with regional anesthesia, thus facilitating delivery of the baby. Its principal disadvantage is that the woman is asleep, so that aspiration of vomitus is a constant threat when the endotracheal tube is not in place.

Induction of anesthesia is achieved by using thiopental 4 mg/kg. In such a dose, thiopental causes minimal depression of the fetus or neonate. It is only when thiopental is administered in a dosage above 6 mg/kg that the baby is delivered with low Apgar scores. Following thiopental injection, a muscle relaxant, usually 1 mg/kg to 1.5 mg/kg succinylcholine, is injected to facilitate intubation. Anesthesia is then maintained with an inhalation anesthetic supplemented with a muscle relaxant. The fetal blood level of muscle relaxants is generally 10% to 40% of the maternal level. The low transmissibility of muscle relaxants across the placenta is due to their low lipid solubility, their high water solubility, and their high ionization. Muscle relaxants in general have no demonstrable harmful effect on the fetus.

The inhalation anesthetic can be nitrous oxide, halothane, enflurane, isoflurane, or similar agents. If these inhalation anesthetics are used in a concentration not exceeding 1 MAC, the neonatal depression is clinically insignificant. In pregnant women the anesthetic requirement is reduced by about 40%, and inhalation anesthetics in a total concentration of 1 MAC produce adequate maternal analgesia and amnesia. After the baby is born, a narcotic, for example 5 mg to 10 mg morphine, can be given intravenously to supplement the anesthesia and to provide for postoperative analgesia. Diazepam 2 mg to 5 mg can also be administered intravenously to potentiate amnesia produced by the inhalation anesthetic.

It must be emphasized that the use of general anesthesia for cesarean section is a major anesthetic technique and that special expertise and skill are essential prerequisites. Endotracheal intubation is a crucial part of the method, and the anesthetist must be qualified not only to make a preanesthetic evaluation as to whether this will be readily feasible, but also to accomplish the intubation with dispatch.

To counter the effects of aspiration if it should occur despite these precautions, a nonparticulate antacid is administered 5 minutes before induction of anesthesia. Other measures that have been suggested, but whose possible fetal effects have not been fully evaluated, are administration of glycopyrrolate to reduce vagal tone, cimetadine to reduce acid secretion, and metaclopropamide to promote emptying of the stomach through the pylorus.

REFERENCES AND RECOMMENDED READING

Abboud TK, Goebelsmann U, Shnider SM et al: Effects of intrathecal morphine analgesia during labor on maternal plasma beta-endorphin levels. Anesthesiology 59:A414, 1983

Abboud TK, Shnider SM, Dailey PA et al: Intrathecal administration of hyperbaric morphine for the relief of pain in labour. Br J Anaesth 54:1351, 1984

Abouleish E: Pain Control in Obstetrics. Philadelphia, JB Lippincott, 1977

Abouleish E: Childbirth: A joy—not a suffering. Philadelphia, Dorrance & Company, 1975

Baraka A: Rapid sequence induction in patients with a full stomach. Anesthesiology 57:543, 1982

Bromage PR: Epidural Analgesia. Philadelphia, WB Saunders, 1978

Datta S, Alpher MH: Anesthesia for cesarean section. Anesthesiology 53:142, 1980

Editorial: Confidential inquiry into maternal deaths. Br J Anaesthes 55:367, 1983

Melzack R, Taenzer P, Feldman P et al: Labor is still painful after prepared childbirth training. Can Med Assoc J 125:357, 1981

PART V

Abnormal Labor

Preterm Labor

Ralph C. Benson

35

Preterm labor is defined as labor that occurs between the end of the 20th week and the end of the 37th week of pregnancy. Neonates weighing less than 2500 g are classified as low-birth-weight infants. The terms *premature labor* (labor before the end of the 37th week that produces an infant weighing less than 2500 g) and *premature infant* (one weighing less than 2500 g and delivered before 37 weeks) have been discarded because the infant's weight and maturity do not necessarily relate to one another or to the duration of pregnancy.

Preterm labor is the most common complication of the third trimester of pregnancy, and the delivery of an undergrown, immature neonate is a clinical crisis that is invariably a threat to the life or health of the newborn and often of the mother as well. Therefore, preterm labor and delivery constitute a high-risk experience for the mother and the infant. Unfortunately, abnormally early labor and delivery occur in 5% to 15% of all pregnancies in developed countries and are considerably more common in the developing nations and among socioeconomically deprived populations.

The undersized neonate, delivered too early, poses some of the most urgent problems of modern medicine. Most of the deaths among newborns are associated with low birth weight. The majority of these infants are preterm. These small for dates and prematures account for the annual loss of more than 60,000 infants in the United States, or nearly two thirds of all deaths during the neonatal period. The death rate of the low-birth-weight neonate is 40 times that of the full-sized infant born at term.

The outstanding causes of disease and death of preterm infants are respiratory distress syndrome, hyaline membrane disease, and intracranial intraventricular hemorrhage. Also, low birth weight, especially if disproportionate to gestational age, is one of the most important risk factors for cerebral palsy. The incidence of cerebral palsy associated with low birth weight may be as high as ten times, mental deficiencies five times, and lethal malformations seven times that of the full-sized infant. Emotional disturbances, social maladjustments, and visual and hearing defects are also multiplied, and medical and custodial costs for these individuals are incalculable.

Pregnancy problems known to predispose a woman to preterm labor should alert the physician to the high-risk status of mother and fetus. With few exceptions, such patients should be cared for and delivered in a maternity hospital unit with consultative and support facilities that are capable of supplying optimal care for mother and infant. It is reprehensible, for example, to permit a woman known to have a multiple pregnancy to deliver in a minimally equipped hospital when she could have been transferred, even in labor, to a center equipped to handle such high-risk situations. This is medical negligence. The referral of twins or triplets to a level-III infant care unit *after* delivery is fraught with danger. The fact that some preterm infants survive such an untimely and hazardous experience is no justification for lack of proper planning and continuity of care. The same admonitions apply to the delivery at term of an infant known in advance to be of low birth weight.

The sex ratio of newborn infants shows a preponderance of males at all stages of antenatal development. The male/female ratio varies from an estimated 170:100 very early in pregnancy to 106:100 at term. However, male fetuses are significantly heavier than female fetuses of equivalent age. Accordingly, among preterm infants born at the same stage of gestation, females weighing less than 2500 g outnumber males of the same weight by a ratio of approximately 110:100. Also, the prognosis for survival of undergrown infants of the same weight favors the female because of greater chronologic age and maturity.

PRETERM LABOR

Causes

Preterm labor occurs in a variety of circumstances; maternal, placental, or fetal factors may be responsible. However, any of these may be coincidental, and mere association does not establish an etiologic role.

The multiple factors involved in the onset of labor at term are outlined in Chapter 31. When a single factor or complication is found to precipitate premature labor in a significant number of cases, it must be presumed that this factor acts by disrupting the balance among the factors that suppress labor and those that stimulate it. In 20% to 30% of the cases of preterm labor, the precipitating factor is premature rupture of the membranes. In about two thirds of the cases, the exact cause of preterm labor can never be determined.

Factors that are known to correlate with the incidence of preterm labor include maternal age (the very young and older women are predisposed); social class (the incidence is higher among the socioeconomically deprived); weight (the malnourished are more often affected); height (women of short stature are prone); prior preterm labors; prior induced abortions; work habits (hard physical work increases the incidence); smoking; and certain pregnancy complications (*e.g.,* hypertension, bacteriuria, and antepartum hemorrhage).

Scoring systems have been devised to identify some of the women who may be at risk for preterm labor (Table 35-1). Such lists are not inclusive, but they direct attention to some of the important features of this problem. The factors described in the following sections may also be involved.

Maternal Problems

Maternal abnormalities that have a recognized relation to preterm labor include medical disorders such as serious cardiovascular or renal disease, severe anemia, cholestasis of pregnancy, marked hyperthyroidism, and poorly controlled diabetes mellitus. Abdominal surgery involving uterine displacement or manipulation (*e.g.,* large bowel resection during advanced gestation) may be inimical to continuation of pregnancy. Maternal injury (*e.g.,* a direct blow to the abdomen, a major fracture, or

Table 35-1
Example of Risk Scoring for Preterm Labor

Score	Personal Data	Past History	Habits	Current Pregnancy
0	0 children at home Excellent SES*	No prior abortions >1 year since last delivery	Light work only Minimum stress	General health good
1	2 children at home Good SES	<1 year since last delivery	Outside work	Unusual fatigue

2	Age < 20 years or
	    >40 years
	Single parent
	Fair SES
		2 prior induced abortions	>10 cigarettes per day
			Unusual anxiety
				Weight gain < 12 lb by
				    32 weeks' gestation
				Proteinuria
				Bacteriuria
				Hypertension

3	Height < 5 feet Weight < 100 lb Malnourished Poor SES	3 prior induced abortions	Heavy work	Breech at 32 weeks Weight loss of 5 lb Head engaged before 34 weeks' gestation Febrile illness Uterine fibroids
4	Age < 18 years	Pyelonephritis		Bleeding after 12 weeks Cervix dilated or effaced Uterus irritable
5		Uterine anomaly Second trimester abortion Previous cone biopsy		Placenta previa Hydramnios
10		Prior preterm delivery Repeated second trimester abortion		Multiple pregnancy Abdominal surgery

* Socioeconomic status.

(From Creasy RK, Liggins CG; Aetiology and management of preterm labour. In Stallworthy J, Bourne G [eds]: Recent Advances in Obstetrics and Gynaecology, Vol 13. London, Churchill Livingstone, 1979)

shock) may terminate gestation early. Preeclampsia–eclampsia may either precipitate labor or necessitate therapeutic intervention and termination of pregnancy. Uterine anomalies (*e.g.,* bicornuate or diminutive uterus) may shorten gestation. Pelvis sepsis or tumors (*e.g.,* appendicitis, large uterine fibromyomas) may cause an increase in uterine irritability. Cervical incompetence may jeopardize containment of the pregnancy. Infection, particularly when associated with hyperthermia (*e.g.,* pyelonephritis, pneumonia, malaria) or localized sepsis (*e.g.,* listeriosis) may terminate pregnancy well before the expected date of confinement.

Untreated Cushing's disease, caused by adrenal or pituitary neoplasm, or by bronchial carcinoma that secretes adrenocorticotropic hormone (ACTH) is associated with spontaneous labor before the 34th week of pregnancy.

Orgasm during pregnancy may be accompanied by palpable uterine contractions and even prolonged uterine spasm. Orgasmic induction of labor, perhaps in part related to the prostaglandin content of semen, has been reported. Although the data are tentative, restriction of coitus may be advisable if there is a history of early termination of pregnancy.

Anecdotal reference is often made to so-called psychogenic or emotionally induced abortion or early labor (*e.g.,* after fright, grief, or anxiety). This was first recorded in the Bible, where note is made (1 Sam. 4:19) that the wife of Phinehas immediately went into labor when she learned of her husband's death.

Finally, the risk of preterm labor is increased by conditions that make careful supervision of pregnancy difficult, by lack of patient information, and by psychosocial stresses. However, none of these factors accounts for the total risk of preterm delivery.

Placental Abnormalities

Gross placental disorders (*e.g.,* preterm separation of the placenta, extrachorial placenta) may be directly responsible for preterm labor. Common histopathologic alterations of the placenta include stasis and edema, infarction, fibrosis, and hematoma formation. Nonetheless, these microscopic alterations may be secondary to general pathologic states associated with early labor.

Fetal Abnormalities

Multiple pregnancy or hydramnios may overdistend the uterus. Congenital adrenal hyperplasia almost always is associated with shortened gestation. Preterm labor is common (about 60%) if the fetus is affected by Potter's syndrome (renal agenesis, pulmonary hypoplasia, characteristic facies). Fetal infection (*e.g.,* rubella, toxoplasmosis) may precipitate preterm labor because of critical fetal disease. As noted before, premature rupture of the fetal membranes is one of the most common causes of preterm labor.

Frequency

Each year approximately 7% of all liveborn infants in the United States are undergrown, and most are delivered after preterm labor. There are important racial differences, however, and the incidence of low birth weight is almost twice as high among nonwhites as whites. The difference between these two groups may be ascribed in part to the lower average weight of the nonwhite fetus at all stages of gestation and to the greater frequency in nonwhites of medical complications (*e.g.,* preeclampsia–eclampsia) that predispose a woman to preterm labor or necessitate therapeutic termination of pregnancy.

In multiple pregnancy, preterm labor is particularly common. The frequency of low birth weight is increased six times in twin gestation, which terminates, on the average, three weeks before the expected date of confinement.

Prevention

Since preterm labor occurs so commonly in socioeconomically deprived populations and among those who are at high risk, it is logical that the incidence would be sharply reduced if the factors leading to both of these circumstances were corrected. However, these problems are largely social and only partly medical.

Preterm labor has a strong tendency to recur and may be a repetitive problem. Normal hygienic measures during pregnancy, including proper diet and rest, avoidance of overwork, and avoidance of excesses of all types (including exercise, temperature, coitus, tobacco, drugs, and alcohol) are recommended as a matter of course. For the patient with a history of repeated preterm labors, it is prudent to restrict work, travel, and exercise and to encourage rest, especially during the last trimester. Except for tobacco, which has been shown to be clearly related to preterm labor, these factors have not been shown definitely to bear a causal relation; admonitions regarding them are intuitive rather than scientific.

Medical, gynecologic, or obstetric complications that predispose a woman to preterm labor must be managed according to the specific requirements of each. Early diagnosis of anemia, hypertension, and other medical problems is important in any plan to achieve fetal maturity. Help at home and increased periods of bed rest should be prescribed for the patient with multiple pregnancy or early hydramnios and for the patient with a demonstrated tendency toward preterm delivery. Acute infection should be treated promptly and aggressively with appropriate chemotherapeutic agents. Routine antepartum examinations, with repeated measurements of the patient's blood pressure and weight and the testing of urine for protein, permit early detection and treatment of preeclampsia; this should reduce the incidence of preterm delivery from this cause. Chronic hypertensive vascular disease is best managed with increased bed rest. Antipressor drugs have not proved valuable for improving fetal survival.

Medical consultation should be sought for the patient with diabetes mellitus, hyperthyroidism, cardiac disease, or other medical complication. Meticulous control of maternal diabetes mellitus, with prevention of acidosis, is of the greatest importance to fetal survival.

The cardiac patient is not likely to deliver early unless cardiac failure develops, which results in fetal hypoxia. Therefore, conservative management is required for maternal survival and fetal survival. Uterine leiomyomas are best treated conservatively during pregnancy. Even if symptoms of degeneration supervene, bed rest and analgesics generally are preferable to surgical intervention because they enhance the chance for the continuation of pregnancy and further fetal growth.

Elective major surgery or extensive dental therapy should be postponed until after delivery, if possible. In an impressive number of patients with cervical incompetence and intact membranes, the onset of premature labor has been averted or postponed by cervical cerclage, which should be done before the cervix has achieved a dilatation of 3 cm or 50% effacement.

A new and increasingly common cause of preterm labor is the multiple pregnancy that often results from the use of clomiphene citrate or human menopausal gonadotropin to promote conception. The evidence that the occurrence of multiple pregnancy following administration of these agents is dose-related emphasizes that these preparations must not be used casually or by those who lack the facilities and experience to apply them with precision and to evaluate their effects.

Diagnosis

Since preterm labor can sometimes be arrested by appropriate management, the diagnosis must be made as quickly as possible and before labor is so far advanced that therapy will be ineffective. A specific time of onset of preterm labor is difficult to pinpoint. However, early rupture of the membranes may be an augury. Increasingly strong and prolonged uterine contractions every five to ten minutes, a cervical dilatation of 3 cm, and 50% cervical effacement, particularly after leakage of amniotic fluid or the passage of blood, strongly suggest that labor is underway. By definition, labor is the occurrence of regular, coordinated, often painful uterine contractions that are accompanied by progressive dilatation of the cervix and often descent of the presenting part and that normally culminate in delivery.

The distinction between contractions of this kind and those of false labor (discussed in Chap. 31) is usually not threatening to fetal welfare at term, but before 37 weeks' gestation it may be urgent. External monitoring devices can help provide objective evidence of the character of the contractions, as well as the condition of the fetus, and they should be applied promptly in all cases in which a woman is admitted in questionable preterm labor. Over a period of time this may help the physician determine the nature of the preterm labor.

Management

When preterm labor is diagnosed with certainty, it is important to decide whether an attempt should be made to stop it or whether the labor should be permitted to

proceed. If the patient is at least 35 weeks' gravid, it is usually advisable to allow labor to proceed.

The following are among the situations in which attempts to arrest preterm labor may be either futile or ill-advised:

1. Advancing, active labor with the cervix dilated 3 cm or more. When labor has advanced to this point, efforts to arrest it are rarely successful.
2. Maternal complications that would be increasingly serious if pregnancy were permitted to continue. Examples are preeclampsia–eclampsia and severe cardiovascular or renal disease.
3. Fetal complications of such nature that continued intrauterine life would be hazardous. Examples are the fetal risk associated with severe preeclampsia and severe maternal diabetes. Fetal death, serious isoimmunization, severe congenital anomalies, and marked hydramnios also weigh against attempts to stop labor. Moreover, if there is any evidence of fetal distress, detected either clinically (*e.g.,* by electronic monitoring) or by laboratory tests for feto–placental insufficiency, no attempt to stop labor should be made. About 6% of low-birth-weight neonates display distress that would be compounded by extension of pregnancy.
4. Ruptured membranes. If this is accompanied by fever or malodorous discharge, the implication is that amnionitis may have developed, and the uterus should be emptied promptly regardless of prematurity. If there is nothing to suggest amnionitis, the risk that it may develop must be weighed against the hazard of prematurity. If the gestational age of the fetus is 28 to 32 weeks and the membranes are ruptured, labor may be postponed for 72 hours. During this time the administration of adrenocorticosteroid therapy to the mother may increase fetal pulmonary maturity. Often, the cervix may be too dilated or effaced for labor to be arrested. The physiological wheel may have turned beyond the point of reversal.

If all patients in whom attempts at the arrest of labor are either contraindicated or futile are excluded, there are only about 20% in whom the attempt may be appropriate and has some chance of success.

A final consideration in the decision of whether to attempt the arrest of preterm labor is the dramatic improvement in survival, and subsequent development, of the very small newborn. Under optimal conditions the outlook for these infants is so favorable that many researchers have questioned whether preterm delivery is really so undesirable that heroic and sometimes hazardous measures should be taken to prevent it.

The following conditions should be present in the woman in whom an effort to arrest labor is to be made:

The fetus should be alive, weigh less than 2500 g, and show no evidence of fetal distress or jeopardy.
The membranes should be intact, and a Bishop score of six or less should be observed.

There should be no obstetric or medical condition that contraindicates continued pregnancy.

The cervix should be dilated less than 3 cm.

Arrest of Preterm Labor

If it is decided to attempt the arrest of preterm labor, the woman should remain at bed rest. An initial pelvic examination is needed to determine the status at the time treatment is begun, but no other pelvic examinations should be made unless they are essential. Fetal heart rate and uterine contractions should be monitored externally. An ultrasound scan should be made to rule out gross malformation or abnormal presentation because the incidence of these is higher in preterm labor, and to permit an estimate of fetal weight, which can be helpful in decisions regarding the conduct of labor and mode of delivery if the effort to arrest labor fails. Amniotic fluid for lecithin/sphingomyelin (L/S) ratio should be obtained from the vaginal pool if the membranes are ruptured or by amniocentesis if they are intact. If an attempt to arrest labor is to be made, the patient should be rapidly hydrated with 5% glucose in water to suppress pituitary oxytocin production. This should be done regardless of which tocolytic drug will be used. After major surgery or trauma, tocolytic therapy may be short term, lasting only until the mother is transferred to a perinatal center. It may be long term if the fetal gestational age is less than 28 weeks.

TOCOLYTIC AGENTS. In individual cases, myometrial-suppressive drugs have stopped labor at least temporarily. However, to prove the true value of tocolytic agents, it must be shown that they result in a greater reduction of perinatal deaths than untreated spontaneous preterm labor. Stated another way, the effectiveness of tocolytic therapy can be measured only by assessing those premature newborns who received treatment rather than by considering the total premature newborn population. Regrettably, a study of this type has not been reported.

However, there seems to have been a slight gradual decline in the perinatal mortality rate after preterm labor without the use of tocolytic agents. Boyland and O'Driscoll have suggested that this may represent a natural improvement in the evolution of the body's ability to correct a problem and better general medical care and not a benefit of drug therapy.

Early diagnosis is essential if tocolytic agents are to be used, because they become increasingly ineffective as cervical dilatation increases beyond 3 cm and effacement exceeds 50%. Most of the agents can suppress uterine contractions and can delay delivery for 12 to 24 hours; but in order to delay delivery for significant periods, they must be used early in labor, when the diagnosis is most difficult to make with certainty and they must be administered continually or repeatedly. It is clear that none of the drugs introduced to date answers the imperative need for an agent that is as safe, as precise, and as predictable in stopping labor as oxytocin and prostaglandins are in starting it. Currently, the Food

and Drug Administration (FDA) is reconsidering the status of all tocolytic agents, and the status of each should be verified before it is used. The agents that have been used, with variable success, include the following:

Progesterone and its derivatives
Ethanol (alone or with adrenergic drugs)
β-Adrenergic (β-mimetic) drugs (isoxsuprine hydrochloride, ritodrine, salbutamol, terbutaline sulfate, fenoterol)
Prostaglandin synthetase inhibitors (aspirin, indomethacin, naproxen, mefenamic acid)
Calcium antagonists (nifedipine and verapamil)
Other drugs (*e.g.,* magnesium sulfate)

PROGESTERONE DERIVATIVES. Although prophylactic progesterone therapy in patients with a history of preterm labor has been reported to be effective in several series of cases, progestogens are not effective in stopping the progress of early labor. In addition, the FDA has prohibited the use of these agents in pregnancy because of data suggesting that they can cause developmental anomalies.

ETHANOL. Ethanol is believed to reduce the secretion of oxytocin from the posterior pituitary, and the drug may also have a direct inhibitory effect on the myometrium. Ethanol has stopped labor for over 72 hours in certain patients and is reported to be effective to some degree in about half of threatened preterm labor cases. Nevertheless, the questions of its contribution, if any, to the fetal alcohol syndrome and its effect on the neonate's respiratory and circulatory adaptation are still unsettled. Because of these questions, plus the drug's extremely unpleasant maternal side-effects and sequelae, the use of ethanol as a tocolytic agent has been abandoned.

Before using tocolytic drugs, the physician should obtain a detailed history; serial measurements of blood pressure, pulse, blood glucose, electrolytes, and hematocrit; and an ECG. In addition, a fluid intake and output chart should be started.

β-MIMETIC AGENTS. The action of the β-mimetic drugs in the suppression of labor is discussed in Chapter 31. β-Mimetic drugs have received extensive trial in the arrest of preterm labor. The cardiovascular side-effects can be distressing: tachycardia occurs with some regularity, maternal hypotension is uncommon but has been reported, and right heart failure and pulmonary edema in women with no history of heart disease have also occurred. Intravenous β-mimetics regularly cause an increase in blood glucose and blood insulin levels; these are of no consequence in normal women but can be important in the presence of diabetes. The agents that have received most attention are isoxsuprine hydrochloride, ritodrine, and terbutaline. The cardiovascular effects of ritodrine appear to be less troublesome than those of terbutaline.

Hypoglycemia in the newborn, which can be observed within 90 minutes of birth, is a predictable consequence of the preterm use of β-mimetic agents among infants who are delivered within five days of the last dose of the agent; it responds promptly to glucose administration. Rare but possibly serious neonatal effects of isoxsuprine (if delivery occurs within 72 hours of the start of the infusion) include respiratory distress syndrome, necrotizing enterocolitis, hypotension, hypocalcemia, and death.

When using isoxsuprine as a tocolytic agent, a loading dose, 50 mg isoxsuprine in 500 ml normal saline solution, is administered intravenously at a rate of 200 to 250 μg/minute. The dosage should be increased by 50 to 75 μg every 15 to 30 minutes until a maximum dosage of 500 μg/minute is reached. If the drug is well tolerated, the clinically effective dose should be continued for six to eight hours. A maintenance dose of 10 to 20 mg isoxsuprine is administered every four to six hours intramuscularly or orally three to four times daily.

Common adverse reactions to isoxsuprine tocolysis include unpleasant cardiovascular, gastrointestinal, and neurologic side-effects. Generally, these reactions are mild with proper dosage, and discontinuation of the drug is not usually necessary.

Ritodrine may be given to suppress labor in a loading dose of 25 mg diluted in 250 ml 5% dextrose in water. (This solution contains 100 mg ritodrine per milliliter.) The intravenous infusion should begin at 50 mg/minute and is given preferably by infusion pump. This rate should be increased by 50 mg/minute every 10 minutes until satisfactory uterine inhibition has been achieved. The maximum intravenous dose, established mainly by tachycardia, is approximately 400 mg/minute. Ritodrine therapy shoud be continued for at least two hours after contractions have ceased. To prevent uterine recovery, therapy should not stop abruptly, but should be reduced gradually over a period of one to two hours. A maintenance dose of 20 to 30 mg ritodrine should be given orally twice daily for at least two weeks.

Adverse reactions to ritodrine tocolysis include hyperglycemia, hyperinsulinemia, and hyperkalemia. All of these reactions are dose-related. Pulmonary edema may occur if ritodrine is given intravenously in isotonic saline solution, especially when overdosage of the drug or prolonged treatment is permitted. Sodium and fluid intake should be restricted to avoid excess hydration.

Terbutaline may be given to inhibit labor in a loading dose of 10 μg/minute in normal saline solution. This dose should be given by infusion pump until a maximum dose of 80 μg is reached. Concomitantly, 30 mEq/liter potassium chloride in normal saline should be administered intravenously.

Terbutaline may also be administered in intravenous boluses and subcutaneously. In intravenous delivery, boluses of 250 μg terbutaline in normal saline should be given. If the dose is well tolerated, the boluses should be repeated at intervals of two to six hours as necessary. An intravenous dose of 30 mEq/liter potassium chloride should also be given slowly during this tocolytic therapy. Terbutaline may be given subcutaneously in a dose of 0.25 mg to 0.5 mg. The injections may be repeated in two to six hours as required.

A maintenance dose of 2.5 mg to 5 mg terbutaline may be given orally either twice or four times a day.

Terbutaline, which has not yet been approved for obstetric use by the FDA, may be the most effective tocolytic agent available, but it is probably the most dangerous. The incidence of acute cardiovascular complications is at least five times as great in terbutaline patients as in those receiving isoxsuprine.

The most serious adverse effect of the terbutaline tocolysis is pulmonary edema, which has been reported in about 5% of gravidas. These patients often have had multiple pregnancy and have received terbutaline by the intravenous or subcutaneous route. Terbutaline-induced pulmonary edema is not caused by left ventricular failure, but is related to flow and pressure changes in the pulmonary vasculature. Treatment consists of stopping the drug, and administering oxygen and small (5-mg to 15-mg) intravenous doses of furosemide. Neither digitalis nor morphine sulfate is routinely required. This complication has not been reported in patients receiving oral terbutaline.

CALCIUM ANTAGONISTS.   Calcium ions are needed for activation of the contractile proteins of the myometrium. Several drugs have been shown to inhibit the passage of calcium through excitable membranes, and extensive clinical use has been made of at least two of them (verapamil and nifedipine) in the treatment of ischemic heart disease. As expected, they have also been shown to reduce uterine motility (see Fig. 31-13). Preliminary studies with verapamil and nifedipine suggest they are effective in arresting preterm labor for periods varying from 3 to 17 days. The side-effects usually are not serious (transient facial flushing and moderate tachycardia). However, in patients with underlying heart disease calcium channel–blocking drugs are contraindicated as tocolytic agents because of the risk of precipitating myocardial ischemia or pulmonary edema.

PROSTAGLANDIN SYNTHETASE INHIBITORS.   There is ample evidence both in lower animals (rat, lamb, sheep) and in humans that prostaglandin synthetase inhibitors are effective in delaying or prolonging labor. When administered to the newborn, they cause the closure of a patent ductus arteriosus, which raised the question of whether they might have similar effects on the fetus if used in an effort to arrest labor. Such effects have been demonstrated in the fetal lamb. A few human cases of arterial pulmonary hypertension resulting from either indomethacin or large amounts of aspirin in late pregnancy have been reported. Prostaglandin synthetase inhibitors are no longer used to suppress premature labor.

MAGNESIUM SULFATE.   Magnesium sulfate is a labor suppressant, but it is less effective than ritodrine or terbutaline. However, it is very safe for mother and fetus.

Magnesium sulfate may be given in an intravenous bolus of 4 g over 10 minutes, followed by an intravenous infusion of 2 g/hour for six to eight hours, with additional fluid by mouth. Deep tendon reflexes and urinary output must be monitored at least hourly and diminution or absence of either indicates the possibility of overdosage (see p. 460). With the recommended program, other serious adverse effects of magnesium administration (*e.g.,* hypotension, sinoatrial or atrioventricular block, or cardiac arrest) are very rare.

GLUCOCORTICOID THERAPY. The use of glucocorticoids to accelerate maturation of the immature fetal lung is discussed elsewhere. The benefits in terms of preventing respiratory distress syndrome appear to be greatest in pregnancies of 29 to 32 weeks' duration. Glucocorticoids are of no benefit after 34 weeks' gestation, or if delivery occurs less than 24 hours or more than seven days after the first injection. If delivery is delayed more than seven days after the first injection, the treatment must be repeated. The agent used by Liggins and Howie is betamethasone (10 mg to 12 mg/24 hours in divided intramuscular injections and continued, if possible, for 48 to 72 hours). Other glucocorticoids given in comparable dosages should be effective also.

Steroid therapy does not seem to lower the incidence of respiratory distress syndrome in neonates born after premature rupture of the membranes, and the occurrence of neonatal sepsis is often thereby increased. In otherwise uncomplicated preterm pregnancy, glucocorticoid therapy has not caused deleterious fetal effects. Psychometric testing of these children at four years of age has shown no intellectual deficits to date.

The use of sympathomimetics, particularly terbutaline, together with glucocorticoids given in a large volume of fluid, has resulted in pulmonary edema in a small percentage of women with normal hearts. Furthermore, although these drugs are primarily β_2-receptor agonists, they do produce some β_1 stimulation, which leads to increased heart rate, cardiac output, and systolic blood pressure, and to decreased diastolic pressure and systemic vascular resistance. These drugs also cause a rise in serum glucose, free fatty acids, and lactate, and a fall in serum potassium.

PROGNOSIS FOR THE INFANT. With good selection of patients, proper dosage, and cautious, well-maintained tocolysis, there should be no negative impact on the neonate in terms of acidosis, respiratory distress syndrome, morbidity, average birth weight, or likelihood of survival. Among preterm labors in which attempts to arrest labor are either unsuccessful or inappropriate, perinatal mortality has declined to levels that only a few years ago were thought to be unattainable. In the Haesslein–Goodlin series, the overall survival of newborn infants weighing 800 g to 1350 g was 65%; in Stewart's series of cases, the mortality for newborns under 1500 g had declined to less than 40%. In 1977 James observed that in a number of institutions in the United States the survival rate for babies weighing less than 1000 g is 40% to 50% (see Fig. 42-8). There has also been a decline in neurologic and intellectual deficits among these babies. Among Stewart's series of 259 children aged 18 months or more who had weighed 1500 g or less at birth, 91.5% had no major handicap. These astonishing advances are due to so many factors that they cannot be listed; all aspects of prenatal, perinatal, and postnatal diagnosis and care have been vastly improved, and each has contributed. If the circumstances are ideal, it is no longer appropriate to consider the tiny fetus as doomed; all whose weight is estimated at more than 600 g should be regarded as patients at risk and must receive active consideration and treatment. However, it must be emphasized that preterm delivery should be carried out in facilities that provide level-III intensive perinatal care. Whenever possible the mother should be transferred to such a unit before delivery; the neonatal results are usually poor when the infant is transported after delivery. Life-threatening maternal complications must be dealt with at once, but heroic measures on behalf of a preterm baby should be taken only in institutions where intensive care for the newborn is immediately available.

THE ROLE OF CESAREAN SECTION. There is general agreement that cesarean section is the method of choice for preterm delivery if monitoring discloses definite fetal distress, if there is a breech presentation (gestational age <34 weeks), or if there is a transverse or oblique lie. Even in the absence of such indications, there is a growing conviction that cesarean section is largely responsible for the lower rates of morbidity and mortality among very low-birth-weight infants (500 g to 1500 g), and most authors consider cesarean section to be far less hazardous to the tiny newborn than vaginal delivery. For preterm cesarean section, the classic incision is usually required, which involves not only the immediate surgical risks but also the added threat of postoperative intestinal obstruction and, in a subsequent pregnancy, uterine rupture. Cesarean section is by no means innocuous, and its risks must be taken into account in deciding the mode of delivery of the preterm fetus.

VAGINAL DELIVERY. If vaginal delivery of the preterm infant is elected, or if it is inevitable, every effort must be made to avoid trauma and to prevent hypoxia. Labor should be conducted with the mother in the recumbent lateral position, nasal oxygen should be administered during labor, continuous fetal monitoring should be started, and systemic analgesia should not be used. Lumbar epidural anesthesia is appropriate if it is needed. Although opinions differ, it is recommended that the membranes be ruptured when the cervix is sufficiently dilated to permit application of an internal monitor. Reliable, efficient monitoring is essential, and the benefits far outweigh the risk of rupturing the membranes. Outlet forceps should be used unless spontaneous delivery occurs as soon as the head reaches the pelvic floor, as may be the case if the fetus is very small. A deep episiotomy should be made to avoid counterpressure on the fetal head.

Oxytocin may be used for stimulation if it is needed, but special surveillance is mandatory. The infusion is started at 1 mU/minute and increased every 10 minutes in increments of 1 mU/minute until a maximum of 10 mU/minute is reached or until laborlike contractions occur every 2.5 to 3 minutes. Prolonged oxytocin stimulation is inadvisable in preterm labor. The infusion should be stopped if effective labor is not established in four to six hours.

After delivery, the infant should be placed at or below the level of the vulva. If breathing occurs quickly, the cord should be cut 30 to 45 seconds after delivery to permit optimal placental transfusion and to allow the passage of placental and cord blood into the expanding pulmonary unit. If breathing is delayed, the cord should be cut 20 to 30 seconds after delivery and the infant transferred immediately to a heated table for resuscitative measures.

REFERENCES

Andersson K: Pharmacological inhibition of uterine activity. Acta Gynecol Scand (Suppl 61)108:17, 1982

Barrett JM, Boehm FH, Vaughn WK: The effect of type of delivery on neonatal outcome in singleton infants of 1,000 g or less. JAMA 250:625, 1983

Bieniarz J, Burd L, Motew M et al: Inhibition of uterine contractility in labor. Am J Obstet Gynecol 11:874, 1971

Boylan P, O'Driscoll K: Improvement in perinatal mortality rate attributed to spontaneous preterm labor without use of tocolytic agents. Am J Obstet Gynecol 145:781, 1983

Brazy JE, Little V, Grimm J et al: Risk–benefit consideration for use of isoxsuprine in treatment of premature labor. Obstet Gynecol 58:297, 1981

Chenoweth JN, Esler EJ, Chang A et al: Understanding preterm labor: The use of path analysis. Aust NZ J Obstet Gynaecol 23:199, 1983

Cotton DB: Effects of terbutaline on acid–base, serum electrolytes and glucose homeostasis during management of preterm labor. Am J Obstet Gynecol 141:617, 1981

Creasy RK, Gummer BA, Liggins CG: System for predicting spontaneous preterm birth. Obstet Gynecol 55:692, 1980

Downey LJ, Martin AJ: Ritodrine in the treatment of preterm labour: A study of 213 patients. Br J Obstet Gynaecol 90:1046, 1983

Elliot JP: Magnesium sulfate as a tocolytic agent. Am J Obstet Gynecol 147:277, 1983

Fedrick J: Antenatal identification of women at high risk of spontaneous preterm birth. Br J Obstet Gynaecol 83:351, 1976

Graham RL, Gilstrap LC, Hauth JC et al: Conservative management of patients with premature rupture of fetal membranes. Obstet Gynecol 59:617, 1982

Gross TL, Sokol RJ: Severe hypokalemia and acidosis: A potential complication of beta-adrenergic treatment. Am J Obstet Gynecol 138:1225, 1980

Guilliams S, Held B: Contemporary management and conduct of preterm labor and delivery: A review. Obstet Gynecol Surv 34:248, 1979

Haesslein HC, Goodlin RC: Delivery of the tiny newborn. Am J Obstet Gynecol 134:192, 1979

Herron MA, Katz M, Creasy RK: Evaluation of a preterm birth prevention program: Preliminary report. Obstet Gynecol 59:452, 1982

Herschel M, Kennedy JL, Kayne HL et al: Survival of infants born at 24 to 28 weeks' gestation. Obstet Gynecol 60:154, 1982

Huddleston JF: Preterm labor. Clin Obstet Gynecol 25:123, 1982

Hurwitz A, Adoni A, Pslti Z et al: Is conservative management of preterm rupture of membranes justified? Int J Gynaecol Obstet 22:131, 1984

Ingemarsson I: Use of β-receptor agonists in obstetrics. Acta Obstet Gynecol Scand (Suppl 61)108:29, 1982

Kauppila O, Grönroos M, Paavo A et al: Management of low birth weight breech delivery: Should cesarean section be routine? Obstet Gynecol 57:289, 1981

Korenbrot CC, Aalto LH, Laros RK, Jr.: The cost effectiveness of stopping preterm labor with beta-adrenergic treatment. N Engl J Med 310:691, 1984

Mabie WC, Pernoll ML, Witty JB et al: Pulmonary edema induced by beta-mimetic drugs. South Med J 76:1354, 1983

Naeye RI: Factors that predispose to premature rupture of the fetal membranes. Obstet Gynecol 60:93, 1982

Neldam S, Osler M: Premature rupture of the membranes and ritodrine treatment. Acta Obstet Gynecol Scand 62:135, 1983

Newton RW, Webster PAC, Binu PS et al: Psychosocial stress in pregnancy and its influence on premature labour. Br Med J 2:411, 1979

Nisell H, Bistoletti P, Palme C: Preterm breech delivery: Early and late complications. Acta Obstet Gynecol Scand 60:363, 1981

O'Driscoll K, Foley M: Correlation of decrease in perinatal mortality and increase in cesarean section rates. Obstet Gynecol 61:1, 1983

Papiernik E, Kaminski M: Multifactoral study of the risk of prematurity at 32 weeks of gestation. J Perinat Med 2:30, 1974

Penney LL, Daniell WC: Estimation of success in treatment of premature labor: Applicability of prolongation index in a double-blind, controlled, randomized trial. Am J Obstet Gynecol 138:345, 1980

Procianoy RS, Pinheiro ACEA: Neonatal hyperinsulinism after short-term maternal beta-sympatheticomimetic therapy. J Pediatr 101:612, 1982

Richards SR, Chang FF, Stempel LL: Hyperlactacidemia associated with acute ritodrine infusion. Am J Obstet Gynecol 146:1, 1983

Schwarz R, Tetzke U: Cardiovascular effects of terbutaline in pregnant women. Acta Obstet Gynecol Scand 62:419, 1983

Skjaerris J, Aberg A: Prevention of prematurity in twin pregnancy by orally administered terbutaline. Acta Obstet Gynecol Scand (Suppl 61)108:39, 1982

Spellacy WN, Cruz AC, Buhi WC et al: The acute effects of ritodrine infusion on maternal metabolism: Measurements of glucose, insulin glucagon, triglycerides, cholesterol, placental lactogen and chorionic gonadotropin. Am J Obstet Gynecol 131:637, 1977

Stedman CM, Crawford S, Staten E et al: Management of preterm premature rupture of membranes: Assessing amniotic fluid in the vagina for phosphatidylglycerol. Am J Obstet Gynecol 140:34, 1981

Stubblefield PG, Heyl PS: Treatment of premature labor with terbutaline. Obstet Gynecol 59:457, 1982

Tchilinguirian NG, Najem R, Sullivan GB et al: The use of ritodrine and magnesium sulfate in the arrest of premature labor. Int J Gynaecol Obstet 22:117, 1984

Van Eyk, Huisjes HJ: Neonatal mortality and morbidity associated with premature breech presentation. Eur J Obstet Gynecol Reprod Biol 15:17, 1983

Ying YK, Tejani NA: Angina pectoris as a complication of ritodrine hydrochloride in premature labor. Obstet Gynecol 60:385, 1982

Dystocia Due to Abnormal Fetopelvic Relations

David N. Danforth

36

Dystocia is defined as abnormal labor. Four "Ps" are concerned in the efficiency of labor: the powers, the pelvis or passage, the passenger, and the psyche. The *powers* are the expulsive forces of the contracting uterus. Both normal and abnormal uterine actions are discussed elsewhere in this book. The influences and effects of the *pelvic architecture* are outlined in Chapter 32. The *passenger* (the fetus) as it passes through the pelvis in the course of labor may, by its size, its presentation, or its position, give rise to abnormalities in labor. The patient's *psyche* may have an important influence on the duration and character of labor.

None of these factors operates independently of the others, and they must all be considered when the physician attempts to determine why a particular labor does not proceed normally. If they are systematically assessed, it should be possible to determine the cause of every abnormal labor.

The position and presentation of the fetus in relation to the pelvis may produce various abnormalities of labor. The problems that arise relate basically to the fact that either the size of the fetus or the diameter of the fetus that presents to the pelvis is such that it cannot readily pass through. The uterus is often very responsive to these minor abnormalities and fails to contract efficiently. Abnormal labor is the result. Some of these problems may eventuate in spontaneous or outlet forceps delivery, and some may require cesarean section. Several can be dealt with satisfactorily by midforceps delivery.

FORCEPS OPERATIONS

Definitions

The following definitions have been approved by the American College of Obstetricians and Gynecologists:

A *low forceps operation* is the application of ob-

stetric forceps to the fetal skull when the scalp is or has been visible at the introitus without separating the labia, the skull has reached the pelvic floor, and the sagittal suture is in the anteroposterior diameter of the outlet of the pelvis.

A *midforceps operation* is the application of obstetric forceps to the fetal skull when the head is engaged, but the conditions for low forceps have not been met. (Many obstetricians object to this definition. An alternative and preferable definition is suggested later.) In the context of this term, any forceps operation that requires artificial rotation, regardless of the station from which extraction is begun, is designated a *midforceps operation.*

A *high forceps operation* is the application of obstetric forceps at any time before the engagement of the fetal head.

The following additional terms are used: *trial forceps operation,* which refers to the circumstance in which the physician recognizes in advance that cephalopelvic relationships are not wholly favorable but considers the possibility of safe vaginal delivery to be great enough that a tentative effort should be made. If any difficulty is encountered, the attempt is immediately abandoned in favor of cesarean section. *Failed forceps operation* is a retrospective diagnosis. The intent is to deliver vaginally, but when undue difficulty is encountered, the physician retreats and delivers by cesarean section. The subject of *outlet forceps* is considered in Chapter 33. No discussion of high forceps is included, since the operation is entirely obsolete and has no place in modern obstetrics.

Midforceps Delivery

The position of midforceps delivery has undergone great change in the past 15 years. Formerly, the operation was uniformly acceptable and was an integral part of obstetric practice. More recently, reviews of midforceps experience have condemned the operation because of the high incidence of neonatal death and, among the survivors, the frequency of long-term intellectual deficits. At present, all agree that the difficult midforceps deliveries of the past are not permissible. However, there is increasing awareness that some midforceps operations can be performed easily and safely.

As currently defined, midforceps delivery encompasses two very different kinds of delivery: difficult and potentially damaging forceps deliveries from a station between 0 and +3, and easy and much safer deliveries from a station between +3 and the level that conforms to the present definition of low forceps delivery. Studies dealing with the safety and propriety of midforceps delivery do not distinguish one from the other. Furthermore, in most of the reviews that condemn midforceps delivery, statements regarding the level of the head at the time of intervention are conspicuously absent. Without such evidence, one reaches the obvious conclusion that most of the poor outcomes occur in forceps deliveries from the higher level.

New definitions are needed if midforceps operations are to be placed in proper perspective. The following are suggested: *Midforceps delivery* is forceps delivery from a station between 0 and +3; *outlet forceps* is forceps delivery after the fetal scalp is or has been visible at the introitus without separating the labia, the skull has reached the pelvic floor, and the sagittal suture is in the anteroposterior diameter of the pelvic outlet; *low forceps delivery* is forceps delivery when the head has reached station +3 or lower but the conditions for outlet forceps have not been met. Use of these definitions would have at least two salutary effects: the term *midforceps* would immediately connote a delivery of more than average risk and difficulty, from a high station; easy forceps deliveries from a low level, including some rotations that should be within the capability of all obstetricians, could be performed without the legally abhorrent and often indefensible stigma of "midforceps."

Indications

Midforceps delivery may be indicated in the following circumstances:

1. Faults in cephalopelvic relations. These include especially malpositions of the head such as persistent occiput posterior or face position, transverse arrest, and a relatively small pelvis that prevents spontaneous advancement of the head regardless of position. In the latter case, it is of vital importance to recognize true disproportion, to know the pelvic diameters in which the traction must be made, and to know the amount of traction that can be safely applied. Happily, the heavy traction of former years is no longer permissible. Cesarean section must be

elected if the head cannot be readily advanced by ordinary traction.
2. Uterine inertia. Uterine inertia is not uncommon in the second stage of labor and may be sufficient to interfere with progress. Occasionally, the quality of the contractions is improved by an oxytocin infusion; but if it is not or if this is not a reasonable procedure in the circumstance, midforceps delivery is indicated, provided the conditions for its performance are favorable.
3. Conditions that threaten the life of the mother. These are unusual, and an inclusive list cannot be given. They include especially circumstances in which the second stage must be shortened, such as advanced heart disease and other cardiopulmonary conditions that produce severe dyspnea.
4. Conditions that threaten the life of the baby. The classic signs of danger are changes in the fetal heart rate (see Chapter 41, Clinical Evaluation of Fetal Status) and, in vertex presentation, the appearance of meconium where none had been present before. Provided the conditions are favorable, delivery should be accomplished without delay. When labor is unusually vigorous, partial separation of the placenta during the second stage is not unusual. It is usually manifested by failure of the uterus to relax completely between contractions, by undue uterine pain and tenderness, and, if the membranes are ruptured, by the passage of port-wine–colored amniotic fluid. Midforceps intervention on behalf of a fetus in jeopardy may require fine clinical judgment as to whether the hazard of forceps delivery is greater than the danger of delay in turning to cesarean section.

Conditions

The conditions for midforceps delivery are as follows:

1. The cervix should be fully dilated. In an extreme emergency forceps may be applied inside a cervix dilated 8 cm (but not less than 8 cm) and Dührssen's incisions made in the cervix at the 10 o'clock and 2 o'clock positions. This is rarely necessary, however, and it is an accepted obstetric principle that full dilatation, except in extraordinary conditions, is requisite for forceps delivery.
2. The membranes must be ruptured. If they are left intact, the forceps will slip, and traction upon the membranes may detach an edge of the placenta. Moreover, the need for forceps delivery cannot be determined with certainty until the membranes are ruptured.
3. The head must be engaged in the pelvis, and there must be no real obstruction to further advancement. Application of forceps to a head that is movable above the pelvic brim is indefensible in modern obstetric practice. Moreover, mere engagement, although it suffices for purposes of definition, is far less favorable

than location of the head below station +2. The higher the station at the time delivery is begun, the greater the risk to mother and baby. If molding is extreme, with large caput succedaneum, the scalp may be almost at the introitus when the biparietal diameter is still at the inlet. One should not apply forceps if the sinciput can be felt above the symphysis.

4. The child must present correctly. All vertex presentations and face presentations with chin anterior are suitable. Chin posterior and brow presentations are not suitable for the application of forceps. No attempt should be made to apply forceps to the breech.

Obstetric Forceps

Types

Two groups of obstetric forceps are available. The so-called classic forceps are those with the standard cephalic and pelvic curves already described in connection with outlet forceps (see Chapter 33). In addition to these, special forceps have been designed for dealing with certain specific problems. Since the invention of the first obstetric forceps, obstetricians have made major or minor modifications of the classic instrument to fit their individual tastes; many have survived, each named for the physician who made the modification. The commonly used forceps are illustrated in Figure 36-1.

Application

Two methods of forceps application are available: pelvic application and cephalic application. *Pelvic application* involves merely placing the forceps in the pelvic cavity and applying the blades to the presenting part so that they will lock, without reference to the position of the head. Mention is made of this application only for its historic interest; except in the most extraordinary circumstances, it is not permissible in modern obstetrics, since it imposes stresses the head can rarely tolerate. If the forceps cannot be accurately applied to

FIG. 36-1. Commonly used forceps. (Douglas RG, Stromme WB: Operative Obstetrics. New York, Appleton-Century-Crofts, 1957)

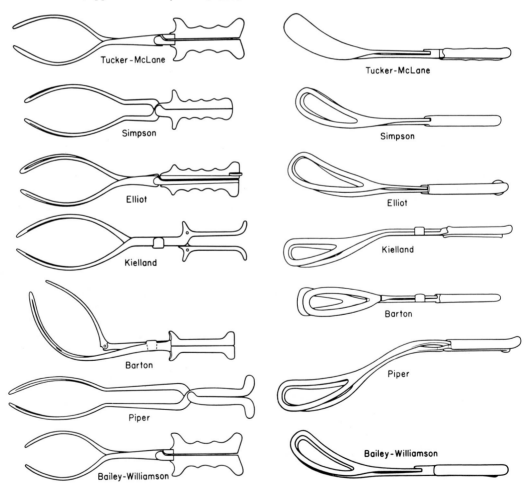

Tucker-McLane

Tucker-McLane

Simpson

Simpson

Elliot

Elliot

Kielland

Kielland

Barton

Barton

Piper

Piper

Bailey-Williamson

Bailey-Williamson

the head, cesarean section is almost invariably the proper alternative. In the *cephalic application,* the blades are applied precisely to the occipitomental diameter of the head. Provided this application is accurate and the movements are made gently, deliberately, and with knowledge of what is to be accomplished, considerable traction can be exerted and any needed rotation performed with safety. Cephalic application of forceps along the occipitomental diameter of the head is possible in several different situations, including the occiput anterior, occiput transverse, and occiput posterior positions and the face presentation (Fig. 36-2). It may also be used for the after-coming head in breech presentations.

FIG. 36-2. Forceps correctly applied along occipitomental diameter in various head positions. (*A*) Occiput anterior. (*B*) Occiput posterior. (*C*) Mentum anterior.

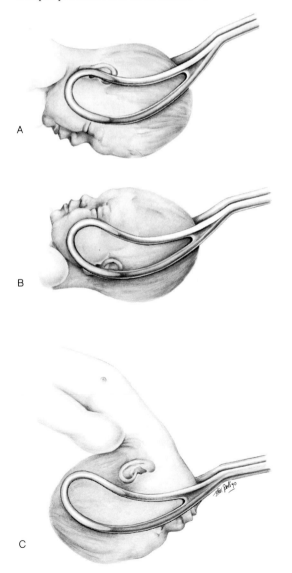

When the forceps are applied to the head in the occiput anterior position, which is most customary, the posterior fontanel should be a fingerbreadth anterior to the plane of the shanks and equidistant from the sides of the blades; the sagittal suture should be perpendicular to the middle of the plane of the shanks in its entirety; and the fenestrations of the blades should be high enough in the pelvis that they can be barely felt or not felt at all.

Choice

For traction to the occiput anterior, most obstetricians in America and the United Kingdom prefer the Simpson instrument or one of its modifications. If this instrument is accurately applied and traction is made in the proper diameters of the pelvis, considerable force may be exerted without injury to the baby. Accordingly, the Simpson or Elliot forceps are considered the safest in ordinary situations when moderate traction is needed.

For rotation from the occiput posterior to the occiput anterior position, most operators prefer the Tucker–McLane instrument, the Luikart modification of the Simpson forceps, or the Kielland forceps. If molding is marked, forceps with a round cephalic curve, such as the Tucker–McLane, may not fit the head well and may in fact cut the infant's cheek at the level of the zygomatic arch, especially if any traction is applied. Hence, forceps with a more elongated cephalic curve (*e.g.,* the Luikart–Simpson) may be preferred. Although the most frequent use of the Kielland forceps is with the fetus in the occiput transverse position, it may also be used with the fetus in the occiput posterior position.

For forceps rotation from the occiput transverse, either the Barton or Kielland forceps can be used. In some cases, especially when there is sufficient space posterior to the head, the Simpson forceps may be applied directly to the transverse, although this is relatively unusual in the classic transverse arrest because of a flat pelvis.

For forceps delivery of the after-coming head, the Piper modification of the Simpson forceps is used in the United States virtually to the exclusion of all others.

In the United Kingdom the Wrigley forceps (a lightened modification of the Simpson instrument with shortened shanks and handles) is extremely popular for low and outlet forceps deliveries and for application to the after-coming head.

Although it is important to select the proper instrument, it must be emphasized that the results depend far more on the skill and judgment of the operator than on the selection of any particular forceps.

Vacuum Extractor (Ventouse)

The vacuum extractor is an instrument that is used to effect delivery by the application of traction to a suction cup attached to the fetal scalp. The instrument consists of the following parts: a flat suction cup that is smaller at the rim than above the rim, to permit the scalp to be anchored in the peripheral reaches of the cup; a chain leading from the cup to a traction handle; and a hose leading from the cup to a suction pump with gauge to measure negative pressure. Several modifications of the instrument have been made since Malmström introduced it in 1954.

In practice, the cup is positioned so that the sagittal and lamboidal sutures are symmetrically palpable at the periphery of the cup. Negative pressure is induced at a rate of 0.2 kg/cm²/2 minutes up to a maximum of 0.6 kg/cm²; from 6 to 7 minutes elapses before the correct pressure is attained. Traction is made in the direction of the curve of Carus coincidently with uterine contractions. The method is considered to have failed if the head is not delivered after 5 such tractions over the course of not more than 15 minutes.

The ventouse has never gained acceptance in the United States as a substitute for obstetric forceps, but in Scandinavia and some other European countries, as well as in Australia, it is used extensively and with excellent results—in some services, vacuum extraction is the only means of instrumental vaginal delivery used. This paradox is not easily explained. However, it does seem clear that, as in all kinds of intervention, there is no substitute for skill and experience. Those who use the ventouse with satisfaction insist that most of the complications result from improper use, such as overlong or incorrectly applied traction, use of excessive negative pressure, failure to prevent cervical or vaginal tissue from entering the cup, overlong application of the cup to the scalp, and failure to recognize circumstances in which use is contraindicated (*e.g.,* cephalopelvic disproportion; breech, brow, or face presentation). The references appended to this chapter provide more detailed information.

ABNORMAL POSITIONS THAT CAUSE DYSTOCIA

Conduct of Labor in Fetopelvic Dystocia

In most cases of dystocia, the possibility of a problem can be suspected within six hours of the onset of labor; the abnormality can usually be diagnosed with certainty in the next six hours, and it should be dealt with, usually by delivery, before 18 hours of labor have elapsed. If the problem is due to fetopelvic dystocia, it can usually be suspected, diagnosed, and dealt with in a much shorter time than if the cause is dysfunctional labor.

In fetopelvic dystocia with vertex presentation, difficulty may be suggested by either (1) excessively slow progress in the first stage (as is not unusual if the fetus is in the occiput posterior position or if the head does not fit well into the lower uterine segment because, for example, of inlet disproportion) or (2) a presenting part that remains at a relatively high station and cannot be easily impressed to deep engagement. In such cases,

x-ray pelvimetry may be of special value, provided it is done by a technique that (1) includes a standing (*not* recumbent) lateral film and a film that shows inlet shape, and (2) permits the obstetrician to obtain a three-dimensional concept of the pelvis at all levels. One such technique is described in Chapter 32. Techniques that do not provide this information (*e.g.,* Colcher–Sussman) are not helpful.

If the labor is to be longer than usual, attention should be given to hydration, regular emptying of the bladder, and sedatives and analgesics as needed.

In conducting the second stage, it is emphasized that the ease and safety of midforceps delivery are much greater if maximum descent and maximum molding have been attained. Moreover, when rotation is incomplete, the lower the head, the greater the likelihood of spontaneous rotation to the anterior. Hence, unless an indication for intervention arises, the second stage should be permitted to proceed as long as progress is made, up to a maximum of 2 hours in the primigravida and 1 hour in the multipara. After a second stage of this duration, there is a risk of uterine rupture and constriction ring dystocia.

The woman's voluntary bearing-down effort may be of great importance in advancing the head to a level from which it can be safely delivered. Her ability to make this effort can be impaired by heavy systemic analgesia or too early use of conduction anesthesia. It can be greatly facilitated by the thoughtful encouragement of the attendant and, in many cases, by two or three deep breaths of 50% nitrous oxide and 50% oxygen at the beginning of each second-stage contraction.

Occiput Posterior Position

When the fetal occiput lies in one of the posterior quadrants of the pelvis, the position is defined as *occiput posterior.* The mechanism of labor and the role of the pelvis in persistent and arrested occiput posterior position are considered in Chapter 32. Suffice it to mention here that the anthropoid pelvis predisposes; that spontaneous rotation may be expected if the transverse diameter of the midpelvis is wide enough to permit the anteroposterior diameter of the head to rotate at this level; that transverse narrowing of the midpelvis because of either convergent sidewalls or prominent spines may prevent spontaneous rotation; and that in the latter case, if the lower sacrum is sufficiently forward, artificial rotation may be needed for delivery. In clinical practice, approximately 70% of fetuses in the occiput posterior position rotate spontaneously, but the rest require artificial rotation or, if the woman's sacrum is far posterior, delivery as direct occiput posteriors.

Diagnosis

As is true of all obstetric complications, it is important that an exact diagnosis be made at the earliest possible time; the intelligent conduct of labor depends on it. Three major factors are concerned in the diagnosis of occiput posterior position: the character of labor, the abdominal contour and the findings on palpation, and the findings on vaginal examination.

CHARACTER OF LABOR. Efficiency of the uterine contractions depends to an important extent on the even fitting of the presenting part to the lower uterine segment. In the occiput anterior position this fitting is optimal, whereas in the occiput posterior position the fitting may be improper. Although there are exceptions to this generalization, when the child is in the occiput posterior position, labor is often desultory and relatively ineffective. Accentuated backache and, in the second stage, gaping of the anus are common. When labor does not progress at the expected rate or when the contractions are of poor quality, the first thought should be the possibility of occiput posterior position.

ABDOMINAL CONTOUR. When the fetus is in the occiput anterior position, the woman's lower abdomen, from umbilicus to vulva, has a gentle convexity, since the fetal head is well flexed and the depression at the nape of the neck is more or less ironed out. When the fetus is in the occiput posterior position, a considerable depression occurs between the fetal chin and the small parts, and this is reflected by a concavity above the level of the symphysis (Fig. 36-3). Although this is not an invariable finding, especially if the fetal head is deeply engaged or the maternal bladder is full, its presence should suggest the possibility of occiput posterior position.

FINDINGS ON VAGINAL EXAMINATION. If the cervix is fully dilated or is so situated and sufficiently pliable that the examiner can readily sweep the examining finger over the head, and if the fetus is in the occiput posterior position, the four suture lines that enter the anterior fontanel will be encountered. (One can rarely reach the posterior fontanel.) This confirms the diagnosis of occiput posterior position. In early labor, or if the cervix is posterior so that this examination would be difficult or painful, the definitive diagnosis may be left for later. If the first two factors are present, however, the physician should make the tentative diagnosis of occiput posterior position and should conduct the labor accordingly. Prior knowledge, either by x-ray films or

clinical examination, of an anthropoid pelvis strengthens the probability of occiput posterior position.

Management of Labor

Since labor is apt to be longer than usual with the fetus in the occiput posterior position, full attention should be given to fetal monitoring, judicious use of sedatives and analgesics, attention to hydration, and in some cases stimulation of labor by oxytocics.

Unless intervention becomes necessary, a full second stage should be permitted to achieve maximum molding and maximum descent of the head.

Management of Delivery

As noted earlier, approximately 70% of fetuses in the occiput posterior position rotate to the anterior spontaneously; delivery in such cases offers no unusual problem. Nor does a special problem arise in cases that are normally destined to deliver face to pubis without rotation. In the monkey, the posterior mechanism and spontaneous delivery face to pubis are the rule. In a woman with a classic anthropoid pelvis and a sacrum directed far posterior, a similar outcome of labor may be expected, and no intervention is required. With such a pelvis, if uterine inertia results in the arrest of the head in the occiput posterior position very deep in the pelvis, the head may be gently delivered in the direct posterior by outlet forceps. In either case, a wide episiotomy is usually required.

Artificial rotation is needed if occiput posterior position persists because of a forward lower sacrum that impedes progress or transverse narrowing of the midpelvis that prevents spontaneous rotation. Two techniques are available: manual rotation and forceps rotation.

The resident in training should master a technique for rotation from the occiput posterior position and should use it with confidence when the circumstances are appropriate. The present trend away from the deliberate performance of a difficult vaginal delivery is entirely correct. However, the trend toward cesarean section in all cases in which the head cannot be readily advanced in the posterior position is clearly not in the best interests of either mother or baby. In most cases rotation from the posterior position is not a difficult pro-

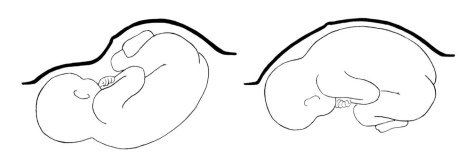

FIG. 36-3. Variation in maternal abdominal contour with fetus in occiput posterior and occiput anterior positions.

cedure, and it can usually be accomplished much more quickly and safely than cesarean section.

MANUAL ROTATION.   Manual rotation is preferred by some obstetricians. Many techniques have been described; one is shown in Figure 36-4. Basically, the head is grasped with the right hand, fingers widely spread, and is elevated above the point of arrest. An assistant pushes the anterior fetal shoulder across the maternal abdomen. The rotation is then accomplished, and forceps are applied for delivery. This technique is especially favored by those who have a small hand. The operator whose hand is large will probably prefer forceps rotation. Both techniques are acceptable and widely used, but the obstetrician should master one and should use it exclusively unless unusual circumstances require a variant.

FORCEPS ROTATION.   Forceps rotation may be carried out after elevation of the head above the level of arrest, at the level of arrest, or by spiral advancement of the head. Spiral advancement of the head is to be eschewed except in the most extraordinary circumstances; it requires much force and is attended by a high probability of both fetal and maternal damage. Rotation at the level of arrest, as in Bill's rotation, is satisfactory if the spines are not prominent and if there is ample transverse space in the midpelvis; however, in most circumstances rotation is easiest if the head is elevated above the level of arrest so that adequate transverse space is ensured. In the standard forceps rotation, classic forceps (preferably the Luikart–Simpson or Tucker–McLean) are applied to the posterior, and the head is then elevated slightly and flexed. By swinging the handles of the forceps in a wide arc so the tips of the blades remain in the same axis, the physician accomplishes rotation in a single sweep or preferably intermittently through short arcs, but in either case with the utmost gentleness (Figs. 36-5 and 36-6). When the rotation to the anterior position has been accomplished, one blade of the forceps is removed, while the other blade is left in place to prevent the head from spinning back to its former position. One blade of a second pair of forceps is applied opposite the splinting blade, the handles are rearranged to lock, the second blade is inserted, and delivery is accomplished as though the position had originally been anterior.

If Kielland forceps are chosen, rotation may be carried out in the axis of the forceps, since this instrument has substantially no pelvic curve. When the rotation is accomplished, classic forceps may be substituted for the Kielland, since the lack of pelvic curve may prevent the use of proper traction.

Brow Presentation

With partial extension of the head, the brow of the infant may become the presenting part. The large (13.5-cm) occipitomental diameter of the head then presents to the pelvis as one diameter, the biparietal

FIG. 36-4.   Manual rotation of head in right occiput posterior (ROP) position. (*A*) Head grasped by whole hand and rotated to anterior position; assistant pushes shoulder toward patient's left. (*B*) Rotation complete; right hand maintains head in position while left blade of forceps is applied. Right hand is used for rotation, regardless of whether from ROP or LOP, and left blade of forceps is always introduced first. (Danforth WC: The treatment of occiput posterior with special reference to manual rotation. Am J Obstet Gynecol 23:360, 1932)

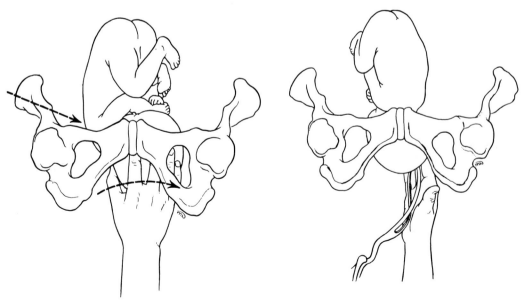

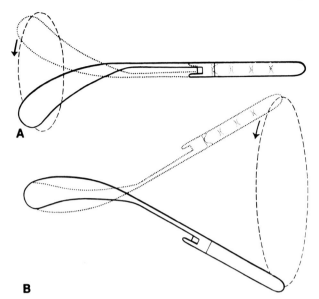

A

B

FIG. 36-5. Forceps rotation of head in occiput posterior position. (*A*) Incorrect technique. (*B*) Correct technique. If handles are rotated in same axis, blades describe wide arc and tear vagina. Handles must be swung widely and tips of blades kept at approximately same point. (Douglas RG, Stromme WB: Operative Obstetrics. New York, Appleton-Century-Crofts, 1957)

remaining as the other. Unless the pelvis is exceptionally large or the baby very small, spontaneous delivery with the head remaining in this position is unlikely; however, it is in these two situations that brow presentation is most frequently encountered. Although loops of cord around the neck or some other anterior neck mass, such as a cystic hygroma, should be looked for as a possible cause, such conditions are seldom found.

Diagnosis is difficult on abdominal examination, although the bony prominence of the occiput may be felt high during palpation downward along the fetal back. Vaginal and rectal examinations are often confusing, but the physician may be alerted to the possibility of brow presentation by the very high station. X-ray films may be needed for diagnosis.

Unless the head is markedly smaller than the pelvis, spontaneous delivery is not to be expected if the head remains in the brow presentation. It may correct spontaneously, converting either to a face presentation by further extension or to an occipital presentation by further flexion. Manual correction may be attempted but should be undertaken only with the membranes intact or at the time of their rupture, and with due awareness that the cord may prolapse before the head. Any such attempt should be quickly abandoned if it is not immediately successful. If conditions appear unfavorable for manual correction and active labor is in progress, it is entirely appropriate to perform cesarean section at once.

Face Presentation

In general, the prognosis for vaginal delivery in face presentation is relatively good insofar as diameters of the head are concerned. It is only when the chin (commonly used as the point of reference in face presentation) and fetal chest point posteriorly that difficulties arise. When the head reaches the upper midpelvis, it is already extended to the maximum degree and cannot negotiate the pelvic curve (see Fig. 32-29).

In many instances, face presentation is the end result of a brow presentation that has undergone further extension. Thus, face presentation is often seen under the same circumstances—a small infant in a large pelvis. In addition, any factors that prevent adequate flexion of the head may result in face presentation; thus, large size of the infant or some relative pelvic disproportion, particularly at the inlet, may favor its development. Abnormalities of the neck, although often mentioned as causes, are seldom found.

The diagnosis can rarely be made on abdominal examination. Vaginal or rectal examination discloses an irregular presenting part, which at once suggests the following possibilities: face presentation, breech presentation (especially footling or full breech), compound presentation, or severe congenital anomaly (especially anencephaly). It is usually necessary to resolve these doubts by x-ray examination, particularly if the baby is large or there is some clinical evidence of relative disproportion.

Since the diameters of the fetal head presenting are not significantly greater than normal, spontaneous delivery or delivery by outlet forceps can be anticipated if the chin is anterior. When the chin remains posterior, forceps or manual rotation is rarely either safe or feasible. A mentum posterior position that persists after labor is established is best managed by cesarean section, regardless of parity or size of the baby.

Transverse Arrest

The term *transverse arrest* refers to the arrest of the fetal head in the transverse position, usually in the midpelvis, rarely at the outlet, with failure of progress for at least 30 minutes. The two major causes are (1) anteroposterior flattening in the midpelvis or lower pelvis, as occurs in the platypelloid or android pelvis, and (2) uterine inertia. The head ordinarily engages in the transverse position, the sagittal suture lying transversely across the pelvis. If there is anteroposterior narrowing in the midpelvis and outlet, the head tends to traverse these levels in the direct transverse position, without anterior rotation. In the gynecoid pelvis, anterior rotation tends to occur in the lower midpelvis. In the latter case, if uterine inertia occurs before the time of internal rotation, progress may cease, the head remaining in the transverse position.

The management of transverse arrest depends upon its cause.

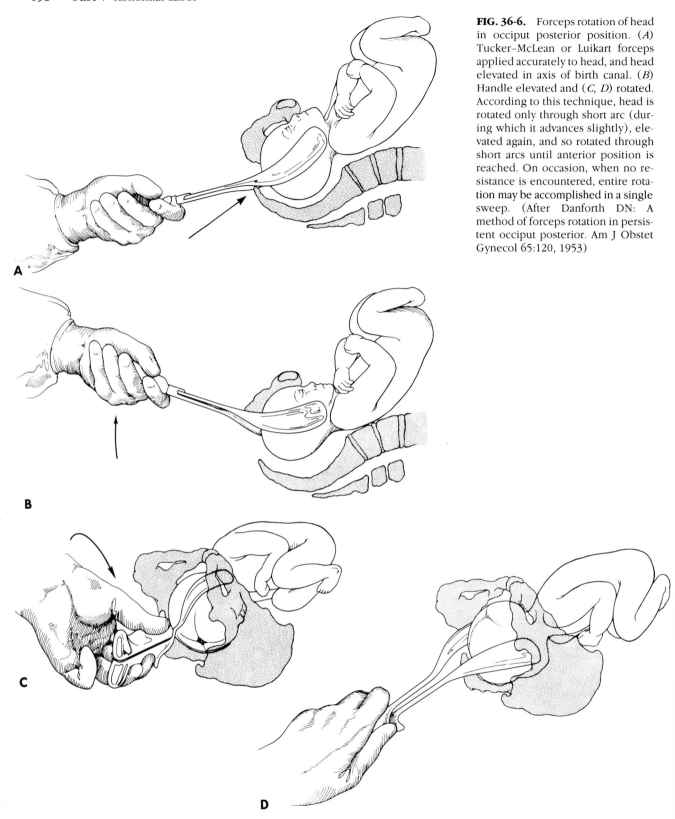

FIG. 36-6. Forceps rotation of head in occiput posterior position. (*A*) Tucker–McLean or Luikart forceps applied accurately to head, and head elevated in axis of birth canal. (*B*) Handle elevated and (*C, D*) rotated. According to this technique, head is rotated only through short arc (during which it advances slightly), elevated again, and so rotated through short arcs until anterior position is reached. On occasion, when no resistance is encountered, entire rotation may be accomplished in a single sweep. (After Danforth DN: A method of forceps rotation in persistent occiput posterior. Am J Obstet Gynecol 65:120, 1953)

If the pelvis is of normal configuration and adequate size, if the arrest occurs at a relatively low level, and if the arrest is believed to have resulted only from desultory second-stage contractions, an oxytocin infusion, administered at a rate that will provide contractions every 2 to 2.5 minutes lasting 30 to 50 seconds, often suffices to induce further descent, anterior rotation, and subsequent delivery either spontaneously or by outlet forceps. As an alternative, if the patient is fatigued, if there has been no progress for 30 minutes, if the head is at a low level, and if the obstetrician is certain the baby can be safely delivered, or if there is an indication for immediate delivery, classic forceps may be applied to the transverse position (or manual rotation may be done at the level of arrest) and the head rotated and delivered.

If the arrest is due to anteroposterior narrowing of the pelvis (a flat or platypelloid pelvis), its management depends on the depth of engagement, the need for prompt vaginal delivery, and the skill and experience of the operator. If progress ceases for 30 minutes or if elapsed time in the second stage requires termination of labor, cesarean section should be elected if the head is not deeply engaged (to or beyond station +3) or if there is any question of the adequacy of the pelvis below the point of arrest. If the head is deeply engaged, if the pelvis is considered adequate, and if the operator's skill and experience permit him to approach this kind of problem with confidence, a trial forceps may be appropriate. The attempt should be promptly abandoned if there is undue resistance.

In *transverse arrest due to flat pelvis,* the head must be advanced in the transverse position until the level for rotation on the pelvic floor is reached. Two techniques are available: one with Kielland forceps and one with Barton forceps. The Kielland forceps were designed originally for application to the head in deep transverse arrest. They have a sliding lock that facilitates application. Knobs are located on the handles; these should point toward the occiput, and before application the physician should face the perineum holding the articulated forceps as they will be applied to the head, with the knobs facing the occiput. In the classic application of the forceps, the anterior blade is introduced anteriorly with the concavity of the cephalic curve looking upward. The blade is then rotated 180 degrees, away from the occiput and toward the knobs, and applies itself to the anterior parietal bone. In modern usage, it is more usual to introduce the anterior blade posteriorly or laterally and to "wander" it around the head until it lies next to the anterior parietal bone. The posterior blade is then introduced and the forceps articulated. Traction is made as an occiput transverse until the head passes the area of anteroposterior narrowing. After anterior rotation, traction with the Kielland forceps must be made with great care because there is no pelvic curve on the forceps. Many operators prefer to substitute classic forceps at this point.

The Barton forceps were originally designed for application to a transversely arrested head at the pelvic inlet. In such instances today, cesarean section delivery is the method of choice for mother and baby, but the Barton forceps may be used for delivery of a head in the occiput transverse position lower in the pelvis (Fig. 36-7). The hinged anterior blade is introduced posterior to the head and is "wandered" over the occiput or face until it lies over the anterior parietal bone. The posterior blade is introduced directly behind the head, and the blades are articulated, again assisted by a sliding lock. The head may be readily advanced in the transverse position, rotated, and classic forceps substituted for delivery. Both instruments are satisfactory for this midforceps operation, and each has its strong supporters. In skilled hands, the use of either instrument can be both easy and atraumatic. However, both types of forceps can be highly damaging if undue force is required to accomplish delivery. Current attitudes are such that in this situation cesarean section is usually elected in preference to use of either Kielland or Barton forceps.

ABNORMAL PRESENTATIONS THAT CAUSE DYSTOCIA

Transverse Lie

When the infant lies in the transverse or one of the oblique diameters of the uterus, rather than presenting either by the breech or by the head, the situation is described as a *transverse lie.* Accurately, this might be described as a transverse presentation, but since the latter term has always been confused with transverse positions of the vertex, the term transverse lie is preferable and is generally used.

Labor with the fetus in transverse lie is fairly efficient so long as the membranes are intact and fit well into the lower pole of the uterus. When they rupture, the needed stimulus is lost, dysfunctional labor results, and full dilatation of the cervix is rarely achieved. Moreover, when the membranes rupture, cord prolapse commonly follows; the baby is now seriously jeopardized.

Etiology

An important cause of transverse lie is the presence of anything in the lower portion of the uterus that prevents engagement of the fetus in longitudinal lie. This is commonly the placenta. Indeed, if the fetus is found to be lying transversely or obliquely, placenta previa or some other lower uterine segment mass, such as a myoma, should be considered. However, most transverse lies are seen in multiparas with lax abdominal walls in which the uterus falls well forward and the fetus simply fails to assume a longitudinal lie.

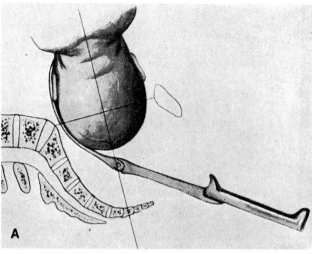

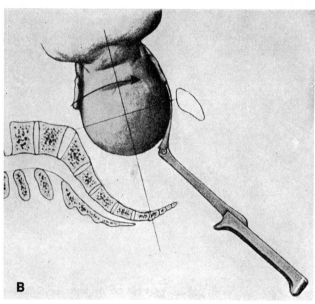

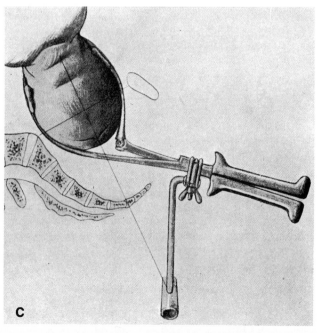

Diagnosis

Leopold's maneuvers (see p. 368) should suggest the diagnosis, for the fetal ovoid lies transversely across the abdomen; neither head nor buttocks occupy the fundal portion of the uterus, and no presenting part can be palpated above the pelvic inlet. The diagnosis is confirmed when vaginal or rectal examination discloses the pelvis to be empty of fetal parts. Similar findings might be offered by a monster of the acardiac type, but this is so rare that the possibility should rest only fleetingly in the examiner's mind. If there should be any doubt, x-ray examination or ultrasound scan gives final information. The most common diagnostic error is to make only a casual abdominal examination and to note that on pelvic examination "the presenting part is not reached." Whenever the presenting part cannot be reached on vaginal or rectal examination, the most searching effort to make an exact diagnosis must be undertaken immediately. In the majority of such cases, the baby is found to be in the transverse lie or in an oblique lie (the head or breech being in the iliac fossa). The latter condition must be approached exactly as though the lie were transverse.

Management

Prior to 36 weeks' gestation, nothing need be done, since the presentation commonly corrects itself to a longitudinal lie. After 36 weeks but before the onset of labor, weekly vaginal examinations should be done to detect the imminence of labor. If the cervix becomes soft, thin, and partially dilated, the patient should be admitted to the hospital and treated as though labor had begun. If the membranes rupture, the baby may be lost because of cord prolapse. Accordingly, if labor is thought to be imminent or has started, cesarean section should be performed immediately. There are only two possible exceptions.

EXTERNAL VERSION. If labor is just beginning, membranes are intact, and the uterus is not unduly irritable, it may be possible to push the head over the pelvic inlet and down into the pelvis. If the head can easily be made to engage, the membranes can be ruptured; as the uterus gains tone, the head will maintain the new position. Management is then the same as with the fetus in a vertex presentation. No anesthesia should

---

FIG. 36-7. Forceps advancement of head in transverse position. (*A*) Introduction of anterior blade of Barton forceps in midline posteriorly. (*B*) Anterior blade "wandered" to position in front of head; advantage of hinged blade is apparent. (*C*) Posterior blade introduced, forceps locked, axis traction handle attached. These illustrations are from original paper on Barton forceps. Head is unengaged. Modern use would require that head be deeply engaged. (Barton LJ, Caldwell WE, Studdiford WE: A new obstetric forceps. Am J Obstet Gynecol 15:16, 1928)

be employed for the external version, and fetal heart tones should be monitored constantly to ensure that cord complications do not occur. If there is any difficulty in accomplishing external version, immediate cesarean section should be elected.

INTERNAL PODALIC VERSION. Internal podalic version is no longer an acceptable method for delivery in transverse lie, regardless of how favorable the conditions may appear to be. In some of the older articles on this kind of management, an infant mortality of 40% and maternal death rate in excess of 5% are reported. If the baby is already dead, the physician may be tempted to deliver by this method to avoid an unproductive cesarean section. However, the maternal risk is so great that most obstetricians elect cesarean sections regardless of the condition of the baby.

Breech Presentation

When the fetus presents with the buttocks toward the pelvis, it is a *breech presentation.* The mortality from vaginal delivery of all infants presenting by the breech, preterm infants included, is about 5.5 times that of infants presenting by the vertex. If preterm infants are excluded, the perinatal mortality in breech presentations is still 3.5 times higher in many large-scale studies. The majority of perinatal deaths in term breech births is accounted for by cord prolapse and other cord complications or by tentorial tears and cerebral hemorrhage during delivery of the after-coming head. Molding, of course, must occur in a matter of moments rather than

hours, and the sudden stresses may be highly damaging to the delicate and vital supporting structures. In the term infant, the primary hazards are those mentioned above; in the preterm infant, the head is usually larger than the breech, and there is the danger of the after-coming head being trapped because the cervix and lower uterine segment are dilated only enough to permit passage of the breech.

In breech presentation, the posture of the lower extremities affects the prognosis of labor. Three major possibilities (Fig. 36-8) are described as follows:

1. *Frank breech* means that the thighs are flexed on the abdomen and the legs are extended; thus, the infant's feet are at the chin.
2. *Complete breech* (full breech) means that the thighs are flexed on the abdomen and the legs are flexed on the thighs so that the infant is sitting tailor fashion and the feet present at the level of the buttocks.
3. *Incomplete breech* (footling breech) means that one or both thighs are extended so that the feet and legs present below the level of the breech. If one leg is completely extended and the other flexed, the presentation is described as a *single footling;* if both legs are extended below the level of the buttocks, it is described as a *double footling.*

Etiology

When the fetus is small in relation to the overall size of the uterine cavity, it tends to move about freely and may assume any presentation. It is only in the latter stages of pregnancy, particularly beyond 32 weeks' ges-

FIG. 36-8. Types of breech presentations. (*A*) Frank breech. (*B*) Complete or full breech. (*C*) Incomplete breech (single footling). (Nursing Education Service, Ross Laboratories)

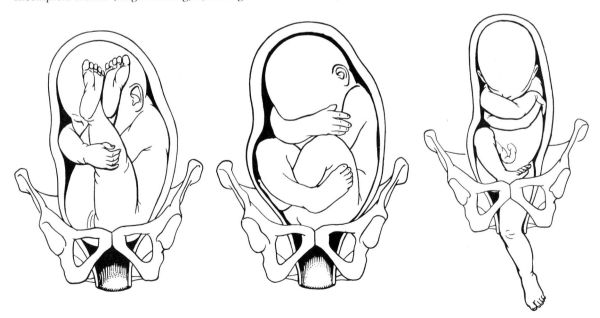

tation, that the fetus accommodates itself to the shape of the uterus. Since the upper portion of the uterus is wider and the lower portion of the uterus and the lower uterine segment are narrower, the wider pole of the fetus tends to accommodate to the larger part of the uterus, and the smaller pole to the less roomy portions. In the preterm fetus, the head is the larger pole and tends to occupy the fundus. At term, however, the breech is the larger and occupies the fundus unless this space is compromised by such factors as a fundal septum, the placenta, or a large fundal fibroid. The incidence of breech presentation at various fetal weights is shown in Table 36-1.

Diagnosis

The Leopold maneuvers for abdominal examination usually, but not always, identify the fetal head in the uterine fundus and the breech in the pelvis. The fetal heart tones are generally best heard above the umbilicus, but this is not a reliable sign. On vaginal examination, the presenting part is usually irregular and may be confused with a face or compound (head and arm) presentation or a cranial abnormality. If there is doubt when the patient is admitted in labor, the diagnosis should be made by x-ray examination of the abdomen. The course of labor and complications to be anticipated depend to a considerable extent on the position of the legs, and efforts should be made to determine whether the breech is frank, complete, or incomplete.

If a breech presentation is diagnosed during pregnancy, external version (see p. 370) has been advocated to substitute the more favorable vertex presentation for the less favorable breech. However, as term approaches, spontaneous conversion to the vertex is likely to occur.

Decision as to Method of Delivery

For a time, the hazard of vaginal breech delivery was considered to be so great that in many services cesarean section was elected for delivery in 85% to 95% of term breech presentations. Since this time, an extensive literature has developed, the consensus of which is that cesarean section is not needed for all cases; careful clinical appraisal should distinguish cases in which vaginal delivery is appropriate from those in which vaginal delivery would be sufficiently hazardous that cesarean section should be elected.

In general, *the factors that are favorable for vaginal delivery* include:

1. Gestational age of more than 36 and less than 38 weeks (If the pregnancy is of *less* than 36 weeks' duration and the baby less than 6 lb, the head is apt to be larger than the breech and may be trapped in the cervix, which is dilated sufficiently for the breech to pass, but not the head.)
2. Estimated fetal weight of more than 6 lb and less than 7 lb
3. Presenting part at or below station 0 at the onset of labor
4. Cervix soft, effaced, and dilated 3 cm or more
5. Ample gynecoid or anthropoid pelvis (in which the after-coming head can be expected to enter the pelvis in the direct occiput anterior position)
6. History of prior breech delivery of baby weighing more than 7 lb or prior vertex delivery of baby weighing more than 8 lb
7. Frank breech presentation

In general, *the factors that are unfavorable for vaginal delivery* include:

1. Gestational age of less than 36 or more than 38 weeks
2. Estimated fetal weight of less than 6 lb or more than 7 lb
3. Presenting part at or above −1 station
4. Cervix firm, incompletely effaced, and less than 3 cm dilated
5. History of difficult prior vaginal delivery or no prior vaginal delivery
6. Android or flat pelvis (In breech, the head approaches the pelvis in the occiput anterior position; in an android or flat pelvis, the head may be required to rotate to the transverse position in order to pass through the inlet, thus causing difficulty in engagement.)
7. Footling or full breech presentation
8. Hyperextension of fetal head (demonstrated by x-ray film—see below)

If vaginal delivery is decided upon, x-ray films are needed to verify the kind of breech presentation and to determine whether the head is extended. *Hyperextension attitudes of the fetal head* (Fig. 36-9) are unusual, but they can be an ominous sign in breech presentation. If the abdominal x-ray film taken on admission reveals hyperextension of 90 degrees or more (the angle between the cervical vertebrae and a line constructed as an upward extension of the main axis of the upper thoracic vertebrae), delivery by cesarean section should be elected. If the angle is less than 90 degrees and all other conditions are favorable for vaginal delivery, this may be pursued; however, a repeat film should be taken later in labor to be sure the extension has not increased. The

Table 36-1
Incidence of Breech Presentation According to Fetal Weight

Fetal Weight (g)	Incidence (%)
1000	23
1500	12
2000	8
>3000	3

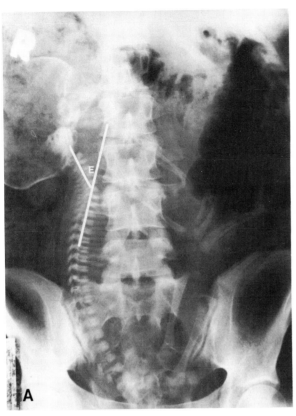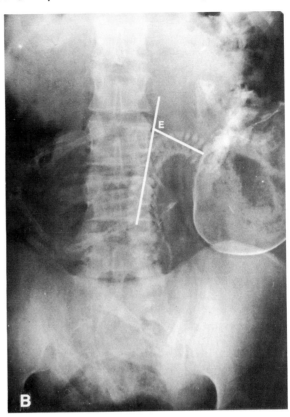

FIG. 36-9. Hyperextension of fetal head. (*A*) Extended head, grade III. Angle of extension (*E*) is angle between cervical vertebrae and upward extension of main axis of thoracic vertebrae. Angle (*E*) in this case is less than 90°. (*B*) Hyperextended head, grade IV; angle (*E*) is more than 90°. (Ballas S, Toaff R, Jaffa AJ: Deflexion of fetal head in breech presentation. Incidence, management and outcome. Obstet Gynecol 52:653, 1978)

cause of hyperextension is not known. Behrman considers most cases to be due to spasm or hypertonus of the neck muscles. Some of the cases appear to be related to Down's syndrome. In others, a cord around the neck has been implicated. Second, an *x-ray pelvimetry* should be performed to determine the details of pelvic configuration as they may bear upon the feasibility of vaginal breech delivery. A suitable technique for x-ray pelvimetry is described by Steer in *Moloy's Evaluation of the Pelvis in Obstetrics.* The three basic films that are needed are a standing lateral film; an inlet film, taken in such a manner as to show the shape of the inlet; and a subpubic arch film, to show the splay of the sidewalls. A technique that provides less than this basic information cannot be expected to be helpful.

The importance of the careful selection of cases and the obstetrician's proficiency in breech delivery must be emphasized. The need for proficiency is illustrated not only by the cases in which there is a choice between vaginal or abdominal delivery, but also by those in which delivery must be vaginal because the breech is already crowning or through the introitus when the

patient is admitted, or because fetal distress or some major maternal complication toward the end of labor makes instant delivery mandatory.

In evaluating fetopelvic relations and the operations necessary for delivery, the physician must be aware of the normal mechanism of labor for breech delivery as outlined in Chapter 32. Each of the three distinct mechanisms (breech, shoulders, and head) must be specifically anticipated with awareness that the longest fetal diameter (the bitrochanteric, the bisacromial, and the suboccipitobregmatic) should traverse the widest part of the pelvis at any given level. Accordingly, the performance of a breech delivery requires not only knowledge that the baby can traverse the pelvis, but also knowledge of the pelvic architecture so the optimal diameters can be utilized.

In summary, the physician should decide at the onset of labor whether the circumstances are favorable and the size of the fetus will permit its ready vaginal delivery through the maternal pelvis. If not, delivery should be by cesarean section. In services in which the policy is for vaginal delivery of favorable cases, between 30% and

50% of breech presentations are found not to be favorable for vaginal delivery and are delivered by elective cesarean section.

It is sometimes said that there can be no trial of labor in breech presentation, but that statement must be qualified. Of the four Ps concerned in the efficiency of labor, early consideration of the pelvis and passenger has already been emphasized. The influence of the powers and the psyche can be assessed as labor progresses. If there is no fetopelvic disproportion, cervical dilatation and descent of the breech should occur progressively. If contractions are inefficient or the presenting part remains unengaged, this may signal unrecognized disproportion. Oxytocin stimulation with a breech presentation after arrest of progress in the active phase of labor has led to poor fetal outcomes and should rarely be used, since such lack of progress often reflects fetopelvic abnormalities. In these contexts, trial of labor does have a place in the management of breech presentation.

The keys to management of labor with the fetus in the breech presentation are (1) early determination of fetopelvic relations and prediction of whether they will permit vaginal delivery, (2) determination of the exact position of the extremities, and (3) observation for prolapse of the umbilical cord. Electronic fetal monitoring should be continuous throughout labor.

INFLUENCE OF FETAL LEG POSITION. The position of the fetal legs considerably influences the course and outcome of labor. In frank breech, the body is splinted by the legs reaching up underneath the chin. Lateral flexion of the fetus may be inhibited, and the breech in this position does not always descend satisfactorily in the pelvis, particularly if the anteroposterior diameters are reduced. It should be noted that the frank breech presentation is most common in the primigravida, whereas complete and incomplete breech presentations are most common in the multipara. Thus, failure of lateral flexion is most common in the first delivery. Dysfunctional labor occurs more often in complete than in frank breech, since the breech does not fit evenly into the cervix and lower uterine segment.

The completely flexed extremities usually occupy the pelvic cavity satisfactorily enough to exclude prolapse of the cord, but this must be determined when the membranes rupture. The incomplete (single or double footling) breech presents a real risk of cord prolapse, since the presenting part tends to fill the pelvis poorly. Such a presentation is more common when the fetus is preterm, compounding the problems of such a delivery.

Management of Delivery

In another era, before cesarean section was used commonly in breech presentation, it was essential that the obstetrician be qualified to deal not only with the "easy" breech delivery, but also with the very serious problems that can occur at each step of the delivery. The earlier references appended to this chapter describe such problems and the means of dealing with them. In addition, this is one area of obstetrics in which the manikin or bony pelvis and fetal doll are by no means obsolete. Those who seek proficiency in vaginal breech delivery will not encounter enough patients so delivered to acquire confidence in their approach to even the most favorable cases. Assiduous practice with a mounted bony pelvis and fetal doll can be immensely helpful. Before a breech delivery, this device can also be valuable in demonstrating to an assistant exactly what he or she is expected to do during delivery of the breech, the shoulders, and the head, so there will be no hesitancy or need for instruction as the delivery unfolds. There are three basic modes of delivery of the breech: spontaneous delivery, assisted breech delivery, and breech extraction. With either of the latter two, the after-coming head may be delivered by manual maneuvers or by forceps.

SPONTANEOUS BREECH DELIVERY. The greatest risk to the fetus occurs in spontaneous breech delivery. The spontaneous and often unattended delivery is commonly preterm, and this, plus precipitous delivery, often with sudden changes in intracranial pressure in the infant, contributes to the high mortality among these babies. Precipitous delivery should be avoided whenever possible by careful observation of the patient, and attempts should be made, even if the mother is exerting strong expulsive force, to guide, control, and prevent too rapid delivery of the head.

ASSISTED BREECH DELIVERY OF BODY. The ideal mode of delivery is assisted breech delivery. The buttocks, or buttocks and feet, of the infant should be crowning, distending the vulva with each contraction. At this point, a generous episiotomy should be made, even if the baby is relatively small, so that extra room is available for any manipulation that may be needed. If episiotomy is deferred until it is really needed, it may be too late. With the next contraction the patient should be urged to bear down and should spontaneously deliver the baby to the umbilicus. Although anesthesia is not a point of discussion here, it should be stated that regardless of what mode of anesthesia is employed, the delivery is facilitated if the patient maintains voluntary abdominal powers until the baby is delivered to the umbilicus. Thus, local or pudendal block and low spinal or epidural anesthesia serve satisfactorily among the regional anesthesias; if a general anesthesia is to be employed, it should ordinarily not be instituted until this point.

In complete breech the legs are already extended. In frank breech it may be necessary to bring down each leg carefully, taking care to sweep them across the fetal flank and gently extract them one at a time.

After delivery of the buttocks, the fetal back *must* be facing the anterior; if the abdomen is permitted to turn anteriorly, the difficulties can be insurmountable unless the position can be readily corrected by the method described by Piper and Bachman. The Prague maneuver, designed to deliver the baby with abdomen anterior and illustrated in many texts, is highly lethal; few babies survive the suggested manipulations.

The mother, if able, should again be urged to bear down, and gentle downward traction (at a 45-degree angle toward the floor) should be made with the baby held with one hand encircling either hip, the fingers on the abdomen, and the thumbs over the fetal sacrum (Fig. 36-10). This traction is facilitated if a sterile towel is wrapped about the body of the infant. A few inches of the umbilical cord should be pulled downward at this time to obviate undue traction on the cord.

Delivery of the baby should continue in a downward direction, and no attempt should be made to deliver the arms until the tip of one scapula can be seen. Continued downward traction may spontaneously deliver the arms and shoulders, but if it does not, the infant, whose back is anterior or in one of the anterior quadrants, should be supported by the obstetrician or by an assistant and the posterior arm delivered first (Fig. 36-11). If the arm has not spontaneously dropped into the hollow of the sacrum, the physician should place two fingers along the humerus as a splint and gently wipe the arm downward over the chest. At this point, the anterior shoulder may drop beneath the symphysis so that the anterior arm will deliver. If it does not, the physician should

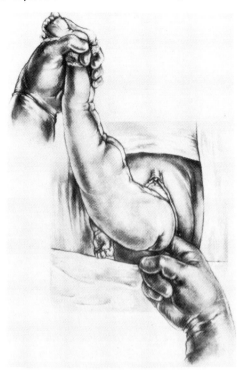

FIG. 36-11. Assisted breech delivery; delivery of posterior arm. (Willson JR: The Management of Obstetric Difficulties, 6th ed. St. Louis, CV Mosby, 1961)

FIG. 36-10. Assisted breech delivery; downward traction on body. (Willson JR: The Management of Obstetric Difficulties, 6th ed. St. Louis, CV Mosby, 1961)

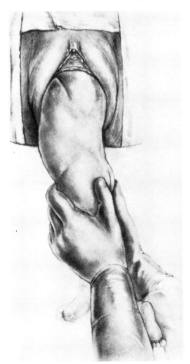

gently rotate the back through 90 to 180 degrees so that the opposite shoulder becomes posterior and the second arm can be delivered. Throughout this time an assistant should be applying gentle downward pressure on the uterine fundus to be certain that the fetal head maintains flexion and satisfactorily follows the shoulders into the pelvis. For ease of delivery it is wise to form a sling of a second sterile towel around the baby's chest and hold the arms to the sides.

DELIVERY OF AFTER-COMING HEAD. At this point it is generally found that the fetal head has maintained good flexion and descended readily into the pelvis so that the chin is near the infant's chest and the face is visible at the perineum. Delivery may be accomplished manually at this point in one of two classic fashions or in a combination thereof. With the infant astride the physician's arm, the physician's index and middle fingers are applied to the malar eminences on the infant's face and pressure is exerted toward the chest so as to maintain flexion of the head. The finger should not be inserted into the infant's mouth, however, as this could cause serious injury. Gentle downward traction is then made by the opposite hand with the index finger hooked over one shoulder and the middle finger over the other (Mauriceau–Smellie–Veit maneuver; Fig. 36-12). Alternatively, the infant may be supported on the obstetrician's arm and flexion of the head maintained as before,

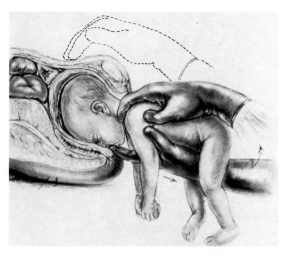

FIG. 36-12. Assisted breech delivery; Mauriceau–Smellie–Veit maneuver. (Willson JR: The Management of Obstetric Difficulties, 6th ed. St. Louis, CV Mosby, 1961)

while the obstetrician applies pressure from above downward on the uterine fundus and the fetal head through the mother's abdomen (Wigand–Martin maneuver). This careful downward pressure may also be maintained by an assistant.

If there is any delay in proper flexion or descent of the head, it is wise to apply forceps to the after-coming head and effect a controlled delivery. The Piper forceps are commonly used in the United States. They have a standard cephalic curve and fenestrated blades, but the shank is joined to the blades at such an angle that the blades remain horizontal beneath the infant's body when properly applied rather than extending at an upward angle as do standard forceps applied to the after-coming

head (Fig. 36-13). In applying the Piper forceps, the physician must remember that the fetal head is tightly held against the vaginal tissues by muscle pressure and surface tension, and inserting a finger laterally will release the head somewhat. If the forceps are to be inserted, it is wise to place four fingers of the opposite hand between the vaginal wall and the fetal head to guide the forceps into place. Because of the angle the shank makes with the blade, the forceps should be inserted with the shank and handles almost horizontal. When the blades are locked, traction can be made and the head delivered by flexion as the physician gradually lifts the handles upward.

BREECH EXTRACTION. Breech extraction is the maneuver in which the physician intervenes before the buttocks have completely passed through the introitus. The procedure is permissible for a second twin that presents by the breech or requires internal podalic version because of a transverse lie.

In singleton pregnancy, full and footling breech usually offer no difficulty; the feet are readily accessible and the legs and buttocks can usually be delivered without incident. Breech extraction in frank breech is another matter. Not only is it one of the most difficult of obstetric maneuvers, but also it imposes great risk on both mother and baby; cesarean section is preferred if this is a reasonable alternative. In modern obstetrics the operation is usually reserved for delivery of a second twin, cases in which the physician is already committed (for whatever reason) to vaginal delivery and the breech cannot be delivered by the mother's voluntary effort, or cases in which instant vaginal delivery is made mandatory by severe fetal distress or some maternal problem in which cesarean section is not feasible.

Breech extraction should not be attempted with the mother under regional or local anesthesia. Deep inha-

FIG. 36-13. Delivery of after-coming head by Piper forceps. Arms and body of infant are held in a towel sling as recommended by Savage. Assistant grasps towel or infant's feet or both. Operator delivers head by flexion, keeping handles below horizontal. (After Dennen EH: Forceps Delivery. Philadelphia, FA Davis, 1964)

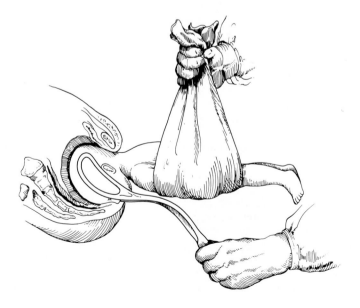

lation anesthesia, usually with halothane, is necessary to provide the required uterine relaxation. When the uterus is sufficiently relaxed, the physician's appropriate hand (the left if the fetal back is to the mother's left) is introduced along the posterior aspect of the fetal legs. If the umbilical cord is found between the legs, it should be disentangled before the extraction is begun. Heavy digital pressure in the popliteal fossa (Pinard's maneuver) causes the knee to flex, making it possible to trigger the fingers over the ankle, to grasp the foot between index and middle fingers, and to deliver it into and through the vagina by downward traction. It is usually desirable that both feet be so delivered at once, but if this is not feasible, traction on the delivered leg toward the mother's thigh causes the buttocks to advance so they are "sitting" on the perineum sacrum posterior. With the help of a finger in the opposite groin, the physician now moves the delivered leg toward the mother's opposite leg, thus bringing the sacrum to the anterior position and permitting delivery of the other leg by upward pressure in the popliteal fossa, then sweeping the leg out across the baby's flank. The remainder of the delivery is conducted as noted in preceding paragraphs.

IMPORTANCE OF PHYSICIAN'S ASSISTANT. A key factor in management of breech delivery is skilled assistance. Hospitals that have made it mandatory for two qualified physicians to be present at every breech delivery have demonstrated a marked reduction in perinatal mortality associated with breech deliveries. The presence of a second physician for consultation and assistance may be expected to decrease the risk if breech delivery is elected.

Shoulder Presentation

Regardless of whether the baby's arm is prolapsed, shoulder presentation is a major complication that must be recognized as early in labor as possible. The shoulder fits quite well into the lower pole of the uterus, and labor usually proceeds apace. This may result in neglect, which inevitably leads to rupture of the uterus. Many such cases are recorded in the earlier literature, and at least 10 of the 90-odd frozen sagittal sections reported near the turn of the century were from women who died from this complication. If shoulder presentation is diagnosed before labor, nothing needs to be done, since the problem will likely resolve spontaneously. If diagnosed in early labor, it should be dealt with at once by cesarean section.

If the diagnosis is made late in labor, the problem is much more serious because of the threat of uterine rupture and the other hazards of prolonged, obstructed labor. If the baby is living, cesarean section must be performed immediately, despite the risk of infection. If the baby is dead and there is a possibility that the uterus has ruptured, delivery must also be by cesarean section; the uterine defect should be repaired if this is feasible or the uterus removed if it is not.

If the baby is dead, the cervix fully dilated, and the uterus intact, the physician must choose between a destructive operation and vaginal delivery, or cesarean section. Those who work in developing countries and have much experience in dealing with obstructed labor are satisfied that, in their hands, the safest and most expeditious means of dealing with such a case is to tie a tape to the prolapsed wrist (so the arm will not be lost), and to decapitate with the Blond–Heidler saw (not a Braun hook or other instrument); the thorax and trunk are readily delivered by traction on the arm, and the head is retrieved by traction in the mouth or by a blunt hook in the foramen magnum. As discussed in Chapter 39, destructive operations of this kind can be extremely difficult, and for the uninitiated cesarean section may offer the safer alternative.

Compound Presentation

Compound presentation refers to prolapse of the fetal hand alongside the presenting breech or vertex, or the foot alongside the head. The combination of hand and vertex is usually least troublesome; as the head advances, the hand tends to remain in place so that it is ultimately out of the way. The combination of hand and breech also tends to resolve spontaneously, but it must be verified that it is the hand and not the foot that is prolapsed (the hand has no heel, and fingers can be readily moved in any direction).

The combination of foot and head may be more serious, and it also tends to be complicated by cord prolapse. If the foot cannot be pushed upward as labor advances, cesarean section is the wisest choice. Version and extraction may be tempting, but this operation carries the same great risks that obtain when it is used for the delivery of an infant in transverse lie.

CEPHALOPELVIC DISPROPORTION THAT CAUSES DYSTOCIA

Cephalopelvic disproportion can produce dystocia in two ways. If the head is too large to pass through the pelvis, it cannot advance beyond the level of obstruction. If this is at the inlet, the problem can usually be recognized early, since the head fails to engage. If the narrowed pelvic diameters are at the midpelvis or outlet, the cephalopelvic relations may be difficult to assess until the head reaches the level in question; often it is wise to wait until full dilatation to note whether sufficient molding may be achieved to permit the head to advance.

Test of labor is a retrospective term, used when the patient has made a good voluntary effort for two hours in the second stage, and the membranes have ruptured, but it is apparent that the baby cannot be safely delivered from below; in this case cesarean section is elected. In this context, the test of labor is rarely applicable in modern obstetrics; absolute disproportion should be diagnosed before two hours of the second stage have elapsed.

Cephalopelvic disproportion also may prevent the proper and even fitting of the presenting part into the lower uterine segment and cervix, one of the requisites for effective contractions in labor. If the head is held up by bony disproportion, it may fit improperly, resulting in irregular or ineffective uterine contractions. This sequence of events occurs most commonly in four situations: (1) in inlet disproportion, in which the head is prevented both from engaging into the pelvis and from settling evenly into the lower pole of the uterus; (2) in the pelvis that is inclined far posteriorly, the symphysis being located almost on a plumb line caudad to the sacral promontory (in this situation the head overrides the symphysis and cannot settle into the lower pole of the uterus; (3) in a severely asymmetric pelvis in which the uterine supports are irregularly placed so that even without true disproportion the fitting of the head may be uneven; and (4) in occiput posterior and similar positions in which the cephalopelvic relations are such that symmetric fitting is prevented. Asynclitism (see p. 636) can produce the same effect. Instead of converting itself, the asynclitism may become permanent during the balance of the labor if a large enough caput succedaneum develops to hold the head in that position.

In all the aforementioned situations, uterine inertia is the result. Some cases can be dealt with by oxytocin stimulation, but if true cephalopelvic disproportion is the cause, it must be recognized at the earliest opportunity and cesarean section performed at once.

A developing caput on the fetal head may be some indication of the strength of contractions and the degree of disproportion. The station of the head is also a helpful sign, since a well-flexed occiput anterior position with the head at the level of the ischial spines indicates that the largest diameter of the fetal head has already entered the inlet. If the head is not at station 0, fundal or suprapubic pressure should be exerted in a downward direction in an attempt to determine whether the head will enter the pelvic inlet. History of previous deliveries may be unreliable, since a baby only slightly larger than those previously delivered may not be capable of passing through the pelvis. If progress is unsatisfactory and evaluation determines this to be due to disproportion, cesarean section delivery gives a lower perinatal mortality than a difficult operative vaginal delivery. Maternal morbidity is also lower.

There is little to be gained by allowing a patient to labor more than two hours in the second stage; indeed, there is great hazard. When, because of inlet contraction, the head fails to engage after one hour in the second stage, cesarean section should be elected. In most cases the problem can be solved before one hour has passed.

SHOULDER DYSTOCIA

Shoulder dystocia is an extremely serious complication of labor that can be highly damaging and even fatal. In Swartz's series of 31 cases, 16% of the babies died; only 18 escaped without injury. Shoulder dystocia occurs when the baby's shoulders are too large to enter the inlet or when they present in an unfavorable diameter. It is to be remembered that the bisacromial diameter is the long diameter and that, when space is at a premium, this longest diameter must adapt to the long diameter of the inlet. As a rule, the shoulders present to the inlet with the bisacromial diameter either in the anteroposterior diameter of the pelvis or in one of the oblique diameters. If the shoulders are large and the anteroposterior diameter of the pelvis is relatively short, the anterior shoulder overhangs the symphysis and fails to engage. The problem is relatively unusual in the anthropoid pelvis, in which the anteroposterior diameter is long; it is more common in the flat pelvis.

Shoulder dystocia may be anticipated if the baby is large or if the inlet is small. It is suspected when, immediately after delivery of the head, the chin is observed to pull tightly back against the perineum, giving the face the appearance of double chin and chubby cheeks. It is diagnosed when slight downward pressure on the head fails to cause the anterior shoulder to stem under the symphysis. In dealing with this problem, it must be remembered that the cervical nerve roots can be seriously damaged by injudicious downward traction to the head in an effort to deliver the anterior shoulder; such traction must be made gently and should be only of sufficient force to cause the advancement of the anterior shoulder that is *already* beneath the symphysis and approaching the subpubic arch.

When the shoulder dystocia is diagnosed, the following steps must be taken at once:

1. The McRoberts maneuver, described by Gonik and co-workers, is tried first and is said to be remarkably effective. The mother's thighs are flexed sharply against her abdomen, thus straightening the lumbosacral angle and rotating the symphysis cephalad, freeing the impacted shoulder as slight traction is made. If this fails,
2. The middle finger of one hand (the right hand if the baby's back is to the patient's left) is placed in the posterior axilla and the heaviest possible traction made in an effort to advance the posterior shoulder into the hollow of the sacrum, thus providing more room for the anterior shoulder to stem beneath the symphysis. Simultaneously, an assistant exerts heavy suprapubic pressure (in an effort to cause the anterior shoulder to engage) and fundal pressure (to cause it to advance). If this fails,
3. Using the same hand as before, and the same abdominal pressure by an assistant, the obstetrician moves the posterior shoulder across the midline so as to bring the bisacromial diameter into an oblique diameter of the pelvis, which may permit the shoulder girdle to advance. If this fails,
4. The posterior shoulder is moved in an arc of 180 degrees so that it now becomes anterior and the previously impacted anterior shoulder is now posterior, but at a lower level so that it may be delivered. This

maneuver, the Woods screw principle, is a modification of Lövset's maneuver for delivery of the shoulders in breech presentation. If this fails,

5. The physician's appropriate hand is introduced posteriorly along the baby's thorax, the posterior forearm is grasped, and the posterior arm is delivered; the anterior shoulder and arm should follow without difficulty. This step is almost invariably successful, but it often produces uterine rupture. It should therefore be omitted if the baby is dead, and the physician should proceed immediately to

6. Cleidotomy, the ultimate solution. Deliberate fracture of the clavicle, although advocated in many texts, is rarely possible; the bone must be cut by heavy embryotomy scissors, preferably through an incision made with the Simpson perforator.

DWARFISM

Dwarfism is not often encountered in obstetric practice, but the problems it poses can be considerable. Among obstetric patients of short stature, the pelvic inclination and configuration are commonly abnormal. Breech presentation is more common in dwarfs than in persons of normal stature. If the head does engage in late pregnancy, respiratory difficulty may be so severe as to preclude vaginal delivery or continuation of pregnancy. Some women of abnormally short stature can and do deliver vaginally, but cesarean section is customary because of either respiratory distress or poor fetopelvic relationships.

REFERENCES AND RECOMMENDED READING

General

Donald I: Practical Obstetric Problems, 5th ed. London, Lloyd–Duke, 1979
Myerscough PR: Monro Kerr's Operative Obstetrics, 10th ed. Baltimore, Williams & Wilkins, 1982
Quilligan EJ, Zuspan F: Douglas–Stromme Operative Obstetrics, 4th ed. New York, Appleton-Century-Crofts, 1982
Steer CM: Moloy's Evaluation of the Pelvis in Obstetrics, 3rd ed. New York, Plenum Medical Book Co, 1975

Forceps Delivery

Bachman C: The Barton obstetric forceps: A review of its use in 55 cases. Surg Gynecol Obstet 45:805, 1927
Barton LJ, Caldwell WE, Studdiford WE: A new obstetric forceps. Am J Obstet Gynecol 15:16, 1928
Danforth DN: Cesarean section. JAMA 253:811, 1985
Danforth DN: A method of forceps rotation in persistent occiput posterior. Am J Obstet Gynecol 65:120, 1953
Danforth DN, Ellis AC: Midforceps delivery—A vanishing art? Am J Obstet Gynecol 86:29, 1963
Danforth WC: The treatment of occiput posterior with special reference to manual rotation. Am J Obstet Gynecol 23:360, 1932

Danforth WC: Forceps. In Curtis AH (ed): Obstetrics and Gynecology, Vol II. Philadelphia, WB Saunders, 1933
Das K: Obstetric Forceps: Its History and Evaluation. St. Louis, CV Mosby, 1929
DeLee JB: The prophylactic forceps operation. Am J Obstet Gynecol 1:34, 1920
Dennen EH: Forceps Deliveries, 2nd ed. Philadelphia, FA Davis, 1964
Dierker LJ, Rosen MG, Thompson K et al: The midforceps: Maternal and neonatal outcomes. Am J Obstet Gynecol 152:176, 1985
Healy DL, Quinn MA, Pepperell RJ: Rotational delivery of the fetus: Kielland's forceps and two other methods compared. Br J Obstet Gynaecol 89:501, 1982
Hughey MJ, McElin TW: Forceps operations in perspective. II. Failed operations. J Reprod Med 21:177, 1978
Hughey MJ, McElin TW, Lussky R: Forceps operations in perspective I. Midforceps rotation operations. J Reprod Med 20:253, 1978
Laufe LE: Obstetric Forceps. New York, Hoeber, 1968
Marin RD: A review of the use of Barton's forceps for the rotation of the fetal head from the transverse position. Aust NZ J Obstet Gynaecol 18:234, 1978
McBride WG, Black BP, Brown CJ et al: Method of delivery and developmental outcome at five years of age. Med J Aust 1:301, 1979
Paintin DB: Midcavity forceps delivery. Br J Obstet Gynaecol 89:495, 1982
Richardson DA, Evans MI, Cibils LA: Midforceps delivery: A critical review. Am J Obstet Gynecol 145:621, 1983
Traub AI, Morrow RJ, Ritchie JWK et al: A continuing use for Kielland forceps? Br J Obstet Gynaecol 91:894, 1984

Vacuum Extractor

Baggish MS: Vacuum extraction. In Iffy L, Kaminetzky HA (eds): Principles and Practice of Obstetrics and Perinatology. New York, John Wiley & Sons, 1981
Berkus MD, Ramamurthy RS, O'Connor PS et al: Cohort study of silastic obstetric vacuum cup deliveries: Safety of the instrument. Obstet Gynecol 66:503, 1985
Greis JB, Bieniarz J, Scommegna A: Comparison of fetal and maternal effects of vacuum extraction with forceps or cesarean deliveries. Obstet Gynecol 57:571, 1981
Leijon I: Neurology and behavior of newborn infants delivered by vacuum extraction on maternal indication. Acta Paediatr Scand 69:625, 1980
Maryniak GM, Frank JB: Clinical assessment of the Kobayshi vacuum extractor. Obstet Gynecol 64:431, 1984
Vacca A, Grant A, Wyatt G et al: Portsmouth operative delivery trial: A comparison of vacuum extraction and forceps delivery. Br J Obstet Gynaecol 90:1107, 1983

Breech Presentation

Ballas S, Toaff R: Hyperextension of the fetal head in breech presentation: Radiological evaluation and significance. Br J Obstet Gynaecol 83:201, 1976
Ballas S, Toaff R, Jaffa AJ: Deflexion of the fetal head in breech presentation. Incidence, management and outcome. Obstet Gynecol 52:653, 1978
Behrman SJ: Fetal cervical hyperextension. Clin Obstet Gynecol 5:1018, 1962
Bowes WA Jr., Taylor ES, O'Brien M et al: Breech delivery:

Evaluation of the method of delivery on perinatal results and maternal morbidity. Am J Obstet Gynecol 135:965, 1979

Brenner WE, Bruce RD, Hendricks CH: The characteristics and perils of breech presentation. Am J Obstet Gynecol 118: 700, 1974

Caldwell WE, Studdiford WE: A review of breech deliveries during a five year period at the Sloane Hospital for Women. Am J Obstet Gynecol 18:623, 720, 1929

Collea JV, Rabin SC, Weghorst GR et al: The randomized management of term frank breech presentation: Vaginal delivery vs. cesarean section. Am J Obstet Gynecol 131:186, 1978

Cruikshank DP, Pitkin RM: Delivery of the premature breech. Obstet Gynecol 50:367, 1977

DeCrespigny LJC, Pepperell RJ: Perinatal mortality and morbidity in breech presentation. Obstet Gynecol 53:141, 1979

Gimovsky ML, Petrie RH, Todd D: Neonatal performance of the selected term vaginal breech delivery. Obstet Gynecol 56:687, 1980

Gimovsky ML, Wallace RL, Schifrin BS et al: Randomized management of nonfrank breech presentation at term: A preliminary report. Am J Obstet Gynecol 146:34, 1983

Karp LE, Doney JR, McCarthy T et al: The premature breech: Trial of labor or cesarean section? Obstet Gynecol 53:88, 1979

Lewis BV, Seniviratne HR: Vaginal breech delivery or cesarean section. Am J Obstet Gynecol 134:615, 1979

Løvset J: Shoulder delivery by breech presentation. J Obstet Gynaecol Br Emp 44:696, 1937

Mann LI, Gallant JM: Modern management of breech delivery. Am J Obstet Gynecol 134:611, 1979

Morley GW: Breech presentation: A 15 year review. Obstet Gynecol 30:745, 1967

O'Leary JA: Vaginal delivery of the term breech. A preliminary report. Obstet Gynecol 53:341, 1979

Piper EB, Bachman C: The prevention of fetal injuries in breech delivery. JAMA 92:217, 1929

Rosen MG, Chik L: The effect of delivery route on outcome in breech presentation. Am J Obstet Gynecol 148:909, 1984

Savage JE: Management of the fetal arms in breech extraction: A method to facilitate application of Piper forceps. Obstet Gynecol 3:55, 1954

Watson WJ, Benson WL: Vaginal delivery for the selected frank breech infant at term. Obstet Gynecol 64:638, 1984

Woods JR Jr.: Effect of low-birth-weight breech delivery on neonatal mortality. Obstet Gynecol 53:735, 1979

Compound Presentation

Ang LT: Compound presentation following external version. Aust NZ J Obstet Gynaecol 18:213, 1978

Shoulder Dystocia

Benedetti TJ, Gabbe SG: Shoulder dystocia. A complication of fetal macrosomia and prolonged second stage of labor with midpelvic delivery. Obstet Gynecol 52:526, 1978

Golditch IM, Kirkman K: The large fetus. Obstet Gynecol 52: 26, 1978

Gonik B, Stringer CA, Held B: An alternate maneuver for management of shoulder dystocia. Am J Obstet Gynecol 145: 882, 1983

Morris WIC: Shoulder dystocia. J Obstet Gynaecol Br Emp 62: 302, 1955

Swartz DP: Shoulder girdle dystocia in vertex delivery. Obstet Gynecol 17:194, 1960

Woods CE: A principle of physics as applicable to shoulder delivery. Am J Obstet Gynecol 45:796, 1959

Dwarfism

Lattanzi DR, Harger JH: Achondroplasia and pregnancy. J Reprod Med 27:363, 1982

Tyson JE, Barnes AC, McKusick VA et al: Obstetric and gynecologic considerations of dwarfism. Am J Obstet Gynecol 180:688, 1970

Dystocia Due to Abnormal Uterine Action

Kent Ueland
Frederick R. Ueland

37

The term *abnormal labor* almost invariably refers to prolonged or dysfunctional labor. However, in some patients labor and delivery occur very rapidly. If this precipitate labor is accompanied by frequent hypertonic uterine contractions and an abnormally high tonus, fetal hypoxia may occur because of decreased oxygen exchange. In addition, rapid descent of the fetus through the pelvis, especially if the delivery occurs unattended, may cause fetal injury and lacerations of the maternal soft tissues. Most commonly, the short labor (less than three hours overall) terminates with the controlled delivery of a normal neonate from a very appreciative mother.

FIRST STAGE OF LABOR

Prolonged Latent Phase

The latent phase of labor is that period from the inception of regular painful uterine contractions to the beginning of the active phase of labor, at 4 cm dilatation of the cervix. Since pinpointing the exact time of onset of labor is frequently difficult and the judgment is purely subjective, assigning an accurate duration to the latent phase may not be possible. Many changes in the cervix that are often associated with labor actually occur during the last few weeks of pregnancy and before the onset of labor. The spontaneous priming of the cervix that occurs in normal late pregnancy involves significant alterations in anatomic, biochemical, and physical characteristics. Consequently the clinical manifestations of these alterations—changes in the consistency, position, effacement, and dilatation of the cervix—are not in themselves certain indicators of labor. However, if a primigravida, for example, continues to have regular uterine contractions with a frequency of at least two every ten minutes and there are definite cervical changes, it can generally be assumed that labor has begun.

The transition from latent phase to active phase may also be difficult to identify. Changes in contractions do not always accompany this transition. The most accurate way of determining the duration of the latent phase is simply to plot a dilatation vs. time graph, usually referred to as a "partogram."

The average length of the latent phase of the first stage of labor is considered to be 6.4 hours in the nullipara and 4.8 hours in the multipara. If the latent phase extends beyond 10 hours in the former and 6 hours in the latter, it should be considered prolonged (Fig. 37-1). The incidence of prolonged latent phase among abnormal labors is high, 30.2% in nulliparous patients and 52.8% among multiparous patients. Figure 37-2 shows how information about frequency, duration, and intensity of uterine contractions is recorded.

Etiology

The primary causes of prolonged latent phase are uterine dysfunction, or a firm, unfavorable cervix at the onset of labor. An episode of false labor can also lead to a diagnosis of prolonged latent phase. Secondary causes of prolonged labor are oversedation, premature administration of anesthesia, and a state of maternal dehydration or fatigue, problems that should rarely be encountered in modern obstetrics.

Management

In general, management of prolonged latent phase is directed at correcting the suspected underlying cause. Treatment for oversedation or prematurely administered anesthesia is to allow the effect of the offending agent to wane. In women in whom false labor is suspected or who have uterine dysfunction or an unfavorable cervix, the one-time administration of intravenous sedation (*e.g.,* 10–15 mg morphine sulfate) may be beneficial.

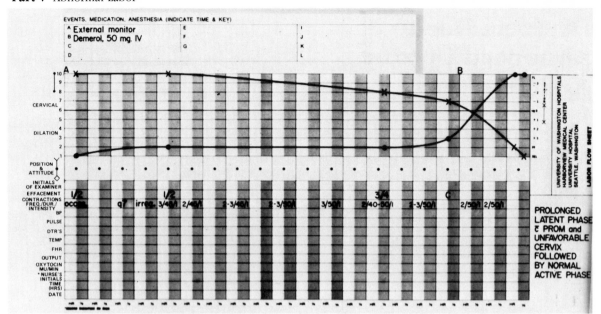

FIG. 37-1. Labor flow sheet (partogram), showing prolonged latent phase, premature rupture of membranes, and unfavorable cervix. The active phase is entirely normal.

This approach allows the patient with an "unripe" cervix to labor in the latent phase in relative comfort. It may convert abnormal uterine contractions to subnormal ones that may in turn be augmented with intravenous oxytocin, thereby overcoming the uterine dysfunction. Oxytocin by itself is of little help in treating primary dysfunctional labor. Ambulation may at times be efficacious. If the contractions cease following sedation, a diagnosis of false labor can be made.

Of patients with prolonged latent phase of labor, 80% to 90% progress to a normal active phase. Less than 10% will require cesarean section.

Protracted Active Phase

The diagnosis of protracted active phase (primary dysfunctional labor) is made if cervical dilatation does not proceed at the expected normal rate of at least 1.5 cm/hour during the active phase of the first stage of labor. Friedman has suggested that primigravidas dilate at a somewhat slower rate (1.2 cm per hour), but Hendricks has shown that in optimal active phase labor, primigravidas and multigravidas dilate at a similar rate. Philpott and Castle, whose belief is that, in the active phase of labor, cervical dilatation should occur at the rate of at least 1 cm/hour, developed a chart for evaluating progress in labor (Fig. 37-3) in order to simplify management of dysfunctional labor.

When cervical dilatation occurs at a slower rate than expected, (Fig. 37-4), the patient should be carefully evaluated. An abdominal examination should be made to determine the frequency, duration, and intensity of uterine contractions. A vaginal examination is performed

to delineate the position and attitude of the presenting part and to determine the configuration and size of the bony pelvis. If cephalopelvic disproportion (CPD) is suspected, computed tomographic digital pelvimetry might be considered if detailed knowledge of pelvic capacity and configuration is needed in delineating therapy. The vaginal examination should be performed during a contraction in order to determine whether or not the presenting part is tightly applied to the cervix. If the examining finger can be readily inserted between the cervix and the presenting part at the peak of the contraction, abnormal (reverse gradient) contractions should be suspected.

Etiology

CPD is an abnormal relationship between the fetal vertex and the maternal pelvis that can, at times, be due to malposition of the presenting part, such as persistent

FIG. 37-2. Method of recording information about frequency, duration, and intensity of contractions.

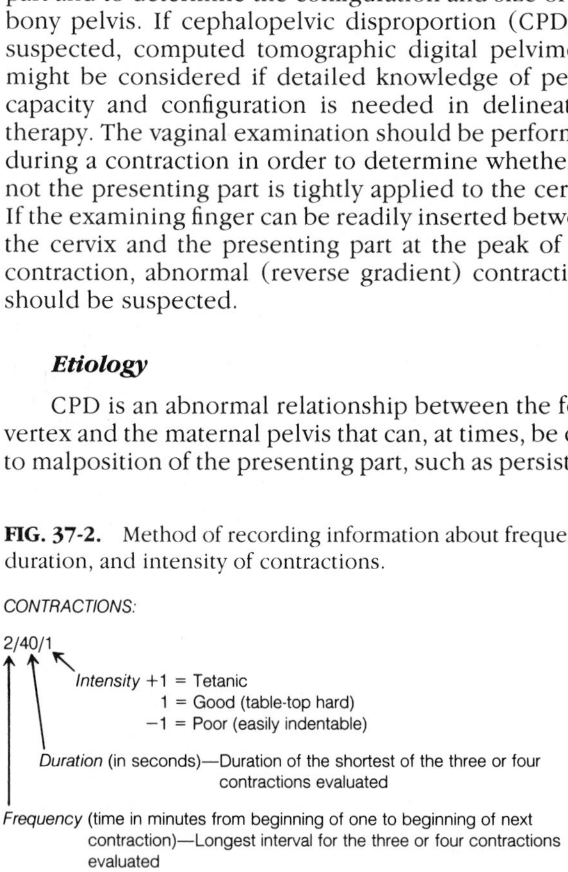

CONTRACTIONS:

2/40/1

Intensity +1 = Tetanic
1 = Good (table-top hard)
−1 = Poor (easily indentable)

Duration (in seconds)—Duration of the shortest of the three or four contractions evaluated

Frequency (time in minutes from beginning of one to beginning of next contraction)—Longest interval for the three or four contractions evaluated

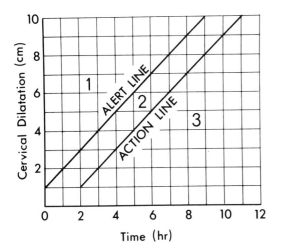

FIG. 37-3. Chart for evaluating progress in active labor. In normal active-phase labor, cervical dilatation will proceed at a rate greater than 1 cm/hour (*Zone 1*). If progress lags, the curve of cervical dilatation will cross the alert line into *Zone 2,* indicating the possibility of dysfunctional labor. Should progress lag even further, the curve will cross the action line into *Zone 3,* indicating the necessity for some form of intervention. (After Philpott RH, Castle WM: Cervicographs in the management of labour in primigravidae. J Obstet Gynaecol Brit Commonw 79:592, 1972)

occiput posterior or extension of the fetal head. These conditions cause an unusually large diameter of the fetal vertex to be presented to the pelvis, which in turn prevents normal descent and may preclude a vaginal delivery. At times, with improved uterine action, spontaneous conversion occurs through rotation and flexion of the head, and vaginal delivery can be safely undertaken.

At other times CPD may be absolute, with the disproportion being due to an unusually large fetus or to a small pelvis. Diabetes, obesity, or excessive maternal weight gain may result in the former, while small maternal stature (*i.e.,* height less than 5 feet) may be responsible for the latter.

CPD is considered a primary cause of protracted active phase. Subnormal uterine contractions and uterine dysfunction (abnormal contractions) are also considered as primary causes of protracted active phase of labor. Secondary factors include oversedation, repeated administration of anesthesia, and, in some cases dehydration or fatigue.

Management

Therapy is aimed at correcting the underlying cause. If secondary causes are evident, such as oversedation, excessive anesthesia, or dehydration and fatigue, they can be promptly corrected. The resultant subnormal

FIG. 37-4. Labor flow sheet, showing a protracted active phase. The rate of cervical dilatation is less than 1.5 cm/hour. The fetus was in vertex occiput posterior (*OP*) position, descent occurred as occiput rotated to anterior (*OA*) position.

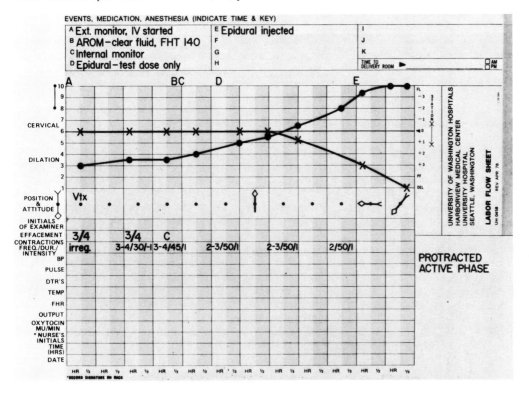

contractions can be managed best by oxytocin augmentation or intravenous fluid administration or both. Patients with abnormal contractions, but without evidence of bony dystocia, may respond to segmental epidural anesthesia followed by oxytocin stimulation. However, it should be emphasized that primary oxytocin stimulation will not help patients with abnormal contractions. Indeed, it may worsen the condition by producing hypertonus and by intensifying abnormal contractions. Minor degrees of bony dystocia in conjunction with malposition and subnormal or mixed subnormal and abnormal contractions can frequently be managed by improving uterine action with amniotomy and oxytocin stimulation. If true bony dystocia exists with protracted cervical dilatation, attempts at augmenting labor are unwarranted and cesarean section is indicated. About 10% of labors with a protracted active phase end in cesarean section.

Controversy has existed through the years over the effect of amniotomy on labor. Some feel that it has no effect, or an unpredictable effect, on the duration of labor. Others suggest it slows labor, whereas still others have stressed the beneficial effect of artificial rupture of membranes. There is some evidence, however, that amniotomy, if performed during the active phase, shortens the first stage of labor in primigravidas. There is no reason to suspect that the same should not hold true for multigravidas as well. Amniotomy may also be useful in improving uterine action in patients having subnormal contractions, regardless of the etiology. However, if amniotomy is to be safely and effectively utilized, it should be performed in the active phase, and only in vertex presentations when the head is fixed in the pelvis or tightly applied to the cervix, in order to avoid prolapse of the umbilical cord. The effectiveness of amniotomy in improving uterine tone and contractility has been variously attributed to decreased uterine volume and shortening of the myometrial cells, to reflex endogenous release of oxytocin and prostaglandins following the increased pressure on the cervix and lower uterine segment by the presenting part, and to reflex stimulation by the central nervous system.

Occasionally, a patient presents with a protracted active phase of labor, frequently superimposed on a prolonged latent phase, in which the underlying cause is a firm, unripe cervix. This condition is known as *cervical dystocia*. In such cases, the resistance of the cervix is sufficient to impede normal progress. If labor is allowed to continue for any length of time in the active phase, the cervix may also become edematous. Attempts at uterine stimulation under these circumstances can be dangerous, since the cervix may tear. Cesarean section is the most appropriate therapy. Cervical dystocia is likely to be associated with unrecognized abnormal uterine activity.

Should secondary arrest of dilatation be superimposed on a protracted active phase of dilatation without any immediately apparent etiology, serious cephalopelvic disproportion must immediately be ruled out.

The majority of these labors terminate with cesarean section.

Secondary Arrest of Dilatation

It is important to emphasize that secondary arrest of dilatation is an abnormal progress of labor in the active phase of first-stage labor. It is most frequently encountered between 6 cm and 8 cm of dilatation. By definition, the diagnosis is made if there is no progress in cervical dilatation for at least two hours.

Etiology

The etiologic factors for secondary arrest of dilatation are similar to those for protracted active phase. The most common underlying cause is, again, cephalopelvic disproportion. Other primary causes include subnormal uterine activity and uterine dysfunction. Oversedation, excessive anesthesia, and fatigue may be secondary causes.

By using a labor graph of cervical dilatation and descent of the presenting part, as shown in Figures 37-5 and 37-6, one can promptly identify the most likely underlying cause of the abnormality. In Figure 37-5 normal descent occurred in the presence of secondary arrest of dilatation. Subnormal uterine activity was suspected clinically, and there was no evidence of CPD. Pitocin augmentation was begun and normal labor followed. In Figure 37-6 the presenting part remained at a high station during the development of secondary arrest of dilatation. Under these circumstances CPD should be the first diagnosis considered. When CPD is documented, cesarean section should be performed.

Management

When evaluating patients who have secondary arrest of dilatation, one should begin by checking uterine contractions. If they are subnormal by abdominal and vaginal palpation, conditions such as conduction anesthesia, excessive sedation, and exhaustion may be the underlying cause of the arrest. If cephalopelvic disproportion can be ruled out by clinical or, on rare occasions, CT pelvic mensuration, an intravenous oxytocin infusion can be safely initiated to augment the subnormal contractions. Under these circumstances, the active phase of labor will usually be rapidly completed (see Fig. 37-5). The often-used policy of allowing the analgesia or anesthesia to wear off seems inconsistent with modern obstetric practice. The anesthesia was used to achieve patient comfort, so augmenting the contractions while the analgesia is still in effect is a much more appropriate approach.

If a minor degree of disproportion is the likely cause, possibly due to fetal malposition, and uterine contractions are subnormal, amniotomy seems indicated if it can be performed safely. This enables internal mon-

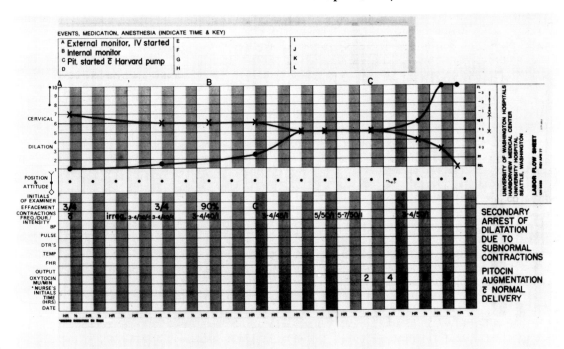

FIG. 37-5. Labor flow sheet, showing secondary arrest of dilatation due to subnormal uterine contractions.

FIG. 37-6. Labor flow sheet, showing secondary arrest of dilatation due to cephalopelvic disproportion. The presenting part remains at high station. Delivery was by cesarean section. *SROM*, spontaneous rupture of membranes.

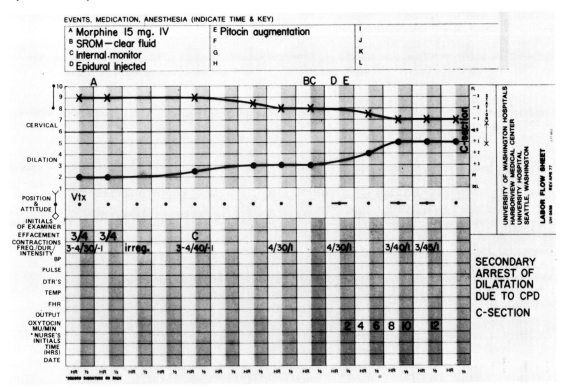

itoring when oxytocin augmentation is begun. Occasionally, the amniotomy itself will induce normal uterine action. Minor degrees of obstruction can frequently be satisfactorily overcome in this manner.

When clinical and CT pelvimetry show evidence of true bony dystocia and the vertex remains at a high station and is associated with abnormal uterine contractions, little can be gained by any of the above procedures, and cesarean section is indicated (see Fig. 37-6). On the other hand, if no bony dystocia exists and the only apparent abnormality is abnormal uterine activity, one may attempt to convert these abnormal contractions with a segmental epidural block at a level of T6 to T12. This procedure often succeeds in converting abnormal to subnormal contractions, which, in turn, can be augmented with intravenous oxytocin to effect normal uterine activity and prompt completion of the first stage of labor. Usually, when one encounters dysfunctional labor, the contractions are a mixture of normal and abnormal or subnormal and abnormal contractions. Rarely are abnormal contractions the only type. Obviously, the higher the proportion of abnormal contractions, the more protracted the labor, since such contractions are ineffective in retracting the lower uterine segment and dilating the cervix.

SECOND STAGE OF LABOR

Protracted Descent

Abnormal labor encountered during the second stage can again be conveniently divided into phases. Abnormalities in this stage of labor are commonly heralded by dysfunctional patterns of dilatation in the active phase of the first stage of labor, such as secondary arrest or protracted dilatation. In protracted descent, the presenting part advances more slowly than the accepted normal rate of 1 cm/hour in nulliparous patients and 2 cm/hour in multiparous patients. Within 10 contractions following complete dilatation and retraction of the cervix, the presenting vertex should normally be on the pelvic floor in all patients. In normal labor with contractions occurring every 2 to 5 minutes, the time for descent should range between 20 and 50 minutes. In fact, approximately 40% of primigravidas do not have a descent phase, as the vertex is already on the pelvic floor at the onset of the second stage of labor. If fetal descent is delayed, clinical evaluation must include uterine contractions. Are they normal, or subnormal? Since abnormal contractions are rare in this stage of labor, they can generally be discounted as a contributing factor. Are the mother's bearing down efforts effective? Bearing down efforts make up 50% of the expulsive force in the second stage. Protruding the abdomen and generating high intra-abdominal and intrauterine pressures while pushing are not necessarily synonymous with effective bearing down, since the effort must be appropriately directed. The bony pelvis must also be reevaluated clinically. CT pelvimetry is inappropriate at this

late stage of labor. The vertex should be carefully palpated to rule out any malposition or abnormality. When evaluating descent one must be careful not to confuse progress with increased molding and caput formation of the fetal head. Thus, when fetal station is being determined, the skull must be palpated carefully; it must not be confused with the soft tissues of the scalp. Figure 37-7 illustrates protracted descent secondary to malposition. Late rotation occurred from occiput right posterior (ORP) to occiput right transverse (ORT) and, finally, to occiput anterior (OA). Epidural anesthesia may have contributed to the delay, although the contractions appeared to be normal.

Etiology

The most common cause for delay in descent is the ineffectiveness of one or both of the expulsive forces. Both contractions and maternal bearing down can be affected by heavy sedation and anesthesia. On occasion, poor bearing down efforts can be attributed to pain as the vertex descends in the vagina, causing the woman to hold back. Other causes of delay in descent can be malposition, a full bladder, and subnormal uterine activity. A more serious problem is that of CPD, particularly during oxytocin administration, which may result in increased molding of the fetal vertex. However, as mentioned previously, this problem appears as an abnormal dilatation pattern during the active phase of labor. It is unusual to have CPD appear as a problem in the second stage of labor without prior warning.

Management

Subnormal contractions can successfully be augmented with intravenous oxytocin. Coaching the patient in bearing down techniques before administering anesthesia can help prevent ineffective pushing after the administration of anesthesia. Even after anesthesia has been administered, coaching can sometimes help. When poor bearing down efforts are the result of pain (an infrequent problem), appropriate anesthesia may be efficacious. Minor malpositions are frequently corrected by improved uterine action and maternal bearing down efforts. The treatment of choice for CPD, even when it is a relative condition, is almost without exception, cesarean section. A difficult midforceps delivery attempted in the presence of bony dystocia invariably ends poorly, causing trauma to the fetus and maternal soft tissues.

Prolonged Pelvic Floor Phase

Once the vertex reaches the pelvic floor it has successfully negotiated the bony pelvis, and the soft tissues of the vulva and perineum offer the only remaining resistance. Rarely do these structures cause obstruction, although occasionally an appropriately timed episiotomy may shorten the pelvic floor phase. Delay in this phase of labor is again mainly attributable to the ineffectiveness

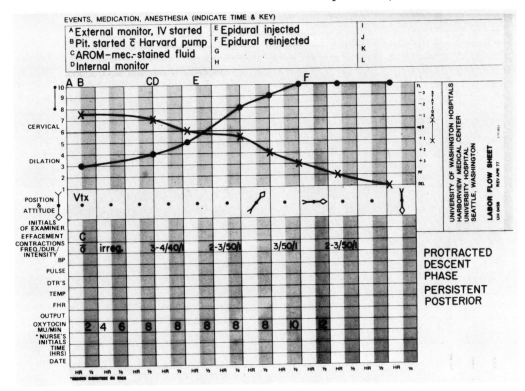

FIG. 37-7. Labor flow sheet, showing protracted descent due to malposition, head advancing as occiput rotates from occiput right posterior (*ORP*) to occiput anterior (*OA*). *AROM,* artificial rupture of membranes.

of the expulsive forces. Subnormal contractions respond well to oxytocin, and it is important to achieve normal uterine activity at this time in order to prepare the uterus for the third stage of labor. Normal contractions before delivery help to shear off the placenta from the uterine wall early and control blood loss after its expulsion by firmly contracting the uterus. If maternal pushing is poor, for whatever reason, delivery can be effected safely with the use of forceps. In fact, many physicians electively use low forceps routinely for delivery.

In all patients, a descent phase of the second stage of labor that lasts more than 10 contractions (20–50 minutes) is considered abnormal.

In primigravidas the pelvic floor phase should last for not more than 20 contractions (*i.e.,* 20–40 minutes). In multiparas this phase of the second stage of labor is negotiated in 10 contractions, or half the time. It is important to consider the second stage of labor in two phases because deviation from normal can then be identified earlier and managed appropriately.

Dystocia Due to Uterine Rings

Three kinds of rings have been described in the uterus: the physiologic retraction ring, the pathologic retraction ring (Bandl's ring), and the constriction ring.

The physiologic retraction ring occurs precisely at the junction of the upper and lower uterine segments. It is a normal and necessary result of the circumferential dilatation and consequent thinning of the lower pole of the uterus that occurs either preparatory to labor or during early labor. These uterine changes are discussed in Chapter 31 (see Fig. 31-32). The ring can be visualized by a high classic cesarean section incision that begins in the lower uterine segment and extends up past the abrupt thickening in the myometrium that characterizes the upper uterine segment. The ring can be readily palpated through a lower-segment cesarean section incision by following the uterine wall upward.

The pathologic retraction ring (Figure 37-8) is an accentuation of the physiologic retraction ring; it also occurs at the junction of the upper and lower uterine segments, but in a neglected, mechanically obstructed second stage of labor. The ring can be felt by abdominal palpation, and it moves cephalad as the neglect continues. Uterine rupture through the lower uterine segment is inevitable unless the obstruction is relieved or the patient is delivered by cesarean section.

Constriction ring (Figs. 37-9, 37-10) is a complication rarely encountered in ordinary obstetric practice. Its mechanics are not well understood. Characteristically, it occurs in prolonged labor with ruptured membranes. Because of the intense incoordination believed to result from "exhaustion," the uterus relaxes poorly and applies itself to the contours of the baby. The

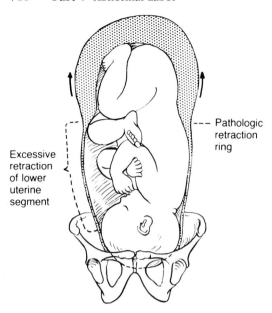

FIG. 37-8. Pathologic retraction ring (Bandl's ring) occurring at the junction of upper and lower uterine segments as a result of obstructed labor.

"rings," therefore, do not go all the way around the uterus, as do the physiologic and pathologic retraction rings, but rather conform to a depression in the baby, such as the neck or abdomen. A cardinal sign is said to be that the presenting part recedes during a contraction. The treatment is cesarean section, using an anesthetic that relaxes the uterus for delivery.

The physiologic retraction ring is a normal, desirable, and almost inevitable anatomic development during the course of normal labor. In contrast, both the pathologic retraction ring and the constriction ring denote severe obstetric pathology; these two rings have in common the fact that they tend to develop only after labor has continued too long against some sort of mechanical obstruction. Fortunately, with earlier recognition and active management of inertial labor, pathologic retraction and constriction rings are becoming a rarity.

AGENTS USED TO STIMULATE LABOR CONTRACTIONS

Oxytocin

Oxytocin, a peptide hormone, that is now commercially synthesized and marketed under a variety of names (Oxytocin, Pitocin, Syntocinon) is a potent myometrial stimulant that has many useful clinical applications. The myometrial response is dose-dependent, and it is therefore imperative that it be administered slowly and with a controlled intravenous infusion device. Excessive doses may result in tetanic contractions or even uterine rupture.

Mechanism of Action

The precise mechanism of action of oxytocin has yet to be delineated. It is thought to bind to receptors on myometrial cell membranes where cyclic AMP is formed. Oxytocin regulates intracellular calcium levels by affecting the sarcoplasmic reticulum and the calcium-magnesium-ATPase system of the myometrial cell membrane. The complicated functional and metabolic coordination includes the formation of gap junctions between myometrial cells along with cellular events, such as changes in concentrations of oxytocin receptors. Oxytocin also stimulates prostaglandin production in the decidua. The suggested cellular mechanisms of oxytocin and parturition are discussed in detail in reviews of the subject by Fuchs and by Huszar.

Pharmacologic Action

Oxytocin infusion results in three primary pharmacologic actions. The best known is the stimulation of uterine contractility. As mentioned previously, this action is dose-dependent. The sensitivity of uterine muscle to oxytocin increases gradually between 20 and 40 weeks of pregnancy and appears to depend on steroid levels and the concentration of myometrial oxytocin receptors. Oxytocin also causes stimulation of breast myoepithelial cells. Again, the response seems to be steroid-dependent. Lastly, oxytocin has an antidiuretic effect similar to, but weaker than, that of vasopressin. Larger doses, not generally indicated for use during pregnancy, may result in an increase in renal free water absorption.

FIG. 37-9. Constriction ring dystocia. The ring conforms to a fetal depression.

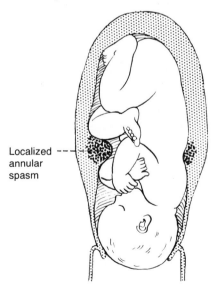

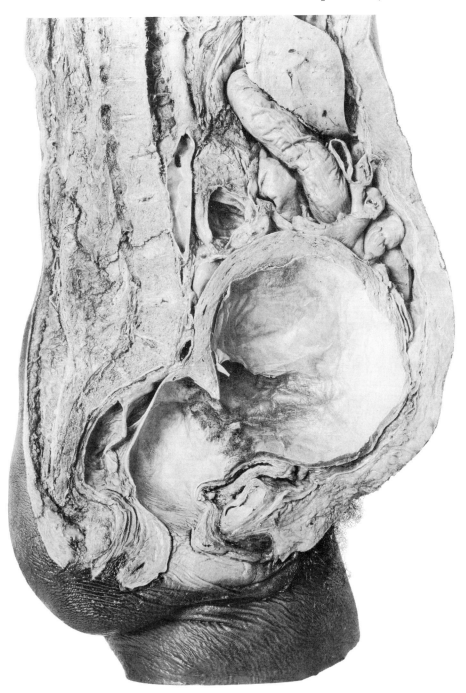

FIG. 37-10. Constriction ring. Frozen sagittal section. The fetus is in occiput anterior position. Death resulted from eclampsia in the second stage of labor. The uterus lay obliquely, slightly to right of midline, causing the left section of the corpus to appear smaller than its actual 8+ months size. Constriction ring projects anteriorly into fetal depression between chain and thorax. (Canton E, Gonzalez JB: Atlas de Anatomia y de Clinica Obstetrica Normal y Patologica, plate XXXV, p 105. Buenos Aires, Pueser, 1910)

Therapeutic Use

Oxytocin is used clinically to induce labor, to augment labor, and to control postpartum blood loss. It is imperative that the patient be examined before oxytocin is used so that fetal position and presentation can be accurately established. The drug should not be used in the presence of known CPD and the fetus should be in a longitudinal lie. Oxytocin administration should be by continuous intravenous infusion using a suitable controlled infusion device, and medical personnel experienced in its use should be present. The infusion should be started at a rate of 0.5 ml to 1 mU/min. If there is clinical evidence of uterine irritability, or if the patient is having contractions, extreme caution must be exercised at the onset of the infusion. The dosage can be safely increased at intervals of 15 to 20 minutes until adequate labor is established. It should *not* be increased and should be reduced or stopped when the contractions are too frequent (a rate of more than five per 10 minutes or an interval between contractions of less than one minute) or when there is increased uterine tonus. Some recommend that the rate of oxytocin infusion should never exceed 16–20 mU/min. However, on rare occasions a higher dose may be necessary. The ideal rate of infusion is one that stimulates normal uterine activity.

During oxytocin infusion continuous electronic monitoring of fetal heart rate is necessary, and direct, continuous, intrauterine pressure measurements are frequently helpful in determining the proper rate of infusion and uterine response. Intravenous infusion with a controlled infusion device is the only recommended route of administration. In the past intramuscular and subcutaneous injections were utilized, but because of unpredictable absorption and response and prolonged activity, these routes are no longer used. Buccal administration results in a much slower response, and one that is also less predictable. These routes of administration should not be used in the presence of a viable fetus.

Contraindications

Uterine stimulation is contraindicated in the presence of an unstable lie (oblique or transverse). Some authors feel that augmentation in the presence of a breech presentation is contraindicated. Others feel that breech alone is not a contraindication. If conditions prevail that would make a vaginal breech delivery safe, gentle augmentation with oxytocin for subnormal uterine activity seems clinically appropriate. Significant CPD, placenta previa, and evidence of hypertonus are all contraindications to oxytocin administration. Oxytocin must be administered with caution in the presence of a uterine scar from, for example, a cesarean section or myomectomy. If the previous surgery was confined to the lower uterine segment and not the muscular corpus, oxytocin can be safely given. It is contraindicated in women who have had a classical cesarean section.

Two additional problems, though rare, are worthy of mention. Large doses of oxytocin, when accompanied by large volumes of electrolyte-free fluid, can result in water intoxication. The vasopressin effect in high doses (50 mU/min or above) is that of an antidiuretic. In the presence of a viable fetus, there are few indications for infusions of such magnitude. Neonatal hyperbilirubinemia has been attributed to oxytocin stimulation, the incidence increasing with prolonged periods of administration. The severity appears to be a function of both time and dosage. This rare complication is self-limiting. An association between neonatal hyperbilirubinemia and oxytocin has been rejected by other investigators, some of whom feel that the hyperbilirubinemia is primarily associated with fetal maturity.

There are well-defined parameters for oxytocin administration. Generally, it is safe when used properly and it is one of the most useful obstetric tools that we have to induce labor and to normalize labor in the presence of subnormal uterine activity. The large molecular weight of oxytocin prevents it from crossing the placenta and it, therefore, has no direct effect on the fetus. The importance of some form of continuous electronic monitoring of both mother and fetus can not be overemphasized when oxytocin is administered.

Prostaglandins

Although not available for routine clinical use in this country, the prostaglandins PGE_2 and $PGF_{2\alpha}$ have had extensive clinical trials in Europe and in many other countries throughout the world, primarily for use in preinduction cervical priming and induction of labor. The intravenous, oral, transbuccal, extra-amniotic, intravaginal and intracervical routes of administration have all been used.

Systemic side effects, such as nausea, vomiting, diarrhea and, occasionally, uterine hypertonus, can occur with the use of these hormones. These effects are related both to dose and to route of administration. For example, when a 0.5-mg dose of PGE_2 is applied intracervically, systemic side effects appear to be nonexistent if the drug is confined to the endocervical canal.

$PGF_{2\alpha}$ appears to be produced in highest concentration in the decidua and is most likely involved in both the initiation and the maintenance of normal contractions in labor. PGE_2 is found in highest concentrations in the cervix and appears to be the hormone responsible for spontaneous cervical priming both late in pregnancy and in the early stages of labor. Local application (intracervically) of PGE_2 produces clinically detectable cervical "ripening" in a time frame as short as six hours. If confined to the endocervical canal it does not induce contractions.

In general, PGE_2 is the compound found most useful clinically for both cervical priming and induction of labor. It has been studied extensively in Sweden in the form of an intracervical gel for cervical priming. When the gel inserted in an unfavorable cervix, the cervical score doubles, there is no increase in uterine activity, and the rate of successful induction with oxytocin improves dramatically. The cesarean section rate for failed induction is also reduced by as much as a half to two thirds.

Other benefits achieved with this method of cervical priming include a shorter time from induction to active labor, a shorter labor, and a shorter time from the onset of induction to delivery. The priming of the cervix results in decreased cervical resistance to dilatation and a marked shortening of the active phase of first-stage labor. These benefits are achieved with normal uterine contractions and are not related to hyperstimulation. Similar benefits are encountered in patients undergoing elective induction of labor with intermittent oral administration of PGE_2 in doses ranging from 0.5 mg to 1.5 mg per hour. There is no statistical difference in labor characteristics between women in spontaneous labor at term and those undergoing elective induction of labor with oral PGE_2.

With an increased understanding of the forces of labor and the endocrinology of parturition, physiologic manipulations of both the expulsive forces and the resistance forces are now possible. Yet to be identified, however, are the factors that trigger the normal labor process, including the role played by the fetus.

REFERENCES AND RECOMMENDED READING

Bargmann W, Scharrer E: The site of origin of the hormones of the posterior pituitary. Am Scient 39:255, 1951

Beazley JM: The active management of labor. Am J Obstet Gynecol 122:161, 1975

Calkins LA: Normal labor. Springfield, IL, Charles C Thomas, 1955

Cefalo RC (ed): Abnormalities of Labor. Clin Obstet Gynecol 25:103, 1982

Federle MP, Cohen HA, Rosenwein MF, et al: Pelvimetry by digital radiography: A low dose examination. Radiology 143:733, 1982

Friedman EA: Labor: Clinical Evaluation and Management, 2nd ed. New York, Appleton-Century-Crofts, 1978

Fuchs AR, Fuchs F: Endocrinology of human parturition: A review. Br J Obstet Gynaecol 91:948, 1984

Hendricks CH, Brenner WE, Kraus G: Normal cervical dilatation pattern in late pregnancy and labor. Am J Obstet Gynecol 106:1065, 1970

Huszar G, Naftolin F: The myometrium and uterine cervix in normal and preterm labor. New Engl J Med 311:571, 1984

Lange AP, Secher NJ, Westergaard JG, Skovgard IB: Neonatal jaundice after labour induced or stimulated by prostaglandin E_2 or oxytocin. Lancet 1(8279):991, 1982

Rayburn WF, Zuspan FP: Drug Therapy in Obstetrics and Gynecology. Norwalk, Appleton-Century-Crofts, 1982

Ulmsten U, Ueland K (eds): The forces of labor: Uterine contractions and the resistance of the cervix. Clin Obstet Gynecol 26:1, 1983

Wetrich DW: Effect of amniotomy upon labor. Obstet Gynecol 35:800, 1970

Transfusions and Shock

David H. Vroon
Sidney F. Bottoms
David N. Danforth

38

Transfusions

David H. Vroon
Sidney F. Bottoms

Blood is a complex substance containing multiple cellular and soluble elements. The transfer of this complex material between unrelated humans is a type of tissue transplantation that, unlike many other surgical procedures, cannot be readily undone. While much has been learned about blood compatibility testing, there remain significant gaps in knowledge. Furthermore, hazards associated with transfusion extend beyond those related to immune phenomena. Transfusion of blood products always presents a risk that must be measured against the potential benefits to the patient. Human blood is also a vital and limited resource that cannot be manufactured; demand frequently exceeds supply. The prescribing physician must be aware of the need to economize this valuable resource and is responsible for actively encouraging volunteer replacement of blood. Unnecessary administration of blood is wasteful and detrimental to patient care.

Indications for blood transfusion generally fall into three categories: to facilitate the delivery of oxygen to tissues, to correct hypovolemia, and to restore adequate circulating levels of cellular or soluble constituents, including hemostatic factors. Since these needs seldom occur simultaneously, routine administration of all components present in fresh whole blood is not appropriate. Infusion of separate cellular or noncellular constituents selected to correct a specific deficiency is always preferable. Component transfusion more effectively corrects the specific deficiency, minimizes untoward reactions associated with unneeded blood constituents, and promotes conservation of a valuable, exhaustible resource (since fractionation of a single donor unit of blood serves the needs of several patients).

High-speed differential refrigerated centrifugation and a closed system of plastic bags allow fractionation and storage of blood components without danger of bacterial contamination and enable preparation of cellular and noncellular blood fractions in hospital and community blood banks. Each blood component has a specific use, produces a specific type of reaction, and has its own half-life both *in vivo* and in the collection container. Effective and judicious use of blood must be based on a thorough knowledge of these characteristics.

ERYTHROCYTE AND VOLUME REPLACEMENT

Red cells are readily stored *in vitro;* they have a shelf life of 35 days at $1°C$ ($34°F$) to $6°C$ ($43°F$) when collected in citrate–phosphate–dextrose–adenine (CPDA-1) anticoagulant cell preservative and probably more than five years when stored at ultralow temperatures. Post-transfusion recovery exceeds 70% for refrigerated and 90% for frozen red blood cells, and the potential post-transfusion life span is essentially normal for stored red blood cells. Nevertheless, specific physicochemical and functional changes incidental to refrigerated storage may have significant consequences for the recipient. These are specifically discussed below with regard to massive red cell transfusions.

Erythrocytes can be replaced by infusion of whole blood, packed red blood cells, or frozen red blood cells. Characteristics of these preparations are summarized in Table 38-1. The need to restore or maintain oxygen-carrying capacity—the most common circumstance in which transfusion is required—is satisfied only by infusion of red blood cells.

Table 38-1
Available Blood Components

Component	Content	Vol (ml)	Indications	Risk	Comments
Whole blood	All components	500	Massive acute blood loss	Hepatitis, volume overload	Consider component therapy
Packed cells	Red cells	200	Blood replacement	Hepatitis, allosensitization	Increases hematocrit 3–5%
Frozen plasma	Clotting factors	200	DIC, factor and immunoglobulin deficiency	Hepatitis	Increase fibrinogen 10 mg/dl per unit infused
Platelet concentrate	Platelets	50	Hereditary and acquired thrombocytopenia	Rh isoimmunization	Increase platelet count 7500/μl per unit infused
Cryoprecipitate	I, V, VIII, XIII	40	DIC, von Willebrand's hemophilia A	Hepatitis	Increase fibrinogen 10 mg/dl per unit
Factor concentrates	VIII, IX	20	Hemophilia A, IX deficiency	Hepatitis	1 U equals factor activity in 1 ml pooled plasma

DIC, disseminated intravascular coagulation.
(American College of Obstetricians and Gynecologists: Blood Component Therapy (ACOG Technical Bulletin 78). Washington DC, ACOG, 1984)

Anemia

Transfusion to correct chronic anemia is indicated primarily for those conditions not amenable to medical therapy, such as congenital hemolytic or aplastic disorders. Patients with anemia secondary to nutritional deficiencies or chronic blood loss are candidates for transfusion only when underlying conditions predispose to heart failure or oxygen deprivation and red cell mass is decreased. Occasionally, a need for immediate general anesthesia and impending labor require transfusion; however, every effort should be made to detect anemia in advance of hospitalization and to correct it with appropriate hematinics.

The majority of patients with anemia do not have a plasma volume deficit; usually there is a plasma volume excess. Therefore, infusion of packed cells is almost always preferable to administration of whole blood in patients with chronic subacute anemia. Packed red cells supply twice as much hemoglobin per unit of volume transfused as does whole blood, thus providing a greater increment in hemoglobin concentration or oxygen-carrying capacity with less danger of circulatory overload. In addition, use of packed red cells minimizes nonspecific reactions due to extraneous cellular and soluble elements that do not contribute to oxygen-carrying capacity. Finally, when frozen red cells are used, the risk of hepatitis is greatly reduced.

In all cases, the decision to transfuse and the amount of the transfusion should be based on clinical judgment rather than solely on arbitrarily selected hemoglobin or hematocrit values. Cause and duration of anemia, as well as activity and cardiopulmonary status of the recipient, are major considerations. Infusion of 1 unit of packed red cells produces, on the average, a 3% increment in recipient hematocrit. Since risk is compounded with multiple-unit transfusions, every effort should be made to limit the number of units used.

Blood Loss

Before a transfusion is given to correct acute blood loss of traumatic, surgical, or spontaneous origin, red cell mass and volume replacement must be considered. Although infusion of whole blood has been accepted as the therapy of choice for acute blood loss, there is growing evidence that the use of crystalloids alone or with packed red blood cells is often advantageous. Massive acute hemorrhage requires erythrocyte replacement. However, acute blood loss, particularly during a surgical procedure, is usually not massive and often does not exceed 1000 ml. Replacement in these cases must be governed by several considerations.

First, the major hazard of acute blood loss is failure to maintain adequate tissue oxygenation. Many adults can tolerate the rapid loss of 1000 ml to 2000 ml blood or up to 40% of blood volume without transfusion if blood pressure and renal blood flow are maintained with volume replacement. Rapid loss of 450 ml blood is insignificant; millions of blood donors experience such a loss every year.

Second, acute blood loss does not automatically mandate replacement of nonerythrocyte cellular and noncellular blood elements. Leukocyte and platelet extravascular reserves are moderately large, and hemorrhage is regularly associated with leukocytosis and thrombocytosis. In contrast, erythrocyte extravascular reserves are minimal and are returned to the circulation over a period of weeks. There are few data to support the concept that plasma protein must be replaced to promote healing and reduce the risk of infection, particularly in surgical patients. Plasma proteins are readily replaced; indeed, repeated weekly removal of 1000 ml plasma from healthy donors for plasmapheresis has no significant effect. In healthy persons as much as 16 g albumin is synthesized each day. Furthermore, albumin distribution throughout the body is such that only 40% exists in the intravascular compartment; loss of as much as 2000 ml blood in an adult results in only a 15% depletion of total body albumin. There is only slightly more total protein present in whole blood than in packed cells (see Table 38-1).

Mild to moderate acute blood loss is well tolerated and usually requires only red blood cell replacement when oxygen-carrying capacity is significantly compromised. Administration of a balanced salt solution augmented by packed red blood cells should therefore be considered the treatment of choice. Whole blood transfusion is indicated to combat extensive hemorrhage.

Emergency Transfusions

Clinical circumstances sometimes mandate blood replacement before the usual compatibility testing has been completed. Communication with the blood bank in these situations must be clear and rational. The risk of a fatal transfusion reaction must be carefully weighed against the risk of irreversible shock or exsanguination. ABO groupings and Rh typing of the patient's blood, selection of donor blood of the same ABO and Rh types, and complete cross-matching require approximately 90 minutes. A dire emergency may warrant abbreviation of this process, and transfusion must never be delayed unnecessarily. Even in an emergency, however, the safest and most expedient compromises must be employed.

Group- and type-specific blood should be administered when time permits analysis of the patient's blood. Previous records must not be accepted as evidence of blood group. When time does not permit grouping and typing of the recipient's blood, group O Rh-negative blood may be administered; however, in such cases, at least 70% of the plasma should be removed before transfusion to avoid subjecting the patient to dangerous levels of antibodies, specifically anti-A and anti-B. In emergency situations, it is preferable to employ packed cells (type specific if there is time for typing; group O, preferably Rh negative, if there is not) and to accomplish additional volume expansion with albumin or plasma

protein fraction preparations that are free of antibodies. In all cases, routine compatibility testing should be initiated in the blood bank. Significant incompatibility can often be detected by the time blood is transported to the patient's bedside. The attending physician should be notified immediately if there is such an incompatibility.

Massive Transfusions

Transfusion of sufficient blood to constitute total volume replacement within 12 to 24 hours presents special problems. In the adult, the amount of whole blood needed is usually 8 to 10 units. Banked or stored whole blood undergoes physical and functional alterations, and its administration in large amounts may produce potentially deleterious changes in hemoglobin affinity for oxygen, clotting mechanisms, and acid–base balance.

Refrigerated storage is associated with a decrease in red cell organic phosphate, particularly 2,3-diphosphoglyceric acid (2,3-DPG), which influences the liberation of oxygen in tissue. Depletion of intracellular 2,3-DPG increases hemoglobin affinity for oxygen and therefore diminishes the erythrocytes' capacity to deliver oxygen to tissues. Loss of 2,3-DPG occurs somewhat more slowly in the CPD-treated blood than in ACD-treated blood; significant decreases are noted after seven to ten days of storage. Restoration of organic phosphates and normal oxygen affinity may require 24 to 72 hours after transfusion of stored cells. Transient changes in recipient oxygen dissociation curves have been demonstrated, although deleterious clinical effects are not well documented. On theoretical grounds, therefore, massive transfusions are associated with significant risk of temporary tissue hypoxia. This can be mitigated by making sure that most of the units given have been stored for less than one week.

Clotting impairments due to rapid deterioration of factors V and VIII and platelets in stored blood are commonly encountered following massive transfusions. All other clotting factors are stable in refrigerated blood. To counteract the effects of depletion of factors V and VIII, 2 units of fresh-frozen plasma should be given after the infusion of the first 8 to 10 units of banked blood; thereafter, 1 unit of fresh-frozen plasma should be given for every 4 units of blood infused. Clotting complications due to platelet depletion are less common; replacement with platelet concentrates should be based on platelet counts.

The problems associated with increased hemoglobin affinity for oxygen and clotting defects can be prevented by the use of fresh whole blood. However, since blood stored for less than 24 hours is usually not obtainable in emergency situations, specific component therapy is often the best alternative.

The addition of acidic preservative solution to stored blood presents the recipient of multiple units with a large acid load. Clinically significant acidosis may occur, particularly in persons who are in shock or who have compromised respiratory or renal function. The acid–base response to multiple transfusions is variable, and administration of sodium bicarbonate may effect an undesirable leftward shift of the oxygen dissociation curve. Bicarbonate administration should be guided by arterial blood gas and pH determinations. Additional storage-related changes, such as increased plasma potassium, reduced ionized calcium, and increased citrate content, are usually significant only in the transfusion of blood in children or in adults with hepatic or renal disease. Plasma constituents can be greatly reduced if packed cells rather than whole blood are given.

Because infusion of multiple units of blood at refrigerated temperatures has been associated with cardiac arrhythmias and even cardiac arrest, blood should be warmed as it is transfused. The use of warm blood also enhances the sensitivity of blood pressure measurement. The heat-exchanging equipment must be carefully monitored, however, since overheated blood may trigger hemolysis with consequent disastrous effects. The practice of warming the entire container of blood at room temperature or in a water bath should be avoided on grounds of inadequate heat exchange and danger of bacterial growth.

PLATELET TRANSFUSION

Platelets facilitate hemostasis by plugging injured small vessels and by releasing a phospholipid, platelet factor 3, which contributes to the coagulation process. The causes of thrombocytopenia are numerous. In obstetric and gynecologic practice, significant acute thrombocytopenia is often associated with abruptio placentae, the infusion of massive quantities of blood, bacterial sepsis, or severe pregnancy-induced hypertension. Replacement therapy should be guided by the platelet count. Active bleeding with a platelet count of less than 50,000/mm^3 is a clear indication for replacement.

Blood platelets retain little hemostatic function after 24 to 48 hours of refrigerated storage. Platelets must be harvested from freshly collected blood. When stored with agitation at room temperature, they remain viable and functional for up to 72 hours. Fresh blood, platelet-rich fresh plasma, and platelet concentrates are sources of functional platelets. Of these, platelet concentrates offer the advantage of providing large numbers of platelets (70–80% of fresh whole blood) in a small volume of plasma (less than 50 ml). After infusion, platelets are hemostatically effective for no more than five days. In a previously sensitized recipient, the beneficial effect of platelet antibodies may be reduced to a matter of hours. An increment of 50,000 platelets/mm^3 can be expected from the transfusion of 1 unit of platelet concentrate per 7 kg of body weight. The increment is substantially less in a patient with sepsis, fever, or active bleeding; however, hemostasis may be achieved in a bleeding patient without a large increase in platelet count. In general, when platelet replacement is indicated in an adult, infusion of platelets harvested from 8 to 10 units of fresh donor blood is required. Volume considerations usually dictate the choice of platelet concentrates rather than fresh whole blood. Since platelets are suspended in plasma and contain small numbers of red blood cells, ABO and Rh compatibility is desirable but not always possible, owing to urgency of need and deficiency of supply. In an Rh-negative patient, infusion of a platelet preparation from Rh-positive donors may result in isosensitization.

TRANSFUSION OF NONCELLULAR PLASMA COMPONENTS

Blood plasma fractions commonly available for replacement of noncellular elements are summarized in Table 38-1. Some of these products are routinely prepared in blood banks; others are available as commercial derivatives. Effective use depends on a thorough knowledge of their specific constituents, indications, advantages, and disadvantages.

Plasma is an effective volume expander, but its possible content of anti-A and anti-B antibodies, aggregated and denatured protein, and the hepatitis virus is a significant disadvantage. Plasma derivatives such as 5% albumin and plasma protein fraction in combination with buffered salt solutions are preferable, since they contain no antibodies and are heat treated to kill hepatitis virus. Concentrated albumin (25% solution) draws about 3.5 times its own volume of extravascular fluid into the intravascular compartment within 15 minutes of administration. Alternative plasma volume expanders include hetastarch (Hespan) and dextran. These synthetic colloids are acceptable to some patients who have religious objection to the use of blood products. Hetastarch is less expensive than albumin or plasma protein fraction. Dextran has anticoagulant effects, can cause erythrocyte agglutination (making cross-matching impossible), and entails a risk of anaphylaxis. It should be avoided in the management of hemorrhage.

Indications for treating hypoproteinemia by infusion of protein solutions are unclear. The widespread practice of treating all degrees of hypoproteinemia is probably without merit. Significant elevation of plasma proteins is obtainable only when 25% albumin is infused.

Clotting disorders due to a deficiency of soluble clotting factors can be alleviated by infusion of fresh-frozen plasma, cryoprecipitate, or single-factor concentrates. All are associated with some risk of hepatitis, the latter two with the highest risk, since they are prepared from plasma pools. Administration of these products should be guided by the results of the basic clotting tests described in Chapter 30.

Congenital deficiencies of individual clotting factors are, for practical purposes, limited to lack of factors VIII, IX, and XI—uncommonly encountered in obstetric and gynecologic practice. Acquired hemostatic defects are usually due to multiple factor deficiencies. Liver disease, ingestion of oral anticoagulants, and hemorrhagic disease of the newborn involve the vitamin K–dependent factors II, VII, IX, and X. Clotting defects associated with massive transfusion of banked blood involve primarily platelets and labile factors V and VIII. Deficiencies secondary to disseminated intravascular coagulation involve primarily platelets, factors V and VIII, fibrinogen, and prothrombin. Administration of fresh-frozen plasma in combination with platelet concentrates is effective in all these conditions when replacement therapy is warranted. Fresh-frozen plasma is often the best agent to replace soluble clotting factors when colloid replacement is also indicated.

Commercial preparations of fibrinogen prepared from plasma pools are no longer available for clinical use because of the unacceptably high incidence of post-transfusion hepatitis associated with them. Fibrinogen replacement is rarely needed, but if it is necessary, adequate fibrinogen levels can be obtained by infusion of cryoprecipitate with significantly less risk of hepatitis transmission. Each bag of cryoprecipitate contains an average of 250 mg fibrinogen; 16 to 20 bags are usually required for replacement therapy. Disadvantages of cryoprecipitate are variability in plasma fibrinogen response and the large volume that must be infused. Acute hemolytic reactions and hemolytic anemia from anti-A or anti-B antibodies are readily avoided by use of blood type–specific cryoprecipitate.

HAZARDS OF BLOOD TRANSFUSION

The transfusion of blood or its components can produce several types of adverse reactions, ranging in severity from life threatening to inconsequential. Some are unavoidable; others are inherent risks of transfusion. Adverse reactions may occur immediately and be readily recognized or be delayed and be unrecognized or blamed on a previous transfusion. It is estimated that untoward reactions occur in more than 5% of transfusions.

Immediate Transfusion Reactions

Immediate adverse effects of transfusion include circulatory overload, air embolism, septicemia, hypothermia, chemical intoxication, and antigen–antibody reactions. Hypothermia and chemical intoxication are discussed under Massive Transfusions. Circulatory overload is the most common immediate complication; minimization of infused volume is a major reason for the use of packed red blood cells rather than whole blood.

Types

Septicemia due to infusion of contaminated blood may be associated with chills, fever, and profound shock requiring emergency measures. Most often gram-negative bacilli capable of growing at 4°C (39°F) are responsible, and they may produce deadly endotoxins. Prevention of transfusion septicemia depends on careful collection and storage of blood. Because a rise in temperature accelerates the growth of any contaminant, storage at room temperature and prolonged infusion must be avoided. Any unit of blood exposed to temperatures over 10°C (50°F) should be considered unusable.

Reactions may occur between donor cellular or protein antigen and recipient antibodies. Less common reactions result from infusion of donor antibodies. Reactions that activate complement and lyse cells are most severe. Vasoactive substances, generated by complement activation and cell destruction, result in the release of hemoglobin and other intracellular proteins, some of which have thromboplastin-like activity. These substances account for the anaphylactic shock, renal failure, and bleeding diatheses observed in severe transfusion reactions.

Immune intravascular destruction of erythrocytes is the most feared complication of transfusion therapy. Shock, bleeding diathesis, and renal failure may occur precipitously and threaten life. Present-day serologic techniques effectively protect against this hazard, but human error is ever present; clerical errors related to misidentification of donor units and recipient account for the majority of acute hemolytic reactions to transfusion. Great care must be taken to ensure that the proper specimen is sent to the laboratory for cross-matching and that the proper unit is administered to the intended recipient.

Immune reactions to leukocytes, platelets, and plasma factors are common causes of less severe transfusion reactions. Because complement activation is minimal, there are no anaphylactic symptoms. Fever and chills are predominant. Leukocyte and platelet antibodies are common in multiparous women and in recipients of multiple transfusions. Modern serologic techniques neither detect incompatibilities nor prevent sensitization to these cellular elements. Reactions are minimized by infusion of packed cells rather than whole blood. However, except for frozen red cells, sufficient plasma and cellular antigens remain in packed cells to effect sensitization. Reactions to plasma proteins are less well documented. Allergic reactions, manifested by itching, erythema, and urticaria, are common. Respiratory symptoms are rare. These reactions tend to occur in patients with an allergic history; the patient with a previous allergic transfusion reaction is likely to experience another. Reactions with anaphylactoid symptoms have occasionally been observed in patients with antibodies to immunoglobulin A (IgA).

A recipient's immune reaction caused by infusion of donor antibodies is usually not severe and may even go unnoticed, owing to immediate dilution of the antibodies in the recipient. However, such a reaction should not be ignored. Infusion of blood or plasma containing platelet or leukocyte antibodies may induce thrombocytopenia or leukopenia in the recipient. Group O blood, platelet concentrates, and cryoprecipitate prepared from pooled blood all contain significant amounts of anti-A and anti-B antibodies. These products, given to a recipient with group A, B, or AB blood, may precipitate an immediate systemic reaction or spherocytic hemolytic anemia. Neutralization by the addition of specific soluble substances A and B is unreliable. For this reason, emergency transfusion of group O blood should be done with packed cells rather than whole blood. When a large amount of platelets or cryoprecipitate prepared from pooled blood is to be infused, group-compatible units should be selected, if possible. If platelet concentrates obtained from pools including Rh-positive donors must be administered to a premenopausal Rh-negative woman, anti-D immune globulin should also be administered to prevent sensitization.

Investigation and Management

Immune reactions to transfusion are almost always associated with chills and fever. Initial manifestations of serious reactions may be indistinguishable from those of inconsequential reactions. Therefore, onset of these symptoms is always reason to stop the transfusion and investigate their cause. Additional transfusions should be avoided until the source of the reaction is identified. All transfusion reactions should be reported to the blood bank and investigated to the extent considered appropriate in consultation with the blood bank director.

The occurrence of chills, fever, back pain, or a drop in blood pressure with oozing of blood from incisions or venopuncture sites suggests a hemolytic reaction. Elevated plasma hemoglobin values, hemoglobinuria, or a positive direct antiglobulin test is confirmatory. All specimens, including blood containers, should be returned to the blood bank for serologic testing. Clerical records should be immediately checked to exclude mistaken identity of either donor blood or recipient. The donor blood should be examined by Gram staining and cultured to exclude bacterial contamination.

Immune, coagulation, and renal disorders associated with acute hemolytic transfusion reactions are life threatening and require vigorous therapy. Mannitol, initially 25 g for adults and up to 150 g per 24 hours, and saline solutions with sodium bicarbonate should be administered immediately to maintain a urinary output of 1 ml to 3 ml/minute. Inability to maintain urine flow is presumptive evidence of acute tubular necrosis, and fluids should then be restricted and the possible need

for dialysis kept in mind. When anaphylactic shock is life threatening, vasopressors are indicated. However, vasoconstriction may contribute to renal damage. Bleeding disorders suggest that defibrination has occurred, which should be confirmed by laboratory tests as discussed in Chapter 30. Intravenous administration of heparin may inhibit intravascular clotting. When replacement therapy is required to control bleeding, platelet concentrates, fresh-frozen plasma, or cryoprecipitate may be employed. Erythrocytes may be transfused as packed cells or whole blood after cross-matching with a fresh specimen from the patient. When ABO incompatibility is the cause of the hemolytic reaction, group O packed cells should be given.

Delayed Complications of Transfusion

Delayed adverse effects of transfusion include sensitization, delayed antigen–antibody reactions, and disease transmission. The frequency and significance of many delayed reactions are not known; more often than not they proceed unrecognized. Occasionally, red blood cell incompatibility occurs with antibody titers too low to be serologically detectable or to cause an immediate reaction. Transfusion of donor cells containing the appropriate antigen may elicit an anamnestic response, with an antigen–antibody reaction occurring several days after transfusion. Systemic manifestations are only occasionally observed; destruction of transfused cells goes unnoticed or masquerades as an autoimmune hemolytic process. A similar situation may occur with platelet antigens; infusion of donor platelets may elicit an immune response that results in thrombocytopenia.

The selection of blood with the same ABO and Rh types as the patient's does not guarantee that recipient isosensitization to one of numerous other red antigens will not occur. Fortunately, most red cell antigens (except ABO, Rh, Kell, and Duffy systems) do not readily elicit an antibody response. Nevertheless, isoimmunization has been estimated to occur in as many as 1% of single-unit transfusions. Transfusion that is free of immediate ill effects may still produce immunization that may interfere with future pregnancies or transfusions. The chances of eliciting antiplatelet or antileukocyte antibodies are even greater, and their production may interfere with future transfusions or organ transplantation.

Infectious diseases transmissible by blood include hepatitis, acquired immune deficiency syndrome, bartonellosis, brucellosis, trypanosomiasis, cytomegalic viral disease, infectious mononucleosis, malaria, and syphilis. Present methods of donor screening and blood processing have eliminated all but the first two of this list as serious clinical problems. The frequency of posttransfusion hepatitis is approximately 7%. Type-B hepatitis accounts for about 10% to 15% of the cases; non-

A and non-B hepatitis account for the remainder. Risk has been shown to correlate with the presence of hepatitis B surface antigen (HBsAg) in donor blood; the proportion of commercial donors; and the number of donor units included in the transfusion volume. Morbidity and mortality from icteric hepatitis in adults are significant; the percentage of blood recipients with anicteric infections who suffer chronic liver damage is unknown.

Elimination of HBsAg-positive donor units cannot totally eliminate posttransfusion hepatitis, but it can help considerably. Further reduction is possible through judicious use of transfusion in general and through selection of component units that carry a low risk of hepatitis. Presently, the only available blood products that have no risk of transmitting hepatitis are immune serum globulin, plasma protein fraction, and albumin preparations. Derivates prepared from plasma pools, such as factor-VIII and -IX concentrates, carry the greatest risk. It is hoped that the use of screening tests will help blunt the developing epidemic of transfusion-acquired acquired immune deficiency syndrome.

Shock

Sidney F. Bottoms
David N. Danforth

Shock is a state of generalized circulatory failure characterized by inadequate tissue perfusion. Inadequate tissue perfusion can be related to diminished circulatory volume, an abnormally enlarged vascular space, or cardiac failure. Given these causes, shock can be classified as hypovolemic, vasogenic, or cardiogenic. Hypovolemic shock includes shock due to fluid loss (*e.g.,* intestinal obstruction) as well as hemorrhagic shock. Vasogenic shock includes anaphylactic shock and neurogenic shock (*e.g.,* total spinal anesthesia) as well as septic shock. Cardiogenic shock includes shock due to cardiac obstruction (*e.g.,* massive embolism) as well as myocardial failure.

Shock begins with a primary (reversible) stage. Increasing severity is accompanied by progressive hypoxia, anaerobic metabolism, and acidosis, followed by injury and necrosis at the cellular level. Hypoxia leads to reduced myocardial contractility and loss of vascular tone, which further compromise tissue perfusion. Secondary (irreversible) shock is the ultimate result of this process.

EVALUATION

Evaluation includes making the diagnosis of shock, evaluating its severity, and determining its cause. The clinical setting is often the key to preliminary evaluation.

For example, postpartum hemorrhage may herald hemorrhagic shock. Similarly, a sudden change in the vital signs of a patient with a large pelvic abscess suggests the possibility of septic shock, and poor color in a postoperative patient with cardiac disease may be the first sign of cardiogenic shock.

The clinical manifestations of shock vary according to the severity of the condition (Table 38-2). Blood pressure and pulse rate are important diagnostic indices for shock, but they must be interpreted with caution. They are influenced by age, pregnancy, posture, anxiety, pain, medications, technique used to measure blood pressure, physical conditioning, and several diseases. Orthostatic changes are more reliable; a postural drop of more than 10 mm Hg in systolic blood pressure or a postural increase in pulse rate of more than 20 beats/minute suggests a 20% to 25% decrease in circulating blood volume. However, postural changes alone are insufficient grounds for the diagnosis of shock; they must be accompanied by evidence of inadequate tissue perfusion such as confusion, oliguria, or diaphoresis.

It may be necessary to begin treatment for shock before the exact cause can be determined. In this situation, emergency management is based on presumptive assignment of the case to one of the three major groups. It is particularly important to exclude the possibility of cardiogenic shock before the institution of treatment based on a presumptive diagnosis of hypovolemic shock; incorrect treatment could precipitate congestive heart failure. Cardiogenic shock should be suspected when there are signs of normal or increased venous return (*e.g.,* jugular vein distention).

Laboratory Studies

In cases of mild shock the cause of which is obvious (*e.g.,* postpartum hemorrhage due to retained placenta, resolved quickly without loss of consciousness or transfusion), extensive laboratory evaluation is not always appropriate. In other cases indicated tests might include blood typing and cross-matching, complete blood count, coagulation studies, serum chemistry analysis (*i.e.,* electrolytes, glucose, calcium, and creatinine levels), arterial blood gas determinations, and urinalysis. Coagulation studies include platelet count, prothrombin time, partial thromboplastin time, fibrinogen, and tests for split products of fibrin. An electrocardiogram is also indicated, even if a cardiac monitor has already been placed. In cases of severe shock, an arterial blood sample may be taken for lactic acid determination; mortality is exceptionally high in association with a lactic acid value greater than 2 mM/ liter.

Additional studies are frequently helpful. A chest radiograph should be obtained if cardiogenic or septic shock is suspected and after central line placement has been carried out. In septic abortion and other cases in which uterine perforation seems possible, roentgenography should be done with the patient in the upright

Table 38-2
Correlation of Clinical Findings and Magnitude of Volume Deficit in Hemorrhagic Shock*

Severity of Shock	Clinical Findings	Reduction in Blood Volume
None	None (normal blood donation)	Up to 20% (500 ml)†
Mild	Minimal tachycardia Slight decrease in blood pressure Mild evidence of peripheral vasoconstriction with cool hands and feet	15–25% (750–1250 ml)
Moderate	Tachycardia, 100–120 Decrease in pulse pressure Systolic blood pressure, 90–100 mg Hg Restlessness Increased swelling Pallor Oliguria	25–35% (1250–1750 ml)
Severe	Tachycardia, over 120 Systolic blood pressure, below 60 mm Hg and frequently unobtainable by cuff Mental stupor Extreme pallor, cold extremities Anuria	Up to 50% (2500 ml)

* Blood volume changes based on clinical observations of Beecher HK, Simeone FA, Burnett CH et al: Surgery 22:672, 1947.

† Based on blood volume of 7% in a 70-kg male of medium build.

(Smith II, Weil MH: In Weil MH, Shubin H (eds): Diagnosis and Treatment of Shock. Baltimore, Williams & Wilkins, 1967)

or lateral recumbent position to determine the presence of free air or a foreign body in the abdominal cavity. Blood and other appropriate cultures are indicated if sepsis is suspected. Prolonged oliguria is an indication for serum and urinary osmalily and urinary electrolyte determinations.

Many of these laboratory studies are useful in providing specific supportive therapy. Hemoglobin and hematocrit values help determine the need for blood transfusion, but they may not reflect acute blood loss for several hours unless plasma volume has been restored with intravenous fluids. A coagulopathy may be encountered with shock as a predisposing factor, or as a side-effect of massive transfusion, or from disseminated intravascular coagulation caused by shock. Coagulation studies identify the specific deficiencies in need of replacement. Arterial blood gas determinations guide both respiratory support and correction of acidosis.

Hemodynamic Assessment

Hemodynamic assessment with central venous pressure or a Swan–Ganz catheter (Fig. 38-1) can facilitate accurate evaluation of the patient in shock. During preliminary evaluation in questionable cases, hemodynamic assessment can usually confirm or rule out a cardiogenic cause of shock. More commonly, this technique is used to evaluate volume replacement therapy.

In hemodynamic assessment for shock, central venous pressure (a measure of the filling pressure for the right side of the heart) or pulmonary artery occlusive (wedge) pressure (a measure of the filling pressure for the left side of the heart) is determined. These pressures are usually low in hypovolemic and vasogenic shock. The pulmonary artery occlusive pressure generally reflects intravascular volume balance more accurately than the central venous pressure, unless these pressures have been equalized by an intracardiac shunt lesion. The pressure is elevated if a central venous pressure is greater than 15 cm H_2O or pulmonary artery occlusive pressure is greater than 20 mm Hg. Diagnostic accuracy is further improved by use of the fluid challenge test, in which these pressures are measured before and after an intravenous fluid challenge of 10 ml to 20 ml/minute is administered for 10 to 15 minutes. An increase of greater than 5 cm H_2O in central venous pressure or greater than 7 mm Hg in pulmonary artery occlusive pressure is significant. A significant increase in these pressures indicates cardiac failure or excessive volume replacement.

A Swan–Ganz catheter also allows measurement of cardiac output and estimation of several other parameters of cardiac function such as cardiac work. These additional capabilities may be useful in the subsequent management of patients with cardiogenic shock or significant ischemic sequelae of other forms of shock. Insertion of a Swan–Ganz catheter is associated with specific risks (cardiac arrhythmias and pulmonary artery rupture, both potentially fatal) and requires special skill

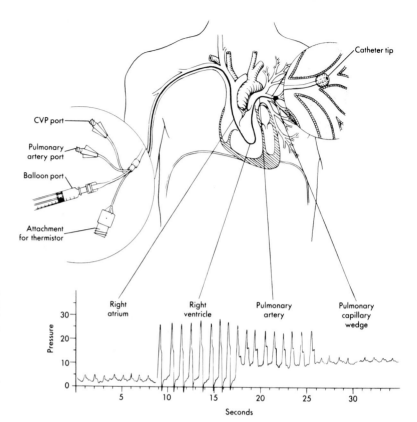

FIG. 38-1. Swan–Ganz catheter placement. Swan–Ganz catheter (7 French) depicting central venous pressure (*CVP*) port, pulmonary artery and balloon port, and attachment for thermistor. During advancement through the right side of heart, characteristic pressure tracings are recorded from right atrial, right ventricular, pulmonary artery, and pulmonary capillary wedge positions. (Bottoms SF: Hemorrhagic shock. ACOG Tech Bull 82:3, 1984)

and monitoring equipment. A specifically trained medical team is necessary for placement, testing, and use of the Swan–Ganz catheter.

The two techniques of hemodynamic assessment share certain limitations. Technical errors related to line placement or equipment are not uncommon; as with blood pressure and pulse, results must be interpreted with caution. Measurement of therapeutic responses (*e.g.,* the fluid challenge test) is more reliable than raw measurements. In the patient with coagulopathy, peripheral insertion of a central venous pressure catheter avoids the significant risk of hemorrhage associated with jugular or subclavian insertion of a Swan–Ganz catheter. Clinical decisions regarding catheter placement should be made on an individual basis according to the considerations outlined above.

MANAGEMENT

The survival of patients with shock depends directly on the duration of shock; many aspects of management need to proceed concurrently (Fig. 38-2). The type of definitive treatment (medical or surgical) that is necessary varies with the cause of the shock, its severity, and the patient's initial response to therapy.

Even when emergency surgery is indicated, a brief attempt at stabilization with blood transfusion or other appropriate medical treatment before surgery is usually

advisable. A team approach and a flowchart should be used if possible. A large-gauge intravenous line should be used to obtain blood for laboratory studies and to provide a reliable route for subsequent therapy. Insertion of a central venous pressure or Swan–Ganz catheter as a second line for more accurate hemodynamic evaluation is usually indicated. An indwelling urinary catheter should be inserted to monitor renal perfusion.

Restoration of tissue oxygenation is the ultimate goal of treatment for shock. Ventilation, oxygen transport capacity, and perfusion must all be adequate to meet this goal. Given that hypoxia is the cause of death in most cases of shock, the administration of supplemental oxygen is recommended. Other respiratory support may also be indicated, and arterial blood gas studies should be obtained. Although there is no substitute for clinical judgment in determining the need for transfusion, maintenance of a minimum hemoglobin level of 10 g/dl to 11 g/dl to ensure adequate oxygen transport capacity is usually a reasonable therapeutic goal for patients in shock.

The first approach used to restore perfusion is to optimize cardiac filling pressures. These pressures are reduced in all forms of shock except cardiogenic shock. Several immediate measures can be used to increase cardiac filling pressures. Elevation of the legs to an angle of about 30 degrees improves venous return while avoiding the risks of the Trendelenberg position (in-

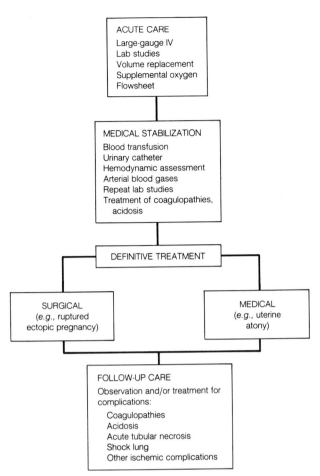

```
┌─────────────────────────────┐
│ ACUTE CARE                  │
│ Large-gauge IV              │
│ Lab studies                 │
│ Volume replacement          │
│ Supplemental oxygen         │
│ Flowsheet                   │
└─────────────────────────────┘
              │
┌─────────────────────────────┐
│ MEDICAL STABILIZATION       │
│ Blood transfusion           │
│ Urinary catheter            │
│ Hemodynamic assessment      │
│ Arterial blood gases        │
│ Repeat lab studies          │
│ Treatment of coagulopathies,│
│   acidosis                  │
└─────────────────────────────┘
              │
     ┌─────────────────────┐
     │ DEFINITIVE TREATMENT │
     └─────────────────────┘
      │                    │
┌──────────────┐    ┌──────────────┐
│ SURGICAL     │    │ MEDICAL      │
│ (e.g., ruptured   │ (e.g., uterine│
│ ectopic      │    │ atony)       │
│ pregnancy)   │    │              │
└──────────────┘    └──────────────┘
      │                    │
┌─────────────────────────────────┐
│ FOLLOW-UP CARE                  │
│ Observation and/or treatment for│
│ complications:                  │
│                                 │
│   Coagulopathies                │
│   Acidosis                      │
│   Acute tubular necrosis        │
│   Shock lung                    │
│   Other ischemic complications  │
└─────────────────────────────────┘
```

FIG. 38-2. Flowchart for the management of hemorrhagic shock. (American College of Obstetricians and Gynecologists: Hemorrhagic Shock (ACOG Technical Bulletin 82). Washington DC, ACOG, 1984)

terference with both cerebral circulation and respiratory efforts). When possible, patients in advanced stages of pregnancy should be placed in the lateral position to avoid compression of the aorta and vena cava. Air-pressurized trousers (MAST) or suits (G-suits) can be applied during transportation of trauma victims to the hospital or of patients with intra-abdominal hemorrhage to the operating room.

The keystone of treatment to increase cardiac filling pressures is volume replacement. If filling pressures fail to respond to rapid infusion of crystalloid fluids (1–2 liters/hour), colloid fluids should be added. Erythrocyte transfusion contributes to volume replacement and is frequently indicated in shock, but this should be reserved for restoration of oxygen transport capacity.

Crystalloid fluids are solutions containing only water and small molecules such as glucose and electrolytes. Not only do crystalloid fluids such as 5% dextrose in lactated Ringer's solution or normal saline maintain acid–base and glucose homeostasis, they also replenish extracellular fluid and electrolytes. In addition, they are immediately available and inexpensive. Formulations such as lactated Ringer's solution minimize electrolyte and acid–base imbalances following rapid administration of large volumes. There is no substitute for serum electrolyte determinations to guide long-term infusions.

Colloid fluids contain larger molecules that cross vascular membranes more slowly than do crystalloids. In plasma colloids help maintain oncotic pressure and thus help prevent edema. Infusion of large volumes of crystalloids without colloid replacement may lead to pulmonary edema. Patients in shock whose previous health was good rarely develop significant deficiencies in colloid concentration before several liters of crystalloids have been infused. Excessive colloid replacement may delay restoration of the extravascular fluid volume, and shock continues until this compartment is adequately replaced. Plasma colloids are usually replaced with albumin or plasma protein fraction to avoid the risk of hepatitis. Fresh-frozen plasma and blood also contain significant amounts of colloid, but they should not be administered for colloid replacement alone.

Vasoconstrictors are generally contraindicated until cardiac filling pressures have been optimized and are often not needed in the management of shock. Although these agents elevate the blood pressure, inappropriate administration can decrease tissue perfusion. If there is continued evidence of poor perfusion (*e.g.,* oliguria) after adequate volume replacement, low-dose dopamine (1–5 μg/minute) can increase cardiac output and dilate the coronary, mesenteric, and renal arteries without causing significant peripheral vasoconstriction. Higher doses (up to 20 μg/minute) produce vasoconstriction and entail a greater risk of cardiac arrhythmias but may be required to maintain circulation to vital organs in severe cases of shock. Ephedrine, like high-dose dopamine, increases cardiac output in addition to causing vasoconstriction. Intravenous administration of 10 mg to 25 mg in divided doses is frequently used for the rapid treatment of hypotension secondary to regional anesthesia. Other vasoactive drugs are rarely needed in the treatment of shock. Isoproterenol (Isuprel) may be used in conjunction with dopamine if it is necessary to increase the cardiac inotropic effect and to decrease pulmonary resistance. If there is intense peripheral vasoconstriction, isoproterenol or isoproterenol with dopamine may be more effective than dopamine alone. Norepinephrine bitartrate (Levophed Bitartrate) may be used if dopamine fails to maintain the arterial pressure; however, both this drug and metaraminol bitartrate (Aramine) have intense vasoconstrictive action and may compromise tissue perfusion. All of the aforementioned agents are potent drugs, and expertise is required in their use and in the measurement and interpretation of their hemodynamic effects.

Shock is usually accompanied by some degree of metabolic acidosis. Severe acidosis (blood *p*H less than 7.2) should be corrected with sodium bicarbonate. Care must be taken to avoid hypercapnia, hypokalemia, fluid overload, and overcorrection of acidosis during administration of bicarbonate. During active hemorrhage or before surgery, any significant coagulopathy other than disseminated intravascular coagulation should be corrected by means of appropriate blood component replacement.

Management subsequent to stabilization and definitive treatment is directed at the detection and treatment of the complications of shock. Severe complications include myocardial infarction, stroke, pituitary necrosis, renal cortical necrosis, and transfusion reaction. Electrolyte imbalance, acidosis, dilutional coagulopathy, acute tubular necrosis, and adult respiratory distress syndrome (shock lung) are among the most frequent complications.

SHOCK AND SHOCKLIKE SYNDROMES

Classifying shock into hypovolemic, vasogenic, and cardiogenic categories is helpful in guiding preliminary diagnosis and management. However, definitive treatment of shock varies with the exact cause. The causes of shock are described more specifically as familiar clinical syndromes.

Hemorrhagic Shock

Hemorrhagic shock may be encountered in pregnancy, delivery, the puerperium, suspected ectopic pregnancy, vaginal hemorrhage, or hemorrhage related to pelvic surgery. Familiarity with the specific causes of hemorrhage makes it possible to identify patients at risk for hemorrhagic shock. Early treatment of predisposing conditions can reduce the incidence of hemorrhagic shock and its complications.

Hemorrhagic shock, a major cause of maternal death, is in part related to the marked increase in blood supply to the genital tract that is associated with pregnancy. The more common obstetric causes of hemorrhage are shown in Table 38-3.

Gynecologic causes of hemorrhage, which are less common than obstetric causes, include genital trauma, uterine leiomyomas, dysfunctional uterine bleeding, ruptured ovarian cyst, and gynecologic malignancy. Patients undergoing pelvic surgery are at risk for hemorrhage, even with the best surgical techniques. Other surgical or medical causes of hemorrhagic shock encountered occasionally in both obstetrics and gynecology incude anticoagulant therapy, idiopathic thrombocytopenic purpura, and ruptured splenic vessel.

Management consists of volume and blood component replacement, control of hemorrhage, and observation and treatment for numerous potential complications. Rapid volume replacement with crystalloids should be started immediately. In critical situations, immediate transfusion using the procedures outlined earlier in this chapter may be preferable to a delay for com-

Table 38-3
Obstetric Causes of Hemorrhage

Disorder	Approximate Incidence
Early Pregnancy	
Ectopic pregnancy	1:150 deliveries
Inevitable and incomplete abortion	1:14 deliveries
Septic abortion	1:200 deliveries
Missed abortion	1:500 deliveries
Gestational trophoblastic disease	1:1500 pregnancies
Late Pregnancy	
Abruptio placentae	1:120 deliveries
Placenta previa	1:200 deliveries
Preeclampsia–eclampsia	1:20 deliveries
Delivery and puerperium	
Cesarean delivery	1:6 deliveries
Inversion of the uterus	1:2300 deliveries
Rupture of the uterus	1:11,000 deliveries
Retained placenta	1:160 deliveries
Placenta accreta	1:7000 deliveries
Postpartum hemorrhage (including uterine atony)	1:20 deliveries
Obstetric lacerations	1:8 deliveries

(American College of Obstetricians and Gynecologists: Hemorrhagic Shock (ACOG Technical Bulletin 82). Washington DC, ACOG, 1984)

plete cross-matching. It is usually advisable to administer crystalloids and colloids at least until type-specific, saline cross-matched blood is available.

Hysterectomy is necessary as a life-saving procedure in some cases of pelvic hemorrhage. The use of prostaglandins to supplement traditional treatment of postpartum uterine atony, as discussed elsewhere, has reduced the need for surgical intervention. In the case of refractory uterine hemorrhage, management by uterine or hypogastric artery ligation (Fig. 38-3) sometimes allows conservation of fertility.

Septic Shock

Septic shock is a clinical syndrome of acute circulatory failure associated with bacteremia. The causative organisms are usually, but not always, gram-negative bacteria. Obstetric causes include infected (septic) abortion, chorioamnionitis, endometritis (especially following cesarean delivery), and pyelonephritis. In gynecology, septic shock may be encountered with tubo-ovarian abscesses (especially ruptured ones), postoperative soft tissue infection, pyelonephritis, malignancy, and the toxic shock syndrome (see p. 987). The importance of early recognition and aggressive treatment of septic shock cannot be overemphasized; in the late 1950s, when less was known of the condition, the mortality ranged from 70% to 90%.

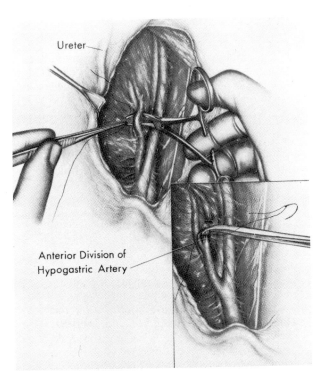

Ureter

Anterior Division of
Hypogastric Artery

FIG. 38-3. Ligation of the right hypogastric artery. The peritoneum is opened lateral to bifurcation of the common iliac artery, and the ureter is reflected medially with a peritoneal flap. There is much variation in the length and points of division of the hypogastric artery into anterior and posterior branches. If possible, the anterior branch should be used for ligation and silk suture placed around it. The *inset* shows anterior division of the hypogastric artery ligated and excised, and a transfixion ligature placed distal to the initial silk tie. (TeLinde RW, Mattingly RF: Operative Gynecology, 4th ed. Philadelphia, JB Lippincott, 1970)

Septic shock is best classified as vasogenic, although diminished intravascular volume and cardiotoxicity may also be involved. In the case of gram-negative organisms, release of endotoxin from disintegrating bacteria may contribute to dilation of the microcirculation, endothelial damage, platelet destruction, leakage of fluid from the vascular to the extravascular space, and varying degrees of disseminated intravascular coagulation and hemolysis. The primary mechanisms may be different for gram-positive septic shock, but the clinical syndrome and its treatment are the same.

Septic shock has an insidious onset more often than hemorrhagic shock and should be considered as a possibility in any febrile patient with chills and hypotension. Initially, the heart may be able to compensate for pooling of blood in the microcirculation, leading to the seemingly paradoxic situation of shock accompanied by increased cardiac output, warm skin, and flushing. Cavanagh and Rao have described the clinical evolution of septic shock in three phases, as described below.

The *early or warm hypotensive phase* is characterized by fever of 38.4°C to 40.6°C (101–105°F); warm, moist skin and flushed face; tachycardia; chills; and hypotension of 85 mm Hg to 95 mm Hg systolic. The sensorium shows no impairment, and urine output is more than 30 ml/hour. This phase may last for several hours, depending on the severity of the infection. The *late or cold hypotensive phase,* which clinically resembles shock due to hemorrhage, is characterized by cold, clammy skin; hypotension on the order of 70 mm Hg systolic or less; cyanosis of the nail beds; subnormal temperature; rapid, thready pulse; impaired sensorium; and oliguria. *Irreversible shock,* the final phase, is characterized by severe metabolic acidosis with sharply elevated levels of blood lactic acid, anuria, cardiac failure, respiratory distress, and coma.

Supportive management for septic shock differs from that for hemorrhagic shock in several ways. The Swan–Ganz catheter is particularly helpful in the hemodynamic assessment of septic shock, since circulating toxins may have direct effects on peripheral vascular resistance and cardiac output. Some patients respond acutely to volume replacement alone, but dopamine is frequently needed. Although the role of pharmacologic doses of steroids (*e.g.,* intravenous methylprednisolone, 30 mg/kg bolus followed by 15–30 mg/kg/day continuous infusion) in the management of septic shock remains controversial, there seems to be general agreement that steroids should be administered if the preliminary response to treatment is poor. Extensive hemolysis requires erythrocyte replacement, but administration of soluble coagulation factors and platelet transfusion may aggravate disseminated intravascular coagulation. Therefore, replacement of coagulation factors and platelets should be avoided unless deficiency appears to be an immediate threat to survival.

Blood cultures should be drawn and repeated at least every 24 hours and whenever the patient has chills or temperature spikes. Cultures and smears from the cervix and uterine cavity (or vaginal cuff) should be obtained if the infection is thought to be of pelvic origin.

Antibiotics should be started intravenously immediately after samples for culture are obtained. Initial coverage for a wide spectrum of organisms is needed for septic shock of pelvic origin. With the proliferation of new antimicrobials, many appropriate combinations are possible. Regardless of the specific agents selected, the spectrum of coverage should be comparable to "triple therapy" with high-dose penicillin (20–30 million units per day in divided doses), an aminoglycoside, and clindamycin. Subsequent doses of aminoglycosides should be guided by determinations of peak and trough blood levels. Shock reduces renal clearance of these agents, thereby predisposing to nephrotoxic and ototoxic side-effects. Death from pseudomembranous entercolitis, a potential complication of wide-spectrum antibiotic administration, can usually be avoided by prompt recognition and treatment of the condition, as discussed in Chapter 13.

In addition to requiring appropriate antibiotics, control of infection frequently requires surgery either for drainage of pus or for removal of the nidus of infection. Therapeutic levels of antibiotics should be administered and hypovolemia should be treated before surgical intervention. If the nidus of infection can be removed surgically, this should be done. Some cases of septic abortion can be cured by curettage, but if only negligible amounts of tissue are obtained or if there is no clear improvement within 3 hours, hysterectomy with bilateral salpingo-oophorectomy and high ligation of the pedicles of the ovarian veins is indicated.

Amniotic Fluid Embolism

Amniotic fluid embolism is usually a cataclysmic event characterized by the sudden onset of dyspnea, chest pain, pulmonary edema, shock, and, sometimes within minutes, death. Most often it occurs in the multigravid patient late in the first stage of labor, when the membranes have ruptured and the fetal head fits snugly into the lower uterine segment. In some documented cases in which there has been no external evidence of ruptured membranes, the amniotic fluid has reached the maternal circulation through a rent in the membranes at a higher level. In this condition, oxytocin may have been used for the induction or stimulation of labor. Under the pressure of uterine contractions, the amniotic fluid flows under the placental margin or to the site of a uterine, cervical, or vaginal laceration, where it gains access to the maternal venous channels; the resulting pulmonary embolization may be massive.

Much study has been devoted to the hemodynamics of the shock that quickly develops. Unfortunately, not all of the data obtained from animal studies are applicable to humans. At present, there is general agreement that pulmonary hypertension, with elevated pulmonary artery pressure and central venous pressure, develops in both animals and humans; however, elevated pulmonary capillary wedge pressure is uniformly seen only in humans, indicating that left ventricular failure is definitely present. The clinical implication of this finding is that circulatory overload may occur with administration of lesser amounts of fluid than would be required if the circulation were normal. Prompt inotropic support is suggested for patients with amniotic fluid embolism. The release of thromboplastin into the maternal circulation culminates, within minutes or hours, in activation of the extrinsic clotting pathway and consequent widespread disseminated intravascular coagulation. An exact diagnosis can be made only by the demonstration of particulate matter of the amniotic fluid (sloughed squamous cells, lanugo hair, meconium, vernix) in the pulmonary vasculature. Not all cases can be so documented, but among those that are diagnosed, it is estimated that death occurs in at least 80%.

The typical clinical picture is catastrophic, with instant collapse and death. Lesser consequences may result from the infusion of smaller quantities of amniotic fluid. Dyspnea, often slight, may be the first sign; its appearance in any patient who is in hypertonic labor after the membranes have ruptured should immediately suggest embolism. Subsequent symptoms may be distress, malaise, a sense of suffocation, agitation, and unexplained cough. Vomiting, chills, and fever occur in some patients. Cyanosis, tachycardia of the order of 140+ beats/minute, and a respiratory rate of 40+/minute occur relatively early and are followed by collapse after a variable period. Sweating, anxiety, and convulsions may be present. Pulmonary edema with pink, frothy sputum usually develops quickly. Fibrin breakdown products can usually be demonstrated, the number of platelets is reduced, and prothrombin time and thrombin–fibrinogen time are increased.

Mulder makes the following recommendations for therapy in suspected cases:

1. Institute positive-pressure oxygen therapy, using an endotracheal tube if feasible.
2. Administer hydrocortisone, 2 g to 4 g intravenously.
3. Attempt to alter bronchospasm and arteriolar spasm with terbutaline sulfate (Brethine), isoproterenol (Isuprel), or aminophylline.
4. Institute general supportive measures such as use of the semi-Fowler position, administration of morphine sulfate, and digitalization with a rapidly acting agent.
5. If possible, measure pulmonary and central venous pressure, preferably with a pulmonary artery flotation catheter.

Hemorrhage, disseminated intravascular coagulation, and uterine atony should be treated according to the principles outlined earlier in this chapter. Peritoneal dialysis or hemodialysis may be needed if the process is sufficiently severe to cause tubular necrosis and anuria.

The only preventive possibilities are avoidance of measures that would tend to produce a tumultuous, driving labor (*e.g.,* injudicious administration of oxytocin or other stimulating agents to a patient whose labor is progressing satisfactorily). Also, after spontaneous or artificial rupture of the membranes, as much amniotic fluid as possible should be allowed to escape vaginally to minimize the likelihood of the fluid's being forced back into the maternal circulation.

Supine Hypotensive Syndrome

The supine hypotensive syndrome is a shocklike state that can occur in advanced pregnancy when the woman assumes a supine posture. First described by McRoberts in 1951, it is characterized by hypotension, reflex bradycardia, sweating, nausea, weakness, and air hunger. The syndrome has been attributed to partial occlusion of the vena cava by pressure of the enlarged pregnant uterus, with consequent reduction of maternal cardiac output. Although cardiac output in late pregnancy is invariably reduced in the supine position, the hypotensive syndrome occurs only in a minority of patients, suggesting that factors other than simple vena cava occlusion may be involved. Bienarz and co-workers have shown that, in addition to producing partial vena cava occlusion, pressure from the gravid uterus compresses the abdominal aorta at the level of the fourth and fifth lumbar vertebrae, which increases arterial pressure in the aortic arch. Milson and Forssman suggest, therefore, that the supine hypotensive syndrome may result from aortocaval compression and subsequent hemodynamic adjustments, and not, as previously thought, from compression of the vena cava alone. They also suggest that, depending on the attitude of the fetus, placement of the patient in the right lateral position may not permit full release of vena cava pressure, given the right-sided location of the vena cava; accordingly, the patient should lie on her left side. Immediate recovery is to be expected.

Postpartum Vasomotor Collapse

Although shock most commonly occurs as a result of acute blood loss and other reductions in the oxygen-transporting mechanism of the blood, changes in electrolyte and steroid metabolism may result in shocklike states, especially in the postpartum period, when there are profound adjustments and alterations in the electrolyte and steroid systems. *Adrenal cortical insufficiency* can result in shock, Addison's disease representing a typical clinical example. Although most patients with Addison's disease can be carried through pregnancy on replacement therapy, the increased stresses of pregnancy, especially when complications such as infection, preeclampsia, or blood loss occur, result in a greater need for hormone substances. Vasomotor collapse and shock can follow a reduction in these substances, and adrenal crises can occur.

Preeclampsia can also result in shock and shocklike states. Such collapse is frequently associated with a marked reduction in the concentrations of sodium and chloride in the serum. In most cases, following delivery, mobilization of the extravascular fluid restores sodium concentration to near normal levels. This syndrome is not common, but it must be considered.

Anesthesia should be mentioned as a cause of postpartum vasomotor collapse. Spinal anesthesia ("spinal shock") as well as overdoses of toxic gases such as cyclopropane have been incriminated. All of these hypotensive reactions are aggravated when anemia or blood loss, chronic or acute, further complicates the picture. In addition, the pregnant patient is much more likely than the nonpregnant patient to develop severe degrees of systemic hypotension as an immediate result of anesthesia. For these reasons, the doses of anesthetic agents given most pregnant patients must be considerably less than those administered to nonpregnant patients.

The manifestations of *amniotic fluid embolism* may first appear after delivery, especially in cases in which there are extensive lacerations of the uterus, cervix, or vagina.

In all cases of postpartum obstetric shock, there is the possibility that Sheehan's disease (pituitary infarction resulting from collapse of the pituitary portal system) may follow. In one case, the pituitary ischemia was found to be selective, limited to the posterior lobe; diabetes insipidus was the result.

Other Causes of Shock

Other potential causes of shock in the pregnant patient include myocardial infarction and cardiac dysrhythmias. Anaphylactoid reactions due to hypersensitivity to various drugs may give rise to shocklike conditions. Cardiovascular abnormalities associated with congenital cardiac defects, coarctation of the aorta, and similar conditions may result in circulatory insufficiency. All such potential causes of shock and shocklike states in pregnancy must be considered and evaluated by the physician both at the time of the patient's initial physical examination and during the course of her prenatal care.

REFERENCES AND RECOMMENDED READING

Alexander MR, Ambre JJ, Liskow BI: Therapeutic use of albumin. JAMA 241:2527, 1979

American College of Obstetricians and Gynecologists: Septic shock. ACOG Tech Bull No 75, 1984

Bienarz J, Crottogini JJ, Curuchet E et al: Aortocaval compression by the uterus in late human pregnancy. Am J Obstet Gynecol 100:203, 1968

Borucki DT (ed): Blood Component Therapy: A Physician's Handbook, 3 ed. Washington, DC, American Association of Blood Banks, 1981

Bottoms SF: Hemorrhagic shock. ACOG Tech Bull No 82, 1984

Campbell JW, Frisse M (eds): Manual of Medical Therapeutics, 24th ed. Boston, Little, Brown, 1983

Cavanaugh D, Rao PS: Septic shock (endotoxin shock). Clin Obstet Gynecol 16(2):25, 1973

Center for Disease Control: Follow-up on toxic-shock syndrome. Morbid Mortal Weekly Rep 29:441, 1980

Clark SL, Cotton DB, Gonik B et al: Hemodynamic alterations associated with amniotic fluid embolism. In Proceedings of the Society of Perinatal Obstetricians, 1985

Cotton DB, Benedetti TJ: Use of the Swan–Ganz catheter in obstetrics and gynecology. Obstet Gynecol 56:641, 1979

Courtney LD: Amniotic fluid embolism. Ob Gynecol Surv 29:169, 1974

Creasy RK, Resnik R: Maternal–Fetal Medicine. Philadelphia, WB Saunders, 1984

Davis JP, Chesney PJ, Wand PG et al: Toxic-shock syndrome: Epidemiologic features, recurrence, risk factors, and prevention. N Engl J Med 303:1429, 1980

McRoberts WA Jr.: Postural shock in pregnancy. Am J Obstet Gynecol 62:627, 1951

Milson I, Forssman L: Factors influencing aortocaval compression in late pregnancy. Am J Obstet Gynecol 148:764, 1984

Monif GRW (ed): Infectious Disease in Obstetrics and Gynecology, 2nd ed. Philadelphia, Harper & Row, 1982

Morrison JC: Blood component therapy. ACOG Tech Bull No 78, 1984

Mulder JI: Amniotic fluid embolism: An overview and case report. Am J Obstet Gynecol 152:430, 1985

Myhre BA: Fatalities from blood transfusion. JAMA 244:1333, 1980

Price TM, Baker VV, Cefalo RC: Amniotic fluid embolism. Three case reports with a review of the literature. Obstet Gynecol Surv 40:462, 1985

Queenan JT (ed): Managing Ob/Gyn Emergencies. Oradell, NJ, Medical Economics Company, 1982

Reid PR, Thompson WL: The clinical use of dopamine in the treatment of shock. Johns Hopkins Med J 137:276, 1975

Schaffner W, Federspiel CF, Fulton ML et al: Maternal mortality in Michigan: An epidemiologic analysis, 1950–1971. Am J Public Health 67(9):821, 1977

Schumer W: Hypovolemic shock. JAMA 241:615, 1979

Schwarz RH: Shock associated with septic abortion. ACOG Tech Bull No 9, 1968

Shands KN, Schmid GP, Dan BB et al: Toxic-shock syndrome in menstruating women: Its association with tampon use and *Staphylococcus aureus* and the clinical features in 52 cases. N Engl J Med 303:1436, 1980

Suratt PM, Gibson RS (eds): Manual of Medical Procedures. St. Louis, CV Mosby, 1982

Swan HJC, Ganz W, Forrester J, Marcus H et al: Catheterization of the heart in man with use of a flow-directed balloon-tipped catheter. N Engl J Med 283:447, 1970

Thompson WL: Blood Substitutes and Plasma Expanders. New York, Alan R Liss, 1978

Weil MH, Shukin H (eds): Diagnosis and Treatment of Shock. Baltimore, Williams & Wilkins, 1967

Wilkins EW Jr. (ed): MGH Textbook of Emergency Medicine. Baltimore, William Wilkins, 1978

Cesarean Section and Other Obstetric Operations

Leo J. Dunn

39

Cesarean Section

The terms *cesarean section, laparotrachelotomy,* and *abdominal delivery* refer to the delivery of a fetus weighing 500 g or more by abdominal surgery that requires an incision through the wall of the uterus. They do not refer to surgery for an abdominal pregnancy, hysterotomy for abortion, or vaginal hysterotomy for delivery. On the basis of history (see Chap. 1) and practical value, cesarean section continues to be one of the most important operations performed in obstetrics and gynecology. Its lifesaving value to both mother and fetus has increased rather than declined over the decades, although specific indications for its use have changed. The initial purposes of preserving the life of a mother with obstructed labor or delivering a viable infant from a dying mother have gradually expanded to include the rescue of the fetus from more subtle dangers. Four major forces that have led to reduced maternal risk from cesarean section include the following: improvement in surgical techniques, improvement in anesthetic techniques, development of safe blood transfusion, and the discovery of antibiotics.

There has been a progressive increase in the incidence of cesarean section in relation to total deliveries. Whereas in the previous decade cesarean section accounted for about 5% of all deliveries, in many hospitals it is now used four to five times as frequently. The reasons for this change include an increase in the number of fetal problems believed to be managed better by abdominal delivery than vaginally, the high incidence of abdominal delivery for those having had a previous cesarean section, and the rise in the ratio of primigravid to multiparous parturients, because primary cesarean section is approximately nine times more common in primigravidas than in multiparas.

INDICATIONS

Cesarean section is indicated when labor is considered unsafe for either mother or fetus, when delivery is necessary but labor cannot be induced, when dystocia or fetal characteristics (*e.g.,* premature breech) present significant risks and contraindicate vaginal delivery, and when an emergency mandates immediate delivery and the vaginal route is not possible or not suitable.

Labor Contraindicated

Under certain conditions, forceful uterine contractions, as in normal labor, constitute a real or potential hazard to mother, fetus, or both. Conditions in which the forces of labor increase the risk to the mother include central placenta previa, previous classic cesarean section, previous myomectomy transecting the uterine wall, previous uterine reconstruction, or previous repair of a vaginal fistula. In such circumstances, normal labor and vaginal delivery may result in uterine rupture, hemorrhage, or serious lacerations of the birth canal and endanger the life or future health of the mother.

Conditions that threaten the fetus and that may be worsened by labor include placenta previa, velamentous insertion of the cord or other forms of vasa previa, and cord presentation. During the past decade, electronic fetal monitoring and fetal scalp pH determinations have been adopted as methods of detecting more subtle dangers involving a relative insufficiency in maternal–fetal exchange that may result in fetal compromise or death. This subject is discussed in Chapter 41.

Delivery Necessary but Labor Not Inducible

In conditions such as isoimmunization, diabetes mellitus, intrauterine growth retardation, and hypertensive disorders, a poor intrauterine environment constitutes an ever-increasing threat to the fetus and preterm delivery may be desirable. If attempts to induce labor are unsuccessful, cesarean section is the alternative. Similarly, when preeclampsia–eclampsia or premature rupture of the membranes with amnionitis threatens maternal well-being and induction of labor is not successful, cesarean section is used. Safe and effective methods of inducing labor earlier for preterm delivery would reduce the need for cesarean section.

The need for preterm delivery has constituted about one half of all cesarean sections because of the incidence of repeated cesarean sections. Repeated cesarean sections are decreasing because more women with previous cesarean section are now being delivered vaginally. The need for early delivery accounts for only 2% of primary cesarean sections.

Dystocia

The historical indications for cesarean section include fetopelvic disproportion, abnormal fetal presentations, dysfunctional myometrial activity, and tumor previa. They represent the mechanical problems of the uterus, fetus, or birth canal that prevent the successful or safe progress of labor and vaginal delivery. Breech presentation, particularly in preterm infants, has assumed increased importance in this category. Cesarean section is being used occasionally for delivery of a second twin if malposition, malpresentation, or a tight cervix or lower uterine segment is encountered.

Dystocia is the stated indication for approximately 26% of all cesarean sections and 54% of all primary cesarean sections.

Maternal or Fetal Emergency

Certain maternal or fetal conditions require immediate delivery of the fetus when vaginal delivery is either impossible or inappropriate. Such circumstances include significant abruption of the placenta, hemorrhage from placenta previa, prolapse of the umbilical cord, active genital herpes and ruptured membranes, or impending maternal death. These conditions account for 19% of all cesarean sections and 38% of all primary cesarean sections.

COMPLICATIONS

Cesarean section is not an innocuous procedure that is without significant maternal or fetal risks. A variety of complications—including unexplained fever, endome-

tritis, wound infection, hemorrhage, aspiration, atelectasis, urinary tract infection, thrombophlebitis, and pulmonary embolism—occurs in 25% to 50% of patients. The frequency of maternal death related to cesarean section varies with the institution and with the condition necessitating the procedure. Accepted maternal death rates range from 1/1000 to 2/1000 operations. As many as 25% of these deaths are related to anesthetic complications.

Abdominal delivery is advantageous only to a fetus who is subject to definite risk from labor or vaginal delivery. Comparison of survival rates and neurologic follow-up of infants delivered by elective cesarean section and infants delivered vaginally shows an approximately twofold increase in death rates and neurologic abnormalities among those delivered by elective cesarean section. Given ideal circumstances for vaginal delivery and for cesarean section, vaginal delivery is more advantageous to both mother and infant than is cesarean section.

Late complications of cesarean section include intestinal obstruction from adhesions and dehiscence of the uterine incision in subsequent pregnancies. Both of these complications are more common when the classic incision rather than a lower uterine segment incision is used. An incision in the lower uterine segment may dehisce prior to labor, but more commonly the scar thins to a transparent "window" that holds during pregnancy but may rupture with uterine contractions. A classic incision ruptures in 1% to 3% of later pregnancies and, compared with a lower uterine segment incision, causes three times as many symptomatic ruptures and most of the maternal deaths that result from rupture.

A rare complication that is not generally appreciated is the lethal combination of uterine infection and classic incision. Invasion of the incision by the infecting organism quickly leads to dehiscence, and the uterine infection then drains freely into the peritoneal cavity. Only prompt surgical intervention by hysterectomy and vigorous antibiotic therapy can salvage the patient.

Although attitudes toward cesarean section have changed radically and indications have become more liberally interpreted, wide variation in the use of cesarean section within the practices of physicians sometimes reflects the status of their knowledge and judgment rather than the nature of their practices. Periodic review of all primary cesarean sections is a useful and desirable function in any hospital that provides maternity care, and can identify physicians whose level of information and competence results in too liberal or too restricted use of the procedure.

Management of Patient with Previous Cesarean Section

The progressive rise in the incidence of cesarean section in the United States must be viewed against the background of an increasing public interest in approximating the most natural circumstances for childbearing that are possible within the limits of safety. These two trends have resulted in more women who were previously delivered by cesarean section expressing interest in vaginal delivery than in the past. The debate about the safety of vaginal delivery following previous cesarean section is not new, and there continues to be a divergence of opinion. However, present data indicate that maternal and fetal risks are sufficiently low, and that labor and vaginal delivery should be considered for all women with previous cesarean sections if no contraindications exist. Contraindications include the presence of a previous classical cesarean section or similar scar of the corpus, evidence of fetopelvic disproportion, or delivery in a facility that is not equipped to handle the emergency of uterine rupture during labor or delivery.

It is the obligation of the physician who electively repeats the cesarean section to procure evidence of fetal maturity. Conversely, it is the obligation of the physician who delivers a fetus vaginally to explore the uterine cavity carefully after delivery to rule out uterine rupture and to be adequately prepared for treatment if rupture occurs.

The dictum that sterilization is absolutely indicated with the third cesarean section has been disproved. However, the integrity of the uterine scar must be evaluated at the time of repeat cesarean section. Both the physician and the patient should have a clear understanding of the possible indications for sterilization before cesarean section is repeated. In practice, however, considering current concepts of family size, repeated incisions in the uterus, and repetitive anesthetic risks, many patients are unwilling to undergo more than three cesarean sections.

TYPES OF CESAREAN SECTIONS

Types of cesarean sections are differentiated by the location and direction of the uterine incision. (The type of incision used to open the abdomen is not used in categorizing the cesarean section.) Uterine incisions are divided into two major types. The first includes incisions made in the upper segment of the uterine corpus (Fig. 39-1). The vertical incision in this location is usually referred to as the *classic incision.* The transverse incision, rarely used in the United States, was originally referred to as the *Kehr's incision.* The second type includes incisions made in the lower uterine segment (Fig. 39-2). These incisions are made in the lower portion of the uterus and require that the bladder be displaced downward in order to expose the appropriate area. The most frequently used is the *transverse (Kerr) incision.* A vertical incision may also be made in this area, but such an incision will involve the upper uterine segment unless the lower segment is quite elongated by labor; this is known as the *Sellheim incision.*

Occasionally, a variation is used, usually because of unanticipated difficulty during cesarean section. Two of these are worth mentioning (Fig. 39-3). They are undesirable and can be avoided by careful assessment and planning of the uterine incision.

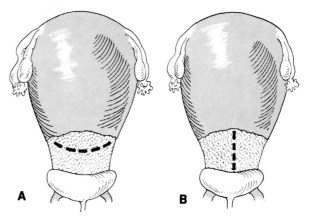

FIG. 39-2. Incisions in lower uterine segment. (*A*) Kerr's incision. (*B*) Sellheim incision.

FIG. 39-1. Incisions in upper segment of uterus. (*A*) Classic incision. (*B*) Kerr's incision.

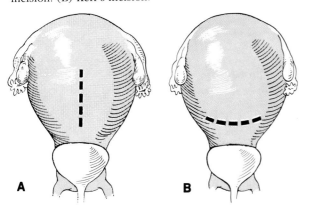

FIG. 39-3. Undesirable variations of uterine incisions. (*A*) J-shaped incision. (*B*) T-shaped incision.

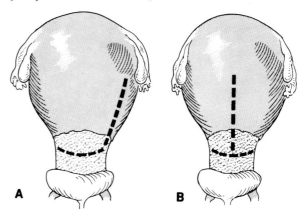

The *J-shaped incision* is made when one begins a transverse lower uterine segment incision and finds that the lower uterine segment is too narrow. The inadequacy of the incision is not realized until delivery is attempted, and then a vertical extension is made surgically from one end to avoid spontaneous extension into the broad ligament. In subsequent pregnancies this incision should be regarded as bearing the risks of a classic incision.

The *T-shaped incision* may be made for the same reasons or in the hasty management of the unexpected finding of placental implantation beneath the area of incision. The operator, having made an inadequate transverse incision, now performs a vertical incision beginning in the center. This incision does not heal well and is even more likely to rupture in subsequent pregnancies than is the classic incision.

Transperitoneal and extraperitoneal cesarean section are the techniques used to reach the uterine wall. The rationale for the extraperitoneal approach was formerly based on the belief that it would reduce the chance of death from peritonitis in a patient with an infected uterus. It has been discarded, however, because it has not proven superior to the less complicated transabdominal lower uterine segment operation. Vaginal cesarean section and vaginal hysterotomy are also of historical interest only.

Other procedures for "peritoneal exclusion," which were originally developed by Frank and Sellheim, are from time to time "rediscovered." The operator first enters the peritoneal cavity and then "excludes" the abdominal cavity by sewing the cephalad edge of parietal peritoneum to the visceral peritoneum and serosa of the uterus after the bladder has been displaced from the lower uterine segment but before the uterus is incised. These procedures are rarely used in contemporary obstetrics.

ANESTHESIA

The choice of anesthetic technique and agents is dictated by a number of factors (see Chap. 43). In summary, a patient with signs of fetal distress, hemorrhage, or shock; with previous injury or surgery to the spine; or with cutaneous infections of the lower back is obviously not a candidate for spinal or epidural anesthetic techniques. Similarly, a patient with active pulmonary disease, such as pneumonia or tuberculosis, is not a candidate for inhalation anesthesia. Under conditions of severe maternal disease, local infiltration may present less maternal risk than either inhalation or regional block.

In the majority of cases, however, there are no clearcut indications or contraindications, and the choice depends on technique and the skills of the anesthetist. Under such circumstances, the relative advantages and disadvantages of regional block and inhalation anesthesia are so similar that, if the anesthetist is clearly more skilled in one than the other, the more familiar technique should be chosen.

Maternal and fetal hemodynamics are markedly affected by maternal position. The dorsal recumbent position, usually used for cesarean section, is disadvantageous primarily because the inferior vena cava is compressed. This decreases venous return and maternal cardiac output, causing hypotension and reduced uterine perfusion referred to as the *inferior vena cava syndrome*. In this syndrome, the weight of the pregnant uterus may have a progressively greater compressive effect upon the aorta as the mean arterial pressure falls, thus reducing blood flow to the pelvis. Obviously, hypotension produced by regional anesthetic techniques compounds this problem. Techniques such as using attachments to the operating table that mechanically displace the uterus laterally, placing inflatable wedges under the patient, or tilting the table to use the effect of gravity to displace the uterus laterally have become common practice as part of preparation for cesarean section, although manual displacement of the uterus to the patient's left is still frequently performed. Rapid intravenous infusion of 1 liter or more of physiologic solution containing sodium immediately before the initiation of regional anesthesia has reduced the incidence of hypotension.

Considerable data support the presumption that the status of the fetus worsens as the time of exposure to anesthesia lengthens. Progressive fetal depression, which is indicated by low Apgar scores, as the induction-to-delivery time is prolonged makes it important to avoid unnecessary delay during the operative procedure. For example, the abdomen should be fully prepared, draped, and ready for the incision before general anesthesia is induced. On the other hand, reckless surgical techniques for rapid delivery of the fetus should be condemned. An induction-to-delivery time of 5 to 15 minutes is reasonable if maternal oxygenation, blood pressure, and displacement of the uterus are monitored and maintained with care.

Anesthetic agents that produce marked relaxation of the myometrium (*e.g.,* halothane) may result in excessive postpartum bleeding.

PROCEDURE

Cesarean section requires the same preoperative care needed for any major surgery and additional consideration for the status of the fetus. A patient who has been in labor for a long period may show signs of dehydration or acidosis, and these should be corrected. Since anemia is relatively common in pregnancy, determination of hemoglobin or hematocrit value before surgery is important. Blood should be available for immediate transfusion because of the ever-present risk of hemorrhage. Because the bladder will be in the operative field, it is necessary to catheterize the patient prior to the procedure with an indwelling catheter. The patient should be given an explanation of the details of the procedure, the risks involved, and the reason it is necessary. The appropriate permission forms should be on record for the procedure, the anesthetic, the administration of blood, and hysterectomy, if it proves necessary.

In a repeat cesarean section in which timing of the procedure is determined electively, evidence of fetal maturity is important. Death or damage from unrecognized low birth weight is always a hazard to the fetus in the elective repeat cesarean section. In the past, a patient was allowed to begin labor before the repeat cesarean section was done in order to reduce the hazard of preterm delivery to a minimum. Today procedures such as diagnostic ultrasound and determination of amniotic fluid lecithin/sphingomyelin (L/S) ratio are reliable indicators of fetal maturity and have reduced fetal death from preterm delivery in repeat cesarean sections. The prudent physician uses the best means available to demonstrate fetal maturity before performing an elective cesarean section.

Preparation

Preparation of the abdomen includes shaving the skin of the abdomen and mons pubis when necessary, scrubbing the area with an antiseptic soap; and preparing the skin with an antiseptic agent such as nonorganic iodide. The abdomen is draped so that the area between the umbilicus and the mons pubis is exposed.

The use of prophylactic antibiotics (see p. 223) is an issue on which opinion is divided. Patients with prolonged rupture of membranes, especially those with associated unsuccessful labor, have a high incidence of post–cesarean section infections. In this instance, cesarean section should be regarded in the same way as other operative procedures in which gross contamination of the operative wound occurs. Use of antibiotics in these patients is indicated and is not prophylactic in the true sense. Those patients undergoing repeat cesarean section without known complication are more clearly the issue. Present studies vary in their conclusions about the advantages and disadvantages of prophylactic antibiotics for patients undergoing cesarean section without antecedent labor. The problems of cost and risk versus benefit are important additional considerations because serious infections often are not prevented by this treatment.

Aspiration of the highly acidic contents of the stomach is a known risk in induction of anesthesia for delivery. The resulting pneumonitis has become known as Mendelson's syndrome. Various techniques are used to prevent aspiration, and an effort is routinely made to increase the pH of the gastric contents in case aspiration occurs. Although the desirability of this goal is widely supported, there are differing opinions about the best method to use. Cimetidine has been advocated by some but criticized by others. A mixture of magnesium and aluminum hydroxides has been used, but some evidence suggests that aspiration of these chemicals has adverse pulmonary effects. Similarly, a magnesium trisilicate mixture has been advocated as being effective and as less likely to have complications if aspirated.

Choice of Uterine and Abdominal Incisions

The transverse incision in the lower uterine segment is the preferred incision for cesarean section. There is no doubt that the classic incision is associated with more immediate and remote morbidity than an incision in the lower uterine segment. Although in subsequent pregnancies a lower segment incision may stretch and become a thin window, or even separate, it generally causes few clinical problems until term or until exposed to the forces of labor. There is no apparent difference in illness or subsequent risk between the transverse and vertical incisions in the lower uterine segment if the upper segment of the corpus is not incised. The classic incision, however, may rupture dramatically at any time from the midpoint of gestation to term and does not tolerate the forces of labor well. The risk to the mother and fetus from this incision is clearly greater. Other considerations regarding choice of incision are discussed in Chapter 63.

The usual abdominal incision is in the midline, although both paramedian and Pfannenstiel's incisions are commonly used in some institutions. Use of the Pfannenstiel incision increases the induction-to-delivery time both in the primary procedure and in subsequent cesarean sections. Furthermore, repetition of this incision in subsequent pregnancies results in a higher incidence of bladder injuries. Despite these concerns, the Pfannenstiel incision is being used more frequently than in the past primarily for the cosmetic benefit.

Technique

The abdomen is opened in layers in a relatively rapid fashion; any large vessels encountered are clamped, but no attempt is made to achieve meticulous hemostasis because it might delay delivery of the fetus. During this portion of the procedure, the anesthesiologist must pay careful attention to the patient's blood pressure so that inferior vena cava compression, previously discussed, does not cause a relative uteroplacental insufficiency and compromise the fetus. If this occurs, the anesthesiologist or an assistant must move the uterus to the patient's left to improve venous return. The abdominal cavity should be inspected briefly to note the direction and degree of rotation of the uterus. Folded, moistened laparotomy pads are placed on either side of the uterus to reduce peritoneal soilage from amniotic fluid, but are not essential. Retractors placed in the abdominal wound and drawn laterally expose the anterior surface of the uterus and the bladder covering the lower uterine segment. With smooth forceps, the operator identifies the

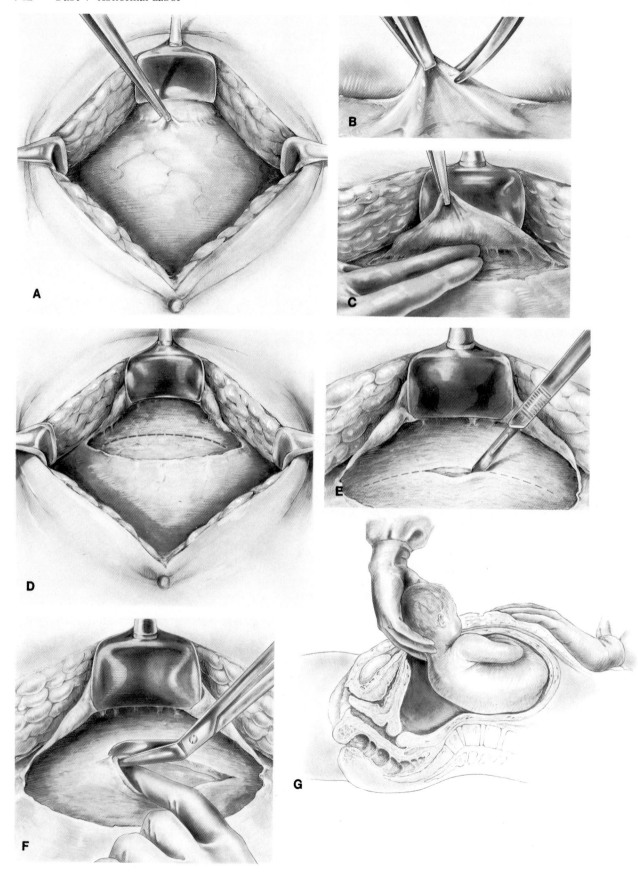

fold of peritoneum between the serosa of the uterus and the serosa of the bladder (Fig. 39-4A). This loose portion of peritoneum is elevated in the midline and incised, allowing entrance into the space between the bladder and the lower uterine segment (Fig. 39-4B). The closed scissors are then bluntly inserted in a lateral direction through this opening beneath the peritoneum, further separating the bladder from the overlying peritoneum. The area of peritoneum over the line of blunt dissection is incised laterally; underlying veins in the broad and cardinal ligaments must be carefully avoided. The operator should now be able to reflect the bladder from the lower uterine segment (Fig. 39-4C, D) using either digital pressure or a folded sponge on a sponge clamp. A small margin of peritoneum can be freed from the serosa of the uterus in the superior portion of the incision to aid in closure of the peritoneum following the delivery of the fetus. If such a peritoneal flap cannot be easily developed at the time, this step should be postponed to avoid unnecessary delay in delivery of the fetus.

The operator should now be looking directly at the fascia covering the lower uterine segment. In the midline, a few centimeters below the peritoneal incision, a small incision in the transverse direction can now be made with a scalpel (Fig. 39-4E). If care is taken in making this incision, the fetal membranes will bulge into the incision without being ruptured. The operator then inserts a finger between the fetal membranes and the overlying wall of the uterus. Using this finger as a guide, the operator inserts the lower blade of bandage scissors into the incision and extends the incision laterally in a gentle upward curve (Fig. 39-4F). The assistant should retract the abdominal wall firmly on the side toward which the operator is dissecting. Under direct vision, the operator should make this half of the incision as far laterally as possible without entering the broad ligament. When this half of the incision has been completed, attention is directed to the opposite side and the procedure repeated. Once this has been completed, a crescent-shaped or curvilinear incision has been formed in the lower uterine segment and the fetal membranes are bulging into the incision.

An alternative method of opening the uterus is to make a shallow curvilinear incision through the pubocervical fascia that extends the full length of the desired opening. The incision is extended through to the fetal membranes in a small area in the center of the wound. Inserting both index fingers into the opening, the operator draws them apart and, with lateral pressure,

bluntly opens the uterus. This method, which works best in a patient with a thin lower uterus segment following labor, has the advantage of reduced bleeding from the incision.

The operator now inserts one hand beneath the lower edge of the uterine wound and over the fetal membranes in order to feel the presenting fetal part. In the case of vertex presentation, the occiput is identified and gently pressed, resulting in increased flexion of the fetal head. The operator's fingers are gradually insinuated between the uterine wall and the fetal head, and, with pressure from this hand, the head can be brought toward the uterine incision (Fig. 39-4G). The membranes can be ruptured and stripped away from the fetal head. The head is then brought into the incision, and the assistant or operator can exert fundal pressure on the fetal buttocks to gently push the fetal head through the incision. Once the head has been delivered, the assistant should suction the mouth and the nares with a bulb suction device while the operator completes the delivery (Fig. 39-5). The fetal shoulders are delivered with gentle traction on the fetal head in a manner similar to that used for vaginal delivery. Specially designed forceps or a vectis may be used instead of the operator's hand in delivering the head through the uterine incision.

Following delivery of the shoulders, the fetus is extracted and should be held in a head-down position to improve drainage of the mouth and nares and to reduce the chance of aspiration. The mouth and nares may again be suctioned, the cord is clamped and divided, and the fetus may now be resuscitated by an assistant, preferably outside the operative field. Special preparations should be made when meconium is known to be present or is anticipated, such as with fetal distress or IUGR. A DeLee trap or other aspiration device should be on the field or already placed in the operator's mouth so that immediate suctioning of the nasopharynx and oropharynx can be done.

The operator now manually removes the placenta, separating it bluntly from the uterine wall with the fingers held extended in a rigid manner and the back of the hand facing toward the uterine wall to prevent injury to the wall by flexed fingertips. A dose of 10 IU oxytocin added to the patient's intravenous infusion helps uterine contractions to reduce the amount of bleeding. Some physicians inject the oxytocin directly into the uterine wall, but this is dangerous; if oxytocin enters the circulation as a bolus, hypotension or cardiac arrhythmias may result. For the same reason, deliberate intravenous injection of an undiluted bolus of oxytocin is hazardous.

FIG. 39-4.   Cesarean section. (A) Reflection of peritoneum from serosa of uterus to bladder is identified. (B) Peritoneal reflection between uterus and bladder is elevated and incised. (C) Bladder is displaced away from lower uterine segment. (D) Bladder is retracted and incision is planned to be 2 cm to 3 cm below peritoneal incision. (E) Small incision is made through uterine wall to fetal membranes. (F) Uterine incision is made in a curvilinear shape, using bandage scissors. (G) Fetal head is elevated through uterine incision by operator's hand.

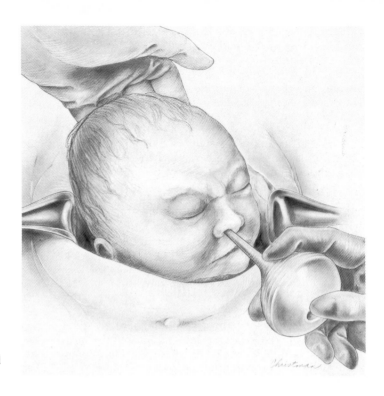

FIG. 39-5. Mouth and nares of infant are suctioned as soon as possible.

The uterine cavity should be inspected for any structural abnormality or retained placental tissue. The surface should then be wiped with a dry laparotomy pad to remove any adherent segments of membranes.

Digital dilatation of the endocervical canal from above is unnecessary and should not be done unless some unusual circumstance suggests nonpatency of the canal.

The cut edges of the uterine wall can now be grasped with Allis clamps, Allis–Adair clamps, T clamps, or other clamps that are noncrushing. These clamps hold the edges for traction and compress bleeding venous sinuses. Crushing clamps should be avoided because they result in devitalized tissue in the uterine incision. It is preferable not to elevate the uterus outside the abdominal cavity for the repair of the incision because this exposes the fallopian tubes to unnecessary trauma.

The first layer of closure (Fig. 39-6*A*) should be of absorbable suture material in a continuous, locked stitch anchored securely at the angle of the incision. The continuous locked suture should be held with firm tension by the assistant throughout the closure. Although the operator should avoid including large segments of the endometrium in the closure, inclusion of a narrow band gives satisfactory results and eliminates the risk of sinuses that may cause postoperative hemorrhage. The second layer of closure (Fig. 39-6*B*) inbricates the first; absorbable suture is used in interrupted stitches in figures-of-eight, in Lembert stitches, or in a continuous suture placed such that the first layer of closure is covered completely. The peritoneum is then reapproxi-

mated with a continuous layer of absorbable suture (Fig. 39-6*C*). If, during the closure, any areas of bleeding are still apparent in the incision line, separate interrupted absorbable sutures in figures-of-eight should be placed in the bleeding area to secure hemostasis.

When the uterus and visceral peritoneum have been reapproximated, the packs are removed from the abdominal cavity and any residual blood or amniotic fluid removed by suction. If meconium soilage or exposure to infected amniotic fluid has occurred, the pelvic cavity should be lavaged with normal saline. Some physicians have advocated irrigation of the uterus or abdominal cavity with antibiotic solutions when infection is known or suspected. However, the efficacy of this procedure rather than the use of intravenous antibiotics is debatable. The ovaries and tubes, and the remainder of the abdominal cavity should be inspected. Prophylactic appendectomy is offered routinely to patients in some institutions, and the complication rate from this additional procedure is relatively small. The abdomen is then closed in layers. The use of mass ligature closure, such as the Smead–Jones technique, for vertical incisions has a lower disruption rate and should be considered especially for patients at high risk of disruption. Postoperative management of the patient should be similar to that of any patient who has undergone major surgery.

The operator should be aware that postpartum patient who has undergone major trauma, including cesarean section, is at high risk for the development of thrombophlebitis and thromboembolism. For that reason, meticulous care of the patient's legs in the operating

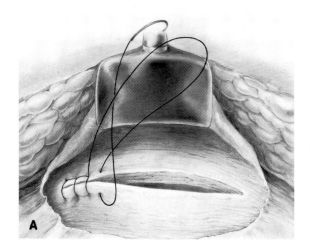

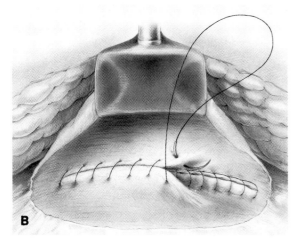

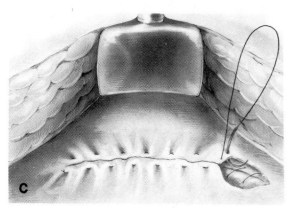

FIG. 39-6. Wound closure. (*A*) First layer of closure. (*B*) Second layer of closure. (*C*) Closure of visceral peritoneum.

postoperative day and can be expected to recover rapidly through the second to fifth postoperative days. Discharge from the hospital can be considered for the average patient any time on the fifth to seventh day, preferably the latter, depending upon the patient's condition and the availability of continued care in her home.

Closure of the Classic Incision

The thickness of the uterine wall may require a three-layer closure to and including the serosa. Continuous suture techniques may be used, but interrupted sutures frequently give a more exact closure. The first layer should include roughly half the thickness of the wall; stitches should be closely spaced and may be simple sutures or figures-of-eight. The second-layer sutures should be placed to avoid leaving a space between the layers and should come close to but not penetrate the serosa. The third layer should close the serosa in a manner that minimizes the raw surface to which the abdominal cavity will be exposed. The closure should be continuous, not locked, with absorbable material. Each bite with the needle should begin on the raw surface of the wound and exit through the serosa a few millimeters from the cut edge. By this technique, the cut edge is infolded and the serosal surfaces are brought over to cover. This is sometimes referred to as a "baseball stitch."

Variations

Under unusual circumstances, the operator may wish to use some variations of the cesarean section technique described.

Following prolonged obstructed labor, the operator occasionally encounters a fetal head deeply impacted in the midpelvis and a greatly elongated and thinned lower uterine segment. Under these circumstances, it may be necessary for an assistant to dislodge the fetal head from the midpelvis with a hand inserted into the vagina either immediately before or during the cesarean section. The manipulations of the fetal head necessary during the delivery, combined with the thinning of the lower uterine segment, may result in a lateral extension of a transverse incision and laceration of the uterine vessels. Under these circumstances, therefore, a vertical incision in the lower uterine segment should be considered. The incision is usually comparable in length to the transverse incision because of the elongated nature of the lower uterine segment, and extension of the vertical is less hazardous to the patient than extension of the transverse incision.

Occasionally (*e.g.*, in the presence of a posterior placenta previa or preterm delivery) the lower uterine segment is so narrow that a transverse incision is inadequate. Under these circumstances a vertical incision in the lower segment is necessary, even if it extends

room is important, and spontaneous movement of the legs and early ambulation following cesarean section are strongly recommended. The urinary catheter may be removed on the first postoperative day. The patient is usually able to tolerate a clear liquid diet by the second

into the upper segment of the uterus. A classic incision may even be necessary under such circumstances. For similar reasons, when the fetus is extremely large, the classic incision may be the best way to avoid extension into the uterine vessels.

Breech presentation after labor usually can be safely managed through a transverse incision in the lower uterine segment, but the operator should be careful to make the incision as wide as possible at first so that delivery of the head is not delayed by the need to extend an inadequate uterine incision.

A transverse lie with the fetal back down or shoulder presentation is usually an indication for a classic incision in the uterus. Attempts to deliver such a fetus through a transverse lower segment incision may result in extension of the uterine incision into the uterine vessels. A transverse lie with the fetal back up (umbrella position) does not need to be managed by a classic incision and can be considered to be similar to a breech presentation.

Occasionally the operator encounters the maternal surface of the placenta when opening the uterus. This can produce considerable anxiety or panic on the part of the operator because of the profuse hemorrhage. Several points are important. First, good suction must be available so that the operative field can be kept reasonably clear for visualization. Second, the operator must move quickly to extend the incision to the full opening believed necessary for delivery of the fetus. Finally, the placenta should not be cut or fractured because disruption of the vessels on the chorionic plate may result in serious fetal hemorrhage. Instead, the placenta should be separated from the uterine wall (as previously described for removal of the placenta) in order to allow access to the fetal membranes. The membranes should be punctured and the fetus delivered through this opening and through the uterine incision. It may be possible to deliver the fetus by the vertex in this situation, but the operator may find it necessary to grasp the feet and deliver the fetus by version and extraction instead. Fetal depression and breathing difficulty, caused by aspiration, should be anticipated. A rare occurrence is the inadvertent displacement of the vertex into the fundus during the initial attempt to deliver the fetus. In most instances this problem is effectively solved by grasping the feet and extracting the fetus as in a breech delivery.

Amnionitis has been considered an indication for the extraperitoneal technique of cesarean section. Experience has shown so little difference in the subsequent maternal illness between the transperitoneal lower uterine segment incision and the extraperitoneal lower uterine segment incision that the extraperitoneal approach has now become passé. Furthermore, in view of the increase in fetal depression with prolonged anesthesia of any type, it seems best not to prolong the induction-to-delivery time by using the extraperitoneal approach.

POSTMORTEM CESAREAN SECTION

The occurrence of circumstances that lead to cesarean birth following the death of the mother is fortunately so rare that most obstetricians never perform such an operation. The principles are relatively simple. Maternal death must be quickly established (on clinical grounds if necessary, but preferably by electrocardiographic or electroencephalographic findings if the patient is being monitored). Aseptic precautions are ignored, and the abdomen and uterus are opened rapidly with vertical and classic incisions, respectively. The fetus is quickly delivered, given immediate resuscitation, and moved to an intensive care nursery as soon as possible. The placenta should be removed manually and the uterus and abdomen closed. Experience suggests that efforts to auscultate fetal heartbeat before deciding upon cesarean section may give erroneous information. The time from apparent fetal death to actual fetal death or serious damage is unknown. The prognostic factors of importance are the length of gestation, the cardiovascular status of the mother prior to death (*e.g.,* prolonged marginal status with septic shock versus excellent status prior to accidental death), and the interval between maternal death and delivery. At best, the prognosis for the fetus is dubious; survival can probably be expected if delivery is accomplished within 10 minutes of apparent maternal death, but the severity of brain damage from cerebral hypoxia is difficult to predict. It has been suggested that, if modern life-support systems are used, the outlook for the fetus may be improved if the cesarean section can be done before the mother's actual death.

Other Obstetric Operations

INDUCTION OF LABOR

Induction of labor is the deliberate initiation of labor prior to its spontaneous onset. The procedure may be either elective or indicated.

Elective induction of labor is defined by the Food and Drug Administration (FDA) as "the initiation of labor for the convenience of an individual with a term pregnancy who is free of medical indications." The most obvious hazard of elective induction is the iatrogenic delivery of a preterm infant. Accordingly, all possible steps must be taken to be certain, regardless of menstrual dates (which are not always accurate), that the fetus is at term and that labor is imminent. Determination of the L/S ratio and prior ultrasound scans can be helpful; in some cases, they are essential. The imminence of labor and the likelihood of successful induction can usually be predicted by the findings on pelvic examination.

Indicated induction refers to the initiation of labor after 20 weeks' gestation when the benefits of delivery to the fetus or the mother exceed the benefits of continuing the pregnancy. Some of the circumstances for which induction of labor may be indicated are premature rupture of the membranes, abruptio placentae, preeclampsia–eclampsia, amnionitis, maternal isoimmunization, certain cases of fetal jeopardy (*e.g.,* fetal growth retardation, postterm pregnancy), certain cases of maternal disease (*e.g.,* diabetes mellitus, hypertensive vascular disease), intrauterine fetal death, and certain other maternal medical problems.

Contraindications to Induction of Labor

Induction of labor is contraindicated in certain situations, such as cephalopelvic disproportion, abnormal presentation, some cases of previous uterine incision (*e.g.,* cesarean section, myomectomy), advanced maternal age, grand multiparity (more than five), multiple pregnancy, certain cases of fetal jeopardy (*e.g.,* as indicated abnormal oxytocin challenge test), and any maternal condition in which labor is contraindicated.

Dangers of Induction of Labor

Regardless of whether oxytocin is used, induced labors tend to be shorter and more vigorous than spontaneous labor, possibly because most candidates for induction have physical signs that are extremely favorable for short labor.

For the fetus, the preeminent risk is prematurity. Other risks are those of either precipitate or prolonged labor; hypoxia due to hypercontractility of the uterus; and, as a consequence of rupture of the membranes, infection and cord prolapse. Hyperbilirubinemia of the newborn has been found to result from prolonged oxytocin infusion, and other fetal consequences have also been postulated. When careful attention is given to selection of patients and technique of induction, however, Niswander, Friedman, and their coworkers found that there is no significant increase in adverse infant outcome from induction of labor.

For the mother, the dangers include such problems as the consequences of tumultuous labor (*e.g.,* rupture of the uterus, premature separation of the placenta, cervical laceration); precipitate or prolonged labor; failure of induction, perhaps necessitating either cesarean section or instrumental delivery; intrauterine infection; postpartum hemorrhage; and amniotic fluid embolism.

Selection of Patients for Induction

The findings on vaginal examination largely determine whether the conditions for induction are favorable, equivocal, or unfavorable. Bishop has emphasized the important factors in making this decision by a scoring system (Table 39-1) in which a score of 0, 1, 2, or 3 is given for each of four designated qualities of the cervix and for station of the fetal head. A total score of 9 or above indicates that labor may be induced with only a small chance of failure. The most favorable case is one in which the head is engaged to station +1 or lower and the cervix is soft, more than 50% effaced, directly in the axis of the vagina, and dilated at least 3 cm. The least favorable case is one in which the head is not engaged and the cervix is firm, posterior, uneffaced, and dilated less than 2 cm. When conditions are favorable, labor should be expected to begin promptly after the induc-

---

Table 39-1
Method for Predicting Success of Induction of Labor

	Rating			
Physical Findings	*0*	*1*	*2*	*3*
Cervix				
Position	Posterior	Midposition	Anterior	
Consistency	Firm	Medium	Soft	
Effacement (%)	0–30	40–50	60–70	80>
Dilatation (cm)	0	1–2	3–4	5>
Fetal Head				
Station	−3	−2	−1	+1>

(From Bishop EH: Pelvic scoring for elective induction. Obstet Gynecol 24:266, 1964)

tion is started and to proceed apace. When they are unfavorable, the attempt at induction may be successful but, if labor does ensue, it can be expected to be protracted and difficult.

Methods

Continuous electronic monitoring of fetal heart rate and uterine contractions should be part of any method for the induction of labor. It should be started 15 minutes before the induction is begun in order to establish baseline characteristics.

Artificial Rupture of the Membranes

Most obstetricians consider amniotomy to be an essential part of any procedure for the induction of labor. If the conditions for induction are especially favorable, rupture of the membranes and drainage of a small amount of amniotic fluid suffice to start labor in about half the cases. According to one technique, preferred by many obstetricians, the patient is admitted to the hospital early in the morning without breakfast, and the membranes are ruptured artificially. Oxytocin is used only if labor has not started within one hour.

Oxytocin Induction

It is important for the physician to understand clearly the indications, contraindications, prerequisites, and techniques of oxytocin use before deciding to induce labor by means of oxytocin. The clinical use of oxytocin in dysfunctional labor is discussed in Chapter 37. The same admonitions apply to its use for induction.

Oxytocin can be very useful for the induction or stimulation of labor. Its misuse, however, creates major maternal and fetal hazards, and the FDA has now prohibited its use in elective induction of labor. Moreover, in medically indicated induction, the FDA stipulates that the drug be given intravenously and that the initial dose be limited to "no more than 1–2 mU/min. This dose may be gradually increased in increments of no more than 1–2 mU/min until the patient experiences a contraction pattern similar to normal labor," that is, contractions of good intensity lasting 40 to 50 seconds and occurring every two to three minutes. The uterus should relax to normal baseline tone between contractions, and the maximum rate of the infusion should not exceed 20 mU/minute. If satisfactory effects are not achieved with a flow rate of 20 mU/minute, higher doses are also unlikely to be effective and can be hazardous. The necessary precision in rate of flow may be obtained with a drip technique, but an infusion pump is preferable. Most of the problems encountered with oxytocin use result from high infusion rates over long periods. When labor is established, the infusion should be slowed and ultimately discontinued.

Some obstetricians prefer to begin induction with an oxytocin infusion, rupturing the membranes only when labor is established. This method avoids the commitment of ruptured membranes, but induction failures are likely to occur more frequently than when the membranes are ruptured as a first step; also, the labors are somewhat longer, and the total oxytocin dose is usually greater.

There is increasing doubt of the propriety of attempted induction when conditions are unfavorable and a long induction-to-delivery time can be anticipated. In one technique that is sometimes used in an effort to avoid cesarean section when delivery is indicated, an oxytocin infusion is run for six to eight hours with the objective of softening and partially dilating the cervix. This is followed by eight to ten hours of rest, and the infusion is then resumed in the hope that delivery can be accomplished vaginally at some time during the second infusion period. Recently, other techniques have been used to initiate cervical changes before oxytocin is considered and to shorten the length of induction. These include the insertion of laminaria the night before the day of induction or the application of prostaglandin gel for cervical softening. Current information indicates that these techniques will have significant effects upon the efficacy of oxytocin induction.

The physician must be aware that oxytocin has definite antidiuretic activity. Urinary output is demonstrably reduced at an infusion level of 20 mU/minute and may be markedly reduced at higher rates. Prolonged or excessive oxytocin administration, coupled with intravenous glucose infusion, has led to water intoxication and maternal death.

Induction by Prostaglandin Administration

At the present time, the uses of prostaglandins E_2 and $F_{2\alpha}$ being investigated continue to include induction of labor. More data must be obtained before the value of these prostaglandins can be clearly established. It is certain that they induce labor at term with an effectiveness that is not radically different from that of oxytocin. The prerequisites for their use are similar to those described for oxytocin. These substances are not entirely without maternal risk, however, as documented by occasional maternal deaths, which are reported to be associated with their use for abortions. The risk of overstimulation and the development of hypertonus also exist. The gastrointestinal side-effects of prostaglandins occur with induction of labor as with the induction of abortion. Direct effects on the fetus that are not attributable to the process of labor have not been established.

Since prostaglandins appear to have a direct effect on cervical ripening (see p. 623), they may be especially useful in cases of indicated induction of labor when the conditions are unfavorable. Several routes have been used to administer them for induction of labor: intravenous, oral, buccal, extra-amniotic, and vaginal or rectal. The protocol developed by Friedman and co-workers is the oral administration of prostaglandin E_2 in a dose of 0.5 or 1 mg hourly until "strong clinical labor" occurs.

The risks of this method of induction are not entirely known, and the FDA has not approved their use if the fetus is alive. However, they have been used extensively for this purpose outside the United States, and most reports are favorable. Some concern has been expressed regarding the fact that hypercontractility and abnormal fetal heart rate patterns sometimes occur, although residual effects in the offspring have not been demonstrated. More recently, the intravaginal use of prostaglandin E_2 in viscous gel (0.2 mg in 10 ml hydroxyethylcellulose gel) has been proposed as an effective agent for softening an unripe cervix in preparation for induction. The current literature indicates that preinduction use of prostaglandins for preparation results in a higher incidence of spontaneous labor, shorter induction time, and lower cesarean section rates.

Other Methods of Induction

Introducing a gloved finger inside the cervix and separating the membranes in a 360° sweep is a technique called *stripping the membranes*. It is an old method that is not very effective unless the patient is near the onset of spontaneous labor. The time interval from procedure to onset of labor is quite variable and unpredictable. The frequency with which this technique is used is difficult to assess because many physicians use it casually during an office examination and do not record it as an attempt at induction. It is not a significant method of induction and, although believed to produce no complications, may be followed by premature rupture of membranes or a dysfunctional latent phase.

Electrical induction of labor remains in the experimental stage. The method is possible, but its practicality as a routine procedure has not been demonstrated in the United States.

Acupuncture is reported to be an effective method of inducing labor, but no carefully performed studies that would yield objective evidence have been done.

If the fetus is dead and uterine enlargement is consistent with a gestation of 16 weeks or more, labor can be induced by the introduction of various substances, such as hypertonic saline, urea, or prostaglandins, into the amniotic sac. Specific techniques are discussed in Chapter 14. (See also Missed Labor, Chap. 29.)

SURGICAL SEXUAL STERILIZATION

Although failure rates of surgical sterilization appear higher when the operations are performed at the time of cesarean section or following vaginal delivery, they should not be delayed for that reason. Tubal ligation adds little time or morbidity to cesarean section and is a much less complicated procedure than hysterectomy. The Pomeroy technique is the most simple sterilization technique, and gives satisfactory results, although the Irving procedure is associated with fewer failures.

Tubal ligation following vaginal delivery can be easily performed by a small transverse infra- or intraumbilical incision. The procedure takes only minutes to perform, has few complications, and does not significantly prolong postpartum recovery.

VERSION AND EXTRACTION

Once a subject for considerable debate and advocated for a variety of obstetric problems, the version and extraction procedure has now been replaced by cesarean section. The major obstetric problem for which version and extraction is sometimes appropriate is for delivery of a second twin, but even in this circumstance, it is permissible only if the conditions are extremely favorable, that is, if the second infant is no larger than the first twin, there is ample pelvic area, and if an anesthetist who is capable of administering an anesthetic that will provide full uterine relaxation is present. Internal podalic version is a formidable obstetric operation, and even in the most favorable circumstances, many modern obstetricians prefer to employ cesarean section for delivery of a second twin in preference to version and extraction, or, indeed, if the head of the second twin does not engage in the pelvis promptly after delivery of the first.

If version and extraction is elected for delivery of the second twin, the following principles should be observed:

1. The procedure should not be done if the membranes have been ruptured for some time and the uterus is firmly contracted around the fetus.
2. The membranes should not be ruptured until a fetal foot or both feet are clearly in the operator's control.
3. Deep anesthesia must be induced, preferably with an agent that has a marked relaxing influence upon the myometrium (*e.g.,* halothane).
4. The fetal head must be displaced to a level above the iliac fossa.
5. Traction should be gentle but sufficient to result in continuous progress in turning and extracting the infant (Fig. 39-7).
6. After delivery, the uterus and birth canal must be carefully inspected for injuries because these are a prime hazard to the mother after this procedure is done.
7. As is true for all other operative obstetric procedures, the patient should be prepared in advance for immediate blood transfusion.

The inexperienced operator will find it difficult to distinguish a foot from a hand during this maneuver.

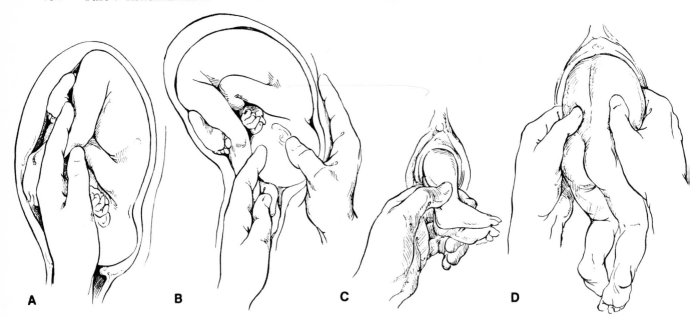

FIG. 39-7.   Version and extraction. (*A*) Feet are grasped. (*B*) Infant is turned; hand on abdomen pushes head toward uterine fundus. (*C*) Feet are extracted. (*D*) Torso is delivered. From this point on, procedure is same as for uncomplicated breech delivery.

This is a critical point, because an error will result in a prolapsed arm with a shoulder presentation. For practice, the physician should feel the hand and foot of a newborn infant and note that when the appendage is straightened into the axis of the leg or arm the heel becomes a definite prominence that has no analogous structure in the hand. A few benign practice sessions can save considerable anxiety at a critical moment.

The technique of breech delivery that completes this procedure is described in Chapter 36.

HYSTERECTOMY IMMEDIATELY FOLLOWING DELIVERY

Indications

Occasionally, hysterectomy must be performed immediately following cesarean section or vaginal delivery. A useful classification is based on emergency indications (uterine rupture, uncontrollable uterine hemorrhage, placenta accreta, uterine infection) and nonemergency indications (sexual sterilization when significant uterine pathology, such as carcinoma *in situ* or uterine leiomyomas, exists).

Emergency Indications

Uterine rupture, especially when it is the dehiscence of a previous cesarean section scar, usually (but not always) mandates immediate hysterectomy. The tear may be repaired if the patient strongly wishes to retain fertility, if her condition is not jeopardized by continued hemorrhage, and if competent repair is technically possible. The wound edge should be debrided before the edges are reapproximated. Suturing techniques are similar to those used for cesarean section repair.

Uncontrollable uterine hemorrhage may result from uterine rupture, uterine atony, placenta accreta, placental site sinusoids following placenta previa, or a coagulation defect. When surgery is indicated to control hemorrhage of uterine origin, the operator must assess the patient's desire to preserve childbearing capacity, as well as the present danger. Nonsurgical management is indicated in such circumstances as uterine atony or coagulation defect.

To stop bleeding, bimanual uterine massage, oxytocin administration, and replacement therapy, including administration of fresh blood, should be employed *before* surgical intervention is considered. Hemorrhage from sinusoids in the lower uterine segment that is associated with placenta previa may be controlled with mattress or figure-of-eight stitches using 2-0 to 0 absorbable sutures placed with an atraumatic needle. If uterine atony is the cause of bleeding and future childbearing is strongly desired, surgical interruption of the arterial flow to the uterus may be tried as the first measure of control. The operator may proceed to bilateral ligation of the hypogastric arteries or the uterine arteries. If this proves efficacious, the problem is solved and the patient's fertility maintained. If not, hysterectomy can be performed.

The lifesaving value of hysterectomy for the treatment of severe uterine infection should be noted. The patient who has experienced a second trimester septic abortion with septic shock, peritonitis, or uterine perforation may be saved by prompt hysterectomy. Clostridial infection, dehiscence of a classic incision with uterine infection, or a severe uterine infection that is unresponsive to antibiotics should also be treated by hysterectomy.

Nonemergency Indications

The risks and benefits of hysterectomy for nonemergency indications are much less certain than for emergency conditions. Hysterectomy performed at term is associated with hemorrhage, infection, thromboembolism, and injury to contiguous organs. Haynes and Martin have shown that the use of hysterectomy has declined, despite an increase in the incidence of cesarean section. This reflects the generally accepted conservative approach in which elective indications for hysterectomy are relatively few, primarily because the complication rate may exceed 50%.

When a less complicated operation is adequate or a safer time can be chosen, the patient's best interest is served by a conservative approach. Tubal ligation is a less dangerous operation at term than hysterectomy. When carcinoma *in situ* must be treated, removal of the entire cervix is much more certain and technically less complicated in the nonpregnant state. These decisions require good judgment, which is based on existing skills, facilities, and the needs of the individual patient.

Procedure

The technique of hysterectomy is described in Chapter 63. Some points are especially pertinent to its performance immediately following cesarean section or vaginal delivery, however.

In general, blood is conserved if the uterine wound for cesarean section is rapidly closed prior to beginning the hysterectomy. The ovaries should be preserved, if normal, and the operator should be aware that the relative shortening of the utero-ovarian ligament at term necessitates extra care in the placement of clamps and sutures in this area. Since the vascular system of the uterus is greatly distended, especially the venous system, considerable care should be taken in the proper placement of clamps and sutures so that a minimum of adjustments will need to be made.

The state of the uterus at term makes it difficult for the operator to determine by palpation the location of the portio of the cervix when performing a hysterectomy. Because of this difficulty, portions of the cervix are sometimes left behind even though the operator's invention is to remove it completely. Figure 39-8 illustrates a method of overcoming this difficulty. While the operator is deciding at what point the specimen is to be

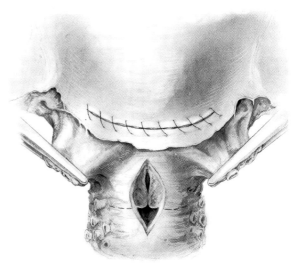

FIG. 39-8. Demonstration of uterine cervix.

transected for removal, a vertical incision can be made in the lower uterine segment and extended caudad until the limits of the cervix can be identified. This incision is essentially bloodless when performed at the proper time. Drainage of the pelvic cavity may be necessary, depending on the adequacy of hemostasis, and is accomplished preferably by suction drains rather than by passive drains such as the Penrose type.

In emergent situations that would be solved by supravaginal hysterectomy, this operation, which is much simpler and quicker, should be selected in preference to total hysterectomy unless there is a compelling reason to remove the cervix.

DÜHRSSEN'S INCISION OF THE CERVIX

Operations that were originally devised to avoid the hazards of cesarean section at a time when the procedure produced high mortality have gradually disappeared. Deliberate incision to open an undilating cervix for the purpose of delivery is almost never done in modern obstetric practice. However, the rare emergency may occur, and knowledge of the procedure can solve a critical problem.

The incisions to open a cervix that has not dilated completely are usually made when the cervix is well effaced and more than 5 cm dilated. The area to be incised is grasped with two empty sponge forceps, and the incisions are made at the 10, 2, and 6 o'clock positions with a pair of sterile bandage scissors (Fig. 39-9).

Incising an incompletely dilated cervix to free the head during the delivery of a preterm fetus in breech presentation may be lifesaving. In this circumstance, visualization and use of ring forceps may not be possible, and the operator must carefully perform the procedure with tactile guidance only.

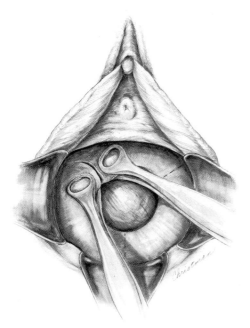

FIG. 39-9. Dührssen's incision at 10, 2, and 6 o'clock positions.

Following the procedure, careful examination should be made to rule out extension of any of the incisions. Repair should be performed under direct vision with absorbable suture material.

DESTRUCTIVE OPERATIONS

The need for destructive procedures on a dead fetus that cannot be otherwise delivered *per vaginam* is so rare that most present-day obstetricians are totally unfamiliar with such procedures. With proper medical care and proper hospital management of labor, the mechanical problem of vaginally delivering a dead fetus whose size or presentation has resulted in a long, obstructed labor is rarely encountered; the fetus who cannot be delivered vaginally is delivered by cesarean section. In developing countries, however, a significant segment of a hospital's clientele often consists of women who are admitted, many of them *in extremis,* with unresolved and very seriously obstructed labor. In such cases, a skillfully performed destructive operation may be far safer and simpler than cesarean section. Every obstetrician should be familiar with the procedures for managing such cases; those who work in areas where they are likely to be encountered should study the papers of Lawson, Lister, and others, who describe such cases in detail and assess the best means of dealing with them. The following discussion is a brief summary of the solutions of some of the clinical problems in which destructive procedures may be appropriate.

Vertex Presentation with Cephalopelvic Disproportion

When hydrocephalus in a dead fetus is the basis for cephalopelvic disproportion and the fetus presents by the vertex, needle aspiration of fetal cerebrospinal fluid can be readily performed before cervical dilatation is advanced. Transvaginal needle or trochar puncture of the fetal head through a partially dilated cervix decompresses the head enough to allow vaginal delivery.

Management of hydrocephalus in a living fetus is now less clear-cut than it has been previously because the availability of shunting techniques after birth enables these infants to survive. Therefore, the application to the living fetus of the techniques described above for the dead fetus is not always appropriate. Currently, hydrocephalus during gestation, which is usually identified by ultrasonography, has been dealt with by efforts to provide decompression by transuterine insertion of shunts into a dilated ventricle. Issues relevant to this treatment include the ability to correlate ultrasonographic measurements of the cortical mantle with prognosis and with other severe anomalies, fetal intracranial infections, and chromosomal abnormalities. Further experience will allow the development of guidelines. Hydrocephalus found during labor now presents treatment dilemmas depending on the degree of severity and associated prognosis. However, the greatly distended head found at term is probably still managed best by decompression and vaginal delivery.

When the fetal head is of normal size, cephalopelvic disproportion may result from an abnormally small pelvic inlet or an unusually large fetus. In either case, the vertex is firmly lodged in the inlet but not engaged. In the usual case, the patient has reached the second stage of labor, and the cervix is fully dilated and retracted. The physician should determine that the fetus is dead and should note any traumatic injury to the vagina from previous attempts at delivery, since a traumatic vesicovaginal fistula sometimes develops. The vagina should also be examined for uterine bleeding and the abdomen should be checked for signs of uterine rupture; evidence of uterine rupture requires immediate laparotomy.

Techniques that involve crushing the fetal skull by means of the cranioclast and cephalotribe have been abandoned by Lister and Lawson, who have had extensive experience with the problem. Instead, a Simpson perforator is pushed through the skull. The operator's other hand should steady the point of the instrument to prevent maternal injury if the instrument slides from the skull when the thrust is made. After the skull is perforated, the instrument's blades are separated widely, turned 90°, and again opened widely. The instrument is advanced to the center of the skull, where the septa are destroyed by rotating and opening the instrument. When the skull contents have been evacuated, the edges of the hole are grasped with four Ochsner clamps and the head delivered by traction.

This technique is apparently quite successful and avoids the use of instruments that are awkward and unfamiliar to the average physician. In spite of this improvement, it is still necessary and important to explore the uterus carefully for evidence of rupture or laceration. Late complications such as fistula entering bladder or rectum may still occur from necrosis.

Breech Presentation and Fetopelvic Disproportion

With a hydrocephalic fetus presenting in breech position, the cerebrospinal fluid can be drained by passing a needle into the fetal head through the maternal abdomen in a manner similar to that used for amniocentesis. As an alternative, the breech and shoulders can be delivered as in the usual breech delivery, and the hydrocephalic head fixed at the inlet by traction on the breech. If a suture is accessible, a needle can be inserted to drain the fluid. If not, a knife laminectomy is performed on the highest accessible vertebrae, and a uterine dressing forceps is pushed through the spinal canal into the head to allow drainage of the cerebrospinal fluid. As the head collapses, it passes into the pelvis and is easily delivered.

When the after-coming head of a normally formed dead fetus is impacted at the inlet, the head is fixed by traction on the trunk, the skull is perforated through any accessible area, the tentoria are destroyed, and the partially collapsed head usually delivers without incident. If it is needed, a blunt hook can be inserted through the opening in the head, with the point of the instrument directed toward the foramen magnum.

Transverse Lie

In the series of neglected cases involving transverse lie, described by Lister, decapitation by the use of the Blond Heidler saw was superior to the use of hooks or scissors. The Blond Heidler saw is similar to other wire saws, except that the outer two thirds is protected by rubber sheaths, leaving only the center third exposed for cutting. This minimizes the maternal risk during use.

Complications

The patient who faces a destructive procedure is likely to be in poor general condition and subject to both immediate and delayed risks. Dehydration, acidosis, infection, and exhaustion are commonly present. Administration of intravenous fluids, electrolytes, and antibiotics should be considered immediately. Antibiotic coverage should be broad and of maximum dose. Blood should be crossmatched and made available for immediate use.

The most serious immediate complication of both the obstetric process and the destructive operation is uterine rupture. In every patient who has delivered vaginally, a thorough manual exploration of the uterine cavity should be done to rule out uterine rupture. If bleeding occurs postpartum, the patient should be reexamined because rupture can be missed with a single examination. Since such women are usually in poor condition, if a rupture is found, it should be dealt with by the simplest and most expeditious means. Hysterectomy is reserved for the cases in which suture of the defect is not feasible or will not control bleeding.

Vesicovaginal or rectovaginal fistulas may be produced by immediate intrapartum injury or may develop later from avascular necrosis. The crushing of the pelvic organs between the presenting fetal part and the bony pelvis produces an injury that may result in a later slough. Constant drainage of the urinary bladder for ten days after delivery is recommended to minimize the stress of bladder distention and to allow healing. If a fistula forms, three months should be allowed before repair is attempted. Some control of urinary leakage can be obtained in the interim by using the Tassette cup with a drainage bag attached to the leg.

REFERENCES AND RECOMMENDED READING

Cesarean Section

Amirikia H, Zarewych B, Evans TN: Cesarean section: A 15-year review of changing incidence, indications, and risks. Am J Obstet Gynecol 140:81, 1981

Arthur RK: Postmortem cesarean section. Am J Obstet Gynecol 132:175, 1978

Browne ADH, Hynes T: Multiple repeat cesarean section. J Obstet Gynaecol Br Commonw 72:693, 1965

Caritis SN, Abouleish E et al: Fetal acid–base state following spinal or epidural anesthesia for cesarean section. Obstet Gynecol 56:610, 1980

Case BD: Cesarean section and its place in modern obstetric practice. J Obstet Gynaecol Br Commonw 78:203, 1971

Crawford JS: Correspondence. Anesthesia 36:641, 1981

Danforth DN: Cesarean section. State of the art review. JAMA 253:811, 1985

Datta S, Alper MH: Anesthesia for cesarean section. Anesthesia 53:142, 1980

Datta S, Ostheimer GW et al: Neonatal effect of prolonged anesthetic induction for cesarean section. Obstet Gynecol 58:331, 1981

DeLee JB: An illustrated history of low or cervical cesarean section. Am J Obstet Gynecol 10:503, 1925

DePalma RT, Leveno KJ, Cunningham FG et al: Identification and management of women at high risk for pelvic infection following cesarean section. Obstet Gynecol 55:185s, 1980

Downing JW, Houlton PC, Barclay A: Extradural analgesia for cesarean section: A comparison with general anesthesia. Brit J Anaesth 51:367, 1979

Farrell SJ, Andersen HF, Work BA, Jr.: Cesarean section: Indications and postoperative morbidity. Obstet Gynecol 56:696, 1980

Fox GS et al: Anesthesia for cesarean section: Further studies. Am J Obstet Gynecol 133:15, 1979

Frigoletto FD, Phillipe M et al: Avoiding iatrogenic prematurity with elective repeat cesarean section without the use of routine amniocentesis. Am J Obstet Gynecol 137:521, 1980

Gilstrap LC, III, Hauth JC, Toussant S: Cesarean section: Changing incidence and indications. Obstet Gynecol 63:205, 1984

Haesslein HC, Goodlin RC: Extraperitoneal cesarean section revisited. Obstet Gynecol 55:181, 1980

Hawrylyshyn PA, Bernstein P, Papsin FR: Risk factors associated with infection following cesarean section. Am J Obstet Gynecol 139:294, 1981

Haynes DM, Martin BJ, Jr.: Cesarean hysterectomy: A twenty-five year review. Am J Obstet Gynecol 134:393, 1979

Loosen PT, Prange AJ, Jr.: Extraperitoneal cesarean sections in the People's Republic of China. Letter to the Editor. N Engl J Med 303:226, 1980

Marshall CM: Cesarean section: Lower segment operation. Baltimore, Williams & Wilkins, 1939

McCaughey W, Howe JP et al: Cimetidine in elective cesarean section. Anesthesia 36:167, 1981

Meier PR, Porreco RP: Trial of labor following cesarean section: A two-year experience. Am J Obstet Gynecol 144:671, 1982

Pedowitz P, Schwartz RM: The true incidence of silent ruptures of cesarean section. Am J Obstet Gynecol 74:1071, 1957

Piver MS, Johnston RA: The safety of multiple cesarean sections. Obstet Gynecol 34:690, 1969

Redick LF: An inflatable wedge for prevention of aortocaval compression during pregnancy. Am J Obstet Gynecol 133:458, 1979

Schreiner RL, Stevens DC et al: Respiratory distress following repeat cesarean section. Am J Obstet Gynecol 143:689, 1982

Stevenson CS et al: Maternal death from puerperal sepsis following cesarean section. Obstet Gynecol 29:181, 1967

Swartz WH, Grolle K: The use of prophylactic antibiotics in cesarean section. J Reprod Med 26:595, 1981

Weber CE: Postmortem cesarean section: Review of the literature and case reports. Am J Obstet Gynecol 110:158, 1971

Induction of Labor

American College of Obstetricians and Gynecologists: Induction of labor. ACOG Tech Bull No. 49, May 1978

Bishop EH: Pelvic scoring for elective induction. Obstet Gynecol 24:266, 1964

Cates W, Jr., Hordaan HVF: Sudden collapse and death of women obtaining abortions induced with prostaglandin $F_{2\alpha}$. Am J Obstet Gynecol 133:398, 1979

Clinch J: Induction of labor: A six-year review. Br J Obstet Gynaecol 86:340, 1979

Department of Health, Education, and Welfare: Food and Drug Administration Bulletin: New restrictions on oxytocin use. Vol 8 No. 5, Oct–Nov, 1978

Flaksman RJ, Vollman JH, Benfield GD: Iatrogenic prematurity due to elective termination of the uncomplicated pregnancy: A major perinatal health problem. Am J Obstet Gynecol 132:885, 1978

Friedman EA, Sachtleben MR, Green W: Oral prostaglandin E₂

for induction of labor at term. Am J Obstet Gynecol 123:671, 1975

Friedman EA, Sachtleben MR, Wallace AK: Infant outcome following labor induction. Am J Obstet Gynecol 133:718, 1979

Hertz RH, Sokol RJ, Knoke JD: Clinical estimation of gestational age: Rules for avoiding preterm delivery. Am J Obstet Gynecol 131:395, 1978

Karim SMM, Amy JJ: Prostaglandins and human reproduction. In MacDonald RR (ed): Scientific Basis of Obstetrics and Gynaecology. Edinburgh, Churchill Livingstone, 1978

Niswander KR, Turoff BB, Romans J: Developmental status of children delivered through elective induction of labor. Obstet Gynecol 27:15, 1966

Patterson SP, White JH, Reaves EM: A maternal death associated with prostaglandin E₂. Obstet Gynecol 54:123, 1979

Prins RP, Bolton RN et al: Cervical ripening with intravaginal prostaglandin E₂ gel. Obstet Gynecol 61:459, 1983

Tylleskar J, Finnstrom O, Leijon I et al: Spontaneous labor and elective induction—a prospective randomized study. I. Effects on mother and fetus. Acta Obstet Gynecol Scand 58:513, 1979

Destructive Operations

Borno RP, Bon Tempo NC, Kirkendall HL, Jr. et al: Vaginal frank breech delivery of a hydrocephalic fetus after transabdominal encephalocentesis. Am J Obstet Gynecol 132:336, 1978

Danforth DN: A method of delivery for hydrocephalus associated with breech presentation. Am J Obstet Gynecol 53:541, 1947

Lawson JB: Obstructed labor. J Obstet Gynaecol Br Commonw 72:877, 1965

Lister UG: Obstructed labor: A series of 320 cases occurring in 4 years in a hospital in southern Nigeria. J Obstet Gynaecol Br Commonw 67:188, 1960

General and Miscellaneous

Baggish MS, Hooper S: Aspiration as a cause of maternal death. Obstet Gynecol 43:327, 1974

Banta HD, Thacker SB: Costs and benefits of electronic fetal monitoring. Washington, DC, National Center for Health Sciences Research, 1978

Bonica JJ: Principles and Practice of Obstetrical Analgesia and Anesthesia, Vol I, Fundamental Considerations. Philadelphia, FA Davis, 1967

Bonica JJ: Principles and Practice of Obstetrical Analgesia and Anesthesia, Vol II, Clinical Considerations. Philadelphia, FA Davis, 1969

Evard JR, Gold EM: Cesarean section for delivery of the second twin. Obstet Gynecol 57:581, 1981

Hill DJ, Beischer NA: Hysterectomy in obstetric practice. Aust NZ Obstet Gynaecol 20:151, 1980

Hobbins JC et al: The fetal monitoring debate. Obstet Gynecol 54:103, 1979

Krebs HB et al: Intrapartum fetal heart rate monitoring: I and II. Am J Obstet Gynecol 133:762, 773, 1979

The Puerperium

William E. Easterling, Jr.
William N. P. Herbert

40

The puerperium is that variable period of six to eight weeks that begins with the delivery of the placenta and ends with the resumption of ovulatory menstrual cycles. The puerperium is less precisely defined in the nursing mother; but, in general, it consists of at least four to six weeks of involutional changes that result in the so-called nonpregnant parous state.

Traditionally, both mother and infant are discharged from the hospital on the third postpartum day; but, with escalating hospital costs and the desire of many women to return home as soon as possible, they are frequently discharged sooner. Normal activities also are resumed earlier than in the past. Ambulation usually begins the day of delivery. Gradually increasing exercise is encouraged, with limitations best judged by the woman herself. Abstinence from intercourse is dictated by perineal tenderness, which generally ceases within three to four weeks. Women planning to begin or resume careers commonly do so six to eight weeks after delivery.

The complete postpartum examination is routinely scheduled six weeks after delivery, because many of the puerperal changes have been completed, or nearly completed, by that time. Communication before that time may be necessary and should be encouraged. The postpartum visit serves several purposes. It provides an opportunity to discuss contraception, lactation, menses, exercise, and other pertinent topics. A thorough physical examination ensures that physiological changes are occurring normally and detects any abnormalities.

PHYSIOLOGY OF THE PUERPERIUM AND CLINICAL MANAGEMENT

Uterus

Involution and Contractions

Following delivery of the placenta and membranes, the uterus lies at a level below the umbilicus, with the fundus resting on the sacral promontory. It is approximately 14 cm long, 12 cm wide, and 10 cm thick (about its size at 15 to 16 weeks' gestation), and weighs about 1000 g. Although the uterus may take a somewhat discoid form as it relaxes, it resumes a globular shape as it intermittently contracts. In the ensuing days, the uterus undergoes a remarkable decrease in size (involution) so that it weighs only about 500 g at the end of the first week, when it once again lies entirely within the true pelvis. Because the increase in myometrium during pregnancy results largely from an increase in the size rather than the number of myometrial cells, involution is associated with a substantial decrease in the amount of cytoplasm and size of the individual cells. Uterine contractions, as measured by intrauterine pressure, increase dramatically in intensity immediately after delivery. Presumably this results from the greatly decreased intrauterine volume around which the myometrium is contracting. Hendricks and colleagues reported that high levels of uterine activity diminish smoothly and progressively and become stable after the first one to two hours postpartum. Thereafter, contractions become increasingly incoordinate with the passage of time, but coordination can be restored by administration of oxytocin or by the application of an apparent oxytocin-releasing stimulus (*e.g.,* suckling). This increased myometrial activity contributes to uterine hemostasis by compressing the intramural vessels, which allows thrombosis to occur. The intense uterine contractions persist throughout the early puerperium, causing *afterpains*. Analgesia may be required, particularly for the severe pain that is sometimes experienced by the multipara. For unknown reasons, afterpains are not usually experienced after the birth of the first child.

Placental Site

Immediately postpartum, the placental site is an elevated, irregular area consisting mainly of thrombosed

755

vascular sinusoids. According to Williams' classic description, the area undergoes an exfoliation because the placental site is undermined by an ingrowth of endometrial tissue. The shedding of this mass of organized thrombi and obliterated arteries prevents scar formation and preserves an intact, normal expanse of endometrial tissue. The superficial layer of decidua surrounding the placental site becomes necrotic during the first few days, and the postpartum vaginal discharge consists of this sloughed tissue with an admixture of serum and leukocytes. The cells of the endometrial glands in the remaining decidua rapidly grow across the denuded surface, and regeneration is completed by the end of the third week.

Cervix

The cervix up to the lower segment persists as an edematous yet thin, fragile tissue for several days. Immediately following delivery, the ectocervix appears ragged, with numerous small but clinically insignificant bleeding points. The tissue appears devitalized and is indeed an optimal site for the development of infection. The lateral margins are often lacerated, and changes in these areas may eventually lead to the typical fish-mouth appearance of the parous cervix. The cervical os, which admits two fingers for the first four to six days of the puerperium, thereafter constricts until it will admit only the smallest curet by the end of the second week. The striking changes that occur in the cervix during the days and weeks after delivery are among the most dramatic of all connective tissue remodeling processes and are equivalent in degree to the cervical changes of labor that allow effacement and dilatation to occur without significant injury. As described in Chapter 31, there is much new interest in these processes, which remain unexplained.

Lochia

The uterine discharge following delivery is termed *lochia*. It is at first bright red, changing in a few days to reddish brown, the *lochia rubra;* this consists mainly of blood, and decidual and trophoblastic debris. After six to eight days, the lochia becomes more serous, the *lochia serosa,* and consists of old blood, serum, leukocytes, and tissue debris. This is followed in several days by the *lochia alba,* a whitish yellow discharge containing serum, leukocytes, decidua, epithelial cells, mucus, and bacteria, which may continue for approximately two weeks after delivery. Lochia rubra that has not abated after two weeks suggests retained secundines or formation of a *placental polyp,* which is an organized fragment of retained placental tissue. This bleeding sometimes responds to ergonovine (0.2 mg orally every 6 hours while awake for 2 days), but curettage is often needed. Clots and frank red vaginal bleeding are not lochia and must be considered in the category of postpartum hemorrhage.

Vagina and Introitus

After delivery, the vagina is a spacious, smooth-walled cavity; it decreases to its nonpregnant size by the end of the sixth to eighth week. Rugae typically appear by the end of the fourth week, but they are never again as prominent as in the nulliparous woman. The vaginal introitus initially appears erythematous and edematous, particularly in the area of the episiotomy or laceration repairs. Careful episiotomy repair should ultimately result in an introitus that is barely distinguishable from that of the nulliparous woman. Care of the perineum consists mostly of good hygiene during the initial two weeks; soap-and-water cleansing, particularly after bowel movements, should be sufficient. Hot baths help to diminish perineal tenderness and promote healing of the episiotomy.

The uterus and lower genital tract require special observation, particularly during the initial hours of the puerperium. Hemorrhage from retained placenta or from uterine atony (suggested by a fundus that refuses to contract in response to gentle massage) and perineal or paravaginal hematomas may develop insidiously.

Urinary Tract

Trauma to the urethra and bladder associated with the passage of the infant through the pelvis leads to predictable changes. The bladder wall is edematous and hyperemic, and there may be small areas of hemorrhage in the muscularis that are not of clinical significance. Secondary to the trauma and enhanced by analgesia, particularly by conduction anesthesia, the bladder may be relatively insensitive to the intravesical pressures that ordinarily initiate the urge to urinate. As a result, urinary retention may develop. Frequent palpation of the bladder in the suprapubic region and insistence that the patient void within the first four to five hours after delivery should prevent overdistention. If the patient is unable to void, the bladder should be catheterized; if the problem persists or if more than 600 ml urine are removed by catheter, an indwelling catheter may be required for the first 24 hours. Following removal of the indwelling catheter, careful checks for residual urine should be made until the volume is less than 100 ml on two occasions.

The glomerular filtration rate remains elevated during the first week after delivery; the urinary output greatly exceeds the fluid intake, often reaching 3 liters/24 hours. This, along with insensible perspiration, accounts largely for the weight loss of about 12 lb during this period. Proteinuria and, less frequently, glycosuria may appear during the first week; but, if they are of the physiologic kind, they disappear within a few days. The pregnancy dilatation of the ureters and renal pelves subsides to normal within six weeks.

Abdominal Wall

The abdominal wall is quite lax during the first one to two weeks after delivery. This may be of great clinical importance in the interpretation of acute surgical disorders that sometimes occur at this time. For example, the abdominal rigidity and guarding, so important in the diagnosis of such diseases as acute appendicitis, do not occur during the early puerperium, and the diagnosis must be made without the assistance of this customary sign. In the average woman, the abdominal wall returns to a nearly nonparous state in about six to seven weeks. During this time, the skin regains its elasticity, although some striae may persist. With proper exercise, the muscles regain significant tonus. Infrequently, with or without an unusually distended uterus, such as in multiple pregnancy, the rectus abdominis muscles remain separated from the median line, a condition termed *diastasis recti abdominis*. Although this defect may be disturbing, surgical correction is seldom necessary, and the separation becomes less evident with the passage of time.

Gastrointestinal Tract

The typical decreased motility of the gastrointestinal tract in the puerperium persists for only a short time, although a return to normal motility may be delayed by excess analgesia or anesthesia. Women with otherwise normal gastrointestinal function may benefit from laxative assistance once or twice during the first few days. If a third- or fourth-degree laceration of the perineum occurs, feces softeners or mild laxatives are indicated.

Circulation

Ueland and Hansen have shown that the cardiac output, which continues to increase in the first and second stages of labor, peaks during the early puerperium. Although the mean values are somewhat lower, the same changes occur in patients delivered under conduction anesthesia. This particular study demonstrated peak increases of 60% to 80% above prelabor levels. This is a value that is somewhat higher than that reported by other researchers. After the first few minutes postpartum, cardiac output decreases to a value that is approximately 40% to 50% above prelabor levels, returning to nonpregnant levels in the ensuing two to three weeks. These changes are primarily caused by appreciable alterations in stroke volume. There is little alteration in blood pressure, and bradycardia occurs fairly consistently regardless of the type of anesthesia employed for delivery. The decrease in heart rate probably accounts in part for the decline in cardiac output. Evacuation of the uterus, with the associated descent of the diaphragm, restores the normal cardiac axis and leads to the normalization of other electrocardiographic features during the early puerperium.

Varicosities of the lower extremities and hemorrhoidal plexus, which are not uncommon during pregnancy, regress promptly after delivery. Varices of the vulva, which are less common, can be seen to empty immediately after delivery. At times, local treatment of hemorrhoids with heat and analgesic creams is necessary, but a decision on surgical correction of all varicosities should be delayed several months because regression is usually complete, or nearly so, by that time.

Puerperal alterations in blood volume depend on several variable factors, including blood loss at delivery, and mobilization and subsequent excretion of extravascular water. Blood loss leads to an immediate but limited decrease in total blood volume. Thereafter, the normal shifts in body water result in a slow decline that ultimately reaches about 10% at the end of the first three days. Subsequently, there is a more gradual decline to nonpregnant levels. During the first 72 hours, there is a disproportionately greater decrease in plasma volume than in cellular components, which results in a slight net increase in hematocrit over the immediate postpartum value.

Puerperal changes in the blood constituents may be clinically confusing unless the physician is aware of them. The leukocytosis of pregnancy is usually about 12,000/cu mm; during the first ten days or two weeks of the puerperium, counts of 20,000 or 25,000/cu mm are not unusual, owing largely to an increase in neutrophils with consequent shift to the left. This, plus a normal increase in the erythrocyte sedimentation rate to 50 or even 60 mm/hour, may confuse the interpretation of acute infections during this time. The red blood count and hematocrit are usually elevated, probably because of the increased red cell mass of pregnancy, which is constricted as the blood volume declines with fluid loss. The coagulation factors I, II, VIII, IX, and X decline within a few days to prepregnant levels. Fibrin split products are elevated during the first week or ten days probably because of their release from the placental site. The total proteins, normally low in pregnancy, return to normal levels during the puerperium, and serum electrolyte concentrations follow a similar course. The plasma lipids, elevated in pregnancy, also decline to normal levels.

Weight Change

Approximately half of the average 25-lb weight gain of pregnancy is lost at delivery. During the initial days of the puerperium, largely as a result of diuresis, an additional six- to eight-lb weight loss can be expected. Most women lose the remaining weight gained at pregnancy over the ensuing weeks and return to their prepregnant weight within several months. Parity alone has very little effect on weight.

General

Shaking chills are not unusual in the first hours after delivery and are usually of no concern. Their exact cause is unknown, but they are usually attributed to heat loss resulting from the delivery of the infant and placenta, and loss of amniotic fluid. A warm blanket can minimize the discomfort.

Fatigue is customary during the first few days after delivery; extra rest and longer periods of sleep are invariably needed. This is easy to arrange in a hospital setting, but special plans should be made if early discharge is contemplated.

Ambulation is encouraged soon after delivery if neither conduction nor general anesthesia was used, or promptly after the effects of anesthesia have subsided. Early ambulation is largely responsible for reducing the incidence of thrombophlebitis (the "milk leg" or "phlegmasia alba dolens" of another era) to almost zero, and it also improves bladder and bowel function.

Diet requirements for nursing mothers are slightly higher than those for nonpregnant women. Special emphasis should be placed on protein (an additional 20 g/day) and calories (an additional 500 cal/day). For those not nursing, the recommendations are the same as those for the nonpregnant woman, as outlined in Chapter 11.

ENDOCRINOLOGY OF THE PUERPERIUM

Lactation

During pregnancy, the breasts are exposed to high concentrations of estrogen and progesterone. The prolactin level also increases markedly but is secondary to estrogen stimulation of lactotroph hyperplasia and reaches the highest point just prior to delivery. Increased levels of insulin and human placental lactogen (hPL) stimulate further breast growth during gestation. It is generally believed that although all the hormonal elements (estrogen, progesterone, thyroid, insulin, and free cortisol) necessary for breast growth and milk production are present in elevated concentrations during pregnancy, the high levels of estrogen inhibit active alveolar secretion by blocking the binding of prolactin to breast tissue, thus inhibiting the milk-producing effect of prolactin on the target epithelium.

Following delivery, estrogen, progesterone, hPL, and insulin blood levels decrease rapidly, followed by diminishing concentrations of prolactin. Milk production and associated breast engorgement begin about three days after delivery with the fall in estrogen, and they are enhanced by suckling and the brisk increase in prolactin secretion that it produces.

Once lactation has been established, suckling is the single most important stimulus for the maintenance of milk production. The conventional concept is that tactile nerve endings in the areola transmit a stimulus to the nuclei of the hypothalamus, resulting in an increase in synthesis and transport of oxytocin to the posterior pituitary and then its release into the circulation; oxytocin then stimulates contraction of the myoepithelial cells surrounding the alveoli, causing milk to be moved into the larger reservoirs beneath the nipple. This may be accompanied by ejection of milk from the breast and is commonly called the *let-down reflex.* Although the concept is well established, the recent studies of Lucas and co-workers have cast some doubt on the belief that oxytocin release is necessarily essential for satisfactory milk flow during breast-feeding. It does seem clear that prolactin is important in the maintenance of lactation. Afferent stimuli from the nipple reach the hypothalamus and initiate a complex response that results in prolactin release. This response is probably mediated through the prolactin inhibiting factor (dopamine), but prolactin-releasing factors may also be concerned. These relationships are considered in more detail in Chapter 46. The net result is a temporary increase in prolactin secretion that stimulates the milk-producing epithelium of the alveoli. The amounts of prolactin released gradually decrease during the first weeks of nursing. After the third or fourth month prolactin returns to normal nonpregnant levels, and, although data suggest continued episodic increases in response to suckling, the factors that maintain milk production remain unclear.

Suppression of Lactation

A mother wishing to stop breast-feeding need only discontinue suckling. Because the release of oxytocin is interrupted, milk accumulates in the alveoli and major ducts, which leads to a cessation of milk formation that is probably secondary to the increase in intra-alveolar and intraductal pressure. The time-honored practice of breast-binding to terminate lactation probably acts by the same mechanism.

When a mother does not want to nurse, simple breast-binding and avoidance of manipulation of the breasts are usually effective measures. A variety of hormonal preparations (estrogens, progestins, testosterone, and others in various combinations) have been used to suppress lactation. Another agent recently approved for use in the United States is bromocriptine, which is a dopamine-receptor agonist that inhibits prolactin secretion. Although it is quite effective, unpleasant side-effects (hypotension, nausea, and headache), an administration schedule lasting 14 days, and occasional rebound lactation limit its usefulness.

Desirability of Breast-feeding

In recent years, the practice of breast-feeding has increased in the United States. Many comparisons have been made between breast-feeding and bottle-feeding with either cow's milk or commercial infant formula.

From a nutritional standpoint, a simple comparison of the specific components of the milk or milk product is not informative because it fails to point out differences in absorption rates and suitability of the various components for the infant. Breast milk contains less protein than cow's milk, but the amino acid composition is more tailored to the metabolism of neonates. Although breast milk and cow's milk have about the same content of iron, the percentage of absorption is greater with breast milk, probably because of different protein-binding properties. The immunologic advantage afforded by breast milk is not found, of course, in other milk products. Immunoglobulins (especially secretory IgA, but also IgG and IgM), lactoferrin, lysozyme, the bifidus factor, and cellular elements protect the neonate against a variety of infections. Breast-feeding may also be more hygienic.

Another significant consideration of breast-feeding is the psychologic aspect. Although close interaction is certainly possible without nursing, the intimacy of nursing can strengthen the bond between mother and infant. On the other hand, social pressure to breast-feed may cause the mother undue anxiety and guilt, making the experience unpleasant to the point of interfering with the normal process of lactation.

Other aspects of comparison between breast milk and other milk products involve economic and contraceptive considerations. Breast-feeding is significantly less expensive than bottle-feeding, and lactation interferes in varying degrees with ovulation, affording some protection against pregnancy. This contraceptive impact is more significant in regard to populations than to individual cases, however; mothers who choose to breast-feed should not rely on lactation to provide complete contraception.

In many ways, breast milk seems superior to other milk products. Therefore, breast-feeding should be encouraged. However, the woman who elects not to breast-feed or who, for some reason, is unable to nurse her child successfully should not be made to feel guilty or anxious.

As a general rule, it should be assumed that any drug ingested by a nursing mother may be present in her breast milk, but the concentrations are usually low compared with blood levels in the mother. Factors that are involved in the transfer of drugs from blood to breast milk include plasma concentration, molecular size, degree of acidity, protein binding, and lipid solubility of the specific agent. Metabolism of a drug by the neonate depends also on the neonate's age and development at the time the drug is administered. Current literature should be reviewed regarding any given drug; however, medications that are believed to be contraindicated for the nursing mother include chloramphenicol, streptomycin, metronidazole, sulfa, antithyroid and some anticancer agents, some diuretics, and, of course, radioactive agents. Data on the use of oral contraceptives during lactation are inconclusive. Both estrogens and

progestins are secreted into breast milk, but in very small amounts, and reports of adverse clinical effects are rare. A shortened duration of lactation, decreased infant weight gain, and slight alterations in milk composition have been reported. Potential long-term effects on reproductive development at puberty and beyond are unclear. If steroid contraceptives are chosen for the nursing woman, low-dose preparations are advised, and lactation should be well established before they are initiated. Until then, barrier methods of contraception are recommended.

It was formerly believed that the incidence of breast cancer was lower among women who had nursed their babies, but it now seems clear that this is not the case.

Hypothalamic–Pituitary–Ovarian Function

The physiology of the hypothalamus, the pituitary, and the ovaries during the puerperium is not well understood. Much information is available concerning the length of postpartum amenorrhea in both nonlactating and lactating women. The observations, summarized by Vorherr, indicate that 40% of non-nursing mothers resume menstruation within 6 weeks after delivery, 65% within 12 weeks, and 90% within 24 weeks. About 50% of the first cycles are ovulatory. In nursing mothers, menstruation returns within 6 weeks in only 15% and within 12 weeks in only 45%. In about 80% of these women, the first ovulatory cycle is preceded by one or more anovulatory cycles.

It has long been held that increased prolactin levels inhibit the release of gonadotropins, thereby reducing ovarian steroid production and accounting for the physiologic puerperal amenorrhea. This inhibitory effect may be more pronounced on the release of luteinizing hormone (LH) than on that of follicle-stimulating hormone (FSH). Jaffe and others have shown that FSH and LH levels are very low in the early weeks postpartum and that the level of FSH increases gradually, followed by an increase in the LH level. Investigating this phenomenon and using synthetic luteinizing hormone-releasing hormone (LHRH), Le Maire and colleagues have demonstrated a temporary pituitary insensitivity to LHRH both in lactating and nonlactating women studied in the first three weeks postpartum. However, the nursing and non-nursing mothers responded in a similar manner to LHRH at six weeks after delivery. Keye and Jaffe have reported that administration of gonadotropin-releasing hormone to non-nursing puerperas resulted in a return of FSH response to early follicular phase levels by the third week and a return of LH response by the fourth week postpartum. It is interesting to note that this response was followed by a period of FSH and LH hyperresponsiveness throughout the remainder of the eight-week study period. This excess reaction to the releasing hormone remains unexplained.

Studying the pituitary–ovarian axis, Zarate and colleagues observed that exogenous gonadotropins (human menopausal gonadotropins) administered in the immediate puerperium had no effect on estrogen, pregnanediol, and pregnanetriol excretion in lactating women. More recently, Andreassen and Tyson reported a significant ovarian output of estradiol in response to LHRH in both nursing and non-nursing women after the 28th day postpartum; no response was noted in either group between postpartum days 4 and 21, suggesting a temporary refractive state in the ovaries. Thus, the genital hypoplasia and infertility characteristic of the lactating mother may be due to pituitary, ovarian, and perhaps hypothalamic suppression, but the exact nature of this changing endocrine milieu is unclear at this time.

ABNORMALITIES OF THE PUERPERIUM

As the new mother enters the puerperium and faces the previously unencountered threats to her health, all those responsible for her welfare must exercise careful observation and provide expert care. Although many abnormalities may occur during the puerperium, only a few are serious or life-threatening. Infection, hemorrhage, and hypertension remain the most common causes of postpartum mortality. It should be remembered, however, that illness unrelated to pregnancy may affect a woman in the puerperium.

Infection

Puerperal infection is defined as infection of the genital tract, sometimes secondarily extending to other organ systems. To assist clinicians and to establish conformity in reported studies, the Joint Committee on Maternal Welfare defined *febrile morbidity* as "a temperature of 100.4°F (38°C) or higher, the temperature to occur on any 2 of the first 10 days postpartum exclusive of the first 24 hours and to be taken by mouth by a standard technique at least four times daily." Extragenital infections such as cystitis, pyelonephritis, or pneumonitis must be excluded. The definition was designed to exclude, as nearly as possible, noninfectious causes of fever. When the definition was prepared, the first 24 hours were excluded because the febrile response to most infections introduced during labor occurs after the first day, whereas fever on the first day suggests an infection that was present before labor. However, this is not always the case; in a recent series, most patients with temperature elevations in the first 24 hours postpartum were found to have genital tract infections. The onset of fever after the tenth postpartum day usually signifies infection of a nonobstetric nature.

Because of the ready availability of antibiotics, puerperal and related infections are regarded with less respect than other infections by some health care per-

sonnel. This may be an ominous development; laxity in aseptic technique is often found to be the explanation for episodic increases in the incidence of maternal infections. This fact, along with the growing number of organisms that are resistant to antibiotics, warns against relaxing any of the well-established standards of asepsis. Particular attention must be given to asepsis in the presence of conditions that predispose the patient to infection, such as premature and prolonged rupture of the membranes, soft tissue trauma and the residual devitalized tissue, prolonged labor, and hemorrhage. The poorly nourished and anemic patient is also much more vulnerable to infection.

The physician's task in the selection of antimicrobial agents increases almost daily because of the ever-increasing number of organisms that are drug-resistant and because of the proliferation of new drugs. Available information changes quickly, but the obstetrician–gynecologist is obligated to maintain an up-to-date working knowledge of the agents themselves, their field of usefulness, their similarities and antagonisms, and their toxic effects. Current monographs can be helpful, and package inserts are a reliable source of prescribing information. (See also Chapter 13.) The final selection of an antimicrobial agent is based on clinical consideration and identification of the organism and its sensitivities. Until this identification is available, a Gram stain of the infected material may provide an important clue to the responsible organism and may greatly narrow the choice of antimicrobial agents.

Microorganisms

With improving techniques in microbial culture and identification, it is becoming clear that the majority of pelvic infections are polymicrobial and involve both aerobes and anaerobes, with anaerobes predominating. Isolation of the organism or organisms specifically responsible for a given infection is difficult because the vagina normally harbors many of the same types of bacteria. Culture specimens, even if properly collected, transported, and inoculated, are of limited usefulness because the same types of bacteria can be identified in patients both with and without infection. A Gram stain may be helpful if a predominant type of organism is identified. Clinical judgment and knowledge of the pathogens that are usually found in specific populations are the best guides to direct therapy.

Anaerobic streptococci (*Peptostreptococcus, Peptococcus*) are the most common pelvic isolates, but aerobic streptococci (α-hemolytic streptococci, β-hemolytic streptococci, and enterococci) are also frequently identified. In recent years, there has been a rising incidence of gram-negative bacterial infections. *Escherichia coli* is the most common offender, followed by *Klebsiella, Enterobacteriaceae,* and *Proteus* species.

Bacteroides fragilis and *Clostridium perfringens,* which are common inhabitants of the normal genital and intestinal tracts, can cause severe infections (including abscess formation) when they have access to devitalized necrotic tissue and blood clots. In particular, clostridial infections can rapidly produce gas gangrene, hemolysis, septic shock, and, in some cases, death. Fortunately, these infections are uncommon.

Uterine infections usually begin in the endometrial cavity. Here bacteria can flourish in the nutrient-rich endometrium, especially in the presence of traumatized and devitalized tissue. Retained placenta, if present, and blood clots further promote microbial growth. Infection can spread deeply within and through the uterine wall to involve the parametrial areas. If the bloodstream is invaded, pelvic thrombophlebitis and distant metastatic abscess can result in prolonged and debilitating illness. Septicemia may be followed by implantation of bacteria on heart valves or by abscess formation in the liver or lungs.

Clinical Manifestations

Postpartum infections of the genital tract are usually insidious in onset; in the early stage, they present the clinician with the uncomfortable and challenging problem of diagnosis by exclusion. Endometritis, the most common form of puerperal infection, may occur without any localizing signs or symptoms. The earliest indication of puerperal sepsis usually occurs two to five days postpartum; but, if the membranes were ruptured for an extended period before delivery, the infectious process may have begun earlier and become manifest sooner. The early indications of infection are malaise, anorexia, and fever. Differential diagnosis must always include urinary tract infections, particularly after operative delivery or catheterization. Operative delivery under general anesthesia must always arouse a high degree of suspicion of respiratory complications. The obstetrician must also watch for the early symptoms of mastitis, which is manifest by tender, indurated, and erythematous areas in the breast. Thrombophlebitis with deep vein tenderness and lower genital tract infection with associated perineal and perirectal pain complete the list of common puerperal infections. It should be emphasized that a febrile course during the puerperium may be a manifestation of any one of a multitude of systemic disorders that may be exacerbated during this stressful time.

Types of Infections

METRITIS. *Endometritis* is more properly termed deciduitis because the superficial layer of the endometrium is involved; this area is the most common site of puerperal infection. In the simplest form, inflammatory changes occur in the superficial layers, with leukocytic infiltration limited to this area and producing the "fruity" odor that is typical of normal lochia. In more severe forms, the infectious process may spread to the adjacent myometrium and, if untreated, may eventually progress to the parametria.

Infection involving the broad ligament adjacent to the uterus is termed *parametritis.* In its mildest form, it may be limited to this region; more often, the tubes, ovaries, and pelvic peritoneum are involved. Isolated parametritis may follow cesarean section, but it is usually associated with endometritis. When the infection is low grade or has been neglected, there may be considerable inflammation, induration, and even abscess formation. With appropriate treatment, severe induration and even small abscesses may resolve to the point of being undetectable on later pelvic examination, and they may not impair subsequent fertility; the outcome, however, is not always this favorable.

Evidence of any of these pelvic infections usually does not appear before 24 hours postpartum and is signaled by sustained temperature greater than 100.4°F (38°C). The patient may complain of mild malaise and anorexia, but report no localizing symptoms. Except in cases of fulminating sepsis, the early signs of infection may be no more than a temperature of 101°F to 102°F (38.3°C to 38.9°C) with a white blood cell count still within the normal range for the early puerperium (10,000 to 15,000/cu mm). Untreated, the minimum changes may persist for 24 to 48 hours, depending on the virulence of the offending organism and the host's resistance. On the other hand, the most severe infections may be associated with chills, extreme lethargy, lower abdominal pain, and fever that spikes to 103°F to 104°F (39.4°C to 40°C) in the early stages. In such instances, there is almost invariably some parametrial involvement, although localized infection with episodic bacteremia may present a similar picture. Generalized peritonitis is rarely associated with metritis. Diffuse direct and rebound tenderness and an associated paralytic ileus, sometimes with vomiting and abdominal distention, are the usual findings. Unless a parametrial abscess ruptures, making emergency surgical intervention mandatory, conservative treatment with antibiotics and supportive measures is recommended.

The diagnosis of metritis should be made only after a complete physical examination, including a careful search for deep vein tenderness and examination of the lungs, abdomen, urinary tract, and pelvis. In women who have had cesarean sections, abdominal tenderness caused by the incision must be distinguished from that caused by infection. Even in severe infections of the endometrium, no significant uterine tenderness may be elicited by abdominal or vaginal palpation. The diagnosis of parametritis is usually obvious. In addition to a clinical picture of severe infection, there is usually significant tenderness lateral to the uterus on both abdominal and pelvic examinations. Moving the uterus to one side or the other also produces pain. If there is associated pelvic peritonitis, signs of peritoneal irritation may be detected low in the abdomen. A sample of intrauterine material may be obtained for culture, but the wide variety of microorganisms that constitute the normal flora of the genital tract frequently obscures the precise cause of infection; therefore, a Gram stain of the material may be the best preliminary guide to the choice of antibiotic. Blood cultures are also indicated when the patient appears disturbingly ill or has an extremely high fever. The generally accepted practice is to obtain urine for examination of the sediment and for culture before instituting treatment, because a urinary tract infection without typical symptoms may be the cause of the fever or may coexist with a uterine infection.

The management of metritis is primarily the administration of antibiotics. The choice of agents is largely empirical because the final results of transcervical cultures may be misleading, as noted earlier. Fortunately, most microorganisms that cause pelvic infection are sensitive to many of the common antibiotics. The selection of antibiotic and route of administration are largely dictated by the severity of the infection. Penicillin, ampicillin, or a cephalosporin is frequently used, alone or in combination with an aminoglycoside (tobramycin, gentamicin), depending on the severity of the clinical manifestations.

Response to antibiotics is usually prompt; but, even so, treatment should be continued for ten days. Lack of response within 36 to 48 hours or worsening of the clinical manifestations requires reevaluation and additional or different antibiotics based on experience and culture results. In addition, pelvic thrombophlebitis should be considered.

Curettage is indicated when retention of placental fragments is suggested by vaginal bleeding, a widely patent cervical os, or passage of tissue resembling the placenta. If curettage is necessary in the acutely ill patient, antibiotics should be given intravenously, preferably two to four hours before surgery. In the most severe cases, when all medical management fails, removal of the infected uterus, tubes, and ovaries may be lifesaving. It is impossible to distinguish clearly between indications for continued conservative management and indications for the more radical surgical approach. Such a judgment depends on the careful assessment of each case.

PERINEAL INFECTIONS. Localized infection of a repaired episiotomy or perineal laceration can occur. These areas are particularly prone to infection in the presence of small, unnoticed hematomas. In most instances, the patient complains of unusual discomfort. Examination of the perineum reveals an edematous, erythematous lesion, usually with purulent drainage, and a tender area of induration in the involved site. Except when associated with hematoma, these infections usually do not produce fluctuant areas early in their course. Significant fluctuance within the first 24 to 48 hours strongly suggests hematoma.

Management of these localized infections, often caused by staphylococci, includes removal of the sutures to enhance drainage. When there is any degree of fluctuance, the wound should be carefully probed with either a large Kelly clamp or a uterine dressing forceps to open any areas of loculation; if a cavity of more than 2 to 3 cm is identified, adequate drainage can be ensured by packing the space loosely with a material such as iodoform-treated gauze to maintain a drainage tract. Sitz baths not only encourage drainage and healing, but also relieve perineal pain. Systemic reaction to the infection (evidenced by fever and leukocytosis) should be treated with antibiotics following culture and sensitivity studies. Such infections should be followed closely, and the perineum should be examined frequently. Persistence of fever and prostration, or enlargement of the infected area suggests necrotizing fasciitis, a rare but often fatal condition. Although antibiotics are important adjuncts, prompt surgical debridement is required when fasciitis is present.

MASTITIS. Infection of the breast is usually caused by coagulase-positive forms of *Staphylococcus aureus*. It is seldom seen during the period of inpatient care; indeed, early discharge has probably contributed to the marked decrease in the epidemic form of mastitis, which in the past posed severe health problems for mothers and newborns.

Unilateral, nonepidemic mastitis occurs in about 1% of nursing mothers. The route of infection is generally believed to be from the infant's nasopharynx through a fissure of the nipple or areola into the periglandular connective tissue of the breast. Soap and water cleansing of the breasts and hands and use of a breast shield until fissures heal will help prevent these infections. Mastitis can develop at any time during lactation, with three to four weeks postpartum being the most frequent time of occurrence.

The onset of mastitis may be sudden, with high fever and malaise. Breast tenderness is often described, but initially it may be overshadowed by the systemic signs. On examination of the involved breast, erythema, induration, and marked tenderness are usually apparent. In the early phase, the induration is relatively brawny; but if the process is left untreated, areas of loculation and abscess may develop.

After cleaning the nipple and surrounding areola thoroughly, a specimen of expressed milk should be obtained for culture. However, the result of the culture may be unreliable because the site of infection may be confined to the periglandular structures. Since the pathogen that most commonly causes mastitis is *S. aureus,* which comprises penicillinase-producing agents, a penicillinase-resistant form of penicillin, such as cloxacillin, is recommended, but erythromycin is an acceptable alternative. Antibiotics should be administered for ten days to prevent recurrence. Rest, fluids, and local heat are important adjuncts. Abscesses require incision and drainage. Nursing from the breast infected with mastitis does not need to be discontinued, although temporary use of a breast pump or periodic manual expression of milk may enable the mother to get much needed rest.

URINARY TRACT INFECTIONS. The relatively high incidence of urinary tract infections in the puerperium is usually attributed to trauma-induced hypotonicity of the bladder and frequent catheterization.

Cystitis, usually characterized by frequent and burning urination, is rarely accompanied by significant fever. Pyelonephritis, which is much more dramatic, is frequently accompanied by shaking chills, spiking fever of 104°F (40°C), and flank pain. The *Murphy punch*, which is a sharp blow over the costovertebral angle, reveals deep-seated tenderness and muscular rigidity. Almost invariably, either the right side only or both sides are involved; unilateral left-sided puerperal pyelonephritis is so unusual that a positive reaction to the Murphy punch on the left side only should prompt the physician to reconsider the diagnosis. The organism responsible is usually *E. coli*. As in other infections, culture and sensitivity studies are essential. Bactericidal agents (penicillins, cephalosporins, aminoglycosides) are usually effective.

Thrombophlebitis and Thromboembolic Disease

Thrombophlebitis and thromboembolic disease occur in fewer than 1% of all puerperas. Nevertheless, they occur significantly more often in the puerpera than in the nonpregnant woman. Incidence data suggest that these disorders may be less common than they were 25 years ago; however, the older data were based on clinical diagnosis only and may have been erroneous. The apparent decline in incidence may also be attributed partly to early ambulation, general improvement in patients' overall health, and fewer instances of traumatic operative delivery. The decrease in the occurrence of pulmonary emboli is attributed not only to these factors but also, more importantly, to current early recognition and treatment of deep vein thrombophlebitis. It is extremely important to recognize deep vein thrombophlebitis in its earliest phases. The obstetrician should maintain a continuing high level of suspicion and should made a daily check of the calves, thighs, and femoral triangles of every patient.

Deep vein disorders in the puerpera have been variously attributed to sluggish circulation in the large sinuses, trauma to pelvic veins secondary to pressure from the fetal head, and estrogen-induced hypercoagulability, perhaps mediated by an increased concentration of antithrombin III. Lastly, pelvic infection may initiate changes that lead to thrombophlebitis in the adjacent veins.

Superficial thrombophlebitis usually involves the saphenous system and is easily diagnosed by the physical finding of tenderness along the course of the vein, often with areas of palpable thrombosis. Skin temperature is usually increased in the involved regions of the lower extremities, but there may be little or no erythema or peripheral edema. Before concluding that the process is limited to the superficial system, the physician must carefully check the deep veins, including examination by Doppler ultrasonography. It must be noted, however, that the Doppler ultrasound technique is more useful above the knee than below it. Limited superficial disease can be managed by bedrest, analgesics, and the use of elastic stockings and a footboard.

Fever, deep vein tenderness, Homans' sign, and venous obstruction as evidenced by swelling of the extremity usually make the diagnosis of deep vein thrombophlebitis apparent. However, it must be strongly emphasized that deep vein disease is clinically unsuspected in a high percentage of cases. Venography is the most reliable diagnostic procedure, but the technique is not a practical approach in all institutions. The Doppler ultrasound technique, which is safer and simpler, can be highly accurate when it is done by those who are skilled in its use.

In deep vein disease, anticoagulation, preferably with intravenous heparin, should be initiated immediately. An initial dose of 5,000 to 7,000 units should be followed by doses of 5,000 to 10,000 units every 4 hours until the activated partial thromboplastin time has increased by a factor of 1.5 to 2 or until the whole-blood clotting time (measured by the method of Lee and White) has doubled or tripled. In the past several years there have been a number of reports supporting the use of continuous intravenous administration of heparin. Many of these studies indicate that this method is safer than intermittent injection, with or without laboratory control, and is no less effective in the prevention of thromboembolism. Constant infusion prevents undesirable fluctuations in anticoagulation. Either activated partial thromboplastin time or whole-blood clotting time should be used to adjust the initial dose ($24,000 \pm 6,000$ units/day). Most authorities favor conversion to sodium warfarin (Coumadin) 10 to 14 days after acute symptoms have subsided and recommend continuing this form of anticoagulation for a two- to six-month postsymptomatic period of treatment. Strict bed rest and physical therapy are important adjuncts in the early management of thrombophlebitis. Thrombolytic therapy with agents such as streptokinase can be used beginning two to four weeks postpartum.

The diagnosis of massive pulmonary embolism is sometimes clear-cut, with the sudden onset of pleuritic chest pain, cough with or without hemoptysis, fever, apprehension, and tachycardia; all of these are warning signs of impending catastrophe. Friction rub and signs of pleural effusion and atelectasis may be present. In the most severe cases, there may be associated hypotension, diaphoresis, electrocardiographic signs of right heart strain, and increasing central venous pressure. Any of these signs are indications for immediate diagnostic procedures. Unfortunately, most pulmonary emboli are not suspected; therefore, the physician must maintain a keen and continuing suspicion of this disorder. If there is a possibility of a pulmonary embolus, a lung scan should be obtained as soon as possible. If the scan is negative, pulmonary embolism is virtually excluded. If the results are equivocal, pulmonary angiography should be done. With a scan or angiogram diagnosis of embolus, immediate anticoagulation, preferably by constant intravenous infusion, results in recovery of the vast majority of these patients. However, recurrent embolization should prompt serious consideration of vena caval and ovarian vein ligation.

Suppurative thrombophlebitis should be managed as described previously, but every effort should be made to identify the responsible microorganism; the patient should be treated with vigorous intravenous administration of the appropriate antibiotics.

Thrombophlebitis may occur in the ovarian veins and other pelvic vessels. When it does, it is termed *right ovarian vein syndrome* or pelvic thrombophlebitis. Patients with this syndrome usually complain of abdominal pain, and it may be difficult to distinguish this pain from pain caused by metritis. Fever is common. A sausage-shaped tender mass may be palpated in the midabdomen, usually on the right side. Pelvic thrombophlebitis should be suspected when patients fail to respond to appropriate antibiotic administration in the first 72 hours after a diagnosis of pelvic infection. Anticoagulation with heparin leads to dramatic improvement in such patients.

Postpartum Hemorrhage

In many cases postpartum hemorrhage can be prevented by meticulous obstetric technique. Avoidance of intrapartum trauma and unnecessarily prolonged anesthesia, prompt repair of lacerations detected by thorough inspection of the cervix and the vagina, and maintenance of adequate tonus of the emptied uterus with prophylactic use of oxytocin are among the important factors.

Uterine Atony

The most common cause of serious postpartum hemorrhage is failure of the uterus to contract satisfactorily. Overextension secondary to hydramnios, large or multiple infants, high parity, prolonged labor, and many general anesthetic agents predispose a woman to the development of uterine atony. On pelvic examination the uterine corpus is soft and "boggy." Atony should be diagnosed as the primary cause of hemorrhage only after other causes of blood loss have been systematically eliminated, because acute blood loss may precipitate atony.

Initial management of uterine atony is fundal massage. It is important not to displace the uterus inferiorly, because displacement may have a tourniquet effect on the uterine veins and provoke further bleeding. Oxytocin can be administered intravenously by injecting 10 to 20 units (1 or 2 ampules) into at least several hundred milliliters of crystalloid and then adjusting the infusing rate to 200 to 250 ml/hour. Concurrently, 10 units of oxytocin can be given intramuscularly for prolonged action. Oxytocin should not be given by intravenous bolus because hypotension may result. Ergonovine or methylergonovine, given in a dose of 0.2 mg intramuscularly, usually causes prompt uterine contractions. The ergot drugs should not be routinely given to hypertensive patients or to any patient by rapid intravenous infusion because hypertension can follow such administration. Prostaglandins are currently being evaluated as agents for the management of uterine atony.

If the uterus does not contract after these measures, placental fragments remaining within the uterus may be responsible. Reexamination of the uterine cavity and curettage with a sharp, large (Hunter) curet should be the next step. In rare instances, hysterectomy or hypogastric artery ligation may be required. Uterine packing is no longer a preferred method of management in patients with uterine atony, although some find this technique helpful, especially until preparations can be made for surgical intervention.

Lacerations

Systematic inspection and palpation of the genital tract is the key to the diagnosis of lacerations. Digital examination of the uterus, and especially of the lower uterine segment, is recommended for all patients by some, but it is definitely indicated for patients with a history of cesarean delivery who subsequently deliver vaginally. However, the discovery of a window defect at the location of the old incision is not an indication for surgery unless there is bleeding from the site. The cervix and vagina should be carefully inspected following all operative deliveries, and this is a routine practice on many obstetric services. The cervix can be visualized easily if a Sims retractor is placed against the anterior vaginal wall and the fingers of one hand are placed against the posterior vaginal wall. Using gentle manipulation with a sponge stick, the entire cervix and vagina can be examined for lacerations. Repair of lacerations is usually accomplished with ease if adequate exposure is maintained. Long, wide retractors and one or two assistants may be needed. A running, interlocking suture of absorbable material is satisfactory.

Careful inspection of the perineum is also important. Extensions of episiotomies or lacerations can be easily and promptly repaired if the anatomy is clearly understood. Undue delay in repair of episiotomies, with or without extensions, can result in significant blood loss. Regardless of the site of the laceration, the repair should begin above the uppermost level of the tear to ensure hemostasis.

If hemorrhage occurs after a woman has left the delivery room, she should be returned there for examination and repair of any lacerations overlooked in the initial postdelivery examination.

Hematomas

Hematomas that occur postpartum are usually located in areas of laceration or episiotomy repair. The perineal pain and obvious mass noted on examination make the diagnosis easy in most instances. Occasionally, a hematoma that is unassociated with interruption of the mucosa develops, presumably secondary to traumatic rupture of a deep vessel. In this case, diagnosis may be more difficult and blood loss more serious. The latter is particularly true when the hematoma tends to dissect superiorly into the broad ligament.

Management of hematomas includes exploration with incision, drainage, and ligation of the bleeding vessel. If the hematoma is evacuated within the first few hours after delivery and good hemostasis is accomplished, the cavity may be closed with figure-of-eight sutures. Otherwise, a drain should be left in the defect. Management of large pelvic hematomas may require laparotomy and, in the rare case of a tear that extends into the broad ligament, hysterectomy.

Other Causes of Postpartum Hemorrhage

When some degree of placenta accreta occurs, all efforts at conservative management, including curettage, may be unsuccessful. Hysterectomy is required in many such cases. Uterine rupture, whether spontaneous or secondary to operative trauma, is a serious complication that necessitates laparotomy either for repairing the defect, if feasible, or for removing the uterus. Preoperative diagnosis of both placenta accreta and uterine rupture is difficult, but these conditions must be suspected when there is no obvious cause for continued uterine bleeding.

A rare, but very serious condition associated with hemorrhage during or immediately following delivery is inversion of the uterine corpus. The acute onset of severe abdominal pain, along with profuse hemorrhage and shock, is characteristic. The outcome is generally good if prompt treatment of shock and replacement of the uterine corpus are accomplished.

Hemorrhage resulting from a defect in coagulation, as seen with amniotic fluid embolism or with pre-eclampsia–eclampsia, can occur in the puerperium. These causes are discussed elsewhere in the text.

Delayed hemorrhage, defined as excessive blood loss occurring more than 24 hours after delivery, is usually caused by retained placental fragments. If a placental fragment is retained for a week or more, necrosis and some degree of organization occur, resulting in the so-called placental polyp. Treatment consists of curettage.

PUERPERAL PSYCHIATRIC DISORDERS

Various psychiatric problems may be encountered in the puerperium, but serious disorders are rare. During the first week, and usually on the third day postpartum, 70% to 80% of women encounter a transient depression, often accompanied by tearfulness. The condition is self-limited and usually vanishes within a few hours or a day. All that is needed is understanding and reassurance. The condition is not easily explained, and its cause probably varies to an extent from one woman to another. The major physiological stresses of the puerperium, including the huge mobilization of water and the endocrine upheaval, may be concerned.

In occasional cases, the postpartum depression may have more significant implications. When the patient shows no tearfulness, a lack of interest in the baby, and undue concern about the problems that will be encountered after she returns home, the obstetrician should consider the possibility of a problem that is more serious than the "baby blues." If it persists for more than 24 hours, the opinion of a psychiatrist may be needed.

In the past, anxiety was common in new mothers during the first weeks at home. This occurred principally among women who had little or no contact with their infant during the hospital stay, who had no firsthand knowledge of the infant's needs or routine care, who were totally dependent on other persons for the decisions and techniques required of them, and who considered themselves to be trapped in an untenable position they had not planned and for which they were wholly unprepared. In the modern era, most women carry an infant to term because they really want a child, and they desire to learn as much about infant care as possible. The educational programs available both during pregnancy and in the hospital are such that most mothers are confident and well prepared, and they do not encounter the profound sense of inadequacy and dependence that was so common 20 and 30 years ago. In addition, the several facets of "family-centered" obstetric care (see Chap. 33) appear to be especially important in achieving a satisfying and lasting family adjustment.

Between the simple, virtually physiologic, mild third day depression and the true psychoses there is a gamut of neuroses that can occur in the puerperium. Some are trivial and self-limited, and do not require special care; in others, the patient is greatly benefited by referral to a psychiatrist. A useful yardstick for the obstetrician in determining the need for psychiatric assistance in these cases is the answer to the question of whether the neurotic manifestations are of sufficient magnitude to interfere with the patient's effectiveness and her ability to cope with the ordinary day-to-day tasks and activities with which she is faced. True psychoses usually occur when the stage for psychosis was set prior to pregnancy; the stress of pregnancy and delivery are precipitating and nonspecific factors.

DISCHARGE INSTRUCTIONS

Some women regain their full strength and vigor more quickly after delivery than others. Periods of rest as needed during the day are desirable, and most women should be advised to avoid, if possible, a return to full employment or a full schedule of household activity for at least one month.

Sitz baths may be helpful if the episiotomy or repaired lacerations are painful. There is no contraindication to tub baths.

Sexual intercourse is permitted as soon as it is comfortable. The six-week period of abstinence formerly recommended is no longer believed to be necessary.

If a woman chooses to breast-feed, oral contraceptives should not be taken for two to three weeks, or until lactation is well established. If she elects to bottle-feed, oral contraceptives may be started several days following delivery. Intrauterine devices, diaphragms, and foams are not recommended until after the puerperium. If the mother is nursing and contraception is desired, condoms may be suitable until the postpartum office visit, when other methods may be considered.

Exercises are probably not needed to restore the tone of the abdominal muscles because the ordinary activity of the puerperium and the normal regression of the pregnancy changes are usually sufficient to accomplish this. However, the process may be hastened to an extent by leg-raising and other exercises that place the rectus abdominis muscles at stress.

POSTPARTUM EXAMINATION

The postpartum examination is usually scheduled for six weeks after delivery. By this time most of the systemic pregnancy changes have receded, the uterus is involuted, the cervix has resumed its nonpregnant contour and appearance, the episiotomy and any perineal lacerations have healed, and the breasts (unless the woman is nursing) have softened to permit easy examination. This is an extremely important visit, not only for evaluation of the woman's physical status, but also to permit the physician to determine whether there are problems requiring additional therapy. Medical or other disorders that complicated pregnancy or delivery and were not of sufficient severity to require earlier follow-up should be specifically evaluated at this time.

In the woman who has experienced an entirely normal pregnancy, labor, and puerperium, the evaluation should consist of a pelvic examination, with specific attention to involution of the uterus and vagina, the pelvic supports, and the cervix; cytologic evaluation of the cervix; investigation of the tone of the abdominal wall; ex-

amination of the breasts; estimation of hemoglobin or hematocrit; urinalysis; blood pressure determination; and weight determination.

Specific inquiry should be made about whether the woman wishes to begin another pregnancy at once, and if she does not, what measures she wishes to take to prevent it. The various methods of contraception should be discussed (see Chap. 14), and she and her physician should select the one that seems to be appropriate for her.

REFERENCES AND RECOMMENDED READING

Andreassen B, Tyson JE: Role of the hypothalamic–pituitary–ovarian axis in puerperal infertility. J Clin Endocrinol Metab 42:1114, 1976

Billewicz WZ, Thompson AM: Body weight in parous women. Br J Prev Soc Med 24:97, 1970

Bowes WA, Jr. (ed): The puerperium. Clin Obstet Gynecol 23:971, 1980

Brockington IF, Kumar R: Motherhood and Mental Illness. New York, Grune and Stratton, 1982

Filker RS, Monif GRG: Postpartum septicemia due to group G streptococci. Obstet Gynecol 53:28S, 1979

Garvey MJ, Tollefson GD: Postpartum depression. J Reprod Med 29:114–116, 1984

Gilstrap LC, III, Cunningham FG: The bacterial pathogenesis of infection following cesarean section. Obstet Gynecol 53:545–549, 1979

Golde S, Ledger WJ: Necrotizing fasciitis in postpartum patients. Obstet Gynecol 50:670–673, 1977

Hendricks CH, Eskes TKAB, Saameli K: Uterine contractability at delivery and in the puerperium. Am J Obstet Gynecol 83:890, 1972

Herbert WNP: Complications of the immediate puerperium. Clin Obstet Gynecol 25:219–232, 1982

Herbert WNP, Cefalo RC: Management of postpartum hemorrhage. Clin Obstet Gynecol 27:139–147, 1984

Jaffe RB, Lee PA: Serum gonadotrophins before, at the inception of, and following human pregnancy. J Clin Endocrinol Metab 29:1281, 1969

Jelliffee DB, Jelliffee EFP: Current concepts in nutrition. Breast is best: Modern meanings. N Engl J Med 297:912, 1977

Josey WE, Staggers SR: Heparin therapy in septic pelvic thrombophlebitis: A study of 46 cases. Am J Obstet Gynecol 120:338, 1974

Keye WR, Jaffe RB: Changing patterns of FSH and LH response to gonadtrophin-releasing hormone in the puerperium. J Clin Endocrinol Metab 42:1113, 1976

Kletzky OA, Marrs RP, Howard WF et al: Prolactin synthesis and release during pregnancy and puerperium. Am J Obstet Gynecol 136:545, 1980

Lawthian JT, Gillard LJ: Postpartum necrotizing fasciitis. Obstet Gynecol 56:661–663, 1980

Leake RD, Waters CB, Rubin RT, Buster JE, Fisher DA: Oxytocin and prolactin responses in long-term breast-feeding. Obstet Gynecol 62:565–568, 1983

Le Maire WJ, Shipiro AG, Riggal F et al: Temporary pituitary insensitivity to stimulation by synthetic LRF during the postpartum period. J Clin Endocrinol Metab 38:916, 1974

Lucas A, Drewett RB, Mitchell MD: Breast-feeding and plasma oxytocin concentrations. Br Med J 281:834, 1980

Monif GRG: Infectious Diseases in Obstetrics and Gynecology. Hagerstown, MD, Harper & Row, 1974

Munsick RA, Gillanders LA: A review of the syndrome of puerperal ovarian vein thrombophlebitis with some original observations on ovarian venous blood flow postpartum. Obstet Gynecol Surv 36:57–66, 1981

Pieri RJ: Pelvic hematomas associated with pregnancy. Obstet Gynecol 12:249–258, 1958

Reynolds SRM: Right ovarian vein syndrome. Obstet Gynecol 37:308, 1971

Salzman EW, Deykin D, Shapiro RM et al: Management of heparin therapy: Controlled prospective trial. N Engl J Med 292:1046, 1975

Stirrat GM: Prescribing problems in the second half of pregnancy and during lactation. Obstet Gynecol Surv 31:1, 1976

Ueland K, Hansen JM: Maternal and cardiovascular dynamics: III. Labor and delivery under local and caudal anesthesia. Am J Obstet Gynecol 103:8, 1969

Vorherr H: The Breast. New York, Academic Press, 1974

Vorherr H (ed): Human lactation. Semin Perinatol 3:191, 1979

Watson P, Besch N, Bowes WA: Management of acute and subacute puerperal inversion of the uterus. Obstet Gynecol 55:12–16, 1980

Welsh JK, May JT: Anti-infective properties of breast milk. J Pediatr 94:1, 1979

Williams JW: Regeneration of the uterine mucosa after delivery with special reference to the placental site. Am J Obstet Gynecol 22:664, 1931

Winikoff B, Baer EC: Translating "breast is best" from theory to practice. Am J Obstet Gynecol 138:105, 1980

Zarate A, Canales ES, Soria J et al: Ovarian refractoriness during lactation in women: Effect of gonadotropin stimulation. Am J Obstet Gynecol 112:1130, 1972

PART VI

The Fetus, Placenta, Membranes, and the Newborn

Clinical Evaluation of Fetal Status

Richard Depp

41

Epidemiologically, it is useful to classify perinatal morbidity and mortality by a number of schemes. The most obvious and frequently used schemes correlate morbidity and mortality with gestational age, which has the strongest relationship to morbidity and mortality, or with birth weight, which is also an indirect means of estimating gestational age. Most causes of complications and death, including respiratory distress syndrome (RDS), hyperbilirubinemia, and intraventricular hemorrhage, result from preterm delivery. Intrauterine growth retardation (IUGR), congenital anomalies, and chromosomal aberrations are also significant factors. A lesser contribution is made by maternal disease, such as preeclampsia and diabetes.

Although correlations of perinatal mortality with gestational age and maternal disease are useful for comparison, they do not allow evaluation of the impact of changing technology in obstetrics and neonatology. More importantly, simple correlations do not allow comparison of populations with different risk characteristics. To accomplish this end, it is useful to classify morbidity and mortality according to preventability; as technology improves, the incidence of "unpreventable" insults should decrease. Much of the morbidity and mortality associated with such events as spontaneous preterm labor, placental abruption, cord accidents, and maternal disease are now considered unpreventable, but new therapeutic protocols may improve the outcomes. Some of the perinatal deaths that are now unpreventable include those associated with congenital anomalies, severe chromosomal abnormalities, and fetal–neonatal developmental abnormalities. The remaining deaths are either potentially or absolutely preventable; many are iatrogenic. In the potentially preventable category, death results from failure either to implement adequate surveillance or to heed ominous warnings; except in retrospect, most are only potentially preventable, given the constraints of current practice. Preventable and iatrogenic complications and death are a continuum that ranges from a neonatal death secondary to RDS in an infant of a diabetic mother who had only marginal indications for delivery to frankly iatrogenic neonatal death following elective induction of labor or repeat cesarean section where fetal maturity was not confirmed. In 1975, up to 8% to 15% of RDS was considered iatrogenic.

Objective clinical evaluation of fetal health status is a primary goal of obstetric care. Considerable progress has occurred in this aspect of obstetric care in the past 15 years. Empiric management, largely employing routine pregnancy interruption at 36 to 37 weeks' gestation, has in many instances been replaced by case determination of the relative risk of intervention versus nonintervention. As a result, both fetal mortality and gestational age–dependent morbidity have been reduced. This change is most noticeable in the insulin-dependent diabetic now commonly delivered at 39 or more weeks' gestation.

The development of amniocentesis in the early 1960s to evalute the pregnancy at risk for isoimmune disease revolutionized obstetric practice and initiated interest in the development of other techniques to evaluate fetal status. Since that time, techniques to determine fetal gestational age and growth, amniotic fluid content, endocrine products of the fetoplacental unit, and fetal heart rate (FHR) antenatally or in labor and to obtain fetal scalp blood samples have become available to the practicing clinician. Most techniques, if properly applied antenatally, allow the physician to delay intervention until maturity is attained. Proper use of instantaneous FHR determinations and scalp blood sampling promotes more selective use of cesarean delivery for fetal distress.

As a result of the availability of these diagnostic tools and superb neonatal care, the measure of clinical success is no longer perinatal mortality, which has been reduced dramatically in many centers, but rather perinatal morbidity.

Perinatal death is primarily the result of the triad of preterm delivery, IUGR, and lethal congenital anomalies. Although there is reason to be hopeful that the incidence of preterm delivery as a result of an incorrect decision may be reduced, there is surprisingly little progress in reducing the incidence of either preterm birth (PTB) or IUGR. To a considerable degree, this results from failure to develop more sensitive means to identify pregnancies that will result in either PTB or IUGR; risk factors can be determined in approximately 50% of cases; the remainder are idiopathic. There is reason for even less optimism relative to lethal congenital anomalies. Two avenues to approach this issue include limiting exposure to drugs and toxic substances (ethanol) and more careful regulation of metabolism in insulin-dependent diabetics during the first trimester.

RISK SCORING

When the mother's condition is stable, therapeutic decisions regarding interruption of pregnancy should be based on the issue of benefit (reduced mortality) versus risk (morbidity and mortality of preterm delivery). Ideally, intervention should occur when the risk of intrauterine demise (detected by some objective technique) outweighs that of neonatal demise, usually from RDS. Since neonatal mortality is clearly linked to gestational age, proper interpretation of clinical data and assessment of risk are often limited by the obstetrician's ability to assign gestational age. The risk of fetal death or neonatal complications may be falsely magnified or reduced if the true gestational age is inappropriately reduced or increased by age assignment error. Diagnostic ultrasound provides the most reliable prediction of fetal gestational age; however, its accuracy decreases rapidly after 26 weeks' gestation. It is thus clear that patient risk identification and management must be undertaken prior to this time. Ideally, a systematic approach should be implemented in the first trimester, when uterine size correlates best with gestational age. A risk identification scheme must be relatively simple and, more importantly, must allow identification of the population of patients who are responsible for the vast majority of cases of perinatal complications and death. It is also essential that the population so identified be of a manageable size, and the percentage of normal outcomes in this group must not be so large that the use of expensive antenatal assessment tools is economically unjustifiable.

Several semiobjective prenatal scoring systems have been developed to identify the patient at risk. Such systems usually consider the impact of five general factors: (1) maternal disease that coexists with pregnancy but is not related to it; (2) maternal disease or complications related to pregnancy; (3) socioeconomic status as measured by income, husband's occupation or education, and race; (4) genetic history; and (5) maternal biologic factors such as height, weight, and age. Recently, objective risk indicators observed in labor have been added to the scoring systems. These systems have the theoretic advantage of assessing the risk of synergistic antenatal, intrapartum, and neonatal factors that predict perinatal morbidity and mortality; and identifying the patient who requires specialized care.

Unfortunately, the interaction of the risk factors is not simple; they may have either cumulative or opposing effects in terms of modifying perinatal outcome. The use of more sophisticated statistical techniques, including covariant or multiple regression techniques, may be necessary. The interaction of such risk factors as nonwhite, low socioeconomic class, minimal education, out-of-wedlock or teenage pregnancy, poor nutrition, extremes of maternal height or weight, stress, fatigue, need to work, and decreased use of contraception is complex and difficult to assess. Furthermore, implementation of a risk-scoring system with appropriate intervention often results in outcome more favorable in the "at-risk" group than observed in the traditional "low-risk" population. Consequently, validation of a more sensitive and specific risk-scoring system may elude us, particularly if the system is tested in traditional academic environments.

Nesbitt and Aubry developed a semiobjective scoring system that assigns a relative score of 0, 5, 10, 15, 20, or 30 to each of a number of risk factors. The total score is determined by subtracting the weighted risk of each identified factor from a perfect score of 100. A score of less than 70 indicates considerable risk. Risk factors with a value of 30 or more points are the following:

Abortions (three or more)
Fetal death (two or more)
Neonatal death (two or more)
Syphilis at term
Diabetes (all)
Hypertension: severe, chronic
Hypertension: nephritis
Heart disease, classes III and IV
Adrenal, pituitary, thyroid disorder
Rh sensitization
Severe obesity
Prior cesarean section
Submucous fibroid
Contracted pelvic plane

The actual outcome of pregnancies in the low-risk versus high-risk groups is depicted in Figure 41-1.

Hobel and co-workers have also devised an expanded scoring system that includes two risk scores. The first, the prenatal score, focuses on problems detected in the history or prenatal period. This score can

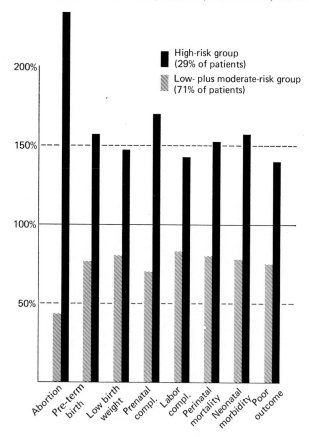

FIG. 41-1. Pregnancy outcome according to estimate of vulnerability based on index score; 100% is average incidence for total group in each category. (After Nesbitt REL, Aubry RH: High risk obstetrics. Am J Obstet Gynecol 103:972, 1969)

fetal factors, such as preterm labor, fetal-monitor abnormality, or abnormal presentation. Assessment of risk in both the prenatal and intrapartum periods yields four possible risk groups (low-low, low-high, high-low, and high-high). Perinatal mortality in one series of patients classified according to this sytem is shown in Table 41-1. The total score is useful to determine the level of care and supervision that is appropriate for the patient under consideration.

Although a risk scoring system identifies a population subset that requires special attention, a critical review of available data shows that predictive ability is limited until the onset of labor. Of total neonatal morbidity and perinatal mortality (Table 41-2), 50% and 39%, respectively, arise from the population who were assessed as low risk during pregnancy. If risk status is reassessed at the onset of labor, the percentage of fetal morbidity and mortality contributed by the low-risk population drops to 30% to 9%, respectively.

The importance of implementing a risk assessment system has been emphasized in a systematic review of 973 perinatal deaths. In that series, 25% of deaths were considered preventable. Avoidable factors were found in 20% of the unpreventable deaths, and multiple errors in management were found in 25% of the cases. Inaccurate assessment of gestational age, failure to detect poor fetal growth, and limited prenatal evaluation of fetal pulmonary maturity and uteroplacental function were common features in the series.

Since most preventable deaths are associated with PTB or IUGR, early identification of patients at risk for either is important. Early identification of risk facilitates prospective planning regarding collection of baseline maternal and fetal data likely to impinge on later decisions, implementation of patient and family education regarding possible outcomes, and recognition of warning signs and need for prophylactic measures such as bedrest and adequate nutrition.

The risk scoring for preterm labor and for intrauterine growth retardation is considered in Chapters 34 and 27, respectively.

be continually updated or recalculated at 32 weeks' gestation. The second, the intrapartum score, overlaps with the prenatal score but focuses largely on problems encountered in late pregnancy or labor, as well as on placental factors, such as placenta previa or abruption, and

---

Table 41-1
Risk Group Characteristics for 1417 Patients Studied Prospectively Between 1969 and 1972

Risk Groups				High-Risk Neonatal Mortality		Perinatal Mortality	
Prenatal	Intrapartal	N	%	N	% of Group	N	% of Group
I. Low	Low	642	45	39	6.1	1	0.2
II. High	Low	233	16	29	12.5	3	1.3
III. Low	High	320	23	72	23.2	17	5.3
IV. High	High	222	16	83	39.9	25	11.3
		1417	100	223	16% of 1417 births	46	3.2% of 1417 births

N, Number of cases.

(Hobel, CJ: In Spellacy WN (ed): Management of the High-Risk Pregnancy. Baltimore, University Park Press, 1976)

Table 41-2
Low Risk vs. High Risk: Relative Contribution (Retrospective) to Total Neonatal Morbidity and Perinatal Mortality*

Period	Risk	No.	Neonatal Morbidity (% Total)	Perinatal Mortality (% Total)
Prenatal	Low	962	111 (50)	18 (39)
	High	455	112 (50)	28 (61)
Intrapartum	Low	875	68 (30)	4 (9)
	High	542	155 (70)	42 (91)
Total		1417	223	46

* Derived from Table 41-1.

(Data derived from Hobel CJ: In Spellacy WN (ed): Management of High-Risk Pregnancy. Baltimore, University Park Press, 1976)

DETERMINATION OF GESTATIONAL AGE

Decisions to intervene or not to intervene in high-risk pregnancy usually hinge on evaluation of maternal and fetal health. When intervention is necessary, it is usually for fetal indications; severe preeclampsia is a notable exception in which deterioration of maternal status is a primary consideration. In all cases, evaluation of gestational age, lung maturity (also estimated indirectly by gestational age), and integrity of the fetoplacental unit are the key variables. Intervention prior to fetal lung maturity should occur only when there is documented evidence of uteroplacental insufficiency (UPI) or significant maternal health deterioration.

Accurate prediction of gestational age is the cornerstone of high-risk pregnancy management. The incidence of patients with suspect dates ranges from 22% to 40%. There may be significant differences in neonatal morbidity and mortality between fetuses estimated to be at 29 to 30 weeks' gestation and fetuses estimated to be 32 to 33 weeks' gestation. Such differences are particularly important in the management of preterm labor and rupture of the membranes before 32 to 34 weeks' gestation. Failure to assign gestational age accurately in patients considered for elective repeat cesarean section at term may result in iatrogenic preterm delivery. The incidence of postterm pregnancy may also be artificially increased by inaccurate menstrual dates; in such instances, the result is often unnecessary antenatal testing for the uncompromised fetus and prolonged and difficult oxytocin inductions. Unfortunately, in many postterm pregnancies, a cesarean section is required after an unsuccessful attempt to induce labor when the cervix is "unripe."

Clinical Estimation

Clinically, a history of regular menses with minimal variation in flow duration or quantity increases the chances that menstrual data will be reliable. Close cor-

relation of fundal height with gestational age prior to 28 weeks' gestation, maternal recognition of fetal movement (quickening) at 18 to 19 weeks' menstrual age, and detection of fetal heart sounds by fetoscope at 18 to 20 weeks' gestation are useful supporting data (Table 41-3). Lack of correlation suggests an incorrect age assignment. Total reliance on these clinical estimators is hazardous in the management of high-risk pregnancy, however. Even when a menstrual history is designated "reliable," one cannot be certain of gestational age. In addition, the detection of fetal heart sounds as a measure of gestational age has limited value unless the patient is seen weekly; otherwise the critical observation point may pass unobserved.

Ultrasound

The increasing use of diagnostic ultrasound has dramatically improved the accuracy of fetal gestational age determinations. The technical aspects of the various tests are discussed in Chapter 15. The following discussion

Table 41-3
Clinical Prediction of Maturity: Time Required for 90% Confidence That Pregnancy is at Least 38 Weeks' Gestation

Indicator	Weeks
Reliable last menstrual period	42
Unreliable last menstrual period	45
First fetal heart sounds	21
Quickening, nulliparas	25
Quickening, multiparas	25

(Data derived from Hertz T, Sokal R, Knoke J et al: Clinical estimation of gestational age: Rules for avoiding preterm delivery. Am J Obstet Gynecol 131:395, 1978)

is intended to provide a perspective of the clinical use of this modality as an aid to the evaluation of fetal status.

The ability of all single-measurement sonographic techniques to predict gestational age or assess growth is limited by both the inherent biologic variation of the part (femur length, crown–rump length) measured and the precision of the technique. Table 41-4 summarizes the predictive range and confidence limits of crown–rump and biparietal diameter measurements (BPD) at various gestational ages. In normal gestation, the rate of growth is probably a function of genetic predisposition. As shown in Figure 41-2, the variance about the mean of BPD measurements increases with advancing gestational age. The fact that fetuses growing in upper percentile limits have more rapid growth rates than those growing in the lower percentile ranks must be considered in the interpretation of all sonographic measurement data. Consequently, sonographic measurement to assign gestational age should be employed with great caution if the first scan is after 26 weeks' gestation because of the variance of plus or minus three weeks.

Since there appears to be significant advantage to early examination by ultrasound, the clinician must develop a selective plan of management that includes ultrasonic estimation of gestational age by fetal cephalometry or femoral length determination prior to 26 weeks' gestation. Pregnancies at risk for altered fetal growth (IUGR) would benefit from additional serial scanning at 31 to 33 weeks' gestation and at regular 10- to 21-day intervals thereafter. Patients at risk for preterm delivery may also benefit from serial scanning, particularly if there is discrepancy between sonographic and menstrual dates. Clinical conditions leading to IUGR or macrosomia that are detectable in early pregnancy include:

Altered fetal growth
    Prior small-for-gestational-age (SGA) newborn

First-trimester bleeding
First-trimester viral infection
Essential hypertension, nephritis
Mitral stenosis, cyanotic heart disease
Diabetes, especially class D or more
Diminished fundal height growth
Family history of hypertension or diabetes
Inaccurate assignment of gestational age
    Irregular menses
    Recent discontinuance of oral contraception
    Discrepancy in fundal height versus last menstrual period
    Late appearance of fetal movement
    Late appearance of fetal heart sounds
    Obesity
    Maternal age over 35 years
Preterm delivery
    Candidate for
        Repeat cesarean section
        Elective induction of labor
        "Indicated" induction
    Prior preterm labor/delivery
    At risk for altered fetal growth
    At risk for multiple gestation
        Family history of twins
        Ovulation induction
    Maternal diethylstilbestrol (DES) exposure
    Uterine anomaly

Unfortunately, this scheme does not include patients who first develop high-risk characteristics in the third trimester that require assessment of gestational age or fetal growth. Common examples include the following:

Preterm labor
Preterm premature rupture of membranes
Hydramnios/oligohydramnios
Poor maternal weight gain

Table 41-4

Prediction of Gestational Age by Ultrasonic Determination of Crown-Rump Length and Biparietal Diameter

Author	Time of Examination	Predictive Range in Determining EDL*	Confidence Limits (%)
Campbell	2nd trimester	±9 days	84
Varma	2nd trimester	±9 days	91
Sabbagha	20–26 weeks	±11 days	90
	27–28 weeks	±14 days	90
	≥29 weeks	±21 days	90
Sabbagha *et al*	GASA†	±1–3 days	95
Robinson and Flemming	Crown–rump, 7–14 weeks	±1–4 days	95

* Paired scans: first at 20–26 weeks, second at 31–33 weeks.

EDL, estimated date of labor; GASA; growth adjusted sonographic age.

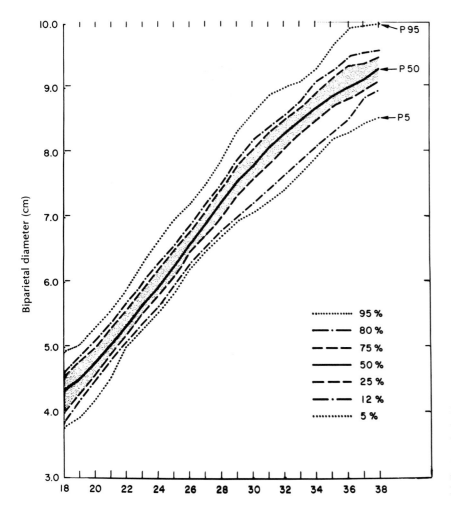

FIG. 41-2. Gestational age as X-coordinate of graph depicting normal growth of the biparietal diameter (*BPD*); maximum separation of large versus small BPDs between 30 and 33 weeks' gestation. (Sabbagha RE, Barton FB, Barton BA: Am J Obstet Gynecol 126:479, 1976)

Poor fundal height growth
Preeclampsia

Other useful indications for ultrasound (see also Chap. 15) include the following:

Confirm normal pregnancy
    Gestational sac (5–6 weeks)
    Fetal development (7th week)
    Fetal echoes (8th week)
Prior to amniocentesis
    Locate placenta, umbilical cord, fetal structures
    Confirm viability
Follow-up of abnormal α-fetoprotein
Assess amniotic fluid volume
Detect fetal anomalies (level-II scan)
    Cephalic: hydrocephalus, microcephaly
    Spina bifida, encephalocele, anencephaly
    Gastrointestinal tract obstruction

Genitourinary abnormalities
Heterozygous achrondoplasia
Assist fetal surgery

Growth-Adjusted Sonographic Age

In certain patients at extremely high risk for UPI, it is important that an attempt be made to determine the actual fetal growth curve and, where possible, to match it to a specific population growth percentile. This is not possible in most instances, unless gestational age has been reliably assigned on the basis of a basal body temperature (BBT) or close correlation of menstrual history and physical findings. Thus, in most cases, one is forced to assign gestational age by matching a single BPD, head circumference (HC), and femur length to a point on an established growth curve arbitrarily at the 50th percentile. Since biologic variation is most marked after 26 weeks' gestation, sonography probably should be used with extreme caution to assign gestational age if the first scan cannot be accomplished prior to 27 weeks' gestation. Although it is often acceptable to predict gestational age within a plus or minus 11-day interval, as may be accomplished by a single scan prior to 27 weeks' gestation, management of many high-risk problems, particularly when preterm delivery is a consideration, requires a more accurate estimation.

Sabbagha has demonstrated that approximately 90% of monkey and human fetuses maintain an apparently predetermined cephalic growth pattern throughout pregnancy. On the basis of this concept, it is possible to assign a growth-adjusted sonographic age (GASA) that predicts gestational age within a plus or minus five-day (95% confidence limit) range; it also allows division of cephalic growth curves into three basic ranks: BPDs greater than 75th percentile; BPDs between the 25th and 75th percentile; and BPDs less than 25th percentile. Variation in the external environment (UPI) may alter the projected course somewhat; however, since cephalic growth is spared (asymmetric retardation) until the late phase in most cases of UPI, this predictable pattern is disrupted in only a few instances prior to 31 to 33 weeks' gestation.

Early onset of symmetric growth retardation may be an exception to this statement. In such instances, cephalic growth may diminish prior to 31 weeks' gestation; as a consequence, fetal age may be overestimated by one week, even when GASA is used. The issue has minimal clinical relevance, however, since the early failure of cephalic and abdominal circumference growth will persist and suggest other causative factors such as "TORCH" complex viral infections, drug exposure, or even simply a normal but constitutionally small fetus. A similar error may develop in approximately 5% of cases in which there is significant early acceleration of cephalic growth, which will result in underestimation of gestational age. Dolichocephaly may also confuse the assignment of age unless cephalic circumference is also determined.

To estimate the GASA, the clinician must order two cephalic measurements, the first at 20 to 26 weeks' gestation and the second at 31 to 33 weeks' gestation. Should the slope of cephalic growth be in excess of the 75th percentile, the fetal BPD is assumed to have been consistently large for gestation. In such a case, the gestational age assigned at the time of the first scan is reassigned to a gestational age consistent with a BPD at the 75th percentile (*i.e.,* earlier gestation) at the time of the original scan; to accomplish this, gestational age is reduced seven days. In contrast, the fetus whose head growth slope is less than the 25th percentile is assumed to have had a BPD at the 25th percentile or lower at the time of the initial scan, and thus the gestational age is increased by seven days. In the event the BPD is at less than the 6th or greater than the 94th percentile, gestational age is advanced or reduced 11 days, respectively. The original assignment is maintained if an average BPD growth slope (25th–75th percentile) is observed.

In practice, we first make an assessment of the reliability of menstrual age. If menstrual age is deemed unreliable, an early scan is ordered (*i.e.,* at 18–24 weeks' gestation). There are benefits to assessment of gestational age at 18 to 20 weeks' gestation, particularly if there is a gross fetal anomaly detectable by a level-I (screening) sonographic examination. However, the practitioner should not be lulled into a false sense of security, since some anomalies may be missed by routine level-I sonographic examination at this time. Should the patient be at special risk for such anomalies, a later level-II scan may be indicated. If there is significant discrepancy (>7 days) between menstrual and early sonographic age or if the pregnancy is at high risk for UPI, GASA is planned and a second scan is scheduled at 31 to 33 weeks' gestation to meet the criteria for GASA.

In those cases complicated by preterm labor or preterm premature rupture of membranes at 27 to 34 weeks' gestation, in which no early ultrasound examination has been performed, menstrual age is generally accepted if menstrual data are felt to be reliable, particularly if the menstrual age falls within the plus or minus three-week gestational age range predicted by sonography. In such cases, it is common to observe a menstrual age that falls at the upper limit of the gestational age range predicted by sonography. This is consistent with the data of Tamura and co-workers who have reported that in such cases both BPD and abdominal circumference (AC) are small when compared with fetal measurements taken at similar points in gestation in cases in which delivery occurs at term. Thus, it may be reasonable to add seven to ten days to the gestational age predicted by the 50th percentile for BPD/HC under such circumstances. That the effect is not solely a function of dolichocephaly is supported by a similar reduction of the AC when corrected for gestational age.

DETECTION OF ABNORMALITIES IN FETAL GROWTH

IUGR may be a function of either intrinsic (chromosomal abnormalities, congenital anomalies, first-trimester TORCH-complex viral infections, or idiopathic) or extrinsic (UPI) factors. Although there are exceptions, growth retardation of the intrinsic type tends to be symmetric, that is, both cephalic and chest–abdominal measurements are 2 or more standard deviations below the mean for gestational age. In contrast, the extrinsic growth retardation tends to be asymmetrically small, that is, cephalic size is proportionately larger. At birth, asymmetric fetal growth retardation is characterized by subcutaneous and organ (especially liver) wasting in the presence of cephalic sparing. Although head growth by population standards may be normal in many cases, it is not known whether final cephalic growth is normal compared with the potential established at conception. We do know, however, that observed fetal growth deviates below that expected on the basis of the observed tendency of the normal population to maintain percentile rankings throughout gestation.

Cephalometry

Although cephalometry is clinically useful to detect slowing of cephalic (BPD and HC) growth, total reliance on serial cephalometry can be misleading. Measurements of the AC or total intrauterine volume may provide additional information. Although serial scanning is theoretically ideal, clinical application may be difficult for a number of reasons. The precision of the serial determinations may vary; clinical problems may not become apparent until after 26 weeks' gestation; cephalic shape may vary (dolichocephaly); slowing of cephalic growth may be a late manifestation of IUGR; and the pattern of fetal growth retardation may vary.

If risk factors for impaired fetal growth do not appear until the third trimester and an early BPD measurement is not available, the clinician must accept the ±14 to 21-day range of prediction for a single scan at 27 or more weeks' gestation. In addition, subsequent evaluation of cephalic growth is limited. Since gestational age is uncertain, growth evaluation is limited to a comparison with the mean population growth rate. Growth should average at least 2 mm per week up to 34 weeks' gestation and at least 1 mm per week measured over a two- to three-week interval, even in the lowest percentile ranking. Because of the slow growth rate and limitations in precision (1.0 mm–1.5 mm) of serial measurements, we require three measurements over a three-week interval (days 0, 7 to 10, and 20 to 21) to assign a "no-growth" designation.

Serial cephalometry, although helpful, has a false-abnormal diagnosis rate of at least 18% (Table 41-5); fetuses with retarded cephalic growth but normal birth weight are thought to be normal. In contrast, approximately 9% of fetuses have normal cephalic measurements in the presence of birth weights below the normal range for gestation. These false-normal cases represent "cephalic sparing"; such fetuses may be at greater risk for intrauterine compromise as a result of UPI.

Growth-Adjusted Sonographic Age, Percentiles

It may be possible to reduce the number of false-normal and false-abnormal results by using GASA in conjunction with AC measurements. GASA allows the physician to compare predicted with observed cephalic growth rather than simply comparing observed growth with a population mean growth rate. In addition, birth weight of less than 3000 g can be predicted in only 5% of fetuses in the greater than 75th percentile, but in 15% of those in the 25th to 75th percentiles and in 52% of those in the less than 25th percentile. Clearly, special evaluation efforts should be focused on fetuses with cephalic growth patterns at less than the 25th percentile. IUGR associated with significant UPI is usually asymmetric. There is subcutaneous and organ (especially liver) wasting in the presence of cephalic sparing. A single BPD may fall within normal gestation-dependent limits for the population but may deviate at 31 to 33 weeks' gestation from that expected if GASA was determined.

Abdominal Circumference

Under normal circumstances, the ratio of the cephalic/abdominal circumference measured at the level of the ductus venosus is greater than 1:1 up to the 35th to 36th week. If gestational age is established precisely, continued cephalic growth in the presence of poor abdominal growth suggests asymmetric retardation; in contrast, persistent cephalic and abdominal growth 2 or more standard deviations below the mean for gestation suggests symmetric retardation.

Table 41-5
Diagnosis of Small-for-Gestational Age Fetus by Serial Ultrasonic Cephalometry

	Cephalic Growth Patterns			
Weight	*Normal* No. (%)*	*Borderline†* No. (%)*	*Retarded‡* No. (%)*	*Total*
Appropriate for gestational age	220 (83)	18 (69)	21 (18)	259
Borderline or small for gestational age	22 (8)	4 (15)	16 (14)	42
Small for gestational age	24 (9)§	4 (15)	77 (68)	105
Total	266 (100)	26 (100)	114 (100)	406

* % is percent of column.

† Distribution of birth weights appears close to that of normal growth rate category.

‡ Difference between birth weights of normal versus retarded categories is highly significant ($P < 0.001$).

§ 9% false-normal secondary to cephalic sparing in a population with asymmetric retardation pattern.

(Modified from Campbell S, Dewhurst CJ: Diagnosis of the small for dates fetus by serial ultrasonic cephalometry. Lancet 2:1002, 1971)

Assessment of Amniotic Fluid Volume

Oligohydramnios accompanies many cases of significant IUGR. As a result, assessment of uterine volume (fetal and placental mass plus amniotic fluid) by measuring transverse and longitudinal diameters of the uterus has recently been advocated as a useful measure in diagnosis of this problem. A value more than 1.5 standard deviations below the mean for gestational age is highly suggestive of IUGR; a value of 1 to 1.5 standard deviations below the mean for gestation is a gray zone in which the diagnosis is less secure. Recently, clinicians have begun to assess amniotic fluid pockets with real-time ultrasound. A pocket of fluid greater than 1 cm in diameter is helpful in ruling out severe oligohydramnios, which may be associated with asymmetric IUGR; it is not necessary to know the precise gestational age as is required for total intrauterine volume determinations.

SIGNIFICANCE OF MECONIUM IN AMNIOTIC FLUID

Antenatal Meconium

For many years, detection of amniotic-fluid meconium was thought to be helpful in assessing antenatal fetal status. However, the discovery of amniotic-fluid meconium before early labor is usually not associated with poor fetal outcome. In fact, 10 perinatal deaths occurred in a series of 392 patients with prolonged pregnancies, although all had clear amniotic fluid at the time of amniocentesis done within seven days of delivery. Furthermore, a finding of meconium in the amniotic fluid cannot be used to distinguish acute and subsequently corrected fetal stress state from either a chronic ongoing one or simply the physiologic passage of meconium. Since antenatal detection of meconium requires amniocentesis or amnioscopy, the potential for complications, such as rupture of membranes, hemorrhage, and infection, that might be encountered at the time of amniocentesis or amnioscopy probably outweighs any potential benefit. The availability of more effective noninvasive tools to assess fetal health has reduced the clinical significance of amniotic fluid meconium detected in the antenatal period.

Intrapartum Meconium

It is generally accepted that the presence of meconium during labor when the fetus is in the vertex presentation is not an indication for intervention. Rather, it is an indication to consider more specific indicators of fetal health such as intrapartum electronic monitoring and, where necessary, scalp blood sampling.

Three explanations for the passage of meconium have been proposed: a normal event that occurs with progressive fetal maturation; hypoxia-induced peristalsis

and sphincter relaxation; and umbilical cord compression–induced vagal stimulation in mature fetuses. There does appear to be a link between gestational age and meconium passage. Meconium passage is infrequent before 32 to 34 weeks' gestation, and there is a significant increase in its passage after the 38th week. The cause of the meconium passage may vary from patient to patient; in some cases it may result from a combination of causes. This may be the reason that no clear relationship has been demonstrated between its passage and fetal outcome.

Meconium, where there are no other indicators of fetal stress, has been reported to be associated with perinatal mortality rates of 4.5% to 8.8%. However, as early as 1962, Fenton and Steer noted that neonatal outcome is good in a great proportion of cases associated with meconium passage and suggested that more specific indicators be developed both to determine the significance of meconium and to diagnose fetal distress. Currently, the approach to management in the presence of meconium involves consideration of three variables: the consistency of the meconium (old and thin versus new and particulate), the time of its appearance (early labor versus late labor), and its relationship to specific monitor patterns. Thick, particulate (fresh) meconium passed for the first time in late labor in association with nonremediable severe variable or late fetal heart rate (FHR) decelerations is clearly ominous, but the presence of meconium alone is not a sign of fetal distress, nor is it predictive of outcome. More specific indicators include nonremediable severe variable or late decelerations of any magnitude (particularly with poor baseline variability) or acidosis confirmed by scalp-blood sampling.

INTRAPARTUM FETAL MONITORING

Before the mid-1970s, the presence of bradycardia, tachycardia, FHR irregularity, passage of meconium in vertex presentations, and falling or low estriol levels were accepted as evidence of fetal distress. Although all are associated with an increased incidence of fetal morbidity and mortality, they are nonspecific indicators; many infants born with these indicators demonstrate no abnormality (false-positive), while many asphyxiated infants are born with no meconium or stethoscopically detected FHR alterations. In the early 1970s, continuous monitoring was commonly employed in a number of centers. Since that time, considerable expertise has evolved in assessing fetal cardiovascular status as reflected by continuous, instantaneous FHR recordings. Surprisingly, however, a consensus definition of "distress" based on objective findings does not exist. Rather, we have criteria for intervention that either predict eventual distress if correction does not occur or suggest early to late transition from compensation to decompensation. Possible decompensation is suggested by progressive loss or absence of baseline variability and absolute or relative tachycardia. However, the evaluation of FHR status is very complex and must consider a large number of factors. Although we cannot objectively define distress and can make only statistical predictions of fetal blood gas status, we have made significant progress in this area.

Indications

The indications for fetal monitoring vary with the attitudes and experience of both the patient and the medical attendant. Since traditional auscultatory techniques are not reliable in evaluating or predicting fetal status, one could logically insist that all patients in labor be monitored routinely. The need for monitoring in the high-risk group is obvious and is generally accepted. In the low-risk group fetal compromise is unusual, but it is also unexpected; fetal monitoring would appear to have special importance in permitting instant diagnosis when it does occur. In both groups of patients, continuous monitoring not only can demonstrate intrauterine conditions that are ominous, but also, when the tracing pattern is normal, can prevent intervention because of presumed problems that do not actually exist. In addition, routine monitoring has other distinct advantages. It eliminates the need for high nurse/patient ratios to maintain continuous surveillance of fetal cardiovascular status; uterine activity can be evaluated retrospectively and immediately when labor progress is found to be abnormal; and a permanent record is available for educational purposes, for peer review, or for review at a later date. Of greatest practical benefit, the technique detects important pathologic patterns that cannot be revealed by traditional methods.

Despite the above-mentioned benefits of routine fetal monitoring, acceptance is not universal. Many patients and physicians insist that routine monitoring cannot be justified because fetal complications are considered unusual in the low-risk population and, furthermore, the technique disrupts the "natural labor processes" and increases the likelihood of intervention, including cesarean section, for presumed fetal distress. Two studies by Haverkamp support these contentions, since it was concluded that electronic monitoring provided no benefit over traditional stethoscopic methods. Both studies involving patients primarily at 30 to 34 weeks' gestation have certain drawbacks that limit the clinical application of the conclusions. Although there were no differences in Apgar scores or in neonatal morbidity and mortality, the studies were conducted with a high ratio of nurses to patients, so high that it is virtually impossible to duplicate in most institutions; the incidence of ominous FHR patterns was higher in the monitored group than in the "blinded" or control group, implying higher initial risk in the monitored women. The validity of the monitoring diagnoses was supported by subsequent low newborn Apgar scores. Furthermore, in the monitored group, there were more cesarean sec-

tions for monitor-independent indications. Banta and Thacker reached conclusions similar to those of Haverkamp. Their study, too, has been seriously challenged.

Nonetheless, the impact of continuous monitoring must be kept in perspective. Neutra, in an extensive appraisal, found that continuous monitoring does reduce neonatal mortality by 1 death for every 1000 births at term. However, the major reduction in intrapartum mortality as a consequence of monitoring is in preterm labor.

Instrumentation

FHR and uterine activity may be monitored by either external (indirect) or internal (direct) methods (Fig. 41-3). The external method provides less information but is noninvasive and has wider clinical application.

Internal monitoring requires that the membranes be ruptured and that the cervix be sufficiently dilated to permit insertion of the intrauterine catheter and application of the fetal scalp electrode. Also, internal monitoring has resulted in such complications as uterine perforation and fetal injury. Amnionitis and postpartum endometritis are both more frequent following internal monitoring, but much of the increased risk results from the indication for internal monitoring (*e.g.,* prolonged rupture of membranes, prolonged induction of labor) rather than from the invasive procedure per se.

For external monitoring, the techniques available for FHR assessment include phonocardiography, abdominal fetal electrocardiography, and ultrasonocardiography; uterine contractions are detected by tokodynamometry. Instruments are applied to the abdominal wall and are held in place by belts. In the past, many patients were kept in the supine posture to maintain quality recordings. However, new autocorrelation techniques facilitate ease of achieving excellent records even when the patient is tilted to one side in an attempt to minimize the risk of supine hypotension-induced UPI. If multiple changes are necessary to reduce cord compression, it may be difficult to obtain adequate external records, and internal monitoring may be necessary. External monitoring also may be impractical when the patient is markedly obese or agitated.

Internal monitoring provides more detailed and more accurate records that are more readily interpreted and unaffected by the patient's position. Uterine activity is measured by means of an open-ended fluid-filled polyethylene catheter inserted through the cervix into the uterine cavity and connected to a strain-gauge transducer. This procedure is not always needed, but it can be especially valuable for monitoring uterine activity when labor is augmented or induced, if the patient is obese or agitated, or if the external record is not clear or appears to be spurious. Fetal scalp electrodes are commonly used to record FHR. They have the same advantages and disadvantages as the intrauterine pressure catheter. Their most important advantage is the

FIG. 41-3. Methods of monitoring fetal heart rate and uterine contractions. (*A*) Indirect method (ultrasonocardiography). Signals derive from external transducers attached to maternal abdomen. (*B*) Direct method. Recordings are made from electrode applied directly to fetus. A transcervical intrauterine pressure transducer is used. Data obtained by direct method are the most precise. (Richard H Paul)

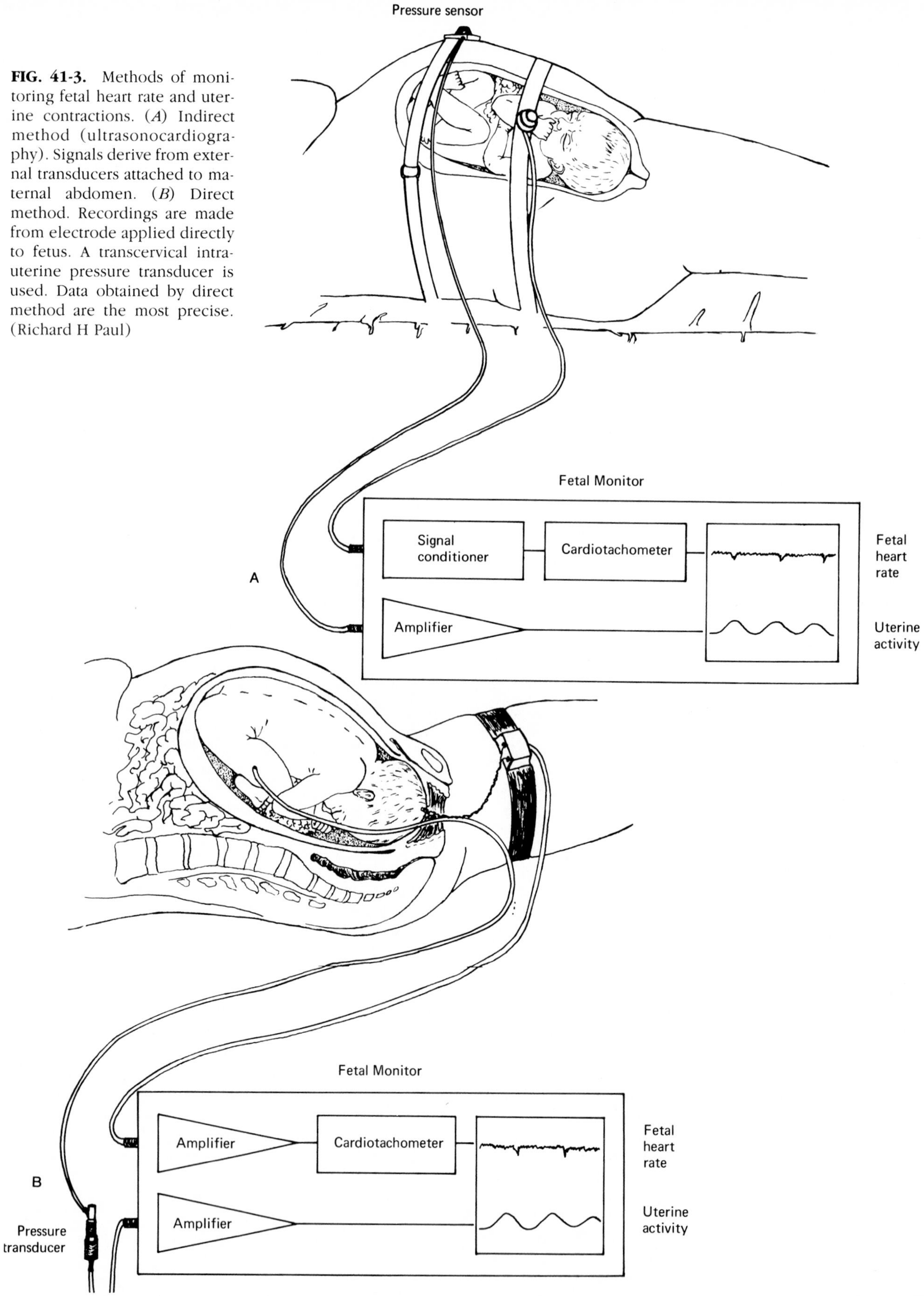

clarity with which short-term FHR variability is recorded, an evaluation that is virtually impossible by external FHR monitoring (Figs. 41-4 and 41-5). In clinical practice, the combination of a fetal scalp electrode and external tocotransducer is commonly used.

Continuous Fetal Heart Rate Monitoring

Traditional auscultatory techniques to evaluate fetal cardiovascular status are no longer acceptable in patients at high risk for asphyxia; few actual measurements are recorded, and the predictive correlation with outcome appears to be poor. In a review of 24,863 labors, Benson and co-workers concluded that there is no single auscultatory indicator of fetal distress, except in the most extreme circumstances.

The technique of continuous electronic FHR monitoring has been developed independently by a number of investigators. The classification proposed by Hon is the most widely accepted in the United States. It is most applicable to intrapartum monitoring; however, it can also be applied to antepartum FHR monitoring, most notably in the oxytocin challenge test (OCT) or contraction stress test (CST) and the nonstress test (NST).

When the fetus is in the nonstressed state, the FHR reflects the intraplay of cardioaccelerator and cardiodecelerator reflexes (Fig. 41-6). Analysis of the FHR involves evaluation of two elements (Fig. 41-7): baseline FHR, which is the portion of the FHR that occurs between uterine contractions or period changes in the FHR; and periodic FHR changes, which are short-term (<10 minutes) alterations in FHR that are associated

FIG. 41-4. Fetal heart rate recorded from electrode applied direct to fetus (*top*) and by indirect ultrasound method (*bottom*). Records were made simultaneously. Precision and accuracy of interval measurement are much greater when direct method is used. (Richard H Paul)

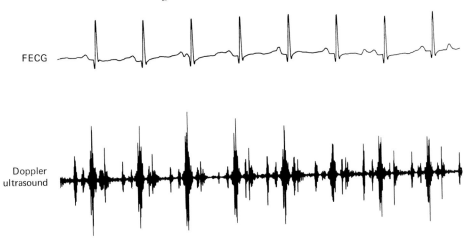

FIG. 41-5. Manner in which fetal heart rate is depicted on monitor chart when recorded by direct (*top*) and indirect (*bottom*) methods. (Richard H Paul)

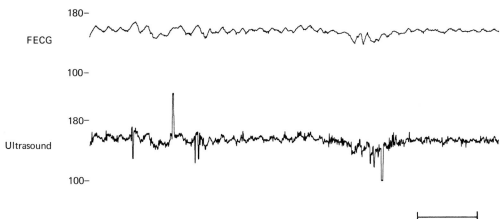

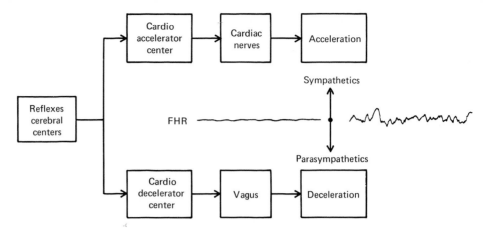

FIG. 41-6. Nervous control mechanisms affecting fetal heart rate (*FHR*). Normal rate at right results from interplay of stimuli from autonomic nervous system. Loss of controlling mechanisms may result from hypoxia and central nervous system damage. (Richard H Paul)

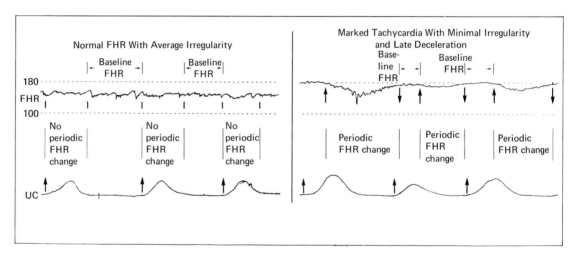

FIG. 41-7. Evaluation of fetal heart rate (*FHR*) is subdivided into control (nonstressed or baseline) and stress (periodic) portions. Baseline rate may correspond to time between contractions (*UC*), as shown at left, or may be only a short interval, as shown at right. (Hon EH: An Atlas of Fetal Heart Rate Patterns. New Haven, Harty Press, 1968)

with uterine contractions or that occur in association with fetal movement.

Baseline FHR

There are two major elements, rate and variability, in the baseline FHR. The baseline rate is established by the predominant rate, independent of decelerations or accelerations, in an observation period of at least ten minutes; a new baseline is established only if a change persists longer than ten minutes. The normal FHR ranges between 120 and 160. Tachycardia is FHR in excess of 160; bradycardia is FHR less than 120. It is uncommon to observe an FHR in excess of 150 at term.

Of the three elements, baseline rate, baseline variability, and periodic change, baseline rate is the least

predictive. The differential diagnosis of fetal tachycardia includes the following:

Immaturity
Prematurity
Maternal fever
Minimal fetal hypoxia
Uterine tachysystole
Drugs (*e.g.,* atropine, scopolamine)
Arrhythmias
Hyperthyroidism
β-Mimetic tocolysis

Tachycardia, either relative or absolute, may be an early manifestation of transition from compensation to decompensation but of itself is not an indicator for intervention. Bradycardia may be seen normally in prolonged pregnancies and occasionally with fetal heart block; with few exceptions, it is not a cause for intervention, particularly in the presence of good baseline variability.

Current fetal monitors record an FHR point on the monitor graph for each cardiac R-R interval, using the formula 60/R-R interval; an R-R interval of 500 msec corresponds to an FHR of 120. When the fetus is in the normal resting state, the duration of the intervals varies; this is termed *short-term* or *beat-to-beat variability.* In addition to short-term or beat-to-beat variability, there is long-term variability, which occurs as reasonably predictable periodic oscillations or irregularities of the FHR with a frequency of 2 to 6 cycles per minute. The magnitude of long-term variability is usually measured by the vertical distance in beats per minute between peak and nadir of the 2 to 6 cycle oscillations. Normal values for short-term and long-term variability are ±2 to 3 beats per minute and 6 to 15 beats per minute, respectively. The following is the differential diagnosis of decreased variability when the long-term variability is less than 6 beats per minute:

Hypoxia (early)
Drugs
    Tranquilizers (diazepam)
    Narcotics
    Atropine, scopolamine
    Barbiturates
    Local anesthetics
    Magnesium sulfate
Prematurity, immaturity
Tachycardia
Physiologic sleep
Uterine tachysystole (prolonged)
Cardiac and central nervous system (CNS) anomalies
Arrhythmias, especially of the nodal type

Periodic FHR Changes

Accelerations and decelerations are included under the general heading *periodic change.* They are of short duration (less than 10 minutes) and must be distinguished from tachycardia and bradycardia. Periodic changes usually occur repetitively in association with contractions or in association with fetal movement. In contrast, tachycardia and bradycardia persist for longer than ten minutes and bear no apparent relationship to contractions or fetal activity.

ACCELERATIONS. Commonly seen in response to fetal movement, periodic accelerations are graphically represented by short-term increases in the heart rate above baseline. Accelerations preceding or following decelerations are frequently called *shoulders.*

DECELERATIONS. In contrast to accelerations, decelerations are represented by periodic slowing of the FHR in association with uterine contractions. The classification of decelerations (Fig. 41-8) is based on evaluation of the uniformity of shape, magnitude, and timing of a series of decelerations versus the shape, magnitude, and timing of a group of uterine contractions. Decelerations are a cardiovascular adaptation to stress. In the case of variable decelerations, the slowing of the heart (diving seal reflex) acts to conserve oxygen consumption and, in conjunction with physiologic preferential shunting of blood to the fetal brain, heart, and adrenal gland, provides protection from an acute asphyxic episode.

Uniform decelerations are of two types, early and late. In both, there is a definite and recurring relationship between the wave form of the uterine contraction and that of the FHR deceleration. The FHR wave form is relatively symmetric, and the onset and offset of the deceleration have a uniform temporal relationship to the onset and offset of the uterine contraction. The descending limb of the FHR curve drops at a rate similar to (or less than) the ascending limb of the associated uterine contraction curve. In general, the magnitude of the deceleration is related to the magnitude of the associated contraction.

Uniform decelerations are subdivided into late and early deceleration categories according to their temporal relationship to the uterine contraction. Deceleration uniformity is more significant in assigning a group of decelerations to a particular category than is the temporal relationship between the peak of the uterine contraction and the nadir or low point of the deceleration. Variable decelerations may bear a late temporal relationship to uterine contractions, but, as the name implies, there are differences in shape, magnitude, or temporal relationship, or in all three.

Early decelerations are uniform decelerations the shape and characteristics of which reflect or mirror the shape and intensity of associated uterine contraction curves. This pattern, which is most commonly observed during the latter half of the first stage of labor, is due to vagal stimulation associated with fetal head compression (Cushing's reflex); the effect is reduced or blocked by administration of atropine. Early decelerations are not common clinically, but they must be distinguished from late decelerations. They are not indicative of significant stress.

Late decelerations are uniform decelerations the shape and characteristics of which, as determined by evaluation of a group of decelerations, reflect the shape and intensity of uterine contraction curves. They begin at or after the peaks of contractions, some 20 to 30 seconds after onset of contractions. Failure to adhere to this rigid definition results in overdiagnosis. The presumed cause is UPI, either acute or chronic.

Variable (nonuniform) decelerations are characterized by a wave form that does not reflect the shape or intensity of associated uterine contraction curves. They may be sporadic, varying in time of onset relative to uterine contractions, and tend to be angular and saw-

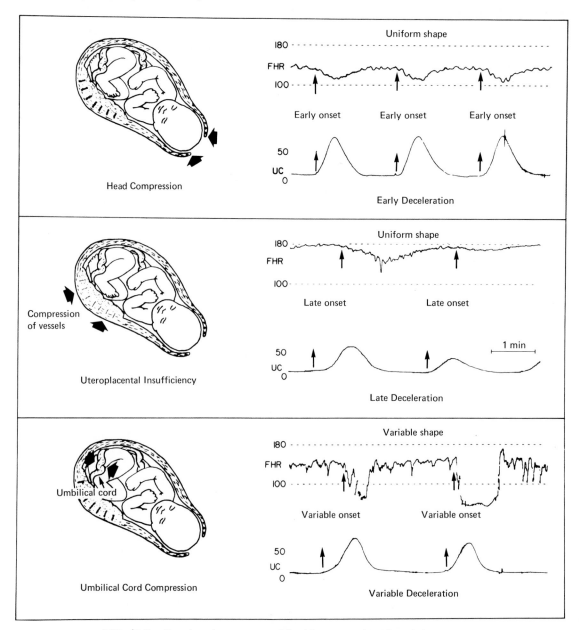

FIG. 41-8. Deceleration patterns of fetal heart rate (*FHR*) and their implied causative mechanisms. Intrauterine pressure (*UC*) is measured in millimeters of mercury. (Hon EH: An Atlas of Fetal Heart Rate Patterns. New Haven, Harty Press, 1968)

toothed in appearance; the descending limb of the deceleration falls faster than the ascending limb of the associated uterine contraction rises. Variable decelerations are presumably the result of umbilical cord compression. Since they are vagally mediated, much of the deceleration may be abolished by the administration of atropine; however, this is not recommended, since the deceleration is a physiologic adaptation to stress that reduces oxygen consumption.

The characteristics of early, late, and variable decelerations are noted in Table 41-6.

Clinical Application

The clinical evaluation of a fetal monitor tracing should begin with an evaluation of uterine activity. Uterine contractions serve as useful reference points for the

Table 41-6
Characteristics of Early, Late, and Variable Decelerations

Early Decelerations	*Late Decelerations*	*Variable Decelerations*
Onset is early (usually first 15 sec) in contracting phase	Onset is late (20–30 sec lag) in contracting phase.	Onset bears a variable time relationship to beginning of the associated contraction; onset may be early or late; however, most are early.
Offset almost coincides with offset of uterine contraction.	Offset is delayed after offset of contraction (latent period).	Offset may be coincidental or delayed with respect to offset of associated contraction.
Duration is usually less than 90 sec.	Duration is usually less than 90 sec.	Duration varies from a few seconds to minutes.
FHR and variability are usually normal.	Baseline FHR is usually in normal or moderate tachycardia range; in terminal phases of asphyxia, baseline may be in bradycardia range.	Baseline FHR is usually in normal range, unless repeated and severe.
FHR usually does not fall below 100 beats/min (variable or combined pattern should be suspected if rate falls to less than 100)		FHR usually falls below 100 beats/min; decelerations to as low as 50–60 beats/min are not uncommon.
Magnitude of drop in FHR should reflect (mirror image) relative intensity of associated contractions when decelerations are viewed as a group.	Magnitude of drop in FHR should, particularly in early stages of appearance, reflect relative intensity of associated contractions when decelerations are viewed as a group.	Magnitude of deceleration does not necessarily reflect relative intensity of associated contractions when decelerations are viewed as a group.
		"Take-off" accelerations frequently precede variable decelerations; a similar "overcompensation shoulder" acceleration frequency marks their conclusion.
		Note: Although decelerations seen in the second stage of labor undoubtedly are associated with head compression, their wave form dictates that they be called variable decelerations.

analysis of FHR response because of their repetitive and stressful nature. Contractions reduce the exchange of carbon dioxide and oxygen between the maternal and fetal compartments and may physically compress the fetal head or compress the umbilical cord between the presenting part and maternal pelvis. In most instances, a fetus can easily tolerate the respiratory stress of three to four contractions per ten-minute interval. The monitor can also provide reassuring signs, which include the following:

Normal baseline rate 100 to 150
Normal baseline variability
Accelerations with fetal movement
Prompt return of variable decelerations to baseline with no evidence of decreasing baseline variability or increasing baseline rate

Uterine tachysystole is a form of excessive uterine activity in which contractions occur at a frequency of five or more per ten-minute interval. Uterine hypertonus is an elevation of resting uterine tone. Both tachysystole and hypertonus impose a fetal respiratory stress. Usually, the resting tonus (measured by intrauterine pressure catheter) is less than 10 mm Hg to 15 mm Hg. Methods that may reduce "relative" or absolute excess uterine activity are listed in Table 41-7.

Variable decelerations also cause fetal respiratory stress; during the deceleration, carbon dioxide tension rises while oxygen tension decreases. Some decelerations are dramatic, dropping 50 or more beats below the baseline. In term pregnancies, such decelerations are of minimal significance unless they repeatedly fall below 70 beats per minutes (probable complete cord compression), last longer than one minute, or are as-

Table 41-7
Management Scheme for Excess Uterine Activity

Possible Cause	Therapy
Oxytocin (excess)	Lower dose; infusion pumps for precision in dose
Lumbar epidural	Fluid preload; avoid supine hypotension
Paracervical block	Low dose and concentration; avoid in fetal acidosis
Contraction coupling and tripling	Lateral position, fluids; if severe, consider β-mimetic or magnesium sulfate

sociated with progressive variability loss. A scheme to evaluate the severity of variable decelerations in pregnancies at term is summarized in Table 41-8.

The clinician should be wary of employing this scheme in preterm labor, since the vagal response is less developed. As a result, the magnitude of the deceleration drop may be less in preterm babies in response to equivalent degrees of cord compression. Reassurance that the fetus is compensating well is provided by serial observations of good baseline variability and the lack of a relative increase in baseline rate. Uterine tachysystole may act in a cumulative manner to aggravate the respiratory insult of variable decelerations. The management scheme frequently used to modify the occurrence or severity of variable decelerations is outlined in Table 41-9.

Late decelerations are the most ominous of all deceleration wave forms. This pattern suggests fetal hypoxia, which may be chronic or acute. Late decelerations associated with chronic UPI (maternal diabetes, preeclampsia, or IUGR) are commonly associated with a lack of baseline variability. In contrast, acute and usually remediable UPI may be observed following prolonged

spontaneous or oxytocin-induced uterine tachysystole. Acute UPI may also be noted in association with maternal supine hypotension or dehydration, or following epidural anesthesia. In such instances, the late decelerations are commonly associated with normal baseline variability. Table 41-10 summarizes clinical observations commonly associated with late decelerations with good variability versus those with poor baseline variability.

Therapy for late decelerations is largely related to prevention. Since most occur as the result of postural hypotension, excessive use of oxytocin, or the administration of epidural anesthesia without intravenous volume loading, implementation of protocols to minimize these complications is extremely important (Table 41-11).

Intervention for fetal "stress" is usually motivated by repetitive, nonremediable, severe variable decelerations or late decelerations that do not respond to classic therapeutic maneuvers. In general, the clinician has 30 minutes in which to modify the observed pattern. Observations that should hasten intervention include prolongation of decelerations or rapidly disappearing baseline variability. In some instances, reassuring signs, such as persistent normal baseline variability, lack of a relative increase in baseline rate, and rapid ascent from the deceleration nadir, may allow delay in intervention, particularly in association with variable decelerations. In contrast, preterm labor or IUGR may hasten intervention, since the fetus has limited reserves.

In considering intervention for late decelerations, the clinician must differentiate late decelerations that are associated with baseline variability (frequently remediable) from those in which there is no variability (nonremediable and usually chronic). In the former instance, position change, hydration, oxygen, and, where possible, reduction of oxytocin infusion is effective. Associated scalp blood pH values may be surprisingly high, but this should not lull the physician into a sense of false security. Without appropriate management, baseline variability will disappear. The presence of late de-

Table 41-8
Scheme to Assist in Evaluating Severity of Variable Decelerations

Nadir of Deceleration	Duration of Deceleration		
	<30 seconds	30–60 seconds	>60 seconds
>80 beats/minute	Mild	Mild	Moderate*
70–80 beats/minute	Mild	Moderate*	Moderate–severe*
<70 beats/minute	Moderate	Moderate–severe*	Severe

* Frequency of fewer than 2 such decelerations in 30 minutes reduces severity one grade.

(After Kubli, FW, Hon EH, Khazin AF et al: Observations on heart rate and pH in the human fetus during labor. Am J Obstet Gynecol 104:1190, 1969)

Table 41-9
Management Scheme for Variable Deceleration

Therapy	Objective
Change maternal position	Reduce cord compression
Decrease uterine activity by decreasing oxytocin, or administering β-mimetic or magnesium sulfate	Increase uteroplacental flow; increase recovery time for oxygen and carbon dioxide exchange
Administer maternal oxygen	Increase maternal-fetal oxygen gradient
Prepare for intervention	Reduce interval from decision to delivery
Elevate presenting part if all else fails	Reduce cord compression temporarily

Table 41-10
Clinical Implications of Goods vs. Poor Baseline Variability with Late Decelerations

Good Baseline Variability	Poor Baseline Variability
Probably normal fetus	Chronic insufficiency (*e.g.*, preeclampsia, diabetes)
Demonstrable insult (CLE, PCB, hypotension, hyperstimulation)	Aggravated by added stress of labor
Usually remediable	Usually not remediable

CLE, continuous lumbar epidural anesthesia; *PCB,* paracervical block.

Table 41-11
Management Scheme of the Fetus with Late Decelerations

Therapy	Objective
Decrease uterine activity	Improve recovery time for oxygen and carbon dioxide exchange
Place mother in lateral decubitus position	Increase uteroplacental blood flow
Provide oxygen, 5–7 liters/min	Increase maternal–fetal oxygen gradient
Maternal blood volume expander	Correct hypotension; increased uteroplacental blood flow
Prepare for operative delivery	Reduce decision–delivery interval

celerations associated with little or no variability (Fig. 41-9) increases the likelihood of fetal metabolic acidosis.

Fetal Scalp Blood Sampling

Although the value of continuous fetal monitoring in predicting outcome is generally accepted, there is justifiable concern regarding the rising incidence of cesarean section for fetal distress that has followed the widespread use of electronic monitoring. A relationship between FHR and scalp blood acid–base values has been recognized, but it may be difficult to predict the pH of a fetus who develops an abnormal FHR pattern. This consideration is perhaps most valid in the presence of late decelerations, ordinarily thought to reflect fetal hypoxemia but found to be associated with normal scalp blood pH values in approximately 50% to 60% of cases.

In some instances, physician response to seemingly dramatic variable decelerations is inappropriately aggressive. It has thus been proposed that fetal scalp blood pH determinations be used to complement electronic fetal monitoring and to assess fetal status more accurately when a monitor pattern suggests possible fetal distress; a reassuring pH value may prevent unnecessary intervention.

The clinical use of scalp blood sampling is based on the assumption that most cases of fetal acidosis are due to asphyxia. In the fetus, pH determination is a better clinical predictor of asphyxia than is fetal oxygen assessment. The normal fetal scalp blood pH in the first stage of labor is 7.25 to 7.45. A value of 7.20 to 7.24 is considered intermediate, whereas a value of less than 7.20 is considered abnormal. In most cases, a scalp pH of less than 7.16 results in a low Apgar score.

Clinically, a value of 7.25 is normal. A repeat sample need not be collected unless the FHR pattern deteriorates. A value of 7.20 to 7.24 requires repeated sampling at 15- to 20-minute intervals, depending on the severity and the trend of the FHR pattern. Decreasing serial pH values are an indication for delivery. A value less than 7.2 is also an indication for delivery unless the FHR pattern is improving. If maternal acidosis is a consideration, maternal blood pH should be measured to rule out maternal contribution to a low fetal pH. A high or low maternal pCO_2 may modify the fetal scalp blood pH. In contrast, accumulation of fixed acids in the maternal compartment has a less dramatic effect, since charged particles (H+) cross the placenta more slowly than does highly soluble CO_2.

Fetal scalp-blood sampling is potentially important when fetal distress is suspected, mild late decelerations

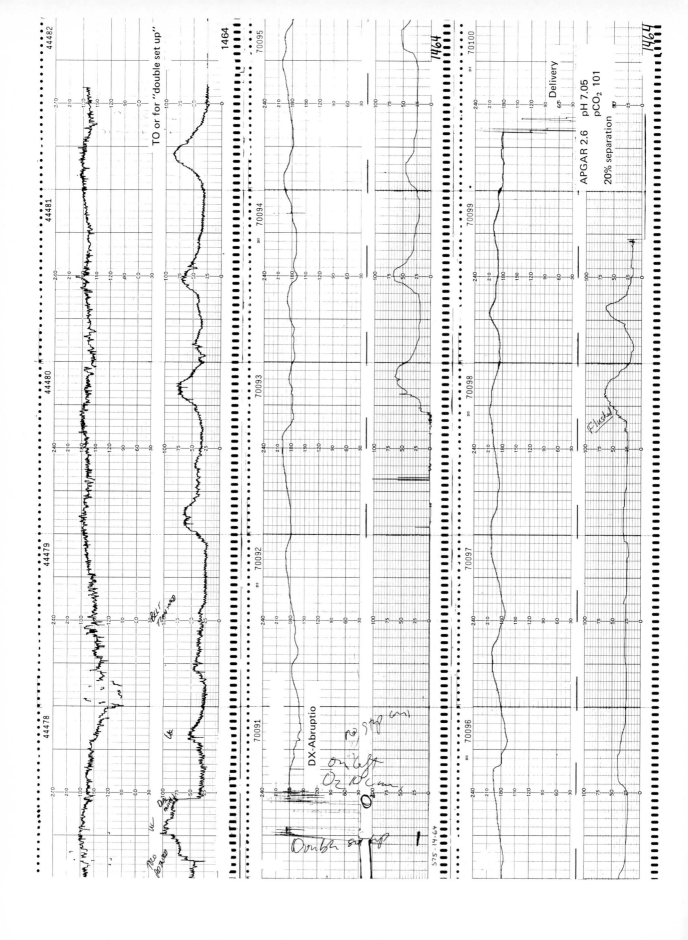

are observed, or there is no baseline variability. In some instances, the fetal *p*H is unexpectedly low. However, the issue is not always clear. Fetal blood sampling is not possible in all cases. A number of conditions must be met: the membranes must be ruptured, the cervix must be at least 2 cm dilated, and the head must be engaged in the maternal pelvis. It may be difficult to procure an adequate sample, particularly when fetal scalp hair is thick. Decisions usually require serial determinations unless a single value is significantly abnormal. Spurious results may occur in association with maternal acidosis or alkalosis, or if there is scalp vasoconstriction or molding. Finally, there is the issue of "monitoring the inevitable." Clearly, electronic monitoring, if properly interpreted, is highly predictive of the blood gas status of the fetus. The correlation of repetitive severe variable or late deceleration patterns with fetal acid–base balance is well established, especially when baseline variability is poor. Abnormal monitor patterns may precede acidosis by a significant period of time. Although a normal scalp blood gas level may allow the clinician to delay a short while, the presence of persistent nonremediable severe variable or late decelerations of any magnitude almost uniformly predicts the eventual development of acidosis.

The clinician must consider the expected interval to delivery, the degree of stress reflected by the pattern, and the presence of unusual risk (preterm labor or IUGR) in making decisions. When there is doubt, measurement of scalp blood gases may be of value. However, as proficiency in evaluating FHR tracings increases, the frequency of cesarean section for fetal stress–distress decreases. The primary cesarean section rate for fetal distress (includes diagnoses of stress, intolerance to labor, and distress) at Prentice Women's Hospital and Maternity Center of the Northwestern University Medical Center is 1.5%. This is consistent with published rates in centers using scalp blood gas evaluation to complement the electronic fetal monitoring assessment.

ANTENATAL FETOPLACENTAL EVALUATION

Fetoplacental status may be assessed in the third trimester by biochemical (estriol or placental lactogen) or biophysical (NST, CST, or OCT and biophysical profile) means. Usually, the result is reassurance that pregnancy can be safely continued. Most reassuring results are associated with favorable outcomes (low false-negative rate); the incidence of false-positive test results (no evidence of fetal or placental disease at delivery following an abnormal test result) ranges from 40% to 60%. Intervention on the basis of a single abnormal result, par-

ticularly in the presence of uncertain fetal pulmonary status, should be unusual unless the maternal status deteriorates.

Fetal assessment tests should be ordered when there is a risk of UPI. By design, these tests provide little or no useful information in the evaluation of pregnancies in which perinatal morbidity and mortality subsequently result from trauma, congenital anomalies, or cord accidents. Since most assays and procedures are expensive, the clinician should ensure that the test to be ordered provides useful information that cannot be gained by other means. Historically, biochemical assay of urinary estriol has been the most commonly used test. In recent years, biophysical assessments of fetoplacental respiratory function (NST, CST, or biophysical profile) have largely replaced biochemical assays. In general, biophysical assessment is considered reliable, can be performed at less frequent intervals, and is less expensive than currently available biochemical measures of fetoplacental function.

Contraction Stress Test (Oxytocin Challenge Test, Nipple Stimulation Test)

Since uterine contractions are associated with a reduction in uteroplacental blood flow, spontaneous (CST), oxytocin-induced (OCT), or nipple stimulation–induced contractions with a frequency of 3 in 10 minutes may be used clinically as a standard test of fetoplacental respiratory function. Stress of this magnitude has been proved clinically to be useful in separating the occasional fetus with suboptimal oxygen reserve from the vast majority of those with normal reserve, and it does not significantly compromise the normal fetus with adequate reserves. In contrast, a fetus who has chronic deprivation (UPI, *e.g.,* as a result of advanced diabetes, preeclampsia, or IUGR) presumably has diminished fetal reserve, which is manifest by repetitive late decelerations associated with most contractions of any frequency.

Common indications for biophysical testing, including the OCT, NST, and biophysical profile, include the following:

Postterm pregnancy (42+ weeks)
Nonreactive NST
Diabetes mellitus
Preeclampsia
Chronic hypertension
IUGR
History of previous stillbirth
Narcotic addiction

FIG. 41-9. Fetal heart rate and uterine contraction data in a patient with placental abruption. Records in top panel were obtained by an external method; those in lower two panels by direct technique. Cesarean delivery. Newborn's condition is indicated at bottom right. (Richard H Paul)

Sickle cell hemoglobinopathy
Chronic pulmonary disease
Organic heart disease
Rh isoimmune disease
Meconium-stained amniotic fluid

Testing is ordinarily initiated at 36 to 37 weeks' gestation in pregnancies at high risk for UPI, but it may begin as early as 28 to 30 weeks' gestation if IUGR is suspected or if maternal cardiovascular status is compromised or as late as 42 weeks' gestation in postterm pregnancies.

Oxytocin is not required if spontaneous uterine activity is sufficient; usually it is necessary to induce uterine activity with intravenous oxytocin, and an infusion pump should be used for this purpose. FHR is recorded for a baseline (nonstress) period of 15 to 20 minutes. If 3 contractions per 10 minutes are observed within this

time interval, oxytocin need not be administered. If 3 contractions are not observed, oxytocin is administered at an initial rate of 0.5 mU per minute and increased by 2 mU increments until 3 contractions occur in a 10-minute interval. It is rarely necessary to exceed 20 mU/minute.

The test results are negative (normal) if there are no late decelerations associated with at least 3 contractions within a 10-minute "window" (Figs. 41-10 and 41-11). Such a result is reassuring; it is associated with a false-normal rate of 1 to 2 per 1000. The procedure is usually repeated weekly, but more frequent testing may be indicated for insulin-dependent diabetics, women with moderate to severe preeclampsia, or women with prolonged pregnancies.

The presence of consistent and persistent late decelerations with most uterine contractions, regardless of their frequency, constitutes a positive CST result (Fig.

FIG. 41-10. Representation of possible contraction stress test (*CST*) outcomes. Upper channel of each strip is fetal heart rate (*FHR*); lower channel reflects uterine contractions (*UC*) in a 10-minute time interval. (Depp R: In Sabbagha RE (ed): Diagnostic Ultrasound Applied to Obstetrics and Gynecology. Hagerstown, Harper & Row, 1980)

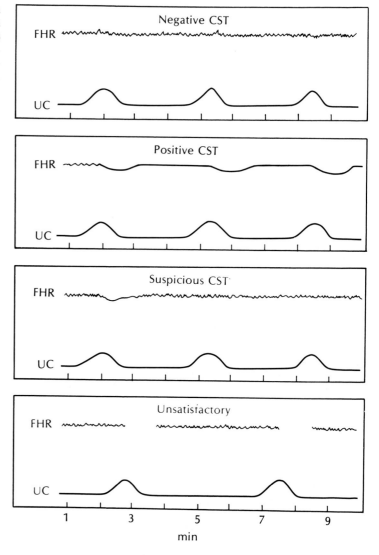

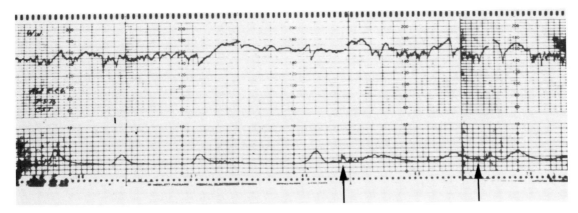

FIG. 41-11. Reactive (negative) result of contraction stress test using abdominal electrocardiogram as source. Lower channel reflects uterine contractions of 40- to 60-second duration. Small superimposed peaks represent fetal movement. Fetal heart rate (*FHR*) baseline (*upper channel*) is 145 to 150. Note accelerations of FHR in response to fetal movement (*arrows*) on lower channel. The estimated magnitude of accelerations is 25 to 30 beats/minute. (Depp R: In Sabbagha RE (ed): Diagnostic Ultrasound Applied to Obstetrics and Gynecology. Hagerstown, Harper & Row, 1980)

41-12). This is often associated with decreased baseline variability and a lack of FHR accelerations with fetal movement. Since positive results on a CST indicate UPI, delivery should be accomplished within a relatively short interval if the fetal lungs are mature. It should be remembered, however, that approximately 30% to 60% of such test results are actually false positive (false abnormal); if allowed to labor subsequently, these patients may demonstrate no further late decelerations. For this reason, it may be safe to attempt vaginal delivery if it is possible to rupture the membranes, apply a direct scalp electrode, and allow the patient to labor in a lateral decubitus position. If not, cesarean section should be considered.

If the lungs are immature, fetal status can also be evaluated by daily determinations of plasma or urinary estriol levels or, more recently, frequent biophysical profile assessment (see below); the pregnancy may be allowed to continue as long as the estriol is stable or rising or the biophysical profile score is at least 6. Although a positive CST result is less predictive (30%–60% false positive) than a negative one (99% true negative), the probability of a true-positive diagnosis is improved if the FHR fails to accelerate with fetal movement. Most women who exhibit a positive CST result accompanied by accelerations with a magnitude of at least 15 beats per minute in response to fetal movement can tolerate labor or some delay until delivery. If there are no accelerations and little or no baseline variability, it is unlikely that the supplemental use of serial estriol measurements will be helpful in allowing the pregnancy to continue until fetal maturity is reached; it is also unlikely that labor will be tolerated without further evidence of late decelerations. As a consequence, it is appropriate to proceed to cesarean section. If no decelerations were noted prior to the CST during baseline observation, it may be appropriate to delay cesarean for a period of time with the patient on her side, well hydrated and oxygenated, until induced contractions decrease in frequency to allow intrauterine resuscitation from the temporary additional stress of the OCT and CST. This resuscitation is reflected by decrease in both the frequency and magnitude of decelerations.

Nonstress Test

Although the CST tests are highly predictive and their results have a very low false-negative rate, they are time-consuming, require intravenous fluids and perhaps oxytocin, and are best performed in a labor unit. These procedures are therefore costly. Since it is unusual to find a positive CST test result if a prior NST result is negative, a negative NST usually suffices for predictive purposes.

A reactive (negative) NST result is characterized by the presence of two or more accelerations of the FHR in 20 minutes or less. The accelerations must be at least 15 beats per minute above the baseline; apparently, it does not matter if the accelerations follow spontaneous movement or are in response to manual stimulation. A nonreactive (positive) NST result is characterized by fewer than two accelerations of at least 15 beats per minute in a 40-minute time interval. If the fetus is not reactive within the first 20 minutes, it should be stimulated artificially and observed for an additional 20 minutes before being designated nonreactive. This minimizes the possibility of lack of activity associated with fetal sleep cycles.

A reactive result on an NST is reassuring. The false-negative rate approximates that of a CST; most series report a false-negative rate of 1 to 3 in 1000. There has

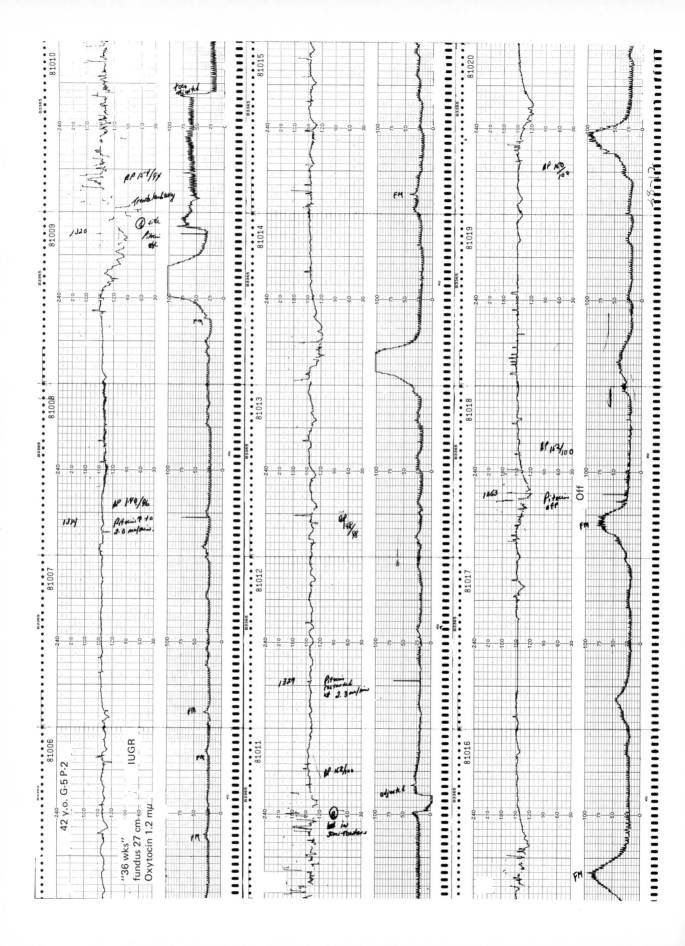

been some concern that a necessary intervention may be delayed if the clinician waits for a nonreactive NST result. This concern does not seem realistic for several reasons. First, the NST appears to be a very conservative indicator of fetal status in that the abnormal rate is about 25% for the NST versus 3% for the CST. This increase in the population judged to be at risk identifies a subset population that may be better served by the CST with the associated lower false-abnormal rate of its results. Second, there appears to be a gradation of nonreaction (decreasing acceleration magnitude, more obvious loss of baseline variability); clearly, the flatter the baseline, the less favorable the outcome. Since these changes are generally observed over time, a CST can be ordered to evaluate fetal status at a very early time in development of the nonreactive state. Third, most CSTs with false-positive results are characterized by a baseline that is reactive. Fourth, there does not appear to be an increase in perinatal mortality when patients who have a reactive NST result are compared with those who have a nonreactive NST result followed by a negative CST result. Finally, from a practical standpoint, the diminished cost and the patient convenience of the NST allow the clinician to assess certain high-risk pregnancies more frequently and less expensively than is realistically possible if the CST is used as the primary test procedure. Recently, however, several investigators have advocated a nipple stimulation CST, which requires no oxytocin and can be completed successfully in 40 minutes in 70% to 90% of patients. Thus, the CST performed in such a manner may no longer have the constraint of cost or time.

The NST is usually used as a screening test. When results are reactive, tests may safely be repeated at weekly intervals; it may be necessary to repeat them more frequently in insulin-dependent diabetics and in patients with preeclampsia, prolonged pregnancies, and cases at high risk for IUGR. Approximately one third of the test results are nonreactive, and such patients require a CST; 80% to 90% of subsequent CSTs show negative results. Even the few who subsequently have a positive CST generally have a good outcome. Most deaths are associated with preterm delivery.

Fetal Activity

Subjective patient assessment of fetal activity has been used by clinicians for many years as an expression of fetal well-being. A sudden increase (cord compression or placental abruption) or a decrease (chronic UPI) in activity may precede fetal demise. Some have suggested that antepartum surveillance of patients with decreased fetal movement would be more beneficial in reducing

perinatal morbidity than simply monitoring all classically high-risk patients. Total reliance on such a scheme seems unreasonable, since patients tend to observe a decrease in fetal movement as gestation progresses; patient reliability also varies. Real-time ultrasound assessment of fetal movement and tone as commonly performed in the biophysical profile may provide more objective data.

Biophysical Profile

Recently, the biophysical profile (see "Ultrasound in Obstetrics and Gynecology" in Chap. 15) has been employed in a number of university centers as an objective biophysical approach to fetal assessment. Its role relative to the NST or CST has yet to be determined. In some centers it is used in the same way as the CST, that is, as a final determinant of fetuses with a nonreactive NST. In other centers, it has been used in a role complementary to the CST when the latter is positive, particularly when the fetus is immature, in hopes of delaying delivery. That the relative role of the biophysical profile is uncertain is not surprising, since one of the five variables of the profile is the NST, which is also highly predictive of CST outcome. The remaining four variables that are assessed by real-time ultrasound include fetal movement, fetal tone, qualitative amniotic fluid volume, and fetal breathing movements (FBM). Each of the five is assigned a score of 0 or 2 on the basis of absence or normal presence during an observation period of up to 30 minutes. With the exception of fetal tone, each has been used separately to assess fetal status. Incorporation of the five variables apparently reduces the false-negative (normal) rate but more importantly reduces the high false-positive (abnormal) rate of each used independently. Like the NST or the nipple-stimulation CST, it can be completed in 20 to 30 minutes in most instances. The minimal contribution by each variable to the total score compatible with favorable outcome is yet to be determined. Recently, Manning has suggested that the NST need not be performed when all four ultrasound-monitored variables are normal. A typical management protocol is summarized in Table 41-12. A normal score of at least 8 points is reassuring, and intervention may be delayed unless maternal health is deteriorating, significant growth retardation is detected, or the cervix is favorable for induction in postterm pregnancies. A score of 6 is equivocal, an indication for repeat testing in 24 hours. An abnormal score (less than 6) is an indication for delivery after 28 weeks' gestation.

Approximately 2% of tests are equivocal; most (82%) are normal on repeat testing within 24 hours. Approximately 1% of tests are abnormal; conversion to normal

FIG. 41-12. Positive response to contraction stress testing, indicating abnormality of fetal heart rate. Baseline FHR is unduly smooth, there is no acceleration associated with fetal movement (*FM*), and late decelerations are clearly evident in third panel (Richard H Paul)

Table 41-12
Management Protocol Using the Biophysical Profile

Score	Interpretation	Management
10	Low risk	Repeat weekly.*
8	Low risk†	Repeat weekly.‡
6	Suspect chronic "stress"	Repeat in 24 hours. Deliver if score ≤6.
4	Suspect chronic "stress"	Deliver if ≥36 weeks. If <36 weeks/surfactant immature: 1. Repeat in 24 hours 2. Deliver if repeat ≤6 or oligohydramnios
0–2	Chronic "stress"	Observe for 2 hours. Deliver if persistent ≤4.

* Repeat twice weekly if insulin-dependent diabetic or prolonged pregnancy.

† If all four real-time ultrasound variables are normal, an NST need not be performed.

‡ If prolonged pregnancy, deliver if there is oligohydramnios or the cervix is favorable.

is apparently rare. To be determined is the long-term physiologic significance of abnormal scores relative to acute versus chronic hypoxia or other causes of abnormal fetal development. Despite the above-described limitations, this technique has great promise and unlike the NST or CST allows more routine "screening" for obvious congenital anomalies independent of a level-II ultrasound examination. A brief summary of two variables used in the biophysical profile, but also used independently to assess fetal status, is presented below.

Fetal Breathing Movement

Fetal chest wall movements were detected as early as 1888. However, it was not until 1970 that Dawes and co-workers were able to document the presence of negative fluctuations of thoracic pressure independent of changes in amniotic fluid pressure in fetal lambs by implanting intratracheal catheters. It was subsequently suggested that antenatal assessment of FBM would eventually prove to be a useful clinical tool. The availability of real-time ultrasound now makes evaluation of FBM a clinical consideration.

Although control of FBM is similar to the control of neonatal respiratory activity, there does appear to be some difference from respiratory control in adults; this may be a function of the maturation of the respiratory control system that occurs after the neonatal period. The most notable exception is the poor responsiveness of the fetal carotid body to hypoxemia and hypercapnia.

Two predominant breathing patterns have been demonstrated in the fetal lamb: a rapid, shallow, regular pattern that accounts for approximately 90% of FBM and a more sporadic pattern characterized by deeper and slower respiratory movements at a rate of 1 to 4 per minute that accounts for approximately 5% of FBM. The rapid pattern appears to be correlated with rapid-eye-movement sleep; the slow pattern appears not to be associated with any particular state of wakefulness or sleep. Additional intermittent positive-pressure fluctuations have been observed in fetal lambs with intratracheal pressure catheters; these movements are thought to be secondary to coughing, gasping, or hiccups.

In the human fetus, FBM may be observed as early as 11 weeks' gestation. It is reliably identifiable at 13 to 14 weeks' gestation. Movements are irregular in early fetal life but become more regular with advancing gestation. Under normal circumstances, FBM can be seen over 30% to 90% of the observation time. Breathing activity rarely occurs continuously for more than 10 minutes; apneic periods of up to 108 minutes have been observed in normal fetuses. The most frequent movements are rapid and of small amplitude. The usual frequency of movements is 30 to 70 per minute.

FBM is probably secondary to diaphragmatic rather than chest wall muscle activity. Control seems to be central, generated within medullary respiratory centers. Physiologic variables that modify FBM in animals also appear to be active in the human fetus. The most significant of these are blood sugar levels, pCO_2 and pO_2 levels, labor activity, fetal presentation, and fetal sleep state. Temperature is of lesser significance, although FBM decreases when temperature is reduced and increases to a panting pattern when temperature is increased. FBM also appears to have a diurnal variation that is independent of blood sugar levels. Factors to consider in interpretation of FBM activity, as based on observations in the lamb fetus, are presented in Table 41-13. Both hypoxia and hypercapnia increase FBM activity; however, when severe or prolonged for greater than one hour, FBM may be arrested and apparently

Table 41-13
Determinants of Fetal Breathing Movements in Fetal Lambs

Determinant	Respiratory Rate	Activity Amplitude
Hypercapnia	↑	↑
Hypoxia	↑	↑*
PaO₂ < 16	Arrest of FBM	
Hypoglycemia	↓	↓
Hyperglycemia	↑†	↑
Labor	Decreased breathing	Periodic apnea

* Slow recovery if hypoxic episode exceeds one hour.

† Excess CO_2 production may be etiology.

↑, increased; ↓ decreased.

does not recover for several hours. Apnea may also develop in advanced labor, apparently a function of maternal hyperventilation-induced hypocapnia and associated fetal hypocapnia. Of interest, FHR variability increases in association with an increase in FBM and activity during labor.

Although pharmacologically induced changes in FBM have been defined in animal models, this has not been possible in human pregnancies. It appears that in general, CNS stimulants increase FBM, while CNS depressants reduce it; the relationship of drug dose to response is not consistent. It has also become apparent that the human fetal CNS is not as sensitive to stimulant or depressant drugs as once thought. Agents that inhibit FBM include methyldopa, nicotine, and alcohol. Although CNS stimulants such as caffeine, epinephrine, isoproterenol, doxapram hydrochloride, and pilocarpine have been found to stimulate FBM in animals, the effects have not been as uniform in the human. The effects of β_2-receptor stimulants are inconsistent; terbutaline sulfate increases FBM, whereas salbutamol appears to have no such effect.

The question of normal criteria has not been totally resolved. Although early studies suggested a cutoff point for high risk at movement during more than 50% of an observation period, several investigators using real-time ultrasound have reported normal outcome with mean FBM incidences of less than 50% in the third trimester. Recent investigators propose that FBM be assessed in a 30-minute interval; the only criterion for normalcy is normal FBM observed in this interval; percent movement time is considered to be of much less importance.

Clinically, most studies indicate that if FBM is seen during more than 50% of an observation period, the mortality is almost zero, whereas the presence of prolonged apnea or only isolated deep breaths increases risk of IUGR and fetal death. Some have correlated FBM changes with pathologic monitor patterns. When FBM occurred during less than 50% of observation time, 15 of 17 fetuses subsequently experienced late decelerations in FHR during labor. Late decelerations were frequently accompanied by gasping activity.

Qualitative Amniotic Fluid Volume

Clinically there is a correlation between diminished fundal height (amniotic fluid, fetus, and placenta) and IUGR. Gohari and co-workers attempted to quantify this relationship more objectively by measuring total intrauterine volume sonographically. Although a correlation was found, the technique was cumbersome. Manning subsequently assessed "qualitative" amniotic fluid volume in a highly selective patient population and observed a relationship between the presence of a fluid pocket of at least 1 cm and absence of IUGR. Subsequent investigators have not observed as strong a relationship but agree that diminished amniotic fluid as evidenced by absence of an amniotic fluid pocket of at least 1 cm to 2 cm increases the risk of asymmetric IUGR and may increase the vulnerability of the umbilical cord to compression. Alternately, oligohydramnios is suggested by marked fetal crowding or poor fetal/fluid interface when scanning.

Table 41-14 summarizes the current assessment of the relationship between IUGR and oligohydramnios. In a highly selected group of patients referred because of a 4-cm fundal height lag and associated 24% incidence of IUGR (Manning and Philipson), oligohydramnios detects 84% of cases and is correct in its classification in more than 90% of cases. However, if the technique is applied to the total population with an assumed 10% incidence of IUGR, it is predicted that only 16% of IUGR cases will be detected.

Table 41-14
Oligohydramnios as Risk Factor for IUGR (SGA)

	Manning *N = 120**	*Philipson* *N = 192†* *Actual*	*Philipson* *N = 2453‡* *Predicted*
IUGR incidence	31 (26)	46 (24)	245 (10)
Oligohydramnios incidence	29 (24)	96 (50)	96 (4)
True positive	26 (90)	38 (40)	38 (40)
Sensitivity	26 (84)	38 (83)	96 (39)§
Specificity	86 (93)	88 (60)	2150 (97)
Anomalies	3‖	0	0

* 120 patients at clinical risk for IUGR; 26/31 had weight less than fifth percentile.

† 96 with oligohydramnios and 96 controlled with 8 (8%) IUGR.

‡ "Calculated" assumes 3.9% oligohydramnios and 10% IUGR (SGA).

§ Assumes 100% true positive.

‖ All had renal agenesis.

For the present, the clinical value of qualitative amniotic fluid volume (QAFV) is to be determined. Indications for assessment include the following:

Diminished fundal height growth
Suspect asymmetric IUGR
Postterm pregnancy
Variable decelerations detected on NST evaluation

However, the clinician should consider the possibility of renal agenesis or that oligohydramnios simply may be an incidental finding of unknown significance suggesting the need for follow-up evaluation of UPI/asymmetric IUGR, including NST or CST, as well as assessment of fetal growth and symmetry and possibly level-II ultrasound. In some instances of moderate oligohydramnios, fetal crowding may result from macrosomia with increased fetal to fluid ratio.

Estriol

Third-trimester biochemical assessment of the fetoplacental unit is most commonly made by measuring either urinary or plasma estriol. Since estriol is the product of fetal and placental compartments, its assay has great theoretic potential. Before the early 1970s, serial urinary estriol assays were the only technique commonly used to evaluate fetal health. There are limitations, however, since factors not strictly related to fetal health may be associated with abnormal values.

As noted in Chapter 19, estriol synthesis is complex. Each site in the synthesis pathway has the potential for disruption. Maternal precursors, largely pregnenolone (21-carbon steroid), serve as a substrate for the fetal adrenal synthesis of the 19-carbon steroid dehydroepiandrosterone sulfate (DHAS). Fetal adrenal function is dependent on interaction between the fetal adrenal and the fetal hypothalamus–pituitary axis and, on occasion, suppression by exogenous steroids. Chronic low-for-gestational-age estriol values may be seen in association with anencephaly (presumed failure of central stimulation) or aplasia of the fetal adrenal.

DHAS undergoes 16α-hydroxylation largely in the fetal liver. This rate-limiting step accounts for approximately 90% of urinary estriol. 16α-Hydroxy-DHAS then undergoes hydrolysis by placental sulfatase to 16α-DHA and is subsequently aromatized (introduction of three double bonds in ring A) to form estriol. Free estriol is conjugated to either the glucuronide or sulfate form in the maternal liver or kidney. Approximately one half of the estriol conjugate is excreted into the enterohepatic circulation by means of bile. Intestinal bacteria hydrolyze the estriol conjugate to free estriol, which is then reabsorbed. As a result, liver or biliary disease or disturbance of gut flora (*e.g.,* by oral antibiotics) may reduce estriol levels detected in the maternal urine.

The analysis of urinary estriol is complex and time consuming. The first step in analysis is acid or enzyme hydrolysis. Significant reduction of recovery occurs in the presence of the urinary antiseptic methenamine. Many laboratories correct for these recovery losses by using an internal standard of radioactive estriol-16-glucuronide; this policy, however, is not widespread.

Clinically, serial estriol determinations are most commonly employed in the management of pregnancy complicated by diabetes, hypertension, suspected IUGR, or postmaturity. Specimens are usually collected on a daily basis with diabetics and two to three times per week with the latter three conditions. Serial determinations are essential; a single value should virtually never be used for assessment or management. In most instances, serial values are compared with a standard curve. Abnormal patterns may be manifest in one of three patterns: progressive downward slope, rapid fall (35%–40% of baseline established by average of values for preceding 3 days), and persistent low values. The clinician must be hesitant in acting immediately on the basis of low values, which can result from failure to collect a true 24-hour specimen, impairment of renal function, or overestimation of gestational age. A high level of urinary glucose or methenamine therapy for cystitis may also be associated with false-abnormal values. Assay of 24-hour urinary creatinine excretion in parallel with estriol provides a reasonable internal standard to determine if 24-hour collection is complete. Some clinicians have favored the calculation of an estriol/creatinine ratio from serial short-term urine collections. Assessment of gestational age and renal function is also helpful.

In those institutions still measuring estriols, the recent trend is toward plasma estriol assay. Plasma estriols may be assayed as unconjugated (free) estriol, which accounts for 8% to 10% of total estriol; total estriol; and immunoreactive estriol. Patient unreliability in collecting a true 24-hour urine specimen and convenience have provided the impetus for the use of plasma estriol assessment. Plasma estriol collection is rapid, simple, and complete. Rising or stable values within normal limits are reassuring. Unfortunately, false-positive results are common.

Plasma unconjugated estriol levels are primarily dependent upon fetoplacental production and secretion rates; they are therefore less affected by disorders of maternal liver or kidney. Distler and co-workers believe that plasma free estriol is the most useful of the plasma tests in the management of the pregnant diabetic. Total plasma estriol includes both the unconjugated and conjugated (glucuronides and sulfates) fractions. The assay includes solvent extraction or enzyme hydrolysis prior to radioimmunoassay. Assay time is six to eight hours.

Some advocate the use of immunoreactive estriol, which reflects approximately 40% of total estriol. This assay has the advantage of eliminating the extraction process; thus, the assay time is considerably less than that for either total or unconjugated estriol. At the present time, clinical use of plasma estriol determinations is not widespread, although some clinicians feel they are useful in the management of prolonged pregnancies.

Human Placental Lactogen

Human placental lactogen (hPL) is a single-chain polypeptide hormone (isolated by Higashi in 1961 and Josimovich and MacLaren in 1962) with a molecular weight of approximately 21,000 daltons and a half-life of approximately 25 minutes. It is produced by the syncytiotrophoblast. Although the precise function of this hormone has not been determined, it does have inherent somatotrophic, lactogenic, mammotropic, and luteotropic activities. As a result, it has also been called *human chorionic somatomammotropin* (see Chap. 19). Immunologically it is similar to human growth hormone.

The clinical significance of hPL is controversial. The level of hPL correlates best with placental weight; however, this is not consistent. The value of hPL in assessing placental integrity is limited. It was originally thought that hPL levels might be useful in predicting the outcome in patients with threatened abortion. However, many patients with low hPL values do not abort; the low values may result from clinical overassessment of gestational age. Real-time ultrasound is probably more accurate in predicting eventual outcome than is hPL; presence of an intact fetal sac or fetal heart motion is also more specific.

Levels of hPL have also been used to assess fetoplacental function in hypertensive diseases of pregnancy, diabetes, and postterm pregnancy, as well as to predict IUGR. There is a high false-positive and false-negative rate when hPL is used to assess these conditions. Furthermore, hPL levels do not necessarily fall before or immediately after intrauterine fetal death. As a consequence, hPL is seldom used clinically, except perhaps as a screening tool for fetal growth retardation.

ASSESSMENT OF FETAL MATURITY

Until the late 1970s, no effort had been made to assess fetal pulmonary maturity or to assess gestational age correctly in up to 8% to 15% of newborns who developed RDS. With more widespread use of early sonography to establish gestational age or amniocentesis to assess surfactant activity, this is no longer a major problem. Spontaneous preterm labor, preterm premature rupture of the membranes, and high-risk pregnancies requiring preterm intervention for maternal–fetal indications presently account for most newborns delivered prior to functional pulmonary maturity.

Amniocentesis

Amniocentesis was first applied to clinical obstetrics as a means to evaluate fetal status in Rh isoimmune disease. It has subsequently been used for a wide range of fetal evaluation procedures and is sometimes performed as early as 14 to 15 weeks' gestation to detect karyotypic or recessive fetal disorders (see Chap. 2). Evaluation of fetal cells contained in the amniotic fluid in the midtrimester allows the clinician to determine fetal sex and chromosome complement. Amniotic fluid may also be assayed for α-fetoprotein levels, either as part of genetic amniocentesis or to follow in abnormal maternal serum α-fetoprotein. Later in pregnancy, usually after 22 to 24 weeks' gestation, amniocentesis is commonly used to evaluate the severity of fetal involvement with Rh isoimmune disease (ΔOD_{450}), as discussed in Chapter 24, and to predict fetal lung maturity (lecithin/sphingomyelin [L/S] ratio, shake test, lung profile) accurately.

Formerly, fetal maturity was assessed indirectly by falling ΔOD_{450} values (0 at 37 weeks' gestation in unsensitized patients), amniotic fluid creatinine greater than 2 mg/dl, decreasing amniotic fluid osmolality, or greater than 30% Nile blue staining of amniotic fluid epithelial cells. At present, the most commonly used indicators of fetal maturity are amniotic fluid L/S, shake test, or lung profile. It is more important clinically to predict functional pulmonary maturity than to predict gestational age at 36 to 37 weeks' gestation, as predicted by the above-mentioned determinations.

Technique

In most institutions, amniocentesis is performed either with ultrasonic guidance to a fluid "pocket" or after a report that indicates the location of a "window" where amniocentesis is most likely to be successful.

The patient is instructed to empty her bladder. The abdomen is then prepared and draped. Local anesthesia is injected into the skin in the anterior abdominal wall at the most appropriate site. Amniotic fluid is aspirated under sterile conditions (Fig. 41-13) through a 20- to 22-gauge needle. Up to 30 ml is withdrawn and centrifuged to separate the fluid into supernatant and cell-rich fractions.

Complications

Complications are infrequent, and the benefits usually far outweigh the slight risk of maternal or fetal damage. Fetal complications include direct fetal trauma, cord hematoma, hemorrhage, preterm labor, and premature rupture of the membranes. Maternal complications include amnionitis, fetomaternal transfusion, and amniotic fluid embolism. Anti-Rh_o globulin is commonly administered to nonsensitized Rh-negative women at the time of amniocentesis; this seems appropriate, especially if the placenta is located on the anterior uterine wall. If the amniotic fluid obtained is significantly bloody, the specimen should be tested to determine if the blood is of fetal or maternal origin. If fetal, the FHR should be evaluated. Prompt delivery may be necessary if distress

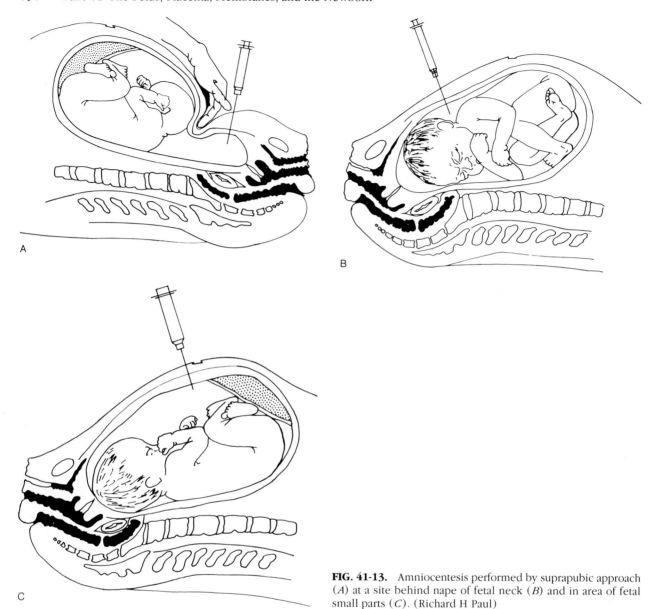

FIG. 41-13. Amniocentesis performed by suprapubic approach (*A*) at a site behind nape of fetal neck (*B*) and in area of fetal small parts (*C*). (Richard H Paul)

is noted at a point in gestation when fetal survival is likely.

Lung Maturation

The changes leading to maturation of the fetal lung are outlined in Chapter 17. Surfactant, released by the lamellar bodies into the amniotic fluid, is a complex mixture of substances that act as a detergent to lower the alveolar surface tension, and so reduce the tendency of the alveoli to collapse. If delivery occurs before the fetal lungs are properly protected by surfactant, the neonate almost inevitably develops RDS (a clinical state of re-

spiratory distress) or hyaline membrane disease (an autopsy finding of a hyaline membrane lining the pulmonary alveoli). The constituents of surfactant can be measured and show characteristic changes in concentration with advancing pregnancy. From 80% to 90% (by weight) of the lipid is phospholipid, of which lecithin constitutes the major portion (70%–80%). Protein (10%–20%) and carbohydrate (1%–2%) account for the remainder of surfactant. Saturated dipalmitoyl lecithin (DPL) accounts for 50% of the total lecithin. Phosphatidylglycerol (PG), phosphatidylinositol (PI), and phosphatidylcholine (PC) are acidic phospholipids that are critically important in stabilizing lecithin in the surfactant layer. Of these, PG seems to be most active; it first appears in the amniotic fluid at 35 to 36 weeks' gestation and rapidly increases thereafter. Acetone-precipitated disaturated lecithin gradually increases as pregnancy advances; PI also increases up to 35 to 36 weeks' gestation, when it peaks, declining thereafter.

L/S Ratio

Under ordinary circumstances, surface-active lecithin begins to appear in the amniotic fluid at approximately 34 to 36 weeks' gestation. Sphingomyelin appears earlier, and its concentrations are higher early in the third trimester. Since sphingomyelin concentrations change very little with advancing pregnancy, they can be used as an internal standard for lecithin by calculating the L/S ratio. Prior to 30 to 32 weeks' gestation in uncomplicated pregnancies, the ratio is generally less than 1.5. At 34 to 35 weeks' gestation, there is a fourfold rise in lecithin, while sphingomyelin remains relatively stable or may decrease at the time of the lecithin surge. An L/S of 2, ordinarily obtained at 35 to 36 weeks' gestation, is clinically accepted as a reliable indicator of functional pulmonary maturity.

The timing of lung maturation may be altered in certain fetal or maternal diseases, and in some cases, the factors that alter surfactant appearance become apparent only after delivery. Class-A diabetes and IUGR are two such factors. Thus, it is not surprising that, in unselected patient series, the L/S ratio may bear no relation to gestational age or birth weight. Hence, the clinician can never reliably predict pulmonary maturity, even when sure of dates. Assessment of surfactant activity is therefore important, regardless of dates, whenever intervention for maternal or fetal indications or inhibition of preterm labor is considered. This may be especially important early in the third trimester, since mature lung function is sometimes found as early as 28 to 30 weeks' gestation. Approximately 19% of women at risk for preterm delivery prior to 38 weeks' gestation and 35% of those who are at risk to deliver between 33 and 36 weeks' gestation demonstrate an L/S ratio in excess of 2.

An L/S ratio in excess of 2 correctly predicts pulmonary maturity in approximately 98% of fetuses; only 2% of those with such a ratio develop RDS (false-mature/false-normal). Most false-mature results are associated with perinatal asphyxia, maternal diabetes, or Rh isoimmune disease. In contrast, an L/S ratio less than 2 is not as predictive; only 37% to 46% of infants born within 72 hours of an L/S ratio less than 2 actually develop RDS (true-abnormal).

Lung Profile

Predictive reliance can usually be placed on the L/S ratio if the value is over 2. In cases in which the L/S ratio is low or intermediate or in which the L/S ratio may give a spurious implication of lung maturity (ges-

tational or class-A to class-C diabetes, Rh disease, perinatal asphyxia), the lung profile, as suggested by Gluck's group, may be extremely helpful in predicting RDS. The profile consists of the L/S ratio and assay of the percentages of disaturated lecithin, PI, and PG. Of these, PG appears to be most important; if it is absent from amniotic fluid, the risk for RDS appears to be high regardless of a low or intermediate L/S ratio; if it is present in concentration of 3% or more, the fetal lung can be considered mature. Disaturated lecithin and PI are added parameters that complete the profile; all may be plotted on a grid (Fig. 41-14), and consistency of the values permits reasonable prediction of lung maturity that is much more reliable than L/S ratio alone in borderline or questionable cases. In a series of cases in which the L/S ratio was less than 2, the profile correctly predicted lung maturity in 14 of 18 fetuses, thus increasing the prediction of true outcome from 68% to 93%.

Surfactant Assessment in High-Risk Pregnancy

The timing of functional maturation (L/S ratio greater than 2) of the fetal lung may vary according to maternal or fetoplacental disease states. Functional maturation evidenced by PG in excess of 3% ordinarily occurs at 35 weeks' gestation. It may occur as early as 28 weeks' gestation in association with class-F and class-R diabetes, pregnancy complicated by severe hypertension–proteinuria syndromes, and prolonged rupture of the membranes. In contrast, maturation is often delayed in class-A diabetics.

The issue of surfactant assessment in pregnancies complicated by maternal diabetes is both controversial and worrisome. The infant of the diabetic mother has a sixfold increase in risk for developing RDS. It is generally accepted that traditional assessment of surfactant by means of the L/S ratio has a false-mature rate of 5% to 6% in diabetics versus an expected rate of 2% in the normal population. A higher incidence of elective cesarean section, prior to onset of labor, asphyxia, and preterm delivery, all of which increase the risk of RDS, may influence the difference in predictability. Furthermore, errors in assignment of gestational age are common in diabetic patients. It appears that the presence of PG in excess of 3% gives better evidence of pulmonary maturity in these patients than does an L/S ratio of 2 or more.

Pregnancy complicated by hypertensive disease, particularly when it is severe and is associated with significant proteinuria or placental infarction, may be associated with accelerated pulmonary maturity, which is manifest by early elevation of the L/S ratio. In some cases, even though the L/S ratio is less than 2, PG may be elevated to a mature 3% level as early as 29 to 30 weeks' gestation. Maturation is generally not accelerated if the hypertension is mild or is of acute onset during pregnancy.

Prolonged rupture of the membranes may be associated with early pulmonary maturation. There is some

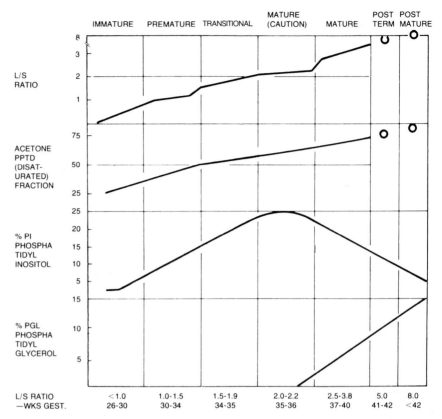

FIG. 41-14. Form used to report lung profile. L/S ratio, acetone-precipitated disaturated lecithin, phosphatidylinositol, and phosphitydylglycerol are recorded at points on curves. Values usually fall within a given grid and lung maturity may be read off at top of form. (Kulovich MV, Hallman MB, Gluck L: The lung profile: I. Normal pregnancy. Am J Obstet Gynecol 135:57, 1979. Copyright ©, Regents of the University of California, 1977)

controversy regarding this issue, since most studies are retrospective and do not control for other factors that may influence surfactant induction. However, when membranes have been ruptured longer than 24 hours and the lung profile has been corrected for gestational age, it has been noted that PG appears earlier (by 1.5 weeks), mean L/S ratios are higher, and a mature L/S ratio is reached earlier.

Shake Test (Rapid Test for Surfactant)

Although the L/S ratio has gained widespread acceptance as a predictor of pulmonary maturity, the assay is slow, complicated, costly, and subject to some errors of precision in the ordinary community hospital. In most institutions, procedures to determine the L/S ratio are performed only during certain hours, and thus surfactant assessment is not always possible when acute conditions require immediate management decisions. As a result, Clements and co-workers have developed the "shake" or "foam stability" test. The procedure requires mixing amniotic fluid with 0.9% saline in various proportions until there is a volume of 1 ml, then adding 1 ml 95% ethanol. The resultant mixture is shaken for 15 seconds and allowed to stand for 15 minutes. A complete ring of stable bubbles in the meniscus of the 1:1 and the 1:2 dilution is a positive result, a stable foam in the

1:1 but not the 1:2 dilution is an intermediate positive result, and a lack of foam in the 1:1 dilution is clearly negative. Although there has been some hesitancy to accept the shake test as a valid measure of pulmonary maturity, the concern appears not to be justified, since the reported false-mature (false-positive) rate is similar to that of the L/S ratio. Positive results reliably predict functional pulmonary maturity; intermediate and negative results indicate increasing risk of RDS.

Clinically, it is equally important to predict pulmonary immaturity as it is to predict pulmonary maturity. False-negative (false-immature) results are common with both the L/S ratio and shake test, even when done within 24 hours of delivery. The usefulness of an intermediate L/S ratio (1.5–2) in predicting the subsequent development of RDS appears to be greater than that of an intermediate shake result (positive in the 1:1 but not the 1:2).

The results of the shake test may be positive in the presence of an immature L/S ratio (false-negative) with subsequent normal neonatal outcome. The shake test therefore complements the L/S ratio, particularly when the L/S ratio is immature. The shake test may actually be able to detect accelerated lung maturity in the presence of an L/S ratio in the 1.5 to 1.9 range. Certainly, a lung profile may show maturity in the presence of an L/S ratio less than 2.

REFERENCES AND RECOMMENDED READING

Risk Scoring

Creasy RK, Gummer BA, Liggins GC: System for predicting spontaneous preterm birth. Obstet Gynecol 55:692, 1980

Galbraith RS, Karchmar EJH, Piercy WN et al: The clinical prediction of intrauterine growth retardation. Am J Obstet Gynecol 133:281, 1979

Harper RG, Sokal MM, Sokal J et al: The high risk perinatal registry: A systematic approach for reducing perinatal mortality. Obstet Gynecol 50:264, 1977

Herron MA, Katz M, Creasy RK: Evaluation of a preterm birth prevention program: Preliminary report. Obstet Gynecol 59:452, 1982

Hobel CJ, Hyvarinen MA, Okada DM et al: Prenatal and intrapartum high-risk screening. Am J Obstet Gynecol 117:1, 1973

Nesbitt REL, Aubry RH: High risk obstetrics. Am J Obstet Gynecol 103:972, 1969

Fetal Gestational Age and Growth Assessment

Battaglia FC, Lubchenco LO: A practical classification of newborn infants by weight and gestational age. J Pediatr 71:159, 1967

Campbell S: The assessment of fetal development by diagnostic ultrasound. Clin Perinatol 1:507, 1974

Campbell S, Dewhurst CJ: Diagnosis of the small for dates fetus by serial ultrasonic cephalometry. Lancet 2:1002, 1971

Campbell S, Newman GB: Growth of the fetal biparietal diameter during normal pregnancy. Br J Obstet Gynaecol 78:513, 1971

Depp R: Dynamics of fetal growth. In Sabbagha RE (ed): Diagnostic Ultrasound Applied to Obstetrics and Gynecology, chap 11. Hagerstown, Harper & Row, 1980

Gohari P, Berkowitz RL, Hobbins JC: Prediction of intrauterine growth retardation by determination of total intrauterine volume. Am J Obstet Gynecol 127:255, 1977

Hertz T, Sokal R, Knoke J et al: Clinical estimation of gestational age: Rules for avoiding preterm delivery. Am J Obstet Gynecol 131:395, 1978

Robinson HP, Flemming JEE: A critical evaluation of sonar "crown-rump length" measurements. Br J Obstet Gynaecol 82:702, 1975

Sabbagha RE: Intrauterine growth retardation: Antenatal diagnosis by ultrasound. Obstet Gynecol 52:252, 1978

Sabbagha RE: Intrauterine growth retardation. In Sabbagha RE (ed): Diagnostic Ultrasound Applied to Obstetrics and Gynecology. Hagerstown, Harper & Row, 1980

Sabbagha RE, Barton BA, Barton FB et al: Sonar biparietal diameter: II. Predictive of three fetal growth patterns leading to a closer assessment of gestational age and neonatal weight. Am J Obstet Gynecol 51:383, 1978

Tamura RK, Sabbagha RE, Depp R et al: Diminished growth in fetuses born preterm after spontaneous labor or rupture of membranes. Am J Obstet Gynecol 148:1105, 1984

Usher R, McClean F, Scott KE: Judgment of fetal age: II. Clinical significance of gestational age and an objective method for its assessment. Pediatr Clin North Am 13:835, 1966

Meconium

Abramovici H, Brandes JM: Meconium during delivery: A sign of compensated fetal distress. Am J Obstet Gynecol 118:251, 1974

Fenton AN, Steer CM: Fetal distress. Am J Obstet Gynecol 83:354, 1962

Green J, Paul R: The value of amniocentesis in prolonged pregnancy. Obstet Gynecol 51:293, 1978

Meis PJ, Hall M III, Marshall JR et al: Meconium passage: A new classification for risk assessment during labor. Am J Obstet Gynecol 131:509, 1978

Miller FC, Sacks DA, Yeh SY et al: Significance of meconium during labor. Am J Obstet Gynecol 122:573, 1975

Intrapartum Monitoring

Continuous Electronic

Banta HD, Thacker SB: Policies toward medical technology: The case of electronic fetal monitoring. Am J Publ Health 69:941, 1979

Benson RC, Shubeck F, Deutschberger L et al: Fetal heart rate as a predictor of fetal distress. Obstet Gynecol 32:259, 1968

Haverkamp AD, Thompson HE, McFee JG et al: The evaluation of continuous fetal heart rate monitoring in high-risk pregnancy. Am J Obstet Gynecol 125:310, 1976

Hobbins JC, Freeman R, Queenan JT: The fetal monitoring debate. Obstet Gynecol 54:103, 1979

Hon EG: An Atlas of Fetal Heart Rate Patterns. New Haven, Harry Press, 1968

Hon EG, Quilligan EJ: The classification of fetal heart rate: II. A revised working classification. Conn Med 31:779, 1967

Neutra RE: Effect of fetal monitoring on neonatal death rates. N Engl J Med 299:324, 1978

Painter MJ, Depp R, O'Donoghue PD: Fetal heart rate patterns and development in the first year of life. Am J Obstet Gynecol 132:271, 1978

Painter MJ, Scott M, Depp R: Neurological and developmental followup of children at six to nine years relative to intrapartum fetal heart rate patterns (abstr). Society of Perinatal Obstetricians, Annual Meeting, Las Vegas, Nevada, January 1985

Paul RH, Hon EG: Clinical fetal monitoring v. effect in perinatal outcome. Am J Obstet Gynecol 118:529, 1974

Paul RH, Khazin SA, Yeh S et al: Clinical fetal monitoring: VII. The evaluation and significance of intrapartum baseline FHR variability. Am J Obstet Gynecol 123:206, 1975

Schifrin BS, Dame L: Fetal heart rate patterns: Prediction of Apgar score. JAMA 219:1372, 1972

Continuous Electronic Monitoring Plus Scalp Blood

Kubli FW, Hon EH, Khazin AF et al: Observations on heart rate and pH in the human fetus during labor. Am J Obstet Gynecol 104:1190, 1969

Wood C, Lumley J, Renou P: Clinical assessment of fetal diagnostic methods. J Obstet Gynaecol Br Commonw 74:823, 1967

Wood C, Newman W, Lumley J et al: Classification of fetal heart rate in relationship to fetal scalp blood measurements and Apgar score. Am J Obstet Gynecol 105:942, 1969

Scalp Blood Gases

Adamsons K, Beard RW, Meyers RE: Comparison of the composition of arterial, venous, capillary blood of the fetal monkey during labor. Am J Obstet Gynecol 107:435, 1970

Beard RW, Morris ED, Clayton SG et al: Foetal capillary pH as an indicator of the condition of the foetus. J Obstet Gynaecol Br Commonw 74:812, 1967

Saling E, Schneider D: Biochemical supervision of the fetus during labor. J Obstet Gynaecol Br Commonw 74:799, 1967

Antenatal Evaluation

Contraction Stress Test

Braly P, Freeman RK: The significance of fetal heart rate reactivity with a positive oxytocin challenge test. Obstet Gynecol 50:689, 1977

Freeman RK: The use of the oxytocin challenge test for antepartum clinical evaluation of uteroplacental respiratory function. Am J Obstet Gynecol 121:481, 1975

Freeman RK, Goebelsman U, Nochimson D et al: An evaluation of the significance of a positive oxytocin challenge test. Obstet Gynecol 47:8, 1975

Pose SV, Castillo JB, Mora–Rojas EO et al: Test of fetal tolerance to induced uterine contractions with a diagnosis of chronic distress. In Perinatal Factors Affecting Human Development, pp 96–103. Washington, DC, Pan-American Health Organization, 1969

Ray M, Freeman RK, Pine S, et al: Clinical experience with the oxytocin challenge test. Am J Obstet Gynecol 114:1, 1972

Trierweiler MW, Freeman RK, James J: Baseline fetal heart rate characteristics as an indicator of fetal status during the antepartum period. Am J Obstet Gynecol 125:618, 1976

Nonstress Test

Evertson LR, Gauthier RJ, Schifrin BS et al: Antepartum fetal heart rate testing: I. Evolution of the nonstress test. Am J Obstet Gynecol 133:29, 1979

Kubli F, Rutgers H: Semiquantitative evaluation of antepartum fetal heart rate. Int J Gynaecol Obstet 10:180, 1972

Lee CY, Diloretto PC, Logrand B: Fetal activity acceleration determination for evaluation of fetal reserve. Obstet Gynecol 48:19, 1976

Nochimson DJ, Turbeville JS, Terry JE et al: The non-stress test. Obstet Gynecol 51:419, 1978

Pratt D, Diamond F, Yen H et al: Fetal stress and nonstress tests: An analysis and comparison of their ability to identify fetal outcome. Obstet Gynecol 54:419, 1979

Rochard F, Schifrin BS, Goupil F et al: Nonstressed fetal heart rate monitoring in the antepartum period. Am J Obstet Gynecol 126:698, 1976

Biophysical Profile and Fetal Activity

Boddy F, Dawes GS: Fetal breathing. Br Med Bull 31:3, 1975

Boddy K, Dawes GS, Robinson JS: In Comline RS, Cross KW, Dawes GS et al (eds): Foetal and Neonatal Physiology, pp 63–66. Proceedings of the Sir Joseph Bancroft Cen-

tenary Symposium, Cambridge, 1972. London, Cambridge University Press, 1972

Boddy K, Robinson JS: External method for detection of fetal breathing in utero. Lancet 2:1231, 1971

Dawes GS, Fox HE, Leduc BM et al: Respiratory movements and paradoxical sleep in the foetal lamb. J Physiol 210:47P, 1970

Hill LM, Breckle R, Wolfgram KR et al: Oligohydramnios: Ultrasonically detected incidence and subsequent fetal outcome. Am J Obstet Gynecol 147:407, 1983

Manning FA: Fetal breathing as a reflection of fetal status. Postgrad Med 61:116, 1976

Manning FA, Hill LM, Platt LD: Qualitative amniotic fluid volume determination by ultrasound: Antepartum detection of intrauterine growth retardation. Am J Obstet Gynecol 139:254, 1981

Manning FA, Morrison I, Lange IR et al: Fetal assessment based on fetal biophysical profile scoring: Experience in 12,620 referred high-risk pregnancies. Am J Obstet Gynecol 151:343, 1985

Manning FA, Platt LD: Fetal breathing movements and the abnormal contraction stress test. Am J Obstet Gynecol 133:590, 1979

Manning FA, Platt LD: Fetal breathing movements and the nonstress test in high-risk pregnancies. Am J Obstet Gynecol 135:511, 1979

Manning FA, Platt LD, Sipos L: Antepartum fetal evaluation: Development of a fetal biophysical profile. Am J Obstet Gynecol 136:787, 1980

Patrick J (ed): Fetal breathing movements. Semin Perinatol 4:249, 1980

Patrick J, Natale R, Richardson B: Patterns of human fetal breathing activity at 34–35 weeks' gestational age. Am J Obstet Gynecol 132:507, 1978

Philipson EH, Sokol RJ, Williams T: Oligohydramnios: Clinical associations and predictive value for intrauterine growth retardation. Am J Obstet Gynecol 146:271, 1983

Sadovsky E, Yaffe H, Polishuk WZ: Fetal movement monitoring in normal and pathologic pregnancy. Int J Gynaecol Obstet 12:75, 1974

Estriol

Diczfalusy E, Mancuso S: Oestregen metabolism in pregnancy. In Klopper A, Diczfalusy E (eds): Foetus and Placenta. Oxford, Blackwell, 1969

Distler W, Gabbe SG, Freeman RK et al: Estriol in pregnancy: V. Unconjugated and total plasma estriol in the management of diabetic pregnancies. Am J Obstet Gynecol 130:424, 1978

Dooley SL, Depp R, Socol ML et al: Urinary estriols in diabetic pregnancy: A reappraisal. Obstet Gynecol 64:469, 1984

Duenhoelter JH, Whalley PI, MacDonald PC: An analysis of the utility of plasma immunoreactive estrogen measurements in determining delivery time of gravidas with a fetus considered at high-risk. Am J Obstet Gynecol 125:889, 1976

Goebelsmann U, Freeman RK, Mestman JH et al: Estriol in pregnancy: II. Daily urinary estriols in the management of the pregnant diabetic woman. Am J Obstet Gynecol 115:795, 1973

Human Placental Lactogen

Higashi K: Studies on the prolactin-like substance in human placenta. Endocrinol Jap 8:288, 1961

Josimovich JB, Kosov B, Mintz DH: Roles of placental lactogen in foetal-maternal relations. In Wolstenholme GEW, O'Connor M (eds): Foetal Anatomy. Ciba Foundation Symposium. London, Churchill, 1969

Josimovich JB, MacLaren JA: Presence in the human placenta and term serum of a highly lactogenic substance immunologically related to pituitary growth hormone. Endocrinology 71:209, 1962

Spellacy WN, Teoh ES, Buhi WC et al: Value of human chorionic somatomammotropin in managing high risk pregnancies. Am J Obstet Gynecol 109:588, 1971

Fetal Maturity

Cher B, Statland BE, Freer DE: Clinical evaluation of the qualitative foam stability index test. Obstet Gynecol 55:617, 1980

Clements JA, Platzker ACG, Tierney DF et al: Association of the risk of the respiratory distress syndrome by a rapid test for surfactant in amniotic fluid. N Engl J Med 286:1077, 1972

Farrell PM, Wood RN: Epidemiology of hyaline membrane disease in the United States: Analysis of national mortality statistics. Pediatrics 58:167, 1976

Frigoletto FD, Phillippe M, Davies IJ et al: Avoiding iatrogenic prematurity with elective repeat cesarean section without the use of amniocentesis. Am J Obstet Gynecol 137:521, 1980

Gluck L, Kulovich MV: Lecithin/sphingomyelin ratios in amniotic fluid in normal and abnormal pregnancy. Am J Obstet Gynecol 115:539, 1973

Gluck L, Kulovich MV, Borer RC et al: Diagnosis of respiratory distress syndrome by amniocentesis. Am J Obstet Gynecol 109:440, 1971

Goldenberg RL, Nelson K: Iatrogenic respiratory distress syndrome: An analysis of obstetric events preceding delivery of infants who develop respiratory distress syndrome. Am J Obstet Gynecol 123:617, 1975

Kulovich MV, Gluck L: The lung profile: II. Complicated pregnancy. Am J Obstet Gynecol 135:64, 1979

Kulovich MV, Hallman MB, Gluck I: The lung profile: I. Normal pregnancy. Am J Obstet Gynecol 135:57, 1979

O'Brien WF, Cefalo RC: Clinical applicability of amniotic fluid tests for fetal pulmonary maturity. Am J Obstet Gynecol 136:135, 1980

Schleuter MA, Phibbs RH, Creasy RK et al: Antenatal prediction of graduated risk of hyaline membrane disease by amniotic fluid foam test for surfactant. Am J Obstet Gynecol 134:761, 1979

The Newborn Infant

L. Stanley James
Karlis Adamsons

42

Survival of the newborn infant depends primarily on prompt expansion of the lungs and the establishment of gaseous exchange. In addition, the infant must regulate body temperature and produce energy from materials obtained from the environment. Most organ systems concerned with homeostasis reach functional maturity prior to term, and several of them, notably the cardiovascular, renal, and skeletomuscular systems, are exercised to some extent during fetal life; those concerned with thermoregulation, on the other hand, are not challenged until after birth.

During the first minutes, hours, and days of life, many alterations in morphology and function take place, perhaps the most dramatic being in the heart and lungs. Although animal experimentation has contributed greatly to our knowledge, our understanding of the many profound changes occurring in the early moments of life is still incomplete.

PHYSIOLOGY OF THE FETUS

Development of Lung and Alveolar Differentiation

During fetal life, the lung has a glandular appearance. Development commences about the 24th day as an outpouching of the gut that branches into the surrounding mesenchyme. Cartilage deposition begins at about the 10th week and continues until the 24th.

The potential air spaces are initially lined by cuboidal epithelium, which begins to flatten between the 16th and 20th weeks, coinciding with capillary ingrowth to establish contact with the epithelium. During this time, the epithelial cells begin to differentiate into two distinct types (type-1 and type-2 cells). Type 1 are vacuolated alveolar cells with some lipoid material; type 2 are nonvacuolated, look more like connective tissue cells, and have lamellar inclusions (see Fig. 17-28).

Production of Fluid by the Lungs

There is a considerable quantity of fluid in the fetal lung prior to delivery. This fluid appears to be an ultrafiltrate of plasma with selective reabsorption or secretion; it is more acidic and has a higher chloride content than plasma. With the onset of respiration, reabsorption of this fluid must be quite rapid. Its low protein concentration, together with the fall in pulmonary artery pressure that occurs when the lung expands, would facilitate this process.

Respiratory Movements

Rhythmic movements of the chest wall and of the diaphragm have been demonstrated to occur in mammalian fetuses at the completion of the first third of gestation. They are associated with relatively large variations in fetal blood flow in the descending aorta and in heart rate. In the well-oxygenated primate fetus near term, these respiratory movements occur 30% to 40% of the time. Respiratory movements are depressed by anesthetic and analgesic agents and by asphyxia. They are reinitiated as gasps in the presence of marked oxygen deprivation. Evidence strongly supports the contention that bronchial and amniotic fluid is not inhaled during regular breathing but only during the deep gasping of asphyxia.

Surface Tension Phenomenon and Lung Function

The normal mature lung contains a surface tension–reducing substance that confers stability during deflation and is responsible for the fine foam formed during acute pulmonary edema. This substance has been identified as a phospholipid together with a specific protein. It can usually be demonstrated by 18 to 20 weeks' gestation, when the fetal lung can be expanded, and its presence coincides with the appearance of lamellar inclusions in the type-2 alveolar cell. The presence of surface-active agent is important in reducing the work required for initial lung expansion and maintaining the stability of the expanded alveolus.

Circulation

Current knowledge of the fetal circulation has been gained principally through the study of lambs delivered by hysterotomy. In this species the uterus does not contract once the fetus is removed, and the placenta remains attached to the uterine wall. Providing the lamb is kept warm and the cord circulation is not interrupted, the fetus will not breathe and the heart can be catheterized, blood samples withdrawn, and radiopaque substances injected.

These studies have shown that arterialized blood from the placenta flows into the fetus through the umbilical vein and passes rapidly through the liver into the inferior vena cava; from there, it flows through the foramen ovale into the left atrium, soon to appear in the aorta and arteries of the head (Fig. 42-1). A portion bypasses the liver through the ductus venosus. Venous blood from the lower extremities and head passes predominantly into the right atrium, the right ventricle, and then into the descending aorta through the pulmonary artery and ductus arteriosus. Thus, the foramen ovale and the ductus arteriosus act as bypass channels, allowing a large part of the combined cardiac output to return to the placenta without flowing through the lungs. Approximately 55% of the combined ventricular output flows to the placenta, while 35% perfuses body tissues, the remaining 10% flowing through the lungs.

The pulmonary arteries and arterioles of the fetus, like those of the systemic circulation, are characterized by a high ratio of wall thickness to the lumen. Pulmonary blood flow is not constant and can be increased up to fivefold by injection of acetylcholine or histamine in microgram quantities into the pulmonary artery. The degree of fetal oxygenation influences pulmonary vascular resistance, pulmonary arterial flow increasing if the mother is given 100% oxygen to breathe. Acute asphyxia of the fetus produces intense pulmonary vasoconstriction, which markedly reduces pulmonary blood flow.

The crista dividens, a structure projecting from the posterosuperior border of the foramen ovale, separates the inferior vena caval flow into two streams before the atria are reached, the stream from the ductus venosus being guided largely into the left atrium. It is improbable that the ductus venosus has any important function in the latter part of fetal life. In the piglet, lamb, and monkey, it is a minute channel at term, and in the foal it is occluded before birth.

Thermoregulation

Under normal conditions, the body temperature of the human fetus is approximately 0.5°C higher than that of the mother. This gradient is determined by the ratio of the heat output of the fetus to the rate of placental perfusion and the direction of flows through the villous capillaries and the intervillous space. The amount of heat dissipated from the body surface into the amniotic fluid is small in comparison with that exchanged across the placenta. Under conditions of hypo- or hyperthermia, the temperature of the fetus parallels that of the mother, although the thermal gradient between fetus and mother increases with the rise in maternal temperature. Oxygenation of the fetus appears to be relatively unaffected as long as fetal temperature does not exceed 41.5°C (107°F). When this limit is exceeded, the fetal circulatory system deteriorates rapidly. In contrast, lowering of fetal body temperature does not interfere with fetal oxygenation even though there is a linear fall in fetal heart rate and blood pressure as fetal body temperature is reduced.

Respiratory Gas Exchange Across the Placenta

Some of the controversy concerning the environment in which the fetus develops has been resolved following the development of techniques for implanting catheters into fetal and maternal vessels for prolonged periods without interrupting pregnancy. These techniques have been successfully employed in sheep, goats, and, more recently, rhesus monkeys. They have enabled serial sampling of arterial and venous blood from the unanesthetized mother and fetus.

As the fetus grows, the functional capacity of the placenta appears to increase to keep pace with the fetus' needs. There are species variations with regard to the relative increase in weight of the fetus and placenta as development proceeds, but the human placenta continues to grow and increase in weight to term. The gradients for hydrogen ion and carbon dioxide tension across the placenta are small (approximately 0.05 pH units and 8 mm Hg, respectively) so that the fetus is neither acidotic nor hypercapnic under normal conditions. Although oxygen tension of fetal arterial blood is low by adult standards, oxygen consumption of the fetal lamb and goat is similar to basal values obtained after birth and appears to remain constant during the third trimester. Hemoglobin concentration and oxygen-carrying capacity of fetal blood during the third trimester are similar to those of the adult animal and do not change as pregnancy advances, unless the animal is subject to stress, such as an operative procedure for blood sampling. Adequate oxygenation of the tissues is probably maintained in the face of a relatively low arterial oxygen tension because of an umbilical vein saturation of 80% to 85% together with a high cardiac output.

Thus, the evidence responsible for the belief that

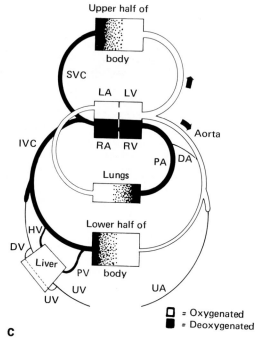

FIG. 42-1. Schematic representations of (*A*) fetal, (*B*) neonatal, and (*C*) adult circulation. *LA, LV, RA, RV* refer to four chambers of heart. *DA,* ductus arteriosus; *PA,* pulmonary artery; *UA,* umbilical artery; *UV,* umbilical vein; *PV,* portal vein; *HV,* hepatic vein; *DV,* ductus venosus; *IVC,* inferior vena cava; *SVC,* superior vena cava. Arrows indicate direction of blood flow.

the fetus has limited control over its oxygen supply and lives under conditions of oxygen deprivation as term approaches can largely be discounted.

PHYSIOLOGY OF THE NEWBORN

Birth Asphyxia

Oxygen levels in the umbilical arterial blood at birth range from 0% to nearly 70% saturation. Even in the most vigorous and healthy infants, the average value is 22%; in nearly one quarter, it is less than 10%. The relatively low oxygen levels are accompanied by varying degrees of hypercapnia and acidosis, the average carbon dioxide pressure being 58 mm Hg and the average pH 7.28 (compared with 40 mm Hg and pH 7.4 in the adult); lower pH and higher carbon dioxide pressure are associated with lower oxygen levels.

These observations suggest that during the final stages of labor and delivery, the exchange of oxygen and carbon dioxide across the placenta is reduced, leading to various degrees of asphyxia at birth. Direct proof of this concept has been provided by the animal experiments described earlier. More recently, sampling of blood from the fetal scalp has shown that, as labor progresses, the fetus gradually becomes acidotic. This latter technique is a most important advance in monitoring the condition of the fetus and is finding increasing clinical application (see Chapter 41).

Several factors can disturb the normal functional relation between fetal and maternal circulations and cause fetal acidosis. Blood flow through the intervillous space is reduced or may stop during strong uterine contractions; it is also reduced if the mother becomes hypotensive as a result of compression of the inferior vena cava or aorta by the uterus. Maternal hyperventilation leading to alkalosis also appears to lead to a reduction in intervillous flow and to fetal acidosis. In addition to these factors, changes in maternal acid–base balance as a result of excessive muscular activity or dehydration during prolonged labor or as a result of respiratory depression from drugs and anesthesia are reflected in the fetus. On the fetal side, cord compression occurs in approximately one third of all deliveries and probably is the most common mechanism to interfere with transplacental exchange.

The composition of cord blood at birth is therefore the result of a disturbance in the functional relation between mother and fetus during labor and delivery, whether this be *per vaginam* or by cesarean section, and does not reflect adaptation to a hypoxic environment *in utero*. Since these changes occur inevitably, considerable limitations are imposed on the interpretation of data relating to the composition of cord blood. This applies not only to respiratory gases but also to all substances that are continuously exchanged between mother and fetus.

Recovery From Birth Asphyxia

During the first minutes after birth, pH continues to fall while lactate levels rise. This occurs as a result of the unloading of acid products from areas that have been underperfused during asphyxia. By 1 to 3 hours of age, pH and lactate levels in the healthy infant are near normal for the adult; however, they remain acidotic for considerably longer in the depressed infant.

Following lung expansion, arterial oxygen tension rises and carbon dioxide tension falls rapidly. Recovery is accomplished initially by pulmonary elimination of carbon dioxide and not by renal excretion of hydrogen ion. By 24 hours, the healthy newborn has reached the same acid–base balance as the mother prior to labor.

A number of factors slow the rate of recovery from birth asphyxia. The most important are preterm delivery and analgesic and anesthetic drugs given before delivery. Delay in recovery is also seen in the more asphyxiated infants, probably because of circulatory impairment and central nervous system depression. This group includes infants who have aspirated meconium before delivery.

An additional factor that delays recovery is a sustained increase in metabolic rate as a result of exposure of the naked newborn to room temperature (Fig. 42-2).

FIG. 42-2. Deep body temperatures (colonic), pH, and excess acid during first two hours of life in two groups of healthy infants. In one group (●) body temperature was maintained by infrared lamp; in other (○), body temperature was allowed to fall while infant was exposed to environmental temperature of 25°C (room temperature).

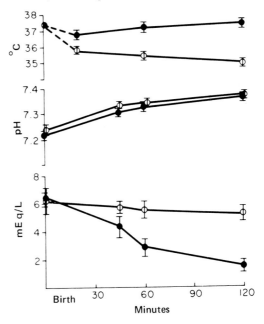

Under these conditions, metabolic acidosis persists, although the vigorous infant achieves a normal pH by increasing carbon dioxide elimination. In the depressed infant, cooling after birth causes a fall in pH and a greater increase in metabolic acidosis. The time at which the cord is clamped following delivery does not appear to influence the newborn's acid–base readjustment.

Several explanations have been offered for the low arterial carbon dioxide pressure (about 32 mm Hg) observed in healthy infants once normal acid–base balance has been achieved. These include hyperventilation due to anoxia or increased levels of organic acids, the influence of progesterone on the respiratory center, the presence of shunts through the fetal channels during the neonatal period, and the respiratory response to mild cold stress noted earlier. At present, it is not known which, if any, of these factors plays the major role.

Respiration

Onset of Breathing

The first breath is in part a continuation of fetal respiratory movements before birth. However, a number of additional factors appear to be important for the initial effort to expand the lungs and for the subsequent maintenance of rhythmic breathing.

Among the stimuli implicated, asphyxia holds a favored position as the principal driving force. There is little doubt that a fall in arterial oxygen tension and pH, accompanied by a rise in carbon dioxide tension, produces gasping *in utero* as well as after birth. Rhythmic breathing may follow an improvement in oxygenation and normalization of acid–base state. The respiratory drive during asphyxia depends on the presence of carotid and aortic chemoreceptors, which are known to be functional in the newborn. However, neither hypoxia nor hypercapnia alone initiates breathing in the experimental animal. This suggests that either the chemoreceptors of the fetus do not respond to hypoxia in the presence of normal pH and carbon dioxide tension or that the state of activity of the respiratory neurons is such that the afferent stimuli from the carotid and aortic chemoreceptors do not lead to a sufficient efferent discharge.

The short time interval between birth and the first breath suggests that the respiratory centers are activated by impulses from peripheral receptors initiated by stimuli other than the relatively slow changes in blood composition. Thermal stimuli immediately after birth must be intense. Calculations based on the rate of fall of skin temperature in the first minutes of extrauterine life indicate that at room temperature the newborn human infant loses about 600 cal/min.

Although thermal stimuli appear to be of particular importance, tactile stimuli do not. Strong stimulation of the fetal lamb by surgical incision produces a gasp, but rhythmic breathing is not initiated. Occlusion of the umbilical cord causes a prompt but transient rise in blood pressure and occasional gasping; however, breathing can occur in the presence of intact umbilical circulation both *in utero* and after delivery.

The First Breath

Most infants make respiratory efforts within a few seconds of being born, and after the first few breaths the lungs are almost completely expanded. This was not the case earlier in the century, when heavy maternal medication and general anesthesia were widely employed for delivery. The onset of breathing was frequently delayed for several minutes, during which tactile and thermal stimuli were applied, often combined with the administration of analeptics.

The first inspiration is usually followed by a cry as the infant expires against a partially closed glottis, creating a positive intrathoracic pressure of up to 40 cm H_2O. Within a few minutes, functional residual capacity reaches about three quarters of final aeration.

Although the intrathoracic pressures recorded during the first breaths are high, it is surprising how often initial lung expansion appears to require little effort. The work for initial lung expansion is undeniably greater than that for quiet breathing, but it is not greater than that performed many times a day during vigorous crying.

Dimensions and Operational Factors of the Lung in the Postnatal Period

Following lung expansion, the functional residual capacity is about 70 ml in the term infant and changes little over the first six days of life. The respiratory rate is approximately 30 per minute in the mature infant and 40 per minute in the preterm infant. Tidal and minute volumes are approximately 20 ml and 600 ml, respectively, for the mature infant and 10 ml and 400 ml for the preterm. There is a significant direct relation between minute volume and weight of the infant, the volume of air breathed being greater by approximately 120 ml/kg body weight in the larger infant.

Basal oxygen consumption values range 4 ml to 5 ml/kg body weight/minute and are approximately 30% higher than those of the adult man. The difference is due to the infant's having a greater proportion of tissues with high metabolic rates in relation to total body weight. The respiratory quotient has limited meaning in the early neonatal period because of disparity between production and output of carbon dioxide. Immediately after birth, the baby is recovering from a metabolic and respiratory acidosis, and if the baby is exposed to room temperature (25°C; 77°F), this problem can be very considerably compounded.

The sensitivity of the respiratory center of the newborn to carbon dioxide is similar to that of the adult. Ventilation increases at least 100% in the vigorous infant when alveolar carbon dioxide tension changes from 40 mm Hg to 50 mm Hg. Ventilation is depressed if the alveolar carbon dioxide tension rises above 80 mm Hg.

The ventilatory response to breathing a gas mixture of low oxygen content is not as pronounced in the newborn infant as in the adult; hyperpnea may not appear, or it may last only a few minutes. Animal experiments indicate that this diminished response can result from cool environmental conditions. If 100% oxygen is substituted for air, there is a temporary decrease in ventilation in the healthy infant but no change in oxygen consumption. On the other hand, administration of higher oxygen mixtures increases ventilation in infants with the respiratory distress syndrome and restores oxygen consumption to normal levels in infants depressed at birth.

Respiratory Responses During and Following Asphyxia

The cardiovascular, respiratory, and biochemical changes that occur during asphyxia under controlled conditions are predictable. Information on this subject is most complete in the newborn monkey. During the initial phase of asphyxia of the unanesthetized newborn animal, respiratory efforts increase in depth and frequency for up to 3 minutes. This period, called *primary hyperpnea,* is followed by primary apnea lasting for approximately 1 minute. Rhythmic gasping then begins and is maintained at a fairly constant rate of about 6 gasps per minute for several minutes. The gasps finally become weaker and slower. Their cessation marks the beginning of secondary apnea.

There is some variation in the duration of gasping (time to the last gasp) in different species, depending on the initial acid–base state, drugs given to the mother, environmental temperature, and degree of maturity of the species at birth. At a given environmental temperature, the principal determinant of duration of gasping in the nonanesthetized animal is the initial arterial *p*H. Narcotics and systemic anesthetic agents administered to the mother can abolish the period of primary hyperpnea and prolong primary apnea; large doses can suppress all respiratory efforts. Gasping is always prolonged at lower body temperatures.

During primary apnea, a variety of stimuli, such as pain, cold, and analeptics, can initiate gasping. Once the stage of secondary apnea has been reached, these stimuli are without effect. Gasping can, however, be reinitiated by artificial ventilation or correction of acidosis by administration of base. There is a linear relation between the duration of asphyxia and recovery of respiratory function after resuscitation. In newborn monkeys, for each minute after the last gasp that artificial ventilation is delayed, there is a further delay of 2 minutes before gasping begins again and of 4 minutes before rhythmic breathing is established (Fig. 42-3). This indicates that the longer artificial ventilation is delayed during secondary apnea, the longer it will take to resuscitate the infant.

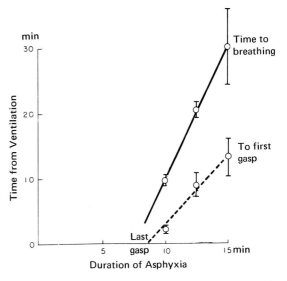

FIG. 42-3. Time from ventilation to first gasp and to rhythmic breathing in newborn monkeys asphyxiated for 10, 12.5, and 15 minutes at 30°C. Mean time from onset of asphyxia until last gasp was 8.42 ± 0.24 (SE) minutes. (Adamsons K Jr., Behrman R, Dawes GS, James LS, Koford C: J Pediatr 65:807, 1964)

Changes in Circulation After Birth

With the onset of respiration and lung expansion, pulmonary vascular resistance falls. This appears to be due largely to the direct effect of oxygen and carbon dioxide on the blood vessels; resistance decreases as oxygen tension rises and carbon dioxide tension falls. Lung expansion per se contributes to lowering of the pulmonary vascular resistance. There then follows a gradual transition from the fetal to the adult type of circulation, the foramen ovale and ductus arteriosus remaining open for varying lengths of time.

Pressure in the left atrium falls in the first few hours of life to levels below those in the normal adult; by 24 hours, it may be less than 1 mm Hg above that in the right atrium. This small pressure difference probably accounts for the persistence of a right-to-left shunt through the foramen ovale for 24 hours or longer.

Pulmonary arterial pressure remains relatively high for several hours. As the pulmonary vascular resistance falls, the direction of blood flow through the ductus arteriosus reverses. In the first hours of extrauterine life, the flow is bidirectional, but the shunt eventually becomes entirely left to right and by 15 hours of age is functionally insignificant.

The ductus arteriosus constricts in response to an increase in arterial oxygen tension. Sympathomimetic amines also cause it to constrict. Hypoxemia can cause a constricted ductus to reopen and at the same time may reestablish the fetal pattern of circulation by increasing pulmonary vascular resistance. This response of the ductus arteriosus to oxygen or hypoxia is thus the opposite of that of the pulmonary arterioles, enabling the right ventricle to contribute a variable fraction of its output to placental perfusion during fetal life. The different reactivity of these vessels during hypoxia, although an asset to the fetus, becomes a liability for the newborn infant. Hypoxic episodes in early neonatal life can lead to a rise in pulmonary vascular resistance and opening of the ductus arteriosus, increasing any residual right-to-left shunt. The reasons for the different responses of these vessels to hypoxia have not so far been determined.

Thermoregulation in the Newborn

Measurements of metabolic rate in the immediate neonatal period have established that newborn human babies, like most warm-blooded mammals, increase their metabolic rate in response to cold; their low thermal stability is due to excessive heat loss rather than to impaired heat production.

The difference in rate of thermal energy dissipation between the newborn and the adult can be explained largely by differences in physical characteristics. At birth, the body mass of the human baby is about 5% that of the adult, while surface area amounts to nearly 15%. The high ratio between body surface and body mass, together with increased curvature of body surfaces, facilitates thermal exchange by convection and radiation. Thickness of skin and subcutaneous fat insulating deeper body structures is significantly less at birth, resulting in greater thermal conductance and a higher skin temperature at low environmental temperatures. As a result of these differences, heat loss per unit of body weight in the term infant is approximately 4 times that in the adult. This value increases further for the preterm infant or the infant of small body size.

In the immediate neonatal period, the body temperature of the human newborn may fall as much as 2°C to 3°C (see Fig. 42-2). It has been calculated that heat losses in the initial minutes following birth may amount to as much as 200 cal/kg/minute under normal delivery room conditions. Several factors are responsible for the high rate of heat loss. At the time of delivery, the deep body temperature of the newborn is about 0.5°C and the skin temperature about 2.5°C higher than that encountered during extrauterine life; there is virtually no thermal gradient between peripheral tissues and deeper structures. Evaporation of amniotic fluid from the skin also contributes to heat loss. Excess heat stored in the peripheral and deeper tissues of the fetus minimizes the impact of the new environment. For the fetus at term, the overall reserve could be as much as 4000 cal.

It remains to be elucidated whether the transient fall in peripheral and deep body temperature that occurs immediately after birth favors or hinders adaptation to extrauterine life. Thermal stimuli might be important in the initiation and establishment of breathing by increasing the state of activity of the reticular system. Cold perception induces cutaneous vasoconstriction and raises systemic vascular resistance, which might be important in the reduction of right-to-left shunting through the patent ductus arteriosus. Prolonged exposure of the naked infant to room temperature, on the other hand, has been shown to lead to progressive metabolic acidosis, particularly in the depressed infant or the infant with impaired pulmonary function.

In homeothermic species, the first line of defense in reducing heat loss consists of cutaneous vasoconstriction, which diminishes the temperature gradient between body surface and environment. Vasoconstriction in response to cold stimuli occurs not only in the term infant but also in the preterm infant from the time of birth. Further reduction in heat loss can be achieved by postural changes that decrease the body surface available for thermal exchange. Increases in metabolic rate in response to cold also serve to maintain body temperature, and the naked newborn responds in this way. Although measurements have not yet been made in the first minutes of life, it is known that infants only 15 minutes old are able to double or even triple their oxygen consumption. A similar response has been documented in preterm infants.

Oxygen consumption in the cold environment is predominantly a function of the temperature gradient between body surface and environment, not of the absolute values of deep body, skin, or environmental temperatures. Basal metabolic rates are observed in healthy mature newborns with varying deep body or skin temperatures as long as the temperature gradient between skin and environment is less than 1.5°C. Once this limit is exceeded, oxygen consumption begins to rise at a rate of approximately 0.6 ml/°C, reaching values up to 15 ml/kg/minute. This compares favorably with maximal heat production of the adult under severe cold stress. From a teleologic point of view, dependence on the thermal gradient rather than the absolute temperature is advantageous because it enables the newborn to reduce oxygen consumption to basal levels as soon as thermal conditions are favorable, allowing a gradual rise in body temperature to normal levels without additional expenditure of energy.

Increased muscular activity probably plays a major role in heat production. However, the metabolic rate can rise without shivering or increased muscular tone, as shown in animal experiments during paralysis of the neuromuscular junction. The brown adipose tissue of the newborn appears to be a source of heat production. The brown fat deposits in the interscapular region, axillae, and perirenal areas, and around large vessels in the chest, are rich in blood and nerve supply and have a high mitochondrial content and a high metabolic rate *in vitro*. Although thermal output of brown fat could make an important contribution to total heat production in certain newborn animals, it is not essential for temperature regulation in all homeothermic species; the newborn piglet, which has virtually no adipose tissue, either white or brown, shows an excellent metabolic response to cold. It is not known to what extent other organs, such as liver and brain, contribute to the increase in total body metabolism during cooling.

The physiological mediator that links perception of cold with increased metabolic activity and thus increased heat production is still unknown. Sympathomimetic amines can increase heat production in the adult, and this response is pronounced in the cold-adapted and in the newborn animal. Increases in oxygen consumption have been observed during intravenous infusion of nor-epinephrine in the human newborn. On the other hand, adrenergic blockade does not alter the increase in oxygen consumption upon exposure to cold, although it does obliterate the response to exogenous noradrenalin.

A variety of factors can interfere with normal homeothermal responses in the newborn. Hypoxia is of particular importance, although sensitivity to oxygen lack varies among species. The newborn human fails to respond to cold when breathing gas mixtures of 15% oxygen. If respiration and adequate oxygenation are not promptly established after birth, the effects of birth asphyxia upon thermoregulation can be rather long lasting. Differences in deep body temperature between asphyxiated and vigorous infants have been detected for up to 20 hours after birth.

Few data are available about the effects of hypnotics, analgesics, anesthetics, and neuromuscular autonomic blocking agents on thermoregulation of the newborn. Administration of meperidine hydrochloride to the mother during labor leads to greater than normal fall in the infant's body temperature in the neonatal period. In the experimental animal, administration of reserpine, a drug known to deplete the body of catecholamine stores, has produced thermal instability in the newborn by interfering with heat conservation. If depression of the newborn is due to excessive maternal medication, it is important to recognize that a fall in body temperature not only potentiates but also prolongs the effect of most analgesic and anesthetic drugs.

RESUSCITATION

The delivery room must be prepared for adequate and prompt treatment of severe asphyxia at birth, regardless of whether it is expected. All members of the delivery room team should be trained in methods of resuscitation, since both mother and baby may be in difficulty at the same time. Indecision or ineffective therapy may lose the few moments during which the baby can be helped.

Every piece of apparatus necessary for emergency resuscitation should be carefully checked before each delivery. There should be suction apparatus, a plastic oropharyngeal airway, a laryngoscope equipped with a pencil handle and a blade, and a plastic endotracheal tube with a stylet. Oxygen should be available. All examinations and needed resuscitation should be conducted on an appropriate table or resuscitator equipped with an overhead source of heat to maintain the baby's body temperature.

Initial Treatment and Appraisal of the Infant

The fetal heart rate should be determined after every contraction during the final stages of labor or, preferably, monitored continuously. The growing use of electronic monitoring of fetal heart rate and biochemical monitoring of fetal acid–base state has enabled earlier recognition of warning signs of fetal distress and allows the obstetrician to take appropriate measures before the infant becomes severely asphyxiated.

Immediately after delivery, the baby should be held head down while the cord is clamped and cut. The infant should then be placed supine on a table, the head kept low with a slight lateral tilt. A nurse or assistant should listen to the heartbeat immediately, indicating the rate by finger movement. If help is not available, the rate can be detected from pulsation of the umbilical cord. A strong beat with a rate of over 100 per minute indicates that there is no immediate emergency. Distant heart sounds or a slow rate indicates severe depression, calling for resuscitative measures. While the nurse is listening to the heart, the physician should aspirate the mouth, the pharynx, and the nose with a catheter. This suction should be brief. From birth to completion of suctioning should take about 1 minute. Slapping the soles lightly frequently aids in initiating a deep breath and crying. More severe methods of stimulation, such as dilating the anal sphincter, hot and cold tubbing, and vigorous backslapping, are traumatic, ineffectual, and a waste of time.

The initial appraisal of the newborn should start at the moment of birth, with particular attention given to the first few breaths and the evenness and ease of respiration. A congenital laryngeal web or choanal atresia can cause complete airway obstruction; both require immediate treatment. A diaphragmatic hernia with abdominal viscera in the chest, abdominal distention from ascites, congenial cystic lungs, or intrauterine pneumonia may all cause respiratory difficulty and may even prevent lung expansion.

The scoring system introduced by Apgar in 1952 is a useful method by which to quantitate the clinical evaluation of the baby (Table 42-1). The score is based on heart rate, respiratory effort, muscle tone, reflex irritability, and color. A score of 0 each is given for no heartbeat, no respiratory effort, no muscle tone, no reflex response to a glancing slap on the soles of the feet, and a pale color. A score of 1 each is given for a slow heartbeat, slow or irregular respiratory effort, some flexion of the extremities, a grimace in response to a glancing slap on the soles of the feet, and a blue coloration. A score of 2 each is given for a heart rate over 100, a good respiratory effort accompanied by crying, a cry in response to the slap on the feet, and a completely healthy coloration. At 60 seconds after birth of the infant, the

Table 42-1
Clinical Evaluation of the Newborn Infant in the Delivery Room by the Apgar Scoring Method

Sign	0	1	2
Heart rate	None	Below 100	Over 100
Respiratory effort	None	Weak cry; hypoventilation	Good; strong cry
Muscle tone	Limp	Some flexion of extremities	Active motion; extremities well flexed
Reflex irritability (response to stimulation of sole of foot)	No response	Grimace	Cry
Color	Pale	Blue	Completely pink

five objective signs are evaluated and each scored as 0, 1, or 2. A score of 10 indicates an infant in the best possible condition. The majority of infants are vigorous, with a score of 7 to 10, and cough or cry within seconds of delivery. No further resuscitative procedures are necessary for them. Mildly to moderately depressed infants form the largest group requiring some form of resuscitation at birth. These infants are pale or blue at 1 minute after delivery; they have not established sustained respirations and may be nearly flaccid. However, their heart rates and reflex irritability are good. Their scores may be 4, 5, or 6. Severely depressed infants are flaccid, unresponsive, and pale; their Apgar scores are 0, 1, or 2.

Immediately after the cord is cut and breathing is established, a drop of 1% silver nitrate is instilled in each eye as prophylaxis against gonorrheal ophthalmia. In some states it is stipulated that silver nitrate be used in all cases; in others the use of less irritating agents, such as penicillin or tetracycline ointment, is permitted.

Treatment of the Moderately Depressed Infant

The time required for recovery, and also the completeness of recovery, are direct functions of the duration of asphyxia (see Fig. 42-3). If initial resuscitative measures have produced no response by 1.5 minutes after delivery, the progressing asphyxia usually leads to diminished muscular tone and a fall in heart rate. A small plastic oropharyngeal airway should then be inserted into the mouth and oxygen applied under pressure of 16 cm to 20 cm H_2O for 1 to 2 seconds. Although this pressure is sufficient to expand the alveoli, some oxygen will reach the respiratory bronchioles. The rise in intrabronchial pressure stimulates pulmonary stretch receptors. This stimulus, added to that of the chemoreceptors, initiates a gasp in about 85% of the cases.

If there is no respiratory effort and the heart rate continues to fall, the infant becoming completely flaccid, the larynx should be visualized with the laryngoscope. This is not a difficult procedure, but skill should be obtained by practice on the stillborn. An ideal method of teaching and learning this technique is by use of an adult cat anesthetized with ketamine hydrochloride.

Intubation is best accomplished with the infant lying supine on a flat surface. A folded towel under the head and slight extension of the neck place the infant in a position resembling a sniffing posture. The head should be steadied with the right hand and kept in line with the body. The laryngoscope is held in the left hand, and the blade is introduced at the right corner of the mouth and advanced between tongue and palate for about 2 cm. As it is advanced, the blade is swung to the midline. This moves the tongue to the left of the blade. The operator looks along the blade for the rim of the epiglottis. The laryngoscope is gently advanced into the space between the base of the tongue and the epiglottis (Fig. 42-4). Slight elevation of the tip of the blade exposes the glottis as a vertical dark slit bordered posteriorly by pink arytenoid cartilages.

If foreign material such as small blood clots, meconium-stained mucus, or vernix obstructs the larynx, quick, brief suction is indicated. When the glottis is seen to be patent, a curved endotracheal tube is introduced at the right corner of the mouth and inserted through the cords until the flange of the tube rests at the glottis. Care must be taken not to intubate the esophagus. The

FIG. 42-4. Sagittal view of mouth and pharynx showing relation of laryngoscope blade to epiglottis.

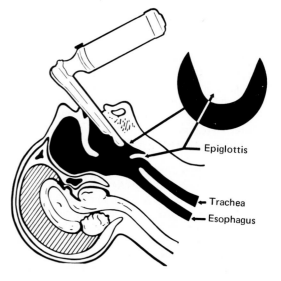

laryngoscope is then withdrawn. Rarely, the glottis is obstructed by a laryngeal web. If this is partial or thin, it may be perforated with a stylet, or the opening may be enlarged with an endotracheal tube. The presence of a thick membrane requires immediate tracheostomy.

If stimuli from these procedures have not initiated a spontaneous gasp, positive pressure should be applied to the endotracheal tube. Brief puffs of air blown through the tube with enough force to cause the lower chest to rise gently usually start spontaneous respiration. If the stomach rises, however, the esophagus has been intubated instead of the trachea, and the position of the tube must be corrected. Pressures between 25 cm and 35 cm H_2O are necessary to expand the alveoli initially and can be applied safely for 1 to 2 seconds. Experience in applying this pressure should be gained by puffing into a spring manometer. Oxygen-enriched gas may be delivered to the infant by placement of a tube carrying oxygen in the operator's mouth.

If the endotracheal tube is fitted with appropriate-sized adapters, it can be connected to a rubber bag of oxygen or oxygen-enriched gas mixture, or to one of the mechanical devices for applying positive pressure.

Artificial expansion of the lungs can initiate a spontaneous gasp. With the first or second application of positive pressure, the infant usually makes an effort to breathe. The endotracheal tube may be withdrawn after the infant has taken five or six breaths.

Treatment of the Severely Depressed Infant

No time should be lost in establishing ventilation. The glottis should be inspected immediately with the laryngoscope. If meconium or thick meconium-stained mucus has been aspirated into the trachea, it must be suctioned out at once prior to inflation of the lungs. It is usually possible to accomplish this within one minute after delivery. These severely depressed infants may require three to eight minutes of artificial ventilation before a spontaneous gasp is taken. The endotracheal tube can be removed as soon as quiet and sustained respiration is established.

Under some circumstances, lung expansion is impossible in spite of proper intubation. There are four conditions in which this occurs: massive aspiration of meconium that cannot be removed by suctioning, intrauterine pneumonia with organization of exudate, large bilateral diaphragmatic hernias with hypoplastic lungs, and congenital adenomatous cysts of the lung. Infants with the first two conditions are usually severely depressed at birth. However, those with hypoplastic lungs may be initially vigorous, scoring as high as 7 at 1 minute of age, and may make strenuous but ineffective respiratory efforts. At present there is no available treatment for this condition. Congenital adenomatous cysts of the lung are associated with hydrops fetalis, a condition that is usually fatal.

Use of Cardiac Massage

Blood pressure and heart rate fall during prolonged asphyxia. If blood pressure is unduly low at the beginning of resuscitation, positive-pressure ventilation is unlikely to be successful unless the heart is massaged. Cardiac massage has been successfully applied through the intact chest wall in human infants.

External manual compression of the heart between the chest wall and vertebral column forces blood into the aorta. Relaxation of pressure allows the heart to fill with venous blood. When combined with proper ventilation, external manual heart compression often maintains blood pressure and adequate oxygenation until spontaneous cardiac activity returns.

The technique consists of intermittent compression of the middle and lower thirds of the sternum 100 to 120 times per minute with the index and middle fingers. Massage is interrupted every 5 seconds to permit two or three inflations of the lung. It should be employed only after the lungs have been well expanded when a heartbeat cannot be detected or the heart rate does not rise promptly. Cardiopulmonary resuscitation is most successful when there has been no evidence of fetal distress.

Use of Analeptics and Drug Antagonists

Analeptics such as nikethamide serve no useful purpose in resuscitation of the newborn. Although they may shorten primary apnea, they are ineffective in secondary apnea (see earlier discussion) and may cause hypotension and convulsions, even if given in the clinically recommended dose.

Naloxone hydrochloride (Narcan) is useful when the depression of respiration in the newborn is due to transplacentally acquired opiates and related compounds. The recommended dose is 0.01 mg per kg of body weight. The drug should be given intramuscularly, intravenously, or subcutaneously after expansion of lungs and the establishment of adequate oxygenation. Although crying and restlessness often follow the administration of Narcan, they are frequently of brief duration and may be followed by even more profound depression of the central nervous system owing to the intrinsic depressant properties of the compound.

The role of epinephrine in the resuscitation of the severely asphyxiated fetus or newborn remains to be determined. Studies with fetal monkeys have demonstrated that large doses of epinephrine (1–5 mμ/kg) administered either intravenously or intra-arterially initiate heart action and restore blood pressure and heart rate to normal in the severely asphyxiated fetus. However, because epinephrine increases pulmonary arterial pressure considerably above normal, there is a distinct risk of increasing filtration of plasma into the alveolar spaces with the resultant clinical picture of pulmonary edema.

Rapid Correction of *p*H

In experimental animals, maintenance of normal *p*H during asphyxia by rapid intravenous infusion of alkali, together with glucose, prolongs gasping and delays cardiovascular collapse. Resuscitation is also facilitated if alkali and glucose are infused at the same time artificial ventilation is started. It has been proposed that the beneficial effects of *p*H correction are derived from prolongation and acceleration of anaerobic glycolysis, restitution of oxygen-carrying capacity of hemoglobin and responsiveness of cardiovascular muscle to sympathomimetic amines, and fall in pulmonary vascular resistance.

Administration of alkali to the asphyxiated newborn has been shown to increase the rate of recovery and responsiveness of the infant. However, the demonstration that alkali administration is associated with intracranial hemorrhage and hypernatremia has caused much concern. These adverse effects of alkali appear to be due to injudicious use, particularly in the presence of impaired carbon dioxide elimination. If the agent is given in too high a concentration, in too great a quantity, and in the presence of severely impaired ventilation, the adverse effects undoubtedly outweigh the benefits.

The most severely asphyxiated infants—those with an arterial *p*H below 7.0—have a base deficit of 26 mEq/liter or greater, in addition to a marked elevation in carbon dioxide tension. By means of artificial ventilation alone, the base deficit can be reduced by approximately 10 mEq/liter in 5 to 10 minutes, provided good alveolar ventilation is achieved and circulatory collapse does not persist. It is advisable initially to attempt to correct half of the residual metabolic component of the mixed acidosis. Thus, a 3-kg infant would receive 8 mEq base. This calculation assumes that the extracellular volume is one third the body weight.

In infants who are so severely asphyxiated that the heart rate does not return after good lung expansion and several episodes of cardiac massage, infusion of alkali or further resuscitation efforts are not recommended.

Use of Hypothermia

There are several reasons why hypothermia might be a valuable adjunct in the resuscitation of the asphyxiated newborn. Metabolic rate could be lowered; increased peripheral vasoconstriction could help maintain blood pressure; carbon dioxide tension could be lowered, owing to increased solubility of carbon dioxide at lower temperature; and *p*H could be elevated, owing to changes in the dissociation constants of water and the other acids. However, the rate of cooling is slow, particularly in the presence of a collapsed circulation, and the rise in *p*H and fall in carbon dioxide tension are small compared with the changes that accompany ventilation.

Experiments in which cooling starts at the same time as asphyxia have no bearing on asphyxia before birth, when the fetus is at a warmer temperature than the mother. Hypothermia as a resuscitative procedure has been tried under controlled experimental conditions in newborn monkeys asphyxiated before cooling; respiration was not reinitiated and brain damage not prevented.

PHYSICAL EXAMINATION IN THE DELIVERY ROOM

As soon as respiration is well established, the physician should carefully examine the newborn to determine the presence of abnormalities, such as tracheoesophageal fistula, duodenal atresia, imperforate anus, or arteriovenous fistula, that require prompt attention. It is also important that less serious defects and birth injuries be discovered first by the physician so that necessary explanations can be made to the mother. The sequence in which various systems of the infant are examined differs somewhat from that customarily employed in the adult.

Skin

The color of the skin is normally pale pink, except for the hands and feet, which may remain cyanotic for more than an hour, even in vigorous infants. Some differential cyanosis of the lower part of the body due to persistence of right-to-left shunting through the ductus arteriosus is often present for the first 30 minutes of life. This is demonstrated more clearly if the infant is given a high concentration of oxygen for 5 to 10 seconds. Persistence of differential cyanosis indicates failure of ductus closure, high pulmonary vascular resistance, or preductal coarctation. These changes are less apparent in infants with pigmented skin. Generalized cyanosis, even with gross cardiac anomalies, after the onset of respiration is rare. Presumably, it is caused by cutaneous vasoconstriction. It is seen in the first few minutes of life in infants who experience difficulties in establishing ventilation.

A generalized pallor indicates either intense vasoconstriction or anemia. The former is present in more axphyxiated infants. The latter should be suspected in the presence of erythroblastosis, placenta previa, or multiple pregnancy, but it can also occur as a result of intraplacental shunts between fetus and mother and, occasionally, with a nuchal cord.

Yellow appearance of the skin and umbilical cord is usually the result of meconium staining and is accompanied by golden coloring of the vernix and meconium in the amniotic fluid. It is also seen in erythroblastotic infants who are severely anemic at birth. Since retention of bilirubin is a late phenomenon in erythroblastosis fetalis, jaundice at birth is rather rare; it may be seen at birth, however, with severe intrauterine infection and hepatitis.

The skin of a normal infant is smooth and elastic. Subcutaneous fat varies in thickness from a fraction of a millimeter in the region of the thorax and scalp to a few millimeters over the abdomen, back, and buttocks. Vernix is usually seen, particularly in the skin folds, and lanugo is present over the back. Diminution of elasticity and subcutaneous fat, together with peeling and wrinkling of the skin, indicate intrauterine malnutrition. In the mature infant, such changes are accompanied by meconium staining. They occur more frequently in the presence of prolonged gestation, or maternal hypertension or preeclampsia. The birth weight of these infants is usually less than expected for gestational age, and they are prone to hypoglycemia in the neonatal period.

Thickening of subcutaneous tissue can be due to edema or fat. The latter is common in infants of diabetic or prediabetic mothers.

Petechiae over the head and neck are seen when there has been a tight nuchal cord or delay in delivery of the body due to shoulder impaction. The presence of pigmented nevi or hemangiomas should be recorded and hemangiomas carefully examined for bruit or pulsation that would indicate an arteriovenous fistula.

Rashes, which are rare, result from viral (varicella, rubella, and cytomegalic inclusion disease) or protozoal (syphilis) infection *in utero*.

Head and Neck

There is considerable variation in the shape of the head as the result of molding during labor and delivery, particularly in the infants of primiparas and in those presenting with the occiput posterior. The head is spherical in infants delivered by the breech or by cesarean section. Excessive elongation should be noted because of the possibility of tentorial tears. Edema of the subcutaneous tissue of the leading parts (usually occiput) is common. Cephalhematoma differs from scalp edema (with or without subcutaneous extravasation of blood) by being confined within the area of one of the cranial bones. Vacuum extractors create a sharply demarcated circular edema that may reach up to 2 cm in thickness; it disappears more slowly than naturally occurring edema. Forceps marks consisting of depressions or edema with erythema and sometimes abrasions frequently signify a traumatic delivery and may be associated with cranial nerve injuries or skull fractures. These should be suspected, particularly in cases of improper application of forceps (face–mastoid). Fortunately, in modern obstetrics, the elimination of most complicated vaginal deliveries in favor of cesarean section has considerably reduced the incidence of these complications.

The anterior fontanel is open and should be palpated for size and tension. Bulging is diagnostic of intracranial pressure and may indicate hydrocephalus or intracranial hemorrhage. The posterior fontanel is closed and is frequently difficult to outline owing to scalp edema. If it is open, hydrocephalus should be suspected. A small or closed anterior fontanel occurs in a condition known as *craniosynostosis* and is not infrequently accompanied by microcephaly or an abnormally shaped head. Soft spots in the skull (craniotabes) are present in about one third of all newborn infants, preferentially located in the parietal area. Rarely, a cranial bone may be missing, indicating osteogenesis imperfecta.

The eyes are usually closed but may be open in postterm infants; in infants with severe asphyxia, they may be wide open and staring. The pupils' size and reactivity to light and the color of the sclera should be noted. Fixed dilated pupils, or anisocoria, indicates severe asphyxia or brain damage. Subconjunctival hemorrhage is occasionally seen following difficult breech or impacted shoulders delivery.

Examination of the position and shape of the external ear is important because malformations are associated with renal anomalies. If the ears are low set or the configuration is deformed, the umbilical cord should be examined to determine if it lacks one umbilical artery, and the infant should be closely observed for the passage of urine.

Saddle deformity of the nose, a pathognomonic sign of congenital syphilis, has virtually disappeared with the advent of antibiotics and improvements in antenatal care.

Since infants prefer nose to mouth breathing, occlusion of the upper airway can cause respiratory difficulties; choanal atresia has resulted in death from asphyxia in infants with no other abnormality of the respiratory tract. Testing for nasal patency is best achieved by occlusion of one nostril and the mouth, rather than passage of a catheter, which can be injurious. Microglossia or underdevelopment of the lower jaw (micrognathia) can also cause obstruction of the airway and can be responsible for difficulties encountered during resuscitation. Slight recession of the mandible is not uncommon in normal infants. Masses in the neck, notably by enlarged thyroid, can cause tracheal compression, which may necessitate tracheotomy. The palate should be inspected with the laryngoscope or palpated. However, even careful palpation is likely to miss posterior defects.

Thorax

The chest must be observed and auscultated for evenness of aeration. In infants 5 minutes of age, adventitious sounds normally remain only over the precordial area. By 20 minutes of age the chest should be clear; persistence of adventitious sounds at this age indicates an aspiration syndrome or intrauterine pneumonia. Sternal or intercostal retraction in term infants is abnormal and indicates airway obstruction or incomplete lung expansion. In preterm infants, some retraction is expected because of the softness of the chest wall and less compliant lung. Prolongation of expiration with or without an audible grunt is also abnormal and frequently is the first sign of incipient respiratory distress syndrome.

Diminished or absent breath sounds on one side are indicative of pneumothorax or diaphragmatic hernia with abdominal viscera in the chest. Percussion usually differentiates the two. Soft or distant heart sounds associated with an increase in heart rate are found with pneumomediastinum. If any of these conditions is suspected, the chest should be x-rayed. (Pneumomediastinum can always be managed conservatively, and pneumothorax usually so; however, if a tension pneumothorax develops, this should be promptly treated by insertion of a blunt needle into the intrapleural space and institution of underwater drainage. Diaphragmatic hernia requires prompt consultation and operative correction.)

The clavicles and ribs should be palpated for fractures, which can be associated with vascular or nerve injuries. This is particularly important if pneumothorax or pneumomediastinum is present. Occasionally, fracture of a rib leads to emphysema of the chest wall, causing crepitus.

The heart is nearly in the midline, and there is frequently marked precordial activity during the first 30 minutes of life, when bidirectional shunting through the ductus arteriosus is maximal. The heart rate following delivery is 160 to 170 beats per minute, which is 15% higher than the rate during labor. By 20 to 30 minutes of age, the rate returns to the previous level. This transient acceleration of heart rate probably represents a response to high levels of catecholamines, as well as various tactile, auditory, and thermal stimuli. Furthermore, increased total cardiac output in the presence of bidirectional shunting is necessary if the rate of tissue perfusion is to remain constant.

A pansystolic crescendo murmur is present in approximately 15% of all infants during the first two hours of life. It is more common in preterm infants and in those recovering from severe asphyxia. Its cause has not yet been determined. Two likely possibilities are shunting through the ductus arteriosus and regurgitation through the mitral or tricuspid valve. Only one third of infants with cardiac malformation have detectable murmurs in the neonatal period.

Abdomen

Before the abdomen is palpated for abnormal masses, the catheter used for oropharyngeal suction during resuscitation should be passed through the mouth and esophagus into the stomach. When the catheter tip is in the proper position, there is usually a bulge in the left upper abdominal quadrant. Even if this is not seen, suction should be applied to the tube and the stomach emptied. Should no secretions be obtained, the position of the catheter should be verified by injection of air

through it during auscultation of the epigastrium. Esophageal atresia or tracheoesophageal fistula must be suspected if difficulties are encountered in the passage of a catheter. The stomach of the newborn contains 4 ml to 8 ml fluid, the volume tending to be greater in infants born by elective cesarean section. Duodenal atresia or other types of upper gastrointestinal tract obstructions are likely to be present if larger quantities of fluid are obtained.

Emptying the stomach is essentially a diagnostic procedure, but it may be therapeutic if the volume of fluid in the stomach is large enough to interfere with movement of the diaphragm. If a soft rubber or plastic catheter is used, there is virtually no danger of visceral injury. Perforation of the stomach in the newborn may occur spontaneously as a result of muscular defects or ulcers.

The liver and kidneys can readily be felt at this time; the liver is relatively large, extending about 3 cm below the costal margin in the midclavicular line.

The anal region should be inspected and the patency of the lower large bowel tested by insertion of the previously used rubber catheter for 8 cm. If anal atresia is present, the bladder should be catheterized and the urine examined for particulate matter, since a rectovesical fistula is frequently associated with this condition.

Genitalia

Examination of the female genitalia is limited to inspection of the labia and clitoris, which is normally hypertrophied. Opaque viscous mucus normally covers the introitus. The urethral meatus is not identified, but patency of the urinary tract can be verified by observation of the passage of urine.

In the male infant, the prepuce is usually adherent and should not be retracted. The position of the testicles should be noted. They are normally in the scrotum, although during the examination they may be retracted toward the inguinal ligament by high tone of the cremaster muscle.

Back and Extremities

The sacrum should be examined for pigmentation and abnormal hair, which is not uncommonly associated with occult spina bifida. Limb position and movement should be observed. Normally, the limbs are flexed and exhibit irregular movement when the infant is stimulated to cry or exposed to cold. Flaccid extension of a limb suggests a nerve injury, which most commonly involves the arm as a result of brachial plexus damage. The extremities should be palpated for fractures. Since such fractures are frequently incomplete, they are not readily detected; if there is reason to suspect one, the limb should be x-rayed. The digits should be counted and examined for webbing.

Neurologic Examination

Usually limited to testing of the grasp and Moro reflexes, neurologic examination is brief. If the infant has had a low Apgar score and remains limp after respiration is established, there is an increased possibility of neurologic impairment. When the infant is asphyxiated at birth, the examiner should evaluate the anterior fontanels and look for signs of brain swelling, such as separation of the cranial sutures. Examination of eyegrounds reveals retinal hemorrhages in most such cases. Because brain swelling secondary to partial or prolonged oxygen deprivation *in utero* requires several hours to develop, its failure to appear immediately after delivery does not exclude the development of this serious complication.

Diagnosis of systemic congenital anomalies such as mongolism may be possible at this time. However, unless the diagnosis is unequivocal, signs should be interpreted with caution, because they may result from birth trauma.

Small-for-Gestational-Age Infant

Infants weighing less than 2500 g may be either truly immature or small for gestational age as a result of impaired intrauterine growth. The use of the graph developed by Lubchenko and associates (Fig. 42-5) is helpful in identifying babies whose weights are inappropriate for gestational age. About one third of low-birth-weight infants fit into the category of small for gestational age. In the remainder, the low weight is appropriate for the preterm delivery. A number of clinical signs are useful in separating the truly immature infant from the one who is small for gestational age. The scalp hair of the truly immature infant is fine and fuzzy, and individual strands are hard to distinguish; in the mature infant, scalp hair is coarse and silky and appears as individual strands. The earlobe of the preterm infant is pliable and has no cartilage. In the infant between 36 and 38 weeks old, there is some cartilage and a brisk rebound. The pigmented area of the breast is approximately 5 mm at 35 weeks' gestation; the breast nodule is not palpable or is lacking in the truly preterm infant, measures 2 mm at 36 weeks, 4 mm at 38 weeks, and 7 mm at term. Sole creases are minimal in the preterm infant; usually only the anterior transverse crease is present. From 34 to 38 weeks, there is an increase in creases over the anterior two thirds of the sole, and at term the sole is covered with creases. In the immature male, the testes are low in the inguinal canal, and the scrotum is small, with few rugae. In the term infant, the testes are in the scrotum, which is pendulous and has extensive rugae.

Placenta and Membranes

The placenta should be inspected for completeness, and its dimensions should be recorded. Increase in placental mass, particularly in its thickness, suggests fetal hyperinsulinemia secondary to intermittent maternal hyperglycemia. Other causes of abnormal placental enlargement are hemolytic diseases of the fetus and fetal syphilis. The maternal surface of the placenta should be inspected for infarcts or attached blood clots. Infarcts often indicate maternal vascular disorder that has resulted in occlusion or thrombosis of the spiral arteriole. An attached blood clot may be diagnostic of hitherto unsuspected premature separation of the placenta, with its implications regarding coagulation disorders.

Brown or green discoloration of the amniotic surface indicates prolonged exposure of the tissue to meconium. Vesicle formation is pathognomonic of renal agenesis. In the case of multiple pregnancy, the placenta and membranes should be examined with special care, with note made of the number of chorionic sacs, vascular anastomoses from one placenta to the other, and the possibility of twin-to-twin transfusion, as described in Chapter 43. Also, zygosity should be determined.

Laboratory Procedures

In all cases of blood incompatibility, blood should be removed from the umbilical cord for typing by Coombs' method and for hematocrit determination. If the infant appears pale, a capillary blood sample should be taken from a heel prick after warming of the limb, and a microhematocrit determination should be done. When the membranes have been ruptured for longer than 12 hours, a section of the cord and surface of the placenta should be removed for microscopic examination, and material for culture should be taken from the amniotic surface of the placenta as well as from the nose and throat of the infant; a sample of the infant's blood should also be cultured. If facilities are available, a blood sample, from either the umbilical vessels or a heel prick, should be obtained in severely asphyxiated infants with a persistent low Apgar score and examined for pH and carbon dioxide pressure. This provides a measure of the degree of the asphyxia before birth and during resuscitation and serves as a guide for therapy. As stated earlier, correction of acidosis facilitates recovery of the asphyxiated experimental animal.

Respiratory Distress Syndrome

The respiratory distress syndrome, also known as *hyaline membrane disease,* is a serious cause of disease and death. It appears to be a failure of the cardiopulmonary system to adapt to extrauterine conditions because of a deficiency of surface active material. The syn-

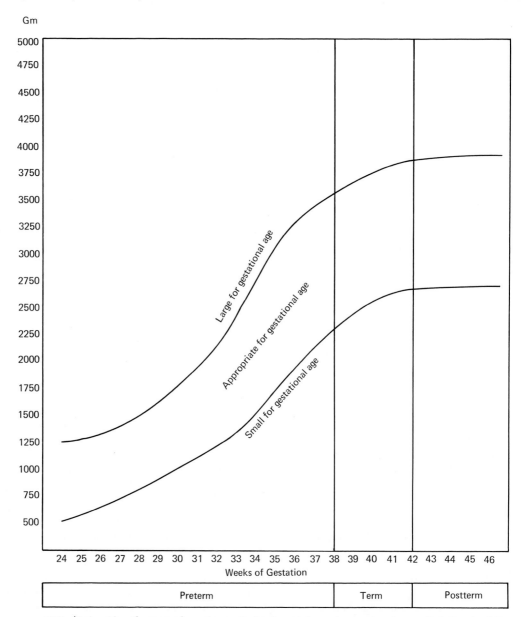

FIG. 42-5. Classification of newborns by birth weight and gestational age. (Lubchenko LO, Hansmann C, Boyd E: Intrauterine growth in length and head circumference as estimated from live births at gestational ages from 26 to 42 weeks. Pediatrics 37:403, 1966)

drome is most common in preterm infants and in those subjected to severe asphyxia during labor and delivery. Prenatal tests of amniotic fluid can determine pulmonary maturity with high accuracy, thus permitting, in cases in which the information is needed, a prediction about the probability that an infant will develop respiratory distress syndrome (see Chapter 41).

Careful observation reveals that these infants are not normal at birth. The onset of respiration is irregular or delayed, some degree of intercostal retraction is usu-

ally present, and expiration is accompanied by phonation in the form of a grunt or cry. Reduced muscle tone and cyanosis are also usually present.

Mildly affected infants gradually recover over the first 6 to 12 hours of life with appropriate warmth and oxygen. In others, cyanosis deepens, respiratory rate rises, and breathing becomes more labored, with marked retraction of the soft tissues around the rib cage and sternal indrawing. These signs reflect decreasing compliance of the lungs due to a combination of atelectasis and congestion. Blood gas analysis reveals low oxygen tension, elevated and rising carbon dioxide tension, and acidosis, partly respiratory and partly metabolic.

Differential diagnosis includes congenital heart disease, aspiration of meconium, diaphragmatic hernia, and pneumothorax. These causes are by comparison rare.

There is a possibility of preventing this syndrome or reducing its severity by accelerating lung maturation through the administration of glucocorticoids. The beneficial effects of accelerated maturation, although controversial, have been demonstrated both in fetal lambs and in humans. Although questions remain as to the complete safety of this therapy, at present there appear to be no adverse effects on the preterm infant in the neonatal and early infant period.

Approximately half of the infants with moderate to severe symptoms in the first six hours of life recover spontaneously. In those who die, respiration and circulation gradually fail. At autopsy, the lungs are solid and airless and have the consistency of liver. Microscopic examination shows widespread atelectasis, with irregular dilatation of bronchial ducts giving the appearance of Swiss cheese. In addition, a pink material, the hyaline membrane, lines the alveolar ducts.

The surface tension of extracts from lungs of infants who have died from the respiratory distress syndrome is higher than expected, indicating that the syndrome is associated with lack or diminution in the amount of surface-active material. The smallest human fetus in whom the presence of surface-active material has been demonstrated weighed only 300 g. This stage of development coincides with the appearance of lamellar inclusions. From animal experiments, it appears that adequate pulmonary circulation is necessary if the integrity of type-2 alveolar cells, which produce the surface-active material, is to be maintained.

Treatment is essentially supportive: assisting ven-

tilation, maintaining oxygenation, and providing adequate fluid and calories. With technical advances in care, mortality from this condition has fallen dramatically in recent years. Artificial surfactant as an adjunct to therapy is currently being investigated.

SURVIVAL AND BRAIN DAMAGE AFTER ASPHYXIA

It is widely believed that the newborn human infant can withstand complete oxygen lack for prolonged periods without serious sequel. This impression stems from reports of infants being delivered alive some time after the mother's death and of successful resuscitation following prolonged apnea at birth. However, reports of difficult resuscitation are rarely, if ever, accompanied by details of long-term follow-up, and a considerable number of liveborn infants in whom the period of asphyxia at birth has not been remarkable demonstrate neurologic impairment at a later age.

Additional support for this contention has been obtained from experiments with small mammals indicating that the tolerance to asphyxia is greater in the newborn than in the adult. Several factors could account for this difference in tolerance to asphyxia. The foremost is the state of development of the central nervous system. Although the degree of maturity at the time of birth varies considerably among species, there is little doubt that metabolic activity of the brain tissue of most newborns is low compared with that of the brain tissue of adults. As a result, the time interval needed to reach a state incompatible with cell survival is longer in the newborn, provided other variables, notably temperature, availability of suitable substrates, and disposition of end products, are identical. A second factor favoring the newborn relates to substrate stores in tissues where energy requirements for maintenance of functional integ-

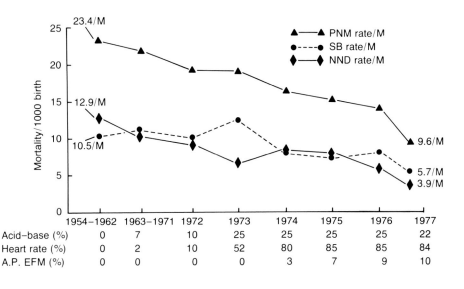

FIG. 42-6. Trends in perinatal mortality (*PNM*), stillbirth (*SB*), and neonatal death rates (*NND*) of infants over 1000 g in relation to fetal heart rate and acid–base monitoring during labor and antepartum stress tests from 1954 to 1977. (Statistics from Columbia Presbyterian Medical Center, New York)

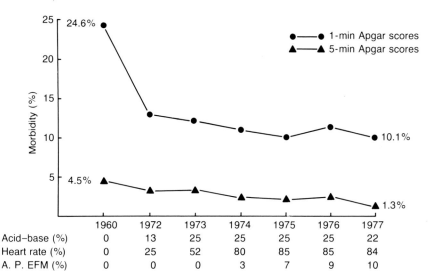

FIG. 42-7. Trends in perinatal morbidity as assessed by 1- and 5-minute Apgar scores ≤ 6 in relation to fetal acid–base and heart rate monitoring from 1960 to 1977. (Statistics from Columbia Presbyterian Medical Center, New York)

	1960	1972	1973	1974	1975	1976	1977
Acid–base (%)	0	13	25	25	25	25	22
Heart rate (%)	0	25	52	80	85	85	84
A. P. EFM (%)	0	0	0	3	7	9	10

rity are high. The glycogen stores in the myocardium are considerably greater in the newborn than in the adult, permitting the circulation of the newborn to be better maintained during asphyxia. Metabolic end products, particularly hydrogen ion, can therefore be distributed between sites of high and low metabolic activity for a longer period. Finally, the fall in body temperature in the newborn after birth may offer additional protec-

FIG. 42-8. Neonatal survival rate by birth weight. (Statistics from Columbia Presbyterian Medical Center, New York)

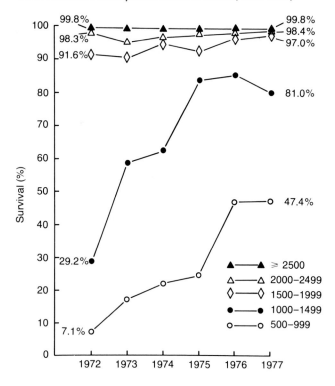

tion because the energy available is expended over a longer time interval.

The only factor not favoring the newborn is the high proportion of total body mass occupied by tissues of high basal metabolic activity. The term infant has about 5 times as much brain tissue per unit of body weight as the adult. Thus, the compartment available for distribution of products formed during anaerobic glycolysis is relatively smaller, resulting in a proportionately greater change in the composition of the internal environment for a given quantity of energy transformed.

The net effect of these four variables determines whether tolerance to asphyxia is greater in the newborn than in the adult.

How long can resuscitation be delayed with safety in the apneic newborn human infant? Asphyxiated newborn monkeys that are resuscitated before the last gasp show little or no permanent cerebral damage. However, prolongation of asphyxia for 4 minutes beyond the last gasp is accompanied by widespread tissue damage and abnormal behavior in the surviving animals. Thus, for the newborn monkey, the "safe" period of anoxia is short if functional integrity is to be maintained. The same may be true for the human newborn. For this reason, and because the duration of asphyxia to which the fetus has been subjected before delivery is not known, no time should be lost in resuscitation of the apneic newborn.

During the last decade there has been a marked decrease in perinatal mortality (Fig. 42-6) and morbidity (Fig. 42-7) in many of the tertiary centers for high-risk patients. This is especially striking in cases involving very low birth weight infants (Fig. 42-8). A number of factors have contributed to this improvement. There has been greater attention to both antepartum and intrapartum surveillance of the fetus by electronic and biochemical monitoring, especially in the low-birth-weight infant. Transitional nurseries have been established in delivery suites, enabling the newest methods of newborn intensive care to be applied with no delay. Improved understanding has led to important advances in the technology of respiratory support and intravenous nutrition. However, it is not known what the relative role of each of these factors has been. The improved survival rate does not so far appear to be associated with an increase in the number of infants with neurologic deficits, but more detailed long-term follow-up observations are necessary before the final outcome can be accurately assessed.

REFERENCES AND RECOMMENDED READING

Adamsons K, Jr., Towell ME: Thermal homeostasis in the fetus and newborn. Anesthesiology 26:5321, 1965

Baum JD, Robertson NRC: Immediate effects of alkaline infusion in infants with respiratory distress syndrome. J Pediatr 87:255, 1975

Bland RD, Clarke TI, Horden LB: Rapid infusion of sodium bicarbonate and albumin into high-risk premature infants soon after birth: A controlled, prospective trial. Am J Obstet Gynecol 124:263, 1976

Dawes GS: Revolutions and cyclical rhythms in prenatal life: Fetal respiratory movements rediscovered. Pediatrics 51:965, 1973

Farrell PM, Avery ME: Hyaline membrane disease. Am Rev Respir Dis 3:657, 1975

Gluck L, Kulovich M, Borer R et al: The interpretation and significance of the lecithin/sphingomyelin ratio in amniotic fluid. Am J Obstet Gynecol 120:142, 1974

Granberg P, Ballard RA, Ballard PL et al: Effect of antenatal beta methasone in preterm infants. Pediatr Res 9:396, 1975

Gruenwald P: Chronic fetal distress and placental insufficiency. Biol Neonate 5:215, 1963

James LS: Physiology of respiration in newborn infants and in respiratory distress syndrome. Pediatrics 24:1069, 1959

James LS: Effect of pain relief for labor and delivery on fetus and newborn. Anesthesiology 21:405, 1960

James LS: Perinatal events and respiratory distress syndrome. N Engl J Med 292:1291, 1975

Johnson JD, Malachowski NC, Grobstein R et al: Prognosis of children surviving with the aid of mechanical ventilation in the newborn period. J Pediatr 84:272, 1974

Karlberg P: Adaptive changes in immediate postnatal period, with particular reference to respiration. J Pediatr 56:585, 1960

Liggins GC, Howie RN: A controlled trial of antepartum glucocorticoid treatment for prevention of the respiratory distress syndrome in premature infants. Pediatrics 50:515, 1972

Liggins GC, Howie RN: Prevention of RDS by maternal steroid therapy. In Gluck L (ed): Modern Perinatal Medicine, p. 415. Chicago, Year Book Medical Publishers, 1974

Lubchenko LO, Hansmann C, Boyd E: Intrauterine growth in length and head circumference as estimated from live births at gestational ages from 26 to 42 weeks. Pediatrics 37:403, 1966

Purvis MJ: Onset of respiration at birth. Arch Dis Child 49:333, 1974

Rey HR, Rootenberg J, Hugh S et al: An on-line data base system and file structure for perinatology. Int J Systems Sci 10:11, 1979

Reynolds EOR, Taghizadeh A: Improved prognosis of infants mechanically ventilated for hyaline membrane disease. Arch Dis Child 49:505, 1974

Simmons MA, Adcock EW, Bard H et al: Hypernatremia and intracranial hemorrhage in neonates. N Engl J Med 291:6, 1974

Stewart A: Follow-up of pre-term infants. In Pre-Term Labour, Proceedings of the Fifth Study Group of the Royal College of Obstetricians and Gynaecologists, 1977

Windle WF: Asphyxial brain damage at birth with reference to the minimally affected child. In Greenhill JP (ed): Year Book of Obstetrics and Gynecology, p 238. Chicago, Year Book Medical Publishers, 1970

Wolstenholme GEW (ed): Somatic Stability of the Newly Born. Ciba Foundation Symposium. London, Churchill, 1961

Abnormalities of the Placenta, Membranes, and Umbilical Cord

Geoffrey Altshuler

43

As more is known of abnormalities of the placenta, membranes, and cord, the information becomes increasingly important in clarification of normal pregnancy changes, as well as in the explanation and documentation of many of the problems associated with pregnancy. Careful examination of these tissues is an important part of the obstetrician's responsibility. In some cases the specimen should be referred to the pathologist for detailed examination.

In 1961, Benirschke outlined important steps in examination of the placenta, membranes, and cord. This paper is still the definitive treatise on the subject. The obstetrician's examination should include inspection of the maternal surface of the placenta after adherent clots have been wiped away, inspection of the fetal surface of the placenta; inspection of the umbilical cord and determination of its approximate length, number of vessels, and site of insertion; and examination of the membranes. If an immediate diagnosis is needed, *e.g.,* when an intrauterine infection is suspected, a segment of placenta and umbilical cord should be submitted for frozen section examination. This enables an immediate histopathologic diagnosis of chorioamnionitis and may also reveal severe cases of villous infection. When there is no urgency, paraffin-embedded sections provide the best material for histopathologic study. Light microscopic diagnoses can be made from placentas that have been refrigerated at 4°C for several days. Placentas should not be stored in freezers, because this produces artifacts that distort the microscopic picture.

Indications for pathologic examination include a maternal history of recurrent reproductive failure (low birth weight or spontaneous abortion in more than one pregnancy), clinically suspected acute or chronic intrauterine infection, growth retardation, dysmorphia, diabetes, multiple births, and erythroblastosis. Gross sur-

gical pathology evaluation in such cases should include inspection of slices made every 2 cm throughout the placenta. At least six blocks of tissue are taken. A minimum of four sections are taken from the placenta proper, including one piece from the area near the insertion of the umbilical cord and one from the lateral aspect, towards the site of rupture of the membranes or any site of apparent hemorrhage or abruption. A sample of membrane roll is taken (Fig. 43-1), as well as a section of the umbilical cord. The inspection to determine the number of vessels in the umbilical cord should be made at least 3 cm distal to the placenta; the normal anastomoses that occur within 3 cm may give a spurious representation of the number of vessels in the cord. Special procedures, outlined by Benirschke, are needed for multiple pregnancy.

GROSS ABNORMALITIES OF THE PLACENTA

Placentomegaly

Normally, the placenta is round or oval. It has a diameter of 16 cm to 20 cm and weighs 450 g to 550 g. Seepage of placental blood or congestion from early cord clamping may significantly alter placental weight. Nevertheless, a weight in excess of 600 g is always pathologic. Although its cause is usually unknown, placentomegaly is often associated with the following conditions: overt or latent maternal diabetes, maternal anemia, maternofetal blood group incompatibility, fetomaternal transfusion, chronic intrauterine infections, fetal malformations (especially of the lung), the twin transfusion syndrome, congenital neoplasms (*e.g.,* neuroblastoma, leukemia, teratoma, and chorioangiomas), and α-thalassemia.

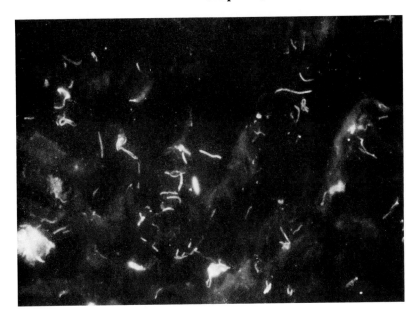

FIG. 43-1. Center of a placental membrane roll, showing bacilli of fusobacteria type with characteristic filamentous and pleomorphic morphology.

Placenta Succenturiata

An accessory placental lobe may be found at various distances from the main disc; the two are linked by vessels coursing across the fetal surface (Fig. 43-2). The accessory lobe may be retained in the uterus following delivery, which can cause postpartum bleeding and infection. If a defect is found in the membranes and vessels terminate abruptly at the placental margin, the uterus should be explored manually to locate and remove the retained accessory lobe.

Extrachorial Placentas

Placentas in which the membranes do not insert at the periphery of the placental disc are described as being either *circummarginate* or *circumvallate* in appearance. If the membranes arise without bulky folding or thickening, the insertion is called circummarginate. If they arise from a cuplike fold or elevation, they are called circumvallate. These abnormalities have been associated with a variety of clinical sequelae but there are no precise correlations. The incidence of spontaneous

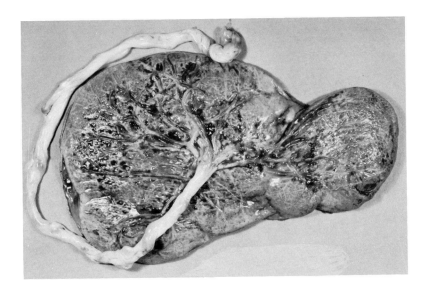

FIG. 43-2. Bilobed placenta. Normal pregnancy, labor, and delivery.

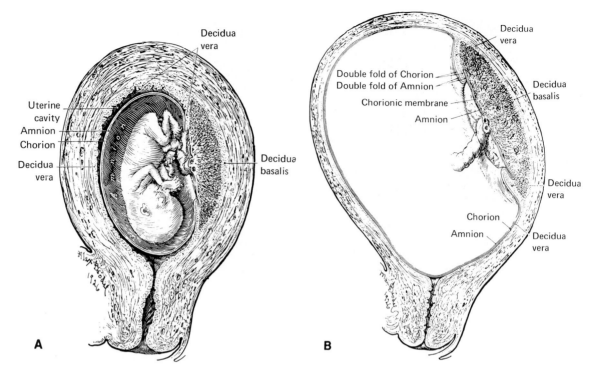

FIG. 43-3.   Placenta circumvallata. (*A*) At 12 weeks' pregnancy, the maternal surface of the placenta is in contact with the decidua basalis. The fetal surface is composed of central chorionic membrane and, at the periphery, an extrachorionic zone covered by decidua. Fetal membranes are reflected at the margin of the central portion, giving rise to circumvallate ring. (*B*) In late pregnancy, well-developed annulus can be seen. Note the relations of chorionic membrane and extrachorionic decidua and the duplication of membranes. (Williams JW: Am J Obstet Gynecol 13:1, 1927)

abortion is said to be increased. Placenta circumvallata can be associated with bleeding in the second and third trimesters that can erroneously suggest placenta previa. Intermittent hydrorrhea and preterm labor may occur. The 1927 paper on placenta circumvallata by Williams is a classic. Figure 43-3 is taken from that paper.

Placenta Membranacea

On rare occasions, a thin membranous placenta is attached to the entire interior uterine surface rather than to a localized area. Bleeding may occur in late pregnancy as the development of the lower uterine segment and effacement of the cervix cause the villi to separate from the decidua in the vicinity of the cervix. During the third stage of labor, spontaneous separation of a membranous placenta may not be complete and manual removal may be difficult. Blood loss in the third stage may be excessive.

Placenta Accreta, Increta, and Percreta

The true incidence of abnormal adherence of the placenta to the uterine wall is unknown. Other than low

implantation, the most common predisposing factor is the presence of a scar from a previous cesarean section. The etiology is a failure of decidualization of the placental bed. When villi are contiguous with myometrium, the abnormality is called placenta accreta. Small foci may not be recognized. In severe or extreme cases, the villi may invade the myometrium (placenta increta) or penetrate to the serosal surface of the uterus (placenta percreta).

Infarcts and Placental Ischemia

Infarcts usually indicate uteroplacental vascular disease, such as a thrombosed or severely degenerate uteroplacental artery (Fig. 43-4). A submucosal uterine myoma or other focal lesion may be the cause, particularly with common, marginally located infarcts. Fresh lesions appear red; older infarcts are grey-white (Fig. 43-5). If the placenta is otherwise relatively normal, a fetus may suffer few ill effects with 30% placental infarction. Although there are associations, there are no precise correlations between placental bed arterial lesions, preeclampsia, hypertension, fetal placental thrombi, and fetal growth retardation.

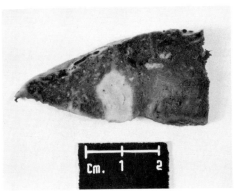

FIG. 43-4. Placental infarct. Cross section of segment of placenta after fixation in formalin. Fetal surface is at top, maternal surface at bottom. A thrombus in a maternal arteriole was demonstrated.

Shrinkage of villi and knotting of syncytiotrophoblasts are characteristic histologic features of severe acute ischemia (Fig. 43-5A). Replacement of villous tissue by fibrinoid material and X-cells is a histologic sign of chronic ischemia or degeneration (Fig. 43-5B). X-cells have a trophoblastic origin. Their function is unknown. They are most abundant in degenerate placentas of term or postmature infants suffering from severe growth retardation. I have therefore postulated that the X-cell is biochemically involved in suppression of the onset of labor.

Placental Cysts

Cysts of all sizes can be found randomly throughout all placentas. Usually they are microscopic, occasionally they are 1 cm in diameter and, rarely, they may have a diameter of 5 cm. They are lined by X-cells and typically contain clear fluid (Fig. 43-6). Sometimes they are altered by hemorrhagic changes.

Placental Calcification

Calcification is common in normal placentas, particularly as pregnancy advances. It progresses pari passu with generalized villous degeneration and ischemia, but its significance is obscure.

MICROSCOPIC ABNORMALITIES OF THE PLACENTA

Decidual Arteriopathy

Fibrinoid degeneration of decidual arterioles and acute atherosis or atherosclerosis often accompany preterm delivery, stillbirth, and fetal growth retardation and are associated with maternal hypertension, preeclampsia, chronic renal insufficiency, and diabetes. These lesions are associated with as many as 30% of placental infarcts and with almost 50% of cases of clinically diagnosed toxemia. The spiral and basal arteries of the placental bed are involved. The etiology is uncertain. Histologic similarities with the vasculopathy of renal transplant rejection and findings of immunofluorescent microscopy suggest that immunologic mechanisms are involved.

Maternal Floor Infarction

Occasionally, placentas have a 3 mm to 6 mm band of fibrinoid tissue across the maternal surface. When this tissue covers more than half of the floor, the placenta is usually severely degenerate. The placentas of 5% of growth-retarded newborns have this abnormality. The pathogenesis is unknown.

Histologic Signs of Fetal Stress

In addition to severe infarction, several other placental signs suggest the possibility of fetal stress.

Meconium Staining

Acute meconium staining is characterized grossly by a green color and microscopically by necrosis of the amniotic epithelium. Chronic meconium staining produces a brownish-green discoloration; histologically, there is reparative proliferation of the amniotic epithelium and there are numerous meconium-laden macrophages. A muddy brown color and meconium-laden macrophages deep within the subamniotic connective tissue indicate that meconium discharge occurred at least four hours before delivery.

Fetal Vasculopathy

Studies of the fetal placental vessels have revealed three major groups of lesions (Fig. 43-7).

Vascular Collapse and Obliterative Sclerosis. These changes are associated with stillbirth and situations in which villous blood flow is reduced or nonexistent.

Thrombotic Lesions. Fetal placental intravascular coagulation can result from hypoxia, acidosis, and infection. The lesions are characterized by the same features that occur in other organs: fibrin deposition, organized thrombi, and recanalized thrombi. These lesions are associated with preeclampsia, fetal growth retardation, stillbirth, and umbilical cord compression.

Endovasculitis. Endothelial inflammatory processes may be proliferative or they may show fibrinoid necrosis or endovascular sclerosis. These lesions are an important

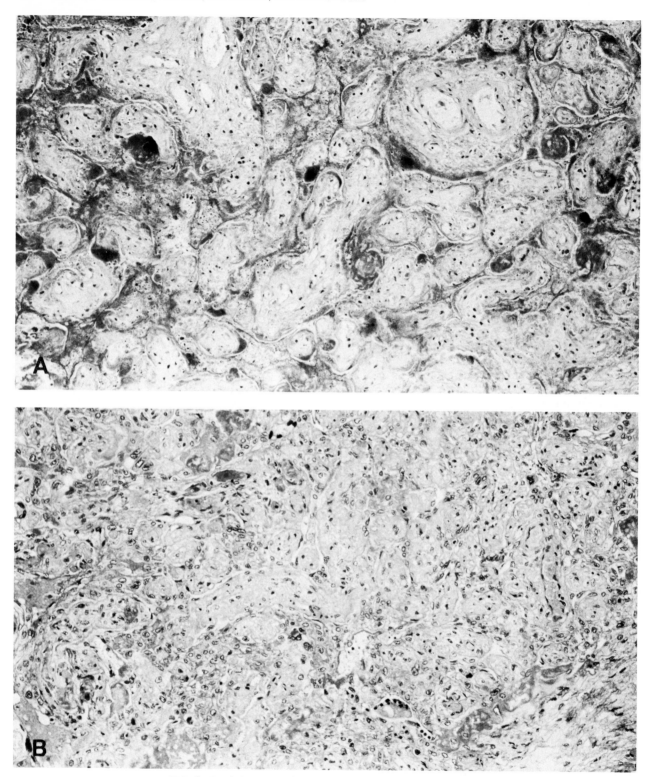

FIG. 43-5. (*A*) Acute placental infarction. Note ghostlike retention of villous architecture and syncytiotrophoblast knots. (H&E, ×180). (*B*) Chronic placental infarction. Placental villi are replaced by X cells and fibrinoid material. (H&E, ×180)

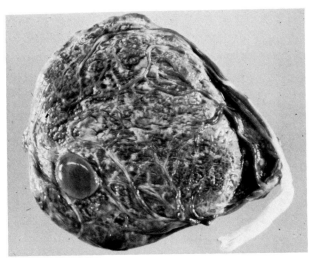

FIG. 43-6. Placenta with X-cell cyst and a velamentous umbilical cord. The cyst at the *bottom left* of the illustration showed hemorrhagic discoloration.

feature of infectious agents that preferentially attack endothelial cells, such as herpes viruses, rubella virus, and *Treponema pallidum.*

Chorangiosis

In chorangiosis, the villi are filled with blood vessels. This entity differs from congestion, in which there is a normal number of vessels in each villus. Chorangiosis is diagnosed by finding ten or more capillaries in ten or more villi in each of ten or more microscopic fields examined with a 10x objective (Fig. 43-8). Fetal stress occurs because of a greatly increased placental vascular bed. The incidence of associated neonatal death is as high as 39% and of major malformations is 42%. Chorangiosis is rare in normal pregnancies but is associated with 5% of the newborns hospitalized in intensive care nurseries. It is also associated with preeclampsia, maternal diabetes, and chronic intrauterine infection. These associations suggest that the cause of chorangiosis may be capillary proliferation resulting from persistent low-grade hypoxemia or the presence of infectious antigens.

Generalized Placental Dysmaturity

The normal placenta develops in three stages that correspond with the gestational trimesters (see Chapter 16). In the first trimester, the placenta is characterized by large hydropic villi bordered by cytotrophoblast and syncytiotrophoblast; in the second trimester, there is proliferation of the stroma or Hofbauer cells; in the third trimester, there is progressive reduction in the size of the villi. Term placentas are characterized by small terminal villi that contain no more than five vascular chan-

nels and that have occasional knots within their syncytiotrophoblastic surfaces.

In some third-trimester placentas, there is a persistent and increased proliferation of Hofbauer cells, a lack of syncytiotrophoblastic knots, and an increase of villous blood vessels. These features indicate placental dysmaturity and chronic stress of the associated fetus. The etiology is usually unknown but often includes chronic intrauterine infection, chromosomal abnormalities, blood group incompatibility, and chronic fetal-maternal transfusion.

Fetal Nucleated Red Blood Cells

In the first trimester, among the fetal placental blood vessels there are normally a few nucleated red blood cells. The presence of such cells in the third trimester is pathologic. Blood group incompatibility, chronic intrauterine infection, chronic fetal-maternal transfusion, and fetal hypoxia may be causative factors.

INFLAMMATION OF THE PLACENTA, MEMBRANES, AND CORD

Bacteria and viruses can reach the contents of the uterus either by the maternal blood stream or by ascent from the vagina and cervix. *Intervillositis* is the name given to the inflammatory reaction surrounding the chorionic villi; it is characteristic of maternal blood-borne infection. *Villitis* (Fig. 43-8) is the term used to describe inflammatory cells within the villi. *Chorioamnionitis* indicates ascending intrauterine infection because it always includes deciduitis and membranitis. With midtrimester spontaneous abortion deciduitis is almost invariably present and chorioamnionitis is extremely common. At midtrimester, the umbilical cord is usually free of inflammation. After 28 weeks of gestation, funisitis commonly accompanies chorioamnionitis. This discrepancy has not been explained.

Placental inflammation is indicative of infection. The causes include aerobic bacteria, mycoplasma, chlamydia, viruses, and anaerobic bacteria that are difficult to culture. Many of the fastidious bacteria that would appear to be bland residents of the maternal genital tract (see Fig. 43-1) can cause deciduitis and chorioamnionitis. The infection *per se* is important, but the inflammatory reaction may also increase prostaglandin synthesis, thereby leading to the onset of premature labor.

There are only two organisms that produce serious perinatal infection in the absence of placental inflammation: group B β-hemolytic streptococcus and herpes simplex virus. When frozen or paraffin-embedded sections of a sick neonate's placenta do not show chorioamnionitis, neonatalogists often terminate antibiotic therapy and investigate non-infectious causes of the patient's condition. A common example is congenital heart disease.

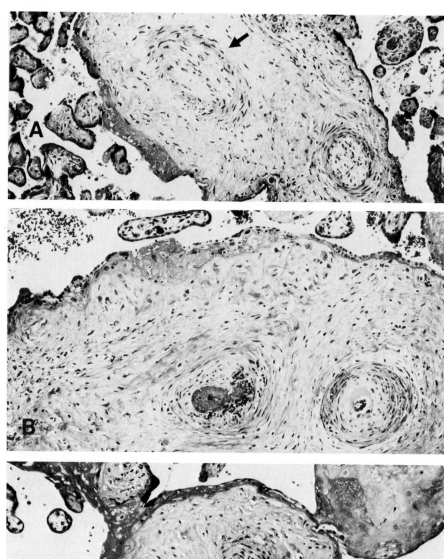

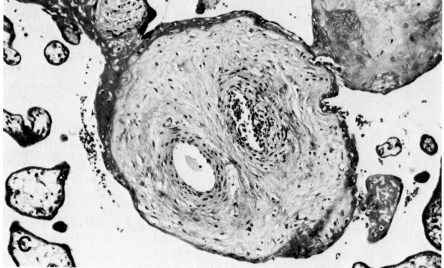

FIG. 43-7. Placental villi, fetal vasculopathy. *A.* Note vascular collapse in three vessels at lower right aspect. Obliterative sclerosis (*arrow*) possibly includes old thrombosis. (H&E, ×180) *B.* Placenta of spontaneous abortion. Presence of fibrin in central vessel indicates that fetal intravascular coagulation preceded fetal death. (H&E, ×180) *C.* Endovasculitis of fetal septal vessel. Inflammatory cell vascular infiltrates are obvious in central vessel. (H&E, ×180)

TORCH Infections

Toxoplasmosis, rubella virus, cytomegalovirus, and herpes simplex virus (TORCH infections), as well as syphilis, produce characteristic placental lesions. In toxoplasmosis, cytomegalovirus, and syphilis, the organisms can be identified by light microscopic examination.

With TORCH infections, the placenta shows dysmaturity and focal villitis. The inflammatory lesions may

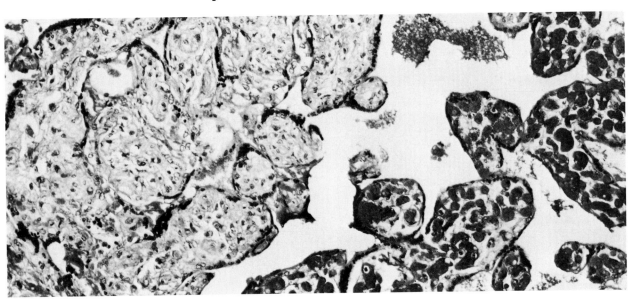

FIG. 43-8. Chorangiosis and villitis. Each villus toward right includes more than ten vascular channels (chorangiosis). Villitis is present in villi toward the left. (H&E, ×180)

be proliferative, necrotizing, or granulomatous. The cell infiltrates include lymphocytes, plasma cells, and lymphohistiocytic cells. As noted before, with cytomegalovirus, rubella, and syphilis, the fetal placental blood vessels typically show endovasculitis or endovascular sclerosis. Deposits of hemosiderin may mark the sites of previous endovascular infection and hemorrhage. In some infections, nucleated red blood cells and erythroblasts may be so profuse as to suggest Rh isoimmunization.

Purulent lesions with numerous polymorphonuclear leuckocytes occur following infection with *Escherichia coli* and *Listeria monocytogenes.* Special stains can be used to identify the bacteria if they are not apparent on routine hematoxylin and eosin staining.

Villitis of Unknown Etiology

Recent publications indicate that 7% to 9% of randomly examined placentas have focal villitis for which the cause is neither pathologically nor clinically apparent. The etiology will remain obscure until cost-effective means are available to differentiate the specific infectious cause in any individual case. In my experience, villitis has been associated with mortality (33%), major congenital anomalies (32%), fetal growth retardation (26%), chorioamnionitis (16%), recurrent reproductive failure (15%), and cytogenetic aberration (9%). Other reported correlations include preterm delivery, stillbirth, and spontaneous abortion. It is difficult to obtain precise incidences. Patient populations differ and there is considerable variation in the extent to which specific infectious causes are investigated and documented.

ABNORMALITIES OF THE MEMBRANES

Stratified Squamous Metaplasia of the Amnion

Placentas often show occasional umbilicated amniotic lesions with a diameter of less than 5 mm. The multilayered epithelial structure of this stratified squamous metaplasia is easily seen on light microscopy. Rarely, the lesions have been associated with a benign dermatosis of black newborns. Of major importance is the immediate need to differentiate the condition from amnion nodosum.

Amnion Nodosum

Elevated amniotic nodules less than 5 mm in diameter are characteristic of amnion nodosum. They may be difficult to detect with the naked eye (Fig. 43-9). On light microscopy the lesions show conglutinated vernix caseosa that makes them easily identifiable. Amnion nodosum is pathognomonic of oligohydramnios. Because of lack of amniotic fluid, sustained compression about the fetal thorax leads to lung hypoplasia. Dyspneic newborns who have low-set ears and so-called Potter's facies may be difficult to ventilate because of severe lung hypoplasia; in this context, the presence of amnion nodosum strongly suggests nonfunctioning kidney syndrome, such as renal agenesis or multicystic renal dysplasia. The other cause of amnion nodosum is oligohydramnios from prolonged leakage of amniotic fluid. There is no relationship between the numerical extent of amnion nodosum and symptomatic disease in the newborn.

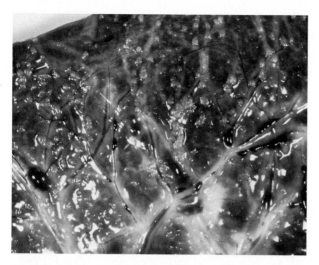

FIG. 43-9. Amnion nodosum. These conglutinated clumps of squames can be easily dislodged. Alternately, lesions of stratified squamous metaplasia appear umbilicated and do not dislodge.

Amnion Bands

Amniotic bands coursing across a part of the uterine cavity have long been known to cause fetal anomalies, such as digital constriction rings, digital or limb amputation, syndactyly, craniofacial defects, and club feet. Their cause is presumed to be separation of amnion from chorion, with repair by mesoblastic proliferation. Despite their severe associations, placental amniotic bands are inconspicuous, and careful inspection is required to find them.

ABNORMALITIES OF THE UMBILICAL CORD

Variations in Length

The average length of the umbilical cord at term is 55 cm. Wide variations are common. Shortness of the cord may cause complications in labor if it interferes with the descent of the fetus. In such cases, marked irregularity and slowing of the fetal heart rate are associated with contractions. Causes of these arrhythmias include hypoxia and increased fetal vagotonia secondary to a cord stretch reflex. Shortness of the umbilical cord may cause premature separation of the placenta and, rarely, inversion of the uterus and cord rupture.

A cord of greater-than-average length is likely to coil about fetal parts. One or more loops of cord are coiled about the fetal neck in one fifth of term deliveries. This occurs too frequently to be considered a complication of labor. Fetal injury can seldom be attributed to looping of the umbilical cord. Before it can be determined that a fetal injury is cord-related, pathologic change must be demonstrated, such as cervical edema associated with cord about the neck.

Infection (Funisitis)

As noted earlier, funisitis is part of the picture of chorioamnionitis and fetal infection. In suspected cases of the amniotic infection syndrome, frozen section of the cord and the placenta may provide a rapid diagnosis. In the example shown in Figure 43-10, chemotaxis is apparent, in the form of orientation of inflammatory cells toward bacteria at the cord surface. This tropism of inflammatory cells does not occur with hypoxia and acidosis, but is characteristic of infection.

Knots

Occasionally, true knots are present in the umbilical cord. Generally, these are loose and are inconsequential to the fetus. If drawn tight, fetal circulation may be obstructed. Obstruction is evidenced by differences in cord diameter and color on either side of a knot and by thromboses within the adjacent umbilical cord and contiguous placental vessels.

Abnormal Insertion

The umbilical cord usually has a paracentral or moderately eccentric insertion into the placental surface. Marginal (battledore) insertion occurs occasionally, and, very uncommonly, the cord inserts velamentously into the placental membranes (see Fig. 43-6). When insertion is velamentous, the fetal vessels may be torn during labor or delivery. Insertio funiculi furcata is an extremely rare anomaly wherein the umbilical cord lacks its protective investment of Wharton's jelly, for a variable distance before its insertion into the placenta. These vessels also are at risk of being torn.

Single Umbilical Artery

In between 0.25% and 1% of deliveries, the umbilical cord has only a single umbilical artery. Anywhere from a quarter to a half of the associated newborns are born with malformations, including renal anomalies, tracheoesophageal fistula, and aberrations of the central nervous system. Follow-up studies in infants with single umbilical artery indicate that if no major malformation is obvious at birth, it is exceedingly unlikely that one will be discovered in later life. Infants of diabetic mothers have an increased incidence of this anomaly, as do twins. Bizarre acardiac monsters of monozygous, identical twinning always have a single umbilical artery; the co-twin is phenotypically normal and has normal umbilical cord vessels.

Umbilical Cord Edema

In about 5% of deliveries, the umbilical cord is edematous. In most of these cases the newborn is unaffected, but some investigators have noted a correlation with

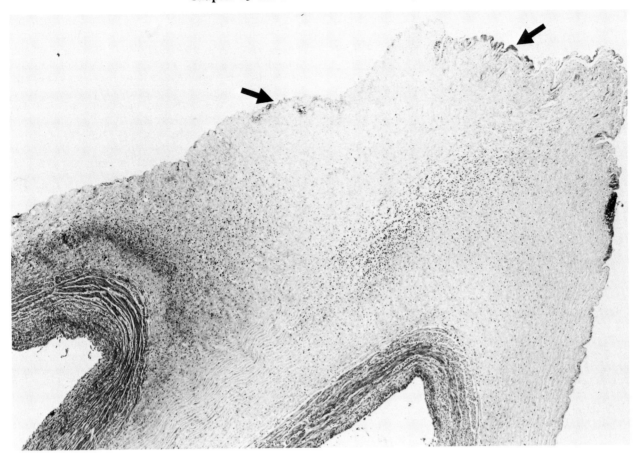

FIG. 43-10. Funisitis, umbilical cord chemotaxis. Bands of polymorphonuclear leukocytes appear selectively attracted toward bacteria (*arrows*) at surface of cord. (H&E, ×50)

preterm delivery and respiratory distress. They have postulated an etiology of low amniotic pressure, increased water content in the fetoplacental unit, and a low red cell mass in the newborn.

Miscellaneous Cord Abnormalities

Varices and hematomas occur occasionally. Severe hematomas may be caused by laceration of vitelline vessels. Associated perinatal mortality has been reported to be as high as 40%. Postmaturity or some other coincidental problem that is also present may contribute to this high mortality rate. Rare cord abnormalities include stricture, calcification, hemangioma, angiomyxoma, myxosarcoma, and teratoma.

NEOPLASMS OF THE PLACENTA

Gestational trophoblastic neoplasia is considered in Chapter 21. Placental neoplasms are otherwise rare.

The reported incidence of hemangiomas (choran-giomas) varies greatly. I have seen grossly identifiable chorangiomas in approximately 1:5000 deliveries. When such cases are reported, they often include mention of hydramnios. Various malformations have also been associated.

Metastatic malignant neoplasms (melanoma, leukemia, lymphoma, and carcinoma of the breast and gastrointestinal tract) are exceedingly rare, as are teratomas.

TWINNING

The incidence of twins varies greatly among nations, from a maximum of 1 multiple birth for every 51 single births in Chile to 1 multiple birth for every 294 single births in Venezuela. In the United States, the Collaborative Perinatal Study found 252 twin births among 21,591 deliveries (1:86) in whites and 317 twin births among 24,126 deliveries (1:76) in blacks.

In animal models, one of the etiologic factors in twinning has been shown to be overripeness of the ovum due to delayed ovulation. In humans, the cause is not clear. For dizygotic twins, it is suggested that the differences in rate of twinning for different countries may be due to differences in pituitary gonadotropin production. The high rate of twinning among women who receive "fertility drugs" is cited as evidence of this possibility.

Twins are either *monozygotic* (identical), resulting from the early division of a single ovum fertilized by a single sperm, or *dizygotic* (fraternal), resulting from fertilization of two ova by separate spermatozoa at the same ovulation (Fig. 43-11). The determination of zygosity is important, and the parents should be given this information as soon as it is available.

Examination of the Placenta

Twin placentas are either *monochorionic* or *dichorionic,* terms that are used to refer, respectively, to the presence of a single chorionic mass and, consequently, a single placenta for both twins, or two placentas, one for each twin. Many of the latter are fused to some extent, some sufficiently so that the placenta may appear to be monochorionic. In such cases, the placenta and the septum dividing the twins must be carefully examined. If there is no septum between the twins, the placenta is monoamnionic and monochorionic; the twins are identical. If a septum divides the twins, but it is made up only of two layers of amnion with no intervening chorion, the placenta is diamnionic and monochorionic; the twins are identical. Sometimes a septum of only two amnions can be recognized immediately by its great transparency, in contrast to the relative opacity of a septum in which chorionic tissue intervenes. Also, since amniotic tissue contains no blood vessels, the presence of any vascular and other chorionic tissue in the septum indicates dichorionic placentation. However, regardless of the gross impression, a microscopic section should be made both for confirmation and for permanent record.

The fetal surface of the placenta should be carefully examined, preferably by means of injection techniques, to note whether the vessels from one side anastomose with those from the other side. In monochorionic placentas, there is free anastomosis of vessels from one side with those of the other; in fused dichorionic placentas, there is no communication between the vessels of the two sides.

The distinction between a mono- and a dichorionic placenta is important. Monochorionic placentation is always diagnostic of monozygosity, which occurs in two thirds of the cases of identical twins. In one third of monozygous twins, splitting of the fertilized ovum occurs very early and there are two separate (dichorionic) placentas; in 10% of the cases of dichorionic placentas, the twins are monozygotic (see Fig. 43-11).

When dichorionic placentas are associated with twins of different sex, no further tests are needed, since the twins are clearly fraternal. If they are of the same sex, zygosity can often be determined by studies of blood groups; if the blood groups are different, the twins are fraternal. If the blood groups are the same, the physician may proceed through the blood types, *e.g.,* Rh, Duffy, Kell, M, N. If all are the same, it is likely the twins are identical. Rarely is it necessary to proceed further, but if ultimate proof were needed, HLA typing and some of the esoteric genetic studies would provide the best evidence currently available. If all turn out the same, it is safe to conclude that the twins are identical.

Twin Transfusion Syndrome

Twin-to-twin transfusion refers to the transfer of blood from one twin to the other through the intraplacental anastomoses of the monochorionic placenta. The donor twin is anemic, pale, and usually smaller and lighter; in addition, this twin's organs may be smaller, as evidenced by a smaller liver and, roentgenographically, a smaller heart. The recipient twin is plethoric, polycythemic, and usually larger. Diamnionic-monochorionic placentas usually have artery-to-artery anastomoses or combina-

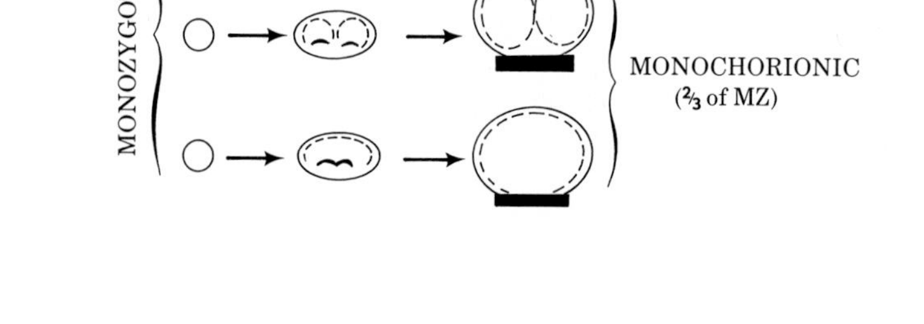

FIG. 43-11. Placentation and incidence data of twins. Monochorionic twins are always monozygous. Dichorionic twins may also be monozygous.

tions of artery-to-artery and artery-to-vein anastomoses. Depending on the kinds and degree of anastomoses, there may be virtually no exchange of blood from one twin to the other, or the transfusion may be of such magnitude as to be fatal to both twins.

Hydramnios is frequently associated with the twin transfusion syndrome. When it occurs, the customary causes of hydramnios (see Chapter 29) are to be considered. If it occurs in multiple pregnancy, some thought should be given to the possibility of twin-to-twin transfusion.

Considerable disparity is sometimes found between twins having dichorionic placentas. In such cases, some cause other than twin-to-twin transfusion must be sought, since there is no anastomosis of vessels from one side to the other in this type of placenta.

REFERENCES AND RECOMMENDED READING

Bejar R, Curbelo V, Davis C, Gluck L: Premature labor: Bacterial sources of phospholipase. Obstet Gynecol 57:479, 1981

Benirschke K, Driscoll SG: The Pathology of the Human Placenta. New York, Springer-Verlag, 1967

Blanc WA: Pathology of Amniotic Infections. In Naeye RL, Kissane JM, Kaufman N (eds): Perinatal Diseases. Baltimore, Williams and Wilkins, 1981

Fox H: Pathology of the Placenta. Philadelphia, WB Saunders, 1978

Heifetz SA: Single umbilical artery: A statistical analysis of 237 autopsy cases and review of the literature. Perspect Pediatr Pathol 8:345, 1984

Ornoy A, Crone K, Altshuler G: Pathological features of the placenta in fetal death. Arch Pathol Lab Med 100:367, 1976

Perrin EDVK (ed): Pathology of the Placenta. New York, Churchill Livingstone, 1984

Abnormalities of the Fetus and Newborn

Geoffrey Altshuler

44

Some abnormalities that occur in the fetus and newborn are iatrogenic, some are of genetic origin, some result from infection, some are due directly or indirectly to incidental complications of pregnancy, and in some the cause is unknown. Among affected babies who survive, it may be difficult or impossible to determine the cause of a given abnormality. Among those who do not survive, the causes may be elusive, and the frequency with which they are found is related directly to the diligence with which they are sought and the expertise of the pathologists who make the search.

In all cases of abnormality in which the cause is not immediately apparent, the placenta, membranes, and cord should be examined with care as outlined in Chapter 43. In all cases of perinatal death, an autopsy should be performed, and it should include careful examination of the brain and its supporting structures and examination of the spinal canal. Lung cultures should be taken for aerobic and anerobic bacteria, *Chlamydia, Mycoplasma,* and viruses. Photography, xeroradiography, and roentgenography are especially important when there are obvious abnormalities, but they may also be rewarding when no abnormalities are evident. For cytogenetic studies, skin is usually satisfactory for fibroblast culture in cases of stillbirth if fetal death occurred less than ten hours earlier or in neonatal death if death occurred less than three days earlier. Even in cases of severe maceration, kidney, lung, and gonad should be examined histologically: observation of glomeruli can help determine gestational maturity; the lungs may show pneumonia; and examination of the gonads will assist in documentation of sex.

Fifty percent of stillbirths are macerated but phenotypically normal. Twenty-five percent are malformed, and the remaining 25% are associated with intrapartum death. In these circumstances, the pathogenesis of death is usually uncertain or unknown. With chromosomal aberrations, it is remarkable that some cases occur as abortions or stillbirths but similar cases survive until the postnatal period.

The results of 100 consecutive liveborn neonatal autopsies are shown in Table 44-1. These autopsies were performed at the Oklahoma Children's Memorial Hospital. Some aspects of the findings are worthy of note. As is generally reported, group-B β-hemolytic *Streptococcus* and *Escherichia coli* were found to be the most common causes of major neonatal infection. Approximately one third of severe anomalies consisted of diaphragmatic hernia. The incidences of necrotizing enterocolitis, major birth injury, and hemolytic disease of the newborn were low, in comparison with statistics universally reported a decade or two ago.

ANOMALIES OF TWINNING

Discordancy of Monozygotic Twins

As noted in Chapter 43, monozygous twins are "identical" in that they arise from the same ovum. However, in some cases they may be very different. A major difference in monozygous twins can result from artery-to-artery and artery-to-vein anastomoses; a marked predominance of the latter can produce the critical and sometimes fatal hemodynamic differences that occur in the twin-to-twin transfusion syndrome (see p. 832). It is also possible for such abnormalities as cleft palate, hypothyroidism, diabetes, skin diseases, coronary heart disease, hypertension, amyotrophic lateral sclerosis, and psychologic and psychiatric disorders to appear in only one monozygotic twin. Genetic aberrations can also occur in only one of monozygotic twins; approximately 15 cases of heterokaryon monozygous twinning have been reported, in which chromosomal nondisjunction

Table 44-1
*Findings of 100 Consecutive Neonatal Autopsies,
Oklahoma Children's Memorial Hospital*

Finding	Number of Cases
Hyaline membrane disease	46
Intraventricular hemorrhage	32
Cerebral germinal matrix hemorrhage	29
Infection*	51
Group-B β-hemolytic *Streptococcus*	8
Escherichia coli	7
Staphylococcus aureus	1
Chorioamnionitis	30
Placental villitis	10
Major anomalies	28
Necrotizing enterocolitis	7
Major birth injuries	2
Hemolytic disease of the newborn	1

* Evidence of infection was obtained from autopsy cultures and from light microscopic features of chorioamnionitis, placental villitis, pneumonia, meningitis, and sepsis.

complicates the twinning process. A twin with Turner's syndrome thus may be partner to a normal twin or to a twin with Down's syndrome.

Mosaicism and Chimerism

A *mosaic* is a person who has cell populations of more than one genotype or karyotype; these are usually derived from a single zygote through somatic mutation, crossing over, or mitotic nondisjunction. A *chimera* is a person who has a mixture of genotypes or karyotypes that results from chorionic vascular anastomoses, transplantation, or double fertilization and subsequent participation of both fertilized meiotic products in one developing embryo. Whenever the clinician diagnoses hermaphroditism, whole body chimerism should be evaluated by complete blood grouping and karyotype studies of several tissues. Whole body chimeras have more than one blood group and more than one karyotype.

Acardiac Monster

The placentas of acardiac monsters are always diamnionic and monochorionic. As such, they always have interplacental anastomoses. Reversal of circulation through these anastomoses probably contributes greatly to the ultimate phenotypic features of these fetuses. Many kinds of acardiac monsters have been described, varying from those with severe malformations but normal skeletal and cerebral structures, to those with no

head or limbs (Fig. 44-1). The umbilical artery is usually single. The sex of the two twins is the same, but karyotypic differences have been reported.

Conjoined Twins

For at least 300 years, numerous kinds of conjoined twins have been reported, more than three quarters of them of the thoracopagus type. The reported incidence is wide, varying from 1 in 2800 to 1 in 200,000, probably as a result of variations in the acquisition of vital statistics. Failure of the yolk sac to split is the most likely cause.

Fetus Compressus and Papyraceus

When a fetus dies, progressive compression produces a condition called *fetus compressus*. The fossil-like form that eventually occurs is referred to as *fetus papyraceus*. This condition occurs most commonly in association with diamnionic–monochorionic placentation, probably as a consequence of fatal twin-to-twin transfusion syndrome.

THE PATHOGENESIS OF TERATOLOGIC ANOMALIES

Six percent of liveborns with serious anomalies have chromosomal abnormalities. The number is only slightly higher when stillbirths are included. Interactions between hereditary and nongenetic influences are considered to cause 20% of anomalies. Environmental factors of ill definable kind may cause as many as 60% anomalies. Numerous infectious agents have also been associated with congenital malformations. The most com-

FIG. 44-1. Acardiac monster.

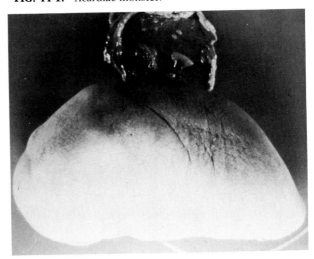

mon are cytomegalovirus, rubella virus, and *Toxoplasma gondii.* About 2% of congenital anomalies result from infection, 1.4% from diabetes, and less than 1% from all other diseases. No more than 3.5% of anomalies are caused by maternal disease. Aspects of teratogenic drugs are discussed elsewhere.

Teratogenic agents produce biochemical cellular paralysis and often cause tissue necrosis or inflammation. Even by the 13th week of gestation, the human fetus is immunologically competent and capable of a severe inflammatory reaction. However, serum immunoglobulin M (IgM) results can not be depended upon to identify these cases; in as many as 50% of cases of culture-proven congenital viral infection, fetal or neonatal serum IgM levels are not elevated. Alternatively, maternal IgG antibody transplacentally causes the fetus to produce IgM. In these circumstances, serum IgM is often elevated in the absence of transplacental infection. The results of light microscopic placental examinations are then very

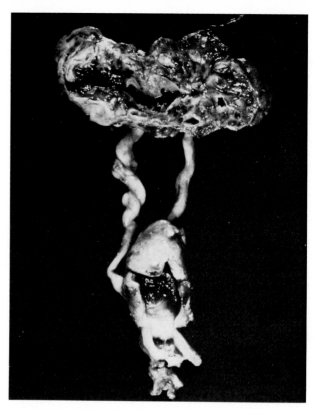

FIG. 44-3. Dysplastic horseshoe kidneys and bladder hypertrophy associated with a clinically diagnosed case of Potter's syndrome.

FIG. 44-2. Cerebral roentgenogram in a full-term newborn showing severe periventricular calcification due to congenital cytomegalovirus infection.

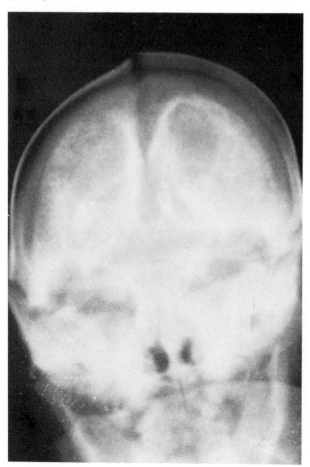

important. Regardless of whether there is brain damage (Fig. 44-2) or other symptomatic disease indicative of congenital cytomegalovirus infection, villitis is always present in the associated placenta.

INTERRELATED TERATOLOGIC ASPECTS OF POTTER'S SYNDROME

There are many syndromes in which a series of pathogenic mechanisms leads to diverse aberrations. Potter's syndrome is a very important example because it occurs commonly (1 in 4000 births) and involves widely disparate abnormalities. When there are absent or severely dysplastic fetal kidneys (Fig. 44-3), severe oligohydramnios results. Lack of amniotic fluid causes fetal compression. This results in lung hypoplasia and talipes. The lack of nutrient amniotic fluid additionally causes placental amnion nodosum, discussed in the previous chapter. Newborns with Potter's syndrome often have low-set ears and abnormal facies (Fig. 44-4). They suffer an early onset of respiratory distress, require large intrapulmonary pressure changes for ventilation, and often develop pneumothorax.

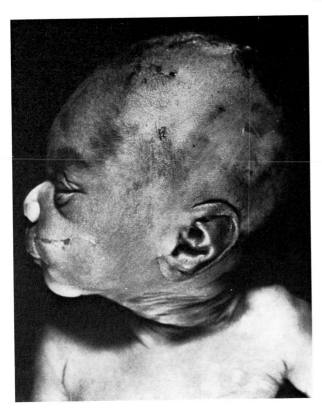

FIG. 44-4. Facies of Potter's syndrome.

CENTRAL NERVOUS SYSTEM MALFORMATIONS

Anencephaly

In anencephaly, a failure of neural tube closure leads to a deficiency of the skull vault (Fig. 44-5). The fetus usually has no hypothalamus but does have a pituitary gland. Deficient hypothalamic fetal hormones results in fetal adrenal atrophy. Lack of this and other trophic hormones may explain why many anencephalic fetuses have prolonged gestation. About 75% of anencephalics are stillborn; the remainder usually die within a few days of birth.

The incidence of this anomaly is highest in Ireland, where it occurs without known cause in 5.9 per 1000 births. Potato blight was considered to be related to anencephaly, but this hypothesis has been disproved. Anencephaly and spina bifida often occur together in singletons, but this concordance is rare in twins. Anencephaly has a high prevalence but low concordance among like-sexed twin pairs.

Although the cause of anencephaly is unknown, a cranial defect (cranioschisis) is presumed to be the primary factor. Brain exposure (exencephaly) results, followed by the progressive cerebral deterioration that characterizes anencephaly.

Arnold–Chiari Malformations

Type-I, type-II, and type-III Arnold–Chiari anomalies resemble one another; in all these types, a conical deformity of the posterior midline cerebellum and the elongated brain stem extend to or even below the foramen magnum. In the type-IV deformity, the cerebellum and brain stem are located within the posterior fossa. A common variant of type IV is the Dandy–Walker malformation, in which a defect in the inferior vermis of the cerebellum is contiguous with a large ventriculocele of the fourth ventricle. Type-II anomalies are characteristically associated with myelomeningocele (Fig. 44-6) and hydrocephalus.

Given that Dandy–Walker and Arnold–Chiari malformations develop at different times in the embryonic period, their causes may differ. Alternatively, there might

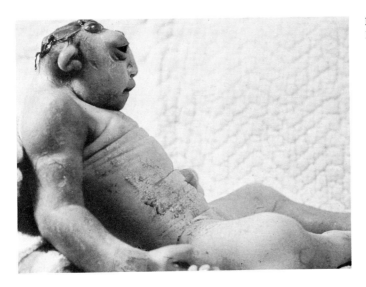

FIG. 44-5. Anencephalic infant shortly after delivery. Note nondevelopment of calvaria. (RA Stander)

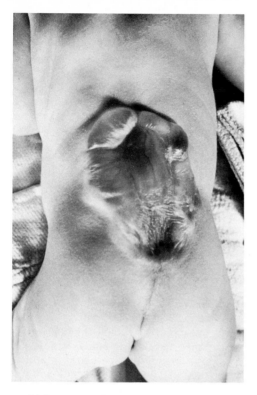

FIG. 44-6. Spina bifida with myelomeningocele. (RA Stander)

be a single cause leading to a spectrum of host responses. It has been shown that administration of reovirus type I in suckling hamsters can produce Arnold–Chiari malformations.

Hydrocephalus

Reovirus type-I inoculation, by both extraneural and intracerebral routes, can produce aqueductal stenosis and hydrocephalus in neonatal hamsters, ferrets, rats, and mice. The following viruses have also been shown to produce hydrocephalus in various animal models: mumps virus, arboviruses, influenza and parainfluenza viruses, adenoviruses, papoviruses, and Rous sarcoma virus. The pathogenesis of human hydrocephalus may involve cicatricial aqueductal stenosis or inflammatory sequelae elsewhere within the ventricular system. Genetically transmitted hydrocephalus in humans has also been occasionally reported. Sometimes there are additional anomalies as well (Fig. 44-7).

CONGENITAL HEART DISEASE

Cardiac anomalies usually occur as isolated defects. Such anomalies do not cause spontaneous abortion, except for rare instances in which closure of the ductus arteriosus results in fetal death. Maternally administered prostaglandin synthetase antagonists, such as acetylsal-

icylic acid and indomethacin, may cause the ductus arteriosus to close. These drugs are potentially hazardous if they are used as tocolytic agents. Hypoplastic left heart syndrome and transposition of the great vessels are common causes of perinatal death whenever the ductus arteriosus closes. Examples of the former include aortic atresia or stenosis, mitral atresia or stenosis, and certain cases of coarctation or interruption of the aortic arch. At least 15% of malformation syndromes include a cardiac anomaly.

GENETIC DEFECTS

Genetic aberrations account for a significant number of malformations. The physician may first be alerted to the possibility of genetic abnormality in an infant by low-set ears and a size that is small for gestational age, features common to many such disorders. Autosomal trisomy syndromes, especially Down's syndrome, trisomy 13–15 (D), and trisomy 18 (Figs. 44-8 and 44-9), are not uncommon (see Chap. 2). Many types of osteochondrodysplasia are known to be genetically transmitted.

FIG. 44-7. Hydrocephalus, bilateral cleft lip and palate, and phocomelia.

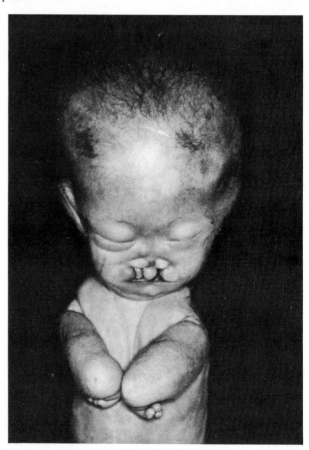

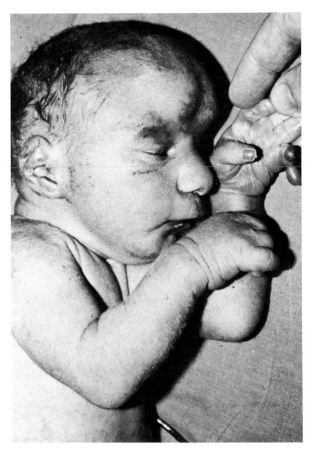

FIG. 44-8. Trisomy 18 (E). Characteristic features include dolicocephaly and micrognathia.

OSTEOCHONDRODYSPLASIA

In 1977 an international nomenclature of constitutional disease of bone was developed under the aegis of the European Society for Pediatric Radiology and the National Foundation–March of Dimes. Twenty-one types of osteochondrodysplasia were classified as being identifiable at birth. Of these, the following are associated with high fetal and neonatal mortality and are likely (unless otherwise indicated) to be genetically transmitted by autosomal recessive means.

Achondrogenesis

Type-I (Parenti–Fraccaro) and type-II (Langer–Saldino) achondrogenesis are invariably lethal. They may be diagnosed *in utero* when hydramnios necessitates fetal roentgenography. Diagnostic features include severe dwarfism, deficient vertebral ossification, and a commonly associated generalized edema. In type-II achondrogenesis, the head is disproportionately large in relation to the trunk, but ossification of the cranial bones is normal. Although there are histopathologic differences between the two conditions, both types show a severe disturbance of echondral ossification.

Thanatophoric Dysplasia

As implied by the Greek word *thanatophoros* ("death bearing"), thanatophoric dwarfism is invariably lethal. Hydramnios and breech presentation are commonly associated with the condition. There are two variants; in one there is a cloverleaf skull deformity (Fig. 44-10),

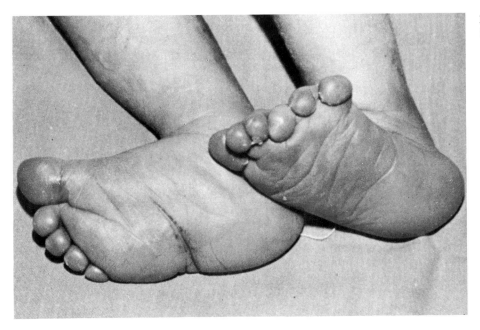

FIG. 44-9. Rocker-bottom feet in trisomy 18.

in the other there is not. In both the trunk is of normal length, the head is large, the chest is small, and there are roentgenographic vertebral features of platyspondylisis with severely widened disk spaces. The histopathology of both types includes markedly reduced enchondral ossification, which results from minimal proliferation, hypertrophy, and alignment of the epiphyseal cartilage.

Lethal Osteochondrodysplasia with Small Thorax and Polydactyly

Jeune's syndrome (asphyxiating thoracic dysplasia), the Ellis–van Creveld syndrome (chondroectodermal dysplasia), and the Majewski and Saldino–Noonan syndromes (short-rib polydactyly) are uncommonly encountered entities of lethal dwarfism.

Homozygous Acondroplasia

The frequently recognized entity of achondroplasia is genetically transmitted in an autosomal dominant manner. Homozygous offspring of achondroplastic parents resemble thanatophoric dwarfs and die early in infancy.

FIG. 44-10. Thanatophoric dwarf with cloverleaf skull.

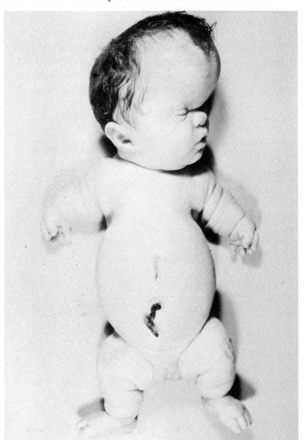

Campomelic Syndrome

Of all the osteochondrodysplasias, the campomelic syndrome is the only one with associated malformations so complex as to include the heart, kidneys, central nervous system, and even cleft palate and tracheomalacia. Skeletal anomalies include bowing of the lower limbs, mesomelic dwarfism, joint dislocations, foot deformities, a bell-shaped thorax, dolichocephaly, and small facial bones.

Osteogenesis Imperfecta

The triad of bone fragility, blue sclerae, and otosclerotic deafness characterizes osteogenesis imperfecta. The condition results from hypoplasia of bone mesenchyme, biochemically evidenced in some cases by alterations in the lysine and hydroxylysine content of collagen. At least four syndromes are associated with this disease; the fatal congenital variety with blue sclerae is transmitted in an autosomal recessive manner. The fetus suffers fractures and, if not stillborn, dies during or shortly after delivery (Fig. 44-11). Normal parents who have had one infant affected with osteogenesis imperfecta congenita are unlikely to give birth to a second affected child.

ABNORMALITIES OF THE EXTREMITIES

Defects of the limbs may occur as isolated minor malformations or may be accompanied by major anomalies that are not overtly apparent. Examples include talipes, polydactyly, and syndactyly. In most of these malformations, cytogenetic studies show no chromosomal anomalies. Examination of the associated placenta can be helpful. Placental amniotic bands, described in Chapter 43, are an occasional cause of amputation stumps, constriction rings, and other abnormalities of the extremities. A newborn with talipes may suffer lung hypoplasia and kidney agenesis or dysplasia, described earlier in this chapter.

ABNORMALITIES OF THE GASTROINTESTINAL TRACT

Tracheoesophageal Fistula and Esophageal Atresia

Several kinds of congenital anomalies of the esophagus occur with a reported incidence of 1 in 800 to 1 in 5000. At least 90% of these anomalies consist of esophageal atresia associated with a fistulous tract from the proximal end of the lower portion of the esophagus to the trachea just above the tracheal bifurcation. The affected newborn regurgitates excessively, and a transnasal or oral catheter cannot be passed. Prompt operative correction produces excellent results.

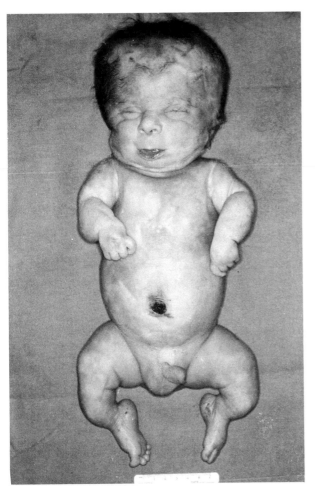

FIG. 44-11. Osteogenesis imperfecta congenita. X-ray films show multiple fractures of the ribs, skull, and extremities.

Neonatal Intestinal Obstruction of Miscellaneous Cause

Bile-stained vomitus is an early sign of acute abdominal obstruction. Causes include Hirschsprung's disease, imperforate anus, malrotation with midgut volvulus, duodenal atresia, intestinal duplications, and meconium ileus. The latter may be a manifestation of cystic fibrosis.

ABNORMALITIES OF THE ABDOMINAL WALL AND GENITOURINARY SYSTEM

Omphalocele

Whereas umbilical hernias are common and usually require no operative treatment, omphaloceles often require two-stage surgical repair. These abnormalities are characterized by a total deficiency of the peritoneal, muscular, and connective tissue layers of the central anterior abdomen.

Cloacal Exstrophy (Vesicointestinal Fissure)

Exstrophy of the lower abdomen is characterized by bladder exstrophy, including external intestine within exposed areas of bladder; bifurcation of the penis or clitoris; imperforate anus; and a short colon. Myelocystocele and omphalocele are often present, as are malformations of the ureters and kidneys.

Prune Belly Syndrome

The prune belly syndrome is caused by lack of abdominal musculature combined with genitourinary anomalies and cryptorchidism (Fig. 44-12). Talipes, hip dislocation, and various musculoskeletal abnormalities are often additionally present. When there are severe urinary tract malformations, resultant oligohydramnios often leads to fatal lung hypoplasia.

BIRTH INJURIES

Because of advances in perinatology, there has been a reduction in the incidence of perinatal birth trauma. Significant injuries continue to occur in 0.5 to 2 per 1000 live births. These injuries include, in order of frequency, facial nerve damage, brachial plexus injury, and fractured clavicle. Causal factors are usually prematurity, breech delivery, midforceps delivery, shoulder dystocia, and prolonged labor. Infants with breech presentation who are delivered vaginally have an eightfold greater incidence of trauma-related death than those with vertex presentation.

Facial Abrasions

The most common birth injury is an abrasion of the face due to the pressure of obstetric forceps. Traction need not be heavy to produce such an abrasion; pressure of the blades against the face as the head is advanced may suffice. Abrasions occur more frequently when the forceps are applied inadvertently to an oblique diameter of the head. When Tucker–McLane forceps are used to apply even slight traction, abrasions almost inevitably are found at the level of the zygomatic arches; accordingly, these forceps are not suited for traction and should be used only for outlet forceps. The abrasions usually heal without incident, but in some cases a scar remains.

Cranial Injuries

Caput Succedaneum

The most frequent cranial injury is caput succedaneum, a diffuse edema and bruising of the scalp layers superficial to the periosteum (Fig. 44-13). The injury results from impaired venous return in the scalp veins

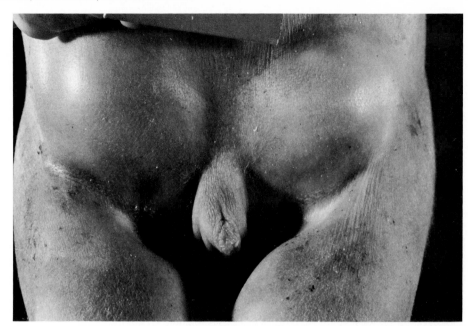

FIG. 44-12. Prune belly syndrome. Cryptorchidism and hypospadias are associated with protuberant abdominal contents. The latter results from cystic kidneys and deficient musculature in the anterior abdominal wall.

caused by pressure due to advancement of the head through the pelvis. The swelling extends beyond the sutures and may extend into the supraorbital tissues and cause periorbital swelling and discoloration. Spontaneous resolution occurs within a few days.

Cephalohematoma

Cephalohematoma is an organized hematoma that separates the periosteum from the underlying bone (Fig. 44-14). It usually overlies the parietal bone and may be bilateral. Cephalohematoma is limited to the area of bone, confined by the sutures. It may enlarge during the first two days of life and remain unchanged for two to three weeks. Many weeks may pass before resolution occurs, but incision or aspiration is contraindicated because of the risk of infection. Some cephalohematomas calcify and convert to bone; a palpable bump remains until the lesion becomes obscured by growth of the underlying calvarium.

Skull Fractures

Linear fractures are typically short and occur in the cleavage lines of the parietal bone at right angles to the sagittal suture. They are usually located beneath a cephalohematoma; however, those hematomas are often unaccompanied by skull fractures. No treatment is required, and no damage to the central nervous system results. Depressed fractures (Fig. 44-15) are usually not true fractures, but rather depressions of the parietal bone that result from prolonged compression against the maternal symphysis pubis or sacral promontory. Normal skull contours are usually regained spontaneously, and

no treatment is needed unless there is evidence of intracranial bleeding.

Intracranial Hemorrhage

Subdural hemorrhage is traumatic in origin. It was a frequent result of the difficult obstetric maneuvers that are no longer used in ordinary practice, and it can result

FIG. 44-13. Caput succedaneum over the vertex. (Potter EL: Pathology of the Fetus and the Infant, 2nd ed. Chicago, Year Book Medical Publishers, 1961)

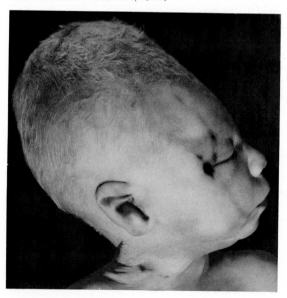

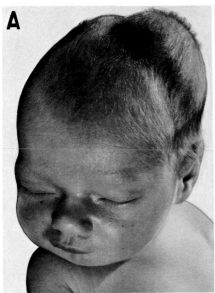 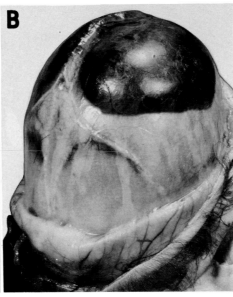

FIG. 44-14. Cephalohematoma over the left parietal bone. (Potter EL: Pathology of the Fetus and Infant, 2nd ed. Chicago, Year Book Medical Publishers, 1961)

from excessive molding. Rupture of the large venous sinuses in the tentorium of falx cerebri causes massive bleeding into the subdural space. The infant is either depressed or stillborn. In the former case the symptoms develop slowly and are characterized by increasing irritability, a bulging fontanel, and sometimes convulsions. Some infants recover completely; some apparently recover but develop long-term sequelae; others have a progressive downhill course terminating in neonatal death.

Intraventricular hemorrhage occurs in as many as 50% of infants who weigh below 1500 g and are hospitalized in intensive care units. Post-hemorrhagic hydrocephalus is an occasional complication. Ninety percent of these cases result from hemorrhagic ischemic necrosis within the paraventricular germinal matrix of the premature brain. Choroid plexus hemorrhage may also be causative. Trauma is rarely causative.

Cerebral Palsy

For many years it was presumed that all cases of cerebral palsy were traumatic in origin; such terms as *brain-damaged* and *minimal brain damage* implied inept and probably traumatic delivery. Eastman was among the first to emphasize the fallacy of this position, suggesting lack of oxygen as a critical factor. Later studies showed that, among women who gave birth to children with cerebral palsy, prenatal maternal bleeding was from 3 to 6 times as frequent as in controls; chronic fetal hypoxia—as may occur in threatened abortion, placenta previa, partial separation of the placenta, preeclampsia, and placental insufficiency—appears to be involved in at least half the cases. Mechanical injury and dystocia are much less often causative.

Nerve Injuries

Facial (Bell's) Palsy

Paresis or paralysis of the facial muscles with inability to close the eye on the affected side (Fig. 44-16) can occur in spontaneous delivery, but it is usually attributed to pressure by the tip of the forceps blade on the facial nerve. The nerve is more superficially situated in neonates than in children or adults and is additionally prone to injury because of lack of protection from the poorly developed mastoid bone. Complete recovery usually occurs spontaneously within two to three weeks; other than protection of the eye to prevent corneal damage, no treatment is needed.

FIG. 44-15. Depressed fracture of the skull in a region of the right parietal bone. (Potter EL: Pathology of the Fetus and Infant, 2nd ed. Chicago, Year Book Medical Publishers, 1961)

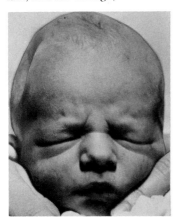

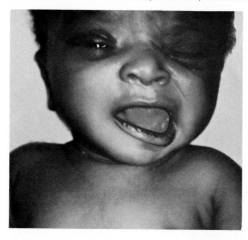

FIG. 44-16. Paralysis of the right side of the face from injury to the right facial nerve. (Potter EL: Pathology of the Fetus and Infant, 2nd ed. Chicago, Year Book Medical Publishers, 1961)

Brachial Plexus Palsy

Brachial plexus damage is usually caused by traction to the plexus during the birth process. Painter and Bergman have succinctly delineated the pathogenesis. The upper plexus is most susceptible to injury when the angle between the neck and shoulder is suddenly and forcibly increased with the arms in an adducted position. This occurs during a vertex delivery when forceful traction is placed on the head in order to deliver the aftercoming shoulder, or when the shoulders are impacted on the pelvic brim and powerful uterine contractions are forcing the head and trunk onward. There are similar hazards during a breech delivery when the adducted arm is pulled forcefully downward to free the aftercoming head, and during a malpresentation when the shoulders are relatively fixed and the head is rotated to achieve an occiput anterior presentation.

The brachial plexus can be damaged when there is difficulty in delivering the after-coming head in breech delivery or when there is extreme lateral flexion of the head in association with shoulder dystocia. The fifth and sixth cervical roots are most commonly involved. In this condition, known as *Erb's* or *Duchenne's palsy* (Fig. 44-17), the arm is limp, rotated medially at the shoulder, and held in extension and abduction. If the seventh and eighth cervical and first thoracic nerves are also injured, the entire arm is affected. In *Klumpke's palsy,* only the seventh and eighth cervical nerves are affected, resulting in wrist drop and paralysis of the muscles of the hand. Usually the injury consists of laceration of the nerve sheath with edema and hemorrhage. If the nerves are not actually severed, the outlook is excellent; recovery follows in one month to two years.

It is important that brachial plexus injury be promptly diagnosed. The arm should be held in abduction with the elbow flexed and the wrist extended. Suitable measures are to tie the infant's arm to the head of the bassinet, to pin a tie to the mattress above the infant's head, or to apply a small airplane splint. Physiotherapy, consisting of light massage and passive movements, is started after a few weeks and is continued for the duration of the disability.

Since the phrenic nerve is derived in part from the brachial plexus, phrenic nerve palsy may occur in conjunction with Erb's palsy. This produces paralysis of one side of the diaphragm, recurrent cyanosis, and dyspnea. Recovery is usually spontaneous but may be slow and can be complicated by pulmonary infection.

Spinal Cord Injuries

Spinal cord injury is rare, occurring in 1 in 25,000 deliveries. It is usually associated with vaginal delivery in a breech position, and the damage most frequently occurs in the lower cervical and upper thoracic areas. Shock, severe respiratory difficulty, Horner's syndrome, flaccidity of the limbs, loss of sensation, and bladder paralysis are characteristic. The differential diagnosis includes myelodysplasia and infantile spinomuscular atrophy.

Fractures

In breech delivery the femur may be fractured during attempts to deliver extended legs, or the humerus may be fractured during delivery of the arm. With shoulder

FIG. 44-17. Erb's palsy resulting from injury of the fifth and sixth cervical roots of the brachial plexus. (Potter EL: Pathology of the Fetus and Infant, 2nd ed. Chicago, Year Book Medical Publishers, 1961)

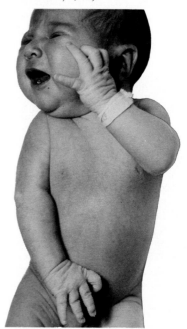

dystocia, fracture of the clavicle may be either sponta-neous or deliberate. Most such fractures are of the greenstick type and heal without incident if appropriate splints are applied.

Muscle Injuries

The most frequent, and potentially serious, muscle in-jury is to the sternocleidomastoid. This muscle can be damaged by excessive traction after delivery of the head in vertex delivery, or after delivery of the shoulders in breech delivery. A palpable hematoma develops in the muscle. Treatment consists of passive stretching of the muscle several times daily. If untreated, the mass may organize, with consequent shortening of the muscle and torticollis. (Most cases of torticollis are due not to this injury, but to congenital maldevelopment of the muscle, and are often accompanied by other congenital abnor-malities.)

NEONATAL CRISES

Hyaline Membrane Disease

More than 40% of cases of perinatal death are attributable to hyaline membrane disease. The disease directly re-sults from deficient surfactant production from a lack of lung alveolar type-II cells. Its most important cause is prematurity. The fundamental pathologic lesion of hya-line membrane disease is diffuse atelectasis. When newborns have survived respiratory distress for four hours or more, the membranes become increasingly obvious and are light microscopically observable along the alveolar ducts.

Perinatal Brain Damage

In all perinatal studies, intraventricular hemorrhage is the most common pathologic finding within the central nervous system. It has been found in more than 30% of our perinatal autopsies and has typically been associated with prematurity. Eighty percent of our neonatal autopsy cases of intraventricular hemorrhage are premature newborns of 32 weeks' gestation or less. The causative lesion is hemorrhagic necrosis within the germinal ma-trix about the lateral ventricles. This immature tissue is not present in term newborns. Soft necrotic foci within the periventricular unmyelinated white matter may be found in at least 30% of neonatal autopsies, depending on the care with which the pathologist seeks to find them. In my experience, 30% of these fetuses with peri-ventricular leukomalacia have had accelerated fibrin deposition in their placentas and a maternal history of urinary tract infection. This may represent maternal en-dotoxemia, a result of infection with *E. coli*. Perinatal asphyxia is often not manifested by anoxic–ischemic neuronal necrosis. Not uncommonly, however, perinatal shock, hypoglycemia, and acidosis are accompanied by neuronal necrosis within the pons and hippocampus. Choroid plexus hemorrhage is found in under 10% of perinatal autopsies, and kernicterus has become even less common.

Perinatal Bacterial Infection

The most common cause of perinatal bacterial sepsis is group-B hemolytic *Streptococcus;* 15 or so years ago it was *E. coli*. Group-B hemolytic *Streptococcus* can be isolated from the cervical cultures of 5% to 30% of asymptomatic pregnant women and from their sexual partners. There are two neonatal clinical pictures. An acute septicemic form occurs in the first few hours or days of life, typically with features of pneumonia. A de-layed meningitic manifestation appears anywhere from the 2nd to the 12th week of life.

E. coli accounts for about 75% of gram-negative perinatal infections. *Staphylococcus* and *Listeria mono-cytogenes* may uncommonly cause pneumonia, men-ingitis, and sepsis, as may many other organisms.

Necrotizing Enterocolitis

The most common surgical emergency in newborns is necrotizing enterocolitis. The incidence of this disorder has risen dramatically in the last ten years, probably be-cause improved obstetric care has permitted the survival of many fetuses who otherwise would have been still-born. Clinical signs of the disease include abdominal distention, vomiting, and gastrointestinal bleeding. The precipitating cause is intestinal ischemia secondary to shock. Despite the name, inflammation is not a primary feature of necrotizing enterocolitis. The intestine shows infarction, most commonly in the ileocecal area. Per-foration, peritonitis, and cicatricial stenotic repair are common sequelae. The fundamental cause of the dis-ease is unknown, but infectious agents and hyperos-molar feedings may be implicated. Breast milk, which contains secretory IgA and leukocytes, may have a par-tially protective effect, but the disease has developed in infants whose diet consisted solely of breast milk.

REFERENCES AND RECOMMENDED READING

Altshuler G: Human morbidity and mortality associated with observations of pathologic placentas. In Ryder O, Byrd M (eds): One Medicine. New York, Springer-Verlag, 1984

Averback P, Wiglesworth FW: Congenital absence of the heart: Observation of human funiculopagous twinning with in-sertio funiculi furcata, fusion, forking and interpositio velamentosa. Teratology 17:143, 1978

Benirschke K, Kim CK: Multiple pregancy. N Engl J Med 288: 1276, 1973

Bergsma D (ed): Birth Defects Compendium, 2nd ed. New York, Alan R Liss, 1979

Bhettay E, Nelson MM, Beighton P: Epidemic of conjoined twins in Southern Africa? Lancet 2:741, 1975

Caviness VS Jr.: The Chiari malformations of the posterior fossa and their relation to hydrocephalus. Dev Med Child Neurol 18:103, 1976

Crosby WM: Trauma during pregnancy: Maternal and fetal injury. Obstet Gynecol Surv 29:683, 1974

Eastman NJ: Mount Everest *in utero*. Am J Obstet Gynecol 67: 701, 1954

Eastman NJ: Editor's note regarding cerebral palsy. Obstet Gynecol Surv 11:381, 1956

Elejalde BR, de Eljalde MM, Gilman M: Analysis of the human fetal skeleton and organs with xeroradiography. Am J Obstet Gynecol 151:666, 1985

Holmes LB: Current concepts in genetics: Congenital malformations. N Engl J Med 295:204, 1977

Illingsworth RS: Why blame the obstetrician? A review. Br Med J 1:797, 1979

James WH: A note on the epidemiology of acardiac monsters. Teratology 16:211, 1977

Johnson RT: Hydrocephalus and viral infections. Dev Med Child Neurol 17:807, 1975

Kalter H, Warkany J: Congenital malformations: Etiologic factors and their role in prevention. N Engl J Med 308:424, 1983

Kosloske AM: Necrotizing enterocolitis in the neonate. Surg Gynecol Obstet 148:259, 1979

McBride WG: Thalidomide embryopathy. Teratology 16:79, 1977

Mueller RF, Sybert VP, Johnson J et al: Evaluation of a protocol for post-mortem examination of stillbirths. N Engl J Med 309:586, 1983

Nakano KK: Anencephaly: A review. Dev Med Child Neurol 15:383, 1973

Niswander KR: The obstetrician, fetal asphyxia, and cerebral palsy. Am J Obstet Gynecol 133:358, 1979

Norman MG: Perinatal brain damage. In Rosenberg HS, Bolande RP (eds): Perspectives in Pediatric Pathology, Vol 4, p 41. Chicago, Year Book Medical Publishers, 1978

Painter MJ, Bergman I: Obstetrical trauma to the neonatal central and peripheral nervous system. Semin Perinatol 6:89, 1982

Pramanik AK, Altshuler G, Light IJ et al: Prune-belly syndrome associated with Potter (renal nonfunction) syndrome. Am J Dis Child 131:672, 1977

Reimer CB, Black CM, Phillips DJ et al: The specificity of fetal IgM: Antibody or antiantibody? Ann NY Acad Sci 254:77, 1975

Remington JS, Klein JO: Infectious diseases of the fetus and newborn infant, 2nd ed. Philadelphia, WB Saunders, 1983

Rimoin DL: International nomenclature of constitutional disease of bone. J Pediatr 93:614, 1978

Shoenfeld Y, Fried A, Ehrenfeld NE: Osteogenesis imperfecta. Am J Dis Child 129:679, 1975

Sillence DO, Rimoin DL, Lachman R: Neonatal dwarfism. Pediatr Clin North Am 25:453, 1978

Warkany J: Congenital Malformations. Chicago, Year Book Medical Publishers, 1971

Wigglesworth J: Perinatal Pathology. Philadelphia, WB Saunders, 1984

Winter RM, Sandin BM, Mitchell RA et al: The radiology of stillbirths and neonatal deaths. Br J Obstet Gynaecol 91: 762, 1984

Yang SS, Heidelberger KP, Brough AJ et al: Lethal short-limbed chondrodysplasia in early infancy. In Rosenberg HS, Bolande RP (eds): Perspectives in Pediatric Pathology, Vol 3, p 1. Chicago, Year Book Medical Publishers, 1976

PART VII

Gynecology

Pediatric and Adolescent Gynecology

Donald Peter Goldstein
Odette Pinsonneault

45

The practice of pediatric and adolescent gynecology differs in many aspects from the care of adult women. Unique gynecologic problems are encountered in this population, especially in children and perimenarchal patients. The gynecologist should, therefore, be familiar with the etiology and the principles of diagnosis and treatment of these conditions. Despite their youth, the optimal evaluation of these patients requires few technical skills beyond the training of most gynecologists.

The gynecologic problems encountered in older adolescents are quite similar to those seen in adults. The distinction between the two groups lies in the emotional instability inherent to the maturing individual. The psychologic impact of the first gynecologic consultation should not be underestimated. The outcome of this experience may have an influence on the care that patient will seek for the rest of her life. There is no doubt that providing gynecologic treatment to adolescents is time-consuming, and the physician with a busy practice may elect to avoid this population. Adolescents need to be seen by a sensitive person who has time to listen to them, give satisfactory explanations, and answer questions, This is the key to gaining their confidence and, accordingly, to improving their compliance.

In this area of gynecologic practice, the attitude of the involved physician is of great importance. Children and adolescents are very sensitive to adults' attitudes. The gynecologist must, therefore, feel comfortable in communicating with these patients and their parents and should have overcome his or her own reticence about performing an adequate pelvic examination on young children and adolescents. Maintaining a nonjudgmental attitude toward their emerging sexuality is also of the utmost importance.

This chapter discusses the most commonly encountered gynecologic problems in the pediatric and adolescent age group. For the most part, those conditions that are shared with the adult population are discussed more comprehensively in other chapters.

HISTORY TAKING AND THE GYNECOLOGIC EXAMINATION

The young child and the perimenarchal patient are most often referred by pediatricians for specific reasons. In these circumstances, a referral note describing the problem, the results of prior diagnostic studies, and prereferral treatment greatly facilitates the history taking. As in other areas of pediatrics, information in this age group is usually obtained from the parents.

Vulvovaginitis and vaginal bleeding are by far the most common complaints that bring these youngsters to the gynecologist. A thorough inquiry about recent infectious disease and antibiotic therapy, hygiene, and use of irritants (bubble bath, perfumed soap, and so on) is essential. The possibility of sexual abuse should always be kept in mind. Vague gynecologic complaints may be used as a pretext to consult for actual or suspected sexual abuse. On the other hand, parents may feel misjudged or threatened if the physician raises this possibility. It is, therefore, essential to approach this matter tactfully.

Older children should also be questioned personally about their symptoms and matters of hygiene. It is sometimes interesting to note how their answers differ from those given by their parents.

The technique of interviewing the teenager is more critical. This first contact is decisive in establishing communication between the patient and her gynecologist. The adolescent is frequently under a tremendous amount of tension during her first examination. She should, therefore, be approached sensitively in a nonjudgmental fashion. It is vital that the physician assure the patient that her confidentiality will be respected and that only those issues agreed upon will be discussed with her parents. Using her first name rather than impersonal terms such as "honey" or "sweetheart" is certainly more likely to make her feel her complaints are being taken seriously.

A complete medical history should be obtained on the first visit. The gynecologic questionnaire (Fig. 45-1) includes a careful assessment of the chief complaint, details of pubertal development and menstrual cycles, and history of *in utero* DES exposure. Straight-

forward questions about sexual activity and the need for contraception are more likely to result in honest answers than an inquiry conducted in a roundabout way. The adolescent who is not sexually active should, however, not be left with the impression that abstinence is abnormal.

Though it is desirable to interview the teenager alone, it is not always possible. When the parents accompany the teenager they may wish to be present while the history is being taken. It is, however, appropriate to ask the parents to leave the room during the physical examination. At this time the patient has the opportunity to express her own concerns, ask questions, and bring up subjects she did not want to discuss in the presence of her parents.

FIG. 45-1. Gynecologic history sheet used at the Gynecology Clinic, The Children's Hospital, Boston, Massachusetts.

GYNECOLOGICAL HISTORY SHEET

THE CHILDREN'S HOSPITAL MEDICAL CENTER, BOSTON, MASSACHUSETTS 02115

REFERRED BY _____   AGE: _____

MENSTRUAL HISTORY

MENARCHE _____

CYCLE _____ DURATION _____ AMT. _____

DYSMENORRHEA _____

INTERMENSTRUAL BLEEDING _____

LMP _____ PMP _____ WKS LMP _____

GYNECOLOGIC HISTORY

LAST PELVIC _____

LAST PAP _____

PREGNANCY TEST _____ RESULTS _____

DYSPAREUNIA _____

POST-COITAL BLEEDING _____

VAGINAL DISCHARGE _____

V.D. _____

MATERNAL STILBESTEROL _____

OBSTETRIC HISTORY

GRAVIDA _____ PARA _____

INDUCED ABS _____ SPONT. ABS. _____

NO. OF LIVING CHILDREN _____

DATE OF LAST DELIVERY _____

NORMAL _____ C SECT _____

CONTRACEPTIVE HISTORY

TYPE _____

DURATION _____

PROBLEMS _____

MEDICAL HISTORY

ANEMIA _____

HEART DISEASE _____

LUNG DISEASE _____

LIVER DISEASE _____

KIDNEY DISEASE _____

HYPERTENSION _____

MIGRAINE HEADACHES _____

THROMBOPHLEBITIS _____

EPILEPSY _____

DIABETES _____

ASTHMA _____

BREAST DISEASE _____

CANCER _____

PSYCHIATRIC CARE _____

SICKLE CELL _____

ALLERGIES _____ _____

CURRENT MEDS. _____

HOSPITALIZATIONS _____

SERIOUS ILLNESSES _____

MAY WE CONTACT YOU AT HOME? ☐ YES ☐ NO

IF NOT, WHERE? _____

16421 01 5C 6 74

Gynecologic Examination of the Young Child

The pelvic examination should always be explained in advance to the mother and the patient. It is important to stress that a properly performed gynecologic examination does not hurt the child and will not compromise her virginity.

A general physical assessment of the child should be carried out, including examination of the head and neck, lungs, heart, breasts, and abdomen. Besides the importance of being thorough, this part of the examination allows the physician to establish physical contact with the patient and gain her confidence. The physician should carry on a conversation with the child about her friends, family, and play so that rapport can be more readily established.

The neonate and infant (0–2 years of age) are best examined either on the table or on the mother's lap, in the so-called "frog-leg position," which is also utilized in some older children. A careful examination of the external genitalia is performed, looking for anatomic abnormalities, signs of infection or inflammation, and presence of lesions, excoriations, or trauma. It is to be remembered that in young children, the clitoris seems disproportionately large compared to the remainder of the vulva. Attention should next be directed to the area of the urethral meatus to look for urethral discharge, a sign of a ureterocele. Hygiene can be assessed by noting the presence of debris and fecal remnants on the perineum. Good visualization of the vestibule and hymen

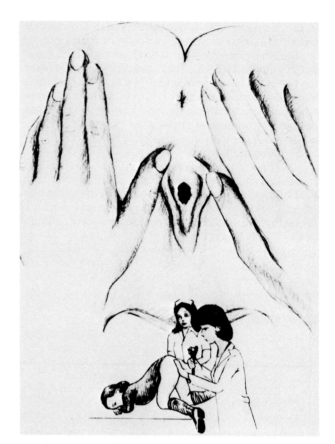

FIG. 45-3. Knee–chest position used for visualization of vagina with otoscope (without speculum).

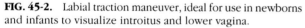

FIG. 45-2. Labial traction maneuver, ideal for use in newborns and infants to visualize introitus and lower vagina.

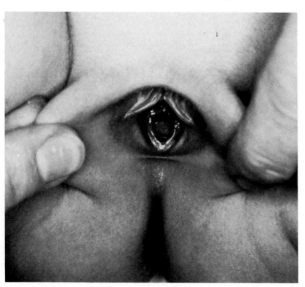

is obtained by gently pulling the labia majora downward and outward, which causes the hymenal ring to gape open, thus allowing inspection of the distal vagina (Fig. 45-2).

The young child (age 2–8 years of age) is best examined in the knee-chest position, with gentle lateral and upward traction being exerted on the buttocks. This maneuver usually opens the hymen enough so that the posterior wall of the vagina and cervix can be completely visualized without the necessity for any vaginal instrumentation. An otoscope (without the speculum) can be used for light and magnification (Fig. 45-3). The vagina should be carefully inspected for the presence of discharge, bleeding, tumors, and foreign bodies. The physician should be aware that, because estrogenization is required, an eye dropper attached to a 4-cm to 5-cm segment of intravenous tubing may be utilized to aspi-poor, the vaginal epithelium in the young child is normally thin, reddened, and friable. For the same reason, the cervix is a small, reddish structure that barely protrudes from the surrounding vaginal mucosa. Several techniques of instrumental vaginoscopy have been described and utilized with success. Capraro presented an excellent step-by-step method of vaginoscopic examination, and the utilization of a veterinary otoscope speculum has been recommended by Billmire and colleagues. In our experience, a satisfactory visualization of the vagina and cervix can be obtained in most instances by examination in the knee-chest position. It is our belief in patients less than eight years old, invasive techniques should *not* be carried out when the patient is conscious. If the knee-chest position proves unsatisfactory, it is preferable to perform the examination under anesthesia.

When vaginal cultures are indicated, they should be obtained at the end of the examination and collected from the deep vaginal fornix. If the size of the hymenal opening permits, a moistened cotton-tipped applicator or a Calgiswab is introduced into the vagina while the child is asked to cough. When several specimens are rate the vaginal contents. This system may also be used for vaginal irrigation when the discharge is not abundant. Five to ten milliliters of sterile, nonbacteriostatic saline are injected in the vagina and then aspirated. Once again, the child should be informed of what will happen, assured that the procedure will "tickle" but not hurt, and allowed to see and handle the material before cultures are taken.

After the examination in the knee-chest position is completed, the patient is placed in the supine position with her knees flexed and heels together, and the pelvic organs are assessed by rectoabdominal examination. In youngsters between one and eight years of age, the only palpable structure is the cervix, which feels like a small nodule behind the anterior rectum. The uterus and ovaries are not palpable in the prepubescent female except during the immediate postnatal period, when the uterus is enlarged owing to the influence of maternal estrogen. Any palpable pelvic structure should prompt a thorough investigation. While the rectal finger is being withdrawn, gentle pressure should be applied against the anterior rectal wall so as to localize any tumor or foreign body and "milk out" any discharge.

Gynecologic Examination of the Older Child and Virginal Adolescent

The older premenarchal patient and the virginal adolescent are approached differently than the younger child since it is possible to have them participate more actively. We have found the use of the mirror to be of great value, since the patient can be distracted by a running commentary while visualizing her anatomy. Many patients in this age group come to their first gynecologic examination already traumatized emotionally by "frightful stories about the torture of the gynecologic examining room." It is, therefore, essential to explain the pelvic examination in detail. All instruments should be shown to the patient, and she should be assured that they are designed especially for young girls. The traditional dorsal-lithotomy position using adjustable stirrups is used for the examination of these patients. The vagina and cervix are best visualized with a Huffman speculum (Fig. 45-4). This instrument is narrow and long (0.5 × 4.5 inches) and conforms nicely to the virginal hymen and vagina. The morphology of the hymenal opening is ascertained, first visually and then by gently introducing a lubricated finger in the vagina. In the presence of a microperforate or septate hymen, attempts to introduce a speculum result in an unsatisfactory examination and only serve to traumatize the patient physically and emotionally. When the utilization of a speculum is made difficult by a rigid hymen or because of involuntary contraction, the postmenarchal patient should be taught how to use tampons and be given an appointment three months later if her problem does not require immediate examination. Otherwise, a pelvic examination under anesthesia and hymenotomy to facilitate future examinations are in order.

When conditions are favorable for the utilization of a speculum, the perineal body is first relaxed by applying gentle pressure against the posterior rectal wall. The finger is then slowly replaced by the warmed speculum. The vagina and cervix are inspected and specimens for culture and Papanicolaou smears are obtained. Asking the patient to distinguish between the normal sensation of pressure and any unnecessary pain contributes to success of this technique.

Internal genital structures are assessed by a rectovaginal examination. At the onset of puberty, the uterus

FIG. 45-4. Huffman speculum. This speculum is especially suitable for use in virginal adolescents because of its narrow gauge and length.

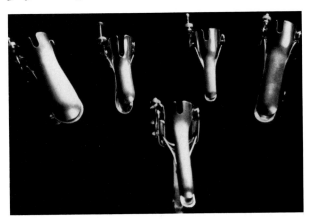

becomes palpable secondary to the rise of serum estrogen levels. In patients complaining of dysmenorrhea or pelvic pain, careful evaluation of the uterine size and shape is mandatory in order to detect the presence of genital tract malformations. The rectovaginal septum and cul-de-sac should also be examined to detect possible endometriosis. It is not unusual to palpate plump, tender ovaries during the premenarchal period. This finding corresponds to the exaggerated follicular activity taking place in the anovulatory ovary and most often regresses after menarche.

GYNECOLOGIC PROBLEMS OF THE NEONATE AND YOUNG CHILD

Vulvovaginitis

The prepubertal child is especially vulnerable to vulvovaginitis because of poor estrogenization of the vaginal epithelium and unsupervised and inadequate perineal hygiene. It is also well known that, compared to older females, these youngsters lack the protection provided by pubic hair and the fatty pads of the labia majora. Contaminants and irritants thus have free access to the sensitive vulvar and vaginal epithelium.

The symptoms of vulvovaginitis are quite variable but most often consist of vaginal discharge, which varies in quantity, color, and odor; vulvar pruritus or burning; and dysuria. Whatever the etiology of the problem, the examination usually reveals edema, redness, discharge, excoriations, and scratch lesions. The presence of fecal remnants and interlabial debris confirms that hygiene is poor.

Physiologic Leukorrhea

Physiologic leukorrhea occurs at both extremes of childhood. During the neonatal period, maternal estrogens stimulate the newborn's endocervical glands and vaginal epithelium. The discharge is characteristically greyish, gelatinous, and sticky. On occasion, a small amount of blood may be present as a result of hormonal withdrawal.

During the 6 to 12 months preceding menarche, rising endogenous estrogen secretion is responsible for the appearance of a whitish discharge not associated with irritative symptoms. After appropriate evaluation, it is of great importance to explain to these young girls that this discharge is part of the normal process of maturation. Unjustified prescription of vaginal cream or antibiotics only serves to make the patient believe that any vaginal discharge is pathologic and eventuates in many unnecessary consultations.

Nonspecific Vulvovaginitis

Nonspecific or mixed vulvovaginitis accounts for a substantial proportion of vulvovaginal infection in young girls approaching menarche. The etiology can most often be traced to poor local hygiene and fecal contamination. Cultures usually grow predominantly *Escherichia coli* and other anal organisms.

General hygienic measures are the first step of treatment. Sitz baths in warm plain water should be given two or three times a day. These should be followed by thorough drying of the vulvar area, for which a hairdryer set at the lowest speed and heat may be helpful. A small amount of unscented talcum powder or corn starch helps keep the vulva dry. Only mild, nonperfumed soap should be used. Bubble baths should be avoided. The patient should also be counseled to wear white, 100% cotton underpants and to avoid tight-fitting clothes, nonabsorbant fabrics, and wet bathing suits. The importance of front-to-back wiping with soft, white, and unscented toilet tissue should also be stressed.

When the patient presents with acute symptoms and excoriation, sitz baths are given more often. No soap or topical medication should be used, since these can increase the inflammatory reaction. Witch hazel pads (Tucks) may be utilized for relief. Antipruritic medication, such as hydroxyzine hydrochloride (Atarax) 2 mg/kg/day in 4 doses or diphenhydramine (Benadryl) 5 mg/kg/day in 4 doses, may occasionally be necessary to prevent the child from scratching. When pruritus remains a problem during the subacute phase, vulvular application of hydrocortisone cream 1% or calamine lotion is useful.

When, despite these measures, symptoms are persistent or recurrent, antibiotic therapy is indicated. Local application of antibacterial cream (AVC, Sultrin, Vagitrol) or oral antibiotics, such as ampicillin 50 mg/kg/day for 10 days, are usually effective. Vaginal douches with povidone-iodine (Betadine) 1% solution administered with a syringe and a small feeding tube or intravaginal application of estrogen cream for two to three weeks may also be helpful. Because most mothers are reluctant to apply an intravaginal medication, compliance is usually better with oral antibiotics.

Specific Vulvovaginitis

GONORRHEA. The reported incidence of gonococcal vulvovaginitis widely varies from author to author. The child may become infected either by contact with contaminated material (fingers, bedding, towels) or secondary to sexual molestation. This issue should always be investigated when gonorrhea infection is diagnosed, and all possible contacts (family, babysitters, and so on) should be cultured. In this age group, the disease remains confined to the vulva and lower vagina and is characterized by purulent vaginal discharge and vulvitis.

Since infection with other types of *Neisseria* (*N. sicca, N. catarrhalis*) are also characterized by intracellular gram-negative diplococci, definitive diagnosis depends on positive cultures. Specimens for pharyngeal and rectal cultures should also be obtained.

Besides general hygienic measures, treatment consists of aqueous procaine penicillin G 100,000 units/kg IM or amoxicillin 50 mg/kg PO (maximum 1 g) in children over two years of age. For patients allergic to penicillin, spectinomycin 40 mg/kg IM is the best alternative. Although less effective, oral erythromycin 40 mg/kg/day divided in 4 doses for 1 week can also be utilized, provided close follow-up is assured. Tetracyline is not recommended in young children because of the possibility of dental staining. Cultures should be repeated 7 to 14 days after the completion of therapy and monthly for three months.

Since gonorrhea infection is highly contagious among children, great care should be taken to avoid contamination of siblings during the acute phase (careful handwashing, disinfection of bath tub and toilet seat, and so on). Since gonorrheal ophthalmia is a possible complication, it is also important to prevent the child from touching her eyes.

CANDIDA ALBICANS. Monilial vulvovaginitis is not common in children and is usually associated with recent antibiotic therapy or diabetes mellitus. The clinical picture is quite characteristic and at the onset consists of erythematous vulva with oozing granulomatous lesions, which later become crusted. Satellite lesions are often present. The cottage-cheese appearance of the vaginal discharge is well known. Diagnosis is made by microscopic visualization of mycelia on KOH preparation of vulvar exudate or vaginal discharge or by positive culture on appropriate medium.

Treatment consists of sitz baths three times daily followed by vulvar application of antifungal preparation. When symptoms persist after two weeks, intravaginal therapy or oral administration of conazole compounds is indicated.

TRICHOMONAS. Although the nonestrogenized vaginal epithelium of the prepubertal child is unfavorable to the growth of trichomonas, this parasite is occasionally responsible for vulvovaginitis. Trichomonas is acquired by direct contact and should lead to consideration of the possibility of sexual abuse, although nonsexual transmission is possible.

The vaginal discharge, characteristically greenish and malodorous, is associated with nonspecific signs of irritation. Treatment consists of oral administration of metronidazole 10–30 mg/kg/day (maximum 125 mg t.i.d.) for 7 days or 1 g in a single dose.

PINWORMS. *Enterobius vermicularis* (pinworm), which is a frequent intestinal parasite in children, may occasionally infect the vagina, giving rise to acute inflammatory symptoms and yellow mucopurulent discharge. Diagnosis is suggested by perianal scratching lesions and confirmed by a positive scotch-tape test, preferably done in the morning.

The parasite is usually eradicated by a single dose of mebendazole (Vermox) 100 mg. All members of the family should also be treated. Pinworm vulvovaginitis is frequently associated with infection by other anal contaminants, which is approached as discussed above.

CONDYLOMATA ACUMINATA. Warty lesions associated with human papillomavirus infection are occasionally found in infants and young children. When these lesions are present, the possibility of sexual molestation should be investigated. Treatment consists of application of 25% podophyllum in benzoin or laser ablation. Visualization of the urinary tract and anal canal is mandatory in cases where recurrence is a problem.

Vulvovaginitis Associated with Other Sites of Infection

In children, vulvovaginitis often follows an episode of infection in another part of the body, especially the upper respiratory tract. β-Hemolytic *Streptococcus, S. pneumonia, Staphylococcus, N. meningitis,* and *Shigella* are all possible causes of vulvovaginal infection and should be treated according to the sensitivity of each organism.

Systemic diseases, such as measles, chicken pox, and scarlet fever, may have vulvovaginal manifestations. Symptoms usually follow the natural history of the primary disease. Scratching and fecal contamination, however, may lead to secondary bacterial infection.

Dermatologic diseases, such as herpes simplex and herpes zoster, eczema, psoriasis, and molluscum contagiosum may also involve the vulvar skin, as may the effects of such irritants as poison ivy.

Vulvovaginitis Associated with Foreign Bodies

The presence of an intravaginal foreign body is suggested by a greenish, bloody, and foul-smelling discharge. The most frequent finding is a small piece of toilet paper or stool. Culture grow mixed flora. Any bloody or malodorous discharge should prompt a thorough vaginal examination.

The foreign body can sometimes be washed out by vaginal irrigation with room-temperature saline using intravenous tubing (Fig. 45-5). When the object is felt by rectal examination, gentle attempts to milk it out or remove it with a bayonet forceps in the knee-chest position may be successful. When the foreign body has

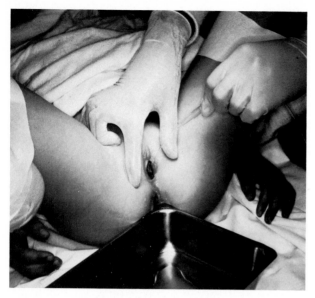

FIG. 45-5. Technique of vaginal irrigation used to wash out foreign bodies and debris. Also applicable in examining small children with perineal and labial tears to assess extent of injury.

been *in situ* for a long time, it is likely to be imbedded in the vaginal wall, and removal under anesthesia is necessary.

Anatomic Causes

In some instances, a microperforate hymen, especially when the opening lies high, near the urethral meatus, may be responsible for pooling of urine in the vagina. Constant maceration of vulvovaginal tissue causes irritation and often secondary infection. In such cases, hymenotomy is curative.

Ectopic Ureters

Ectopic ureters are usually diagnosed before adolescence. In some instances, children with ectopic ureters are erroneously believed to be incontinent or to have enuresis or chronic vaginitis. Work-up should consist of pelvic ultrasound studies, intravenous pyelography, and cystoscopy.

Labial Adhesions

Labial adhesions occur most commonly in young girls six months to six years of age. The cause is unknown but may be related to an irritation that erodes the vulvar epithelium, causing the labia to stick together. Occasionally, the vaginal orifice is completely covered,

causing poor drainage of vaginal secretions and sequestering of urine in the vagina (Fig. 45-6). Mothers often become alarmed because the vagina appears to be absent.

In mild cases no treatment is necessary because the labia will separate completely with estrogenization at puberty. In cases where vaginal or urinary drainage is impaired, an estrogen-containing cream should be applied nightly for three weeks, and then as necessary. A repeat course of therapy is sometimes needed. Forceful separation is generally contraindicated because it is traumatic for the child and may cause the adhesions to form again. When estrogen therapy fails, separation is best performed under general anesthesia. This is followed by application of a bland ointment (such as Desitin or White's A&D) and gentle separation at regular intervals.

Vaginal Bleeding

Most girls have their first menstrual period sometime between the age of 9 and 16 years. Except for hormone withdrawal bleeding during the first week or two of life, genital bleeding before the age of nine years is not normal, and is most likely due to organic causes. Therefore, this sign should always be taken seriously and carefully assessed.

FIG. 45-6. Labial adhesions in a four-year-old with only small opening at the level of the urethra. The patient complained of recurrent pain and discharge, which were due to sequestering of urine in the vagina.

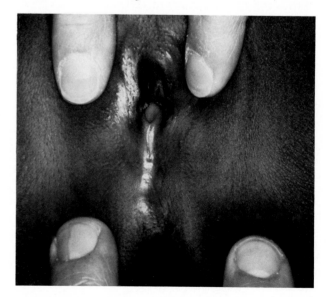

Classically, vaginal bleeding in childhood is divided into two types: (1) that associated with signs of isosexual precocity, and (2) that *not* associated with signs of isosexual precocity. However, we find it more useful to classify the problem on the basis of etiologic factors as follows:

I.   Infection
        Primary
            Bacterial
            Fungal
            Parasitic
            Viral
        Secondary
            Foreign body
            Reflux of urine
            Pelvic abscess
            Fistula
II. Trauma
        Accidental
        Sexual
III. Endocrine Abnormalities
        Newborn bleeding due to maternal estrogen withdrawal
        Isosexual precocity
        Exogenous hormone ingestion
        Hypothyroidism
IV. Anatomic Abnormalities
        Prolapse of urethral mucosa
        Vaginal or uterine prolapse
        Cervical ectropion
        Ectopic ureter
V.   Idiopathic
        Vulvar dystrophy
        Vulvitis secondary to irritants
        "Premature endometrial activity"
        Self-induced
VI. Neoplasms
        Benign
        Malignant
VII. Blood Dyscrasias
        Coagulopathy
        Hematologic neoplasms

Vulvovaginitis with or without the presence of a foreign body was the most common cause of vaginal bleeding in 63 patients under nine years of age who presented at the Gynecology Clinic of The Children's Hospital, Boston, between January, 1974, and December, 1983 (Table 45-1). When a young child presents with vaginal bleeding it is mandatory to perform a thorough investigation to rule out presence of malignancy, just as one would do in a patient in the postmenopausal age group. It has been our policy to perform an anesthesia examination as part of the initial work-up unless we are completely content that full visualization of the

Table 45-1
Causes of Vaginal Bleeding in 63 Children Under Nine Years of Age, The Children's Hospital, Boston, 1974–1983

Cause	Patients	
	Number	*Percent*
Infection	41	65
Trauma	10	16
Endocrine abnormalities	3	
Anatomic abnormalities	3	
Blood dyscrasias	3	19
Idiopathic	2	
Neoplasms	1	

cervix and vagina were possible during the outpatient examination.

GYNECOLOGIC PROBLEMS OF THE ADOLESCENT

Acute Adolescent Menorrhagia

Abnormal menstrual bleeding is one of the most common reasons for gynecologic consultation in adolescents. The spectrum of complaints ranges from minor deviations from the average menstrual pattern to life-threatening hemorrhage. Whatever the seriousness of symptoms, abnormal bleeding is usually a subject of great concern for both the patient and her parents and it deserves attentive consideration.

Since the subject of dysfunctional bleeding is discussed thoroughly in Chapter 46, only the acute problems seen in the postmenarchal period are dealt with here.

Acute menorrhagia usually occurs quite dramatically and requires prompt management. The classic picture is that of a pale, anxious teenager who presents at the emergency ward with heavy bleeding of several days' or weeks' duration.

Since dysfunctional uterine bleeding, by definition, occurs on the basis of anovulatory cycles, the teenager in the first years of her menstrual life is the most susceptible candidate. Gantt and McDonough reported a 55% to 82% incidence of anovulatory cycles during the first two postmenarchal years, 30% to 55% during the next two years, and 0% to 20% at 4 to 5.5 years.

DIFFERENTIAL DIAGNOSIS. The differential diagnosis of acute adolescent vaginal hemorrhage is summarized as follows:

I. Anovulatory Uterine Bleeding (dysfunctional uterine bleedng)
II. Pregnancy-Related Complications
    Spontaneous abortion
    Complications of pregnancy termination procedures
    Ectopic pregnancy
    Gestational trophoblastic diseases
    Bleeding of the third trimester of pregnancy
III. Local Genital Tract Conditions
    Benign and malignant tumors (vagina, cervix, uterus, ovary)
    Infection
    Intrauterine contraceptive devices
    Trauma
    Intravaginal foreign bodies
IV. Systemic Causes
    Coagulation disorders
    Thyroid dysfunction
    Diabetes mellitus
    Nutritional disorders, iron deficiency
    Hepatic diseases
    Renal diseases
V. Causes of Chronic Anovulation

Although dysfunctional (anovulatory) uterine bleeding accounts for the largest number of these cases, other causes of abnormal genital bleeding should be systematically ruled out.

Pregnancy-related complications are common in adolescents and should be excluded, even in a supposedly virginal patient. These include spontaneous abortions, complications of elective pregnancy termination procedures, ectopic pregnancy, and gestational trophoblastic disease. Occasionally, young patients present with third-trimester bleeding in a previously undiagnosed pregnancy.

Though rare, benign and malignant conditions of the genital tract may be responsible for severe hemorrhage. Sarcoma botryoides, which most often occurs in the young child, will present during adolescent years. Bleeding vaginal adenosis, clear-cell adenocarcinoma, extensive ectropion, and cervical or vaginal polyps or hemangiomas may be found on pelvic examination. Other uterine neoplasms and endometrial polyps are rarely encountered in this age group. Estrogen-secreting ovarian tumors can also cause endometrial hyperplasia, which leads to heavy bleeding, as it can during the perimenopausal age group. Pelvic inflammatory disease with associated endometritis and intrauterine contraceptive devices may induce heavy vaginal bleeding. Traumatic conditions, either postcoital or self-imposed, and the presence of intravaginal foreign bodies should also be considered.

Coagulation disorders are probably the most common systemic condition associated with acute menor-

rhagia. In 1981, Claessens and Cowell reported a 19% incidence of such defects among 59 patients hospitalized for a first episode of hemorrhagic menstrual bleeding. Their findings included cases of idiopathic thrombocytopenic purpura, von Willibrand's disease, Glanzmann's disease, thalassemia major, and Fanconi's anemia. Leukemia, effects of radiation and chemotherapy, and some drugs (anticoagulants, aspirin, hepatotoxic drugs) are also possible causes of deficient coagulation mechanisms.

Other systemic conditions possibly associated with menorrhagia are thyroid dysfunction, diabetes mellitus, nutritional disorders, and hepatic and renal diseases.

Patients who present with acute menstrual hemorrhage in late adolescence should be investigated for other causes of chronic anovulation.

WORK-UP.   A complete history should be obtained, insisting on the description of recent events as well as premenarchal development. In cases of acute menorrhagia it is difficult to assess the amount of blood loss because the frightened patient and her overanxious mother are too nervous to be objective. Questions about the number of perineal pads or tampons utilized, degree of saturation, the quantity and size of blood clots, and presence of orthostatic symptoms facilitate estimation of blood loss. The normal volume of menstrual bleeding averages 30 ml to 40 ml and corresponds to 10 to 15 moderately soaked pads or tampons. Information pertinent to all possible causes of vaginal hemorrhage should also be obtained.

A complete physical examination should be performed. Special attention must be paid to signs of hypovolemia and anemia, namely, pallor, low blood pressure and orthostatic hypotension, tachycardia, and the presence of a functional heart murmur. The abdomen should be carefully palpated for the presence of a mass, localized pain, or peritoneal signs. A speculum examination is mandatory to evaluate the amount of bleeding and to rule out any vaginal abnormality and visualize the cervix. In the presence of a tight hymen, blood clots may accumulate and distend the vagina. The finding of as much as 500 ml coagulated blood in the vagina is not unusual. This retrograde accumulation of clots may also account for cervical dilatation, which can be erroneously attributed to a spontaneous abortion. Internal genital structures are assessed by rectovaginal examination looking for the presence of uterine enlargement and adnexal masses or tenderness.

The laboratory work-up should consist of hemoglobin, hematocrit, platelet count, blood type and cross match, and basic clotting studies, including prothrombin time (PT), partial thromboplastin time (PTT), and bleeding time. These specimens should be drawn before the institution of any hormonal therapy or transfusion.

Serum β-hCG or another highly sensitive pregnancy test and a cervical culture for gonorrhea should be obtained in every patient. Determination of blood sugar, thyroid function tests, and urinalysis are also recommended but are not essential before treatment is instituted. In certain instances, a pelvic sonogram may be indicated for evaluation of an enlarged uterus or adnexal mass. The need for additional diagnostic studies depends on the clinical assessment of each patient.

MANAGEMENT. The aims of the therapy of acute adolescent menorrhagia are to control bleeding, restore adequate intravascular volume and correct anemia, treat underlying conditions when present, and prevent recurrence. Method and intensity of therapy obviously depend on the severity of hemorrhage. The adolescent in whom the bleeding is mild to moderate without signs of hypovolemia can be treated on an outpatient basis, provided close follow-up and good complicance are assured. These patients often have moderate anemia caused by prolonged bleeding. In the presence of severe hemorrhage or anemia (hemoglobin less than 8 g %) or when the patient is hypovolemic, admission is mandatory.

The initial treatment is medical rather than surgical in most patients. Since bleeding is primarily due to unstable endometrium that is caused by fluctuating estrogen levels, the rationale of therapy is to stop the hemorrhage by administering estrogen and to stabilize the endometrium with progestogens. We have used birth-control pills containing 2 mg of norethindrone and 100 μg of mestranol very effectively in this situation. These are administered at the rate of one pill every 4 hours until the bleeding subsides. If bleeding does not stop within 24 to 36 hours, other causes of bleeding should be seriously considered. In the presence of acute, severe hemorrhage, intravenous conjugated estrogens (Premarin, Ayerst) administered at a dosage of 25 mg every 4 hours for not more than four doses may be utilized in addition to the oral progestogens. The major side effect of oral progestogen and intravenous estrogen use is nausea and vomiting, for which we use antinausea medications prophylactically. Blood replacement is used when necessary.

Once the bleeding has stopped or decreased appreciably, oral contraceptives are tapered gradually over a period of seven days and then continued at a rate of one pill daily for 21 days. Withdrawal bleeding will follow the discontinuation of treatment. The patient should be informed that this may be heavy but is self-limiting.

Dilatation and curettage is reserved for those cases where medical treatment fails to control the bleeding within 24 to 36 hours. Approximately 20% of patients require surgical intervention to control bleeding. In most instances where medical management has failed, endometrial hyperplasia is present. Occasionally, curettings will be scant as a result of a complete endometrial slough.

We have encountered two patients who did not respond to dilatation and curettage. In both instances bleeding was controlled by uterine packing. This was carried out using an iodoform gauze, which was left in place for 24 hours and then withdrawn slowly. Prophylactic antibiotic coverage should be given in this unusual situation. The only patient who required hysterectomy was a 20-year-old girl with artificial heart valves who was anticoagulated.

FOLLOW-UP. Close follow-up of these patients is essential to prevent recurrence and provide adequate emotional support. After the initial phase of therapy, the patient may remain anovulatory. It is, therefore, advisable to continue these patients on low-dose birth-control pills for a period of at least three months. The adolescent in need of birth control can be continued on low-dose oral contraceptives. When the risk of unwanted pregnancy is not a concern, the best approach is to start the patient on basal body temperature charts and administer oral progestogens cyclically if the temperature curve is monophasic. A rational regimen is to induce withdrawal bleeding every six weeks with a 10-day course of medroxyprogesterone acetate (Provera), 10 mg daily. This treatment is usually adequate to prevent endometrial hyperproliferation. Since it does not suppress the hypothalamic-pituitary-ovarian axis, it allows the teenager to develop regular, ovulatory cycles on her own. When this occurs, the patient may menstruate spontaneously between Provera courses.

Long-term follow-up includes correction of anemia with iron supplements and nutritional counseling, and surveillance for spontaneous occurrence of ovulatory cycles. Patients presenting with acute menorrhagia in the perimenarchal period are at greater risk of chronic anovulation, infertility, and endometrial carcinoma.

The emotional aspects of this problem should not be underestimated. For these youngsters, a hemorrhagic event of this type is a very sad way to begin their active reproductive life. Adequate explanation, reassurance, and psychologic support during the acute episode and over the subsequent months will serve to guide these teenagers through their menstrual problems optimistically.

Persistent Hypermenorrhea

Cyclic heavy menses is also a frequent complaint in adolescents. These patients usually present with more or less regular menstrual cycles, ranging from four to six weeks, but characterized by excessive bleeding, either in amount or duration.

Although anovulation is the leading cause of recurrent hypermenorrhea in this population, other causes such as uterine pathologies, coagulation defects, and systemic diseases must be considered.

Besides a thorough history and physical examination, the basic work-up of these teenagers should consist of hemoglobin, hematocrit, and platelet count determination, screening clotting studies, and thyroid function tests.

Therapy depends on the degree of the bleeding abnormality. Patients with mildly increased menstrual flow in whom there is no secondary anemia can be managed expectantly. In these cases, basal body temperature recording confirms the diagnosis of anovulation. Prostaglandin inhibitors may also be used to decrease the amount of bleeding. Adolescents in need of birth control obviously benefit from oral contraception. When treatment is required because of the degree of the flow or associated anemia, medroxyprogesterone acetate is prescribed to regularize cycles and induce a progestational effect on the endometrium. In this situation, 10 mg medroxyprogesterone acetate daily is administered from the 15th to the 25th day of each cycle. For most of these young patients, a calendar month schedule (treatment for the first 10 days of each month) is understood more easily. After three to six months, therapy is discontinued and the patient is observed for spontaneous occurrence of ovulatory cycles. Failure of hormonal therapy is an indication for dilatation and curettage.

Persistent Polymenorrhea

The complaint of too-frequent periods is also common among adolescents. Anovulation, once again, is the most frequent cause of polymenorrhea in this age group. In some patients, this menstrual abnormality may also originate from a short follicular phase or corpus luteum dysfunction, which usually is self-limiting when the hypothalamic-pituitary-ovarian axis matures.

The physician should, however, be aware of the fact that very often this complaint is unjustified. A thorough history frequently brings to light that the patient calculates her intermenstrual interval from the last day of one period to the first day of the next. The recording of a menstrual calendar and information about normal physiology are usually sufficient to reassure these adolescents.

When cycles are shorter than 21 days, therapy with medroxyprogesterone acetate administered as described above, is indicated. With very short intermenstrual intervals, it may be necessary to start the treatment on the 10th day of the cycle for a period of 15 days.

Acute and Chronic Pelvic Pain in the Adolescent

Acute and chronic pelvic pain accounts for a substantial number of consultations for gynecologists who deal with the adolescent age-group. The reasons are simple: first, there is a tendency to attribute a gynecologic etiology to all pain "below the umbilicus" in perimenarchal and postmenarchal females. Second, most physicians are reluctant to perform a pelvic examination in the young patient.

The differential diagnosis of pelvic pain, in fact, includes a wide variety of gynecologic, nongynecologic, and functional or psychosomatic causes, and these must be thoroughly investigated.

Acute Pelvic Pain

Acute pelvic pain necessitates aggressive management because of the intensity of symptoms and the possibility that a life-threatening condition may exist.

DIFFERENTIAL DIAGNOSIS. The differential diagnosis of acute pelvic pain in adolescents is summarized as follows:

I. Gynecologic Causes
       Infection
            Pelvic inflammatory disease
       Rupture
            Follicular cyst
            Corpus luteum cyst
            Endometrioma
            Tumor (rare)
       Torsion
            Ovarian cyst
            Tube
            Hydatid of Morgagni
II. Nongynecologic Causes
       Gastrointestinal
            Appendicitis
            Meckel diverticulitis
            Gastroenteritis
            Mesenteric adenitis
            Intestinal obstruction
       Urinary
            Cystitis
            Pyelonephritis
            Calculi

The gynecologic causes can be divided into three categories: infection, rupture, and torsion. In general, symptoms associated with infection usually develop progressively over a few days. In cases of rupture or torsion, pain occurs suddenly. Nongynecologic etiologies involve mainly the digestive or the urinary tract.

HISTORY AND PHYSICAL EXAMINATION. The history should define, as exactly as possible, the sequence of events, the pain location and its radiation, and associated gastrointestinal, urinary, and systemic symptoms. A careful menstrual, contraceptive, and sexual history is also mandatory.

A complete physical examination should, of course, be performed. Special attention is paid to the abdomen to localize the pain, determine whether a mass is present, and identify peritoneal signs or evidence of bowel obstruction. A pelvic examination must be performed on every patient in order to determine the size, shape, and symmetry of the uterus and the presence of adnexal or cervical tenderness and to identify adnexal masses or thickening.

DIAGNOSTIC STUDIES. The basic laboratory workup should include a complete blood count with differential, a determination of erythrocyte sedimentation rate, a complete urinalysis, a urine culture, a pregnancy test, and a cervical culture.

The finding of a high white blood cell count or sedimentation rate suggests the presence of either an infectious or inflammatory process or some kind of ischemia, usually in association with adnexal torsion or bowel obstruction. Hemoglobin and hematocrit values are usually poor indicators of bleeding, since in acute hemorrhage hemodilution may not have occurred. Depending on the type of pregnancy test utilized, it should be remembered that a negative result does not always rule out an early or an ectopic pregnancy.

A pelvic ultrasound may be valuable to confirm the presence of a mass, to identify the presence of free fluid in the cul-de-sac, and to identify an intrauterine pregnancy.

MANAGEMENT. After the first diagnostic steps have been taken, the patient can be placed into one of the following categories:

1. There is a definite surgical emergency that prompts immediate laparotomy. In this case the suspected diagnosis is usually an acute hemoperitoneum, a ruptured tubo-ovarian abscess, acute appendicitis or ruptured appendix, or other gastrointestinal surgical emergencies.
2. The patient suffers from a medical condition and adequate treatment is started. Conditions of this kind include urinary tract infection, gastroenteritis, pelvic inflammatory disease.
3. The suspected problem needs further investigation (*e.g.,* urinary calculi).
4. The problem remains undiagnosed. The question in this case usually is: "Does this patient have pelvic inflammatory disease, an ectopic pregnancy, appendicitis, a ruptured or torsioned ovarian cyst?"

At this point, laparoscopy becomes an invaluable diagnostic tool. The potential risk of a surgical diagnostic procedure remains a concern for many physicians. In fact, laparoscopy provides an immediate diagnosis that allows for appropriate medical or surgical treatment. It is also more cost-effective to perform an immediate laparoscopy than to subject the patient to a long period of inpatient observation during which a surgical catastrophe, such as a ruptured appendix or ectopic pregnancy, remains a possibility. In cases of ruptured ovarian cysts or hemorrhagic corpus luteum in which there is no more active bleeding, it is possible to aspirate free blood and clots and ensure hemostasis by fulgurating bleeders. This technique saves the patient several days of agonizing pain and usually allows her to be discharged within 12 hours of the procedure.

In our judgment, the advantages of laparoscopy certainly outweigh the minimal surgical risk in these generally healthy teenagers.

Chronic Pelvic Pain

Chronic pelvic pain (CPP) in adolescents is a frequent complaint and an important source of frustration for the patient, her parents, and her physician. CPP can be defined as three months or more of constant or intermittent, cyclic or acyclic pelvic pain, or at least three separate visits to a physician for this problem, without a definite diagnosis. Symptoms can be characterized by dull or severe pain, dysmenorrhea, dyspareunia, or vaginal pain. Very often these teenagers have been absent from school frequently, going from doctor to doctor, have undergone a number of radiologic examinations, have tried a variety of analgesics without success, and have been referred for psychiatric evaluation.

Guzinski has drawn an excellent picture of the CPP patient with whom it is difficult to deal. After having been told, often more than once, that nothing is wrong with her, she may come to you desperate, with a considerable amount of anger and frustration. It is, therefore, important to assure her that all efforts will be made to sort out her problem and that she will not be abandoned and her symptoms dismissed.

DIFFERENTIAL DIAGNOSIS. The differential diagnosis of CPP in adolescents is summarized as follows:

I.   Gynecologic Causes
     Dysmenorrhea (primary, secondary)
     Mittelschmertz
     Endometriosis
     Chronic pelvic inflammatory disease
     Ovarian cyst
     Genital tract malformation
     Pelvic congestion
     Pelvic serositis

II. Gastrointestinal Causes
    Constipation, bowel spasms
    Appendiceal fecaliths
    Bowel inflammatory diseases
    Dietary intolerance (lactose)
III. Urinary Causes
    Urinary tract infection
    Hydronephrosis
    Urethral stricture
    Urethral caruncle
    Urinary retention
IV. Orthopedic Causes
    Lordosis, kyphosis, scoliosis
    Herniation of intervertebral disk
V. Adhesions
    Postoperative
    Post pelvic infection
VI. Psychogenic Causes

The differential diagnosis includes many systems that can be responsible for pelvic symptoms either directly or by referred pain, as well as those of psychogenic etiology.

An efficient approach to the problem depends on a thorough history and physical examination as well as the judicious use of diagnostic studies.

HISTORY AND PHYSICAL EXAMINATION. It is essential to review the complete history of the problem, including description, location, and radiation of the pain, exacerbating and relieving factors, and association with the menstrual cycle or with gastrointestinal, urinary, and musculoskeletal symptoms. The past medical and surgical history may also yield important clues. All prior diagnostic procedures and trials of treatment should be recorded and, when possible, old medical records should be obtained. The familial and social history, as well as the association of the pain episodes with stressful events, should be detailed.

A complete physical examination should be performed, the abdomen being carefully palpated in search of any masses, tender areas, or organomegaly. Special care should be taken to differentiate deep pain from abdominal wall tenderness, especially in patients who underwent prior surgical procedures. It is also of great importance to perform a skeletal assessment to identify any orthopedic abnormality that may be the cause of referred pelvic pain or be associated with a congenital reproductive tract anomaly. A speculum examination should be included to identify any vaginal or cervical anomaly and obtain cultures and cytology. The bimanual recto-vaginal-abdominal palpation evaluates the pelvic structures and localizes tender areas. The posterior cul-de-sac should also be assessed for pain and nodularity.

DIAGNOSTIC STUDIES. The minimal laboratory work-up in these patients consists of a complete blood count with differential and erythrocytic sedimentation rate, a urine analysis and culture, and a cervical culture. Other hematologic and biochemical studies are ordered depending on clinical indications.

Pelvic ultrasonography may be useful to define a mass, provide information about a suspected genital tract malformation, or screen patients in whom a satisfactory pelvic examination is impossible. Routine sonography in every patient is probably not advisable. In a study of 96 adolescents evaluated for CPP at The Cleveland Clinic, Gidwani reported that of 15 patients in whom a pelvic mass was detected by ultrasonography, only five were actually found to have a mass at laparoscopy.

No specific rules can be given regarding radiologic examinations. It is certainly not advisable to submit all these teenagers to pelvic radiation without clinical indications. Gastrointestinal, urologic, and orthopedic studies should be ordered on the basis of the diagnostic impression after a thorough history, physical examination, and laboratory work-up.

LAPAROSCOPY. Laparoscopy is an invaluable tool in the diagnosis of CPP. It can be used to diagnose or confirm the presence of organic disease that cannot be demonstrated by physical, radiologic, and sonographic examination. It allows the surgeon to obtain appropriate biopsies and to perform minor surgical procedures, such as fulguration of endometriosis, lysis of adhesions, and aspiration of ovarian cysts. Negative findings at laparoscopy may equally be valuable in reassuring the patient that no organic disease is present and help her accept the idea that she might have a functional problem that requires medical or emotional treatment.

Indications for laparoscopy in the evaluation of adolescents with CPP can be summarized as follows:

1. Dysmenorrhea unresponsive to the usual therapy with prostoglandin inhibitors or ovulation suppression
2. Confirmation or exclusion of clinically suspected endometriosis, chronic pelvic inflammatory disease, pelvic adhesions, appendiceal fecaliths, ovarian cysts, and pelvic serositis
3. Evaluation of undiagnosed pain after appropriate work-up

Between July, 1974, and December, 1983, 282 patients ranging in age from 9 to 21 years underwent a diagnostic laparoscopy at The Children's Hospital because of chronic pelvic pain. Most of these adolescents had been referred to our Gynecology Service after a negative gastrointestinal and urinary tract work-up or because of dysmenorrhea unresponsive to the usual therapy with prostaglandin inhibitors or oral contraceptives. Many of these patients had undergone psychiatric evaluation because of persistent and undiagnosed pain. Cases of chronic pelvic inflammatory disease were not included in the data because this condition is usually suspected on the basis of the past history and the finding of positive cervical culture or elevated erythrocyte sedimentation rate.

Table 45-2 summarizes the diagnosis in these patients. Three quarters of the patients were found to have intrapelvic pathology. Endometriosis was the most frequent finding and was diagnosed in 45% of the cases. In most instances, the disease was mild to moderate, with implants located in the posterior cul-de-sac, on the ovaries, and on the lateral pelvic walls. The next most common finding was postoperative adhesions, which occurred in 13% of patients and were, for the most part, secondary to appendectomy or ovarian cystectomy.

One of the most puzzling laparoscopic findings was the presence of pelvic serositis in 5% of the patients. This was characterized by hyperemia and granuloma-like lesions of the pelvic peritoneum and uterine serosa. Peritoneal biopsies revealed the presence of mesothelial hyperplasia with hemosiderin deposits. Peritoneal culture and cytology were normal. The significance of these changes remains unclear. Do they signify the appearance of very early endometriosis, a reaction to repeated hemoperitoneum secondary to a leaking corpus luteum, a viral infection, or an incidental finding? These patients have proven to be very difficult to treat. Owing to the small number of cases, no uniform therapy has emerged. Some patients respond to therapy with long-term prostaglandin inhibitors, others to ovulation suppression, and others to therapy with adrenal steroids. Long-term follow-up will hopefully better define this entity.

Table 45-2

Laparoscopic Findings in 282 Adolescents with Chronic Pelvic Pain, The Children's Hospital, Boston, 1974–1983

Finding	Patients	
	Number	*Percent*
Endometriosis	126	45
Postoperative adhesions	37	13
Serositis	15	5
Ovarian cyst	14	5
Uterine malformation	15	5
Others*	4	2
No pathology	71	25

* Ileitis, infarcted hydatid of Morgagni, pelvic congestion.

Other findings in patients with CPP included ovarian cysts, uterine malformations of the obstructive type, cases of ileitis, infarcted hydatids of Morgagni, and pelvic congestion.

No organic disease was documented in 25% of the patients. In this group, pain was attributed to functional bowel disease or to psychogenic factors. Despite apparently normal bowel function, many teenagers with CPP improve when placed on a regimen of stool softeners and increased dietary fiber. The value of a negative laparoscopy should also not be underestimated. In many instances, the assurance that their pelvic structures are normal is sufficient to improve the condition of these adolescents. Goldstein and colleagues reported that 74% of these patients were symptomatically improved after a negative laparoscopy. In a few, adjunctive psychologic or behavioral modification therapy is necessary.

For the years 1980 to 1983, the results were broken down into age-groups (Table 45-3). It is interesting to note that the incidence of endometriosis among adolescents complaining of CPP increases progressively with age, from 12% in the 11- to 13-year-old group to 54% in patients aged 20 and 21 years. Pelvic serositis, on the other hand, was encountered mostly in the 11- to 15-year-old group. Other findings remained fairly constant in all age groups.

ADNEXAL MASSES IN CHILDREN AND ADOLESCENTS

Over the past decade, gynecologists have been consulted more frequently about the problem of ovarian masses during childhood and adolescence. The true incidence of this condition has probably not changed but the increasing use of ultrasound by pediatricians and family practitioners has led to the detection of many functional cysts that previously would have gone undetected. Even though most of these masses are functional and require only reassurance, it is imperative that true ovarian neoplasms receive immediate attention and therapy. It is, therefore, important that gynecologists feel comfortable in the evaluation of a child or teenager with an adnexal mass.

Differential Diagnosis

The differential diagnosis of adnexal masses includes enlargement of other reproductive structures as well as masses of extragenital origin.

Every type of ovarian tumor seen in the adult can also be encountered in children and adolescents. The relative incidence of each entity is quite different, however. For example, functional masses are much more common in adolescents because of the high incidence

Table 45-3

*Age-Related Incidence of Laparoscopic Findings in 129 Adolescents with Chronic Pelvic Pain,
The Children's Hospital, Boston, 1980–1983*

	Number of Patients				
Finding	Age 11–13	Age 14–15	Age 16–17	Age 18–19	Age 20–21
Endometriosis	2 (12%)	9 (28%)	21 (40%)	17 (45%)	7 (54%)
Postoperative adhesions	1 (6%)	4 (13%)	7 (13%)	5 (13%)	2 (15%)
Serositis	5 (29%)	4 (13%)	0 (0%)	2 (5%)	0 (0%)
Ovarian cyst	2 (12%)	2 (6%)	3 (5%)	2 (5%)	0 (0%)
Uterine malformation	1 (6%)	0 (0%)	1 (2%)	0 (0%)	1 (8%)
Others	0 (0%)	1 (3%)	2 (4%)	1 (3%)	0 (0%)
No pathology	6 (35%)	12 (37%)	19 (36%)	11 (29%)	3 (23%)

of anovulatory cycles. In this age group, neoplastic tumors are more likely to be of germinal rather than of epithelial origin.

Fortunately, in children and adolescents, only one in ten ovarian tumors is malignant. It is difficult to obtain accurate statistics about the frequency of functional cysts because most studies are based on surgical reviews. Since a large number of patients with functional adnexal enlargement are treated expectantly and never undergo surgery, they are not included in published series.

Lack and Goldstein presented their experience with 242 children and adolescents operated upon for ovarian masses. The results of this study are summarized in Table 45-4. Thirty-one percent of the patients were found to have a tumor-like condition including follicle, corpus luteum, and simple and endometriotic cysts. Of the 166 cases of primary ovarian tumors, there were 118 (71%) germ-cell tumors, of which 78 (66%) consisted of benign mature teratomas. Of 27 epithelial tumors, 85% were benign. Twenty-one (13%) of their patients had a sex cord-stromal tumor, which is generally considered to be a low-grade malignancy. These results are comparable to those in other reports.

Signs and Symptoms

Many ovarian tumors are asymptomatic and are discovered fortuitously during a routine pelvic examination. Since most young patients do not consult for periodic pelvic examinations, ovarian masses are often picked up when they become large enough to cause symptoms or to be felt by abdominal palpation. Smaller ovarian enlargements are frequently found incidentally at the time of an ultrasound examination performed for an unrelated symptom, such as pain. Findings of this kind account for a large proportion of the consultations for masses that prove to be physiologic.

Symptoms are usually related to the size of the mass or to mechanical accidents, such as rupture, torsion, or hemorrhage. In the young prepubertal girl, pain is abdominal because of the reduced pelvic capacity and the

Table 45-4

Pathologic Diagnosis of 242 Ovarian Tumors Treated Surgically at Children's Hospital Medical Center (Boston) 1928 to 1982

	Tumor	
Diagnosis	Number	Percent
Tumor-Like Enlargements	76	(31%)
Primary Ovarian Tumors	166	(69%)
Germ cell tumors	118	(71%)
Mature teratoma	78	
Immature teratoma	17	
Endodermal sinus tumor	14	
Dysgerminoma	8	
Choriocarcinoma	1	
Epithelial tumors	27	(16%)
Serous	14	
Mucinous	12	
Mixed	1	
Sex cord—stromal tumors	21	(13%)
Granulosa	10	
Sertoli-Leydig	7	
Thecoma	2	
Fibroma	1	
Unclassified	1	

(Adapted from Lack EE, Goldstein DP: Primary ovarian tumors in childhood and adolescence. Curr Probl Obstet Gynecol, no. 10, 1984)

fairly high position of the ovaries. In the older patient, symptoms are more often pelvic. Bladder and ureteral compression may also be encountered •with larger masses. Malignant tumors that infiltrate the surrounding tissue may induce bowel obstruction. In mechanical accidents, symptoms develop acutely and are usually characterized by severe pain and peritoneal signs, including nausea and vomiting. In hormone-producing tumors, precocious puberty, menstrual irregularities, or virilization may lead to the diagnosis.

On pelvic examination, the mass can usually be palpated by rectoabdominal examination with the patient in the lithotomy position. As mentioned previously, ovarian tumors in children are often intra-abdominal rather than pelvic and should be considered in the differential diagnosis of abdominal masses. Other physical findings depend on the degree of invasion of the tumor and its hormonal activity.

Diagnostic Work-Up

Ultrasound is an invaluable tool in the diagnosis of ovarian masses. It provides information about the size, location, and consistency of the tumor, (*i.e.,* whether it is cystic, solid, or complex). Ultrasound is also useful to determine the presence of free peritoneal fluid and ascites. A flat plate of the abdomen will reveal the presence of calcifications, which suggest a diagnosis of dermoid cyst. This information can, however, also be obtained by ultrasonography.

The remainder of the work-up depends on the clinical picture. If the tumor is solid or hormonally active, blood should be drawn for assessment of levels of hCG, alpha-fetoprotein, CA-125, and estradiol. FSH and LH levels may help to differentiate a true precocious puberty responsible for a functional cyst from an estrogen-secreting tumor inducing a pseudoprecocious puberty. When hirsutism or signs of virlization are present, a testosterone level should be obtained. When malignancy is suspected, a preoperative metastatic work-up should be done, including chest x-ray; CT scan of brain, chest, and abdomen; and liver function tests.

Management

Postmenarchal Adolescent

In the postmenarchal patient, ovarian masses are approched in much the same way as in the young adult. Figure 45-7 summarizes the management of ovarian tumors in this age group. Upon the finding of an ovarian mass, an ultrasound study should be obtained to confirm the diagnosis and further define the tumor's characteristics. Due to the high incidence of functional masses, an asymptomatic, purely cystic tumor with a diameter of 6 cm or less is observed for two or three cycles for spontaneous regression. In patients with functional masses, the use of oral contraceptives to inhibit ovarian function may accelerate regression and prevent the appearance of new functional enlargement. Cystic masses that do not decrease in size over a period of three months, that enlarge, or that are larger than 6 cm initially should be operated on. A laparoscopy may be performed prior to laparotomy to confirm the diagnosis. When the cyst appears to be functional and is less than 6 cm in diameter, puncture aspiration may be performed. All fluid obtained should be sent for cytologic examination.

Solid and complex tumors should be removed without delay. A laparoscopy may be performed as the initial procedure in order to establish the diagnosis, help to decide on the optimal incision, and, in cases of unexpected malignancy, allow the surgeon to discuss the extent of the proposed surgery with the parents.

Laparotomy should be performed through an incision large enough to allow excision of the tumor without rupture and according to the principles of ovarian surgery (*i.e.,* peritoneal lavage, complete abdominal exploration, frozen section, and periaortic node dissection when indicated).

Premenarchal Child

In the premenarchal child, since the presence of a functional enlargement is unlikely, all ovarian tumors should be explored surgically. There are, however, two exceptions to this rule. The first of these occurs in the neonatal period, when both withdrawal from estrogen and progesterone, which results in a transient secretion of gonadotropins by the newborn female, and the influence of maternal hCG can cause follicle cysts to develop. These cysts are usually of a fairly large size. In 16 cases of follicle cysts in infants six months of age or younger reported by Lack and Goldstein, the average diameter was 8.3 cm (range: 3–16 cm). In these situations, management depends on the size of the mass. When it is large enough to cause obstruction of the digestive or urinary tract, the cyst should be excised. Healthy ovarian tissue should be preserved if at all possible. Smaller cystic ovarian enlargements in the newborn can be observed for spontaneous regression, providing there is no evidence of torsion, hemorrhage, or rupture.

The second period of childhood during which functional cysts may be encountered is the premenarchal period. In the premenarchal child in whom sexual development has begun, an ovarian mass proved to be completely cystic by ultrasound can be safely managed according to the same protocol as described for postmenarchal patients.

All solid or complex masses, no matter what the age of the patient, and all cystic tumors occurring at any time during childhood except the neonatal and prepubertal periods should be managed surgically.

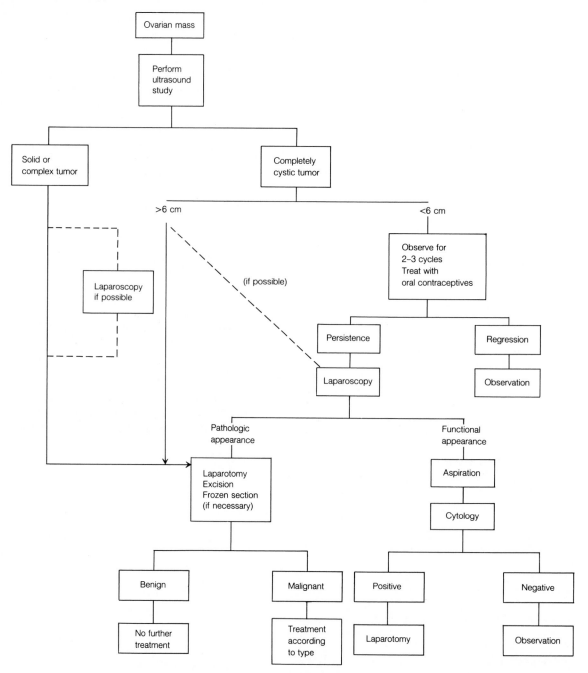

FIG. 45-7. Management of ovarian tumors in the postmenarchal adolescent.

CONGENITAL ABNORMALITIES

A large proportion of congenital abnormalities of the female genital tract remain undiscovered until adolescence. These are usually diagnosed either when symptoms occur, especially menstrual disorders and coital difficulties, or simply because most patients undergo their first pelvic examination at this time.

Although some congenital malformations are obvious at first glance, the diagnosis of many of these defects requires a high index of suspicion. A thorough understanding of the nature of these anomalies is essential to gynecologists who deal with the teenage group. Early diagnosis, adequate treatment, and appropriate psychologic support and counseling assure the preservation of reproductive function when feasible and allow these adolescents to develop a serene attitude toward their sexuality.

Vulva

Labial Adhesions

In adolescents, labial synechia secondary to hypoestrogenism are quite infrequent. When they occur, the problem is approached as for younger children. During adolescence, the most commonly encountered type of labial adhesion is an epithelial bridge between either the labia majora or minora. These bridges may be congenital or posttrauma and since they may be easily torn, surgical incision is advisable.

Labial Minora Hypertrophy or Asymmetry

In some instances, one or both of the labia minora are unusually large and the patient consults because she notices the anomaly or because of symptoms of irritation associated with exercise. In most of these cases, simple reassurance is all that is necessary. Comparison with asymmetry or hypertrophy of other parts of the body may help the patient to accept this peculiarity. Improved hygiene and avoidance of tight clothes are usually sufficient to relieve discomfort. When these measures prove to be ineffective, or in the presence of a troublesome cosmetic problem, surgical reduction is in order.

Imperforate Hymen

Although the diagnosis of an imperforate hymen should be made long before adolescence as part of routine neonatal and pediatric examinations, it is not uncommon to see a teenager present with the typical picture of primary amenorrhea, cyclic or acyclic pelvic pain, bulging hymen, hematocolpos, hematometra, or hydrocolpos.

The surgical therapy consists of hymenotomy, which often reveals a large accumulation of blood (Figure 45-8). The central part of the hymen should also be excised to allow further unobstructed menstrual flow. We have found that needle-tip electrocautery facilitates hemostasis on the hymenal edge. This technique avoids the need for many sutures and minimizes the likelihood of secondary retraction. The use of a Yankauer suction tip inserted high into the vagina or through the dilated cervix into the uterus facilitates evacuation. Prophylactic antibiotic therapy is not required.

Microperforate, Cribriform, and Septate Hymen

Microperforate, cribriform, and septate hymenal openings are most often asymptomatic. Quite frequently, however, patients with these anatomic variants consult because of unsuccessful attempts at inserting a

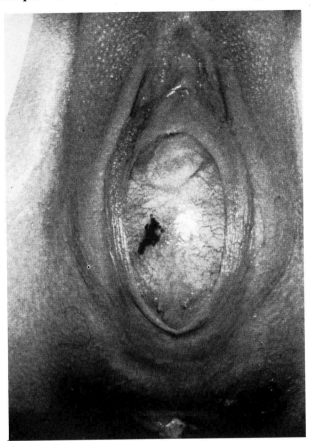

FIG. 45-8. Bulging imperforate hymen in a 12-year-old girl with amenorrhea, abdominal pain, and a large pelvic mass.

tampon or coital difficulties. With a microperforate hymen, the adolescent may also complain of postmenstrual vaginal spotting or malodorous discharge secondary to incomplete obstruction. In these situations, hymenotomy is indicated.

When the diagnosis is made fortuitously, the patient should be told about this structural anomaly and informed of the necessity of surgical correction. Performing the procedure during the early teens allows the adolescent to use tampons without difficulty and may avoid later conflictual situations when the patient desires to become sexually active.

Vagina

Congenital Absence of Vagina

Patients with congenital absence of the vagina usually consult in their mid teens because of primary amenorrhea. In most of them, the uterus is also absent and either Mayer-Rokitansky-Kuster-Hauser syndrome (müllerian agenesis) or testicular feminization will ultimately be diagnosed. In some instances, vaginal agenesis coexists with a functioning uterus; adolescents with this anomaly present at an earlier age with obstructive symptoms.

The pelvic examination of these patients reveals the absence of the vagina, and a particular feature is the small space separating the urethral meatus from the anus. The outer part of the vagina may be present as a blind vaginal canal of variable depth. This finding is more likely to be associated with testicular feminization syndrome. In a series presented by Bryans, 7 out of 11 patients with testicular feminization had a vaginal depth of 3 cm or more at the time of presentation, whereas in 13 of the 19 patients with Mayer-Rokitansky-Kuster-Hauser syndrome, the vaginal length before therapy was less than 1 cm. The presence or absence of a uterus is ascertained by rectoabdominal examination. External genitalia are usually of normal appearance. In cases of testicular feminization, characteristic stigmata can usually be observed.

The work-up should consist at least of pelvic ultrasound to confirm the presence or absence of a uterus, renal echography or intravenous pyelography to detect urinary tract anomalies (found in approximately one third of patients with müllerian agenesis), assessment of plasma testosterone level, which will be in male range in case of testicular feminization syndrome, and a karyotype.

Therapy of vaginal agenesis aims at creating a vaginal canal to allow satisfactory sexual function and to establish adequate menstrual drainage when a functioning uterus is present. Therapeutic management should be individualized for each patient.

When obstruction to menstrual flow is not a concern, therapy is best delayed until the patient desires it and has acquired enough maturity to comply with the demanding postoperative care that is the key to a successful outcome. In patients who already have a vaginal depth of 3 cm or more, treatment is not always needed, since coital activity may be enough to induce vaginal deepening. When a rudimentary vagina is present, the nonsurgical Frank method, which consists of progressive vaginal dilatation using dilators, should be attempted first. When surgical creation of a neovagina is indicated, the preferred technique at our institution is the McIndoe procedure, which utilizes a split-thickness skin graft placed in a space created between the urethra and the rectum. Following this operation, in order to avoid postoperative stenosis, a vaginal stent (such as the Youngs vaginal dilator) must be used until the patient has regular coital activity. The patient's motivation, therefore, plays an important role in the timing of surgery. The Williams' vulvovaginoplasty is an acceptable therapeutic alternative. This technique offers the advantages of a shorter operative time, does not necessitate a skin graft, and entails less risk of permanent stenosis if the patient does not comply with postoperative dilatation. The Williams' procedure is most often performed

to lengthen a preexisting rudimentary vagina or when the result of a McIndoe procedure is not satisfactory.

When a functioning uterus and cervix are present, treatment cannot be delayed, because menstrual flow will be obstructed. In such cases, the principal problem is the young age at which surgical correction is necessary. When a neovagina is created, use of a stent that is centrally opened to allow drainage of menstrual blood and that is left in place for four to six months decreases the likelihood of irreversible stenosis.

Transverse Vaginal Septum

Transverse vaginal septa are most often located at the junction of the upper and middle third of the vagina but can be encountered at any level along the vaginal canal. Such septa may vary from a narrow annular ring to a completely obstructive membrane and also vary widely in thickness.

Symptoms depend on both the width and the location of the anomaly. A narrow annular septum usually is a fortuitous finding of no clinical significance and does not require any treatment. On the other hand, primary amenorrhea and early symptoms of obstruction occur in cases of complete septum, and surgical excision is then imperative. When the upper and lower vagina communicate only by a small fistulous tract through the septum, the clinical picture is sometimes quite puzzling. These patients may present with dysmenorrhea, irregular vaginal spotting, or purulent discharge because of partial obstruction and accumulation of blood above the defect. Secondary pelvic inflammatory disease due to anaerobic infection may also be the initial mode of presentation. A septum lying low in the vagina is frequently the cause of dyspareunia. Infertility and soft tissue dystocia are unusual presentations of this malformation in the adolescent group.

Surgical correction consists of complete excision of the septum and anastomosis of the upper vagina to the lower vagina. The use of a stent may be necessary when the septum involves a long vaginal segment and primary anastomosis is impossible.

Longitudinal Vaginal Septum

Longitudinal vaginal septa most often occur in association with abnormalities of uterine fusion but may sometimes be an isolated malformation. Such septa divide the vagina sagittally in two equal or unequal parts for its entire length or partially. Surgical excision is indicated when dyspareunia becomes a problem or when childbearing is anticipated.

In some instances the septum fuses with the lateral vaginal wall and creates a blind vaginal pouch, giving rise to obstructive symptoms. This entity will be discussed together with obstructing uterine fusion anomalies.

Cervix and Uterus

Cervical Agenesis

Congenital absence of the cervix can occur in association with vaginal agenesis or with a normal vagina. This rarity causes early obstructive signs and symptoms characterized by hematometra, tubal regurgitation of menstrual blood, and secondary endometriosis.

Attempts to preserve fertility by creation of a fistulous tract between the endometrial cavity and the vagina have been very disappointing. A conservative surgical approach usually leads to repeated operations, and only two successful pregnancies are reported in the literature. Furthermore, Niver and colleagues reported that of 18 patients in whom conservative surgery was attempted, 2 died of sepsis. The recommended therapy of cervical agenesis, therefore, remains hysterectomy with ovarian conservation, when possible.

Obstructing Uterine and Vaginal Duplication

Abnormalities of uterovaginal fusion that are diagnosed during adolescent years are mostly of the obstructing type. These anomalies can be divided into three categories according to the site of obstruction. In our experience at The Children's Hospital with 16 cases of uterine or vaginal obstructing duplication, the most commonly encountered anomaly is a didelphic uterus with unilateral vaginal obstruction secondary to a blind vagina. Unicornuate uterus with a contralateral blind horn, either rudimentary or of normal size, is second in frequency. Finally, a small number of patients present with cervical obstruction of one horn of a bicornuate uterus associated with an ipsilateral blind vaginal pouch. Fistulous tracts of various types may connect the blind vagina to a septate cervix or to the main vaginal cavity. Intercervical fistulas have also been discovered.

Signs and symptoms depend on the type of the abnormality. Since, in these cases, the obstruction is present only on one side, primary amenorrhea is not a feature. By far the most common presenting complaint is pelvic pain, either cyclic or acyclic, which is the consequence of unilaterally obstructed menstrual flow and secondary endometriosis. Abnormal vaginal bleeding and purulent discharge are also common and are usually associated with a fistulous tract connecting the obstructed to the unobstructed side. A blind vagina may become distended with menstrual blood, giving rise to vaginal pain or the sensation of pressure. On physical examination, masses corresponding to distended pelvic structures or abnormal uterine shape and discharge from possible fistulas can usually be visualized or palpated.

In these patients the minimal work-up should include a combined pelvic and renal sonogram and an intravenous pyelography. In our series, unilateral renal agenesis was found in 9 patients. Associated vesicoureteral reflux has also been reported. Laparoscopy and hysterosalpingogram should also be performed to determine the exact nature of the anomaly.

Therapy aims to preserve the reproductive function. For a unilaterally blind double vagina, the only treatment needed is a vaginal septectomy. In the case of a blind uterine horn, the type of surgery depends on the size of the obstructed horn and consists of either unification metroplasty or hemihysterectomy. For combined cervical obstruction, blind vaginal pouch, and fistulous tracts, vaginal septectomy should be performed. Furthermore, a unification procedure with complete removal of the cervical septum should also be performed to remove the cervical obstruction. Associated endometriosis should be treated adequately when necessary.

BREAST MASSES

Breast masses occur infrequently in adolescent females and often pose a problem in management. Virtually all breast masses are either benign tumors that require removal or physiologic swellings that regress spontaneously. Though malignancy is rare, patients and parents are concerned about any breast abnormalities and the cosmetic aspects of breast surgery.

Between January, 1972, and December, 1983, we performed 102 surgical procedures in 86 female adolescents ranging in age from 8 to 19 years (mean 16.3 years) for persistent or enlarged breast masses (Table 45-5). Puncture aspiration should be performed on all cystic masses. When fluid is obtained, no surgery is indicated unless the cyst recurs and is symptomatic or enlarged. Mammograms are not indicated. Surgery should be recommended when the mass is firm, not decompressible, persistent, or enlarging.

Fourteen patients underwent repeat procedures for recurrence. Bilateral lesions were present in 11% of patients. Only five procedures were done on an inpatient basis; two because of an intercurrent medical condition, two because of the size of the mass, and one because of associated inflammatory signs. General anesthesia was used in approximately three quarters of the patients. The lesion was excised through a circumareolar incision in 51% of the cases. During the last year of the study, this type of incision was utilized in 70% of the procedures. There were no operative complications.

The pathologic diagnosis of 100 biopsy specimens are listed in Table 45-6. Fibroadenoma was the predominant pathologic finding (83%).

This series confirms the previously reported high incidence of fibroadenomas and the rarity of malignancy associated with breast masses in adolescent females. However, although they are extremely rare, malignant tumors do occur in adolescents. Farrow and Ashikari reported one case of primary breast carcinoma among 237 patients aged 10 to 20 years, for an incidence of 0.4%. Haagensen reported that 0.02% of breast carci-

Table 45-5
*Summary of 102 Breast Procedures in
86 Adolescent Females*

Procedure Type	Number of Procedures
Type of Surgery	
Excisional biopsy	99 (97%)
Incision and drainage	1 (1%)
Incision and drainage and excisional biopsy	1 (1%)
Needle aspiration	1 (1%)
Repeat Procedures	16 (16%)
2 procedures: 13 (15% of patients)	
4 procedures: 1 (1% of patients)	
Site of Lesion	
Unilateral	91 (89%)
Bilateral	11 (11%)
Hospital Status	
Ambulatory	97 (95%)
Inpatient	5 (5%)
Type of Anesthesia	
General	74 (73%)
Local	28 (27%)
Type of Incision	
Circumareolar	52 (51%)
Curvilinear	30 (29%)
Unspecified	20 (20%)

nomas were found in women younger than 25 years. In Norris and Taylor's study of 5000 cases of breast cancer, 23 patients (0.46%) were under 25 years of age, and one (0.02%) was under 20.

All physicians dealing with adolescent females should be familiar with the physiology of breast development. Very often, a perimenarchal patient consults for the presence of a unilateral or bilateral tender subareolar mass. In these circumstances, the normally developing breast bud should be recognized. It is a firm button-shaped structure approximately 1 cm in diameter. Excision or biopsy will lead to dramatic and inexcusable iatrogenic amastia or breast deformity.

In general, pathologic masses are eccentric in location. Fibroadenomas are characterized by an asymptomatic firm, rubbery, mobile mass sometimes irregular in shape. They vary in size from a few millimeters to huge masses and may be multiple and bilateral. In fibrocystic disease, cysts tend to be tender and to vary in size and location with menstrual cycles. These patients should be placed on a caffeine-free diet. Brooks and associates demonstrated an 88% improvement in symptoms, a 91% reduction in palpable nodularities, and an 85% improvement in graphic thermal patterns after six months of caffeine restriction in patients with fibrocystic

breast disease. When of cystic consistency, the mass should be aspirated using a 23-g needle. This procedure is usually well tolerated by adolescents and does not necessitate anesthesia. Very often, the cyst collapses following this procedure and does not recur. All fluid obtained should be sent for cytologic examination, and the patient should be carefully observed in order to diagnose any recurrence.

A breast mass in an adolescent should certainly be observed for three to six menstrual cycles. This allows some masses to regress spontaneously and avoids unnecessary procedures. Furnival and colleagues demonstrated the accuracy of clinical diagnosis in 70 women aged 17 to 25 years presenting with breast symptoms. They used a conservative approach and found that fewer than half of their patients with a palpable mass on initial examination eventually needed biopsy because of persistence.

Indications for surgical excision are as follows: All persistent or rapidly growing breast masses should be excised, since it is the only accurate means of obtaining a definite diagnosis. Furthermore, even though benignity is almost certain, the presence of a persistent mass is a tremendous source of anxiety for the patient, which in itself represents a sufficient surgical indication. The presence of nipple discharge is also an indication for surgery because of its possible association with an intraductal papilloma, a cystosarcoma phylloides, or other malignant lesion.

Table 45-6
Pathologic Diagnosis of 100 Breast Biopsy Specimens

Pathology	Number of Patients
Fibroadenoma	83 (83%)
Adult	58
Juvenile	19
Giant	2
Cellular	2
Papillary	1
Fibroadenoma with mixed stroma	1
Fibrocystic Mastopathy	8 (8%)
Fibrocystic disease	4
Simple cyst	2
Fibrocystic mastopathy	1
Stromal sclerosis	1
Other	9 (9%)
Chronic mastitis	2
Epidermal inclusion cyst	1
Adenomatous hyperplasia	1
Intraductal hyperplasia with focal secretion	1
Capillary hemangioma	1
Fat necrosis	1
Normal fat and breast tissue	1

When proceeding with surgery, one should give consideration to the cosmetic results. In recent years, we have tried to excise as many masses as possible through circumareolar incisions, which result in almost invisible scars. It is generally accepted that one half of the areolar circumference can be incised without the blood supply being compromised. Even when the mass is located quite far from the areola, it can usually be reached by raising an areolar flap and dissecting under the skin. Use of electrocautery for dissection and a meticulous hemostasis reduces the risk of postoperative hematomas. A small Penrose drain may be utilized when necessary. In our experience, fibroadenomas as large as 10 × 10 cm have been excised through this type of incision without complications. When the circumareolar route is judged unacceptable because of the size or location of the mass, efforts should be made to respect the natural skin folds and avoid radial incisions. The defect created in the deep breast tissue should be carefully closed in order to avoid postoperative deformity. For skin closure, a fine subcuticular suture gives good results. However, because of the curvature of the circumareolar incision, we feel that the use of interrupted 4-0 nylon sutures that are removed on the third or fourth postoperative day gives the best cosmetic results.

It must be remembered that fibroadenomas frequently prove to be either lobulated or larger than appreciated at the time of preoperative palpation. Therefore, the surrounding breast tissue should be carefully inspected after excision to ensure that no small parts or lobules of the lesion are left behind.

The vast majority of breast procedures in adolescents can be carried out on an ambulatory basis, which is certainly less emotionally disturbing and less expensive for the patient. The choice of the type of anesthesia depends on the adolescent's ability to cooperate and on the extent of the dissection that will be required. In these young patients, in whom the anesthetic risk is usually very low, it seems preferable to proceed under general anesthesia through a circumareolar incision than to sacrifice the cosmetic result by using a more direct peripheral incision under local anesthesia.

Although the pathologic diagnosis of adolescent breast masses does not usually create any therapeutic controversy, the surgeon should be careful in interpreting a pathologic report mentioning cytosarcoma phylloides. As mentioned by Oberman, this term suggesting the presence of a malignant tumor is, in fact, used to describe a wide variety of benign and malignant lesions ranging from cellular juvenile fibroadenoma to fibrosarcoma. This pathologic diagnosis should, therefore, always prompt a pathologic consultation in order to avoid over or under interpretation.

Finally, no discussion of breast masses would be complete without a few words about self-examination. Hein and colleagues, in a study of 95 teenagers admitted for a breast mass, found that 77 (81%) of the lesions had been self-detected. Although it was not known whether the patients had been previously instructed in breast self-examination, this report certainly proves that adolescents are concerned with their own health and that teaching them breast self-examination is worth the effort.

IN UTERO EXPOSURE TO DIETHYLSTILBESTROL

During the 1950s and early 1960s, diethylstilbestrol (DES) and other nonsteroidal estrogens were given to pregnant women with the aim of preventing miscarriages. In 1971 Herbst and colleagues reported an association between maternal use of DES and the later development of clear cell adenocarcinoma of the vagina and cervix in female offspring. More recently adenosis, the presence of glandular (columnar) epithelium of müllerian origin in the vaginal wall (which is normally stratified squamous epithelium), has been described in 36% to 90% of exposed young women. Although adenosis is a benign lesion, the proximity of areas of adenosis to adenocarcinoma in several patients has necessitated the follow-up of all patients exposed to DES.

The number of exposed young women is estimated to range from at least several hundred thousand to perhaps several million. Reliable histories are often difficult to obtain and thus all patients (prepubertal and postpubertal) who have abnormal bleeding should have a vaginal examination regardless of history. What should the general physician do?

1. Determine the maternal drug history on all patients.
2. Refer for gynecologic exam at menarche or age 14 all patients with a known maternal history of ingestion of any amount of DES or other nonsteroidal estrogen.
3. Be available for counseling and discussion of the importance of gynecologic follow-up.

This last point is particularly important, because it is not unusual for mothers to feel extremely guilty about having taken the medication. Some desire to have their daughters checked under some other pretense. The adolescent girl may express great anger toward her mother for making her body imperfect. However, in general, it is much less destructive to a teenager to deal with these issues openly rather than to allow the physician and mother to have a "secret." Although mothers and daughters are usually seeking reassurance that the vagina is "clean," the high frequency of adenosis indicates that this is not possible. Although the carcinoma risk is minimal (probably less than 4/1000) the long-term risk of the presence of adenosis is unknown.

What constitutes the gynecologic exam of the teenager exposed *in utero* to DES?

1. Careful palpation of the vagina
2. Speculum examination with Papanicolaou smear and Schiller's stain of the vagina
3. Biopsies as indicated by the Schiller's stain

If colposcopy is available, follow-up is greatly facilitated. The colposcope allows the whole spectrum of atypia, dysplasia, and carcinoma to be identified. Photos should be taken and then reviewed at subsequent visits. Colposcopy detects more cases of adenosis (80–90%) than visual exam (less than 30%) or Schiller's stains (40–80%).

Adenocarcinoma

Although sporadic cases of clear cell adenocarcinoma of the cervix and, less commonly, the vagina had been reported prior to the 1960s, the incidence has dramatically risen since 1966. Of the 170 initial cases collected by Herbst and colleagues, information on maternal medication was obtained in 146. This was as follows:

Stilbestrol, dienestrol, or hexestrol	84
Above, plus progestational agent	11
Hormone medication of unknown type for bleeding	19
Progestational agent alone	1
No history of above medications	31

The data showed a wide range of dosage and duration of DES therapy; some mothers had an extremely short course of low-dose DES. In all cases, nonsteroidal estrogens were started before the 18th week of pregnancy.

At the time of diagnosis, patients presented most commonly with bleeding or discharge, but 28 patients were asymptomatic. Several of these asymptomatic patients were discovered to have cancer on routine examination done solely because of a positive maternal history; all these patients are now living. The Papanicolaou smear was reported as positive or suspicious in 76%; in 11 patients, the Papanicolaou smear was the first clue to diagnosis. However, it should be noted that 20 patients with cancer had a negative smear, indicating that a negative Papanicolaou smear cannot be considered reassuring in patients exposed to DES *in utero*

The average age at diagnosis was 17.5 to 18 years; however, it is unclear whether this age will increase as time elapses or whether it reflects an actual age of greatest risk. Cases have occasionally occurred in prepubertal girls, but all had symptoms of bleeding for weeks to months prior to the diagnosis.

The current recommendation of Herbst and co-workers for therapy of stage I and stage II tumors is radical hysterectomy. Metastatic disease is common and implies a poor prognosis.

Adenosis

In contrast to the rare occurrence of adenocarcinoma, adenosis is a common finding in young women exposed *in utero* to DES, being reported in 36% to 90% of patients. Adenosis is the presence of glandular epithelium of müllerian origin (resembling the endocervix and endometrium) in the vaginal wall. Exposure to DES appears to have interfered with normal differentiation and development of the cervix and vagina. Several typical gross lesions have been described including (1) "vaginal hood"—a circular fold that partially covers the cervix; (2) cock's comb appearance of the cervix—an irregular peak on the anterior border of the cervix; (3) erythroplakia—reddish areas that may give the cervix or vagina a "strawberry" appearance.

Herbst and colleagues studied two populations of young women, an "exposed to DES" group and a "control" group. The examiners were not told which group patients belonged to. The results were as follows:

	Exposed to DES	Control
Nonstaining vagina	56	1
Nonstaining cervix	95	49
Adenosis	35	1 (1 case with inclusion cyst)
Erosion	85	38
Vaginal or cervical fibrous ridges	22	0

The observation that adenosis is commonly found adjacent to foci of clear cell adenocarcinoma necessitates careful follow-up of this lesion. No form of treatment for adenosis has been determined, although there is good evidence that spontaneous healing occurs. At this time the most prudent course appears to be follow-up examinations every six to twelve months.

PRECOCIOUS PUBERTY

A thorough understanding of the normal progression of puberty is essential in the evaluation of patients with precocious puberty, premature thelarche, and premature adrenarche. It should be recalled that in normal adolescence, estrogen is responsible for breast development, for maturation of the external genitalia, vagina, and uterus, and for initiation of menses. An increase in adrenal androgens is associated with the appearance of pubic and axillary hair. Excess androgens of either ovarian or adrenal origin may cause acne, hirsutism, voice changes, increased muscle mass, and clitoromegaly. Thus, precocious puberty in females can be divided into two categories: isosexual precocity, in which the patient has normal pubertal development, including menses; and heterosexual precocity, in which the patient has evidence of virilization with or without changes characteristic of a normal puberty.

Premature thelarche is defined as the appearance of breast development in the absence of other signs of puberty. Premature adrenarche is defined as the appearance of pubic hair (or axillary hair, or both) without signs of estrogenization. Since, in normal puberty, there may be a dissociation between the time of appearance of sexual hair and breast development, premature the-larche or adrenarche may be the first sign of a true precocious puberty. Because most cases of precocity require special endocrine studies, referral to an endocrinologist is often necessary. However, the gynecologist can usually initiate the investigation of precocious puberty and can diagnose and follow cases of premature thelarche and adrenarche.

Isosexual Precocious Puberty

In true isosexual precocity, the stimulus for development arises in the hypothalamus and pituitary gland. In response to rising levels of luteinizing hormone (LH) and follicle-stimulating hormone (FSH), the ovaries produce estrogen. The young girl develops breast and pubic and axillary hair and begins menstruation, sometimes not in the usual sequence. With the establishment of the cyclic midcycle LH peak, the child becomes potentially fertile.

In isosexual pseudoprecocity, an ovarian tumor or cyst or adrenal adenoma produces estrogen autonomously. The fluctuating estrogen levels result in sexual development and anovulatory menses.

In over 80% of patients with isosexual precocious puberty, the hypothalamic-pituitary axis is activated prematurely for unknown reasons. Approximately 80% of patients with idiopathic precocious puberty have abnormal encephalograms; this suggests that a neuroendocrine dysfunction may contribute to precocious puberty.

Despite the relatively high incidence of constitutional or idiopathic precocious puberty, this diagnosis cannot be made without a thorough evaluation and exclusion of some of the following organic causes:

1. Cerebral disorders (5–10% of cases)
2. Ovarian tumors (5% of cases)
3. Adrenal disorders (rare)
4. Gonadotropin-producing tumors (rare)
5. Hypothyroidism (rare)
6. Iatrogenic disorders (rare)

Patient assessment by the gynecologist prior to referral to an endocrinologist should include a careful history and physical examination as well as a family history. As noted above, it is important to perform appropriate studies to rule out cerebral disorders and ovarian tumors, which are the two most common organic causes of this condition.

Laboratory tests should include the following:

1. Skull x-ray films or CT scan of the brain
2. Hand and wrist x-ray films for bone age
3. Vaginal smear or urocytogram for estrogenization
4. Electroencephalogram
5. Serum FSH, LH, estradiol, dehydroepiandrosterone sulfate (DHAS), testosterone, and 17-hydroxyprogesterone levels
6. Pregnancy test
7. 24-hour urine specimen for 17-ketosteroids and 17-hydroxycorticosteroids

Treatment and follow-up depend on the diagnosis. Ovarian tumors and CNS tumors require surgical intervention. Idiopathic and CNS-induced precocity can be treated with medroxyprogesterone acetate (Depo-Provera), 150 mg IM every other week for 2 to 4 years or until the age of 8 years. Although such therapy results in cessation of menses and initial regression of breast development, the accelerated rate of bone maturation and the ultimate height are unchanged.

Even if the diagnosis of idiopathic precocious puberty is made, follow-up must continue at least every six months to exclude the possibility of organic disease not originally evident. It should be remembered that children with sexual precocity do not automatically manifest intellectual or psychosocial precocity. In fact, the degree of psychologic maturity of a young girl is more likely to be related to the life experiences she encounters and transacts.

Heterosexual Precocious Puberty

Heterosexual precocity arises from excess androgen production from an adrenal or ovarian source, which results in acne, hirsutism, and virilization. The differential diagnosis includes (1) congenital adrenocortical hyperplasia (CAH); (2) Cushing's syndrome; (3) adrenal tumors; (4) ovarian tumors, such as arrhenoblastomas, lipoid-cell, and Sertoli cell tumors; and (5) rarely, familial precocious puberty with isolated elevation of LH.

As is true with isosexual precocity, patients should undergo careful history and physical examination. Laboratory tests should include determinations of levels of serum FSH, LH, estradiol, dehydroepiandrosterone (DHA), DHA sulfate (DHAS), testosterone, and adrostenedione. A 24-hour urine collection should be assayed for 17-ketosteroids, 17-hydroxycorticosteroids, and pregnanetriol.

The treatment and follow-up of heterosexual precocious puberty is based on the diagnosis. Ovarian and adrenal tumors should be surgically excised, if possible. Patients with congenital adrenal hyperplasia should receive glucocorticoid replacement. Follow-up should include careful monitoring of urinary 17-ketosteroids, serum 17-hydroxyprogesterone, and growth every three months or so. If the bone age is not too advanced, breast development in patients with congenital adrenal hyperplasia may regress with treatment.

Premature Thelarche

Premature thelarche is most commonly seen among young girls one to four years of age. Occasionally, neonatal breast hypertrophy fails to regress within six months after birth. This persistent breast development is also characterized as premature thelarche. The typical child with premature thelarche has bilateral breast buds of 2 cm to 4 cm with little or no change in the nipple or areola. The breast tissue feels granular and may be slightly tender. In some cases, development is quite asymmetric; one side may develop 6 to 12 months before the other. Growth is not accelerated, and the bone age is normal for height age. No other evidence of puberty appears; the labia remain prepubertal without obvious evidence of estrogen effect.

Although it was originally thought that premature thelarche was caused by an increased end-organ sensitivity to low levels of endogenous estrogen, the fact that serum estrogen levels are at least transiently elevated suggests that small luteinized or cystic graafian follicles may be responsible in some cases. The usual clinical course of regression, or at least lack of progression, of breast development would then correlate with the waning of the estrogen levels as the follicles become atretic.

Treatment consists mainly of reassurance and careful follow-up to confirm that the breast development does not represent the first signs of precocious puberty.

Premature Adrenarche

Most patients with premature adrenarche have a slight increase in urinary 17-ketosteroid production and increased plasma DHA and DHAS levels, suggesting that hormone biosynthesis in the adrenal gland undergoes maturation prematurely to a pubertal pattern. Although production of these androgens is suppressible by dexamethasone and therefore dependent on adrenocorticotropic hormone, the mediator for the change at puberty and in premature adrenarche is unknown.

The assessment of the patient with premature adrenarche is similar to that for heterosexual precocious puberty. The important findings are the presence of pubic hair and the *absence* of breast development, estrogenization of the labia and vagina, and virilization.

The laboratory tests that should be obtained include an x-ray film of the wrist for bone age, vaginal smear, a 24-hour urine test for 17-ketosteroids and 17-hydroxysteroids, and tests for serum DHAS, estradiol, testosterone, and 17-hydroxyprogesterone. The differential diagnosis must exclude early precocious puberty, congenital adrenal hyperplasia, and an adrenal or ovarian tumor.

Treatment of premature adrenarche is reassurance and follow-up. The child should be examined every six months to confirm the original diagnostic impression. In general, pubertal development at adolescence can be expected to be normal.

REFERENCES AND RECOMMENDED READING

Billmire MD, Farrell MK, Dine MS: A simplified procedure for pediatric vaginal examination: Use of veterinary otoscope specula. Pediatrics 65:823, 1974

Bongiovanni AM (ed): Adolescent Gynecology: A Guide for Clinicians. New York, Plenum Pub., 1982

Brooks PG, Gait S, Heldfond AJ et al: Measuring the effect of caffeine restriction on fibrocystic breast disease. J Reprod Med 26:279, 1981

Capraro VS: Gynecologic examination in children and adolescents. Pediatr Clin North Am 19:511, 1972

Claessons EA, Cowell CA: Acute adolescent menorrhagia. Am J Obstet Gynecol 193:377, 1981

Dewhurst CJ: Practical Pediatric and Adolescent Gynecology. New York, Marcel Dekker, 1980

Emans SJH, Goldstein DP: Pediatric and Adolescent Gynecology, 2nd ed. Boston, Little, Brown and Co, 1982

Furwival CM, Irwin JRM, Gray GM: Breast disease in young women—When is biopsy indicated? Med J Austr 2:167, 1983

Gantt PA, McDonough PG: Dysfunctional bleeding in adolescents. Barwin BN, Belish S (eds): Adolescent Gynecology and Sexuality, p 59. New York, Masson Pub USA, 1982

Gidwani GP: Laparoscopy for diagnosis of chronic pelvic pain. Transitions Dec, 1981

Goldstein DP, DeCholnoky C, Emans SJ et al: Laparoscopy in the diagnosis and management of pelvic pain in adolescents. J Reprod Med 24:251, 1980

Guzenski G: A new approach to chronic pelvic pain. Fem Patient 8:32, 1983

Haagensen CD: Diseases of the Breast. Philadelphia, WB Saunders, 1974

Heald FP (ed): Adolescent Gynecology. Baltimore, Williams & Wilkins, 1966

Hein K, Dell R, Caten M: Self-detection of a breast mass in adolescent females. J Adolesc Health Care 3:15, 1982

Herbst A: A prospective comparison of exposed female offspring with unexposed controls. New Engl J Med 292:334, 1975

Herbst A: Clear cell adenocarcinoma of the vagina and cervix: Analysis of 170 registry cases. Am J Obstet Gynecol 119:713, 1974

Herbst A, Ulfelder HJ, Poskanzer CP: Adenocarcinoma of the vagina. New Engl J Med 284, 878, 1971

Huffman JW, Dewhurst CJ, Capraro VJ: The Gynecology of Childhood and Adolescence, 2nd ed. Philadelphia, WB Saunders, 1981

Jones HW Jr., Heller RH: Pediatric and Adolescent Gynecology. Baltimore, Williams & Wilkins, 1966

Kreutner, AKK, Hollingsworth DR: Adolescent Obstetrics and Gynecology. Chicago, Year Book, 1978

Lack EE, Goldstein DP: Primary ovarian tumors in childhood and adolescence. Curr Probl Obstet Gynecol October, 1984

Norris HJ, Taylor HB: Carcinoma of the breast in women less than thirty years old. Cancer 26:953, 1970

Oberman HA: Breast lesions in the adolescent female. Pathol Annu 14:175, 1979

Disorders of Menstrual Function

Daniel H. Riddick

46

Menstrual dysfunction is a symptom of some underlying abnormality of the reproductive system. The abnormality may be developmental, organic, or endocrinologic. An appreciation of the pathophysiologic conditions underlying abnormalities of menstruation and a rational approach to evaluation and therapy require a full understanding of the normal anatomy, embryology, and endocrine interrelationships of the reproductive system. This chapter deals with the pathophysiology of menstrual function. Where appropriate, basic physiology is referred to, but it is not discussed in any detail.

The symptoms of menstrual dysfunction are considered in terms of the systems whose malfunction gives rise to them. Amenorrhea, dysfunctional uterine bleeding, and anovulation are not disorders but symptoms needing to be diagnosed. Treatment depends entirely on the underlying cause of the symptom.

PRIMARY AMENORRHEA

Primary amenorrhea is defined as the failure to begin menstruation by an appropriate age determined by individual differences in the age of initiation of sexual development. Menarche is discussed in detail in the chapter dealing with adolescent reproductive function and development, but in general, it would be expected to occur at the earliest at approximately age 10 if pubertal development begins at age 8 and by age 17 if pubertal development begins at the latest normal age of 14. The evaluation of sexual development is, therefore, crucial to the appropriate evaluation of the underlying causes of primary amenorrhea and to the determination of whether amenorrhea as a pathophysiologic process exists at all. Thus, a young woman whose pubertal development began at age 13 might well present to the physician complaining of failure to menstruate at age 14. The events responsible for the orderly development of

the reproductive system with endometrial proliferation to the point of menstruation would not be expected to have been completed in this short period of time. This patient and her family need education about the normal developmental sequence and the expected time of appearance of various manifestations of this development rather than an expensive and time-consuming endocrine or other medical evaluation. Thus, the first and most important decision to be made by the physician is whether an abnormality exists at all or whether the patient is fearful that there may be an abnormality and only needs reassurance of her normalcy. The approach to patients with the complaint of primary amenorrhea is heavily dependent upon a carefully obtained developmental history and a physical examination directed initially toward establishing the presence and degree of secondary sexual development.

Absent or Arrested Sexual Development

When secondary sexual development fails to begin by age 14 or when development began at an appropriate age but ceased to progress completely, the underlying abnormality may involve hypothalamic dysfunction, pituitary dysfunction, or failure of the ovaries to respond to normal gonadotropic stimulation. The end result of failure of any of these three systems will be the failure of the ovarian follicle to produce estradiol, resulting in failure to stimulate the secondary sexual target organs. Each of these primary systems will be considered only briefly, since they are discussed in more depth in the chapters dealing with pubertal development.

Hypothalamic Dysfunction

Destructive processes involving the hypothalamus at the time of onset of puberty or after its initiation will result in failure of GnRH production and secondary failure of the pituitary gland to release sufficient FSH and LH for ovarian stimulation. Tumors of the hypothalamus, such as hamartomas, or other central nervous system tumors involving the hypothalamus, such as craniopharyngiomas, may result in failure of normal pubescence with failure to begin menstruation. Infiltrative or infective disorders, such as sarcoidosis and encephalitis, may also be associated with hypothalamic failure.

A *developmental malformation* involving olfactory bulb hypoplasia and anosmia is also associated with presumed abnormalities in the central nervous system regulation of hypothalamus function. This condition, which has been described in both men and women, results in failure of normal hypothalamic GnRH production with secondary failure of pituitary FSH and LH production (Kallmann's syndrome). Pituitary response to exogenously administered GnRH is normal in these individuals.

Significant changes in body *weight*—either excessive weight gain or excessive weight loss—may also be associated with failure of normal sexual development and primary amenorrhea. The initiation of menstrual function requires a critical mass of body fat; at age 13 the mass required is equivalent to approximately 17% of body weight. Similar calculations relating different heights, ages, and ideal body weights to normal or abnormal menstruation can also be made. Extreme weight loss from inadequate caloric intake associated with an abnormal body image and other psychiatric disturbances is referred to as *anorexia nervosa*. This condition can occur during pubertal development, resulting in primary amenorrhea, and may cause death if not recognized and appropriately treated. A variant of this disorder, *bulimia,* is manifest by alternating binges of eating and fasting that result in wide weight swings and amenorrhea.

Severe *psychologic stress,* such as the death of a parent or rape at a critical time in development, may also result in failure to institute menses. The mechanism for hypothalamic suppression in these disorders is not understood at the present time.

The chronic physical exercise programs of young *athletes,* such as gymnasts, long distance runners, skaters, and ballerinas, have all been associated with delayed or failed menstruation. Various mechanisms have been proposed to explain this association, including diminished body fat, hyperprolactinemia, "stress," and endorphin excess. None of these explanations is satisfactory by itself, however. The end result is failure of the hypothalamus to produce enough GnRH for normal pituitary release of FSH and LH.

Two additional syndromes of hypothalamic dysfunction resulting in incomplete pubertal development and the associated amenorrhea are the Prader-Willi syndrome and the Laurence-Moon-Biedl syndrome. Hypothalamic dysfunction in the Prader-Willi syndrome is associated with massive obesity, carbohydrate intolerance, hypotonia, and mental retardation. The abnormalities associated with the Laurence-Moon-Biedl syndrome are polydactyly, obesity, mental retardation, and

retinitis pigmentosa. Both syndromes are transmitted as an autosomal recessive trait.

A final group of patients will display delayed onset of normal pubertal development and menstruation without any definable cause for the hypothalamic dysfunction. These patients have what is referred to as *constitutional delay* of normal puberty and menstruation and are discussed in more detail under pubertal development.

Pituitary Dysfunction

Disorders of the pituitary gland resulting in failure of normal FSH and LH production are categorized either as pituitary tumors or as pituitary failure.

When a pituitary tumor arises during pubertal development, normal progression of puberty is usually arrested and primary amenorrhea results. The most common pituitary tumor is composed primarily of lactotrophs, which produce the protein hormone *prolactin*. Prolactin in excessive amounts feeds back to the hypothalamus, inhibiting GnRH production. This results in failure of pituitary gonadotropin production. Elevated prolactin levels in mature women are often associated with galactorrhea and will be discussed in greater detail under the category of secondary amenorrhea. It is important to note here, however, that if breast development is inadequate due to an arrest of pubertal development, the effect of prolactin on the breast glandular system will not be manifest and galactorrhea will be found uncommonly. The absence of galactorrhea in no way indicates the absence of a prolactin-secreting pituitary adenoma in these patients. Prolactinomas are almost always benign tumors that cause their effect by their increasing size or by the hormonal effects of prolactin.

Growth-hormone-producing pituitary tumors also occur in this age group and are associated with amenorrhea and physical signs of growth hormone excess. In the pubertal patient, growth hormone excess results in excessive long-bone growth, producing the condition known as *gigantism*. Gigantism occurs in this age group because the long-bone epiphyses have not yet been closed by adequate estrogen exposure.

Finally, *ACTH*-secreting pituitary tumors have been described in this age group. These tumors are discussed in the chapter on disorders of adrenal function.

Pituitary failure can be either idiopathic, in which an underlying etiology cannot be determined, or due to a destructive process within the pituitary gland, such as a large pituitary tumor, a craniopharyngioma growing from embryonal rests in Rathke's pouch, or the consequences of previous head and neck radiation therapy for the treatment of an unrelated tumor of that region. Regardless of the cause, FSH and LH production is lost as pituitary failure develops. Loss of growth hormone and thyroid-stimulating hormone occurs somewhat later in the destructive process. Usually the last trophic hormone to be lost is ACTH. The hypoadrenalism that follows loss of ACTH production is life-threatening because the adrenal gland is unable to respond with cortisol output to traumatic or infectious stress.

Ovarian Failure

Ovarian failure occurs whenever follicles no longer exist that are capable of producing estradiol in response to gonadotropin stimulation. Such loss of follicular function may be the result of a rapid deterioration of follicles that begins during embryonic life and results in the absence of follicles by infancy or early childhood, the result of a more rapid than normal loss of follicles during puberty or in the decade following puberty, or the result of radiation or chemotherapeutic damage during the treatment of malignancy. When follicular loss occurs before the onset of puberty, there will be no sexual development and, of course, no menarche. Follicular dysfunction may also occur partway through puberty, giving rise to an arrest of pubertal development and primary amenorrhea. Similarly, the signs and symptoms associated with radiation and chemotherapy will depend on the stage of pubertal development when the follicles were destroyed. In each of these instances, estradiol production will either not occur or will cease prematurely, resulting in a failure of endometrial proliferation and, consequently, the failure to institute menses.

Gonadal dysgenesis is the result of an accelerated loss of ovarian follicles occurring during embryogenesis or in the first few years after birth. In the absence of follicles, the ovaries are composed only of ovarian stromal tissue that appears as fibrous bands, which are referred to as streak gonads (Fig. 46-1). The most common form of gonadal dysgenesis is caused by the absence of one of the X chromosomes in all of the cells of the body. This condition is referred to as *Turner's syndrome* (Fig. 46-2). In addition to gonadal dysgenesis,

Turner's syndrome is associated with short stature (adult height of less than five feet), webbed neck, a high-arched palate, coarctation of the aorta, a shield-shaped chest, widely spaced nipples, increased carrying angle of the upper extremities (cubitus valgus), shortened fourth metacarpal bones of the hand, a low hairline on the neck, and a variety of renal abnormalities. It is unusual for all of these signs to occur in any one patient; in many patients, in fact, only one or two may be evident. The diagnosis is made either at birth following the finding of lymphedema of the lower extremities or during adolescence when puberty and menarche fail to appear. The majority of fetuses affected with this condition are aborted during the first trimester of pregnancy; other than trisomy, 45 XO is the most common genetic abnormality found in first-trimester abortuses.

A less common form of gonadal dysgenesis occurs in a phenotypically normal female with streak gonads and a 46 XY karyotype (*Swyer's syndrome*). Such individuals are perfectly normal-appearing females who do not undergo pubertal development or menarche. Since the streak gonads do not produce testosterone in spite of the XY karyotype, phenotypic genital development proceeds along female lines.

Premature ovarian failure before complete pubescence and menarche is not uncommon; it results in incomplete pubescence and amenorrhea. Genotypically and phenotypically, individuals with premature ovarian failure are entirely normal. The ovaries resemble postmenopausal ovaries rather than the streak gonads of ovarian dysgenesis. The condition is almost always permanent.

Radiation therapy to the pelvis, particularly in the treatment of lymphatic malignancy, is usually associated with permanent loss of ovarian follicles unless particular care is taken to shield the ovaries from the radiation. Such shielding requires an operative procedure to move

FIG. 46-1. Streak gonads. The ovary is composed of stroma without evidence of follicles.

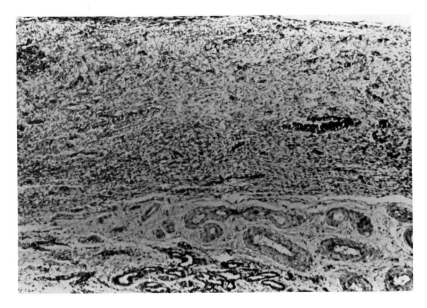

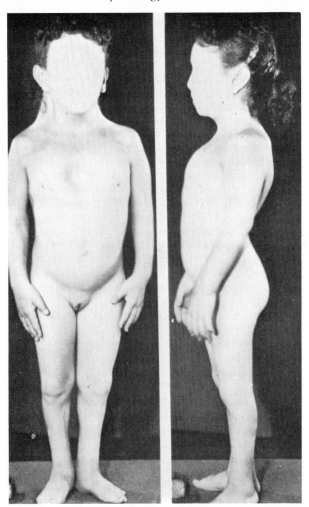

FIG. 46-2. Patient with gonadal dysgenesis. Note the short stature (42 inches final height); webbing of the neck; multiple nevi; low-set hairline and ears; lack of secondary sex characteristics; wide-spaced nipples; and edema of the feet and hands. (Federman DD: Abnormal Sexual Development: A Genetic and Endocrine Approach to Differential Diagnosis. Philadelphia, WB Saunders, 1967)

the ovaries out of the radiation field. Even so, ovarian failure often occurs.

Chemotherapy is associated with the only form of apparent ovarian failure that often is reversible. Following chemotherapy for malignancy follicular anatomy is normally disrupted for a number of years. The granulosa cells of the follicle often regenerate, with resumption of pubertal development or with menarche when the chemotherapy was used during pubescence.

Diagnosis

History

A carefully taken history will often point to the major dysfunction resulting in primary amenorrhea. Of particular importance is the developmental sequence and the age at which pubertal development began. From this information it is possible to determine whether the onset of puberty was simply delayed or whether pubertal development was arrested before completion. A previous history of central nervous system infection, neurologic symptoms, or anosmia is suggestive of hypothalamic dysfunction. Patients with pituitary tumors, on the other hand, rarely have central nervous system symptoms other than headaches or visual disturbances. Galactorrhea may be complained of if sufficient breast development occurred before the development of hyperprolactinemia, and the symptoms associated with excess of growth hormone or cortisol may be reported. The patient with pituitary gland failure of either an idiopathic or a destructive nature frequently complains of generalized weakness, fatigue, and cachexia. If the failure is due to a destructive lesion, such as a craniopharyngioma, other central nervous system symptoms may be present depending on the specific area of involvement by the tumor. A history of previous irradiation of the head and neck, even though it may have occurred many years previously, should increase the index of suspicion of impending pituitary failure.

In many patients with primary ovarian failure, no specific history may be forthcoming other than failure to undergo complete pubertal development and menarche. This is particularly true when ovarian failure occurs partway through pubertal development. Clearly, a history of radiation therapy to the pelvis or chemotherapy before or during pubertal development greatly increases the likelihood that ovarian failure is the underlying cause of the amenorrhea. A history of growth rate below the tenth percentile is one of the most important historical facts related to gonadal dysgenesis of the Turner's variety. Other than streak gonads, short stature is the most common symptom of Turner's syndrome and is present in virtually all patients suffering from it. With pure gonadal dysgenesis (XY), on the other hand, the growth rate is generally entirely normal except for the lack of a pubertal growth spurt. Here again, only the failure of normal pubescence would point to the disorder.

Physical Examination

The physical examination is of particular importance in identifying the presence of abnormal pubertal development and will often suggest the specific etiology of the problem. Of special importance is the development of secondary sexual characteristics, including pubic and axillary hair, and breast development. The age of onset of sexual development should be ascertained and the actual and expected development since that time should be compared. Tanner's classification of breast and pubic hair development (discussed in the chapter on adolescent development) is often of help in objectifying these physical findings. A careful neurologic examination should be performed to look for signs of central nervous system dysfunction. Any abnormality found should be pursued aggressively with additional appropriate studies. Another important part of the evaluation of these patients is an assessment of the body habitus in which the span from fingertip to fingertip with the arms extended is compared with the height from crown to floor. In patients with pure gonadal dysgenesis, the long bones continue their slow, progressive growth, giving rise to long arms, long legs, and a eunuchoid body habitus. This reflects the failure to produce enough estrogen to close the epiphyses and stop long-bone growth. Other specific physical findings, such as short stature, webbed neck, and the other findings associated with Turner's syndrome should be carefully sought during the physical examination. Similarly, the physical findings associated with growth hormone excess and gigantism or cortisol excess and Cushing's syndrome should be sought.

Laboratory Investigation

The laboratory investigation of primary amenorrhea in the absence of complete pubertal development is directed in part by the findings of the history and physical examination. Specific findings will dictate specific studies to confirm the suspected diagnosis. The most critical laboratory study in the evaluation of this group of patients is the determination of the plasma FSH and LH concentration. In patients with ovarian failure from any cause, estradiol will not be produced in sufficient quantities to produce negative feedback on gonadotropin production by the pituitary gland. In the absence of estradiol production during puberty, the FSH and LH levels will continue to rise until menopausal levels (in the range of 70–120 mIU/ml) are achieved. If the gonadotropin concentrations are within the normal reproductive age range or, as is more likely in these patients, below the normal range, ovarian follicular function can be assumed to be normal, and the underlying abnormality will lie either in hypothalamic or in pituitary function.

When ovarian failure is diagnosed and gonadotropin levels are elevated, a karyotype study should be done. This will identify the specific karyotype of the individual, such as 45 XO in Turner's syndrome, 46 XY in pure gonadal dysgenesis, and 46 XX in idiopathic premature ovarian failure. Should idiopathic ovarian failure be the final diagnosis, the presence of autoantibodies against the thyroid gland, the adrenal gland, and the ovary should be tested for, since these are commonly associated findings and may indicate additional endocrine gland failure yet to come. Whether such circulating autoantibodies against the ovary are the cause of the premature ovarian failure or simply an associated finding is not yet known.

If the gonadotropin determination suggests an abnormality of the hypothalamus or pituitary gland, a peripheral karyotype study need not be done. Rather, one must pursue a diagnostic course that will eliminate the specific abnormalities that might be present, leaving one with a diagnosis of dysfunction of the hypothalamus or pituitary gland of unknown etiology. A prolactin determination, the most important single hormonal assay,

will indicate a wide variety of abnormalities within the central nervous system that ultimately interfere with the production of dopamine (PIF). If the production of dopamine is decreased, its inhibitory effect on the pituitary lactotrophs is lost and hyperprolactinemia will appear. Specific trophic hormone assays such as growth hormone, ACTH, and TSH assessments will be indicated by the physical examination and are not routinely performed. When impending pituitary gland failure is considered, a TRH stimulation test is probably the most important initial test for the diagnosis. Patients with impending pituitary failure will have a markedly blunted release of prolactin in response to 200 μg TRH given intravenously, with prolactin sampling occurring over the hour following injection. The prolactin level will rise to levels between 30 ng/ml and 100 ng/ml within 30 minutes of the injection when pituitary function is normal and will rise little or not at all in patients with pituitary failure. Radiographic evaluation of the central nervous system for tumor or other destructive lesions of the hypothalamus or pituitary gland is carried out by computed tomography (CT). If there is any doubt about the presence of a central nervous system neoplasm, this evaluation is mandatory. The CT scan has largely replaced the more dangerous and traumatic techniques of arteriography and pneumoencephalography except under very specific conditions.

Treatment

The treatment for primary amenorrhea is diagnosis-specific; that is, it is directed at the underlying cause and not at the symptom of amenorrhea. Tumors involving the hypothalamus will ordinarily require neurosurgical therapy. Prolactinomas of the pituitary gland, on the other hand, will usually respond to medical therapy utilizing bromocriptine, a dopamine agonist. This treatment is discussed in more detail under the category of secondary amenorrhea, in which such tumors are far more common. Other adenomas of the pituitary gland may well require transsphenoidal hypophysectomy to avoid craniotomy.

Surgical therapy for patients with ovarian failure depends on the presence or absence of a Y chromosome in the karyotype. If a Y chromosome is present, the risk of development of a gonadal neoplasm is 20% to 25%. The most common tumors are the *gonadoblastoma* and, less frequently, the *dysgerminoma*. In patients with a Y component to the karyotype and streak gonads, neoplasia may develop at a relatively early age, so that bilateral gonadectomy is indicated at whatever age the diagnosis is made. In the absence of a Y chromosome, no surgical intervention is normally indicated.

Patients with irreparable hypothalamic dysfunction due to destructive processes or to developmental abnormalities such as Kallmann's syndrome should be treated with cyclic estrogen and progesterone therapy to induce pubertal development. Later in life, at the time of desired childbearing, such individuals may respond to the pulsatile administration of GnRH via a pump similar to an insulin pump for the stimulation of pituitary FSH and LH production and ovulation induction. If irreparable damage has occurred to the pituitary gland or total hypophysectomy has been necessary, estrogen and progesterone therapy is indicated to induce puberty and then to maintain estrogen-dependent tissues and cyclic menstrual function. All patients with ovarian failure will require estrogen and progesterone replacement therapy for the completion of pubertal development and induction of cyclic menstrual bleeding. Ovarian function may resume spontaneously in patients who have received chemotherapy in the past. In these patients spontaneous ovarian function should be evaluated by intermittent withdrawal of estrogen therapy during the teenage years.

The last group of patients with primary amenorrhea are the young athletes in whom all other causes of failure to complete pubertal development have been ruled out. These patients, in general, will undergo complete pubertal development and menarche but at a later age than their nonathletic peers. Estrogen and progesterone replacement therapy may be indicated for psychosocial reasons if for none other. Management must be individualized, but for many young women of commitment and talent, cessation of athletic activity to achieve menarche is probably not wise. It cannot be overemphasized, however, that the diagnosis of physical-stress-related amenorrhea must be one of exclusion rather than an assumption based on history alone.

Primary Amenorrhea with Sexual Development

Normal Phenotypic Secondary Sexual Development in Sequence

In persons with primary amenorrhea, when a careful history and general physical examination have demonstrated the development of apparently normal secondary sexual characteristics with a normal developmental sequence except for the absence of menarche, the *pelvic examination* becomes the most important part of the evaluation. If the examination shows the external genitalia, uterus, and adnexa to be within the normal range, hypothalamic, pituitary, or ovarian dysfunction become the most important considerations. The differential diagnosis of abnormalities involving the hypothalamus and pituitary glands as well as the various causes of ovarian failure must be considered in these patients in exactly the same way as in those who have primary amenorrhea in the absence of sexual development or with incomplete pubescence. The only difference between these two groups of patients is in the timing of the onset of the process that ultimately interrupts the normal developmental sequence. Thus, the differential diagnosis must include central nervous system tumors, pituitary tumors, physical and emotional stress, and premature ovarian failure. Again, a determination of the concentration of circulating FSH and

LH will direct one either to the central nervous system or to the ovary, depending on whether the values obtained are in the postmenopausal range or in the low normal range. These results will also determine the direction of further laboratory investigation in the same fashion as described above.

When phenotypic secondary sexual development and sequence is normal but the pelvic examination is abnormal, the abnormality is most likely to lie in an incomplete development of the müllerian system. As described in detail elsewhere, the fallopian tubes, uterus, cervix, and upper two thirds of the vagina develop embryonically from the müllerian structures. These bilateral structures fuse in the midline with absorption of the central portion beginning with the uterine fundus, forming a single uterine fundus and cavity when normally developed. Additionally, there will be a single vaginal canal extending to the level of the hymenal ring. The hymenal ring marks more or less the lowest extent of the müllerian system where it communicates with the invagination of the urogenital sinus, which is of nonmüllerian origin. When fusion fails to occur, a double or bicornuate uterus results. When fusion occurs but the central portion of the fused müllerian ducts is not absorbed, the external appearance of the uterus will be normal but the uterine cavity, cervix, and vagina may all be divided into two portions. Failure of normal embryonal development of any of these processes may result in dysplastic or noncommunicating structures and amenorrhea. The etiology of *müllerian dysgenesis* is unknown. Whatever the cause, it often affects the development of the renal system as well, resulting in a variety of *renal anomalies*.

When failure of communication between the müllerian ducts and the urogenital sinus occurs, the result is an *imperforate hymen*. This defect prevents the discharge of the menstruum, so that old blood accumulates on a monthly basis. Patients with imperforate hymen usually complain of progressive pelvic pain that is accentuated on a monthly basis and primary amenorrhea with otherwise apparently normal development. The pelvic examination reveals entirely normal external genitalia and a short vaginal pouch that ends blindly at the level of the hymenal ring. Often the blind pouch will be distended and bluish in color, reflecting the accumulation of blood behind it. Rectal examination often reveals a palpable mass indenting the rectum from above and occupying the expected space of the vagina. Ultrasonic evaluation will reveal a large fluid-filled vaginal space, confirming the diagnosis. Such patients should be treated promptly by excision of the hymen, which may be 0.5 cm or more in thickness. It is often helpful to insert, under anesthesia, a large-bore needle through the vaginal wall into the presumed blood-filled vagina (hematocolpos). The appearance of thick, dark-brown material will confirm the diagnosis and the needle provides a guide for entering the space with the scapel. This procedure is usually curative with an imperforate hymen, but patients are at increased risk for pelvic endometriosis because of the retrograde efflux of menstruum through the fallopian tubes and into the pelvic cavity. Patients who have persistent pelvic pain following successful drainage of the hematocolpos should be laparoscoped to establish the presence or absence of endometriosis if laparoscopy was not done at the time of the initial surgical procedure. Medical suppression of endometriosis as described elsewhere should be considered in patients with this additional diagnosis.

A spectrum of other forms of müllerian dysgenesis is seen extending all the way from partial *vaginal agenesis* to complete müllerian dysgenesis, in which the upper two thirds of the vagina are entirely absent and only fibrous remnants represent what would have been the uterus and fallopian tubes. It is of great importance to be certain of the degree of müllerian dysgenesis before making any decision about surgical management. If vaginal agenesis is present with a normal cervix and uterus, the clinical presentation may be very similar to that of an imperforate hymen. On ultrasonography or laparoscopy, such patients will show a large accumulation of blood within the uterus (hematometra) and often within the pelvic cavity as well. The surgical therapy for such patients involves dissection of the potential space between the hymen and the cervix and usually the placing of a split-thickness skin graft obtained from the buttocks to provide continuity between the cervix and the lower vagina. Once adequate healing has occurred and postoperative constriction has been prevented by the use of a vaginal stent for three to six

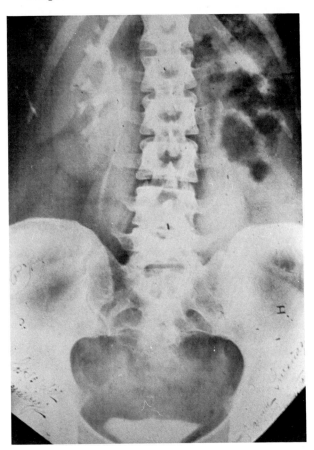

FIG. 46-4. Intravenous pyelogram of a patient with müllerian dysgenesis. Note the complete absence of the left kidney and collecting system.

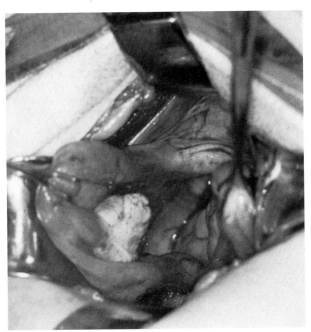

FIG. 46-3. Müllerian dysgenesis. Note normal ovaries and fibrous band held by Babcock clamp representing the müllerian remnants.

months postoperatively, the newly created vagina will take on the appearance of a perfectly normal vagina and be entirely functional. These patients may be expected to have normal pregnancy and delivery.

More commonly, however, when vaginal agenesis is encountered there will be *complete müllerian dysgenesis* affecting cervix, uterus, and fallopian tubes (Fig. 46-3). Such patients usually do not have abdominal pain unless a small amount of endometrium, representing the dysgenetic müllerian system, is present within the fibrous tissue. There will be no palpable mass on rectal examination except in patients in whom the renal anomaly is a pelvic kidney. All patients with müllerian dysgenesis should have an evaluation of the renal system by intravenous pyelogram before any operative intervention (Fig. 46-4). Laparoscopy in a patient with a pelvic kidney is fraught with hazard. Similarly, attempts to excise a retroperitoneal mass at laparotomy may obliterate the blood supply to the mass before it is realised that the mass represents a pelvic kidney. The incidence of renal abnormalities in association with müllerian dysgenesis approaches 50%. The remainder of the management of patients with total müllerian dysgenesis includes the creation of a vagina by skin grafting, as described above, in which the dissection in the potential vaginal space between the bladder and the rectum is carried out to the depth of the peritoneum. A vagina created by this technique is sexually functional, but childbearing is, of course, not possible. If a patient has experienced pain in addition to her symptom of primary amenorrhea, laparotomy and removal of the müllerian remnants may be indicated, since such symptoms often indicate the presence of functional endometrial tissue within the remnants that will result in progressive pain.

It is important to remember that in all patients with müllerian dysgenesis who have normal secondary sexual development, the ovaries are entirely normal. Cyclic follicular stimulation with estradiol production and ovulation occurs normally, and no hormonal supplementation is required. In an occasional patient with total müllerian dysgenesis, the cyclic pain experienced may represent the pain associated with ovulation (*mittelschmerz*) rather than pain from retained functional endometrial tissue in the müllerian remnants. These two possibilities can be differentiated quite simply by using a basal body temperature curve to determine whether the onset of pain occurs with the temperature rise or at the conclusion of the temperature rise and of the ovarian cycle. Finally, individuals with normal secondary sexual development, primary amenorrhea, and müllerian dysgenesis do not need additional laboratory investigation, and particularly they do not need a karyotype, since all will be 46 XX individuals.

Abnormal Secondary Sexual Development or Sequence

In the patient with primary amenorrhea, when a careful history reveals that secondary sexual development did not follow the usual pattern, two additional diagnostic categories must be considered. One category is made up of patients in whom nonphysiologic sex hormone production or ingestion has occurred. Although these patients are discussed in detail elsewhere, the major categories of concern involve *neoplasia* of the ovary or the adrenal gland, the major sex-hormone-producing glands. If the major secretory product of such neoplasms is estrogen, estrogenically induced secondary sexual development will occur in an accelerated fashion, resulting in thelarche without significant adrenarche and the onset of vaginal bleeding before the degree of overall sexual development would lead one to expect it. Should the neoplasm produce primarily androgens, then the predominant secondary sexual symptom will be that of secondary sexual hair growth. If the process continues, signs of generalized hirsutism, masculinization, and defeminization will appear. Abnormalities of adrenal gland steroidogenesis secondary to genetically acquired enzymatic deficiencies may also produce abnormal levels of biologically active androgens that induce the same signs and symptoms as androgens produced by neoplastic processes. The details of diagnosis and treatment of these disorders are discussed elsewhere in this text.

The other diagnostic category of importance in patients with abnormal secondary sexual development comprises the *androgen insensitivity syndromes*. Embryologically, both external and internal genital development proceed along phenotypically female lines in the absence of exposure to testosterone or dihydrotestosterone. Patients with androgen insensitivity are *46 XY individuals* with varying degrees of inability to respond biologically to normal levels of testicular androgen. The spectrum of androgen insensitivity syndromes runs from complete insensitivity, where phenotypically the external genitalia are female in appearance, to varying degrees of incomplete insensitivity, where the external genitalia will be ambiguous, with a greater tendency toward masculinized external genitalia as the degree of adrogen insensitivity lessens.

Complete androgen insensitivity is a sex-linked recessive trait in which sisters of an affected individual have a one in three chance of having the disorder and female offspring from a normal sister of an affected individual have a one in six chance of having the disorder. Thus, both a careful family history and genetic counseling to the parents and sisters of affected individuals are critical. Frequently, however, there is no positive family history, indicating the likelihood of a new mutation.

The most common form of androgen insensitivity is the complete form, formerly referred to as testicular feminization (Fig. 46-5). This latter terminology should be dropped from usage not only because it is inaccurate but also, and more importantly, because it is upsetting to the patient and her family. Patients with complete androgen insensitivity have normally functioning testicles both in terms of testosterone production and production of müllerian inhibiting factor. Thus, the müllerian system will be resorbed embryologically in such patients, with the result that the fallopian tubes, uterus, and upper two thirds of the vagina will be absent. The vagina thus ends in a short vaginal pouch at the hymenal ring. The *testicles* may be found anywhere *intra-abdominally* along the path of the spermatic cords and not infrequently are present in inguinal hernias. This diagnosis should always be entertained in phenotypic female children with bilateral inguinal hernias and evaluated prior to correction of the hernias. As will be discussed later, the testicles should not be removed in these individuals until the completion of pubertal development.

In patients with complete androgen insensitivity, pubertal development will reflect only estrogenic changes. Thus, there is normally *full breast development* and the development of female body contours. Pubertal development requiring androgen stimulation—that is, the development of pubic and axillary hair—will be absent. The presenting complaint of persons with this disorder is either primary amenorrhea or the failure to de-

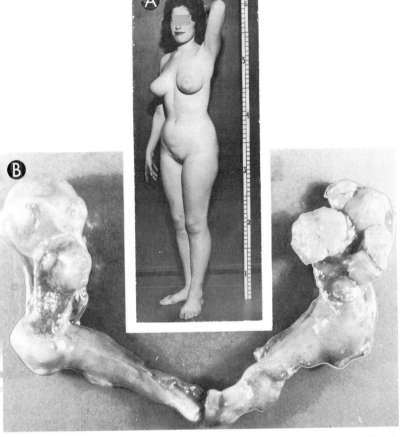
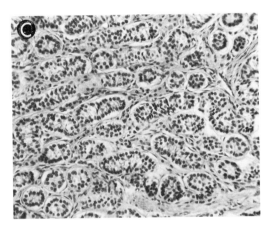

FIG. 46-5. (*A*) Androgen insensitivity in 18-year-old apparent female with primary amenorrhea, minimal sexual hair, large breasts and areolae, but small nipples. FSH before surgery: over 13, less than 52 mouse uterine units; 17-ketosteroids, 21 mg/24 hours; 17-ketogenic steroids, 5.5 mg/24 hours; pregnanetriol, 1.2 mg/24 hours. (*B*) Gonads and rudimentary uterine structures removed from patient in *A*. Note nodular appearance of gonad. (*C*) Photomicrograph of gonad. Immature testicular tubules are lined principally by primitive germ cells with some Sertoli cells present. Note marked resemblance to fetal testis. (Morris JM, Mahesh VB: Am J Obstet Gynecol 87:731, 1963)

velop pubic hair. The underlying genetically induced abnormality in complete androgen insensitivity is the failure to induce the formation of the cytosolic androgen receptor necessary for the translation of circulating testosterone into a biologic effect. Thus, although circulating testosterone levels are in the normal male range during puberty, there is no evidence of cellular recognition of its presence, and *secondary sexual hair* does not develop. It is not known whether the estrogenically induced pubertal changes are the result of intracellular conversion of testosterone to estrogen or of the total absence of any antagonistic effect of testosterone on circulating estrogen in the body. Diagnosis of this condition is usually quite simple in the individual with good breast development and female habitus without sexual hair. The diagnosis is confirmed by a pelvic examination

demonstrating a blind vaginal pouch and a 46 XY karyotype.

The *clinical management* of patients with complete androgen insensitivity differs from that of all other phenotypically female patients bearing a Y chromosome in their genetic makeup. Patients with complete androgen insensitivity should be allowed to undergo complete pubertal development with their gonads in place. Normal pubertal development is more satisfactorily and simply achieved by this approach. Such an approach is possible because *neoplastic changes* in intra-abdominal testicles usually do not develop until the *midtwenties*. Thus, it is possible to allow full pubertal development to occur and then perform gonadectomy with hormonal replacement with estrogen. A sexually functional vagina may be created either surgically or by progressive dilation of the blind vaginal pouch in the manner described for patients with müllerian dysgenesis. Individuals with complete androgen insensitivity can function entirely satisfactorily as normal women with the exceptions that they cannot bear children and do not have menses.

The success or failure of the management of patients with this disorder depends as much on the sensitive education of the patient and her family as on her medical care. The use of such terms as testes, testicular feminization, and male karyotype is not only unhelpful but destructive. Long-term counseling may be required to help the young woman adjust to her condition, particularly if it was initially presented to her in an insensitive fashion. The terms *androgen insensitivity, abnormal ovarian development,* and *genetic abnormality* should be substituted for the inflammatory terms discussed above.

ABNORMAL UTERINE BLEEDING

Once the normal hypothalamic-pituitary-ovarian interaction has been established, the production of sufficient estrogen to induce endometrial proliferation will result in the onset of menstrual bleeding. A variety of abnormalities of uterine bleeding may occur thereafter. The cessation of menses is usually preceded by a time of abnormal uterine bleeding that reflects a dysfunction in mechanisms of menstruation. Abnormalities of uterine bleeding ultimately reflect either an abnormality in the orderly sequence of estrogen production by the ovarian follicle followed by progesterone production after ovulation or the presence of undiagnosed organic pathology, whether benign, neoplastic, or pregnancy-related. Like amenorrhea, abnormal uterine bleeding is a symptom not a diagnosis. The efforts of the physician must be directed first at establishing a *specific diagnosis* toward which appropriate *specific therapy* can be directed. It is only by this approach that successful therapy can be achieved and serious pathology discovered.

As discussed elsewhere in this text, normal menstruation requires the orderly production of estrogen from the developing ovarian follicle resulting in both the proliferation of the endometrium and the formation of receptors for progesterone to be produced by the corpus luteum following ovulation. Additionally, a critical level of estrogen is necessary for the maintenance of the endometrium. An acute decrease in plasma estrogen below this critical level will result in endometrial breakdown and bleeding. If estrogen exposure is prolonged without subsequent ovulation and progesterone production, the endometrium will continue to proliferate and will require still more estrogen to maintain its growth. If this process continues, the endometrium outgrows its blood supply, resulting in breakdown of the tissue and bleeding.

In the normal menstrual cycle, the production of progesterone begins shortly before ovulation and continues in increasing amounts through the first week following ovulation. The effect of progesterone is to convert the previously proliferated endometrium into an endometrium in which both the glandular and the stromal components become secretory in nature. Glandular secretory activity is evident histologically, and it is now known that the endometrial stroma produces a wide variety of apparently locally acting protein hormones, one of which is identical to pituitary prolactin. This secretory activity during the first week of the luteal phase of the cycle is in preparation for implantation of the early embryo.

The changes brought about in the endometrium by progesterone exposure after an adequate proliferation of the endometrium by estrogen are universal in that most of the endometrium undergoes this biologic transition rather than only a portion thereof. The endometrium from the lower uterine segment seems to be less affected by progesterone than the remainder. In the absence of pregnancy, progesterone production by the corpus luteum begins to decline approximately one week before the onset of menstrual bleeding. The decline in progesterone is associated with cyclic vasoconstriction of the spiral arterioles and the progressive release of prostaglandins from the endometrium as it becomes anoxic and necrotic owing to the vasoconstriction. These changes are generalized throughout the endometrium and ultimately result in generalized tissue death and shedding of the endometrium in an orderly and self-limited fashion. Thus, in the absence of pregnancy, the proliferative effects of estrogen on the endometrium are biologically concluded by the action of progesterone. Unopposed estrogen stimulation resulting in endometrial hyperplasia and neoplasia is thereby avoided.

Abnormalities of uterine bleeding may occur as changes in frequency, amount, or duration of flow. The various terms used to describe these variations from the normal pattern are as follows:

Oligomenorrhea—bleeding occurring at intervals, usually irregular, of 40 days or more.
Polymenorrhea—bleeding occurring at regular or irregular intervals of less than 22 days.
Menorrhagia—bleeding occurring at regular intervals that is excessive in both amount and duration.
Metrorrhagia—bleeding occurring at irregular intervals that is usually normal in amount.
Menometrorrhagia—bleeding occurring at regular or irregular intervals that is excessive in amount and prolonged in duration.
Hypomenorrhea—bleeding occurring at regular intervals that is decreased in amount.
Intermenstrual bleeding—bleeding occurring between what is otherwise regular menstrual bleeding.

Considered in its broadest categories, abnormal uterine bleeding occurs either in conjunction with ovulatory cycles or in the setting of anovulation. When abnormal uterine bleeding is interspersed with what is otherwise regular cyclic ovulatory uterine bleeding confirmed either by basal body temperature curve or the determination of plasma progesterone, attention must be focused primarily on organic pathology. If the abnormal bleeding is associated with anovulation, the underlying etiology will more often than not be endocrinologic.

Ovulatory Abnormal Uterine Bleeding

Abnormal uterine bleeding in a patient who has previously had normal, regular cycles is often associated with *complications of pregnancy*. Such bleeding may be the result of retained gestational tissue either from a known previous pregnancy or from the incomplete abortion of a current pregnancy. The other major complication of early pregnancy associated with abnormal uterine bleeding is ectopic pregnancy. Abnormal uterine bleeding often is associated with ectopic pregnancy as the endometrial lining begins to degenerate secondary to inadequate hormonal support from the developing ectopic trophoblast. Abnormal bleeding may be the first symptom of ectopic pregnancy, occurring before significant pain or the more serious sequelae of rupture and hematoperitoneum. Only when the index of suspicion is high will the diagnosis of ectopic pregnancy be established prior to rupture.

The other major causative factor in ovulatory forms of abnormal bleeding is *organic disease* involving the uterus or vagina. Such benign disorders as adenomyosis, endometriosis, endometrial polyps, and endometritis may all present as abnormal bleeding superimposed on a background of normal ovulatory cycles. Bleeding from endometriosis may occur secondary to cervical or vaginal lesions or present as premenstrual spotting, which is often associated with pelvic endometriosis.

The possibility of abnormal uterine bleeding secondary to *blood dyscrasias,* such as idiopathic thrombocytopenic purpura, von Willebrand's disease, or leukemia, should always be considered when ovulatory abnormal bleeding occurs.

Iatrogenic causes of abnormal bleeding, such as the ingestion of sex steroid hormones—either estrogenic or progestational—or of anticoagulants, and bleeding secondary to an intrauterine device must be considered and can usually be identified from the patient's history.

One of the more common forms of ovulatory abnormal uterine bleeding is that which occurs at or just before the time of ovulation. This bleeding may occur in every cycle, or may occur intermittently at *midcycle.* Bleeding at the time of ovulation results from the physiologic fall in circulating estrogen levels occurring just before the LH surge. The diagnosis is established by the appearance of light bleeding precisely at midcycle and by the lack of other evident causes for bleeding. The bleeding is also frequently associated temporally with unilateral sharp pelvic pain resulting from ovulation (*mittelschmerz*). The use of a basal body temperature curve to establish these temporal relationships is of great benefit.

Another abnormality often associated with varying degrees of menstrual dysfunction in ovulatory patients is the *inadequate corpus luteum* or the luteal phase defect. This defect often precedes anovulation. A normally functioning corpus luteum requires adequate LH stimulation following ovulation. As described in detail elsewhere, the ability of LH to stimulate the luteinized granulosa cells is dependent on the action of FSH and follicular estrogen in stimulating LH receptor protein and thus assuring an adequate LH receptor concentration within the granulosa cell membrane by the time of ovulation. The biologic effect of LH on these preconditioned granulosa cells is to stimulate steroidogenesis and progesterone production during the 14 days following ovulation. If progesterone production is adequate and the endometrium is capable of responding to progesterone, a series of well-defined histologic changes occur that allow the accurate dating of the endometrium relative to the time of ovulation and subsequent menses. A discrepancy of two or more days between the actual date of onset of menses and the date predicted on the basis of the histologic maturation observed on endometrial biopsy is the *sine qua non* for the diagnosis of luteal insufficiency. If progesterone production occurs for fewer days than normal, the luteal phase of the cycle will be shortened and the menstrual frequency will increase. Often, however, the duration of progesterone production is entirely normal but the rate of production is diminished, resulting in a cycle of normal length but an inadequately stimulated endometrium. Patients with disorders of luteal function may present with abnormalities of uterine bleeding or with infertility resulting from an endometrial bed that is inadequate for implantation. Inadequate corpus luteum may also result in habitual abortion.

Abnormal luteal function may result from abnormal FSH stimulation of the preovulatory follicle secondary to hypothalamic-pituitary dysfunction, from interference with gonadotropin stimulation of the follicle by increased levels of circulating androgens, or from inadequate or inappropriate LH stimulation during and following ovulation. Rarely, abnormal luteal function may be caused by an inability of the endometrium to respond to normal progesterone production during the luteal phase. Luteal phase abnormalities occur commonly during the perimenarchal and especially the perimenopausal years, at which times the reproductive system is in a state of, respectively, "physiologic" immaturity or postmaturity. Thus, luteal phase inadequacy may be the harbinger of total follicular failure either at the normal menopausal age or prematurely. The other common clinical situation in which inadequate corpus luteal function is observed is in the anovulatory infertile patient undergoing ovulation induction. Luteal phase abnormalities may be the result of inadequate follicular stimulation by the ovulatory inducing agents or may follow high doses of clomiphene citrate, at which, possibly, the antiestrogenic properties of the drug are manifest at the follicular or endometrial level. This circumstance is discussed in greater detail in the chapter on ovulation induction and infertility.

Finally, irregularities of endometrial shedding are occasionally due to shortening of either the follicular or luteal phases of the cycle or to a persistence of the corpus luteum called Halban's disease. Each of these abnormalities is best diagnosed by a careful examination of a basal body temperature curve and the elimination of the other likely causes of abnormal bleeding by the history and physical examination. The conditions are benign and self-limited unless they reflect early changes in hypothalamic-pituitary-ovarian interrelationships due to a developing endocrinopathy.

Anovulatory Abnormal Uterine Bleeding

Anovulatory abnormal uterine bleeding occurs either as a prelude to secondary amenorrhea or in pathophysiologic conditions in which the synchrony of events necessary for ovulation does not occur but adequate follicular stimulation by gonadotropins persists, resulting in normal but tonic estrogen production by the ovary. After menarche, hypothalamic-pituitary disorders of the kind described under hypothalamic and pituitary causes of primary amenorrhea may present initially as anovulatory abnormal bleeding. Thus, organic disease involving the hypothalamus and pituitary gland must be considered in the evaluation of the patient as well as psychogenic and other stress factors, such as excessive athletic exertion. Ingestion of illicit drugs or exogenous sex steroids, such as oral contraceptives, may also produce anovulatory abnormal bleeding.

Endocrine disorders involving the adrenal gland or thyroid gland commonly present as abnormalities of menses in association with anovulation. The underlying mechanism of anovulation in patients with abnormalities of the thyroid or adrenal glands is an alteration in the feedback regulatory control of estrogens and androgens at the level of the hypothalamus and pituitary gland. In disorders of the thyroid gland this abnormality is due to alterations in liver metabolism that lead both to changes in binding proteins for sex hormones and to abnormalities in enzymes involved in the metabolism of sex hormones. Abnormalities of the adrenal glands produce biologically active sex steroids in abnormal quantities. In general, hypothyroidism will be associated with menometrorrhagia, hyperthyroidism with oligomenorrhea, hyperfunction of the adrenal gland with oligomenorrhea and signs of excess adrenal androgen or cortisol production, and hypofunction of the adrenal gland with oligomenorrhea and ultimately amenorrhea. These disorders involving other endocrine organs are discussed in detail in other sections of this text.

Destructive lesions involving the *ovary* may also be associated with anovulation and the associated abnormal uterine bleeding. These destructive processes may involve inflammatory or infectious disease, such as chronic salpingo-oophoritis or neoplastic lesions of the ovary, whether hormonally functional or not. They may also be the harbinger of premature ovarian failure.

Finally, *functional disturbances* in the production of gonadotropins reflecting a not fully mature hypothalamic-pituitary-ovarian relationship in the perimenarchal years or reflecting a decline in both sensitivity and number of ovarian follicles in the perimenopausal years are usually associated with aberrations of menses and anovulation. Oligomenorrhea associated with multiple follicular cysts of the ovary and a thickened ovarian capsule, anovulation, mild androgen excess, and mild-to-moderate obesity is referred to variously as the polycystic ovary syndrome or the Stein-Leventhal syndrome. The disorder, which is of unknown etiology, is discussed in detail in the section on androgen excess syndromes. The initiating abnormality in hypothalamic-pituitary-ovarian dysynchrony and function can undoubtedly vary, but the end result of anovulation is the same. These patients have tonic stimulation of multiple ovarian follicles resulting in a tonic production of androstenedione, estradiol, and peripherally formed estrone. There may in addition be a mild abnormality of androgen production by the adrenal gland as well. The result of this abnormal hormonal milieu is an abnormal production of FSH and LH, with LH predominating. Such individuals produce more than sufficient estrogen for endometrial proliferation, and periodic menstrual bleeding occurs as the endometrium, stimulated by unopposed estrogen, exceeds its blood supply. Ovulation—and consequently progesterone production—does not occur. Such patients have uterine bleeding that occurs less frequently than normal but is heavy and prolonged. In addition, because of the tonic unopposed estrogen stimulation, they are at greatly increased risk for endometrial hyperplasia and neoplasia if the condition remains uncorrected.

Diagnosis of Abnormal Uterine Bleeding

History

The first step in establishing a specific diagnosis of the cause underlying abnormal uterine bleeding is a carefully obtained patient history. The conditions under which abnormal bleeding occur are of great importance, often pointing to trauma, pregnancy, or hypothalamic-pituitary dysfunction. The preceding menstrual history is also of importance because it enables the clinician to place the dysfunction in the context of an acute change rather than a chronic change. Symptoms of other glandular dysfunction, such as those associated with androgen excess or thyroid or adrenal dysfunction, should be sought. The investigator should carefully determine whether the abnormal bleeding is occurring in conjunction with normal cyclic bleeding or is totally irregular. This will help designate the bleeding as either ovulatory or anovulatory in nature. Symptoms of progesterone production, such as breast swelling and tenderness, fluid retention, and dysmenorrhea with vaginal bleeding, should also be sought. Finally, a history of drug or sex steroid ingestion, intrauterine device usage, or easy bruisability and bleeding gums may point to the correct diagnosis. At times, it may be helpful to monitor the patient with a basal body temperature curve so that the episodes of uterine bleeding can be related to ovulation.

Physical Examination

The physical examination is also of great importance in evaluating abnormal uterine bleeding. The general physical examination is directed at identifying signs suggesting dysfunction of the thyroid, adrenal, or other endocrine glands as well as signs of central pathology interfering with normal hypothalamic and pituitary function.

The pelvic examination is directed first at determining the source of the bleeding. It is often difficult for a patient to know whether the bleeding she observes is of uterine, vaginal, rectal, or urethral origin. The external genitalia are examined for the presence of labial trauma, varicosities, or other signs of inflammation or neoplasia. Similarly, the rectum and urethral meatus are carefully inspected. The vagina is then examined for the presence of trauma, foreign bodies, vaginal infections, including trichomonas and monilia, and neoplasia or adenosis. Lesions of the cervix and cervical erosion should be noted as well. Abnormal uterine bleeding following coitus often reflects cervical or vaginal pathology and may be the first sign of cervical carcinoma. Cervical trauma associated with an attempted self-induced abortion, or cervical dilatation with tissue appearing in the cervical os will point toward pregnancy-associated bleeding. The bimanual examination should be directed particularly toward the palpation of any uterine enlargement or irregularity that might be associated with uterine myomas or pregnancy. Bilateral adnexal tenderness and thickening may reflect a chronic pelvic inflammatory process, whereas unilateral adnexal enlargement and tenderness suggest either a neoplastic ovarian process or a tubal gestation. Finally, a rectovaginal examination not only will detect bleeding from a rectal lesion but also will allow the complete examination of the posterior pelvis and cul de sac, where uterosacral ligament thickening or cul-de-sac irregularity may point either to pelvic endometriosis or pelvic neoplasia.

Laboratory Investigation

Laboratory studies are of secondary importance in the diagnosis of the causes of abnormal uterine bleeding and usually only substantiate a diagnosis already determined by the findings of the history and physical examination. The two most important laboratory tests are a β-hCG assay, which should be done whenever the possibility of a pregnancy-related condition arises, and a prolactin determination, since hyperprolactinemia may present initially as ovulatory dysfunction or anovulation and abnormal uterine bleeding. The history and physical examination normally indicate whether or not specific thyroid, adrenal, or androgen studies are needed. In the absence of historical or physical findings consistent with endocrinopathy involving the thyroid or adrenal glands, laboratory testing will rarely, if ever, be helpful.

In considering the possible causes of abnormal uterine bleeding, it is often helpful to think in terms of *the reproductive life* of the individual. Thus, in *adolescent* patients the most common causes of abnormal uterine bleeding are vaginal trauma associated with either athletics or early sexual exposure and hypothalamic-pituitary dysfunction occurring physiologically as this system matures in its interaction with the estrogen production of the ovaries. The possibility of a pregnancy-associated condition not volunteered in the history must also be considered.

Patients in the *active reproductive* portion of their lives more commonly exhibit pregnancy-associated abnormalities, endocrine-related abnormal uterine bleeding associated with anovulation, and organic pathology. Finally, the predominant causes of abnormal uterine bleeding in *perimenopausal* patients are organic pathology, neoplasia, and follicular dysfunction. In these patients, endometrial sampling by aspiration endometrial biopsy or diagnostic dilatation and curettage finds its greatest and most important use.

Treatment

Treatment of abnormal uterine bleeding is best considered in the same age-related fashion as etiology. In adolescents, specific abnormal findings associated with the abnormal bleeding should, of course, be treated specifically. Mild traumatic lesions may require no specific therapy, but occasionally a vaginal laceration will require suturing. The vast majority of adolescents with abnormal uterine bleeding, however, suffer from hypothalamic-pituitary-ovarian immaturity and are more in need of reassurance and education than medication. If the frequency, duration, or degree of bleeding is sufficient to warrant therapy, the simplest and most effective therapy is to replace the progesterone that is lacking in such individuals because of the anovulatory state. Progesterone given as 10 mg medroxyprogesterone acetate daily for 5 days every 60 days if bleeding has not intervened will provide periodic interruption of the proliferative effects of unopposed estrogen and predictable vaginal bleeding. As the system matures and ovulatory function begins, bleeding will occur spontaneously at intervals shorter than 60 days so that the patient will stop taking the progesterone accordingly.

The treatment of abnormal uterine bleeding that is related to pregnancy or organic pathology during the reproductive years is specific and depends on the underlying cause. Similarly, the treatment of an underlying endocrinopathy will depend on its etiology. The treatment of the patient with polycystic ovarian disease depends on whether pregnancy is desired or not. When pregnancy is desired, the induction of ovulation with clomiphene citrate is highly effective. When pregnancy is not desired, treatment with a combined estrogen and progestin oral contraceptive will interrupt the unopposed estrogen proliferation of the endometrium, provide regular predictable menses, and diminish both the elevated androgens and their biologic effects.

Occasionally, the uterine bleeding associated with anovulation and relatively high tonic estrogen stimulation may be heavy and acute or prolonged. Bleeding of this kind is more common in younger patients than in patients of reproductive age. Such patients must be treated promptly and aggressively. Intravenous conjugated estrogens, 25 mg every 4 to 6 hours for four to six doses will usually control the hemorrhage promptly. This therapy should be followed by a medium-dose estrogen–progestin oral contraceptive, one tablet four times each day for one week followed by one tablet each day for the next 21-day cycle. Following withdrawal menses at the conclusion of this therapy, three additional cycles of combination estrogen and progestin at the usual dose, one tablet per day, should be provided. Withdrawal menses should occur between cycles. Following such therapy, if oral contraception is not desired, intermittent medroxyprogesterone acetate given as described above may be instituted. In the occasional patient who does not respond to this medical regimen, diagnostic curettage is indicated both for temporary arrest of the bleeding and, more important, for diagnostic purposes. It should be understood clearly that curettage does not affect the underlying pathophysiology that caused the bleeding and will interrupt it only temporarily, if at all. If definitive therapy or regular control of endometrial proliferation either by cyclic oral contraceptives or by intermittent medroxyprogesterone is not instituted, recurrence of the problem may be anticipated. In the patient with a history of prolonged and continuous uterine bleeding in which a minimal amount of endometrium might be expected to be present, treatment should start with stimulation of endometrial proliferation with a conjugated estrogen, 1.25 mg daily for 25 days, for the last 10 days of which 10 mg medroxyprogesterone acetate is added. Following a withdrawal menses, the patient may be treated either with a combination estrogen and progestin oral contraceptive or with medroxyprogesterone acetate as described previously.

Abnormal uterine bleeding that occurs in conjunction with oral contraceptive usage is discussed in detail elsewhere in this text. In most patients with this disorder, bleeding occurs because the ratio of estrogen to progesterone is too low for that patient's individual endometrial needs, and endometrial instability results. Such patients are best treated by the addition of a conjugated estrogen, 0.625 mg daily, to be taken concurrently with the oral contraceptive for two or three cycles. Endometrial proliferation will be increased, and this will correct the bleeding for many months following the cessation of the additional estrogen. Doubling the dose of the oral contraceptive is not usually effective, because the ratio of estrogen to progestin is not changed, and it appears that it is the ratio that is important for endometrial stabilization.

The treatment for patients with luteal phase defects, as for those with anovulation, is determined by the wishes of the patient concerning pregnancy. Most patients with this disorder will, in fact, suffer from either infertility or repeated pregnancy wastage. The approach to treatment may consist either in attempting to further stimulate normal folliculogenesis using either clomiphene citrate or menopausal gonadotropins or in adding progesterone in the form of vaginal suppositories, 25 mg twice each day beginning two to three days after apparent ovulation and continuing until menses begin or the eighth week of pregnancy has been reached. Patients not desiring pregnancy may require no therapy if the bleeding abnormality is minor, or they may be treated by administration of a progestin in the second half of each cycle or by oral contraceptive therapy.

In summary, in patients with abnormal uterine bleeding, the source of the bleeding must be determined. A careful search, directed primarily by a thorough history and physical examination, must be made for underlying pathophysiologic conditions of both an endocrine and organic nature. Treatment should be directed to the specific underlying cause whenever possible. Some underlying causes are much more common in one age group than in another, which greatly facilitates diagnosis. A significant number of patients, however, will have no determinable underlying cause for their anovulatory bleeding. In these patients the treatment of choice is the arrest of the acute bleeding episode and prevention of recurrence with restoration of cyclic menses utilizing either medroxyprogesterone acetate or a combined oral contraceptive. Ovulation should be induced only in patients who wish to become pregnant immediately. The use of ovulation-inducing agents to "test the system" for future reference has no place in modern reproductive endocrinology and often results in an unwanted pregnancy.

SECONDARY AMENORRHEA

Secondary amenorrhea is the cessation of menses for six or more months. The choice of a six-month time period is rather arbitrary but is based on the fact that people often miss several cycles for a variety of known and unknown causes that resolve spontaneously. When amenorrhea has persisted for six months, however, the likelihood that it is caused by underlying persistent abnormality is greatly increased. On first contact with a patient complaining of amenorrhea, sufficient information should be obtained, regardless of the duration, to determine whether specific signs and symptoms of underlying conditions, such as hirsutism, galactorrhea, or pregnancy, are present. The presence of any such signs or symptoms indicates that further evaluation is needed.

The first and most important step in the evaluation of a patient with secondary amenorrhea is to *rule out* the presence of a *pregnancy.* In most patients, β-hCG concentration should be determined. The young adolescent may be reluctant to communicate the likelihood of pregnancy. Still other patients may have had temporary amenorrhea that resolved spontaneously with ovulation and no intervening menses. Such an individual may have been amenorrheic for two or three months and then conceived, never having had a menstrual period in the interim. Thus, a history of many months of amenorrhea does not exclude an early intrauterine pregnancy.

Causes

The basic requirements for the initiation of menstrual bleeding are also necessary for its continuance. Thus, many of the underlying causes of primary amenorrhea must also be considered in secondary amenorrhea. Emphasis is placed in this section on the more common causes of secondary amenorrhea as well as on those not discussed in detail under primary amenorrhea.

Secondary amenorrhea is often the end point in a spectrum of abnormalities of menses, as described previously. Menses often do not stop abruptly but first become irregular, then less frequent, and finally cease altogether. Therefore, much of the discussion of abnormal uterine bleeding that precedes this section is pertinent also to secondary amenorrhea.

Following a careful history and physical examination, the first step in the evaluation of patients with secondary amenorrhea is to *distinguish between hypothalamic-pituitary dysfunction, ovarian failure,* and *endometrial failure.* The FSH and LH levels will be in the menopausal range for patients with ovarian failure and in the normal or low-normal range for patients with hypothalamic-pituitary dysfunction and endometrial failure. Since prolactin concentrations are elevated in a wide variety of hypothalamic-pituitary disorders, laboratory studies of prolactin levels should be obtained. If the level is elevated, further studies should be done. If concentrations of gonadotropins and the level of prolactin are normal, the next important consideration is dysfunction of the endometrium itself.

Endometrial Failure (Asherman's Syndrome)

Asherman's syndrome is a condition caused by an obliteration of most of the functioning endometrial tissue in the uterine cavity. In the absence of sufficient endometrium, particularly in the presence of an inflammatory process, collagen will replace endometrial tissue and obliterate all or part of the endometrial cavity. This condition may lead to obstruction to the outflow of the menstruum or there may be so little endometrial tissue that bleeding is insignificant. Almost always there will be a *clear history* of a dilatation and curettage (D&C) performed for postpartum bleeding several days after delivery, of a D&C performed in the presence of an infected abortion, or of several D&Cs performed in close approximation to one another for abnormal uterine bleeding. The hallmark of this diagnosis is a history of absent or markedly diminished menstruation following the D&C. Additional outpatient studies are an estrogen-progestin challenge test and a hysterosalpingogram, which will often show the absence of an endometrial cavity or severe deformity and obliteration of parts of the cavity. The rationale for the estrogen-progestin challenge test is based on the fact that the only requirement for withdrawal menses following estrogen and progestin stimulation is the presence of endometrial tissue. Thus, a patient in whom pregnancy has been ruled out who is treated with 2.5 mg of conjugated estrogen daily for 21 days, during the last 10 of which 10 mg medroxyprogesterone acetate is added, will undergo withdrawal menses if endometrium is present in the uterine cavity.

Optimal treatment for Asherman's syndrome involves the *hysteroscopic lysis* of the intrauterine adhesions (synechiae). The treatment prior to the advent of the hysteroscope was blind attempt to lyse the intrauterine adhesions during a D&C. Not infrequently a second operative treatment is required to completely restore the endometrial cavity. An intrauterine device is inserted into the uterine cavity following the operative procedure to keep the uterine cavity open, and the patient is treated for two to three months with high-dose estrogen (5 mg conjugated estrogens daily) with a progestin added for the last 10 days. The intrauterine device is removed at the time of withdrawal menses and a repeat hysterosalpingogram is performed approximately one month thereafter. Restoration of regular menses and fertility can be anticipated in two thirds of patients so managed.

Ovarian Failure

When a patient's gonadotropin concentrations are in the menopausal range, ovarian follicles will be lost, as in the patient with primary amenorrhea. In general, premature ovarian failure is the loss of follicles before the age of 35. The underlying causes of premature ovarian failure are similar to those discussed in the section on primary amenorrhea. Although most patients will have idiopathic ovarian failure, a *karyotype* should be obtained in all cases. The predominant abnormal chromosomal pattern in patients with secondary amenorrhea is sex chromosome mosaicism. There will almost invariably be a 46 XX pattern in some of the cells in addition to a 45 XO or 46 XY pattern or an aberration in the structure of the X chromosome resulting in functional failure. Any combination of sex chromosome patterns may be seen. The only pattern of clinical importance is that containing a Y chromosome. *Gonadectomy* should be performed in all patients in whom a Y chromosome is present. As discussed previously, patients with idiopathic ovarian failure should undergo immunologic testing for antiovarian and other endocrine antibodies and testing of the thyroid and adrenal gland for impending failure.

Patients treated with *chemotherapy* for malignancy after menarche will usually develop secondary amenorrhea lasting for variable periods of time. Overall, the younger the patient, the more likely she is to resume regular spontaneous menses as the follicular cells regenerate. Women over 30 years of age have a high incidence of permanent ovarian failure, however. *Radiation* damage to the ovaries is irreversible.

All patients with premature ovarian failure should be treated with *estrogen and progesterone replacement* therapy as previously described. Replacement is required both to maintain the secondary sexual organs and for prophylaxis against osteoporosis.

Hypothalamic-Pituitary Dysfunction

Abnormalities involving the hypothalamic stimulation of the pituitary gland and pituitary gland abnormalities *per se* may result in the cessation of menses. Tumors, central nervous system infection, physical or psychologic stress, and significant fluctuations in body weight may all induce secondary amenorrhea, just as they may induce primary amenorrhea. Young women who have just gone to college often develop secondary amenorrhea due to the radical change in life patterns and the stress of new-found independence. This benign secondary amenorrhea usually resolves spontaneously.

On the other hand, serious fluctuations in weight, such as those associated with anorexia nervosa or bulimia usually result in secondary amenorrhea. These conditions are discussed in detail in another section of this text. Inadequate body weight is becoming a more and more common cause of secondary amenorrhea in older women. The emphasis in today's culture on physical fitness, low-calorie diets, and "youth forever" is carried to the extreme by some individuals, resulting in secondary amenorrhea. The diagnosis of this cause of amenorrhea rests on the patient history and the elimination of other serious causes of amenorrhea.

Patients with hypothalamic amenorrhea from all causes will have *gonadotropin* concentrations in the *normal to low-normal* range. Additionally, if organic pathology is infiltrating or destroying the hypothalamus, the prolactin level will be elevated due to loss of hypothalamic dopamine in the normal inhibitory control of pituitary prolactin release. In patients with hypothalamic amenorrhea and elevated prolactin levels, computed tomography is clearly indicated. Even when the patient's prolactin level is normal, any signs or symptoms of central nervous system pathology should be further investigated.

Treatment of patients with hypothalamic amenorrhea will depend on the pathology involved and on the desires of the patient. If body weight is abnormal, a simple correction to within a few percent of the ideal body weight may be all that is required. If pregnancy is desired, stimulation of ovulation with clomiphene citrate or menopausal gonadotropins is the appropriate treatment. Patients with very low levels of circulating estrogen may require estrogen supplementation if the underlying pathology cannot be corrected. In patients with normal estrogen levels, intermittent progestin withdrawal bleeding both to provide regular menstruation and to interrupt the uninhibited estrogenic proliferation of the endometrium is indicated. In patients desiring contraception, however, the use of a low-estrogen oral contraceptive may be the treatment of choice.

Pituitary gland dysfunction is very common as an underlying cause of secondary amenorrhea and has received much attention over the last few years because of changing concepts in both diagnosis and management. Since pituitary dysfunction, particularly hyperprolactinemia, occurs most commonly in the setting of secondary amenorrhea, a detailed discussion of this disorder follows.

Hypofunction of the pituitary gland may result either from pituitary necrosis following postpartum hemorrhage (*Sheehan's disease*) or from pituitary necrosis from septic embolization secondary to puerperal infection (*Simmonds's disease*). Patients with hypofunction of the pituitary gland fail to lactate postpartum, often fail to regrow normal pubic hair when it was shaved as part of the delivery preparation, and undergo a slow, progressive development of cachexia and lethargy. Occasionally, pituitary failure will not be complete, and consequently each trophic hormone and its respective target organ should be evaluated. Diagnosis of this condition is based on the *history* and the evaluation of trophic hormone production and target organ function. Pituitary failure is most accurately diagnosed by a *TRH stimulation test* as described for pituitary failure earlier in this chapter.

Abnormalities of the pituitary gland that produce elevated levels of trophic hormones are similar to those previously discussed and are discussed in more depth in other chapters. In brief, a pituitary tumor occurring after menarche that produces growth hormone results in *acromegaly* rather than gigantism since the epiphyses will be closed or nearly so. Thus, bony proliferation is evidenced in increased bone thickness, particularly on bony prominences of the face and lower jaw. An excess of *ACTH* production from functioning pituitary tumors results in *Cushing's syndrome,* which is discussed elsewhere.

Pituitary dysfunction resulting in *hyperprolactinemia* has been recognized for many years. These abnormalities have been categorized as those occurring following pregnancy (Chiari-Frommel syndrome), those occurring in nulliparous women with no evidence of a pituitary tumor (Ahumada-Del Castillo syndrome), and those in which an evident pituitary tumor is present (Forbes-Albright syndrome). When a tumor was present, it was referred to as a *chromophobe adenoma,* because the cells failed to stain specifically for secretory granules, which suggested that the tumor was nonfunctioning. It is now known that virtually all chromophobe adenomas are, in fact, prolactin-secreting tumors, and they are now referred to as *prolactinomas.* The earlier categorization of syndromes is of historical interest only, since there is much overlap between the conditions they describe.

Prolactin as a discrete hormone had been studied in various animal species but was not separated from growth hormone as a discrete peptide hormone until the pioneering work of Henry Friesen in the early 1970s. The studies of Dr. Friesen and others showed that prolactin exists in the human being as in other animal species as a peptide hormone without saccharide or other components and has a molecular weight of approximately 20,000. The amino acid sequence of human prolactin has subsequently been described. Our knowledge of how pituitary prolactin production is controlled has also expanded greatly in the last few years. The conceptual substance PIF, or prolactin inhibiting factor, is now known to be either identical to or very closely related to dopamine, which acts to inhibit synthesis and release of prolactin by pituitary lactotrophs. The amenorrhea associated with increased prolactin levels is believed to be due to the negative effect of prolactin on hypothalamic GnRH production. Suppression of GnRH results in a suppressed production of pituitary FSH and LH and the appearance of the subsequent low-estrogen form of amenorrhea.

Prolactin concentrations in the circulation are usually less than 25 ng/ml in normal men, women, and children. The most common cause of elevated circulating prolactin concentrations is pregnancy. Amniotic fluid also contains extremely high concentrations of prolactin (in the microgram range). The other physiologic state in which prolactin is elevated is during lactation.

It should be clear that any pharmacologic substance that interferes with normal hypothalamic dopamine levels will result in an alteration in prolactin production. Almost all of the psychotropic medications have been implicated in abnormal prolactin secretion and in the clinical symptoms of galactorrhea and oligoamenorrhea. Dopamine agonists, such as bromocriptine (Parlodel), suppress prolactin production by the lactotrophs which results in a diminution in the concentration of circulating prolactin.

Prolactin has a normal diurnal variation analogous to that of growth hormone but differently timed, with a peak rise in concentration in both men and women during the late night hours of sleep between 3 A.M. and 5 A.M.

Estrogen, which is known to be mitogenic to pituitary lactotrophs, is a strong stimulator of prolactin production by the pituitary gland. This effect is seen most notably during pregnancy, when the high levels of estrogen augment the normal diurnal variation of prolactin production. The other major stimulator of prolactin production is hypothalamic TRH. TRH acts on pituitary lactotrophs through a mechanism involving the dopaminergic pathways. This mechanism is different from that through which TRH exerts its effect on pituitary TSH production, which appears to be nondopaminergic.

Stimulation of casein, the primary milk protein, is the only specific action so far attributed to prolactin in the human being. Suckling greatly stimulates the release of pituitary prolactin, and this effect can be completely inhibited by the presence of the dopamine agonist bromocriptine.

Pathophysiology

A wide variety of abnormalities, both organic and pharmacologic, result in elevated circulating levels of prolactin and consequent amenorrhea and galactorrhea (Fig. 46-6). Almost all the psychomimetic drugs that affect hypothalamic catacholamine levels have been associated with elevations in prolactin concentration, amenorrhea, and galactorrhea. It should be kept in mind that patients receiving psychomimetic drugs may also have an expanding central nervous system lesion that is causing both the abnormal psychiatric state and the elevated prolactin levels. Physical stress and recent food intake may also temporarily increase prolactin concentrations. The most common cause of amenorrhea and galactorrhea is pregnancy, however, and this must always be excluded.

FIG. 46-6. Causes of hyperprolactinemia.

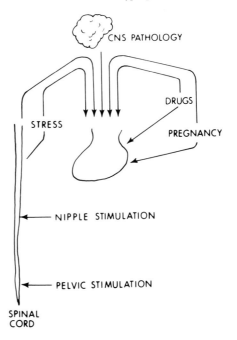

The major central nervous system abnormality other than prolactin-producing adenomas that can result in elevations of prolactin is central nervous system tumors or nonprolactin-producing pituitary tumors that physically interfere with the portal system that joins the hypothalamus with the pituitary gland in a functional sense. The result of such organic pathology is a loss of the normal dopaminergic inhibition of pituitary prolactin production. Thus, the equivalent of pituitary stalk sectioning occurs. The most common nonpituitary tumor producing this effect is the craniopharyngioma, which is a tumor originating in Rathke's pouch. Tumors of this kind characteristically calcify and thus are evident on plain lateral skull x-ray.

An uncommon but nevertheless important cause of increased levels of circulating prolactin is hypothyroidism with elevated TRH concentrations. This condition should always be considered in patients with amenorrhea and galactorrhea and is most easily detected by determining the TSH level.

The modern diagnosis of pituitary tumors began with the development of a sensitive radioimmunoassay for human prolactin in the early 1970s. The normal circulating concentration of prolactin in the nonpregnant state is less than 25 ng/ml. Any patient with any aberration of menses, amenorrhea, or galactorrhea should have a serum prolactin assay. If the prolactin level is elevated, further diagnostic studies should be obtained to evaluate the pituitary gland for a possible tumor. In general, the prolactin concentration and tumor size correlate fairly well, but large tumors have been reported with only modest elevations of prolactin (30–60 ng/ml).

A variety of dynamic pituitary tests have been studied over the past several years in an attempt to distinguish between functional states and tumors, both of which may result in elevated prolactin concentrations. None of these dynamic stimulation or suppression tests has proven of value on an individual patient basis.

The classic signs and symptoms of amenorrhea and galactorrhea associated with prolactin producing-pituitary tumors are well known. Most patients with pituitary tumors will demonstrate both amenorrhea and galactorrhea, but either symptom alone may be associated with a tumor and should be evaluated accordingly. The pathophysiologic relationship between elevated prolactin concentrations and depressed FSH and LH concentrations is not fully understood. It was felt for many years that the amenorrhea associated with pituitary tumors was the result of a large tumor mass compressing the normal pituitary gland and diminishing its physiologic function. This explanation has not withstood the more recent finding of amenorrhea and galactorrhea in patients with extremely small prolactin-producing tumors. It is now believed on the basis of recent studies in primates that the amenorrhea of hyperprolactinemic states is the result of diminished GnRH production caused by the effect of prolactin on the hypothalamus.

The amenorrhea of pituitary tumors is a low-estrogen form of amenorrhea that manifests in most patients as either failure of withdrawal menses following progesterone challenge or a vaginal maturation index shifted in the direction of parabasal cells. This hypoestrogen state requires time to develop, however, so that not all patients with pituitary tumors will demonstrate hypoestrogenemia. As the pituitary tumor expands and grows upward, the optic chiasm is compressed, leading to the classic finding of bitemporal hemanopsia. Findings of visual field abnormalities were common before the advent of more sophisticated methods of diagnosis. With early diagnosis and treatment of small tumors, changes in the visual fields have become uncommon.

Pituitary tumors arise as more or less well defined accumulations of the specific cell types of the pituitary gland from unknown underlying causes. The tumors are almost always benign, although malignant varieties have occasionally been reported. The tumors are characteristically slow to develop and the signs and symptoms are often mild or vague for many years.

Diagnosis

When an elevated prolactin level has been found and physiologic and pharmacologic causes for its elevation have been ruled out, appropriate radiographic studies of the sella turcica should be obtained. Great strides have been made in the past ten years in the ability to detect prolactin-producing microadenomas of the pituitary gland in very early stages of development. The progress is due to the introduction of assays of circulating levels of prolactin and refined radiographic techniques for visualizing the sella turcica. The three basic radiographic techniques in use are the coned-down view of the sella, hypocycloidal polytomography, and computed tomography (CT).

Coned-Down Sella Turcica X-Rays

To be visible on a coned-down view of the sella turcica, a tumor must be 10 mm or more in diameter. Such a tumor will result in an overall increase in the volume of the sella ($>16 \times 13$ mm), a double floor of the sella resulting from asymmetrical depression of the floor due to tumor growth, erosion of the floor of the sella, thinning of the dorsum sellae, and occasionally a soft tissue density in the sphenoid sinus if the tumor is large. Total skin dose of radiation exposure by this technique is less than 0.5 rad.

The major disadvantages of the technique are that approximately 75% of patients with surgically proven small adenomas will have normal coned-down views and that anatomic variations as sphenoid septae, indentations by the carotid artery, and minor developmental asymmetries cannot be distinguished from a tumor by this technique.

Hypocycloidal Polytomography

Hypocycloidal polytomography is a technique in which complex movements of the x-ray tube with 1 mm to 2 mm "slices" produce very sharp views of small areas of the sella turcica and a blurring of the surrounding structures that increases markedly the sensitivity of the technique. Tumors of 4 mm to 5 mm in size produce demonstrable changes in the sella that can usually be appreciated with this technique. It will reveal localized abnormalities, the earliest possible point at which tumor development can be detected, and is currently the best guide for the surgical exploration of the sphenoid sinus and sella turcica in the neurosurgical management of the disorder. Abnormalities seen include a localized blistering of the anterior lateral portion of the sella and localized thinning or erosion of the floor or dorsum of the sella (Fig. 46-7). The technique distinguishes between anatomic variations and tumors more precisely than does the cone-down approach. Lateral views are the most sensitive, and anterior views are rarely necessary. There is an extremely high correlation between abnormalities seen by this technique and the presence of surgically proven tumors when the radiographic changes occur in conjunction with an elevated serum prolactin concentration.

The disadvantages of this technique are that the radiation exposure is relatively high (up to 20–23 rad) and that approximately one third of normal women will show minor changes in the sella on polytomography. Thus, the high correlation between the presence of a tumor and abnormalities on polytomography depend

FIG. 46-7. Hypocycloidal polytomography of the the sella turcica revealing microadenoma (*arrow*).

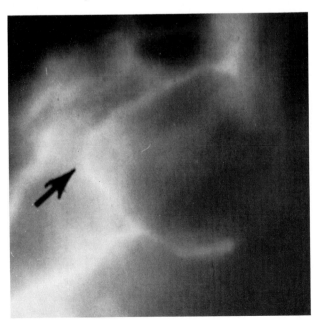

on the additional finding of elevations in the serum prolactin level. Another potential disadvantage has been the possible association between polytomography and the development of cataracts of the lenses. This should be an avoidable complication if the eyes are properly shielded, exposure is limited to the lateral view, and studies are performed only when clinically indicated.

Computed Tomography

Computed tomography has greatly increased the ability to define abnormal changes throughout the central nervous system and the other organs of the body. The basic principle is to feed information obtained by tomographic x-ray slices into a programmed computer to develop a three-dimensional picture of the structure under consideration. Among the major advantages of the CT scanner are that it demonstrates the actual tumor rather than bony changes of the sella and that it can reveal suprasella extension of the tumor. Contrast-medium enhancement has further improved the value of the scanner and has virtually eliminated the need for combined tomography and pneumoencephalography for evaluation of suprasellar lesions or the empty sella syndrome.

The new generation of CT scanners provide resolution equivalent to that of polytomography, but it must be remembered that the greater the degree of resolution, the greater the amount of radiation exposure necessary for sharp delineation of the structure. Thus, resolution comparable to that of polytomography requires radiation equal or in excess of that used in lateral polytomography. Spatial resolution remains limited and high-frequency artifacts are frequently seen.

The particular diagnostic technique used depends to some degree on the clinical presentation and on the anticipated therapeutic approach to the adenoma. Patients with visual field defects or other neurologic symptoms will undoubtedly have a tumor large enough to be clearly diagnosed on a simple coned-down view of the sella. Patients with amenorrhea and galactorrhea of relatively short duration and an elevated serum prolactin level will probably need polytomography or high-resolution CT scanning to diagnose the presence of a small tumor. If there is an abnormality of the polytomography, CT scanning of the suprasellar region is important to determine the full extent of the adenoma.

Occasionally, the pituitary fossa will appear enlarged but empty (*empty sella syndrome*). The endocrine studies in patients with the empty sella syndrome are usually normal; however, if the prolactin level is elevated in such patients, a pituitary tumor should be strongly suspected.

Treatment

Once the diagnosis of a pituitary tumor has been confirmed, the various choices of therapy must be considered. Modern *surgical* treatment of pituitary adenomas began with Schloffer's successful partial adenomectomy by the transsphenoidal route in 1907. The development of transsphenoidal hypophysectomy utilizing image intensification has allowed the selective removal of very small pituitary tumors with sparing of the normal gland. This approach has markedly diminished the morbidity associated with open craniotomy. Selective adenomectomy has been performed in this fashion on many patients in the past few years. Preliminary results suggest that it may be possible by early treatment to avoid some of the sequelae of pituitary tumors seen in earlier years. Since pituitary tumors probably develop very slowly over many years, long-term follow-up of various treatment modalities will be necessary before it will be possible to evaluate the success or failure of any treatment modality. Long-term follow-up studies to date indicate that recurrence rates following adenomectomy for microadenomas (<1 cm in diameter) approach 50% to 60% and for macroadenomas (>1 cm diameter) may approach 90%. Transient diabetes insipidus, hypopituitarism, and, occasionally, neurologic deficits are the only significant sources of morbidity following transsphenoidal surgery. Operative death is rare. Large tumors involving the optic chiasm may require a transfrontal approach with its inherent increased morbidity and mortality.

Radiation therapy has been used in the past as ad-junctive therapy to pituitary surgery in patients in whom it was felt that the tumor had not been completely removed or when signs and symptoms of persistence of the tumor existed following surgery. More recently, proton beam therapy has been used as primary therapy for pituitary tumors in a few centers. The long-term results of such therapy are not yet known. The major side effect of radiation therapy is the slow development of panhypopituitarism, which may occur over as much as ten years and results from the inability to treat the adenoma only. The other drawback to radiotherapy is the relative radioresistance of many of these tumors.

The recent availability of bromocriptine, a dopaminergic agonist, has offered the possibility of *medical* therapy for pituitary tumors. Bromocriptine suppresses the synthesis and release of prolactin from both tumorous and nontumorous cells. It has proven quite effective in reversing the amenorrhea-galactorrhea syndromes in which no tumor has been demonstrable. There have been numerous recent reports of patients with prolactin-producing pituitary tumors treated over an extended period with bromocriptine with the subsequent finding of tumor regression and apparent cure (Fig. 46-8). Upon stopping the medication, however, most patients will have a recurrence of hyperprolactinemia, suggesting that bromocriptine suppresses but does not obliterate the adenoma. Thus, long-term medical treatment should be

FIG. 46-8. Computed tomography of a pituitary adenoma with suprasellar extension before and after treatment with bromocriptine. (Thorner MO et al: Rapid regression of pituitary prolactinomas during bromocriptine treatment. J Clin Endocrinol Metab 51:438, 1980. Copyright © 1980)

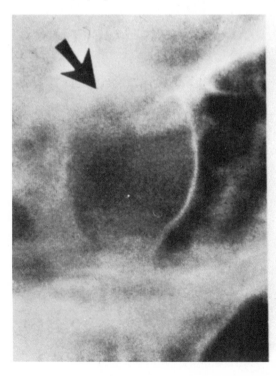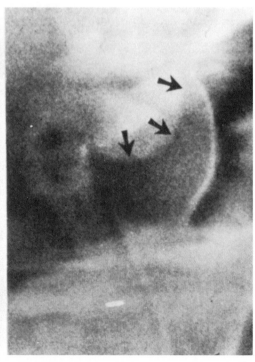

anticipated. The use of bromocriptine for the treatment of overt pituitary tumors is now under intensive clinical investigation. Microadenomas of the pituitary gland have been diagnosed only since the advent of hypocycloidal polytomography and prolactin radioimmunoassay. Whether these small lesions represent true adenomas or hyperplasia secondary to hypothalamic-pituitary dysfunction is unknown. Thus, the natural history of microadenomas and their clinical course is not known, and this greatly complicates decisions about the choice of therapy or even about whether therapy should be suggested at all. Proper treatment of microadenomas will ultimately be determined when five-year and ten-year follow-up studies of patients left untreated, treated with surgical therapy, and treated with medical therapy are reported.

After the surgical or radiation *treatment* of pituitary tumors, patients should be followed with assays of prolactin concentrations at six-month intervals. Pituitary and adrenal testing along with selective polytomography of CT scans should be performed on an annual basis if menses do not return and prolactin concentrations do not return to normal. In patients who resume normal menses and who cease lactation, routine follow-up can safely be provided. Since the initial growth of pituitary tumors occurs over a prolonged period, one might expect that recurrence of the disease would not appear for a number of years. Therefore, such patients should always be followed expectantly, and any reappearance of endocrine dysfunction should raise the index of suspicion of a recurrence or of persistence of the original tumor.

Patients treated with radiation therapy should be followed on an annual basis so long as regular menses occur and lactation ceases. The insidious development of panhypopituitarism in patients treated with radiation therapy requires long-term follow-up and investigation of any symptoms that might reflect the development of pituitary failure.

The proper treatment of recurrence or persistence of disease is unknown, but long-term treatment with bromocriptine should be the initial approach. Radiation therapy of the pituitary gland has also been used successfully in some patients.

Since ovulatory cycles resume during bromocriptine therapy in patients with functional hyperprolactinemia as well as with demonstrable pituitary tumors, there is a growing experience with pregnancy in the presence of pituitary tumors. Because of the high estrogen levels occurring during pregnancy and the known stimulatory effect of estrogen on the pituitary gland, there has been much concern as to the effect of pregnancy on pituitary tumors. There have been many case reports describing both good and poor outcomes in patients with suspected or known but untreated pituitary tumors who have become pregnant. Two large series of patients have been reported providing some overall understanding of the issue. It would appear from these studies that the vast majority of patients who become pregnant with active

pituitary tumors require no therapy whatsoever during pregnancy and suffer no permanent sequelae when they are followed conservatively and receive treatment only when symptoms demand. Patients with untreated microadenomas have approximately a 5% risk of developing significant complications during pregnancy. Pregnancy wastage in such patients is within the normal expected range for a control population, and the patients are no more prone to obstetric risks than their normal counterparts. In addition, in a series of nearly 1,500 infants exposed to bromocriptine there was no detectable difference in fetal anomalies or other abnormalities.

Other Endocrine Dysfunction

Abnormalities of thyroid or adrenal gland function may cause secondary as well as primary amenorrhea. The basic evaluation and treatment of these disorders is discussed elsewhere and will not be elaborated further here. A careful history and physical examination will usually point toward dysfunction of one of these glands.

One final consideration is what has been referred to as "*post-pill amenorrhea*". Much controversy has existed concerning secondary amenorrhea following cessation of oral contraceptive ingestion. The preponderance of data would indicate that the ingestion of oral contraceptives does not cause secondary amenorrhea. Secondary amenorrhea is often observed following oral contraceptive ingestion, because pathologic process that either preceded the initiation of oral contraceptive therapy or began during contraceptive therapy continues to progress while the pill is being taken. Regular cyclic menses resulting from the action of estrogen and progesterone on the endometrium continue unaltered regardless of the pathology existing and progressing in other parts of the reproductive system. Thus, a patient with a large pituitary tumor will have regular cyclic menses while taking oral contraceptives. It is because of this masking effect of oral contraceptives that the cessation of menses following the pill was thought to be secondary to its ingestion. Thus, any patient with amenorrhea lasting longer than six months following cessation of oral contraceptives or in whom signs and symptoms of other pathology are evident sooner than six months should be evaluated in the same way as all other patients with secondary amenorrhea.

CONCLUSION

Amenorrhea, whether primary or secondary, and other abnormalities of uterine bleeding are symptoms of some underlying pathology, either endocrinologic or organic. A specific approach to the diagnosis of the underlying condition includes a detailed and careful history and physical examination. A determination of pituitary gonadotropin levels allows the investigation to focus on specific organ systems: elevated levels indicate ovarian failure whereas normal or low levels indicate hypothalamic-pituitary dysfunction. The presence of functional endometrial tissue is easily determined by a estrogen-progestin challenge test after pregnancy has been specifically ruled out of consideration. Thus, the particular area of dysfunction is identified and the differential diagnosis within that organ system is considered. This approach not only leads to the establishment of a prompt and correct diagnosis, but follows a logical sequence predicated on an understanding of the normal physiology of the reproductive system.

REFERENCES AND RECOMMENDED READING

Aksel S, Jones, GS: Etiology and treatment of dysfunctional uterine bleeding. Obstet Gynecol 44:1, 1974

Archer DF, Lanttanzi DR, Moore EE et al: Bromocriptine treatment of women with suspected pituitary prolactin-secreting microadenomas. Am J Obstet Gynecol 143:620, 1982

Arronet GH, Arrata WSM: Dysfunctional uterine bleeding. Obstet Gynecol 29:97, 1967

Carr DB, Bullen BA, Skrinar GS et al: Physical conditioning facilitates the exercise-induced secretion of beta-endorphin and beta-lipotropin in women. N Engl J Med 305:560, 1981

Claessens EA, Cowell CA: Acute adolescent menorrhagia. Am J Obstet Gynecol 139:277, 1981

Cooper DS, Jacobs LS: Apomorphine inhibits the prolactin but not the TSH response to thyrotropin releasing hormone. J Clin Endocrinol Metab 44:404, 1977

Coulam CB, Annegers JF, Abboud CF et al: Pituitary adenomas and oral contraceptives: A case-control study. Fertil Steril 31:25, 1979

Davies AJ, Anderson ABM, Turnbull AC: Reduction by naproxen of excessive menstrual bleeding in women using intrauterine devices. Obstet Gynecol 57:74, 1981

Ehara Y, Siler TM, Yen SSC: Effects of large doses of estrogen on prolactin and growth hormone release. Am J Obstet Gynecol 125:455, 1976

Frank RT: Formation of artificial vagina without operation. Am J Obstet Gynecol 35:1053, 1938

Fries H: Secondary amenorrhea, self-induced weight reduction and anorexia nervosa. Acta Psychiatr Scand (Suppl) 248:5, 1974

Frisch RE, McArthur JW: Menstrual cycles: Fatness as a determinant of minimum weight for height necessary for their maintenance or onset. Science 185:949, 1974

Gemzell C, Wang CF: Outcome of pregnancy in women with pituitary adenoma. Fertil Steril 31:363, 1979

Goldfarb JM, Little AB: Current concepts. N Engl J Med 302:666, 1980

Griffin JE, Wilson JD: The syndromes of androgen resistance. N Engl J Med 302:198, 1980

Hodgson SF, Randall RV, Holman CB et al: Empty sella syndrome. Med Clin North Am 56:897, 1972

Hsu LKG, Crisp AH, Harding B: Outcome of anorexia nervosa. Lancet 1:61, 1979

Jacobi J, Lloyd HM, Meares JD: Onset of oestrogen-induced prolactin secretion and DNA synthesis by the rat pituitary gland. J Endocrinol 72:35, 1977

Jacobs HS, Knuth UA, Hull MGR et al: Postpill amenorrhea—cause or coincidence? Br Med J 2:940, 1977

Jones GS: Luteal phase defects. In Behrman SJ, Kistner RW

(eds): Progress in Infertility, p 299. Boston, Little, Brown & Co, 1968

Kilbanski A, Neer RM, Beitins IZ et al: Decreased bone density in hyperprolactinemic women. N Engl J Med 303:1511, 1980

Lloyd HM, Meares JD, Jacobi J: Effects of estrogen and bromocryptine on *in vivo* secretion and mitosis in prolactin cells. Nature 255:497, 1975

Maciulla GJ, Heine MW, Christian CD: Functional endometrial tissue with vaginal agenesis. J Reprod Med 21:373, 1978

Macleod RM, Lehmeyer JE: Studies on the mechanism of the dopamine-mediated inhibition of prolactin secretion. Endocrinology 94:1077, 1974

Magyar DM, Marshall JR: Pituitary tumors and pregnancy. Am J Obstet Gynecol 132:739, 1978

Manuel M, Katayama KP, Jones Jr HW: The age of occurrence of gonadal tumors in intersex patients with a Y chromosome. Am J Obstet Gynecol 124:293, 1976

March CM, Israel R, March AD: Hysteroscopic management of intrauterine adhesions. Am J Obstet Gynecol 130:653, 1978

Noyes RW, Hertig AT, Rock J: Dating the endometrial biopsy. Fertil Steril 1:3, 1950

Post DK, Biller BJ, Adelman LS et al: Selective transsphenoidal adenomectomy in women with galactorrhea–amenorrhea. JAMA 242:158, 1979

Rebar RW, Erickson GF, Yen SSC: Idiopathic premature ovarian failure: Clinical and endocrine characteristics. Fertil Steril 37:35, 1982

Schenker JG, Margolioth EJ: Intrauterine adhesions: An updated appraisal. Fertil Steril 37:593, 1982

Sheehan HL: The incidence of postpartum hypopituitarism. Am J Obstet Gynecol 68:202, 1954

Sherman BM, Harris CE, Schlechte J et al: Pathogenesis of prolactin-secreting pituitary adenomas. Lancet 2:1019, 1978

Smith NJ: Excessive weight loss and food aversion in athletes simulating anorexia nervosa. Pediatrics 66:139, 1980

Spark RF, Baker R, Beinfang DC et al: Bromocriptine reduces pituitary tumor size and hypersecretion: Requiem for pituitary surgery? JAMA 247:311, 1982

Stein IF, Leventhal ML: Amenorrhea associated with bilateral polycystic ovaries. Am J Obstet Gynecol 29:181, 1935

Stone TW: Further evidence for a dopamine receptor stimulating action of an ergot alkaloid. Brain Res 72:177, 1974

Swanson JA, Chapler FK: Renal anomalies in the XY female. Obstet Gynecol 51:237, 1978

Syvertsen A, Haughton VM, Williams AL et al: The computer tomographic appearance of the normal pituitary gland and pituitary microadenomas. Radiology 133:385, 1979

Tagatz G, Fialkow PJ, Smith D: Hypogonadotropic hypogonadism associated with anosmia in the female. N Engl J Med 283:1326, 1970

Thomas AE, McKay DA, Cutlip MB: A nomograph method for assessing body weight. Am J Clin Nutr 29:302, 1976

Thorner MO, Besser GM: Bromocriptine treatment of hyperprolactinaemic hypogonadism. Acta Endocrinol (Suppl Kbh) 216:131, 1978

Toaff R, Ballas S: Traumatic hypomenorrhea-amenorrhea (Asherman's syndrome). Fertil Steril 30:379, 1978

Tolis G, Ruggere D, Popkin DR et al: Prolonged amenorrhea and oral contraceptives. Fertil Steril 32:265, 1979

Tucker HS, Grubb SR, Wigand JP et al: Galactorrhea-amenorrhea syndrome: Follow-up of 45 patients after pituitary tumor removal. Ann Intern Med 94:302, 1981

Tulandi T, Kinch RA: Premature ovarian failure. Obstet Gynecol Surv 36:521, 1981

Turkalj I, Braun P, Krupp P: Surveillance of bromocriptine in pregnancy. JAMA 247:1589, 1982

Tyson JE, Friesen HG: Factors influencing the secretion of human prolactin and growth hormone in menstrual and gestational women. Am J Obstet Gynecol 116:377, 1973

van Bogaert, L-J: Diagnostic aid of endometrium biopsy. Gynecol Obstet Invest 10:289, 1979

Varga L, Lutterbeck PM, Pryor JS et al: Suppression of puerperal lactation with an ergot alkaloid—a double blind study. Br Med J 2:743, 1972

Vaughn TC, Haney AF, Wiebe RH et al: Spontaneous regression of prolactin-producing pituitary adenomas. Am J Obstet Gynecol 136:980, 1980

Vigersky RA, Andersen AE, Thompson RH: Hypothalamic dysfunction in secondary amenorrhea, associated with simple weight loss. N Engl J Med 297:1141, 1977

Wallach EE (ed): Dysfunctional uterine bleeding. Clin Obstet Gynecol 13:363, 1970

Walsh PC, Madden JD, Harrod MJ et al: Familial incomplete male pseudohermaphroditism, type 2. N Engl J Med 291:944, 1974

Warren MP: The effects of exercise on pubertal progression and reproductive function in girls. J Clin Endocrinol Metab 51:1150, 1980

Wentz AC: Abnormal uterine bleeding. Primary Care 3:9, 1976

Wilkins L: Diagnosis and Treatment of Endocrine Disorders in Childhood and Adolescence, 2nd ed. Springfield, IL, Charles C Thomas, 1967

Wilson JD, Harrod MJ, Goldstein JL et al: Familial incomplete male pseudohermaphroditism, type 1. N Engl J Med 290:1097, 1974

Androgen Excess

Marc A. Bernhisel
Charles B. Hammond

47

Androgen excess is a pathologic state in women manifested primarily by masculine somatic changes. Hirsutism, the most common finding associated with androgen excess, is an excessive growth of hair of characteristically dark color and coarse texture found in the androgen-dependent areas of the skin. Hirsutism is frequently accompanied by the development of acne vulgaris, a consequence of androgen stimulation to the pileosebaceous unit. The parameters of excess hair growth are often measured by a culturally or ethnically determined norm. Androgen excess resulting in increased hair growth may also result in ovarian dysfunction, manifested by menstrual abnormalities and infertility.

Virilization, the most severe form of androgen excess, is characterized by the regression of female secondary sexual characteristics and the acquisition of male characteristics. Signs and symptoms of virilism include severe hirsutism, male-pattern hairline recession, acne, increased muscle mass, clitoromegaly, and deepening of the voice. Virilism is associated with a pathologic state of severe androgen excess and is often associated with neoplasia.

This chapter attempts to review the synthesis and metabolism of the androgenic steroids, their role in normal and abnormal physiology, and the clinical diagnosis and treatment of androgen excess states.

ANDROGENS

Androgens are a unique group of steroid molecules that function to stimulate primary and secondary male sexual characteristics as well as some female secondary sexual characteristics. Androgenic function is integral in the development of the male reproductive tract *in utero*. This development occurs in response to androgen secretion from the embryonic testes beginning at six weeks' gestation. The wolffian (mesonephric) duct,

stimulated by androgens, develops to form the epididymis, vas deferens, and seminal vesicles. Continued androgen elaboration from the fetal testicular Leydig cells results in differentiation of the bipotential genital tubercle and urogenital sinus into the penis, scrotum, and penile urethra.

At puberty, androgens function in both sexes to initiate pubarche (sexual hair development). In the male, the androgens testosterone and dihydrotestosterone (DHT), which are primarily secreted from the testes, complete maturation of the male reproductive tract, both morphologically and physiologically. These and adrenal androgens stimulate pubertal hair growth in the male. In the female, who lacks testes, androgens are primarily produced in the zona reticularis of the adrenal as a by-product of the enzymatic conversion of cholesterol to cortisol or of the conversion of adrenal steroidal precursors that occurs in peripheral tissues. The androgens so produced stimulate pubertal hair growth in the mons pubis and axilla. Androgens also function in the ovary as obligate precursors to the synthesis of estrogens.

STEROIDOGENESIS

Steroidogenesis occurs in specialized tissues, largely in response to specific regulatory hormones. For example, adrenocorticotropic hormone (ACTH), the pituitary regulatory hormone of adrenal cortisol production, has a high binding affinity to an adrenal plasma membrane receptor and reacts there with adenyl cyclase to activate cyclic adenosine monophosphate (AMP) formation. This ultimately results in the production of free cholesterol. In the ovary, a specific membrane receptor binds the cholesterol–lipoprotein complex (low density lipoprotein; LDL) and converts it into free cholesterol (or its esterified storage form). Cholesterol is the basic structural molecule of all steroid classes (glucocorticoids, mineralocorticoids, and sex steroids). Cholesterol is converted into steroids in both the adrenal and the ovary in an enzyme-dependent, hormone-regulated manner. These enzymatic modifications of the cholesterol molecule occur in the cytosol, mitochondria, and microsomes of the specialized tissue cells.

Androgens are C-19 modifications of cholesterol. Sites C-17, C-3, and C-5 on the androgen molecule determine androgenic potency and effect (Fig. 47-1). At the C-17 position, the conversion of this 17-ketogroup of androstenedione (Δ^4A) to the 17β-hydroxyl complex of testosterone increases the androgen potency sevenfold. Dehydroepiandrosterone (DHA) is changed to the more potent Δ^4A by the formation of a ketogroup at C-3. The introduction of a hydrogen atom in the α-plane at C-5 increases the cytosol binding (and therefore potency) of DHT over its precursor, testosterone.

Androgens are distributed in serum by a number of binding proteins, which are important in androgen metabolism as well as in the regulation of androgen effect. They include albumin, cortisol-binding globulin, acid α_2-glycoprotein, and testosterone estrogen–binding globulin (TeBG). TeBG binds the largest portion of plasma testosterone and largely determines the amount of free or active testosterone that is available to diffuse into the target cell from the intervascular space, eventually affecting androgen-sensitive tissues. TeBG is produced in the liver. Its synthesis is diminished by circulating androgens and by menopause, obesity, and hypothyroidism. The synthesis of TeBG is increased by circulating estrogen and by hyperthyroidism.

The manifestation of androgen effect has been shown to be dependent on both the steroid production rate and tissue responsiveness. Male and female fetuses at 12 to 22 weeks' gestation have an equal potential to develop masculine sexual characteristics on the basis of tissue responsiveness and an equal ability to convert testosterone to DHT (via 5α-reductase), the trophic hormone of the genital tubercle. The male is thus differentiated from the female by testicular production of testosterone. In the absence of testosterone, female genitalia develop despite the chromosomal complement. The female retains the ability to respond to androgen stimulation after birth. The skin, muscles, larynx, and urogenital system may be masculinized by supraphysiologic androgen levels, but complete phallic masculinization does not occur.

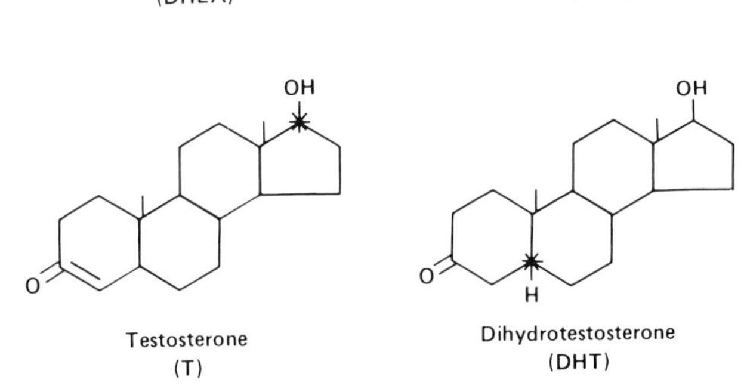

HAIR PATTERNS

The hair follicles and sebaceous glands (pilosebaceous unit) are skin appendages and are androgen sensitive. Hair follicles may produce vellus and terminal hair in humans. Vellus hair is light, finely textured, and short. Terminal hair is dark and coarse and may grow long. High levels of androgens, found normally in men, stimulate the terminal conversion of vellus hair in the sexual hair regions, including the face, sternum, back, and upper abdomen. Ambisexual hair is found at puberty in both males and females. It includes the hair in the axilla, lower pubic triangle, forearms, and legs. This hair is responsive to the lower androgen levels that are seen in normal females. Nonsexual hair includes eyebrow and scalp hair and is largely independent of a stimulatory androgen effect. Except in these androgen-independent areas, follicles must be exposed to androgens for a long period of time before terminal hair is produced. Conversely, terminal hair growth persists after androgens are removed, albeit at a slower rate.

Hair growth is a cyclic rather than a continuous process occurring through three phases of hair follicle activity. The growth phase of the hair follicle is termed *anagen,* the resting phase *telogen,* and the intermediate phase (between resting and growth) *catagen.* All follicles continuously cycle through all three phases of activity, and thus there is continuous growth and shedding of hair. The length of time a hair follicle spends in each phase depends on its anatomic location. The relatively short hair of the extremities, eyebrows, and eyelashes is the result of a short anagen phase and a longer telogen phase. Conversely, the long hair of the scalp has an extended anagen phase of 1 to 6 years and a short telogen phase.

During the anagen phase there is proliferation of the basal epithelium of the hair shaft downward toward the bulb of the hair follicle in the dermis. Matrix cells grow rapidly toward the skin surface, and superficial matrix cells differentiate to form a keratinizing column. The bulb of the hair follicle forms around the dermal papilla until the bulb sheds, marking involution (catagen). The follicle remains at this stage if it is not stimulated to grow further (telogen). During the resting

FIG. 47-1. Major serum androgens. *Asterisk* indicates sites affecting androgen potency.

Dehydroepiandrosterone
(DHEA)

Androstenedione
(Δ^4A)

Testosterone
(T)

Dihydrotestosterone
(DHT)

phase the hair is loosely attached to the follicle and easily shed.

SOURCES OF ANDROGENS AND THEIR METABOLISM

The principal androgens are DHT, Δ^4A, DHA, and dehydroepiandrosterone sulfate (DHAS).

DHT is the most potent androgen, having approximately twice the potency of testosterone in bioassays. It is largely derived from the peripheral conversion of Δ^4A in serum. It may be directly secreted in the plasma by the ovary and the adrenal. There is no significant menstrual change in plasma DHT levels.

Testosterone is the second most potent androgen. Approximately 1% of testosterone in normal women and 3% in normal men circulates freely. In cycling women, approximately half of daily testosterone production is carried out by the ovaries and the adrenals. The ovarian contribution is between 5% and 20%, depending somewhat on the stage of the menstrual cycle; the adrenal produces between 1% and 38% of total testosterone. The other 50% of testosterone is produced by the peripheral conversion of Δ^4A, which primarily occurs in the liver, skin, fat, and skeletal muscles. Serum testosterone levels show only slight diurnal variation, paralleling cortisol secretion.

Δ^4A is the obligate intermediate of esterone (E_1) but has the potential to be converted to testosterone. It is responsible for approximately 20% of the androgenic activity of testosterone. The Δ^4A production rates of the ovary and the adrenal are approximately equal; about 10 percent is derived from the peripheral conversion of DHA. Δ^4A has a diurnal secretion that can vary as much as 50% in parallel with cortical secretion from ACTH stimulation. It also changes to a smaller degree from increased ovarian secretion at midcycle.

DHA and DHAS are weak androgens, having only 3% of the potency of testosterone. They are thought to be derived from peripheral conversion into more potent androgen forms. Both DHA and DHAS are secreted directly from the adrenal (85% and 95%, respectively) with only small contributions from the ovary. Serum DHA levels vary with cortisol circadian rhythmicity much more than do DHAS levels. Both steroids are the major precursors of urinary 17-ketosteroids (17-KS).

ANDROGEN EXCESS SYNDROMES

The development of hirsutism and acne from androgen stimulation to the pilosebaceous unit is one of the earliest signs of hyperandrogenism. Approximately 90% of hirsute women produce greater than normal amounts of one or more of the androgens. Various causes of hyperandrogenism are listed below:

Ovarian Causes
Functional
    Polycystic ovarian syndrome
    Hyperthecosis
    Hyperandrogenism–insulin resistance–acanthosis
Neoplastic
    Sertoli–Leydig cell tumor
    Hilus cell tumor
    Luteoma
    Other

Adrenal Causes
Functional
    Congenital adrenal hyperplasia
    Acquired adrenal hyperplasia
Neoplastic
    Adrenal adenoma
    Adrenal carcinoma
    Cushing's syndrome

Mixed Adrenal–Ovarian Causes

Miscellaneous Causes
Acromegaly
Congenital porphyria
Hurler's syndrome
Trisomy E syndrome

Ovarian Causes

Functional

Polycystic ovarian syndrome (POS) is the most common cause of ovarian androgen excess and probably the most common cause of hirsutism. Nearly a 70% incidence of hirsutism has been found in women with POS. It is also likely that POS is the endpoint in a spectrum of physiologic abnormalities.

Clinical manifestations of hirsutism, anovulation, and infertility are found in more than 50% of women with polycystic ovaries. Other symptoms found with varying frequency are obesity, virilism, and dysfunctional bleeding. Histologically, the classic ovarian finding in POS is multiple small follicular cysts with poor granulosa cell development. The follicles are surrounded by a thickened, luteinized theca.

The biochemical parameters of POS remain ill defined. Patients with the syndrome are often found to have modestly elevated levels of testosterone, DHAS, and prolactin. They often demonstrate a reversal of the normal estradiol:estrone (E_2:E_1) ratio, and frequently their ratio of luteinizing hormone (LH) to follicle-stimulating hormone (FSH) is equal to or greater than 3:1. Several theories have been advanced to explain the biochemical abnormalities found in POS in light of the unique anatomic and physiologic findings. LH is generally elevated in POS patients which may reflect greater pulse frequency or pulse amplitude in response to gonadotropin-releasing hormone (GnRH) from the hypothalamus. Chronically elevated estrogen levels can sensitize the pituitary to GnRH stimulation. This stimulation is reflected by increased LH secretion and by preferential inhibition of FSH secretion. FSH may also be affected directly by the ovary through a protein inhibin–like secretion from multiple follicular cysts. The consequence of this abnormal LH:FSH ratio is an LH-induced excess of $\Delta^4 A$ and testosterone from ovarian theca and stroma cells. Without requisite FSH levels, normal granulosa cell aromatization of $\Delta^4 A$ to E_2 is reduced in POS. However, ovarian analogs are peripherally converted to E_1, which is chronically elevated in noncyclic, anovulatory POS patients. The cycle is completed, according to this theory, by the continued stimulation of pituitary LH from E_1 through the hypothalamus. Alternatively, deficiencies of enzymes required for E_2 synthesis—3β-hydroxysteroid dehydrogenase and aromatase—have been found in *in vitro* studies of POS ovaries. Erickson and colleagues have reported a lack of estrogen production in granulosa cells cultured from characteristically small polycysts found in the POS ovaries. Relatively diminished FSH levels, coupled with elevated androgen secretion from degenerating follicles, may indicate that the primary cause of POS is ovarian.

A recently described variation in the POS spectrum includes hyperandrogenism, insulin resistance, and acanthosis nigricans. The insulin resistance in this syndrome is positively correlated with the quantity of androgen excess. Insulin resistance occurs in a state of normal pancreatic β–islet cell reserve in response to high circulating levels of insulin. High levels of androgen may increase the peripheral insulin resistance. Insulin in turn may increase gonadal androgen production by direct or indirect follicular stimulation. Acanthotic changes are usually found in the skin areas over the neck, in the axillae, and beneath the breasts. Acanthosis nigricans is also associated with other insulin-resistant endocrinopathies as well as with additional benign and malignant processes. High circulating levels of insulin or peptides (*e.g.,* melanocyte-stimulating hormone, ACTH) may initiate acanthotic changes.

Hyperthecosis is a syndrome that has many of the clinical features of POS but characteristically is associated with more severe hirsutism and often with virilism. Histologically, hyperthecosis and POS overlap to a large degree. However, hyperthecotic ovaries are found to have numerous islands of luteinized cells scattered throughout the stroma, often in proximity to the hilum. Induction of ovulation in patients with hyperthecosis is extremely difficult because of elevated androgen levels; testosterone levels are frequently in the tumor range. Therapy for patients with hyperthecosis has often consisted only of wedge resection of the ovaries or bilateral oophorectomy.

Neoplastic

Ovarian neoplasms causing hyperandrogenism are rare. In women of reproductive age, they are frequently manifested by amenorrhea and rapidly progressive hirsutism or virilism.

The most common masculinizing ovarian tumors are the gonadal stromal group; the Sertoli–Leydig (arrhenoblastoma) cell tumor is the most frequently found neoplasm. This tumor typically presents in women between the ages of 20 and 30 years. However, it has also been reported in a 2½-year-old girl and in a 70-year-old woman. Women with this tumor generally report a cessation of menstrual periods and rapid hair growth. The tumor characteristically is unilateral, frequently is palpable by pelvic exam, and produces high amounts of testosterone. Peripheral testosterone serum concentrations often exceed 200 ng/dl (normal male levels). The hilus cell (Leydig) tumor is another potentially masculinizing neoplasm derived from the gonadal stroma. This tumor is frequently nonpalpable and may be manifested in postmenopausal women by the development of hirsutism.

Other tumors that may stimulate stromal activity and lead to excessive production of androgens include dysgerminomas, teratomas, Brenner tumors, serous cystadenomas, and Krukenberg tumors. All of these tumors may be associated with an increase in $\Delta^4 A$ production. Ovarian luteoma of pregnancy is a rare and potentially masculinizing tumor that may affect both mother and fetus. It is a solid, frequently bilateral neoplasm that has some of the same histologic cellular features as the theca lutein cyst of pregnancy. Virilism or hirsutism in pregnancy may occur with any of the tumors described above.

Adrenal Causes

The adrenal gland, alone or in combination with the ovary, has been implicated in several studies as the major source of hyperandrogenism in hirsute women. The high occurrence rate of hyperandrogenism suggests a different pathophysiology from that of congenital adrenal hyperplasia (CAH) or adrenal neoplasm in producing the state of androgen excess. Anatomic enlargement of the zona reticularis has been suggested from biopsies obtained from normal-sized adrenals of hyperandrogenic patients.

Congenital Adrenal Hyperplasia

The most common congenital enzyme deficiency of the adrenal causing androgen excess is 21-hydroxylase. This deficiency is usually manifested at birth by varying degrees of genital ambiguity but may be characterized by severe salt loss resulting in hypotension and shock. The defect results from the inability of the adrenal to catabolize glucocorticoids or mineralocorticoids. As a result, ACTH levels are high, causing overproduction of adrenal prehormones. 17α-Hydroxyprogesterone (17-OHP) is the prehormone of cortisol and of the androgens. Diagnosis of 21-hydroxylase deficiency is based on levels of 17-OHP greater than 5 ng/ml. This deficiency is commonly associated with an increase in both DHA and DHAS levels.

11β-Hydroxylase deficiency is the next most common congenital cause of androgen excess. As in 21-hydroxylase deficiency, the failure is a conversion blockage that diminishes the production of cortisol and results in increased ACTH stimulation of the glucocorticoid and mineralocorticoid prehormones as well as of androgens. 11-Deoxycorticosterone (DOC), a potent mineralocorticoid, is produced in excess and is frequently associated with salt retention and hypotension in the neonate. The finding of an elevated serum 11-deoxycortisol level is diagnostic of 11β-hydroxylase deficiency.

Reduction in levels of the 3β-hydroxysteroid dehydrogenase 4-5 isomerase enzyme results in diminished production of glucocorticoids, mineralocorticoids, and sex steroids. This rare defect leads to the clinical manifestations of salt wasting and inadequate masculinization in the male newborn. The female who survives childhood will not develop secondary sex characteristics owing to deficiency in E_2 production but may develop hirsutism because of the overproduction of DHA.

Acquired Adrenal Hyperplasia

Adrenal androgens may be produced in excess owing to functional derangement of the adrenal gland following pubertal maturation. Late-onset CAH appears from HLA linkage studies to be an allelic variant of perinatal CAH. Late-onset CAH is diagnosed by elevated 17-OHP response to ACTH stimulation. 11β-Hydroxylase or 3β-hydroxysteroid dehydrogenase deficiencies appearing after childhood have not been associated by HLA studies with classic CAH. However, both enzyme-deficient states have been documented in patients with androgen excess after childhood. The true incidence of late-onset CAH has not been established. The incidence in hirsute women has been estimated at anywhere from 0% to 30%. A particular problem in establishing frequency has been a lack of uniform diagnostic criteria for the mild enzyme deficiencies and lack of an established cause and effect of the deficiency with androgen excess. Heterozygote carriers of 21-hydroxylase enzyme deficiency demonstrate diminished hydroxylase activity but do not appear to be at a higher than normal risk for hirsutism.

Neoplastic Disorders

Cushing's syndrome is most frequently caused (70%) by an ACTH-secreting pituitary tumor. This tumor is associated with bilateral adrenal hyperplasia, cortisol elevation, and commonly, hirsutism or virilization. Less frequently (20%), Cushing's syndrome is caused by a cortisol-secreting adenoma or carcinoma of the adrenal gland. The remaining causes are secondary to ectopically secreted sources of ACTH. The clinical signs and symptoms of Cushing's syndrome include muscle weakness, ecchymosis, abdominal striae, central obesity, osteoporosis, and hypokalemic alkalosis.

Severe hirsutism and virilism due to adrenal causes are usually seen in patients with androgen-secreting adrenal adenomas or carcinomas. They are often found in prepubertal or postmenopausal females. These tumors generally produce the Δ 5 androgens DHA and DHAS, with levels often exceeding 20 ng/ml and 900 ng/ml, respectively. Normal levels are generally less than 5 ng/ml and 2500 ng/ml, respectively. These tumors are not usually suppressed by dexamethasone administration. Rarely, a testosterone producing tumor with the characteristics of an ovarian rest (including responsiveness to human chorionic gonadotropin) is found in the adrenal gland and manifests itself clinically by rapid virilism.

Mixed Adrenal–Ovarian Causes

Excess androgen production by both the adrenal gland and the ovary has been found in several studies of adrenal and ovarian vein catheterization or dexamethasone suppression. Kirschner and co-workers found that in 30% of hirsute patients, androgen excess had both adrenal and ovarian sources. Abraham and colleagues reported a 39% incidence. Adrenal androgens putatively affect the ovary either indirectly, by increasing E_1 conversion and thus increasing LH stimulation of ovarian androgens, or directly, by inhibiting 3β-hydroxysteroid dehydrogenase and aromatase enzymes, thereby causing inadequate follicular maturation and increased androgen production.

CLINICAL EVALUATION OF ANDROGEN EXCESS

Endocrinologic evaluation is mandatory in females presenting with prepubertal hirsutism, hirsutism of rapid onset, or onset of virilization at any age. The development of hirsutism in association with menstrual abnormalities (e.g., in POS) may warrant evaluation to rule out more serious processes.

A thorough history should be obtained from the hirsute patient, and note should be made of the time of onset and speed of hair growth. A history of rapid hair growth, often with virilism, suggests a neoplasm of adrenal or ovarian origin. Patients with features of POS, including chronic anovulation and hirsutism, have usually noted a gradual onset of excess hair growth beginning two to three years after the onset of menarche. Eumenorrheic women with androgen excess frequently have an adrenal source of hyperandrogenemia.

A patient presenting with primary amenorrhea and

hirsutism should be evaluated with a leukocytic karyotype to exclude a Y-bearing dysgenetic gonad. The prepubertal female presenting with hirsutism should be evaluated for CAH and adrenal or ovarian neoplasia. Finally, iatrogenic causes of excess hair growth should be investigated. The androgen danazol, frequently used in the treatment of endometriosis and benign cystic breast disease, may cause hirsutism and acne. Similarly, some of the nor-testosterone progestogens used in oral contraceptives have also been reported to cause hirsutism and acne.

The drugs diphenylhydantoin, penicillamine, and diazoxide may produce hypertrichosis, defined as excess growth of nonsexual hair. This condition is also seen in patients with anorexia nervosa, dermatomyositis, and hypothyroidism.

The physical examination is used to quantify the signs of androgen excess. Hair morphology and distribution should be graded. Various scoring methods have been suggested for quantifying hirsutism. Perhaps the most functional is that proposed by Abraham. According to his categorization, *mild hirsutism* is defined as the presence of fine pigmented hair over the extremities and the face (sideburns and chin, but not with a com-

plete beard), chest, abdomen, and perineum; *moderate hirsutism* is defined as the presence of coarse, pigmented terminal hair over the extremities, face (but not with a complete beard), chest, abdomen, and perineum; and *severe hirsutism* is defined as coarse, pigmented hair over the whole beard area, the proximal interphalangeal joints, in the ears, and over the nose. Other indications of androgen excess, such as acne and signs of hypercorticolism (Cushing's syndrome), should be carefully evaluated. Abdominal and pelvic examinations are used to investigate adrenal and ovarian neoplasms. A unilateral androgen-producing ovarian tumor is palpated approximately 60% of the time.

Laboratory evaluation of the hirsute woman is outlined in Figure 47-2. The evaluation is more specific and sensitive if serum rather than urinary assays are used in the initial evaluation. Serum testosterone, prolactin, and DHAS levels should be initially obtained. If the DHAS level is greater than 9000 ng/ml, the possibility of an adrenal tumor must be excluded by computed tomography (CT). If the serum testosterone concentration is more than 2 times normal, the possibility of an ovarian tumor must be excluded. Percutaneous venous catheterization may be used to identify the androgen-

FIG. 47-2. Suggested flowchart for the diagnosis of hirsutism. *DHEAS,* dehydroepiandrosterone sulfate; *T,* testosterone; *PRL,* prolactin; *NI,* normal; *PCOS,* polycystic ovarian syndrome; *17-OHP,* 17α-hydroxyprogesterone; *CAH,* congenital adrenal hyperplasia.

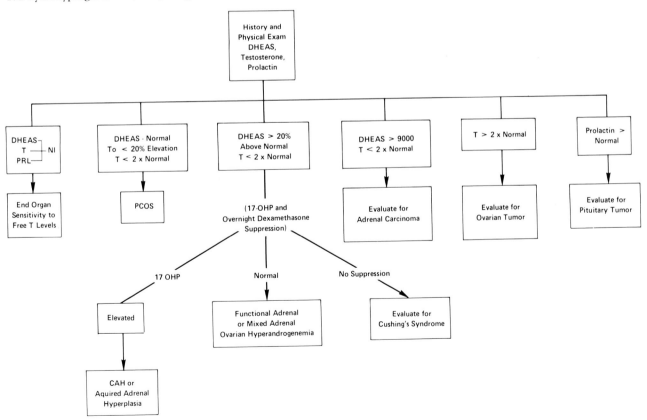

secreting ovary (or adrenal) responsible for androgen secretion, particularly if this cannot be identified by a physical examination or CT scan.

An elevation of DHAS greater than 20% above normal but to less than 9000 ng/ml and a normal to slightly elevated testosterone level may be found in patients with POS, late-onset CAH, or Cushing's syndrome. An elevated 17-OHP level establishes the diagnosis of CAH. The diagnosis of Cushing's syndrome is detailed in Figure 47-3. An overnight 1-mg dexamethasone suppression test is used to rule out cortisol elevation. If cortisol val-

ues exceed 5 μg/dl, a urinary free cortisol (UFC) or a low-dose dexamethasone suppression test (0.5 mg every 6 hours for 4 days) should be administered. The normal UFC level is less than 15 μg/24 hours. Falsely elevated levels may be observed in patients with intercurrent infection, psychiatric stress, or posttraumatic or postsurgical stress. The low-dose dexamethasone test uses the measurement of urinary 17-hydroxycorticosteroids (17-OHC). If the UFC is above 50 μg/24 hours or the urinary 17-OHC is more than 3 mg/24 hours, a high-dose dexamethasone suppression test (2 mg every 6

FIG. 47-3. Suggested flowchart for the diagnosis of Cushing's syndrome. *CT,* computed tomography; *ACTH,* adrenocorticotropic hormone. (After London SN, Hammond CB: Hirsutism. Post Grad Obstet Gynecol 3:1, 1983)

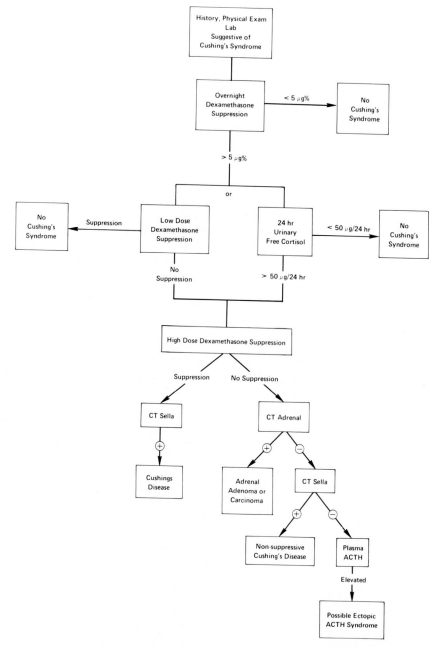

hours for 4 additional days) is performed. A reduction of urinary 17-OHC to less than 50% of baseline defines suppression.

Elevation of serum testosterone and DHAS below the neoplastic range, combined with historical features of prolonged anovulation and gradually increasing hirsutism, suggests POS.

Hyperprolactinemia has been associated with elevated levels of DHA and DHAS; 40% of chronically hyperprolactinemic women have some androgen abnormality. The precise mechanism of androgen elevation by prolactin is unknown; however, treatment by surgery (of pituitary lactotrophic hyperplasia) or administration of bromocriptine is associated with decreasing DHA and DHAS levels. Moderate prolactin elevation is frequently associated with POS and can affect pituitary gonadotropin function as well as adrenal androgen production.

It has been proposed that hirsutism of unknown cause is due to hypersensitivity of the hair follicle to normal levels of circulating androgens.

TREATMENT OF ANDROGEN EXCESS

Treatment of the hirsute woman is based on the cause and source of the androgen excess. Surgical extirpation of an ovarian, adrenal, or pituitary tumor is required when such a neoplasm is identified. A combination of glucocorticoid and mineralocorticoid is used to diminish the ACTH drive in CAH. This will lower the ― 5 androgens DHA and DHAS. Cyclic ovulation, which may have been previously suppressed during the state of androgen excess, usually follows such therapy.

The treatment of POS is primarily based on suppressing the LH drive of ovarian androgens. This is accomplished with a combination estrogen–progesterone oral contraceptive. The estrogen component also stimulates hepatic synthesis of TeBG, which in turn decreases free testosterone levels. Oral contraceptives may also lower adrenal androgen secretion, presumably by diminishing pituitary stimulation of the adrenal. If oral contraceptives cannot be used, oral medroxyprogesterone treatment may be attempted. Medroxyprogesterone, 10 mg to 20 mg, suppresses LH secretion and increases hepatic clearance of serum testosterone.

If hyperandrogenemia is suppressed by dexamethasone but not by oral contraceptives, the source of the androgen excess is most likely adrenal, and the condition can be treated with low-dose dexamethasone (0.5 mg at bedtime). Caution should be used with dexamethasone, however, since chronically administered doses, particularly over 0.5 mg per day, may result in cushingoid changes. Conversely, serum levels of cortisol should be measured every morning to ensure that they are equal to or greater than 3 μg/dl; anything lower than that can lead to impairment of the pituitary–adrenal axis.

Cyproterone acetate (CA), which was originally developed as a progestogen, has a powerful antiandrogen property. CA competes directly with testosterone to block androgen at the cellular level in the pilosebaceous unit. Additionally, CA is a potent ACTH inhibitor with significant potential to suppress adrenal androgens (and glucocorticoids). Because it can produce adrenal insufficiency and other side-effects, CA has not been approved for use in the United States.

The histamine H_2 receptor agonist cimetidine is reported to interfere with DHT binding to cytosol androgen receptors. In divided doses, 1500 mg cimetidine diminishes hair growth without affecting peripheral androgen levels.

Spironolactine, an antihypertensive agent that competes with aldosterone at the distal renal tubule, has an antiandrogen effect that has been used in the treatment of hirsutism. The mechanism of this antiandrogen action is unclear. It may result from reduction of androgen synthesis by enzymatic blockage of the 17-20 desmolase and 17-hydroxylase enzymes, or from competitive binding of androgen receptors of the pilosebaceous unit, or from both. The usual dosage of spironolactone is 100 mg to 200 mg per day. Side-effects are related to a mild, transient diuresis. Serum potassium levels should be monitored periodically, since spironolactone is a potassium-sparing mineralocorticoid antagonist.

Synthetic GnRH, agonists, and antagonists have been shown to have ovarian suppressive effects and may have future clinical utility in the suppression of ovarian androgen production.

As new hair growth is reduced, electrolysis can be used to destroy existing hair follicles. Depilatories, bleaching agents, and shaving may also be used as androgen reduction therapy proceeds. Plucking hairs, however, often results in scarring and should be avoided.

Induction of ovulation in the patient who has chronic anovulation but desires pregnancy may be accomplished with clomiphene citrate. Preliminary reports indicate that the efficacy of clomiphene may be increased when the agent is used in combination with low-dose dexamethasone. If prolactin levels are elevated, bromocriptine may be used with clomiphene citrate to induce ovulation.

REFERENCES AND RECOMMENDED READING

Abraham GE, Maroulis GB, Buster JE et al: Effect of dexamethasone on serum cortisol and androgen levels in hirsute patients. Obstet Gynecol 47:395, 1976

Axelrod LR, Goldzieher JW: The polycystic ovary. III. Steroid biosynthesis in normal and polycystic ovarian tissue. J Clin Endocrinol Metab 22:431, 1961

Barbieri RL, Ryan KJ: Hyperandrogenism, insulin resistance and acanthosis nigrans syndrome: A common endocrinopathy with distinct pathophysiologic features. Am J Obstet Gynecol 147:90, 1983

Carter JN, Tyson JE, Warne GL et al: Adrenocortical function in hyperprolactinemic women. J Clin Endocrinol Metab 45:973, 1977

Chetkowski RJ, DeFazio J, Shamonki I et al: Incidence of late-onset congenital adrenal hyperplasia due to 21-hydroxylase deficiency among hirsute women. J Clin Endocrinol Metab 58:595, 1984

Crapo L: Cushing's syndrome: A review of diagnostic tests. Metabolism 28:955, 1979

Erickson GF, Hsueh AJW, Quigley ME et al: Functional studies of aromatase activity in human granulosa cells from normal and polycystic ovaries. J Clin Endocrinol Metab 58:595, 1984

Garcia-Bunuel R, Berek JS, Woodruff JD: Luteomas of pregnancy. Obstet Gynecol 45:467, 1975

Givens JR: Androgen metabolism. In Sciarra JJ (ed): Gynecology and Obstetrics, pp 1–10. Philadelphia, JB Lippincott, 1983

Hammerstein J, Meckies J, Leo-Rossberg I et al: Use of cyproterone acetate (CPA) in the treatment of acne, hirsutism, and virilism. J Steroid Biochem 6:827, 1975

Hatch R, Rosenfield RL, Moon HK, Tredway D: Hirsutism: Implications, etiology and management. Am J Obstet Gynecol 140:815, 1981

Ireland K, Woodruff JD: Masculinizing ovarian tumors. Obstet Gynecol Surv 31:81, 1976

Kirschner MA, Zucker IR, Jespersen D: Idiopathic hirsutism—An ovarian abnormality. N Engl J Med 294:637, 1976

Lee PA, Gareis FJ: Evidence for partial 21-hydroxylase deficiency among heterozygote carriers of congenital adrenal hyperplasia. J Clin Endocrinol Metab 41:415, 1975

Lobo RA, Wellington LP, Goebelsmann U: Serum levels of DHEA-S gynecologic endocrinology and infertility. Obstet Gynecol 57:607, 1981

London SN, Hammond CB: Hirsutism. Post Grad Obstet Gynecol 3:1, 1983

Loriaux DL: Spironolactone and endocrine dysfunction. Ann Intern Med 85:630, 1976

Maroulis GB: Evaluation of hirsutism and hyperandrogenemia. Fertil Steril 36:273, 1981

Meikle AW, Stringham JD, Wilson DE, Dolman LI: Plasma 5-alpha-reduced androgens in men and hirsute women: Role of adrenals and gonads. J Endocrinol Metab 48:969, 1979

Vaughn TC, Hammond CB: Diagnosing and treating the hirsute woman. Ortho Forum 1:13, 1981

Vigersky RA, Mehlman I, Glass AR, Smith CE: Treatment of hirsute women with Cimetidine. A preliminary report. N Engl J Med 303:1042, 1980

Wu CH: Plasma free and protein-bound testosterone in hirsutism. Obstet Gynecol 60:188, 1982

The Climacteric

Steve N. London
Charles B. Hammond

48

The *menopause* is defined as the last episode of physiologic uterine bleeding. The menopause is just one event in the *climacteric,* which the First International Congress on Menopause has defined as that phase in the aging process of women which marks the transition from the reproductive stage of life to the nonreproductive stage. Although these definitions are exact, the terms *menopause* and *climacteric* are often used interchangeably. The *perimenopause* is defined arbitrarily to include the first few years of the climacteric and the first year after the menopause.

HISTORY

The menopause has been a popular subject for medical authors from early times. Aetius of Amida in the 6th century A.D. described the symptoms of the menopause and related their onset to the time of year as well as to the patient's habits, physical traits, diet, and general health. The subsequent 12 centuries saw many theories come and go. Popular remedies during this time included purgatives, enemas, leeches, and phlebotomies.

It was not until the 1920s that scientific investigation began to replace many of the unsupported theories and remedies for menopausal symptoms. During that decade estrogens were finally isolated and characterized as distinct hormonal compounds. Use of these compounds in 1935 allowed Mazer and Israel to report successful treatment of vasomotor symptoms.[1] Davies described improvement of atrophic vaginitis with estrogens.[2] Later, Albright and colleagues observed that estrogens had a beneficial effect on osteoporosis.[3] These findings led to an increase in the use of estrogens to treat menopausal symptoms during the latter part of the first half of the 20th century.

While the use of estrogens rapidly increased, some prominent gynecologists had serious reservations. In the American Journal of Obstetrics and Gynecology of 1940, Emil Novak stated, "There is perhaps no gynecologic disorder in which the indication for organotherapy is more rational than in the treatment of typical climacteric symptoms . . . The question of the possible hazard of inciting malignancy in cancer-susceptible individuals cannot be described too arbitrarily in the present state of our knowledge."

Despite these cautions, estrogen use in the climacteric continued to increase. In 1966, in the book *Feminine Forever,* Robert A. Wilson referred to the menopause as a "curable disease state."[4] Following this, estrogen sales increased approximately 400% between 1960 and 1975.

In December of 1975, two articles and an editorial were published linking exogenous replacement therapy to an increased risk of endometrial cancer.[5-7] Several other articles with similar conclusions soon appeared, and the use of estrogens dropped dramatically. Only in the past few years have studies concerning the potential gains versus the hazards of replacement therapy appeared. As a result of these studies, physicians have again developed a more positive attitude toward the postmenopausal patient and estrogen replacement therapy.

EPIDEMIOLOGY

Average age at the climacteric has apparently remained unchanged since the 6th century A.D., while age at the onset of puberty has steadily declined; the average age of women at menopause in the Netherlands is now 51.4 years, with a standard deviation of 3.8 years.[8]

Age at menopause appears to be unaffected by race, socioeconomic status, education, physical characteristics, alcohol consumption, age at menarche, or date of last pregnancy. Only cigarette smoking appears to affect it. In a study conducted in Göteborg, Sweden, 50-year-old women were asked whether they were cigarette smokers and whether they had undergone menopause.[9] The investigators found 50% of the women who had undergone menopause were smokers, compared with 26% in the premenopausal group. Several theories have been advanced to explain why menopause occurs earlier among smokers than among nonsmokers. One theory proposes that nicotine has a direct effect on the central nervous system or the gonad and that the content of cigarette smoke causes certain changes in hepatic enzymes that affect the metabolism of steroid hormones.

During the last century human longevity has increased dramatically. Women in the United States can now expect to live to the age of 80, which means tht the population of postmenopausal women is increasing. Current U.S. census figures indicate that at some point in the 1980s there will be over 50 million women over the age of 50 in this country. These 50 million women can expect to spend about one third of their lives with reduced ovarian function. A recent review estimates that 75% to 85% of these women will develop symptoms secondary to estrogen deficiency and that in 15% these symptoms will be so severe as to require physician intervention.[10]

CAUSE

At present there is no single all-inclusive theory to explain the menopause. However, although the exact mechanism is unknown, there is no doubt that the ovary is primal to the menopause. The follicular unit and its inevitable demise are ultimately responsible for the reduction of estrogen secretion and the cessation of menses.

As noted in Chapter 5, the ovary develops on the medioventral border of the urogenital ridge, adjacent to the kidney and the primitive adrenal. Until approximately 42 days' gestation, the gonads are indifferent, *e.g.,* on a morphologic basis the ovary and testis are indistinguishable. This indifferent gonad is formed from proliferation of the mesodermal coelomic epithelium, the mesenchymal cell mass on the urogenital ridge, and mesonephric elements. Additionally, the indifferent gonad contains large primordial germ cells that migrated from the yolk sac to the genital ridge during the fifth week of embryonic life.

By 42 days' gestation, 300 to 1300 primordial germ cells have seeded the indifferent gonad. These cells will become either oogonia or spermatozoa. In females they undergo mitosis to form oogonia. The oogonia replicate so that there are approximately 600,000 by the eighth week of gestation and 6 to 7 million by the 20th week of gestation.

Between the 8th and 13th weeks of gestation, under the influence of a meiosis-inducing substance secreted by the rete ovarii, meiosis is initiated. The initiation of meiosis converts the oogonia to *primary oocytes,* some

of which become surrounded by precursors of granulosa cells, thus creating *primordial follicles.* Conversion of oogonia to primary oocytes and the formation of primordial follicles is not completed until the sixth month after birth. Primary oocytes that do not form primordial follicles degenerate. It has been estimated that of the 6 million oogonia present in the fetal ovaries at 20 weeks, only 700,000 to 2 million will survive to form primordial follicles. Furthermore, there is no evidence that additional oocytes ever arise from germinal epithelium postnatally. Thus, the human female has a variable but finite number of follicles.

The 2 million primordial follicles that are present at birth are lost from the ovary either by ovulation or by *follicular atresia,* which is the physiologic degeneration of the oocyte and its surrounding stroma. Atresia begins as early as the fifth month of fetal life and continues throughout the menstrual years. Extensive studies have shown atresia occurs throughout the menstrual cycle, at all stages of follicular development, and even during pregnancy. What selects and causes a primordial follicle to undergo atresia or go on to ovulate is unknown. The total number of oocytes at puberty and the efficiency of the atretic process determine age at menopause. Variations in these two factors can account for the differences among individuals.

Although the exhaustion of hormonally responsive primordial follicles is responsible for the menopause, there are usually still some primordial follicles in the ovaries of postmenopausal women. This suggests that the more functionally normal follicles (either in their sensitivity to gonadotropin stimulation or in their ability to withstand atresia) are depleted first. Thus, as a woman ages she is left with more resistant, less hormonally active follicles. This concept helps explain the signs and symptoms of the climacteric.

The dramatic changes in follicle number and function cause the ovary to undergo several gross and microscopic changes (Fig. 48-1). One of these changes is a decline in ovarian weight from 14 g in the fourth decade to approximately 5 g postmenopausally. Microscopic examination of the postmenopausal ovary usually reveals some primordial follicles, but any visible developmental changes in them are typically those of atresia. The ovarian stroma undergoes hyperplasia, particularly in the hilar region, and there is an overall increase in the number of medullary stromal and interstitial cells.

SYSTEMIC CHANGES WITH AGING

Senescence is the process or condition of aging. The term *disease* is defined as a morbid process with a characteristic train of symptoms. Senescence produces its own symptoms and in a young person is considered a disease. Physicians have been unable to accept involution and the symptoms aging produces as a natural and inevitable phase of life. Since the menopause is the

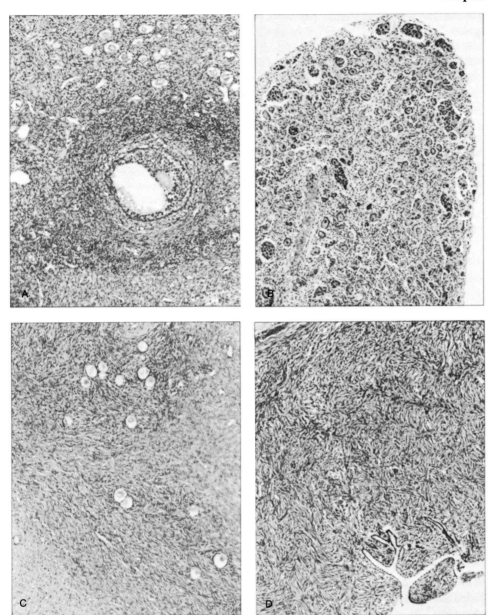

FIG. 48-1. Ovaries in various stages of development. (*A*) Newborn ovary. Compared with the fetal ovary, this specimen shows fewer follicles and an increased amount of stroma. A mature follicle has developed, apparently under the influence of maternal hormones. (*B*) Fetal ovary, 36 weeks gestational age. Abundant primordial follicles (germ cells surrounded by primitive granulosa cells) are present within a stroma or spindle-shaped mesenchymal cells. The surface epithelium is artificially absent because of specimen handling and processing. (*C*) Mature ovary. Primordial follicles are scattered in the ovarian stroma. The lower portion of this photomicrograph contains apparent "enzymatically active stromal cells," which probably contribute to steroid production. (*D*) Postmenopausal ovary. A dense ovarian stroma without follicles is seen. Ovarian surface mesothelium, protected from artifactual denudement by being in a menopausal crypt, is demonstrated. (Magnification of *A–D* ×100) (Photomicrographs courtesy of Kenneth J Fortier, M.D., Duke University Medical Center)

most obvious sign of senescence in women, many signs and symptoms as well as diseases have been incorrectly attributed to gonadal failure. Many organ systems are affected by the aging process independently of gonadal failure. Changes in those systems are briefly outlined below, and hormonal changes are shown in Table 48-1.

Nervous System

Neural cells reach maturity and stop dividing in infancy. With normal aging, the brain loses 5% to 10% of its gross weight, and the total number of brain cells decreases 20% to 50%.[11] Aging brain cells also show a decline in functional ability. There is a significant slowing in the transmission of impulses between neurons, although intraneuronal depolarization remains almost normal. Cerebral blood flow may decline 30% to 40% with age. This decrease does not correlate with alterations in cognitive functions. All persons show some deterioration in short-term memory with age even in the absence of organic brain disease. Other changes include difficulties with thermoregulation and a decline in sensitivity of sight, hearing, smell, taste, and touch. The sense of taste shows a particularly dramatic decline with age. A 75-year-old person may have only 20% of the ability to taste as a 20-year-old.

Cardiovascular System

With regard to the cardiovascular system, it is often difficult to tell when normal aging ends and disease begins.

Certain changes occur so frequently that they may be normal. Physical changes include hypertrophy of the myocardium and calcification of the heart valves. There is a decrease in maximal oxygen consumption that parallels a decrease in cardiac output. This decline is at the rate of 1% per year starting in the third decade. The aging heart usually functions well for everyday activities but has significantly diminished reserves for stress.

Respiratory System

Emphysema is a normal change due to age. The alveolar septal membranes become weak and break down, leaving dilated alveoli. Normal aging also causes the collagen in the septa to become rigid owing to cross-linking. This rigidity causes a restrictive limitation on pulmonary functions. With age there is a diminution in vital capacity, a decrease in maximum breathing capacity, and an increase in residual volume. In persons 75 years of age, maximum inspiratory and expiratory pressures may have dropped 50% and voluntary ventilation by 60%.[12]

Urinary Tract

The decrease in the ability of the aging kidney to clear medications and toxic substances may be a reflection of a decrease in cardiac output and consequent decrease in renal plasma flow. The kidney may also lose the ability to concentrate urine. On microscopic examination the aging kidney will show evidence of interstitial fibrosis, tubular atrophy, and glomerular degeneration.[13,14]

Table 48-1
Hormonal Changes During Aging

Hormone	Serum Concentration	Response to Physiologic or Pharmacologic Stimulation	Metabolic Disposal Rate	End-Organ Sensitivity
Antidiuretic hormone	No change	Increased		
Growth hormone	Decreased	Decreased		Decreased
Thyrotropin (TSH)	No change	No change	No change	No change
Thyroxine (T4)	No change	No change	Decreased	
Triiodothyronine (T3)	No change			
Parathyroid hormone (PTH)				
Intact	Decreased			Increased
C-terminal fragment	Increased			
Cortisol	No change	No change	Decreased	
Adrenal androgens	Decreased	Decreased		
Aldosterone	Decreased	Decreased	Decreased	
Insulin	No change	Decreased	No change	No change
Glucagon	No change	No change		

(Gregerman RI, Bierman EL: Aging and hormones. In Williams RH (ed): Textbook of Endocrinology, 6th ed. Philadelphia, WB Saunders, 1981)

Gastrointestinal System

Few structural changes occur in the gastrointestinal tract, but digestive disorders are common among the elderly. There is age-related atrophy of the intestinal mucosa and marked reduction in gastric secretions. This results in an increased incidence of gallstones, gastrointestinal cancer, and diverticulosis with advancing age.

Immune System

The immune system shows a steady decline in function from adolescence to death. The reasons for this are unknown. Anatomically there is a decrease in stem cells in the bone marrow, an increase in B cells in the spleen and lymph nodes, and a decrease in circulating lymphocytes. Functionally there is a decrease in antibody response of B cells to antigens, an increase in autoantibodies, a decrease in proliferative responses of T and B cells, and changes in modulators to include B-cell suppression and helper T-cell function.[15,16]

Skin and Musculoskeletal System

The skin loses its subcutaneous fat and elasticity with age. This results in skin that is easily traumatized and slow to heal. The increased incidence of arthritis in elderly persons is in part due to degenerative changes in the articular surfaces and perichondrial margins of the joints.

Endocrine System

With the exception of the gonads, the endocrine glands undergo very little change with aging. The pituitary loses 20% of its volume by the ninth decade of life.[17] However, despite this reduction in size, the pituitary maintains normal concentrations of growth hormone, adrenocorticotropic hormone, and thyroid-stimulating hormone.

Anatomically, the thyroid gland undergoes progressive fibrosis with age. In persons older than age 50, concentrations of triidothyronine are diminished by 25% to 40%. Still, elderly patients remain clinically euthyroid.[17]

Albright in 1942 suggested that there was an "adrenopause" as well as menopause. He made this statement on the basis of a 20% and a 40% decrease in dehydroepiandrosterone sulfate (DHAS) levels and dehydroepiandrosterone (DHA) levels, respectively, in postmenopausal women. Estrogen replacement produces a twofold increase in DHAS values. Therefore, the magnitude of the diminished concentrations of the two androgens is probably due to estrogen deprivation.[18] Serum cortisol concentrations remain unaffected by estrogen therapy. *In vitro* data suggest that estrogen is a noncompetitive inhibitor of 3β-hydroxysteroid dehy-

drogenase, and a relative block at this site would augment DHA production.

Beta-cell degeneration of the pancreas progresses with age. By age 65, 50% of patients have chemically abnormal responses to the glucose tolerance test. However, frank diabetes is clinically evident in only 7%.

The progressive decline in the number of primordial follicles in the ovary results in diminished steroid production from the ovary and adrenal glands. This loss of hormone production results in perturbations in feedback dynamics (Fig. 48-2). Despite their interdependence in the endocrine system, the hormones will each be discussed individually.

Gonadotropin-Releasing Hormone

Currently there is no appropriately sensitive or specific assay for measuring gonadotropin-releasing hormone (GnRH) concentration in the sera of humans. Thus, there are no controlled studies on the role of GnRH in the climacteric. In reproductive-age women GnRH is released in pulses every 60 to 90 minutes. The amplitude and pulse frequency of GnRH are determined primarily by circulating levels of estradiol. In rhesus monkeys, increasing serum estradiol levels produce a reduction in GnRH-stimulated gonadotropin release. In the few published reports on circulating concentrations of GnRH in postmenopausal women, GnRH has been found to be increased. This may be due to diminished circulating estradiol concentrations and therefore diminished negative feedback on GnRH.

Gonadotropins

Changes in gonadotropins occur long before the menopause (Fig. 48-3). One of the earliest signs of the climacteric is an elevation in follicle-stimulating hormone (FSH) concentration. This may be due to increased FSH stimulation being required in the premenopause because the remaining follicles are relatively resistant to FSH stimulation. Alternatively, it may be caused by a decrease in the production of inhibin.

The follicular phase is prolonged as fewer and fewer follicles become available for maturation and it takes progressively longer to achieve preovulatory estrogen levels. When the preovulatory estrogen level is not attainable, an anovulatory cycle results. During this time, FSH values of 40 mIU/ml or more are found. Values of greater than 100 mIU/ml almost certainly indicate follicular exhaustion. Luteinizing hormone (LH) concentrations are elevated but are more variable than FSH levels and, for the first time since premenarchal times, the FSH:LH ratio is greater than 1.

These increases in FSH and LH concentrations (18 and 3 times, respectively, as compared with premenopausal follicular phase levels) are reached two to three years after the menopause. Gonadotropin concentrations over the next five decades remain stable or decrease slightly. In contrast, surgical menopause (castration)

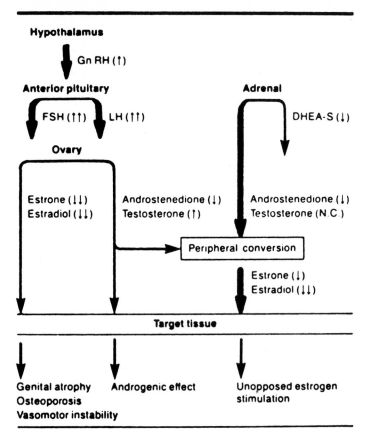

FIG. 48-2. Schematic diagram of hormonal changes after the menopause. *Arrows* refer to menopausal hormone concentration. ↑, increased; ↓, decreased; *N.C.,* no change; *GnRH,* gonadotropin-releasing hormone; *FSH,* follicle-stimulating hormone; *LH,* luteinizing hormone; *DHEA-S,* dehydroepiandrosterone sulfate. (After Hammond CB, Maxson WS: Physiology of the Menopause. Monograph in Current Concepts. Kalamazoo, MI, Scope Publications, 1983)

results in rapid and dramatic changes in FSH and LH values. By 20 days after oophorectomy, FSH values are usually greater than 70 mIU/ml, and LH values are greater than 50 mIU/ml. Maximal concentrations are reached by 40 days.[19,20]

The pulse frequency and clearance rate of the gonadotropins also change during the climacteric.[21,22] FSH in premenopausal women is secreted with little minute-to-minute variation and no evidence of periodicity. LH in premenopausal women has large minute-to-minute variation and has a periodicity of every 1 to 2 hours in the follicular phase and every 4 hours during the mid-luteal and late luteal phases. In postmenopausal women, pulses of both LH and FSH occur approximately every 1 to 2 hours. There is also extreme minute-to-minute fluctuation that is not coincident with the major pulse. The metabolic clearance rate of LH is about twice that of FSH, despite similar production rates in postmenopausal women. This may account for the greater pulse amplitude of LH than of FSH.

Estrogens

The principal circulating estrogen of the premenopausal woman is 17β-estradiol. The serum concentration of 17β-estradiol fluctuates in relation to maturation and involution of the ovarian follicle and the corpus luteum.

Estradiol is produced either by direct ovarian secretion or by peripheral conversion of testosterone and estrone. The exact percentages of total estrogen production from each source vary with the phase of the menstrual cycle and the age of the woman. The adrenal gland has not been shown to secrete estradiol directly in any significant quantities.

Oophorectomy in premenopausal women reduces circulating estradiol concentrations from a mean of 120 pg/ml to 18 pg/ml (Fig. 48-4). This suggests that up to 95% of circulating estradiol is derived from the ovary. Estradiol production in the ovary is achieved by the synergistic actions of the granulosa and theca cell components. According to the "two-cell" theory, theca provides C-19 steroids, which are converted to estrogens by the aromatase system in the granulosa cells. The granulosa cells are stimulated by FSH and estradiol, while the theca and stromal cells respond to LH. As follicular exhaustion progresses, estrogen concentration gradually decreases. As the age of the patient increases, fewer and fewer follicles remain, and estradiol concentrations approximate those in oophorectomized premenopausal women.

The predominant estrogen of the postmenopausal woman is estrone, the biologic estrogenic potency of which is only one third that of estradiol. As with estradiol, virtually no estrone is produced by the postmeno-

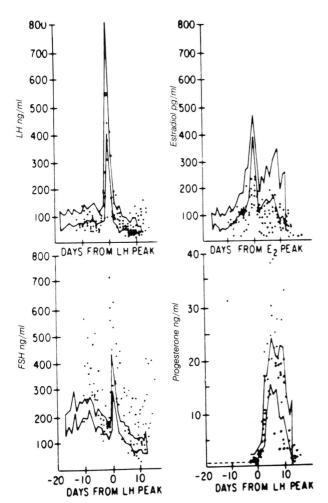

FIG. 48-3. Luteinizing hormone (*LH*), follicle-stimulating hormone (*FSH*), estradiol, and progesterone levels in premenopausal women 46 to 56 years old (*dots*) and women 18 to 20 years old (*enclosed area,* mean ± 2 SEM values). (Sherman BM et al: The menopausal transition: Analysis of LH, FSH, estradiol, and progesterone concentrations during menstrual cycles of older women. J Clin Endocrinol Metab 42:629, 1976. © 1976, The Endocrine Society)

premenopausal women, whose production rates of estrogens vary with the ovarian cycle, postmenopausal women have fairly constant circulating levels of estrone and estradiol. The concentration of estrone rises to 4 times that of estradiol after the menopause. Both estrone and estradiol are inactivated by the sulfotransferase enzymes. Interestingly, estrone sulfate has an average concentration of 128 pg/ml, compared with only 35 pg/ml for estrone. Thus, the inactive conjugated form may be a pool from which biologically active estrogens can be produced.

Androgens

With the loss of follicles at menopause, the only remaining active steroidogenic element of the ovary is the stroma. The stroma lacks the aromatase enzyme needed for conversion of the major androgens (androstenedione and testosterone) to estrogens.

Androstenedione, the most extensively produced androgen in reproductive-age women, declines in the climacteric. Androstenedione production decreases from 1500 pg/ml in premenopausal women to 800 pg/ml to 900 pg/ml in postmenopausal women. The

FIG. 48-4. Hormone levels following bilateral oophorectomy in premenopausal women. (Judd HL: Hormonal dynamics associated with the menopause. Clin Obstet Gynecol 19:775, 1976)

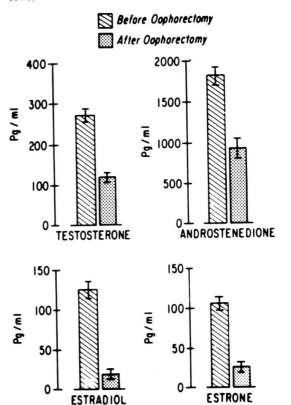

pausal ovary or adrenal gland. Oophorectomy in postmenopausal women produces no discernible change in circulating estrone or estradiol levels (Fig. 48-5). Most estrone is formed by the peripheral conversion of androstenedione by an extraglandular aromatase enzyme; this enzyme has been identified in liver, fat, and certain hypothalamic nuclei. The activity of this extraglandular aromatase enzyme is age and weight dependent and increases twofold during the perimenopause.[23,24]

Essentially all estradiol in postmenopausal women can be accounted for by the conversion of estrone to estradiol. Even though testosterone production in the postmenopausal woman remains constant, only about 0.1% of testosterone is converted to estradiol. Unlike

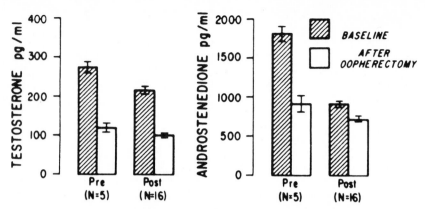

FIG. 48-5. Hormone levels following bilateral oophorectomy in postmenopausal women. (Judd HL, et al: Effect of oophorectomy on circulating testosterone and androstenedione levels in patients with endometrial cancer. Am J Obstet Gynecol 118:793, 1974)

remainder of the circulating androstenedione is produced by the adrenal glands. Overall, the ovary contributes approximately 20% of circulating androstenedione.

In the premenopausal woman, circulating testosterone is derived from three sources: the ovary (25%), the adrenal gland (25%), and extraglandular conversion from androstenedione (50%). The postmenopausal ovary produces a larger percentage of testosterone than does the premenopausal ovary, yielding about 50% of circulating concentrations (Fig. 48-6).

The adrenal androgens DHA and DHAS decrease in the climacteric. This is part of a generalized decline in adrenal androgen production, which may result from a decrease in ovarian estrogen precursors.[18]

FIG. 48-6. Androgen production after oophorectomy in premenopausal and postmenopausal women. (Judd HL: Hormonal dynamics associated with the menopause. Clin Obstet Gynecol 19:775, 1976)

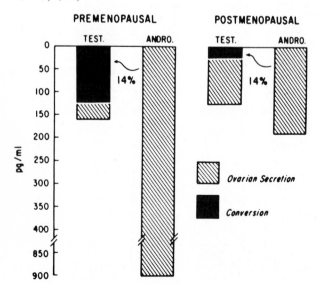

MANIFESTATIONS OF ESTROGEN DEPRIVATION

Although many signs and symptoms of the menopause are attributable to aging, several important symptom complexes are related specifically to estrogen deprivation and menopause. These changes occur in patients of any age following ovarian failure (natural or surgical) and can be classified as either specific hormone-related problems or probable hormone-related problems.

Specific Hormone-Related Problems
Genitourinary atrophy
Vasomotor instability
Osteoporosis

Probable Hormone-Related Problems
Blood lipid changes
Atherosclerotic cardiovascular diseases
Insomnia
Psychosexual symptoms

Genitourinary Atrophy

Large numbers of estrogen receptors are found in the vagina, vulva, urethra, and trigone of the bladder. This is not surprising, since müllerian and mesonephric structures arise in close embryonic proximity. Thus, these structures are sensitive to a decrease in circulating estrogen.

Not all genitourinary tissues atrophy at the same rate. The atrophy begins with diminished estrogen levels and continues over many years.

The *vulva,* although not derived from müllerian structures, undergoes atrophy following the menopause. There is thinning of hair of the mons and shrinkage of the labia minora. The labia majora flatten as the subcutaneous fat and elasticity of the structure diminish. Although vulvar dystrophies are most common in the climacteric, estrogen deprivation does not appear to be the primary causal factor.

With estrogen loss, the *vagina* becomes pale and its epithelium thins, resulting in diminished distensibility and reduced secretion. The vagina is easily traumatized; vaginal trauma may account for as much as 15% of all postmenopausal bleeding. The vaginal pH rises from between 4.5 and 5 to between 6 and 8. Such an alkaline environment predisposes the vagina to colonization by a multitude of bacterial pathogens, so that the incidence of vaginitis increases during the postmenopausal years. Estrogen administered systemically or intravaginally reverses the thinning of the vaginal mucosa and decreases vaginal pH.[25,26] Treatment must be continuous for one to three months; then only intermittent therapy is necessary to maintain the effect.

Although the incidence of descensus, cystocele, and rectocele of the *uterus* are increased in the climacteric, there is little evidence to suggest that estrogen deprivation is the cause. Probably the increase in incidence is due to estrogen loss coupled with the age-related slowing of cell division and decrease in elasticity of tissue.

The *urethra* is also affected by estrogen loss. The distal urethra may become rigid and inelastic and undergo thinning of the epithelium. This predisposes to the formation of ectropion (urethral caruncula), diverticula, and urethrocele. The "urethral syndrome," a nonbacterial, recurrent urethritis, is more common in postmenopausal than in premenopausal women owing to the above-mentioned urethral changes. This condition is treatable by estrogen therapy, urethrotomy, or, less frequently, urethral dilatation. Despite the changes in the urethra and supporting pelvic fascia, there does not appear to be any increase in the incidence of true stress urinary incontinence in postmenopausal women compared with premenopausal women.

Bacteriuria may be found in 7% to 10% of postmenopausal women but in only 4% of premenopausal women. The higher incidence in postmenopausal women may be due to mucosal atrophy and increased vaginal contamination due to lowering of the external urethral orifice onto the anterior vaginal wall (caused by vaginal foreshortening). Estrogen therapy frequently improves urinary frequency, dysuria, nocturia, urgency, postvoiding dribbling, and to some extent stress urinary incontinence.[27] Additionally, estrogen causes proliferation of the vaginal epithelium and a return to vaginal acidity with resultant relief of symptoms of vaginitis and frictional dyspareunia.

Vasomotor Symptoms

Hot flashes are experienced by 75% to 85% of women following natural menopause and 37% to 50% of premenopausal women after bilateral oophorectomy. Vasomotor symptoms are most common in the early menopause. Seventy-five percent of women have hot flashes within 12 months of their last menstrual period. The symptoms persist for at least one year in 82% and for at least five years in approximately 50%. The hot flash is described as a warmth that begins in the face and spreads to the chest, and it is often accompanied by a visible red flush. The hot flash is episodic rather than continuous and is frequently associated with nausea, dizziness, headache, palpitations, diaphoresis, and night sweats.

Meldrum and associates have standardized a technique for measuring changes in skin temperature during hot flashes and have noted a mean interval of 54 ± 10 minutes between hot flashes.[29] These investigators also found that the subjective sensation of flushing precedes any changes in skin temperature and is over before the maximal peripheral change is measured. Thus, the subjective experience of a hot flash is not likely to be due to a peripheral disturbance.

Hot flashes do not occur in women with gonadal dysgenesis who have not been exposed to exogenous estrogens. This finding prompted several investigators to see whether hot flashes are correlated with changes in circulatory steroid peptide hormone levels. Several investigators have found no difference in FSH:LH and total estrogens between patients with vasomotor symptoms and patients without symptoms. Meldrum and co-workers also failed to identify any significant change in estrone or estradiol at time of reported hot flashes.[29] Interestingly, increases in DHA, androstenedione, and cortisol were noted 10 to 20 minutes after observed hot flashes. The significance of these observations is unknown.

In independent studies Meldrum and associates and Casper and colleagues noted a close temporal relationship between each hot flash and a pulse of LH (Fig. 48-7).[30,31] These data suggest that either LH itself or factors initiating the release of LH are responsible for hot flashes in patients with gonadal failure. To determine which is responsible, Meldrum and co-workers studied women with pituitary insufficiency and found both subjective and objective evidence of hot flashes.[30] Thus, it seems that LH elevation per se is not responsible for the hot flash (Fig. 48-8).

All of these studies suggest that hypothalamic factors that stimulate LH release are responsible for the hot flash. The hypothalamic centers that control thermoregulation are located in the preoptic and anterior hypothalamic (POAH) nuclei. The four neurotransmitters active in these nuclei are gonadotropin-releasing hormone (GnRH); norepinephrine, dopamine, and β-endorphin, all of which affect gonadotropin secretion. Because dopamine and β-endorphin exert inhibitory influences on gonadotropin secretion and GnRH and norepinephrine exert stimulatory influences, the latter are most likely to play a role in hot flashes. Given that hot flashes occur in patients with Kallmann's syndrome following discontinuation of estrogen replacement, GnRH itself is probably not primal to the initiation of the hot flash. In ovariectomized rats there is an increase

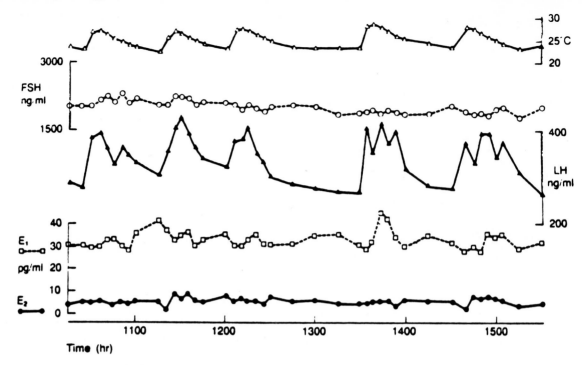

FIG. 48-7. Cortisone (*C*), follicle-stimulating hormone (*FSH*), luteinizing hormone (*LH*), estrone (*E_1*), and estradiol (*E_2*) during a hot flash in a menopausal woman. (Meldrum DR et al: Gonadotropins, estrogens and adrenal steroids during the menopausal hot flash. J Clin Endocrinol Metab 50:685, 1980. © 1980, The Endocrine Society)

FIG. 48-8. Serial measurements of skin temperature, resistance, and serum follicle-stimulating hormone (*FSH*) and luteinizing hormone (*LH*) in a woman who had been treated for a pituitary adenoma. *Arrows* mark the onset of subjective hot flashes. *E_1*, estrone; *E_2*, estradiol. (Meldrum DR, Erlik Y, Lu JKH, Judd HL: Objectively recorded hot flashes in patients with pituitary insufficiency. J Clin Endocrinol Metab 52:684, 1981. © 1981, The Endocrine Society)

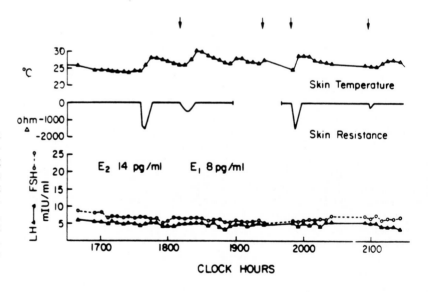

in the concentration and turnover of hypothalamic norepinephrine. In humans clonidine (an α-adrenergic agonist/antagonist) can treat hot flashes fairly effectively. Therefore, one possible explanation of the origin of the hot flash is that gonadal failure may increase hypothalamic norepinephrine with increased pulsatile GnRH and subsequent LH secretions. This increase in norepinephrine then results in activation of the neuroeffector pathways that control thermoregulation.

Experimental evidence suggests that estrogen deficiency is the primary abnormality affecting the hypothalamic neurons that produce the hot flash. Although serum concentrations of estrogen are similar in women with and in women without symptoms, there appears to be a difference between the two groups in bioavailable estrogen (Fig. 48-9).[32] Animal studies have shown that only estrogen not bound to sex hormone–binding globulin (SHBG) is available to be transported across the blood–brain barrier into the brain tissue. Erlik and co-workers were able to predict which women would have hot flashes on the basis of non–SHBG-bound estradiol concentrations.[32]

Estrogen has traditionally been the drug of choice to relieve hot flashes. However, a number of alternatives have recently been shown to effectively suppress hot flashes. Medroxyprogesterone acetate, 10 mg orally daily or 100 mg injected monthly, is also effective. Bellergal, an ergot alkaloid, has been found to be somewhat effective in the treatment of hot flashes. Clonidine, 0.1 mg to 0.2 mg twice a day, is also effective. However, in nonhypertensive patients, side-effects are common.

Osteoporosis

Osteoporosis is defined as an abnormal rarefaction of bone due to failure of the osteoblasts to lay down bone matrix. Thus, the term refers to a generalized group of diseases that have multiple etiologies. *Disorders commonly associated with osteoporosis* are calcium deficiency, long-term heparin treatment, hyperadrenocorticism, hypogonadism, adult hypophosphatasia, immobilization, malabsorption, metabolic bone disease, systemic mastocytosis, scurvy, and thyrotoxicosis. Other disorders associated with osteoporosis include alcoholism, diabetes mellitus, epilepsy, malnutrition, Menkes' syndrome, chronic obstructive pulmonary disease, and rheumatoid arthritis. *Heritable disorders of collagen metabolism associated with osteoporosis* are cystathionine synthetase–deficiency homocystinuria, Ehlers–Danlos syndrome, Marfan's syndrome, and osteogenesis imperfecta. *Types of osteoporosis not associated with other diseases* include idiopathic (juvenile and adult), postmenopausal, and senile osteoporosis.[33]

Fuller Albright was the first to associate osteoporosis with postmenopausal and oophorectomized women. Bone loss is accelerated following the menopause or oophorectomy regardless of age. In both sexes maximal skeletal mass is attained by age 35. By age 50 both men and women have begun to experience a generalized loss of bone that may reach as much as 15% by age 80. Women have significantly less bone mineral content than do men of similar race and age. Following oophorectomy, bone loss averages 3.9% per year for the first six years after surgery and then 1% per year thereafter. Overall bone loss after natural menopause averages 1% to 2% per year. By the age of 80, some untreated white women have lost 30% to 50% of their bone mass. The exact incidence of osteoporosis is unknown. However, 25% of all white women over the age of 60 have spinal compression fractures. Forearm fractures are 10 times more common among 60-year-old women than among men of the same age. Vertebral fractures have occurred in 50% of women aged 75 (Fig. 48-10). Hip fracture, the most serious sequela of osteoporosis, occurs in 20% of women by age 90, and 80% of postmenopausal women with hip fractures are found to have significant preexisting osteoporosis.

The problem with hip fractures in women is that the immobilization required for treatment results in complications leading to death in about 15% of cases. In 1983 it was estimated that 300,000 people suffer hip

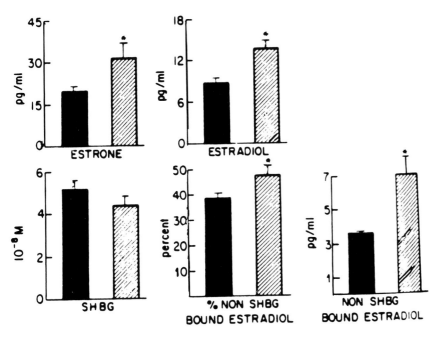

FIG. 48-9. Non-sex-hormone–bound estradiol in women with and without hot flashes. Values are mean ± SE in 24 women with hot flashes (*solid bars*) contrasted with 24 asymptomatic subjects (*striped bars*). *Asterisk*, statistical significance between the two groups. (Erlik Y, Meldrum DR, Judd HL: Estrogen levels in postmenopausal women with hot flashes. Obstet Gynecol 59:405, 1982. Reprinted with permission from The American College of Obstetricians and Gynecologists)

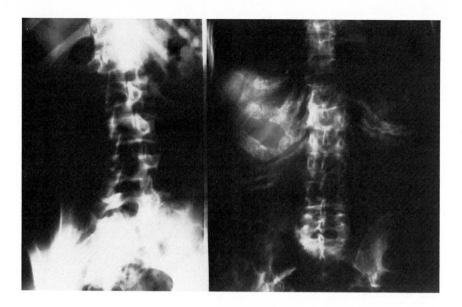

FIG. 48-10. Lumbar spine x-ray films of a normal individual (*left*) and a patient with severe postmenopausal osteoporosis (*right*). (Hammond CB, Ory SJ: Endocrine problems in the menopause. Clin Obstet Gynecol 25: 19, 1982)

fracture yearly. The financial impact of this injury is staggering. Femoral neck fractures currently cost an estimated $1.4 billion per year in acute health care costs, and this may rise to $3 billion by the end of this decade. According to additional estimates, more than 20,000 individuals will die within three months of their hip fractures and a further 50,000 will require long-term care.

Clinical Features Associated with Increased Risk

In general, bone density seems to parallel skin pigmentation, being greatest in blacks and least in whites. Persons with a family history of osteoporosis and early menopause (either natural or surgical), as well as persons whose weight is low for their height, are in a high-risk group. Diet can also affect the rate of osteoporosis. Heaney and associates demonstrated that calcium intake in the United States is well below the level of calcium lost from the body.[34] In the average postmenopausal woman, there is a negative calcium balance of 40 mg per day, a loss equivalent to a 1% to 2% annual reduction in skeletal mass as measured in cortical bone.

Much more confusing are the roles of cigarette smoking, caffeine, and alcohol on osteoporosis. All of these factors are usually associated with other possibly pathogenic factors that may confound studies.

The place of general activity in the development and prevention of osteoporosis is intriguing. It has long been known that inactivity produces muscular and skeletal degeneration. Astronauts on long space missions who did not exercise showed a significant loss of bone mineral content. Interestingly, exercise was found to prevent this loss. Unfortunately, the type of exercise that will produce a positive bone balance has yet to be defined.

Calcium and Bone Metabolism[35-38]

Bone is in continuous transition between bone deposition and bone resorption. On the average, 1 mg to 2 mg (0.02–0.04%) of the skeleton is formed and resorbed daily. This "*bone remodeling*" is affected directly by parathyroid hormone, vitamin D, and calcitonin. Bone remodeling is also indirectly influenced by gonadal steroids.

Two cells, the osteoblast and the osteoclast, are responsible for bone remodeling. Bone deposition is controlled by the osteoblast, which deposits an amorphous organic matrix called *osteoid* in a mesh of collagen fibrils. The precipitation of calcium and phosphate to form hydroxyapatites that crystallize results in hardening of the osteoid. The rate of mineralization is dependent on the extracellular concentrations of calcium and phosphorus, which may be regulated locally by the osteoblast. Bone resorption is modulated by the osteoclast. Located on either the periosteal or endosteal surfaces, osteoclasts can cause rapid release of calcium and phosphorus into the circulation to maintain peripheral calcium homeostasis. The organic matrix is more slowly degraded through the action of hydrolases and collagenases. The degradation of collagen results in the presence in the urine of hydroxyproline, which can serve as a marker of increased bone resorption.

Calcium plays a crucial role in the maintenance of skeletal integrity. Of the 1 kg to 2 kg of calcium in the body, 98% is contained in bone. Yet with gonadal failure, calcium homeostasis goes awry. Heaney's five-year calcium balance study in 168 perimenopausal women showed that the calcium intake requirement of premenopausal and hormonally treated postmenopausal women is 0.99 g per day, whereas that of untreated postmenopausal women is 1.504 g per day.

Parathyroid hormone (PTH) may be the critical

modulator of calcium balance. In response to hypocalcemia, PTH exerts three main effects:

1. Stimulation of renal mitochondrial 1α-hydroxylation, which converts 25-hydroxyvitamin D to the biologically active form 1α,25-dihydroxyvitamin D.
2. Direct action on bone causing rapid release of calcium from bone within several minutes. Bone remodeling is a late effect that occurs several hours after PTH infusion, during which time osteoclasts increase in number and activity.
3. Reduction in the renal calcium clearance rate with augmented tubular reabsorption of calcium after glomerular filtration.

Whereas PTH is responsible for rapid replacement of peripheral calcium, general calcium maintenance is through 1α,25-dihydroxyvitamin D. Vitamin D is a hormone derived from 5,7 diene steroids. The parent compounds is acquired from dietary sources, or photobiosynthesis in the skin. Vitamin D exists in three forms with varying biologic activities. Vitamin D, the weakest form, is first hydroxylated in the liver to another, relatively inactive, form, 25-hydroxyvitamin D. The second hydroxylation, to 1α,25-dihydroxyvitamin D, occurs in the kidney and produces the most active form of vitamin D. The hydroxylase enzyme in the kidney is under the trophic influence of PTH. 1α,25-Dihydroxyvitamin D stimulates the absorption of both calcium and phosphorus from the intestinal lumen into the circulation.

With declining estrogen levels, calcium homeostasis changes. As estrogen levels decline, circulating calcium remains constant but serum phosphorus levels increase. This may be due to a measurable decrease in serum 11,25-dihydroxyvitamin D. A relative deficiency in the 1α hydroxylase enzyme has been implicated. These reduced levels of 1α,25-dihydroxyvitamin D may cause the decline in calcium absorption that occurs with age. Urinary calcium excretion may increase 20% in postmenopausal patients. Hydroxyproline levels are also increased after menopause. Unfortunately, measurement of neither urinary calcium excretion nor hydroxyproline has been able to predict who will develop osteoporosis.

Diagnosis

Bone mass in both males and females peaks at age 30. After age 30, bone loss is almost universal for both sexes. Females lose cortical bone at a rate of 0.5% per year, and the rate increases at the menopause or after oophorectomy. The rate of bone loss after ovarian failure is 1% to 3% of cortical bone and may be as high as 10% to 15% in the axial skeleton. Nevertheless, only 30% to 35% of women develop pathologic osteoporosis (skeletal fragility and atraumatic fracture).

Thus, one of the physician's most difficult tasks is to differentiate between patients with osteopenia (age-related bone loss) and patients destined to develop pathologic osteoporosis. Routine x-ray films are of little value, since at least 30% of bone must be lost before

obvious changes are radiographically demonstrable. Despite the inaccuracy of routine x-ray films, two indices have been developed to diagnose osteoporosis from plain films. The first is the *Singh index,* in which trabecular bone patterns in the proximal femur are graded. However, because this index is based on bone structure and not mineral content, its use is limited. The *Barnett-Nordin index* uses radiogrametry to evaluate cortical and total bone volume. Both indices provide useful information in large-scale clinical trials but are generally not particularly helpful in the identification of bone loss in an individual patient. Bone biopsy is currently the best way to evaluate osteoporosis. However, the process is painful and expensive, and most patients are unwilling to undergo the series of biopsies required for evaluation.

Single-beam photon absorptiometry has become the most generally accepted technique for obtaining reliable and reproducible measurements of cortical bone mineral mass.[39] Single-photon scans accurately measure only peripheral bone, which is mostly cortical bone. Unfortunately, variable relationships have been found in comparisons of mineral content in the axial skeleton (where osteoporosis generally strikes first) and the appendicular skeleton. Dual-beam photon absorptiometry can accurately measure bone mineral content in the lumbar vertebrae. This technique is promising, but the equipment is expensive and not widely available.

The most promising technique for measurement of the axial skeleton is computed tomography (CT). The accuracy and reproducibility of CT are about 100%, and this technique can detect loss in trabecular bone density as early as six months after oophorectomy.[40] *In vivo* neutron activation analysis offers the additional advantage of measuring the central skeleton in both the trunk and thigh areas, which are the regions most often affected by osteoporosis. However, this method is so cumbersome and expensive that it is likely to remain in clinical research centers and have little direct application for the clinician.

It is important in diagnosing osteoporosis not to forget that other entities besides aging can produce decreased bone density. Although the most common cause of osteoporosis is aging, we recommend that the initial evaluation of a patient with suspected osteopenia include measurements of serum calcium, inorganic phosphate, creatinine, alkaline phosphotase, electrolytes, glucose, serum glutamic-oxaloacetic transaminase (SGOT), bilirubin, albumin, and total protein; serum protein electrophoresis; complete blood count with differential; and routine urinalysis and 24-hour urine collection for measurement of calcium and creatinine. In some patients, an iliac crest bone biopsy may be necessary to establish a definitive diagnosis.

Ovarian Failure and Bone Loss[41,42]

The rapid loss of bone mineral content following gonadal failure suggests that ovarian steroids may exert a direct effect on bone turnover. However, several studies have failed to demonstrate estrogen receptors in bone. Therefore, estrogen must work through some indirect mechanism to reduce bone loss (Fig. 48-11).

Estrogen therapy causes several biochemical changes in hypogonadal women. Usually there is a reduction in urinary calcium and hydroxyproline within seven days. This reaction, which has been documented by assessment of biopsy material in estrogen-treated patients, suggests diminished osteoclast function. There is also increased calcium absorption from the gut in women on estrogen therapy.

The mechanism by which estrogens produce these changes is unknown. One hypothesis suggests that estrogen increases the level of bioactive PTH. This would increase gut absorption of 1,25 dihydroxyvitamin D, which would increase gut absorption of calcium, which in turn would diminish bone catabolism. A more attractive hypothesis is that estrogen either directly or indirectly stimulates calcitonin production. Increased cal-

citonin would reduce bone turnover, and the reduction in bone turnover would reduce serum calcium, thereby stimulating PTH production; this would increase 1,25 hydroxyvitamin D levels and increase calcium absorption from the gut. Evidence is slowly accumulating that increased calcitonin production is the primary effect of estrogen on bone metabolism.

Estrogen Replacement Therapy[43–48]

Although the exact mechanisms by which estrogens prevent bone loss are unknown, several large clinical studies have demonstrated a causal relationship between estrogen deprivation and accelerated bone loss. In a ten-year, double-blind prospective study by Nachtigall, a dramatic difference in bone mineral density was found between estrogen-treated and placebo-treated patients if estrogen therapy was begun within three years of the loss of ovarian function. More important, there was a

FIG. 48-11. Estrogen and bone mineral metabolism. Theoretical interactions between estrogen and other factors in the development of osteoporosis. *PTH,* parathyroid hormone. (Spencer H: Osteoporosis: Goals of therapy. Hosp Pract 4:131, 1982. Original illustration and adaptation by Nancy Lou Gahan)

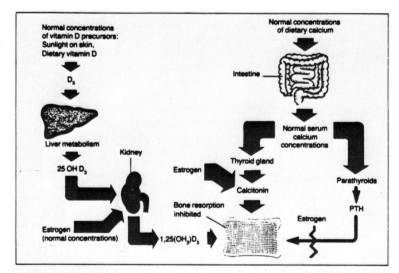
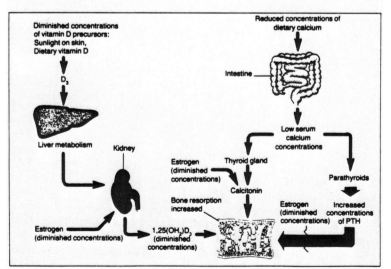

significant difference in number of fractures between estrogen-treated and placebo-treated patients. In this study, 7 of the 62 placebo-treated patients but none of the 67 estrogen-treated patients had fractures.

Cessation of estrogen therapy results in rapid and progressive loss of bone mineral content (Fig. 48-12). Lindsay and co-workers reported a 2.5% per year average rate of loss of bone mineral content among women whose estrogen replacement therapy had been stopped.[49] This rate of bone loss is comparable to the rate of bone loss during the first two years following bilateral oophorectomy. In Lindsay's study, four years after cessation of estrogen therapy, total bone mineral content in formerly treated patients was equivalent to that in women who had never received treatment.

Although it is known that estrogens given to early menopausal women can retard bone loss, the role of estrogen in the treatment of established osteoporosis is less clear. Two large uncontrolled studies suggested that estrogen reduced the rate of fractures in patients who had at least one osteoporotic fracture at the start of therapy. The results suggest that estrogen may be useful in the treatment of established disease. However, the doses used for treatment are higher than those used for prevention and thus may be associated with more side-effects.

The dosage of estrogen necessary to prevent bone loss depends on its type and route of administration. Currently most work is done with conjugated estrogens, of which 0.625 mg per day provides adequate protection against the development of severe osteoporosis. Various

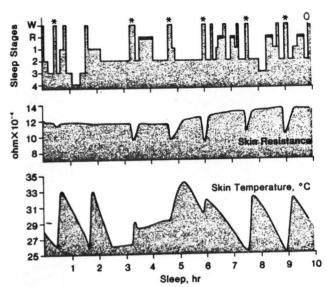

FIG. 48-13. Sleepgram of an estrogen-deficient patient. *Asterisks* mark hot flashes. *Open circle* indicates arousal of the patient at the end of the study. (Erlik Y et al: Association of waking episodes with menopausal hot flashes. JAMA 245:1742, 1981. Copyright © 1981, American Medical Association)

combinations of estrogen, androgen, vitamin D, sodium fluoride, calcitonin, PTH, and growth hormone have been tried, but the ideal combination (if there is one) has not yet been determined.

Psychologic and Sexual Problems

Sigmund Freud characterized the menopausal woman as "quarrelsome and obstinate, petty and stingy, sadistic, and anal-erotic." Wilson in 1966 popularized this notion by stating that "the menopausal syndrome is based on an erratic disorientation of the woman's entire frame of mind." However, there is little evidence for the role of estrogen deprivation in the pathogenesis of most of the psychologic disorders and symptoms ascribed to the menopause.

Insomnia and fatigue affect 30% to 40% of all post-menopausal women. Recent evidence indicates these symptoms may be related to estrogen deficiency. In a study using sleep polygraphs, a close relationship was found between hot flashes and waking episodes (Fig. 48-13). Thus, some estrogen-deficient women may suffer chronic sleep deprivation. Two double-blind studies found insomnia to be specifically reduced by estrogen.

Estrogen may also alleviate psychosocial problems of the climacteric through its effects on catecholamine metabolism. In 1972 Klaiber and colleagues noted decreased plasma monoamine oxidase activity in patients with depression who had been given a daily dose of 5 mg to 20 mg conjugated estrogens.[50] Estrogens may also modify dopamine and serotonin metabolism, accounting

FIG. 48-12. Bone loss after cessation of estrogen therapy. (Lindsay R, Hart DM, MacLean A et al: Bone response to termination of oestrogen treatment. Lancet 1:1325, 1978)

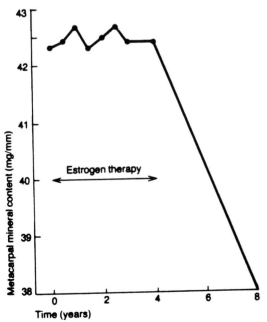

for the "mental tonic" effect. However, estrogen also exerts a strong placebo effect in the relief of the psychologic symptoms seen in postmenopausal women.

There is a prevalent notion that "sex doesn't matter in old age." However, in a study of sexual activity of single women between 50 and 69 years of age, both previously married subjects and subjects who had never been married clearly maintained sexual activity, including masturbation (59% and 44%, respectively), coitus (37% and 25%), and orgasmic dreams (35% and 52%).[51] The studies of Masters and Johnson have shown that all four stages of sexual response are diminished postmenopausally.[52] Specifically, the vasocongestive increase in breast size during the excitement phase is reduced or absent. Generalized myotonic contraction is decreased, and the sexual flush is less frequent and more limited. Vaginal lubrication diminishes, and the vagina is less expansive. Some women also experience painful uterine contractions with orgasm.

Estrogen deficiency has been suggested as a possible cause for the change in libido and sexual response in the menopause. It is hypothesized that disinterest may occasionally be a consequence of dyspareunia from an atrophic vaginal mucosa, introital stricture, and decreased vaginal distensibility. However, dyspareunia occurs in under 8% of postmenopausal patients. Additionally, oophorectomy in the premenopausal patient apparently does not affect libido unless the uterus is also removed. There is no direct evidence to support hormonal deprivation as a cause of reduction in sexual activity. Dean adequately summarizes the sexual decline as being one of circumstance, not of potential.[53]

Atherosclerosis and Lipids

Atherosclerosis is a special type of arteriosclerosis that is often associated with aneurysm formation, embolic phenomena, and vascular occlusion. Factors that increase an individual's risk for atherosclerosis include hypertension, diabetes mellitus, hyperlipidemia, smoking, and obesity. However, there is tremendous variation in susceptibility to atherosclerosis.

The level of circulating lipid correlates fairly consistently with an individual's risk of developing atherosclerosis. There is augmented risk of coronary artery disease when cholesterol concentration exceeds 220 mg/dl to 250 mg/dl.[54] These elevated cholesterol levels are associated with increased concentrations of low density lipoproteins (LDL). High density lipoproteins (HDL), which carry cholesterol, seem to protect against the development of atherosclerosis. The association of atherosclerosis, lipids, and the menopause was inevitable when it was noted that men younger than 55 are 5 to 8 times more likely to have coronary artery disease than women of similar age.[55] Estrogens have multiple effects on blood lipids. "Natural" estrogens (including conjugated equine estrogens) depress serum LDL and elevate HDL,[56] theoretically protecting against athero-

sclerotic heart disease. Synthetic estrogens (including ethinyl estradiol in oral contraceptives) create a reverse pattern. Synthetic estrogens also appear to increase serum triglyceride concentrations, whereas natural estrogens do not.[57]

There is no conclusive evidence that estrogen therapy reduces the risk of coronary artery disease, nor is there justification for the use of estrogen therapy as prophylaxis for myocardial infarction. Conversely, the use of natural estrogens in low doses does not appear to significantly increase the risk of coronary artery disease.

POTENTIAL RISKS OF ESTROGEN THERAPY

As previously discussed, estrogen therapy is beneficial in cases of genitourinary atrophy, vasomotor instability, osteoporosis, and possibly atherosclerotic cardiovascular disease and psychosexual symptoms. However, the benefits of estrogen replacement therapy must be weighed against the risks. Definite risks of estrogen therapy are endometrial hyperstimulation, endometrial neoplasia, and cholelithiasis. Possible risks are hypertension, glucose intolerance, breast cancer, and thrombophlebitis.

Endometrial Carcinoma

The endometrium of both pre- and postmenopausal women can become hyperplastic when subjected to prolonged stimulation by estrogens in the absence of progesterone. Prospective studies in the United Kingdom suggest that between 18% and 32% of postmenopausal women treated with unopposed estrogens will develop hyperplasia. Approximately one third of the hyperplasias will be of the adenomatous variety.[58] This type of hyperplasia is significant, since 12% of cases of adenomatous hyperplasia become malignant after 18 months and 30% become malignant within ten years.[59]

Numerous studies indicate that the relative risk for uterine cancer is 1.7 to 12.5 in women who receive estrogen-only replacement therapy. In general, this augmented risk appears to be related to both the dosage and the duration of estrogen therapy.[58,60]

The upsurge in estrogen therapy between 1960 and 1970 was associated with an increased incidence of endometrial adenocarcinoma but not of patient mortality. This is primarily because uterine carcinoma in patients on estrogen therapy tends to be minimally invasive and extremely well differentiated and is usually diagnosed at an earlier stage than in similar controls. The five-year survival rate of patients who are diagnosed as having uterine cancer during estrogen replacement therapy is approximately 95%. This is significantly better than that in women who develop uterine cancer and are not undergoing estrogen therapy.[61]

The largest factor in the development of uterine cancer in women using estrogen seems to be the lack of progestin. Progestational agents have three potential mechanisms by which they protect against the development of endometrial carcinoma: they inhibit replenishment of the estrogen receptor while creating a pseudodecidual response; they induce the enzyme estradiol dehydrogenase, which converts the potent estrogen estradiol to estrone; and they cause the endometrium to shed.[62,63]

As mentioned, histologic studies have revealed an 18% to 32% incidence of hyperplasia with chronic estrogen treatment alone. The addition of a progestin for 7 days reduces this rate to 4% and for 10 days reduces it to 2%. When progestin was given for 12 to 13 days, the incidence of hyperplasia was zero.[64] The incidence of endometrial carcinoma is similarly reduced not only below the rate recorded with unopposed estrogen but also below the rate seen in an untreated population.

Breast Cancer

The potential role of estrogen in the generation of breast neoplasia comes primarily from the ability of estrogen to induce mammary tumors in animals, particularly mice. In humans, estrogen's role is much less clear; some patients with metastatic breast carcinoma respond beneficially to endocrine ablative surgery, whereas others have remission with estrogen therapy. Breast cancer must be considered a multifactorial disorder in which genetic factors, endocrine relationships, oncogenic factors, and environmental factors all play a part.

Several investigators have examined the relative risk ratios of patients taking unopposed estrogens for endometrial and breast cancer. In all of these studies, the association between estrogen and breast cancer was very weak if present at all.[65–67] Relative risk ratios are usually reported only in epidemiologic case control studies, in which cases of breast cancer are matched with controls and as many variables as possible are studied. Such studies cannot establish true cause-and-effect relationships, only associations. A relative risk ratio of 5 does not mean that the incidence of the disease was found to be 5 times higher than normal; rather, it means that the use of estrogen was 5 times greater in the group with the disease than in the controls. A report of relative risk ratios greatly magnifies the association between hormones and cancer.

The addition of a progestin to estrogen replacement therapy decreased the rate of breast cancer in several prospective studies. In Nachtigall's study there were 4 breast cancers among 84 placebo users and none in the 84 estrogen–progestin group.[65] In the Wilford Hall studies of Gambrell, the estrogen–progestin users had a significantly lower incidence of breast cancer (67.3:100,000) than the control group (350.6:100,000).[66] This significance held up when compared with data of the Third National Cancer Survey (incidence, 188.3:100,000) and the National Cancer Institute SEER data (incidence, 229.2:100,000).

Although the results are not conclusive, it appears that the prognosis for breast cancer, like that for endometrial cancer, may be better for estrogen users than for nonusers. At Wilford Hall, from 1972 to 1981, 256 postmenopausal women developed breast cancer. Overall mortality was 30.5%. Mortality for estrogen users was 16%, compared with 35.8% for nonusers. Similar findings were reported in a study from Vanderbilt University. Whether the improved survival rate resulted from increased surveillance or from a protective effect of the hormone remains open to speculation.

Thromboembolism

High-dose estrogen compounds (particularly synthetic estrogens), both in men and in women, have been associated with an increased incidence of thromboembolus formation. The incidence of thrombophlebitis and thromboembolism associated with oral contraceptives increases with dosage and patient age. There is clinical laboratory evidence of a mild "hypercoagulable state" in postmenopausal women receiving estrogen replacement therapy. However, there is no evidence that the doses of estrogen (particularly the "natural" estrogens) used for postmenopausal estrogen replacement therapy are associated with any significant increase in clinically apparent thrombophlebitis or thromboembolism.[68] Nevertheless, until more long-term studies are performed, estrogens should be used with caution for patients with significant risk factors for thrombosis formation or those with a past history of this problem.

Hypertension

The synthetic estrogen in oral contraceptives has been associated with a mild (5–6 mm Hg systolic and 1–2 mm Hg diastolic) increase in blood pressure that is reversed upon discontinuation of the steroid. The association between natural estrogens and hypertension is less clear; it appears unlikely that low-dose natural estrogen therapy causes significant hypertension. Nevertheless, because idiosyncratic hypertension is occasionally reported in women taking estrogen, all women on estrogen therapy should receive routine blood pressure measurements at regular intervals.

Alterations in Glucose Tolerance

Alterations in glucose tolerance have been reported in some studies of patients receiving conjugated estrogens, ethinyl estradiol, mestranol, and quinestrol. However, other studies in which similar doses of these estrogens were used showed no alterations in glucose tolerance. In a prospective study by Thom, 1.25 mg conjugated estrogen did not produce any negative effect on glucose tolerance.[69] It would therefore appear that estrogens may have a mild deleterious effect on glucose tolerance but are unlikely to cause frank diabetes. Although estrogens are not contraindicated in diabetic patients, frequent glucose monitoring would be prudent.

Cholelithiasis

The Boston Collaborative Drug Surveillance Program indicated a relative risk of 2.5 for gallbladder disease in postmenopausal women taking estrogen. The annual incidence in women aged 45 to 49 was 87 per 100,000 for women not on estrogen, compared with 218 per 100,000 for estrogen users. The exact mechanism for this increase is unknown, but estrogens probably induce alterations in lipid balance or bile salt content in the gallbladder that favor stone formation.

Abnormal Uterine Bleeding

Abnormal uterine bleeding is one of the most serious side-effects of unopposed estrogen therapy in post-menopausal women. The occurrence of bleeding appears to be dose related. Lauritzen demonstrated a 2% to 12% increase of uterine bleeding in patients receiving 1.25 mg conjugated estrogen (only) per day, compared with a 1% to 4% incidence at a dosage of 0.625 mg per day.[70] The occurrence of abnormal uterine bleeding requires endometrial sampling to rule out neoplasia.

ESTROGEN PHARMACOLOGY

Estrogens are C-18 steroids derived from the cyclopentanophenanthrene steroid nucleus. Estrogens circulate in three forms: free, conjugated, and protein bound. Free estrogen, the bioavailable form, is lipophilic. This allows it to freely traverse many cell membranes. Free estrogens may be rendered biologically inactive in the liver by addition of a sulfate or glucuronide molecule. The conjugated estrogens are water soluble and are excreted in the urine or bile. The sulfated form of estrogen may serve as a reservoir for the free form. Sulfatases can cleave the sulfate molecule to convert the inactive sulfated form to the biologically active free form. Unconjugated estrogens circulate primarily bound to albumin or SHBG.

The potency of a particular estrogen varies with the end point, *i.e.*, the effect of that estrogen in a given assay system (Table 48-2). For example, diethylstilbestrol is a potent estrogen if assessed by its ability to cornify the mouse vagina, but it is a weak estrogen if assessed by its ability to inhibit LH secretion. Potency estimates must consider duration of exposure as well as molar quantities. For example, estriol occupies the nucleus only one to four hours and thus has a weak uterotropic effect in the rat bioassay. However, if estriol is infused or given by repetitive injection, a uterotropic effect similar to that of estradiol can be obtained.

Many estrogen preparations are available for clinical use. Comparative potency has been difficult to determine because there is no single uniform bioassay for estrogens, and variation of the dose, route, and frequency of administration can turn a "weak" estrogen into a potent one. Estrogens in clinical use are listed below:[71]

Conjugated Steroidal Estrogens
Estrones
   Conjugated equine estrogens
   Esterified estrogens
   Piperazine estrone sulfate
Estradiols
   Estradiol cypionate
   Estradiol valerate
   Micronized 17β-estradiol
Estriols
   Estriol
   Estriol hemisuccinate

Nonconjugated Steroidal Estrogens
17-ethinyl-estradiol
17-ethinyl-estradiol-3-methyl ether (mestranol)
17-ethinyl-estradiol-3-cyclopentoether (quinestrol)

Table 48-2
Relative Strength of Estrogen in Varying Assay Systems

Hormone	Vaginal Cornification (%)	Antigonadotropin (%)	Anti-implantation (%)	Antiovulation (%)
Estradiol	100	100	100	100
Estrone	30	30	70	150
Estriol	3	10	12	15
Ethinyl estradiol	150	300	70	170
Mestranol	10	100	20	85

(Hammond CB, Maxson WS: Current status of estrogen therapy for the menopause. Fertil Steril 37:5, 1982. Reproduced with permission of the publisher, The American Fertility Society)

Synthetic Estrogen Analogs (Nonsteroids)
Stilbene derivatives
    Benzestrol
    Chlorotrianisene
    Dienestrol
    Diethylstilbestrol
    Hexestrol
    Promethestrol diproprionate
Naphthalene derivative
    Methallenestril

In the United States conjugated estrogens are the most commonly prescribed estrogens for therapy of the menopause. These estrogens, obtained from the urine of pregnant mares, contain 48% estrone sulfate, 26% equilin sulfate, 15% 17α-dihydroequilin sulfate, and smaller amounts of many other conjugated estrogens.[72] The major circulating estrogen in women receiving conjugated estrogens is equilin (Table 48-3). In humans equilin is both potent and long lasting (owing to storage and slow release from adipose tissue). According to the mouse uterine weight bioassay, the relative potencies of diethylstilbestrol, equilin sulfate, and estrone sulfate are 2.5, 2, and 0.4, respectively. Currently, there is no evidence that equilin has detrimental effects in humans, other than those inherent to all estrogen therapy. The effects of conjugated estrogens on a particular organ system are dose and time dependent. The gonadotropins FSH and LH can be suppressed by as little as 0.3 mg and 0.625 mg conjugated estrogen, respectively. Interestingly, in postmenopausal women 1.25 mg conjugated estrogen given daily will not suppress FSH and LH to normal premenopausal levels.[73,74] This dosage is capable of increasing vaginal cornification and relieving vasomotor symptoms, so its failure to suppress the gonadotropin is surprising. A possible explanation is that estrogen may contribute significantly to negative feedback on gonadotropins but other substances such as inhibin are required for complete suppression.

Comparison of the biologic potencies of the clinically available estrogen compounds in humans is diffi-cult owing to methodologic problems. Estrogen potency in humans can be analyzed by observation of the maturation index, endometrial proliferation, and cervical mucus fern. The minimal doses of estrogens required to achieve similar biologic effects are estradiol, 5 mg; diethylstilbestrol, 5 mg; conjugated estrogens, 3.75 mg; mestranol, 0.08 mg; and ethinyl estradiol, 0.05 mg.[75]

Estradiol cannot be absorbed through the gut without chemical modification. The addition of an ethinyl group at the 17- position results in almost complete absorption following oral administration. Another way to allow gut absorption of estradiol is to micronize the estradiol. In this form, 80% of the particles are 20×10^6 M or less, which allows effective oral, sublingual, and vaginal absorption.[76] Conjugated estrogens are effectively absorbed either orally or intravaginally.

A daily dose of 1.25 mg intravaginal conjugated estrogen raises total circulating estrogen to 93 pg/ml, a level comparable to that achieved with 0.625 mg oral conjugated estrogen.[77] Oral administration of micronized estradiol and conjugated estrogens results in an estrone:estradiol ratio of greater than 1. This is due to the rapid conversion of estradiol to estrone in the mucosa of the small intestine.[78] Intravaginal administration of micronized estradiol results in an estrone:estradiol ratio of less than 1 because of bypassing of the 17-ketosteroid reductase of the intestinal mucosa. After 15 days of intravaginal micronized estradiol cream at a dosage of 0.2 mg per day, estradiol and estrone levels of 61 pg/ml and 37 pg/ml, respectively, are reached.[79,80] Vasomotor and genitourinary symptoms diminish by day 15 of administration of intravaginal micronized estradiol.

Therefore, physiologic levels of estrogen may be achieved with a variety of estrogenic preparations given through various routes. With the exception of intravaginal estradiol, estrone levels exceed estradiol levels. The clinical significance of this reversal of the estrone:estradiol ratio is not known. Currently, there is no evidence that one form of estrogen is therapeutically superior to another, nor that one is more likely to cause major side-effects than another (if relative dose is considered).

Table 48-3
Serum Concentrations (Means) of Estrogens at a Dose of 1.25 mg Conjugated Equine Estrogen

Estrogen	Pretreatment	Treatment (3–23 weeks)	Posttreatment (13 weeks after withdrawal)
Equilin (pg/ml)	0	1082–2465	143
Estradiol (pg/ml)	48	82–170	77
Estrogen (pg/ml)	45	125–197	47

(Hammond CB, Maxson WS: Current status of estrogen therapy for the menopause. Fertil Steril 37:5, 1982. Reproduced with permission of the publisher, The American Fertility Society)

MANAGEMENT OF ESTROGEN THERAPY IN THE MENOPAUSE

Estrogens are contraindicated in patients with: known or suspected estrogen-dependent neoplasia; undiagnosed, abnormal genital bleeding; a history of phlebitis; acute liver disease; and stroke.

The specific indications for administration of estrogen to a patient must be well defined and balanced against the potential risks. This is especially true in patients with the following, who possess relative contraindications to estrogen therapy: a family history of estrogen-dependent neoplasia, uterine leiomyomata, severe varicose veins, a history of liver disease, diabetes mellitus, porphyria, and severe hypertension.

Conditions in which the benefits outweigh the risks of estrogen therapy include vasomotor symptoms, genitourinary atrophy, and osteoporosis. Vasomotor symptoms often last only two to three years following the menopause. Therapy should be with the smallest dose of estrogen that controls the symptoms. After two to three years, the dose may be tapered or stopped. Genitourinary atrophy can usually be treated with 0.625 mg to 1.25 mg conjugated estrogens. An increase in superficial cells is usually observed within one month of initiation of therapy. In one study utilizing 0.625 mg oral conjugated estrogen per day, the maximum effect on the index was observed by the end of the first month of therapy.

The smallest dose of conjugated estrogens that will prevent bone loss depends on the type of estrogen used and the route of administration. One cannot assume that an "equivalent" amount of a synthetic estrogen will prevent bone loss. While it is impossible to measure exact equivalent potency in the human body, it seems that 0.625 mg conjugated estrogen equals 5 mg ethinyl estradiol. Yet 15 μg ethinyl estradiol or 20 μg mestranol is necessary to prevent bone loss.[81] For optimal protection, the estrogen should be supplemented with 1000 mg calcium daily and an exercise program. Because rapid bone loss follows discontinuation of estrogen therapy, estrogen therapy should be continued until the patient is in her 80s or beyond. Women receiving calcium supplementation should have periodic checks of serum calcium and phosphorus initially to detect otherwise asymptomatic hyperparathyroidism.

All estrogen is best administered in a cyclic fashion, 25 days on and 5 days off. A progestin must be added for the last 10 to 14 days of the cycle for all patients with a uterus. An estrogen-free period is useful to allow the progestin to down-regulate the estrogen receptors in the endometrium and to allow shedding to occur. It is not known whether the use of progestin for 10 to 14 days each month will completely protect the endometrium if the estrogen is given continuously.

Since the data by Gambrell suggests that progestin may protect against breast cancer, it is probably wise to use progestins with estrogen therapy even in women without a uterus.[59] The progestins most commonly used are medroxyprogesterone acetate, 10 mg, and norethindrone acetate, 10 mg. These doses may cause weight gain, breast tenderness, edema, and depression in some patients. If a patient becomes symptomatic, the dose may be reduced to 5 mg. The exact dosage of medroxyprogesterone acetate needed to suppress endometrial receptor activity is not well defined. However, some data suggest that 2.5 mg medroxyprogesterone acetate may provide adequate endometrial protection for patients also taking 0.3 mg and 0.625 mg conjugated estrogens. Medroxyprogesterone acetate, 5 mg, may effectively protect against endometrial hyperplasia in patients also taking 1.25 mg of conjugated estrogen. Other progestins such as norethindrone (2.5 mg) or norgestrel (150 μg) may be used, but the effect of these progestins on LDL and HDL is unknown.

If a patient develops breakthrough bleeding, sampling of the endometrium is mandatory. Whether periodic endometrial sampling is necessary for patients on estrogen plus progestin therapy is controversial. Authorities recommend sampling every one to three years, despite its lack of cost effectiveness and the patient discomfort it causes.

REFERENCES

1. Mazer C, Israel SL: Symptoms and treatment of the menopause. Med Clin North Am 19:205, 1935
2. Davies ME: Treatment of senile vaginitis with ovarian follicular hormone. Surg Gynecol Obstet 61:680, 1935
3. Albright F, Smith PH, Richardson AM: Postmenopausal osteoporosis: Its clinical features. JAMA 116:2465, 1941
4. Wilson RA: Feminine Forever. New York, Mayflower-Dell, 1966
5. Smith DC, Prentice R, Thompson DJ, Herrmann W: Association of exogenous estrogen and endometrial carcinoma. N Engl J Med 293:1164, 1975
6. Weiss NS: Risks and benefits of estrogen use. N Engl J Med 293:1200, 1975
7. Ziel HK, Finkle WD: Increased risk of endometrial carcinoma among users of conjugated estrogens. N Engl J Med 293:1167, 1975
8. Jaszmann LJB: Epidemiology of the climacteric syndrome. In Campbell S (ed): Management of the Menopause and Postmenopausal Years. Lancaster, MTP Press, 1976
9. Jick H, Porter J, Morrison A: Relation between smoking and age of natural menopause. Lancet 1:1354, 1977
10. Subcommittee of Council of Medical Women's Federation of England: Investigation of menopause in 1000 women. Lancet 1:106, 1933
11. Comfort A: The Biology of Senescence, 3rd ed, p 265. New York, Elsevier, 1979
12. Norris A, Mittman C, Shock NW: Changes in ventilation with age. In Cander L, Moyer JH (eds): Aging of the Lung, pp 136–142. New York, Grune & Stratton, 1964
13. Cole WH: Medical differences between the young and the aged. Am J Geriatr 18:589, 1970
14. Elwood CM: The management of surgery in the patient with renal insufficiency. In Siegel JH (ed): The Aged and High Risk Surgical Patient, p 199. New York, Grune & Stratton, 1976

15. Finkelstein MS: Unusual features of infection in the aging. Geriatrics 37:65, 1982
16. Leech SH: Cellular immunosenescence. Gerontology 26:330, 1980
17. Gregerman RI, Bierman EL: Aging and hormones. In Williams RH (ed): Textbook of Endocrinology, 5th ed, p 1059. Philadelphia, WB Saunders, 1974
18. Abraham GE, Maroulis GB: Effect of exogenous estrogen on serum pregnenolone, cortisol, and androgens in postmenopausal women. Obstet Gynecol 45:271, 1975
19. Monroe SE, Jaffe RB, Midgley AR Jr.: Regulation of human gonadotropins: XXXI. Changes in serum gonadotropin in menstruating women in response to oopherectomy. J Clin Endocrinol 34:420, 1972
20. Ostergard DR, Parlow AL, Townsend DZ: Acute effect of castration on serum FSH and LH in the adult woman. J Clin Endocrinol 31:43, 1970
21. Kohler PO, Ross GT, Odell WD: Metabolic clearance and production rates of human luteinizing hormone in premenopausal and postmenopausal women. J Clin Invest 47:38, 1968
22. Coble YD, Kohler PO, Cargille CM, Ross GT: Production rates and metabolism clearance rates of human follicular stimulating in premenopausal and postmenopausal women. J Clin Invest 48:359, 1969
23. Vermeulen A, Verdonck L: Sex hormone concentrations in postmenopausal women: Relation to obesity, fat mass, age and years postmenopause. Clin Endocrinol 9:59, 1978
24. MacDonald PC, Rombaut RP, Siiteri PK: Plasma precursors of estrogen. I. Extent of conversion of plasma androstenedione to estrone in normal males and nonpregnant normal, castrate and adrenolectomized females. J Clin Endocrinol Metab 27:1103, 1967
25. Rakoff AE, Nowroozi K: The female climacteric. In Greenblatt RB (ed): Geriatric Endocrinology, p 165. New York, Raven Press, 1978
26. Notelovitz M: Gynecologic problems of menopausal women. I: Changes in genital tissue. Geriatrics 33:24, 1978
27. Corlett RC Jr.: Urologic problems in menopause. Female Patient 4:30, 1979
28. Notelovitz M: Gynecologic problems of menopausal women. Part 3: Changes in extragenital tissues and sexuality. Geriatrics 33:51, 1978
29. Meldrum DR, Shamonki IM, Frumar AM et al: Elevations in skin temperature of the finger as an objective index of postmenopausal hot flashes: Standardization of the technique. Am J Obstet Gynecol 135:713, 1979
30. Meldrum RD, Erlik Y, Lu JKH, Judd HL: Objectively recorded hot flashes in patients with pituitary insufficiency. J Clin Endocrinol Metab 52:684, 1981
31. Casper RF, Yen SSC, Wilkes MW: Menopausal flushes: A neuroendocrine link with pulsatile LH secretion. Science 205:823, 1979
32. Erlik Y, Meldrum DR, Judd HL: Estrogen levels in postmenopausal women with hot flashes. Obstet Gynecol 59:403, 1982
33. Hammond CB, Maxson WS: Physiology of Menopause. Monograph in Current Concepts. Kalamazoo, MI, Scope Publications, 1983
34. Heaney RP, Recker RR, Soville PD: Menopausal changes in calcium balance performance. Lab Clin Med 92:953, 1978
35. Krane SM, Potts JT Jr.: Skeletal remodeling and factors influencing bone and bone mineral metabolism. In Isselbacher KJ, Adams RD, Braunwald E et al (eds): Harrison's Principles of Internal Medicine, 9th ed, p 349. New York, McGraw-Hill, 1980
36. Cryer PE, Kissane JM: Osteopenia. Am J Med 69:915, 1980
37. Gallagher JC, Riggs BL, De Luca HF: Effect of estrogen on calcium absorption and serum vitamin D metabolites in postmenopausal osteoporosis. J Clin Endocrinol Metab 51:1359, 1980
38. Utian WH: Menopause in Modern Perspective: A Guide to Clinical Practice. New York, Appleton-Century-Crofts, 1980
39. Cameron JR, Sorenson JA: Measurement of bone mineral in vivo: An improved method. Science 142:230, 1963
40. Cann CE, Genont HK, Ettinger B, Gordon GS: Spinal mineral loss in oopherectomized women: Determination by quantitative computerized tomography. JAMA 244:2056, 1981
41. Lindsay R, Coutts, JRT, Hart DM: The effect of endogenous estrogen on plasma and urinary calcium and phosphate in oopherectomized women. Clin Endocrinol 6:87, 1977
42. Nordin BEC, Peacock M, Crilly RG et al: Summation of risk factors in osteoporosis. In De Luca HF, Frost HM, Jee WSS et al (eds): Osteoporosis: Recent Advances in Pathogenesis Treatment, p 359. Baltimore, University Park Press, 1981
43. Aitken JM, Hart DM, Lindsay R: Oestrogen replacement therapy for prevention of osteoporosis after oopherectomy. Br Med J 3:515, 1973
44. Recker RR, Saville PD, Heaney RP: Effect of estrogens and calcium carbonate on bone loss in postmenopausal women. Ann Intern Med 87:649, 1977
45. Lindsay R, Hart DM, Aitken JM et al: Long-term prevention of postmenopausal osteoporosis by estrogens. Lancet 1:1038, 1976
46. Lindsay R, Hart DM, Forrest C, Baird C: Prevention of spinal osteoporosis in oopherectomized women. Lancet 2:1151, 1980
47. Nachtigall LE, Nachtigall RH, Nachtigall RD, Beckerman EM: Estrogen replacement therapy: A 10-year prospective study in the relationship to osteoporosis. Obstet Gynecol 53:277, 1979
48. Lindsay R, Fogleman I, Hart DM: Minimum effective dose of estrogen for protection against postmenopausal bone loss. Am Soc Bone Mineral Res (Abstr), 1982
49. Lindsay R, MacLean A, Kraszowski A et al: Bone response to termination of oestrogen treatment. Lancet 1:1325, 1978
50. Klaiber EL, Broverman DM, Vogel W, Kobayashi Y: The use of steroid hormones in depression. In Psychotrophic Actions of Hormones: Proceedings of the First World Congress in Biologic Psychiatry, Buenos Aires, Argentina. New York, Spectrum, 1974
51. Christenson CV, Johnson AB: Sexual patterns in a group of older, never-married women. J Geriatr Psychiatry 7:80, 1973
52. Masters VH, Johnson VE: Human Sexual Response. Boston, Little, Brown, 1966
53. Dean SR: Discussion (of the paper by Pfeiffer, Verwoedt and Vans, 1972). Am J Psychiatry 128:1267, 1972
54. Fredrickson DS: Atherosclerosis and other forms of arteriosclerosis. In Adams RD, Braunwald E, Isselbacher KJ et al (eds): Harrison's Principles of Internal Medicine, 7th ed, p 1225. New York, McGraw-Hill, 1974
55. Ober KP, Miller EC: Medical aspects of the menopause. In Eskin BA (ed): The Menopause: Comprehensive Management, p 129. New York, Masson Publishing, 1980
56. Coronary Drug Project Research Group: The coronary drug

project: Initial findings leading to modifications of its research protocol. JAMA 214:1303, 1970

57. Philips GB: Sex hormones, risk factors and cardiovascular disease. Am J Med 65:7, 1978

58. Whitehead MI, King RJB, McQueen J, Campbell S: Endometrial histology and biochemistry in climacteric women during oestrogen/progestin therapy. J R Soc Med 72:322, 1979

59. Gusberg S: The individual at high risk for endometrial carcinoma. Am J Obstet Gynecol 126:535, 1976

60. Siiteri PK, Hemsell DR, Edwards CL, MacDonald PC: Estrogens and endometrial cancer. In Scow RO (ed): Proceedings of the Fourth International Congress on Endocrinology, p 1237. Amsterdam, Excerpta Medica, 1973

61. Chu J, Schweid AI, Weiss NS: Survival among women with endometrial cancer: A comparison of estrogen users and nonusers. Am J Obstet Gynecol 143:569, 1982

62. Tseng L, Gurpide E: Effect of progestins on estradiol receptor levels in human endometrium. J Clin Endocrinol Metab 41:402, 1975

63. Tseng L, Gurpide E: Induction of human estradiol dehydrogenose by progestins. Endocrinology 97:825, 1975

64. Studd JWW, Thom MH, Paterson MEL, Wade-Evans T: The prevention and treatment of endometrial pathology in postmenopausal women receiving exogenous oestrogens. In Pasetto N, Paoletti R, Ambrus JL (eds): The Menopause and Postmenopause, p 127. Lancaster, M.T.P. Press, 1980

65. Nachtigall LE, Nachtigall RH, Nachtigall RB et al: Estrogen replacement. II: A prospective study in the relationship to carcinoma and cardiovascular and metabolic problems. Obstet Gynecol 54:74, 1979

66. Gambrell RD Jr.: Role of hormones in the etiology and prevention of endometrial and breast cancer. Acta Obstet Gynecol Scand (Suppl) 106:37, 1982

67. Hammond CB, Jelovsek FR, Lee KL et al: Effects of long-term estrogen replacement therapy. II: Neoplasia. Am J Obstet Gynecol 133:537, 1979

68. Studd J, Dubiel M, Kakkar VV et al: The effect of hormone replacement therapy on glucose tolerance, clotting factors, fibrinolysis and platelet behavior in postmenopausal women. In Cooke ID (ed): The Role of Estrogen/Progestin in the Management of the Menopause, p 41. Baltimore, University Park Press, 1978

69. Thom M, Chahravarti S, Onam DH, Studd JWW: Effect of hormone replacement therapy on glucose tolerance in postmenopausal women. Br J Obstet Gynecol 84:776, 1977

70. Lauritzen CH: The female climacteric syndrome: Significance, problems, treatment. Acta Obstet Gynecol Scand (Suppl) 51:47, 1976

71. Hammond CB, Maxson WS: Current status of estrogen therapy for the menopause. Fertil Steril 37:5, 1982

72. Adams WP, Hasegawa J, Johnson RN, Haring R: Conjugated estrogens bioequivalence: Comparison of four products in postmenopausal women. J Pharmacol Sci 68:986, 1979

73. Geola FL, Freeman AM, Tataryn IV et al: Biological effects of various doses of conjugated equine estrogen in postmenopausal women. J Clin Endocrinol Metab 51:620, 1980

74. Schiff I: Effects of conjugated estrogens on gonadotropins. Fertil Steril 33:333, 1980

75. Martinez-Manatau J, Rudel HW: Antiovulatory activity of several synthetic and natural estrogens. In Greenblatt RB (ed): Ovulation, p 243. Philadelphia, JB Lippincott, 1969

76. Hammond CB, Soules MR: Clinical significance of estrogen metabolism and physiology. Contemp Obstet Gynecol 11: 41, 1978

77. Deutsch S, Ossowski R, Benjamin I: Comparison between degree of systemic absorption of vaginally and orally administered oestrogens at different dose levels in postmenopausal women. Am J Obstet Gynecol 139:967, 1981

78. Ryan KJ, Engell L: The interconversion of estrone and estradiol by human tissue slices. Endocrinology 52:287, 1953

79. Martin PL, Yen SSC, Burnier AM, Hermann H: Systemic absorption and sustained effects of vaginal estrogen creams. JAMA 242:2699, 1979

80. Rigg LA, Hermann H, Yen SSC: Absorption of estrogens from vaginal creams. N Engl J Med 298:195, 1978

81. Whitehead MI, Townsend PT, Pryse-Davies J et al: Effects of estrogens and progestins on the biochemistry and morphology of the postmenopausal endometrium. N Engl J Med 305:1599, 1981

Infertility

Kamran S. Moghissi
Tommy N. Evans

49

Barren marriages have played an important historical role, affecting the fate of nations and empires. Most women have a strong desire to bear children. Failure to do so may be tragic for some women and can result in unhappiness, marital discord, and ill health. Approximately 10% to 15% of married couples in the United States are infertile.

The terms *sterility* and *infertility* are often used interchangeably. However, *sterility* is better applied to describe the woman who can never become pregnant because of a congenital anomaly, disease, or operation. *Infertility* is used to describe the presumably normal patient who is unable to conceive during a specific period of time, usually 1 year. Primary infertility exists where there has been no prior conception. Secondary infertility may follow one or more previous pregnancies.

In determining the cause of infertility and in treating it, the physician must consider the couple together. Although it is usually the woman who initiates an infertility investigation, simultaneous investigation of the husband is important, a fact that is often difficult for a husband to accept. Approximately one third of barren marriages are due to some defect in the husband, one third to disorders in the wife, and one third to abnormalities in the couple.

Diagnosis of infertility should not be based on an arbitrary period of inability to conceive. Over 60% of fertile couples initiate a pregnancy within 3 months of trying to do so and almost 85% do so within the first 12 months. Approximately 80% of the couples in the United States practice contraception at some period during their marriages. Contraception *per se* probably does not increase infertility, but the incidence of infertility shows a distinct progression with advancing age. The peak of fertility is between 20 and 25 years of age; fertility decreases after 30 in women and after 40 in men. Older couples, although married only briefly, deserve early investigation. Instruction and reassurance may be all that is required. Spermatozoa are in the fallopian tubes during midcycle in healthy young women who experience coitus three times or more weekly without contraception.

Among couples who seek medical aid because of infertility, about 45% subsequently conceive. In another 40%, the cause of sterility is found but cannot be corrected, so pregnancy is impossible. In the remaining 15%, no pregnancy occurs even though there is no detectable cause of infertility. In-depth evaluation of the couple is more likely to detect and correct the causes of infertility.

CAUSES OF INFERTILITY IN THE FEMALE

Female fertility depends upon (1) normal ovarian function, (2) endocrine preparation of a normal uterus for implantation, (3) cervical mucus favorable for sperm transport, (4) normal anatomic development permitting coitus, (5) lack of obstruction, and (6) normal tubal function (Fig. 49-1). Physiologic infertility occurs during that period of the cycle remote from the time of ovulation, during pregnancy, after menopause, and, frequently, during lactation.

Vaginal Abnormalities

Vaginal obstruction to intromission may result from a rigid hymen or a small hymenal orifice. Less commonly, it is due to an intact hymen or congenital abscence of the vagina. Psychogenic vaginismus may also occur. Pregnancy is rarely achieved when the ejaculate is deposited at the vaginal introitus without intromission.

Adequacy of vaginal secretions may be important. Normal vaginal fluid is acid (pH 3–5) and inactivates spermatozoa in a short time. Seminal fluid is alkaline

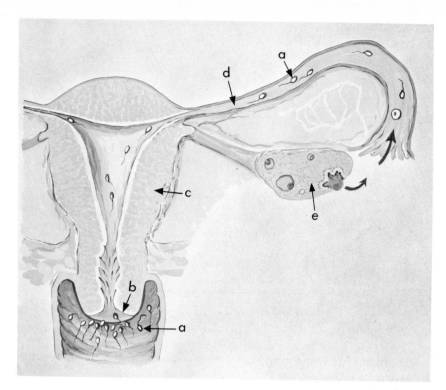

FIG. 49-1. Causes of infertility. (*a*) Defective or inadequate sperm. (*b*) Cervical abnormality. (*c*) Uterine abnormality. (*d*) Tubal abnormality. (*e*) Ovarian abnormality (anovulation).

and, together with cervical mucus and vaginal sweating during sexual excitation, provide a buffering system that renders the pH of the upper vagina more alkaline. Such a medium seems to be essential for normal sperm transport. Vaginitis may cause dyspareunia and reduce fertility. However, conception can occur despite severe vaginal infection.

Cervical Abnormalities

The uterine cervix and its secretions have an important function in reproduction. Cervical mucus is receptive to spermatozoa at or near the time of ovulation and impedes their penetration at other times. The cervix and its mucus secretion also act as a sperm reservoir, protect the sperm cells from the hostile environment in the vagina, filter out abnormal and unsuitable spermatozoa, protect sperm from phagocytes, and may play a role in sperm capacitation. Nutrients found in cervical mucus supplement the energy requirements of spermatozoa.

Cervical mucus is a complex secretion produced by the secretory cells of the endocervix. It contains 92% to 98% water. The principal constituent of cervical mucus is a carbohydrate-rich glycoprotein of the mucin type. Other constituents include serum type proteins, lipids, enzymes, and inorganic salts.

Secretion of cervical mucus is regulated by the ovarian hormones; estrogens stimulate production of copious amounts of watery mucus, while progesterone inhibits and alters the secretory activity of cervical epithelial cells. Many cyclic changes occur in cervical mucus (Fig. 49-2). At midcycle, near the time of ovulation, cervical mucus becomes more profuse, thinner, alkaline, and acellular; it also exhibits a good spinnbarkeit (Fig. 49-3) or stretchability (5 cm or more). Mucus collected near the time of ovulation and dried reveals a characteristic crystallization pattern or ferning on microscopic examination (Fig. 49-4). Progestational agents and pregnancy changes prevent ferning and abolish spinnbarkeit. A viscous plug of inspissated mucus effectively obstructs sperm penetration. Chronic infection of the endocervix may also impair penetration. However, conception can occur, and frequently does, in patients with extensive cervical erosions and chronic cervicitis. Obstetric, thermal, or surgical injuries of the cervix (*e.g.,* lacerations, trachelorrhaphy, amputation, or deep cauterization) may interfere with conception. Hostile cervical mucus may be demonstrated by placing a drop of midcycle mucus on a coverslip with a drop of normal semen adjacent to it (Miller-Kurzrok test). Failure of penetration of the mucus by spermatozoa suggests unfavorable cervical mucus. Other *in vitro* tests, such as the capillary tube test (Kremer test), may provide additional information on the ability of the sperm to penetrate cervical mucus.

Malpositions, such as elongation and anterior placement of the cervix with retrodisplacement of the uterus, advanced uterine descensus, and a pinhole cer-

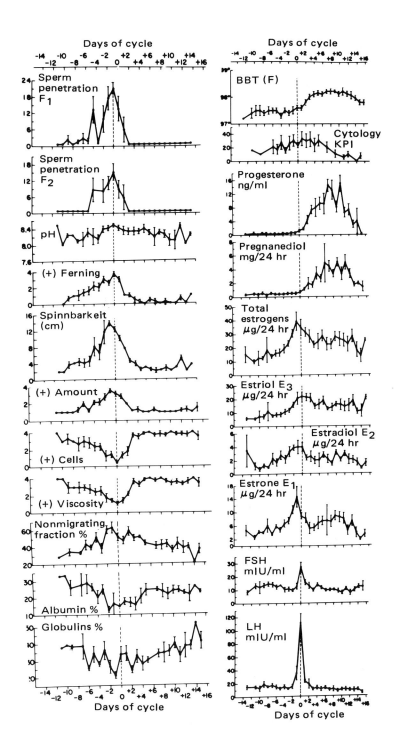

FIG. 49-2. Composite of serum gonadotropin and progesterone levels, urinary estrogen and pregnanediol values, basal body temperature (*BBT*), karyopyknotic index (*KPI*) of vaginal cytology, and cervical mucus properties throughout menstrual cycle in 10 normal women. Day 0 is day of luteotropic hormone (*LH*) peak (*dotted line*). Vertical bars represent 1 standard error of the mean. F_1 and F_2 indicate number of sperm in first and second microscopic fields (×200) from interface, 15 minutes after start of *in vitro* test of cervical mucus penetration by sperm. (Moghissi KS et al: A composite picture of the menstrual cycle. Am J Obstet Gynecol 114:405, 1972)

vical os, may also interfere with conception. Retroversion of the uterus alone is rarely a cause of infertility. Occasionally, the epithelium of the endocervix is totally destroyed as a result of deep conization, extensive or repeated cauterization, or cervical amputation. The resultant dry cervix is not compatible with normal function and may cause infertility.

Uterine Abnormalities

Hypoplasia of the uterus may reflect endocrine disturbance. Prognoses regarding future pregnancy based on uterine size are often in error. With correction of an underlying endocrine imbalance, normal maturation of the uterus may occur.

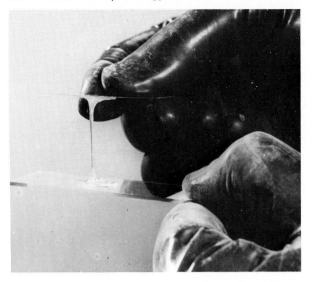

FIG. 49-3. Technique for determining spinnbarkeit (fibrosity) of cervical mucus.

Inadequate progestational stimulation or inadequate secretory response of the endometrium may prevent nidation of the ovum.

Endometritis, particularly the chronic granulomatous type (*e.g.,* tuberculosis), may affect sperm transport as well as implantation of the fertilized ovum. Amenorrhea and intrauterine synechiae (Asherman's syndrome) may result from inflammatory destruction of the endometrium or, more frequently, from uterine curettage during the postpartum period or after incomplete abortion.

Uterine tumors, especially polyps and myomas, may cause infertility by distorting the uterine cavity and producing obstruction. Usually, submucous myomas or large intramural tumors are involved. Interference with vascularity and nutrition of the endometrium may explain infertility associated with myomas even when there is no significant anatomic displacement. Pregnancy may occur after myomectomy unless there is a demonstrable distortion of the uterine cavity or fallopian tubes. However, myomas are often of secondary importance in infertility, since they in turn may be associated with anovulation, hyper- and polymenorrhea, and endometrial hyperplasia. Myomas are not common in young women. They are usually found after the age of 35, a period of declining fertility.

Congenital malformations of the uterus are usually associated with abortion and preterm labor rather than infertility.

Prostaglandins are substances found in large amounts in semen, in both male and female generative tracts, and in many other human tissues. They alter uterotubal activity, but their precise role in sperm transport, ovulation, and fertilization is not yet defined.

Tubal and Peritoneal Abnormalities

Peritubal and periovarian adhesions following peritonitis from appendicitis or from postabortal or puerperal sepsis may interfere wth ovum pickup by the fimbriae of the fallopian tube or obstruct entrance of the ovum into the fimbriated end of the tube. Inflammatory damage may interfere with tubal motility, secretions, and ciliogenesis of the endosalpinx, blocking or interfering with sperm migration and ovum transport. Probably 20% to 40% of female infertility is due to tubal obstruction. This often follows previous salpingitis but may occur secondary to transient tubal spasm or endometriosis. Endometriosis is more common among infertile women. Both ovarian and parovarian tumors can obstruct the fallopian tube and affect ovulation and entry of the ovum into the tube. Rarely, marked elongation and other congenital defects involving the fallopian tubes are responsible for infertility.

FIG. 49-4. (*A*) Typical ferning of cervical mucus at midcycle. (*B*) Incomplete (atypical) ferning during early secretory phase of cycle.

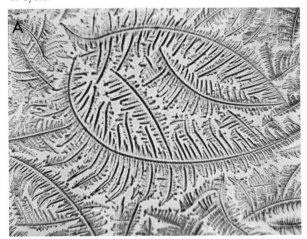

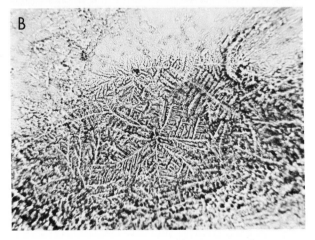

Ovarian Abnormalities

Anovulatory cycles are common during the first few years after menarche and for several years prior to menopause. Otherwise, ovulation usually occurs in women who are menstruating normally and regularly. Approximately 15% to 20% of infertile women have ovulatory defects. Oligomenorrhea and amenorrhea are frequently associated with oligoovulation (infrequent ovulation) or anovulation (lack of ovulation), usually secondary to hypothalamic, pituitary, or ovarian deficits. Less commonly, ovarian tumors, hyper- and hypothyroidism, adrenal dysfunction, and systemic disease prevent ovulation. Even with evidence of continuing ovulation, severely debilitating diseases can lower fertility.

Recent investigations have emphasized the importance of the intrafollicular environment in the regulation of ovulation. The antral fluid of the preovulatory follicle contains relatively large amounts of estradiol and progesterone, low physiologic levels of prolactin, low levels of androgens, and concentrations of LH and FSH that approach 30% and 60%, respectively, of those found in the plasma. Additionally, nonsteroidal ovarian factors such as folliculostatin (inhibin) may play a role. Disturbances of the intrafollicular hormonal environment, such as a decrease in estrogen concentration or an increase in the androgen or prolactin level, may lead to anovulation. Hyperprolactinemia (with or without amenorrhea) and galactorrhea may be associated with anovulation or luteal phase defects. In cases of galactorrhea-amenorrhea, particularly when associated with hyperprolactinemia, pituitary adenoma must be suspected and investigated. Other causes of ovulatory defects may be faulty nutrition, metabolic dysfunction, and psychogenic disturbances.

A variant of the abnormal ovulatory process that leads to infertility is a luteal phase defect. There are several types of luteal phase abnormalities: (1) an inadequate luteal phase that is associated with deficient corpus luteum function and inadequate progesterone production, (2) a short luteal phase, defined as a luteal phase of less than 12 days, and (3) an aluteal phase in which the luteal deficiency is so severe that it may be confused with anovulation. Luteal phase defects may be due to abnormal stimulation of the graffian follicle or to a defective intraovarian milieu, *e.g.*, hyperandrogen states or increased prolactin levels.

Psychogenic Sexual Disturbances

Vaginismus, dyspareunia, and frigidity in the female, and impotence in the male, nearly always are psychogenic. Misapprehension and guilt reactions to normal sexual urges occur. Frequent coitus, masturbation, nocturnal orgasms, and continence have no demonstrable physical ill effects except those secondary to the patient's psychologic reaction. Some patients attribute infertility to lack of libido or orgasm. Although normal sexual response may promote conception, pregnancy does occur without orgasm. Some women who have borne many children deny that they have ever had an orgasm. Dyspareunia and frigidity may be incidental factors when there is no genital disease. Both may reduce fertility by reducing the frequency of coitus. Escape of seminal fluid after coitus probably is of little consequence; only a small amount of seminal fluid in the proper place is required. Furthermore, large numbers of sperm are known to penetrate cervical mucus shortly after ejaculation. Infrequently, apareunia and dyspareunia associated with anxiety and apprehension may be associated with tubal spasm and infertility.

Coitus at 24- to 48-hour intervals during the period of fertility is desirable for conception. Too frequent coitus occasionally impairs fertility, but prolonged abstinence does not necessarily increase fertility.

CAUSES OF INFERTILITY IN THE MALE

Developmental abnormalities such as testicular hypoplasia, cryptorchidism or late descent of the testicles, and testicular dysfunction may cause infertility in the male.

Pituitary gonadotropin stimulates the germinal cells lining the seminiferous tubules to produce spermatozoa and the interstitial cells to secrete androgens. Failure of these functions can result from hypopituitarism and hypothalamic disorders. Spermatogenesis may be deficient or lacking (azoospermia) in an otherwise normal male. Virility and libido are regulated by androgens produced by Leydig cells, are unrelated to sperm production, and are usually unaffected even in azoospermic men. While male fertility often declines after 40, it may persist into old age. Orchitis due to mumps, tuberculosis, syphilis, or other inflammatory disease may alter spermatogenesis. Inflammatory disease of the epididymis and ductus deferens can result in obstructive infertility. Infection of the seminal vesicles and the prostate may alter the quality, volume, and pH of seminal fluid, which serves as a vehicle for spermatozoa and serves other protective and nutritive functions. Gonadal damage resulting from trauma, surgery, or radiation may cause oligospermia or azoospermia. Exposure of the testicle to heat reduces spermatogenesis. Varicocele is not a common abnormality, but it may be associated with infertility. Fertility is sometimes restored after ligation of the spermatic vein. In some cases, tight "jockey shorts" can raise scrotal temperatures sufficiently to impair sperm production.

As in the female, systemic debility and stress in the male may reduce fertility. Occupations may be a contributing factor. Fertility appears to be higher among rural than urban people and among manual laborers than those whose work involves intellectual pursuits. Probably, the difference in age at the time of marriage is more important than the social class distribution. Relative frequency of intercourse may also be a factor. Nutritional status of the male is probably not of major importance except when it is prolonged or associated with some endocrine disturbance, such as hypopituitarism or Fröhlich's syndrome. Certain drugs (alkylating agents, sex steroids, alcohol) depress spermatogenesis, and others (*Rauwolfia* derivatives) can depress libido.

In its contribution to infertility, Klinefelter's syndrome (usually sex chromatin-positive) is comparable to Turner's syndrome or ovarian dysgenesis (sex chromatin-negative) in the female. Degenerative changes in the seminiferous tubules may result from torsion of the testes, herniorrhaphy, or a large varicocele or hydrocele. Strictures involving the ejaculatory apparatus may contribute to infertility. The penile urethra and accessory glands concerned with ejaculation may be underdeveloped. Usually, such underdevelopment is associated with generalized hypogonadism. Hypospadias or the much less common epispadias not only can prevent proper deposition of the seminal fluid but also can dissipate the ejaculatory force.

INVESTIGATION OF THE INFERTILE COUPLE

Any couple who seeks medical aid to accomplish pregnancy deserves attention, regardless of the duration or apparent extent of the problem. Not all such couples require full-scale investigation. Anxiety about imagined rather than real infertility may be the only problem. As a general rule, formal infertility study may be deferred until after about 1 year of ordinary effort to achieve pregnancy. Both husband and wife should undergo tests at approximately the same time, and neither should be subjected to extensive investigation without being aware that comparable information is being obtained about the spouse as the investigation progresses. Early in the investigation, the couple should be apprised of anticipated procedures, duration of investigation, and cost involved. Overall management of the couple by one physician (*i.e.,* gynecologist or reproductive endocrinologist) is encouraged. At least 10 months may be required for investigation, therapy, and evaluation of results.

Detailed medical histories and general physical examinations aid in the exclusion of medical and gynecologic disease associated with infertility. *The medical history of the woman* should include information about (1) the patient's age and duration of infertility; (2) duration of marriage and previous marital and sexual history, including pregnancies; (3) pubertal development; (4) previous inflammatory disease and all prior medical treatment; (5) previous surgery, particularly involving the genitourinary system; (6) previous infertility studies and results; (7) marriage compatibility (elicited by indirect questioning); (8) constitutional and metabolic disease; and (9) duration of contraception and methods employed. *The history of the man* should include information about (1) age; (2) pubertal onset and development; (3) general physical status; (4) previous endocrine disease, gonadal trauma, or exposure to radiation; (5) delay in descent of testicles; (6) previous orchitis or prostatitis; (7) previous genital surgery; and (8) past severe illnesses. Separate questioning of the couple is desirable to permit corroboration and to encourage confidential disclosures. Questioning can also provide information regarding the frequency and technique of coitus and the couple's awareness of the fertile time in the menstrual cycle.

During the interviews, the physician can acquire some idea about the motivation of the couple, as well as their fitness, for parenthood. Physical examination of the wife should include a careful pelvic examination, and that of the husband should include examination of the genitalia for the presence of developmental or organic anomalies. Examination may reveal systemic disease that would contraindicate pregnancy. Consciously or subconsciously, the physician's investigation and treatment may be influenced by such judgments. After the first few office visits, enough information may have been obtained to warrant recommending psychiatric evaluation.

Preliminary tests should include urinalysis, complete blood count, and screening tests for venereal disease, *e.g.,* culture for gonorrhea and serologic test for syphilis, on both wife and husband. Additional laboratory tests such as thyroid function tests (for suspected hypo- or hyperthyroidism); assay of serum androgens; determination of gonadotropin and prolactin values (for amenorrhea or anovulation); and chromosomal studies (for genetic disorders) may be performed when indicated.

Successful diagnosis of the cause of infertility and its proper management depend to a large extent on a well-organized and logical workup of the infertile couple. For the male, the basic infertility survey includes history, physical examination, laboratory tests, and semen analysis. For the female, it involves history; physical examination; laboratory tests; evaluation of the cervix, uterus, tubes, and peritoneum; detection of ovulation; assessment of immunologic compatibility; and evaluation of psychogenic factors. Procedures commonly used in the evaluation of female infertility are

Evaluation of cervix
Assessment of quantity and quality of cervical mucus
Postcoital test of interaction between sperm and cervical mucus
In vitro test of cervical mucus penetration by sperm

Evaluation of uterus
Hysterosalpingography
Endometrial biopsy
Hysteroscopy

Assessment of tubal patency
    Rubin test
    Hysterosalpingography
    Pelvic endoscopy (culdoscopy, laparoscopy)

Assessment of peritoneum
    Culdoscopy
    Laparoscopy

Detection of ovulation
    Recording basal body temperature
    Assessment of quantity and quality of cervical mucus
    Cytologic examination of material from vaginal smear
    Determination of serum progesterone level
    Endometrial biopsy

Evaluation of immunologic compatibility
    Franklin–Dukes test
    Sperm agglutination tests
    Sperm immobilization tests

Many of these procedures must be performed at a specific time of the menstrual cycle. Some of the studies may be combined, and the order in which they are performed can be altered for the convenience of the patient or to suit specific circumstances.

Semen Analysis

Even in a sophisticated laboratory, semen analysis provides only a rough measure of the functional ability of sperm. When infertility is persistent, semen analysis should always be repeated. The usual procedure is to obtain at least two or three semen analyses at 2- to 3-week intervals in order to establish a pattern for various

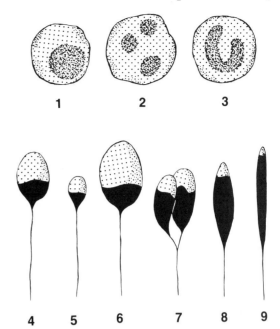

FIG. 49-5. Morphologic variations of spermatozoa. (*1, 2*) Immature cells. (*3*) White blood cell (for comparison with immature cells). (*4*) Oval sperm (normal). (*5*) Small (microcytic) sperm. (*6*) Large (macrocytic) sperm. (*7*) Double-headed (bicephalic) sperm. (*8, 9*) Tapering forms.

semen characteristics. A specimen obtained shortly after intercourse may be deceptively low in sperm count. Semen collected in a clean wide-mouth container either by masturbation or coitus interruptus after two to five days continence usually permits an accurate evaluation. A condom should not be used for semen collection, since most condoms are treated with spermicidal chemicals that interfere with sperm viability. For those males who are unable to provide a sample by masturbation, an untreated seminal collection device (HDE Corporation, Mountainview, California) is available. The specimen should be kept at room or body temperature and examined within 1 hour. Table 49-1 shows the information that is usually contained in a semen analysis report. The morphologic variations in spermatozoa are shown in Figure 49-5.

There is no general agreement on a standard quality of semen consistent with fertility. Obviously, a high sperm count, good motility, and a large percentage of normal sperm in an ejaculate that liquefies promptly and is devoid of exogenous cells, debris, immature sperm cells, and agglutination all increase the likelihood of subsequent pregnancy. It is difficult to evaluate the fertility potential of a specimen in which one or several parameters are below average, however. Even with counts below 10 million, provided other semen characteristics (motility and morphology) are not grossly abnormal, pregnancy may occur.

Table 49-1
Standard Semen Analysis

Parameter	Average Values
Consistency	Fluid (after liquefaction)
Color	Opaque
Liquefaction time	≦20 min
pH	7.2–7.8
Volume	2–6 ml
Motility (grade 0–4)	≦50%
Count (millions/ml)	20–100
Viability (eosin)	≦50%
Morphology (cytology) cell types	≦60% normal oval
Cells (white blood cells, others)	None to occasional
Agglutination	None
Biochemical studies (*e.g.,* fructose, prostaglandins, zinc), if desired	

To assess more accurately the fertility potential of sperm, attempts have been made to assay certain sperm acrosomal enzymes, such as acrosin, that are concerned in the fertilization process and to study sperm fertilizing capacity. In the latter technique, the ability of spermatozoa to initiate *in vitro* fertilization of zona-free hamster eggs is used as an index of their fertilizing potential. These experimental methods, although not yet available for routine clinical use, indicate the need for more refined techniques to assess male fertility potential.

Volume of less than 1 ml and a total count of less than 50 million are usually associated with infertility, but neither excludes the possibility of impregnation. Except in rare instances, aspermia is uncorrectable. Sometimes a surgically removable obstructive lesion coexists with normal spermatogenesis, but this is not true aspermia. Testicular biopsy aids in the diagnosis of normal spermatogenesis associated with obstructive azospermatosis. Seminal deficiency may be attributed to hypopituitarism, nutritional deficiency, debilitating illness, metabolic disease, trauma, radiation, gonadotropic inadequacy, obstructive lesions of the epididymis and the vas deferens, and congenital defects such as Klinefelter's syndrome. Determination of serum testosterone value, gonadotropin assays, and testicular biopsy may be required individually or collectively to arrive at the cause of male infertility. An elevated FSH level (above 40 m IU) is usually indicative of testicular failure and would be a contraindication to further therapy in the male.

Evaluation of the Cervix

Survival of spermatozoa within the reproductive tract of the female depends on their prompt penetration of the cervical mucus. Interaction between cervical mucus and sperm is determined by the Sims-Huhner (postcoital) test, which consists of examination of mucus aspirated from the cervical canal two to eight hours following coitus near the time of ovulation. The quantity and quality of cervical mucus (spinnbarkeit, ferning, viscosity, cellularity, and pH) are evaluated. When cervical mucus is suitable and the semen of good quality, there should be at least 10 to 15 sperm per highpower field in a specimen of endocervical mucus six to eight hours after coitus. This finding (a positive result) suggests normal cervical mucus with adequate estrogenic response, a potentially fertile husband, and satisfactory coital technique. Presence of less than 5 active sperm per highpower field (a negative result) is indicative of oligospermia, unsuitable cervical mucus, or faulty coital practices. In the latter instance, a repeat test after a shorter interval following intercourse is recommended.

A postcoital test alone is not sufficient to assess male fertility and should not replace semen analysis. Occasionally, vaginitis and cervicitis cause an erroneous interpretation of this test. A negative result on the Sims-

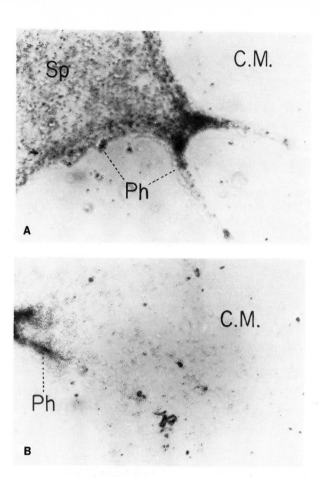

FIG. 49-6. *In vitro* test of cervical mucus penetration by sperm. Phalanx (*Ph*) formation. Spermatozoa (*Sp*) fanning out from apex of phalanges and penetrating cervical mucus (*CM*). (Moghissi KS et al: Mechanism of sperm migration. Fertil Steril 15:15, 1964)

Huhner test should be followed by an *in vitro* test of cervical mucus penetration by sperm using either the slide test (Fig. 49-6) or capillary tube test. A recent development is the availability of standardized bovine estrus cervical mucus (PeneTrak, Sorono Diagnostics, Braintree, Massachusetts) to test in the laboratory the ability of the sperm to penetrate normal cervical mucus. Bovine cervical mucus is biophysically and biochemically similar to human cervical mucus and is readily penetrated by human sperm.

On rare occasions, the presence of antisperm antibodies in cervical mucus may cause immobilization of sperm in cervical mucus.

A dry cervix with no evidence of mucorrhea at midcycle and cervical stenosis is usually associated with a history of trauma (conization, cauterization, or amputation). The diagnosis is easily made by inspection of the cervix. Hematometra may be associated with severe cervical stenosis.

Evaluation of the Uterus

Anatomic abnormalities of the uterus are usually recognized by pelvic examination. For a precise diagnosis, hysterography is often required. Polyps, submucous myomas, uterine synechiae, and congenital deformities are recognized by hysterography (Fig. 49-7). Hysteroscopy using fiberoptic equipment may be useful in the recognition of intrauterine disorders.

Examination of an endometrial biopsy (Fig. 49-8) obtained at the end of the luteal phase is an integral part of an infertility survey. Its purpose is not only to confirm ovulation, but also to assist evaluation of corpus luteum function. Morphologic dating of endometrium should coincide with the day of the cycle on which the specimen was obtained (Fig. 49-9). An immature or out-of-phase endometrium is incompatible with normal fertility and indicates inadequacy of corpus luteum function or improper end-organ response.

Assessment of Tubal Patency

Tubal patency can be assessed by the passage of gas or contrast material through the cervix, uterine cavity, and fallopian tubes. Another method is direct endoscopic visualization of indigo carmine solution escaping from the fallopian tubes after injection through a uterine cannula. Simultaneous observation of the pelvic structures by means of culdoscopy, colpotomy, or laparoscopy can be of adjunctive value. Probably the safest time to carry out a tubal patency test is following menstruation and before ovulation, since at this time there is no risk that a fertilized ovum will be displaced.

FIG. 49-7. Hysterosalpingograms. (*A*) Normal uterus and fallopian tubes with peritoneal spill. Note outline of ovarian beds and leakage into proximal part of vagina. (*B*) Loculation of contrast material in inflammatory pockets at distal ends of tubes. (*C*) Didelphic uterus with double vagina. (*D*) Large filling defect in uterine cavity due to submucous myoma. Note incomplete tubal filling and absence of peritoneal spill.

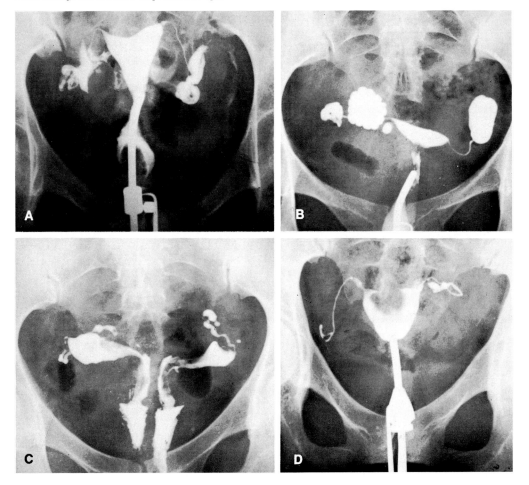

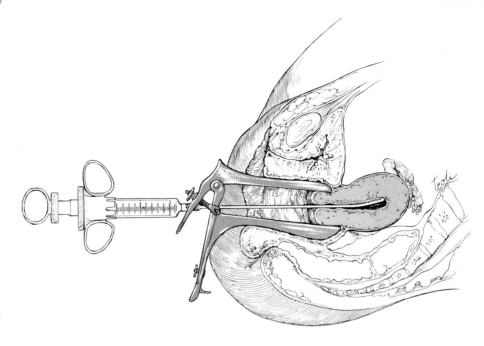

FIG. 49-8. Technique of endometrial biopsy with Novak suction curet.

Rubin Test

The Rubin test involves insufflation of the uterus and tubes with carbon dioxide under pressure after a tightly fitting cannula has been inserted into the cervical os. This test is associated with a relatively high rate of false negative and false positive results and has been abandoned by most physicians.

Hysterosalpingography

Hysterosalpingography is discussed in Chapter 61. Congenital malformations of the uterus and distortions produced by submucous myomas and endometrial polyps can be visualized by this technique. Also, the exact points of obstruction can be identified, and the feasibility of tubal reconstruction assessed. Radiopaque contrast material, such as iodized oil or a water-soluble material, is injected and its dispersion visualized by roentgenography. An abnormal diffusion pattern suggests previous pelvic inflammatory disease with residual peritubal and periovarian adhesions.

Hysterosalpingography may be of therapeutic as well as diagnostic value. The reason for this is uncertain. Pregnancy following hysterosalpingography has been attributed to a therapeutic effect of the iodine in the contrast material, to the penetration of filamentous tubal adhesions, and to the stimulating effect of x-radiation.

Hazards of Tubal Patency Tests

Extreme pain and patient anxiety may necessitate carrying out tubal patency tests under anesthesia. However, this is seldom necessary and, indeed, severe pain and anxiety should probably be the signal to discontinue the test. Carbon dioxide gas rather than air should be used for the Rubin test, as fatal air embolism has been reported when air was used. Embolism with contrast material may also occur but seldom is associated with morbidity. Both the Rubin test and hysterosalpingography can ignite a subacute pelvic inflammatory process. Specific anaphylactic reactions to contrast material (*e.g.*, iodine sensitization) may occur. After the use of iodized oil, penetration of uterotubal vessels with subsequent microembolization in the lungs and granulomas in the fallopian tubes and endometrium have been reported. Abortion can result from a tubal patency test during pregnancy; however, many pregnancies have survived such procedures. A tubal patency test is probably contraindicated within 24 hours of the end of the menstrual period, immediately after uterine curettage, following recent pelvic inflammatory disease, and during pregnancy.

Pelvic Endoscopy

Although pelvic endoscopy was established at the turn of the century, widespread use of procedures for visualizing the pelvic and abdominal viscera did not become popular until sophisticated endoscopic devices were developed. Modern optical systems, such as high-intensity fiberoptic light sources, have greatly enhanced the safety and popularity of pelvic endoscopy for detection of causes of infertility and other pathologic conditions.

Pelvic endoscopy is indicated when hysterosalpingography suggests tubal or peritoneal abnormality and the patient fails to become pregnant, when ovarian disease or endometriosis is suspected, and when a com-

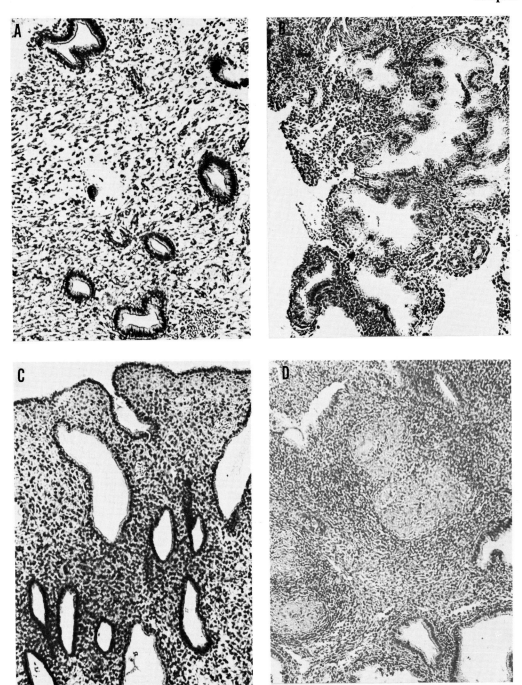

FIG. 49-9. Endometrial biopsies. (*A*) Proliferative phase with low gland epithelium and central nuclei. (*B*) Secretory phase with compact stroma, round cell infiltration, and convoluted or sawtooth glands with basal nuclei. (*C*) Proliferative pattern in biopsy obtained during anovulatory cycle three days before menstruation. (*D*) Tuberculous endometritis in infertile patient with epithelioid tubercles with Langhans' giant cells and round cell infiltration.

plete infertility survey reveals no abnormality. In a significant proportion of patients in the latter category, endoscopy reveals unsuspected tubal or ovarian disease, such as endometriosis and peritubal adhesions. Pelvic endoscopy is mandatory before certain surgical operations such as tuboplasty, conservative operations for suspected endometriosis, or wedge resection of ovaries for polycystic ovarian disease (Stein-Leventhal syndrome). Wedge resection is now rarely required, since ovulation usually can be induced with clomiphene citrate or sequential gonadotropins.

Laparoscopy

The technique is described in Chapter 63. The procedure is usually performed with the patient in the modified lithotomy position and under general anesthesia. An insufflation cannula is placed in the cervix to be used for uterine manipulation and for the subsequent injection of indigo carmine dye to test tubal patency. After a special needle has been inserted through an infraumbilical incision, the peritoneal cavity is distended with several liters of carbon dioxide or nitrous oxide. A trocar is then introduced, and a fiberoptic laparoscope placed through the trocar shield. This permits a detailed examination of pelvic as well as other abdominal structures (Fig. 49-10). Introduction of a probe through a second incision facilitates manipulation of the uterus, ovaries, and fallopian tubes. Patency of the fallopian tubes can be evaluated by injecting an indigo carmine solution through the insufflator and any area of obstruction identified. The procedure also enables the operator to sever adhesions, fulgurate endometrial implants, obtain ovarian biopsies, and perform other minor procedures.

FIG. 49-10. Schematic view of pelvic structures as observed through laparoscope.

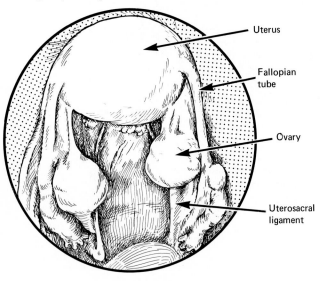

Uterus

Fallopian tube

Ovary

Uterosacral ligament

Detection of Ovulation

Development of new techniques of hormone assay has led to more accurate methods of ovulation detection and prediction. The only direct proof of ovulation is pregnancy or recovery of an ovum from the fallopian tube. All other tests are either indirect or presumptive (see Fig. 47-2). The most practical methods for assessing ovulation are (1) basal body temperature (BBT) recordings (Fig. 49-11); (2) examination of daily vaginal smears; (3) demonstration of characteristic changes in the cervical mucus (increase in volume and spinnbarkeit; decrease in viscosity with fern formation near ovulation, followed by decrease in amount, disappearance of ferning, and spinnbarkeit; and increase in viscosity and cellularity during the luteal phase); and (4) evidence of secretory change in endometrial biopsies obtained during the latter part of the luteal phase. Mittelschmerz and midcycle spotting are only presumptive evidence of ovulation and are not reliable.

Vaginal smears show a high maturation or karyopyknotic index coinciding with the time of ovulation. Occasionally, vaginal cytology can be difficult to interpret because similar changes are associated with anovulatory follicular maturation.

Radioimmunoassay demonstrates a surge of serum luteinizing hormone (LH) in midcycle, and ovulation is believed to occur usually within 24 hours after the LH peak. Serum and urinary estradiol values reach a peak approximately 1 day before the LH surge. Both serum progesterone and urinary pregnanediol (a metabolite of progesterone) levels begin to rise with ovulation and reach a peak about 1 week later (see Fig. 49-2). A single assay of serum progesterone performed during the midluteal phase may provide presumptive evidence of ovulation without indicating the actual time it occurred.

Endometrial biopsy is an office procedure that usually can be performed with minimal or no analgesia just before or at the onset of menstruation. Typical secretory change in an endometrial biopsy obtained just before or at the onset of menstruation is presumptive evidence of ovulation (see Fig. 49-9). Endometrial histology can be misleading if the patient has ingested a progestogen which produces secretory changes comparable to those associated with ovulation. Endometrial biopsy is also used by most clinicans for the diagnosis of luteal phase defect. For this purpose, the biopsy should be obtained just before or at the onset of menses and histologically dated.

Immunologic Incompatibility

The possibility that immune mechanisms may be responsible for some cases of infertility has provoked intense study in recent years. These relationships are considered in Chapter 12. Relevance of the agglutination tests to immunologic infertility has been questioned,

A

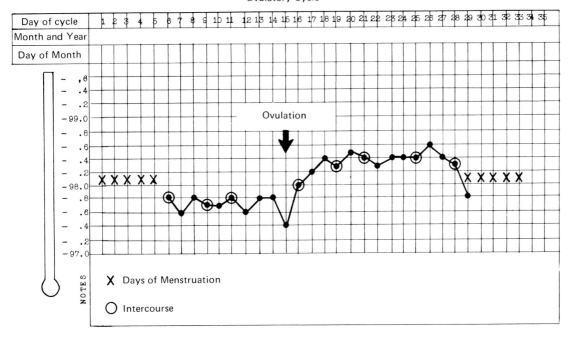

B

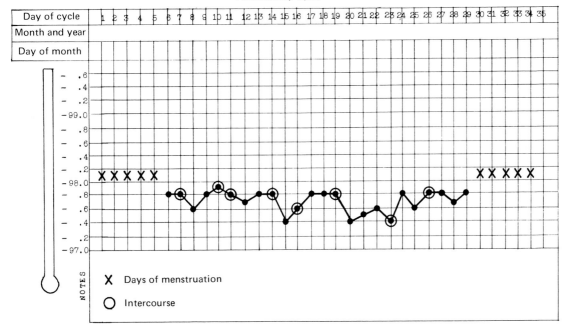

FIG. 49-11. Basal body temperature records suggesting (*A*) ovulatory and (*B*) anovulatory cycles. As a rule, intercourse on day 16 (*A*) would be expected to be fruitful; but, as is shown here, this is not always the case.

since it has been shown that the active serum protein fraction causing head-to-head agglutination in this test system may be a steroid-binding β-lipoprotein (Fig. 49-12).

TREATMENT

After the investigation of both husband and wife has been completed, a specific therapeutic program can be outlined. If no abnormalities have been found, the couple may need only information with respect to the probable time of ovulation and appropriate coital technique and frequency. When abnormalities have been detected, treatment should be directed toward the correction of specific disorders. Improvement of general health, correction of obesity, and avoidance of stress, extreme fatigue, excessive smoking, and alcohol consumption should be emphasized.

Treatment of the Male

Genetic and anatomic disorders may lead to severe oligo- or azoospermia. The prognosis is poor if spermatogenesis does not occur or is inadequate. Deficient sperm in the seminal plasma secondary to obstruction of the vas deferens or epididymis can sometimes be corrected surgically. Prevention of male infertility is abetted by early surgical or endocrine treatment of cryptorchidism and appropriate prophylaxis or treatment of orchitis. In recent years, several therapeutic modalities have evolved to correct disorders of spermatogenesis caused by hypothalamic-pituitary malfunction with occasional success. These include (1) administration of testosterone (100–200 mg weekly for 3–4 months), which usually results in a decrease in sperm count followed in some instances by rebound or subsequent increase; (2) administration of clomiphene citrate, to which a patient with a reduced or low-normal output of gonadotropic hormone may show a favorable response; (3) administration of human chorionic gonadotropin (hCG) to stimulate endogenous testosterone production; (4) administration of human menopausal gonadotropin (hMG) and hCG as a source of follicle-stimulating hormone (FSH) and LH when clomiphene citrate therapy has been unsuccessful or when a selective gonadotropin deficiency is demonstrated. Consistent improvement has not been observed with any one of these therapeutic regimens. This is in part due to the lack of knowledge of the process of spermatogenesis and inability to evaluate and diagnose intratesticular derangement, particularly in cases of so-called idiopathic oligospermia.

The single most important advance in the field of male infertility during the last two decades has been recognition of varicocele as a cause of oligospermia and asthenospermia. High ligation of the internal spermatic vein in a patient with varicocele and a sperm count consistent with the condition may be followed by improvement in sperm motility and other parameters of semen

FIG. 49-12. Sperm agglutination. (*A*) In rabbit serum containing antibodies to human sperm. (*B*) In human serum containing sperm-agglutinating and sperm-immobilizing antibodies.

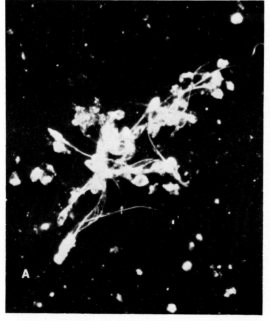
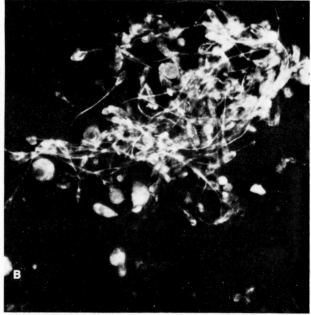

quality. In patients with varicocele, recent studies suggest that, within an average of eight months after the operation, a pregnancy rate of approximately 40% to 50% may be expected.

Glucocorticoid therapy for male infertility is justified only in those patients with a frank endocrinopathy, such as adrenal hyperplasia. Thyroid preparations administered to a euthyroid male are of no value. Recently some pregnancies have been reported to result from *in vitro* fertilization of oocytes by sperm from oligospermic males. In this procedure, semen samples containing about half a million healthy, motile sperm may be sufficient to bring about fertilization and pregnancy.

Treatment of the Female

Treatment of Cervical Abnormalities

When a properly timed postcoital test produces a negative result, penetrability of cervical mucus should be investigated by placing ovulatory mucus on a glass slide adjacent to a specimen of semen and examining the mucus-sperm interaction under the microscope (Miller-Kurzrok test). Alternatively, sperm migration may be observed in a capillary test tube. To determine whether cervical mucus or sperm is abnormal, sperm of known fertility and donor ovulatory mucus may be used in cross testing.

Lack of sperm in cervical mucus in an otherwise normal couple may be due to dyspareunia, apareunia, or, occasionally, severe cervical prolapse. Appropriate management of these conditions should restore fertility.

Chronic endocervicitis is best treated with systemic administration of antibiotics after cultures have identified the responsible organism.

Hostile cervical mucus may reflect inadequate estrogenic stimulation, inadequate response of the cervical epithelium, or anovulation. Cervical mucus in these instances remains viscous and somewhat cellular with low spinnbarkeit and atypical ferning. A mildly acid pH may persist throughout the cycle. These abnormalities can usually be overcome by the administration of 0.1 mg stilbestrol or 10–20 μg ethinyl estradiol daily from day 7 through day 15 of the cycle. In patients with documented anovulation or abnormal ovulation, induction of normal ovulatory cycle is usually associated with mucorrhea and improved quality of cervical mucus. Efforts to make the vaginal environment more favorable for spermatozoa by precoital alkaline douching are of dubious value.

When cervical mucus abnormalities are not responsive to the above treatments or when cervical epithelial secretory function is destroyed (*e.g.,* after conization or amputation of the cervix), intrauterine insemination may result in pregnancy. In this procedure, the semen sample is centrifuged and the spermatozoa are washed, suspended in a special buffer, and injected into the uterine cavity.

Treatment of Uterine Abnormalities

Congenital anomalies of the uterus, such as bicornuate or septate uterus, that are associated with infertility or repeated abortion may be treated surgically by means of a unification procedure (metroplasty). Endometrial polyps can easily be removed by dilatation of the cervix and curettage. Uterine synechiae (Asherman's syndrome) are best treated by surgical debridement through a hysteroscope, insertion of an intrauterine device, and estrogen therapy. Myomectomy may be warranted when hysterosalpingography or hysteroscopy demonstrates tumor encroachment on the uterine cavity or fallopian tube ostia, provided other causes of infertility have been excluded.

Inadequate luteal endometrial phase or inadequate progestational preparation of the endometrium may be improved by the use of ovulation-inducing agents or postovulatory cyclic progesterone therapy.

Chronic endometritis due to tuberculosis or other infections requires appropriate antibiotic and chemotherapeutic management.

Anterior displacement of the retroverted uterus with a Smith-Hodge pessary may rarely be effective when the elongated cervix of a retroposed uterus is far removed from the seminal pool or when the male semen volume is small.

Treatment of Fallopian Tube Disease

Unilateral or bilateral tuboplasty to remedy obstruction may be indicated when other causes of infertility have been ruled out. Endoscopic examination of the tubes and other pelvic structures to evaluate the nature and extent of tubal disease should precede tuboplasty.

At the time of operation for tubal obstruction, salpingolysis may be indicated if peritubal adhesions are present. During the past few years, considerable progress has been made in tubal surgery. Improved operative techniques, including the use of inert material such as polyglycolic sutures, and microscopic or other magnifying devices, have significantly increased the success rate of reconstructive tubal operations. With the use of microsurgical techniques for salpingoplasty, pregnancies have been reported in as many as 60% of patients. In the presence of advanced tubal pathology, however, even these techniques yield poor results. Patient selection is of critical importance in successful tubal surgery.

Salpingostomy is reserved for fimbrial occlusion. If the obstruction is medial and the fimbriae normal, surgical correction by reimplantation of the patent portion of the tubes into the uterus or by an end-to-end anastomosis may be feasible. Implantation of the ovary into the uterus (Estes' operation) is probably ill-advised; it is associated with an increased risk of uterine rupture, and the few pregnancies that have occurred after such an operation have rarely gone to term.

In the presence of minimal tubal abnormality (*e.g.,*

fimbrial stenosis), hydrotubation (repeated intrauterine instillation of a hydrocortisone solution during the follicular phase of the cycle) has been suggested but is of doubtful value.

Recently, the technique of *extracorporeal (in vitro) fertilization* has been advocated as a last resort for patients whose fallopian tubes have been completely destroyed or removed but who have a normal uterus and at least one functioning ovary. The technique is rather involved and consists of (1) stimulating ovulation to induce the development of several follicles, (2) harvesting ova at the time of ovulation by laparoscopy or by ultrasound–directed probes, (3) *in vitro* fertilization in a special culture medium, (4) culture of the fertilized egg until the blastula reaches the 4- to 8-cell stage, and (5) transcervical implantation of the embryo into the uterine cavity. The procedure is currently being performed in many university and medical centers in the United States and other countries. In the largest and best-established centers, successful induction of pregnancy in 20 to 25% of patients has been reported. This procedure is one of the most rapidly advancing fields of reproductive medicine and opens a new avenue for research and patient management. It is anticipated that with increasing experience and better understanding of the technology for the oocyte recovery, fertilization, and implantation processes, the pregnancy rate will improve.

Treatment of Anovulation

In the presence of anovulatory cycles with or without amenorrhea, the diagnostic approaches outlined in Chapter 46 are applicable to the management of infertility. Judicious management of ovulation failure requires the establishment of the precise cause of anovulation by means of hormone assays, and other diagnostic procedures.

CLOMIPHENE CITRATE. A synthetic compound related to chlorotrianisene (TACE), clomiphene citrate is a weak estrogen. It is indicated for the treatment of ovulatory failure when there is evidence of follicular function with adequate endogenous estrogen production but no cyclic stimulation by pituitary gonadotropin. Clomiphene is a potentiator of gonadotropin, which causes an increase in ovarian secretion of estrogen. Peripherally, this compound has antiestrogenic properties. An intact hypothalamic–pituitary–ovarian axis, even though functionally inadequate, is necessary for the drug to act.

In properly selected cases, clomiphene citrate is successful in inducing ovulation in approximately 70% followed by pregnancy in 40%. It is the drug of choice for the treatment of anovulation due to polycystic ovarian disease (Stein–Leventhal syndrome), oligoovulation, post-pill amenorrhea, and in some cases of amenorrhea-galactorrhea. Patients with premature menopause, ovarian dysgenesis, or pituitary destruction are not responsive to clomiphene citrate.

A usual course of clomiphene citrate consists of a dose of 50 mg once or twice daily for five days (a total of 250–500 mg) starting on the fifth day of the cycle. (Larger doses of clomiphene have been used when there are specific indications and when the usual regimen has failed to induce ovulation.) In the presence of amenorrhea and a normal level of estrogen, endometrial bleeding is provoked by progesterone, 100 mg intramuscularly on two successive days, or medroxyprogesterone acetate (Provera), 10 mg daily for seven days. Clomiphene citrate is then started on the fifth day after the bleeding starts. During the administration of clomiphene, there is at first a transient rise in circulating gonadotropins, followed quickly by a return to normal. Approximately one week following the conclusion of the five-day course of treatment, there is a dynamic burst in circulating gonadotropins to levels characteristic of ovulation. Hence, the optimum time for intercourse is five to ten days after completion of the five-day course. Up to six courses may be required.

The gonadotropin burst that attends the use of clomiphene citrate acts as a marked stimulus to the ovaries, and significant ovarian enlargement and multiple ovulations may result. Ovarian enlargement is rarely troublesome; but, in a sensitive patient, it can be sufficient to cause pain, ovarian hemorrhage, torsion, or rupture. It is therefore important that a pelvic examination be performed before every course of clomiphene citrate, and immediately if abdominal pain occurs. If the ovaries are found to be enlarged, clomiphene citrate should be discontinued until there is complete regression; subsequent doses should be smaller than those that produced the enlargement. If marked ovarian enlargment occurs, large doses of an oral contraceptive will cause rapid regression.

Side effects of clomiphene citrate occur with sufficient frequency that the patient should be warned of them. She should be instructed to call the physician immediately if she experiences abdominal pain, severe bloating or fullness, or the "chair syndrome" (pain on sitting down in a chair). Other bothersome, but usually less serious, side effects include hot flashes, depression, transient photophobia and blurring of vision, breast discharge, and mastalgia.

If ovulation has not occurred after six courses of clomiphene citrate, several other devices may be tried: (1) the LH surge resulting from clomiphene citrate may be supplemented by administration of hCG (a single intramuscular dose of 5000–10,000 IU, on the 7th day after completion of five days of clomiphene citrate); (2) if the pretreatment endogenous estrogen level is judged subnormal, a salutary effect may be achieved by administration of conjugated estrogens (1.25 mg daily) for ten days before a five-day clomiphene citrate course and hCG 7 days after the course of clomiphene citrate is completed; (3) if this fails after three courses, and no untoward effects have been observed up to this time, the clomiphene citrate dose may be increased to a maximum of 50 mg four times daily for five days (1000 mg) followed seven days later by a single injection of hCG; (4) if no pregnancy follows, clomiphene citrate may be abandoned and the use of hMG considered.

HUMAN MENOPAUSAL GONADOTROPIN. hMG (Pergonal) is a potent preparation that causes intense stimulation of the ovaries. Its use is not without hazard; hyperstimulation and multiple ovulations may result, and special precautions and special facilities for the appraisal of its effects are mandatory. The only indication for the use of hMG as primary treatment without prior trial of clomiphene citrate is pituitary failure or ablation confirmed by the lack of endogenous gonadotropins.

Contraindications to the use of hMG include (1) a high level of endogenous FSH, indicating primary ovarian failure; (2) overt thyroid or adrenal dysfunction; (3) an intracranial tumor, *e.g.,* pituitary tumor; (4) abnormal uterine bleeding of undetermined cause; and (5) any cause of infertility other than anovulation.

Women vary widely in their sensitivity to hMG. Even the same woman may demonstrate variable sensitivity during different treatment cycles. The therapeutic objective is to stimulate the ovary so that follicular maturation occurs and to produce estrogens in amounts equivalent to those normally present in the immediate preovulatory phase. Exactly at this point (not before, not after), the administration of 10,000 IU hCG as a single injection or in divided doses over two to three days usually results in ovulation. HCG is derived from the urine of pregnant women and produces an effect similar to the midcycle LH surge in the normal cycle.

Because of the variable response, the time at which the appropriate level of estrogen production will occur cannot be anticipated. Frequent, preferably daily, tests must be made to determine estrogen levels. Cervical mucus ferning, spinnbarkeit, and the nature of the vaginal smear can provide adequate evidence of response in early phases of the induction, but they are not sufficiently precise for evaluation of the hMG response in the late follicular phase. An acceptable method is to monitor the patient's response until 4+ ferning of the cervical mucus is achieved. Thereafter, daily assay of total urinary estrogens or serum estradiol levels is required. In the normal 28-day ovulatory cycle, the value for total urinary estrogens averages 60 μg–70 μg/24 hours, with normal variations from 20 μg–100 μg.* HCG is administered immediately when the total urinary estrogen value reaches 100 μg/24 hours. Ovulation usually follows one or two days after the hCG injection. Serum estradiol assays may be used in lieu of urinary estrogens to monitor the hMG effect.

HMG is supplied in ampules containing 75 IU FSH and an equal amount of LH. A workable schedule is to

* The level of urinary estrogens varies with the methods used and from one laboratory to another. Each laboratory should establish its own norms.

administer one ampule each day for three successive days; if the urinary estrogen level is less than 50 μg/24 hours, two ampules each day may be given for the next three days, and the amount similarly increased every three days until the urinary estrogen level is 50 μg–100 μg/24 hours or serum estradiol reaches 500–1000 μg/ml (exact levels depend upon the type of assay). Then hMG is discontinued and hCG administered. It is hazardous and usually futile to persist if pregnancy has not been achieved after three such courses. A recent addition to the technique of monitoring follicular development is the assessment of the number of mature follicles and their diameter by a sector scan ultrasound. Ideally, a single dominant follicle with a diameter of 18 mm to 22 mm should be observed before the administration of hCG. Many centers now use a combination of estrogen assay and ultrasound monitoring for induction of ovulation with hMG–hCG.

In addition to daily assessment of total urinary or serum estrogen level, vaginal examinations should be performed daily and cervical mucus or vaginal cytology studied. Moderate enlargement of the ovaries occurs in 7% to 10% of patients. Most cases of significant enlargement of the ovaries, sometimes with ascites, and most cases of multiple pregnancy occur when the total urinary estrogen level rises to 100 μg–200 μg/24 hours or serum estradiol level exceeds 1000 pg/ml. Rapid enlargement of the ovaries sometimes begins during hMG treatment, but maximum ovarian stimulation occurs seven to ten days after ovulation (hCG administration). If the ovaries are palpably enlarged during treatment, hMG should be stopped; if they are palpably enlarged at the end of the hMG course, hCG should not be given (Fig. 49-13).

BROMOCRIPTINE. Bromocriptine (Parlodel) is a dopamine receptor agonist and activates postsynaptic dopamine receptors. The drug is a semisynthetic peptide alkaloid and is believed to act by stimulating the release of prolactin-inhibiting factor from the hypothalamus, thus regulating the release of prolactin from the anterior pituitary. Bromocriptine itself is also a potent inhibitor of the synthesis and release of prolactin by the pituitary gland, although it has little or no effect on other pituitary hormones. Bromocriptine is indicated for the treatment of anovulation associated with hyperprolactinemia with or without the galactorrhea–amenorrhea syndrome (Fig. 49-14). It may also be effective in patients who have luteal phase deficiency resulting from hyperprolactinemia. When there is no demonstrable pituitary tumor, bromocriptine therapy initiates ovulatory menstrual cycles and suppresses galactorrhea in about 75% of anovulatory patients with galactorrhea–amenorrhea (Fig. 49-15).

Patients selected for bromocriptine therapy should be screened carefully for pituitary adenoma. Only those found to have an elevated prolactin level (above 20 ng/ml) should be considered for treatment. The usual dosage is 2.5 mg to 7.5 mg/day taken with meals

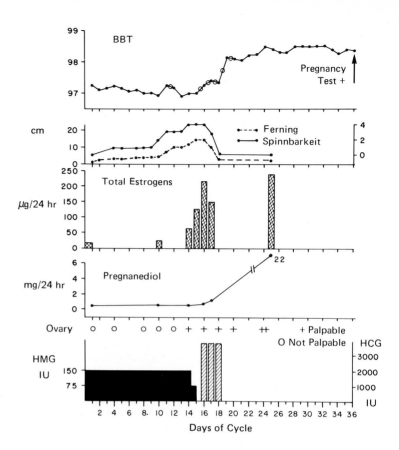

FIG. 49-13. Induction of ovulation with hMG and hCG, leading to single fetus pregnancy and normal term delivery. This patient had primary amenorrhea and did not respond to clomiphene citrate. Induction cycle was monitored by urinary estrogen assay.

in divided doses until normal ovulatory menstrual cycles are established. Duration of treatment should not exceed six months. It is recommended that treatment be initiated with 2.5 mg daily and be increased to therapeutic doses within the first week. Adverse reactions in decreasing order of frequency include nausea, headache, dizziness, fatigue, abdominal cramps, nasal congestion, and constipation.

GONADOTROPIN-RELEASING HORMONE (GNRH). Gonadotropin releasing hormone (GnRH) is a synthetic decapeptide that causes the release of FSH and LH from the anterior pituitary gland. However, continuous administration of GnRH brings about a suppression and exhaustion of pituitary gonadotropes and results in the phenomenon of "down-regulation." Experimental studies have shown that when GnRH is administered in a pulsatile fashion (10–15 μg every 90 minutes) through a miniaturized pump, ovulation may be induced in properly selected patients and pregnancies will result. GnRH is particularly suitable in patients with hypothalamic amenorrhea and anovulation. Preliminary clinical experience indicates that pregnancy rates with this drug may be similar to that with hMG–hCG.

WEDGE RESECTION OF OVARIES. Bilateral ovarian wedge resection is reserved for the rare patient with polycystic ovary disease who does not respond to clo-

miphene citrate or gonadotropin therapy. The operation may adversely affect fertility by inducing postoperative adhesion.

OTHER MODES OF TREATMENT. Both hyper- and hypothyroidism may be associated with anovulatory cycles. Correction of thyroid dysfunction usually produces ovulation unless the disorder has been of long duration.

Hydrocortisone and its derivatives induce ovulation in women with hyperfunction of the adrenal cortex or those with a deficiency of enzymes involved in adrenal steroidogenesis (*e.g.,* a 21-hydroxylase defect).

Treatment of Immunologic Infertility

The only available treatment for infertility caused by sperm-agglutinating or sperm-immobilizing antibodies consists of an attempt to reduce the antibody titer in the woman's reproductive tract by use of condoms for six to twelve months. Pregnancy may occur when use of condoms is discontinued. The effectiveness of this treatment has not been critically evaluated. (See Chap. 12) The use of large doses of glucocorticoids (prednisolone) in patients with sperm antibodies has been suggested, but their effectiveness has not been adequately documented.

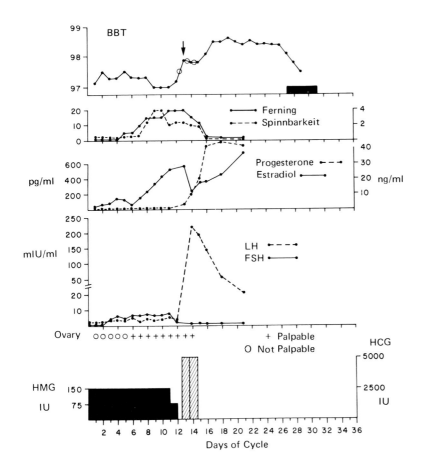

FIG. 49-14. Induction of ovulation with hMG and hCG. This patient had primary amenorrhea and was unresponsive to clomiphene citrate. Induction cycle was monitored by radioimmunoassay of serum estradiol levels. Note biphasic BBT and rise of serum progesterone after hCG administration, indicating ovulation.

Artificial Insemination

Artificial insemination may be accomplished using either the husband's sperm (AIH, homologous insemination) or semen from a donor (AID heterologous insemination).

Homologous insemination is rarely successful when the cause of infertility cannot be determined or when there is sperm deficiency. Artificial techniques are hardly an improvement over normal coitus unless there is some developmental anomaly preventing intromission or normal ejaculation. Hypospadias and epispadias may be indications. Other rare indications include dyspareunia, impotence, a displaced cervix far from the seminal pool in the posterior vaginal fornix, small seminal volume (less than 1 ml), and retrograde ejaculation.

A special technique that has produced relatively encouraging results is that of split-ejaculate insemination. The husband is instructed to supply a semen sample, after 2 days abstention, by masturbation into two separate containers. The first portion of the ejaculate usually contains 75% of all spermatozoa and may be used for insemination. The procedure is particularly useful in patients who have a large semen volume, liquefaction defects, or sperm motility disorders.

Insemination with donor semen is still controver-

sial. There are many religious and legal implications. Both husband and wife should unequivocally support heterologous insemination before it is considered by the physician. If either has reservations about it, such a procedure is contraindicated. It is preferable that the initial proposal come from the couple rather than the physician. Arguments against artificial insemination with donor semen are (1) reactions of the couple to a child thus produced are not predictable, (2) the legal status of the child is uncertain, (3) it sometimes is difficult to be certain that the husband is and will remain sterile, (4) it contravenes some religious precepts, and (5) the child may be disinherited at the whim of the husband. Nevertheless, artificial insemination with donor semen is rapidly becoming more common, and pioneering efforts are being made in some states to legalize artificial insemination and to legitimize the status of the babies conceived in this manner.

Before insemination, the following should be determined: (1) the probable time of ovulation, (2) tubal patency, (3) lack of a medical contraindication to pregnancy, and (4) evidence that the patient is not already pregnant. Within 1 hour of collection, a few milliliters of semen are drawn into a sterile syringe, and 0.5 ml to 1 ml is instilled within the cervical canal. The remainder of the specimen is sprayed over the cervix and into the

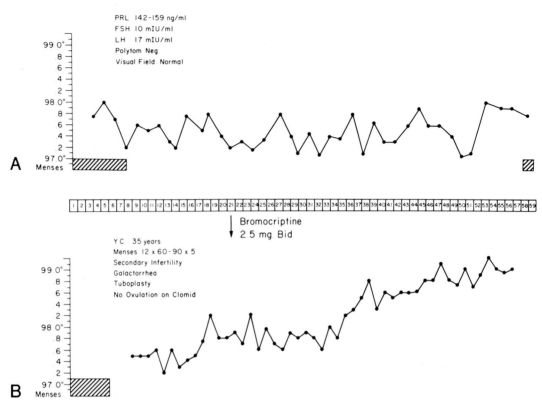

FIG. 49-15. Induction of ovulation and pregnancy with bromocriptine in an anovulatory woman with hyperprolactinemia. (*A*) Anovulatory cycle characterized by monophasic basal body temperature. (*B*) Ovulation and pregnancy (elevation and sustained rise of basal body temperature resulting from bromocriptine therapy).

proximal vagina. Insemination of unwashed sperm within the uterine cavity may precipitate uterine contractions and expulsion of the semen. The donor should be carefully selected with respect to race, blood type compatibility, physical appearance, general health, and genetic background. Anonymity must be preserved.

UNEXPLAINED INFERTILITY

Unexplained, or idiopathic, infertility refers to the failure of a couple to conceive in whom no definite cause for infertility can be identified. The average incidence of unexplained infertility is approximately 15% among infertile couples who have been thoroughly evaluated. Since these patients are under considerable emotional distress, they deserve special consideration. The salient features of management of these patients consist of (1) assessment of previous infertility studies to detect any

omission or misinterpretation, (2) reevaluation of those factors that may have changed since initial studies, and (3) initiation of studies to detect uncommon causes of infertility, *i.e.*, immunologic infertility, luteal phase defect, and defects in sperm fertilizing ability.

Psychotherapy

Psychotherapy helps some infertile couples. Occasionally, serious psychogenic problems are not apparent on the surface and can be fathomed only after repeated consultation. The couple's motivation is important. Becoming pregnant may be obsessional from the time it is first suspected that pregnancy is not possible. Need for ego support and proof of sexual identification may underlie the desire for pregnancy. After intensive infertility investigation and treatment followed by a single pregnancy, some women practice contraception indefinitely or even request sterilization.

PROGNOSIS

Some patients become pregnant in spite of, not because of, the investigation and treatment employed. This fact dictates caution in interpretation of the efficacy of specific therapeutic procedures. Prolonged and piecemeal therapy can produce considerable emotional harm, create serious tensions, and even disrupt the marriage. Tact is needed when informing a couple about the prognosis for future pregnancy. Unless the husband is a castrate or the wife has undergone hysterectomy, it is probably ill-advised to tell any couple that a successful pregnancy is impossible.

The prognosis for infertility patients, in general, has considerably improved in the last decade. Depending on the cause or causes of infertility, pregnancy will occur in 30% to 70% of couples who have been adequately evaluated and treated.

ADOPTION

When pregnancy seems improbable, adoption may be proposed by the couple. It should be suggested only indirectly by the physician. The suitability of the couple for parenthood with respect to physical and economic status, as well as emotional stability must be considered. Women are generally more enthusiastic about adoption than are their husbands. Contrary to general belief, adoption of a baby probably does not enhance fertility.

REFERENCES AND RECOMMENDED READING

Beer A, Neaves WB: Antigenic status of semen from the viewpoint of the female and male. Fertil Steril 39:3, 1978

Behrman SJ: Artificial insemination. Clin Obstet Gynecol 22: 245, 1979

Belsey MA, Eliasson R, Gallegos AJ et al: Laboratory Manual for Examination of Human Semen and Semen-Cervical Mucus Interaction. Geneva, World Health Organization, 1980

Cohen MR: Laparoscopy, Culdoscopy and Gynecography. Philadelphia, WB Saunders, 1970

Corson SL: Use of the laparoscope in the infertile patient. Fertil Steril 32:359, 1979

Edwards RG, Steptoe PC: Current status of *in vitro* fertilization and implantation of human embryos. Lancet 2:1265, 1983

Garcia CR, Mastroianni L: Microsurgery for treatment of adnexal disease. Fertil Steril 34:413, 1980

Hafez ESE, Evans TN (eds): Human Reproduction—Conception and Contraception, 2nd ed. Hagerstown, Harper & Row, 1980

Horwitz ST: Laparoscopy in gynecology. Obstet Gynecol Surv 27:1, 1972

Jones GS: Luteal phase insufficiency. Clin Obstet Gynecol 16: 255, 1973

Lobo RA, Gysler M, March CM et al: Clinical and laboratory predictors of clomiphene response. Fertil Steril 37:168, 1982

MacLeod J: Human male infertility. Obstet Gynecol Surv 26: 335, 1971

Miller DS, Reid RR, Cetel NS et al: Pulsatile administration of low dose gonadotropin releasing hormone. JAMA 250: 2937, 1983

Moghissi KS: The function of the cervix in human reproduction. Curr Probl Obstet Gynecol vol 7, March 1984

Moghissi KS (ed): Current concepts in infertility. Clin Obstet Gynecol 22:9, 1979

Moghissi KS, Sacco AG, Borin K: Immunologic infertility. I. Cervical mucus antibodies and postcoital test. Am J Obstet Gynecol 136:941, 1980

Moghissi KS, Syner FN, Evans TN: A composite picture of the menstrual cycle. Am J Obstet Gynecol 114:405, 1972

Moghissi KS, Wallach E: Unexplained infertility. Fertil Steril 39:1, 1983

Shulman JF, Shulman S: Methylprednisolone treatment of immunologic infertility in the male. Fertil Steril 38:591, 1982

Siegler A: Hysterosalpingography. Fertil Steril 40:139, 1983

Steinberger E, Rodriguez-Rigau LJ: The infertile couple. J Androl 4:111, 1983

Sweeney WJ: Pitfalls in present day methods of evaluating tubal function: II. Hysterosalpingography. Fertil Steril 13:124, 1962

Taymor ML: Evaluation of anovulatory cycles and induction of ovulation. Clin Obstet Gynecol 22:145, 1979

Wallach EE: Evaluation and management of uterine causes of infertility. Clin Obstet Gynecol 22:43, 1979

Wu CH: Monitoring of ovulation induction. Fertil Steril 30: 617, 1978

The Urinary Tract as It Is Related to Gynecology

J. Andrew Fantl

50

The clinical involvement of the gynecologist in the management of disorders of the bladder and urethra stems from the nature of gynecologic practice. The genital and lower urinary tracts in females cannot be artificially separated, since they are closely related anatomically and physiologically. Dysfunctions and diseases of the lower urinary tract represent 5% to 6% of the reasons for gynecologic consultations. Pathology of bladder or urethra may produce genital symptoms and vice versa. It is the purpose of this chapter to review those aspects of bladder and urethral pathology most commonly encountered by gynecologists.

ANATOMIC AND PHYSIOLOGIC CONSIDERATIONS OF THE FEMALE BLADDER AND URETHRA

Embryology

The bladder and urethra are derived from an endodermal structure, the cloaca. A mesodermic ventral growth, the urorectal septum, divides the cloaca into the urogenital sinus (ventral) and the rectum (dorsal). The proximal segment of the urogenital sinus becomes the vesicourethral canal, which forms the bladder and proximal urethra. The distal segment of the urogenital sinus differentiates into pelvic and phallic portions. The pelvic portion becomes the remainder of the urethra, periurethral glands, and lower vagina, while the phallic portion develops into the vestibule in the female (Fig. 50-1). These relationships are considered in more detail in Chapter 5.

Anatomy

The bladder is a hollow, muscular viscus located behind the symphysis pubis and covered only superiorly and anteriorly by peritoneum. Its muscle is a meshwork of interdigitating smooth muscle fibers and is referred to as the *detrusor*. There is controversy as to whether the detrusor ends at the vesicourethral junction or whether inner fibers are continuous with the inner longitudinal muscle layer of the urethra. The meshwork distribution of the muscle fibers of the detrusor suits its function. Its contraction results in a coordinated simultaneous reduction of all the diameters of the bladder. The trigone is a distinct portion of the bladder identified between both ureteric orifices and the bladder neck. It is of mesenchymal origin, and its muscular wall is continuous with that of the ureters. Superficial and deep trigonal muscle layers are recognized. The superficial one continues into the posterior urethral wall while the deep one does not.

The female urethra is a 4-cm to 4.5-cm long tubular structure that communicates the bladder to the exterior. It is located under the symphysis pubis and pierces the pelvic diaphragm anterior to the vagina. The urethral walls contain smooth and striated muscle fibers as well as elastic and connective tissue. A rich submucosal vascular plexus is present. An internal longitudinal and an external circular smooth muscle layer have been described, but there is no well-defined circular smooth muscle sphincter at the proximal urethra. The origin, disposition, and relationship of the striated urethral musculature is controversial. Modern investigators indicate that a well-defined striated muscle sphincter is present within the urethral wall. This sphincter is located primarily in the midurethra and is thicker anteriorly. Its fibers are independent and separate from the periurethral musculature, which represents medial fibers of the levator ani muscle. The urethral mucosa is transitional (urothelium) and squamous epithelium. The latter responds to hormone stimulation and is seen primarily in the distal third of the urethra. Compound racemose glands are present in the posterolateral wall of the distal

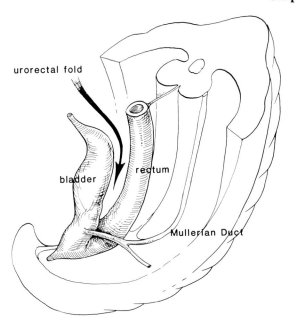

FIG. 50-1. Urogenital sinus is separated from the rectum by the urorectal fold.

urethra. They open into the urethral lumen or into the vestibule around the external meatus. The proximal urethra is supported by fibromuscular condensations (*pubourethral ligaments*) that attach the proximal urethra to the posterior aspects of the symphysis.

Neurology

Central and peripheral nervous systems are responsible for the appropriate neurologic control of bladder and urethral function. Specific cortical, pontine–mesencephalic, and cerebellar centers have been described. Details of their function are beyond the scope of this chapter but can be summarized as facilitating or inhibiting medullary reflexes. Both autonomic and somatic peripheral nervous systems participate in the innervation of bladder, urethral, and periurethral musculature. The detrusor receives primarily cholinergic innervation, whereas the bladder neck and urethra have predominantly adrenergic receptors. The urethral striated sphincter and the periurethral musculature are independently innervated by somatic fibers (Fig. 50-2). Sensory impulses from the bladder and urethra are proprioceptive (tension) or exteroceptive (pain, temperature, touch). Proprioceptive impulses originate in receptors present in collagen fibers around muscular fibers. Exteroceptive impulses originate in free nerve endings that are present in the submucosa and mucosa. Proprioception travels toward the sensory cortex in the posterior column accompanied by the sensation of touch. Pain and temperature sensations ascend by means of the spinothalamic tract.

Function

The bladder and urethra should be considered a functional unit. Two phases of lower urinary tract function can be described: the storage phase of urine collection and the micturition phase of urine evacuation. During storage, the urine excreted by the kidneys is transported through the ureters to the bladder, where it is collected. The rate of urine production varies with fluid intake as well as with physiologic, environmental, and psychologic factors. The urine fills the bladder intermittently, and the detrusor adapts to the increased volume without significant intravesical pressure increment. This phenomenon is called *accommodation*. During the collection phase, the detrusor of the normal continent adult does not contract. This characteristic is referred to as *detrusor stability*. It is an acquired behavior and is absent at birth and early infancy. A newborn empties its bladder periodically through involuntary detrusor contractions triggered by critical volumes. Stability of the detrusor results from behavioral learning (toilet training), which inhibits spontaneous bladder contractions and renders the detrusor stable. Cortical inhibitory impulses acting over sacral reflexes are thought to represent the neurologic mechanism that results in detrusor stability. During storage, the urethra acts in its entirety as the sphincter of the bladder. Such sphincteric function maintains the pressure in the urethra higher than in the bladder. The urethral resistance at rest (intrinsic) is the result of the action of its various anatomic components. The striated musculature, the smooth musculature, and the fibrolastic tissue together with the vascular plexus contribute to a similar extent to the urethral resistance. During exertion, intra-abdominal pressure increases and is transmitted to the bladder. Such an increase in vesical pressure challenges the sphincteric competence of the urethra. Two protective mechanisms augment urethral resistance during exertion: pressure transmission capacity and striated muscle contraction. The first is based on transmission of intra-abdominal pressure to the proximal urethra and occurs as long as the bladder neck remains above the pelvic diaphragm. The second is a reflex contraction of the urethral striated sphincter and periurethral striated musculature and is triggered by an abrupt increase in intra-abdominal pressure (*e.g.,* cough, sneeze).

The micturition phase is represented by a series of events leading to the complete emptying of the bladder's contents. Voiding occurs normally when a set of circumstances is given. These are related to the sensation of bladder fullness, convenience of time, place, and environment. The act of micturition is voluntary, and in this regard the detrusor represents the body's only smooth muscle organ under volitional control. The adult not only has command over the motor (contractile) activity of the detrusor but also can voluntarily suppress sensory inputs from the bladder. The ability to inhibit the need to void until convenient time and place is familiar to all. Voiding results from the establishment of

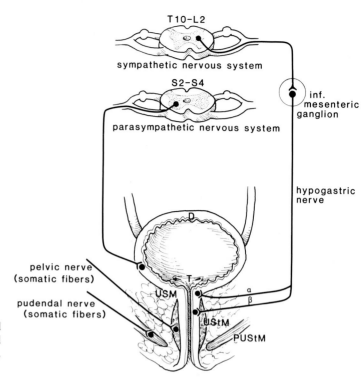

FIG. 50-2. Schematic representation of the peripheral innervation of the lower urinary tract. *USM,* urethral smooth muscle; *UStM,* urethral striated muscle; *PUStM,* periurethral striated muscle; *D,* detrusor; *T,* trigone.

a pressure gradient now higher in the bladder than in the urethra. Intravesical pressure rises as a result of a detrusor contraction, and intraurethral pressure decreases because of active urethral relaxation. On occasion, voluntary abdominal contraction occurs independently or in conjunction with the detrusor contraction. Rarely, voiding occurs solely as a result of urethral relaxation.

TERMINOLOGY

To allow appropriate clinical interpretation of symptoms, signs, and laboratory testing, terminology should be specific. For many years, clinicians and investigators have been handicapped by lack of consensus in the terms used. Recently, through efforts of organizations such as the International Continence Society and the Urodynamic Society, more uniformity in definitions and terms has been reached. Some of these are discussed in this section.

Symptoms

Urinary frequency indicates the episodes of voluntary micturition occurring between rising and falling asleep (diurnal frequency). It is variable in the normal population and can be influenced by such factors as fluid intake, psychologic stress, and environmental changes. Most adults void between six and eight times while

awake. The perception of change probably has more clinical significance than the actual number of micturitions. Central nervous system as well as renal parenchymal disorders may alter urinary frequency and should also be considered when evaluating this symptom.

Nocturia represents voiding as a result of being awakened from sleep by the desire to empty the bladder (nocturnal frequency). Nocturia increases with age and may have little significance in the elderly. Patients with difficulty sleeping or other medical conditions may be awakened from sleep because of pain or for other reasons not representing nocturia. Increased nocturnal diuresis may result in nocturia and can be caused by chronic renal or cardiac disease.

Urgency indicates a strong desire to void and is usually described as the sensation that voiding is imminent and unavoidable. On occasion, patients refer to concomitant suprapubic or perineal pain. Urinary urgency may be associated with a detrusor contraction (motor urgency), or it may represent solely a sensory symptom (sensory urgency).

Dysuria indicates painful urination. It is usually perceived as a burning sensation during micturition. One should differentiate "urethral" from "vulvar" dysuria. In the first instance pain arises from urethral tissues, whereas in the latter the discomfort is caused by contact of urine against affected vulvar skin.

Hematuria refers to the presence of blood in the urine. In some cases the blood is a contaminant, and catheterization is needed to be certain that it arises from the urinary tract. The presence of 1 to 5 red blood cells per high-power field is not necessarily abnormal and usually needs no inquiry unless there are urinary tract symptoms or findings. The presence of microscopic hematuria of more than five red blood cells per high-power field is termed *microhematuria* and indicates a need for formal urologic evaluation.

Urinary incontinence is defined as "a condition in which involuntary loss of urine is a social or hygienic problem and is objectively demonstrated." Adult females may suffer occasional involuntary urine loss without significantly impairing their social or occupational activities. On the other hand, minimal incontinence may affect persons with specific conditions of employment or social environment. Ultimately, it is the impact of the incontinence on the person that dictates the clinical significance of the condition. Differences in sociocultural characteristics and hygienic standards should call for specific clinical judgment of each case. Objective demonstration of incontinence is necessary to establish the diagnosis. Urinary incontinence may be confused with excessive vaginal or urethral discharge or even with excessive perineal perspiration. Cases have occurred in which incontinence was used for psychologic or financial gain.

Stress incontinence is a symptom, not a condition. It indicates the occurrence of involuntary urine loss in association with physical exertion. Various mechanisms can be responsible for the symptom of stress incontinence.

Urge incontinence represents a symptom complex. It indicates the occurrence of involuntary urine loss in association with the symptom of urgency. It is described as urgency just prior to or simultaneous with the episode of incontinence. Like stress incontinence, urge incontinence does not represent a disease or condition but constitutes a symptom that may be present in various clinical situations.

Physical Examination

A gynecologic examination should not be considered complete unless the lower urinary tract has been evaluated. The urethral meatus and anterior vaginal wall become visible and accessible to palpation with the use of a Sims' speculum (Fig. 50-3*A*). If the patient is requested to strain, the degree of anterior vaginal wall relaxation can be properly ascertained. Anterior relax-

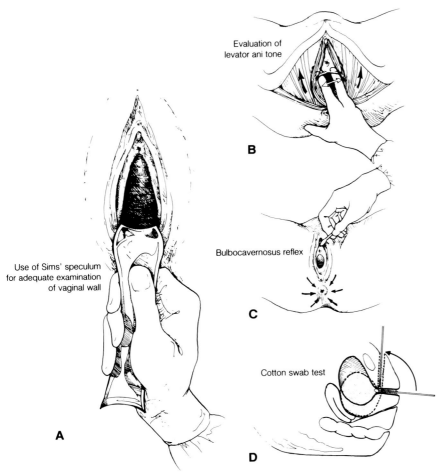

Evaluation of levator ani tone

Use of Sims' speculum for adequate examination of vaginal wall

Bulbocavernosus reflex

Cotton swab test

A   B   C   D

FIG. 50-3. (*A*) Use of a Sims' speculum allows for proper assessment of anterior and posterior vaginal walls. (*B*) Pelvic muscle tone can be ascertained by requesting the patient "squeeze" while the examiner palpates the margins of the levator ani. (*C*) Integrity of the sacral reflex S2-4 can be determined by eliciting the bulbocavernosus reflex. Gentle clitoral stroke should produce anal sphincter contraction. (*D*) Mobility of a cotton swab inserted in the urethra determines axial mobility during straining.

ation may or may not represent a cystocele. A cystocele in itself does not predispose to recurrent urinary tract infections unless urethral kinking induces obstruction. Palpation and stripping of the urethra is an often neglected step. Urethral secretions, induration, pain, or cystic or solid masses may be discovered and lead to or confirm a suspected diagnosis. Bimanual examination may disclose a distended bladder or help in its identification as the source of pelvic pain. Rectal examination should be routine in any gynecologic examination. Decreased or absent anal sphincter tone may be present in neuropathic conditions. Fecal impaction can represent a reversible cause of urinary incontinence due to obstruction and overflow. The levator muscle tone (Fig. 50-3*B*), integrity of the sacral reflex S2–4 (Fig. 50-3*C*), and degree of urethral mobility (Fig. 50-3*D*) can be easily determined.

Laboratory and Urodynamic Evaluations

Urine Analysis and Bacteriologic Assessment

Urine analysis and urodynamic evaluations represent the most common urinary tract evaluations performed in gynecologic practice. The analysis of urine and microscopic evaluation of its sediment provide a variety of information, but their most common application is in the evaluation of infection. Urinary tract infection encompasses a spectrum of diseases the common denominator of which is the microbial invasion of the urinary tract. *Pyuria* refers to the presence of five or more white cells per high-power field or centrifuged urine. It indicates inflammation, which may or may not represent infection. Pyuria without urinary tract infection can be observed in cases of genital infection, urinary stones, or conditions leading to tissue necrosis. When persistent pyuria remains unexplained, special cultures should be taken for fastidious organisms and for tuberculosis.

Bacteriologic Assessment

Urinary tract infection almost always results in bacterial colonization of the urine; this is referred to as *bacteriuria.* Because bacteriuria may be the result of contamination during collection or storing, the concept of *significant bacteriuria* was introduced. Quantification of bacteriuria is accomplished by counting colonies of bacteria per milliliter of urine. When the urine is collected by the clean-catch, midstream technique, 100,000 (10^5) or more colonies per milliliter indicate significant bacteriuria. This is a statistical concept. A colony count of 10^5 or more bacteria per milliliter has 80% probability of representing a urinary tract infection. Two consecutive observations of significant bacteriuria increase the probability of infection to 96%. Colony counts of less than 10,000 organisms per milliliter of urine have a 98% chance of representing contamination, whereas counts of 10,000 to 100,000 indicate infection in approximately 5% of cases. Lesser counts may be clinically significant when specimens are obtained transurethrally, but any growth is significant if suprapubic aspiration is used. Sources of error in quantitative bacteriologic assessment of urine include improper collection or storage, equipment contamination, vigorous diuresis, frequent voiding, urinary acidification, complete obstruction, or concomitant antimicrobial therapy. One should be flexible in the clinical interpretation of colony counts; consideration should be given to symptomatology and collection technique as well as to bacteriologic characteristics.

A cotton swab used to obtain a Gram stain and culture from the meatus provides an opportunity to evaluate the characteristics of organisms and cells present in the distal urethra. The female urethra always harbors bacteria in its distal end and as much as 50% of the time in its proximal end. Saprophytic bacteria are most common, but pathogenic organisms such as *Escherichia coli* may be recovered. *Chlamydia trachomatis* and *Mycoplasma hominis* may also be cultured from the urethra. Such organisms may on occasion be responsible for lower urinary tract infections with no evidence of significant bacteriuria. Trichomonads may be identified on a wet mount. Their presence is frequently but not always associated with vaginal infestation. Although *Neisseria gonorrhoeae* may be cultured from the urethra, it is more commonly recovered from the cervical canal. Cytologic evaluation of cells present at the external meatus allows evaluation of hormonal status. A cellular count determining the percentage of superficial, intermediate, and parabasal cells provides an index of estrogenic effect on the urethra.

Urinary Cytology

The cells present in bladder washings or fresh midstream urine can be fixed and evaluated for malignant changes. Experience in cytologic screening is needed, since only minimal differences may be present between benign and malignant transitional cells.

Endoscopy

Visualization of the urethral and bladder walls (urethrocystoscopy) is invaluable in the clinical investigation of the lower urinary tract. The mucosa of the urethra and bladder can be evaluated for tumors, bleeding sites, inflammation, foreign bodies, diverticula, or fistulas. Under appropriate anesthesia and operating room conditions, tissue biopsies can be obtained through surgical endoscopes. Endoscopy of the bladder and urethra is a delicate procedure demanding training and experience.

Cystometry

Cystometry evaluates the behavior of the bladder during filling. It provides information on bladder sensation, detrusor stability, and the relationship between intravesical pressure and bladder volume (compliance). Various methods of performing this evaluation have been described. They vary as to the route and medium of bladder filling as well as the sophistication of the pressure recording system. Abnormalities of bladder sensation have been noted in patients with peripheral neuropathy (diabetes) or neurologic disease (multiple sclerosis). Surgical denervation (radical hysterectomy) or cord trauma may also result in altered bladder sensation. Detrusor instability may be transient or chronic. Neuropathic or inflammatory conditions as well as urethral obstruction may be the cause. In females usually there is no demonstrable reason. Low compliance is usually noted when normal distensibility of the bladder wall is affected (radiation cystitis).

Urethral Pressure Profile

The urethral pressure profile evaluates urethral sphincter function, which can be evaluated at rest (passive urethral pressure profile) and during exertion (dynamic urethral pressure profile) (Fig. 50-4).

FIG. 50-4. (*A*) Passive urethral pressure profile. Simultaneous pressure recording of intraurethral and bladder pressure allows for the determination of the urethral closure pressure by electronic subtraction. *MUCP,* maximal urethral closure pressure; *FUL,* functional urethral length. (*B*) Dynamic urethral pressure profile. Determination of the urethral closure pressure during coughing. The closure pressure proximal to the maximal urethral closure pressure does not become negative during forceful coughing. This usually indicates urethral sphincter competence.

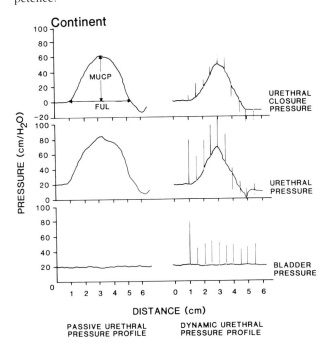

Uroflowmetry and Pressure Flow Studies

Uroflowmetry and pressure flow studies investigate the emptying phase of lower urinary tract function. Uroflowmetry allows for the determination of the volume of urine expelled through the urethra per unit of time. If intravesical, intraurethral, and intra-abdominal pressures are monitored simultaneously, pressure flow studies are obtained. In addition, striated muscular activity can be determined through simultaneous electromyography of the pelvic floor.

Although urodynamic assessments provide specific objective measurements of lower urinary tract function, clinical judgment must always be used when interpreting results. Most patients seen in gynecologic practice do not need complex urodynamic assessment, but physicians should be familiar with the available techniques as well as the information they can provide and the indications for their use.

DISEASES OF THE URETHRA

Caruncle

A urethral caruncle is a polypoid reddish lesion present at the external meatus. It is commonly seen in postmenopausal women and although usually asymptomatic may lead to pain, bleeding, and dysuria. The cause is unknown but may be related to hypoestrogenism. Histologically, it represents granulation tissue with a hemangioma-like vascular pattern. Diagnosis should include histologic confirmation if the lesion bleeds or ulcerates or if there is notable enlargement between examinations. Estrogen or symptomatic treatment may be sufficient but excision is sometimes necessary.

Mucosal Prolapse

Prolapse of the urethral mucosa presents as a dusky reddish lesion encompassing the entire circumference of the external meatus (Fig. 50-5). It sometimes occurs in children five to ten years of age but is primarily observed in postmenopausal women. Clinically, the lesion is not painful, but symptoms include bleeding, dysuria, and a clear watery discharge. Although insidious onset is common, the lesion may appear abruptly after an injury or an episode of severe, repetitive coughing. Biopsy may be necessary for diagnostic confirmation. On occasion, thrombosis may occur and the mucosa may become secondarily infected. Symptomatic mucosal prolapse may be treated by excision, cauterization, or suture amputation.

Urethral Trauma

Lacerations, transections, or even partial or total destruction of the urethra may occur as a result of accidents, placement of foreign bodies, urethral coitus, or surgical

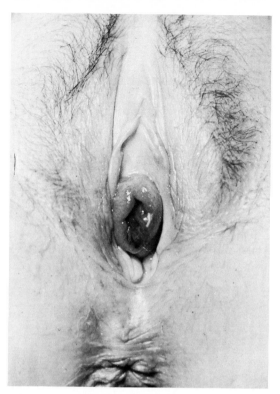

FIG. 50-5.   Urethral mucosal prolapse. (Haines M, Taylor CW: Gynaecological Pathology. London, Churchill, 1962)

injury. The degree, location, and extension of the injury should be carefully determined, if necessary through radiography or urethroscopy. Treatment will vary with the location and extent of the injury. Simple bladder drainage or suturing may be all that is needed for uncomplicated lacerations. More complex injuries may need reconstructive surgery or implantation of an artificial sphincter.

Polyps

Inflammatory polyps of the proximal urethra or bladder neck are usually not true polyps, but rather inflammatory mucosal tags. They have been associated with chronic inflammation of the urethra or bladder, but their significance is not known. Usually no treatment is required. A true benign polyp of the distal urethra is differentiated clinically from the caruncle by the color of the urethral mucosa, its mobility, and its long stalk. Tissue diagnosis is required for confirmation. Management includes treatment of the underlying infection and resection or cauterization of the polyp.

Urethral Stricture

A stricture is a constriction of the urethra that leads to mechanical obstruction. Strictures are usually fibrous bands located at the external meatus. Most are the result

of chronic urethritis and periurethritis, but they may also be observed in association with urethral diverticula. Midurethra or bladder neck strictures are rare and result usually from surgery (postdiverticulectomy). The syndrome is that of recurrent urinary tract infection, sensation of incomplete voiding, residual urine, and low flow rate. Urethral dilatation with concomitant treatment of an infective or atrophic process is the management of choice. Meatal fibrous rings may be treated by external urethrotomy.

Urethritis

The term *urethritis* indicates urethral inflammation that is usually produced by urethral infection. Symptoms include urinary urgency, frequency, nocturia, hesitancy, and, on occasion, dyspareunia. Palpation of the urethra produces pain, and urethral stripping may sometimes produce a purulent secretion. Gram-negative bacteria, which are responsible for most bladder infections, may affect the urethra concomitantly. The gonococcus does not characteristically affect the bladder, but it can infect the urethra. Other microorganisms that may affect the urethra and periurethral glands include fastidious organisms (prolonged incubation with 7% CO_2), *C. trachomatis, M. hominis,* and trichomonas. Unless clinical and laboratory precautions are taken to identify these organisms, the diagnosis will not be confirmed. Viral infection may also occur in the urethra. Herpetic lesions can affect the meatus or its vicinity. Condylomata acuminata may be found isolated in the urethra, but most commonly they are associated with similar genital lesions and tend to clear when the genital lesions are adequately treated. Urethral inflammation may also be caused by trauma (during intercourse) or by chemicals such as deodorants, detergents, and soaps (*e.g.,* bubble bath). Hypoestrogenism can induce urethral inflammatory changes (atrophic urethritis). For many years, the term *urethral syndrome* was used as a "catch-all" diagnosis for patients who presented with symptoms of urethrocystitis but whose standard urinary bacteriology revealed nonsignificant bacterial growth. Many such cases would now be diagnosed as one of the specific infections described above. In some patients a specific diagnosis is never made, in which case the condition is referred to as *sensory urgency syndrome.* Identification of the organisms involved directs specific therapy. Estrogen supplementation significantly reduces symptoms due to atrophy.

Urethral Diverticulum

Diverticulum of the urethra represents a suburethral or periurethral, fibrous cystic mass that communicates with the urethral lumen. The wall does not contain muscle, and seldom can any epithelium be identified. This lesion occurs in 1% to 4% of patients, and although congenital diverticula have been described, most are acquired. Infection of periurethral glands with cystic formation and subsequent rupture into the urethral lumen appears to be the most common pathogenesis. Patients may have no symptoms, or they may complain of urgency, frequency, dysuria, dyspareunia, or incontinence. The diagnosis is usually suspected by examination (Fig. 50-6), but it should be confirmed by radiography or urethroscopy. Only symptomatic cases should be treated surgically, since complications may be significant. Surgery may include total or partial excision or marsupialization.

Malignant Lesions of the Urethra

Both primary and secondary malignant lesions of the urethra have been described. The most common primary lesion is the epidermoid carcinoma. Secondary lesions may derive from lesions in the genital tract. Symptoms may include frequency, dysuria, hematuria, or urethral mass. Endoscopy and biopsies are essential. Management and prognosis are determined by the nature and extent of the lesion.

DISEASES OF THE BLADDER

Cystitis

Cystitis is microbial invasion of the bladder. The incidence in females is higher than in males, and it increases with age. About 1% of school-age girls are affected, and 10% have had this infection by the age of 60. The pres-

FIG. 50-6. Distal urethral diverticulum.

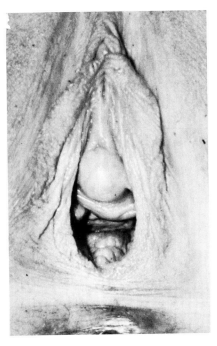

ence of significant bacteriuria in asymptomatic females may be as high as 6% to 8%. This figure becomes clinically relevant during pregnancy. Pregnant women with significant bacteriuria are likely to develop acute upper urinary tract infections (pyelitis or pyelonephritis). In addition to the possibility of parenchymal damage, upper urinary tract infections in pregnancy may lead to premature labor. Symptoms of cystitis include urinary urgency, frequency, nocturia, and dysuria. There is usually hesitancy and sensation of incomplete voiding. Occasionally, urinary incontinence may occur. Bimanual examination may reveal a tender bladder. Diagnostic confirmation requires bacteriologic assessment of the urine. Less than 10^5 organisms per milliliter of urine may be of clinical significance in symptomatic patients if organisms other than gram-negative enterobacteria are found.

Fever is unusual in mild cystitis, but in severe cases temperatures of the order of 100.2°F (37.8°C) may be present. Temperatures above 101°F (38.3°C) suggest infection of the upper urinary tract.

In cases of uncomplicated cystitis it is permissible to prescribe urinary tract antiseptics without performing tests other than the initial urinalysis that makes the diagnosis and the follow-up urinalysis. Appropriate regimens are nitrofurantoin, 100 mg orally 4 times daily for 5 days, or nalidixic acid, 1 gm orally 4 times daily for 5 days. If infection persists or if the symptoms do not abate or if cystitis recurs, a formal evaluation should be made.

So-called hemorrhagic cystitis is the most common cause of hematuria in women, and it results from intense engorgement of the bladder mucosa by the same organisms that cause simple, nonhemorrhagic cystitis. If the onset of hematuria is accompanied by the classic symptoms and urinary findings of cystitis, it is permissible to treat the initial episode as above without any tests other than follow-up urinalysis after the conclusion of therapy. If the symptoms do not resolve promptly, if hematuria or pyuria persists, or if they recur, a formal evaluation is indicated. Hematuria may result from such lesions as cancer of the bladder, polyps, or renal tumors. Accordingly, hematuria is never to be taken lightly.

URINARY INCONTINENCE

Symptoms of involuntary urine loss, together with those of cystitis, represent the most common lower urinary tract problems for which gynecologists are consulted. Occasional loss of urine may occur in up to 50% of young, healthy women. The clinical significance of the condition depends, therefore, on the patient's own perception of disability.

Criteria for the classification of urinary incontinence have varied. A review of conditions that lead to involuntary loss of urine is presented below.

Causes of Urinary Incontinence in Females
Without urothelial defect
   Genuine stress incontinence
   Detrusor instability

Others
    Urethral instability
    Unconscious abdominal contractions
    Bladder hernia
With urothelial defect
    Fistulas
    Ectopic ureter and other congenital anomalies
    Diverticula and trauma

Urinary Incontinence Without Urothelial Defect

Genuine Stress Incontinence

Genuine stress incontinence (GSI) occurs when the intravesical pressure exceeds the urethral resistance in the absence of a detrusor contraction. It implies incompetence of the urethral sphincter mechanism due to a rise in intra-abdominal pressure. The many factors that can contribute to induce a reversal of the pressure gradient between the urethra and the bladder are listed below. It is of utmost clinical relevance to determine which factors are involved in each patient.

Factors Contributing to Genuine Stress Incontinence
Increased abdominal pressure
    Abdominopelvic tumors
    Obesity
    Chronic pulmonary disease
Bladder overdistention (overflow incontinence)
Urethral incompetence
    Decreased or absent pressure transmission capacity
    (urethral hypermotility)
    Decreased intrinsic sphincter mechanism
        Hypoestrogenism
        Periurethral fibrosis
        Denervation
        α-Adrenergic blockade
        β-Adrenergic stimulation
        Trauma

Decreased pressure transmission capacity due to urethral hypermobility is the most common single factor. The proximal urethra is found below the pelvic diaphragm, and abdominal pressure is transmitted unequally to the bladder and urethra. Urethral hypermobility does not always result in GSI. In the presence of a satisfactory resting (intrinsic) urethral resistance and an effective striated muscle reflex contraction, a hypermobile urethra may remain competent. On occasion, a relatively competent urethra is overcome by excessive vesical pressure. These conditions include abdominopelvic tumors, chronic cough, obesity, and vesical overdistention (overflow incontinence). The urethral intrinsic sphincter mechanism may be affected by hypoestrogenism, α-adrenergic blocking agents, β-adrenergic stimulating agents, and other drugs. In addition, trauma and fibrosis may alter the elastic connective tissue and also affect intrinsic function.

Stress incontinence, of course, is the primary symptom. Leaking occurs as a "spurt" during exertion. Sensory symptoms such as urgency, frequency, and nocturia may coexist but are somewhat less common than in other forms of incontinence. The observation of a spurt of urine occurring through the urethra at the time of exertion remains a very helpful diagnostic observation. Unfortunately, in many cases direct observation may not be possible (erect position) or doubt exists as to whether leakage occurred at the exact time of the exertion or shortly afterward.

The symptom of stress incontinence may be present in conditions other than GSI. These include detrusor instability, urethral instability, small fistulas, diverticula, and ectopic ureter. The diagnostic workup should rule out these conditions and confirm the diagnosis of GSI. In addition, the factors contributing to GSI in each patient should be determined. The urethral pressure profile (passive and active) (Fig. 50-7) may help in the definitive diagnosis. If hypermotility of the urethra is the major contributing factor, surgery directed toward reposition of the proximal urethra within the abdominal cavity should cure more than 90% of patients. If the intrinsic sphincter mechanism is affected (urethral fibrosis), obstructive procedures or even artificial sphincter placements might be needed.

Detrusor Instability

It has been mentioned that in the continent adult the detrusor remains stable during bladder filling. It

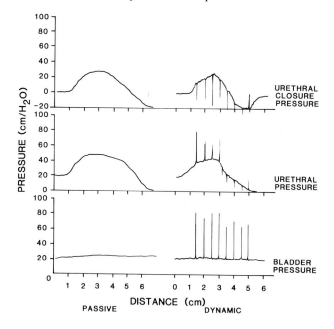

FIG. 50-7. Passive and dynamic urethral pressure profiles in a patient with GSI. A low passive urethral closing pressure and a dynamic closing pressure profile that becomes negative during coughs are demonstrated. These observations are compatible with urethral sphincter incompetence.

does not contract involuntarily at rest nor after provocative maneuvers such as coughing or jumping. The detrusor is unstable in about 25% to 30% of women with urinary incontinence. In these patients incontinence occurs as a result of a bladder contraction and not because of urethral sphincter deficiency. In most cases (over 90%) the reason is unknown; hence, the designation idiopathic detrusor instability (IDI). Known conditions that may also lead to an unstable bladder include upper motor neuron lesions, irritation of the lower urinary tract (*e.g.,* infections, trauma), and urethral obstruction. Diminished cortical inhibition of sacral reflexes is thought to be the pathophysiologic mechanism leading to instability. The clinical syndrome includes sensory symptoms such as urinary frequency, urgency, and nocturia. Dysuria is uncommon. Incontinence occurs in 70% to 75% of patients with instability. Some patients without incontinence may complain of sensory symptoms despite an unstable detrusor. In addition, some patients with few or no sensory problems may be incontinent as a result of involuntary bladder contractions. The diagnosis is confirmed only through cystometry (Fig. 50-8). Treatment of instability should be directed to the cause. Most cases of idiopathic instability

can be managed with behavior modification techniques. The objective of this form of therapy is to regain cortical control over sacral reflexes. It is accomplished through therapeutic programs of voluntary scheduled voidings. Anticholinergic or musculotropic agents and denervating surgical procedures may also be helpful in selected cases.

Other causes of urinary incontinence that occur in the absence of urothelial defect are described below.

Urethral Instability

It has been noted that in some instances abrupt decreases in urethral pressure result in incontinence. They occur at various bladder volumes, spontaneously or after provocation. The phenomenon is independent of detrusor contractions, and it seems not to be voluntarily induced. The etiology and pathogenesis are unknown.

Unconscious Abdominal Contractions

Rarely, incontinence may be induced by voluntary, though seemingly unconscious, contractions of the abdominal musculature. Simultaneous monitoring of intra-abdominal pressure is diagnostic. These patients exhibit psychologic symptoms, have multiple somatic complaints, and usually have undergone many surgical procedures. A psychiatric condition is suspected.

Incisional Bladder Hernias

Hernia of the bladder can occur through postoperative fascial abdominal wall defects. Patients may present with diffuse lower abdominal discomfort, sensory symptoms of the lower urinary tract, and urinary incontinence. The mechanism of incontinence is poorly understood. Repositioning of the bladder and correction of the hernia result in resolution of symptoms.

Causes of Urinary Incontinence With Urothelial Defect

Fistulas

Genitourinary fistulas are abnormal communications between the genital and the urinary systems. The most common fistula locations are shown in Figure 51-15 and are discussed on page 970.

Ectopic Ureter and Other Congenital Anomalies

The presence of an ectopic ureter is usually associated with a congenital duplication of renal units. The ureteric opening is usually in the distal urethra. Although more commonly seen in the young, adults have become symptomatic after vaginal surgical procedures or deliveries. Constant incontinence may occur and resemble a genitourinary fistula. If the ureteral orifice is small,

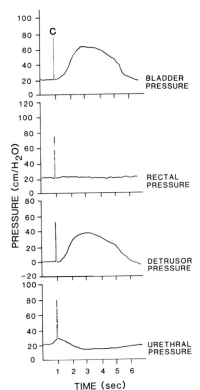

FIG. 50-8. Cystometry demonstrating detrusor instability. The detrusor pressure (intravesical minus intra-abdominal pressure) increases after a cough. It represents an involuntary bladder contraction triggered by a cough. The patient is unable to inhibit the contraction, and incontinence occurs.

the symptom of stress incontinence can mimic GSI. The diagnosis is usually made by ultrasonography as the proximal ureter is dilated. Intravenous pyelography may be misleading, since the ectopic parenchyma may be hypofunctional. Other congenital anomalies leading to incontinence include bladder extrophy and epispadias.

Urethral Diverticula and Trauma

Diverticulum of the urethra may cause involuntary loss of urine. Emptying of the diverticulum's contents may occur during exertion or intercourse, or a posturinary dribble may be present. The urethra can be injured during pelvic trauma or surgical intervention. Incontinence may be the result of fistula formation, injury to the sphinteric mechanism, or both. Specific anatomic and functional assessment should be made before attempting surgical correction.

THE UPPER URINARY TRACT

From a purely clinical standpoint, the gynecologist is rarely concerned directly with upper urinary tract pathology. From a surgical standpoint, it is of utmost relevance that the gynecologist be knowledgeable of the topographic anatomy of the ureters and be technically capable of tracing them intraoperatively. Obstruction of the ureters may occur in various gynecologic conditions such as endometriosis, invasive carcinoma of the cervix (Fig. 50-9), or massive pelvic tumors. During pregnancy ureteral dilatation occurs as the result of uterine compression and the effect of progesterone on ureteral smooth musculature. This may predispose to upper urinary tract infection, especially in patients with bacteriuria. Parenchymal renal disease may alter diuresis and lead to nocturia and urinary frequency. Renal tumors, although rare, must always be considered in the differ-

FIG. 50-9. Bilateral hydronephrosis and hydroureter due to carcinoma of the cervix. (Kelly HA: Operative Gynecology, vol 2. New York, Appleton, 1899; drawing by Max Brödel)

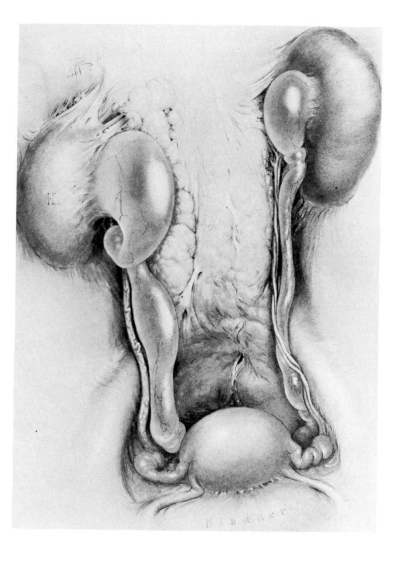

ential diagnosis of hematuria. The possible pelvic location of the kidney (pelvic kidney) is an important congenital condition to remember in the differential diagnosis of pelvic masses. If this condition is suspected, intravenous pyelography should be performed prior to surgical exploration.

REFERENCES AND RECOMMENDED READING

Embryology

Campbell MF: Development anatomy of the urinary system. In Youssef AF (ed): Gynecological Urology. Springfield, IL, Charles C Thomas, 1960

Ostergard DR: Embryology and anatomy of the female bladder and urethra. In Ostergard DR (ed): Gynecologic Urology and Urodynamics: Theory and Practice. Baltimore, Williams & Wilkins, 1980

Anatomy

Goslin JA et al: A comparative study of the human external sphincter and periurethral levator ani muscles. Br J Urol 53:35, 1981

Zacharin RF: Investigation of vesicourethral anatomy. In Zacharin RF (ed): Stress Incontinence of Urine. Hagerstown, Harper & Row, 1972

Neurology

Andrew J, Nathan PW: The cerebral control of micturition. Proc R Soc Med 58:553, 1965

Bradley WE, Scott FB, Timm GW: Innervation of the detrusor muscle and urethra. Urol Clin North Am 1:69, 1974

Function

Turner–Warwick R: Observations on the function and dysfunction of the sphincter and detrusor mechanisms. Urol Clin North Am 6:11, 1979

Terminology and Clinical Evaluation

Abrams P, Feneley R, Torrens M: Patient assessment. In Chisolm GD (ed): Urodynamics. New York, Springer–Verlag, 1983

Stanton SL (ed): Clinical Gynecologic Urology. St. Louis, CV Mosby, 1984

Lesions of the Urethra

Pratt JH, Malek RS: Lesions of the female urethra. In Slate WG (ed): Disorders of the Female Urethra and Urinary Incontinence. Baltimore, Williams & Wilkins, 1982

Urinary Tract Infections

Kunin CM: Detection, Prevention and Management of Urinary Tract Infection, 3rd ed. Philadelphia, Lea & Febiger, 1979

Genuine Stress Incontinence

Fantl JA: Genuine stress incontinence. In Sciarra JJ (ed): Gynecology and Obstetrics. Philadelphia, Harper & Row, 1984

Stanton SL: Urethral sphincter incompetence. In Stanton SL (ed): Clinical Gynecologic Urology. St. Louis, CV Mosby, 1984

Stress Incontinence. In Asmussen M, Miller A (eds): Clinical Gynecologic Urology. London, Blackwell Scientific Publications, 1983

Detrusor Instability

Cardozo LD et al: Biofeedback in the treatment of detrusor instability. Br J Urol 50:250, 1978

Fantl JA: Urinary tract incontinence due to detrusor instability. Clin Obstet Gynecol 27:474, 1984

Structural Defects and Relaxations

Harold M. M. Tovell
David N. Danforth

51

CONGENITAL ANOMALIES

Congenital anomalies of the female reproductive tract are considered in detail in Chapter 5. They are myriad in type, depending on the degree and kind of involvement, and occur at any level from the fimbriated end of the fallopian tubes to the vaginal introitus and external genitalia. They may take the form of absence (agenesis), imperfect development with consequent narrowing (atresia), or duplication of any part of the uterus or vagina due to a failure of fusion of the müllerian duct system. Occasionally the persistence of an embryonic state may be seen, as in certain cases of fused labia minora and imperforate hymen. Maternal ingestion of androgenic hormones or poor perineal hygiene in infancy may result in fused labia minora, which may interfere with the normal urinary stream or obstruct coitus later in life. Daily application of an estrogenic cream frequently suffices to separate the labia and restore the normal relationships of the external genitalia.

The hymen separates the internal from the external genitalia and may vary from a complete wall of mucous membrane (imperforate) to complete absence. The hymenal opening varies in size and shape and may be crescentic, fringed, biperforate, or cribriform. The imperforate hymen presents a clinical problem only after menarche, when the accumulation of menstrual blood may result successively in hematocolpos, hematometria, and hematosalpinx. The patient presents with a history of menstrual molimina and periodic pelvic pain without evidence of external bleeding. Examination reveals a thin, fluctuant, bluish black, bulging septum, frequently under great tension. A radial or cruciate incision and removal of one or more segments of the membrane allow the thick, chocolate-colored liquid to escape slowly.

When a congenital anomaly of the internal genitalia is found, a thorough investigation of both the genital and urinary tracts shoud be made, since other anomalies of the müllerian (paramesonephric) and wolffian (mesonephric) systems frequently coexist. Knowledge of these defects may be of significant clinical importance in the management of a subsequent pregnancy or in the evaluation of a gynecologic problem.

ACUTE INJURIES

Most acute injuries and lacerations of the vulva, vagina, and uterus occur at parturition, and their management is an obstetric problem. Nonacute injuries incurred to the supporting structures of the uterus and vagina during childbirth may become a gynecologic problem later in life and are discussed later in this chapter.

Nonobstetric injuries include those resulting from falls, coitus, sexual assault, and a variety of miscellaneous trauma. They vary in extent from a simple bruise of the vulva or perineal area or a small abrasion of the vestibular mucous membrane to an enormous hematoma involving the entire half or more of the perineal area (Fig. 51-1) and horrendous lacerations of the vulva, pelvic floor, and vagina. In managing an acute injury it is necessary to observe the following order of procedure:

1. An accurate history of precisely how the injury occurred should be carefully recorded. Medicolegal problems may exist in any case of genital tract injury regardless of the patient's protestations to the contrary. (The procedure to be followed in the case of alleged rape is outlined in Chap. 9).
2. A careful inspection is made of the vulva and vestibule under a good light, with the patient in the lithotomy position, on a gynecologic examination table with her legs in stirrups. A photographic record of the injury might be considered with the patient's permission.
3. A gentle, single-digit vaginal examination should be performed to note any vaginal wall hematoma or lac-

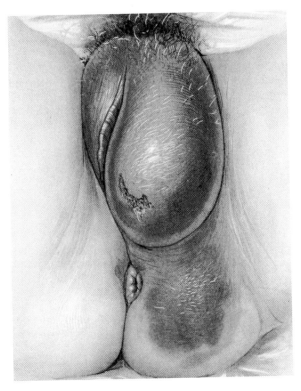

FIG. 51-1. Hematoma of the vulva occupying the left labium majus and extending downward out of the perineum. The vaginal outlet is discolored, and all surrounding parts are distorted and infiltrated with blood. Below is an abrasion of the skin. The patient fell astraddle in a chair. (Kelly HA: Operative Gynecology. New York, Appleton, 1898; drawing by Max Brödel)

eration or the presence of any foreign body. A speculum examination, if feasible, should also be performed to confirm any findings or to determine any injury above the introitus.

4. A rectal examination is made to determine any injury to the sphincter or rectal wall or the presence and extent of a perineal hematoma.

Superficial abrasions and lacerations will granulate and heal well and require no sutures. Arterial bleeding, however, may require ligation of the offending vessel; otherwise, gentle pressure suffices to control any ooze. Irrigation and lavage with an aqueous antiseptic solution are essential.

Large, painful hematomas may develop and may be extremely frightening to the patient. They absorb slowly and seldom become infected. They are best managed by hot compresses or sitz baths.

Extensive injuries, including larger lacerations of the vulvar appendages, vagina, and perineum, require prompt repair, usually in an operating room environment. Good exposure and assistance with blood replacement and general anesthesia may be required. The possibility of injury to the urethra or bladder, or both, and to the anal sphincter and canal or rectum should always be considered. An indwelling bladder catheter should be inserted for one or two days or longer if the urethra or bladder has been injured. No permanent damage results from acute or traumatic injuries to the vulva, vagina, or perineum if sound surgical principles and management are undertaken in their repair. Subsequent weakness and prolapse may develop, however, if the pelvic diaphragm (levator muscles and fascia) is torn. Depending on the nature of the injury, prophylactic antibiotic and anti-tetanus vaccine should be considered.

VAGINAL ATRESIA DUE TO INJURY

The most common causes of acquired vaginal atresia are childbirth injury, overzealous vaginal plastic operation, and the intravaginal use of radium.

Atresia following childbirth injury may occur at any level in the vagina, usually along a lateral wall in the upper third. It is felt as a sharp annular constricting band of tissue and may result from a faulty repair of a laceration or failure to perform a needed repair. No treatment is necessary unless dyspareunia exists. Some annular bands may require a simple incision in one or more places. Graduated obturators may be used to dilate the constricting bands in the lower third of the vagina.

Not infrequently, vaginal atresia may occur following an anterior and posterior colporrhaphy with resulting dyspareunia or a complete inability to have intercourse. Excessive removal of redundant anterior or posterior vaginal wall skin or excessive tightening of the levator ani muscles during the posterior wall repair and perineorrhaphy contributes to this distressing potential medicolegal problem. The gynecologist should be constantly aware of this danger when performing any vaginal plastic procedure.

Vaginal atresia following radium treatment for cervical cancer is a frequent occurrence when preventive measures are not taken. The vault is narrowed within a month after removal of the radium, and the anterior and posterior walls become adherent within two months, making intercourse unsatisfactory or totally impossible and the cervix completely inaccessible for follow-up examination. To prevent this distortion, the patient may be instructed in the regular use of a vaginal obturator commencing shortly after removal of the radium, or the gynecologist or radiotherapist can digitally break down any adhesions and expose the cervix at weekly intervals until the vaginal walls have healed or until intercourse is resumed.

CERVICAL INJURIES

The majority of cervical injuries are obstetric in nature and occur when the cervix is retracting over the advancing head in the terminal phase of the first stage of labor. Less obvious or concealed injuries to the cervix are usually functional in nature and may be iatrogenically produced at the time of dilatation and curettage in a young, nulliparous girl with a congenitally atretic or stenotic cervical canal (Fig. 51-2).

Obstetrically acquired cervical lacerations usually occur at the lateral angles of the external os and may extend to or beyond the vaginal vault into the lower uterine segment. They should be repaired immediately upon completion of the third stage of labor.

Uncomplicated lacerations that are not repaired result in the so-called fish mouth type of cervix in which one or both lateral angles of the external os have a deep cleft. Old stellate lacerations are sometimes seen. They are usually shallow lacerations that result from multiple tears around the circumference of the cervix during labor and delivery.

Uncomplicated cervical lacerations, when properly repaired at the time of delivery, are of no clinical importance. If they are not repaired they heal poorly, and two important clinical problems result. First, the columnar epithelium of the cervical canal grows out onto the ectocervix, forming an ectropion from which a severe chronic cervicitis and leukorrhea may result. The second problem results from a laceration that occurs high in the canal. Poor healing and scar tissue interrupt the continuity of the fibrous cervical ring such that it cannot withstand the stresses placed on it as pregnancy progresses, and a late abortion inevitably occurs. Such concealed lacerations in the cervical canal, whether produced at childbirth or at the time of dilatation and curettage, produce an incompetent cervix.

RELAXATION OF PELVIC SUPPORTS

The term *relaxation* is used to describe the weakening effects of the lengthening and attenuation of the fascial supports of the urethra, bladder, uterus, upper posterior wall of the vagina, and lower anterior wall of the rectum. Although relaxation may occur in both young and old

FIG. 51-2. (*A*) Concealed cervical injury. The cervix feels normal, and speculum examination does not disclose defect. (*B*) Deep left cervical laceration seen on speculum examination. (Danforth DN: Cervical incompetency. In Davis CH, Carter B: Obstetrics and Gynecology. Hagerstown, Prior, 1953)

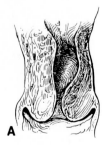
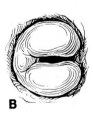

A   B

virginal women, the great majority of cases are the delayed but direct result of childbirth. If injury to the supports is extensive, evidence of relaxation may appear soon after delivery. More often the symptoms and signs of pelvic relaxation appear in the menopausal and postmenopausal era, when the tonic effect of the ovarian hormones is lost and atrophic changes in the fascial supports begin. Pelvic relaxation should be regarded in the same way as hernia elsewhere in the body. Both are produced by a weakness of the supporting tissues and are progressive in nature, and no amount of exercise or rest will correct the problem or restore the normal anatomic relationships.

Anatomic Considerations

For a proper understanding of the clinical problems and the surgical management of pelvic relaxations, a detailed knowledge of the functional anatomy of the bony, ligamentous, and fascial supports is required. The student is urged to review the appropriate sections described in Chapter 3. The following, simplified, clinical concepts of the various structures involved in normal pelvic supports are stressed.

The *pelvic diaphragm,* formed by the bilaterally situated, fan-shaped levator ani muscles extending in the central pelvis between the peripheral anterior and posterior bony segments and lateral pelvic walls, effectively supports the pelvic structures directly over the pelvic outlet. As depicted in Figure 3-12, the muscles blend together in the mid-line where they surround and support the three openings in the pelvic floor through which the terminal portions of the urinary, reproductive, and intestinal tracts pass. Sometimes called the *levator sling,* the thick, striated muscle and its overlying fascia provide the necessary support for the pelvic viscera and yet allow considerable expansion to meet the functional demands of a normal vaginal delivery and bowel evacuation. Any congenital or acquired weakness eventually results in the widening of the opening and the subsequent herniation of the pelvic viscera through the floor of the pelvis.

The perineal musculature composed of the more superficially located muscles of the perineum is depicted in Figures 3-27 and 3-28. The perineal musculature consists of the paired ischiocavernosus, bulbocavernosus, and deep and superficial transverse perineal muscles together with the external anal sphincter and musculofascial tissues of the urogenital diaphragm. Together these form a second layer of support but are seldom effective in preventing the eventual downward displacement of the bladder, vagina, or rectum once the levator muscles have been seriously weakened.

The endopelvic fascia is the fibroareolar connective tissue that fills the space below the pelvic peritoneum and above the upper fascial sheaths of the levator ani muscle. With varying degrees of thickness, depending on functional requirements for support, it covers the bladder, vagina, cervix, uterus, rectosigmoid, and anal canal, in addition to forming fascial sheaths for vessels and nerves passing through the pelvis. A diagrammatic representation of the fibroareolar connective tissue lining the pelvic walls and viscera is depicted in Figure 3-10. The tissue is loosely arranged in areas where no stress is encountered, as in the paravesical and pararectal spaces. In other areas, where greater degrees of support are required to withstand the stress incurred during the functional activity of the organ involved, the loose meshwork of fascial tissue is condensed into thick, fibrous bands forming the vesicouterine, cardinal, and uterosacral ligaments and the fascial sheaths surrounding the pelvic organs.

In essence, the function of the endopelvic fascia is to provide both ligamentous and fascial supports for all pelvic viscera, nerves, and blood vessels and to fill the empty spaces between the viscera and the pelvic side walls below the peritoneum and above the levator ani muscles.

The following major supports of the uterus and vagina are of concern in the surgical repair of pelvic relaxations.

The cardinal ligaments, or transverse cervical or Mackenrodt's ligaments, which pass medially from the lateral pelvic wall to the paracervical fascia on the lateral aspect of the cervix, are the primary supports of the uterus and upper vagina. They contain the blood vessels, lymphatic channels, and nerves for the central pelvic viscera and are sometimes referred to clinically as the lateral parametria.

The uterosacral ligaments extend from the presacral or perirectal fascia to the paracervical and upper paravaginal fascia, where they are incorporated with the cervical and vaginal attachments of the cardinal ligaments. Their primary function is to maintain the uterus in anteversion and the cervix at right angles to the vaginal axis, and to assist in suspension of the uterus and upper vagina. They also carry blood vessels, lymphatic channels, and nerves to the central pelvic viscera and are sometimes referred to clinically as the *posterior parametria.*

The pubocervical fascia includes the pubovesical and vesicouterine components of the endopelvic fascia and extends from the posterior aspect of the symphysis pubis, passing beneath the urethra and bladder; it is incorporated with the paracervical fascia anteriorly and laterally, where it blends into the cervical attachments of the cardinal ligaments. It is the primary support of the anterior vaginal wall and bladder.

The paravaginal and perirectal fascia maintain the integrity of the lower posterior two thirds of the vagina. This endopelvic fascial sheath surrounds the vagina and rectum and is fused in the lower one half or two thirds of the vagina, below the peritoneum, in the deepest point of the pouch of Douglas and above the hymenal ring at the vaginal introitus. Further support in this area is given by the strong muscular bellies of the levator muscles and their overlying fascia.

Symptoms of Pelvic Relaxation

Symptoms of pelvic relaxation generally relate to the particular structure or structures involved, such as the urethra, bladder, uterus, cul-de-sac, or rectum. The patient may refer to them as a swelling, a protrusion, a pulling or dragging sensation, fatigue, or a pressure feeling. Low backache, although frequently associated with pelvic relaxations, is probably secondary, if related at all, to the postural adjustments made by the patient in an attempt to reduce the primary symptoms.

Back strain may result from unaccustomed postural attitudes. Symptoms that suggest a structural defect, a uterine displacement, or both include urinary incontinence with stress, pelvic pain or pressure, or a feeling of fullness in the pelvis, particularly after prolonged periods of standing or with deep penetration during coitus. Finally, the longer the structural defects have been present, the more progressive they become and the more accentuated the symptoms are by the time the patient seeks relief.

Types of Pelvic Relaxations

Weakness in the supports of the reproductive tract is clinically referred to according to the anatomic site or organ involved. *Urethrocele, cystocele, uterine prolapse, enterocele,* and *rectocele* are terms commonly used to describe the pelvic hernias or types of pelvic relaxations. In addition, such entities as perineal lacerations and uterine displacements are encountered in clinical practice and are included in any discussion of pelvic relaxations.

Urethrocele

A urethrocele is caused by the herniation of the pubocervical and paravaginal fascia under the urethra, producing a bulging into the vaginal canal. The patient may be asymptomatic or she may complain of a vaginal mass or protrusion and incontinence of urine on stress if the weakness involves the fascial supports in the region of the posterior urethrovesical angle. Any bulge in this area may be mistaken for a urethral diverticulum or redundant vaginal skin and should be carefully distinguished at the time of examination.

Cystocele

A cystocele is any bulging of the anterior vaginal wall beneath the floor of the bladder (Fig. 51-3). It is caused by the loss of support in the area that is normally maintained by the pubocervical or paravaginal fascia and the permanent stretching of the oblique tunnel of the levator sling through which the vagina passes. The patient may complain of a bearing-down sensation, a vaginal protrusion, and urinary stress incontinence if there is a coexisting urethrocele. The weakness in the anterior

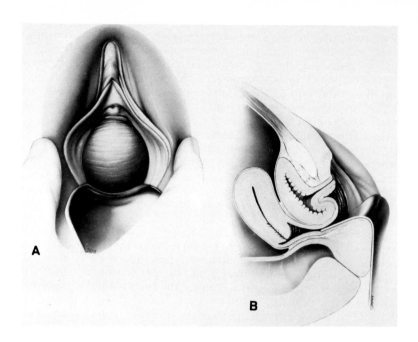

FIG. 51-3. Cystocele. (*A*) Exposed by a Sims' speculum. (*B*) Sagittal view. The patient has been asked to bear down and cough. (Drawing by L. Dank)

vaginal wall can be readily palpated or the bulging accentuated with stress such as by coughing, straining, or bearing down. If the posterior wall of the vagina is depressed with a Sims' speculum, the bulging of the anterior vaginal wall below the bladder will be readily observed. If a significant portion of the bladder lies below the urethrovesical opening, urine retention with recurrent episodes of urinary frequency, urgency, and cystitis and ascending urinary tract infections may also be a problem.

Uterine Prolapse

Uterine prolapse occurs when the primary supporting ligaments of the uterus, namely the cardinal ligaments, are attenuated or injured, thus permitting the uterus to drop as shown diagrammatically in Figure 51-4. For clinical staging and descriptive purposes, three degrees of uterine prolapse are recognized. First-degree prolapse is the presence of some descent of the uterus, but the cervix has not reached the vaginal introitus. Second-degree prolapse is when the cervix alone or with part of the uterus passes through the vaginal introitus (Fig. 51-5). Third-degree prolapse or procidentia (Fig. 51-6) is the protrusion of the entire uterus beyond the vaginal introitus; the examining fingers can be brought together at the introitus, above the uterine fundus. Because the bladder is normally adherent to the cervix above the vaginal vault, it is brought down with the uterus (Fig. 51-7). Similarly, the peritoneal pouch of Douglas is also elongated in marked degrees of uterine prolapse. In advanced cases of uterine prolapse there exists either a potential or real cystocele and enterocele that require attention at the time of surgical repair. The symptoms of uterine prolapse are due to the discomfort and inconvenience as well as to the irritation of the exposed cervix and vaginal epithelium. Frequently the cervix is markedly elongated and eroded, producing bleeding and discharge.

Procidentia is a complex anatomic distortion. Anteriorly the bladder, including the trigone area, has advanced with the uterus. Not only are the ureters exposed for easy surgical injury, but kinking or edema may already have given rise to chronic obstruction and hydroureter. Renal damage may be an associated problem. Posteriorly, advancement of the pouch of Douglas with a consequent enterocele places loops of small bowel

FIG. 51-4. Uterine prolapse or descensus. Schematic representation shows the supporting influence of the transverse cervical ligaments. When these are attenuated or lengthened, gravity and intra-abdominal pressure bring the uterus to a lower level in the pelvis. (Modified from Kelly HA: Gynecology. New York, Appleton, 1928)

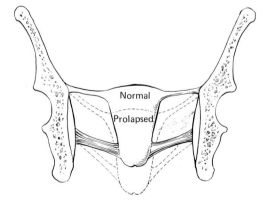

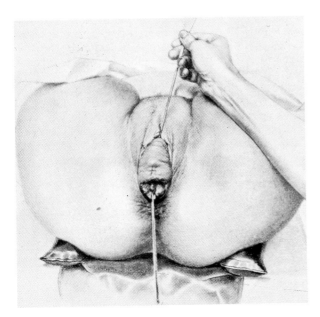

FIG. 51-5. Partial prolapse of the uterus and vagina. Sound is introduced into the bladder to show altered direction of urethra. The light spot on the anterior vaginal wall plainly shows the position of the end of sound in the bladder. (Kelly HA: Operative Gynecology. New York, Appleton, 1898; drawing by Max Brödel)

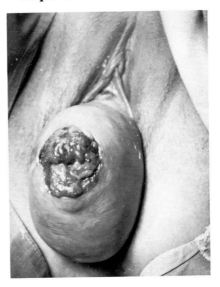

FIG. 51-6. Procidentia, with marked decubitus ulceration and granular erosion of the cervix. The bladder is on the anterior aspect of the mass. The pouch below the cervix contains loops of small bowel.

within easy reach of the surgeon's knife. It should be evident that the repair of a third-degree prolapse and maintenance of a functional vagina is no easy task and requires a thorough knowledge of the existing and correct anatomic relationships and careful attention to the restoration of the pelvic supports.

In long-standing cases severe edema may develop in the prolapsed structures such that they cannot be easily replaced. Firm and sometimes prolonged circumferential pressure often reduces the size of the prolapsed structures so that, beginning with the most dependent portion, reduction can be accomplished. If this is not effective, keeping the patient in bed for 24 hours, with the hips, and particularly the prolapsed structure, elevated, will generally lessen the edema sufficiently to permit easy reduction.

Enterocele

An enterocele is a herniation of the investing fascia of the posterior vagina above the deepest point in the pouch of Douglas between the uterosacral ligaments and below the cervix (Fig. 51-8). It may be caused by a congenital weakness of the fascial supports in this area, which produces a narrow-necked peritoneal sac associated with a deep cul-de-sac. More frequently it is acquired through obstetric trauma, and the sac is wider but shorter. Since it lies above the rectovaginal septum, the sacculation contains loops of small bowel and occasionally omentum, but not rectum. Depending on its

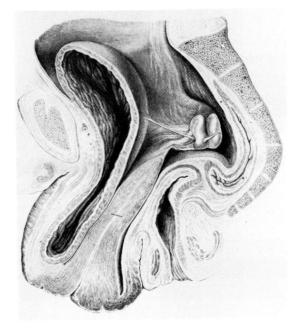

FIG. 51-7. Drawing in parasagittal section shows approximate relations of the procidentia illustrated in Figure 51-6. (Halban J, Tandler J: Anatomie und Ätiologie der Genitalprolapse beim Weibe. Vienna, Braumüller, 1907)

size and extent, there may be no symptoms or there may be a dull dragging sensation and low backache; rarely a deep pelvic pain may be present. If an enterocele is large, protrusion through the introitus can be very troublesome.

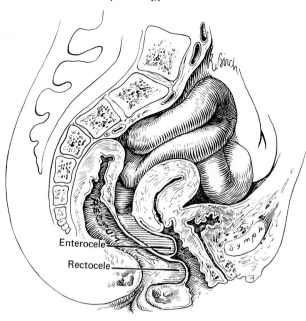

FIG. 51-8. Sagittal section demonstrates relative position of enterocele and rectocele. (Te Linde RW, Mattingly RF: Operative Gynecology, 4th ed. Philadelphia, JB Lippincott, 1970)

A common error in gynecologic surgery is failure to recognize and correct either a potential or existing enterocele. All too often the bulge in the posterior vaginal wall is interpreted as a large or high rectocele. Examination for an enterocele is best accomplished with an anterior vaginal wall retractor held in place and a finger in the rectum. If the upper portion of the vaginal

sacculation fails to admit the examining finger, an enterocele most likely exists. In any operation undertaken to correct a prolapse of the uterus or rectocele, the possibility of an enterocele should be considered and looked for and, if it is present, the necessary steps taken to correct it. It is emphasized that no rectocele repair has ever repaired an enterocele and that the failure to repair an enterocele at the time of surgery for symptomatic prolapse may fail to cure the patient's complaints. This can be the source of great chagrin when the gynecologist discovers the persisting vaginal hernia at the time of the postoperative visit.

Rectocele

A rectocele is a herniation of the anterior rectal wall through the relaxed or ruptured pararectal and paravaginal fascia in the rectovaginal septum (Figs. 51-8 and 51-9). The supports are weakened and attenuated by childbirth and further weakened with straining at the time of defecation.

A slight to moderate rectocele is asymptomatic, but as the hernia increases in size the fecal column tends to be pushed into the sacculation, which protrudes into the vaginal canal. A not infrequent complaint is that defecation can be accomplished only with digital pressure applied vaginally against the sacculation.

Prolapse of the Vagina

Prolapse of the vagina is an uncommon but very distressing condition both to the patient and gynecologist; it occurs after the abdominal or vaginal removal of the uterus. It is usually associated with an enterocele and cystocele and often results from a failure to rec-

FIG. 51-9. Rectocele. (*A*) Exposed by lateral traction. (*B*) Sagittal view. The patient is straining as if passing stool. (Drawing by L. Dank)

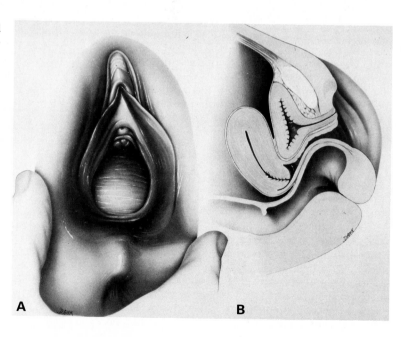

ognize and correct a potential or existing enterocele at the time of hysterectomy, or a failure to reattach the vaginal vault to the uterosacral and cardinal ligaments and pubocervical fascia following removal of the uterus. Rarely, a debilitating disease, including obesity, old age, and chronic malnutrition, or some combination of these conditions plays a role in this distressing form of hernia.

Chronic Perineal Lacerations

Old or chronic lacerations of the perineum result from a failure to repair or an improper repair of an acute second- or third-degree perineal laceration during childbirth.

An old second-degree laceration involves the substance of the perineal body but not the sphincter ani. The thickness of the perineum between the distal portion of the vagina and the vestibule and the anal canal is greatly reduced so that the vaginal opening gapes. A rectocele is usually present. The symptoms may be negligible, but often there is a loss of sexual sensation for both partners at the time of intercourse. A surgical repair may be indicated if the patient's complaints are valid.

An old third-degree laceration is one in which the sphincter ani is divided and retracted sufficiently to cause incontinence of both feces and flatus (Fig. 51-10). The perineal body and lower inch or two of the midportion of the posterior vaginal wall may be totally absent and the vaginal opening widely gaping. Surgical repair is

FIG. 51-10. Complete tear of the perineum. Note well-defined sphincter pits and retraction and thickening of the muscle, with a deep dimple behind it. A vaginal cyst due to inclusion of vaginal mucosa in the healing process is seen in the right sulcus in the scar area. (Kelly HA: Operative Gynecology. New York, Appleton, 1898; drawing by Max Brödel)

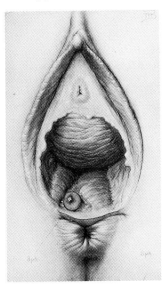

essential to relieve the patient's distressing and embarrassing symptoms.

Principles of Treatment

Pelvic relaxations of varying types and degrees are normally found in all women who have delivered children vaginally. Although symptom-producing pelvic relaxations may occur in any age group, they most often occur after the climacteric. They should always be treated surgically, preferably when the patient has completed her family, unless strong contraindications exist to required anesthesia for the surgical repair, such as chronic debility, severe cardiopulmonary disease, or extreme age of the patient that outweighs the risk of the operative procedure involved.

The more common indications for treatment are a sensation of a protruding mass, recurrent cystitis, urinary stress incontinence, difficulty with defecation, vaginal protrusion, and loss of sexual feeling. In the case of uterine descensus, protrusion and such symptoms as pelvic discomfort or sensations of pressure or bearing down may constitute the indications for repair. Occasionally the lack of sensation at time of coitus may indicate a needed repair in properly selected patients.

Surgical Therapy

The operative procedures employed to correct symptomatic relaxations of the vagina and uterine prolapse are beyond the scope of this chapter. The interested student is encouraged to review any one of several gynecologic surgery texts listed in the references and recommended reading.

Suffice it to emphasize that the successful repair of any vaginal or uterine prolapse depends on the ability and skill of the gynecologic surgeon to dissect the various uterine and vaginal supports and to reconstruct the structural relationships that will provide a deep and well-supported vagina and its adjacent structures. Palliative surgical procedures such as colpocleisis or vaginectomy are performed only in rare instances in which the medical status of the patient contra-indicates any extensive procedure and the maintenance of vaginal function is of no importance.

Nonsurgical Therapy

Several types of pessaries (Fig. 51-11) are useful for the patient with symptomatic pelvic relaxation who, for one reason or another, is unable to undergo a surgical repair. A pessary can be effective when the uterus prolapses with the bladder but may be useless if there is no support at the vaginal outlet.

The choice of pessary must be individualized. Ring pessaries are effective for prolapse of the uterus but are of little use for a cystocele. The rubber doughnut or plastic types of pessaries with a collapsible ring or the

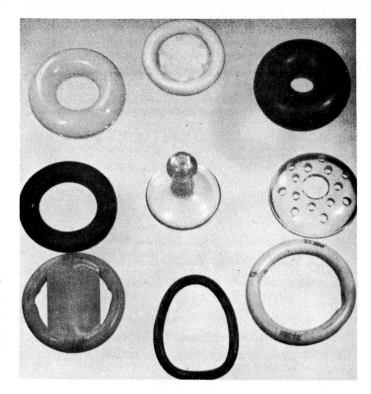

FIG. 51-11. A collection of various types of pessaries. Clockwise, beginning with the 12 o'clock position, they are (1) round solid ring, plastic, (2) rubber doughnut, (3) plastic disk with perforation, (4) collapsible ring, (5) Smith–Hodge pessary, (6) Gellhorn pessary (center), (7) collapsible ring with central support, (8) solid rubber ring, (9) rubber doughnut, inflatable. (Parsons L, Sommers S: Gynecology. Philadelphia, WB Saunders, 1962)

Smith–Hodge pessary (Fig. 51-12) is useful when a cystocele exists (Fig. 51-13). Soft, pure gum rubber, cubed-shaped pessaries with concave surfaces on all sides and of various sizes are also beneficial in appropriately selected patients (Fig. 51-14).

Any physician who inserts a pessary assumes responsibility for its care. The patient must be advised that the pessary should not be painful or uncomfortable. If it is or should become uncomfortable, it probably has

become displaced and should be checked and another size or different type inserted. If the patient is unable to remove the pessary and reinsert it periodically, she should be examined at two- or three-month intervals for any vaginal irritation. All postmenopausal patients in whom a pessary has been placed should be given oral or topical estrogen therapy to improve the tone and resistance of the vaginal epithelium to infection.

DISPLACEMENTS OF THE UTERUS

The anatomic position of the uterus as it relates to the axis of the vagina is one of anteversion and gentle antiflexion as it rests on the collapsed bladder, inclined toward the symphysis.

In about one third of women, the uterus is retroverted or inclined posteriorly toward the sacrum and gently retroflexed. The term "flexion" refers to the angle between the axis of the cervical canal and the long axis of the uterine cavity. When the uterus is "displaced," it is either in a midposition, retroverted, or displaced laterally. Many displacements may be of no clinical significance, although at other times they may indicate significant pelvic disease.

The most common of simple displacements of the uterus is retroversion. It may be congenital in origin, acquired following childbirth, or the result of cul-de-sac pathology, in which it is usually part of a disease process and may be of clinical significance. Lateral dis-

FIG. 51-12. Smith–Hodge pessary.

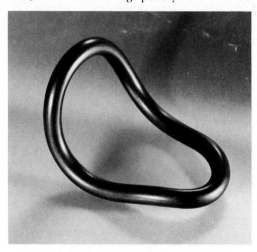

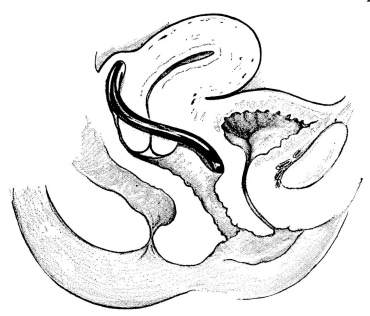

FIG. 51-13. Sagittal view of a Smith–Hodge pessary in place. Observe how the uterus is held up in the normal position. It should be comfortable and the vagina checked regularly for irritation. (Parsons L, Sommers S: Gynecology. Philadelphia, WB Saunders, 1962)

placements of the uterus may occur in association with adnexal pathology, in which the uterus is either pushed aside by a large adnexal mass on the opposite side or pulled to the side of the disease process by inflammatory adhesions or scars.

Retroversion of the Uterus

Congenital retroversion of the uterus is seldom, if ever, of any clinical importance. Though a variety of pelvic symptoms have been attributed to a congenitally retroverted uterus, including dysmenorrhea, dyspareunia, infertility, back pain, and menorrhagia, the position of the uterus in the pelvis has never been established as the sole cause of these symptoms. The uterus is freely mobile and can be anteverted manually during pelvic examination or tilted forward if the patient assumes the knee–chest position. A movable symptom-producing retroverted uterus can be held in an anteverted position with a Smith–Hodge pessary (see Fig. 51-13).

The indications for using the Smith–Hodge pessary to antevert a congenitally retroverted uterus include the following: (1) to assist the uterus to rise out of the pelvis more easily in early pregnancy and possibly relieve back pain; (2) to achieve a more favorable relationship between the ejaculate and external cervical os in an occasional infertile couple in whom all studies are negative; and (3) to relieve deep pelvic dyspareunia or dysmenorrhea in some patients in whom no other therapeutic management has been successful. If the painful symptoms are completely relieved for three months while the pessary has maintained the uterus in an anteverted position and if they recur after removal of the pessary, a uterine suspension procedure might be considered.

Acquired Retroversion

Acquired retroversion of the uterus most often follows childbirth and results from an attenuation of the two sets of ligaments most responsible for maintaining the uterus in anteversion, namely, the uterosacral and round

FIG. 51-14. Pure gum rubber cube pessary, which comes in various sizes. Support is provided by suction action of six concave surfaces. The pessary is self-positioning after insertion and provides effective support in vaginal prolapse. (Milex Products, Chicago)

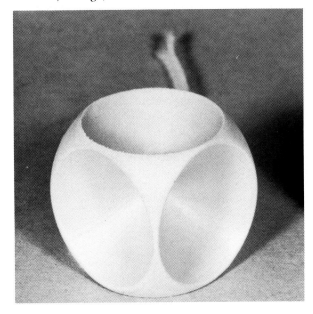

ligaments, during pregnancy and delivery. Normally, most uteri return to an anterior position within two months following delivery, and approximately one third will remain retroverted.

Fixed retroversion results from traction on the corpus from adherent pelvic and especially adnexal lesions, notably those due to chronic salpingo-oophoritis and endometriosis. Large myomata of the uterus may also cause the uterus to become retroverted. Pelvic symptoms are due to the underlying pathology. In the course of corrective surgery aimed at preserving or improving fertility, mobilization of the uterus and adnexa and their maintenance in an anterior position, away from old and potential new sites of adherence, are probably the most valid single indication for a uterine suspension operation.

Symptoms of Retroversion

Uncomplicated uterine retroversion is rarely symptomatic. Occasionally a patient may have difficulty conceiving because the cervix points toward the anterior vaginal wall, away from the seminal pool left in the posterior fornix after coitus in the supine position.

Backache is not a symptom of an uncomplicated uterine retroversion. More often, low back pain is caused by spasms of the small muscles of the back, often associated with an abnormality of the bony spine. Faulty posture, poor general health, and obesity may be contributing factors, but the retroverted uterus is not responsible.

Chronic pelvic congestion syndrome, a condition usually associated with a retroverted uterus, has been described as a cause of chronic deep pelvic and low back pain. At operation the pelvic veins may be engorged and tortuous and the uterus and cervix enlarged and congested in the retroverted position. The ovaries are frequently enlarged and prolapsed and often contain many follicular cysts. Menstrual abnormalities may exist, and frequently the syndrome associated with premenstrual tension may be exaggerated. The clinical syndrome, most frequently seen in the white population, may also be associated with chronic cystic mastitis. Heavy psychologic overtones are often present, and the diagnosis of pelvic congestion syndrome must be made with caution.

Symptoms associated with fixed uterine retroversion, as noted above, are due to the associated condition maintaining the uterus in the retroverted position. Deep pelvic pain and low backache, dysmenorrhea, dyspareunia, and menstrual irregularities are the most commonly encountered complaints.

Inversion of the Uterus

Inversion of the uterus is a phenomenon that usually occurs in the third stage of labor; the uterus turns inside out such that the endometrium lining the fundus extends through the dilated cervix. If the inversion is complete, the entire uterus is turned inside out through the cervix into the vagina, and the adnexa are carried into the inversion cup with the uterine fundus. The condition may be spontaneous or result from excessive fundal pressure and traction upon the umbilical cord in an effort to expel the placenta attached to the uterine fundus. Although the condition is rare, it must be recognized and treated immediately when it is encountered. The management of this condition in its acute stage is an obstetric problem and is considered in Chapter 38.

Polypoid submucous fibroids arising on a wide stalk from the fundus may grow and distend the lower pole of the uterus, giving rise to silent uterine contractions that ultimtely expel the tumor through the external cervical os. The fundus follows, and inversion may be produced by heavy traction on the polypoid tumor presenting at the external os. Occasionally vaginal hysterectomy may be necessary, and the gynecologist should be prepared to undertake this operation when a large polypoid submucous fibroid is to be removed vaginally either by excision or by avulsion.

In chronic uterine inversion, infection and edema of the exposed endometrium are the rule. Excessive bleeding and shock are common as a result of infection and failure of the endometrial hemostatic mechanisms. In addition, the adnexa within the inversion cup are usually congested and adherent both to one another and to the uterine serosa. A pulling, abdominal discomfort may be present as a result of the adnexal congestion as well as of the prolonged tension on the infundibulopelvic ligaments and round ligaments.

Uterine inversion of long duration should be treated surgically. Unless an effort must be made to preserve childbearing potential, hysterectomy is the definitive procedure. In long-standing cases, the prolapsed structure should be treated by antiseptic vaginal douches before operation. An abdominal approach is necessary, and the correction is accomplished after an incision is made through the posterior aspect of the cervix, extending into the posterior vaginal vault. An assistant pushes the fundus upward from below until the normal relationships are restored. The defect may then be repaired or a hysterectomy may be performed.

Fistulas

A fistula is an abnormal or unnatural communication from one hollow viscus to another or from a hollow viscus to the skin. In the female reproductive tract, fistulas may result from a congenital anomaly, trauma, gynecologic surgery, obstetric injury, cancer, radiation therapy, or infection. The most common sites for fistulas are shown in Fig. 51-15.

Enterovesical, enterouterine, and enterovaginal fistulas generally involve the sigmoid colon or rectum and result from malignant disease, diverticulitis, pelvic abscess, or tuberculosis. Rectovaginal fistulas may also result from a surgical injury during a colpoperineorrhaphy operation or an episiotomy. Fistulas resulting from injury or infection are usually amenable to surgical closure,

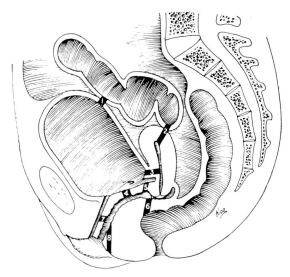

FIG. 51-15. The most common sites for fistulas: (1) vesicocolic, (2) uterocolic, (3) vesicouterine or vesicocervical, (4) vesicovaginal, (5) ureterovaginal, (6) rectovaginal, (7) urethrovaginal, (8) vaginoperineal. (Jeffcoate TNA: Principles of Gynaecology, 3d ed. London, Butterworths, 1967)

ureter, hydroureter, hydronephrosis, and ultimate loss of the kidney if the lesion is not dealt with in time.

In addition to the above, postoperative urinary or fecal drainage may occur through an abdominal incision. An abdominal wall urinary tract fistula results almost invariably from inadvertent suture placed in the bladder at the time of closure of the abdominal incision or an unrecognized incision into the bladder when the abdominal cavity is entered. These fistulas rarely close spontaneously. Recognition of the injury at the time it is made is of utmost importance. If 5 ml indigo carmine is instilled into the bladder before operation, there is instant spill of blue dye and instant diagnosis if the bladder is injured. This simple, harmless test for a bladder fistula should be routine in all patients in whom there is a remote possiblity of bladder injury.

Fecal fistulas involving the small intestines and draining either vaginally or through an abdominal incision are rare and usually occur when there has been much dissection of adherent adnexal masses, as in extensive endometriosis, residues of pelvic inflammatory disease, carcinoma of the ovary, and pelvic radiation therapy, with denudation of bowel serosa and peritoneum. Small bowel fistulas rarely close spontaneously, and their surgical repair is usually required.

but those associated with malignant disease, radiotherapy, or both are not.

Fistulous openings from the urinary tract into the vagina are urethrovaginal, vesicovaginal, or ureterovaginal. Urethrovaginal fistulas are almost invariably the result of an inept attempt at vaginal delivery with forceps; fortunately, such injuries are now rare. Vesico-vaginal fistulas may result from an obstetric injury, a traumatic pelvic fracture if bone spicules perforate the bladder, a pelvic cancer, or an injury during gynecologic surgery. Ureterovaginal fistulas are usually the result of injury at the time of either a simple or radical hysterectomy.

In the case of surgical injuries of the ureters or bladder, the defect is usually not evident until the local edema begins to subside and the sutures give way, seven to ten days after the operation; at this time urinary incontinence becomes evident. Examination of the patient in the knee–chest position, with a Sims' speculum holding the posterior vaginal wall away, may permit diagnosis of a urinary tract fistula. If not, three large pledgets of cotton may be placed in the vagina, one above the other, and methylene blue solution run into the bladder. If only the lowest pledget stains, the fistula is urethral; if the middle or upper pledget stains, the fistula is vesical; if none of the pledgets stains but the upper one is wet with urine, the fistula is ureteral. A cystoscopic examination may also be helpful in localizing the site and determining the size of the fistula.

It is of special importance that the exact nature of a urinary tract fistula be determined. A small traumatic vesicovaginal fistula may close spontaneously without incident. The outlook for a uretero-vaginal fistula is more dismal, since if the drainage does stop, the closure of the fistula is generally accompanied by stenosis of the

REFERENCES AND RECOMMENDED READING

Allen WA: Chronic pelvic pain. Am J Obstet Gynecol 109:198, 1971

Baden WF: Vaginal relaxation. Clin Obstet Gynecol 15, no. 4: 1033, 1972

Capraro VJ, Greenberg H: Adhesions of the labia minora: A study of 50 patients. Obstet Gynecol 39:65, 1972

Goff BH: The surgical anatomy of cystocele and urethrocele with special reference to the pubocervical fascia. Surg. Gynecol Obstet 87:725, 1948

Green TH Jr.: Gynecology, 2nd ed. Boston, Little, Brown & Co, 1971

Greenhill JP: Surgical Gynecology, 3rd ed. Chicago, Year Book Medical Publishers, 1963

Kinzel GE: Enterocele: A study of 265 cases. Am J Obstet Gynecol 81:1166, 1961

Mattingly RF: TeLinde's Operative Gynecology, 6th ed. Philadelphia: JB Lippincott, 1985

Meigs JV: Enterocele. In Meigs JV, Sturgis SH (eds): Progress in Gynecology, vol. 11. New York, Grune & Stratton, 1956

Nichols DH, Randall CL: Vaginal Surgery, 2nd ed. Baltimore, Williams & Wilkins, 1983

Porges RF, Porges JC, Blinick G: Mechanisms of uterine support and the pathogenesis of uterine prolapse. Obstet Gynecol 15:711, 1960

Taylor HC Jr.: Chronic pelvic congestion. Am J Obstet Gynecol 57:211, 1949

Tovell HMM, Dank L: Gynecologic Operations. Hagerstown, Harper & Row, 1978

Ulfelder H: The mechanisms of pelvic supports in women: Deductions from a study of the comparative anatomy and physiology of the structures involved. Am J Obstet Gynecol 72:856, 1956

Watson BP: Complete tear of perineum. In Meigs JV, Sturgis SH (eds): Progress in Gynecology, vol. 1. New York, Grune & Stratton, 1946

Pelvic Infections

David A. Eschenbach

52

The various types of pelvic infections are assuming increasing importance because they represent the most common condition that the gynecologist treats. There has been a dramatic increase in the recognition of pelvic infections because of new microbiologic and serologic techniques, because of educational efforts that have increased physician awareness, and because of a rapid increase in the prevalence of sexually transmitted infections (Table 52-1).

The impact of pelvic infections on the physical condition of women ranges from minor annoyance to serious illness, and in some instances, even death. The cost of treating pelvic infections is enormous if direct medical costs and indirect costs, including time lost from work, are calculated. For example, it has been estimated that by the year 2000, one of every two women who reached the reproductive age in the 1970s will have had an episode of pelvic inflammatory disease (PID). Of women with PID, 25% will have been hospitalized, 25% will have had major surgery, and 20% will be sterile.

All genital sites—the vulva, vagina, urethra, cervix, endometrium, fallopian tubes, and ovaries—are susceptible to infectious organisms. Certain agents preferentially infect certain sites and give rise to characteristic symptoms; other agents cause little symptomatology until major pathologic changes occur. Still other organisms are not recognized until congenital neonatal infection occurs or a male partner becomes infected. The gynecologist should have special knowledge of the infections caused by *Neisseria gonorrhoeae, Chlamydia trachomatis, Treponema pallidum,* genital mycoplasma, *Mycobacterium tuberculosis,* and anaerobic bacteria, which may act alone or together to produce pelvic infections ranging from mild vaginitis to severe PID.

GONORRHEA

Gonorrhea is caused by *Neisseria gonorrhoeae,* a gram-negative diplococcus. The bacteria that attach by pili to columnar or transitional cells are rapidly engulfed by pinocytosis. The organism attracts leukocytes, giving rise to the commonly associated purulent discharge. Gonorrhea is usually sexually transmitted, although it can be acquired by the newborn after passing through an infected cervix, causing gonorrheal ophthalmia.

Course of the Disease

N. gonorrhoeae first attaches to tissues of the lower genital tract that are not covered by stratified squamous epithelium: the urethra, the Bartholin glands, and the endocervix. The anus and rectum can also be infected either by colonization from cervical infection or during anal coitus. Urinary frequency, dysuria, and a purulent vaginal discharge are the first symptoms, usually appearing two to five days after exposure. Many women do not seek medical attention if these symptoms are mild. Occasionally the discharge is locally irritating and causes edema, erythema, and soreness of the vulva. Pharyngitis may result from *N. gonorrhoeae* pharyngeal infection. In 2% of infected women, disseminated gonococcal infection occurs, causing fever, septicemia, dermatitis, arthritis, endocarditis, or meningitis, in various combinations.

In about 20% of women with untreated gonorrhea, the organisms ascend to produce upper genital tract infection or acute PID (Fig. 52-1). Acute PID is the most common and serious sequel of gonorrhea. The mechanical and antibacterial properties of cervical mucus probably provide a barrier against upward extension; during menstruation the mucus barrier is lost and *N. gonorrhoeae* can be disseminated in a rich menstrual blood medium to the uterus and fallopian tubes. A transient endometritis occurs as the organisms pass through the uterine cavity and reach the fallopian tubes, where they produce an acute and usually bilateral, inflammatory reaction of the tubal mucosa. The tubes characteristically

Table 52-1
Sexually Transmitted Infections

Organisms	Diseases
Bacteria	
Neisseria gonorrhoeae	Gonorrhea
Chlamydia trachomatis	Chlamydial infection
Treponema pallidum	Syphilis
Hemophilus ducreyi	Chancroid
Calymmatobacterium granulomatis	Granuloma inguinale
Gardnerella vaginalis, anaerobes	Vaginitis
Group B β-hemolytic Streptococcus	Group B infection
Mycoplasmas	
Mycoplasma hominis	Mycoplasma infection
Ureaplasma urealyticum	Mycoplasma infection
Viruses	
Herpesvirus hominis	Genital herpes
Cytomegalovirus (CMV)	CMV infection
Hepatitis B virus	Hepatitis
Human Papillomavirus	Condyloma acuminatum
Molluscum contagiosum virus	Molluscum contagiosum
Protozoa	
Trichomonas vaginalis	Vaginitis
Fungi	
Candida albicans	Vaginitis
Parasites	
Sarcoptes scabiei	Scabies
Phthirus pubis	Pediculosis pubis

become swollen and reddened as the muscularis and serosa are inflamed. If exudate drips from the fimbriated ends of the tubes, a pelvic peritonitis is produced that ultimately can give rise to the filmy peritoneal adhesions typical of healed salpingitis. The swollen and congested fimbriae may adhere to one another and produce tubal occlusion.

The process may take any of the following courses:

1. With prompt, appropriate antibacterial therapy the infection may subside with little damage to the reproductive tract.
2. The swollen and congested fimbriae may adhere to one another or to the ovary, trapping the exudate in the tube and giving rise to pyosalpinx or, if the ovary becomes infected, to a tubo-ovarian abscess.
3. The mucosal folds may adhere to one another, forming glandlike spaces that are filled, at first, with exudate and later, as the process becomes chronic, by watery secretion, which is the so-called follicular salpingitis (Fig. 52-2).

4. If the infection subsides after agglutination of the fimbriae and closure of the peripheral end of the tube, watery secretion accumulates and distends the tube forming a hydrosalpinx, which is a retort-shaped structure resembling pyosalpinx (Fig. 52-3).

Hydrosalpinx was formerly regarded as the end stage of pyosalpinx, but the intact, atrophic epithelium and the absence of chronic inflammatory reaction suggest that the primary pathology is closure of the fimbriated end of the tube.

Symptoms and Signs

In the primary stage when gonorrhea is first acquired, and when it is most infectious, at least 50% of women have no symptoms. The most common symptoms, when they occur, are dysuria, urinary frequency, and a purulent vaginal discharge. Except for the discharge, which may be milked from the urethra or is present in the vagina, there are few signs of the acute gonococcal infection.

In the stage of acute salpingitis, bilateral, severe lower abdominal pain and pyrexia are common. Pelvic, usually not generalized, peritonitis is present. Direct and rebound tenderness; muscle guarding, which prevents abdominal palpation in the lower quadrants; and tender adnexa are present on bimanual examination. Movement of the cervix causes pain. However, a sizable proportion of women experience either mild or no symptoms in this primary stage.

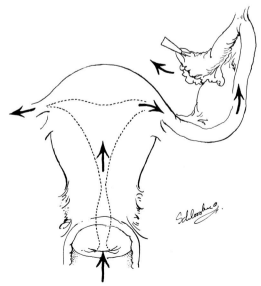

FIG. 52-1. Mode of transmission of gonococcal pelvic infection. Portal of entry is external genitalia. Organism enters cervix, following mucous membrane, passes up through uterine cavity, and attacks fallopian tube. Pelvic peritonitis results from escape of pus from tubal fimbria. (Wharton LR: Gynecology and Female Urology, 1st ed. Philadelphia, WB Saunders, 1943)

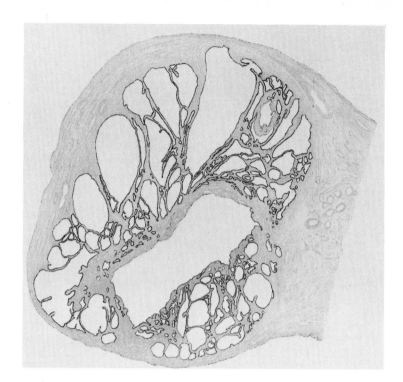

FIG. 52-2. Follicular salpingitis, an end stage of gonorrheal salpingitis. Mucosal folds adherent, giving rise to innumerable round or irregular cystlike cavities lined by cuboidal epithelium. (Kelly HA: Operative Gynecology, Vol 2, plate XI. New York, Appleton, 1898; drawing by Max Brödel)

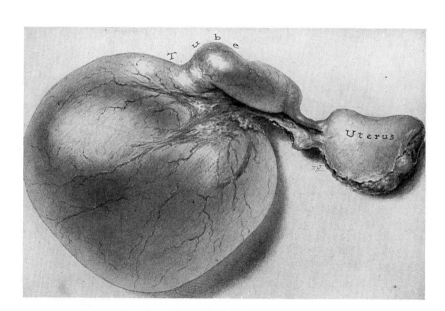

FIG. 52-3. Hydrosalpinx. (Curtis AH, Huffman JW: A Textbook of Gynecology, 6th ed. Philadelphia, WB Saunders, 1950)

In the stage of subacute salpingitis, the infection continues, but the signs and symptoms are less overt than are those of the acute stage.

In the end stage of salpingitis, the uterus and the adnexa are usually fixed by pelvic peritoneal adhesions. The adnexa are often either adherent to the posterior aspect of the uterus or are prolapsed in the cul-de-sac, which pulls the corpus uteri into a retroverted position. Notable features are dyspareunia, sterility, and chronic,

aching pelvic pain that increases before menstruation and subsides to an extent after menstruation.

Diagnosis

The diagnosis of gonorrhea depends on a culture of *N. gonorrhoeae*. Among symptomatic women during the initial phase of gonorrhea, the finding of intracellular gram-negative diplococci in the exudate from the cervix or urethra points to gonorrheal infection. Gonococcal cultures should be performed on women when Gram stains are positive; when symptoms suggest gonorrhea (women with undiagnosed vaginal discharge or dysuria); when other sexually transmitted diseases are present; when bartholinitis or skenitis is present; when acute lower abdominal pain suggests acute salpingitis; when suspected disseminated gonococcal infection is suspected; and when women are contacts of males with gonorrhea.

The sites to be cultured are, in order of importance, the cervix, the anal canal, the urethra, and the pharynx. Vaginal discharge should be wiped away from the cervix before obtaining either a culture or Gram stain. Genital samples must be cultured on Thayer–Martin or similar media containing antimicrobial agents that inhibit growth of the normal bacterial and fungal flora. Because 40% to 50% of women with gonorrhea also have chlamydia, patients with gonorrhea should also receive a test for chlamydial infection.

Serologic tests for active gonococcal infection have such a low predictive value that they are almost without benefit.

Since gonorrhea is a sexually transmitted disease, it follows that gonorrhea is also usually present in the male partner. The importance of identifying and treating male sexual contacts is emphasized by the fact that more than 40% of the male contacts of women with gonorrhea are asymptomatic carriers who would otherwise not seek treatment.

Treatment

Drug Therapy

Recent changes have been made in the recommended treatment for both complicated and uncomplicated gonorrhea. The current Center for Disease Control Recommended Treatment Schedules—1982 are detailed in the following sections.

UNCOMPLICATED LOWER GENITAL TRACT GONORRHEA. The drug regimens used to inhibit gonorrhea and chlamydial infections have changed to include either tetracycline, in a dosage of 500 mg 4 times daily, or doxycycline, in a dosage of 100 mg twice daily for 7 days. Tetracycline should not be used by pregnant women. Three other effective regimens are aqueous procaine penicillin G (APPG), 4.8 million units injected intramuscularly at two sites, with 1 g of probenecid by mouth; ampicillin 3.5 g with 1 g probenecid by mouth; or amoxicillin 3 g with 1 g probenecid by mouth. Patients who are allergic to penicillin should receive tetracycline, which must be given one to two hours after meals because food and milk products interfere with absorption. Women who cannot tolerate tetracycline may be treated with spectinomycin 2 g in one intramuscular injection.

Penicillin-resistant strains of *N. gonorrhoeae* that elaborate penicillinase continue to be present in some isolates, making it mandatory that all gonorrhea patients have posttreatment cultures three to seven days following therapy and that any posttreatment isolates be tested for penicillinase production. Patients who fail penicillin treatment should receive spectinomycin 2 g, cefoxitin 2 g with probenecid, or cefotaxime 1 g intramuscularly.

Patients with gonorrhea who also have incubating syphilis (seronegative, without clinical signs of syphilis) are likely to be cured by all of the above regimens except spectinomycin. In patients treated with spectinomycin, an initial as well as a six-week follow-up serologic test for syphilis should be performed.

ACUTE GONORRHEAL SALPINGITIS. Hospitalization is appropriate in the following situations: uncertain diagnosis, in which surgical emergencies such as appendicitis and ectopic pregnancy must be excluded; suspicion of pelvic abscess; severe illness; pregnancy; inability of patient to follow or tolerate an outpatient regimen; or failure to respond to outpatient therapy.

The following antimicrobial regimens are appropriate for outpatients: Cefoxitin 2 g IM followed by doxycycline 100 mg twice daily for 10 days; or APPG 4.8 million units intramuscularly, ampicillin 3.5 g, or amoxicillin 3 g, each with 1 gram probenecid in one dose followed by doxycycline for 10 days. Tetracycline should be avoided in pregnant patients, but the other drugs may be used.

For hospitalized patients, intravenous administration of one of the following three combination regimens may be used: cefoxitin 8 g daily with doxycycline 200 mg daily; Metronidazole 2 g daily with doxycycline; or gentamicin 240 mg daily with clindamycin 2400 mg daily. Upon discharge, oral doxycycline or clindamycin should be administered for a total of ten days. The tetracycline regimen should not be used in pregnant women.

Surgery

Laporoscopy may be helpful either for diagnosis or to define the extent of the disease. Surgery may be indicated in the case of a ruptured pyosalpinx or ovarian abscess; colpotomy drainage is usually preferable if the lesion is accessible. For example, if laporotomy is performed with a presumptive diagnosis of appendicitis and acute salpingitis is found instead, the procedure should be limited to the taking of a tubal culture and closure of the abdomen. If laporotomy is needed for such problems as an unresolved abscess or an adnexal mass that does not subside, surgery should be limited to the most conservative procedures that will be effective. Unilateral abscesses respond to unilateral salpingo-oophorectomy if appropriate antibiotic regimens are used; routine hysterectomy and bilateral salpingo-oophorectomy are rarely needed in young women with limited disease.

When chronic pain occurs, surgery should be deferred as long as possible to allow maximum healing. Mild analgesics (opiates should be avoided if possible) and heat may suffice until the swelling and fixation are reduced. Surgery may be indicated for persistent pain that does not respond to conservative measures, for recurrent attacks of pelvic pain, or for a pelvic mass that does not resolve. Laparoscopy with lysis of adhesions usually suffices, but occasionally adnexectomy or even hysterectomy is required. If sterility is the outstanding symptom, surgery may be indicated if the tubal lesion is determined to be amenable to surgical repair.

CHLAMYDIA

Chlamydia trachomatis is a sexually transmitted organism that is often associated with gonorrhea. Chlamydia infects the same tissues—the urethra, cervix, fallopian tubes, and Bartholin's glands—and produces the same spectrum of symptoms and diseases as gonorrhea. Analogous to gonococcal infection, transmission to males produces both symptomatic and asymptomatic urethritis. Chlamydia causes urethritis, bartholinitis, cervicitis, endometritis, and salpingitis, including Fitz-Hugh–Curtis perihepatitis. Lymphogranuloma venereum is a chlamydial infection. Neonates born of mothers with genital chlamydia infection have a 40% risk of developing chlamydial conjunctivitis and a 10% to 20% risk of developing chlamydial pneumonia.

C. trachomatis is an obligate intracellular bacteria. After attachment to columnar or transitional epithelial cells, it is engulfed by pinocytosis. The intracellular organisms remain within a phagosome membrane that protects them from host defense mechanisms, and they replicate until they replace most of the cell and ultimately cause the cell to rupture. The infective particles are released into the extracellular space and the process is repeated. The replication time is relatively slow, explaining the characteristically long latent period between the time of exposure and the onset of symptoms, which ranges from weeks to months.

Chlamydial infections are assuming increasing importance among the sexually transmitted diseases (STD). In most western societies *C. trachomatis* is three to five times more common than *N. gonorrhoeae*. The diagnosis is difficult because routine cultures for *C. trachomatis* are not performed among asymptomatic individuals, and hence, it is not often identified until overt infection occurs. The precise attack rate of chlamydial salpingitis is unknown, but it may approximate that of gonorrhea.

Diagnosis of chlamydial infections can be made by culture or by a newly developed direct monoclonal antibody slide test. Samples should be taken from both the cervix and the urethra because in many cases organisms will be identified in only one site. Other sites that are obviously infected should also be cultured. Since the organisms are obligate intracellular bacteria, tissue-culture methods similar to those used for virus recovery are required. The culture should contain cellular material; exudate alone is not sufficient. Serologic diagnosis by microimmunofluorescent methods is possible, but it is not widely available. Pap smears of genital material detect only 40% of infections.

Tetracycline and erythromycin (0.5 g four times daily for 7 to 10 days) are the most effective drugs in the treatment of chlamydial infections. Sulfa and sulfatrimethoprim preparations and chloramphenicol are also effective. Penicillins and clindamycin are less effective than these antibiotics. Cephalosporins and aminoglycosides do not cure chlamydial infections.

SYPHILIS

Although most women who have syphilis are asymptomatic and have only serologic evidence of infection, physicians must constantly be aware of the possibility of syphilitic infection. Spirochetes rapidly enter lymphatics after exposure, but a primary lesion, the *chancre,* usually takes about three weeks to develop. The classic primary ulcer is painless and firm, with sharply defined, raised edges; however, the majority of syphilitic ulcers are atypical. Therefore, any suspicious genital ulcer should be studied by dark-field examination. Serous material expressed from the ulcer base is mixed with saline, and because *Treponema pallidum* is an anaerobe, this must be immediately placed under a cover slip whose edges are occluded by Vaseline. The identification of typical spirochetes by dark-field microscopy establishes the diagnosis of primary syphilis. Serologic tests are usually nonreactive when the chancre first appears but become reactive one to four weeks later.

Secondary syphilis appears six or more weeks later and is characterized chiefly by a symmetric, macular, papular, or papulosquamous rash and generalized, nontender lymphadenopathy. *Condylomata lata* (Fig. 52-4) are highly infectious, hypertrophied, wartlike lesions of secondary syphilis that may occur in moist areas such as the vulva or perineum and must be distinguished from other vulvar lesions. Superficial, painless mucosal erosions of the mouth or vagina, called *mucous patches,* develop in one third of patients. Systemic symptoms of fever, weight loss, or malaise may occur. Serologic tests are positive.

Untreated patients then enter a latent phase of syphilis during which clinical and physical manifestations are absent. Diagnosis is established by serologic tests. Intermittent spirochetal bloodstream invasion may occur during the early latent phase of the first four years. In pregnancy, the risk of congenital infection of the fetus in the primary and secondary phases of syphilis is 80% to 95%; the risk during the early latent phase is 70%. During the late latent phase, immunity develops, which reduces blood invasion, and the risk of congenital syph-

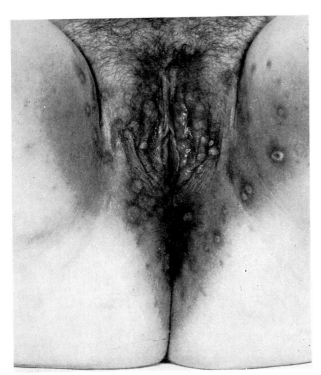

FIG. 52-4. Condylomata lata of vulva and perineum. (Curtis AH, Huffman JW: A Textbook of Gynecology, 6th ed. Philadelphia, WB Saunders, 1950)

ilis decreases to 10%. About one third of patients with untreated late syphilis manifest central nervous system or cardiovascular symptoms of tertiary syphilis.

Venereal Disease Research Lab (VDRL) and fluorescent treponemal antibody (FTA) serology should be performed for any patient who has a suspicious lesion; if it is nonreactive or if spirochetes cannot be demonstrated in the discharge, the tests should be repeated in one month.

VDRL antibody is a nontreponemal, nonspecific reagin antibody. The antibody can be titrated, and the titer either falls or disappears after therapy of early or secondary syphilis. Accordingly, the VDRL test can be used to judge the activity either of a first episode or of reacquired infection in a patient known to have had syphilis in the past. Treated patients with latent syphilis, however, may retain high, stable VDRL titers. Acute bacterial or viral infections can give rise to acute false-positive reactions that last up to six months. Several conditions such as aging, addiction to drugs, autoimmune disease, and pregnancy may give rise to chronic, nonspecific, false-positive VDRL reactions. False-positive VDRL titers are usually 1:8 or less. The FTA antibody is a specific antitreponemal antibody, and false-positive FTA reactions are rare. A patient with a positive VDRL should have a confirmatory FTA test to exclude a false-positive VDRL reaction. Patients with a false-positive VDRL will have a negative FTA test. In patients with syphilis, FTA antibody remains positive indefinitely, and since the test is not titrated, it is unnecessary to repeat FTA testing in a known positive patient.

Treatment

The treatment schedules for syphilis that are currently recommended by the U.S. Public Health Service Center for Disease Control are as follows.

Early Syphilis

Early syphilis is defined as primary, secondary, or latent syphilis of less than one year's duration. The drug of choice is benzathine penicillin G (2.4 million units total, intramuscularly) because it provides effective treatment in a single visit. Alternative choices include APPG, 4.8 million units total: 600,000 units by intramuscular injection daily for 8 days or, for patients who are allergic to penicillin, either tetracycline hydrochloride 500 mg 4 times daily by mouth for 15 days, or erythromycin (stearate, ethylsuccinate, or base) 500 mg 4 times daily by mouth for 15 days.

Syphilis of More Than One Year's Duration

Benzathine penicillin G is the drug of choice, 7.2 million units total: 2.4 million units intramuscularly each week for 3 successive weeks. Alternative choices include aqueous procaine penicillin G, 9.0 million units total: 600,000 units intramuscularly daily for 15 days or, for those who are allergic to penicillin, tetracycline hydrochloride 500 mg 4 times daily by mouth for 30 days, or erythromycin 500 mg 4 times daily by mouth for 30 days. As noted elsewhere, tetracycline must not be used in pregnancy.

Patients with syphilis of more than one year's duration require a spinal tap to exclude asymptomatic neurosyphilis.

Syphilis in Pregnancy

The treatment is the same as for the corresponding stage of syphilis among nonpregnant women except that tetracycline is not used and special follow-up is required. The Jarisch–Herxheimer reaction commonly occurs, and pregnant women should be hospitalized in anticipation of this possibility. The reaction is ascribed to the sudden massive destruction of spirochetes by antibiotics, and it is indicated by fever, myalgia, tachycardia and, occasionally, hypotension. Treatment is stopped if symptoms become severe. The reaction usually begins within 24 hours and subsides spontaneously in the next 24 hours of penicillin treatment.

GENITAL MYCOPLASMAS

Genital mycoplasmas have often been thought of as organisms in search of a disease because they are ubiquitous and not highly virulent. Two genital mycoplasmas are important: *Mycoplasma hominis,* which has been recovered from the vagina in 15% to 70% of women, and *Ureaplasma urealyticum* (formerly called T-strain mycoplasma), which has been recovered from 40% to 95% of women. The importance of a third isolate, *Mycoplasma genitalium,* is not yet known. The phylogenic position of the organism is between bacteria and viruses.

The most convincing role formycoplasmain human female infections is as a pathogen in salpingitis and postpartum fever. Mycoplasmas can be recovered from the tubes of 5% to 15% of women with salpingitis. In primate model studies, *M. hominis* produces an adnexitis but not salpingitis. Mycoplasmas have been recovered from the blood of 10% to 15% of women with postpartum fever, and antibodies to *M. hominis* have been demonstrated in 50% of such women.

The presence of the organism in the mother has also been associated with low birth weight and chorioamnionitis in the infant. Mycoplasmas have been recovered from the fetal tissue of midtrimester spontaneous abortuses, which suggests a relationship between the organism and abortion. The overall importance of mycoplasmas for the antepartum patient is unknown.

The organism's role in fertility is not settled. In some studies mycoplasmas have been isolated more frequently from infertile than fertile women, and in some studies women treated with antibiotics had higher fertility rates than did untreated controls. However, other investigators have failed to confirm these observations.

FIG. 52-5. Mode of transmission of tuberculous pelvic infection. Tubercle bacillus invades pelvic organs by way of blood stream from distant focus in lung or other organ. (Wharton LR: Gynecology and Female Urology, 1st ed. Philadelphia, WB Saunders, 1943)

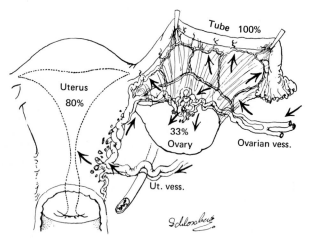

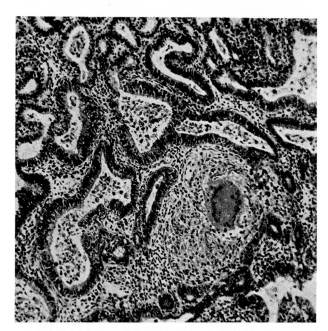

FIG. 52-6. Tuberculosis of fallopian tube. (Original magnification ×105). (Curtis AH, Huffman JW: A Textbook of Gynecology, 6th ed. Philadelphia, WB Saunders, 1950)

Both mycoplasmas are sensitive to tetracycline. Erythromycin inhibits *U. urealyticum* but not *M. hominis.* Both are sensitive to aminoglycosides and chloramphenicol, but not to sulfa.

GENITAL TUBERCULOSIS

Female genital tuberculosis is relatively uncommon in the United States, and fewer than 1% of salpingitis infections can be attributed to *Mycobacterium tuberculosis.* The reason for this is not entirely clear, because pulmonary tuberculosis remains a problem in many impoverished areas. Although it has been demonstrated that spread of tuberculosis from the primary pulmonary complex to the pelvis usually occurs early during tubercular infection, early detection is rarely feasible. Approximately 10% of patients with pulmonary tuberculosis also develop genital tuberculosis.

Pathogenesis

Virtually all genital infections are secondary to a pulmonary infection, which usually spreads by means of the bloodstream from the lung focus to the vascular wall of the fallopian tube, generally within one year of the primary pulmonary infection (Figs. 52-5, 52-6). Direct extension then occurs from the tube in several directions: to the pelvic peritoneum, to the endometrium, to the cervix, and to the ovary. Less commonly, lymphatic extension to genitalia can occur from abdominal sources or by direct extension from the intestinal tract. Genital tuberculosis is rarely caused by an ascending infection from a sexual partner with tuberculous epididymitis.

The initial tubal lesion may remain localized for a considerable period, in some cases years, or it may extend to the interior tubal mucosal surface. The endosalpingitis results either in an exudative phase with ulcer formation at the site of caseous degeneration, which produces the typical moth-eaten pattern seen on hysterosalpingography; or an adhesive phase in which large tubercles are present within the tubes (dense perisalpingeal adhesions are characteristic). In contrast to bacterial salpingitis, tubal occlusion, particularly fimbrial closure, does not occur early in tuberculous disease, and the tubes may remain patent despite relatively marked destruction of the tubal wall.

Tubal infection is present in virtually all women with genital tuberculosis. Endometrial infection is present in 50% to 80% of cases. Because of menstrual sloughing, infected endometrium is shed monthly; after menstruation, the endometrium is again infected by seeding from the tubes. Myometrial infection can occur, but only in the most advanced cases. Cervical infection occurs in only 10% to 25% of patients, resulting in either an ulcerative lesion that can grossly resemble cervical carcinoma, or a papillomatous lesion.

Clinical Forms

Latent Genital Tuberculosis

In this form, tuberculosis appears to be partially or completely arrested following an initial tubal infection, and the patient has few or no pelvic complaints. Pelvic physical findings are normal. The diagnosis is made in the course of an investigation of infertility (endometrial biopsy or dilatation and curettage) or by chance during laparotomy. In these cases a precarious balance exists between the disease and the host defense mechanisms. Active but latent infections have been documented 30 years following an initial infection.

Tuberculous Salpingitis

This is a more advanced infection that may develop immediately after the primary hematogenous tubal spread, or it may follow a prolonged latent phase. The tubes are grossly enlarged by the inflammatory reaction. Although the symptoms and findings can be identical to those of acute bacterial salpingitis, the clinical manifestations are usually more indolent and prolonged. Additionally, tuberculous salpingitis does not respond to the antibiotic therapy used for other forms of salpingitis. Despite these differences, tuberculosis is often discovered only by histologic examination of an excised tube.

Tuberculous Peritonitis

In this form, widespread infection of all peritoneal surfaces produces ascites, adhesions, and innumerable small nodules (tubercles) throughout the abdomen. Usually the serosal surfaces of the pelvic organs are involved, and the tubes are often patent. This form results from hematogenous or lymphatic spread.

Diagnosis

A history of pulmonary tuberculosis can often be elicited from patients with genital tuberculosis, but simultaneous active pulmonary infection is uncommon. A normal chest film does not exclude genital tuberculosis, because pulmonary lesions are found in only 30% to 50% of cases. The most common complaints are sterility and pelvic pain. Deteriorating health and menstrual abnormalities can also occur. Menorrhagia may be associated with the abdominal pain, but amenorrhea or oligomenorrhea may occur among patients with tuberculous peritonitis. Most women with genital tuberculosis are seen in the second and third decades of life, but because of the frequent tendency for long latency periods, the disease may become active even after menopause. It must be reemphasized that the clinical picture of tubal tuberculosis can be similar to that of acute bacterial salpingitis. In some cases the clinical picture can be very bizarre and in such cases Kelly's classic admonition comes to mind. When one is confronted with a pelvic problem that does not conform to expected rules, the first consideration should be ectopic pregnancy and the second should be pelvic tuberculosis. If the signs and symptoms of salpingitis occur in a woman who is considered to be virginal, pelvic tuberculosis should be strongly considered.

A first-strength tubercular skin test is important because a negative test virtually rules out the possibility of tuberculosis. Diagnosis can be established best by an endometrial biopsy; this should be performed during the week preceding menstruation, when the endometrium is thickest and is most likely to contain tubercles. A portion of the specimen should be cultured, and the remainder should be submitted for histologic examination. Repeated cultures of the menstrual flow have also been utilized with success by some investigators. If cultures of either biopsy specimens or menstrual blood are negative, a curettage may be productive. If tubercle bacilli are recovered by culture, antimicrobial susceptibility testing should be performed to predict drug resistance.

Endometrial biopsy, curettage, and culture of menstrual flow or endometrial tissue can provide an exact diagnosis of genital tuberculosis if they are positive, but, if negative, the presence of the disease cannot be excluded. If these measures fail to verify a diagnosis in a patient whose history and pelvic findings suggest genital tuberculosis, diagnostic laparotomy is justified. Diagnostic laparoscopy may be performed if there is minimal likelihood of tuberculous peritonitis, but caution must be used because of the possibility of perforating a loop of adherent bowel. Hysterosalpingography may reveal characteristic tubal patterns, but it may also cause severe exacerbation of pelvic tuberculosis and should not be used if there is a likely possibility that this disease is present.

The incidental discovery of reproductive tract tuberculosis, perhaps in the course of an infertility survey, may be the first indication that the patient has tuberculosis. In such patients an effort must be made to determine if other sites (*e.g.,* lungs, urinary tract, bone, and gastrointestinal tract) may also be infected.

Treatment

The therapy currently recommended is isoniazid 300 mg daily and ethambutol 1200 mg daily for 18 to 24 months. Patients without adnexal masses should have an endometrial biopsy for culture and microscopic examination 6 and 12 months after the onset of therapy. Persistent organisms should be susceptibility-tested to identify drug-resistant strains. Laparotomy is performed if adnexal masses persist for four months; rifampin or streptomycin should be given preoperatively. Bilateral salpingectomy and removal of other tuberculous foci may be performed in young women with minimal disease, but bilateral salpingo-oophorectomy and total hysterectomy are indicated in those who have advanced disease or are of advanced age. Pregnancy following tubal tuberculosis is rare, even among women with minimal disease. If the tubes are damaged by genital tuberculosis, efforts to improve fertility by tubal plastic operations are usually futile.

ANAEROBIC BACTERIA

Anaerobic bacteria are being associated with an increasing number of pelvic infections. The application of modern anaerobic culture techniques has accounted for most of this increased recognition of these infections. Typically, multiple anaerobic species, usually together with one or more aerobic bacteria, combine to form a polymicrobial infection. Intra-abdominal abscess, postoperative pelvic inflammatory disease, and bacterial vaginosis (nonspecific vaginitis) infections are currently the most important examples of anaerobic bacterial infection.

Anaerobic bacteria are part of the normal cervicovaginal flora. Although many of the mechanisms by which anaerobic bacteria become pathogenic and unknown, two mechanisms known to cause anaerobic infection are tissue trauma that occurs following surgery, which reduces the redox potential, and antibiotic selection that preferentially inhibits aerobic bacteria. The clinician can virtually assume the presence of anaerobes

when infection is associated with a foul-smelling odor and abscess formation; only anaerobes produce odorous metabolic products. Anaerobes are virtually always isolated from an abscess if modern anaerobic techniques are used before antibiotic therapy is begun. Anaerobic infections also commonly produce gas formation and thromboembolism.

The anaerobic bacteria most commonly found in genital infections include anaerobic gram-positive cocci (Peptococcus and Peptostreptococcus), gram-negative rods (Bacteroides species—*B. fragilis, B. melaninogenicus, B. bivius*—and Fusobacterium species), and anaerobic gram-positive rods (Clostridium and Enbacterum species).

The organism should be cultured before the institution of antimicrobial therapy. Because anaerobes are part of the normal flora, deep tissue cultures that are not contaminated by surface bacteria are required. Unfortunately, 48 or more hours are required for anaerobe recovery, and treatment is usually begun based upon clinical signs. Anaerobic infection should be particularly suspected with abscess formation, a foul odor, gas formation, tissue necrosis, "sterile" cultures from obviously infected sites, and thromboembolism. Antibiotic sensitivity testing is only a rough guide for an organism's susceptibility, but *in vitro* and *in vivo* experience has shown that clindamycin, metronidazole, second- and third-generation cephalosporins, and extended-spectrum penicillin are also very effective in treating anaerobic infections.

VULVITIS

Herpes

Today herpes simplex virus (HSV) infection is the most common cause of vulvar ulcers and is one of the most common viral genital infections. Typical HSV genital infection occurs three to seven days after exposure. Primary (first) genital infections typically consist of multiple vesicles that rapidly produce coalescent ulcerations of the vulva, which may be exceedingly painful. The vagina and cervix may also be involved, producing profuse leukorrhea. External dysuria is common and bilateral inguinal lymphadenopathy is usual. Vulvar lesions may last three or more weeks but after this time heal completely. Constitutional symptoms of fever, malaise, headache (aseptic meningitis), and urinary retention (myelitis) may persist for one week. Primary infection may also result in few or no noticeable ulcers.

Following the primary infection, latent HSV infection usually occurs in the sacral ganglion and perhaps locally in the dermis. The virus is rarely transmitted during the latency period when there are no symptoms and no physical evidence of infection. However, most patients develop a secondary (recurrent) infection from the latent virus weeks to months after the primary infection. The lesions of the secondary infection are usually less painful, more localized, and last a shorter time (three to seven days) than those of the primary infection. Systemic reactions are unusual in secondary HSV.

The infection is caused by *Herpesvirus hominis.* From 75% to 85% of genital infections are caused by type-2 *H. hominis;* the remainder of genital infections are caused by type-1 *H. hominis,* which is the primary cause of lip and perioral infections. The two types of herpes are clinically indistinguishable. The vesicles and ulcers of HSV infection contain many virus particles that are highly infectious, and viral shedding occurs until the lesions reepithelialize. Therefore, genital contact with a person who has either genital or oral lesions leads to a high attack rate. Transmission usually occurs from contact with symptomatic lesions, but the virus can be isolated from asymptomatic lesions. It is rarely present in normal-appearing vulvar and cervical tissue.

The diagnosis of herpes can be made clinically if typical, painful, multiple vulvar ulcers are present. Laboratory confirmation of atypical lesions and lesions that appear during pregnancy is best attained by virus isolation, which usually can be achieved within 48 hours. Pap smears or other cytologically examined material can identify intracellular inclusions and multinucleated cells, but unfortunately the cytologic method is only 40% as sensitive as culture in identifying HSV infections. Accordingly, a negative cytologic search in no way excludes HSV infection. Complement fixing and neutralizing antibodies appear within one week of the onset of infection; failure of an experienced laboratory to identify antibodies within three weeks is evidence against HSV infection. High antibody levels do not protect against recurrent or neonatal HSV infection.

The increased frequency of herpes infection and its serious fetal effects have caused HSV to assume increasing importance in pregnancy. This is discussed in Chapter 30.

HSV infection has been associated with cervical cancer. Women with cervical cancer have a higher incidence of antibody and usually a higher antibody titer than do controls without cancer. HSV has caused nongenital animal tumors; however, these circumstantial reports suggesting a relationship between herpes and cancer are not sufficient to establish a direct effect of HSV in causing human cancer. Nevertheless, women with HSV infection should receive frequent Pap smears and colposcopic examinations.

Local therapy of genital herpes is limited to the relief of pain. Most of the local treatment modalities either do not penetrate to virus-containing cells or are administered after the damage has occurred. They neither shorten the duration of symptoms nor prevent recurrent infection. Many local antiviral compounds have been used, but rigorous double-blind and well-controlled studies have shown most of them to be ineffective. Local symptomatic therapy is often helpful (*e.g.,* a 10-minute Sitz bath 3 to 4 times daily, followed by drying with a bulb light or a hair dryer). Corticosteroids and antibacterial and antifungal ointments are not only without

benefit but tend to prevent drying, and as a result may delay healing. The most promising treatment alternative is systemic antiviral therapy such as acyclovir, which reduces the ulcerative phase and, if used continually, reduces recurrences. However, it is not effective enough to warrant routine use.

Condyloma Acuminatum

The genital wart (Fig. 52-7) is caused by a DNA virus of the papovavirus group which is distinct from the papovaviruses that cause the common warts. This virus thrives in the moist genital area and is usually sexually transmitted. The incubation period averages three months. Warts are most commonly located on the labia and posterior fourchette. They originally appear as individual lesions although, if neglected, large confluent growths up to several centimeters in diameter can occur. Vaginal and cervical warts are common. When white warts are found on the cervix, they may be atypical and biopsy or colposcopy may be needed to exclude cervical neoplasia; if so, treatment should be delayed until the nature of the lesion is determined. Recently, a flat-wart variant has been discovered that typically causes koilocytosis in Pap smears, and small lesions are usually only visible by colposcopy. The flat wart has also been associated with cervical dysplasia and cancer. More information is required on the therapy of this wart, but women with flat warts should have frequent Pap smears.

Genital warts must be differentiated from the less verrucous, more flat growths of syphilitic condyloma latum (see Fig. 52-4) and carcinoma *in situ* of the vulva; punch biopsies may be required to exclude these lesions. Small to medium-sized verrucous lesions can usually be treated with 25% podophyllin in tincture of

FIG. 52-7. Condylomata acuminata of vulva.

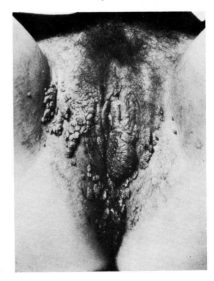

benzoin, which the patient must wash off after four hours. Small amounts (0.25 ml) should be used to prevent severe burns; the drug should not be used at all during pregnancy. Large amounts have produced coma in the adult and even fetal death in pregnant women. Atypical lesions should be biopsied before therapy because podophyllin causes bizarre histologic changes that persist for months. Liquid nitrogen, trichloroacetic acid, or cryocautery should be used if the lesions do not respond to podophyllin or if the woman is pregnant. Recurrence often results from reinfection by an untreated partner or from failure to treat vaginal and cervical lesions.

Furunculosis

The hair follicles of the mons and vulva may become infected by staphylococci, giving rise to pustules. This must be distinguished from herpetic and syphilitic lesions. The diagnosis can be made by culture or by the finding of gram-positive cocci in Gram stains of pus taken from the hair follicle. If only a few small lesions are present, they can be treated with hot, wet compresses or hexachlorophene scrubbing. Larger areas require antistaphylococcal antibiotics.

Bartholinitis

Two stages of Bartholin gland infection occur. The first is an acute infection of the duct and lining of the gland, usually by either *N. gonorrhoeae* or *C. trachomatis*. If unchecked, obstruction of the duct results, leading to the second stage, abscess formation. Anaerobic bacteria can be isolated from the majority of such abscesses. Rarely, synergistic vulvar gangrene has resulted from bartholinitis.

Cultures and a Gram stain of material expressed from the duct may identify gonococci. Cervical gonococcal cultures and chlamydial tests should be obtained, and if the patient is in the initial stage of gonococcal infection ampicillin or tetracycline should be administered for seven to ten days, as discussed previously in this chapter. Patients in the second stage usually require abscess marsupialization or incision with placement of a drain for three to six weeks. Simple incision and drainage usually lead to recurrent abscess formation. Recurrent infection from vaginal flora and mucus cyst formation are frequent sequelae of bartholinitis.

Chancroid

The soft chancre infection characteristically causes a painful ulcer with a ragged, undermined edge and a raised border. In contrast, the syphilitic chancre is painless and indurated. "Kissing ulcers" on apposing surfaces of the vulva may occur. Tender, unilateral adenopathy is common, and suppuration occurs in about 50% of women with lymphadenopathy.

The incubation period of this uncommon, sexually transmitted disease is two to five days. The infection is caused by *Hemophilus ducreyi*, gram-negative bacteria that form a school-of-fish pattern when seen in the Gram-stain preparation. The organism is fastidious, and it is best recovered by using newly developed media to culture aspirated lymph nodes or the chancre.

The differential diagnosis includes syphilis, which can be excluded by dark-field examinations of the lesion on at least three separate days. Chancroid may also resemble genital herpes and lymphogranuloma venereum. Treatment with sulfisoxazole is preferred so that dark-field and serologic studies of syphilis are not obscured; tetracycline therapy has also been successful.

Granuloma Inguinale

This chronic granulomatous infection is rare in temperate climates. The organism is usually considered to be sexually transmitted, although gastrointestinal transmission may occur in some cases. The initial papular lesion typically ulcerates and develops into a soft, red, painless granuloma that may be covered by a thin gray membrane. The granuloma may spread over the course of many months to involve the anus and rectum (Fig. 52-8). Lymph nodes are moderately enlarged and painless, but they do not suppurate. Long-standing disease may cause not only genital scarring and depigmentation, but also lymphatic fibrosis with consequent genital edema. Malignancy has been reported in granulomatous areas, but this is unusual.

The infection is caused by a gram-negative bacillus, *Calymmatobacterium granulomatis,* which is difficult to culture because it is an intracellular parasite. The identification is usually made from scraped or biopsied material obtained from the periphery of the lesion. Bipolar staining bacteria are best identified within mononuclear cells (*Donovan bodies*) by Wright or Giemsa staining.

The differential diagnosis includes syphilis, chancroid, and lymphogranuloma venereum. Two to three weeks of ampicillin, tetracycline, or erythromycin is the therapy of choice.

Lymphogranuloma Venereum (LGV)

The incubation period for LGV is two to five days. Thereafter, a transient, primary, painless genital or anorectal ulcer develops. Multiple large, confluent inguinal nodes develop two to three weeks later and eventually suppurate. Acute infection may cause generalized systemic symptoms. If untreated, the infection enters a tertiary phase that can lead to extensive lymphatic obstruction that, together with continued infection, causes fistulas and ulceration of the anal, urethral, or genital area.

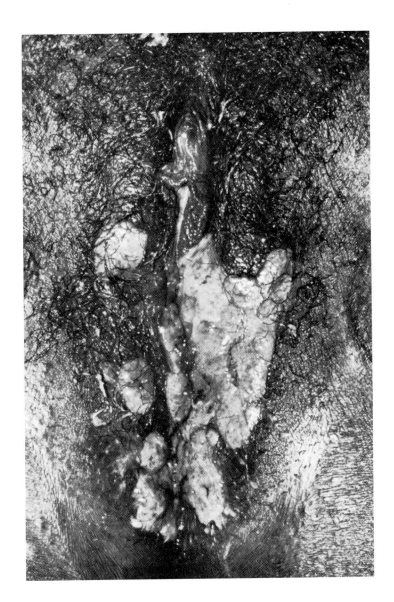

FIG. 52-8. Vulval granuloma inguinale of relatively recent origin. Some lesions are separate, others confluent. Margin of lesion is raised and scrolled; base is granular and covered imperfectly by thin, gray slough. (Demis DJ, Crounse RG, Dobson RL, McGuire J [eds]: Clinical Dermatology, Vol 3. Hagerstown, Harper & Row, 1972)

Women with LGV are particularly susceptible to rectal stricture. Edema and elephantiasis of the external genitalia and lower extremities are serious sequelae.

The infection is caused by the sexually transmitted organism *C. trachomatis*, an intracellular bacterium. Usually only L_{1-3} chlamydia immunotypes, which produce accelerated *in vitro* tissue destruction, cause LGV. The diagnosis can be made by culturing Chlamydia from genital lesions or lymph nodes. Cell culture methods are required to recover the organism. Indirect serologic methods are available. The most specific and sensitive serologic test is the microimmunofluorescent antibody test in which the specific immunotype and titer are identified. Complement fixation (CF) tests are positive in 95% of patients with LGV, but the CF test lacks specificity; it is often falsely positive in patients without LGV because of to their exposure to other chlamydial infec-

tions. The intradermal Frei test is no longer used because it reacts positively if there are other prior or concurrent chlamydial infections.

The disease responds to tetracycline, erythromycin, and sulfonamide drugs. Large lymph nodes should be aspirated to prevent chronic drainage. Surgical excision of scarred areas may be necessary.

ACUTE URETHRAL SYNDROME

It is well recognized that no more than one half of women with symptoms of dysuria and urinary frequency have acute cystitis, which is defined by pyuria and midstream urine cultures that contain greater than 10^5 organisms per milliliter of coliform or staphylococcal organisms. Until recently, the cause of symptoms in the remaining women was unknown. Some women will have vaginitis. Women with external dysuria consisting of labial pain with urination and a vaginal discharge often are found to have candidal vaginitis. Women with recent onset of internal dysuria and urinary frequency who do not have vaginitis or 10^5 organisms per milliliter in the urine cultures, are usually considered to have an acute urethral syndrome. The infectious causes of acute urethral syndrome among females has been recently analyzed. About one half of women with acute urethral syndrome have less than 10^5 coliforms or *Staphylococcus saprophyticus* per milliliter isolated from urine obtained by suprapubic aspirates or urethral catheterization. Virtually all of these women have pyuria, defined as eight or more leukocytes per HPF of urine. An additional one fourth of patients with this syndrome have "sterile" pyuria; *C. trachomatis* can be isolated from two thirds of these women with pyuria. Usually no organisms are isolated from the remaining one fourth of patients without pyuria or bacteriuria. Although women who have recently acquired gonorrhea often develop transient dysuria, gonorrhea is only occasionally isolated from a general group of women with dysuria.

Therapy of acute urethritis consists of therapy for the infectious agent, whether it is coliform, *S. saprophyticus,* or Chlamydia.

A more chronic form of urethritis, which consists of periurethral gland inflammatory reaction that has responded to some degree to urethral dilatation, has been identified by cystoscopy. However, this entity has not been well studied bacteriologically, and it is unknown how many of these patients have a chlamydial or a low-bacterial-count coliform type of urethritis.

VAGINITIS

Vaginal infections are the most common gynecologic complaint. Infectious vaginitis can produce symptoms of increased vaginal discharge, vulvar irritation and pruritus, external dysuria, and a foul odor. Women with infectious vaginitis have either abnormal organisms (Trichomonads), or a quantitative increase in the normal flora (Candida, *G. vaginalis,* anaerobes). At least four entities of infectious vaginitis have been identified; candidal; trichomonal; bacterial vaginosis (nonspecific vaginitis); and, in children, gonococcal. Every effort should be made to establish the diagnosis of one of these specific infections and to avoid the diagnosis of unspecified vaginitis. The establishment of a specific diagnosis is mandatory because the selection of effective therapy depends on a correct diagnosis.

Other conditions that may cause excessive vaginal discharge include cervicitis, a cervical erosion or ectropion, vaginal foreign bodies (most commonly retained tampons), and allergic reactions to douching or vaginal contraceptive agents. The atrophic "vaginitis" among postmenopausal women may produce burning and dys-

pareunia; an infectious etiology has not been established.

A small amount of vaginal discharge may be normal, particularly at the midcycle when large amounts of cervical mucus production may produce a clear vaginal discharge. A normal vaginal discharge should not have a foul odor, nor should it be pruritic.

Examination

The external genitalia may be normal, or they may be edematous, erythematous, and excoriated to the point of fissure formation. Occasionally local primary vulvar disease must be excluded from a secondary effect of vaginitis.

On speculum examination the vaginal mucosa may be erythematous or edematous. Discharge characteristics that are important to observe are the viscosity of the discharge, the presence of floccular elements, the color, and the odor. Vaginal discharge should be examined for the *p*H; in addition, a potassium hydroxide (KOH) odor test and a microscopic exam consisting of a normal saline and 10% KOH wet mount should be done. A drop of each solution is mixed with the discharge. Before placing a cover slip over the two separate drops, the KOH portion is tested for the presence of a fishy amine odor. Microscopic examination of the KOH portion is made for hyphae under the 100× objective, and examination of the saline portion is made for trichomonads and clue cells under the 400× objective. Multiple causes of vaginitis are frequent.

Vaginal cultures are not particularly helpful except when used selectively to identify candidal or trichomonal infection. Microscopy, the most specific diagnostic method, is only 80% sensitive in identifying various types of vaginitis. Therefore, when infectious vaginitis is suspected among patients who do not have specific diagnoses established, a repeat examination should be performed several days later.

Candida

The most prominent symptom of candidal vaginitis is intense vulvar and vaginal pruritus. External dysuria is common. A curdlike vaginal discharge and vulvar pain may also occur. Vulvar signs of edema, geographic erythema, and fissures may be present. Classically, the vagina is dry and it has a bright red color mottled by adherent white, curdy plaques. However, many women with candida have little discharge and no erythema.

Candida albicans causes more than 90% of vaginal yeast infections. Other Candida and Torulopsis species can also cause infection. These saprophytic fungi can be isolated from the vagina in 15% to 25% of asymptomatic women. Therefore, the mere presence of vaginal Candida does not identify an infection, but an overgrowth of these organisms can lead to symptomatic vaginitis. An overgrowth is produced by a change in host resistance or in the local bacterial flora, which allows the organisms to proliferate. Several host factors have been associated with candidal infection, the most widely accepted of which are pregnancy, diabetes, and the administration of immunosuppressive drugs and broad-spectrum antibiotics. Because cellular, and not humoral, immunity is required for resistance to fungal infections, pregnant women and patients receiving immunosuppressive drugs that decrease the cellular immunity are predisposed to excessive fungal growth. Overgrowth is also favored by high urine glucose levels; pregnant women and diabetics with elevated blood glucose levels are susceptible. Women treated with broad-spectrum antibiotics may develop candidal vaginitis as a result of antibiotic suppression of the normal gastrointestinal and vaginal bacterial flora, thereby allowing fungal overgrowth. The role of oral contraceptives in candidal infection remains controversial. These compounds do cause both carbohydrate metabolic alterations and an increased prevalence of Candida in the vagina. However, the rate of symptomatic candidal infection among oral contraceptive users is no higher than among nonusers. A small subset of users, however, may develop recurring infections. It is not necessary to discontinue oral contraceptives if candidal infection occurs only infrequently, unless recurring infections occur.

The most practical means of diagnosing candidal vaginitis is by microscopic examination of wet mount. Vaginal plaques, vaginal discharge, or vulvar scrapings from the edge of the erythematous border is mixed with 10% potassium hydroxide (Fig. 52-9). The mycelial form that usually is found only during an infection can be identified in this preparation in 80% of the cases. The Gram stain, which also identifies the blastospore forms of both noninfectious and infectious states, is more sensitive than wet mounts in identifying fungi. Fungi can be readily recovered on a variety of media. Because they are part of the normal vaginal flora, the recovery of fungi by culture does not necessarily diagnose an infection. Cultures should be limited to patients with suspected candidal vaginitis, including those with unidentified pruritus or suspicious signs that cannot be identified by examination of the wet mount.

In most cases of candidal vaginitis the organisms can also be cultured from the rectum. Since antifungal preparations are not absorbed from the intestinal tract, local vaginal therapy is required. Two imidazole agents, miconazole nitrate and clotrimazole, are more active than nystatin against Candida *in vitro*. The vaginal insertion of boric acid capsules may also be effective. These agents should be administered to women with primary and repeated candidal vaginitis because they are more likely than nystatin to completely eradicate fungi from the vagina and also to prevent recurrent infection. Although imidazole drugs are not absorbed to any degree from the vagina, there is some concern over the possibility of fetal teratogenicity; their use in pregnancy should, therefore, be limited to the last 20 weeks. The preparations are inserted vaginally once nightly for seven days or twice daily for seven doses. More prolonged therapy may be necessary in certain cases. About 15% of male sexual contacts of women with candidal vaginitis have symptomatic balanitis. It is unclear whether the male infection causes or results from vaginal candidiasis. However, males should be identified and treated to prevent recurrent female infection. Oral antifungal administration to decrease gastrointestinal colonization does not improve therapeutic cure rates or diminish recurrence rates.

The patient who develops frequent recurrences represents the most difficult problem in the treatment of candidal vaginitis. Extended two- to three-week vaginal therapy, treatment of the male, and reduction of sugar intake are at present the only ways to limit these often frustrating infections. A glucose tolerance test should be performed in recurrent or resistant cases to exclude unrecognized diabetes. Also, some women with candidal infection have additional concurrent vaginal infections; a repeated physical and wet-mount examination may clarify the problem.

Gentian violet (1% aqueous solution) has a limited place in the treatment of resistant or recurrent infection. It may cause local edema, and leaves an indelible stain on clothing and linens.

Trichomonas Vaginitis

The characteristic symptoms of Trichomonas infection are a profuse, malodorous, often uncomfortable and sometimes frothy vaginal discharge, internal and exter-

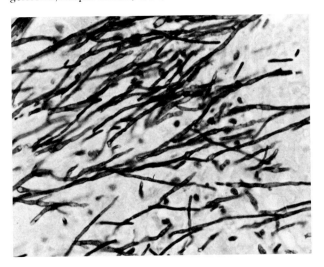

FIG. 52-9. *C. albicans* growing as hyphae and pseudohyphae within infected tissue (Original magnification ×320). (Monif GRG: Infectious Diseases in Obstetrics & Gynecology. Hagerstown, Harper & Row, 1974)

nal dysuria, and vulvar pruritus. This is probably one of the most common sexually transmitted organisms; it is present in 3% to 15% of asymptomatic women and in 20% to 50% of women who attend clinics for sexually transmitted disease. The organism is most likely to be identified among symptomatic women who have recently acquired the infection. However, over 50% of women with trichomonas are asymptomatic. Most male contacts of women with trichomoniasis asymptomatically carry the organism in the urethra and prostate.

The classic vaginal discharge is present in only about one third of women. The vulva may be edematous and moistened by the discharge. Subepithelial hemorrhage of the cervix ("strawberry cervix") is sometimes seen with the naked eye; smaller hemorrhagic areas are usually identified colposcopically. Women with symptomatic trichomoniasis have a discharge that has a *p*H of greater than 4.5 and forms amines with 10% potassium hydroxide. Motile trichomonads are demonstrated in the saline wet-mount (Fig. 52-10) smear. Trichomonads are larger than white blood cells, and they are identified by their rapid, jerking motility. The wet mount usually also contains many polymorphonuclear leukocytes. Nonmotile trichomonads can sometimes be identified by a Pap smear by their characteristic flagellate appearance. Although the wet mount may identify trichomonads with 80% sensitivity among symptomatic women, overall less than 50% of women with trichomoniasis have the organisms identified by a wet mount.

FIG. 52-10. Characteristic configuration of a trichomonad seen in wet smear at high-power magnification. (Monif GRG: Infectious Diseases in Obstetrics & Gynecology. Hagerstown, Harper & Row, 1974)

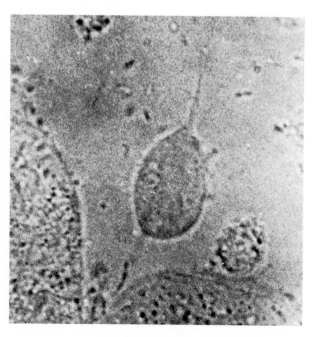

The organism, *Trichomonas vaginalis,* is an anaerobic protozoan. A culture of *T. vaginalis* is easy to perform but, unfortunately, because a freshly prepared medium is needed, culture has limited practicality, and its current use is limited to cases in which the diagnosis is suspected, but the organism cannot be identified in the wet mount or in a Pap smear. Screening cultures of asymptomatic women are not presently recommended except for certain high-risk populations. Women with trichomoniasis should also be cultured for *N. gonorrhoeae,* because as many as 60% of women with proved gonorrhea also have been found to have trichomoniasis. Trichomoniasis frequently causes the symptom that led the patient with gonorrhea to present for care.

T. vaginalis resides not only in the vagina, but also in the urethra, bladder, and Skene's glands; therefore, systemic rather than local therapy is required. Metronidazole is effective in treating trichomoniasis; the preferred regimen is 2 g in one dose because of complete patient compliance and high effectiveness. Extended seven-day metronidazole therapy of 500 mg 3 times daily does not increase the 95% cure rate of a single dose. Simultaneous treatment of the male sexual partner is recommended. Recurrent trichomoniasis is usually attributable to a lack of drug compliance or reexposure to untreated sexual partners. The organism usually remains very sensitive to metronidazole *in vitro,* but some organism insensitivity is being reported.

Metronidazole therapy is controversial because of questions of its possible tumor-causing potential in humans. In animals, large doses (equivalent to 350 to 1000 human doses) cause tumors. The drug has also been shown to cause bacterial mutation of the kind associated with a drug's carcinogenic potential. In small series of women evaluated for up to ten years following metronidazole therapy for trichomoniasis, no increased tumor rates were found. However, these data are only slightly reassuring that the drug does not cause cancer. Because of these concerns, the drug should be avoided in pregnancy, particularly during the first 20 weeks. Unfortunately, other drugs that may be used during pregnancy lack efficacy, and the iodine preparations, which may be somewhat effective, should not be used because the iodine is absorbed in high enough levels to suppress the fetal thyroid. For nonpregnant women, the short-term use of a drug with at most a minimal carcinogenic potential seems justified, especially because this is the only agent that eradicates the disease.

Candidiasis and trichomoniasis often coexist. Persistent discharge after adequate treatment for trichomoniasis should lead to repeated cultures for both candidiasis and gonorrhea.

Bacterial Vaginosis (Nonspecific Vaginitis)

The term *bacterial vaginosis* is now used to identify the vaginitis that results from an overgrowth of both anaerobic bacteria and the organism formerly referred to as *Hemophilis vaginalis,* but now renamed *Gardner-*

ella vaginalis in recognition of Herman Gardner, who first described the syndrome and identified the organism. Both anaerobes and *G. vaginalis* are normal inhabitants of the vagina, but their overgrowth results in the appearance of a thin, homogeneous, foul-smelling (hence vaginosis), yellow-gray vaginal discharge that adheres to the vaginal walls and is present at the introitus. In contrast to most other kinds of vaginitis, the vaginal epithelium appears normal and white blood cells are not usually present. The "fishy," foul odor that is caused by amines produced by the anaerobes is accentuated when 10% potassium hydroxide is added to the discharge.

The diagnosis of bacterial vaginosis is based on a pH greater than 4.5, the characteristic homogeneous appearance of the discharge, a fishy amine odor with the addition of 10% KOH, and the presence of clue cells. Clue cells are vaginal epithelial cells to which gram-negative organisms are attached. These cells are epithelial cells that are stippled with adherent bacteria; typically, the cell border is so obscured by adherent bacteria that it cannot be identified. In bacterial vaginosis, 2% to 50% of the epithelial cells show this distinctive marking, but as mentioned, polymorphonuclear leukocytes and lactobacilli are notably absent. Gram stains can also be used for diagnosis. Small curved rods called *Mobiluncus* found on Gram stain are highly associated with this entity. Cultures are not helpful because anaerobes and *G. vaginalis* can be recovered from normal women. In fact, up to 40% of asymptomatic normal women carry *G. vaginalis*. Although the number of colonies of both organisms is higher among women with bacterial vaginosis than among normal women, quantitative culture methods are cumbersome and they add only slightly to the specificity of diagnosis.

The factors that lead to an overgrowth of *G. vaginalis* and anaerobes have not been identified. Sexual transmission of the infection has long been considered a risk factor, but this has not been proven. *G. vaginalis* can usually be recovered from the urethra of the male sexual contact, but treatment of the male does not prevent recurrence of the infection.

Metronidazole (500 mg twice daily for 7 days, or as a 2-gram STAT dose) is the most effective drug for bacterial vaginosis. Ampicillin administered orally (500 mg every 6 hours for 7 days) cures 60% of the cases. The difference in response between these two drugs has not been explained. Metronidazole is usually effective only against the anaerobes, although metronidazole metabolites do inhibit *G. vaginalis*. Tetracycline, sulfonamides, and erythromycin are ineffective. At the present time, the treatment of the male with ampicillin can only be advocated when bacterial vaginosis recurs.

Toxic Shock Syndrome

Toxic shock syndrome is a newly described acute illness caused by the toxin-producing *Staphylococcal aureus* species. About 6% of women carry *S. aureus* in the vagina, but only 2% of women have *S. aureus* bacteriophage types that are capable of producing the toxin. The syndrome is highly associated with menstruation, and probably with tampon use, but it has also occurred following delivery and abdominal operations. Characteristic features include a high fever ($\geq 38.9°C$), a diffuse rash, hypotension, skin desquamation (usually one to two weeks later), and a wide variety of systemic effects such as gastrointestinal (vomiting, diarrhea), muscular (myalgia), mucous membrane (hyperemia), renal (elevated blood urea nitrogen or creatinine levels), hepatic (enzyme abnormalities), dermatologic (thrombocytopenia), and brain (disorientation, coma) abnormalities. The case-to-fatality ratio has been reduced from 15% to 3%. Vaginal cultures recover *S. aureus*. Blood, throat, and cerebrospinal fluid cultures, together with serologic tests for Rocky Mountain spotted fever, leptospirosis and measles, are usually indicated to exclude diseases with similar presentations.

The vaginal tampon, if present, should be removed. Patients should be hospitalized and, when indicated, given large fluid volumes for blood pressure maintenance. β-Lactamase–resistant antibiotics are recommended, and if other causes of bacterial sepsis such as meningococcemia cannot be excluded, additional antibiotics are given. Other life-supporting measures such as intubation, vasopressor administration, and dialysis are often necessary. Antibiotics are not of proven benefit in the acute illness stage, but they do reduce recurrence rates from 30% to 5%.

Although the effectiveness is uncertain, it is prudent for all women to avoid the prolonged and overnight use of tampons or intravaginal contraceptive devices. It is recommended that postpartum women not wear tampons of any kind for six to eight weeks after delivery. Women who have had toxic shock syndrome should be advised against resuming tampon use and warned of recurrence.

CERVICITIS

The majority of hysterectomy specimens contain an area beneath the squamocolumnar junction that is infiltrated by plasma cells and lymphocytes. In the presence of such cells, the pathologist is obliged to make a diagnosis of chronic cervicitis. Unless the inflammatory reaction is extensive, there are no symptoms, and cultures recover either no organisms or only organisms that are part of the normal vaginal flora. This condition is not of clinical importance. To qualify as a pelvic infection, the inflammatory reaction must result from the effects of pathogenic organisms or established infection. The common causes of acute cervicitis are *N. gonorrhoeae*, *C. trachomatis*, and puerperal infection. The organisms penetrate the columnar epithelium or areas denuded by obstetric or surgical injury. Symptoms are usually limited to a profuse purulent vaginal discharge or intermenstrual bleeding. In more than three fourths of women who have a purulent or mucoid cervical discharge, *N. gonorrhoeae* or *C. trachomatis* can be isolated separately or in combination from the endocervix. The diagnosis can be established by the presence of white or yellow cervical mucus or by more than ten white blood cells per high-powered microscopic field. Associated findings include cervical bleeding, erythema, and edema. Tetracycline therapy is recommended.

Infectious ulcers of the cervix caused by herpes virus, syphilis, and chancroid must be distinguished from erosion and the other conditions described in Chapter 56. Depending on the nature of the lesion, Gram stain, Pap smear, culture, dark-field examination, colposcopy and, in some cases, biopsy may be required.

ENDOMETRITIS

Scattered lymphocytes and occasional neutrophils normally appear in the endometrium in the second half of the menstrual cycle, and their presence does not necessarily constitute endometritis. In some cases of abnormal bleeding, they may appear, and they may represent an abnormal inflammatory reaction. In at least one report, chronic endometritis was related to the isolation of genital mycoplasma from the endometrial cavity.

For the most part, endometritis is an ill-defined entity that produces uncertain symptoms, and it should not be diagnosed unless plasma cells or a specific etiologic factor is found. Endometritis may occur in the following situations: puerperal endometritis (see Chap. 40), gonococcal or chlamydial endometritis occurring among patients with PID, endometritis following instrumentation or surgery, tuberculous endometritis, purulent endometritis occurring in pyometra caused by a cervical stricture or following radium insertion, and endometritis that characteristically occurs in the presence of a tailed intrauterine device (IUD).

The chronic endometritis that is associated with the use of IUDs is well documented. It is clear, however, that it is not the foreign body per se that leads to chronic inflammation, but rather the tail of the IUD, which acts as a wick for organisms to reach the endometrium from the vagina. Transfundal endometrial cultures of hysterectomy specimens from women who had used tailed IUDs for more than a few weeks uniformly recovered bacteria, and the cultures from women who had used tailless IUDs or no IUD were sterile. The organisms that can be recovered are usually of low pathogenicity, but some more virulent intrauterine bacteria undoubtedly cause the malodorous discharge and the salpingitis that occur more frequently among IUD users than among non-IUD users. In addition, an anaerobe, *Actinomyces israelii,* has been found in Pap smears from about 5% of women using IUDs, but not among non-IUD users. This organism may colonize the endometrium of IUD users, and when it is found in the Pap smear, the IUD should be removed and penicillin should be prescribed for 20 days.

SALPINGITIS

Acute primary salpingitis is a bacterial infection that begins as endosalpingitis when pathogenic organisms invade the fallopian tube. *N. gonorrhoeae, C. trachomatis,* genital mycoplasma, and normal flora aerobic and anaerobic bacteria cause the overwhelming majority of tubal infections. Virtually all primary salpingitis occurs among sexually active, menstruating, nonpregnant women. Tuberculous, parasitic, or fungal salpingitis is rare in industrialized countries. Salpingitis usually occurs spontaneously without instrumentation or trauma to the genital tract; however, approximately 15% follows instrumentation (*e.g.,* IUD insertion, dilatation and curretage, abortion, hysterosalpingography, or tubal insufflation). Salpingitis can also begin as a perisalpingitis secondary to acute appendicitis or other interabdominal bacterial infection, but this kind of infection accounts for less than 1% of the cases of salpingitis.

Acute salpingitis is a common event. Approximately 1% of women between 15 and 39 years of age develop salpingitis annually. Young, sexually active women between 15 and 24 years of age have the highest rate of infection. As noted at the opening of this chapter, this rate of infection has tremendous national consequences. It is estimated that at least one billion dollars is required to treat the 800,000 women who develop acute salpingitis in the United States annually.

Epidemiology

In most women, but certainly not all, the infection is caused by sexually transmitted organisms. The rate of salpingitis is increased fivefold among women with multiple sexual partners. The rate among younger women may be higher because they are more likely to have multiple partners, or they may be more susceptible to infection because they have less acquired immunity against these organisms than do older women. Previous salpingitis predisposes a woman to the development of subsequent salpingitis, perhaps because a mucosa damaged by a prior infection is more susceptible to infection than normal tissue. In addition, patients with previous uncomplicated gonorrhea have a high rate of subsequent salpingitis, either because women who have once had gonorrhea are likely to have a second gonorrheal infection, or perhaps because in some women infection that may have appeared to be clinically uncomplicated may actually have been a subclinical tubal infection. Subclinical tubal infection would be expected to predispose a woman to the development of clinical salpingitis.

The presence of an IUD is an independent factor in the development of salpingitis. Women using an IUD have a rate of salpingitis that is increased two- to fourfold compared to women not using an IUD. The highest rate of salpingitis among IUD users occurs within a few weeks of insertion, at which time cervical bacteria are introduced into the endometrial cavity along with the IUD. However, most infections among IUD users occur long after insertion, probably because bacteria "wick" along the IUD tail leading from the vagina to the uterus. Such a mechanism for IUD-associated salpingitis is supported by the isolation of intrauterine bacteria at the time of hysterectomy only among users of tailed IUDs, but not among users of tailless IUDs or women without an IUD. Other mechanisms of IUD infection are possible, such as the enhancement of anaerobic bacterial growth, the presence of a chronic inflammatory reaction, or the production of microulcers by the IUD.

The IUD seems to be a greater factor in producing salpingitis among nulliparous than multiparous women. Also, IUD-induced salpingitis is more commonly nongonococcal than gonococcal. Women using barrier or oral contraceptive methods have a lower than expected rate of salpingitis. The protective effect of oral contraceptives on ascending infection may be due to changes in the cervical mucus, the periodic scanty withdrawal bleeding from an inactive endometrium, or decreased myometrial activity at the times of periodic uterine bleeding.

Socioeconomic factors also influence the rates of salpingitis, which are estimated to be 4% among women of low socioeconomic status and 1% among women of higher socioeconomic status. Women in the former group tend to have a higher rate of sexually transmitted disease; they are less apt to seek medical care for local symptoms and are more apt to have an untreated infectious partner than women of higher socioeconomic status. Other reasons for this difference must be elucidated.

The role of males with untreated gonococcal or chlamydial urethritis is often ignored by gynecologists. More than 75% of male contacts of women with gonococcal salpingitis have not been treated by the time the female develops symptomatic infection. Of the male contacts with infectious gonococcal urethritis, more than one half are asymptomatic. Among asymptomatic male contacts of women with gonococcal salpingitis, *N. gonorrhoeae* is isolated from 40%. Males with chlamydial, nongonococcal urethritis would also be expected to be a reservoir for chlamydial salpingitis. To reduce the rate of new and recurrent salpingitis, male contacts of women with either gonococcal or nongonococcal salpingitis should be examined and cultured. If infectious organisms are found, they should be appropriately treated. To prevent subsequent PID, it is also important that culture and appropriate therapy be provided to the male contacts of *asymptomatic* women identified as having gonorrhea or chlamydia.

Bacteriology

N. Gonorrhoeae

Formerly *N. gonorrhoeae* was believed to cause the majority of infectious salpingitis. This is no longer true, and in the United States today gonorrhea has assumed a less important position. In most studies N. gonorrhoeae can be recovered from only 40% to 50% of

women with acute gonococcal salpingitis. However, gonococcal prevalence varies greatly: *N. gonorrhoeae* is isolated from less than 20% of the cases of salpingitis in Sweden, and it is isolated from 80% of salpingitis cases in certain populations in the United States. Among women with both cervical gonorrhea and salpingitis, *N. gonorrhoeae* is the most frequent intra-abdominal isolate, but it is the sole isolate in only 30% of these cases. In the remainder, either no organisms can be isolated or other organisms are isolated either alone or together with *N. gonorrhoeae*. In recent studies, over half of the women with gonorrhea also had *C. trachomatis* in their tubes, cervix, or both. Positive gonococcal cultures are usually obtained during the early stages of infection. During the later stages of infection, the organisms are either present only within epithelial cells or they are inhibited by leukocytes, two factors that make it difficult to isolate the organism.

Chlamydia

It is now evident that sexually transmitted *C. trachomatis* is as important an organism as the gonococcus in causing acute salpingitis. In some reports, from 20% to 36% of women with acute salpingitis have cervical *C. trachomatis,* but recent data indicate that over 50% of women with salpingitis have chlamydial infections, and in most of these women the organism can be isolated from the fallopian tube. The organism produces an analogous salpingitis among primates. We have only recently appreciated that women with mild symptoms and signs can have salpingitis and that these women often have severe tubal damage. Chlamydia often produces only mild symptoms compared to gonococcal salpingitis, and previously the chlamydial salpingitis was undiagnosed.

Mycoplasmas

Genital mycoplasmas have been recovered from the abdomen in 2% to 16% of patients with salpingitis. In addition, more than 20% of patients with salpingitis have mycoplasmal antibody changes suggestive of invasive infection. These organisms lack the virulence of the gonococcus and chlamydia, and they probably play a lesser role in salpingitis.

Nonsexually Transmitted Aerobic and Anaerobic Bacteria

The fourth group of causative organisms of salpingitis are the nonsexually transmitted aerobic and anaerobic bacteria that are normally present in the cervical and vaginal flora. These organisms can be a direct cause of salpingitis, but more commonly they cause secondary infection in combination with sexually transmitted organisms, IUD use, or instrumentation. In salpingitis caused by these organisms, polymicrobial infection is the rule; infection caused by a single organism is unusual. In such cases, many different gram-positive and gram-negative aerobic organisms have been isolated as well as anaerobic organisms, particularly peptostreptococci and bacteroides species, including *B. fragilis*. Anaerobic organisms are particularly common in serious infections, and they are almost always found in the presence of abscess formation. The complex relationships that exist between gonococci, chlamydia, and these organisms have not been solved, but it is evident that they commonly invade tissues that have previously been infected by sexually transmitted organisms.

Pathogenesis

Salpingitis occurs when the uterus and fallopian tubes are infected by bacteria that are usually confined to the cervix and vagina. The ascent of bacteria from the cervical location to the fallopian tubes probably occurs most commonly during menses. The association between infection and menstruation is most striking among women who develop gonococcal salpingitis in whom abdominal pain occurs within seven days of the onset of menses in one half to two thirds of patients, suggesting that gonococci are disseminated from their cervical location at the time of menstruation. Virulent gonococci proliferate at menstruation, and less virulent gonococci are present at other times of the cycle. As noted earlier, the cervical mucus possesses properties that cause it to act as a barrier against the ascent of organisms into the uterus between menstrual periods, but the barrier is lost at menstruation. The movement of organisms from cervix to tubes occurs most commonly during the first menstrual period after the cervical infection is acquired. In addition to menstruation, other risk factors are operative. Virulent bacteria in the cervix are more likely to cause salpingitis than are nonvirulent bacteria. Endotoxin-producing *N. gonorrhoeae* and *C. trachomatis* are two virulent organisms that are capable of causing salpingitis, but virulence occasionally is also evidenced by mycoplasma and organisms of the normal flora.

The bacterial virulence can be lessened if the patient develops specific antibodies to the organism. From 10% to 17% of women identified to have cervical gonorrhea develop clinically recognized salpingitis, and probably most of these women develop the tubal infection during the first one or two menstrual periods after the cervical infection is acquired, before specific bactericidal antibodies have developed. A failure to develop antibodies may be associated with an increased risk of salpingitis.

The usual route of infection is the contiguous spread of organisms ascending from the cervix to the endometrial cavity and fallopian tubes. Lymphatic or hematogenous dissemination of organisms from the uterus to the adnexa is uncommon among nonpregnant women except, perhaps, in those with mycoplasma or IUD infections. When the bacteria reach the uterus, they commonly invade the fallopian tubes by contiguous spread along the mucosa (see Fig. 52-1), although it is possible that organisms may be transported to the fallopian tubes by cilia or even carried by their attachment to spermatozoa.

The Fitz-Hugh–Curtis Syndrome

Perihepatitis, consisting of capsular inflammation without involvement of the liver parenchyma, that has been associated with gonococcal salpingitis is referred to as the Fitz-Hugh–Curtis syndrome. The swelling of the liver capsule gives rise to inspiratory pain, usually in the right upper quadrant. Early in the inflammatory process, a purulent or a fibrinous collection appears on the capsular surface. "Violin-string" adhesions form between the liver capsule and the anterior abdominal wall, undoubtedly representing a late end-stage manifestation of the earlier acute capsular inflammation.

Perihepatitis of this kind was formerly believed to be caused solely by *N. gonorrhoeae*, which travel transperitoneally from the fallopian tubes. Recently, culture, serologic, and experimental data have been reported which suggest that *C. trachomatis* also causes this syndrome. It has also become apparent that organisms may reach the liver by lymphatic and hematogenous routes, as well as by the more widely accepted transperitoneal migration. The syndrome occurs virtually exclusively among women, although two men with this syndrome have been reported. Salpingitis is almost invariably the source, but the syndrome has also followed appendicitis and other causes of peritonitis.

The Fitz-Hugh–Curtis syndrome is frequently misinterpreted as cholecystitis, viral pneumonia, or pyelonephritis. Liver enzyme levels may be mildly elevated, and the gallbladder may not visualize on oral cholecystogram. The syndrome may cause symptoms in 5% to 10% of women with salpingitis, but in another 5% of women the perihepatitis is asymptomatic and the violin-string adhesions may only be recognized as an incidental finding when the surgeon makes his routine exploration of the upper abdomen in the course of laparotomy. Although many women with Fitz-Hugh–Curtis syndrome note the onset of lower abdominal pain before or at the same time as the upper abdominal pain, in some the upper abdominal pain may be so severe that they fail to complain of lower abdominal pain. Given the frequency of salpingitis and the infrequency of acute cholecystits among young women 15 to 30 years of age, the Fitz-Hugh–Curtis syndrome is a more likely cause of upper quadrant pain than cholecystitis and should be suspected in any woman with pleuritic upper quadrant pain who also has physical signs of salpingitis. Laparoscopy is a specific diagnostic tool for unclear cases.

Diagnosis

A tremendously broad spectrum of clinical severity results from salpingitis. Patients without abdominal pain and those with mild manifestations are often not iden-

Table 52-2

Laparoscopic Observations in Patients with a Clinical Diagnosis of PID

Diagnosis	Jacobson and Weström	Chaparro and Colleagues	Sweet and Colleagues	Total (%)
Salpingitis	532	103	25	661 (62)
Normal findings	184	51	0	235 (22)
Ovarian cysts	12	39	0	51 (5)
Ectopic pregnancy	11	27	1	39 (4)
Appendicitis	24	2	1	27 (3)
Endometriosis	16	0	0	16 (1)
Other	35	1	1	37 (3)
Total				1066 (100)

PID, pelvic inflammatory disease.
(Eschenbach DA: Epidemiology and diagnosis of pelvic inflammatory disease. Obstet Gynecol 55:142S, 1980)

tified. Although severe manifestations are usually recognized, they occur in only 30% of patients. The insistence upon rigid criteria such as fever, severe tenderness, leukocytosis, and an elevated sedimentation rate leads to a failure of diagnosis in nonovert cases. In fact, a clinical diagnosis of salpingitis which relies upon the history, physical examination, and nonspecific laboratory tests is plagued by large false-negative and false-positive errors. Several studies have demonstrated that a clinical diagnosis of salpingitis is confirmed by laparoscopy in only two thirds of patients (Table 52-2); about 20% of patients had no disease, and another 10% had other pelvic conditions, most commonly an ovarian cyst, ectopic pregnancy, appendicitis, or endometriosis. An additional 10% of patients who had a clinical diagnosis of other conditions had salpingitis demonstrated by laparoscopy.

History

The important points in the history of patients with presumed pelvic inflammatory disease are listed in Table 52-3. Lower abdominal pain is the most consistent symptom among women with overt salpingitis, although in 6% of patients it may be mild or even absent. The pain of an acute attack is present for less than 15 days in 85% of patients who present with PID. Women with gonococcal salpingitis usually have acute onset of pain during menses; in chlamydial salpingitis the onset of pain is usually insidious and is not associated with menses. The abdominal pain is usually continuous, most severe in the lower quadrants, and equal bilaterally. It is increased by movement, the Valsalva maneuver, and intercourse. Abnormal vaginal bleeding occurs in 35% of women with salpingitis. Problems such as appendicitis and ectopic pregnancy are more likely to occur if there is no recent history of vaginal discharge and dysuria. The risk of sexually transmitted disease can also be helpful in forming a tentative opinion: women who have had multiple sexual partners, gonorrhea, PID, or

some other sexually transmitted disease, or a male partner having symptoms of such a disease have an increased risk of PID.

Physical Examination

Patients with salpingitis usually have lower abdominal, cervical, and bilateral adnexal tenderness. However, none of these findings is specific; patients with other disease or with no apparent disease may have similar physical findings, and other associated findings may lack the sensitivity to be useful. For example, although a temperature of 38°C or higher is present more often in patients with than without salpingitis, only 65% of patients with laparoscopically confirmed salpingitis have a temperature of more than 38°C. The clinical findings in 204 patients with a final diagnosis of pelvic inflammatory disease are shown in Table 52-4.

Table 52-3

Historic Data Useful in Patients with Pelvic Inflammatory Disease

Age	Contraceptive used
Marital status	Gravidity, parity
Date last menstrual period	Last sexual exposure
Date onset of pain	No. of partners last month, 6 months
Characteristics of pain	History of previous gonorrhea, PID
Fever, chills	History of previous STD
Vaginal discharge	Symptoms in sexual partner
Nausea, vomiting	

PID, pelvic inflammatory disease; STD, sexually transmitted disease.
(Eschenbach DA: Epidemiology and diagnosis of pelvic inflammatory disease. Obstet Gynecol 55:142S, 1980)

Table 52-4
Clinical Findings in 204 Women with a Diagnosis of Acute PID

Finding	Percent with Cervical N. gonorrhoeae Gonococcal PID (N = 91)	Percent with No Cervical N. gonorrhoeae Nongonococcal PID (N = 113)	P
Abdominal tenderness	99	99	
Severe abdominal tenderness	37	29	
Abdominal rebound tenderness	76	66	
Liver tenderness	33	19	<.05
Purulent vaginal discharge	42	32	
Purulent cervical exudate	47	19	<.0005
Cervical tenderness	98	96	
Adnexal tenderness	100	100	
Unilateral adnexal tenderness	8	6	
Adnexal mass > 6 cm diameter	26	23	

Patients population has been previously reported. *PID,* pelvic inflammatory disease.
(Eschenbach DA: Epidemiology and diagnosis of pelvic inflammatory disease. Obstet Gynecol 55:142S, 1980)

Laboratory Tests

Such nonspecific tests as the white blood cell count and the sedimentation rate can be helpful only if the results are abnormal; unfortunately, they are often normal. Of the patients with laparoscopically confirmed salpingitis, 50% have a normal white blood cell count and 25% have a normal sedimentation rate. C-reactive protein levels may be somewhat more useful.

Specific laboratory tests such as a cervical Gram stain can be helpful. Properly obtained specimens free of vaginal discharge are 67% sensitive in the diagnosis of women with gonococcal salpingitis. Thus, if one half of the tested patients have gonococcal salpingitis, one third of all patients could have the diagnosis established by cervical Gram stain alone.

It is mandatory to obtain a culture for gonorrhea and a test for chlamydia. However, cervical culture for other organisms has not been of benefit.

Culdocentesis

Culdocentesis is helpful if fluid that contains white blood cells (indicative of PID) or nonclotting blood (indicative of intra-abdominal bleeding) is obtained. A Gram stain of aspirated fluid may suggest a causative organism. A culture of the fluid will be helpful in predicting antibiotic response.

Ultrasound and Computed Tomography

Ultrasound can be used to distinguish the presence of an abscess from an inflammatory mass within an ad-nexal mass. It may also be helpful in defining a mass in the very obese or if bimanual examination is unsatisfactory because of muscle guarding. In some cases it may be valuable for follow-up measurement of a mass that is believed to be resolving. More recently, computed tomography has been used successfully for the same purposes; it may be especially helpful if ultrasound is difficult to perform, as it is in the presence of peritonitis or a recent abdominal incision. For the most part these tests are not needed; a skillfully performed vaginal examination usually provides the necessary information.

Laparoscopy

Laparoscopy should be used without hesitation when the diagnosis is unclear. The accuracy of this method of diagnosis should approach 100%. It is estimated that for every 100 times a clinical diagnosis of pelvic inflammatory disease is made without visual confirmation, four patients with ectopic pregnancy and three patients with appendicitis are treated for pelvic inflammatory disease, resulting in a critical delay in the correct diagnosis. As noted earlier, about 20 of 100 women with a clinical diagnosis of pelvic inflammatory disease will be found to have no abnormality. In all cases in which laparoscopy is performed, regardless of the findings, cultures should be taken from the fimbriated ends of the tubes.

The pain and tenderness resulting from acute pelvic inflammatory disease should be expected to abate three or four days after antibiotics are started. If it does not begin to resolve or if it should worsen, laparoscopy is indicated both for confirmation of the diagnosis and direct culture for both aerobic and anaerobic organisms.

Examination of the Male Partner

Examination of the male sexual partner may be helpful in establishing the diagnosis in a woman suspected of having pelvic inflammatory disease. At least 80% of male contacts of women with PID will not have been identified as infectious by the time pelvic inflammatory disease occurs in the female partner. If there is no urethral discharge, urethral material for culture and Gram stain can be obtained using a calcium alginate swab.

Treatment

Adequate treatment of salpingitis includes an assessment of severity, antibiotic therapy, additional general health measures, close patient follow-up, and treatment of the male sex partner. Most patients, except for those with the mildest manifestations, should be hospitalized. Specific indications for hospitalization exist for those who have severe manifestations of salpingitis (severe peritonitis, severe nausea, or temperature higher than 38°C), a suspected abscess, outpatient antibiotic failure, or an unclear diagnosis of salpingitis.

After treatment is started, all patients should be examined within 2 to 3 days and again at 7 and 21 days to verify a satisfactory response. Ideally, the antibiotic should be selected according to the organism that is recovered from the fallopian tube, but in many cases empiric therapy must be used. The treatment regimens recommended by the CDC were designed to treat gonococcal and, to varying degrees, chlamydial and anaerobic salpingitis. Nongonococcal salpingitis responds to these regimens more slowly than do those caused by *N. gonorrhoeae*. The recommended agents must be used in full doses because subacute salpingitis frequently follows the use of lower doses.

Hospitalized patients who have peritonitis but no adnexal abscess usually respond rapidly to the regimens. In the presence of an adnexal abscess, even if the systemic manifestations are mild, antibiotics should be selected that inhibit *B. fragilis* because 80% of pelvic abscesses contain this organism. A combination of aminoglycoside and clindamycin, or doxycycline and metronidazole should be used to treat a known or suspected pelvic abscess. Cefoxitin also has been shown to be effective against this and other anaerobes.

If an IUD is in place, it should be removed 24 to 48 hours after therapy is started.

The position of surgery in dealing with PID is generally as considered earlier in the discussion of gonorrhea.

Other aspects of this problem are considered in Chapter 14.

OOPHORITIS

Oophoritis may occur without accompanying salpingitis in infections such as mumps, septicemia, or other generalized systemic illness. Oophoritis of this type is not common, and usually results only in lower abdominal pain that lasts for a few days during the course of an acute infectious illness. The ovarian infection usually subsides without incident, although abscesses can occur. If bimanual examination is not satisfactory, ultrasound scans or polytomography may be used to determine its presence.

Most cases of oophoritis are secondary to salpingitis. The ovary becomes infected by the purulent material that escapes from the fallopian tube. If the tubal fimbriae are adherent to the ovary, the tube and ovary together may form a large retort-shaped, tubo-ovarian abscess. Antibacterial therapy, as previously outlined and also discussed in Chapter 13, is immediately indicated, and surgery is mandatory if the mass is considered to be leaking or ruptured, or if it fails to resolve.

REFERENCES

Angerman NS, Evans MI, Moravec WD et al: C-reactive protein in the evaluation of antibiotic therapy for pelvic infection. J Reprod Med 25:63, 1980

Bartlett JG, Moon NE, Goldstein PR et al: Cervical and vaginal bacterial flora: Ecologic niches in the female lower genital tract. Am J Obstet Gynecol 130:658, 1978

Brunham RC, Paavonen J, Stevens CE et al: Mucopurulent cervicitis: The ignored counterpart in women of urethritis in men. N Engl J Med 311:1, 1984

Curran JW: Economic consequences of pelvic inflammatory disease in the United States. Am J Obstet Gynecol 138: 848, 1980

Eschenbach DA, Buchanan TH, Pollock HM et al: Polymicrobial etiology of acute pelvic inflammatory disease. N Engl J Med 293:166, 1975

Eschenbach DA, Holmes KK: Acute pelvic inflammatory disease: Current concepts of pathogenesis, etiology, and management. Clin Obstet Gynecol 18:35, 1975

Gall SA, Kohan AP, Ayers OM et al: Intravenous metronidazole or clindamycin with tobramycin for therapy of pelvic infections. Obstet Gynecol 57:51, 1975

Gardner H: *Hemophilus vaginalis* after twenty-five years. Am J Obstet Gynecol 137:385, 1980

Goldman P: Drug therapy. Metronidazole. N Engl J Med 303: 1212, 1980

Gorbach SL, Bartlett JG: Anaerobic infection. N Engl J Med 290:1177, 1237, 1289, 1974

Hager WD, Brown ST, Kraus SJ et al: Metronidazole for vaginal trichomoniasis. Seven-day vs single-dose regimens. JAMA 244:1219, 1980

Holmes KK: The *Chlamydia* epidemic. JAMA 245:1718, 1981

Holmes KK, Counts LW, Beaty HN: Disseminated gonococcal infection. Ann Intern Med 74:979, 1971

Insler V, Bettend FG (eds): The Uterine Cervix in Reproduction, p 71. Stuttgart, Thieme, 1977

Jacobson I, Weström L: Objectivized diagnosis of acute pelvic inflammatory disease. Am J Obstet Gynecol 105:1088, 1969

Johannisson G, Löwhagen G-B, Lycke E: Genital *Chlamydia trachomatis* infection in women. Obstet Gynecol 56:671, 1980

Josey WE: The sexually transmitted infections. Obstet Gynecol 43:467, 1974

Koehler PR, Moss AA: Diagnosis of intra-abdominal and pelvic abscesses by computerized tomography. JAMA 244:49, 1980

Lal S, Nicholas C: Epidemiological and clinical features of granuloma inguinalae. Br J Vener Dis 46:461, 1970

Mårdh P-A, Ripa I, Svensson I et al: Role of *Chlamydia trachomatis* infection in acute salpingitis. N Engl J Med 296:1377, 1977

McCormack WM, Stumacher RJ, Johnson K et al: Clinical spectrum of gonococcal infection in women. Lancet i:1182, 1977

McIntosh K: Recent advances in viral diagnosis. Arch Pathol Lab Med 104:3, 1980

Nahmias AJ, Roizman B: Infection with herpes simplex viruses 1 and 2. N Engl J Med 289:667, 719, 1973

Ohm MJ, Galask RP: Bacterial flora of the cervix from 100 prehysterectomy patients. Am J Obstet Gynecol 122:683, 1975

Paavonen J, Kiuiat N, Browning RC et al: Prevalence and manifestations of endometritis among women with cervicitis. Am J Obstet Gynecol 152:280, 1985

Pheifer TA, Forsyth PA, Durfee MA et al: Nonspecific vaginitis: Role of *Haemophilus vaginalis* and treatment with metronidazole. N Engl J Med 298:1429, 1978

Plummer FD, D'Costa LJ, Nsanze H et al: Epidemiology of chancroid and *Haemophilus ducreyi* in Nairobi, Kenya. Lancet ii:1293, 1983

Potterat JJ, King RD: A new approach to gonorrhea control. The asymptomatic man and incidence reduction. JAMA 245:578, 1981

Richart RM (ed): Ovarian abscesses in IUD wearers. Contemp Ob/Gyn 17:141, 1981

Schacter J: Chlamydial infections. N Engl J Med 298:428, 490, 540, 1978

Schaefer G: Female genital tuberculosis. Clin Obstet Gynecol 19:223, 1976

Shands KN, Schmid GP, Blum DBB et al: Toxic shock syndrome in menstruating women: Association with tampon use and *Staphylococcus aureus* and clinical features in 52 cases. N Engl J Med 303:1436, 1980

Spence MR, Gupta PK, Frost JK et al: Cytologic detection and clinical significance of *Actinomyces israelii* in women using intrauterine contraceptive devices. Am J Obstet Gynecol 131:295, 1978

Spiegel CA, Amsel R, Eschenbach D et al: Anaerobic bacteria in nonspecific vaginitis. N Engl J Med 303:601, 1980

St. John RK, Brown ST, Tyler CW: Pelvic inflammatory disease, 1980. Am J Obstet Gynecol 138:845, 1980

Stamm WE, Running K, McKevitt M et al: Treatment of the acute urethral syndrome. N Engl J Med 304:956, 1981

Tam MR, Stamm WE, Handsfield HH et al: Culture-dependent diagnosis of *Chlamydia trachomatis* using monoclonal antibodies. N Engl J Med 310:1146, 1984

Taylor–Robinson D, McCormack WM: The genital mycoplasmas. N Engl J Med 302:1063, 1980

Thompson SE, III, Hager WD, Wong K-H et al: The microbiology and therapy of pelvic inflammatory disease in hospitalized patients. Am J Obstet Gynecol 136:179, 1980

U.S. Public Health Service Center for Disease Control: Sexually transmitted disease treatment guidelines, 1982. MMWR 31:35S, 59S, 1982

Wang S-P, Eschenbach DA, Holmes KK et al: *Chlamydia trachomatis* infection in Fitz-Hugh–Curtis syndrome. Am J Obstet Gynecol 138:1034, 1980

Weström L: Incidence, prevalence, and trends of acute pelvic inflammatory disease and its consequences in industrialized countries. Am J Obstet Gynecol 138:880, 1980

Endometriosis

James A. Merrill

53

Endometriosis is a common and protean pathologic entity that is responsible for much disability. It is unique to patients with a uterus, although it has been reported twice in the male bladder. This lesion is characterized by the presence and proliferation of endometrial tissue outside the uterus. It is a benign lesion with certain characteristics of malignancy. The ectopic tissue shows the ability to grow, infiltrate, spread, and even disseminate in a manner similar to malignant tissue. Histologic changes of malignancy are rare; only then is endometriosis truly malignant in the sense of interfering with vital functions or causing death. Indeed, endometriosis may be reversible and regress following cessation of ovarian activity. It is a noninfectious process with a similar response of inflammation, fibrosis, and adhesion formation, which may be cause, effect, or both. The ectopic endometrial tissue is usually responsive to gonadal steroids. This is the basis of medical therapy, and menstrual-type bleeding is important in the pathology and symptomatology of the disease. Endometriosis has a definite, although poorly understood, adverse effect on fertility. In this discussion, the term *endometriosis* designates only lesions that exist in sites other than the endometrial surface or myometrium. These include the subperitoneal lesions on the serosal surface of the uterus, which react in all respects similarly to lesions elsewhere, but not adenomyosis.

INCIDENCE AND IMPORTANCE

The exact incidence of endometriosis is difficult to determine because lesions exist in many patients without causing symptoms. Endometriosis accounts for many days of disability from pain and frustration from infertility. It is found at about 20% of gynecologic operations, and with more liberal use of laparoscopy, the operative incidence, at least in selected groups, appears to be higher. However, the operative diagnosis is not confirmed pathologically in at least 8% of cases. Endometriosis is a significant finding in only about one third of the patients in whom it is found at surgery. Endometriosis has been reported to be most common in patients between the ages of 30 and 40, rare in postmenopausal patients, and unusual in patients under 20 years of age. The use of laparoscopy, however, has revealed endometriosis to be more common in teenage patients than previously indicated. Teenage patients represent 4% to 9% of the cases. Endometriosis has been found by laparoscopy in 20% to 50% of selected teenage patients.

Since endometriosis is usually responsive to gonadal steroids, the lesions commonly regress following cessation of ovarian activity. Although it is rare in postmenopausal patients, there are well-documented cases of endometriosis becoming active and even symptomatic many years following the menopause. It has been stated that endometriosis improves with pregnancy, but this impression is difficult to document.

Traditionally, endometriosis is considered more prevalent among private, white patients than among indigent nonwhite patients. The patients have been described as educated, motivated achievers with fastidious habits. Certainly, there is no difference in incidence related to race alone. It is difficult to prove a relationship between social status and incidence, although differences in diet influence steroidogenesis, which may influence endometriosis. It is possible that a need to receive attention makes persons in higher socioeconomic classes more likely than persons in lower classes to visit a doctor and thus is responsible for earlier and more frequent diagnosis in the former group.

It is also possible that selectivity accounts for the apparent relation between endometriosis and infertility. Infertility is a common reason for patients with endometriosis to seek medical care. However, infertile patients receive careful evaluation, including surgical exploration leading to a diagnosis of endometriosis, more often than do fertile patients with the disease.

PATHOLOGY

Location of Lesions

Endometriosis has been described in unusual and remote sites in the body, but the majority of lesions are limited to the pelvis (Fig. 53-1). The ovary is the most common site, and involvement is usually bilateral. The next most common site is the peritoneum of the cul-de-sac or pouch of Douglas. Such lesions may extend to involve the rectovaginal septum. The uterosacral ligaments may be involved with or without involvement of the peritoneum of the pouch of Douglas. The round ligament, oviduct, and peritoneal surface of the uterus are next in frequency of occurrence. The rectosigmoid can be involved either as an isolated lesion or as extension from ovarian or uterosacral lesions. Far less common are isolated lesions of the ileum, cecum, appendix, bladder, ureter, cervix, and vagina. Endometriosis is not uncommon in pelvic lymph nodes of patients with pelvic lesions. Unusual sites of endometriotic involvement include the umbilicus, laparotomy scars, episiotomy scars, arms, legs, pleura, lungs, diaphragm, kidneys, spleen, and spinal canal.

Gross Appearance

Endometriosis takes the form of multiple tiny, puckered, hemorrhagic foci referred to as "mulberry spots" or "powder-burn spots." They are usually surrounded by stellate scars and are frequently associated with dense adhesions. The degree of fibrotic reaction is variable. In the ovary, involvement may also exist as typical cysts or *endometriomas,* rarely larger than 10 cm and filled with thick chocolate syrup–like material composed of blood and blood pigment, the so-called chocolate cysts of the ovary. Not all blood-filled cysts of the ovary are due to endometriosis, however. The adhesions associated with endometriosis of the ovary are far denser than those found with salpingitis or other pelvic inflammatory processes. For this reason endometrial cysts are often ruptured during surgical removal.

Involvement of the peritoneum of the cul-de-sac or pouch of Douglas consists of the puckered bluish red nodules. Surrounding scar tissue often makes them large enough to be palpated rectovaginally. Lesions in this location occlude the posterior cul-de-sac, fixing the uterus in retroversion. At times the lesions are completely scarred and lose their blue, hemorrhagic appearance. Even in the absence of blood-filled cysts or puckered spots, dense adhesions involving the posterior surface of the uterus and broad ligament should alert the physician to the probability of endometriosis.

Lesions in the large bowel rarely penetrate the mu-

cosa. The main pathologic change is fibrotic thickening of the outer coats of the bowel sometimes associated with stricture formation. In this location endometriosis is easily mistaken for carcinoma or diverticulitis of the rectosigmoid. In addition to small lesions in the bladder-flap peritoneum, endometriosis may produce fibrotic nodules in the wall of the bladder, which rarely protrude into the lumen.

Microscopic Appearance

Microscopically, the lesions consist of endometrial glands and stroma, frequently with hemorrhage into the stroma and adjacent tissue. This hemorrhage may result in the accumulation of large numbers of hemosiderin-laden macrophages or pseudoxanthoma cells (Fig. 53-2). The endometrial glands and stroma usually show a response to the menstrual cycle comparable to that of the uterine endometrium. Occasionally the ectopic endometrium shows a poor secretory response to progesterone. Pregnancy may be accompanied by a typical decidual response of pelvic endometriosis, although the finding of extrauterine decidua alone is not pathognomonic of endometriosis. Decidua without glands occurs in nonpregnant women and during pregnancy may be a mesenchymal response to the pregnancy hormones.

Hemorrhage into the lumen of the endometrial cyst frequently results in pressure atrophy and obliteration of recognizable endometrial tissue in the wall. Such cysts are lined only by granulation tissue, hemosiderin-laden macrophages, and occasionally cholesterol crystal clefts with appropriate foreign body reaction.

There may be a remarkable degree of fibrous proliferation surrounding endometriotic lesions. This is particularly true in the bowel (Fig. 53-3). Because of the reactive phenomena, there are many cases of unquestioned gross endometriosis seen at the operating table in which the removed tissues show no evidence of microscopic endometriosis. Microscopic confirmation of gross endometriosis may be increased if the lesions are marked with a suture by the surgeon before removal.

Malignant Change

Malignant change in endometriosis is extremely rare. Meticulous search of the lesions has revealed, in a few cases, evidences of atypical or adenomatous hyperplasia that might be considered precancerous. Of the endometrioid carcinomas demonstrated to have originated in endometriosis, adenoacanthomas and well-differentiated adenocarcinomas occurred with relatively high frequency, rather more so than among endometrioid carcinomas in general; also, the prognosis appears to be somewhat better. Other malignancies reported rarely to arise in endometriosis are mucinous adenocarcinoma, clear cell carcinoma, mixed mesodermal sarcoma, and

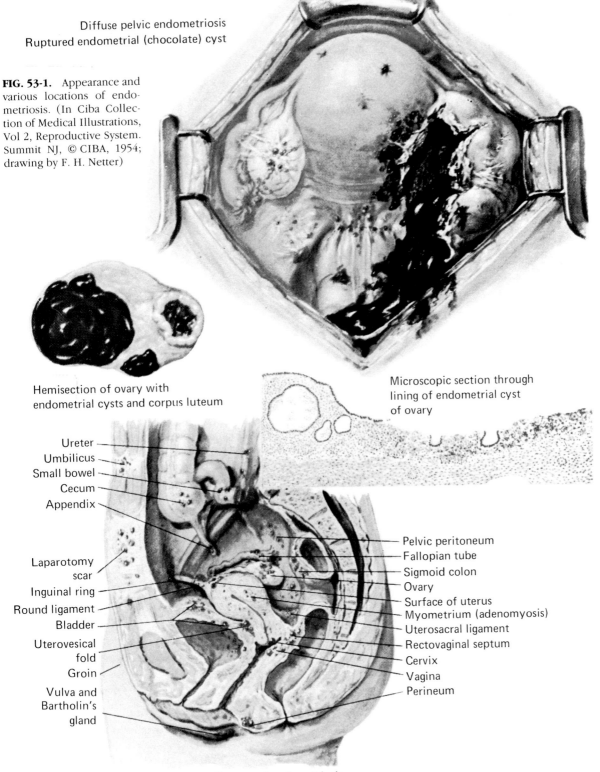

Diffuse pelvic endometriosis
Ruptured endometrial (chocolate) cyst

FIG. 53-1. Appearance and various locations of endometriosis. (In Ciba Collection of Medical Illustrations, Vol 2, Reproductive System. Summit NJ, © CIBA, 1954; drawing by F. H. Netter)

Hemisection of ovary with endometrial cysts and corpus luteum

Microscopic section through lining of endometrial cyst of ovary

Ureter
Umbilicus
Small bowel
Cecum
Appendix

Laparotomy scar
Inguinal ring
Round ligament
Bladder
Uterovesical fold
Groin
Vulva and Bartholin's gland

Pelvic peritoneum
Fallopian tube
Sigmoid colon
Ovary
Surface of uterus
Myometrium (adenomyosis)
Uterosacral ligament
Rectovaginal septum
Cervix
Vagina
Perineum

Possible sites of distribution of endometriosis

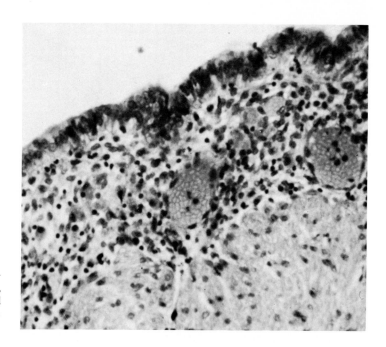

FIG. 53-2. Microscopic appearance of lining of endometrial cyst composed of endometrial epithelium, stroma, and hemosiderin-filled macrophages. Dilated capillaries are characteristic of active lesions of endometriosis.

FIG. 53-3. Endometriosis in submucosal region of large bowel.

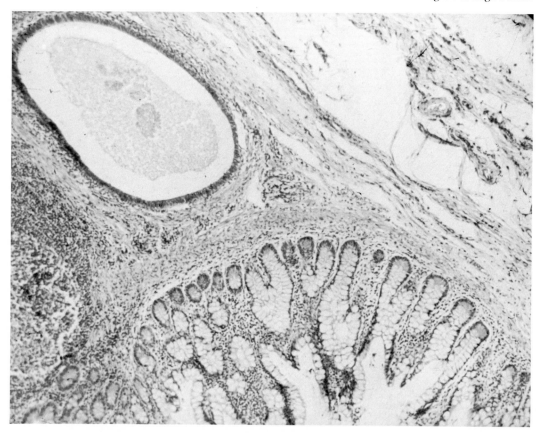

carcinosarcoma. In addition to the ovary, the sites have been the cervix, rectovaginal septum, vagina, and pleura.

The relationship of endometriosis to the later development of cancer has been reviewed by Mostoufizadeh and Scully. An important consideration to which they call attention is the possible risk of estrogen replacement in women with proven endometriosis, since there is no means of monitoring the changes that may occur in retained endometrial tissue.

ETIOLOGY

The etiology of endometriosis is not certain, although there are many speculations. Endometriosis is almost always limited to women with menstruating endometrium and possibly occurs more often in women with some acquired or congenital obstruction to the outflow of menstrual discharge. Indeed, endometriosis may improve following removal of the uterus.

Experiments suggest that ovarian steroids may not be necessary for the initiation of endometriosis but are necessary for its survival and growth. The very rare examples of endometriosis occurring in postmenopausal women, women who have undergone hysterectomy, and males are attributed to the stimulating effect of estrogen. The higher than usual incidence in Japanese women may be attributed to different estrogen metabolism (estriol is the predominant ovarian metabolite). The low incidence in women of low socioeconomic class may result from differences in steroidogenesis consequent to deficient diet.

Although race was once thought to be important, there is no evidence that endometriosis occurs with different incidence in the black and white populations.

Surgical trauma to the endometrium may have the same etiologic importance as menstruation, as suggested by the occurrence of endometriosis in wounds and rare distant sites after surgery.

Experimental and clinical observations have linked irritation, such as radiation and infection, to the disease. Disseminated endometriosis has been observed in monkeys receiving total body irradiation. Inflammation is as likely to be the result as the cause of endometriosis.

Heredity may have causal significance. Investigators have found endometriosis to exist with increased incidence in the close family relatives of patients with endometriosis.

Such possible etiologic factors suggest considerations for prevention, which might include correction of anatomic abnormalities, decrease of menstruation by pregnancy and steroid contraception, avoidance of intrauterine manipulation, and proper nutrition.

HISTOGENESIS

There are three major theories of histogenesis of endometriosis: transportation, formation *in situ,* and a combination of these.

Transportation

Sampson's theory suggests that endometriosis is caused by retrograde tubal flow of menstrual fragments, *implantation* and growth on the ovary and peritoneal surfaces, followed by secondary seedings from the new foci. Vascular metastasis has also been suggested. Endometrial tissue is found in lymphatics and pelvic lymph nodes. This offers the best explanation for the rare distant sites of endometriosis. Direct transplantation of endometrium has been suggested by the observation of lesions in incisional scars following surgery involving the uterus and in vaginal incisions such as episiotomies. A composite theory of the histogenesis of endometriosis includes direct extension into the myometrium or endosalpinx, exfoliation and implantation of endometrial cells at menstruation or during curettage, lymphatic spread, venous spread and hematogenous metastases to distant organs, and secondary lesions from foci already established.

Formation *In Situ*

Metaplasia or differentiation of celomic epithelium, possibly triggered by inflammatory or hormonal alterations, has been suggested. This theory gains support from embryologic studies, observations of differentiation of surface epithelium of the ovary into the various cell types of the müllerian duct, and the decidual reaction seen frequently in tissues beneath the pelvic peritoneum during pregnancy. Lesions of endometriosis have been reported to contain tubal and endocervical epithelium. Growth of celomic epithelium, including downward extension into the ovarian cortex and other subsurface connective tissue areas of the pelvis, is observed at sites of irritation and inflammation. A variety of irritants cause metaplasia and growth of celomic epithelium. The theory of embryonic cell rests in the production of endometriosis has been discarded.

Combination (Induction)

Hertig and Gore proposed that endometriosis could develop following the formation of a fibrinopurulent exudate, organization of such exudate, and eventual development of metaplastic celomic epithelium with a glandular pattern. A theory of induction has been proposed in which chemical-inducing substances may be liberated from transported endometrium and activate undifferentiated mesenchyme to form endometrial epithelium and stroma.

The theory is supported by Merrill's experimental observations of endometrial tissue that develops in connective tissue adjacent to cell-free extracts of endometrium and adjacent to diffusion chambers containing autologous or heterologous endometrium; such chambers prevent escape of cellular material but allow dispersion of noncellular material from the endometrium. Endometrial tissue also developed adjacent to diffusion chambers containing endometrium from histoincompatible donors. Absence of nuclear sex chromatin was observed in the endometrial tissue that developed in experiments in which males were the recipients, indicating induction, not growth. Such an induction theory combines both the transportation and metaplasia theories and appears to be the most likely.

Comment

Many observations strongly support the concept that transportation of endometrial fragments by one means or another is important in the development of endometriosis. Menstrual fragments have been observed in the lumen of the oviduct as well as in the peritoneal cavity, and endometrial fragments appear in lymphatic and venous channels of the uterus. Menstrual endometrium is viable in tissue culture, but menstrual fragments shed from intraocular transplants in the monkey do not survive or form endometriosis. Transplantation of fragments of endometrium is followed by endometriosis, and diversion of menstrual flow into the peritoneal cavity or anterior abdominal wall is followed by endometriosis. Even human endometriosis has been found following experimental subcutaneous injection of menstrual discharge.

None of these experiments conclusively proves that the transported endometrial fragments have grown. It is equally possible that they degenerate and in the process induce differentiation in the adjacent mesenchyme. Moreover, the influence of irritation, inflammation, and hormonal alteration on such metaplasia and inclusion cyst formation is noteworthy.

At present it seems likely that no one theory satisfactorily explains all of the lesions of endometriosis, that each may play a role, and that this interesting entity may arise from combinations of influences.

SYMPTOMS

Endometriosis may be extensive without producing any symptoms whatsoever, and the frequency and degree of symptoms are poorly related to extent of the disease. Indeed, many patients with very few small lesions are severely disabled.

Pelvic pain is the most significant symptom of endometriosis. In many, this takes the form of *acquired dysmenorrhea* beginning in the 20s or early 30s and gradually progressing in severity. The pain is described as dull aching or cramping lower abdominal and back pain, occurring with menstruation and diminishing gradually after the onset of flow. Not all patients have pain that is characteristically related to menstruation. Many complain of vague aching, cramping, or bearing-down sensation in the pelvis or low back, which may or may not become worse during the menstrual period and be somewhat relieved following menstruation. Less

often, patients complain of *dyspareunia,* particularly when the uterus is fixed in retroversion and when endometriotic lesions are found in the region of the uterosacral ligaments or the posterior fornix of the vagina. Upon direct questioning, one may obtain a history of *pain with defecation* during menstruation, particularly if the lesions involve the area of the rectovaginal septum.

The mechanism of pain is not altogether clear. Dyspareunia and pain with defecation are related to pressure on distended lesions or to stretching of adhesions. Pelvic pain and dysmenorrhea may be related to hemorrhagic distention of an endometrial cyst that is restricted by fibrosis or to escape of bloody discharge into the peritoneal cavity. Dysmenorrhea may also be related to increased local concentration of prostaglandins. Rupture of an endometrioma may cause acute peritoneal irritation.

Abnormal uterine bleeding is the presenting symptom almost as often as pain. It has no specific pattern and may be excessive, prolonged, or frequent. One study reported anovulation in 11% of patients with endometriosis. Inadequate function of the corpus luteum in patients with endometriosis is a controversial concept. The endometrium is usually normal morphologically, and bleeding may be the result of the frequent association with other pelvic pathology, such as myomas.

Infertility may bring a patient with endometriosis to the physician. It is impossible to determine the true incidence of infertility in patients with endometriosis or the incidence of endometriosis in patients with infertility. Infertility has been reported in 20% to 66% of patients with endometriosis. Endometriosis has been reported in 8% to 77% of infertile patients studied by endoscopy. Also, it is difficult to explain exactly how endometriosis may interfere with fertility. However, it is probable that endometriosis is associated with at least a relative infertility. Certainly, distortion and fixation of the oviducts, fixation of the uterus, and pain during intercourse may be significant factors.

The oviducts usually are patent, although microscopic salpingitis was reported in 33% of 87 cases. Although ovulation usually is not interrupted, abnormal ovulation is offered as a possible factor, including misplaced corpus luteum, absent stigmata, decreased production of progesterone (luteal phase defect), and inoperative hormonal feedback mechanism with respect to luteinizing hormone. Related reports by investigators are contradictory, however. Altered peritoneal fluid in patients with endometriosis appears as the most favored explanation for infertility in patients with minimal disease. The alterations might affect gamete survival and transport, fertilization, and tubal motility. There have been reports of increased volume, increased prostaglandin and prostanoid concentrations, increased macrophages, and decreased sperm recovery. None of these observations has been confirmed by all investigators. Evidence has been introduced for an autoimmune response to antigens in the desquamated ectopic endometrium with consequent formation of antiendometrial antibodies that might interfere with implantation.

An increase in early abortion rate (32%) has been reported in patients with mild, untreated endometriosis but not in those with more extensive, treated endometriosis. An increase in local prostaglandin concentration has been suggested as the cause.

Unusual symptoms related to involvement of the gastrointestinal tract or urinary tract result from obstruction or interference with function of these organs. Rectal bleeding occurs in approximately 20% of patients with endometriosis of the bowel. Pain and tenderness in the umbilicus, scars, or inguinal region accompany lesions in these locations. Hemoptysis occurring at the time of menstruation has been described in the rare cases of endometriosis involving the lung or bronchus. Cyclic subarachnoid hemorrhage with hemiparesis has been reported with endometriosis in the spinal canal and cyclic sciatica with endometriosis in the sciatic notch.

PHYSICAL FINDINGS

The most important clinical finding is multiple tender nodules palpable along the uterosacral ligaments or above the posterior fornix of the vagina. Such nodules are noted to enlarge and become much more tender during menstruation. Often the uterus is fixed in retroposition. Attempts to move it are accompanied by severe pain. Thickening and nodularity of the adnexa may be similar to, and suggestive of, pelvic inflammatory disease. Endometrial cysts of the ovary are rarely movable and usually closely adherent to the uterus, with adjacent induration and tenderness. In rare cases, blue cystic areas may be seen at the umbilicus, in adbominal wound scars, on the cervix or vagina, or elsewhere. These appear or enlarge during menstruation. The lesions of endometriosis have been seen during cystoscopy but are rarely observed during proctosigmoidoscopy.

DIAGNOSIS

Endometriosis should be considered in the young woman with acquired dysmenorrhea, intermittent or constant pelvic pain, dyspareunia, and menstrual abnormality, who has a tender, fixed, retroverted uterus and palpable nodules in the region of the uterosacral ligaments. Endometriosis should be considered in patients with similar symptoms who have unilateral or bilateral adnexal thickening or adnexal masses.

Certainly, the diagnosis of endometriosis should be considered when infertility has no other apparent cause. Laparoscopy with visualization of the typical foci is of great value in confirming the diagnosis and commonly is indicated in the evaluation of the infertile woman. A positive diagnosis is important if expensive therapy is to be considered. The increased use of laparoscopy to evaluate patients with pelvic pain, abnormal uterine bleeding, and infertility has resulted in more, and more accurate, diagnoses of endometriosis. Biopsy of externally visible lesions, lesions of the cervix or vagina, or lesions seen at cystoscopy confirms the diagnosis.

Endometriosis should be a part of the differential diagnosis of malignant disease of the ovary, chronic salpingo-oophoritis, carcinoma of the rectum and colon, diverticulitis, causes of intestinal obstruction, tumors of the umbilicus, inguinal swellings, and causes of hematuria. It is impossible to palpate all small endometriotic lesions, but remembering the protean manifestations of endometriosis may increase the frequency (approximately 20%) of accurate diagnosis.

TREATMENT

The treatment of endometriosis must be influenced by the facts that it is predominantly a disease of women of childbearing age, that infertility is often a presenting complaint, and that accurate diagnosis is difficult without surgical exploration. Since endometriosis is to some extent responsive to cyclic ovarian hormones, removal of the ovaries and uterus relieves symptoms in the majority of patients. However, such treatment is not compatible with desire for future childbearing and can be recommended only for those patients who have completed their families. For the most part, treatment should be designed to produce maximal symptom relief with minimal interference with childbearing function, or it should actually increase fertility potential.

Evaluation of various methods of treatment is complicated by the difficulty in accurate diagnosis and the inherent selection of patients. It is, for example, difficult to compare the results of surgical therapy and hormone therapy if the diagnosis of patients treated surgically is established by pathologic examination and the diagnosis of patients treated with hormones is based only on clinical findings. Similarly, it is difficult to assign a fertility-promoting effect to therapy when the only patients under study are women under 35 years of age who seriously desire pregnancy, who have limited endometriosis allowing conservative therapy, and who have no other cause of sterility. Such selection, which is common in the management of endometriosis, must be considered when evaluating therapy.

A difficult problem in comparing the results of treatment with various modalities is created by the fact that different series contain patients with different degrees of severity of the disease. For this reason, a number of investigators have proposed classification systems for endometriosis. The factors used to indicate *increase* in the severity of the disease are (1) adhesions, (2) ovarian cysts, (3) scarring and retraction, (4) fixation of pelvic structures, and (5) obliteration of cul-de-sac. The classification proposed by the American Fertility Society (AFS) is shown in Figure 53-4. Staging is accomplished by systematic clockwise or counterclockwise inspection of the pelvis and assignment of points according to the findings. A modification of the system proposed by Acosta is less complex and may be more applicable (Table 53-1).

Although many investigators have shown a direct relationship between extent of endometriosis and suc-

THE AMERICAN FERTILITY SOCIETY
REVISED CLASSIFICATION OF ENDOMETRIOSIS

Patient's Name _____ Date_____

Stage I   (Minimal) - 1-5
Stage II (Mild)   - 6-15
Stage III (Moderate) - 16-40
Stage IV (Severe) - >40

Laparoscopy_____ Laparotomy_____ Photography_____
Recommended Treatment_____

Total_____

Prognosis_____

PERITONEUM	**ENDOMETRIOSIS**	<1cm	1-3cm	>3cm
	Superficial	1	2	4
	Deep	2	4	6
OVARY	R Superficial	1	2	4
	Deep	4	16	20
	L Superficial	1	2	4
	Deep	4	16	20

	POSTERIOR CULDESAC OBLITERATION	Partial	Complete
		4	40

	ADHESIONS	<1/3 Enclosure	1/3-2/3 Enclosure	>2/3 Enclosure
OVARY	R Filmy	1	2	4
	Dense	4	8	16
	L Filmy	1	2	4
	Dense	4	8	16
TUBE	R Filmy	1	2	4
	Dense	4*	8*	16
	L Filmy	1	2	4
	Dense	4*	8*	16

*If the fimbriated end of the fallopian tube is completely enclosed, change the point assignment to 16.

Additional Endometriosis: _____   Associated Pathology: _____
_____   _____
_____   _____
_____   _____

To Be Used with Normal
Tubes and Ovaries

L   R

To Be Used with Abnormal
Tubes and/or Ovaries

L   R

For additional supply write to: The American Fertility Society, 2131 Magnolia Avenue,
Suite 201, Birmingham, Alabama 35256

A

EXAMPLES & GUIDELINES

STAGE I (MINIMAL)	STAGE II (MILD)	STAGE III (MODERATE)

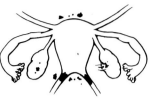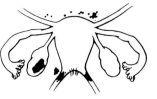

PERITONEUM
  Superficial Endo – 1-3cm - 2
R. OVARY
  Superficial Endo – < 1cm - 1
  Filmy Adhesions – < 1/3 - 1
        TOTAL POINTS   4

PERITONEUM
  Deep Endo – >3cm - 6
R. OVARY
  Superficial Endo – < 1cm - 1
  Filmy Adhesions – < 1/3 - 1
L. OVARY
  Superficial Endo – < 1cm - 1
        TOTAL POINTS   9

PERITONEUM
  Deep Endo – >3cm - 6
CULDESAC
  Partial Obliteration - 4
L. OVARY
  Deep Endo – 1-3cm - 16
        TOTAL POINTS   26

STAGE III (MODERATE)	STAGE IV (SEVERE)	STAGE IV (SEVERE)

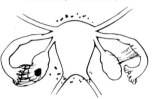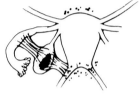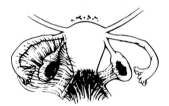

PERITONEUM
  Superficial Endo – >3cm - 3
R. TUBE
  Filmy Adhesions – < 1/3 - 1
R. OVARY
  Filmy Adhesions – < 1/3 - 1
L. TUBE
  Dense Adhesions – < 1/3 - 16*
L. OVARY
  Deep Endo – '<1 cm -4
  Dense Adhesions – < 1/3 -4
        TOTAL POINTS   29

PERITONEUM
  Superficial Endo – >3cm - 3
L. OVARY
  Deep Endo – 1-3cm - 32**
  Dense Adhesions – < 1/3 - 8**
L. TUBE
  Dense Adhesions – < 1/3 - 8**
        TOTAL POINTS   51

*Point assignment changed to 16
**Point assignment doubled

PERITONEUM
  Deep Endo – >3cm - 6
CULDESAC
  Complete Obliteration - 40
R. OVARY
  Deep Endo – 1-3cm - 16
  Dense Adhesions – < 1/3 - 4
L. TUBE
  Dense Adhesions – >2/3 - 16
L. OVARY
  Deep Endo – 1-3cm - 16
  Dense Adhesions – >2/3 - 16
        TOTAL POINTS   114

Determination of the stage or degree of endometrial involvement is based on a weighted point system. Distribution of points has been arbitrarily determined and may require further revision or refinement as knowledge of the disease increases.

To ensure complete evaluation, inspection of the pelvis in a clockwise or counterclockwise fashion is encouraged. Number, size and location of endometrial implants, plaques, endometriomas and/or adhesions are noted. For example, five separate 0.5cm superficial implants on the peritoneum (2.5 cm total) would be assigned 2 points. (The surface of the uterus should be considered peritoneum.) The severity of the endometriosis or adhesions should be assigned the highest score only for peritoneum, ovary, tube or culdesac. For example, a 4cm superficial and a 2cm deep implant of the peritoneum should be given a score of 6 (not 7). A 4cm

deep endometrioma of the ovary associated with more than 3cm of superficial disease should be scored 20 (not 24).

In those patients with only one adnexa, points applied to disease of the remaining tube and ovary should be multiplied by two. **Points assigned may be circled and totaled. Aggregation of points indicates stage of disease (minimal, mild, moderate, or severe).

The presence of endometriosis of the bowel, urinary tract, fallopian tube, vagina, cervix, skin etc., should be documented under "additional endometriosis." Other pathology such as tubal occlusion, leiomyomata, uterine anomaly, etc., should be documented under "associated pathology." All pathology should be depicted as specifically as possible on the sketch of pelvic organs, and means of observation (laparoscopy or laparotomy) should be noted.

B

FIG. 53-4. (*A*) Revised classification of endometriosis, American Fertility Society, 1985. (*B*) Reverse side of classification form, to show guidelines and examples in use of form. (American Fertility Society: Revised American Fertility Society Classification of Endometriosis, 1985. Fertil Steril 43:351, 1985. Reproduced with permission of the publisher, The American Fertility Society)

cess of pregnancy following treatment, others have shown no relationship, specifically not with the AFS classification. Buttram found no relationship between extent of endometriosis and duration of infertility or between extent of endometriosis and symptoms of dyspareunia and dysmenorrhea.

In general, treatment consists of observation and symptom palliation, surgery, and hormone therapy.

Observation

Observation, reassurance, mild analgesia, and antiprostaglandins are effective in many patients and should be the initial management of young patients whose symptoms are not severe or incapacitating. If the lesions are small and multiple and are producing few symptoms, it may be best to leave them alone. Indeed, they sometimes become inactive after a while. Time is often helpful, and some procrastination is justified. Indeed, there are reports that active treatment of mild disease has no demonstrated effect upon the rate of achieved pregnancies. An expectant course should *not* be followed if large masses are palpated or if the differential diagnosis includes more significant disease. The clinical diagnosis of endometriosis is often inaccurate.

Surgery

When symptoms are severe, incapacitating, or acute, surgery is indicated. Surgery is indicated if symptoms become worse under medical management and may be indicated if infertility persists and no cause other than endometriosis is found. Endometrial cysts of the ovary are indications for surgery if they are larger than 6 cm to 8 cm in diameter. When surgery is undertaken, every effort should be made to accomplish a conservative procedure that will preserve childbearing function, if this is desired. The extent of surgery also depends on the extent and location of the lesions and the surgeon's judgment.

Severe symptoms of endometriosis may be dealt with *radically* if the woman is approaching the menopause or has completed childbearing. Bilateral salpingo-oophorectomy and hysterectomy relieve symptoms without risking injury to bowel or other structures by attempting to excise every fragment of endometriosis. Even constricting lesions of the bowel or urinary tract may regress following this therapy.

Hysterectomy alone may afford relief of symptoms while maintaining the advantages of ovarian function, even in the presence of some residual areas of endometriosis. Apparently ablation of cyclic menstruation and possible repeated regurgitation of menstrual fragments results in quiescence of remaining areas of endometriosis. Thus, hysterectomy with removal of as many foci of endometriosis as is easily achievable, but conservation of all or part of the ovarian tissue, has been recommended for the young woman with sufficiently severe symptoms to warrant surgery, who has completed her family and is not desirous of future childbearing. Many gynecologists, however, recommend the addition of bilateral salpingo-oophorectomy in this circumstance with immediate replacement of estrogen. Estrogen has been given safely to patients following hysterectomy and oophorectomy and can be controlled easily if there is evidence of recurrence. The risk of malignant change in residual endometriosis may exist but is extremely small, substantially less than with an intact uterus.

Table 53-1
Classification of Endometriosis

Extent of Disease	Findings
Mild	Scattered, superficial implants on structures other than uterus, tubes, or ovaries; no scarring
	Rare, superficial implants on ovaries
	No significant lesions
Moderate	Involvement of one or both ovaries with multiple implants or small endometriomas (<2 cm)
	Minimal peritubular or periovarian adhesions
	Scattered, scarred implants on other structures
Severe	Large ovarian endometriomas (>2 cm)
	Significant tubal or ovarian adhesions
	Tubal obstruction
	Obliteration of cul-de-sac, major uterosacral involvement
	Significant bowel or urinary tract disease

(Modified from data from Acosta AA et al: A proposed classification of pelvic endometriosis. Obstet Gynecol 42:19, 1973)

Less radical procedures ("conservative surgery") are indicated in the majority of patients. This generally means excision of all gross endometriosis with preservation of the uterus, tubes, and as much ovarian tissue as possible. This may mean unilateral oophorectomy, resection of endometrial cysts from one or both ovaries, excision of peritoneal lesions, release of adhesions, and resection of portions of rectal or bladder wall. It is possible to excise even fairly large endometrial cysts and conserve functioning ovarian tissue. The CO_2 laser has been used to treat endometriosis. Small endometrial cysts, peritoneal lesions, and adhesions can be safely removed by tissue vaporization, *possibly* with less reaction than accompanies traditional surgery.

Some gynecologists recommend suspension of the uterus and presacral neurectomy. A segmental resection and reanastomosis of bowel may be required if castration is not indicated. The results of conservative surgery with regard to relief of symptoms are good. With remaining ovarian function and residual endometriosis, progression is possible, however. The recurrence rate varies from 2% to 47%. The reoperation rate varies and is proportional to the frequency with which conservative surgery is the first-chosen treatment. The difficulty in evaluating the effect on fertility is discussed above; the frequency of subsequent pregnancy may be as high as 70%; however, the average is about 55%, and most pregnancies occur in the first year after surgery.

Hormone Administration

The use of steroid hormones has been recommended for the patient with symptoms not relieved by reassurance and mild analgesics, who desires subsequent pregnancy, and in whom surgery is either contraindicated or not acceptable, and in the patient with recurrence of symptoms following conservative surgery. The variety of hormones used includes estrogens, androgens, and progestins, in various dose schedules. Danazol now is preferred to the other steroids, and gonadotropin-releasing hormone (GnRH) agonists are being evaluated as another means of abolishing ovarian function. It is of interest that almost all doses and combinations of hormones have been successful in the hands of their advocates, almost all of whom report relief of symptoms in approximately 80% of cases. This is about the same percentage of success obtained in selected patients who were not treated. In the majority of cases the relief appears to be temporary and the medication is often associated with annoying side-effects. The long-term use of expensive medication should not be undertaken without accurate diagnosis.

Estrogen, in the form of stilbestrol, has been recommended in small doses for the purpose of ovulation suppression and in large doses for the purpose of producing pseudopregnancy, and the beneficial effects have been considered equivalent to those of pregnancy. At present it is generally agreed that this therapy is ineffective because the symptoms and objective findings soon return and intermenstrual bleeding, edema, and nausea may be annoying side-effects.

Testosterone and methyltestosterone have been used and reported to be effective in relieving the symptoms of endometriosis. Methyltestosterone linguets, 5 mg to 10 mg daily, have been recommended. The 5-mg dose may be given continuously. Relief of symptoms is reported in 80% of patients, with subsequent pregnancy in 11% to 60% of those complaining of infertility. Side-effects of hirsutism, acne, and increased libido are reported. The effect of androgens is thought to be suppression of ovulation through the hypothalamus, but there must be a direct effect on the lesions as well, since ovulation is not always suppressed in patients receiving benefit from the therapy.

Progestin–estrogen treatment is based on ovulation suppression and the production of pseudopregnancy, with decidual reaction in the endometriotic lesions, atrophy of the glands, eventual fibrosis, and obliteration of the endometriotic lesion (Fig. 53-5). All of the synthetic progestins, in combination with estrogens, have been used in doses that cause months of amenorrhea. The estrogen–progestin oral contraceptives are recommended. Starting with a dose of one tablet daily, the dosage is increased to two tablets after two to three weeks. If breakthrough bleeding occurs, the dose is increased by one table daily and maintained. Medroxyprogesterone acetate (Depo-provera), 100 mg intramuscularly every two weeks for four doses and then 200 mg each month for an additional four- to six-month period, has been used. Estrogen is given for breakthrough bleeding. Treatment is continued up to nine months and symptomatic improvement in 85% to 89% of patients has been reported. Subsequent pregnancy has been reported in 30% to 47% of infertile patients. Complaints of nausea, restlessness, edema, irregular uterine bleeding, and excess weight are made by a significant number of patients. The need for surgery after pseudopregnancy is reported in 11% to 51% of patients. Improvement in the endometriosis following therapy persists for varying intervals, but in many cases the findings and symptoms return. Improvement is overestimated when compared with surgical findings. Some gynecologists believe that there is no evidence that synthetic progestin–estrogen actually cures endometriosis, and that the use of such agents should be considered a temporizing measure for specially selected cases. The use of progestin–estrogen for five to eight weeks prior to contemplated surgery may make the lesions more easily identifiable and may soften the usually dense adhesions.

A synthetic derivative of 17α-ethinyl testosterone (danazol) has replaced in large part the use of other steroid hormones. This drug was initially thought to act mainly as a gonadotropin suppressant at the hypothalamic–pituitary level. However, there is evidence that danazol may act partly by competitive inhibition at the level of estrogen, progesterone, and androgen receptors as well as directly influencing the function of certain steroidogenic enzymes. Thus, danazol may have some suppressive effects at each level of the hypothalamic–

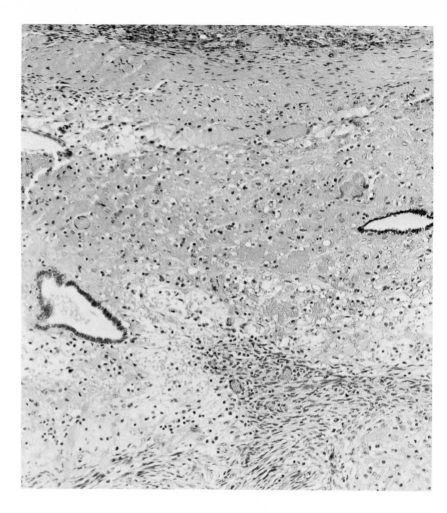

FIG. 53-5. Microscopic section of endometriosis of ovary following 6 months' treatment with synthetic progestins. Stroma demonstrates marked decidual reaction with beginning fibrosis; remaining glands show moderate atrophy. ×100. (Kistner RW: Chap VII-1. In Meigs JV, Sturgis SH (eds): Progress in Gynecology IV. New York, Grune & Stratton, 1963)

pituitary–ovarian–endometrial axis. Treatment induces a state of "pseudomenopause" with anovulation and atrophy of endometrial tissue.

Recommended treatment is 800 mg (divided) per day, although 400 mg to 600 mg daily may be adequate; in some patients 200 mg daily is sufficient. It is recommended that patients with mild disease be treated for three to four months, moderate disease six to eight months, and severe disease for greater than eight months or until palpable lesions disappear. The medication is expensive and is not used if the diagnosis of endometriosis is only presumptive.

There are reports of 70% to 100% relief of symptoms during treatment and corrected pregnancy rates as high as 80%. Overall pregnancy rates are approximately 50%, which compare favorably with pregnancy rates following conservative surgery. The relief of symptoms occurs early in the course of therapy, in contrast to pseudopregnancy. Controlled laparoscopic studies reveal regression of lesions in 3 to 18 months. However, recurrence rates of 23% at one year and 39% at three years have been reported. In successfully treated patients, most pregnancies occurred in the first year following treatment. Side-effects of acne, hot flashes, edema,

weight gain, hirsutism, and muscle cramps are reported. The value of danazol in the treatment of infertility patients with mild endometriosis has been questioned. In a cooperative study, pregnancy rates (28%) were no greater than for untreated patients.

Continuous administration of synthetic GnRH agonist to patients with endometriosis produces gonadotropin suppression and anovulation. Such therapy effectively eliminates ovarian function with consequent low levels of estrogen and androgen. Investigators using intermittent daily injections or intranasal spray have reported disappearance of endometriosis lesions after six months of treatment without significant side-effects. Pregnancies have been reported after cessation of the medication. Treatment schedules vary from 200 μg to 400 μg of the agonist 2 to 3 times daily for 6 to 8 months. Amenorrhea occurs usually after the first month. This is a promising new medical approach to therapy; experience with it is limited, however.

X-Ray Treatment

In recurrent cases after failure of conservative surgery, roentgenographic suppression of the ovaries may be effective. The x-ray dose required is not large, but care must be taken to avoid damage to normal structures that are fixed by the dense adhesions. This is rarely, if ever, recommended.

CONCLUSION

Just as there is no final agreement regarding the etiology and histogenesis of endometriosis, there is no agreement regarding the most successful mode of treatment. Each case must be treated individually, based on the physician's experience and the desires of the patient. Hysterectomy, removal of the adnexa and other tissue containing endometriosis is the optimal treatment for patients who have no desire for fertility and who have significant symptoms. Conservative surgery most often is the recommended treatment for young patients complaining of infertility. Young patients not currently desiring pregnancy may be satisfactorily managed with observation, reassurance, and mild analgesia. Danazol may be used for this group and also for those with recurrence following conservative surgery.

The treatment of the asymptomatic patient is probably not indicated.

REFERENCES AND RECOMMENDED READING

Acosta AA et al: A proposed classification of pelvic endometriosis. Obstet Gynecol 42:19, 1973

Badawy SZA et al: Autoimmune phenomena in infertile patients with endometriosis. Obstet Gynecol 63:271, 1984

Barbieri RL, Evans S, Kistner RW: Danazol and the treatment of endometriosis: Analysis of 100 cases with a 4 year follow-up period. Fertil Steril 37:373, 1982

Bergman H, Friedenberg RM: Endometriosis: Urologic manifestation. NY State J Med 72:1152, 1972

Brosset A: Value of irradiation therapy in the treatment of endometriosis. Acta Obstet Gynecol Scand 36:209, 1957

Butler L et al: Collaborative study of pregnancy rates following Danazol therapy of stage I endometriosis. Fertil Steril 41: 373, 1984

Buttram VC: Surgical treatment of endometriosis in the infertile female: A modified approach. Fertil Steril 32:635, 1979

Buttram VC, Belue JB, Reiter R: Interim report of study of danazol for the treatment of endometriosis. Fertil Steril 37:478, 1982

Chang SH, Mattox WA: Adenocarcinoma arising within cervical endometriosis and invading the adjacent vagina. Am J Obstet Gynecol 110:1015, 1971

Chatman DA, Ward AB: Endometriosis in adolescents. J Reprod Med 27:156, 1982

Cheesman KL et al: Alterations in progesterone metabolism and luteal function in infertile women with endometriosis. Fertil Steril 40:590, 1983

Czernobilsky B, Morris WJ: A histologic study of ovarian endometriosis with emphasis on hyperplastic and atypical changes. Obstet Gynecol 53:318, 1979

Gould SF, Shannon JM, Conha GR: Nuclear estrogen binding sites in human endometriosis. Fertil Steril 39:520, 1983

Guzick DS, Rock JA: A comparison of Danazol and conservative surgery for the treatment of infertility due to mild or moderate endometriosis. Fertil Steril 40:580, 1983

Hammond CB, Haney AF: Conservative treatment of endometriosis. Fertil Steril 30:497, 1978

Hertig AH, Gore H: Endometrial cystoma, benign and malignant. In Tumors of the Female Sex Organs, Part 3, p 105. Washington, D.C., Armed Forces Institute of Pathology, 1961

Kempers RD, Dockerty MB, Hunt AB et al: Postmenopausal endometriosis. Surg Gynecol Obstet 111:348, 1960

Kistner RW, Siegler AM, Behrman SJ: Suggested classification of endometriosis. Fertil Steril 30:240, 1978

Labay GR, Feiner F: Malignant pleural endometriosis. Am J Obstet Gynecol 110:478, 1971

Levander G, Normann P: Pathogenesis of endometriosis. Acta Obstet Gynecol Scand 34:366, 1955

McArthur JW, Ulfelder H: The effect of pregnancy upon endometriosis. Obstet Gynecol Surv 20:709, 1965

Malick JE: The etiology of endometriosis. JAMA 81:407, 1982

Meigs JV: Endometriosis: Etiologic role of marriage age and parity: Conservative treatment. Obstet Gynecol 2:46, 1953

Merrill JA: Endometrial induction of endometriosis across millipore filters. Am J Obstet Gynecol 94:780, 1966

Mostoufizadeh M, Scully RE: Malignant tumors arising in endometriosis. Clin Obstet Gynecol 23:951, 1980

Muse KN, Wilson EA: How does mild endometriosis cause infertility? Fertil Steril 38:145, 1982

Oliker HA, Harris AE: Endometriosis of the bladder in a male patient. J Urol 106:858, 1971

Panganiban W, Corwog JL: Endometriosis of the intestine and vermiform appendix. Dis Colon Rectum 15:253, 1972

Pittaway DE, Wentz AC: Endometriosis and corpus luteum function. J Reprod Med 29:712, 1984

Ridley JH: The histogenesis of endometriosis. Obstet Gynecol Surv 23:1, 1968

Rodman MH, Jones CW: Catamenial hemoptysis due to bronchial endometriosis. N Engl J Med 266:805, 1962

Shaw RW, Fraser HM, Boyle H: Intranasal treatment with luteinizing hormone releasing hormone agonist in women with endometriosis. Br Med J 287:1667, 1983

Stillman RJ, Miller LC: Diethylstilbestrol exposure in utero and endometriosis in infertile females. Fertil Steril 41: 369, 1984

Stuart WW, Ireland GW: Vesical endometriosis in a postmenopausal woman: A case report. J Urol 118:480, 1977

Wheeler JM, Johnston BM, Malinak LR: The relationship of endometriosis to spontaneous abortion. Fertil Steril 39: 656, 1983

Wheeler JM, Malinak LR: Recurrent endometriosis: Incidence, management, and prognosis. Am J Obstet Gynecol 146: 247, 1983

Yeh TJ: Endometriosis within the thorax: Metaplasia, implantation or metastasis? J Thorac Cardiovasc Surg 53:201, 1967

Young EE, Gamble C: Primary adenocarcinoma of the rectovaginal septum arising from endometriosis. Cancer 24: 597, 1969

Gynecologic Malignancy: General Considerations

Felix N. Rutledge

54

All physicians should have a broad knowledge of medicine to recognize disease of any body site or organ system. This is a goal of the education and training of medical students and residents. Regardless of the field of specialization, this core of knowledge should emphasize basic gynecologic cancer. Any physician who treats women (the physician need not be a gynecologist or gynecologic oncologist) eventually encounters a need for this knowledge, since gynecologic cancers are common and the size and symptoms may mimic disease of other organs. A basic understanding of gynecologic oncology among physicians in general should help in the early detection of these diseases, because gynecologic cancers are often visible, palpable, and easy to study by means of biopsy. It is possible for physicians in many diagnostic specialties as well as surgical specialties to recognize gynecologic cancer and to direct the patient for proper treatment.

Proper treatment includes definitive therapy, posttreatment surveillance for recurrence, and treatment of recurrences should they develop. This often involves a team of specialists such as gynecologic oncologists, radiotherapists, and chemotherapists. Good management of the first treatment ranks next to early detection in importance for long-term survival. The first treatment offers the best chance for cure, and this opportunity must not be lost as a result of inappropriate or inadequate treatment methods, limited surgical training, or the lack of radiotherapists and their modern, versatile equipment.

One of the major advances in gynecologic cancer has been the creation of the subspecialty of gynecologic oncology, which identifies those physicians who have additional training and knowledge about treatment methods, who are prepared to deal with the complications of treatment should they occur, and who are able to provide posttreatment surveillance. These specialists also serve as consultants to physicians managing patients with an earlier stage cancer that does not need referral for its simpler treatment.

Counseling patients about the treatment of cancer is part of the practice of obstetrics and gynecology; therefore, basic knowledge of gynecologic cancer with a frequent update of new methods is essential to this role. An overview of the basic gynecologic oncology and current treatment trends should be of interest to the student of obstetrics.

Usually, we think of four major sites of gynecologic cancer: endometrium, ovary, cervix, and vulva. Cancer of the vagina, seemingly increasing in frequency, may reach major status. Endometrial cancer has displaced cervical cancer as the most common invasive gynecologic cancer. This would not be true if intraepithelial lesions were counted. Early detection methods have lowered the incidence of invasive cancer of the cervix, while an older age female population and estrogen use (although debatable) have increased the risk of endometrial cancer. The frequency of cancer of the ovary seems stable, and the incidence of invasive cancer of the vulva is declining. The combined incidence of gynecologic cancers is still lower than the incidence of cancer of the breast or colon.

In terms of mortality, cancer of the ovary is the number-one killer, a fact that has not changed with advances in radiation treatment or the introduction of chemotherapy. Although it occurs less frequently than endometrial cancer, cancer of the ovary causes more deaths. Unlike endometrial cancer, cancer of the cervix is suitable for early detection; one half to one third of the patients have intraepithelial lesions when discovered.

AGE

The age distribution of various gynecologic cancers is worth noting, since the relationship helps diagnostically, and some interesting changes have occurred in recent years. The peak incidence of cancer of the cervix is about 40 years, but the appearance may extend from late adolescence to old age, a span that covers a major part of a woman's life. Some of the youngest gynecologic oncology patients have cancer of the cervix. Approximately 10% of the invasive cervical cancers occur in women younger than 35 years; however, 50% of the intraepithelial cancers of the cervix are in those younger than 35 years of age.

Cancer of the endometrium occurs in menopausal and postmenopausal women; only 10% of patients or fewer are below 40 years of age. The diagnosis of endometrial cancer may be made in younger women, but a decision for treatment as cancer should be considered very carefully. Severe endometrial hyperplasia and endometrial cancer in youth may be indistinguishable histologically, with the odds favoring benign disease.

Cancer of the ovary, a devastating disease, may strike the young woman seemingly at the peak of her career or family commitment, or it may wait until she and her husband are enjoying their retirement. This cancer is currently our greatest concern, since it is the leading cause of death among gynecologic cancers and the fourth among causes of death due to cancer among women in the United States. Only cancer of the breast, cancer of the large intestine, and cancer of the lung are more lethal. The age for development is predominantly in the fourth, fifth, and sixth decades of life. Some special types of ovarian cancer occur in children.

Among gynecologic cancers, cancer of the vulva is the least frequent, accounting for 3% to 5% of all cases. This cancer is primarily a disease of older women, the average patient being in her 50s.

ETIOLOGY

Cancer of the cervix occurs predominantly in sexually active women, especially those who began coitus at an early age. Multiparity increases the occurrence, and involvement with multiple sex partners seems to be a contributing factor. At present, a venereal–viral agent is suspected, but evidence is still needed to prove that this agent plays a causal role. The viruses that cause herpetic infections and condylomatous warts are suspected, especially the papillomavirus. Because in some families a mother–daughter sequence for cancer of the cervix has been observed, heredity is theoretically deemed a contributing factor. Epidemiology shows geographic and ethnic variability; for example, blacks and Latin Americans have a higher incidence of cancer of the cervix than Jewish women, and in the Middle East there is a relatively low incidence.

Carcinoma of the endometrium may be associated with estrogen excess, especially if the estrogen is unopposed by progesterone. Estrogen excess occurs in obese patients by the production of estrone in the peripheral fat by the conversion of androstenedione, which

is produced by the adrenals even after menopause. Exogenous estrogen given for replacement therapy may also have a small role in carcinogenesis. Estrogens are not the only carcinogenic agents; many patients with cancer of the endometrium do not fit any of these conditions. Evidence is accumulating that some adenocarcinomas of the endometrium have estrogen-related causes while others do not. Some of these patients are not overweight, and many have never received hormone therapy. Also, the cancers may differ histologically and in prognosis. Estrogen-related ones are better differentiated histologically and more superficially invasive, and they have a better prognosis.

Least understood is the cause of cancer of the ovary. The epidemiology of this cancer fails to point out any significant role for environment, social behavior, fertility, or hereditary factors. No ethnic or environmental group is protected. Occasionally a family history is notable for the development of ovarian cancer among the female members, but a significantly greater risk population cannot be identified at present.

Similarly, the cause of cancer of the vulva remains a mystery. Some gynecologists believe there has been a recent increase in the frequency of intraepithelial carcinoma of the vulva, and the reason may be similar to that behind the high frequency of intraepithelial carcinoma of the cervix, a venereal-transmitted virus. Transmission of the agent is assisted by recently liberalized attitudes toward multiple sex partners, which increases contact among persons harboring the virus. This theory of viral etiology is apparently lacking proof and, if true, may apply only to intraepithelial cancers, since most invasive vulvar cancer occurs in older women in whom the histology shows no signs of having progressed through a condyloma or intraepithelial phase. Although cancer of the vulva occurs more frequently among patients with condylomata acuminata, granulomatous disease of the vulva, syphilis, and dysplastic vulvar disease, at present it is uncertain whether viral infections are causative or merely associated.

Increased frequency of cancer of the vagina is not due to intrapartum exposure to diethylstilbestrol, since this type of cancer of the vagina is extremely rare. The rising incidence of vaginal carcinoma is probably a function of earlier detection and improved distinction from cancer of the cervix, which may be impossible to make in later-stage disease.

DIAGNOSTIC METHODS

For cancer of the cervix, vaginal cytology (Papanicolaou [Pap] smear) has proven to be highly accurate for the detection of afflicted patients even without symptoms. The Pap smear has revealed cervical cancer and its precursors in very early developmental stages, making early treatment possible and causing a decline in the incidence of invasive cervical cancer. Nevertheless, patients with advanced cancers of the cervix are still encountered, perhaps owing to patients' neglect or rapidly growing types of cancer. In a few cases the test may be at fault; the Pap smear can fail to detect a lesion, and vaginal cytology is most likely to be false-negative when the cancer is advanced. Approximately one half of advanced cancer patients have a negative Pap smear because large cervical cancers with associated infection produce abundant necrotic debris, serous exudate, and hemorrhage, diluting the number of neoplastic cells on the smear. A suitable smear is more difficult to obtain if a cancerous lesion is clinically evident on the cervix; thus, the patient should also have the cervix inspected.

This inexpensive test for cancer of the cervix has proven effective in underdeveloped countries where the facilities for cancer detection are extremely limited. An example of this is the marked decline in the incidence of cancer of the cervix in the People's Republic of China following the institution of a comprehensive program of cancer detection with Pap smear. Some 20 years ago there was optimism that eventually the Pap smear would eliminte cervical cancer entirely by detecting cervical dysplasia or intraepithelial carcinoma and permitting institution of simple treatment. Although the Pap smear has contributed enormously toward the control of the cancer, success has been incomplete.

Cancer of the endometrium can be detected by vaginal cytology, but there is a high incidence of false-negative tests. Cells collected from the external os of the cervix average a 50% accuracy when there is endometrial cancer in the fundus. When cells are collected from the uterine cavity or high endocervical canal, the accuracy improves to 70%. Cytology of the uterine cavity has the least false-negative interpretation. The best diagnostic test for endometrial cancer is a specimen collected within the uterine cavity. Many new instruments have been perfected recently for collecting these specimens. Since these tests can be performed as an office procedure or in an outpatient clinic, a costly hospital admission is avoided.

Cancer of the ovary may be indicated by palpation, sonography, or computed tomography (CT) scanning. These studies may identify an abnormal pelvic or abdominal mass. However, the diagnosis requires histologic confirmation, which usually means entering the abdomen for the specimen. Cells from the peritoneal cavity obtained by needle puncture through the vagina or through the anterior abdominal wall may establish the presence of intraperitoneal carcinoma, but such a test does not determine the organ of origin. As a practical matter, laparotomy is usually required to establish the histologic diagnosis and to provide the abdominal cavity search for metastasis that is necessary for accurate staging before institution of treatment. Laparoscopic examination may provide some of this information, but for treatment planning needs, this information is incomplete. Regrettably, early detection of asymptomatic cancer of the ovary is not possible. Occasionally an early-stage lesion is discovered by chance. However, ovarian cancer usually grows and metastasizes rapidly; thus, the time

period for early discovery is short. Disappointingly, development of immunodiagnostic methods has been slow and has had little impact on control of this disease.

Cancer of the vulva should be easy to find and diagnose. Unfortunately, patients often conceal the lesions, and physicians sometimes mistake them for benign lesions or treat symptoms without examination. There are multiple causes for needless delay in treatment of cancer of the vulva. In recent years more physicians have become aware of intraepithelial lesions. Intraepithelial cancer of the vulva has no typical appearance, although localized areas of color differences due to increased pigmentation, hyperkeratosis, wartlike lesions, and shallow ulcerations are often indicative. Physicians who have good illumination for inspection of the vulva, who search the region carefully, and who perform frequent biopsies are most likely to find early vulvar cancers among their patients.

GROWTH AND PATTERN OF SPREAD

Gynecologic cancers generally advance into the surrounding tissues and to regional lymph nodes before spreading to establish distant metastases. An exception to this is intraperitoneal spread, notable in cancer of the ovary and occasionally in cancer of the endometrium. The predictability for cancer of the cervix and cancer of the vulva to enlarge locally and progress in a stepwise manner as nodes become involved along the lymphatic pathway is a basis for the design of surgery for these cancers. Cancer of the endometrium may bypass the pelvic nodes and go directly to the para-aortic nodes. Cancer of the ovary spreads intraperitoneally once the ovarian surface is penetrated. However, metastasis to the pelvic nodes and aortic nodes by ovarian carcinoma also occurs.

For the past few years, the mechanics of cancer metastasis have been investigated extensively, and the findings will ultimately alter our theories about how metastases occur and what determines how a particular site is selected by the cancer. These concepts may ultimately influence our ideas on the role of regional lymph node dissection. Current theories on metastases include tumor heterogeneity and the interaction of the tumor with the host to produce substances that encourage the permeation of the cells into adjacent tissues as well as blood and lymphatic vessels. While regional lymph nodes have long been considered a screen or sieve for floating cancer cells from gynecologic cancer, the patterns of spread are not always consistent with this function. Additionally, some patients develop distant metastasis without involvement of the regional nodes. The importance of the regional nodes in preventing metastasis is established, but they are not the only battleground for the lymphocytes to destroy cancer cells. Differences among patients for resisting metastasis are well known, but the influencing factors are not understood. We recognize that the body's defenses are enhanced by good nutrition and are depressed by chronic infection, radiation treatment, and radical surgery. These clinical observations are now being explained through the actions of mononuclear cells that are capable of spontaneous or natural immunity. Cells that have been identified in this category include macrophages, natural killer (NK) cells, and lymphokine-activated killer (LAK) cells. The body fluids of cancer patients have been found to have both blocking and enhancing effects on mononuclear cell–mediated cytotoxicity. The role of immune complexes as a prognosticator is still controversial.

At some point, the host's immune system will be overwhelmed by the effects of the tumor and possibly the cumulative effects of therapy itself. A very complex interaction of the above factors may determine the rate and growth and progression of the cancer, as has been shown in animal models.

These demonstrations have now become very important for the clinician because some of these factors can be measured quantitatively for women. We will soon be in an era when the metastatic event can be determined, predicted, and, it is hoped, avoided. Our capacity to augment the defenses with various immunomodulating agents that enhance killer cell activity is growing.

Treatment of metastases to the inguinal, femoral, external iliac, the obturator, the hypogastric, and to some of the other lower common iliac nodes is successful. When only a few nodes are involved by small deposits, about one half of patients can be cured. Excision and radiation therapy are usually equally effective as treatments. There is little success for treating para-aortic lymph node metastasis. Knowledge of the growth and spread pattern is essential for treatment.

TREATMENT MODALITIES

Surgical excision is the most successful treatment for gynecologic cancers that develop at either end of the genital tract. These are cancers of the ovary, uterus, and vulva. Advanced cancers of the cervix and vagina are less suitable for surgery because an adequate margin of cancer-free tissue cannot be excised without resection of the nearby bladder or rectum.

Cancer of the endometrium tends to remain confined to the corpus and is thus eminently suitable for resection. Seventy-five percent of endometrial cancer patients are in stage I, and many are cured by hysterectomy alone. However, 75% of patients with endometrial cancer are postmenopausal, and for this age group, medical and physical impediments to surgery are common. The treatment for some of these patients must be solely radiation therapy. When there is spread beyond the uterus, hysterectomy is still done to remove the primary growth, and the metastases are dealt with by radiation therapy or chemotherapy. Hysterectomy is the most effective single-treatment method for endometrial cancer. However, irradiation also plays an important role.

Operations for cancer of the ovary range from conservative hysterectomy with bilateral salpingo-oophorectomy for small, localized lesions confined to the ovary to resection of segments of intestine and omentectomy. Because most cures are accomplished by resection, an aggressive surgical attack on advanced cancer of the ovary is warranted. While resection may not remove all of the cancer, if the total tumor burden can be significantly lowered and especially if the size of the remaining tumor mass is less than 2 cm, the effect of either chemotherapy or irradiation therapy is improved.

Surgical resection excels over other methods of treatment for carcinoma of the vulva because these cancers are conveniently positioned for surgical removal and the range needed for resection is minimally restricted by neighboring organs. The bladder and rectum create a limitation when the cancer is extensive; when they are involved, an exenteration is required. If this extensive resection is not feasible, radiation therapy, either before or after vulvectomy, is an alternative. Irradiation for carcinoma of the vulva has been slow to gain popularity because of a long-standing belief that the skin of the perineum tolerates irradiation poorly. With the development of new x-ray machines that lessen the severity of radiation dermatitis, external radiation treatment is being advocated as an adjunct to vulvectomy when complete resection is difficult.

For early carcinoma of the cervix there are two effective treatment methods: extended hysterectomy and full-dose radiation therapy. Extended hysterectomy may be preferred because the abdominal exploration provides a more accurate staging, treatment failures due to radioresistance are eliminated, the side-effects of irradiation on the bladder and rectum are avoided, and the mucosa of the vagina is less damaged. Extended hysterectomy is preferred for young patients to preserve ovarian hormone production. Hysterectomy combined with radiation therapy is used for patients who have a localized but unusually large bulk of cancer, abnormal anatomic variations that block placement of radium, histologic types that are considered to be radioresistive, and a physical condition such that surgery poses a lesser risk than irradiation. Of the most common treatments for cancer of the cervix—primary surgery, combinations of surgery and irradiation, and irradiation alone—the last suits the most patients.

Chemotherapy is a major advance for treatment of epithelial cancer of the ovary, fallopian tube cancer, germ cell tumors of the ovary, and trophoblastic disease, replacing external irradiation as the better treatment for inoperable disease. Chemotherapy has had little effect on cancer of the endometrium, cervix, vagina, and vulva, except for progestin therapy for some endometrial cancers. Progress in chemotherapy has plateaued for the past ten years since the discovery of cis-platinum. While some of the older drugs may be preferred for some tumors, cis-platinum is the major anticancer agent in gynecologic oncology. Usually cis-platinum is combined with other therapeutic drugs. For the late-stage epithelial cancer of the ovary, there will be fewer chemotherapy cures than anticipated ten years ago. Many long-term remissions are produced, but the attrition due to recurrence and death over long-term observation is disappointing. On the other hand, chemotherapy as an adjunct to surgical resection in earlier stage epithelial cancer of the ovary seems to reduce postoperative recurrence.

The success of chemotherapy for trophoblastic disease continues to be an outstanding accomplishment, although a 100% cure rate is not possible. Perhaps the greatest recent advance in chemotherapy and gynecologic oncology is in the treatment of germ cell tumors of the ovary. This treatment induces dramatic tumor regression (some patients seem cured) and obviates the need for radiation treatment, which was used before the advent of chemotherapy.

RESULTS OF TREATMENT

The overall results of treatment of gynecologic cancer are based on averages calculated after a period of observation and do not reflect major deviations for some persons or differences between one patient and another within the group. These differences include variations in virulence of tumors, sensitivity of tumors to irradiation or chemotherapy, host resistance to tumors, and the patient's ability to withstand the therapy indicated. The FIGO system for staging gynecologic cancer reflects the prognosis. The University of Texas M. D. Anderson Hospital and Tumor Institute's statistics are used here to illustrate what is expected for five-year survival of the various invasive gynecologic cancers.

The results of treatment of cancer of the cervix by irradiation are as follows: stage Ib, 91%; stage IIa, 82%; stage IIb, 65%; stage IIIa, 54%; and stage IIIb, 40%. Radical hysterectomy is used for selected patients with stage-I carcinoma of the cervix, and results are the same as with radiation treatment.

Carcinoma of the endometrium is usually treated by hysterectomy with preoperative irradiation (intracavitary radium or radiation therapy, or both). The five-year survivals are stage I, 77.7%; stage II, 53.9%, stage III, 18.9%; and stage IV, 3%. A more precipitous drop is noted between stages II and III than for carcinoma of the cervix. This is because stage-III endometrial cancer usually involves intraperitoneal metastasis.

Cancer of the ovary shows a wide difference between stages I and II. The five-year survival figures are stage I, 71.7%; stage II, 25.8%; stage III, 12%; and stage IV, 0%.

The five-year survivals for carcinoma of the vulva, as collected from the literature, shows stage I, 89.7%; stage II, 79.6%; stage III, 47.9%; and stage IV, 15.2%.

ACCURATE STAGING

It is surprising that the FIGO staging functions so well, since its inaccuracies are well known. Laparotomy subsequent to clinical staging often reveals undetected metastasis. The inaccuracy of staging, on which radiotherapists depend, has been criticized by those who advocate surgical treatment whenever feasible.

For the past 15 years oncologists have been increasingly insistent on accurate staging, to the extent of performing a diagnostic and assessment laparotomy prior to radiation treatment. Even when laparotomy was performed, the true extent of spread was often undetected as the result of an incomplete search of the abdominal cavity. Carcinoma of the ovary is a good example of this. For years the 25% recurrence in stage-I disease was baffling, since seemingly the cancer was confined to the ovary and could be excised. The reason should have been obvious; there must have been unrecognized metastases that were not excised. Not until a search was made for subclinical-sized peritoneal implants and free cancer cells were they found in about the same frequency as the recurrence incidence. Viewing of less accessible peritoneal spaces, biopsy of normal-appearing peritoneum, and biopsy of aortic lymph nodes established the correct stage.

Pretreatment laparotomy for more precise staging of cancer of the cervix has been performed at some centers for cancer treatment. Several large series of patients have been investigated, and metastases above the field of radiation treatment have been discovered. To achieve a cure, it is obviously paramount to have all the cancer treated, including that above the pelvis. Unfortunately, enlarging the field of external irradiation has been poorly tolerated and added very few cures. Still, the principle of accurate staging is sound, since in time an effective therapy of remote metastases will be discovered.

This same trend toward first learning as far as possible the limits of cancer is also developing in the treatment of endometrial carcinoma. Many treatment centers prefer to perform laparotomy with hysterectomy and from this information to decide whether adjunctive radiation treatment is needed.

New techniques have helped find metastases and may sometimes substitute for laparotomy. Lymphangiography is very useful and well tolerated, and it is now a routine pretreatment study for all stage-II through stage-IV carcinomas of the cervix. Other cancers are also suited for this test. Its use in the investigation of the retroperitoneal nodes is limited, but it may be more accurate than CT scan for small-sized metastases in lymph nodes. Development of aspiration biopsy with the long, thin needle has been a successful sequel to localization of enlarged nodes by lymphangiography or CT scan. Thin-needle aspiration can confirm cancer histologically. Passage of this needle through organs en route to the suspected retroperitoneal mass is safe.

CT and ultrasonography can complement lymphangiography with better measurements of size. Also, they may identify masses not involving the lymphatics, such as intraperitoneal masses. These tests are not performed routinely for all new patients but are used when there is a special need.

Peritoneoscopy provides a view of the abdominal cavity, but not of all parts, and not of the retroperitoneal areas. A view of the ovaries, uterus, omentum, liver, diaphragm, cul-de-sac, and paracolic gutters may provide valuable staging information, and peritoneoscopy may replace laparotomy for this purpose. It is least useful for investigating cancer of the cervix. The technique may be helpful in some endometrial cancer patients if there is a mass outside the uterus and in some patients with cancer of the ovary.

MONITORING TREATMENT AND SURVEILLANCE FOR RECURRENCE

Except for β–human chorionic gonadotropin, the recovery of cancer products from the blood, peritoneal fluid, spinal fluid, or vaginal secretions has only recently found clinical usefulness. The identification of carcinoembryonic antigen (CEA) and its commercial production have alerted clinicians to the potential for cancer monitoring and has intensified research for other tumor products.

The intensive search for a tumor-specific antigen during the past 10 to 15 years has been frustrated by the difficulty of separating a specific tumor antigen from other tissue antigens. However, clinically useful substances that are not tumor specific have been made from earlier products produced by the tumor cells. Quantitative determination of these substances reflects the presence and, to a degree, the amount of neoplasia.

In gynecology and urology, α-fetoprotein is produced in excess in germ cell tumors of the ovary and in some testicular tumors. It can be measured in the patient's serum and can be used to produce monoclonal antibodies, which can be used in differential immunologic staining. Labeled antibody to α-fetoprotein can localize metastasis and recognize recurrence.

The development of monoclonal antibodies to tumors has added greater specificity and sensitivity to tests for cancer. An example is the anti–colon carcinoma monoclonal antibody, which has had some clinical trial. There is optimism that the monoclonal antibody will soon be used for monitoring a variety of tumors and be used to transport therapeutic agents to the site.

Some gynecologic tumors such as the mucinous ovarian cancers produce an abundance of CEA. Labeled anti-CEA monoclonal antibodies allow imaging of small-sized cancers and have clinical usefulness. Immunoscintigraphy still has some technical problems, but it will be adopted clinically when they are corrected.

THE TERMINAL CANCER PATIENT

There is a great deal of emotionalism in the management of the terminally ill patient, and it is easy to find fault with medical management. Criticism by compassionate friends may be more severe than that from the loving immediate family. The doctor is often the subject of this criticism, being accused of excessive prolongation of life, failure to allow the patient to die with dignity, failure to support emotionally the patient who has developed a dependence on the doctor who has managed the cancer treatment, failure to control the patient's pain, and abandonment of the patient.

The gynecologic oncologist should be prepared by specialty training to manage the terminal care of patients with uncontrollable cancer. However, because of logistics, the local physician may acquire this role. Thus, all physicians need some training in this area. The scientific journals contain articles about new drugs and new technology for administering the drugs. The subject is much larger than can be discussed here; however, a brief mention may stimulate more study.

Care of the terminally ill patient is as much the physician's responsibility as is the provision of proper therapy. Too frequently the physician turns his back when it is clear that the outlook is hopeless. Support for both the patient and her family is essential at this time. The social, economic, and emotional turmoil can be overwhelming. The physician who possesses compassionate understanding will make regular visits and provide assurance that medical needs such as pain control will be met.

Modern cancer therapies have produced a greater need for effective relief from pain. Incomplete remissions or failing remissions after chemotherapy leave a patient alive and functional, but the cancer pain remains. Analgesic drugs are available, but for some patients the associated side-effects such as drowsiness and depressed responses are incapacitating.

It is estimated that 60% to 80% of cancer patients suffer pain in the final stages of the disease. Eventually the pain is continuous and more intense. Almost all of these patients can be maintained in comfort and relatively free of pain if due thought is given to the selection of the drugs that are used. In the beginning of the program to control pain, the mildest, most effective drug should be used. For analgesia, aspirin, acetaminophen, and propoxyphene are sometimes completely effective and should be used first in a dose of 650 mg every three to four hours. Codeine, 30 mg to 60 mg, may be added if necessary, but a mild laxative may also be needed to counteract the constipating effect. If this is inadequate or unsatisfactory, one may advance to oxycodone/acetylsalicylic acid–phenacetin–caffeine (APC), which may be more effective and better tolerated. For severe pain, one of the variants of "Brompton's mixture" is usually suitable. It has the advantage of an oral medication that can be readily used at home and can be adjusted to the needs of the patient. A 20-ml dose (which may be needed every three to four hours) contains the following: cocaine, 10 mg; morphine, 10 mg; grain alcohol, 2.5 ml to 5 ml; flavoring syrup; and chloroform water to make 20 ml. The alcohol may be omitted if the patient has stomatitis. The morphine content may be increased, if needed, up to 120 mg, or chlorpromazine can be added to potentiate the narcotic effect. A commercial preparation of oral morphine sulfate (10 mg/5 ml) is now available and appears to be just as effective as Brompton's mixture. After the first several doses the patient may sleep for prolonged periods; this may be interpreted as due to excessive dosage, but it more likely results from relief from pain and exhaustion. A customary dose is 20 mg morphine solution every four hours; some patients require doses of up to 75 mg.

Tranquilizers and mood elevators are useful; however, they may induce somnolence when combined with narcotics. They may also aggravate respiratory depression or cause confusion and dizziness. For patients who are agitated or depressed, diazepam, 2 mg 3 times per day, may be prescribed for daytime, or haloperidol, 10 mg, may be given at bedtime. These drugs may reduce the need for analgesia. The phenothiazines are difficult to use with narcotics because of extrapyramidal effects. Nausea is a common problem among patients, and for this drugs such as promethazine, prochlorperazine, and trimethobenzamide hydrochloride may be helpful.

Analgesics are best administered by the oral route, but intractable nausea may eventually make this route impractical. Morphine is well absorbed following intramuscular injection, but when pain becomes severe and chronic, this method carries risk for hematomas. Also, the medication peaks in effect.

A new development is the administration of morphine via Ommaya reservoir placed into the ventricles of the brain, which can be recharged by needle puncture through the scalp. This requires an operation and thus is not advised until the pain is very severe and cannot be controlled by simpler methods.

Utilizing special catheters, a technique for long-term intravenous administration of analgesics, has been successful for pain control. To prevent infection, trained staff must maintain the catheter. The method, therefore, is not ideal for home care.

New developments in portable infusion pumps that distribute the narcotic evenly over a period of time may be used for morphine or hydromorphone hydrochloride (Dilaudid) to control refractory pain. The same injection site may be used for two to three days before another must be found.

The mistakes of the past have been withholding medication until pain returns (administration of narcotics on a schedule that avoids return of pain is more merciful and reduces the amount required over 24 hours); trying to avoid narcotics addiction even when the cancer is out of control; and early administration by injection when the oral route is available.

CONCLUSIONS

Management of gynecologic cancers is changing to become more conservative and more cost efficient. There are also new concerns for the patient's quality of life after treatment. Older philosophies that insisted on a standard treatment applied according to the diagnosis and without regard for unique prognostic factors are being altered for more individualized therapy. The treatment of endometrial cancer illustrates these changes. Twenty years ago the accepted treatment for endometrial cancer was preoperative irradiation, sometimes external therapy, and administration of intracavitary radium followed by hysterectomy. This plan was employed even for grade-I and superficially invasive lesions. Over the past ten years preoperative radiation has been omitted for the patient with a favorable grade and degree of infiltration. The trend may ultimately be to discontinue preoperative irradiation for all patients with this diagnosis.

Very high doses of radiation for all gynecologic cancers have had a trial and are being moderated. Dogged attempts to sterilize tumors with more and more ionizing energy have proven catastrophic. We now realize that the worst compliction of treatment is not necessarily failure to destroy all the cancer; the complications caused by ultraradical treatment may be even worse. The gynecologist has also learned the lesson of radical resection and the excesses of using both irradiation and surgery to their maximum.

Although control of cancer has progressed very little during the past 20 years in terms of cures, we believe that we understand better what the problems are and why progress is so slow. Even in the area of early detection, which we should be able to accomplish in all but cancer of the ovary, we still have not eliminated delay in discovery of late-stage disease. Many symptoms are still neglected, and women with late-stage disease still appear for initial treatment. We have been disappointed in our hope of 20 years ago that earlier detection and cancer-screening programs would, by today, have led to the control of gynecologic cancer.

REFERENCES AND RECOMMENDED READING

Miller N: Terminal care of the gynecologic cancer patient. Obstet Gynecol 4:470, 1954

Rutledge F, Boronow RC, Wharton JT: Gynecologic Oncology. New York, John Wiley & Sons, 1976

Lesions of the Vulva and Vagina

J. Donald Woodruff

55

Benign Lesions of the Vulva

The vulvar skin is of ectodermal origin, and consequently it is subject to diseases that are common to the skin elsewhere as well as to infectious processes that are more or less specific to the genital area.

Benign lesions of the vulva may be classified as follows:

I. Inflammatory lesions
   A. The common dermatitides
      1. Reactive (not allergic)
      2. Intertrigo (seborrheic dermatitis)
      3. Psoriasis
      4. Candidiasis
      5. Tinea (various types)
      6. Vestibular (major and minor) gland infections
   B. Viral diseases
      1. Herpes simplex
      2. Condyloma acuminatum
      3. Molluscum contagiosum
   C. Ulcerative lesions
      1. Venereal (syphilis, lymphogranuloma, chlamydia), and granuloma inguinale (B. Donovania)
      2. Behçet's disease
      3. Crohn's disease
      4. Nonspecific (hidradenitis, ecthyma, folliculitis, factitious, decubitus) lesions
II. Traumatic lesions
   A. Hematomas
   B. Lacerations

III. White lesions (excluding neoplasms)
   A. Absence of pigment
      1. Leukoderma or vitiligo
   B. Hyperkeratotic
      1. Inflammatory lesions
      2. Benign neoplasms
   C. Dystrophies
      1. Hyperplastic
         a. Typical
         b. Atypical (mild, moderate, marked)
      2. Lichen sclerosus
         a. Typical (et atrophicus)
         b. Atypical?
      3. Mixed dystrophies (hyperplasia and lichen sclerosus)
         a. Typical
         b. Atypical (mild, moderate, marked)
IV. Benign neoplasms
   A. Solid tumors: granular cell myoblastoma, aberrant breast, lipoma, fibroma, hemangioma, hidradenoma, nevus, condyloma, acrochordon (fibroepithelial polyp), endometrioma, pyogenic granuloma
   B. Cystic lesions: inclusion, Bartholin duct, mucous, canal of Nuck (hydrocele)

Since cancer of the vulva may be associated with ulcerative, erythematous, proliferative, or hyperkeratotic lesions, biopsy must be used freely if malignancy is to be diagnosed in its early or even precursory stages. The instruments shown in Figure 55-1 are used for single or multiple biopsy of all suspicious or controversial lesions in order to prove the true histologic nature of the disease with the knowledge that one can expect no concomitant spread of malignancy from the procedure and the patient can be afforded an accurate evaluation and therapy.

The use of 1% toluidine blue as a local nuclear stain

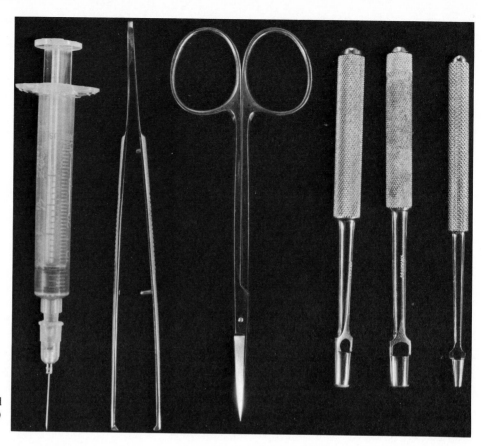

FIG. 55-1. Instruments used for biopsy of vulva. (*Right*) Keyes dermatologic punches.

may assist in selecting sites for biopsy. The vulva is painted with this agent and then washed for two to three minutes with 1% acetic acid. The stain is removed from normal tissues by the latter agent, but remains as a mark of cellular atypia or ulceration in those areas with retention of the dye. It must be appreciated that there are many false-negative and false-positive results from the use of this diagnostic technique. Acute excoriative processes (*e.g.,* reactive dermatitis) produce superficial ulcerations, and the underlying exposed nuclei will absorb the stain; consequently, such processes should be treated and, if nonhealing, erythematous, or ulcerative foci remain, the stain should be applied and suspicious areas biopsied. Conversely, white, hyperkeratotic lesions may *not* absorb the dye and must be biopsied regardless of the results of the toluidine blue study.

INFLAMMATORY LESIONS OF THE VULVA

Vulvitis due to infectious agents is discussed in Chapter 52. The following lesions, in which there is an inflammatory reaction, also should be noted.

The most common benign affliction of the female external genitalia is contact dermatitis. This was formerly called eczema or eczematoid dermatitis; however, the

great majority of such dermatoses are caused by local irritants, such as tight underclothing that retains moisture, aerosol sprays, bubble bath and bath oils, colored toilet paper, detergents used in washing underclothing, perfumed soaps and powders, and a variety of other agents to which the vulva is commonly exposed. Obviously, the treatment is to eliminate the irritant and to use local fluorinated hydrocortisones. The latter agents are extremely powerful and should be used sparingly in strengths of 0.025% to 0.1%. Furthermore, they should be used only for symptomatic relief. Prolonged usage may produce systemic reaction or local fibrosis.

Intertrigo and seborrheic dermatitis are commonly seen in the diabetic patient. The elimination of moisture by the use of cornstarch and the topical use of fluorinated hydrocortisone creams or lotions for the pruritus are the appropriate approaches to the acute problem. The classic agents used for "dandruff" elsewhere may be applied to the vulva; however, elimination of moisture and local irritants and the use of antipruritic agents are usually sufficient. The chronic hyperkeratotic alterations are "white lesions," which are discussed later in this chapter.

Psoriasis is usually multifocal. The classic picture on extragenital skin is characterized by "silver scales" and associated redness with linear excoriation. On the moist vulva, however, psoriasis appears as an erythematous patch without scales. Consequently, it is most important that the entire patient be examined, not just the vulvar area, if the appropriate diagnosis is to be made.

Candidiasis of the vulva is commonly associated with a vaginal infection, as noted in Chapter 52. Diabetes often accompanies such lesions.

Tinea cruris is usually sharply marginated, affects the adjacent skin surfaces, and is often found elsewhere on the body. Accentuation of the skin markings occurs in the more chronic situations. Lotrimin is most commonly used in the treatment of such lesions. Tinactin is also effective.

Infection in the major vestibular (Bartholin) gland is well known, and if an abscess develops, it should be incised. Minor vestibular glands are superficial and lie just external to the hymenal ring. Infection in the latter produces dyspareunia. Excision may be necessary to alleviate the pain.

ULCERATIVE LESIONS

Among the ulcerative lesions, special note should be made of Crohn's disease (Fig. 55-2). It is not well appreciated that approximately 25% of patients with classic enteritis also have draining sinuses, fistulous tracts in the perineum, or fissuring at the outlet and edema. Unless this relationship is appreciated, inappropriate therapy may be instituted. Simple incision and drainage of the sinuses may lead to rectovaginal fistula or even breakdown of the perineum. Prednisone is the classic treatment, usually in doses of approximately 40

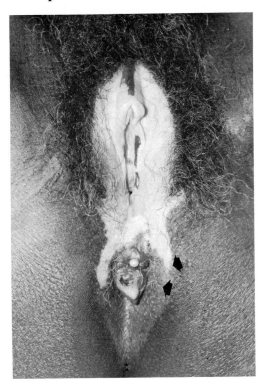

FIG. 55-3. Leukoderma with differential pigmentation on labia minora and prepuce. Patient had pruritus at perianal area, and small areas of depigmentation caused by chronic dermatitis (vitiligo) are apparent, particularly at *arrows.*

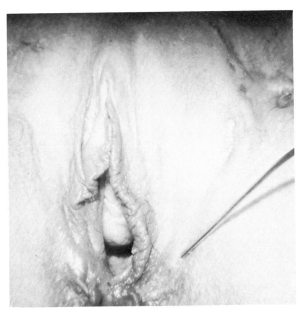

FIG. 55-2. Patient with Crohn's disease (regional enteritis) and concomitant draining sinus. Probe in fistulous tract.

mg/day. The addition of metronidazole, 1000 mg to 1500 mg daily, to the therapeutic regimen has made it possible to reduce the dosage of cortisone. Treatment with corticosteroids should be continued indefinitely. The metronidazole should be continued if surgery is contemplated.

Behçet's disease, probably an autoimmune disease, is characterized by ulcerations on the vulva and adjacent perineum, associated with similar lesions on the buccal mucous membrane. The third member of this "triple symptom syndrome," iritis, is not commonly recognized. Nevertheless, it should be appreciated that iritis is the most serious manifestation of all because it may progress to fatal neurologic disease. The fundamental treatment is prednisone 40 mg/day, reduced if possible at the end of one month. There are many theories about the origin of this disease, and thus many therapies have been instituted. Spontaneous regressions and recurrences are common and constitute a major difficulty in the management of this disease.

WHITE LESIONS

Leukoderma, also called vitiligo, is common on the vulva, often appears at the time of puberty, and is seldom symptomatic (Fig. 55-3). Associated depigmented areas are often found elswhere on the body. When symptoms arise in this context, they generally are related to a superimposed dermatitis.

Vitiligo, acquired loss of pigment, is also extremely common and is usually associated with local inflammatory disease (Fig. 55-4). Such alterations are often transitory and migratory. The café-au-lait spots associated with neurofibromatosis (von Recklinghausen's disease) are rare on the vulva.

Hyperkeratotic lesions may be recognized in a variety of circumstances. Increased deposition of keratin (hyperkeratosis) is a protective phenomenon noted particularly on traumatized skin and, therefore, may be associated with any irritation, varying from chronic inflammatory disease to carcinoma. The white or grayish-white appearance of the skin in such situations is due to the absorption of moisture by the keratin. Intertrigo, probably the most frequent dermatitis in which hyperkeratosis develops on the vulva, is found most commonly in the interlabial and crural folds and is extremely difficult to combat, particularly in the obese diabetic woman, in whom it is commonly found. Seborrhea (seborrheic dermatitis) is a corollary of intertrigo and is also extremely common in the moist atmosphere of the vulva. Chronic dermatitis results from a variety of locally irritative conditions and similarly produces a thick, protective layer of keratin. The acuminate wart in its initial state is brown or reddish brown and microscopically shows superficial parakeratosis; however, in its later stages it is characterized by the development of hyperkeratosis. Thus, the chronic irritative lesion, regardless of etiology, may eventually produce the superficially protective keratin coat.

FIG. 55-4. Vitiligo.

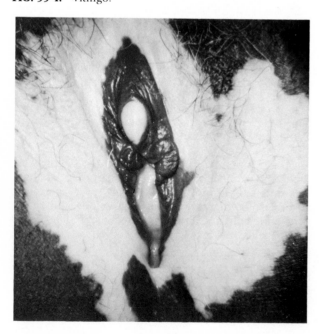

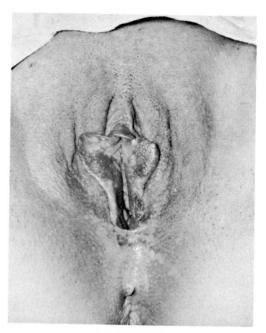

FIG. 55-5. Lichen sclerosus with foci of whitish alterations on labia minora and at fourchette.

Dystrophy means simply a disorder resulting from "abnormal nutrition" and thus has been applied to describe those lesions that are characterized by a keratin layer of varying thickness (accounting for the white or grayish white color), an abnormal thinning or thickening of the epithelial layer, an underlying chronic inflammatory infiltrate, and varying degrees of change in the subepithelial connective tissue. The latter may, in truth, relate to nutritional deficiencies, as noted by the vascular patterns. These dystrophies are probably the most common lesions, previously diagnosed as leukoplakia.

The term *leukoplakia* means a white patch and has been applied to almost every white lesion on the vulva. It is therefore highly nonspecific and should be eliminated from the terminology of vulvar disease.

In addition to leukoplakia, a variety of other terms demand careful evaluation and modifications. Kraurosis is a clinical designation meaning shrinkage. The microscopic correlate is lichen sclerosus. Thus, as a specific lesion, the term "kraurosis valvae" should be eliminated in favor of more specific clinical and histopathologic interpretations.

Lichen sclerosis (et atrophicus) has been recognized on the vulva in all age groups (Fig. 55-5). Girls in the first decade of life have been afflicted with this nonspecific, patchy, white alteration of the labial skin. Most of these patients improve at the time of the menstruation; however, the lesion may occur throughout the menstrual years, usually beginning as small, bluish white papules with eventual coalescence into white plaques. In its initial phases, lichen sclerosus is asymptomatic and demands no therapy. It assumes major significance in the postmenopausal patient, in whom it is commonly associated with severe and recalcitrant pruritus. Malignancy may develop in 2% to 3% of these patients if pruritus is not controlled.

In the prepubertal patient, relief of symptoms is most important. Local hydrocortisone is usually effective. Testosterone is not recommended in such patients; however, 2% progesterone cream may be used if needed for symptomatic relief. It is in the postmenopausal patient that long-term treatment with topical testosterone is most effective. Because persistent therapy with topical fluorinated hydrocortisone may produce fibrosis and scarring of the subepithelial tissues, steroids should be used primarily for symptomatic relief in the acute case but not as constant therapy over a long time. Clitoral enlargement and increased libido are associated with the use of testosterone in approximately 20% of the patients.

"Primary senile atrophy" and "atrophic vulvitis" should be eliminated as diagnoses because most of these lesions are variations of lichen sclerosus.

The microscopic picture of lichen sclerosus is characterized by moderate hyperkeratosis, a thinning of the epithelium with a loss of the rete pegs, underlying collagenization, and inflammatory infiltrate (Fig. 55-6). Similar changes may be seen in the so-called kraurosis; however, the latter term fundamentally means shrinkage and is thus a gross clinical, rather than a microscopic, diagnosis. The later stages of lichen sclerosus are commonly associated with dyspareunia caused by constriction of the outlet and fissure formation at the fourchette.

Hyperplastic dystrophy is characterized by gross lesions that are white or grayish-white and may be either diffuse or focal. The patches are firm and often cartilaginous on palpation (Fig. 55-7). They simulate the general appearance of the lesions previously diagnosed as leukoplakia. Histologically, the keratin layer is usually thicker than that seen with lichen sclerosus and the epithelium is more proliferate, with elongated and often blunted rete pegs. In typical hyperplasia there is an increase in the cellular elements of the epithelium, but no abnormality of maturation. Underlying chronic inflammatory infiltrates vary in degree. Many such alterations are simply caused by chronic dermatitis, and thus treatment should be symptomatic. Biopsy must be used freely to eliminate the possible coexistence of cellular atypia. As noted above, local fluorinated hydrocortisone is the best of the antipruritic agents. Occasionally, very hypertrophic and often atypically pigmented areas may not respond to either local or systemic hydrocortisones, but the subcutaneous injection of such preparations may be dramatically effective. Small areas of 2 cm to 3 cm may be injected with 2 ml to 3 ml of fluorinated hydrocortisone, (*e.g.,* Triamcinolone or Kenalog), producing dramatic results not only in elimination of the symptoms but in restoration of the normal coloration. Local measures to eliminate irritation are similar to those described previously and, regardless of the pathology, all patients should be instructed to observe these rules. On occasion these conditions are solitary and can be locally excised. However, multicentric foci must be eliminated by thorough investigation of the adjacent tissue. Diagnosis must be confirmed in all cases by biopsy. Multiple specimens are necessary in most instances because various patterns often coexist.

Atypical hyperplastic dystrophy is usually a white lesion, but red or pigmented lesions may show similar alterations. The latter do not simulate the epithelial changes described for cervical neoplasia. Atypical maturation and intraepithelial "pearl" formation are the hallmarks of atypical hyperplastic dystrophy and often occur adjacent to invasive vulvar cancer (Fig. 55-8).

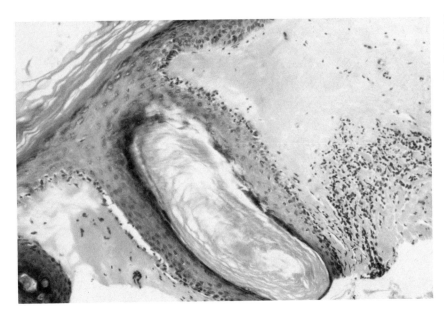

FIG. 55-6. Classic microscopic appearance of lichen sclerosus. Thin epithelieum with underlying collagenation, inflammatory infiltrate, and follicular plugging.

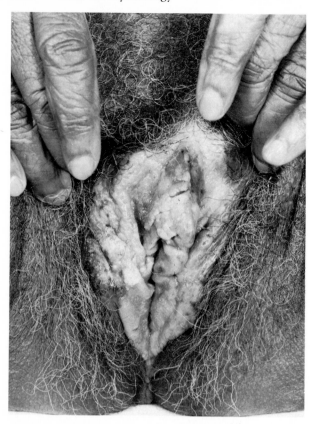

FIG. 55-7. Thick, white hyperkeratotic changes may be associated with hyperplastic dystrophy. Biopsy must be used freely in these cases to rule out malignancy.

Thus, it is imperative to recognize the differences between cervical and vulvar neoplasia in both the *in situ* and invasive stages. Finally, it must be noted tht histologic abnormalities may be associated with severe viral disease (human papilloma [HPV] and herpetic lesions). These undoubtedly account for the so-called reversible atypias that have been described recently.

Mixed dystrophy is a combination of lichen sclerotic changes and hyperplasia. Biopsy is important in identifying the malignant potential of such lesions and must be used liberally. Colposcopy and cytology have not been helpful in differentiating the degrees of cellular atypia. Biopsy is simple and essentially painless if the area is infiltrated with a local anesthetic agent, and the Keyes dermatologic punch is used to remove the tissue (see Fig. 55-1).

The basic treatment of all irritative lesions of the vulva must begin with a positive diagnosis; consequently, biopsy is imperative. Assuming that no major atypia is discovered, the next step is to eliminate the irritation. It seems quite possible that the chronic alterations associated with scratching may be most important in the genesis of neoplasia. The treatment includes the use of topical fluorinated hydrocortisones to control the symptoms and reduce the local inflammatory reaction, the use of estrogen intravaginally in the postmenopausal patient, the treatment of any associated intravaginal infection, and the elimination of local irritants as noted previously. In the more persistent case, after these treatments have failed to control the symptoms, alcohol injection of the external genitalia will eliminate the symptoms and not only afford relief to the patient, but will allow the skin to recover from the persistent

FIG. 55-8. Atypical hyperplastic dystrophy.

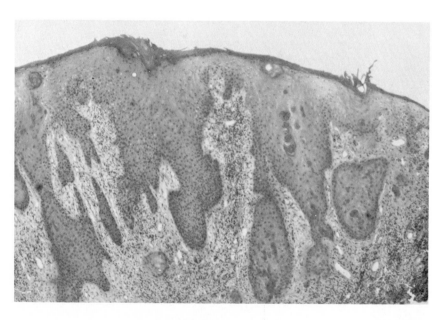

scratching. This procedure should be used with caution, since slough of tissue may result from too deep an injection. The previously suggested subcutaneous injection should be used prior to alcohol, since it is effective in 80% to 85% of the cases and can be performed in the office.

SOLID TUMORS

The majority of benign solid tumors (*e.g.,* lipoma and fibroma) occur only rarely on the vulva and are similar to such lesions elsewhere; thus, they need no special discussion here. All varieties of vascular tumors on the external genitalia have been described; however, the congenital variety deserves special note. Appearing at two to three months of age, it produces remarkable distortion of the vulva but generally needs and should receive no therapy unless excessive bleeding occurs because such lesions disappear spontaneously. Small, elevated, hemorrhagic nodes are sometimes mistaken for hemamgiomas but are, in truth, tiny varicosities that may produce an occasional episode of irregular bleeding. Varicosities may attain great size and a varicocele, similar to that of the male, develops in the vulva. Such lesions are almost always unilateral and are much less common than those that develop as the result of obstruction in the vessels of the spermatic cord. The hidradenoma is a rare lesion that, because of the intricate adenomatous

pattern, has been confused with malignancy. Malignant alterations are extremely uncommon and the lesion, rarely more than 1 cm in its largest dimension, can be treated by local excision (Fig. 55-9).

A variety of pigmented lesions are seen on the vulva. An irritative focus of chronic dermatitis may be pigmented, as may carcinoma *in situ* and the "spreading melanoma." Again, as noted previously, biopsy is imperative to evaluate accurately the histopathology of such lesions.

Both intradermal and compound nevi occur frequently and should be removed for positive diagnosis. The malignant potential of the primary lesion is essentially nil. Nevertheless, malignancy cannot be ruled out without excision and careful histopathologic study. More ominous patterns such as atypical melanocytic hyperplasia (melanoma *in situ*) are not grossly differentiated from the benign pigmented lesions.

A variety of papillary lesions have been noted on the vulva. The common acuminate wart, which is of viral origin, constitutes a recurring therapeutic problem and may be a precursor of malignancy. The fibroepithelial polyp or acrochordon is common in all areas subjected to irritation and needs no treatment other than accurate diagnosis.

Of special interest to both pathologists and clinicians is the granular-cell myoblastoma. This benign lesion arising from the nerve sheath is associated with extensive, overlying pseudoepitheliomatous hyperpla-

FIG. 55-9. (*A*) Hidradenoma on right inner labium majus. Rectocele is also visible inside introitus. (*B*) Photomicrograph of hidradenoma of vulva. (Novak ER, Woodruff JD: Gynecologic and Obstetric Pathology. Philadelphia, WB Saunders, 1962)

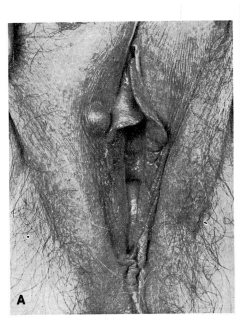
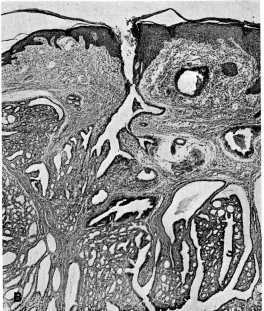

sia, often misdiagnosed as carcinoma *in situ* or even early invasive cancer. Careful investigation of the underlying tissue is important in order to make an accurate evaluation and institute the appropriate therapy. The finding of large cells with prominent eosinophilic granules makes the accurate diagnosis. Finally, the myoblastoma is not a well localized tumor and, therefore, is subject to local recurrences. Nevertheless, malignant myoblastomas are uncommon. Although multicentric foci arising in diverse areas in the body are not infrequent, they should not be interpreted as metastases.

Vulvar endometriosis is uncommon and occurs most commonly in areas subjected to trauma. The incision or excision of the chronically infected Bartholin gland seems to be an ideal precursory event for the development of such lesions. Furthermore, episiotomy sites are not uncommon foci for implantation of the "stimulus" leading to the development of endometriosis. As usual, the characteristic feature is cyclic swelling and pain. Such lesions also develop in the inguinal canal and adjacent mons.

CYSTIC LESIONS

The sebaceous cyst or, more accurately, "epidermal inclusion," is the most common cystic lesion of the vulva (Fig. 55-10). Although a majority of these lesions result from occlusion of the sebaceous gland on either labia minora or labia majora, microscopically they are *epidermal* inclusion cysts and in the chronic, quiescent

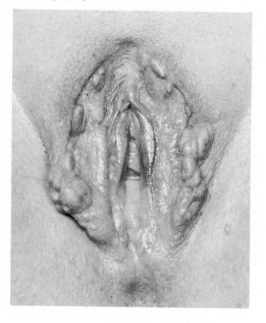

FIG. 55-10. Multiple sebaceous cysts of vulva. (Woodruff JD: Tumors of the Female Genitalia. In Pack GT, Ariel IM [eds]: Treatment of Cancer and Allied Diseases, Vol 6. New York, Hoeber, 1962)

state are lined by stratified epithelim. Before the actual development of such lesions, the swelling contains only sebaceous material and thus is not a true cyst. These lesions need no treatment unless they become infected, at which time simple incision and drainage are usually sufficient. If they are recurrently infected, excision may be done; however, recurrences are common.

Cystic dilatation of the main Bartholin duct (Fig. 55-11*A* and *B*) may be caused by chronic inflammatory reactions with scarring and occlusion or by trauma from lacerations or incisions in the area. For the most part, these cysts are asymptomatic and therapy is unnecessary. If symptomatic, the use of the indwelling Word catheter requires only local anesthesia and can be carried out as an office procedure. Excision is necessary only if marsupialization is unsuccessful in controlling the infection or if the diagnosis of malignancy is entertained.

Dysontogenetic (mucous) cysts are found at the introitus and adjacent labia minora. These cysts contain mucoid material and possibly represent the residua of incomplete separation of the cloaca by the urorectal folds; thus, they represent dilatations in rectallike tissue. They may, as noted above, originate by occlusion of the minor vestibular glands that ring the outlet at the introitus. Regardless of origin, these lesions are benign.

Cysts that appear high in the labium majus (hydrocele of the canal of Nuck) simulate the hydrocele in the male. Since the round ligament has an investment of peritoneum, the latter may be occluded in the inguinal canal and allow the accumulation of fluid along the round ligament as it inserts into the labium majus. It is important to discover the origin of such lesions, because simple incision and drainage leads to prompt recurrence. Furthermore, the lesions may indicate hernias, and any portion of bowel that is present in the sac must be removed.

Benign Lesions of the Vagina

Benign lesions of the vagina include inflammatory reactions (Chap. 52), "leukoplakia" (hyperkeratosis resulting from chronic irritation such as that associated with total prolapse of the uterus), cystic lesions, and solid tumors.

CYSTIC LESIONS

Benign cystic lesions of the vagina are inclusion cysts, Gartner's duct cysts, endometriosis, adenosis, and vaginitis emphysematosa.

The inclusion cyst is extremely common and occurs most frequently near the outlet at the site of previous lacerations or episiotomy scar. It seldom attains sufficient size to become symptomatic, and associated inflam-

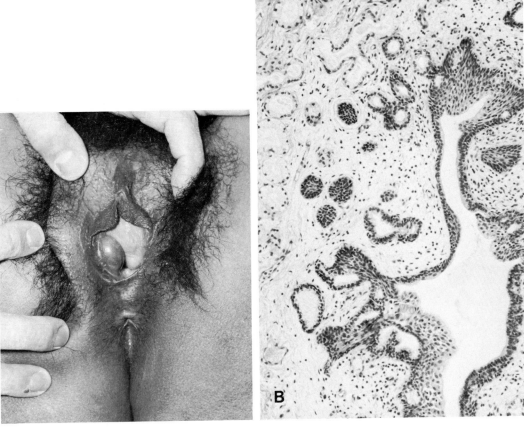

FIG. 55-11. (*A*) Bartholin duct cyst projecting into introitus. (*B*) Various epithelia present in Bartholin gland, primarily transitional in center with mucous-secreting acini.

matory reaction is uncommon. Thus, excision or incision and drainage are rarely necessary. The cyst is filled with desquamated cellular material from the stratified squamous epithelial lining.

Gartner's (mesonephric) duct may be the origin of multiple tiny cystic dilatations or, on rare occasions, a large solitary cyst. The former are palpable only as fine elevations on the mucosal surface in the vaginal fornices or along the course of the mesonephric duct. They are common and rarely symptomatic. The latter may develop in the midline of the anterior vault and simulate a cystocele (Fig. 55-12). Recognition of the nature of the lesion is important in determining therapy. Removal is usually not needed unless they present symptoms. Although no harm is done if the cyst is inadvertently opened during removal, the surgeon may be dismayed if he erroneously believes he has incised the bladder. Malignancy rarely develops in these mesonephric remnants, although the "mesonephroma" described 40 or 50 years ago probably represents such a lesion.

Endometriosis usually develops as a penetration of cul-de-sac disease, and as such appears in the posterior fornix of the vagina where it is characterized grossly by a bluish discoloration produced by the old blood. If penetration is incomplete, the associated nodular induration extending from the uterosacral ligaments into the vagina may simulate cancer. To rule out the latter, the vaginal lesion should be biopsied to establish the diagnosis. Nevertheless, recognizing that most of the vagina is of paramesonephric origin, endometriosis could arise in sites other than the cul-de-sac. If the lesion is asymptomatic and is the only abnormality present, no therapy other than accurate evaluation is indicated. Otherwise, appropriate treatment for endometriosis, either medicinal or surgical, should be instituted.

Adenosis varies in gross appearance from diffuse granular thickenings to an irregular, rugose, mucoid lesion. The frequency of adenosis is difficult to assess; however, Sandberg suggests that more than 40% of all women demonstrate such subepithelial adenomatous structures. Any area of the vagina may be involved, but most commonly it is the anterior or posterior wall of the upper half of the vault. Probably arising from aberrant ectopic cervical-type "glands" (Fig. 55-13), the lesion is rarely symptomatic and thus therapy is unnecessary. Recently, interest in adenosis vaginae has increased with the appearance of these adenomatous elements in the vaginas of young women whose mothers had received

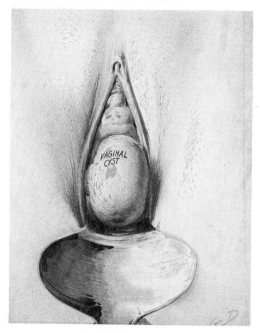

FIG. 55-12. Cyst of anterior vaginal wall. Cyst protrudes through vulva when exposed with speculum. (MacLeod D, Read CD: Gynaecology, 5th ed. London, Churchill Livingstone, 1955)

diethylstilbestrol (DES) during pregnancy. The physician may be alerted to this group of lesions by the occasional presence of a transverse septum in the upper third of the vagina or the more frequent occurrence of a collarlike structure around the cervix (Fig. 55-14). Ap-

proximately 500 adenocarcinomas have been reported from the population at risk. Such neoplasms develop most commonly in the menarcheal years. Nevertheless, the lesions have been reported in a seven-year-old child, although admittedly the number of occurrences in those younger than 14 years of age is extremely small. Conversely, such malignancies have been discovered in the midthird decade of life, the oldest patient at present being 30 years of age. Of importance is the magnitude of this at risk population, which now must approximate more than one million young women. Methods of investigation of this special group have challenged the profession. At present, the basic question is whether the young woman at risk will develop mesonephroid carcinoma of the vagina, and the answer currently must be "rarely," or less than 0.1%. The follow-up of the patient at risk should consist of careful palpation of the tissue with inspection and cytopathologic evaluation. Colposcopy has not been helpful in identifying the early adenocarcinoma. Most cases of clear cell or mesonephroid carcinoma are found during the first study. However, at least four cases have been discovered in the follow-up study of initially benign adenosis; one of these was a multifocal lesion. It should be appreciated that in at least 25% of the cases of vaginal adenosis, there is no definable history of the maternal ingestion of either DES or other hormones.

Of concern in the future may be the development of epidermoid neoplasia at the many squamocolumnar junctions produced by the change in the embryology of the area. Stafl, in his colposcopic studies, has commented on this variety of histologic alteration. Nevertheless, there is no evidence that "multiple squamocolumnar junctions" place the patient at greater risk for

FIG. 55-13. Vaginal adenosis, showing surface-stratified epithelium with underlying glands, one of which contains metaplastic epithelium.

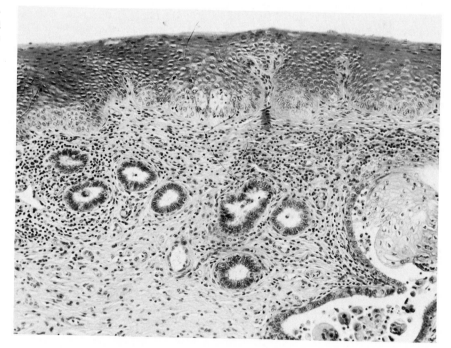

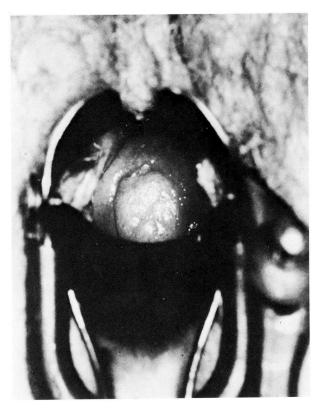

FIG. 55-14. Photograph of cervix of 22-year-old DES-exposed offspring demonstrating complete cervical collar and polypoid structure of central portion of cervix. Note that anterior portion of collar is slightly peaked, giving rise to a deformity referred to as a "cockscomb." (Townsend DE: In Herbst AL [ed]: Intrauterine Exposure to Diethylstilbestrol in the Human, p 26. Chicago, American College of Obstetricians and Gynecologists, 1978)

the development of neoplasia than does one. Stafl notes that benign adenosis can be demonstrated colposcopically in over 90% of the young women at risk. Nevertheless, the incidence of such alterations depends largely upon the stage of the pregnancy at which therapy was instituted. For example, if treatment was begun prior to the tenth week of gestation, adenosis occurs in approximately 90% of the female progeny. Conversely, if medication was instituted after the 16th week of gestation, the risk factor is no greater than that for the female population at large. Microscopic examination of the adenomatous lesion reveals that the epithelia characteristic of the paramesonephric system (*i.e.,* mucinous, endometroid, and endosalpingeal) may be found in many cases; however, the mucinous or endocervical variety is the most common.

Another cystic lesion that is rarely diagnosed is vaginitis emphysematosa. Characterized by widespread submucosal cyst formation, this uncommon lesion is found in the pregnant woman or in the severely decompensated cardiac patient. The blebs are filled with carbon dioxide, and definitive infecting agents have not been recovered from the contents. Therapy should be directed toward the associated vaginitis, commonly found to be trichomonal in the pregnant woman. Complications have not been reported. Microscopically, the lining of the cavities is characterized by the presence of irregular, "reactive" giant cells (Fig. 55-15).

SOLID TUMORS

Benign solid tumors of the vagina include fibromyoma, polyps, papilloma, and condyloma.

Fibroma (fibromyoma), a rare solid tumor, may arise *de novo* from the connective tissue and smooth muscle

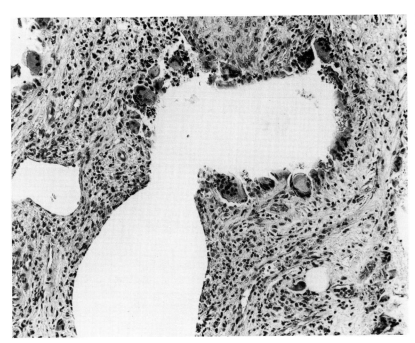

FIG. 55-15. Microscopic appearance of vaginitis emphysematosa, showing cystic spaces lined by giant cells.

elements of the vaginal wall. However, many of these lesions are intraligamentary uterine fibromyomas that have become divorced from the fundus and have dissected into the paravaginal area. These lesions, whether primary or secondary, are rarely symptomatic, and the incidence of sarcomatous change is negligible. Of major concern is the overdiagnosis of both the leiomyoma and the polyp. Because of edema and degenerative changes, these lesions may be misconstrued as stromal malignancies. Excision usually is a minor procedure; however, the uterine vessels or the ureter may be encountered if dissection is extensive. If any question exists about the nature of the tumor, excision must be done, because the treatment of vaginal malignancy is complicated by the necessity for radical surgery or technically difficult radiation. Local excision is often followed by recurrence despite "benign histology."

True papillary tumors other than condylomata acuminata are rare. Most of these lesions are, in truth, fibroepithelial tags (acrochordon). Although vaginal polyps are uncommon, they nevertheless have been classically misinterpreted because of the edematous nature of the lesion. A diagnosis of sarcoma botryoides is often made on the basis of these histologic features. In the follow-up of such cases, it is noteworthy that although the polyp may recur, malignancy has not been reported.

Condylomata acuminata are common in the vagina and are associated classically with extensive condylomatosis of the vulva (Figs. 52-4, 55-16). The urethra, cervix, and perianal areas are frequently involved. These lesions may become exuberant, particularly during pregnancy. In pregnancy they present major complications because of associated vascularity, edema, and inflammatory reaction. The customary treatment, podophyllin, should not be used during pregnancy. The trauma of delivery may result in vaginal laceration and extensive bleeding. Nevertheless, since the acuminate wart is of viral origin, the lesion may spontaneously regress postpartum with the institution of good local hygiene and the elimination of associated infection. It should be noted, however, that laryngeal papillomas in the newborn have been associated with vaginal condylomatosis in the mother. Although these lesions are benign, they do present problems in the care of the neonate. Currently, cesarean section may be recommended for extensive vaginal condylomatosis, not because of the possibility of infection of the newborn, but because of the bleeding that may accompany the trauma of vaginal delivery.

In the nonpuerperal state, general cleanliness often results in reduction in the size of the lesion. Podophyllin should be used sparingly in the vagina because local reactions may be severe. Anaphylactic shock has been reported as a complication of the injudicious use of this cauterizing solution. Local application to the individual lesion followed by vaginal douche within two hours of the application has rarely resulted in any unfavorable reaction. Although the small individual warts may be treated in this way, extensive involvement of the vagina

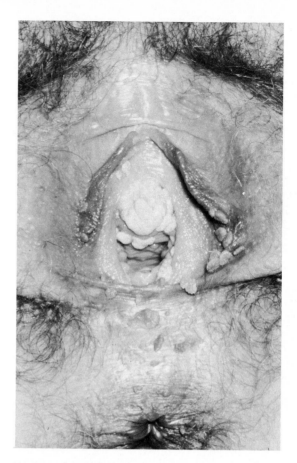

FIG. 55-16. Condylomata acuminata affecting urethra, vagina, and external genitalia.

may require excision under general anesthesia. In resistant cases, 5-fluorouracil (Efudex) is often effective. Laser therapy has been used with satisfactory results.

Malignant Tumors of the Vulva

Vulvar anaplasia comprises 3% to 4% of all primary malignancies of the genital canal. Despite the availability of these lesions for early investigation, there is a longer interval between the appearance of symptoms and the establishment of diagnosis of carcinoma of the vulva than for any other primary malignancy of the female genitalia. Much of this delay may result from the reluctance of the elderly patient to seek medical advice; however, the 30% to 35% of cases in which the physician is at fault may be related to the commonplace nature of the initial symptom—pruritus. Too often, treatment is suggested over the telephone before thorough study has been carried out.

As noted previously, the dystrophies may show a variety of histologic alterations, which are described as typical or atypical hyperplasias. Atypia and dysplasia are also used to describe atypical hyperplasia. In many series the lesions are found because of the preexistence of cervical neoplasia (multifocal disease).

Vulvar malignancies may be classified as follows:

I. Primary malignancy
  A. Carcinoma *in situ*
    1. Bowen's disease
    2. Erythroplasia of Queyrat
    3. Atypical pigmentation (pigment incontinence)
  B. Paget's disease
  C. Invasive cancer
    1. Squamous-cell lesions—Well differentiated, others
    2. Basal-cell carcinoma (histologic variations)
    3. Bartholin gland lesions
      a. Squamous-cell lesions
      b. Transitional lesions
      c. Cribriform (adenocystic) lesions
    4. Verrucous carcinoma—This tumor is locally invasive but not metastasizing. The histology is identifiable and the treatment is wide excision. Recurrences are common and often locally destructive.
  D. Other malignancies—Including melanoma (melanotic and amelanotic), sarcoma, lymphoma, embryonal rhabdomyosarcoma, and breast cancer
II. Secondary malignancy

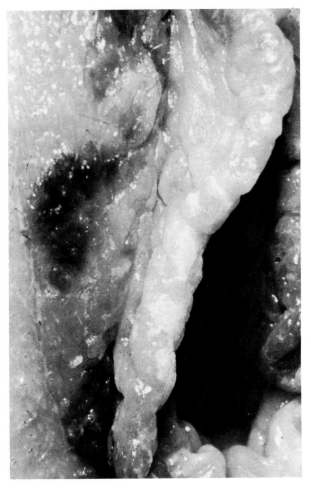

FIG. 55-17. Carcinoma *in situ* of vulva. (*Right*) Multiple whitish foci. The intervening areas are reddish.

CARCINOMA *IN SITU*

Carcinoma *in situ* occurs at any age, but frequently during the third and fourth decades of life. Although a common complaint is pruritus, the lesion may present as a lump or may be relatively asymptomatic. These lesions are found adjacent to invasive cancer, but the cases that result from dystrophy and carcinoma *in situ* to invasive disease are few and far between. The gross appearance varies greatly. The Bowenoid lesion is scaly and characterized by a red background dotted with white hyperkeratotic islands (Fig. 55-17). Other lesions are almost entirely white, red (erythroplasia of Queyrat), or a combination of these patterns (Fig. 55-18). Others are irregularly pigmented, with a diffuse but hazy background of hyperkeratosis (Fig. 55-19). These variable and bizarre patterns demand that many lesions be biopsied to determine their true nature. The increased frequency with which multiple areas of anaplastic change are found in the lower genital canal and perianal areas (the anogenital area) is noteworthy. Such alterations demand thorough study of the entire region, both initially and at follow-up examinations. Microscopic sections demonstrate variations in atypical cellular maturation (Figs. 55-20, 55-21) in one and the same lesion, thus justifying the term "carcinoma *in situ*" in preference to a specific designation such as "Bowen's disease."

Of major interest are the variations in the histologic patterns adjacent to invasive cancer and those described as marked atypical hyperplasia or carcinoma *in situ*. It seems quite possible that viral disease may produce histologic patterns indistinguishable from carcinoma *in situ,* representing the cases of so-called reversible atypia.

If multiple foci of malignancy are carefully excluded by use of toluidine blue and random biopsies, wide local excision of the lesion is the acceptable treatment. Thus, although vulvectomy has been the proposed therapy, it is obvious that more conservative approaches are indicated in most young patients. Conversely, it seems apparent at the present time that carcinoma *in situ* occurring in the patient over the age of 60 years may be an

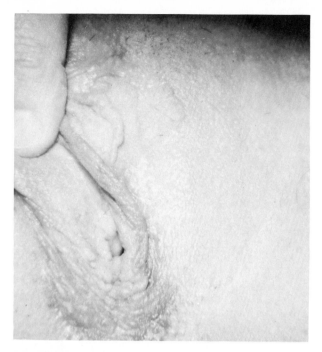

FIG. 55-18. Carcinoma *in situ* of vulva. Reddish lesion at fourchette; white lesion at left vulva.

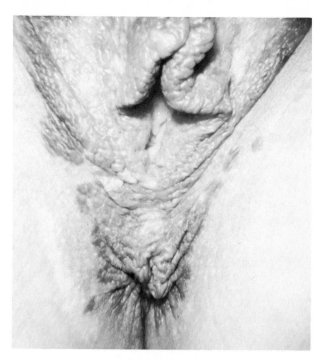

FIG. 55-19. Pigmented carcinoma *in situ* of vulva.

FIG. 55-20. Carcinoma *in situ* of vulva showing intraepithelial pearl formation and individual cell anaplasia.

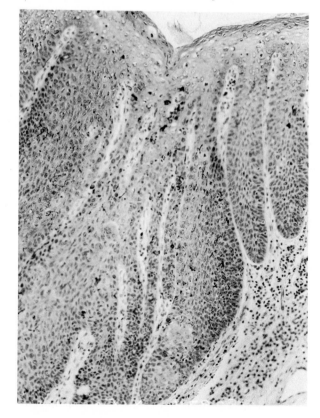

entirely different disease, and thus vulvectomy is more appropriate in such instances unless an isolated focus can be identified. Careful follow-up is essential in either case, because simple excision does not remove the precipitating agent and the potentiality of recurrence always exists, regardless of whether the surgery is radical or simple. The use of topical chemotherapeutic agents (*e.g.,* 5% fluorouracil cream) have been used with success rates of approximately 60% to 75%. Nevertheless, the magnitude of the local irritation precludes the use of such agents. In most instances, the erythroplastic lesion seems to respond favorably. Recently an immunologic approach has been used successfully in recurrent, especially pigmented, lesions. The patient is sensitized to dinitrochlorobenzene (DNCB), and the agent is applied locally to the lesions. A severe reaction may occur, and it is essential to evaluate carefully the strength of the agent needed for each individual patient. Finally, laser therapy has been used effectively in the treatment of intraepithelial neoplasia. The basic treatment is wide local excision with careful histopathologic study. Laser therapy has been effective, but it does not allow for careful histologic evaluation. Vulvectomy is contraindicated in patients 45 years of age or younger unless they are immunosuppressed.

Paget's Disease

Like its counterpart on the breast, vulvar Paget's disease (Fig. 55-22) is characterized grossly by a fiery red background mottled with white hyperkeratotic islands and,

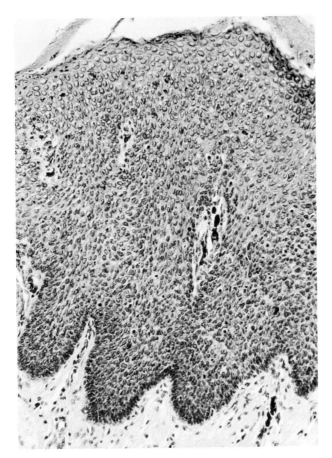

FIG. 55-21. Another pattern of intraepithelial vulvar carcinoma characterized by increase in basal and parabasal cells.

a thorough study of every patient should be made to rule out a mammary lesion.

Invasive Carcinoma

The common vulvar malignancy is a skin cancer and thus should be classified as squamous-cell, not epidermoid, carcinoma (Figs. 55-24, 55-25). Approximately 65% to 70% are mature "pearl-forming" tumors, and the remainder are poorly differentiated or a mixture of patterns. At present there is no difference in survival between these histologic variants. The average age of all patients with vulvar cancer is 60 to 65 years. Approximately 10% of these malignancies are found in the third and fourth decades of life.

The primary symptom is pruritus, especially if the preceding disease is of the dystrophic type; however, many patients have noted a lump or local irritation for many years. Patients with chronic granulomatous disease or a long-standing benign tumor that has undergone malignant alteration usually complain of a mass, local discomfort, and bleeding. Diagnosis is made on examination of the biopsy material. Diagnostic problems lie in differentiating benign proliferating tumors and chronic granulomatous disease from their malignant counterparts.

Classification and Staging

The Fédération Internationale de Gynécologie et Obstetrique (FIGO) has accepted the following classification of vulvar cancer. We feel that the TNM portion

in this respect, simulates Bowen's disease. Unlike the mammary lesion, which is usually associated with an underlying malignancy, the vulvar disease is intraepithelial in 75% of cases. Nevertheless, the tendency to recur locally makes the neoplasm a constant threat. Despite this threat, a rare case of malignancy has been reported to follow the initial intraepithelial lesion.

Microscopically, the characteristic large, pale cells of apocrine origin are found initially in the basal layer but eventually involve the entire surface epithelium as well as that of the underlying appendages (Fig. 55-23). The positive reaction of the cells to mucicarmine stain serves to differentiate the lesion from Bowen's disease and melanoma.

Therapy primarily demands simple vulvectomy to determine the extent of involvement of the underlying tissues. If invasive disease is recognized in the removed specimen, inguinal and femoral lymph node dissection is indicated. In view of the frequency of recurrence, careful follow-up is mandatory. Radiation has been of little value for the local or metastatic disease. The association with Paget's disease of the breast has been recorded in several studies, and, although uncommon,

FIG. 55-22. Paget's disease of vulva. Darker areas are grossly red; white patches are evident.

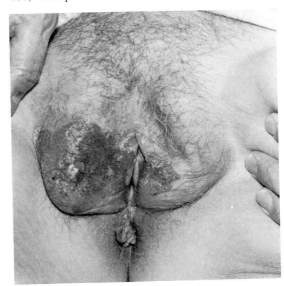

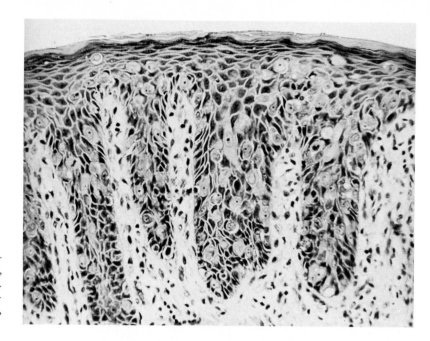

FIG. 55-23. Paget's disease of vulva. Epidermis shows maturation, enlarged rete pegs, and Paget's cells with pale cytoplasm (×185). (Haines M, Taylor CW: Gynaecological Pathology. London, Churchill Livingstone, 1962)

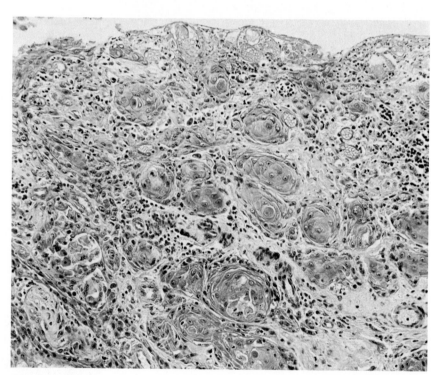

FIG. 55-24. Invasive cancer characterized by pearl formation without overlying, full-thickness, epithelial changes.

of the classification (tumor, nodes, metastases) is cumbersome and would be wisely eliminated. The final grouping of the FIGO classification, clinical staging, seems sufficient.

Clinical staging of invasive carcinoma of the vulva

1. Stage I: (TI NO; TI NI)
   a. Tumor confined to vulva, 2 cm or less in largest diameter; no nodes palpable or, if groin nodes palpable, they are mobile, not enlarged, and not clinically suspicious of neoplasm
2. Stage II: (T2 NO; T2 NI)
   a. Tumor confined to vulva and more than 2 cm in largest diameter; status of nodes as in stage I
3. Stage III: (T3 NO; T3 NI; T3 N2; TI N2; T2 N2)
   a. Tumor of any size confined to vulva, with palpable

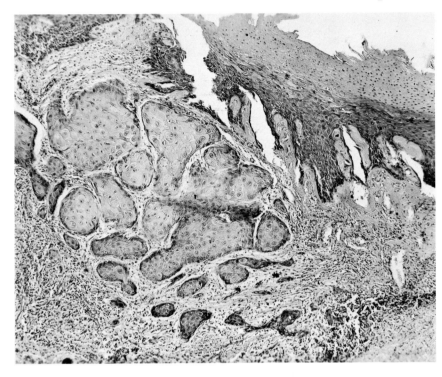

FIG. 55-25. (*Left*) Invasive carcinoma with atypical maturation of invasive epithelium. (*Right*) Abnormal changes are characterized by parakeratosis and irregular rete pegs with collagenation (leukoplakia).

nodes in groin which are enlarged, firm, mobile, and clinically suspicious of neoplasm

  b. Tumor of any size with adjacent spread to urethra, vagina, perineum, or anus with or without suspicious, mobile nodes in groin

4. Stage IV: (TI N3; T2 N3; T3 N3; T4 N3; T4 NO; T4 NI; T4 N2; all other conditions containing M1a or M1b)

  a. Tumor of any size or extent with fixed or ulcerated nodes

  b. Tumor of any size infiltrating mucosa of bladder, rectum, or urethra, or fixed to bone

  c. Tumor of any size with palpable deep pelvic lymph nodes or other distant metastases

Treatment

Treatment is fundamentally surgical, with removal of the vulva and the superficial and deep inguinal and femoral nodes. The lymphatic drainage of the vulva is shown in Figure 55-26. It has been suggested that there is cross-lymphatic circulation and thus a bilateral lymphadenectomy should be carried out in most cases (Fig. 55-27). Nevertheless, current studies suggest that unilateral lesions do not have contralateral nodal metastases if the ipsilateral nodes are not involved. Thus, in specific cases unilateral node sampling may eliminate the need for the more extensive operation, which carries a predictably high postoperative morbidity. Extraperitoneal lymph node dissection is unwarranted today. Its place may be taken by pelvic irradiation if the superficial nodes are positive. An 85% to 90% salvage may be expected if

FIG. 55-26. Lymphatic spread of carcinoma of vulva. Note possible contralateral spread of cancer, especially from anterior vulva and clitoris with possible direct metastasis to Cloquet's node rather than initial involvement of inguinal node. (From Traut HF, Benson RC: Cancer of the Female Genital Tract, 2nd ed. New York, American Cancer Society, 1957)

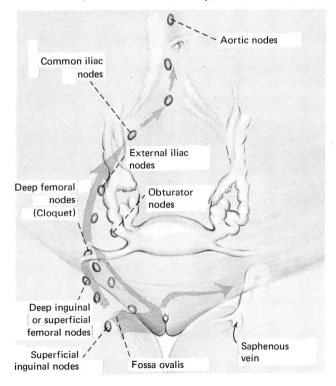

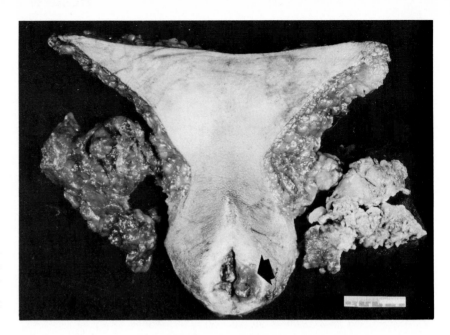

FIG. 55-27. Specimen from radical vulvectomy with inguinal and femoral node dissection. Carcinoma may be seen at *arrow.* Surrounding tissue shows hyperkeratosis with changes consistent with lichen sclerosus.

nodes are uninvolved; however, even with metastasis to these regional sentinels, five-year survival rates approximate 30% to 35%. Various classifications have been proposed, but the features noted above are of fundamental importance in determining prognosis. Those interested in more information may refer to the works listed under References and Recommended Reading.*

The term *microinvasive cancer of the vulva* demands careful evaluation, because it is not the same as the similar lesions on the cervix. Among 58 cases with invasion to a depth of less than 5 mm treated by various surgical techniques, 5 patients (9%) later died as the result of recurrent or metastatic disease.

Local recurrence is a major threat. Approximately 80% of all patients with vulvar malignancy die from direct invasion of local organs. These lesions may be "reoccurrences" rather than recurrences and suggest the possible presence of a persistent carcinogen or the lack of host resistance.

Verrucous carcinoma is unique. In spite of the massive local tumor, metastases to the regional nodes do not occur; therefore lymphadenectomy is unnecessary. Radiation therapy is contraindicated. Local recurrences are common and should be managed surgically.

Basal cell carcinoma comprises 5% of all vulvar cancers. Like its counterpart on the skin elsewhere, it is a locally invasive but rarely metastasizing lesion. Wide local excision is the treatment of choice for these tumors.

Although Bartholin's gland is an uncommon site

---

* Recently there has been a resurgence of interest in the use of radiation therapy, particularly for the massive lesion in the elderly patient with medical contraindications to extensive surgery. Results suggest that excision of the tumor mass with follow-up external-beam therapy to the nodes may be an alternative to surgery, particularly in the patient who has positive inguinal nodes, specifically Cloquet's. Radiation should not be given to vulvar skin!

for the origin of malignancy, tumors arising in the gland present a wide variety of patterns. The common squamous-cell cancer develops at the orifice of the duct and represents a variant of primary vulvar carcinoma; thus, it should not be classified as a Bartholin's gland tumor. The transitional type arises from the characteristic urogenital epithelium of the duct. The true Bartholin gland cancer is a mucoid, cribriform adenocarcinoma developing from the acini of the gland (adenoid cystic tumor). This variety deserves special mention, because it is classically slow-growing, indolent, and locally invasive; however, late metastases occasionally appear in the lungs. The last type usually presents as an indurated mass in the deep recesses of the perineum, whereas the former types grossly simulate the common vulvar malignancies. Wide local excision is the treatment for the adenoid cystic lesion, but local recurrences are common.

Other Primary Malignancies

As noted earlier, the vulva is the site of origin of approximately 2% to 3% of malignant melanomas in women. Since both the spreading and nodular varieties are difficult to differentiate from many of the benign pigmented lesions, biopsy should be used freely. Early diagnosis is of obvious importance. The survival is related directly to the depth of invasion, which is differentiated into five levels. Levels 1 and 2 (involvement of the intrapapillary ridges) are associated with essentially 100% five-year survival; conversely, the salvage in level-5 tumors (involvement of the subcutaneous fat) is an unimpressive 0% to 20%. Surgery is the treatment of choice, and at the present time radiation and chemotherapy have added little to the salvage rate. Current thought suggests that there is no need for radical surgery in patients with involvement of only the epithelium and the rete ridge. Breslow has suggested depth measurement as a more accurate determinant of prognosis. For lesions less than 0.75 mm (Clark's level 1) five-year survival is 100%, only the rare patients with lesions extending from 0.75 to 1.5 mm (Clark's levels 1 and 2) are found to have nodal involvement. Therapy of the future may well be wide local excision with elective lymph node dissection.

Procrastination in treatment is often due to misdiagnosis or lack of follow-up after a suspicious area is biopsied. Biopsy is the method of diagnosis, and there is no validity in the opinion that every such lesion must be excised because of the danger of spread induced by biopsy. Furthermore, there is no evidence that the prognosis is worse for lesions that are diagnosed during pregnancy.

Rare cases of fibrosarcoma have been reported arising primarily in the external genitalia. Surgery is the treatment of choice, although triple chemotherapy has been suggested by some authors.

Lymphoma and embryonal rhabdomyosarcomas have been reported on the external genitalia. These cases classically arise in young people, and the former often represents the superficial demonstration of an underlying lesion.

Secondary Malignancies

Most of these lesions arise in the adjacent area and affect the vulva by direct extension; malignancies of the cervix and rectum are common offenders. Adenocarcinoma of the endometrium and choriocarcinoma show a predilection for metastasizing to the external genitalia, and on occasion the diagnosis of trophoblastic malignancy is first made on examination of biopsy material from the vulvar metastasis. Obviously, extension from the cervix, vagina, or rectum may occur.

Malignant Tumors of the Vagina

Primary malignancy arising in the vagina makes up 2% to 15% of all anaplastic disease arising *de novo* in the genital canal.

Vaginal malignancies may be classified as follows:

I. Primary malignancy
   A. Carcinoma
      1. Epidermoid carcinoma
         a. *In situ*
         b. Invasive
      2. Adenocarcinoma
         a. Clear cell (mesonephroid carcinoma arising in adenosis)
         b. Other—Adenocarcinoma in endometrium

   B. Sarcoma
      1. Sarcoma botryoides
      2. Others
         a. Fibro- and leiomyosarcoma
         b. Rhabdomyosarcoma and lymphoma
   C. Melanoma
II. Secondary malignancy, arising from primary lesion in cervix, endometrium, ovary, bowel, vulva, or urinary tract.

The currently accepted FIGO staging for primary carcinoma of the vagina is as follows:

Stage 0:   Carcinoma *in situ*
Stage I: Carcinoma limited to vaginal wall
Stage II: Carcinoma involving subvaginal tissues but not extending to pelvic sidewall
Stage III: Carcinoma extending to pelvic sidewall
Stage IV: Carcinoma extending beyond true pelvis or involving mucosa of bladder or rectum (extension by bullous edema per se does not permit stage IV classification)

IN SITU EPIDERMOID CARCINOMA

In situ carcinoma of the vagina has been described as occurring in three different situations: with other similar lesions in the lower genital canal (regional response to a carcinogen), as residua after incomplete surgery for carcinoma *in situ* of the cervix, and following radiation for invasive carcinoma of the cervix. Preinvasive changes may be grossly evident prior to the development of invasive disease, but such cases are obviously in a minority. Although asymptomatic, these lesions can be recognized early if routine cytology is performed on all patients and if the possibilities of multicentric foci of origin and postirradiation neoplasia are kept in mind.

Similar to invasive disease, *in situ* malignancy can be treated by surgery and radiation. Because the lesion is superficial, removal is the treatment of choice; however, if the patient is in the third or fourth decade of life, such ablative surgery should be avoided unless the vagina is reconstituted. The latter can be accomplished by immediate covering of the denuded vaginal cavity by skin graft (McIndoe procedure). This procedure has been performed successfully in six consecutive cases in our clinic. Recently the use of local chemotherapeutic agents (topical 5-fluorouracil) has provided a successful and more conservative approach to such lesions. The advantage of 5-fluorouracil is that it "seeks out" the abnormally metabolizing areas. Laser therapy has been used successfully for isolated foci of neoplasia. The keratinized tumor and those previously treated with irradiation or other scarifying procedures do not seem to respond as well to the local chemotherapeutic agents as the more classic epidermoid variety.

INVASIVE EPIDERMOID CARCINOMA

This type of cancer is the most common invasive neoplasm of the vagina. Approximately two thirds of all patients are over the age of 50 years. The common symptom is a bloody vaginal discharge and in many series total vaginal prolapse has been an associated finding (Fig. 55-28). In the more extensive cases, urgency and pain on urination and defecation occur. Diagnosis is confirmed by biopsy. Differential diagnosis lies between primary and secondary malignancy, adenosis, endometriosis, and chronic proliferative inflammatory processes.

Radiotherapy is the most widely accepted treatment for invasive cancer. Intravaginal application of radium or a similar agent plus external radiation are combined as for cervical malignancy, but complications, particularly rectal and vesical, are more common. The use of radium needles has been reported to be effective but should be the option of the radiotherapist in consultation with the clinician.

When invasive carcinoma involves the lower third of the vagina, the nodes involved are more commonly those of cancer of the vulva (Fig. 55-29). Conversely, if the lesion is in the upper vagina, the lymphatic pathways are similar to those of the cervix. If inguinal nodes are involved, management is usually the same as that for cancer of the vulva, that is, radical surgery. Exenterative procedures may be necessary because of frequent involvement of the rectum, bladder, or urethra, or of all three structures. Treatment should be continued indefinitely.

ADENOCARCINOMA

Primary adenocarcinoma is rare. As noted earlier, interest in recent years has been concentrated on that variety of adenocarcinoma arising in adenosis and developing

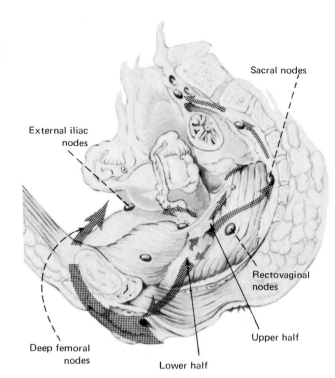

FIG. 55-29.   Lymphatic spread of carcinoma of vagina. Extension of cancer of upper half of vagina is similar to that of carcinoma of cervix, while cancer in lower half spreads like vulvar cancer. (From Traut HF, Benson RC: Cancer of the Female Genital Tract, 2nd ed. New York, American Cancer Society, 1957)

most commonly in the young woman (aged 7 to 27 years) whose mother received nonsteroidal estrogen therapy during pregnancy. These malignancies are difficult to diagnose in the early stages because of the infrequency with which the cells are shed from the deeper glandular elements. Colposcopy has not been able to determine the early malignant alterations. In view of the rarity of malignant change in such cases (400 cases from a countrywide survey now reside in the registry), it seems that the wisest approach to the patient at risk is careful observance with routine examinations and multiple cytologic and colposcopic studies (Figs. 55-13, 55-30).

If malignancy does arise in the context of adenosis, the treatment most commonly advocated has been surgery. Unfortunately, the latter involves removal of much of the vagina, the uterus, and pelvic lymph nodes. If extension to the bladder or rectum is present, even more extensive surgery is necessary. Radiation has been used in a few cases, with reportedly good results. Nevertheless, with only relatively few cases upon which to base judgment, it is difficult, at present, to establish the ideal form of treatment. Preventive measures have been instituted, consisting mainly of the elimination of estrogen therapy to the pregnant woman. Currently, five-year sur-

FIG. 55-28.   Invasive carcinoma of vagina with total prolapse.

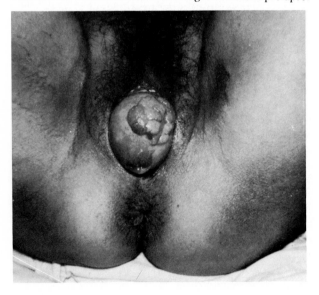

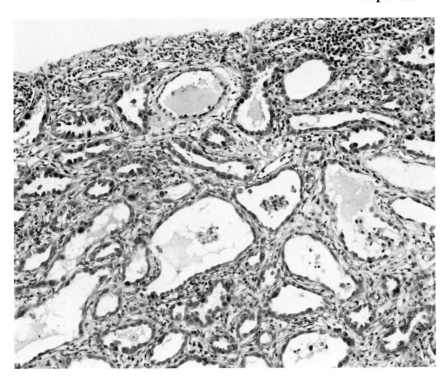

FIG. 55-30. Classic mesonephroid carcinoma in vaginal adenosis of 17-year-old girl. Note hobnail pattern.

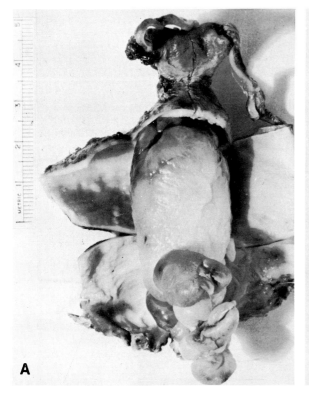

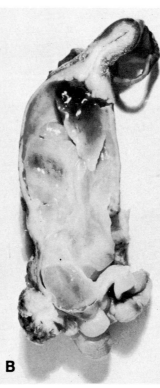

FIG. 55-31. Sarcoma botryoides, juvenile form. (*A*) Gross surgical specimen of lesion from 16-month-old infant. Tumor arose in vagina and invaded pelvic tissues. Vagina has been split posteriorly to show uterus and tumor. Patient was not given roentgenotherapy, but was treated with aminopterin, a folic acid antagonist. She was alive and well eight years later. (*B*) Midsagittal section of specimen in *A*. Note lack of involvement of uterus. AFIP Acc. Nos. 218754–693 and 218754–694 (Specimen courtesy of Dr. Sidney Farber). (Hertig AT, Gore H: Tumors of the Female Sex Organs. Part 2. Tumors of the Vulva, Vagina and Uterus. Washington, DC, Armed Forces Institute of Pathology, 1960)

vival is approximately 75%. Finally, in about 30% of the cases, there is no history of hormone ingestion by the mother.

SARCOMA BOTRYOIDES

Although rare, this grapelike polypoid lesion arising from the lower end at the müllerian tubercle is very aggressive, and the number of patients who survive is low. Occurring in the first decade of life (two cases have been reported in the newborn), the initial symptom is a bloody vaginal discharge. The gross appearance is almost unmistakable, although foreign bodies and acuminate warts may simulate the botryoid sarcoma. The microscopic picture is characterized by edematous blebs lined by a thin, stratified epithelium. The loose stroma gives the false impression of benignity; however, the elongated, malignant mesodermal elements that surround the rhabdomyoblast can be discerned by careful study.

Therapy has not been satisfactory; however, recently salvage has improved with the use of exenterative surgery (Fig. 55-31), a loathsome procedure in these young children. Chemotherapy may be a hope for the future.

OTHER PRIMARY MALIGNANCIES

Fibro- and leiomyosarcomas are rare primary malignancies of the vagina, as is the malignant melanoma, although all such lesions have been reported. Prognosis depends upon the extent of the lesion at the time of initial therapy. It should be noted that most of the fibro–leiomyosarcomas in young people are locally aggressive and recurring, but rarely metastasize. The converse is true for the older patient.

Primary endodermal sinus tumors have been reported as primary lesions in the vagina. Fewer than 20 cases have now been reported. The vagina actually represents an area close to the terminal portion of the line in the embryo, and thus it should not be surprising to see germ-cell tumors in this area. It is important to note their presence, because triple chemotherapy has been effective in controlling these tumors in the ovary and

should be instituted for similar lesions in the vagina. Conversely, surgery, as performed for sarcoma botryoides, is certainly not the treatment of choice, and irradiation has been classically unsatisfactory for the similar lesion in the ovary.

SECONDARY MALIGNANCY

Whereas primary neoplasia of the vagina is uncommon, secondary involvement by malignancies arising in the adjacent area is not. Direct extension from the cervix, rectum, or ovary may be found in the areas adjacent to the primary tumor. Metastases from endometrial cancer appear in the subepithelial lymphatics. Uterine choriocarcinoma may involve the vagina as a metastatic or locally invasive lesion.

REFERENCES AND RECOMMENDED READING

Buscema J, Woodruff JD: The significance of the histologic alterations adjacent to invasive vulvar carcinoma. Am J Obstet Gynecol 137:902, 1980

Buscema J, Woodruff JD, Parmley TH et al: Carcinoma in situ of the vulva. Obstet Gynecol 55:225, 1980

Friedrich EG: Reversible vulvar atypia. Obstet Gynecol 39:173, 1972

Friedrich EG: Vulvar Disease. Philadelphia, WB Saunders, 1983

Friedrich E, Kaufman R, Gardner H, Woodruff JD: The vulvar dystrophies, atypias, and carcinomata in situ: An invitational symposium. J Reprod Med Vol. 17, No. 3, September, 1976

Gardner HL, Kaufman RH: Benign Lesions of Vulva and Vagina. Boston, GK Hall & Co, 1982

International Society for the Study of Vulvar Disease: New nomenclature for vulvar disease. Obstet Gynecol 47:122, 1976

Japaze H, Garcia–Bunuel R, Woodruff JD: Primary vulvar neoplasia: A review of in situ and invasive carcinoma, 1935–1972. Obstet Gynecol 49:404, 1977

Kaufman RH, Gardner HL, Brown DJ et al: Vulvar dystrophies: An evaluation. Am J Obstet Gynecol 120:363, 1974

Woodruff, JD: Novak's Obstetric and Gynecologic Pathology, 9th ed. Philadelphia, WB Saunders, 1984

Woodruff JD, Julian CG, Puray T et al: The contemporary challenge of carcinoma in situ of the vulva. Am J Obstet Gynecol 115:677, 1973

Lesions of the Cervix Uteri

James A. Merrill
Saul B. Gusberg
Philip J. DiSaia
Gunter Deppe
Adolf Stafl

56

Benign Lesions

James A. Merrill

The nonmalignant unhealthy cervix is a common entity. In addition to being a source of gynecologic symptomatology, benign lesions have a role as precursors of cervical malignancy and may contribute to infertility and pregnancy wastage. Attention has been focused on the relationship between cervical infection and a variety of disorders. The cervix is readily accessible for diagnosis and therapy.

ACUTE CERVICAL DISEASE

Constantly exposed to trauma and irritation, the cervix is a common site of inflammation. However, identification of clinically significant inflammatory changes is difficult, requiring an understanding of the physiologic and anatomic changes that occur throughout a woman's reproductive life. It may be difficult to differentiate exposed normal columnar epithelium from cervicitis. Infectious inflammation also must be distinguished from reaction to physical and chemical trauma. The cervix may be involved when there is vaginitis.

Acute cervicitis is characterized by edema, erythema, exposed columnar epithelium (ectopy), and mucopurulent (rarely bloody) endocervical discharge. Although acute cervicitis may be the result of use of irritating vaginal medication, use of tampons, cryotherapy, cautery, or surgical trauma, infection is the most common cause. *Chlamydia trachomatis, Neisseria gon-*

orrhoeae and herpes simplex virus (HSV) are the principal recognized pathogens, in descending order of frequency. Indeed, *C. trachomatis* infection has been found in over 50% of women seen with clinically apparent mucopurulent cervicitis. Although patients may complain of discharge, pain, bleeding, or dysuria, many are asymptomatic. Herpes infection, already described for the vulva, may involve the cervix with resultant shallow ulcers. The diagnosis of herpes infection of the cervix, often unsuspected, may be established by routine cervical cytology. Rare infections include *chancroid, tuberculosis, actinomyces,* and *syphilis.*

Mucopurulent cervicitis, which has been given little attention in the past, must be appropriately diagnosed and treated.

CHRONIC CERVICAL DISEASE

Chronic cervicitis and related changes most commonly are reactions to the trauma and minute lacerations associated with parturition. They may also be the result of other trauma or instrumentation, acute infection, or epithelial atrophy associated with estrogen deficiency. Chronic cervicitis is associated with changes in the size, shape, and appearance of the cervix and the cervical os. If one bases the diagnosis on microscopic evidence of inflammation, chronic cervicitis is present in over 90% of parous women.

Clinical Picture

Few symptoms can be considered specific. The most common symptom is a mucopurulent vaginal discharge; pelvic pain, backache, and dyspareunia are uncommon.

Genital spotting or bleeding after douching or intercourse suggests cervical disease. However, although this may be a symptom of cervicitis, it is more common with malignant than benign disease. Infertility is also sometimes attributed to cervical factors.

Visible and palpatory findings are more reliable than symptoms and serve as the primary basis for diagnosis. The cervix may be hypertrophied and there may be single, bilateral, or multiple lacerations. A tenacious mucopurulent discharge is often seen exuding from the endocervical canal. There may be red areas about the os, occasionally denuded of squamous epithelium. This so-called erosion assumes various sizes and shapes but tends to be irregular. Nabothian cysts, which result from mucous distention of endocervical glands or clefts, appear as blue, slightly raised 1-mm to 3-mm nodules on the surface of the cervix. Healed cervical lacerations often expose portions of the endocervical canal, producing a granular red area termed *eversion. Erosion, eversion,* and *ectropion* commonly refer to lesions of the exocervix covered by columnar epithelium. Exposed endocervical epithelium frequently exists during pregnancy and in women using oral steroid contraception.

Chronic cervical disease may cause tenderness of the cervix or adjacent parametrium. Microscopic examination of the endocervical mucus aids diagnosis. Normal mucus is essentially free of leukocytes; in the presence of cervicitis, leukocytes are abundant. It is important to emphasize that all of these findings often are present without producing symptoms.

Pathology

Polymorphonuclear or mononuclear leukocytes are collected in the cervical stroma beneath the squamous epithelium and adjacent to endocervical glands. The endocervix may be thrown up into papillary folds, the tips of which are densely infiltrated with leukocytes. There is proliferation of young capillaries, and the surface epithelium is absent in erosion (Fig. 56-1). With eversion, the endocervical columnar epithelium extends onto the portio.

As a result of inflammation or hormonal variation, the columnar epithelium of the endocervix may be replaced by stratified squamous epithelium, and endocervical glands may become filled with squamous cells. This process is called *epidermidalization, squamous metaplasia, prosoplasia,* and *reserve-cell hyperplasia. Epidermidalization* refers to the upward growth of squamous epithelium replacing the columnar epithelium. *Squamous metaplasia* implies an *in situ* differentiation of columnar cells into squamous cells (Fig. 56-2), resulting in stratified epithelium with superficial columnar cells and basal cells of squamous appearance. *Reserve-cell hyperplasia* or *prosoplasia* implies growth of cuboidal subcolumnar cells at the squamocolumnar junction that retain the bipotential of differentiation into either columnar or squamous cells. Thus, there is con-

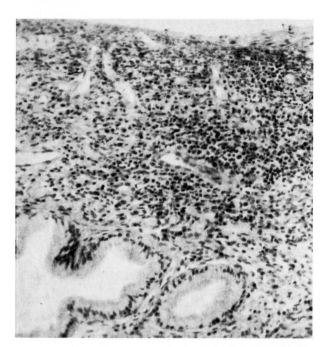

FIG. 56-1. Cervical erosion. Surface squamous epithelium is absent, and the stroma is densely infiltrated with inflammatory cells.

stant but irregular regression of the squamocolumnar junction toward the cervical os throughout early adult life. The area between the original and the new squamocolumnar junction is known as the *transformation zone,* which may contain islands of metaplastic epithelium. The so-called reserve cells can be identified in the infant cervix and remain throughout adult life. Some authors have suggested that these cells are important in the histogenesis of cancer of the cervix.

A less common pathologic finding is *adenomatous hyperplasia,* an accumulation of closely packed endocervical glands lined by cuboidal epithelium rather than by the typical columnar cells. This lesion, which also involves the subcolumnar reserve cells, has been observed in patients taking oral steroid contraceptives. Because of the apparent immaturity of the glands in this situation, the lesion may be mistaken for adenocarcinoma.

Papovirus infection is associated with morphologic changes referred to as *koilocytotic atypia;* these changes are described in the section on Condylomata Acuminata.

Relation to Cancer

There is evidence suggesting some possible relation between benign cervical disease and subsequent malignancy. Seroimmunologic studies have suggested a relation between HSV infection and cervical cancer. However, there is inadequate evidence to establish HSV as

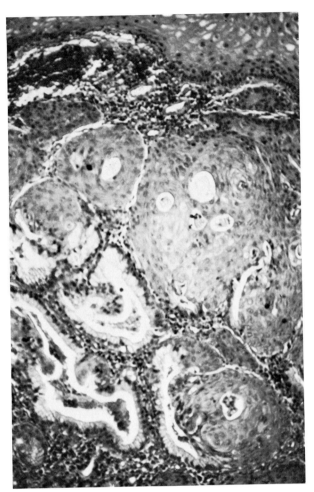

FIG. 56-2. Squamous metaplasia of endocervical glands. Some glands are completely filled with squamous cells; in others, transition from columnar to squamous cells is apparent.

a primary carcinogen for cervical cancer. The presence of human papillomavirus in invasive cancer of the cervix and related studies of precursor lesions suggest the possibility that papillomavirus infection may be causally related to carcinoma of the cervix. Chlamydial infection also has been associated with malignant and premalignant lesions of the cervix, although there are reasons for this association other than carcinogenesis. Carcinoma of the cervix is uncommon in patients who have not been long exposed to chronic inflammation or irritation or who have received adequate treatment for nonmalignant lesions. This all suggests the importance of diagnosis and adequate treatment of nonmalignant lesions.

Treatment

What and how to treat is in some measure a matter of philosophy. It is agreed that a patient with symptoms thought to be caused by an unhealthy cervix should be treated. Because evidence suggests a relationship between benign cervical disease and subsequent malignancy, many physicians extend the policy of treatment to include the patient with an unhealthy cervix not causing symptoms and continue treatment until the portio is entirely covered with intact squamous epithelium.

Logically, the treatment of chronic cervical disease should begin with prevention. Careful management of the obstetric patient, prompt attention to cervical injuries at delivery, careful postpartum treatment of the cervix, and adequate treatment of cervical infections reduce the incidence of chronic cervicitis. Traditional times at which to treat the cervix are during postpartum follow-up and family planning visits. Adequate measures must be taken to exclude malignant disease. Cervical cytology and careful inspection of the cervix, often including application of iodine (the Schiller test), colposcopy, and biopsy of abnormal areas should be done at the first examination.

We prefer to begin with simple treatment and progress, as needed, to more vigorous forms of therapy. Frequently the diagnostic measures (cervical biopsy) in themselves stimulate adequate healing. During pregnancy and in the puerperium, the use of acid douches or jellies may be all that is necessary, since lesions that appear at this time often heal by physiologic repair mechanisms. Use of antibiotics should be limited to the treatment of specific isolated pathogens. If cervical disease is coincident with postmenopausal atrophic vaginal changes, topical or systemic administration of estrogen is important.

Over the years, numerous methods have been utilized to destroy abnormal cervical epithelium and promote growth of healthy epithelium. These have included chemical cauterization, electrocauterization, cryotheraphy, and laser therapy. Each has been enthusiastically applied with success. Chemical cauterization has limited value in the treatment of relatively minor chronic cervicitis. Negatol or silver nitrate solution may be applied once or twice weekly; a single application is usually without value. Electrocauterization is accomplished by radial cauterization of the entire surface of the cervix to remove all diseased tissue. Although effective, electrocauterization was replaced by cryotherapy. The latter technique is more technically convenient and better accepted by patients. It is performed as an outpatient procedure without anesthesia or analgesia.

In cryotherapy liquid freon, carbon dioxide gas, or nitrous oxide is used as the refrigerant. A probe is chosen that approximates the anatomic configuration of the cervix. Lateral spread of the ice ball usually begins within 10 to 15 seconds after the refrigerant has been circulated. It is important to make certain that the ice extends at least 4 mm to 5 mm onto normal-appearing epithelium. Some recommend only a freeze–thaw cycle; others freeze, partially thaw, and then refreeze. A profuse, watery discharge is common for four to six weeks following cryotherapy. The carbon dioxide laser is the most current method of treating the unhealthy cervix. This has the advantage of precisely vaporizing abnormal epithelium, carefully monitored by colposcopy, and is easily accomplished in an outpatient setting. Laser therapy is more costly than the other methods mentioned above.

ALTERED EPITHELIUM

Congenital erosion is a misnomer for a physiologic process that appears as a symmetric, red, velvety area surrounding the os. The surface may be slightly elevated, in contrast to the shallow depression of the acquired erosion. This condition, common in babies and children, consists of areas of columnar epithelium extending from the cervical canal, over the external os, and onto the portio. Most of these lesions resolve spontaneously. However, a few remain into adult life and result in a clear mucous discharge or become secondarily infected and produce a mucopurulent discharge. The lesion may be encountered at the time of premarital examination. Treatment is seldom necessary but could include cryotherapy.

Adenosis describes proliferation of endocervical columnar epithelium in the vagina. These lesions, which are probably of müllerian duct origin, appear as small, slightly raised, red foci. Islands of columnar epithelium are commonly found beneath the lining squamous epithelium of the vagina. Similar lesions may be seen in the portio vaginalis of the cervix. More often, the lesions are seen as extensions of the endocervical mucosa onto all or most of the portio vaginalis, producing a pseudopolyp within a hood or collar-like structure (see Fig. 55-14). Thus, there is similarity to so-called congenital erosions. Adenosis in young women is linked to prenatal exposure to diethylstilbestrol (DES) or similar nonsteroidal estrogens. Adenosis of the vagina or cervix has been found in as many as 80% of young women so exposed. Clear cell adenocarcinoma may arise in such areas but is extremely rare. Adenosis probably requires no therapy and usually resolves by epidermidalization or squamous metaplasia before the age of 30. Certainly young women with adenosis should be carefully examined at frequent intervals to establish that clear cell carcinoma or squamous atypia is not present. Adenosis of the vagina is discussed in Chapter 55.

Leukoplakia describes one or more white, tenacious patches on the portio vaginalis. These cannot be wiped away. Microscopic examination shows surface keratinization of the squamous epithelium with varying degrees of epithelial hyperplasia. In the cervix, leukoplakia is not considered premalignant; however, there may be associated dysplasia. All white plaques should be adequately biopsied and studied microscopically. Specific treatment is not needed, but the lesion should be followed and biopsied again if progression is evident.

CYSTS

A *nabothian cyst* forms as a result of obstruction of the mouth of an endocervical gland and subsequent distention of the gland with mucus. Such cysts rarely produce symptoms or require treatment. They may be evacuated with the electrocautery at the time of surface cauterization or by cryosurgery.

Endometriosis rarely occurs in the cervix. It produces small, red or blue, slightly raised cysts 1 mm to 2 mm in diameter. They may result from seeding at the time of prior curettage. They are pathologic curiosities and require no treatment unless they produce symptoms.

Cysts arising from *remnants of the mesonephric duct* occur in the lateral aspects of the cervix. They are rare and usually measure less than 2.5 mm in diameter. The diagnosis is based on microscopic examination. The cysts are lined by a low columnar or cuboidal epithelium without intrinsic stroma. Treatment, if necessary, consists of simple excision.

TUMORS

Aside from chronic inflammation, *polyps* are the most common lesions of the cervix, found in women of all ages, but most often during the reproductive years. They are soft, velvety red lesions, usually pedunculated, protruding from the cervical os. Commonly arising from the lower end of the endocervix, they may arise from the portio vaginalis. They vary in size from a few millimeters to rarely more than 2 cm in diameter. The base is usually narrow. Polyps probably develop as the result of inflammatory hyperplasia of endocervical mucosa.

Symptoms are similar to those of chronic cervicitis; the most common is genital bleeding, usually following trauma such as coitus or douching. The diagnosis is made easily by inspection of the cervix. Since many polyps are asymptomatic, genital bleeding should stimulate investigation beyond the polyp for a more significant cause.

Microscopically, the surface is lined by columnar epithelium with areas of ulceration or squamous metaplasia. The stroma frequently is congested and infiltrated by inflammatory cells.

Unless the stalk is large, treatment consists of avulsion of the polyp as an office procedure; however, if the patient has a history of recent abnormal bleeding, she should have endometrial biopsy or curettage. Polyps should be submitted to the laboratory for pathologic examination to exclude coexisting malignancy, although this is uncommon.

Once thought to be uncommon in the cervix, *condylomata acuminata* in their various histologic types are not rare. Condylomata, which are caused by papillomavirus infection, have a reported incidence in England as high as 35 per 100,000 women. More than half the lesions are located on the cervix. This is particularly true of flat condylomata, which are often subclinical. The incidence of condyloma virus isolated from women screened for cervical cancer has been reported at between 1% and 2% in all women, and higher in young women. The florid papillary condyloma is a soft, gray or red, papillary lesion with a broad base (Fig. 56-3).

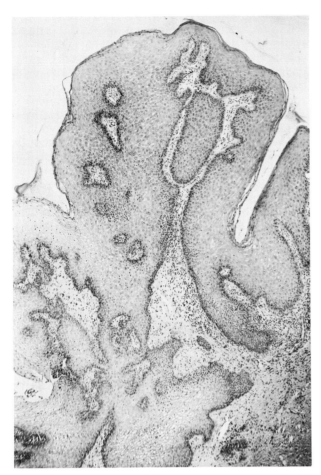

FIG. 56-3. Papillary condyloma. (Kistner RW, Hertig AT: Papillomas of the uterine cervix: Their malignant potentiality. Obstet Gynecol 6:147, 1955)

The three varieties of flat condylomata are usually not visible to the naked eye but appear as white epithelium with or without a "spiked" surface. The surface of condylomata is usually hyperkeratotic, and the surface layers contain many koilocytes—cells with large perinuclear cavitation, irregular edges, and dense cytoplasm in the area surrounding the perinuclear cavity. These lesions may show cytologic atypia, including abnormal mitotic figures. Papillary condylomata have finger-like stalks of fibrous stroma, which may be congested and infiltrated with inflammatory cells. Biopsy may remove a single condyloma. It is recommended that patients with these papillomavirus lesions receive the same careful evaluation and treatment usually afforded women with cervical dysplasia and cervical intraepithelial neoplasia. Conservatism and observation are indicated during pregnancy.

Cervical *myomas* and *fibromas* are rare. They appear as smooth, firm masses of varying sizes, replacing a portion or all of the cervix. Large myomas may distort the bladder and produce pressure symptoms. Such tumors are of most concern during pregnancy, when they may interfere with normal vaginal delivery. If a tumor is pedunculated, it may be removed through the vagina; more commonly, the tumor must be mamanged the same as a uterine myoma.

Hemangioma, lipoma, and *ganglioneuroma* are other rare tumors found in the cervix. Treatment, dependent on size and symptomatology, is usually surgical.

STENOSIS

Stenosis of the cervix may follow chronic cervical infection, treatment for endocervicitis, cauterization or conization of the cervix, cryosurgery, radium therapy, and senile atrophy. Stenosis is usually asymptomatic but may cause abnormal genital bleeding, dysmenorrhea, and infertility. Since stenosis may follow diagnostic conization of the cervix, cervical patency should be ensured by sounding of the cervical canal at postoperative examinations. When the stenosis is complete or almost complete, accumulation of cervical or uterine secretions may cause distention of the uterine cavity and secondary infection. Such distention of the uterus with blood (*hematometra*), fluid (*hydrometra*), or exudate (*pyometra*) may be asymptomatic for long periods or may produce cramping abdominal pain. Differential diagnosis incudes the soft or cystic tumors occurring in the pelvis. Diagnosis is established by initial inability to pass a uterine sound or small probe and subsequent release of fluid when the canal is opened. It may be necessary to sound the cervical canal with the patient under anesthesia. Many gynecologists believe that a gentle attempt to sound the uterine cavity should be a routine part of each pelvic examination. Treatment consists of cervical dilatation and maintenance of patency with a drain.

REFERENCES AND RECOMMENDED READING

Ahern JK, Allen NH: Cervical hemangioma. J Reprod Med 21: 228, 1978

Brunaham RC et al: Mucopurulent cervicitis—The ignored counterpart in women of urethritis in men. N Engl J Med 311:1, 1984

Evans AS, Monaghan JM, Beattie AB: Carbon dioxide laser treatment of cervical warty atypias. Gynecol Oncol 17: 296, 1984

Farrar HK Jr., Nedoss BR: Benign tumors of the uterine cervix. Am J Obstet Gynecol 81:124, 1961

Ferenczy A: Anatomy and histology of the cervix. In Blaustein A (ed): Pathology of the Female Genital Tract. Berlin, Springer-Verlag, 1982

Fluhmann CF: The Cervix Uteri and Its Diseases. Philadelphia, WB Saunders, 1961

Fluhmann CF: Histogenesis of acquired erosions of the cervix uteri. Am J Obstet Gynecol 82:970, 1961

Gardner HL: Cervical endometriosis, a lesion of increasing importance. Am J Obstet Gynecol 84:170, 1962

Hellman LM: Changes in cervical epithelium during pregnancy. Prog Gynecol 3:433, 1957

Henderson PH, Buck CE: Cervical leukoplakia. Am J Obstet Gynecol 82:887, 1961

Herbst AL, Bern HA (eds): Developmental Effects of Diethylstilbestrol (DES) in Pregnancy. New York, Thieme-Stratton, 1981

Huffman JW: Mesonephric remnants in the cervix. Am J Obstet Gynecol 56:23, 1948

Kyriakos M, Kempson RL, Konikov NF: A clinical and pathologic study of endocervical lesions associated with oral contraceptives. Cancer 22:99, 1968

Meisels A, Morin C, Cassas-Cordoro C: Human papilloma virus infection of the uterine cervix. Int J Gynecol Pathol 1:75, 1982

Melody GF: Obstructed cervix: A study of 100 patients. Obstet Gynecol 10:190, 1957

Okagaki T et al: Identification of human papilloma virus DNA in cervical and vaginal intraepithelial neoplasia with molecularly cloned virus-specific DNA probes. Int J Gynecol Pathol 2:153, 1983

Zuna RE: Association of condylomas with intraepithelial and microinvasive cervical neoplasia. Histopathology of conization and hysterectomy specimens. Int J Gynecol Pathol 2:364, 1984

Malignant Lesions of the Cervix Uteri

Saul B. Gusberg
Philip J. DiSaia
Gunter Deppe

The unique accessibility of the cervix uteri to cell and tissue study and to direct physical examination has permitted the intensive investigation of incipient uterine cancer and has enabled us to learn a great deal about the histogenesis of cervical and endometrial cancer. While this knowledge is as yet incomplete, it has taught us that most of these tumors have a gradual, rather than explosive, onset and that their precursors may exist in a reversible form that is followed by a stage of surface, or *in situ,* development for some years. While these phases may be asymptomatic, they are detectable by methods now available, and wide use of these techniques undoubtedly has contributed much to the declining incidence rates for invasive cervical cancer noted in the past 30 years. This developmental concept of uterine cancer has convinced many gynecologists that complete control of these diseases will be possible in the foreseeable future; we can expect to eradicate death from uterine cancer by the diagnostic and therapeutic techniques now at our command.

EPIDEMIOLOGY

The epidemiology of cervical neoplasia has been studied in great detail and several studies have shown that the disease is found more often in women of low socioeco-nomic status, women with early age of first coitus, female prostitutes, women having coitus with many partners, and possibly women who are infected with herpesvirus type 2 or the papilloma virus. The occurrence rate of squamous carcinoma of the cervix is very low among Jewish women when compared with non-Jewish women—a ratio of about 1:5. Similarly, carcinoma *in situ* is one-sixth as common in Jewish as in non-Jewish women. In the opposite direction, black women have twice the occurrence rate of invasive carcinoma of the cervix and twice the rate of *in situ* cancer when compared with white women, but poverty has proven more important than race. Possibly both genetic and socio-economic factors are operative. Since squamous cell carcinoma is practically never encountered in virgins, it would appear that the carcinogen, or promoting factor, whatever its nature, is transmitted by coitus and that cervical neoplasia may be a form of venereal disease. The prevalence and incidence of carcinoma *in situ* and preclinical cancer are shown in Figures 56-4 and 56-5.

PRECURSORS OF SQUAMOUS CELL CARCINOMA

Those lesions in which the full thickness of the epithelium is composed of undifferentiated neoplastic cells are referred to as *carcinoma in situ* (Fig. 56-6), and the term *dysplasia* is used for all other precancerous disorders of the epithelium which are subdivided into mild, moderate, and severe grades (Fig. 56-7). Because of the lack of sharp divisions, these early forms have been called CIN—*cervical intraepithelial neoplasia*—and are divided into three grades: CIN 1 (mild dysplasia), CIN 2 (moderate dysplasia), and CIN 3 (severe dysplasia and carcinoma *in situ*).

FIG. 56-4. Carcinoma *in situ,* British Columbia, 1955–1980. (Benedet L: Obstet Gynecol 60:540, 1982. Reprinted with permission from The American College of Obstetricians and Gynecologists.)

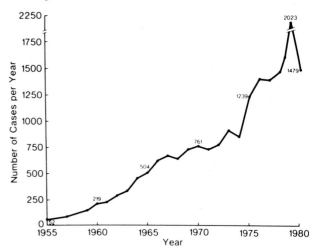

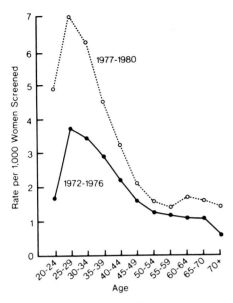

FIG. 56-5. Rates of preclinical carcinoma of the cervix in British Columbia. (Benedet L et al: Obstet Gynecol 60:541, 1982. Reprinted with permission from The American College of Obstetricians and Gynecologists.)

Gross Appearance

In this early period the squamous epithelium that harbors the incipient tumor has no features discernible by the naked eye that distinguish it from normal squamous epithelium. However, the application of Schiller's iodine solution to the portio of the cervix reveals the area involved by cervical intraepithelial neoplasia in 80% of cases (Fig. 56-8). Schiller's iodine stains normal mucosa dark brown by virtue of its reaction with the glycogen

in the cytoplasm of the normal, mature squamous cells. In contrast, the cells in CIN contain less glycogen and fail to stain with the iodine, leaving an unstained region, usually sharply demarcated from the surrounding normal epithelium. The unstained area is referred to as *Schiller-positive.* It is important to emphasize that not all Schiller-positive areas on the portio of the cervix are neoplastic tissue. The majority are benign lesions such as leukoparakeratosis, erosions, or ectropion. Thus, the usefulness of the Schiller test lies not in its diagnostic ability but in its ability to outline the area that must be biopsied. With the increased practice of colposcopy the nonspecific Schiller's test is being used less frequently in the diagnosis of cervical neoplasia.

CIN is usually found at the junction of the portio squamous epithelium and the columnar mucous epithelium of the endocervix. The fact that the earliest stage of cancer of the cervix is located at the squamocolumnar junction is of great interest theoretically and of great importance practically. This implies that squamous carcinoma of the cervix *usually arises* in the squamous epithelium at this junction between the two different epithelial types. It is noteworthy that the histologic squamocolumnar junction is not always located at the external os of the cervix. In some patients with CIN, the squamocolumnar junction is often located out on the portio, owing to eversion of the endocervix or erosion near the os. This spilling out of columnar mucous epithelium onto the portio places most dysplasia within the direct vision and reach of the gynecologist during vaginal examination. However, occasionally, and especially in older patients, the squamocolumnar junction is above the external os, within the endocervical canal, and cannot be directly visualized. Care must be taken in any biopsy method to sample the squamocolumnar junction regardless of its gross anatomic location.

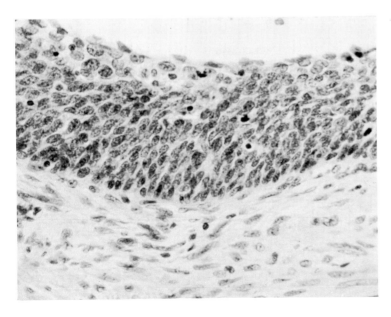

FIG. 56-6. Carcinoma *in situ* of cervix. Spindle-shaped, dark-staining epithelial cells rise to surface layers. (McKay DG, Terjan B, Poschyachinda D, Younge PA, Hertig AT: Obstet Gynecol 13:2, 1959)

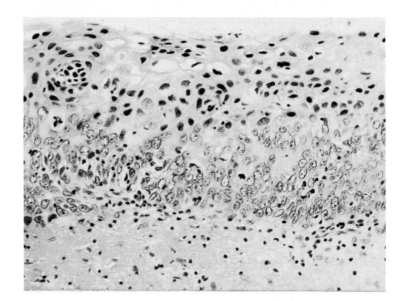

FIG. 56-7. Dysplasia of cervix. This microscopic view shows hyperchromatism and pleomorphism of nuclei of upper half of epithelial layer and evidence of increased growth rate in basal half. This lesion shows CIN 2 (moderate dysplasia). (McKay DG, Terjan B, Poschyachinda D, Younge PA, Hertig AT: Obstet Gynecol 13:2, 1959)

Histologic Characteristics

Since the unaided eye and the Schiller test are inadequate to establish the diagnosis, the identification of CIN depends entirely upon microscopic examination. Three microscopic methods are available for establishing the diagnosis: (1) biopsy with histologic examination, (2) cervical smear with cytologic examination, and (3) colposcopic examination.

Histologic examination is the definitive diagnostic tool. CIN is, in essence, a disturbance of growth, and the cellular changes are predominantly in the nuclei. Nuclear changes are the hallmarks of neoplasia in most tissues of the body.

NUCLEAR PLEOMORPHISM.   The nuclei of all layers of the squamous epithelium are variable in size and shape. Many nuclei are enlarged and vesicular, some are small, and the nuclear membrane is irregular and wrinkled rather than rounded and smooth. The enlargement of the nucleus results in an increase in the nucleocytoplasmic ratio.

HYPERCHROMATISM.   The nuclear material is usually clumped into coarse granules, giving the cell a darker staining quality. Often the nucleus is pyknotic, consisting of one dense ball of DNA in which no nuclear details can be discerned. These pyknotic cells are found in greatest number in the surface layers.

MULTINUCLEATION.   Cells containing two nuclei are abundant in dysplasia. Cells with as many as ten nuclei in a syncytium are common and are essentially tumor giant cells.

MITOSES.   Not only is there an increased number of normal mitoses, but abnormal mitoses are frequent. The latter may have three of four spindles but often take

the form of multiple giant chromosomes scattered irregularly throughout the cytoplasm of the cell. These polyploid mitoses are responsible for the appearance of the multinucleated giant cells. From its point of origin at the squamocolumnar junction CIN spreads out onto the epithelial surfaces. It appears to spread more readily into the endocervix, destroying and replacing the columnar mucous epithelium as it advances. It spreads along the actual lining of the canal, but also grows downward into endocervical glands and may ultimately completely replace the mucous epithelium of the gland (Fig. 56-9). The tumor may spread over a large area and involve many endocervical glands before it invades connective tissue, although the extent varies from patient to patient and some small tumors may invade early. Only the inability to penetrate the basement membrane and to invade the stroma differentiates CIN grade 3 carcinoma *in situ* from an invasive cancer.

OTHER CHANGES.   In addition to the changes in individual cells there are changes in the relations of cells to each other. This is best seen in the basal layer, which shows a disturbance in polarity, with cells growing haphazardly in every direction instead of having the normal palisaded arrangement. Also, the basal layer, instead of being one cell thick, is usually several cells thick; this change is referred to as *basal cell hyperplasia.* Another abnormality in CIN is the appearance of cornification at the epithelial surface. There may be a thick layer of anuclear cells or a persistence of pyknotic nuclei in cornified cells. This hyperkeratosis and parakeratosis led to the term *dyskeratosis* as a synonym for this condition.

Cytologic Characteristics

The Papanicolaou stain of cervical smears is primarily used as a screening test for the detection of neoplasia. Overall, it has a false negative rate of 10% to 30%. How-

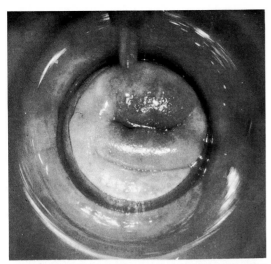

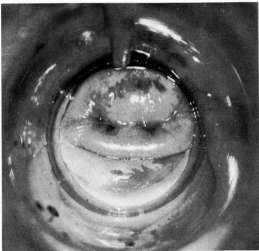

FIG. 56-8. Cervix with cervical intraepithelial neoplasia (CIN). (*Top*) Natural appearance. (*Bottom*) Stained with Schiller's iodine. Neoplastic focus is outlined as geographic, irregular Schiller-positive area.

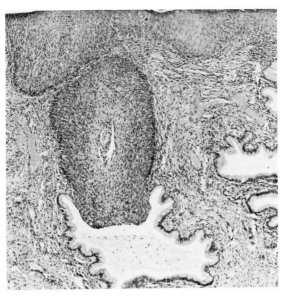

FIG. 56-9. Carcinoma *in situ* of cervix with involvement of endocervical gland.

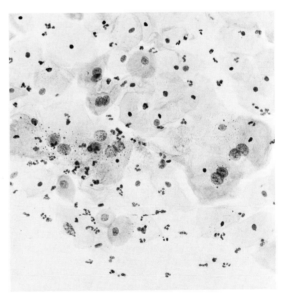

FIG. 56-10. Exfoliated cells from cervical intraepithelial neoplasia (CIN). Neoplastic cells are binucleate, and nuclei are considerably larger than those of surrounding normal squamous cells. (Takeuchi A, McKay DG: Obstet Gynecol 15: 134, 1960)

ever, the false negative rate may approach 50% in invasive disease where the serous and seropurulent effusion of the lesion dilutes the cytologic preparation. CIN can be identified by alterations in the nuclei, such as enlargement and irregularity, hyperchromatism and pyknosis, and multinucleated cells (Fig. 56-10). The subclassification of cervical neoplasia into grades can be accomplished by using a cell-counting technique that is based upon the histologic definition of the stages of cervical intraepithelial neoplasia. It relies on the fact that the greater the degree to which the epithelium is replaced by undifferentiated cells, the more likely such cells are to exfoliate and to be found in the smear. In CIN grade 2, 10% to 20% of the atypical cells are of basal type and in CIN grade 3, 30% or more of the atypical cells are of basal type.

Colposcopic Characteristics

By using a microscope with epiillumination that is capable of magnifying from 6 to 40 times, one can observe the histologic appearance of the surface layers of the epithelium of the cervix in the living patient. The use of the colposcope and interpretation of the findings are discussed later in this chapter.

Development of Invasive Carcinoma from Cervical Intraepithelial Neoplasia

The cervical cancer precursors form a continuum without clearly identifiable subsets. Different grades are often found adjacent to each other, and one stage of the disease seems to merge into the next. Spontaneous regressions in the absence of biopsy or other types of therapy are unusual. The course of cervical intraepithelial neoplasia in individual patients is unpredictable.

Richart followed 557 women ascertained as having dysplasia by three abnormal pap smears using only cytology and colpomicroscopy as diagnostic procedures. He found that the progression rate increases with increasing grade of CIN and that the transit time to carcinoma *in situ* was approximately 85 months for very mild dysplasia, 38 months for moderate dysplasia, 12 months for severe dysplasia, and 44 months for all of the dysplasias combined.

Progression rates to invasive cancer are higher in CIN grade 3 (carcinoma *in situ*) than in earlier states.

The great practical importance of cervical intraepithelial neoplasia is obvious, since recognition at this stage of development permits complete cure of the disease by appropriate treatment.

Invasive carcinoma of the cervix is associated with a high degree of aneuploidy. All grades of CIN may have an aneuploid chromosome distribution pattern and an abnormal nuclear DNA content. These findings support the view that CIN is a preinvasive neoplasm.

Microinvasion

Utilizing the most widely accepted definition of early stromal invasion as "microinvasion"—less than 3 mm depth of invasion from the basement membrane, no vascular or lymphatic space involvement, and no confluent tongues of the invasive process implying bulk disease—one has many options for therapy. The incidence of lymph node involvement or other extrauterine disease in this subset of patients should be less than 1%. With this in mind, simple hysterectomy (after thorough review of a cervical conization specimen) appears to be adequate therapy for most patients. Indeed, many clinicians feel that conization itself may be sufficient therapy in most patients, especially in pregnancy, where further therapy precipitates many other decisions relative to the fetus and mother.

INVASIVE CARCINOMA

The neoplastic process becomes potentially dangerous to the patient only when the tumor breaks from its intraepithelial confines and invades the stroma of the cervix. Early invasion occurs predominantly from *in situ* carcinoma on the portio of the cervix or in endocervical glands. Early invasion may occur from several sites simultaneously. Long strands or cords of tumor cells may extend for relatively long distances in the cervical connective tissue and, here and there, break their way into lymph vessels and venules. It is curious to note that at the point of invasion the cells tend to become well differentiated. In the *in situ* stage, growth is rapid and little or no differentiation occurs, but invasion of stroma is associated with the development of abundant acidophilic cytoplasm, a forerunner of the "epidermoid pearl" so common in well-developed carcinomas. It may be necessary to take many, even serial, sections of a cervix to find one or two foci of early invasion. Patients with true early stromal invasion have survived for a long time with no evidence of recurrence after simple total hysterectomy or even a cone biopsy.

Histologic Characteristics

Squamous cell carcinoma of the cervix makes up 90% to 95% of cervical cancers and can be arbitrarily classified into three basic histologic grades:

GRADE I. Well-differentiated squamous cell carcinoma is composed of sheets and cords of cells with abundant acidophilic cytoplasm, clearly visible intercellular bridges, and often the production of variable amounts of keratin. The formation of the epidermoid pearl is characteristic of these well-differentiated tumors, and relatively few mitoses are found. Grade I tumors constitute about 5% of squamous cell cancers of the cervix.

GRADE II. This is the most common variety and is characterized by masses and cords of spindle-shaped squamous cells with elongated nuclei and scant cytoplasm. There may be a few areas in which the cells have become enlarged and well differentiated to form pearls, but in general there are no intercellular bridges and little keratin formation. Mitoses are frequent (Fig. 56-11); 85% of squamous cell carcinomas are in this category.

GRADE III. Undifferentiated tumors have a rapid growth rate, with numerous mitoses and cells with closely crowded nuclei and scant cytoplasm. These tumors are difficult to recognize as having originated in squamous cells and constitute approximately 10% of cervical squamous cell tumors.

In general, a tumor is diagnosed according to its best-differentiated portion and graded according to the least-differentiated part. Histologic grading has been used for prognosis and prediction of radiation sensitivity of a given tumor. In practice, histologic grading is useful in describing the variants of cervical cancer for purposes of pathologic diagnosis but is less useful than clinical staging in prognosis or in selection of therapy. Lymphatic penetration and attraction of a collar of lymphocytes can serve as indices of tumor virulence.

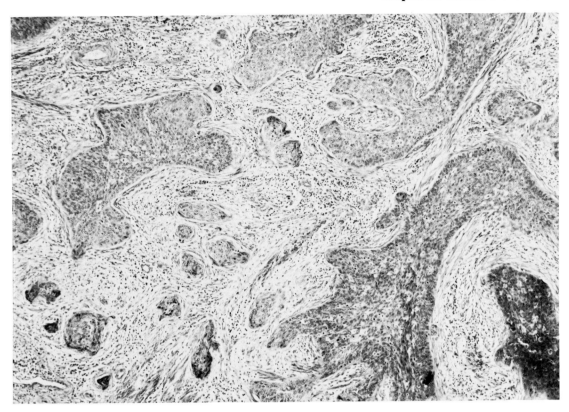

FIG. 56-11. Grade-II invasive squamous cell carcinoma of cervix.

Gross Appearance

As the neoplasm invades, it expands locally and grows out onto the portio and into the stroma of the endocervix. Growth may be predominantly in one of three directions. Exophytic tumors are more common (64%) than the endophytic or ulcerative lesion. A friable, granular, red and yellow fungating mass centering on the external os or causing destruction of the entire portio is characteristic. The lesion may be ulcerated and covered with a patchy necrotic surface, or it may have a purulent, sanguineous, or serous exudate. It usually bleeds readily following slight trauma (Fig. 56-12). Endophytic tumors may be very deceptive on vaginal examination and present only an enlargement of the cervix with no ulceration or apparent damage to the portio epithelium. Lesions confined to the uterus are classified as stage I.

Spread of Tumor Beyond the Cervix

Possible sites of direct extension of cervical cancer to adjoining organs or regional nodes are shown in Figure 56-13.

VAGINAL EXTENSION. The friable fungating tumor may spread outward onto the fornices and down the vaginal wall. If this is the only location in which the tumor has grown beyond the cervix and it does not involve the lower third of the vagina, it corresponds to stage IIA of the international classification.

LATERAL EXTENSION. Extension into one or both cardinal ligaments is frequent. If one or both cardinal ligaments are involved and yet the tumor does not extend to the lateral wall of the pelvis, the tumor corresponds to Stage IIB.

ENDOMETRIAL EXTENSION. Direct growth upward into the endometrial cavity occurs, but is not common.

LYMPHATIC SPREAD. Lymphatic vessels are invaded even by early tumors. The tumor tends to accommodate itself to the lumen of the lymph channel and propagate along it by direct extension. Tiny fragments of the tumor break off and lodge in the next lymph node, where they die or continue to grow and destroy the lymph node. Tumor emboli are then cast off to the lymph node lying next in the lymphatic chain or, in the case of obstruction to the flow of lymph in the first node, retrograde metastases occur. Although there is considerable variation from one case to the next, the most frequently involved nodes are the paracervical, hypogastric, obturator, and external iliac, which are called the primary lymph nodes. The secondary nodes—the sacral, common iliac, aortic,

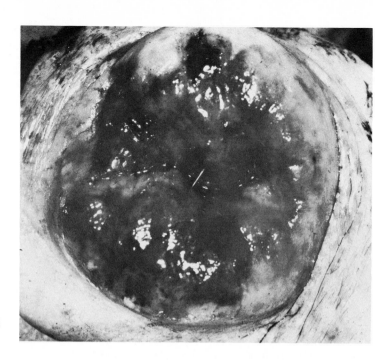

FIG. 56-12. Gross appearance of squamous cell carcinoma of cervix.

and inguinal—are less frequently involved. Lymph node metastases are found in approximately the following incidence: stage I, 15%; stage II, 30%; stage III, 50%; and stage IV, over 60%.

If, at the time of discovery, a tumor extends to the lateral pelvic wall either by continuous involvement of the broad ligaments or by nodular implants on the wall,

FIG. 56-13. Possible sites of direct extension of cervical cancer to adjoining organs or regional nodes.

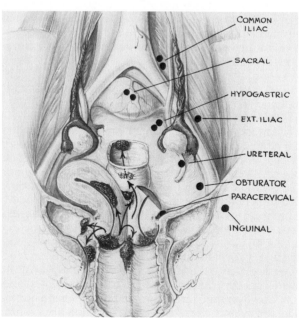

COMMON
ILIAC

SACRAL

HYPOGASTRIC

EXT. ILIAC

URETERAL

OBTURATOR

PARACERVICAL

INGUINAL

it corresponds to stage IIIB of the clinical international classification. A less common variant, corresponding to stage IIIA, is a tumor involving the lower third of the vagina. Ureteral obstruction as manifested by a staging intravenous pyelogram, in and of itself requires a stage III classification.

BLOOD VESSEL INVASION. Blood vessel invasion occurs with lymphatic invasion and may be seen even in early tumors, although it is more extensive in the later stages. Arteries are seldom involved; most blood vessel invasion is into venules or veins. Invasion of blood vessels and lymphatics allows spread to distant parts of the body. Approximately 30% of patients dying of cervical cancer have metastases in the liver, lungs, spleen, and, rarely, other viscera.

When a cervical cancer has spread to distant lymph nodes and to other viscera, it corresponds to stage IVB of the clinical international classification. A tumor is classified as stage IVA when it invades the bladder or rectum, in which case vesicovaginal or rectovaginal fistula may result.

It should be emphasized that the international classification is a clinical preoperative or pretreatment evaluation of the extent of the tumor and may not delineate the actual pathologic or anatomic extent found at the time of surgery or autopsy.

DIAGNOSIS OF CERVICAL CANCER

It is important for us to remember and also to educate our patients about the importance of irregular or noncyclic uterine bleeding, including postcoital spotting, intermenstrual bleeding, and postmenopausal bleeding, since these phenomena may indicate a cervical lesion. The direct transmission of the blood through the vaginal canal to the body surface makes these symptoms apparent to the patient promptly, but we must teach her to consult her physician for diagnostic evaluation. These considerations are of crucial importance in the management of this disease, since the conventional constitutional symptoms of pain and weight loss can make no contribution to the salvation of patients with uterine cancer; these latter symptoms are present in advanced, usually inoperable, disease only.

Preinvasive Phase (Cervical Intraepithelial Neoplasia)

The lesions of cervical intraepithelial neoplasia are asymptomatic. The median age for CIN is about 10 years younger than the age for invasive cancer of the cervix. Since these cell disturbances do not cause ulceration of the cervix, patients do not exhibit abnormal uterine bleeding. In some, the lesion causes enough fragility of the epithelium to result in bleeding on contact, so that an alert patient may note staining after douching, examination, or coitus. Sixty percent of patients with carcinoma *in situ* are completely asymptomatic, and more than one-half of the remainder harbor other pelvic abnormalities probably responsible for the symptoms.

The physical examination is not usually helpful in the diagnosis of carcinoma *in situ,* since there is no characteristic feature of palpation or inspection of the cervix. Intraepithelial carcinoma may be present in a cervix that appears perfectly healthy and epithelialized on speculum examination (Fig. 56-14), or it may be present in an innocent-appearing, so-called erosion or ectropion. In unusual instances one may detect some minimal changes, such as exuberance or florid convexity in an erosion, or a whitish leukoplakic cast to the epithelium, but these are uncommon.

Cell Smear

Faced with the problem of detecting these important lesions in patients who are asymptomatic and in whom no significant changes are detectable on examination, one can understand readily the enormous benefit that accrues from the cytologic study method of Papanicolaou. This method may indeed be responsible for the ultimate control of cervical cancer. Certainly, it outstrips by far any therapeutic advance made in the past three decades. The reasons for its unique significance are:

1. It is a simple clinical test; obtaining the sample is easy for the physician and free of discomfort to the patient.
2. It is applicable to asymptomatic women as a screening measure, since no lesion need be present to sample. It is a general uterine epithelial sample, in a sense.
3. As a stimulus to biopsy it has enabled tissue documentation of the earliest development of cervical cancer.
4. Its detection efficiency of 90% or more permits treatment at a stage when cure is almost certain. Many women already owe their lives to this method.

Taking the sample of uterine secretion is direct and easy but requires several precautions. The smears must be obtained before bimanual vaginal examination or introduction of lubricating jelly, which distorts the morphologic picture. A clean, dry speculum should be introduced into the vagina and samples taken of secretion from the portio of the cervix at the squamocolumnar junction or transformation zone and from the endocervical canal; we prefer to take the first with an Ayre spatula and the second with a pipet or saline-moistened cotton-tipped swab. Since the cervical cancer precursors have been shown to be a continuum, the designation cervical intraepithelial neoplasia (CIN) grades 1, 2, and 3 has increasingly been utilized in cytologic and histologic classifications of cervical cancer precursors.

A classification introduced by Richart is as follows:

Normal or atypical benign
CIN grade 1 (mild dysplasia)
CIN grade 2 (moderate-severe)
CIN grade 3 (severe dysplasia and carcinoma *in situ*)
Invasive squamous cell carcinoma
Adenocarcinoma
Atypical cells present; repeat to rule out
Specimen insufficient for diagnosis

The cytologic screening method has been implemented by mass surveys of adult asymptomatic women

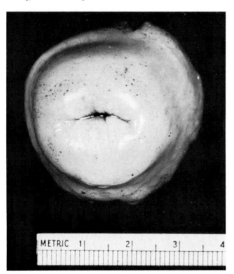

FIG. 56-14. Carcinoma *in situ* in healthy-appearing cervix. Congestion is operative distortion.

in various parts of the country. These surveys show a prevalence rate of 0.3% to 1.6% for cervical cancer, the disparity depending upon the type of population sampled. Since increasing age and lower socioeconomic status, together with some ethnic considerations, are associated with a higher incidence of cervical cancer, these differences in case finding are readily understandable.

Biopsy

Since treatment cannot be instituted solely on the basis of a cytologic specimen, an abnormal smear test result must be followed by a cervical biopsy to establish tissue documentation. Most patients with intraepithelial neoplasia have a cervix that is normal in appearance or harbors an innocent-looking erosion; thus, certain techniques are used to select the locations from which punch biopsies will be taken. The biopsies can be taken as an outpatient procedure (no anesthesia required), utilizing the Schiller iodine staining method or colposcopy to define areas of abnormality. Unfortunately, the columnar epithelium of the erosion so commonly present in the multiparous cervix also fails to take the Schiller stain, so that when that technique is used, the precise area of malignant transformation may be obscured by normal epithelium. Where extensive disease (extending up the endocervical canal and out of vision) is identified colposcopically, a more efficient and definitive tissue sampling is achieved by a circumferential (cone) biopsy that encompasses the entire squamocolumnar junction

FIG. 56-15. Kevokian biopsy instruments characteristic of those used by most centers. Upper instrument is the endocervical curette used to obtain an endocervical curettage. The lower instrument is a sharp alligator-jaws–type used for cervical punch biopsies.

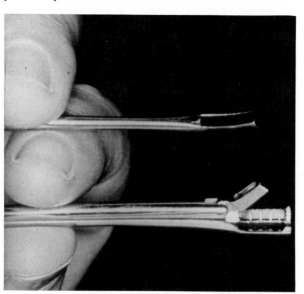

and the lower portion of the cervical canal. Office or outpatient biopsies are performed in many centers utilizing both a cervical biopsy instrument of the alligator type (Fig. 56-15) and an endocervical curette (Fig. 56-15). The physician must obtain at least one biopsy from each area to ensure that an occult invasive lesion is not missed. A very experienced colposcopist, seeing no extension of disease into the endocervical canal, may elect to omit the endocervical curettage, but, in general, this second sample is prudent.

Colposcopy

Colposcopy (described later in this chapter) has gained a firm position as the step between an abnormal result of cell study and final diagnosis. It enables localization of the lesion so that a "directed" biopsy can be obtained. Its use may save the patient the expense of hospitalization and anesthesia if dysplasia only is disclosed, but cone biopsy under anesthesia is generally preferred as the definitive diagnostic procedure if the local biopsy discloses later forms of CIN; in this way invasive carcinoma can be ruled out.

Invasive Phase

Since the patient usually arrives for diagnostic appraisal with a history of abnormal bleeding, one may expect to find an ulcerated or friable lesion on the cervix. Certainly, the presence of a red, raised, friable lesion demands immediate biopsy. No reassurance can be offered such a patient without the completion of diagnostic tests.

Bimanual examination permits an appraisal of cervical infiltration, tumor protrusion, or vaginal extension. Speculum examination allows visual confirmation of this palpation, and rectovaginal examination offers the best appraisal of parametrial infiltration.

Results of cytologic examination are positive except in the unusual massively necrotic lesion whose cell exfoliation is so morphologically disturbed that smear clarity cannot be attained.

Biopsy can be accomplished with a variety of sharp instruments. No anesthetic or other preparation is necessary for such a biopsy and significant bleeding is unusual. Furthermore, there need be no fear of disseminating the cancer, for it is the extruded surface of the tumor that is approached. Precise appraisal of the extent of the lesion is mandatory before staging can be meaningful and therapy properly applied.

CLINICAL STAGING

An international convention of staging permits comparison of results of treatment between institutions and definition of codes of treatment within an institution. *Stage* refers to the clinical extension of disease, *class* to the cytologic smear reading, and *grade* to the differentiation of the tumor by histologic examination.

The staging of cancer of the cervix is a clinical appraisal, preferably confirmed under anesthesia; it is not changed if later findings at surgery or subsequent treatment reveal further advancement of the disease. It is appropriate to consider that stage I lesions may already have microscopic metastases to the pelvic lymph nodes in some instances, but the gross clinical findings alone are used for the stage designation, in accordance with the international classification. The stage designations for cancer of the cervix are diagramed in Figure 56-16.

The revised FIGO classification is as follows:

Stage 0   Carcinoma *in situ,* intraepithelial carcinoma

Stage I   The carcinoma is strictly confined to the cervix (extension to the corpus should be disregarded)

Stage IA   Microinvasive carcinoma (early stromal invasion)

Stage IB   All other cases of stage I; occult cancer should be marked "occ"

Stage II   The carcinoma extends beyond the cervix, but has not extended to the pelvic wall; it involves the vagina, but not as far as the lower third

Stage IIA   No obvious parametrial involvement

Stage IIB   Obvious parametrial involvement

Stage III   The carcinoma has extended to the pelvic wall. On rectal examination, there is no cancer-free space between the tumor and the pelvic wall. The tumor involves the lower third of the vagina. All cases with hydronephrosis or nonfunctioning kidney are included.

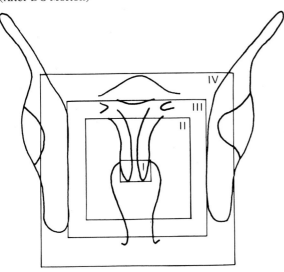

FIG. 56-16. Clinical stages of carcinoma of cervix. (*I*) Cervix only. (*II*) Involvement of parametrium or upper two thirds of vagina. (*III*) Extension to pelvic sidewalls or involvement of lower third of vagina. (*IV*) Extension outside reproductive tract. (After DC Morton)

Stage IIIA   No extension to the pelvic wall

Stage IIIB   Extension to the pelvic wall and/or hydronephrosis or nonfunctioning kidney

Stage IV   The carcinoma has extended beyond the true pelvis or has clinically involved the mucosa of the bladder or rectum. A bullous edema as such does not permit a case to be allotted to stage IV.

Stage IVA   Spread of the growth to adjacent organs

Stage IVB   Spread to distant organs

QUALIFICATIONS IN STAGING CERVICAL CANCER. Stage IA (microinvasive carcinoma) represents those cases of epithelial abnormalities in which histologic evidence of early stromal invasion is definite. The diagnosis is based upon microscopic examination of tissue removed by biopsy, conization, portio amputation, or removal of the uterus. Cases of early stromal invasion should thus be allotted to stage IA.

The remainder of stage I cases should be allotted to stage IB. As a rule, these cases can be diagnosed by routine clinical examination.

Occult cancer is a histologically invasive cancer that cannot be diagnosed by routine clinical examination. As a rule, it is diagnosed on a cone specimen, the amputated portio, or on the removed uterus. Such cancers should be included in stage IB and should be marked "stage IB, occ." Stage I cases can thus be indicated in the following ways:

Stage IA   Carcinoma *in situ* with early stromal invasion diagnosed on tissue removed by biopsy, conization or portio amputation, or on the removed uterus.

Stage IB   Clinically invasive carcinoma confined to the cervix.

Stage IB occ   Histologically invasive carcinoma of the cervix which could not be detected at routine clinical examination but which was diagnosed on a large biopsy, a cone, the amputated portio, or the removed uterus

As a rule, it is impossible to estimate clinically whether a cancer of the cervix has extended to the corpus or not. Extension to the corpus should, therefore, be disregarded.

A patient with a growth fixed to the pelvic wall by a short and indurated but not nodular parametrium should be allotted to stage IIB. It is impossible at clinical examination to decide whether a smooth and indurated parametrium is truly cancerous or only inflammatory. Therefore, the case should be placed in stage III only if the parametrium is nodular on the pelvic wall or if the growth itself extends to the pelvic wall.

The presence of hydronephrosis or nonfunctioning kidney due to stenosis of the ureter by cancer permits a case to be allotted to stage III even if, according to the other findings, the case should be allotted to stage I or stage II.

The presence of bullous edema, as such, should not permit a case to be allotted to stage IV. Ridges and furrows into the bladder wall should be interpreted as signs of submucous involvement of the bladder if they remained fixed to the growth at "palposcopy" (*i.e.,* examination from the vagina or the rectum during cystoscopy). Finding malignant cells in cytologic washings from the urinary bladder requires further examination and a biopsy from the wall of the bladder.

TREATMENT OF CERVICAL CANCER

Preinvasive Phase

The early forms of CIN may be completely removed by biopsy or may be destroyed by cautery, cryosurgery, or laser surgery.

The treatment of cancer *in situ* of the cervix is based on the reproductive requirements of the patient (Fig. 56-17). Surgery is, in general, preferred to radiotherapy, since morbidity is lower, preservation of normal tissues greater, preservation of ovarian function common, and the problem of radiation resistance nonexistent. If the patient is still in her childbearing years, with her family incomplete, and if her equanimity and responsibility permit her to remain under observation, conization of the cervix is recommended. This coning excision of the transformation zone about the histologic external os and lower canal usually causes the cytologic smear to become negative and preserves the competence of the cervix for childbearing.

Cryosurgery has been recommended for the treatment of some cases of cervical dysplasia and carcinoma *in situ*. The main disadvantage of this kind of treatment is the absence of a complete tissue sample for histologic study, as can be obtained in the cone specimen. Cryosurgery should be used only after expert colposcopic evaluation and sampling of the most abnormal lesion by colposcopically directed biopsy. The squamocolumnar junction must be fully visualized, the endocervical curettage must be negative, and there must be no colposcopic, histologic, or cytologic suspicion of invasive cervical cancer. Also, cryosurgery for CIN 3 should be used only in patients who are reliable and agreeable to long-term follow-up. Even with these precautions the physician using cryosurgery to deal with cervical carcinoma *in situ* always takes a calculated risk that the lesion will recur or that an invasive lesion was missed in the preliminary evaluation.

More recently the *carbon dioxide laser beam* has been utilized for the treatment of early cervical neoplasia. This has the advantage of precise destruction of small lesions without destruction of normal tissue. Preliminary results are encouraging, but further study is needed. Tissue sampling must be complete.

The constant surveillance required when such conservative treatment is offered makes it questionable for

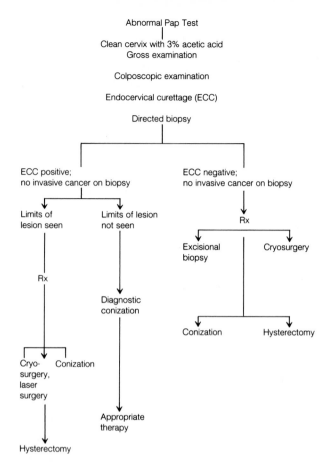

FIG. 56-17. Method of evaluation and management of abnormal cytology. Patients with an abnormal Pap smear are given a colposcopic examination, and areas consistent with dysplasia or more advanced disease must be biopsied and an ECC performed. Further therapy is determined on the basis of these results.

a patient whose family is complete. In such a patient preferred treatment is cervical conization or hysterectomy with preservation of the ovaries as indicated. Although following hysterectomy an individual is also best subjected to regular periodic examination, the cure rate is virtually 100% and vaginal vault recurrences are uncommon.

CARCINOMA *IN SITU* IN PREGNANCY. Routine cytologic smear examinations in pregnant women permit detection of asymptomatic lesions and, occasionally, carcinoma *in situ* in this younger group. When a positive smear is encountered, colposcopy and directed biopsy are indicated if invasive disease is suspected. Here too, the expertise of the colposcopist may influence the degree of sampling. Very experienced colposcopists often are capable of ruling out invasive disease short of any biopsies and follow the patient with repeat cytologic smear until a postpartum evaluation. Patients with all degrees of intraepithelial neoplasia are allowed to continue to term and deliver vaginally. Definitive therapy should be decided upon in the postpartum period after a fresh reevaluation of the patient's status.

Invasive Phase

In considering the principles of treatment of cancer of the cervix, one must remember that clinical staging does not strictly define the limits of the disease. For example, stage I cancer of the cervix is associated with microscopic metastases to lymph nodes in 15% of cases, and that incidence is higher in more advanced stages. This does not vitiate the importance of staging in the management of this disease, but it does underline the importance of treatment to the entire pelvis, including the cervix, parametria, and other support ligaments, as well as the draining lymph nodes.

There are now two excellent modes of treatment for invasive cancer of the cervix, and a brief historical review is necessary to place in context the choice of one modality or the other for the individual patient. Simple total hysterectomy, performed first by Freund in 1878, was quickly found to be ineffectual in the treatment of cervical cancer. In 1895, Ries and Clark, in the United States, and Wertheim, in Vienna, began to perform the radical operation that was intensively studied by Wertheim and came to bear his name.

X-rays also were discovered in 1895 and were applied shortly to all types of external cancer, but it remained for the introduction of the Coolidge tube in 1913 to make radiotherapy constant and reliable. Radium, discovered in 1898, was employed by 1903 for the treatment of cancer of the cervix and by 1920 radiotherapy was well defined by the group headed by Regaud and working at the Curie Institute in Paris. Thereafter, radiotherapy gained widespread popularity, because it appeared to be more efficient than surgery in the cure of cancer of the cervix and had a much lower morbidity and negligible mortality. In the next 25 years this method was considered to be the standard one for the treatment of this disease in most large clinics throughout the world. In only a few centers did radical hysterectomy retain its popularity.

The renaissance of radical hysterectomy in this country was initiated by Meigs of Harvard University in 1944, and in a very short period the procedure was adopted by many clinics throughout the United States. Dissatisfaction had been expressed with the limitations of radiotherapy because (1) some lesions were not radiosensitive, (2) some patients with limited clinical disease already had microscopically disseminated disease in the lymph nodes which was alleged to be radioresistant, (3) radiation injuries were apparent, and (4) gynecologists were, by definition, surgeons rather than radiotherapists and felt more comfortable with surgery.

With the introduction of modern techniques of surgery, modern anesthesiology, antibiotics, and greater understanding of electrolyte balance, it appeared that the enormous morbidity once attendant upon radical hysterectomy could be strikingly reduced.

In the succeeding decade it became apparent that radical hysterectomy in skilled hands was a relatively safe operation. Several other factors, however, introduced a new balance in the consideration of radiotherapy versus surgery: it was demonstrated that the number of radiation-resistant lesions was relatively small, that radiation injury in skilled hands was limited, and that while the mortality from radical surgery was reducible, there seemed to be an irreducible number of injuries attendant upon this operation, especially with respect to ureterovaginal fistula. With increasing confidence that radiotherapy could deal with disease in lymph nodes as well as the primary lesion, even harder decisions were required. During this decade it was apparent that if radical hysterectomy was confined to patients who were relatively young, lean, and in otherwise good health, and was done in a good hospital by a skilled surgical team, an excellent cure rate could be obtained; the place of this operation in the therapeutic armamentarium was clearly established. If radiation therapy was reserved for the remaining patients who were not suitable for operation, it was obvious that these poorer quality patients would have a poorer rate of cure even for same-stage disease. However, when attempts were made to select patients impartially for surgery or radiotherapy, it became evident that without rigid selection in favor of surgery, radiotherapy would attain an equal rate of cure. It was then clear that a choice for the individual patient could be based upon the therapist's experience or training or on the biologic nature of the tumor.

Although the majority of cervical cancers are radiosensitive and radiotherapy is more or less standard today in most clinics, surgery is preferable in an early lesion in a young, otherwise healthy woman, since this form of treatment will leave her tissues in a better state of preservation over the years. In the United States, the choice between radical hysterectomy and radiotherapy (see Chapter 62) applies only to stage I or stage IIA lesions. More advanced stages are best initially approached by radiotherapeutic methods. Where the two options for therapy realistically exist, the patient must be advised as to the method and possible complications of both, and her preference must be heavily weighed. Factors that may influence the decision for radical surgery include, a previous history of PID or inflammatory disease of the bowel, coexistence of early pregnancy, previous pelvic surgery that may have caused small bowel to become adherent and fixed in the radiation field, and relative youth. The decision to advise the radiotherapeutic approach may be based on the patient's advanced age, obesity or serious medical illnesses.

Radical hysterectomy is a difficult operation requiring seasoned surgical judgment in addition to conventional technical skill because it involves removal of the uterus, tubes, ovaries, upper third of the vagina, and all of the parametrium on each side (Figs. 56-18 to 56-20), as well as pelvic lymph node dissection encompassing the four major pelvic lymph node stations: ureteral, obturator, hypogastric, and iliac. The magnitude and complexity of this procedure may be judged by the knowledge that these tissues are bordered and constrained by vital structures such as the bowel, the bladder, the ureters, and the great vessels traversing the pelvis.

Late-stage disease presents the problem of a high percentage of aortic lymph node involvement. The treatment of positive aortic nodes by radiotherapy has been associated in some series with an increase in complications, without a proportionate increase in cure. Ultimate management of this group of patients might necessitate the addition of a systemic treatment such as chemotherapy or immunotherapy. Despite the availability of chemotherapeutic agents for many years, chemotherapy has been minimally tested in the treatment of carcinoma of the cervix. The use of chemotherapeutic agents for patients with cervical cancer initially being treated with extensive surgery with or without radiotherapy is difficult because of decreased pelvic tissue vascularity, decreased renal function due to ureteral in-

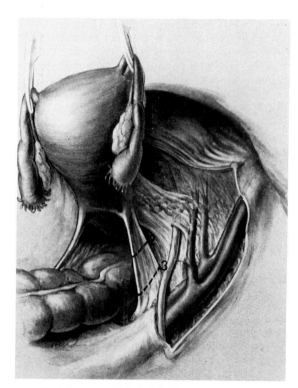

FIG. 56-18. *Broken lines* identify the point of transection of the cardinal ligaments in class-II and -III radical hysterectomy. (Courtesy Gregorio Delgado, M.D., Georgetown University School of Medicine, Washington, DC)

FIG. 56-19. *Broken lines* identify the point of transection of the uterosacral ligaments in class-II and -III radical hysterectomy. (Courtesy Gregorio Delgado, M.D., Georgetown University School of Medicine, Washington, DC)

FIG. 56-20. *Broken lines* illustrate level of vaginal removal in class-II and -III radical hysterectomy. (Courtesy Gregorio Delgado, M.D., Georgetown University School of Medicine, Washington, DC)

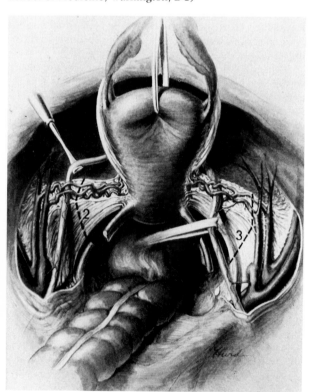

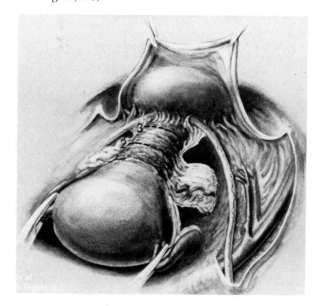

volvement, and compromised bone marrow secondary to previous therapy. A further problem is pelvic scarring, which does not allow adequate measurement of disease and evaluation of response. Recent clinical trials with cisplatinum (II) diamminedichloride show that it is an active drug against squamous cell carcinoma of the cervix and may be beneficial to patients with advanced disease.

In the case of central disease that has failed to respond to radiation, pelvic exenteration may offer the possibility of cure to a patient whose local disease is so massive that it threatens disaster by ureteral compression and uremia, and yet is confined to the pelvis without distant metastases. This massive surgical approach is more applicable to those with so-called *geographic spread*—that is, a more or less local tumor with accidental, so to speak, involvement of bladder and rectum—than to those with the unfortunately more conventional biologic spread by way of lateral parametrial lymphatic permeation to sidewall fixation. Pelvic exenteration, which usually includes removal of the bladder, uterus, and vagina, and sometimes the rectum also, should be reserved for carefully selected patients with true central persistence as confirmed at exploratory laparotomy (Fig. 56-21). Patients must be good candidates

for cure since, because of the morbidity and disability associated with it, use of the procedure as palliation is not justified. Approximately 50% of carefully selected patients can expect to remain free of disease.

The management of cervical cancer in pregnancy introduces special problems, considered in Chapter 29.

PROGNOSIS FOR CERVICAL CANCER

The outlook is highly favorable for patients with early cervical cancer. Indeed, a cure rate of 100% can be expected for stage 0 lesions. Prognosis is less hopeful for more advanced lesions, but with appropriate modern treatment the following cure rates can be expected: stage I, 85%; stage II, 50% to 60%; stage III, 30%; and stage IV, 5% to 10%. Clearly, the earlier the lesion is diagnosed and treated, the better are the prospects for cure.

RECURRENCE PATTERNS AND CAUSES OF DEATH FROM CERVICAL CANCER

Ninety percent of all recurrences in cervical cancer occur within 24 months of therapy. The most frequent sites for a recurrence of this neoplasm are pelvis, periaortic nodes, liver and lung. After therapy, surveillance should include periodic examinations of the pelvis (including Papanicolaou smear), abdomen, and chest. Cervical cancer causes death by uremia, infection, or hemorrhage. Uremia is caused by compression of the ureter by cancer and fibrous tissue, which produces hydronephrosis and pyelonephritis (see Fig. 50-9). This is the most common cause of death, not only in untreated patients with cervical cancer (60%) but in treated patients as well (50%). Infection, the second most common cause of death, may be a local pelvic abscess or may spread to the peritoneum or bloodstream, causing death from bacterial endotoxin shock. Infection is responsible for approximately 40% of deaths. Most of these patients are also suffering from severe inanition. Uncontrollable hemorrhage causes death in approximately 2% to 7% of patients.

FIG. 56-21. Five steps in the evaluation of patients for an exenterative procedure. (Courtesy A. Robert Kagan, M.D., Los Angeles, California)

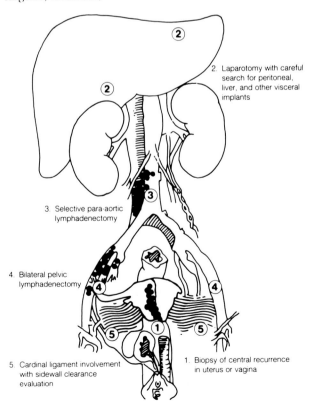

2. Laparotomy with careful search for peritoneal, liver, and other visceral implants

3. Selective para-aortic lymphadenectomy

4. Bilateral pelvic lymphadenectomy

5. Cardinal ligament involvement with sidewall clearance evaluation

1. Biopsy of central recurrence in uterus or vagina

ADENOCARCINOMA

Approximately 5% to 10% of cervical cancers arise from the columnar mucous epithelium lining the endocervical canal and endocervical glands and have the histologic pattern of adenocarcinoma. Grossly, the tumors usually arise within the endocervix and grow in a papillary or ulcerative fashion. Occasionally, they develop into polyps. They tend to grow deep into the cervical stroma before they erode onto the portio and may remain clinically silent until late in the life of the tumor. Growth into the endocervical stroma produces enlargement and often fragility of the cervix. Microscopically, the tumor is usually a mucinous adenocarcinoma as-

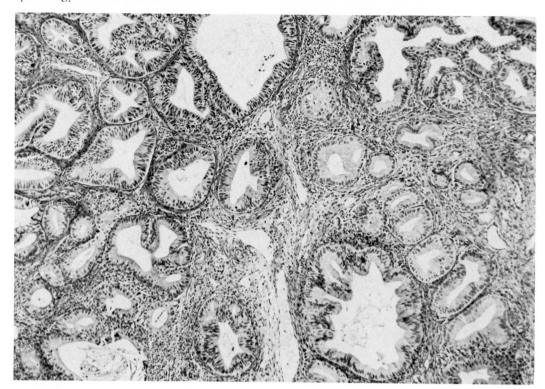

FIG. 56-22. Adenocarcinoma of endocervix.

sociated with papillae and neoplastic glands (Fig. 56-22). As the tumor grows, it becomes less well differentiated and grows in solid sheets of mucin-containing cells with few remnants of its previous glandular architecture. Adenocarcinoma of the cervix has approximately the same prognosis and general clinical behavior as squamous cell carcinoma.

REFERENCES AND RECOMMENDED READING

Abdulhay G, Rich WM, Reynolds J et al: Selective radiation therapy in stage IB uterine cervical carcinoma following radical pelvic surgery. Gynecol Oncol 10(1):84, 1980

Averette HE, Denton RC, Ford JH Jr.: Exploratory celiotomy for surgical staging of cervical cancer. Am J Obstet Gynecol 113:1090, 1972

Baggish MS: High-power density carbon dioxide laser therapy for early cervical neoplasia. Am J Obstet Gynecol 136:117, 1980

Barron BA, Richart RM: A statistical model of the natural history of cervical carcinoma based on a prospective study of 557 cases. J Nat'l Cancer Inst 41:1343, 1968

Bassan JS, Glaser MG: Bony metastasis in carcinoma of the uterine cervix. Clin Radiol 33(6):623, 1982

Berek JS, Castaldo TW, Hacker NF et al: Adenocarcinoma of the uterine cervix. Cancer 48:2734, 1981

Bruckner HW, Cohen CJ, Deppe G et al: Chemotherapy of gynecological tumors with platinum II. J Clin Hematol Oncol 7:619, 1977

Cohen CJ, Deppe G, Castro-Marin CA et al: Treatment of advanced squamous cell carcinoma of the cervix with cisplatinum (II) diamminedichloride (NSC 119875). Am J Obstet Gynecol 130:853, 1978

DiSaia PJ: Surgical aspects of cervical carcinoma. Cancer 48:548, 1981

Fisher HAG, Bonnet AH, Rivard DJ et al: Nonoperative supravesical urinary diversion in obstetrics and gynecology. Gynecol Oncol 14(3):365, 1982

Flint A, Terhart K, Murad TM, Taylor PT: Confirmation of metastases of fine needle aspiration biopsy in patients with gynecologic malignancies. Gynecol Oncol 14(3):382, 1982

Fuller AF, Elliot N, Kosloff C et al: Lymph node metastasis from carcinoma of the cervix, stages IB and IIA: Implications for prognosis and treatment. Gynecol Oncol 13:165, 1982

Gusberg SB: Cancer of the cervix: Cancer in situ and pathogenesis. In Gusberg SB, Frick HC, II (eds): Corscaden's Gynecologic Cancer. Baltimore, Williams & Wilkins, 1978

Gusberg SB: Cancer of the cervix: Diagnosis and principles of treatment. In Gusberg SB, Frick HC, II (eds): Corscaden's Gynecologic Cancer. Baltimore, Williams & Wilkins, 1978

Hinselmann H: Verbesserung der Inspektionsmöglichkeit von Vulva, Vagina und Portio. Munch Med Wochenschr 77:1733, 1925

Kolstad P, Stafl A: Atlas of Colposcopy. Baltimore, University Park Press, 1972

Nelson JH Jr., Macasaet MA, Lu T et al: The incidence and significance of para-aortic lymph node metastases in late invasive carcinoma of the cervix. Am J Obstet Gynecol 118:749, 1974

Piver MS, Rutledge FN, Smith PJ: Five classes of extended hysterectomy of women with cervical cancer. Obstet Gynecol 44:265, 1974

Prempree T, Patanaphan V, Scott R: Radiation management of carcinoma of the cervical stump. Cancer 43:1262, 1979

Richart RM, Barron BA: A follow-up study of patients with cervical dysplasia. Am J Obstet Gynecol 105:386, 1969

Richart RM: Cervical intraepithelial neoplasia: A review. In Sommers SC (ed): Pathology Annual. New York, Appleton-Century Crofts, 1973

Sorbe B, Frankendal BO: Combination chemotherapy in advanced carcinoma of the cervix. Cancer 50:2028, 1982

Symmonds RE, Pratt JH, Webb MJ: Exenterative operations: Experience with 198 patients. Am J Obstet Gynecol 121:907, 1975

Thigpen T, Shingleton H: Phase II trial of cis-Platinum (II) diamminedichloride in treatment of advanced squamous cell carcinoma of the cervix (abstr). Am Soc Clin Oncol 19:332, 1978

Thigpen T, Shingleton H, Homesley H et al: Cis-platinum in the treatment of advanced or recurrent squamous cell carcinoma of the cervix. Cancer 48:899, 1981

Townsend DE, Ostergard DR, Mishell DR Jr. et al: Abnormal Papanicolaou smears: Evaluation by colposcopy, biopsies and endocervical curettage. Am J Obstet Gynecol 108:429, 1970

UICC/American Joint Committee for Cancer Staging: Classification and staging of malignant tumors in the female pelvis. ACOG Technical Bulletin, No. 47, June 1977

Wasserman TH, Carter SK: The integration of chemotherapy into combined modality treatment of solid tumors. VIII. Cervical Cancer. Cancer Treat Rev 4:25, 1977

Wertheim E: Radical abdominal operation in carcinoma of the cervix uteri. Surg Gynecol Obstet 4:1, 1907

Wharton JT, Jones HW, Day TG et al: Preirradiation celiotomy and extended field irradiation for invasive carcinoma of the cervix. Obstet Gynecol 49:333, 1977

Zender J, Baltzer J, Lohe KJ et al: Carcinoma of the cervix. An attempt to individualize treatment: Results of a 20-year cooperative study. Am J Obstet Gynecol 139:752, 1981

Colposcopy

Adolf Stafl

Colposcopy was developed by Hinselmann in 1925, and although it was used extensively in German-speaking countries and in South America, it made relatively little impression in the English-speaking world, except in Australia. The delay in adoption of colposcopy in Great Britain and the United States was due mainly to Hinselmann's highly technical and difficult terminology, most of which originated from visual impressions not necessarily related to the underlying histopathologic processes. The development of diagnostic exfoliative cytology also delayed the introduction of colposcopy in English-speaking countries. Learning how to take an adequate cervical smear is certainly much easier than learning how to use the colposcope. Training in col-

poscopy is time consuming, but without adequate training adequate results are impossible.

Colposcopy and cytology were long considered competitive methods of early cancer detection. The fact is, however, that each method has its particular limitations and strengths in cancer detection and the two methods complement one another. Cytology is a laboratory method of detection; colposcopy is a clinical method. Each deals with a different aspect of neoplasia. Cytology evaluates the morphologic changes in the exfoliated cells; colposcopy evaluates the changes in the terminal vascular network of the cervix that reflect the biochemical and metabolic changes in the tissue.

In recent years colposcopy has attracted a wide interest in the United States and is used by an increasing number of physicians. Its acceptance has been stimulated by new colposcopic terminology, new concepts in the natural history of cervical neoplasia, the change in priorities in the clinical application of colposcopy, and the improvement of training in the method's use.

TECHNIQUE

The colposcope (Fig. 56-23) is basically a stereoscopic microscope by which the cervix can be visualized in bright light at a magnification of 6 to 40 times. The examination technique is rapid, requiring little more time than inspection of the cervix with an unaided eye. After a specimen for cell study has been obtained, the mucus is carefully removed from the cervix by means of a swab

FIG. 56-23. Zeiss colposcope.

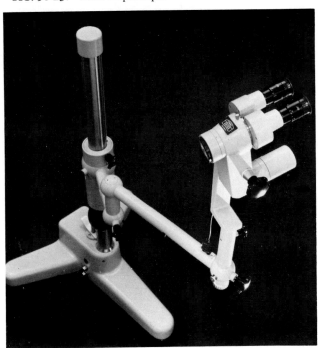

of dry gauze. Cottonwool swabs should be avoided because they leave fibers behind. The colposcope is then focused on the cervix. During inspection the surface of the cervix should be moistened with normal saline; a dry epithelial surface is insufficiently transparent and allows only a poor view of the vascular pattern. In routine colposcopic examination, a magnification of 16 is used. Optimal contrast of the vessels is achieved by insertion of the green filter. After inspection of the saline-moistened cervix, a generous amount of 3% acetic acid is applied to the cervix. The acetic acid helps coagulate the mucus, which can then be easily removed from the clefts and folds of columnar epithelium. After the application of acetic acid, areas of columnar epithelium stand out as typical grapelike structures. At the same time, the acetic acid causes the tissue to swell and the transparency of the tissue is greatly reduced. Metaplastic, dysplastic, and carcinoma *in situ* epithelium assumes a whitish appearance over a fairly well demarcated area. The effect of the acetic acid lasts only a few minutes, but the cervix may again be soaked with acetic acid if further examination is desirable.

TERMINOLOGY

In 1978 during the Third World Congress for Cervical Pathology and Colposcopy in Orlando, Florida, a new colposcopic terminology was adopted. Colposcopic findings are divided into four groups: normal, abnormal, unsatisfactory, and other. These are described below.

Normal Colposcopic Findings

Original Squamous Epithelium

Original squamous epithelium is the smooth, pink featureless epithelium originally established on the cervix and vagina. No remnants of columnar epithelium are identified, such as mucus-secreting epithelium, cleft openings, or nabothian cysts (Fig. 56-24).

FIG. 56-24. Original squamous epithelium. Superficial spiderlike network of capillaries is barely visible. (×16; Kolstad P, Stafl A: Atlas of Colposcopy. Oslo, Universitetsforlaget, 1972)

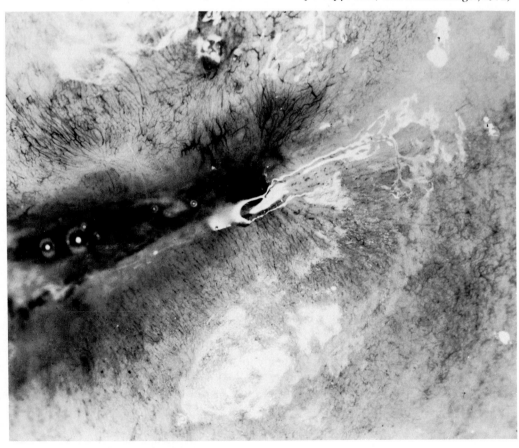

Columnar Epithelium

Columnar epithelium is a single layer of tall, mucus-producing epithelium that extends into the endocervix from the original squamous epithelium or the metaplastic epithelium. The area covered with columnar epithelium has an irregular surface, with long stromal papillae and deep clefts. After application of acetic acid, this epithelium has a typical grapelike structure. Columnar epithelium may be present on the portio or may extend into the vagina (Fig. 56-25).

Transformation Zone

The transformation zone is the area between the original squamous epithelium and the columnar epithelium in which metaplastic epithelium of varying degrees of maturity is identified. Components of a normal transformation zone include islands of columnar epithelium surrounded by metaplastic epithelium, gland openings, and nabothian cysts. In a normal transformation zone, there are no colposcopic findings suggestive of cervical neoplasia (Fig. 56-26).

Abnormal Colposcopic Findings

Atypical Transformation Zone

An atypical transformation zone contains one or more of the following findings, which are suggestive of cervical neoplasia:

1. *White epithelium.* A focal, abnormal colposcopic lesion seen after application of acetic acid. The white epithelium is a transient phenomenon seen in the area of increased nuclear density (Color Plate 56-1).
2. *Punctation.* A focal abnormal colposcopic lesion with a stippled vascular pattern caused by capillary loops in stromal papillae. The vascular changes are sharply demarcated against normal epithelium (Fig. 56-27).
3. *Mosaic.* A focal abnormal colposcopic lesion in which the tissue has a mosaic pattern. The fields of mosaic are separated by reddish borders (Fig. 56-28).
4. *Hyperkeratosis.* A focal colposcopic pattern in which hyperkeratosis or parakeratosis appears as an elevated whitened plaque. This whitened plaque is identified before the application of acetic acid. At times, hyperkeratosis may be identified outside the transformation zone.
5. *Abnormal blood vessels.* A focal abnormal colposcopic pattern in which the blood vessel pattern appears not as punctation, mosaic, or delicately branching vessels, but rather as irregular vessels with abrupt courses appearing as commas, cork-screw capillaries, or spaghetti-like forms running parallel to the surface (Fig. 56-29).

Suspect Frank Invasive Cancer

Suspect frank invasive cancer is colposcopically obvious invasive cancer that is not evident on clinical examination (Fig. 56-30).

Unsatisfactory Colposcopic Findings

The designation of unsatisfactory colposcopic findings is applied when the squamocolumnar junction cannot be visualized.

Other Colposcopic Findings

Other colposcopic findings include the following conditions:

1. *Vaginocervicitis.* In this condition there is a diffuse colposcopic pattern of hyperemia in which the blood vessels appear in a stippled pattern that is similar to the vascular pattern in punctation (Fig. 56-31).
2. *True erosion.* In this condition colposcopic examination reveals an area denuded of epithelium. The condition is usually caused by trauma.
3. *Atrophic epithelium.* Atropic epithelium is an estrogen-deprived squamous epithelium in which the vascular pattern is more readily identified owing to the relative thinness of the overlying squamous epithelium.
4. *Condyloma and papilloma.* These are exophytic lesions that may be inside or outside the transformation zone.

CORRELATION OF COLPOSCOPIC AND HISTOLOGIC FINDINGS

Table 56-1 correlates the colposcopic terminology with the colposcopic appearance and the expected histologic changes. Normal colposcopic findings show, histologically, original cervical epithelium (either squamous or columnar) or metaplastic squamous epithelium. In patients with normal colposcopic findings when the squamocolumnar junction is fully visible, cervical neoplasia should not be present in the tissue.

The most common abnormal colposcopic findings are white epithelium, punctation, and mosaic. Since the pathogenesis of these patterns is similar, combinations of these findings are common. The histologic counterparts of these patterns range from minimal dysplastic changes to carcinoma *in situ*. For prediction of histopathologic changes in directed biopsy, it is not important whether the lesion viewed colposcopically appears as

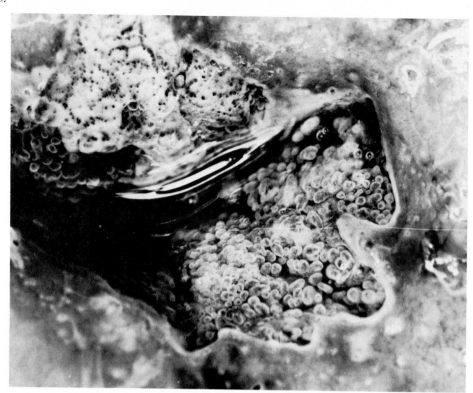

FIG. 56-25.   Normal columnar epithelium. On the posterior lip there is an area covered with columnar epithelium, with typical grapelike structure visible after application of acetic acid. (×16; Kolstad P, Stafl A: Atlas of Colposcopy. Oslo, Universitetsforlaget, 1972)

FIG. 56-26.   Normal transformation zone. Islands of columnar epithelium, tongues of squamous metaplasia, and gland openings are visible. (×25)

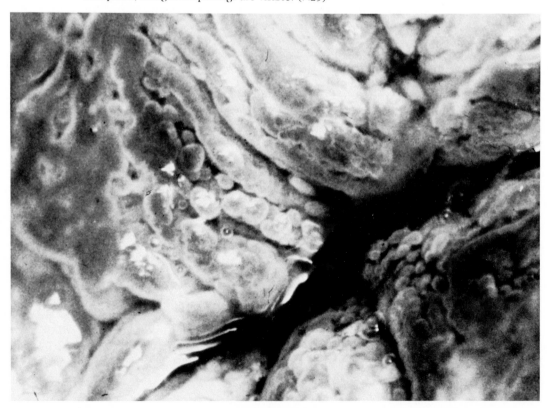

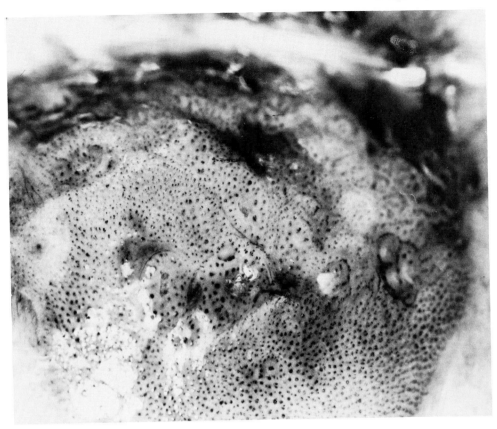

FIG. 56-27. Punctation. Sharply demarcated lesion on posterior lip of cervix with punctation vessels. Biopsy from this area showed carcinoma *in situ* (×16; Kolstad P, Stafl A: Atlas of Colposcopy. Oslo, Universitetsforlaget, 1972)

white epithelium, punctation, or mosaic; however, the histopathologic changes can be predicted by reference to the following easily observable colposcopic features: (1) vascular pattern, (2) intercapillary distance, (3) surface pattern, (4) color tone, and (5) clarity of demarcation.

The *vascular pattern* is one of the most important diagnostic features. Changes in the vascular pattern correspond closely to the degree of histologic changes. It is generally accepted that the first change in carcinogenesis is at the cellular biochemical level and can be detected only by very sophisticated laboratory methods that are not clinically applicable. During the first stage of carcinogenesis, the morphology of the tissue is unaltered. The blood vessels, however, react to these changes in tissue metabolism and cell biochemistry, and such vascular alterations constitute the first morphologic abnormality in the development of cervical neoplasia. These changes are clearly visible through the colposcope but are not detectable in routine histologic sections. For a detailed description of the different patterns of vessels and their diagnostic significance, the reader is referred to the colposcopic literature.

Intercapillary distance refers to the amount of cer-

vical tissue that separates blood vessels. During a colposcopic examination, the intercapillary distance in a colposcopically abnormal lesion can be estimated by comparison with that of the capillaries in the adjacent normal epithelium. In cervical neoplasia, the intercapillary distance increases as the stage of the disease advances.

The colposcope provides a stereoscopic magnification that greatly facilitates the study of the *surface contour,* which can be described as smooth, uneven, granulated, papillomatous, or nodular. Normal squamous epithelium or minimal dysplasia has a smooth surface; carcinoma *in situ* and particularly early invasive cancer have an uneven, slightly elevated surface.

Colposcopic lesions show different *color tones,* varying from white to deep red. The difference between the surface color of the cervix before and after the application of acetic acid is diagnostically significant. When there is a marked change from deep red to white after application of acetic acid, a more severe histologic lesion may be expected (Color Plate 56-2). It is, therefore, very important to examine the cervix colposcopically both before and after application of acetic acid.

An important feature of a colposcopically abnormal

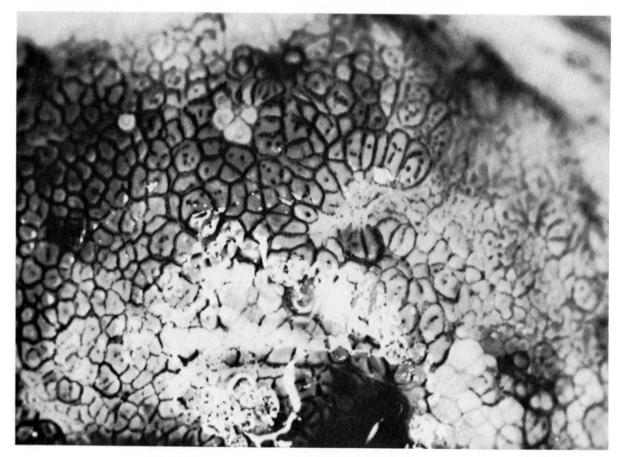

FIG. 56-28. Mosaic pattern. Coarse mosaic with significantly increased intercapillary distance. Biopsy from this area showed carcinoma *in situ*. (×16; Kolstad P, Stafl A: Atlas of Colposcopy. Oslo, Universitetsforlaget, 1972)

lesion is the border between the lesion and the adjacent normal tissue. The borderline between normal squamous epithelium and inflammatory changes or minimal dysplasia is quite diffuse and irregular. Severe dysplasia or carcinoma *in situ* usually produces a lesion with sharp borders that distinctly demarcate it from the adjacent normal epithelium.

CLINICAL APPLICATIONS OF COLPOSCOPY

In recent years clinical use of colposcopy as a screening procedure for cervical cancer has declined, and the method has assumed a more important role in the evaluation of patients with abnormal cell studies. In Europe, colposcopy has been promoted primarily as a cancer-detection technique, placing it in competition with cytologic examination. Each method has its particular lim-

itations and strengths in cervical cancer detection; these are summarized in Table 56-2. Without doubt, cell study is the better method for cervical cancer screening. Cervical smears can be obtained by any trained medical personnel, and their examination can detect lesions in the endocervical canal; moreover, such smears are economical. The limitations of cell study include the fact that inflammation, atrophy, and folic acid deficiency may produce suspicious changes in cell morphology that are not related to cervical neoplasia. Also, the many procedural steps between the patient and the cytopathologist may lead to diagnostic errors. The diagnostic accuracy of cell study has been exaggerated. Reports from the literature show a false-negative rate of 2% to 5%. However, these rates are obtained by the best cytologists under specially controlled research conditions that cannot be reproduced in routine practice. The practical false-negative rate for a study of a single Papanicolaou smear is estimated at 15% to 20%. The true false-negative

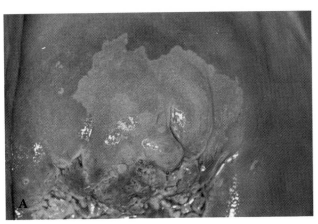 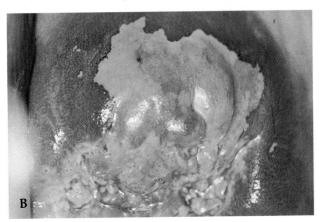

COLOR PLATE 56-1. White epithelium. (*A*) Sharply demarcated area of white epithelium visualized after application of acetic acid. Borders are irregular. Biopsy from this area showed mild dysplasia. In lower portion of picture, normal columnar epithelium is present. (*B*) Same cervix after Schiller test. Neither area covered with white epithelium nor area covered with columnar epithelium takes iodine stain. Thus, the Schiller test cannot distinguish between dysplasia and normal columnar epithelium.

COLOR PLATE 56-2. White epithelium with punctation. (*A*) Cervix before application of acetic acid. Lesion is darker than surrounding normal epithelium and punctation vessels are visible. (*B*) Cervix after application of acetic acid. Note remarkable change in color. Lesion is much whiter than surrounding normal epithelium. Biopsy from this area showed severe dysplasia.

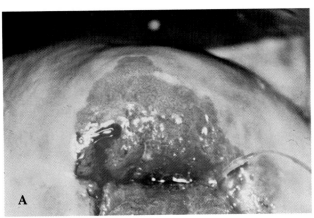 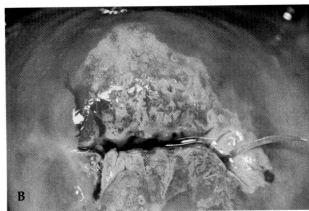

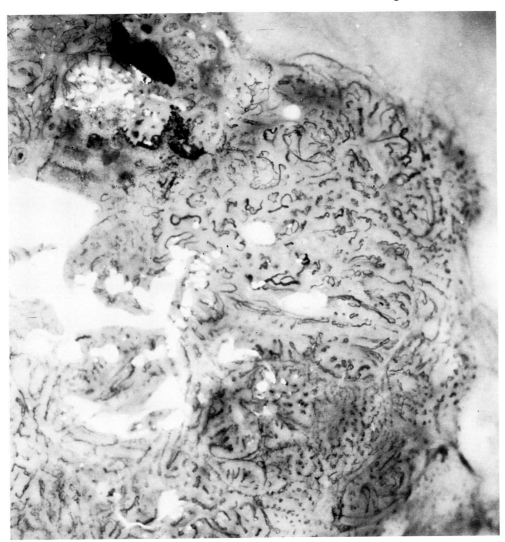

FIG. 56-29. Atypical vessels. Terminal vessels are irregular in size, shape, and arrangement. Biopsy showed microinvasive carcinoma. (×16; Kolstad P, Stafl A: Atlas of Colposcopy. Oslo, Universitetsforlaget, 1972)

rate of cell study is difficult to determine, because a cervix that appears normal and has normal cells is not examined further. Theoretically, the only accurate way of evaluating the false-negative rate of cell study is to perform a cervical conization biopsy in all patients, including those whose cells are normal, and to study the cones in serial sections. For obvious reasons, such an evaluation cannot be done. Any other method is a compromise associated with varying degrees of inaccuracy.

Many studies have compared the accuracy of colposcopy and cell study, and there is general agreement that a combination of the two methods increases the diagnostic accuracy over that of either method separately. Navratil, who simultaneously applied both methods to a series of 55,000 patients, of whom 838 had cervical carcinomas, found that 87% of the neoplastic lesions were diagnosed by cell study and 79% by colposcopy. With the simultaneous use of both methods, 98.8% of lesions were recognized on initial examination.

Although routine colposcopy might detect cervical neoplasia missed through cytologic screening, it is doubtful whether the time and effort involved would justify its use. Even in populations with a relatively high prevalence of cervical neoplasia, it would be necessary to examine 2000 patients by colposcopy to detect a single case of cervical neoplasia missed by cell study. This

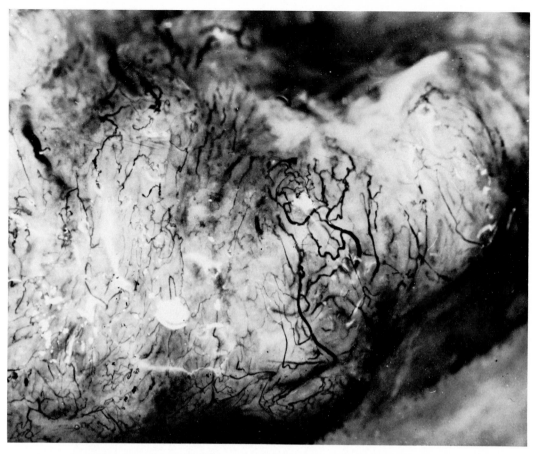

FIG. 56-30.   Suspect frank invasive cancer. Atypical branching and network vessels are compatible with frank invasive cancer. Biopsy confirmed diagnosis. (×16; Kolstad P, Stafl A: Atlas of Colposcopy. Oslo, Universitetsforlaget, 1972)

FIG. 56-31.   Original squamous epithelium with inflammatory changes. Terminal vessels in *Trichomonas* infection may give colposcopic picture resembling punctation; however, capillaries are diffusely distributed over both ectocervix and vaginal wall. (×16; Kolstad P, Stafl A: Atlas of Colposcopy. Oslo, Universitetsforlaget, 1972)

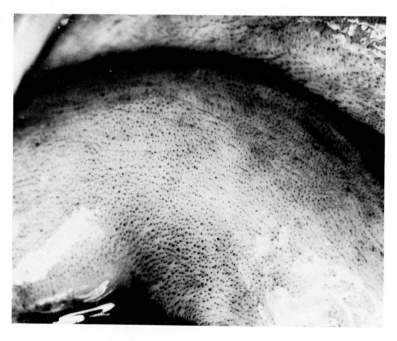

Table 56-1
Correlation of Colposcopic and Histologic Findings

Colposcopic Term	Colposcopic Appearance	Histologic Correlate
Original squamous epithelium	Smooth, pink Indefinitely outlined vessels No change after application of acetic acid	Squamous epithelium
Columnar epithelium	Grapelike structures after application of acetic acid	Columnar epithelium
Transformation zone	Tongues of squamous metaplasia "Gland openings" Nabothian cysts	Metaplastic squamous epithelium
White epithelium	White, sharp-bordered lesion visible only after application of acetic acid No vessels visible	From minimal dysplasia to carcinoma *in situ*
Punctation	Sharp-bordered lesion Red stippling Epithelium whiter after application of acetic acid	From minimal dysplasia to carcinoma *in situ*
Mosaic	Sharp-bordered lesion Mosaic pattern Epithelium whiter after application of acetic acid	From minimal dysplasia to carcinoma *in situ*
Hyperkeratosis	White patch Rough surface Already visible before application of acetic acid	Usually hyperkeratosis or parakeratosis; seldom carcinoma *in situ* or invasive carcinoma
Atypical vessels	Horizontal vessels running parallel to surface Constrictions and dilatations of vessels Atypical branching, winding course	From carcinoma *in situ* to invasive carcinoma

application of colposcopy is, therefore, still questionable, both because it is not economical and because few physicians are trained in the technique. In the future, however, this situation may change. By including colposcopic training in most residency programs or by training paramedical personnel in basic colposcopy, it may be possible to achieve the ideal goal of examining all patients both cytologically and colposcopically. Routine colposcopy requires almost the same amount of time as the visual examination of the cervix and does not significantly prolong the gynecologic examination.

At present, the main value of colposcopy is in the evaluation of patients whose cell studies are abnormal and who are at high risk (owing to intrauterine exposure to diethylstilbestrol or clinical evidence of adenosis). Colposcopy makes it possible to localize the lesion, evaluate its extent, and obtain a directed biopsy from which the histopathologic diagnosis can be established. Colposcopy is very accurate in differentiating invasive from noninvasive lesions and inflammatory atypia from neoplasia. In patients with abnormal cells, colposcopy can immediately differentiate between inflammatory and neoplastic changes. The limitation of colposcopy is its inability to detect a lesion deep in the endocervical canal. However, in this latter situation, results of the colposcopic evaluation are not negative but rather unsatisfactory because the squamocolumnar junction is not visible. Further diagnostic steps are required. The frequency of unsatisfactory colposcopy findings in premenopausal women is 12% to 15%. After menopause, the frequency of unsatisfactory colposcopy rises significantly, so that the value of colposcopy in the evaluation of the cervix of postmenopausal women is somewhat more limited. However, in patients whose squamocolumnar junction is fully visible, the false-negative rate of colposcopy is very low. This was demonstrated by Stafl and Mattingly from the results of the Wisconsin Colposcopy Program, in which the false-negative rate of directed biopsy was 0.3%.

Clinical diagnosis of lesions demonstrated to con-

Table 56-2
*Advantages and Disadvantages of
Colposcopy and Cell Study*

Advantages	Disadvantages
Cell Study	
Ideal for mass screening	Cannot localize lesion
Economical	
Specimen can be obtained by any medical personnel	Inflammation, atrophic changes, folic acid deficiency may produce suspicious changes
Detects lesions in endocervical canal	Many steps between patient and cytopathologist allow misdiagnosis
Detects adenocarcinoma	Value of single smear is limited
Colposcopy	
Localizes lesion	Inadequate for detection of endocervical lesions
Evaluates extent of lesion	Difficult training
Differentiates between inflammatory atypia and neoplasia	
Differentiates between invasive and noninvasive cervical lesions	
Enables follow-up	

tain abnormal cells should be done only by an experienced colposcopist; not every gynecologist should attempt to master the technique. Such an effort is uneconomical and time consuming, and an individual physician is unlikely to see enough candidates for colposcopy to maintain his expertise at a high level. It is more reasonable to train a few physicians in a community or region to whom patients with abnormal cytologic results can be referred for colposcopic consultation.

The increased interest in colposcopy carries the potential danger of unrestricted use and abuse of the technique. Like every diagnostic method, colposcopy has limitations that must be fully recognized. The importance of adequate training and experience cannot be overemphasized. Inexperience can lead to serious mistakes in the diagnosis and management of cervical cancer that might significantly discredit colposcopy. The limitation of colposcopy in the diagnosis of lesions in the endocervical canal should be fully appreciated, and when the squamocolumnar junction is not fully visible, other methods of evaluation (endocervical curetting, conization) must be used. It should also be recognized that although the diagnosis of carcinoma *in situ* is often relatively easy, the proper evaluation of vascular changes

suggesting invasion requires much longer experience. When used intelligently with a thorough understanding of all the morphologic details, colposcopy is an important diagnostic tool, both for clinical practice and research.

REFERENCES AND RECOMMENDED READING

Bolten KA: Practical colposcopy in early cervical and vaginal cancer. Clin Obstet Gynecol 10:808, 1967

Bolten KA, Jacques WE: Introduction to Colposcopy. New York, Grune & Stratton, 1960

Coppleson M, Pixley F, Reid BL: Colposcopy: A Scientific and Practical Approach to the Cervix in Health and Disease. Springfield IL, Charles C Thomas, 1971

Hinselmann H: Verbesserung der Inspektionsmoglichkeit von Vulva, Vagina und Portio. Munch Med Wochenschr 77: 1733, 1925

Kolstad P, Stafl A: Atlas of Colposcopy. Baltimore, University Park Press, 1972

Mestwerdt G, Wespi HJ: Atlas der Kolposkopie, 3rd ed. Stuttgart, Fischer, 1961

Stafl A: Use of the azocoupling method for identification of alkaline phosphatase in study of the capillary network of the cervix uteri. Cesk Morfol 10:336, 1962

Stafl A: The clinical diagnosis of early cervical cancer. Obstet Gynecol Surv 24:976, 1969

Stafl A, Dohnal V, Linhartova A: Uber kolposkopische, histologische und Gefassbefunde an der Krankhaft veranderten Portio. Geburtshilfe Frauenheilkd 23:437, 1963

Stafl A, Friedrich EG Jr., Mattingly RF: Detection of cervical neoplasia: Reducing the risk of error. Clin Obstet Gynecol 16:238, 1973

Stafl A, Linhartova A: Die Umwandlungszone und ihre Genese. Arch Gynaekol 204:228, 1967

Stafl A, Linhartova A, Dohnal V: Das kolposkopische Bild der Felderung und seine Pathogenese. Arch Gynaekol 199:223, 1963

Stafl A, Linhartova A, Dohnal V: Das kolposkopische Bild des Grundes, des papillaren Grundes, der atypischen Umwandlungszone und deren Pathogenese. Arch Gynaekol 204:212, 1967

Stafl A, Mattingly RF: Isoantigens ABO in cervical neoplasia. Gynecol Oncol 1:26, 1972

Stafl A, Mattingly RF: Colposcopic diagnosis of cervical neoplasia. Obstet Gynecol 41:169, 1973

Stafl A, Mattingly RF: Vaginal adenosis: A precancerous lesion? Am J Obstet Gynecol 120:666, 1974

Stafl A, Mattingly RF: Angiogenesis of cervical neoplasia. Am J Obstet Gynecol 121:845, 1975

Stafl A, Mattingly RF, Foley DV, Fetherston WC: Clinical diagnosis of vaginal adenosis. Obstet Gynecol 43:118, 1974

Tredway DR et al: Colposcopy and cryosurgery in cervical intraepithelial neoplasia. Am J Obstet Gynecol 114:1020, 1972

Lesions of the Corpus Uteri

James A. Merrill
William T. Creasman

57

Benign Lesions of the Corpus Uteri

James A. Merrill

BENIGN LESIONS OF THE ENDOMETRIUM

The growth and development of the endometrium reflect accurately the aging process and hormonal changes in women. This is observed best during the phases of the menstrual cycle and in the changes occurring during intrauterine or extrauterine pregnancy. Likewise, the endometrium may reflect abnormal endocrine states and is responsible to the exogenous administration of hormones, occasionally with the production of pathologic conditions.

Irregular Shedding and Ripening

Irregular shedding of the endometrium indicates a specific clinicopathologic syndrome characterized by prolongation of regular cyclic menstrual bleeding, which is often increased in amount. The diagnosis is substantiated by curettage of the uterus done beyond the fifth or sixth day of menstrual flow. Microscopic examination of endometrial curettings shows areas of typical postovulatory menstrual endometrium as well as areas of early proliferative endometrium.

This abnormality of endometrial growth is apparently produced by prolonged or excessive output of progesterone by the corpus luteum. A cystic corpus lu-

teum or a corpus luteum cyst occasionally is associated. Both the clinical symptoms and the endometrial pathology have been produced by administration of progesterone during the premenstrual phase of the cycle. Time and the curettage of the uterus required for diagnosis are usually therapeutic.

A somewhat related condition is referred to as *irregular ripening* of the endometrium. Microscopic examination of endometrium removed during the postovulatory phase of the menstrual cycle reveals a patchy mixture of proliferative and secretory endometrium. Such a diagnosis requires that the histologic changes be observed in the superficial layer of the endometrium. The symptoms and treatment are similar to those of irregular shedding and it is possible that the two conditions are the same.

Endometrial Hyperplasia

Endometrial hyperplasia is a common pathologic finding in patients with excessive, irregular, or prolonged menstruation. It also occurs in patients without symptoms or signs and may cause or accompany postmenopausal bleeding. Progressive changes of endometrial hyperplasia may lead to malignancy. The pathologic physiology is thought to be excessive or continued and unopposed estrogen activity. Estrogen production need not be excessive if it is prolonged and unopposed by progesterone from a corpus luteum. Anovulation is the most common cause of such altered hormone production, although anovulatory cycles are not always associated with endometrial hyperplasia or with abnormal bleeding. Thus, hyperplasia is encountered most commonly at the two extremes of menstrual life, postpuberty and the menopause, since both of these epochs are associated with failure of ovulation. Hyperplasia of the endometrium may also result from excess estrogen production from such sources as functioning ovarian tumors, polycystic ovary disease, and abnormalities of the adrenal cortex and possibly other endocrine glands. Administration of hormones or medications with a hormonally active metabolite may cause hyperplasia; digitalis, for example, is known to result in estrogen activity. A careful history should be taken to exclude all sources of exogenous hormone, especially in menopausal or postmenopausal women. Recently, endometrial hyperplasia has equalled or exceeded carcinoma as a cause of postmenopausal bleeding.

The actual mechanism of uterine bleeding is not clear. In addition to increased volume of tissue, there may be altered vasculature including fibrosis and elastosis of spiral arterioles that may interfere with their contraction. It is apparent, however, that the frequency and extent of the bleeding are not dependent upon the degree of hyperplastic change. Profuse bleeding may occur with minimal hyperplasia.

Pathology

The uterus may be enlarged, but commonly is of normal size. The endometrium may be enormously thickened and polypoid (Fig. 57-1), even to the point of being confused with carcinoma. Endometrial curettings are abundant, soft, and succulent. Friability suggests malignancy, but may occur with hyperplasia. Occasionally the curettings are not abnormal grossly. Endometrial hyperplasia is often associated with endometrial polyps, myomas, and adenomyosis.

The most common type of endometrial hyperplasia is *cystic hyperplasia* (Fig. 57-2). Microscopically, the endometrial glands are dilated, increased in number,

FIG. 57-1. Gross appearance of marked polypoid hyperplasia of endometrium.

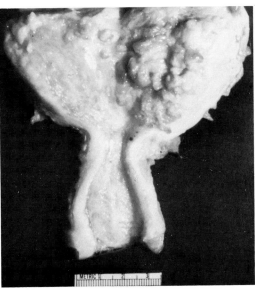

and lined by pseudostratified, regular columnar epithelium, without evidence of secretory activity. The cells are tall, but not atypical.

The degree of cystic dilatation is quite variable. The stroma, consisting of cells with little cytoplasm, is dense and contains focal collections of lymphocytes and thin-walled vascular channels. Mitoses are numerous in the epithelium and stroma. During the bleeding phase, areas of necrosis and thrombi are seen.

Adenomatous hyperplasia, which represents a more active or advanced phase of hyperplasia, is characterized by an abundance of closely packed glands, some of which are cystically dilated, with small outpouchings. An aggregation of "daughter" glands may surround a larger gland, or there may be a cluster of varying-sized glands with little or no intervening stroma (Fig. 57-3). The stromal proliferation is similar to that described for cystic hyperplasia. However, unlike cystic hyperplasia, the epithelium may show cellular irregularities or be stratified, producing papillary projections into the lumina of the glands.

Atypical adenomatous hyperplasia, or *anaplasia,* is a further exaggeration of this with larger cells, rounded vesicular nuclei, abundant pale-staining cytoplasm, and further glandular crowding. It has been suggested that atypical adenomatous hyperplasia be termed "dysplasia."

Cystic endometrial changes occur in postmenopausal women, probably as the result not of estrogen stimulation but of atrophy, with occlusion of gland mouths and accumulation of secretion within the glands. The endometrium is thin, consisting of many thin-walled, dilated glands and scant stroma. Indeed, the stromal cells and epithelial cells show more atrophy than proliferation. We refer to this lesion as *cystic atrophy* instead of including it as one of the hyperplastic lesions of the endometrium.

Progestational hyperplasia refers to the glandular changes that occur in the endometrium in early pregnancy. In the usual nonpregnant menstrual cycle, endometrial glands and stroma show regressive changes commencing about days 21 to 23 of the cycle. If pregnancy occurs during that cycle, regression does not occur and there is continued growth and proliferation. This growth may be so exuberant as to be misinterpreted as a pathologic hyperplasia. Furthermore, occasionally in early pregnancy, atypical glandular cellular changes are observed. These pregnancy changes have been misinterpreted as malignancy, particularly clear cell carcinoma. Such findings are likely to be observed in endometrial curettings obtained from women with abnormal uterine bleeding in whom pregnancy is not suspected. This has been described specifically in patients with ectopic tubal gestation (the Arias–Stella reaction). The atypical changes are entirely physiologic. In a small number of patients receiving high doses of synthetic progestins, atypical stromal changes may be seen. In these endometria, atypical glandular components are not present.

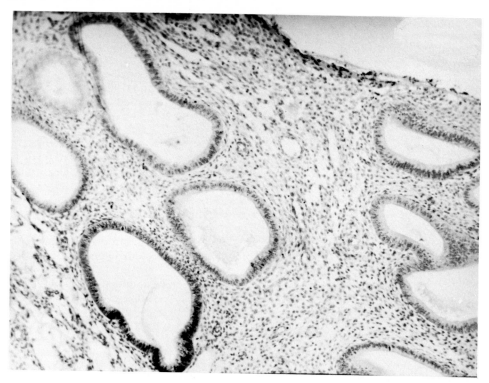

FIG. 57-2. Cystic hyperplasia of endometrium. In addition to glandular changes, stroma contains numerous thin-walled vascular channels, which may partially explain excessive menstrual bleeding in this condition.

FIG. 57-3. Adenomatous hyperplasia of endometrium. Note intraluminal papillary projections and ''daughter'' glands. (Kistner RW: Clin Obstet Gynecol 5:1166, 1962)

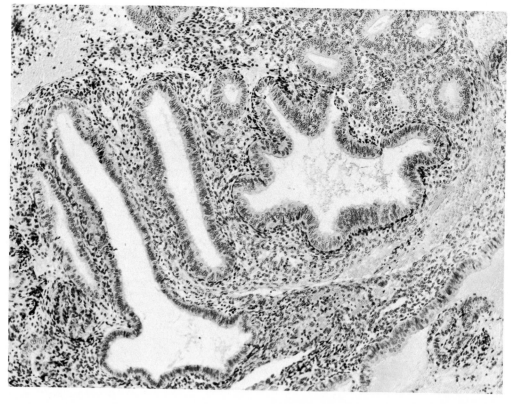

Relation to Cancer

In the majority of cases, the microscopic pattern of hyperplasia is clearly benign. In a few, there is marked proliferative activity and even atypia of cellular detail and growth pattern. In these cases, the interpretation of curettings is not easy and the criteria of malignancy vary considerably among pathologists. The severity of endometrial hyperplasia is often overdiagnosed. Despite alarming conclusions from retrospective studies, prospective studies have revealed progression of endometrial hyperplasia to adenocarcinoma in only 1% to 14% of all cases. However, the neoplastic potential may be greater in postmenopausal women. Regression of the hyperplasia is certainly much more common than progression to neoplasia. The risk of developing adenocarcinoma varies with the morphology, being small with cystic hyperplasia, greater with adenomatous hyperplasia and substantial with atypical hyperplasia. Carcinoma is likely to develop only when hyperplasia has persisted or progressed under observation. In these cases the risk is as high as 40%. The physician should become familiar with the meaning of the diagnostic terms used by the pathologist. The hyperplastic abnormalities go by various terms, and intelligent management of the patient necessitates an awareness of each. As we use the terms, *cystic hyperplasia* and usually *adenomatous hyperplasia* are considered benign. Adenomatous hyperplasia with areas of atypia is viewed with suspicion. However, such lesions may be reversible and should not be considered categorically as premalignant. *Carcinoma in situ* of the endometrium is used by us to indicate the lesion that is probably not reversible. The same lesions may be referred to by other names in other clinics. *The terminology is not important, as long as you know what your pathologist means by it.* Occasional difficulties in the pathologic evaluation of hyperplastic lesions make the gynecologist's decision regarding treatment a difficult one. Cytologic and chemical studies of endometrial hyperplasia have not been consistent enough to offer reliable prognostic significance and are not as helpful as follow-up with repeat endometrial sampling. The relation of cancer to hyperplasia is discussed later in this chapter.

Treatment

Diagnosis is established by endometrial sampling. Traditionally this has been by curettage of the uterus, which results in immediate cure in a substantial number of patients. Some gynecologists are of the opinion that suction endometrial biopsy is an adequate diagnostic procedure for most patients. Expense is minimal and sensitivity and reliability are comparable to results obtained with curettage.

Both initiation of ovulation and progestin therapy correct the pathophysiology of endometrial hyperplasia, effectively and have been successful in causing regression, including adenomatous and atypical hyperplasia. If the patient is receiving exogenous estrogen, this should be discontinued and repeat endometrial sampling should be done after two to four months. Progestin therapy is indicated for adenomatous hyperplasia or atypical hyperplasia. It may not be necessary for cystic hyperplasia but is not harmful. Medroxyprogesterone acetate, 10 mg daily for seven to ten days each month is an appropriate medication. The medication also may be given daily in continuous fashion. In either case, a medication-free interval of approximately four weeks should be allowed before repeat endometrial sampling is done. The advantage of second endometrial sampling after two to four months is that it permits an *active* assessment of the biologic behavior of the process rather than a *static* one, avoids unnecessary hysterectomy, and places the patient at no risk. In those cases in which the process regresses to nonhyperplastic endometrium, further management requires only observation and discontinuation of estrogen therapy. When the hyperplastic process shows evidence of progression, hysterectomy is indicated. If there is no change in the morphologic appearance of the hyperplasia, management should depend on any underlying endocrinopathy and the degree of hyperplasia. Persistent adenomatous hyperplasia may be considered an adequate indication for hysterectomy in the postmenopausal patient.

Endometrial Polyps

Endometrial polyps are sessile or pedunculated projections of the endometrium (Fig. 57-4). They develop as solitary or multiple soft tumors, frequently composed of hyperplastic endometrium. Diffuse endometrial hyperplasia may consist of multiple polypoid projections. The cause of most endometrial polyps is best explained as similar to that of endometrial hyperplasia.

Most polyps are asymptomatic, and it is difficult to determine which symptoms actually are due to endometrial polyps, since they are frequently associated with leiomyomas of the uterus and endometrial hyperplasia.

FIG. 57-4. Endometrial polyp. This polyp has a long pedicle and has protruded through cervical os; as a result, tip of polyp was hemorrhagic and necrotic.

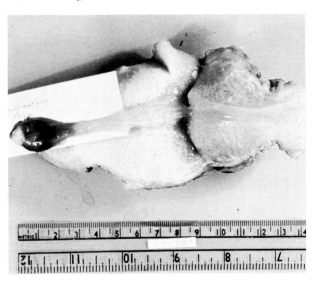

Polyps are often an incidental discovery at the time of curettage or hysterectomy. When symptoms do exist, the clinical picture is one of nonspecific abnormal uterine bleeding. Endometrial polyps occasionally cause postmenopausal bleeding. It is not clear that polyps bear any relation to endometrial cancer, except possibly those found in postmenopausal women.

Incidence

These lesions are common, but their exact incidence is not known. The age range is from 12 to 81 years, although they are most frequently found in women between 30 and 59 years of age.

Pathology

Polyps vary in size from a local elevation of the endometrium to a growth filling the endometrial cavity. They may be sessile or pedunculated. Most arise in the fundus or cornua of the uterus, but may protrude through the cervix. These are usually firmer and less red than cervical polyps. In the majority of cases the polyp is made up of endometrium similar to that seen in the basalis and does not show secretory changes. Less than one third of the polyps contain functional endometrium, similar histologically to the endometrium from which they arise. Polyps frequently show a microscopic picture of cystic hyperplasia and, less commonly, one of adenomatous hyperplasia. The tip of the polyp may be necrotic and inflamed, particularly if it is long and protrudes into the cervix (Fig. 57-5). Squamous metaplasia of the lining surface has been observed.

Diagnosis and Treatment

The diagnosis is usually established at the time of curettage or hysterectomy. Occasionally a polyp may protrude through the cervical os and be mistaken for a cervical polyp. Polyps may be diagnosed from hysterosalpingograms, in which they produce a depression in the outline of the uterine cavity. Polyps are often missed at curettage unless the curettage is accompanied by the insertion of a grasping instrument in the uterine cavity. For this reason, no curettage should be considered complete unless a polyp forceps is introduced prior to and following the actual curetting.

Endometrial polyps are benign, although carcinoma of the endometrium coexists with them in about 10% of postmenopausal women. However, the carcinoma is usually not in the polyp. Thus, polyps require no special treatment other than removal, although in postmenopausal women there must be a curettage of the endometrium.

BENIGN LESIONS OF THE MYOMETRIUM

Endometritis

Acute and chronic endometritis are discussed in Chapter 51. Rarely, chronic endometritis may be diagnosed at the time of uterine curettage as the cause of abnormal uterine bleeding. Adhesions may be a consequence and lead to cessation of menses and infertility (Asherman's syndrome). This condition is treated by separation of the adhesions, administration of exogenous estrogen,

FIG. 57-5. Submucous myoma, cystic atrophy of endometrium, and endometrial polyp with cystic hyperplasia and slight congestion of tip. These were unexpected findings in uterus removed from postmenopausal patient.

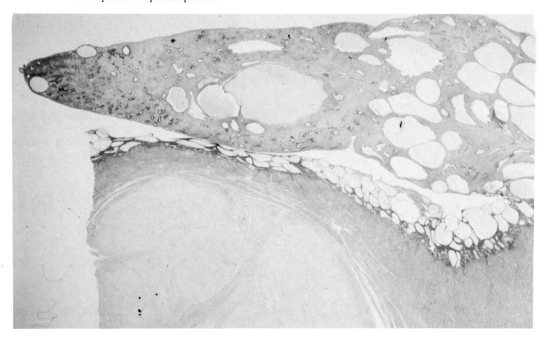

and temporary placement of an inert device to prevent reformation of adhesions.

If endometritis causes obstruction of the cervical canal, the uterine cavity may become distended by exudate (*pyometra*) or blood (*hematometra*). Most often, however, these are complications of malignant disease.

Leiomyomas

A leiomyoma is a well-circumscribed, but nonencapsulated, benign uterine tumor, composed mainly of smooth muscle but with some fibrous connective tissue elements. The tumor is also called myoma, fibromyoma, fibroma, and fibroid. The term "fibroid" has been firmly established in medical parlance by usage, although "myoma" is more accurate.

Incidence

The exact incidence of leiomyomas is uncertain; however, they constitute the most common pelvic tumor, and it has been estimated that one out of every four or five women over the age of 35 years has a uterine myoma. Although most myomas produce no symptoms, it has been estimated that 60% of all pelvic laparotomies in women are done for the reason (or excuse) of myomas. The lesion is most frequently found in the fourth and fifth decades of life and more commonly in black than in white patients. Interestingly enough, however, the incidence of myomas among African blacks is reported to be very low, suggesting causative factors other than heredity.

Location

Myomas are classified according to their location in the uterus. *Intramural* tumors, which are most common, are situated in the muscle wall without close proximity to either the mucosa or the serosa. With growth, these tumors distort the cavity as well as the external surface of the uterus. Single large intramural tumors may pro-

duce symmetric enlargement of the uterus. *Subserous* tumors (Fig. 57-6) are located directly beneath the serosa and project from the external surface of the uterus, producing the typical knobby configuration of the fibroid uterus. With growth, the subserous tumor may become pedunculated, attached to the uterus by a broad or long thin pedicle. On occasion such a pedunculated tumor may become attached to adjacent viscera, peritoneum, or omentum, lose its primary blood supply, and develop a secondary blood supply from the adherent structure. These tumors are referred to as *parasitic;* fortunately, they are rather rare. *Intraligamentous* tumors result from growth of a subserous tumor into the broad ligament. These may impinge on the ureter or even the pelvic blood vessels. They have special significance with respect to difficulty of surgical removal. *Submucous* tumors are present just beneath the endometrium (Fig. 57-7). With growth, they displace and thin the endometrium over their surface, which may become the site of necrosis and infection. Submucous tumors may also become pedunculated and eventually protrude into the cervical canal or the vagina. In this situation, infection is common.

Pathology

The corpus is the most common site of origin of myomas. They are usually multiple, of various sizes, and distort the contour of the uterus (Fig. 57-8). A single myoma may produce a rather uniform enlargement of the uterus simulating pregnancy.

Tumor size varies from the small 1-cm seedling myomas to those weighing as much as 147 lb. They are firm and well demarcated from the surrounding myometrium. On sectioning, the tumor bulges from the surface and the pseudocapsule, produced by compression of adjacent myometrial tissue, becomes readily apparent. The surface is smooth, glistening white with a whorled and fasciculated pattern.

Microscopic examination discloses bundles of smooth muscle arranged in interlacing patterns, sepa-

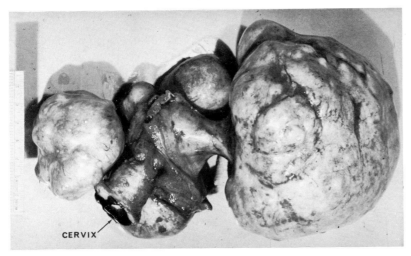

FIG. 57-6. Uterus containing numerous pedunculated subserous myomas. Tumors of this sort may be mistaken for ovarian neoplasms.

CERVIX

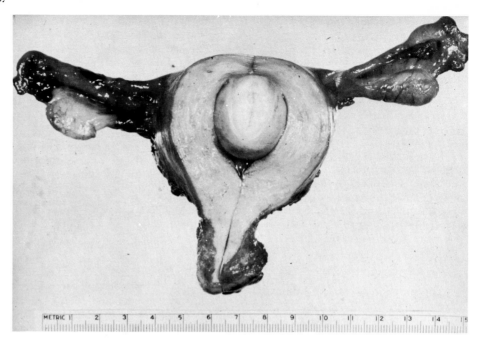

FIG. 57-7. Uterus containing submucous myoma that completely fills uterine cavity.

rated by fibrous connective tissue. There are relatively few blood vessels. The arrangement in bundles allows groups of smooth muscle cells to be seen variously in cross section or longitudinal section, giving a typical microscopic appearance (Fig. 57-9). The tumors have

no true capsule. At the margin there is usually an area of compressed myometrium forming a pseudocapsule. The artifact of fixation results in a space between the myoma and the adjacent compressed myometrium. Mitoses are rarely seen.

Histogenesis

Although myomas are common, their origin and development are not well understood. The tumors undoubtedly arise from smooth muscle within the myometrium. It has been suggested that they arise from persistent small, embryonic cell rests. Evidence has been offered that the tumors arise from the smooth muscle of blood vessel walls within the myometrium. It has further been suggested that myomas develop in response to estrogen stimulation; the evidence for this theory is far from convincing. The most impressive observation is that the tumors occur most commonly during the reproductive years and usually undergo regression, often complete, following the menopause. Oral contraceptives may cause myomas to enlarge. Also, it is generally held that leiomyomas increase in size during pregnancy, when estrogen production is high. However, Randall and Odell found little evidence that these tumors actually proliferate during pregnancy.

Degeneration and Complications

Myomas are subject to a variety of degenerative phenomena (Figs. 57-10, 57-11). Some have clinical significance, but most are pathologic findings unrelated to the clinical picture. The majority of these degenerative changes result from alteration in the blood supply of the tumor occurring with rapid growth, pregnancy,

FIG. 57-8. Large submucous myoma. Great distortion of uterine cavity shows futility of attempted curettage in such circumstance (Drawing by M. Brödel). (In Kelly HA: Operative Gynecology, Vol 2. New York, Appleton, 1903)

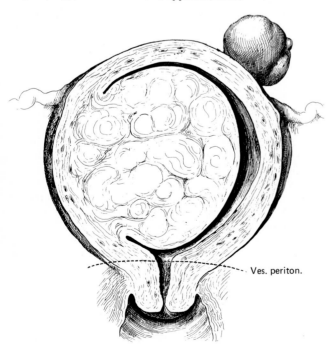

Ves. periton.

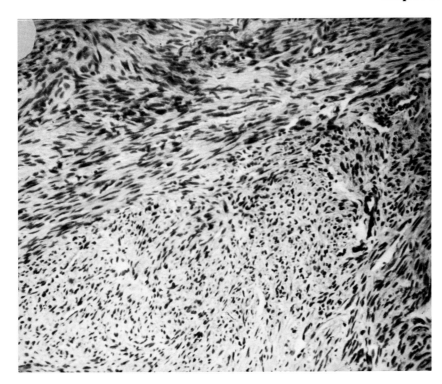

FIG. 57-9. Microscopic section of benign myoma. Smooth muscle cells are seen in cross-section and longitudinal section.

mechanical accident, or postmenopausal atrophy. The most common type of degeneration is *hyalinization*. A great many myomas, even small ones, reveal some degree of hyaline change. On cut section, the surface appears homogeneous and has lost some of the whorled, fascicular pattern. Microscopically, broad zones of hyaline connective tissue replace the smooth muscle cells. Somewhat less common is *cystic degeneration*. Small or large areas undergo liquefaction and myxomatous change resulting in cystic foci. When these are present to a substantial degree, the consistency of the tumor is soft, and on section, the cystic areas are obvious grossly. *Calcification* of myomas is an interesting degenerative change occurring more commonly in the postmenopausal woman (Fig. 57-12). The areas of calcification may be scant or diffuse. When diffuse, the tumor may be visualized roentgenographically. Occasionally such a myoma is an incidental finding during radiographic examination of the abdomen. Rarely, there is heterotopic bone formation. *Fatty degeneration* of myomas is observed usually as an incidental microscopic finding. *Necrosis* may result from torsion or twisting of a pedunculated myoma and may be associated with abdominal pain, tenderness, fever, and leukocytosis. This may occur as an acute accident. A special variety of necrosis is *carneous* or *red degeneration*. This is said to occur in 8% of tumors complicating pregnancy. The change is due to aseptic necrosis associated with hemorrhage into the substance of the tumor and subsequent hemolysis. Grossly these tumors become beefy red and soft and clinically produce pain and tenderness.

Infection of a myoma may occur in association with adjacent pelvic inflammatory disease but is most common in the submucous pedunculated myoma, which becomes necrotic first and inflamed secondarily.

Degeneration is important in two respects: (1) it may produce symptoms and signs that require treatment, including surgery, and (2) on the basis of gross appearance, a benign, degenerated leiomyoma may be confused with a sarcoma. Sarcomatous transformation of a myoma does occur, but the incidence is less than 1% and, in general, should not influence the clinical management of patients with leiomyomas.

Physical Signs

A presumptive diagnosis of leiomyoma of the uterus may be made by abdominal palpation if the uterus is displaced out of the pelvis or if the tumors are large. They are palpated as firm, irregular nodules arising from the pelvis and extending into the lower abdomen. Generally, the nodular mass is movable. If tumors are pedunculated they may be moved separately. If the tumor mass fills the pelvis, mobility is restricted, and similar restriction may result from associated inflammatory involvement of the supporting tissues.

Bimanual pelvic examination is more revealing. Diagnosis is relatively simple if the uterus can be outlined easily and its contour is distorted by multiple smooth, round nodules. These masses may be small irregularities on the surface of the uterus, no larger than 1 cm, or masses that fill the pelvis and lower abdomen. The examination should be done carefully to make certain that the masses are part of the uterus. A normal uterus may

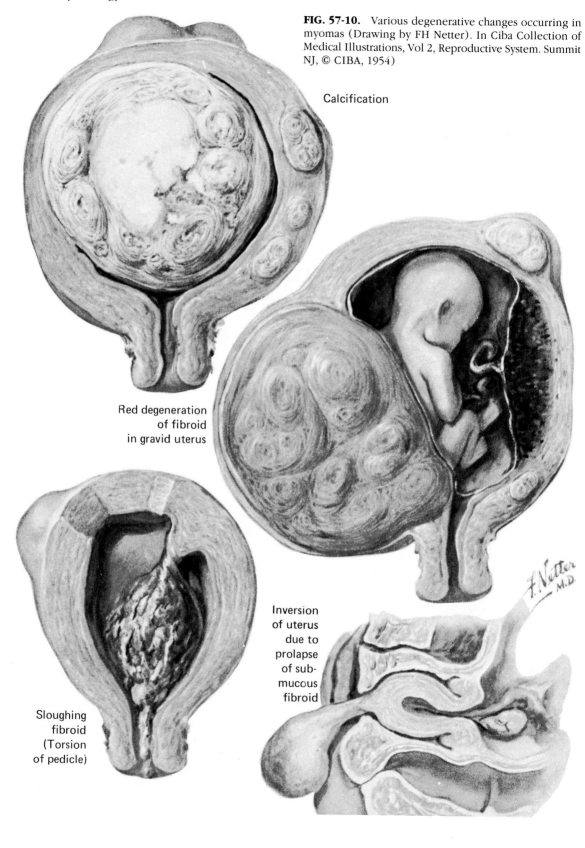

FIG. 57-10. Various degenerative changes occurring in myomas (Drawing by FH Netter). In Ciba Collection of Medical Illustrations, Vol 2, Reproductive System. Summit NJ, © CIBA, 1954)

Calcification

Red degeneration of fibroid in gravid uterus

Sloughing fibroid (Torsion of pedicle)

Inversion of uterus due to prolapse of sub-mucous fibroid

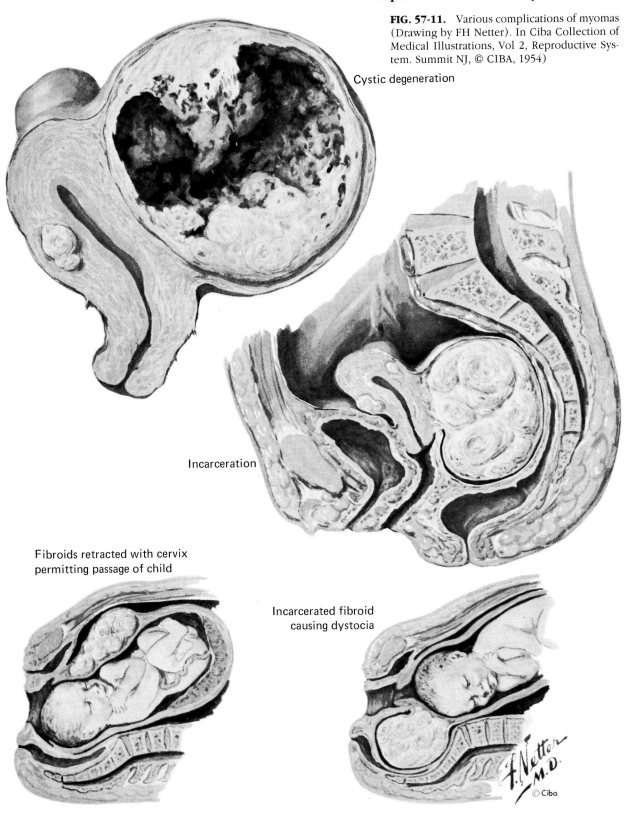

FIG. 57-11. Various complications of myomas (Drawing by FH Netter). In Ciba Collection of Medical Illustrations, Vol 2, Reproductive System. Summit NJ, © CIBA, 1954)

Cystic degeneration

Incarceration

Fibroids retracted with cervix permitting passage of child

Incarcerated fibroid causing dystocia

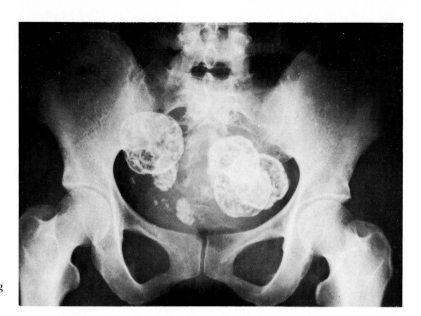

FIG. 57-12. Radiograph of abdomen showing many calcified uterine myomas.

be displaced posteriorly by a solid ovarian tumor. Sounding the uterus gives the direction of the uterine cavity and its depth. Frequently the uterine cavity is enlarged by myomas and directed toward the myomas. If the cavity is of normal size and deviated away from the masses, an extrauterine tumor must be considered. It is possible, of course, for a solitary myoma to displace the major portion of a normal-sized uterus. A pedunculated, submucous myoma may be seen protruding from the cervical os as a grayish-pink smooth mass. If there is infection or necrosis, the surface may be red and friable. It is possible to diagnose a submucous myoma at the time of uterine curettage. An irregularity of the cavity is felt by the uterine sound or by the curet when it is brought down the anterior or posterior wall. One should not mistake the cornual areas for myomas, however.

Symptoms

Most myomas, even large ones, produce no symptoms. Indeed, many more are discovered as an incidental finding than are associated with symptoms, despite the great frequency with which such tumors are removed in the operating room. The mere presence of uterine myomas does not mandate active treatment.

The asymptomatic tumor may present a problem in differential diagnosis. Symmetric enlargement of the uterus may be confused with pregnancy. Usually the menstrual history and typical changes in the cervix and vagina make the pregnancy apparent. The myomatous uterus has a firm consistency as opposed to the soft, pregnant uterus. An hCG test for pregnancy should be done if any doubt exists. If the tumor is pedunculated, it may be difficult to distinguish from an ovarian tumor; indeed, the distinction may be impossible and exploratory surgery may be required to exclude ovarian neoplasm, particularly in postmenopausal patients. Adnexal

inflammatory masses and endometriosis can usually be distinguished from a solitary subserous or pedunculated myoma on the basis of symptoms and associated findings of pelvic scarring or fixation. Ultrasound may help to make the distinction.

BLEEDING. Any pattern of abnormal uterine bleeding may occur, but the most common is excessive or prolonged menses. This may produce a rather profound anemia. It is important to remember that the patient with myomas may have abnormal uterine bleeding from causes other than the myomas. The patient's endocrine status and endometrium must be carefully evaluated.

The exact mechanisms by which myomas of the uterus cause bleeding abnormalities are not altogether clear. In many cases bleeding is probably due to associated endocrine disorders such as anovulation. Indeed, such underlying abnormalities in endocrine function may have a causal relation to the tumors themselves. In one study, 36% of myomatous uteri were found to have endometrial hyperplasia. Submucous myomas may produce bleeding because of congestion, necrosis, and ulceration of the surface. Excess bleeding may result from the increased surface area of the endometrium when tumors enlarge and distort the endometrial cavity. The surface area of the normal uterine cavity is about 15 cm². In the presence of the multiple myomas it may be as great as 225 cm². Large tumors also may produce mechanical interference with the blood supply to the endometrium, and the presence of intramural tumors may interfere with the ability of the uterus to contract and effectively occlude blood vessels at the time of menstruation. Large vascular channels are frequently seen in the endometrium adjacent to myomas.

PRESSURE. Pressure on the bladder produces urinary frequency, urgency and, rarely, inability to void.

Constipation results from pressure on the rectum. With extremely large tumors, pressure on the pelvic vessels may result in edema or varicosities of the legs. Rarely, ureteral pressure produces hydroureter or hydronephrosis.

PAIN.   Pain and tenderness may result from degeneration of the myoma. The onset is gradual and the pain intermittent. A dull aching soreness is usual, but the pain may be colicky. Fever and leukocytosis accompany severe degeneration. A tumor with a long pedicle may twist and produce acute pain, tenderness, nausea, and signs of peritoneal irritation. The pressure of large tumors on adjacent viscera may result in pain. With growth, stretching of old inflammatory adhesions may result in bilateral pelvic discomfort. Cramping pain may be associated with attempts at passage of a submucous tumor from within the uterine cavity. Intramural tumors may aggravate or produce dysmenorrhea, although other sources of dysmenorrhea should be considered first. The most common type of discomfort, particularly with large tumors, is a sensation of pelvic heaviness or "bearing down."

DISTORTION OF THE ABDOMEN.   The patient herself may notice the presence of a tumor by self-examination or noticeable alterations in girth and abdominal contour.

INFERTILITY.   Myomas are sometimes found in the process of evaluating infertile patients. Their presence should not be interpreted immediately as having a causal relation to the infertility. Myomas *may* impair fertility, particularly if they occlude the endocervical canal, sufficiently distort the isthmic portions of the oviducts, or cause sufficient thinning and change in the endometrium to impair proper implantation. However, many patients, even those with sizable uterine tumors, are normally fertile and maintain pregnancy to term. Other causes of infertility should always be sought.

PREGNANCY COMPLICATIONS.   Uterine myomas may present symptoms only during pregnancy. The management of this special situation is considered below.

Treatment

OBSERVATION AND REASSURANCE.   In many, if not most, cases treatment is not necessary when a diagnosis of uterine myoma is made, particularly if the patient is asymptomatic, has small tumors, or is postmenopausal. These patients should be carefully examined every three to six months to check for unusual growth or complications. Abnormal uterine bleeding due to myomas requires diagnostic curettage, but if no malignancy is found, it often can be controlled by appropriate supportive therapy and endocrine management. This is recommended for the patient who is approaching the menopause. If the bleeding can be controlled for a short time, it will cease spontaneously at the menopause and the myomas will regress.

Treatment may be indicated for patients with asymptomatic tumors if the differential diagnosis includes another lesion of greater significance (such as an ovarian tumor), if the tumor is unusually large (particularly if it produces abdominal distortion), and possibly if infertility is present with no other apparent cause. How large is a "large" tumor? Many consider a myomatous uterus larger than a three-month pregnancy an indication for treatment. Sudden growth of a tumor, particularly in a postmenopausal woman, is indication for treatment.

SURGERY.   For patients with significant symptoms, surgery is the preferred method of treatment. Myomectomy (the removal of tumors) can be done to preserve the uterus for future childbearing. This is accomplished through the vagina in cases of pedunculated submucous myomas, employing a wire loop and electrocautery. Myomectomy is more commonly done by the abdominal approach. A single pedunculated subserous tumor can be removed easily, but it is also possible at one time to remove a great many intramural and even submucous tumors from the uterus. Myomectomy is the operation of choice when the indication is infertility or when a tumor is to be removed because its location is likely to interfere with normal delivery. Occasionally myomectomy is indicated because the patient has a strong desire to retain menstrual function, although future childbearing is not a special consideration. Multiple myomectomy has a high frequency of postoperative complications in terms of adhesions and bowel obstruction, and there is a relatively high incidence of recurrence. Thus, removal of a single pedunculated tumor may be of value, but multiple myomectomy should be done only in selected young, otherwise fertile patients who are desirous of having more children.

For the majority of patients with symptoms thought to be related to myomas, the treatment should be total hysterectomy. If the tumors are small, the hysterectomy may be done vaginally, particularly if there is associated pelvic relaxation. Most often we prefer the abdominal approach for ease of operating and ability to inspect the remainder of the pelvis carefully. Since large tumors and intraligamentous tumors may distort the ureters from their usual course and make them more liable to surgical trauma, catheters should be placed in the ureters before surgery to enable the surgeon to locate the ureters and avoid accidental injury. There is no reason to remove the ovaries when doing a hysterectomy for uterine myomas. *Hysterectomy should not be done without prior curettage of the uterus to rule out intercurrent endometrial or cervical disease.*

RADIATION.   In the past, radiation has been used for the treatment of myomas. It is mentioned here only to be condemned, since radiation has no place in the treatment of uterine myomas.

Myomas in Pregnancy

Reports indicate that the incidence of uterine myomas during pregnancy varies from 0.3% to 7.2%. The tumors almost always precede the pregnancy, although they may not become apparent until pregnancy occurs. During the course of pregnancy myomas usually increase in size. However, this is largely due to edema and degeneration and probably does not represent true proliferation of the tumor. The frequency of spontaneous abortion is increased in patients with uterine myomas. No treatment is indicated during the pregnancy; moreover, it is difficult to predict which cases will proceed without mishap. Fortunately this is not a common cause of abortion.

During the second and third trimesters, increase in the size of tumors may produce or increase pressure symptoms. Degeneration of intramural tumors due to alterations in blood supply or twisting of pedunculated tumors produces symptoms of gradual or acute pain, usually associated with localized tenderness. This may be difficult to distinguish from other acute intraabdominal accidents or inflammation, and surgery may be necessary for this reason. However, in the majority of patients, degeneration rarely constitutes an indication for surgical intervention. The patient is best treated by bedrest, symptom relief, and careful observation. Myomectomy, which is indicated rarely, is followed by an increased incidence of abortion and premature labor.

During late pregnancy and delivery, myomas may produce fetal malpresentation, uterine inertia, or mechanical dystocia, depending upon the number, size, and location of tumors. A large tumor in the lower uterine segment or cervix may actually block descent of the head into the pelvis (see Fig. 57-11). Fortunately, most such tumors rise out of the pelvis as pregnancy progresses. Dystocia is more likely to occur with true cervical myomas. Such situations require expert obstetric judgment and, on occasion, cesarean section. If cesarean section is accomplished, myomectomy is not advisable at the same operation.

Postpartum hemorrhage is more likely when the uterus contains myomas. This complication should be anticipated and appropriate precautions taken to avoid unnecessary blood loss or to combat it if it occurs. Because of the sudden change in the shape and position of the uterus, twisting or vascular accidents of pedunculated tumors may complicate the puerperium.

The management of a pregnant patient with myomas is essentially no different from the management of a normal pregnant woman. Close observation is necessary; hospitalization, analysis and, rarely, surgery may be needed, but in the majority of cases a safe vaginal delivery can be anticipated.

Adenomyosis

Adenomyosis is a benign disease of the uterus characterized by areas of endometrial glands and stroma within the myometrium. There is usually no direct connection between these heterotopic foci and the endometrium lining the uterine cavity. The lesion is not a tumor, but a hyperplastic growth, and may be localized or diffuse. *Adenomyoma* refers to a localized tumorlike mass composed of hyperplastic smooth muscle admixed with foci of endometrium. While adenomyosis has certain morphologic similarities to endometriosis, it is not, in the author's opinion, truly related to endometriosis, nor should it be considered to be part of the endometriosis complex. The term "endometriosis interna" should not be used to refer to adenomyosis. Endometriosis is not commonly found in association with adenomyosis.

Clinical Picture

Adenomyosis is usually diagnosed by the pathologist as an incidental finding in a uterus removed because of functional symptoms, intractable abnormal bleeding, or suspicion of myomas. Adenomyosis is found in approximately 20% of removed uteri and probably is of more clinical significance than is generally recognized. In one study, adenomyosis was found to be diagnosed correctly before surgery in only 10% of cases. This disease is observed most commonly in women during the fifth and sixth decades; classic manifestations are progressively heavy menstrual bleeding, increasingly painful dysmenorrhea, and a gradually enlarging, tender uterus. Adenomyosis does not produce symptoms following the menopause. All or part of this classic symptom complex occurs with other more common or more readily diagnosed conditions. Moreover, adenomyosis and uterine myomas frequently coexist, and some believe that endometrial hyperplasia commonly occurs in the same uterus. Myomas are a much more common cause of uterine enlargement than is adenomyosis, and endometrial hyperplasia is a more common cause of abnormal bleeding. Even endometrial hyperplasia, if marked, may cause a diffuse enlargement of the uterus. Secondary dysmenorrhea, a common complaint of women with adenomyosis, is more common in patients without definite pelvic disease and in those with endometriosis.

Thus, adenomyosis should be considered when a patient in her 40s complains of prolongation and increase of menstrual flow and dysmenorrhea, and is found to have a globular, firm, tender uterus that is one or two times enlarged. It should be apparent, however, that only a few such patients will be proved to have adenomyosis. Increased awareness may increase the frequency with which an accurate diagnosis is made, but it should not constitute a reason for increasing the frequency of hysterectomy or neglecting a careful search for other important disease.

Pathology

The uterus is firm, enlarged, and somewhat globular. On section, the myometrium is greatly thickened and the cut surface irregular, with a somewhat knobby appearance. There may be tiny foci of translucent tissue protruding from the cut surface. Microscopic examination shows areas of endometrial glands and stroma scattered throughout the myometrium (Fig. 57-13). By tradition, the diagnosis is made when such foci are separated from the basal layer of lining endometrium by more than one low-power microscopic field. The ectopic endometrium is rarely responsive to cyclic ovarian hormones and usually resembles nonsecretory basal endometrium. In this regard the appearance is like the endometrium found in endometrial polyps. There are occasional examples of cystic hyperplasia in adenomyotic foci. Occasionally during pregnancy the areas undergo a decidual change, and rarely a typical response to the progestational phase of the menstrual cycle is seen.

An adenomyoma may be difficult to distinguish grossly from a myoma. The cut surfaces reveal the nodule to be poorly demarcated from the surrounding myo-metrium, and it does not bulge above the myometrium as the typical myoma does. There is no cleavage plane or pseudocapsule. Microscopically, the adenomyoma resembles a myoma with foci of endometrium.

Histogenesis

There are numerous theories of histogenesis, none of which is proved. It is commonly accepted that adenomyosis arises by downward extension of the basal portion of endometrium into the underlying myometrium. This explains the infrequency with which adenomyosis shows cyclic response to ovarian hormones. The mechanism of symptom production is similarly difficult to explain and is often related to coexisting pathologic conditions of the uterus or ovary. Prolonged or excessive menstrual flow has been explained by interference with

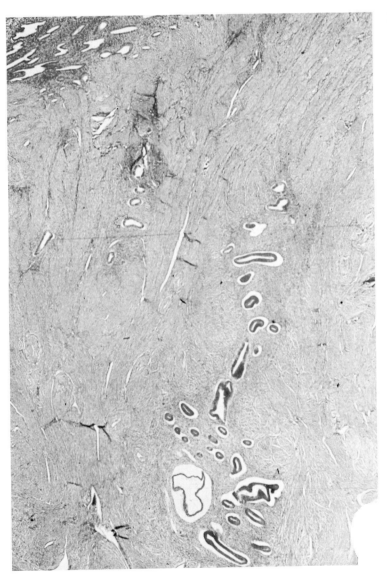

FIG. 57-13. Microscopic section of uterus with adenomyosis. Foci of endometrium are present deep to endometrium within myometrium.

adequate myometrial contraction. Conversely, the adenomyotic foci have been credited with irritation of uterine muscular contractility and resultant dysmenorrhea. Areas of adenomyosis are rarely the sites of malignant change, although this has been described. In cases of well-differentiated adenocarcinoma of the endometrium, it may be difficult to differentiate areas of adenomyosis from areas of myometrial invasion.

Treatment

Hysterectomy is the treatment of choice for the patient with symptomatic adenomyosis, even though it is frequently undertaken on the basis of an incorrect preoperative diagnosis.

Stromal Adenomyosis

This lesion is variously referred to as *endolymphatic stromal myosis, stromatosis, stromal endometriosis,* or *stromal adenomyosis.* Some examples are actually endometrial sarcoma or mixed müllerian tumors. The truly benign variety is morphologically similar to adenomyosis, except that the ectopic areas consist only of endometrial stroma without glands. The gross appearance of the benign condition is no different from that of adenomyosis. Microscopic examination demonstrates multiple foci of compact endometrial stromal cells, similar to those seen in the proliferative phase of the menstrual cycle, throughout the myometrium. Sometimes these foci extend into lymphatic or venous channels. No specific clinical picture is associated with stromal adenomyosis. The exact diagnosis rests upon the pathologist's interpretation of microscopic findings. In the truly benign variety—without vascular involvement—hysterectomy is adequate treatment.

Unusual Tumors

Other benign tumors of the uterus are hemangioma, lymphangioma, lipoma, and cysts of mesonephric origin. Few cases of each have been reported. There are no specific clinical syndromes and the precise histogenesis of these tumors is not known. They are usually noted as incidental findings or mistaken for myomas. Hysterectomy is the usual treatment.

Lymphangiomas may resemble soft myomas. They are usually small, circumscribed nodules composed of a maze of lymphatic channels with a background of fibrous connective tissue. Lymphangiomas must be distinguished from lymphangiectatic changes in a myoma. They are very rare indeed. *Hemangiopericytoma* is a rare tumor composed of nonneoplastic capillaries surrounded by collars of neoplastic capillary pericytes. It is usually found incidentally, sometimes confused with stromal adenomyosis, and the prognosis is good. *Lipo-*

mas are lobulated, encapsulated yellow growths consisting of adult adipose tissue. It is usually possible to distinguish a myoma with fatty degeneration from a lipoma by the remaining areas of smooth muscle in the former. Cysts or small adenomatous growths in the lateral wall of the uterus are rare. These lesions presumably arise from remnants of the mesonephric duct or tubules. Even more rarely such lesions give rise to malignant neoplasms.

Subinvolution of the Uterus: Fibrosis Uteri

Subinvolution of the uterus, or fibrosis uteri, is a diffuse, symmetric enlargement of the uterus occasionally found in multiparous women and credited with various symptoms, notably abnormal uterine bleeding. Some believe this to be a significant abnormality of the uterus resulting from incomplete puerperal involution, with retention or deposition of excess elastic connective tissue. For whatever reason, parous women have larger uteri than nonparous women. This condition *per se* has no clinical importance, is never an indication for surgery, and should be disregarded in a consideration of diseases of the uterus.

REFERENCES AND RECOMMENDED READING

Benign Lesions of the Endometrium

Bergman P: Traumatic intra-uterine lesions. Acta Obstet Gynecol Scand 40(Suppl 4):1 1961

Buttram VC, Riter RC: Uterine lyomyomata: Etiology, symptomatology and management. Fertil Steril 36:433, 1981

Cohen CJ, Gusberg SB: Screening for endometrial cancer. Clin Obstet Gynecol 18:27, 1975

Gambrell RD: The prevention of endometrial cancer in postmenopausal women with progestogens. Maturitas 1:10, 1978

Gusberg SB, Kaplin AL: Precursors of corpus cancer. Am J Obstet Gynecol 87:662, 1963

Hathcock EW, Williams GA, Englehardt SM et al: Office aspiration curettage of the endometrium. Am J Obstet Gynecol 120:205, 1974

Hertig AT, Sommers SC: Genesis of endometrial cancer. One study of prior biopsies. Cancer 2:946, 1949

Holstrom EG, McLennan CE: Menorrhagia associated with irregular shedding of the endometrium. Am J Obstet Gynecol 53:727, 1947

Katayama KP, Jones HW: Chromosomes of atypical hyperplasia and carcinoma of the endometrium. Am J Obstet Gynecol 97:978, 1967

Kistner RW, Gore H, Hertig AT: Carcinoma of the endometrium: A preventable disease? Am J Obstet Gynecol 95:1011, 1966

Overstreet EW: Clinical aspects of endometrial polyps. Surg Clin North Am 42:1013, 1962

Sutherland AM: Tuberculosis of the endometrium. J Obstet Gynaecol Br Commonw 63:161, 1956

Benign Lesions of the Myometrium

Baruah BD, Barkakati D: Endometrial changes in uterine myoma. J Obstet Gynecol India 12:246, 1961

Buttram VC Jr, Reiter RC: Uterine leiomyomata: Etiology, symptomatology and management. Fertil Steril 36:433, 1981

Miller NF, Ludovici PP: On the origin and development of uterine fibroids. Am J Obstet Gynecol 70:720, 1955

Molitor JJ: Adenomyosis: A clinical and pathological appraisal. Am J Obstet Gynecol 110:275, 1971

Parks J, Barter RH: The myomatous uterus complicated by pregnancy. Am J Obstet Gynecol 63:260, 1952

Randall JH, Odell LD: Fibroids in pregnancy. Am J Obstet Gynecol 46:349, 1943

Schwarz O: Benign diffuse enlargement of the uterus. Am J Obstet Gynecol 61:902, 1951

Stearns HC: A study of stromal endometriosis. Am J Obstet Gynecol 75:663, 1958

Strassman EO: Plastic unification of double uterus. Am J Obstet Gynecol 64:25, 1952

Tavassoli F, Kraus F: Endometrial lesions in uteri resected for atypical endometrial hyperplasia. Am J Clin Pathol 70:77, 1978

Vellios F: Endometrial hyperplasia. Gynecol Oncol 2:152, 1974

Wentz WB: Progestin therapy in endometrial hyperplasia. Gynecol Oncol 2:362, 1974

Winkler E et al: Pitfalls in the diagnosis of endometrial neoplasia. Obstet Gynecol 64:185, 1984

Malignant Lesions of the Corpus Uteri

William T. Creasman

CARCINOMA OF THE ENDOMETRIUM

Cancer of the uterine corpus is the most common malignancy found in the female pelvis in the United States today. According to the American Cancer Society, 39,000 new cases were expected in 1984. This lesion, therefore, occurs more than twice as frequently as carcinoma of the cervix and ovary. The American Cancer Society, in reviewing the incidence of this disease for the decade of the 1970s, noted that the actual number of patients with endometrial cancer was 1.5 times the predicted figure. Reasons for the apparent increase in the incidence of endometrial cancer are as follows: (1) a greater availability of medical care, resulting in more cancers being detected; (2) more women than ever reaching the critical age for developing endometrial cancer; (3) a broadening of the criteria for the diagnosis of endometrial cancer by inclusion into the cancer registry of severe dysplasia, atypical adenomatous hyperplasia,

carcinoma *in situ,* and so-called well-differentiated cancers, and (4) a worldwide increase in endometrial cancer due at least in part to environmental and demographic factors. An increase in the use of exogenous estrogen has also been implicated. However, in Czechoslovakia and Norway, a 50% to 60% increase in endometrial cancer has occurred despite the fact that estrogens are rarely prescribed or are not generally available in those countries. Regardless of the reasons for its increasing incidence, the management of corpus cancer becomes increasingly important in the health care of the female patient.

Total abdominal hysterectomy and bilateral salpingo-oophorectomy remain the keystone of therapy. Although various forms of radiation have been advocated, many studies in the literature note that, at least in certain circumstances, combined therapy does not give significantly better results than surgery alone. Although selected studies have shown a 90% or better survival rate in stage-I carcinoma of the endometrium, the last report from the Fédération Internationale de Gynécologie et Obstetrique (FIGO) notes only a 75% five-year survival. This chapter identifies risk factors in this malignancy and advocates adjunctive therapy in addition to hysterectomy and removal of the adnexa to improve survival rates in patients with additional risks.

Epidemiology

Although endometrial cancer may appear at any time during the reproductive and menopausal years, it is found primarily in women who have experienced cessation of menses. The median age of patients with corpus cancer is 61.1 years. The age range extends from the second to the ninth decade, but only 5% of patients are under 40 years of age and less than 25% of cases are diagnosed before menopause.

Obesity, nulliparity, and late menopause are three factors classically associated with endometrial cancer and, therefore, qualify as "risk factors." Obese women 21 to 50 pounds overweight develop endometrial cancer with three times the frequency of normal-weight women; for those who are 50 pounds overweight, the frequency is increased 10 times. Unfortunately, screening limited to the obese population would diagnose only 50% of endometrial cancers. The main reason advanced to explain why obesity should be a contributing factor is that obese women apparently have an increased peripheral conversion of androstenedione to estrone in the fat tissues.

Approximately one fourth of patients with endometrial cancer are nulliparous. The nulligravida's risk of developing endometrial cancer is twice as high as that of women who have had one child and to three times as high as that of women who have had five children. In some nulliparous women, ovarian dysfunction may contribute to the development of the endometrial carcinoma as well as being the cause of the nulliparity. Endometrial cancer has been reported to occur in 25% of patients with polycystic ovary disease (Stein-Leventhal syndrome), in whom the endometrium is exposed to unopposed estrogen. In these women, induction of a progestational endometrium may reduce this risk.

Late menopause is associated with an increased risk of endometrial cancer. Women who reach menopause after age 52 have a risk about 2.4 times greater than women reaching menopause before age 49.

Hypertension and diabetes mellitus are frequently associated with endometrial cancer. Diabetes has been reported in as many as 40% of patients with endometrial cancer. Hypertension is prevalent in the elderly obese population, but it does not appear to be a significant factor by itself, even though 25% of patients with endometrial cancer do have hypertension or arteriosclerotic heart disease.

Estrogens in Endometrial Cancer

The possible relationship between estrogen and endometrial cancer has received increasing attention in the last decade. Experiments of nature have provided us with information that implicates estrogen as a possible contributing factor in the development of endometrial cancer. The role of polycystic ovary disease has already been mentioned. For many years it has been known that endometrial cancer can occur in patients with hormone-secreting tumors, particularly of the ovary. In patients with so-called feminizing ovarian tumors or polycystic ovaries, the endometrial cancers that do develop are usually stage-I, grade-1 lesions that have less myometrial involvement and better survival than adenocarcinomas that develop without these associated entities. In this, the cancers resemble adenocarcinomas of the endometrium developing in patients who have taken exogenous estrogen, which might indicate a common etiologic link.

Estrogen-induced neoplasias have been reported in experimental animals. The cancers produced appear to be characteristic of the species itself rather than of the estrogen given. Exogenous estrogen can induce endometrial cancer in rabbits, but the malignancy also occurs naturally in this animal. Primates are remarkably resistant to the possible carcinogenic effect of estrogen even after extremely long periods of exposure.

Beginning in the mid-1970s there appeared, in rapid succession, several articles indicating a substantial increase of endometrial cancer among patients receiving exogenous estrogen, the risk factor being from 1.8 to 28 times that of a control population. As a result, replacement estrogen therapy, which had been enjoying considerable popularity, experienced a very rapid decline in use. As the data were more thoroughly evaluated it became apparent that those who took estrogen and developed cancer of the endometrium had a preponderance of well-differentiated, superficially invading cancers that were highly curable: more than 90% of the

patients survived for five years or longer. It now appears that with optimal care, if a woman takes estrogen and develops a cancer of the endometrium, her chance of dying from it is 1 in 4,500 to 1 in 20,000; her chance of survival is therefore equal to or better than a woman of similar age who never took estrogen and never developed endometrial cancer. Several studies have indicated that the addition of progestins to estrogen as replacement therapy has a protective effect against the development of endometrial cancer, and hormone replacement therapy of this kind is now accepted as standard. The benefits of estrogen replacement therapy are significant and well known and are appreciably more important to the patient than the possible risks.

Preinvasive Cancer

Adenomatous hyperplasia of the endometrium (in its most severe form it is sometimes called carcinoma *in situ* or stage-0 endometrial cancer), like dysplasia and *in situ* carcinoma of the cervix, is a preinvasive lesion. Some investigators prefer the term adenomatous hyperplasia or stage-0 endometrial carcinoma to carcinoma *in situ* of the endometrium because of the difficulty of defining morphologically a noninvasive endometrial cancer in an area in which stromal replacement is such an imperfect criterion of malignancy. Whatever the term used, the lesion's biologic implication as a cancer precursor is clear, and developmental phases can be defined. One prospective study disclosed development of invasive endometrial cancer from adenomatous hyperplasia in 12% of the patients in a relatively short (5–10 years) follow-up period. Other studies have reported cancer developing in 15% to 25% of patients with this lesion. The highest incidence of adenomatous hyperplasia occurs in patients between the ages of 45 and 50 years, about 10 tens younger than the age of peak incidence of frank cancer of the endometrium. Indeed, the epidemiologic profile of adenomatous hyperplasia is very similar to that of endometrial carcinoma.

Treatment of adenomatous hyperplasia or stage-0 lesions depends on the age and reproductive needs of the patient. In young women, for whom preservation of the uterus is important, restoration of ovulation or creation of a gestational endometrium by endogenous or exogenous means can reverse the pattern of hyperplasia. In women with dysfunctional bleeding of the menopause, a scheme of treatment may be developed that relieves the presenting symptoms and, in addition, effects prophylaxis. The specifics of treatment are based on the histologic characteristics of the endometrial sample obtained at the time of diagnostic curettage. Observation or endocrine manipulation of patients with adenomatous hyperplasia who are beyond their reproductive years is both illogical and radical and should be carried out only under special circumstances. Often a diagnosis of adenomatous hyperplasia derived from a curettage specimen is followed by a diagnosis of frank invasive cancer of the endometrium when the hysterectomy specimen is reviewed. Thus, the treatment of choice for patients with this premalignant lesion who are beyond their reproductive years is hysterectomy.

Pathology

Carcinoma of the endometrium may start as a focal, discrete lesion, as, for example, in an endometrial polyp, or it may be diffuse, appearing in several different areas and involving much, or in some cases, most of the endometrial surface. Most adenocarcinomas are preceded by the predisposing lesions (adenomatous or atypical hyperplasia) described earlier on page 1069. As the lesion progresses, the affected endometrium becomes thickened and thrown up into folds of very friable, yellow-tan tissue that is easily dislodged (Fig. 57-14). In advanced stages, the tissue may be sufficiently luxuriant to fill the uterine cavity. In such cases the uterus is clinically enlarged, and multiple sections of the myometrium usually show evidence of invasion, which may be

so extensive as to penetrate the entire thickness of the uterine wall (Fig. 57-15). The curettings are very copious; sometimes bits of tissue roll out spontaneously as the cervical dilators are withdrawn, even before the curette is used. The abundant, friable fragments are characteristic of endometrial cancer. Nevertheless, one must not be trapped into believing that a gross diagnosis is possible, for luxuriant, benign secretory curettings may strongly resemble those of endometrial carcinoma.

Microscopic Findings

In most cases the diagnosis of endometrial carcinoma is based on an appraisal of the general architecture of the lesion. It may be substantiated by the bizarre cytologic details that usually characterize malignancy, that is, pseudostratification, differences in size, shape, and staining reaction, and abundance of normal and abnormal mitotic figures in the glandular lining cells; however, the autonomous, highly abnormal endometrial ar-

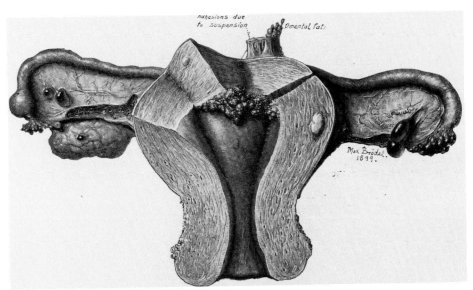

FIG. 57-14. Adenocarcinoma arising in the fundus. The remainder of the endometrium is normal. Adhesions due to prior uterine suspension are noted. (Kelly HA: Gynecology. New York, D Appleton & Company, 1928. Drawing by Max Brödel. Kelly attributes specimen to TS Cullen.)

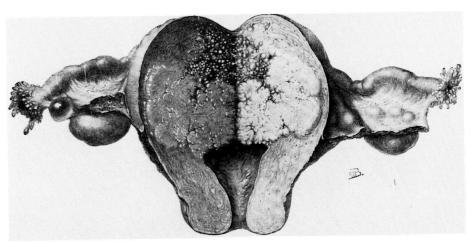

FIG. 57-15. Advanced adenocarcinoma of the endometrium showing deep myometrial invasion and metastatic nodules in the broad ligament. (Kelly HA: Gynecology. New York, D Appleton & Company, 1928. Drawing by Max Brödel. Kelly attributes specimen to WW Russell.)

chitecture, as seen with the scanning or low-power objective, usually provides the evidence of cancer.

Adenocarcinoma of the endometrium is categorized in three groups, according to the degree of differentiation. It is this grouping that forms the basis for *grading.* The groups are not necessarily separate and distinct; one may merge imperceptibly with another, and examples of two or sometimes all three of the groups may be found in the same tumor. Grade is assigned according to the pattern that is dominant.

Grade-1 lesions (Fig. 57-16) are highly differentiated. The number of glands is greatly increased, such that they often are apposed to one another (the so-called "back-to-back" pattern). There is little or no intervening stroma, and stromal cells are inconspicuous. Pseudostratification is present, and the overgrowth of the columnar epithelium results in budding, or papillary projections into the gland lumina. In some grade-1 adenocarcinomas, the glandular cells appear to be more or less normal; in others the columnar cells are enlarged, the nuclei are deeply basophilic and somewhat enlarged, and normal and abnormal mitoses are frequent. Focal and superficial areas of ulceration, necrosis, and inflammatory reaction are often present, and the delicate vasculature of the matrix and papillary projections is opened by the advancing tumor. This last finding is what accounts for the fetid vaginal discharge and bleeding that characterize this tumor.

Grade-2 lesions (Figs. 57-17, 57-18) are described in the FIGO staging system as "differentiated adenomatous carcinomas with partly solid areas." They are otherwise known as "moderately" differentiated lesions. The glands are highly irregular in form, and the proportion of epithelial cells that show the marked variation and atypia characteristic of neoplasia is higher than in grade 1 lesions. Sheets of such cells, in which the glandular pattern is lost, are found either apparently isolated in the more abundant matrix or in continuity with glandular epithelium.

Grade-3 lesions (Fig. 57-19) are described in the FIGO staging system as "predominantly solid or entirely undifferentiated carcinomas." The sheets of neoplastic cells are larger and more abundant than in grade-2 lesions, and the glandular pattern is scarcely evident.

As noted elsewhere, *myometrial invasion* is more apt to be associated with the more aggressive, grade-3 lesions. However, it also occurs in grade-1 and grade-2 lesions, especially those that are of advanced stage.

Spread

Endometrial carcinoma advances to involve the surrounding endometrium and, if allowed to progress, usually invades the myometrium to greater or lesser extent. When the entire thickness of the myometrium is penetrated, the tumor may appear under the serosa as nodules, single or clustered, that are yellow-white in color. As the tumor advances into the myometrium, lymph channels are opened, and extension to the regional lymph nodes follows the distribution of the lym-

FIG. 57-16.   Well-differentiated (grade 1) adenocarcinoma of the endometrium. (Gompel C, Silverberg SG: Pathology in Gynecology and Obstetrics, 3rd ed. Philadelphia, JB Lippincott, 1985)

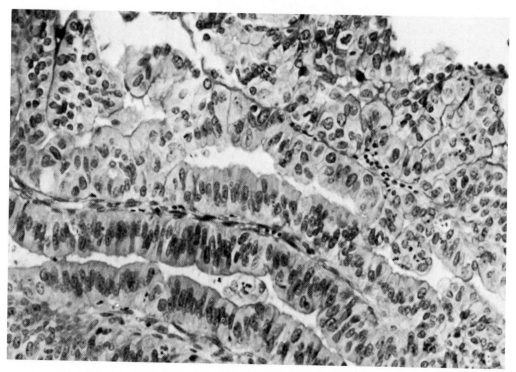

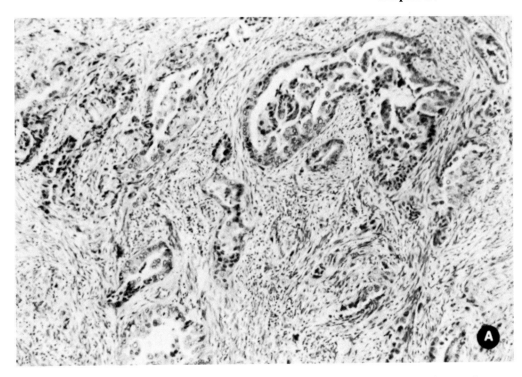

FIG. 57-17. Slightly differentiated (grade 2) adenocarcinoma of the endometrium. (Gompel C, Silverberg SG: Pathology in Gynecology and Obstetrics, 3rd ed. Philadelphia, JB Lippincott, 1985)

FIG. 57-18. Slightly differentiated adenocarcinoma of the endometrium; detail of a gland. (Gompel C, Silverberg SG: Pathology in Gynecology and Obstetrics, 3rd ed. Philadelphia, JB Lippincott, 1985)

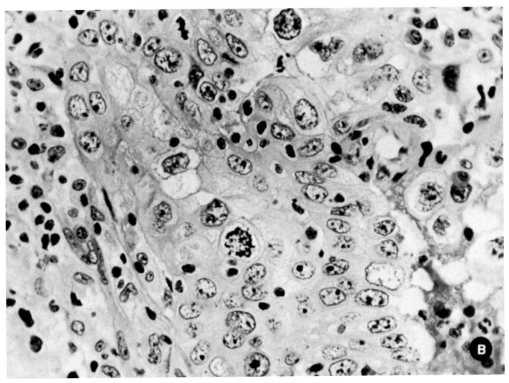

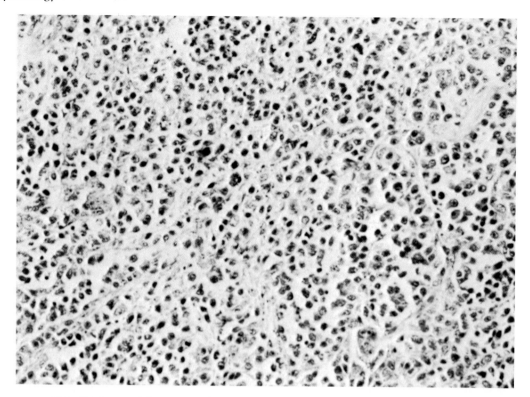

FIG. 57-19. Undifferentiated (grade 3) adenocarcinoma of the endometrium. (Gompel C, Silverberg SG: Pathology in Gynecology and Obstetrics, 3rd ed. Philadelphia, JB Lippincott, 1985)

phatic drainage from the corpus (Fig. 57-20). The ovary, which is quite close to the uterus along this route, is one of the principal sites of metastasis.

If the cancer extends inferiorly to involve the cervix (stage II), new routes for metastasis become available (see Fig. 56-13). Accordingly, in cases of stage-II cancer of the endometrium, therapy must also be directed to the areas that must be considered in invasive cancer of the cervix. (For example, radical hysterectomy, which is not helpful in cancer limited to the corpus, may be an important measure in dealing with endometrial cancer involving the cervix.)

Vascular spread is a late manifestation of endometrial cancer. It may account for certain remote metastases, as in the lungs and liver.

Seeding from spill of viable tumor cells may follow spontaneous perforation of the uterus, with resulting implants in various portions of the pelvic or upper abdominal peritoneum. Malignant cells may also find their way to the vagina; implants on the intact vaginal mucosa are extremely unusual, but cancerous cells are sometimes identified on a Papanicolaou smear.

Diagnosis

Abnormal uterine bleeding is the most important symptom of endometrial cancer. Certainly, any patient with uterine bleeding after the menopause must be evaluated for endometrial cancer, even though only 20% of these patients are found to have a genital malignancy. As age increases there is an increasing likelihood that postmenopausal bleeding is due to endometrial cancer. The perimenopausal patient with bleeding must also be critically evaluated. Women at this age may attribute abnormal bleeding to the approaching menopause. However, the menstrual periods during this time of life should become progressively lighter and less frequent. Any other type of bleeding must be evaluated for an adenocarcinoma of the endometrium. Endometrial adenocarcinoma in many instances is more difficult to identify in the premenopausal patient. Heavy and prolonged menstrual periods as well as intermenstrual spotting may be indicative of a cancer, and endometrial sampling is advised. Most younger patients with endometrial cancer are obese and in many instances considerably so. Irregular bleeding in such patients is also an indication for endometrial sampling.

The routine cervical Papanicolaou smear is much less helpful in detecting endometrial cancer than in diagnosing early cervical disease; only one third to one half of patients with endometrial cancer have abnormal Papanicolaou smears on routine screening. However, if malignant cells indicative of adenocarcinoma do appear on the routine Papanicolaou smear, further investigation is indicated.

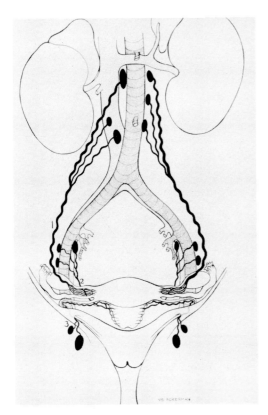

FIG. 57-20. Schematic representation of lymphatics of uterine corpus showing (*1*) uteroovarian pedicle, (*2*) external iliac pedicle, and (*3*) round-ligament pedicle leading to inguinal lymph nodes. Del Regato JA, Spjut HJ: Ackerman and Del Regato's Cancer Diagnosis, Treatment and Prognosis, 5th ed. St Louis, CV Mosby, 1977)

Historically, the fractional dilatation and curettage has been the definitive procedure for ruling out endometrial cancer. However, outpatient procedures have been suggested as an alternative for over half a century. Biopsy curettage of the endometrial cavity may be performed by using small curettes or suction instruments. The overall accuracy of the curette biopsy approaches 90%, and that of vacuum curettage approaches 100%. One advantage of the vacuum technique appears to be its ability to diagnose precursor lesions. Cytologic sampling of the endometrial cavity, when used independently, has not been as successful as the biopsy technique. Some investigators have suggested combining cytologic and histologic evaluation of the endometrial cavity as the ideal method of evaluating abnormal uterine bleeding. Endocervical curettage at the same time rules out cervical involvement and obviates the need for fractional curettage. Any cytologic or histologic abnormality short of invasive cancer mandates formal fractional curettage to rule out a small focus of invasive disease. All patients in whom symptoms persist despite normal cytology and outpatient biopsy should have a fractional curettage as well.

Staging

As in other cancers, staging of endometrial carcinoma is intended to provide a measure of prognosis, and it is essential in designing therapy. It also enables comparison of the effectiveness of various therapeutic protocols both within a particular institution and in different institutions. The FIGO staging of endometrial cancer is shown in Table 57-1. Endocervical curettage is an essential part of staging, since it is needed to differentiate stage I from stage II. (Curettage is sometimes misleading, and it may be impossible to determine whether the cervix is involved except by examination of the hysterectomy specimen.) Routine hematologic studies and clotting profiles are obtained in all patients. The preliminary evaluation, before therapy, is completed by chest x-ray, ECG, intravenous urogram, and metabolic profiles; other studies are omitted unless specifically indicated.

Unlike ovarian cancer (which is staged after *all* of the data are assembled, including the results of abdominal exploration, peritoneal washings, and appropriate biopsies), carcinoma of the endometrium is staged according to the clinical findings *before* any therapeutic measures are taken. In this context, an endometrial cancer assigned to stage I before laparotomy would remain in this stage even if laparotomy disclosed metastases in the ovary; however, a presumed stage-I lesion would immediately be transferred to stage IV if pulmonary metastases were found on the preoperative chest x-ray film. The value of staging as a predictor of prognosis in endometrial cancer is compromised to an extent because of the large number of cases (approximately 75% of all cases of endometrial cancer) that are categorized into stage I. As noted later, this is a very heterogeneous group, and the outlook for a given patient may be greatly altered by a number of factors that are not taken into account in determining the stage of the lesion.

Grading provides a measure of the aggressiveness of the tumor, and it is an essential part of the staging of stage-I lesions. FIGO now recognizes three grades. The higher the grade, the more rapid is the clinical course and the higher is the incidence of myometrial invasion and metastases (Table 57-2). The decision as to grade is made by examination of the curettings.

Prognostic Factors

There are several factors that affect the outlook for a given case of endometrial cancer. They also may have a direct bearing on the selection of therapy.

Stage and Grade of Tumor

The higher the stage of a particular lesion, the poorer is the outlook (Table 57-3). As noted earlier, grading provides a measure of the aggressiveness or virulence of a tumor. As noted in Table 57-3, the higher grades in both IA- and IB-lesions are accompanied by a significantly higher incidence of lymph-node metastasis.

Table 57-1
FIGO Staging of Endometrial Carcinoma

Stage	Description
Stage I	The carcinoma is confined to the corpus
IA	The length of the uterine cavity is 8 cm or less
IB	The length of the uterine cavity is more than 8 cm
	Stage I cases should be subgrouped with regard to the histologic type of adenocarcinoma as follows:
	G1: Highly differentiated adenomatous carcinoma
	G2: Differentiated adenomatous carcinoma with partly solid areas
	G3: Predominantly solid or entirely undifferentiated carcinoma
Stage II	The carcinoma involves the corpus and cervix
Stage III	The carcinoma extends outside the corpus but not outside the true pelvis (it may involve the vaginal wall or the parametrium but not the bladder or rectum)
Stage IV	The carcinoma involves the bladder or rectum or extends outside the pelvis

G, tumor grade.

Table 57-2
Risk of Lymph Node Metastasis, Deep Muscle Invasion, and Recurrence in Stage-I Endometrial Cancer by Tumor Grade

Grade	Lymph Node Metastasis	Deep Muscle Invasion	Recurrence
1	2%	4%	4%
2	11%	15%	15%
3	27%	39%	42%

Table 57-3
Pelvic and Aortic Node Metastasis in Stage-I Endometrial Carcinoma by Tumor Grade

Stage and Grade	Pelvic Metastasis	Aortic Metastasis*
IA		
Grade 1	1/63 (1.6%)	1/46 (2.2%)
Grade 2	5/45 (11.1%)	4/31 (12.9%)
Grade 3	4/22 (18.2%)	4/17 (23.5%)
IB		
Grade 1	1/30 (3.3%)	0/24 (0.0%)
Grade 2	5/43 (11.6%)	2/23 (8.7)
Grade 3	7/19 (36.8%)	6/16 (37.5%)

* Indicates only patients whose paraaortic nodes were sampled.

Age

Younger patients tend to have have early, well-differentiated lesions without myometrial invasion, and are apt to be in better general health than older patients. Older patients may have some intercurrent chronic disease, and tend to have more advanced, poorly differentiated lesions with greater myometrial invasion. In addition, immunocompetence may be reduced with advancing age. It therefore follows that the outlook is usually better when the disease occurs in younger women. Also, in some older patients with debilitating intercurrent disease, rigorous definitive therapy may be impossible, making it necessary to resort to palliative rather than curative measures.

Pathologic Subtypes of Adenocarcinoma

Prognosis may be altered in some of the pathologic subtypes of endometrial cancer (Table 57-4). In *adenoacanthoma* (adenocarcinoma with a benign squamous component), reports differ as to the outlook; current consensus is that prognosis is the same as for "pure" adenocarcinoma, varying only with the grade of the adenomatous component (Fig. 57-21). The outlook in *adenosquamous carcinoma* (Fig. 57-22), in which the squamous component also shows evidence of malignancy, appears to be less favorable than in pure adenocarcinoma and, like adenoacanthoma, to depend on the grade of the adenomatous component. Although more data are needed, it has been suggested that this lesion has a rather poorer prognosis than simple adenocarcinoma: its virulence (as judged by grade, tendency to vascular invasion, and extrauterine extension) is greater; its course is more rapid; and the lesions are usually more advanced at the time of detection. Although unusual, *clear cell carcinoma* has a generally poor outlook: the lesion tends to occur in the elderly, often in an advanced form. *Papillary carcinoma of the*

Table 57-4

Five-Year Survival Rates in Patients with Stage-I Endometrial Cancer by Histologic Subtype (I)

Subtype	Number of Patients	Survival Rate (%)
Adenoacanthoma	192	87.5
Adenocarcinoma	501	79.8
Papillary	34	67.6
Adenosquamous	49	53.1
Clear cell	43	44.2

endometrium is also unusual, and there are few reports in the literature. Prognosis appears to be intermediate between that of pure adenocarcinoma and clear cell carcinoma. So-called *secretory adenocarcinoma* is another rare subtype and occurs as a well-differentiated adenocarcinoma with secretory changes. The prognosis is much the same as that of pure adenocarcinoma.

Uterine Size

FIGO recognizes uterine size as a prognostic factor in endometrial cancer. However, there is not full agreement that uterine size per se is necessarily related to prognosis. Uterine enlargement that is due only to en-

dometrial cancer is obviously an unfavorable factor. However, if it is due largely to fibroids or adenomyosis, then mere size would appear to be irrelevant.

Myometrial Invasion

When the tumor invades the myometrium, the likelihood of involvement of both the myometrial vasculature and the lymphatics is increased (Table 57-5). Accordingly, the mere presence of myometrial invasion causes the prognosis to be less favorable.

Peritoneal Cytology

If the tumor appears to be confined to the uterus, the presence of malignant cells in the washings is an important prognostic sign. Immediately after the abdomen is opened and before any manipulation is done, 100 ml normal saline is distributed about the pelvis, aspirated, and sent to the laboratory for cytologic examination.

Lymph Node Metastasis

Pelvic lymph node metastases are present in approximately 10% of stage-I cases of carcinoma of the endometrium. The incidence of metastasis to para-aortic nodes in stage I is also approximately 10%. However, since total abdominal hysterectomy and bilateral sal-

FIG. 57-21. Adenoacanthoma of the endometrium. (Gompel C, Silverberg SG: Pathology in Gynecology and Obstetrics, 3rd ed. Philadelphia, JB Lippincott, 1985)

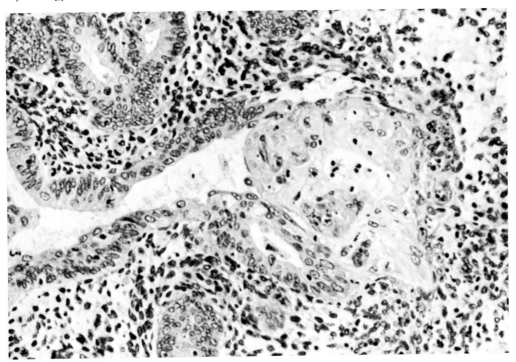

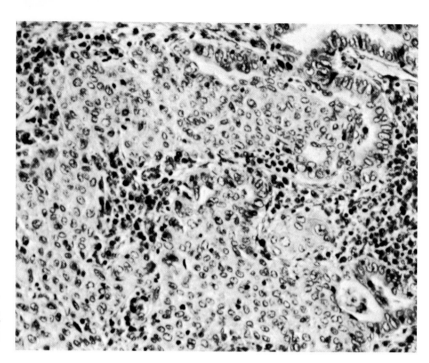

FIG. 57-22. Mixed adenosquamous carcinoma of the endometrium. (Gompel C, Silverberg SG: Pathology in Gynecology and Obstetrics, 3rd ed. Philadelphia, JB Lippincott, 1985)

pingo-oophorectomy have long been considered sufficient therapy for stage-I lesions, the lymph nodes are not routinely evaluated. The estimates, therefore, may be too low. The incidence of lymph node involvement correlates well with stage and grade of the tumor, depth of myometrial invasion, and location of the lesion within the uterus. In stage-II carcinoma of the endometrium, lymph node metastases are present in approximately 35% of cases.

Adnexal Metastasis

Occult microscopic adnexal metastases (usually in the ovary) are present in approximately 10% of patients with clinical stage-I disease. Adnexal involvement correlates well with depth of myometrial invasion and level of the primary lesion in the uterus. The incidence of positive peritoneal washings and lymph node metastasis is higher in the presence of adnexal metastasis, and the prognosis is less favorable.

Significance of the Prognostic Factors

As noted earlier, the current FIGO staging of endometrial cancer does not take into account the presence of extrauterine metastases unless they are diagnosed before any therapeutic measures are taken. It is therefore evident that the stage-I cases are a heterogeneous group, and that the mere designation of a lesion as stage I gives no indication either of the extent of the disease or the outlook for a given case. It is hoped that the FIGO committees that are concerned with staging will recognize this important defect and will adjust the method of staging to conform to that of ovarian cancer, in which *all* data bearing on the extent of the disease are taken into account. In the meantime, in order to arrive at a prediction of the course of a given case of stage-I disease, one is left with consideration of the aforementioned prognostic factors as they may bear upon the outlook. In an effort to determine the relative importance of these factors, a combined study of 222 stage-I lesions was made by the gynecologic oncology divisions of Duke University, the University of Mississippi, and the University of Southern California. Pelvic lymph nodes were sampled in all cases, and aortic lymph nodes were sampled in 157 cases. Among these patients, the following factors were found to correlate directly with the incidence of extrauterine metastases to adnexa or lymph nodes and, consequently, with survival: depth of the

Table 57-5
Rate of Pelvic and Aortic Node Metastasis from Endometrial Cancer by Extent of Invasion

Maximal Invasion	Pelvic Metastasis	Aortic Metastasis*
Endometrium only	2/92 (2.1%)	1/68 (1.4%)
Superficial muscle	4/80 (5.0%)	5/55 (9.0%)
Intermediate muscle	3/17 (17.6%)	1/8 (12.5%)
Deep muscle	14/33 (42.4%)	10/26 (38.4%)

* Indicates only patients whose para-aortic nodes are sampled.

uterine cavity; grade of the lesion; extent of the myometrial invasion; presence of malignant cells in the peritoneal washings; and the level of the lesion in the corpus uteri—the lower the lesion in the uterine cavity, the higher the incidence of metastases in the adnexa or lymph nodes. When these factors are considered it is apparent that some patients in stage I are at very low risk; for others, depending on the weight of the variable factors, the risk is very high indeed.

Treatment

The early literature dealing with the treatment of endometrial cancer is extensive. It is also confusing, perhaps especially so because some series of cases must have been weighted with greater or lesser numbers of risk factors that were not taken into account in evaluating the results. The names of Cullen, Kelly, Healy, and Heyman are prominent in this early literature, and their varied management of endometrial cancer foreshadowed the differences that were to follow for many years. In the intervening years, several different regimens were recommended. Recognizing that the lymph nodes are often involved in endometrial cancer, Javert and R. G. Douglas recommended hysterectomy, bilateral salpingo-oophorectomy, and pelvic lymphadenectomy if abdominal exploration revealed no metastases; selective lymphadenectomy was advised if obvious metastases were found, since this information might help in assigning prognosis. In a later review of the M. D. Anderson experience, Rutledge concluded that the low (10% to 12%) incidence of nodal disease in stage I disease did not justify routine lymphadenectomy; but he did suggest that selective lymphadenectomy may be important in determining adjunctive therapy for patients at greater risk for nodal disease (*i.e.,* those with grade-2 or grade-3 lesions and those showing myometrial invasion).

Surgery

In stage-I lesions, most agree that the details of the surgical procedure should be based on the grade of the lesion, as determined preoperatively from examination of the curettings. In stage-I, grade-1 lesions, total abdominal hysterectomy, bilateral salpingo-oophorectomy, and cytologic examination of peritoneal washings are considered sufficient. In stage-I, grade-2 and grade-3 patients, who are at much higher risk, selective pelvic and para-aortic lymphadenectomy are also performed to determine the need for adjunctive therapy. Management in stage-1 lesions is summarized in Figure 57-23.

Removing the uterus as part of the initial surgery has the special advantage that one can verify that indeed one is dealing with stage-II disease; at fractional curettage, the finding of malignant tissue in the endocervix is sometimes merely spill from the lesion higher in the uterus, giving the spurious implication that the cervix is involved. In a retrospective review, Onsrud found that of 174 cases originally considered to be stage II, the hysterectomy specimen showed the cervix to be involved in only 56% of the cases.

After surgery, a sample of the tumor should be sent for assay of estrogen and progesterone receptors. This information may be of benefit if progestin or chemo-

FIG. 57-23. Primary surgical management of stage I adenocarcinoma of the endometrium. ^{32}P, radioactive phosphorus. (DiSaia PJ, Creasman WT: Clinical Gynecologic Oncology. St. Louis, CV Mosby Co., 1984. Reproduced by permission)

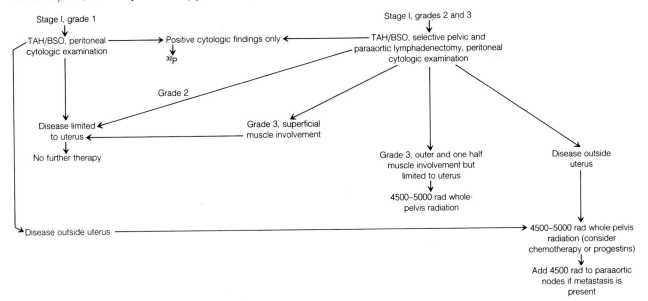

therapy should be needed later to deal with any recurrent (see below).

Adjunctive Therapy

RADIATION.   Since the early 1900s, radiation in one form or another has played an important role in the treatment of cancer of the endometrium. Its exact position is still unsettled, and the number of suggested methods approaches the number of articles written on the subject. The articles of Jones, Rutledge, and Patterson are helpful in bringing the various attitudes into perspective. The several options and techniques are discussed in Chapter 62, including the preoperative application of radium, postoperative external radiation, the timing of hysterectomy after radiation, the postoperative application of radium to the vaginal vault, and the radiation treatment of recurrent endometrial cancer.

A suggested protocol for the treatment of stage-I lesions, including the position of radiation, is shown in Figure 57-23. If pathologic review of the surgical specimen reveals occult cervical disease that was not appreciated earlier, then postoperative radiation is given in the same manner as for stage-I, grade-2 and grade-3 lesions. Equivalent radiation is also used for stage-II lesions if pelvic lymphadenectomy was not performed.

PROGESTINS.   Progestins have been used for many years in the treatment of recurrent endometrial cancer, and approximately a third of patients respond favorably. Patients with well-differentiated tumors have a higher response rate than those with moderately or poorly differentiated lesions. Recently, the role of specific estrogen/progesterone receptors in recurrent endometrial cancer has been evaluated. Receptor content appears to vary from tumor to tumor, and both estrogen and progesterone receptors appear in higher concentrations in well differentiated tumors than in those that are poorly differentiated. Although the exact role of receptors in management is not clear, preliminary data suggest that responsiveness of recurrent tumor to progestins is related to the content of estrogen and progesterone receptors in the tumor; if both receptors are present the likelihood of a favorable response is good regardless of tumor grade or extent or presence of other unfavorable prognostic factors; if the concentration of receptors is low, it is unlikely that the recurrent tumor will respond to progestins.

It is important that regardless of the apparent response or the lack of it, the initial series be continued for 12 weeks; in some patients at least this length of time is required before any response can be noted.

For reasons that are not apparent, progestins appear not to be helpful in the primary management of endometrial cancer. Prophylactic progestins are therefore not recommended. However, the question does arise whether their selective use in patients at special risk for recurrence could be helpful if estrogen/progesterone receptor status of the tumor were taken into account.

CHEMOTHERAPY.   Kauppila has recently provided evidence that the response to combined cytotoxic chemotherapy may also be a function of estrogen/progesterone receptor status of the tumor: patients with low values for estrogen or progesterone receptor or both had a significantly more favorable response to this therapy than did those with higher receptor values. Additional data are needed, but the study does provide new emphasis that receptor assay may be extremely important in determining optimal therapy for this group of patients.

In general, the effects of cytotoxic agents in recurrent endometrial cancer have been disappointing. Adriamycin is considered to be the treatment of choice for this tumor, yet only about 10% of patients so treated have had a completely favorable response; survival of those who had only a partial response was the same as for those who had no response. Cis-platinum, as a single chemotherapeutic agent, has been reported to show activity in this tumor, but the reported experience is very limited.

A large, prospective randomized study was carried out under the aegis of the Gynecologic Oncology Group, in which the combinations of melphalan, 5-fluorouracil, and megace were evaluated against the combination of Adriamycin, 5-fluorouracil, cyclophosphamide (Cytoxan), and megace. An objective response occurred in approximately one third of both treated groups; however, the favorable response continued for only about six months, and the mean survival for both groups was approximately ten months. Moreover, the toxicity from both regimens was appreciable. One concludes that the optimal drug or combination of drugs for this disease has yet to be determined.

OTHER MALIGNANCIES OF THE CORPUS UTERI

Sarcomas of the uterus are rare, constituting only 3% to 5% of all uterine tumors. These lesions arise primarily from two tissues: endometrial sarcomas from endometrial glands and stroma, and leiomyosarcomas from the uterine muscle itself. Other sarcomas, such as the angiosarcoma and fibrosarcoma, arise in supporting tissues. A classification of these tumors is shown in Table 57-6. The tumors that are "pure" are composed of one cell type only, whereas mixed tumors have more than one cell type. Homologous tumors contain tissue elements that are indigenous to the uterus, whereas heterologous tumors are defined as those that contain tissue elements foreign to the uterus, such as rhabdomyosarcomas or chondrosarcomas.

Patients with sarcomas are usually postmenopausal. Leiomyosarcomas appear most frequently in patients in their mid-50s, whereas mixed mesodermal sarcomas (MMS) and endometrial sarcomal sarcomas (ESS) most commonly occur in patients 10 years older. In patients with uterine sarcomas, an abdominal mass and pain are

Table 57-6
Ober Classification of Uterine Sarcomas

Type	Homologous	Heterologous
Pure	Stromal sarcoma (endolymphatic stromal myosis)	Rhabdomyosarcoma
	Leiomyosarcoma	Chondrosarcoma
	Angiosarcoma	Osteosarcoma
	Fibrosarcoma	Liposarcoma
Mixed	Carcinosarcoma	Mixed müllerian tumors (mixed mesodermal tumor)

(Di Saia PJ, Morrow CP, Townsend DE: Invasive Cancer of the Endometrium. In Quilligan EJ (ed): Synopsis of Gynecologic Oncology. New York, John Wiley & Sons, 1975)

frequent occurrences. An enlarging uterus is common; in the postmenopausal woman this should not be considered to be a myomatous uterus, and a sarcoma must be ruled out. Vaginal bleeding may occur, and friable, polypoid mass may extend through the dilated cervix.

When symptoms of this nature are present, histologic evaluation of the uterus is warranted. Tissue, of course, is readily available if a tumor protrudes through the cervix, but if it is a leiomyosarcoma, the lesion is usually high in the uterus. About 50% of all uterine sarcomas are clinical stage I. However, as many as one third of these patients are found to have extrauterine disease at the time of surgery.

Leiomyosarcoma

The diagnosis of leiomyosarcoma is made histologically mainly by the mitotic count of the tumor. The so-called cellular myomas and bizarre leiomyomas may appear to be malignant, but if there are fewer than 5 mitoses per 10 high-power fields, the lesion is considered to be benign. Those with more than 10 mitoses per 10 high-power fields are, in fact, malignant. Some investigators feel that 5 to 10 mitoses indicates malignancy, while others are somewhat more reserved in their evaluation. The main reason for the variation in this determination is that very few patients have 5 to 10 mitoses per 10 high-power fields. If there is vascular invasion or if disease is found outside the uterus, the prognosis is very poor.

Mixed Müllerian Sarcoma

Patients included in this category are those with homologous malignant mixed müllerian tumors, and heterologous malignant mixed müllerian tumors. Both a sarcoma and a carcinoma must be identified. Tumors in the heterologous group must also have histologic evidence of tissue not normally found in the uterus, such as bone, cartilage, or skeletal muscle.

These tumors tend to be aggressive, and they spread early to regional lymph nodes and adjacent tissues. Microscopic invasion of blood vessels and lymphatic channels is common. As many as one third of patients with stage-I mixed müllerian sarcomas have metastasis to the pelvis lymph nodes. Hematogenous spread, particularly to the lung and liver, is common.

Endometrial Stromal Sarcoma

Endometrial stromal tumors are the rarest of the sarcomas. They are usually divided into two groups: *endolymphatic stromal myosis* and *endometrial stromal sarcoma*. The former usually follows an indolent course and is considered a low-grade stromal sarcoma. It can have an infiltrative growth pattern, and can project from the cut surface in a wormlike fashion that may also be seen in blood vessels of the broad ligament. Microscopically, there is very little cellular atypia and few, if any, mitoses. The clinical course is very slowly progressive, and treatment by surgery alone is adequate. Endometrial stromal sarcoma, on the other hand, has a more aggressive course with frequent and early metastases and a poor prognosis. The differentiation between these two lesions depends on the number of mitoses per 10 high-power fields. Usually 10 mitoses per 10 high-power fields should be present in order to categorize the tumor as endometrial stromal sarcoma.

Treatment

Total abdominal hysterectomy and bilateral salpingo-oophorectomy should be considered the first line of treatment of patients with uterine sarcoma. Because of the propensity of these lesions to metastasize to the pelvic or para-aortic lymph nodes, some authorities have suggested selective sampling in these areas. It should be noted that even in clinical stage-I disease, a large number of these patients will at the time of surgery have disease outside of the uterus; in such cases the prognosis is extremely grave. The value of radiation therapy either preoperatively or postsurgery is still under debate. Some researchers have found fewer local recurrences when radiation is given; however, there does not appear to be a difference in overall survival between those treated with surgery only and those who have had surgery and radiation. This is true whether the lesion is Stage I or more advanced. There also does not appear to be any difference in survival between the different cell types when corrections for stage of disease have been made.

The treatment failure rate appears to be higher in mixed müllerian sarcoma and endometrial stromal sarcoma than in leiomyosarcoma. When recurrences do appear, they are apt to be multiple, and isolated pelvic occurrence is very rare. These recurrences are extremely difficult to treat.

Because of the poor prognosis of sarcomas, adjuvant chemotherapy has been attempted. A large prospective randomized study was conducted by the Gynecologic Oncology Group (GOG). Patients with stage-I and stage-II sarcoma in which all gross tumor was removed were treated with surgery alone, or surgery plus doxorubicin (Adriamycin). No statistical difference in progression-free interval or survival was found between the two groups.

Patients with recurrent disease do poorly. The GOG evaluated doxorubicin versus doxorubicin plus DTIC in 240 patients with stage-III, stage-IV, and recurrent sarcomas of the uterus. No difference in response was noted between the two regimens. Patients with leiomyosarcomas did have a significantly longer survival than those with the other cell types, but there was no real advantage for either regimen. In another GOG protocol, doxorubicin with and without cyclophosphamide was evaluated in 104 patients with primary stage-III, stage-IV, or recurrent sarcoma of the uterus. Response rate was identical for both treatment arms, and the median survival was less than one year. Additional regimens are being evaluated, but optimistic results are lacking.

REFERENCES AND RECOMMENDED READING

Badib AO, Vongtama V, Kurohaha SS et al: Radiotherapy in the treatment of sarcomas of the corpus uteri. Cancer 24:724, 1969

Creasman WT, McCarty KS Sr, McCarty KS Jr: Clinical correlation of estrogen, progesterone binding proteins in human endometrial adenocarcinoma. Obstet Gynecol 55:363, 1980

Creasman WT, Boronow RC, Morrow CP et al: Adenocarcinoma of the endometrium; its metastatic lymph node potential: A preliminary report. Gynecol Oncol 4:239, 1976

Creasman WT, Weed JC Jr: Cancer of the Endometrium. Current Problems in Cancer 5(2). Chicago, Year Book Medical Publishers, 1980

DiSaia PJ, Castro JR, Rutledge FN: Mixed mesodermal sarcoma of the uterus. Am J Roentgenol 117:632, 1973

DiSaia PJ, Morrow CP, Boronow RC et al: Endometrial sarcoma: Lymphatic spread pattern. Am J Obstet Gynecol 130:104, 1978

Donegan WL, Wharton JT: Carcinoma of the endometrium: A survey of practice. Am Coll Surg Bull 69:5, 1984

Frick HC II, Munnell EW, Richart RM et al: Carcinoma of endometrium. Am J Obstet Gynecol 115:663, 1973

Greenblatt RB, Stoddard LB: The estrogen-cancer controversy. J Am Geriatr Soc 26:1, 1978

Heyman J: The so-called Stockholm method and the results of treatment of uterine cancer with Radiumhemmet. Acta Radiol 16:129, 1935

Javert C, Douglas R: Treatment of endometrial carcinoma. Am J Roentgenol 75:580, 1956

Jones HW: Treatment of adenocarcinoma of the endometrium. Obstet Gynecol Surv 30:147, 1975

Kauppila A, Janne O, Kujansuu E et al: Treatment of advanced endometrial adenocarcinoma with combined cytotoxic therapy. Cancer 46:2162, 1980

Kempson RL, Bari W: Uterine sarcoma: Classification, diagnosis, and prognosis. Hum Pathol 1:331, 1970

Kohorn EI: Gestagens and endometrial carcinoma. Gynecol Oncol 4:398, 1976

Lewis B, Stallworthy JA, Cowdell R: Adenocarcinoma of the body of the uterus. J Obstet Gynaecol Br Comm 77:343, 1970

Norris HJ, Taylor HB: Mesenchymal tumors of the uterus. I: A clinical and pathological study of 53 endometrial stromal tumors. Cancer 19:755, 1966

Omura GA, Major FJ, Blessing JA et al: A randomized study of Adriamycin with and without dimethyl riazenoimidazole carboxamide in advanced uterine sarcoma. Cancer 52:626, 1983

Onsrud M, Kolstad P, Normann T: Postoperative external pelvic irradiation in carcinoma of the corpus stage I: A controlled clinical trial. Gynecol Oncol 4:222, 1976

Onsrud N, Aalders J, Abeler V et al: Endometrial carcinoma with cervical involvement (stage II). Prognostic factors in value of combined radiological surgical treatment. Gynecol Oncol 13:76, 1982

Patterson E, Spratt D, Tomkiewicz Z et al: Management of stage I carcinoma of the uterus. Obstet Gynecol 59:755, 1982

Perez CA, Askin F, Baglan RJ et al: Effects of irradiation on mixed müllerian tumors of the uterus. Cancer 43:1274, 1979

Piver MS, Barlow JJ, Lurain JR et al: Medroxyprogesterone acetate (Depo-Provera) versus hydroxyprogesterone caproate (Delalutin) in women with metastatic endometrial adenocarcinoma. Cancer 45:268, 1980

Rutledge FN: The role of radical hysterectomy in adenocarcinoma of the endometrium. Gynecol Oncol 2:331, 1974

Salazar OM, Bonfiglio TA, Patten SF et al: Uterine sarcomas: Analysis of failures with special emphasis on the use of adjuvant radiation therapy. Cancer 42:1161, 1978

Salazar OM, Bonfiglio TA, Patten SF et al: Uterine sarcomas: Natural history, treatment and prognosis. Cancer 42:1152, 1978

Silverberg SG: Leiomyosarcoma of the uterus. Obstet Gynecol 38:613, 1971

Taylor HB, Norris HJ: Mesenchymal tumors of the uterus. IV: Diagnosis and prognosis of leiomyosarcomas. Arch Pathol 82:40, 1966

Thigpen JT, Buchsbaum HJ, Mangan C et al: Phase II trial of Adriamycin in treatment of advanced or recurrent endometrial carcinoma. Cancer Treat Rep 63:21, 1979

Underwood PB, Lutz MH, Kreutner A et al: Carcinoma of the endometrium: Radiation followed immediately by operation. Am J Obstet Gynecol 128:86, 1977

Lesions of the Fallopian Tube

James A. Merrill

58

BENIGN LESIONS

A variety of cysts and tumors arise in the pelvic supporting structures and fallopian tubes (oviducts). Such lesions are usually benign and originate from peritoneal inclusions or embryonic remnants. The embryologic development of the oviducts and broad ligament accounts for mesonephric and paramesonephric derivatives capable of causing cystic structures. The majority are small, multiple, not associated with any clinical syndrome, and without clinical significance. An awareness of them is important, however, because they are often encountered at the time of pelvic surgery, and intelligent management requires an appreciation of their nature. Occasionally a cystic structure in the broad ligament reaches sufficient size to be palpated or to produce symptoms from pressure on adjacent structures, twisting of a pedicle, rupture, or hemorrhage. Under these circumstances, the lesion is often mistakenly thought to be of ovarian origin. Surgical removal is required.

Cysts of the broad ligament are of mesonephric or paramesonephric origin. They may be intraligamentous or pedunculated, but the location is not diagnostic of origin. Most broad ligament cysts can be classified by the character of their lining epithelium. Pedunculated cysts of the broad ligament are common and are referred to as *hydatids of Morgagni* (Fig. 58-1). The cyst is small and translucent, with a long, slender pedicle attached near the fimbria of the oviduct, frequently bilaterally. It rarely exceeds 1 cm in diameter. Intraligamentous cysts may be small or may reach 10 cm to 15 cm or more in diameter. They are thin-walled and unilocular. These cysts are commonly referred to as *parovarian cysts* because of their location. The ovary is intact and separate from the cyst, and the oviduct is stretched across the circumference. If large, such intraligamentous cysts should be removed. Malignant change is rare and can

be ignored. The student is referred to the excellent review by Gardner and colleagues for further discussion of the microscopic pathology.

The most common tumorlike lesions of the oviduct are Walthard's cell rests (Figs. 58-2, 58-3). They are seen on the peritoneal surface of the oviduct and adjacent broad ligament as multiple, small (1 mm to 2 mm), glistening, soft, waxlike cysts. They are benign and probably arise from inclusions of surface celomic epithelium. At times, they must be differentiated from tubercles. This is usually possible because of their typical glistening, noninflamed appearance. Microscopic examination reveals subperitoneal nests of squamouslike epithelial cells, some of which show central cystic change.

Salpingitis isthmica nodosa is an uncommon lesion of the oviduct that is characterized by one or more nodular thickenings of the isthmus (Fig. 58-4). Microscopically, there is a thickening of the smooth muscle surrounding the isthmic lumen of the oviduct. Within the smooth muscle are discrete acini, or glandlike spaces, lined by immature tubal-type epithelium. Unlike the epithelium of the major portion of the oviduct, this epithelium tends to be cuboidal rather than columnar. The lesion can be distinguished easily from endometriosis of the oviduct. Opinions differ as to its genesis. Many consider it to be an aftermath of inflammation of the oviduct; others favor a congenital origin from embryonic rests. We believe that the lesion arises from downgrowth of the epithelium of the oviduct in a manner similar to that which occurs in adenomyosis. Salpingitis isthmica nodosa rarely requires treatment. Excision of the isthmic portion of the oviduct with microreanastomosis has been advocated in the treatment of infertility. The diagnosis may be suspected on hysterosalpingogram.

Accessory oviducts or diverticula of the oviducts are developmental anomalies that may be confused with

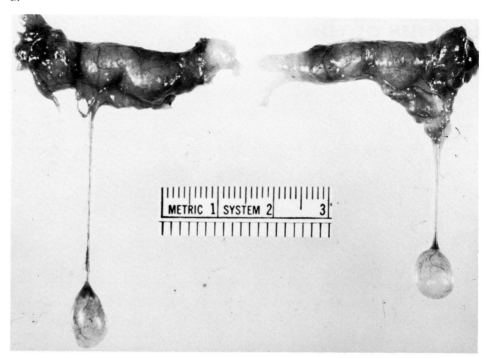

FIG. 58-1. Hydatids of Morgagni attached to mesosalpinx of each oviduct.

FIG. 58-2. Numerous Walthard's cell rests on surface of oviduct and mesosalpinx.

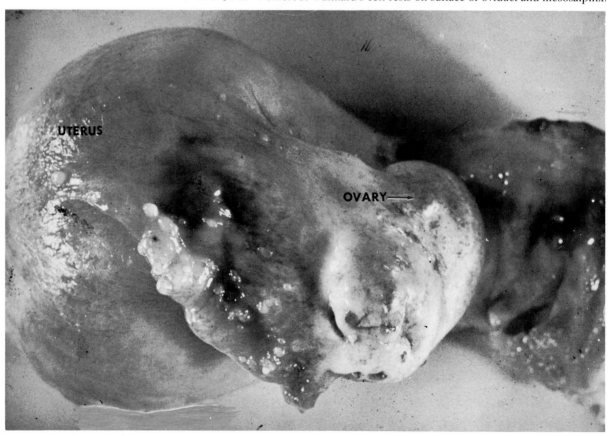

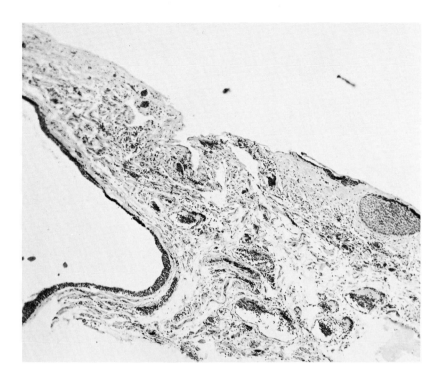

FIG. 58-3. Microscopic section of meso-salpinx showing Walthard's cell rests. One on surface is solid mass of cells; other shows cystic change.

FIG. 58-4. Microscopic section of oviduct with salpingitis isthmica nodosa. Central lumen is intact; smooth muscle oviduct wall contains numerous glandlike spaces.

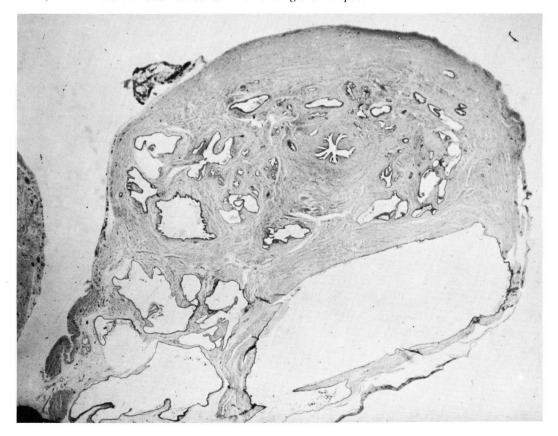

broad ligament cysts or salpingitis isthmica nodosa. The microscopic pattern of typical tubal plicae and epithelium is diagnostic.

Several rare benign tumors of the oviduct have been described: dermoid cysts, hemangiomas, lymphangiomas, leiomyomas, and adenomatoid tumors. The adenomatoid tumors are the most common and are usually small and circumscribed, confined to the muscular wall (Fig. 58-5). They are composed of small, glandlike spaces lined by cells of mesothelial, endothelial, or epithelial appearance. There is no agreement about their origin. They are usually incidental findings, and all such tubal lesions reported to date have been benign.

Myomas arise in the round ligament (Fig. 58-6). They commonly become pedunculated and pose the problems of treatment and differential diagnosis described in Chapter 57. In gross and microscopic appearance they resemble myomas of the uterus.

Adrenal rests are found in the broad ligament (Fig. 58-7). In a review of autopsy material from 98 infants and children, broad ligament or mesovarian adrenal rests were present in three. This is explained by the proximity of the anlage of the adrenals to the genital ducts. Adrenal rests may be grossly visible but are more often microscopic. They are small nodules that are firm, smooth, and yellow. Microscopic appearance is typical of adrenal cortical tissue. It is extremely rare that adrenal rests produce endocrine symptoms.

Endometriosis frequently involves the broad ligament, oviducts, and uterosacral ligaments. It is discussed in Chapter 55.

MALIGNANT LESIONS

Cancer of the fallopian tube is uncommon; it constitutes less than 1% of all cancer of the female genital tract. The recorded cases of cancer of the oviduct—less than 1000—suggest the probability of three cases per million women per year. Furthermore, this malignancy is difficult to diagnose. In at least two cases (Mitchell; Starr) very early tubal cancers were found accidentally on microscopic examination of tubal fragments resected for postpartum sterilization.

Suspected tumor of the ovary or uterus is the usual reason for surgery in the patient with cancer of the oviduct; in many cases, both tube and ovary are involved, and less often tube and endometrium. Thus, it may be difficult to decide which site is primary. It has been suggested that some of these multiple lesions represent multicentric foci of origin. As is true of other cancers, the success of treatment is directly correlated to the extent of the disease at the time of treatment. Unfortunately, because of the difficulty of diagnosis, many tubal neoplasma are diagnosed late.

More than 90% of the primary cancers of the oviduct are carcinoma. Leiomyosarcomas, mixed tumors, and trophoblastic tumors rarely arise in the oviduct.

FIG. 58-5. Microscopic section of adenomatoid tumor of oviduct.

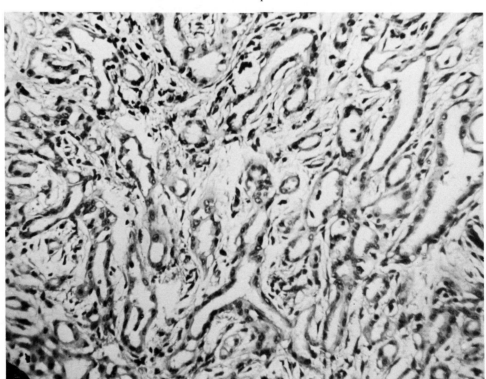

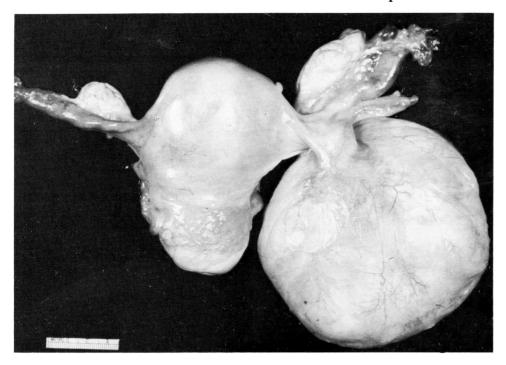

FIG. 58-6. Myoma of round ligament. Uterus, oviducts, and ovaries are normal.

FIG. 58-7. Section of ovary, mesosalpinx, and oviduct from newborn infant. Mesosalpinx contains well-defined adrenal rest surrounded by remnants of wolffian duct. (Merrill JA: Ovarian hilus cells. Am J Obstet Gynecol 78:1258, 1959)

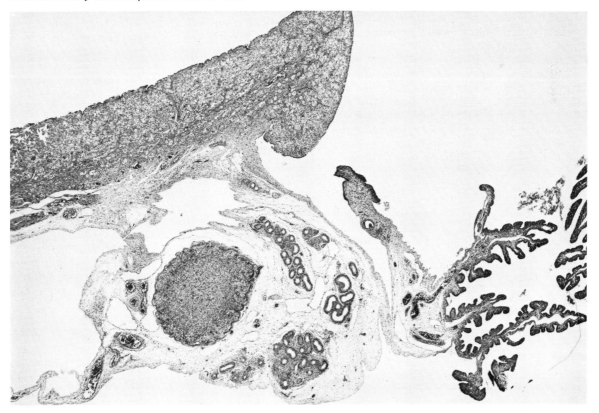

Primary Carcinoma

Most primary tubal carcinomas are papillary adenocarcinoma, although squamous cell carcinoma, carcinoma *in situ,* and even adenomatous hyperplasia, can arise from the tubal epithelium.

Age

The age reported for patients with primary tubal carcinoma ranges from 17 to 80 years. The highest incidence of this disease occurs during the fifth decade of life. Women with carcinoma of the oviduct are frequently infertile.

Symptoms

Symptoms are rare in patients with early tubal carcinoma. About 20% of all patients have no symptoms. In those who do have symptoms, the most common are vaginal discharge, abnormal vaginal bleeding, irregularities of menstruation, and pain. The discharge is often yellow or slightly blood-tinged (honey-colored). A classic, but rare, symptom of episodic vaginal discharge known as *hydrops tubae profluens* has been described with both carcinoma of the oviduct and hydrosalpinx. In this circumstance, cramping pelvic pain and an adnexal mass disappear with a sudden serous or serosanguineous discharge.

Diagnosis

An adnexal mass is the most common physical finding in a patient with tubal carcinoma. However, 50% of women have no palpable pelvic mass. Carcinoma of the fallopian tube is rarely diagnosed before surgery. Most tubal carcinomas are found in patients undergoing surgery for a preoperative diagnosis of ovarian neoplasm, uterine myoma, or tubo-ovarian inflammatory disease. Laparotomy may disclose a rare early lesion not suspected on the basis of preoperative pelvic examination. The triad of pain, discharge, and adnexal mass occurs in about 50% of patients. The possibility of carcinoma of the oviduct should be considered in a postmenopausal nulliparous woman with a serous or serosanguineous discharge and an adnexal mass. Some cases have been suspected when cytologic examination of vaginal smears repeatedly showed abnormal cells even though material obtained from cervical biopsies and endometrial curettings was normal. However, the reported accuracy of cytologic examination of vaginal smears as a diagnostic procedure for carcinoma of the oviduct is disappointingly low, varying from 0% to 60%.

Laparoscopy and hysterosalpingography have been suggested as aids in the diagnosis of carcinoma of the oviduct.

Pathology

At surgery, an oviduct harboring a carcinoma frequently resembles a subacutely or chronically infected tube with pyosalpinx or hydrosalpinx. The tumors are bilateral in 15% to 30% of cases. Ascites is a rare associated finding. Adhesions to adjacent peritoneal surfaces are often less tenacious than the adhesions usually associated with pelvic inflammatory disease. The appearance of the opened tube, packed with friable papillary excrescences, is characteristic. Less often there is a localized, soft, friable tumor mass. There may be soft, yellow areas of necrosis or soft, red-brown areas of hemorrhage. In some situations, the entire lumen is filled with tumor, some of which may protrude from the fimbriated end. The carcinoma in the oviduct may be continuous with an ovarian neoplasm. In these circumstances, it is impossible to say whether the tumor first appeared in the tube or the ovary.

The microscopic pattern is that of a papillary adenocarcinoma (Fig. 58-8). Well-differentiated tumors are composed of delicately branched processes covered by a thin layer of columnar epithelial cells. The pattern may resemble that of a papillary serous cystadenocarcinoma of the ovary. Less well-differentiated tumors have a trabecular or alveolar pattern. The muscular wall of the tube is usually invaded, and the tumor may completely fill the lumen of the tube and replace all normal tubal epithelium. For certain diagnosis of primary carcinoma of the oviduct, the lesion should be confined to the endosalpinx and there should be a microscopically identifiable transition between the anaplastic epithelium of the malignant neoplasm and the adjacent benign tubal epithelium (Fig. 58-9).

The adenomatous salpingitis that characterizes tuberculosis of the oviduct may, on occasion, be confused with tubal carcinoma. However, in the case of inflammation, the cellular characteristics of neoplasia are absent. The presence of typical granulomatous inflammation makes the diagnosis of malignancy doubtful.

Squamous carcinoma, adenoacanthoma, and transitional-cell carcinoma have been reported to occur in the tube.

Associated Disease

Because carcinoma of the oviduct grossly resembles hydrosalpinx and pyosalpinx, and because carcinoma of the tube is often found in association with healed or subacute salpingitis, it has been suggested that chronic inflammation may be a predisposing factor. The observation of a relatively high incidence of infertility among patients with carcinoma of the fallopian tube further suggests preexisting tubal disease in these patients. It is possible, of course, that the tubal inflammation seen at the time carcinoma of the oviduct is diagnosed is secondary to necrosis and infection within the tumor itself.

Spread

Carcinoma of the oviduct metastasizes by lymphatics to regional lymph nodes, by direct extension to adjacent pelvic viscera, and by seeding to omental and peritoneal surfaces. Involvement of para-aortic nodes was reported

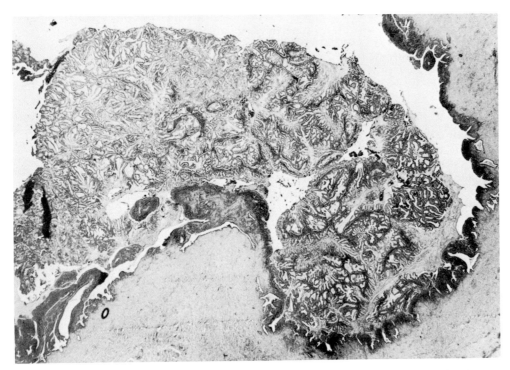

FIG. 58-8. Papillomatous growth pattern of primary adenocarcinoma of fallopian tube (×50).

FIG. 58-9. Early primary papillary adenocarcinoma of fallopian tube (×10).

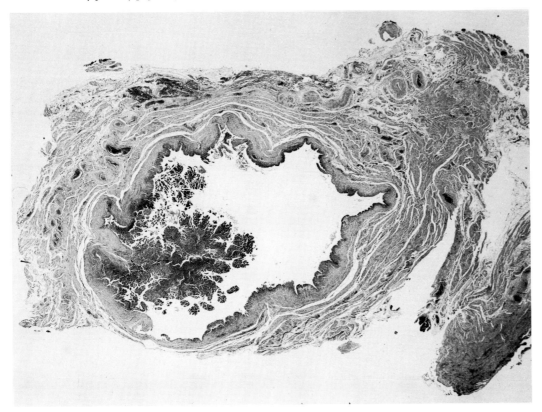

in one third of cases in one series (Tamimi). Distant metastasis is infrequent, and the biologic behavior is similar to that of epithelial cancer of the ovary. Peritoneal implants may occur with an intact tube, with the tubal lumen patent through the fimbriated end.

Staging

As in all malignant tumors, staging is essential for comparison of cases and evaluation of therapy. Because the *Fédération Internationale de Gynécologie et Obstetrique* (FIGO) has not yet addressed this question for tubal carcinoma, no uniform staging has been adopted. Several have suggested, and used, a staging system similar to that for carcinoma of the ovary. A simpler staging system, also used by several authors, is as follows:

Stage I: Carcinoma limited to the tube; no extension to the serosa
Stage II: Carcinoma extending to the tubal serosa or adjacent viscera
Stage III: Carcinoma extending beyond the pelvis, but still confined to the abdominal cavity
Stage IV: Extra-abdominal metastases

Treatment

The usual treatment for carcinoma of the oviduct is total abdominal hysterectomy, bilateral salpingo-oopherectomy, and omentectomy. Peritoneal cytology and pelvic and para-aortic lymph node sampling should be done for staging and prognosis. More extensive procedures than these may be indicated if the lesion has spread to adjacent organs or structures. The value of extensive procedures and cytoreductive surgery cannot be stated because they have not been performed often enough to permit valid assessment of the results. Postoperative adjunctive chemotherapy and, rarely, pelvic-abdominal external beam radiation are recommended. This course of treatment is given in a manner similar to that described in Chapter 59 for the treatment of ovarian epithelial cancer. Progestins and antiestrogens have been used with success. The endosalpinx and endometrium are functionally similar. Intraperitoneal insertion of colloidal isotopes has been used.

Prognosis

The prognosis for survival depends on the extent of the malignancy. If spread beyond the tube is grossly apparent, the prognosis is extremely poor. The five-year survival rates vary from 0% to 44%. Bilateral tubal carcinoma is associated with a poorer prognosis than is unilateral disease. There appears to be little correlation between prognosis and the microscopic differentiation of the tumor, although solid tumors seem to have a worse prognosis than papillary ones. The presence of tumor in capillarylike spaces correlates with lymph node metastasis.

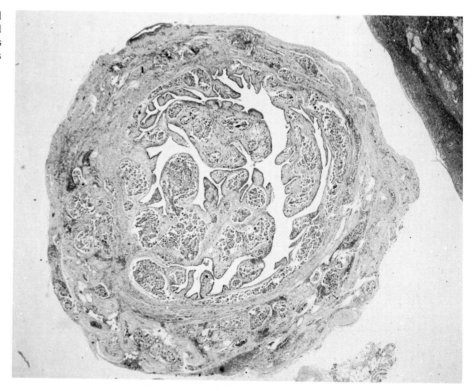

FIG. 58-10. Secondary tubal carcinoma showing intact tubal epithelium and carcinoma areas in lymphatics. Primary cancer was located in endometrium (×20).

Metastatic Cancer

Cancer metastatic to the oviducts occurs much more commonly than primary carcinoma. Indeed, metastasis or direct extension from lesions arising in the adjacent organs accounts for 80% to 90% of malignancies found in the oviduct. Most of these tumors originate in the ovary or uterus. Metastases from the breast or gastrointestinal tract also have been reported. Metastases may extend along the serosa, through subepithelial or subserosal lymphatics, or directly along the lumen of the endosalpinx. The histologic pattern, which shows conspicuous lymphatic involvement and intact tubal epithelium (Fig. 58-10), is easily distinguished from primary tubal carcinoma.

When both tube and ovary are involved, the salvage is worse than if only one or the other were involved, regardless of which was the primary site of the neoplasm.

Rare Malignant Tumors

Sarcoma

A few cases of primary sarcoma (usually leiomyosarcoma) of the oviduct have been reported. The prognosis is poor, similar to that for sarcomas elsewhere. Treatment primarily is surgical.

Mixed Müllerian Tumor

A primary, malignant, mixed müllerian tumor has occasionally been seen in the oviduct. The clinical findings and gross pathology are similar to those of primary adenocarcinoma of the oviduct. Microscopically, the lesions, which have been bilateral in one third of cases, are similar to tumors in the myometrium with various types of neoplastic immature connective tissue and epithelium. Treatment is similar to that for primary tubal carcinoma.

Trophoblastic Tumors

Rare primary tubal choriocarcinoma has been reported. The tumor presumably has followed ectopic tubal pregnancy. Success with chemotherapy is similar to that for gestational choriocarcinomas arising in the uterus.

REFERENCES AND RECOMMENDED READING

Anbrokh YM: Histological characteristics and questions concerning histogenesis of cancer of the fallopian tubes. Neoplasms 17:631, 1970

DeQueiroz AC, Roth LM: Malignant mixed Müllerian tumor of the fallopian tube. Report of a case. Obstet Gynecol 36: 554, 1970

Dowdeswell RH, Pratt–Thomas HR: Benign teratoma of the fallopian tube. Obstet Gynecol 39:52, 1972

Ebrahimi T, Okagaki T: Hemangioma of the fallopian tube. Am J Obstet Gynecol 115:864, 1973

Federman Q, Toker C: Primary transitional cell tumor of the uterine adnexa. Am J Obstet Gynecol 115:863, 1973

Gardner GH, Greene RR, Peckham B: Normal and cystic structures of the broad ligament. Am J Obstet Gynecol 55:917, 1948

Hertig AT, Gore H: Tumors of the Female Sex Organs, Part 4. Washington DC, Armed Forces Institute of Pathology, 1961

Mazzarella P et al: Teratoma of the uterine tube. A case report and review of the literature. Obstet Gynecol 39:381, 1972

Moore SW, Enterline HT: Significance of proliferative epithelial lesions of the uterine tube. Obstet Gynecol 45:385, 1975

Okagaki T, Richard RM: Neurilemoma of the fallopian tube. Am J Obstet Gynecol 106:929, 1970

Palomaki JF, Blair OM: Hilus cell rest of the fallopian tube. A case report. Obstet Gynecol 37:60, 1971

Roberts JA, Lifshitz S: Primary adenocarcinoma of the fallopian tube. Gynec Onc 13:301, 1982

Salazar H et al: Ultrastructure and observations on the histogenesis of mesotheliomas, "adenomatoid tumors," of the female genital tract. Cancer 29:141, 1972

Sedlis A: Carcinoma of the fallopian tube. Surg Clin N Am 58: 121, 1978

Starr AJ, Ruffalo EH, Shenoy BV et al: Primary carcinoma of the fallopian tube: A surprise finding in a postpartum tubal ligation. Am J Obstet Gynecol 132:344, 1978

Tamimi HK, Figge DC: Adenocarcinoma of the uterine tube: Potential for lymph node metastasis. Am J Obstet Gynecol 144:132, 1981

Woodruff JD, Pauerstein CJ: The Fallopian Tube. Baltimore, Williams & Wilkins, 1969

Young JA, Kossman CR, Green MR: Adenocarcinoma of the fallopian tube: Report of a case with an unusual pattern of metastasis and response to combination chemotherapy. Gynec Onc 17:238, 1984

Lesions of the Ovary

James A. Merrill
Charles Zaloudek
Fatteneh A. Tavassoli
Robert J. Kurman

59

Benign Lesions

James A. Merrill

Abnormalities of ovarian development result in an array of intersex problems and endocrine disorders. Abnormalities of ovarian function are associated with menstrual disorders and reproductive failure. Inflammatory disease of the ovary is uncommon, and usually it is associated with the more significant infections of the oviduct. These benign lesions are described in other chapters of this book. This chapter deals with abnormalities characterized by ovarian enlargement.

SIGNIFICANCE OF OVARIAN ENLARGEMENT

The consideration of ovarian neoplasms has always stirred great interest among gynecologists. The very history of modern gynecology begins with Ephraim McDowell's successful removal of a large ovarian tumor in 1809, which is described on page 19. This, the first successful removal of an abdominal tumor, was a landmark in abdominal surgery. Equally fascinating has been the wide variety of histologic patterns found in ovarian neoplasms and the corresponding array of clinical findings.

More than any other gland or organ in the body, the ovary has the potential of producing an unusual number of neoplasms of both epithelial and connective tissue origin. Knowledge of the physiology and anatomy of the ovarian cycle is required for correct evaluation of the pathologic nature of an ovarian enlargement, and the immediate treatment and ultimate prognosis depend upon the pathologic interpretation. The mature ovary is a complex gland consisting of different types of connective tissue as well as cells with specific differentiation and function. Moreover, the adult ovary contains embryonic remnants, in addition to cells, capable of differentiation into various morphologic and functional types. The cyclic growth, enlargement, and subsequent atresia of follicles form the basis for most nonneoplastic enlargements of the ovaries.

The embryonic gonads develop in the genital ridge, ventral to the mesonephros and adjacent to the primordial adrenal. In the ovary, these intimate relations result in embryonic rests that persist past fetal life. We should expect to find neoplasms in the ovary arising from these structures and, indeed, such tumors are present. The gonad develops from a mass of specialized mesenchyme. Differentiation of this mesenchyme results in the follicular apparatus of the ovary (granulosa and theca cells) and components of the tubular apparatus of the testis. This bipotential capacity of the embryonic gonad is best demonstrated in the ambiguous gonads of intersex patients. In the mature ovary this specialized mesenchyme persists as the ovarian cortical stroma and probably retains some of its original potential for differentiation, accounting for the hormone-producing, mesenchymomas composed of "female-directed" or "male-directed" cells. The surface epithelium of the ovary, so-called *germinal epithelium,* is derived from celomic epithelium and has the same potential for development as the primitive müllerian duct. Cystic neoplasms arising from these cells result in the most common of ovarian tumors, composed of various epithelia. The oocytes migrate to the embryonic gonad and exert an organizing effect on the stroma. These primordial germ cells retain a vast potential for differentiation, and an almost limitless variety of tissues arises from neoplastic growth of these cells.

These observations form the basis for the many theories of histogenesis of ovarian neoplasms.

Many ovarian neoplasms are asymptomatic and many functional cystic enlargements of the ovary are found, and unfortunately removed, incident to abdominal surgery for other indications. It is not uncommon for a surgeon operating for appendicitis to find an ovary that appears "cystic" or contains a "cyst." Failure to understand the significance of such findings results in sacrifice of the ovary or a portion thereof. Efforts should be made to diagnose true ovarian neoplasms early and at the same time recognize the functional nature of non-neoplastic ovarian enlargements.

Ovarian tumors have been described in patients of all ages, including intrauterine fetuses, newborn infants, children, and nonagenarians. However, they are most prevalent during the reproductive years, and benign tumors occur most often in women in their 40s. Ovarian tumors are likely to be malignant when they occur in youngsters and women past 50 years of age.

SYMPTOMS

Many ovarian tumors are asymptomatic, and even when symptoms do appear, they are notoriously late in doing so. This is true of benign and malignant tumors alike. Ovarian enlargement or neoplasia may be discovered first during a premarital or prenatal examination, a school or employment physical examination, or a periodic health examination. With a few notable exceptions, what symptoms are present are not characteristic of any specific tumor.

Pressure

An enlarging tumor may press on the bladder, producing overflow incontinence or urinary frequency. Occasionally a tumor becomes impacted in the pelvis and obstructs either the urethra or the ureters. Similarly, a tumor, particularly a solid tumor, may press on the rectum and produce constipation. More commonly, a sizable tumor or cyst produces an ill-defined pressure sensation or "heaviness" in the pelvis. When tumors reach great size they interfere with venous and lymphatic drainage from the lower extremities, resulting in edema of the legs or varicosities. They may also produce venous distention over the abdomen and elevate the diaphragm enough to cause shortness of breath.

Size

Occasionally a very large tumor produces as its only symptom an increase in girth (Fig. 59-1). The patient describes a progressive increase in the size of her abdomen and the frequent need to buy new clothes or to

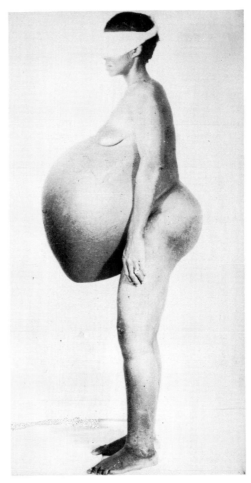

FIG. 59-1. Patient with huge benign cystadenoma of ovary. Cyst weighed 128 lb; following removal, patient weighed 126 lb. There was marked edema of lower extremities. (JW Kelso)

let out the waist of old ones. Often this is erroneously accredited to middle-age spread.

In infants and children, ovarian tumors are often noticed by parents at the time of bathing or changing clothes. In the rare instances of tumors diagnosed in the newborn, suspicion is aroused solely by the obvious appearance of an abdominal mass.

Pain

Pain is a rare symptom of an uncomplicated ovarian tumor, even one of considerable size. Pain may result from rupture, torsion of the pedicle, or distention of a cyst through rapid enlargement or hemorrhage. Ovarian pain is a constant aching referred to the ipsilateral iliac or inguinal region and into the inner aspect of the upper thigh. Pain occasionally radiates into the vulva. An ovarian tumor may produce dyspareunia, particularly if it is situated deep in the cul-de-sac. Pain may result from adhesions to or pressure on adjacent structures. However, most pain is the result of some acute accident or complication.

Gastrointestinal Abnormalities

Vague gastrointestinal complaints, such as mild nausea, epigastric discomfort, and anorexia are not rare with ovarian neoplasms, particularly if associated with ascites. Such symptoms tend to be overlooked and rarely lead to the diagnosis of ovarian neoplasm.

Menstrual Abnormalities

Tumors with endocrine function are often the cause of menstrual abnormalities. Estrogen-producing tumors may cause oligomenorrhea or amenorrhea, followed by irregular, excessive, or prolonged menses. The masculinizing tumors are often associated with amenorrhea or oligomenorrhea. Certain tumors not ordinarily regarded as having functional potential may be accompanied by endocrine activity, menstrual aberrations, and endometrial hyperplasia; this is related to functional activity of the stroma of such tumors as cystadenomas, Brenner tumors, and adenofibromas. However, abnormal bleeding is more often unrelated to the ovarian neoplasm.

Hormone Changes

In addition to menstrual abnormalities, some tumors with endocrine function are associated with other clinical manifestations of hormone production. Ovarian mesenchymomas, which include granulosa–theca-cell tumors, Sertoli–Leydig tumors, and lipid tumors, may be associated with feminization or masculinization. In the prepubertal girl, feminization is manifested as sexual precocity, with menstrual flow and breast development. In the postmenopausal woman, the only significant finding is often return of uterine bleeding. Feminizing tumors in women of childbearing age may cause alterations in secondary sex characteristics, but commonly the symptoms are related to overstimulation of the endometrium and lower genital tract. The same tumors may produce masculinization, characterized by hirsutism, enlargement of the clitoris, anovulation, amenorrhea, breast atrophy, and deepening of the voice. Tumors derived from adrenal rests may produce some of the symptoms of Cushing's disease, and an interesting but rare tumor, struma ovarii, may produce symptoms of hyperthyroidism.

These symptoms are usually dramatic, but the tumors that produce them constitute a small portion of the total number of ovarian neoplasms.

Infertility

Ovarian tumors can be associated with infertility. Except in conditions related to polycystic ovary disease, there is seldom a direct relation between the ovarian enlargement and the infertility.

COMPLICATIONS

The most dramatic symptoms occurring with ovarian neoplasms are the result of secondary changes or complications. This is particularly true of benign tumors.

Vascular Accident

Hemorrhage into a cyst is usually a slow process producing gradual distention and minimal symptoms. If the hemorrhage is sudden and large in amount, it produces acute abdominal pain with typical ovarian radiation and signs of peritoneal irritation. The tumor is tender, and motion of the cervix or uterus produces pain. Hemorrhage from a cyst may escape into the peritoneal cavity, resulting in abdominal distention, tenderness, and rebound tenderness. If the cyst has collapsed, the diagnosis is difficult unless its presence was suspected earlier. Rarely, necrosis occurs, more commonly in malignant than in benign ovarian neoplasms.

Torsion

Many of the benign tumors, both cystic and solid, develop a tenuous pedicle which is triradiate—the infundibulopelvic ligament, the utero-ovarian (suspensory) ligament and oviduct, and the mesosalpinx (Fig. 59-2). Neoplasms that rise out of the pelvis and are not large enough to be fixed in position may undergo complete or partial torsion of the pedicle. In one study, torsion was found to be present in 12% of patients operated on for tumors. If the torsion is incomplete, the result is congestion and enlargement of the neoplasm with thrombosis of vessels. If the torsion is complete and obstructs the arterial blood supply, gangrenous necrosis results. Thus, the symptoms may be gradual pain and tenderness in the region of the tumor or the abrupt onset of pain typical of an acute abdominal condition. Torsion occurs somewhat more commonly in pregnant women and in children. In the latter it is frequently confused with acute appendicitis.

Rupture

As a result of hemorrhage or torsion, an ovarian cyst may rupture and spill its contents into the peritoneal

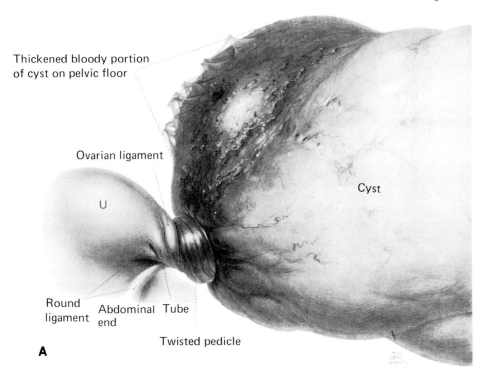

Thickened bloody portion
of cyst on pelvic floor

Ovarian ligament

U

Cyst

Round
ligament   Abdominal   Tube
            end

Twisted pedicle

A

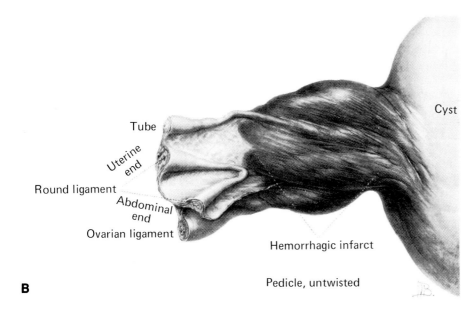

Tube

Uterine
end

Round ligament

Abdominal
end

Ovarian ligament

Cyst

Hemorrhagic infarct

Pedicle, untwisted

B

FIG. 59-2. (*A*) Left ovarian cyst with twisted pedicle, including uterine tube, ovarian ligament, and round ligament. (*B*) Pedicle untwisted to show its anatomic elements, extent to which round ligament is involved, and hemorrhagic infarct. (Drawing by Max Brödel. In Kelly HA: Operative Gynecology, Vol 2. New York, Appleton, 1903)

cavity. This results in intensification of the symptoms or occasionally a temporary reduction if the symptoms have been the result of distention of the cyst. Rupture may also occur as a result of trauma, such as a fall, a blow to the abdomen, or intercourse. Rupture of small, thin-walled ovarian cysts is not rare following vigorous bimanual examination, particularly when this is done under anesthesia. When the cyst contains serous fluid there may be few or no symptoms. If a benign cystic teratoma (dermoid) ruptures, the irritating sebaceous material produces an intense chemical peritonitis. Pseudomyxoma peritonei produces a specific diffuse accumulation of tenacious mucinous material throughout the abdomen.

Infection

Ovarian neoplasms rarely become infected. If they do, it is usually secondary to necrosis, hemorrhage, or salpingitis. It is often impossible to distinguish an infected ovarian tumor from a tubo-ovarian abscess.

PHYSICAL FINDINGS

The physical findings in patients with ovarian neoplasms vary with the nature of the tumor: its consistency, surface contour, position, mobility, and benign or malignant nature. Most benign tumors are unilateral, separate from the uterus, and freely movable. Bilaterality or fixation should arouse suspicion of malignancy. The majority of benign tumors are cystic and pedunculated. They are palpated as smooth, tense masses, readily movable, frequently from one side of the pelvis to the other. Since the pedicles are sometimes long, the neoplasm may be palpated on the side of the pelvis opposite its origin and is often found in different locations at different examinations. The external surface of benign cystic tumors is usually smooth and regular, but there may be nodular areas, irregularities, or even solid portions. Benign solid tumors are similarly smooth, also with occasional bosses, but of firm consistency. Some cystic tumors, the benign cystic teratoma (dermoid) in particular, often rise out of the pelvis and are palpated in the abdomen. Most benign tumors are movable, but a tumor may be fixed because it fills the available space in the pelvis or because the pedicle is very short. Small tumors, either cystic or solid, may be palpated best by rectal examination, noting the mass within the cul-de-sac. Presence of definite nodules on the surface of an ovarian tumor is uncommon if the tumor is benign.

It may be difficult to distinguish a huge cyst from ascites. If the abdominal distention is due to an ovarian cyst, there may be distention of veins over the lower abdomen and an absence of the shifting dullness characteristic of ascites. Percussion is dull over all of the abdomen except the flanks, where the displaced intestines lie. The percussion note does not change with changes in position. Distortion of the uterus with displacement of the cervix behind the symphysis pubis and elongation of the vagina is suggestive of a large ovarian cyst. Ascites may be present with small, benign ovarian tumors. *Meigs's syndrome* consists of ascites and hydrothorax in association with fibroma or thecoma of the ovary. In fact, the ascites may make it difficult to accurately palpate a small tumor. Nonneoplastic cystic enlargement of the ovaries may make the ovaries readily palpable but not otherwise abnormal and difficult to distinguish from true cystic neoplasms.

DIAGNOSIS

Although the presence of an ovarian neoplasm is sometimes suggested by one or more symptoms, particularly those of acute or sudden onset, the most important factor in diagnosis is the interpretation of an enlargement or mass in the region of the ovary. The diagnosis may be made with reasonable certainty in many cases. However, the differential diagnosis of an adnexal mass must include distended bladder, redundant sigmoid or low-lying cecum, pelvic abscess, ectopic pregnancy or hydrosalpinx, uterine myoma, desmoid tumor or urachal cyst, impacted feces, carcinoma of the sigmoid, diverticulitis of the sigmoid, adherent bowel or omentum secondary to surgery or infection, pelvic kidney, retroperitoneal neoplasm or abscess, hematoma of the rectus muscle, ascites, and bicornuate uterus with pregnancy in one horn.

The examination must be done with care. The bladder always should be empty. Many gynecologists have observed the rapid disappearance of an apparent ovarian cyst following catheterization of the bladder. Likewise, the rectum should be empty, and on occasion it may be advisable to repeat the examination following an enema. It is sometimes helpful to examine the patient in the knee–chest position. In this position an ovarian tumor on a pedicle may be easily displaced out of the pelvis, whereas a uterine myoma or a fixed inflammatory mass of either adnexal or bowel origin will not be displaced. If the mass is high on either side, not adjacent to the uterus, particularly if mobility is limited, a lesion of the sigmoid or cecum should be suspected. Ascites should be suspected if it is difficult to outline the contour of the supposed ovarian cyst and especially if there is a demonstrable fluid wave or shifting dullness. A history of systemic disease that might result in ascites is helpful. Sounding the uterus may be helpful in distinguishing ovarian enlargement from uterine enlargement. A small uterus, markedly displaced, suggests an ovarian enlargement whereas a deep endometrial cavity might suggest uterine enlargement.

Laboratory studies, imaging techniques, and laparoscopy will not substitute for careful history and pelvic examination. If there is any doubt at the first examination, the patient should be reexamined, possibly under anesthesia. Ultrasonography, CT scan, and laparoscopy usually are of limited value unless there is a question about actual ovarian enlargement.

X-Ray Examination

X-ray studies are of value in the diagnosis of ovarian neoplasms. Roentgenography may reveal calcification or formed teeth within a benign, cystic teratoma. Diffuse calcification in an ovarian neoplasm should arouse suspicion of a malignant, serous cystadenocarcinoma (containing psammoma bodies). Intravenous urography (IVP) is usually indicated in the management of a patient with ovarian enlargement, first to identify kidney position (to eliminate the possibility of ectopic pelvic kidney) and second to identify any ureteral displacement or distortion, which might complicate the surgical approach to a tumor. Barium enema is helpful in detecting displacement of the bowel and in excluding primary bowel lesions as the source of a presumed ovarian enlargement. Computed tomography (CT) may be helpful, but for the majority of ovarian enlargements such a study is not necessary. Its use is limited to those cases in which findings on physical examination are uncertain, and it is less often applicable than sonography.

Ultrasound

Ultrasound is rarely necessary in the evaluation of ovarian enlargement. Although it can localize pelvic and intraabdominal masses, distinguish cystic from solid tumors, and discriminate between uterine and adnexal masses (see Chapter 63), such determinations rarely, if ever, influence the proper management of the patient in whom an ovarian enlargement has been palpated. O'Brien's study revealed sonography to be inferior to clinical evaluation and pelvic examination. Sonography should not be used routinely; it should be reserved for specific indications such as uncertain physical findings, obesity, uncooperative patient, and so on. It may be used to distinguish pregnancy from ovarian enlargement.

Endocrine Studies

Endocrine assays that may be of some value in the diagnosis of hormone-producing ovarian lesions are studies of levels of pituitary gonadotropins, chorionic gonadotropins, estrogens, and androgens, and studies of thyroid function.

TREATMENT

The management of actual or suspected ovarian neoplasms is basically surgical. Operation is indicated for the relief of symptoms, and when there are no symptoms, surgery is performed to exclude malignancy. Indeed, it is not unrealistic to consider every ovarian neoplasm to be potentially malignant. The likelihood of malignancy of all ovarian neoplasms is between 15% and 25% and is even greater among children and postmenopausal women. Therefore, the need for accurate diagnosis is clear. Occasionally it is possible to differentiate benign from malignant tumors on the basis of history and physical examination, but usually an accurate diagnosis can be made only following gross and microscopic examination of the tumor.

Exploratory operation is essential for all patients in whom an ovarian neoplasm is suspected. This concept should *not* be extended to include all patients with an enlargement of the ovary, since many ovarian enlargements simply represent extensions of the normal cystic response of the ovary to changing physiology. Which patients need surgery has to be decided rather arbitrarily.

Many gynecologists rely upon the size of the ovarian enlargement. We consider ovarian enlargements greater than 7 cm in diameter as probably neoplastic and those under this size as probably nonneoplastic; 7 cm is an easy size to remember because it is exactly the diameter of a new tennis ball. Other gynecologists draw the line at 6 or 5 cm. According to one study, 93% of ovarian cysts less than 5 cm in diameter were nonneoplastic. For many gynecologists the presence of a palpable ovary in a postmenopausal woman (indicative of enlargement) is sufficient reason for surgery because of the possibility of ovarian malignancy.

Since the probability of malignancy is greater in solid than in cystic tumors, we prefer to operate on most patients with solid tumors, even those smaller than 7 cm. It is often of value to reexamine the patient and note changes in the size of an ovarian enlargement. A patient found to have a mass about 7 cm in diameter should be reexamined in several weeks. Attention should be given to the phase of the ovarian cycle, for the enlargement of a corpus luteum prior to menstruation may not be apparent in the postmenstrual phase. If follow-up examination reveals gradual enlargement of a cystic mass, even though it is smaller than 7 cm, neoplastic growth should be suspected. If the tumor regresses in size or disappears, it is safe to assume the enlargement was functional.

Oral contraceptives have been recommended to accelerate involution of nonneoplastic ovarian enlargement. Since most of these cysts are gonadotropin-dependent, the inhibitory effect of ovarian steroids on the release of pituitary gonadotropins diminishes the stimulus to cyst formation and persistence. Spanos studied patients with unilateral cystic adnexal masses. Oral contraceptives were prescribed and the mass disappeared in 72% of patients reexamined in 6 weeks. All patients with a persistent mass were found to have a neoplasm at laparotomy.

A plan of observation and follow-up is not applicable to the infant or young girl. In these patients, any enlargement mandates surgical exploration. The same is true for the postmenopausal woman. The probability of malignancy increases sharply after the age of 50 years, and all ovarian enlargements in postmenopausal women should be investigated surgically. In the young woman, however, careful repeat examination may show surgery to be unnecessary.

When surgery is the treatment of choice, the type and extent needed can only be determined at the operating table on the basis of the pathologic findings considered in the light of the patient's age, general health, and desire for future childbearing. Treatment may consist of (1) nothing; (2) excision of the lesion, preserving the remainder of the ovary; (3) unilateral removal of the adnexa; (4) bilateral removal of the adnexa with hysterectomy; or (5) more radical procedures. We are opposed to tapping large ovarian cysts to reduce their size to make removal less difficult. Even when the greatest caution is exercised, cells may be spilled into the peritoneal cavity and cause irritation and metastatic implantation.

Differentiation of Ovarian Enlargement

The findings at surgery will permit identification of the nonovarian causes of a pelvic mass. These should be dealt with according to their nature.

Much depends upon gross diagnosis. For practical purposes ovarian enlargements may be classified as (1) functional or nonneoplastic, (2) obviously malignant, (3) probably benign, and (4) questionable.

Functional Cystic Enlargements

At the outset it is essential to distinguish functional enlargements from neoplasms. Functional enlargements tend to be multiple, small, smooth, thin-walled, filled with clear fluid, and bilateral (Fig. 59-3). The corpus luteum is recognized by its characteristic shape and yellow color. Functional cysts rarely require surgical treatment, unless there is associated bleeding, as may occur from a corpus luteum or corpus luteum cyst. These may be managed by suture of the rupture site or excision of the cyst.

Obviously Malignant Tumors

Many malignant neoplasms of the ovary can be diagnosed accurately by inspection of the tumor, the peritoneal cavity, and the relation of the tumor to adjacent structures. The characteristics of malignant tumors and their management are discussed later.

Probably Benign Tumors

Some benign ovarian neoplasms can be diagnosed accurately at the time of surgery by gross inspection, section of the tumor and, occasionally, microscopic examination of frozen sections. This is so for the unilocular, thin-walled, simple serous cystoma and some of the nonpapillary cystadenomas. The benign cystic teratoma (dermoid) is easily diagnosed on the basis of its smooth, gray exterior and an interior filled with sebaceous material, hair, and sometimes calcified matter or teeth. Benign fibroma may be suspected if the tumor is unilateral, very firm, and has a glistening gray external surface and a compact, smooth, cut surface. Microscopic examination of a frozen section confirms the suspicion. A conservative operative approach is indicated if the woman is in the reproductive years and especially if she is young and desirous of further childbearing. If significant normal ovarian tissue is present, the lesion may be excised alone. In the majority of cases it is preferable to remove the entire ovary containing the cyst or tumor.

Neoplasms of Questionable Nature

Unfortunately, it is often difficult to determine the malignant or benign nature of an ovarian neoplasm without histologic examination. Leads can be gained from examination of the external surface and interior of a tumor. Solid tumors, particularly of a soft or semisolid consistency, are more likely to be malignant than are completely cystic tumors. Bilateral tumors should arouse suspicion of malignancy. The presence of papillary excrescences on the surface of a cystic tumor commonly indicates malignancy. However, if the papillary processes are firm, broad-based, and not friable, they may be part of a benign process; thus, they cannot be considered absolute indications of malignancy. Fixation of the neoplasm to adjacent tissues should be taken as evidence of probable malignancy.

All ovarian neoplasms should be opened in the operating room and examined by the surgeon or the findings reported to him by a pathologist. The external surface of a neoplasm may appear benign, whereas the interior reveals obvious evidences of malignancy. Hemorrhage, areas of necrosis, or small, friable papillary excrescences within the interior of a cyst suggest malignancy, as does a coarsely granular, fleshy, or semisolid cut surface. The finding of sebaceous material suggests a benign cystic teratoma (dermoid). The presence of tenacious mucinous fluid indicates a mucinous neoplasm, which has a relatively low incidence of malignancy. Solid areas within an otherwise cystic tumor should arouse suspicion of malignancy. A biopsy for frozen-section examination should be taken from any solid or otherwise suspicious area. However, frozen-section examination is often of limited value. Unfortunately, microscopic distinction between malignant and benign neoplasms is most difficult in the very cases for which a frozen section is most indicated: that is, neoplasms whose nature is not apparent on gross examination.

Conservative Approach

If the lesion is thought to be benign, the opposite ovary and the uterus may be conserved if they are normal. Most physicians prefer to remove the opposite ovary and uterus in postmenopausal patients. A conservative approach is justified in the management of the questionable lesion if the patient is young and wants additional children. Simple oophorectomy is done, and further decisions regarding therapy are reached following the final pathologic interpretation of the specimen. If the patient is premenopausal or postmenopausal, questionable lesions should be treated by bilateral salpingo-oophorectomy and hysterectomy.

The decision to conserve the opposite ovary is dependent upon its being normal and not the site of a second neoplasm. This is particularly true when the gross diagnosis of the primary tumor is in question. The

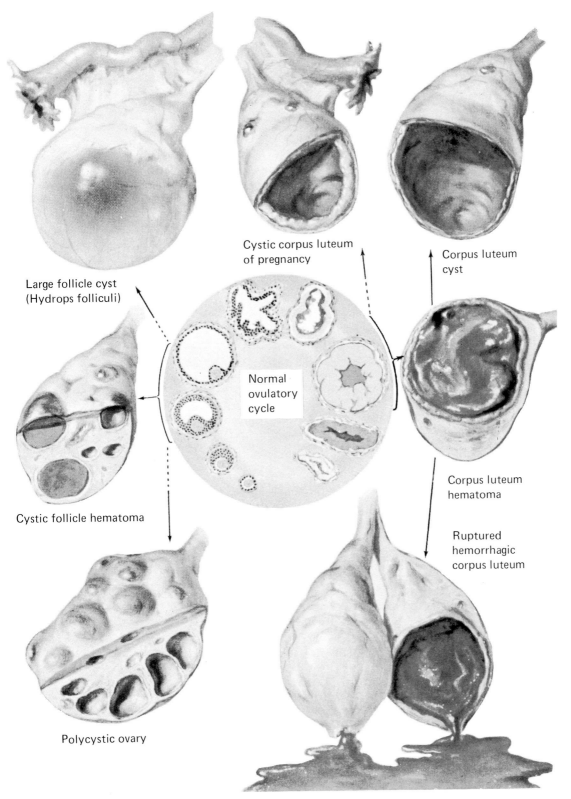

Large follicle cyst
(Hydrops folliculi)

Cystic corpus luteum
of pregnancy

Corpus luteum
cyst

Normal
ovulatory
cycle

Corpus luteum
hematoma

Cystic follicle hematoma

Ruptured
hemorrhagic
corpus luteum

Polycystic ovary

FIG. 59-3. Physiologic, nonneoplastic cystic enlargements of ovaries. (Drawing by FH Netter. In Ciba Collection of Medical Illustrations, Vol 2, Reproductive System. Summit NJ, © CIBA, 1954)

external surface should be carefully examined. If the primary neoplasm is thought to be a benign cystic teratoma (dermoid), a serous cystadenoma, or a predominantly solid tumor, it is advisable also to split the opposite ovary and inspect the interior. The frequency of bilateral occurrence of these tumors warrants this approach. If evidence of another neoplasm is found, the tumor should be excised or the ovary removed.

If an ovary is sectioned for inspection, the incision should be made in the sagittal plane, which allows for examination of the ovary down to the hilus, where certain tumors originate. Not everyone recommends such examination of the opposite ovary, however. This procedure is followed by adhesion formation, which may interfere with pregnancy in the very patients for whom a conservative operation is elected to permit further child bearing.

HISTOGENESIS

The most common enlargements of the ovary are those arising from physiologic cystic proliferation of the normal follicular apparatus of the ovary; these are not true neoplasms. Sometimes they represent a failure of normal regression or involution.

In general, the benign true neoplasms of the ovary arise either from normal constituents of the ovary or from congenital rests or heterotopic implants. The tumors developing from structures of the ovary are (1) the majority of the cystic tumors, which arise from the surface (germinal) epithelium; (2) the hormone-producing tumors, which arise from the specialized stroma of the ovarian cortex; (3) the rare tumors also found in sites other than the ovary, which arise from the nonspecialized connective tissue of the ovary; and (4) the benign and malignant teratomas, which arise from the germ cells. Tumors arising from congenital rests or heterotopic implants include adrenal tumors, hilus-cell tumors, and mesonephric and metanephric rest tumors.

CLASSIFICATION

Classifications of tumors or enlargements of the ovary have evolved through a need to understand the origin and function of these lesions and their clinical significance. As more is learned about the physiology and metabolism of the ovary, it becomes apparent that all of the classifications have serious shortcomings. Nonetheless, some form of organization is necessary to permit an orderly discussion of the varieties of ovarian enlargements. The following outline serves this purpose:

A. Functional cysts
   1. Follicle cyst
   2. Corpus luteum cyst
   3. Theca lutein cyst
B. Hyperplasias
   1. Polycystic ovary
   2. Hyperthecosis
   3. Luteoma
C. Endometrial cysts
D. True neoplasms
   1. Common surface epithelial neoplasms
      a. Germinal inclusion cyst
      b. Serous cystadenoma
      c. Mucinous cystadenoma
      d. Cystadenofibroma
      e. Endometrioid tumor
      f. Brenner tumor
   2. Sex chord–mesenchymal tumors (gonadal stromal tumors)
      a. Granulosa cell tumor
      b. Theca cell tumor
      c. Sertoli–Leydig cell tumor (androblastoma)
      d. Gynandroblastoma
      e. Hilus cell tumor
      f. Lipid cell tumor
   3. Nonintrinsic connective tissue tumors
      a. Fibroma
      b. Rare tumors
   4. Germ cell tumors
      a. Mature teratoma
         1) Cystic teratoma (dermoid)
         2) Struma ovarii
         3) Carcinoid tumor
      b. Immature teratoma
      c. Embryonal teratoma
      d. Extraembryonal teratoma (endodermal sinus tumor)
      e. Germinoma
      f. Gonadoblastoma
      g. Choriocarcinoma
   5. Tumors of uncertain origin
      a. Adrenal tumor
      b. Mesonephroma (clear cell)
      c. Lipid cell tumor
   6. Metastatic tumors
      a. Krukenberg
      b. Breast
      c. Other

FUNCTIONAL OVARIAN CYSTS

Follicle Cyst

Mature or atretic follicles that become distended with pale, straw-colored fluid are frequently found in the ovary. Enlargement of atretic follicles to the point of producing grossly visible cystic changes is common during infancy and childhood and may, rarely, enlarge one or both ovaries. Following puberty, grossly cystic follicles are less common but still constitute the most frequently seen cystic enlargement of the ovary.

Follicle cysts are the result of failure of ovulation,

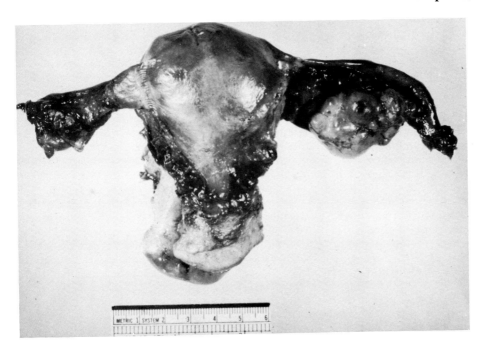

FIG. 59-4. Uterus and ovaries. Note numerous small follicle cysts on surface of right ovary.

with continued growth of the follicle. They are usually multiple and occur in both ovaries (Fig. 59-4). Follicle cysts only occasionally attain a diameter larger than 3 cm. Follicle cysts causing marked enlargement of the ovaries are rare complications of hyperstimulation from exogenous gonadotrophins used to induce ovulation. They do not always alter the external surface of the ovary but may produce yellow blebs on the surface. When cut, they are seen to be thin-walled and filled with a clear serous fluid. Microscopically, the cystic space is lined by a layer of granulosa and underlying theca cells, occasionally flattened or obliterated by the intracystic pressure (Fig. 59-5).

Follicle cysts rarely produce symptoms unless they are large or complicated by rupture or hemorrhage, as reported in cases of hyperstimulation from exogenous gonadotrophins. However, they are often associated with endometrial hyperplasia and uterine myomas. The cysts vary in size from time to time and may disappear between examinations. A diagnosis is usually made at the

FIG. 59-5. Microscopic section of wall of follicle cyst showing lining granulosa cells.

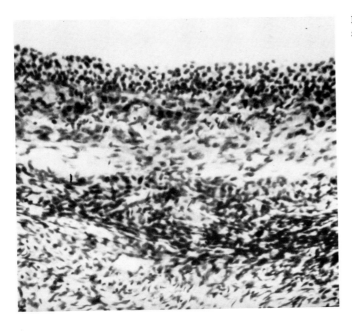

operating table, and treatment consists of nothing, puncture of the cyst, or excision of the cyst if it is large or hemorrhagic.

Corpus Luteum Cyst

The corpus luteum that develops following ovulation is normally a cystic structure, albeit small and often only potentially cystic. During pregnancy, with growth and continued function, the corpus luteum becomes truly cystic and at times sufficiently large to be palpated on bimanual pelvic examination. This cystic corpus luteum is not difficult to diagnose or explain. In the absence of pregnancy, the corpus luteum normally collapses and in due time is replaced by hyaline connective tissue to form the corpus albicans. Occasionally, in the nonpregnant state, the corpus luteum becomes cystic as a result of either unusual continued growth or of hemorrhage into the lumen.

Such cystic enlargement rarely exceeds 4 cm in diameter but has been observed as large as 11 cm. Grossly, the cyst protrudes from the contour of the ovary and the wall appears convoluted, with yellow-orange areas alternating with the usual gray surface. If the cyst is filled with blood, a dark red or purple discoloration is seen. Microscopically, all elements of the corpus luteum are present in the cyst wall. Depending on the age of the cyst and the degree of intracystic pressure, luteinized granulosa and theca cells may be easily recognizable or may be distorted. The center of the cyst contains blood, serous coagulum, and some connective tissue organization.

Symptoms are related to large size or complications of torsion, rupture, or hemorrhage. The greatest clinical significance of a corpus luteum cyst is that it can simulate ectopic pregnancy. Continued hormone production may cause amenorrhea and subsequent irregular uterine bleeding. In such cases, the ovarian enlargement may be difficult to distinguish from swelling of the oviduct. Sudden hemorrhage into the cyst can produce pelvic pain of an aching or colicky type. If the cyst ruptures, the associated findings of intra-abdominal hemorrhage complete the picture of ectopic gestation. More commonly, cystic corpora lutea and corpus luteum cysts produce no symptoms and undergo absorption or regression.

If the symptoms warrant operation, treatment usually consists of excision of the cyst and conservation of the remainder of the ovary.

Theca Lutein Cyst

During pregnancy, atretic follicles are numerous in the ovaries. Occasionally they undergo cystic enlargement. Bilateral ovarian enlargement due to multiple theca lutein cysts occurs in 50% to 60% of women with hydatidiform mole, 5% to 10% of women with choriocarci-

noma, and a few women who have multiple gestation. Cyst formation is best explained as a response to the increased production of chorionic gonadotropin.

The cysts are almost always bilateral, and the enlargement may exceed 15 cm. The external surface of the ovary is slightly lobulated, smooth, and blue or gray. The cut surface discloses many thin-walled, clear-fluid-filled cystic spaces with a gray lining. Microscopically, the cysts are lined by theca cells showing varying degrees of luteinization and a central layer of fibrous connective tissue (Fig. 59-6). Granulosa cells may be present but usually are not. Central to the zone of fibrous connective tissue there may be organized blood.

Theca lutein cysts rarely produce symptoms of their own and are usually found incidentally in a patient with hydatidiform mole (Fig. 59-7). Indeed, the finding of bilaterally enlarged ovaries offers strong support to the diagnosis of hydatidiform mole. These cysts may undergo the same complications as other ovarian enlargements. Despite the occasional enormous size of theca

FIG. 59-6. Microscopic section of wall of theca lutein cyst showing vertically arranged luteinized theca cells. There is slight fibrosis of central lining.

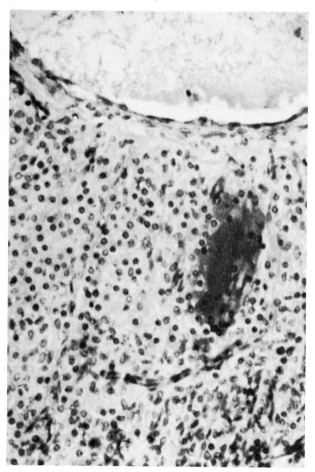

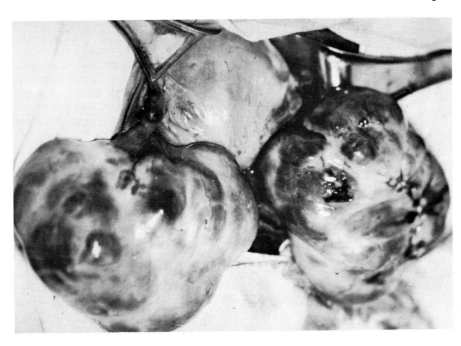

FIG. 59-7. Bilateral theca cysts associated with hydatidiform mole.

lutein cysts, they are physiologic and should be removed only when this is dictated by the nature of the intrauterine pathology. Following evacuation of a hydatidiform mole or termination of a pregnancy, complete regression of the cysts and return of the ovary to normal size may be anticipated.

HYPERPLASIAS

Polycystic Ovary

Bilateral polycystic enlargement of the ovaries is found in adolescent girls and young women with a complex of symptoms and endocrine abnormalities related to anovulation (Fig. 59-8). These ovaries are enlarged, tense, and oval. The external surface is smooth and white, sometimes revealing subcapsular cysts. The tunica is thick, tough, and white. The ovarian cortex is represented by a thick fibrous capsule surrounding ovarian stroma containing multiple follicle cysts (Fig. 59-9). Microscopically, the follicle cysts demonstrate prominent hyperplasia of the theca interna cells, which are frequently luteinized (Fig. 59-10). Atretic follicles are numerous, with similar hyperplasia and luteinization of theca cells surrounding the lumen. Primordial follicles are not present in the thickened tunica but are commonly aligned immediately beneath this zone in the ovarian stroma. Evidence of present or prior ovulation is usually not seen.

These ovarian changes may result from a specific type of ovarian insufficiency without clearly demonstrable causes outside of the ovary. Indeed, in 1935 Stein and Leventhal reported seven cases of a possible syndrome consisting of bilateral polycystic ovarian en-

largement, amenorrhea or irregular menses, infertility, and often masculinization. Similar cystic ovarian enlargement is not uncommon in patients with various types of adrenal hyperplasia and has been observed with pituitary and hypothalamic tumors, increased intracranial pressure, adrenal tumors, and chronic inflammatory disease of the pelvis. Moreover, similar changes have been observed in ovaries containing small, masculinizing mesenchymomas. The ovaries of prepubertal girls from 10 to 15 years old are morphologically similar to the polycystic ovaries just described. All of these observations suggest that the microscopic morphology of the polycystic ovary is specific only of *anovulation*. Furthermore, the similarity between the morphology of the polycystic ovary in the abnormal postpubertal woman and the normal prepubertal girl, as well as certain features of the clinical findings in the former patients, suggest that the clinical syndrome of the polycystic ovary is related to acyclic hypothalamic activity and failure to initiate regular ovulation at puberty.

For many years there has been interest in *polycystic ovary disease* and its variations, and there have been efforts to explain the altered ovarian physiology. As a result of this enthusiasm, the polycystic ovary syndrome has, in general, become more elusive and hard to define. If we eliminate the nonovarian causes of anovulation and related symptoms of amenorrhea, infertility, and possibly hirsutism, we may describe a complex that warrants the designation syndrome (Stein–Leventhal or polycystic ovary syndrome). Characteristically, these young patients, who may still be in adolescence or slightly beyond, have never developed regular ovulatory cycles. A few have never menstruated, but most have had irregular menstrual periods that have gradually be-

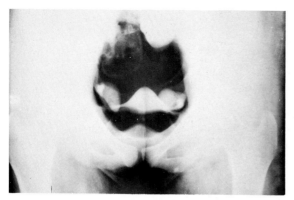

FIG. 59-8. X-ray gynegram of adolescent patient demonstrating bilateral polycystic enlargement of ovaries.

come more abnormal. In some cases this menstrual abnormality is first manifested by excessive or prolonged bleeding due to endometrial hyperplasia. Eventually, the periods may become infrequent, scanty, or absent. Infertility exists and is commonly the most serious problem among the patients who are married. There may be hirsutism but rarely, if ever, true masculinization. Obesity is sometimes noted. Ovarian enlargement, while common, may be absent or unilateral. This may be demonstrated by pelvic examination, ultrasonography, laparoscopy, or exploratory laparotomy. The uterus and breasts are said to be frequently hypoplastic, although this has not been common in our experience. The endocrinologic aspects of this syndrome and its diagnosis and treatment are considered in Chapter 47.

Hyperthecosis

A somewhat related ovarian abnormality is *hyperthecosis*. The clinical manifestations may resemble those of the polycystic ovary syndrome, usually with more marked

hirsutism and even true masculinization. The ovaries show varying degrees of enlargement. The characteristic histologic finding is extreme hyperplasia of theca cells throughout the ovarian stroma; some of the cells are luteinized. These morphologic findings may be present with or without the other histologic changes characteristic of the polycystic ovary. The cause of this lesion is unknown, but in all probability it is related to either polycystic ovary disease or adrenal hyperplasia.

Luteoma

Luteomas are hyperplastic nodules of large, pale, polyhedral lutein cells in the stroma in one or both ovaries. Such lesions may be discrete, as large as 3 cm, yellow, brown, or white. They have been reported in perimenopausal and postmenopausal women in association with androgen manifestations. In this circumstance they may be classified with the lipid-cell tumors. Luteoma of pregnancy is a specific hyperplastic entity that develops during pregnancy and involutes following delivery. These lesions probably arise from hyperplasia of luteinized theca cells of atretic follicles. The lesions are bilateral in as many as half of the cases and may reach large sizes (20 cm). In approximately one quarter of cases, patients have evidenced androgen manifestations. However, in most cases the lesions are asymptomatic incidental findings. The lesions regress rapidly following termination of pregnancy and should only be removed if the diagnosis is unknown or uncertain.

ENDOMETRIAL CYSTS

Endometriosis (detailed in Chap. 53) is mentioned here because it may produce single or multiple cysts (*endometrioma*) in the ovary that may reach significant proportions. Endometriosis has a specific symptom

FIG. 59-9. Gross appearance of cut surface of bilateral polycystic ovaries.

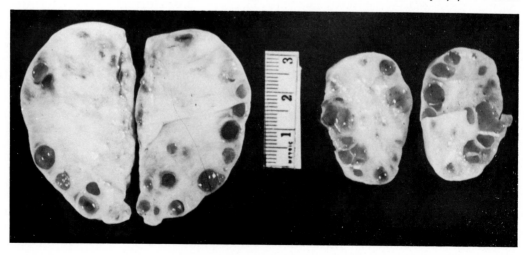

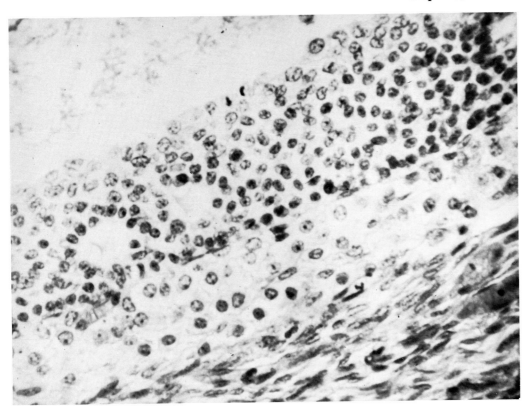

FIG. 59-10. Polycystic ovary. Microscopic section of follicle cyst with inner lining of granulosa cells and outer zone of hyperplastic luteinized theca cells. Theca cells are large with abundant pale cytoplasm. Note Call–Exner body in granulosa layer.

complex, but the large endometrial cysts alone may produce symptoms similar to those of other ovarian cysts and tumors.

TRUE OVARIAN NEOPLASMS

Common Surface Epithelial Neoplasms

Germinal Inclusion Cyst

Germinal inclusion cysts are common microscopic findings in the ovaries of menopausal or postmenopausal women. They are superficial, beneath the surface epithelium, and unilocular. The lining epithelium is usually columnar with elongated basophilic nuclei. Cilia are occasionally present. Since this is the characteristic epithelium of serous cystomas, cystadenomas, and cystadenocarcinomas, it is probable that inclusion cysts are the forerunners of more significant cystic tumors of the ovary. Somewhat similar lesions are seen in ovaries with surface inflammation or adhesions, in which an actual infolding of the surface epithelium is observed. A similar process of epithelial inclusion is probably the mechanism by which all cystic epithelial ovarian tumors are formed.

Serous Cystadenoma

The serous cystadenoma and the mucinous cystadenoma are the most common benign ovarian neoplasms. Serous tumors constitute 15% to 25% of all benign ovarian tumors. Serous cystadenomas occur most commonly between the ages of 20 and 50 years and reach their peak incidence in the third and fourth decades of life. The reported frequency of bilaterality varies from 12% to 50%. Those with papillary projections are more often bilateral. Most serous cystic tumors are benign; however, an indefinite number (32% to 45%, according to various studies) are malignant. This does not indicate the frequency with which a histologically benign serous cystadenoma becomes malignant, but does indicate a significant potential for malignancy. The frequency of malignant change, like bilaterality, is greater in those tumors with papillary processes.

The serous cystadenoma (Fig. 59-11) is a unilocular, parvilocular, or multilocular cystic neoplasm derived from the surface epithelium of the ovary and lined by epithelium that resembles the mucosa of the oviduct. The external surface is smooth or lobulated, gray or bluish-gray, and darker if there has been hemorrhage into the cyst. External papillary projections occur in 10% to 30% of tumors. They are firm, white, and broad-based.

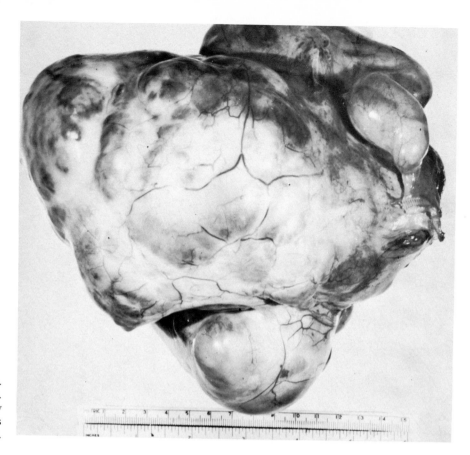

FIG. 59-11. Serous cystadenoma. Surface is lobulated and glistening. Tumor has assumed shape of bony pelvis with growth. Hydrosalpinx is attached to superior surface of cyst.

Softness and friability suggest malignancy. The benign serous cystadenoma is usually of moderate size and varies from 5 to 15 cm in diameter; occasionally it fills the entire abdomen. The cut surface reveals a single or multiple loculi that have a smooth gray lining and contain clear, yellow fluid. The majority are unilocular and thin-walled. Less common are those with multiple loculi and numerous thin septa. Papillary processes similar to those described on the external surface may be present. It is not rare to find solid portions, but this should suggest malignancy. Occasionally one or more of the loculi contains blood.

Microscopically, the epithelial lining of a serous cystadenoma varies from simple cuboidal to tall columnar with elongated nuclei, resembling the epithelium of the oviduct (Fig. 59-12). Cilia are observed in some cases. The stroma varies from an edematous to a densely fibrous type and is variable in amount. The papillary processes are broad, fibrous, and covered by a single layer of epithelium (Fig. 59-13). Occasionally small calcific concretions, known as *psammoma bodies,* are found in the stroma adjacent to the epithelium. These deposits, if present in large numbers, may be visible on x-ray examination of the abdomen.

The microscopic evaluation of malignancy in this group of tumors may pose considerable difficulty. Indeed, in some tumors of a borderline nature a piling up of epithelial cells and slight degrees of dedifferentiation make it impossible to distinguish between a benign and a malignant process. In these cases (which are also referred to as "tumors of low malignant potential") only the clinical course indicates the biologic nature of the tumor. The problem of borderline malignancy is discussed elsewhere.

No symptoms are specific for this tumor. The diagnosis is commonly made after pelvic examination in a patient who is asymptomatic or has noticed gradual abdominal enlargement.

Treatment must be planned with knowledge of the frequency of bilateral involvement, the potential for malignancy, and the fact that papillary processes and hemorrhage suggest malignancy. In patients past the childbearing age, treatment should consist of bilateral salpingo-oophorectomy and hysterectomy. Conservatism is recommended for most others.

Mucinous Cystadenoma

Mucinous cystadenomas are unilocular or multilocular cystic ovarian tumors occurring as often as, or more often than, the serous cystadenoma. According to various studies, they constitute 16% to 30% of all benign ovarian neoplasms. Unlike the serous tumors, they are bilateral

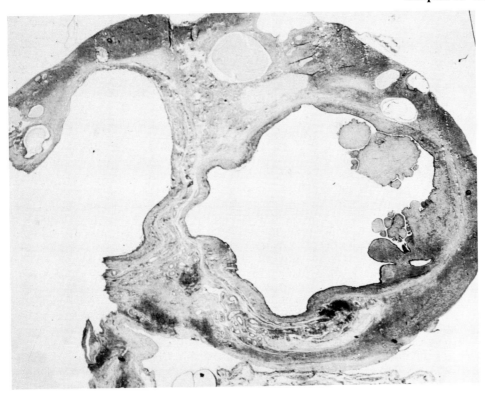

FIG. 59-12.   Microscopic view of papillary serous cystadenoma. Tumor did not enlarge ovary and was not visible externally. Papillary processes are blunt and broad-based, lined by single layer of epithelium. This lesion represents early phase in histogenesis of serous tumor of ovary.

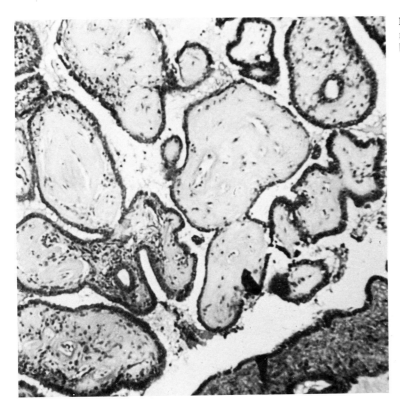

FIG. 59-13.   Microscopic section of papillary serous cystadenoma. Papillae are small and delicate but lined by single layer of epithelium.

in only 5% to 7% of cases. Moreover, the incidence of similar tumors appearing later in the conserved opposite ovary is extremely low. These tumors rarely become malignant. Mucinous cystadenomas occur most frequently during the third and fifth decades of life, and only occasionally (10%) after the menopause. They may complicate pregnancy.

There are two theories of histogenesis. The most commonly accepted is an origin from the surface epithelium of the ovary with differentiation to the endocervical type of müllerian duct epithelium. The other theory holds that the epithelium is intestinal in type and arises from a monophyletic teratoma in which only one type of tissue persists. It is possible that the cysts arise in both fashions.

Mucinous tumors are often much larger than the serous cystadenoma and usually account for the legendary huge cysts that are reported. They range from 1 to 50 cm in diameter, with the majority being 15 to 30 cm. Ordinarily they are completely cystic and multilocular. The external surface is smooth, occasionally lobulated, pinkish-gray, and without extracystic papillar growths (Figs. 59-14, 59-15). The cut surface shows individual cysts or locules, varying in size and containing a sticky, slimy, or viscid material. The interlocular septa are very thin. Intracystic papillary processes are present in 10% to 25% of cases, and as is true for the serous tumor, are even more common in the malignant variety.

Microscopically, the locules and cysts are lined by a typical tall columnar "picket-fence" type of cell, with a basally situated nucleus and superficial accumulation of mucin within the cytoplasm (Fig. 59-16). The cell resembles the secretory cell of the endocervix and intestine. Argentaffin cells also may be present. Dense connective tissue stroma is scant and forms a capsule.

The usual treatment for the obviously benign mucinous cystadenoma is unilateral oophorectomy. In older women bilateral oophorectomy and hysterectomy is preferable.

Pseudomyxoma peritonei is a complication that may result if the contents of a mucinous cyst are spilled into the peritoneal cavity by rupture, extension, or at surgery. This is a good reason not to tap or aspirate ovarian cysts at operation. Fortunately, pseudomyxoma does not always develop with spillage. Moreover, pseudomyxoma peritonei has been reported in the presence of intact ovaries and ovarian cysts. The process is biologically malignant, although it is histologically benign. Diffuse implants develop on all the peritoneal surfaces, with tremendous accumulation of mucinous material within the peritoneal cavity. Rarely is there spread beyond the peritoneum or invasion of vital structures. Microscopic examination of the implants reveals the morphology of a benign mucinous tumor. In fact, areas of epithelium are scant and hard to find. The clinical course is usually progressive malnutrition and emaciation. The fluid is difficult to remove because of its viscosity, and repeated laparotomies may be required. The interesting association of mucinous cysts of the ovary and *mucocele of the appendix* has been reported.

FIG. 59-14. Mucinous cystadenoma. Surface is bosselated and a solid portion is present in lower pole.

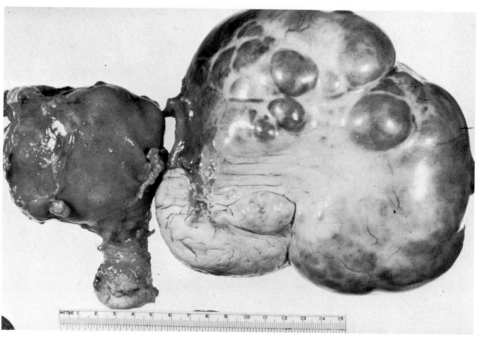

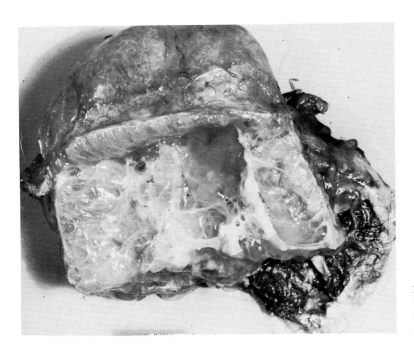

FIG. 59-15. Mucinous cystadenoma coexisting with cystic teratoma (dermoid). Coexistence of these two tumors supports theory of origin of mucinous tumors from benign teratomas.

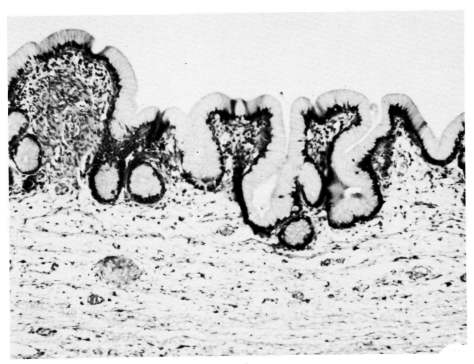

FIG. 59-16. Microscopic appearance of lining of mucinous cystadenoma. "Picket-fence" epithelium is characteristic of this tumor.

Cystadenofibroma

The cystadenofibroma is a variant of the serous cystadenoma and much less common. This tumor is partially cystic and partially solid. The age distribution is similar to that of the serous tumors. It is usually benign and unilateral.

The external surface is gray or white, composed of multiloculated cystic areas and lobulated solid portions with broad papillae or deep sulci. The papillae are firm and nonfriable. The cut surface reveals numerous amber fluid-filled cysts within firm, glistening grayish-white lobules. Microscopically, the solid areas are composed of whorls of fibrous connective tissue containing various amounts of ovarian stroma and are lined by typical surface or germinal epithelium. The cystic spaces are similar to those of serous cystadenoma. The cystadenofibroma can be distinguished from a fibroma with cystic degeneration by the papillary or gyrated character of the surface. Similar gross and microscopic findings are not uncommon in normal-sized postmenopausal ovaries.

Treatment varies with age and associated findings.

Endometrioid Tumor

Ovarian tumors with a pattern resembling endometrial tumors have been reported to occur with significant frequency. In the past, these tumors have been considered to arise from areas of endometriosis. It seems probable that they more often arise *de novo* just as the serous and mucinous tumors do. The majority are malignant.

Brenner Tumor

The Brenner tumor is a fibroepithelial tumor with gross characteristics similar to the fibroma. It constitutes approximately 1% to 2% of all ovarian tumors and is rarely malignant. Brenner tumors have been reported in patients 6 to 81 years of age; however, approximately one half the patients are over the age of 50 years. One study indicates that approximately 13% of the tumors are bilateral; figures as low as 5% have been given by others.

According to the most widely accepted theory of histogenesis, Brenner tumors arise from Walthard's cell rests, which themselves are a modification and inclusion of the surface epithelium (germinal epithelium) of the ovary. Brenner tumors and mucinous cystadenomas occasionally coexist. This is explained as metaplasia either of the mucinous epithelium to the squamoid type or of the epithelial nests of the Brenner tumor to a mucinous type. The association of these two tumors is compatible with a theory of origin from the surface epithelium of the ovary. Coexistence of other genital tumors has been reported.

The tumors vary from microscopic size to 30 cm in diameter. The average tumor is between 10 and 15 cm in diameter. They are usually solid but may be partially cystic. The surface is smooth and grayish-white, with irregular lobulation. The cut surface is grayish-white and whorled. The cystic areas vary in size and contain clear serous fluid. Microscopically, the solid portion of the tumor consists of abundant fibrous connective tissue and typical nests of squamous-like epithelial cells with characteristic longitudinal grooving of the nucleus (Fig. 59-17). Frequently the centers of these nests become cystic. The cells lining the central cavity are cuboidal, low columnar, or occasionally typical of mucinous epithelium.

A few Brenner tumors have been associated with postmenopausal bleeding, and it has been suggested that they occasionally contain hormonally active stroma. In common with the fibroma and thecoma, Meigs's syndrome of ascites and hydrothorax occurs with Brenner tumors.

Treatment usually consists of simple excision or oophorectomy.

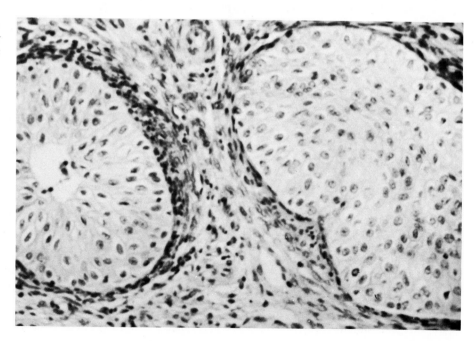

FIG. 59-17. Microscopic appearance of cell nest in Brenner tumor. Note beginning cystic change in one of the cell nests.

Sex Cord–Mesenchymal Tumors (Gonadal Stromal Tumors)

The *mesenchymomas* constitute a group of tumors frequently demonstrating endocrine function. They all have certain morphologic similarities, and each probably arises from ovarian cortical stroma (or embryonic gonadal stroma) or its follicular wall derivatives. Recently there has been a trend to refer to these tumors simply as *feminizing mesenchymomas* (granulosa and theca cell tumors) and *masculinizing mesenchymomas* (androblastoma, hilus cell tumor, lipid tumors), depending on histology. It is apparent that the morphology is often amazingly similar and that tumors of each morphologic type may demonstrate clinical features of estrogen or androgen production and, on occasion, both. The granulosa cell tumor, which is generally feminizing, has been reported to produce masculinization. The theca cell tumor, which also is usually feminizing, may produce virilization; hyperplasia of the theca cell in the polycystic ovary syndrome is often associated with features of androgen activity. The masculinizing tumors (arrhenoblastoma, androblastoma, or Sertoli–Leydig cell tumors) have rarely been associated with estrogen activity. Thus, any attempt to limit the production of specific hormones to a specific cell or a specific tumor of the ovary is not realistic in the light of clinical findings or present knowledge of steroid biosynthesis in the ovary. *Any cell or tissue that is capable of steroid biosynthesis is capable of producing progestrone, estrogens, and androgens.* The predominance depends on the rates of biosynthesis and the enzymes required for the various steps thereof. It is postulated that all of these tumors arise from the mesenchymal ovarian stroma, which retains most of its embryonic multidifferentiating potential. This potential may be exploited both in degree and direction by tumorigenic stimuli. Abnormal hormone production probably occurs as a result of subsequent imbalance of normal enzyme activity and disruption of the usual steroid metabolic pathways.

In considering the clinical importance of this group of hormonally active tumors, it is impossible to stress too strongly the fallacy of emphasizing the histology rather than the metabolic activity of the tumor. However, histologic classification remains a handy means of considering the pathology of these tumors and is a necessity in deciding the malignant potential.

Granulosa Cell Tumor

These tumors, composed predominantly of granulosa cells, commonly produce menometrorrhagia, menopausal bleeding, postmenopausal bleeding, and enlargement of the breasts. Occurring at any age, about 50% are found in postmenopausal patients. They may occur in youngsters and must be distinguished from constitutional precocity. Except in young women and children, treatment should consist of bilateral salpingo-oophorectomy and hysterectomy. Increasingly, gyne-

cologists are recommending a conservative approach in women desiring future childbearing, if the tumor is intact. Possibly one third of these tumors have proved to be biologically malignant (see Figs. 59-43, 59-44).

Thecoma

Most granulosa cell tumors contain varying amounts of theca. There are tumors, however, composed principally or entirely of theca cells (12% of the feminizing mesenchymomas). Thecomas constitute about 2% of all ovarian tumors. They occur at all ages from 1 to 92 but are uncommon in women under the age of 35. They are most often found in postmenopausal women.

The evidence is good that thecomas arise from the ovarian cortical stroma. Indeed, transition from cortical stromal hyperplasia to thecoma has been observed, and it is not uncommon to find cortical stromal hyperplasia in the opposite ovary.

Theca cell tumors are unilateral and practically never malignant; fewer than 20 cases of malignant thecoma have been reported. The encapsulated tumor may be so small that the external contour of the ovary is unaltered, or it may become as large as 15 to 20 cm in diameter. The external surface is firm, ovoid or round, smooth, and gray, occasionally streaked with yellow. The cut surface is firm, uniform, and gray, frequently showing yellow foci which represent luetinization with fat deposition (Figs. 59-18, 59-19). Microscopic examination reveals interlacing bands of plump, spindle-shaped theca cells with intervening zones of hyalinization (Fig. 59-20). Fat stains frequently reveal the presence of fat within the cells. Occasional tumors show marked luteinization. Thecomas have been found within polycystic ovaries. The similarity between the two suggests a common endocrine pathogenesis.

Symptoms are related to estrogen production. However, it has been stated that in 25% of cases there is no evidence of hormonal activity. Since the tumors are most common in the postmenopausal period, the most frequent symptom is postmenopausal uterine bleeding. Menopausal bleeding or hypermenorrhea with endometrial hyperplasia are less common symptoms. A small but significant number of patients with thecomas (often luteinized) show evidence of excess androgen production. An unusual associated finding is ascites and hydrothorax (Meigs's syndrome) without metastasis or implants.

Treatment usually consists of removal of the involved ovary in young patients, and bilateral salpingo-oophorectomy and hysterectomy in older patients.

Sertoli–Leydig Cell Tumor (Androblastoma)

Androblastoma is a rare tumor of the ovarian stroma that recapitulates phases in the development of the male gonad and is composed of cells that resemble Sertoli and Leydig cells with varying degrees of differentiation (see Fig. 59-45). Well-differentiated tumors are usually

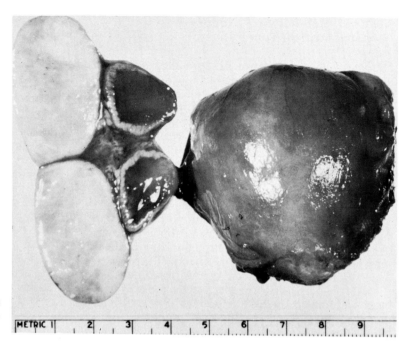

FIG. 59-18.   Thecoma of ovary. Cut surface is white streaked with yellow. Note also hemorrhagic corpus luteum.

FIG. 59-19.   Section through polycystic ovary containing well-circumscribed luteinized thecoma. Note follicle cysts in cortex of ovary. Patient's symptoms included hirsutism, oligomenorrhea, and infertility.

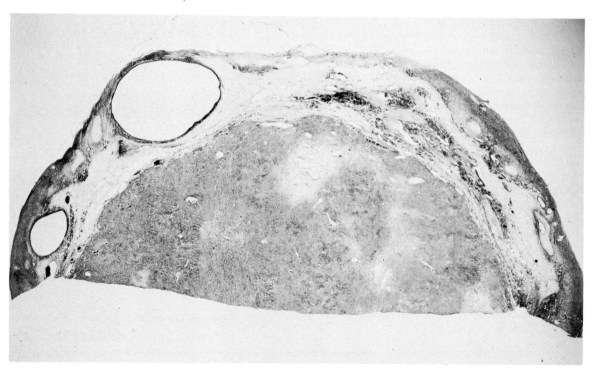

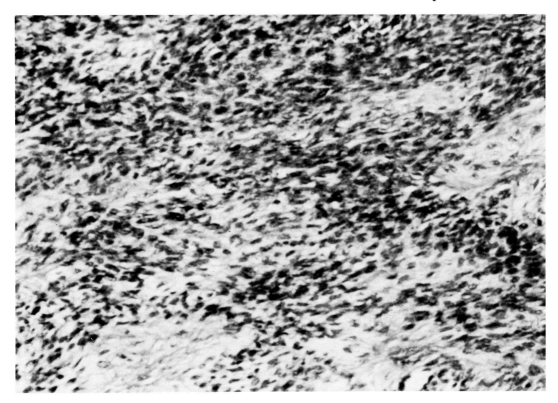

FIG. 59-20. Microscopic view of thecoma. Fat stain reveals fat within cystoplasm of plump, spindle-shaped cells.

androgenic, producing virilization, but some cases have been predominantly estrogenic. Although the overall malignant potential of these tumors is about 25%, most well-differentiated tumors behave in a benign fashion. Like granulosa cell tumors, androblastomas are commonly solid and soft with occasional cystic areas that may contain blood. The well-differentiated tumor (adenoma of Pick) consists of tubules lined by small columnar cells and rare islands of Leydig cells, containing lipid. Less differentiated tumors show a wide variety of morphologic features and estrogenic activity is rarely seen.

Gynandroblastoma

Gynandroblastoma is an extremely rare tumor described by Meyer in 1930. Its ability to produce both masculinizing (hirsutism, hypertrophy of the clitoris, voice change) and feminizing (vaginal bleeding due to endometrial hyperplasia) effects is attributed to the mixed and varied histologic pattern in which elements of both Sertoli–Leydig and granulosa cell tumor may be present side by side or intermixed. This suggests that granulosa cell tumors and Sertoli–Leydig cell tumors probably have a common origin.

Hilus Cell Tumor

Hilus cell tumors are extremely rare; approximately 50 have been described in the literature. The tumors are small and produce relatively little enlargement of the ovary. They have been discovered most often in menopausal women with hirsutism who have had menstrual abnormalities (oligomenorrhea and amenorrhea), infertility, enlargement of the clitoris, and related features of masculinization (Fig. 59-21). Hilus cell tumors produce high levels of testosterone. Only one malignant tumor has been described.

Grossly, they are circumscribed, solid, soft, and yellow or brown (Fig. 59-22). Microscopically, they consist of nonencapsulated sheets or cords of polyhedral cells similar to the normally occurring hilus cells of the adult ovary (Fig. 59-23). The cytoplasm contains lipochrome pigment and eosinophilic crystalloids.

Unilateral oophorectomy is recommended. It may be necessary to bisect the ovary to discover the tumor.

Lipid Cell Tumor

Because it is difficult to distinguish between hilus cell tumors, luteinized thecomas, adrenal-like tumors, and pure Leydig cell tumors, pathologists increasingly

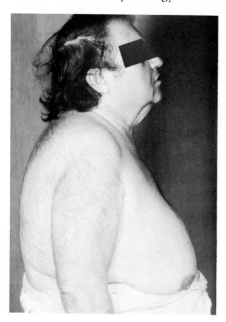

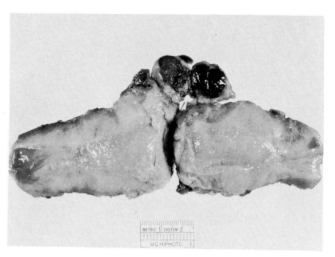

FIG. 59-21.   Patient with marked masculinization resulting from hilus cell tumor. Same appearance may be associated with other masculinizing tumors of ovary.

FIG. 59-22.   Uterus and ovary containing hilus cell tumor. Ovary was not enlarged. (Merrill JA: Am J Obstet Gynecol 78: 1258, 1959)

FIG. 59-23.   Ovarian hilus cell tumor. Microscopic section from edge of tumor demonstrates lack of encapsulation and nests of cells comprising growth. (Merrill JA: Am J Obstet Gynecol 78:1258, 1959)

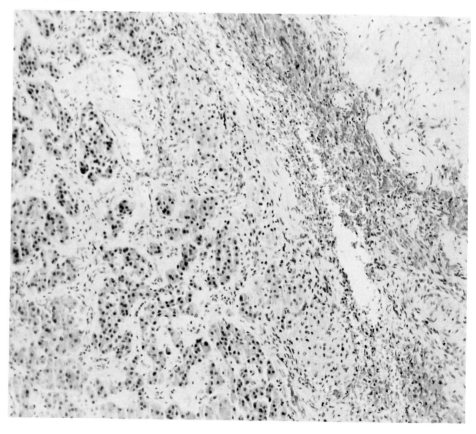

favor the use of the designation *lipid cell tumor* for this group of masculinizing tumors. The pregnancy luteoma is sometimes included, although this is probably a nonneoplastic hyperplasia of luteinized theca cells, at least during pregnancy.

Nonintrinsic Connective Tissue Tumors

Fibroma

The ovarian fibroma is a connective tissue tumor composed of fibrocytes and variable amounts of collagen. The fibroma occurs most frequently in middle age, with an average age incidence of 48 years. These tumors probably arise from the nonintrinsic connective tissue of the ovarian cortical stroma, although they may represent the inactive end stage of thecomas. The frequency of bilaterality is between 2% and 10%.

The average size of ovarian fibromas is 6 cm, with 5% of the tumors larger than 20 cm. At operation the tumor is firm or hard and smooth; the external and internal surfaces are grayish-white and glistening (Fig. 59-24). The cut surface is composed of homogeneous fibrous tissue, but may contain cysts. Microscopically, the tumor consists of small, thin, spindle-shaped cells arranged in bundles, giving an overall fasciculated appearance. Small tumors are usually cellular; large tumors more fibrous. As mentioned, differentiation from thecoma may be difficult.

There are no specific symptoms other than the occasional finding of ascites and less often hydrothorax. The explanation of this occurrence with benign solid tumors is not clear and of no special relevance. The effusion disappears following removal of the tumor.

Simple removal of the tumor is adequate therapy for this group of findings, which is known as *Meigs's syndrome.*

Other benign mesenchymal tumors such as leiomyoma, hemangioma, and lipoma, for example, are very unusual indeed.

Germ Cell Tumors

Benign Cystic Teratoma (Dermoid Cyst)

Dermoid cysts are relatively common, probably derived from primordial germ cells, and composed of any combination of well-differentiated ectodermal, mesodermal, and entodermal elements. They are slightly less common than the serous and mucinous cystadenomas, probably making up 18% to 25% of all ovarian neoplasms. The tumors may occur at any age, but the peak incidence is reported between 20 and 40 years. The tumors are almost always benign. In the unusual cases of malignancy, the malignant element is usually squamous epithelium.

Dermoids are bilateral in approximately 12% of patients, and most measure 5 cm to 10 cm in diameter. At operation the tumors are round, with a smooth, glistening gray surface. At body temperature they have the consistency of other tensely cystic tumors. Outside the body they have a soft pultaceous consistency. On sectioning, they are usually unilocular and filled with thick sebaceous material and tangled masses of hair (Fig. 59-25). There is often a solid portion at one pole of the cyst which contains the bulk of the cellular elements and the various dermal structures. In possibly 30% to 50% of cases the cyst contains formed teeth. Microscop-

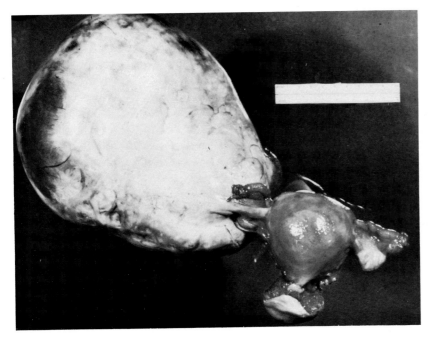

FIG. 59-24. Fibroma of ovary. External surface is firm, smooth, and white.

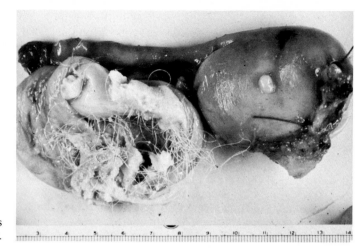

FIG. 59-25. Benign cystic teratoma of ovary. Tumor has been sectioned; sebaceous material and hair are apparent.

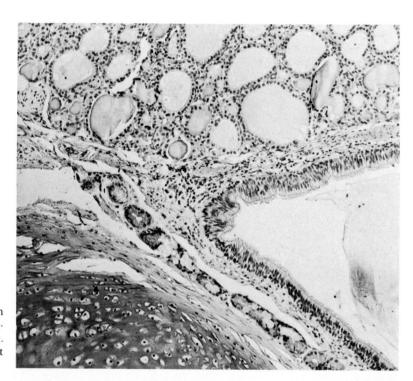

FIG. 59-26. Microscopic section of benign cystic teratoma showing thyroid tissue, respiratory epithelium, salivary glands, and cartilage. This section duplicates structures of anterior part of neck.

ically, a wide variety of tissues are found (Fig. 59-26). Most common are tissues normally found above the diaphragm: skin, sweat glands, respiratory epithelium, cartilage, salivary glands, and nervous tissue. Ectodermal structures are almost always present, with mesodermal and entodermal structures only slightly less frequent.

Because teeth are commonly present, x-ray of the abdomen may aid in diagnosis. Moreover, a dermoid cyst often has a long pedicle, allowing it to be palpated in the abdomen or anterior to the uterus. The frequency of torsion is relatively great. Since the tumors occur in young patients, treatment usually consists of excision of the cyst, conserving the remaining portion of the ovary. Some recommend that the opposite ovary be incised and inspected for a second tumor, although this is controversial.

Struma Ovarii

Struma ovarii is a unique benign cystic teratoma, in which thyroid tissue constitutes the entire, or nearly entire, cellular portion of the neoplasm. In external appearance this tumor is not distinguishable from a dermoid cyst. On sectioning, loculi of typical colloid may be seen (Fig. 59-27). The loculi are of various sizes and and have a yellowish-brown color. Microscopically, well-differentiated thyroid tissue is seen.

About 5% of strumas produce symptoms or signs of thyrotoxicosis, and possibly 10 patients have been reported with evidence of hyperthyroidism that was relieved by removal of the ovarian tumor. Rarely, thyrotoxicosis is unrelieved by thyroidectomy but finally is relieved when a struma ovarii is detected and removed.

Equally rare are carcinoid tumors that may have symptoms of the carcinoid syndrome. These tumors are of low-grade malignancy.

Gonadoblastoma

Gonadoblastoma is an unusual tumor that recapitulates the embryonic development of the gonad. It is usually a unilateral, soft, solid tumor, small in size, composed of large germ cells, sex chord elements, calcific concretions, and cellular stroma resembling Leydig or theca cells. Gonadoblastomas are found principally, but not always, in dysgenetic gonads of phenotypic females with a Y chromosome in the karyotype. The tumors themselves are almost invariably benign, but the germ cell component may give rise to highly malignant germ cell tumors including dysgerminoma, endodermal sinus

tumor, and embryonal carcinoma. Consequently, even in the absence of a palpable tumor it is advisable to remove the gonads of phenotypic females with gonadal dysgenesis and a Y chromosome in the karyotype. If a Y chromosome is absent, the risk of gonadoblastoma is extremely small; however, among the approximately 100 reported cases of this tumor, one occurred in a patient with a 45,XO karyotype and three in patients with 46,XX pattern.

Adrenal Rest Tumor

The adrenal rest tumor, often referred to by other terms, is one of the group of lipid masculinizing tumors of the ovary related in morphology and symptomatology to the hilus cell tumor, the luteinized thecoma, and the Sertoli–Leydig tumor. It resembles the cortical tissue of the adrenal, grossly and microscopically. According to a survey of 56 adrenal rest tumors reported in the literature, the tumors were usually unilateral and varied in size from 1 to 30 cm (42% were 5 cm or less in diameter, and 81% were 11 cm or less). They occurred in patients aged 6 to 71 years, the average age being 32 years. About 21% were considered malignant.

The most likely theory of histogenesis supposes an origin from embryonic rests of adrenal cortex in the ovary. Adrenal rests are relatively common in the ovaries and mesovarium of newborns but tumors are very rare in the adult.

Grossly, the tumors are usually encapsulated and lobulated. They are solid, rubbery, and usually yellow. Microscopically, the cells are typically those of the adrenal cortex and are arranged centripetally in strands separated by capillary networks. The cytoplasm contains lipid and brown pigment granules.

Essentially all patients have some features of masculinization including voice change, hypertrophied clitoris, atrophy of the breasts, and amenorrhea. Of the 56 patients reported in the literature, 30 had one or more features of Cushing's syndrome.

Treatment is oophorectomy.

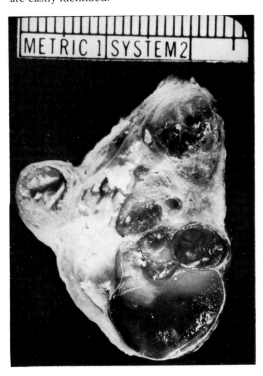

FIG. 59-27. Gross section of struma ovarii. Locules of colloid are easily identified.

REFERENCES AND RECOMMENDED READING

Aimen J, Edman C, Worley RJ et al: Androgen and estrogen formation in women with ovarian hyperthecosis. Obstet Gynecol 51:1, 1978

Anderson WR et al: Granulosa-theca cell tumors: Clinical and pathologic study. Am J Obstet Gynecol 110:32, 1971

Arey LB: Origin and form of the Brenner tumor. Am J Obstet Gynecol 81:743, 1961

Babaknia A, Calsopoulos P, Jones HW Jr.: The Stein–Leventhal syndrome and coincidental ovarian tumors. Obstet Gynecol 47:223, 1976

Barber HRK: Gynecological tumors in childhood and adolescence. Obstet Gynecol Surv 28:357, 1973

Barber HRK, Graber EA: The postmenopausal palpable ovary syndrome. Obstet Gynecol Surv 28:357, 1973

Barclay DL, Forney JP, Yellios F et al: Hyperreactio luteinalis:

Postpartum persistence. Am J Obstet Gynecol 105:642, 1969

Beck RP, Latour JPA: Review of 1019 benign ovarian neoplasms. Obstet Gynecol 16:478, 1960

Beck RP, Latour JPA: Atypical fibromas and thecomas of the ovary. Obstet Gynecol 19:228, 1962

Caspi E et al: Ovarian lutein cysts in pregnancy. Obstet Gynecol 42:388, 1973

Chalvardjian A, Scully RE: Sclerosing stromal tumors of the ovary. Cancer 31:664, 1973

Colgen TJ, Norris HJ: Ovarian epithelial tumors of low malignant potential. Int J Gynecol Pathol 1:367, 1983

Danforth DN: The cytological relationship of the Walthard cell rest to the Brenner tumor of the ovary and to the pseudomucinous cystadenoma. Am J Obstet Gynecol 43:948, 1942

De Bacalao EB, Dominquez I: Unilateral gonadoblastoma in a pregnant woman. Am J Obstet Gynecol 105:1279, 1969

Doss N, Leverich EB, Kemmerly JR: Covert bilaterality of mature ovarian teratomas. Obstet Gynecol 50:651, 1977

Dunnihoo DR et al: Hilar cell tumors of the ovary: Report of two new cases and review of the world literature. Obstet Gynecol 27:703, 1966

Emig OR, Hertig AT, Rowe FJ: Gynandroblastoma of the ovary: Review and report of a case. Obstet Gynecol 13:135, 1959

Farber M, Tran TH, Millan VG et al: Lipoid cell tumor of the ovary. Obstet Gynecol 54:576, 1979

Fox H: Human ovarian tumors: Classification, histogenesis, pathogenesis and criteria for experimental models. In Murphy ED, Beamer WG (eds): Biology of Ovarian Neoplasia, Page 22. Geneva, UICC, 1980

Gusberg SB, Danforth DN: Clinical significance of struma ovarii. Am J Obstet Gynecol 48:537, 1944

Kutsube Y, Berg JW, Silverberg SG: Epidemiologic pathology of ovarian tumors. Int J Gynecol Pathol 1:3, 1982

Marcus CC, Marcus SL: Struma ovarii. Am J Obstet Gynecol 81:752, 1961

Meigs JV: Pelvic tumors other than fibromas of the ovary with ascites and hydrothorax. Obstet Gynecol 3:471, 1954

Merrill JA: Morphology of the prepubertal ovary: Relationship to the polycystic ovary syndrome. South Med J 56:225, 1963

Norris HJ, Taylor HB: Virilization associated with cystic granulosa tumors. Obstet Gynecol 34:629, 1969

Novak ER, Long JH: Arrhenoblastoma of the ovary: A review of the ovarian tumor registry. Am J Obstet Gynecol 92:1082, 1965

O'Brien WS, Buck DR, Nash JD: Evaluation of sonography in the initial assessment of the gynecological patient. Am J Obstet Gynecol 149:598, 1984

Pedowitz P, Pomerance W: Adrenal-like tumors of the ovary. Obstet Gynecol 19:183, 1962

Randall CL, Hall DW: Clinical considerations of benign ovarian cystomas. Am J Obstet Gynecol 62:806, 1951

Scully RE: Tumors of the Ovary and Maldeveloped Gonads. Washington DC, Armed Forces Institute of Pathology, 1979

Spanos WJ: Preoperative hormonal therapy of cystic adrenal masses. Am J Obstet Gynecol 116:551, 1973

White KC: Ovarian tumors in pregnancy. Am J Obstet Gynecol 116:544, 1973

Yoonessi M, Abel MR: Brenner tumor of the ovary. Obstet Gynecol 54:90, 1979

Young RH, Scully RE: Ovarian sex cord–stromal tumors: Recent progress. Int J Gynecol Pathol 1:101, 1982

Malignant Lesions

Charles Zaloudek
Fatteneh A. Tavassoli
Robert J. Kurman

Cancer of the ovary presents a significant diagnostic and therapeutic challenge to the gynecologist. It is the most frequent cause of death among all cancers of the female genital tract and affects females of all ages. Although the five-year survival rate is still only 30%, significant progress has been made in the diagnosis and treatment of this disease. Clinicopathologic studies have provided an improved understanding of the pathology and natural history of most types of ovarian cancer. In particular, the recognition that there is a pathologically and clinically distinctive group of epithelial tumors of low malignant potential ("borderline" malignancy) has been an important development permitting the identification of a favorable prognostic group. Increased knowledge about the patterns of spread of ovarian cancer has permitted a more rational approach to staging. Improved methods of treatment using combination chemotherapy are now available for certain types of ovarian cancer, especially germ cell tumors. Finally, new diagnostic techniques such as sonography, computed tomography (CT), and measurement of serum oncofetal proteins permit more effective monitoring and assessment of therapy. Despite these advances, the practicing gynecologist plays a key role in the management of this disease, since early detection remains the single most effective method of improving prognosis.

CLASSIFICATION

More than 30 types of neoplasms have been identified in the ovary, and as a consequence, the classification of ovarian tumors is complex. Most of the neoplasms that arise in the ovary fall into one of three broad categories: neoplasms derived from the ovarian surface epithelium ("epithelial tumors"), neoplasms derived from the gonadal stroma ("gonadal stromal tumors"), and neoplasms derived from germ cells ("germ cell tumors"). A few rare tumors fall outside of these groups; the gonadoblastoma, for example, contains both germ cell and gonadal stromal elements, and soft tissue sarcomas of various types occasionally arise from mesenchymal elements that constitute the supportive framework of the ovary.

A useful classification of malignant ovarian tumors, widely accepted in the United States and throughout the world, has been put forward by the World Health

Organization. We advocate the use of this classification, which is based mainly on currently accepted concepts of the histogenesis of ovarian neoplasms. The classification is shown below:

Classification of Malignant Neoplasms of the Ovary

I. Epithelial tumors
   A. Serous tumor
      1. Low malignant potential
      2. Carcinoma
   B. Mucinous tumor
      1. Low malignant potential
      2. Carcinoma
   C. Endometrioid tumor
      1. Low malignant potential
      2. Carcinoma
   D. Clear cell tumor
      1. Low malignant potential
      2. Carcinoma
   E. Brenner tumor
      1. Proliferating
      2. Carcinoma
   F. Mixed mesodermal tumor
      1. Adenosarcoma
      2. Malignant mixed mesodermal tumor
   G. Undifferentiated carcinoma
II. Germ cell tumors
   A. Dysgerminoma
   B. Yolk sac (endodermal sinus) tumor
   C. Teratoma
      1. Immature
      2. Malignant tumor developing in benign teratoma
      3. Monodermal or highly specialized teratoma
   D. Embryonal carcinoma
   E. Choriocarcinoma
   F. Mixed germ cell tumor
   G. Gonadoblastoma
III. Sex cord–stromal tumors
   A. Granulosa tumor
   B. Sertoli tumor
   C. Sertoli–Leydig tumor
   D. Lipid cell tumor
   E. Gynandroblastoma
   F. Unclassified
IV. Soft tissue tumors not specific to ovaries
V. Lymphoma/leukemia
VI. Unclassified tumors
VII. Metastatic tumors

EPIDEMIOLOGY AND ETIOLOGY

Cancer of the ovary is the most frequent cause of death from genital cancer in women. In the United States, 18,500 new cases of ovarian cancer are detected each year, and more than 11,500 women die from it. Cancer of the ovary ranks as the fifth most frequent type of cancer in women, and it is the fourth leading cause of cancer deaths, exceeded only by cancer of the breast, lung, and large intestine.

There is considerable worldwide variation in the incidence of ovarian cancer. It is most frequent in the industrialized countries of Western Europe and in the United States. The highest age-adjusted death rate for ovarian cancer is 11 per 100,000 women per year in Scandinavia. In the United States, the annual death rate is 7 per 100,000 women for whites and 6 per 100,000 for blacks. Ovarian cancer is comparatively infrequent in most third-world countries and in Japan, where the age-adjusted annual death rate is less than 2 per 100,000 population.

Ovarian cancer is predominantly a disease of peri- and postmenopausal women, with an average patient age of 50 to 59 years. Most ovarian cancers that occur in children are malignant germ cell tumors; epithelial neoplasms are uncommon in this age group. The incidence of ovarian cancer increases with age, reaching a peak annual incidence of 70 cases per 100,000 population aged 75. Epithelial neoplasms are by far the most frequent type of ovarian cancer in adults, accounting for more than 90% of cases. Gonadal stromal tumors account for approximately 2% of ovarian malignancies in adults, but malignant germ cell tumors are rare in women over age 40. The incidence of all types of ovarian cancer has remained relatively constant over the last 30 years.

Little is known about the cause of ovarian cancer. The relatively high incidence in industrialized countries suggests that environmental factors or diet may play a role in its etiology. Asbestos and talc have been proposed as possible causative agents, but to date there is no proven link between these substances, or any others, and the development of ovarian cancer.

Genetic factors have been implicated in the etiology of some ovarian neoplasms. Occasional families have been reported in which several members have serous carcinoma, and most female patients with the Peutz–Jeghers syndrome (hamartomatous polyps of the gastrointestinal tract and mucocutaneous melanin pigmentation) have an unusual gonadal stromal tumor, referred to as a *sex cord tumor with annular tubules*.

Hormones may play a role in the etiology of ovarian cancer. Compared with controls, patients who develop ovarian cancer are more frequently nulliparous, have their first pregnancy at a later age, and have smaller families. The international variation in the incidence of ovarian cancer may be related to this factor; ovarian cancer is less common in poor countries, where birth control is rarely practiced and pregnancy at an early age and a large family are the norm, than in richer countries. The observation that patients with breast cancer have a twofold increase in the risk of developing ovarian cancer further supports the concept that hormones play a role in the etiology of ovarian cancer. However, there is no evidence that oral contraceptives or other exogenous hormones cause ovarian cancer; in fact, the incidence of ovarian cancer appears to be lower in women with a history of oral contraceptive use than in women who have not used oral contraceptives.

DIAGNOSIS

Symptoms

Early diagnosis of ovarian cancer is difficult because symptoms are often absent or vague until the neoplasm has attained a large size and metastasized. Even large tumors usually produce nonspecific symptoms. Seventy percent of patients have metastases outside the pelvis at diagnosis.

Early symptoms include vague sensations of pelvic or abdominal discomfort, urinary frequency, and alterations in gastrointestinal function. When a neoplasm attains a diameter of about 15 cm, it rises into the abdominal cavity, which leads to feelings of abdominal fullness or distention and early satiety. Abdominal enlargement can also be secondary to ascites. About 15% of patients experience abnormal vaginal bleeding. Finally, hemorrhage into a tumor or torsion of an ovary containing a neoplasm can produce sudden pain and other symptoms of an acute abdomen.

Patients with gonadal stromal tumors or malignant germ cell tumors sometimes present with symptoms that specifically suggest the presence of an ovarian tumor. For example, granulosa tumors often produce estrogen, so postmenopausal women may experience abnormal bleeding secondary to endometrial hyperplasia. Sertoli–Leydig tumors frequently secrete testosterone, resulting in virilization in 50% of patients. Choriocarcinoma and embryonal carcinoma generally produce human chorionic gonadotropin (hCG), leading to oligomenorrhea or amenorrhea and, in premenarchal girls, to isosexual precocious pseudopuberty.

Physical Findings

Ovarian tumors are almost invariably detected by pelvic examination. The ovaries are usually not palpable in postmenopausal women and premenarchal girls, and since nonneoplastic cysts are rare in these age groups, palpation of an adnexal mass requires further evaluation. In menstruating women, follicular and luteal cysts can cause transient ovarian enlargement. Menstruating women with small (less than 5 cm in diameter) unilateral adnexal masses should be carefully followed for two to three months. Functional cysts should involute during this period, whereas neoplastic masses can be expected to remain the same size or enlarge. A persistent mass or one larger than 5 cm diameter requires evaluation and laparotomy.

Preoperative Evaluation

Preoperative evaluation should include a plain film of the abdomen, a chest film, a complete blood count, and serum chemistries, including liver function studies. An intravenous pyelogram provides information about renal function and the status and location of the ureters, and it delineates any important anatomic abnormalities of the urinary system (*i.e.,* pelvic kidney). Between 5% and 10% of malignant adnexal masses prove to be metastatic tumors in the ovaries. The most common primary site for such metastases is the large bowel, so a barium enema should be performed preoperatively. In women with symptoms referable to the upper gastrointestinal tract or in high-risk groups, such as women of Japanese descent, an upper gastrointestinal study is important to rule out stomach cancer. Finally, since multiple cancers of the female genital tract may occur, a Papanicolaou (Pap) smear should be performed to evaluate the cervix, and women with abnormal vaginal bleeding or uterine enlargement should have a fractional dilatation and curettage.

Neither ultrasonography nor CT is recommended as part of the routine preoperative evaluation of patients with adnexal masses, since the findings rarely alter the treatment. CT and ultrasound may be useful in the evaluation of patients with advanced or recurrent cancer, but both techniques sometimes fail to demonstrate even extensive intra-abdominal disease.

Percutaneous fine-needle aspiration, using sonographic or CT guidance if necessary, is an accurate method of diagnosing a variety of tumors. It should not be used for the initial diagnosis of an ovarian tumor, however, since such a neoplasm should be treated by surgical excision regardless of the results of fine-needle aspiration, and there is some risk that a cystic neoplasm will rupture when aspirated. Fine-needle aspiration can sometimes be used to provide morphologic documentation of recurrent carcinoma, obviating the need for laparotomy.

STAGING

Clinical studies reveal that patients with stage-I epithelial cancers have a long-term survival rate of 60% to 70%. Prior to the use of combination chemotherapy, patients with certain types of stage-I germ cell tumors had survival rates of only 15%. These observations imply that occult metastases are present at diagnosis in many patients. Studies conducted during the past ten years have shown that metastatic carcinoma can be detected at sites that were not formerly evaluated in patients thought to have stage-I or stage-II cancer of the ovary. For example, 16% of patients with epithelial cancers have metastatic deposits on the inferior surface of the diaphragm, 12% have para-aortic lymph node metastases, 4% have omental metastases, and 32% have malignant cells in peritoneal washings. In addition, metastatic deposits in more readily visualized portions of the abdominal and pelvic cavities can be overlooked unless the staging procedure is conducted in a careful, systematic fashion.

The stage is the single most important determinant of prognosis and method of treatment (Fig. 59-28). Staging is based predominantly on the gynecologist's observations at laparotomy and the pathologist's evaluation of specimens submitted for histologic and cytologic study. Introduced by the International Federation of Gynecology and Obstetrics (FIGO) in 1974, the system that is presently in use is summarized below:

Staging of Carcinoma of the Ovary
Stage I
Growth limited to the ovaries
  Ia Growth limited to one ovary; no ascites
    (i) No tumor on the external surface; capsule intact
    (ii) Tumor present on the external surface and/or capsule ruptured
  Ib Growth limited to both ovaries; no ascites
    (i) No tumor on the external surface; capsule intact
    (ii) Tumor present on the external surface and/or capsule ruptured
  Ic Tumor either Ia or Ib, but with obvious ascites present or positive peritoneal washings
Stage II
Growth involving one or both ovaries with pelvic extension
  IIa Extension and/or metastasis to the uterus and/or tubes

  IIb Extension to other pelvic structures, including the peritoneum and the uterus
  IIc Tumor either IIa or IIb, but with obvious ascites present or positive peritoneal washings
Stage III
Growth involving one or both ovaries with intraperitoneal metastases outside the pelvis and/or positive retroperitoneal nodes
Tumor limited to the true pelvis with histologically proven malignant extension to small bowel or omentum
Stage IV
Growth involving one or both ovaries with distant metastasis; parenchymal liver metastases
Special Category
Unexplored cases that are thought to be ovarian carcinoma

Proper staging requires that the patient be explored through a vertical midline incision. The presence and character of ascitic fluid should be noted and an initial sample submitted for cytologic evaluation.

Once a diagnosis of carcinoma is established by visual examination or intraoperative frozen section, the incision should be extended above the umbilicus to permit adequate exposure of the abdominal cavity. The surgeon should note whether the carcinoma is unilateral or bilateral, whether the capsule is intact or ruptured, and whether or not excrescences are present on the surface. The subsequent course of the operation depends on the gynecologist's initial assessment of the extent of tumor spread. If widespread extrapelvic metastases are present, the gynecologist can proceed with the treatment phase of the operation. If the carcinoma

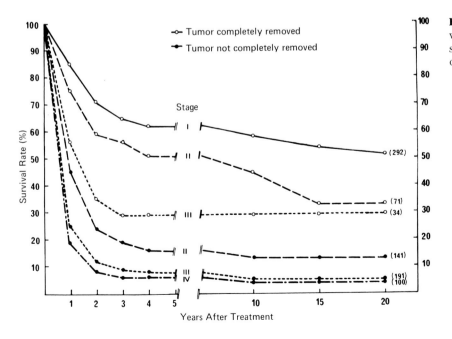

FIG. 59-28. Survival rates for patients with ovarian carcinoma in relation to stage and operability of tumor. Numbers of patients are given in parentheses.

appears localized (stage I or II), a systematic staging procedure should be completed before the neoplasm is resected. If the ovarian neoplasm is so large that it interferes with adequate visualization of the abdomen and pelvis, or if the surgeon judges that there is a risk of rupture, the neoplasm can be resected prior to completion of abdominopelvic exploration.

The gynecologist should keep the potential metastatic pathways of ovarian cancer in mind while conducting the exploration. Cytologic specimens should be obtained from the right inferior surface of the diaphragm, the left and right paracolic spaces, and the pelvis. Each site is lavaged with 100 ml of saline, which is then aspirated and sent for cytologic evaluation. The undersurface of the diaphragm, especially its right leaf, and the surfaces of the liver are palpated and visualized and any raised or roughened areas biopsied. All abdominal and pelvic peritoneal surfaces, including the serosa of the large and small intestines, the bladder, and the mesentery, are examined and any red, roughened, or nodular areas excised. The omentum is carefully palpated and omentectomy performed to permit detection of microscopic metastases. Adhesions between an involved ovary and adjacent structures should be excised and submitted for histologic examination. The para-aortic and pelvic lymph nodes should be carefully evaluated and any enlarged or firm nodes excised for histologic study. Occult primary cancers in other organs can give rise to large metastatic deposits in the ovaries, so the stomach, pancreas, and small and large intestines must be carefully palpated.

The stage is ultimately assigned after all available evidence is correlated. This includes the results of clinical and radiographic examinations, the gynecologist's observations at laparotomy, including the size and location of residual tumor deposits and whether any of them exceeds 2 cm in diameter, and the pathologist's findings.

DISSEMINATION

Ovarian cancer can spread by several pathways (Fig. 59-29): The neoplasm can *directly invade* adjacent organs such as the small intestine, rectosigmoid, colon, peritoneum, omentum, uterus, fallopian tube, and broad ligament. Alternatively, spread can occur *by way of the peritoneal fluid,* malignant cells implanting throughout the pelvis and abdominal cavity, including the omentum, posterior cul-de-sac, infundibulopelvic ligaments, paracolic gutters, right hemidiaphragm, and capsule of the liver. Transabdominal dissemination, the most common form of spread, accounts for the fact that many ovarian cancers are stage III at the time of diagnosis. Ascites often develops with peritoneal metastases, and fluid may pass through lymphatics in the right hemidiaphragm. In this manner, malignant cells can implant on the pleura and produce a malignant pleural effusion. Dissemination may also occur *through lymphatics* to the pelvic and para-aortic lymph nodes (Fig. 59-30). The pelvic and para-aortic lymph nodes are involved in approximately 10% of patients initially thought to have stage-I or stage-II carcinoma. The frequency is higher in patients with advanced disease, where it approaches 50%. Metastases may occasionally be detected in distal sites such as supraclavicular or inguinal lymph nodes. The least common method of spread is *hematogenous dissemination.* Hematogenous metastases occur in the liver parenchyma, the skin, and the lungs.

Field carcinogenesis has been proposed as a likely explanation for the synchronous or sequential development of carcinoma at separate sites in the female genital tract. The high frequency of bilaterality in ovarian carcinoma can be explained by this mechanism, since the carcinoma usually has the appearance of a primary neoplasm in both ovaries. Similarly, the frequent association of endometrioid carcinoma of the ovary with endometrial carcinoma could be due to a field effect. Field carcinogenesis has recently been invoked as a possible explanation for the long-term survival of patients with stage-III serous tumors of low malignant potential. In most patients, the peritoneal "implants" are *in situ* proliferations histologically identical to the tumor in the ovary. If the "implants" are separate primary noninvasive peritoneal proliferations, the favorable prognosis is understandable. Patients whose death is attributed to stage-III serous tumors of low malignant potential usually have peritoneal "implants" which, in contrast to the ovarian tumor, exhibit an invasive pattern of growth.

FIG. 59-29. Four mechanisms of dissemination of ovarian cancer cells. (Cole WH, McDonald GO, Roberts SS, Southwick HW: Dissemination of Cancer. New York, Appleton-Century-Crofts, 1961)

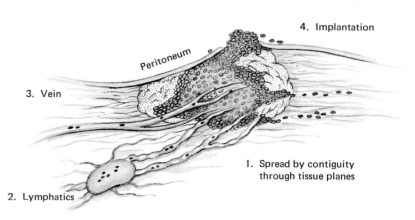

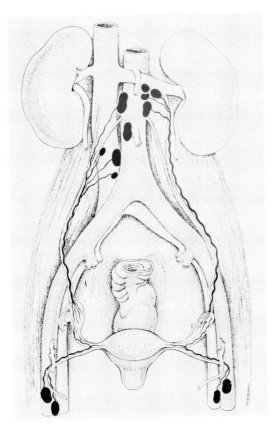

FIG. 59-30. Diagram of lymphatics of the ovary showing drainage by para-aortic lymph nodes. There is inconstant drainage toward the external iliac nodes.

EPITHELIAL TUMORS

Epithelial tumors constitute more than 60% of neoplasms arising in the ovary and more than 90% of the malignant ones. These are consequently the most important group of ovarian tumors.

Most epithelial tumors are derived ultimately from the ovarian surface epithelium, a specialized type of mesothelium. Inclusions develop when surface epithelium is introduced into the cortex at the time of ovulation or when the ovary is involved in a pelvic inflammatory process. Fluid may accumulate within inclusions, producing cysts, and the lining may undergo metaplasia to various types of müllerian epithelium; tubal metaplasia is most frequent. Most carcinomas are cystic neoplasms that are thought to arise from epithelial inclusions within the cortex. A minority arise on the surface of the ovary, where they grow as surface papillary tumors.

Epithelial tumors are classified according to the predominant pattern of histologic differentiation. There are five main types: serous, mucinous, endometrioid, clear cell, and Brenner (transitional cell). In addition, mixed mesodermal tumors of the ovary are thought to be derived from the surface epithelium and subjacent stroma and are also considered to be epithelial tumors. Some malignant epithelial tumors are so poorly differentiated that they cannot be accurately placed into any of the above categories and are therefore classified as undifferentiated carcinomas.

Epithelial tumors are also classified as benign, as of low malignant potential, or as carcinoma, depending on the degree of cellular proliferation and atypia and the presence of stromal invasion. Epithelial tumors of low malignant potential ("borderline" epithelial tumors) account for 10% to 15% of epithelial neoplasms. Tumors of low malignant potential, which have gained widespread recognition as distinct tumor types only in the last decade, have morphologic features intermediate between those of a cystadenoma and a carcinoma. Clinicopathologic studies of patients with epithelial tumors of low malignant potential illustrate the importance of this group of neoplasms. In contrast to patients with epithelial carcinoma, more than 70% of women with epithelial tumors of low malignant potential have localized disease at presentation. The prognosis is favorable. In the most detailed study of mucinous tumors of low malignant potential, patients with stage-I tumors had an actuarial five-year survival rate of 96%. In a study of serous tumors of low malignant potential, it was observed that no patient with a stage-Ia, -Ib, or -IIa neoplasm died of metastases and that only half of the patients with stage-IIb and -III tumors were dead at last follow-up; the mean survival of those patients who ultimately died of tumor was 8.9 years. These results are dramatically different from those obtained with patients with invasive epithelial carcinomas; they indicate that patients with epithelial tumors of low malignant potential, even those with advanced-stage neoplasms, have a more favorable prognosis and much longer survival and require different therapy from patients with invasive carcinoma.

Serous Tumors

Serous carcinoma, which accounts for 35% of malignant epithelial tumors, is the most common type of ovarian cancer. It occurs twice as frequently as serous tumors of low malignant potential. Together these neoplasms constitute 45% to 50% of all malignant epithelial tumors of the ovary.

Serous tumors are frequently bilateral. Approximately 35% of serous tumors of low malignant potential are bilateral, whereas 40% to 60% of serous carcinomas involve both ovaries. Extraovarian spread at diagnosis is frequent. Thirty percent of patients with serous tumors of low malignant potential have extraovarian tumor at presentation, usually in the form of peritoneal implants. As many as 85% of patients with serous carcinoma present in stages II to IV. Stage III is the most frequent stage at diagnosis, accounting for about 50% of cases.

Serous tumors are composed of epithelial cells that resemble, to a variable degree, the cell types seen in

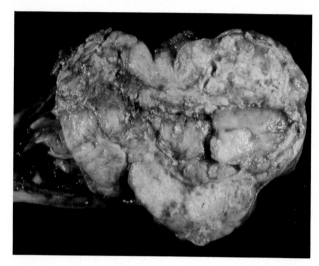

FIG. 59-31. Serous carcinoma. Solid portions of this neoplasm are white and fleshy, with extensive chalky areas of necrosis. A cystic component is visible at left.

the fallopian tube. The similarity to normal fallopian tube epithelium is greatest in benign serous tumors, which are composed of ciliated and nonciliated columnar cells with oval, basal nuclei, and least in serous carcinoma.

Gross Pathology

Low-malignant-potential and malignant serous tumors have similar appearances. They are both large, uni- or multilocular cystic neoplasms. Half of them exceed 15 cm in diameter, and most of the remaining ones range in size from 5 cm to 15 cm. Cut section reveals coarse papillae projecting into and sometimes filling cystic lumina. Papillary excrescences are frequently present on the exterior of both low-malignant-potential and malignant serous tumors. Solid areas, hemorrhage and necrosis, invasion through the cyst wall, and adhesions to adjacent structures are features that suggest that a neoplasm is a carcinoma rather than a tumor of low malignant potential (Fig. 59-31).

Microscopic Pathology

Serous tumors of low malignant potential have architectural features intermediate between those of a cystadenoma and those of a carcinoma. The coarse papillae seen grossly are covered by stratified epithelial cells that form micropapillary tufts from which individual cells and small clusters of cells bud into the cystic lumina (Fig. 59-32). There is usually mild to moderate nuclear atypia, and occasionally mitotic figures are present. Psammoma bodies, which are small, whorled, calcified bodies arising as products of cellular degeneration, are characteristic of serous tumors, and are present in 50% of tumors of low malignant potential. The key distinguishing feature between a serous tumor of low malignant potential and a serous carcinoma is the absence of stromal invasion in the former.

Well-differentiated serous carcinomas contain papillae covered by stratified epithelial cells showing variable degrees of cytologic atypia and mitotic activity (Fig. 59-33). Most serous carcinomas are poorly differentiated (grade-2 or -3) neoplasms characterized by trabecular and solid patterns of growth, papillae being present only focally. Psammoma bodies are found in many serous carcinomas and in their metastases.

FIG. 59-32. Serous tumor of low malignant potential. Coarse papillae are covered by one to two layers of mildly atypical columnar epithelial cells. Cells are shed into the cystic lumen both individually and in clusters.

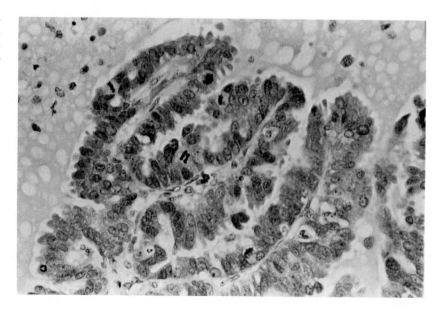

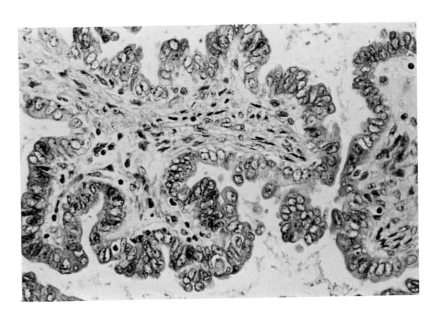

FIG. 59-33. Serous carcinoma. Papillae are covered by stratified low columnar epithelial cells. Note the high nucleus/cytoplasm ratio and the presence of numerous mitotic figures. (×250)

Mucinous Tumors

Mucinous tumors of low malignant potential and mucinous carcinomas account for 10% to 20% of all malignant epithelial tumors of the ovary. Each type constitutes 5% to 10% of all malignant epithelial tumors. The average age of patients with mucinous tumors is 50 to 55 years, approximately the same as that of patients with other types of epithelial tumors, but there is a bimodal age distribution, and a significant number of patients are of reproductive age. Conservative treatment of mucinous tumors by unilateral salpingo-oophorectomy is thus a frequent consideration. Stage-I mucinous tumors are bilateral in fewer than 10% of cases, and a stage-I tumor of low malignant potential or a stage-Ia(i) grade-1 mucinous carcinoma can be adequately treated by unilateral salpingo-oophorectomy. Extraovarian spread at diagnosis is less frequent than in patients with serous tumors. Approximately 15% of mucinous tumors of low malignant potential and 40% of mucinous carcinomas are detected in stages II to IV.

Gross Pathology

Mucinous tumors of low malignant potential and mucinous carcinomas have similar appearances. They are usually large neoplasms, the average diameter being 16 cm to 17 cm. Examples of these neoplasms are among the largest ovarian tumors. They are multilocular cystic tumors filled with thick, viscous mucin. Papillae are occasionally noted, but more commonly the cysts have a smooth lining. Solid areas, hemorrhage, and necrosis (Fig. 59-34) are more frequent in mucinous carcinoma, but they occur with sufficient frequency in mucinous tumors of low malignant potential that their presence or absence is of no diagnostic value. Invasion through the cyst wall with growth on the external surface of the ovary is infrequent and is generally an indication of carcinoma.

Microscopic Pathology

Light and electron microscopic study of the proliferating epithelium in a mucinous tumor of low malig-

FIG. 59-34. Mucinous carcinoma. Partially cystic, this large neoplasm has a fleshy, mucoid cut surface. (×160)

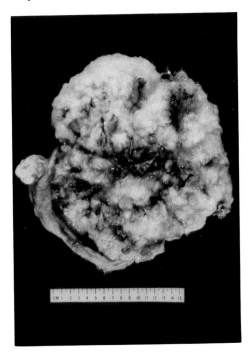

nant potential reveals an admixture of endocervical-type columnar mucinous cells with basal nuclei and intestinal-type cells, including columnar cells with eosinophilic cytoplasm, goblet cells, and basal endocrine cells. The epithelial lining of the cysts is proliferative, forming secondary cysts and micropapillary processes. Although there is cell stratification, the epithelium is usually limited to two to three cell layers. Mild to moderate cytologic atypia and moderate numbers of mitotic figures are present. There is no stromal invasion.

Mucinous carcinoma is composed almost entirely of intestinal-type cells. Glands, cysts, and papillae vary markedly in size and shape and may be arranged back to back, with no intervening stroma (Fig. 59-35). They are lined by atypical cells that have large, hyperchromatic nuclei and prominent nucleoli. Mitotic figures are usually numerous, especially in poorly differentiated carcinoma. Mucin production is prominent in well-differentiated carcinoma but scanty and focal in poorly differentiated tumors. The criterion on the basis of which the diagnosis of mucinous carcinoma is made is the presence of stromal invasion. This may be manifested as irregular, small malignant glands infiltrating the stroma and eliciting a desmoplastic response, as a back-to-back arrangement of glands, as a solid or cribriform growth pattern often accompanied by necrosis, or as marked cellular stratification (four or more layers).

Unlike most other epithelial tumors of the ovary, mucinous tumors vary markedly in their histologic appearance from area to area. Some mucinous carcinomas, for example, contain areas that are indistinguishable from a tumor of low malignant potential or even a mucinous cystadenoma. Extensive sampling for microscopic examination is therefore necessary for an accurate pathologic diagnosis. This can compromise the accuracy of intraoperative frozen sections, which can be used only to study limited areas of a tumor.

Pseudomyxoma Peritonei

Pseudomyxoma peritonei is a rare condition characterized by the progressive accumulation of mucin within the abdominal cavity. It occurs in women who have a mucinous tumor of the ovary, mucocele of the appendix, or both. Pseudomyxoma peritonei appears to develop when there is slow leakage of mucin and tumor cells from a mucinous tumor (usually of low malignant potential). The tumor cells implant on the peritoneum, where they grow autonomously and secrete large quantities of mucus. Pseudomyxoma is usually present when the patient is initially operated upon and does not appear to develop as a consequence of rupture of a mucinous tumor at operation.

Because pseudomyxoma peritonei can also be secondary to a mucocele of the appendix, an appendectomy should be performed in all cases. If mucinous tumors of the ovary and appendix are both present, histologic study may reveal whether the pseudomyxoma is secondary to leakage from the ovarian or appendiceal tumor, but in many instances the source of the condition cannot be determined.

It is difficult to eradicate all of the mucinous epithelium present on the peritoneum, so mucus frequently reaccumulates, requiring repeated surgical procedures to remove it. Treatment with systemic alkylating agents has proven beneficial in some cases. About half of all patients with pseudomyxoma succumb to the condition, usually after a long illness.

Endometrioid Tumors

Endometrioid carcinoma has a histologic appearance identical to that of a typical adenocarcinoma of the endometrium. Endometrioid carcinoma constitutes 15% to 20% of malignant epithelial tumors of the ovary, mak-

FIG. 59-35. Mucinous carcinoma. Infiltrating, crowded glands are lined by tall columnar cells with pale cytoplasm. Note the atypical, stratified nuclei. (×160)

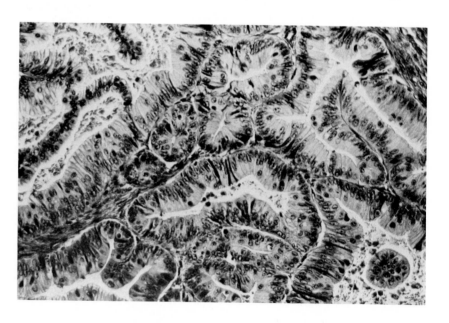

ing this the second most frequent type of carcinoma of the ovary.

The histologic similarity to endometrial carcinoma raises the question of whether endometrioid carcinoma originates in ovarian endometriosis. Pathologic studies reveal that 5% to 10% of endometrioid carcinomas do in fact originate in endometriosis and that endometriosis is present in the involved ovary in an additional 10% to 15% of cases. Most endometrioid carcinomas, however, develop by neoplastic transformation of surface epithelium–derived cells.

Endometrioid carcinoma is bilateral in 20% to 30% of all patients but in only 15% of patients with stage-I neoplasms. Extraovarian spread is seen at diagnosis in 40% to 50% of cases.

Fifteen to twenty percent of patients with endometrioid carcinoma have a synchronous adenocarcinoma of the endometrium. The endometrial carcinoma is usually small and superficial and associated with hyperplastic changes in the adjacent endometrium. In this setting, the endometrial and ovarian carcinomas are regarded as separate primary neoplasms. The survival of patients with endometrioid carcinoma and a small, synchronous endometrial carcinoma is similar to that of patients with endometrioid carcinoma not associated with endometrial pathology. Endometrial carcinoma can metastasize to the ovary, but in such instances the endometrial neoplasm is usually large, deeply invasive, and poorly differentiated.

Gross Pathology

Endometrioid tumors do not have a specific macroscopic appearance. Some neoplasms are entirely solid, with soft or firm gray tan cut surfaces. Others are partially or largely cystic, and have gray tan solid areas admixed with the cysts. Foci of hemorrhage and necrosis are often present.

Microscopic Pathology

Endometrioid tumors of low malignant potential are rare, and most of them are cystadenofibromas. The proliferative epithelium, which resembles that seen in atypical hyperplasia of the endometrium, is surrounded by dense fibrous stroma. Squamous differentiation of the epithelium is present in half the cases. Stromal invasion is not identified, nor are there extensive back-to-back arrangements of glands or sheets of tumor cells. There are no reported instances of death from well-documented endometrioid tumors of low malignant potential, so it is uncertain whether such neoplasms should be regarded as proliferative, but clinically benign, neoplasms or as carcinomas of low malignant potential, as the World Health Organization definition suggests.

Well-differentiated endometrioid carcinoma is characterized by glands lined by stratified columnar cells with moderate amounts of eosinophilic or lightly basophilic cytoplasm and large, hyperchromatic nuclei (Fig. 59-36). Mitotic figures are readily identified. The glands are arranged in a cribriform pattern with no intervening stroma. Solid growth patterns are present in moderately or poorly differentiated neoplasms. Squamous differentiation is present in 25% to 50% of endometrioid carcinomas. If the squamous epithelium is histologically benign, which is most often the case, the neoplasm may be referred to as an *adenoacanthoma;* if malignant, it may be called an *adenosquamous carcinoma.*

Clear Cell Tumors

Clear cell carcinoma accounts for 5% to 10% of malignant epithelial tumors of the ovary. In the past this tumor was termed *mesonephric* or *mesonephroid carcinoma,* but it is now recognized that clear cell carcinoma is of

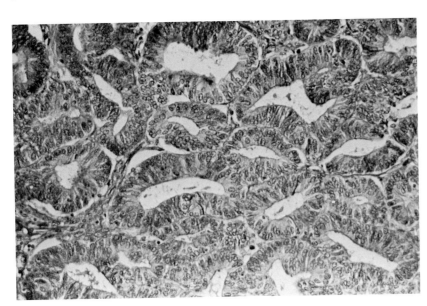

FIG. 59-36. Endometrioid carcinoma is composed of glands arranged back to back and lined by stratified malignant cells. It is histologically similar to an adenocarcinoma of the endometrium. (×160)

surface epithelial derivation and closely related to endometrioid carcinoma. Up to 25% of patients with each of these types of neoplasms have pelvic endometriosis, and both types of neoplasms occasionally develop in ovarian endometriosis. In addition, mixed epithelial tumors having both clear cell and endometrioid components are relatively common.

The relatively favorable overall prognosis in clear cell carcinoma is due to the fact that 60% to 70% of patients present with stage-I tumors. Fewer than 5% of patients with stage-I disease have bilateral tumors, and the contralateral ovary is involved in only 10% to 15% of patients with advanced disease.

Gross Pathology

Clear cell carcinomas are large (10–20 cm in diameter) and have a variable gross appearance. Most are cystic neoplasms, the lumina of which contain papillae, polyps, or fleshy, gray tan, solid nodules, but a significant proportion are entirely solid. Hemorrhage and necrosis are common, and in about a third of the neoplasms there is invasion of the cyst wall.

Microscopic Pathology

Rarely, a clear cell tumor can be classified as being of low malignant potential. Such neoplasms are typically cystadenofibromas in which glands, tubules, or cysts are lined by cytologically atypical clear cells. Stromal invasion is not present. All well-documented examples have had a benign clinical evolution.

Clear cell carcinoma has a varied histologic appearance with a mixture of cell types and growth patterns being present in most neoplasms. Two cell types are characteristic. The first is the clear cell, which has a round, centrally placed nucleus and abundant clear cy-

toplasm (Fig. 59-37). Histochemical stains reveal that the cytoplasm is clear because it contains abundant glycogen. The second cell type is a columnar cell with an apical hyperchromatic oval or fusiform nucleus that bulges into gland lumina, producing a "hobnail" appearance. The clear cells are arranged in sheets, or they and the hobnail cells line papillae, tubules, or cysts.

Other Types of Epithelial Tumors

Brenner tumors contain epithelium that resembles the transitional epithelium lining the urinary tract and a fibrous stroma. Malignant Brenner tumors are rare. Their epithelial component resembles a high-grade transitional cell carcinoma of the bladder. The tumor cells grow in sheets and invade the stroma. The nuclei are large, pleomorphic, and hyperchromatic, and mitotic figures are numerous. Hemorrhage and necrosis are usually present.

An intermediate (low-malignant-potential) type of Brenner tumor characterized by pathologists is usually referred to as a "proliferating" Brenner tumor, since all reported examples have followed a benign clinical course. The epithelium in this neoplasm is proliferative transitional epithelium similar to that seen in low-grade transitional cell carcinoma of the bladder. Marked degrees of epithelial proliferation are sometimes present with a papillary growth pattern, but there is no stromal invasion, and the tumor cells lack the cytologic features of malignancy observed in the malignant Brenner tumor.

Malignant mixed mesodermal tumors are biphasic neoplasms that are histologically identical to mixed müllerian tumors of the uterus. Their epithelial component is a carcinoma, frequently of the endometrioid type, and their stromal component is a sarcoma. A wide variety of sarcomatous elements have been described,

FIG. 59-37. Clear cell carcinoma. Tumor cells are polygonal, with central nuclei and abundant clear cytoplasm. (×250)

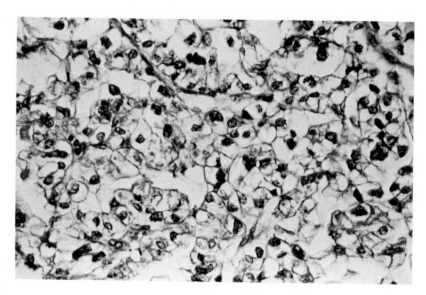

including endometrioid stromal sarcoma, leiomyosarcoma, fibrosarcoma, rhabdomyosarcoma, and chondrosarcoma. An *adenosarcoma* is a low-grade variant of the mixed mesodermal tumor in which the epithelial component is histologically benign while the mesenchymal component is sarcomatous.

In most studies of ovarian carcinoma, between 5% and 10% of epithelial tumors are too poorly differentiated for the pathologist to classify them into one of the specific types described above. These neoplasms, which are bilateral in 50% of cases, are called *undifferentiated carcinomas*.

Treatment

Surgery

All of the histologic types of ovarian carcinoma are treated in the same way. The standard surgical procedure for carcinoma of the ovary is total abdominal hysterectomy and bilateral salpingo-oophorectomy. A partial or complete omentectomy should be performed, and in advanced disease an attempt should be made to resect as much metastatic tumor as possible. The contralateral ovary and fallopian tube are removed unless conservation of fertility is important. The contralateral ovary is resected because it has been shown to contain an occult metastasis or primary carcinoma in 5% of cases. Moreover, there is a small, but significant, chance that a second primary carcinoma will subsequently arise in a retained ovary. There are several reasons for performing a hysterectomy. First, carcinoma of the ovary frequently implants on the uterine serosa and can also spread to the uterus through lymphatic channels or the fallopian tube. Second, there is an increased frequency of endometrial hyperplasia or carcinoma in patients with certain types of epithelial tumors of the ovary (mainly endometrioid carcinoma). In addition, all patients with carcinoma of the ovary are at increased risk of developing a second primary malignancy of the genital tract. Finally, removal of the uterus facilitates evaluation of the pelvis during follow-up.

Conservative treatment by unilateral salpingo-oophorectomy for a stage-Ia(i) tumor can sometimes be recommended for a young woman who wants to retain her fertility. Reliable follow-up must be possible, and the tumor must be an epithelial tumor of low malignant potential or a low-grade adenocarcinoma. Careful staging, with visual examination and wedge biopsy of the contralateral ovary, must confirm that the patient's neoplasm is confined to one ovary. It should be encapsulated, unruptured, and not adherent to adjacent structures. A patient with ascites does not qualify for conservative treatment, nor does one in whom malignant cells are detected in peritoneal washings.

In cases of advanced cancer, the surgeon must determine the appropriate treatment after exploring the patient's abdomen. Some patients have unresectable cancer. In such instances the surgeon should attempt to establish the diagnosis by excising an involved ovary; if this is not feasible, a biopsy should be obtained from the ovary or a metastasis. Several studies have revealed that survival in stage-II or -III ovarian cancer is improved when all visible cancer is completely resected or significantly reduced in volume, leaving no individual deposits larger than 1.5 cm to 2 cm in diameter. Radiation therapy is ineffective when there are large residual tumor masses, and treatment with many chemotherapeutic regimens is also most successful when residual tumor volume is minimized. Gynecologic oncologists accordingly advocate removal of as much tumor as possible, even in instances in which not all cancer can be resected, with the most radical surgery reserved for those patients in whom all, or nearly all, visible disease can be resected. This type of surgery has been referred to as *cytoreductive surgery*. In addition to improving survival, cytoreductive surgery can relieve symptoms produced by pressure from large tumor masses and relieve intestinal obstruction, and in some instances ascitic fluid does not accumulate as rapidly.

A *second-look laparotomy* is performed in patients who have received a complete course of chemotherapy and who are in complete clinical remission. The purpose of the laparotomy is to determine whether there is any residual visible or microscopic tumor. Laparoscopy may be helpful in the evaluation of patients who are candidates for a second-look laparotomy, since the need for laparotomy is obviated if recurrent carcinoma is detected or if malignant cells are present in peritoneal washings. Chemotherapy can be discontinued if no tumor is detected. If present, tumor is usually found at sites where there was residual tumor after the initial surgery. Patients who presented with advanced cancer frequently have residual carcinoma, but the tumor deposits are usually decreased in size and may be amenable to resection. Resection of all visible residual tumor at the second-look operation appears to improve the prognosis. If residual tumor is present, chemotherapy must be continued, but different agents are administered.

Chemotherapy

The patient whose neoplasm has spread beyond the ovary is a clear candidate for chemotherapy, even if all tumor has been resected. Chemotherapy is usually advocated for women with stage-I disease as well, except for those with stage-Ia(i) well-differentiated carcinoma, the hope being that it will improve on the 70% to 80% five-year survival rate achieved by surgery alone. Survival rates exceeding 90% have been reported, but there is no controlled study demonstrating a statistically significant improvement in survival among stage-I patients as a result of adjuvant chemotherapy. Patients with localized (stage-I or -IIa) epithelial tumors of low malignant potential have an excellent prognosis and do not require adjuvant therapy. The treatment of patients with more advanced disease is not agreed upon, but most such patients receive single-agent chemotherapy.

A variety of drugs are active against ovarian cancer. Of these, melphalan (Alkeran) has emerged as the drug of choice for single-agent chemotherapy. Melphalan is most effective in an adjuvant setting for patients with no visible residual tumor after surgery. It has also been used to treat patients with minimal residual tumor (tumor masses less than 2 cm in diameter) and to treat patients with more advanced disease who cannot tolerate more toxic combination chemotherapy regimens. When used as adjuvant therapy for patients in stages I to III in whom all visible tumor has been resected, melphalan appears to be as effective in preventing recurrences as radiotherapy. A five-year survival rate of approximately 70% can be anticipated in this group, with the best results in patients with stage-I disease. Combination chemotherapy is more effective than single-agent chemotherapy in patients with minimal residual tumor, but it is also more toxic. Acute leukemia is an infrequent, but significant, complication of chemotherapy.

Advanced cancer is treated by chemotherapy, since radiation therapy is ineffective in patients with extensive residual disease. Multiagent chemotherapy appears to be more effective than single-agent chemotherapy; most current regimens include doxorubicin (Adriamycin) and cisplatin in combination with other drugs, such as cyclophosphamide and hexamethylmelamine. Modern combination chemotherapy can achieve a complete clinical remission in 40% to 60% of patients and complete or partial remission (greater than 50% reduction in tumor) in as many as 90% of patients.

Radiation Therapy

RADIOISOTOPE THERAPY. Chromic phosphate containing ^{32}P is currently used for radioisotope therapy. ^{32}P emits β-particles (electrons) with an average energy of 0.69 MeV and an average tissue penetration of 2 mm to 3 mm. Its half-life is 14.3 days. A colloidal suspension of radioactive chromic phosphate is introduced into the abdomen through catheters placed in the pelvis and over the liver at the time of surgery for ovarian cancer. The usual dose is 15 mCi, which is instilled, together with a volume of fluid sufficient to facilitate intra-abdominal distribution, when the patient has recovered from surgery.

Five-year survival rates of approximately 90% have been reported in several small studies of patients with stage-I ovarian cancer treated with ^{32}P. This is an improvement over historical results, but there are no controlled studies comparing ^{32}P therapy with other treatment modalities. Radioisotopes at least theoretically treat the entire peritoneal cavity, but because of minimal tissue penetration and uneven distribution throughout the abdominal cavity, ^{32}P is generally used only in treatment of stage-I ovarian cancer.

EXTERNAL-BEAM RADIOTHERAPY. External-beam therapy can be used to administer a more uniform dose of radiation than radioisotope therapy, and it treats the pelvic and para-aortic lymph nodes. It has been amply demonstrated that pelvic irradiation alone is insufficient treatment for ovarian cancer, even in stage I, so if external beam therapy is to be used without complementary chemotherapy, the entire abdomen, including the diaphragm, must be irradiated. Radiation is administered by the open-field or moving strip technique. The pelvic dose is 4500 rad to 5000 rad, and 2250 rad to 2800 rad are delivered to the abdomen. The effectiveness of external-beam radiation is limited by the inability of the abdominal organs to tolerate large doses of radiation.

External-beam abdominopelvic irradiation is most successful when all visible tumor has been surgically resected or when there are only small (less than 2 cm in diameter) residual deposits. In such circumstances, five-year survival rates of 70% to 80% have been reported for patients with disease in stages I to III. Abdominopelvic irradiation is contraindicated when a large volume of unresectable tumor is present, since treatment is rarely successful and is associated with significant morbidity.

Overall, the results obtained with external-beam therapy have been disappointing. In a large study conducted at M. D. Anderson Hospital, comparable results were obtained in patients treated with abdominopelvic irradiation and with melphalan chemotherapy. There was less morbidity in patients treated with chemotherapy, and this method of treatment cost significantly less than external-beam therapy. Only interim results of this study were reported in 1975, however, and there have been only a few confirmatory studies from other institutions. In spite of the paucity of controlled comparative trials, most oncologists advocate chemotherapy as the most appropriate postoperative therapy for patients in stages I and III. Pelvic irradiation followed by systemic chemotherapy remains the most accepted treatment of stage IIb, but this technique has not been compared in a randomized study with chemotherapy alone.

GERM CELL TUMORS

Germ cell tumors represent 15% to 20% of all ovarian neoplasms. Approximately 4% are malignant, and within this category are some of the most aggressive ovarian tumors, which until recently were almost uniformly rapidly fatal. Malignant germ cell tumors occur primarily in children and young women. In patients under 20 years of age, nearly 60% of ovarian tumors are of germ cell origin, and in children under 10 years of age, 84% of these are malignant.

Because of their rarity, malignant germ cell tumors have until recently been poorly understood. Their separation into pure histologic types led to the recognition that each type has a distinctive biologic behavior and that the treatment for each differs accordingly. The classification of ovarian tumors by the World Health Orga-

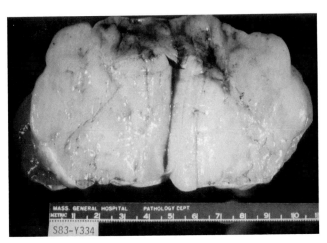

FIG. 59-38. Dysgerminoma. The homogoneous fleshy, tan cut surface is characteristic of this neoplasm. (Courtesy of Robert E Scully, MD)

Microscopic Pathology

The tumor is composed of aggregates of large polygonal cells with vesicular nuclei having one or more nucleoli (Fig. 59-39). The cytoplasm is clear or lightly granular and contains abundant glycogen. Delicate fibrous septa surround lobules of tumor cells, and if densely fibrous areas are present, the tumor cells have a cordlike arrangement. Dysgerminomas are often infiltrated by lymphocytes and foreign body giant cells; epithelioid cells and granulomas are present in 20%.

Syncytiotrophoblastic giant cells are present in some dysgerminomas, and immunoperoxidase methods have demonstrated the presence of hCG. Dysergerminomas containing syncytiotrophoblastic giant cells are associated with elevated serum hCG levels. The presence of only syncytiotrophoblasts does not warrant the diagnosis of choriocarcinoma.

Prognosis and Treatment

The five-year survival of patients with dysgerminoma ranges from 96% for stage-Ia tumors to 63% when tumor has extended beyond the ovaries. At the time of laparotomy, nearly three quarters of all patients have stage-I disease, but in contrast to other malignant germ cell tumors, dysgerminoma is occasionally bilateral. Ten percent of dysgerminomas are visibly confined to both ovaries at the time of operation (Stage Ib). Five percent of patients with a tumor that appears to be confined to one ovary have occult microscopic dysgerminoma in the contralateral ovary. For this reason, if unilateral salpingo-oophorectomy is considered, a biopsy of the opposite ovary must be performed even if it appears grossly normal. Dysgerminoma is unique among germ cell tumors in that it is highly radiosensitive. When indicated, postoperative treatment consists of radiation therapy.

nization established standard nomenclature and histologic criteria, thereby permitting accurate assessment of the clinical behavior of these neoplasms. Coincident with these developments was the discovery that cellular elements within the neoplasms produce oncofetal proteins, or so-called tumor markers. Among these, alpha-fetoprotein (AFP) and human chorionic gonadotropin (hCG) have the greatest utility. Identification of these markers in tissue sections assists in the histologic diagnosis, and measurement of the markers in serum provides a highly sensitive method for monitoring response to treatment.

Dysgerminoma

Dysgerminoma is the most common malignant germ cell tumor of the ovary, accounting for nearly 50% of this group and 2% of all malignant ovarian neoplasms. Three quarters of the patients are between 10 and 30 years of age, and only 4% are over 40; the median age is 22 years. Patients generally present with a pelvic or abdominal mass, abdominal enlargement, or pain. The duration of symptoms ranges from one month to two years, with a median of four months. About 2% of non-pregnant women have positive pregnancy tests, and children may present with precocious puberty.

Gross Pathology

Dysgerminoma is a solid, fleshy tumor with a smooth exterior surface; the median diameter is 15 cm. The cut surface is fleshy and has a uniform tan to pink color (Fig. 59-38). Hemorrhagic or cystic areas suggest the presence of admixed elements of choriocarcinoma, endodermal sinus tumor, and teratoma.

Yolk Sac (Endodermal Sinus) Tumors

Endodermal sinus tumor, the second most common malignant germ cell tumor, constitutes about 1% of all ovarian malignancies. Patients with these tumors are almost invariably younger than 40 years of age. The clinical presentation is frequently sudden; half of the patients have had symptoms for one week or less. Three quarters of the patients have abdominal pain and nearly all have a large abdominal or pelvic mass. At the time of surgery, 70% of patients appear to have stage-Ia disease; involvement of the contralateral ovary is rare except in cases of disseminated peritoneal spread.

Gross Pathology

The neoplasms are soft, with a smooth exterior and a median diameter of 15 cm. The cut surface is predominantly solid, with cysts of variable size throughout producing a honeycomb appearance. Large areas of hemorrhage and necrosis are common (Fig. 59-40).

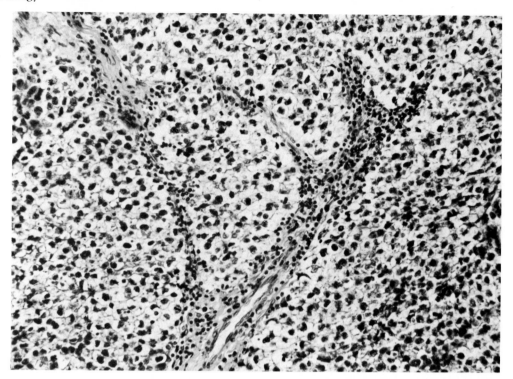

FIG. 59-39. Dysgerminoma. Nests of large polygonal cells with a clear cytoplasm are surrounded by fibrous septa containing lymphocytes.

Microscopic Pathology

A wide range of patterns are frequently admixed. Occasionally, one pattern may dominate to the exclusion of the others. Five patterns have been described in detail.

FIG. 59-40. Yolk sac (endodermal sinus) tumor. The neoplasm has both cystic and solid portions, with the latter predominating. Hemorrhage and necrosis are present. (Armed Forces Institute of Pathology Photograph)

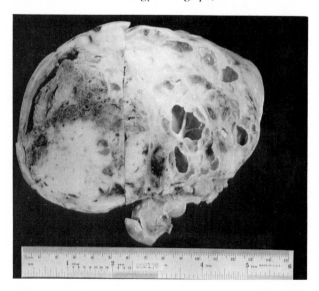

The most common is the *reticular,* or microcystic, pattern, characterized by a loose meshwork of spaces and channels lined by flattened or cuboidal cells with scant cytoplasm and indistinct borders (Fig. 59-41). Hyaline droplets are common in this pattern. The typical endodermal sinus, or *festoon,* pattern is characterized by the presence of perivascular structures (so-called Schiller–Duval bodies) composed of a central capillary core surrounded by a mantle of primitive cells. These structures are thought to recapitulate the endodermal sinus of the yolk sac. The rarer *polyvesicular vitelline* pattern is characterized by multiple cysts and vesicles with flattened to columnar epithelial cells with clear cytoplasm. The *alveolar–glandular* pattern is composed of cystic spaces containing papillary processes covered by cuboidal epithelium. The rarest form is the *solid* pattern, composed of sheets of undifferentiated (embryonal) cells. There are no prognostic differences among the various microscopic patterns.

Prognosis and Treatment

Before the use of modern chemotherapy, 84% of patients with stage-Ia tumors died, in spite of treatment with surgery and adjuvant radiotherapy. It is therefore likely that in most cases occult metastases are present at the time of diagnosis. Adjuvant combination chemotherapy is consequently administered even when there is no visible residual tumor. A survival rate of greater than 80% has been reported in patients with

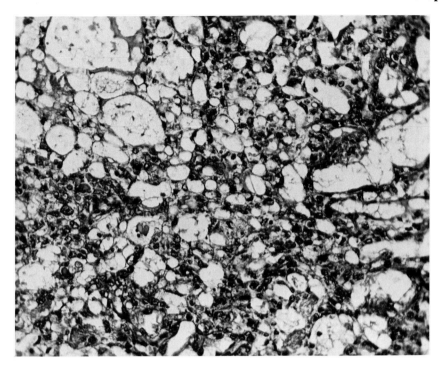

FIG. 59-41. Yolk sac (endodermal sinus) tumor. In the microcystic pattern illustrated here, a loose meshwork of spaces is lined by malignant germ cells. (×180) (Armed Forces Institute of Pathology Photograph)

stage-I disease treated with chemotherapy, and greater than 50% of patients with advanced disease are successfully treated. Young patients with stage-Ia disease may be treated by unilateral salpingo-oophorectomy followed by adjuvant chemotherapy. Successful pregnancy has been reported following this form of treatment.

Teratoma

The vast majority of ovarian teratomas may be divided into two broad categories, immature and mature, depending on the appearance of their component tissues. Immaturity in a teratoma reflects the degree to which the neoplastic tissue resembles embryonic tissue. The potential for recurrence is directly related to the amount of immature tissue present. Immaturity should not be confused with malignant transformation occurring in a mature teratoma; such neoplasms, although they are malignant, develop within mature tissue. Only immature teratomas are considered in this discussion.

Immature teratomas, the third most common malignant germ cell tumor, represent nearly one quarter of all malignant ovarian germ cell tumors in patients under 15 years of age. The median patient age is 18 years. Twenty percent of patients are prepubertal, and the oldest patients are less than 40 years of age. Symptoms are nonspecific and usually of short duration. Three quarters of patients have a palpable abdominal or pelvic mass, frequently accompanied by pain.

Gross Pathology

Immature teratomas are usually large unilateral tumors with a median diameter of 18 cm. The external surface is smooth, and the cut surface is soft, gray to pink, with hemorrhage, necrosis, and large cysts in one third of cases. Hair is present in 20% of tumors. Bone, cartilage, or calcified areas are usually visible.

Microscopic Pathology

These neoplasms contain varying proportions of immature tissue derived from the three germ layers (Fig. 59-42). Neural tissue is the most common immature element and the easiest to grade. The criteria for grading are as follows:

Grade 0: Mature tissue only.
Grade 1: Abundant mature tissue but some immaturity; neuroepithelium is absent or limited to 1 low-power field (×40) per slide.
Grade 2: More than 1 low-power field per slide of neuroepithelium, but not exceeding 3 low-power fields.
Grade 3: Extensive areas of immature tissue are present; neuroepithelium is found in four or more low-power fields per slide.

In addition to neural elements, mesoderm-derived tissues such as cartilage, bone, lymphoid tissue, and smooth muscle may be encountered. Striated muscle is rare. Endodermal elements include respiratory and gastrointestinal epithelium. Immature teratomas typically contain a variety of tissues showing varying degrees of immaturity, but it is the most primitive areas that have the propensity the metastasize and consequently play the most important role in grading.

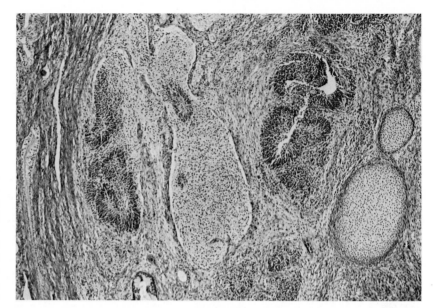

FIG. 59-42. Immature teratoma. Neuroepithelium (*center left and right*) is almost invariably present in an immature teratoma; the amount is directly related to the grade of the tumor. Immature cartilage (*lower right*) is also seen in this photograph. (×40) (Zaloudek CJ: The ovary. In Gompel C, Silverberg SG (eds): Pathology in Gynecology and Obstetrics, 3rd ed, Philadelphia, JB Lippincott, 1985)

Prognosis and Treatment

Approximately 70% of immature teratomas are stage Ia. Bilateral involvement (stage Ib or Ic) does not occur without peritoneal spread, but about 5% of contralateral ovaries contain a benign cystic teratoma. Early spread is by direct extension to the adjacent pelvic tissues and by peritoneal implantation. Lymphatic invasion and extra-abdominal metastases are rare. For stage-I disease, prognosis is related to the grade of the tumor. In advanced-stage disease, the grade of the metastases is the major prognostic determinant. Before the use of modern chemotherapy, all patients with grade-0 metastases survived, whereas patients with grade-1 or -2 metastases had only a 40% to 50% survival rate. No patients with grade-3 metastases survived. More recently, patients with advanced-stage high-grade tumors who have received triple-agent chemotherapy have survived long term (3–6 years). Pathologic examination of residual disease resected at second-look operation following multiple courses of chemotherapy revealed grade 0 (mature teratoma) exclusively. On the basis of these findings, it appears reasonable to treat patients with stage-Ia grade-1 disease by unilateral salpingo-oophorectomy only. Patients with higher grade stage-I neoplasms and all those whose tumors have ruptured require adjuvant chemotherapy. Patients with advanced-stage disease require maximal surgical resection for therapy and for accurate grading. If the metastases are all grade 0, and the primary tumor is no worse than grade 1, no further treatment is necessary. Patients with higher grade metastatic tumors (grade 1, 2, or 3) and those whose primary tumors are grade 2 or 3 require adjuvant chemotherapy.

Embryonal Carcinoma

Embryonal carcinoma is relatively rare, accounting for only 5% of malignant germ cell tumors. The median patient age is 15 years. As with other germ cell tumors, the majority of patients present with an abdominal or pelvic mass, and half have abdominal pain. Symptoms tend to be of short duration; the mean duration is three weeks. Signs of precocious puberty are present in almost half of the prepubertal girls. Amenorrhea or vaginal bleeding is found in one third of the women in the reproductive-age group. Pregnancy tests are usually positive, and serum levels of hCG are elevated.

Gross Pathology

The tumors are large (median diameter, 17 cm) and soft. The cut surface is gray yellow and variegated with extensive hemorrhage and necrosis. Cysts are common.

Microscopic Pathology

Embryonal carcinoma is composed of large, primitive, pleomorphic cells with amphophilic, slightly vacuolated cytoplasm and vesicular nuclei with one or more nucleoli. The cells are usually arranged in solid sheets, but glandlike spaces and papillary processes also occur. Syncytiotrophoblastic giant cells are frequently present in embryonal carcinoma.

Prognosis and Treatment

Before the use of modern chemotherapy, the five-year survival was 50% for stage-I disease and 39% for all stages combined. Therapy is the same as for endodermal sinus tumors and consists of excision of all visible tumor and postoperative adjuvant chemotherapy. Since occult metastasis to the opposite ovary rarely occurs, unilateral salpingo-oophorectomy can be performed for stage-I tumors.

Choriocarcinoma

Choriocarcinoma rarely occurs in pure form. Most non-gestational choriocarcinoma of the ovary occurs admixed with teratoma, endodermal sinus tumor, embryonal carcinoma, or dysgerminoma and is best placed in the mixed germ cell category. This is important, because if choriocarcinoma is pure, it is more likely to be of gestational than of germ cell origin. An unequivocal diagnosis of pure choriocarcinoma of germ cell origin can be made only in a prepubertal child. In a review of published cases of both pure and mixed choriocarcinoma, the age range was 7 months to 35 years, with a mean of 13 years. Half of the patients with germ cell tumors containing choriocarcinoma present with abdominal enlargement and pain, and half the premenarchal girls have signs of precocious puberty.

Gross Pathology

Choriocarcinoma is soft and characteristically hemorrhagic. Other gross features depend on the presence of additional germ cell elements.

Microscopic Pathology

The tumor is composed of a dimorphic population of cytotrophoblast and syncytiotrophoblast. Both elements must be present for a diagnosis of choriocarcinoma. Viable tumor is typically scanty, as hemorrhage and necrosis are usually extensive.

Treatment

These neoplasms are treated by surgical excision and combination chemotherapy.

Mixed Germ Cell Tumors

Germ cell tumors that contain two or more of the previously described pure types are referred to as *malignant mixed germ cell tumors;* they represent 8% of malignant germ cell tumors. Patients with such neoplasms range in age from 5 to 33 years, with a median age of 16 years. One third of the children with these tumors present with signs of precocious puberty, and 40% of nonpregnant patients of reproductive age have positive pregnancy tests.

Gross Pathology

Mixed germ cell tumors are large neoplasms with a median diameter of 15 cm. Their exterior is smooth. The appearance of the cut surface depends on the type and amount of the various elements present in the neoplasm. Solid, fleshy, tan areas correspond to dysgerminoma, mucoid cystic areas generally represent teratoma, and hemorrhagic and necrotic areas reflect endodermal sinus tumor or choriocarcinoma.

Microscopic Pathology

The most common element is dysgerminoma, found in 80% of tumors, followed by endodermal sinus tumor in 70% and embryonal carcinoma in 15%. Only two malignant elements are present in two thirds of mixed germ cell tumors. The most frequently encountered mixture is dysgerminoma and endodermal sinus tumor.

Prognosis and Treatment

At laparotomy two thirds of patients are found to have stage-Ia disease. In a retrospective study in which the majority of patients were not treated with adjuvant combination chemotherapy, the prognosis for patients with stage-I tumors appeared to depend on the size and histologic composition of the neoplasm. Patients with tumors that were larger than 10 cm and more than one third endodermal sinus tumor, choriocarcinoma, or grade-3 teratoma had a poor prognosis. In contrast, patients with tumors composed exclusively of combinations of dysgerminoma, embryonal carcinoma, or grade-1 or -2 teratoma, as well as patients with tumors that contained less than a third of endodermal sinus tumor, choriocarcinoma, or grade-3 teratoma had a more favorable prognosis. A recent study in which adjuvant chemotherapy was used did not show these differences. Surgical treatment of stage-Ia tumors may consist of unilateral salpingo-oophorectomy, but the contralateral ovary should be biopsied, since there may be occult involvement of a visibly normal ovary in patients with mixed germ cell tumors containing dysgerminoma.

Gonadoblastoma

Gonadoblastoma is the most common neoplasm of abnormal gonads, in which it arises almost exclusively. Patients with gonadoblastoma range in age from 1 to 40 years and typically have congenitally abnormal gonads associated with sexual maldevelopment. The gonadal abnormalities observed include bilateral streak gonads, a streak on one side and a testis on the other, or abnormal gonads of indeterminate type. The development of a gonadoblastoma in an individual with maldeveloped gonads has been shown to depend on the presence of a Y chromosome. Thus, although 80% of patients with gonadoblastoma are phenotypic females, 90% have a Y chromosome. Gonadoblastomas occurring in normal women with a 46XX karyotype who have become pregnant and have had normal offspring are rare, as are gonadoblastomas occuring in true hermaphrodites. Some such patients may be hidden mosaics, and in others the gonadoblastoma may have arisen as a hamartomatous malformation in a polyovular follicle.

Some patients with gonadoblastoma are virilized, and it has been shown that the tumors can synthesize both androgens and estrogens. Steroid production appears to be independent of the presence of Leydig cells, since in some instances the tumor may elaborate androgens in the absence of these cells.

Gross Pathology

Gonadoblastomas vary from being a few millimeters in size to being large, solid masses, which may be soft, firm, or gritty, depending on the degree of calcification and the extent of a germinomatous component, if one is present. Dystrophic calcification is common and may be recognized in abdominal roentgenograms before surgery.

Microscopic Pathology

Gonadoblastoma is composed of a mixture of germ cells resembling dysgerminoma cells and gonadal stromal cells. The latter most closely resemble Sertoli cells. They surround individual germ cells or are aligned around the periphery of clusters of germ cells. Stromal cells also surround spaces containing eosinophilic material, creating a microfollicular pattern. Cells that are identical to luteinized ovarian stromal cells or testicular Leydig cells, but that do not contain crystals of Reinke, are present in the stroma in two thirds of gonadoblastomas.

Approximately half of gonadoblastomas are overgrown by germinoma. Rarely, endodermal sinus tumor, embryonal carcinoma, or choriocarcinoma develops in a gonadoblastoma instead of or in addition to a germinoma.

Prognosis and Treatment

Any patient with gonadal dysgenesis and a Y chromosome runs a high risk of developing a germ cell tumor, particularly a gonadoblastoma. One third of gonadoblastomas are bilateral, and they may be small enough as to be detectable only microscopically. If unresected, the gonadoblastoma tends to be overgrown by malignant elements; the median incidence of malignant germ cell tumors in patients with gonadal dysgenesis and a Y chromosome is 25%. Consequently, total abdominal hysterectomy and bilateral salpingo-oophorectomy are indicated in patients with gonadoblastoma, virtually all of whom have gonadal dysgenesis and an abnormal contralateral ovary. Surprisingly, metastases from germinoma arising in gonadoblastoma are uncommon even when the tumor is large and bilateral. In contrast, other neoplasms arising in gonadoblastoma, such as endodermal sinus tumor, embryonal carcinoma, or choriocarcinoma, have been fatal within 1.5 years. Further treatment is therefore determined by the histologic nature of the malignant germ cell elements.

Tumor Markers

Detection of oncofetal antigens in tissue sections by immunocytochemical methods has shed light on the histogenesis of germ cell tumors and has provided a functional correlation with the traditional morphologic classification. Although several different oncofetal and placental proteins have been identified, systematic correlation of serum marker levels and their immunocytochemical localization in tissue have been performed only for AFP and hCG.

Serologic and immunohistochemical studies have shown that there is a close correlation between serum level and tissue localization of AFP and hCG and that AFP and hCG serum levels are an accurate reflection of the histologic composition of the tumor. The current management of germ cell tumors is therefore based on the measurement of both of these markers in the serum with radioimmunoassay techniques and on their localization in tissue sections with immunocytochemical methods. Elevation of either AFP or hCG in the serum of a child or young woman with an adnexal mass strongly suggests the presence of a malignant germ cell tumor. Normal levels do not exclude the possibility of dysgerminoma and immature teratoma, since these tumors are generally not associated with the production of AFP or hCG. In contrast, endodermal sinus tumors are almost invariably associated with high levels of AFP. Embryonal carcinoma may be associated with elevated levels of both markers, depending on the degree of differentiation along yolk sac (AFP secretion) or trophoblastic (hCG secretion) lines.

Although AFP and hCG are of value in diagnosis, their most effective use is in monitoring response to therapy and detecting recurrence early, when the tumor is small (markers are often positive months before other clinical parameters) and can be most effectively eradicated by chemotherapy. The activity of the disease can be accurately monitored after initial therapy by the use of serial determinations of serum AFP and hCG. The pattern of serum marker levels following surgery has been referred to as *concordant* if AFP and hCG rise and fall in a parallel fashion and as *discordant* if they do not. The patterns of marker production following chemotherapy are a reflection of the response of heterogeneous populations of cells to chemotherapy, since each marker is synthesized by a different cell type. Chemotherapy may interfere with marker production without destroying the cells or may selectively destroy marker-producing and non–marker-producing cells. Moreover, marker levels may be negative if the tumor has differentiated into mature tissue that does not produce a marker, such as mature teratoma, or if the tumor has reverted to an undifferentiated embryonal carcinoma that is incapable of marker synthesis. Tumor markers provide a functional tool to assess the presence and extent of germ cell neoplasms quite distinct from the traditional anatomic studies used to follow the course of most tumors.

GONADAL STROMAL TUMORS

Gonadal stromal tumors constitute approximately 6% of all ovarian neoplasms; nearly 90% of them fall into the granulosa tumor or thecoma category.

The histogenesis of gonadal stromal tumors is controversial, since the origin of the cells from which they are derived is uncertain. The functioning gonadal stroma may originate either from coelomic epithelium or from subcoelomic mesenchymal cells of the gonadal ridge.

The term *sex cord–stromal tumor* is also used for this category of ovarian neoplasms because of uncertainty regarding the origin of granulosa and Sertoli cells. The current classification of ovarian gonadal stromal neoplasms has evolved gradually.

All gonadal stromal tumors have the potential for steroid hormone production; they account for 85% to 90% of functioning ovarian tumors. Each gonadal stromal cell type may produce multiple steroids concomitantly, particularly in the neoplastic state. As a result, although each tumor type is associated with a specific endocrine effect, deviations from the typical clinical presentation are common. The clinical effect depends on what predominant steroid is produced by the tumor and the extent of peripheral conversion of androgens to estrogen.

Granulosa Tumors

Granulosa tumors are relatively rare, accounting for 1% to 3% of all ovarian neoplasms. They occur over a wide age range; cases have been reported in newborn infants as well as in postmenopausal women. Approximately 40% of granulosa tumors occur after the menopause, but only 5% develop before puberty.

A majority of patients present with symptoms of a functioning ovarian tumor, an abdominal mass, or both; under 5% are asymptomatic. The tumor or associated ascites causes abdominal distention in 10% of patients. Acute abdomen due to hemorrhage into or rupture of a cystic neoplasm is the presenting event in 5% of patients.

Granulosa tumors are capable of synthesizing a variety of steroid hormones, resulting in clinical symptoms in about three quarters of patients. Most have symptoms caused by estrogenic hormones. The clinical presentation varies and is dependent on the patient's age. In prepubertal girls, granulosa tumors usually produce isosexual precocious puberty; they account for at least 10% of cases of precocious puberty. In women of reproductive age, menstrual irregularities, menorrhagia, and amenorrhea (due to inhibition of ovulation as a result of high estrogen levels) are common. In postmenopausal women, vaginal bleeding, not infrequently due to endometrial hyperplasia or carcinoma, is a common presenting symptom. The frequency of endometrial hyperplasia has been reported to be as high as 50% in some series, and endometrial adenocarcinoma occurs in 10% of patients. Menopausal and postmenopausal women are more than twice as likely as young women to have hyperplasia or carcinoma of the endometrium. Endocrine-related endometrial carcinomas are well differentiated, are often confined to the endometrium, and have little malignant potential.

Gross Pathology

Granulosa tumors are circumscribed and have a smooth or lobulated external surface. The cut surface is solid with focal cystic areas (Fig. 59-43). The tumors vary from firm and rubbery to soft and fleshy. The color is usually yellow but may be tan, gray, pink, or brown. Areas of hemorrhage and necrosis are common, partic-

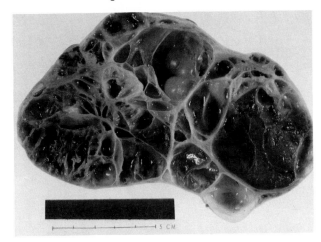

FIG. 59-43. Granulosa tumor. This neoplasm is multiloculated and largely cystic. Some of the cystic spaces are filled with blood. (Armed Forces Institute of Pathology Photograph)

ularly in larger tumors. Occasionally a granulosa tumor is a unilocular or multilocular cyst resembling a cystadenoma.

Microscopic Pathology

Granulosa cells are small and round or polygonal to spindle-shaped with scant cytoplasm and indistinct cell membranes. The nuclei are round or ovoid and characteristically have a longitudinal groove and a small nucleolus (Fig. 59-44).

Because most granulosa tumors contain variable numbers of theca cells, they are frequently termed *granulosa–theca tumors*. However, most pathologists believe that the term *granulosa tumor* is more appropriate, since the theca cells are thought not to be neoplastic but rather to reflect a response of the ovarian stroma to the granulosa cell proliferation. When granulosa tumors metastasize, theca cells are not present in the metastatic deposits.

A variety of histologic patterns have been described, including microfollicular, with its characteristic Call–Exner bodies (see Fig. 59-44), macrofollicular, trabecular, insular, moire silk, and diffuse (sarcomatoid). Although one pattern may dominate, an admixture of patterns is generally present. The sarcomatoid variant, regarded by some as the most aggressive form, is the least differentiated and may contain numerous mitoses.

The *juvenile* granulosa tumor is an unusual variant that is encountered predominantly in children. Two histologic patterns are encountered in this tumor: a lobular macrofollicular pattern and a solid form characterized by a disorderly admixture of granulosa and theca cells. Numerous mitotic figures, cytologic atypia, and extensive luteinization are typically present. Despite the ominous histologic appearance, only 15% of juvenile granulosa tumors metastasize.

The *cystic* granulosa tumor is another unusual variant. This type of granulosa tumor usually occurs in children or young women who present with hirsutism or

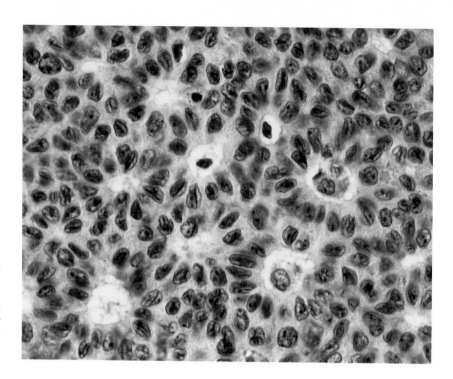

FIG. 59-44. Granulosa tumor. The granulosa cells have monotonous, small vesicular nuclei. Many nuclei are lobulated or longitudinally grooved. This photograph illustrates a microfollicular growth pattern with Call–Exner bodies (granulosa cells around clear spaces). (×250)

virilization. The tumor is composed of monomorphic granulosa cells lining large cystic spaces. None of the reported cases has metastasized.

Prognosis and Treatment

Granulosa tumors are neoplasms with a potential for malignant behavior. The most important prognostic factor is the stage of the tumor. Almost 90% of granulosa tumors are stage Ia. No single histologic feature reliably identifies neoplasms with a high risk of recurrence. Capsular invasion, a high level of mitotic activity, nuclear atypia, and vascular invasion reflect increased malignant potential, but tumors without these features may also recur. Additional unfavorable prognostic factors include patient age at diagnosis over 40 years, large tumor size, bilaterality, and rupture of the tumor.

Survival at ten years is 86% to 96% for patients with stage-I disease but only 26% to 40% for patients with more advanced neoplasms. The reported overall ten-year survival for all stages ranges from less than 60% to over 90%. With long periods of follow-up, a progressive decline in survival has been documented. Recurrences have been reported as long as 30 years after the initial diagnosis, so long-term follow-up is required.

Hysterectomy and bilateral salpingo-oophorectomy are the standard treatment. Unilateral salpingo-oophorectomy is justifiable in young women in whom preservation of reproductive function is a consideration, if the tumor is confined to one ovary. Surgical resection and irradiation have been successful in managing isolated recurrences, which generally develop in the pelvis. Chemotherapy has been used in a small number of patients with advanced disease. On the basis of the available data, it appears that some of the best responses have been obtained with melphalan, doxorubicin (Adriamycin), and a combination of dactinomycin (Actinomycin D), 5-fluorouracil, and cyclophosphamide.

Sertoli Tumors

Patients with Sertoli tumors range in age from 7 to 79 years, with a median age of 33 years. They usually present with a pelvic or abdominal mass. Sertoli tumors are functional in more than 60% of cases. Estrogenic manifestations, reflected by endometrial hyperplasia, predominate, but androgenic and progestational effects also occur. Prepubertal girls may present with isosexual precocious pseudopuberty.

Gross Pathology

Sertoli tumors typically present as unilateral, well-circumscribed, solitary masses. The cut surface is solid, fleshy, and yellow tan. In a recent study of 28 Sertoli tumors, 13 were 10 cm or larger in size.

Microscopic Pathology

The Sertoli tumor has distinctive growth patterns, designated as *simple tubular, complex tubular,* and *folliculome lipidique* (Fig. 59-45). These are often admixed, but one may be dominant. Areas of solid (diffuse) Sertoli cell proliferation are generally present as well. Intracytoplasmic lipid is present in most neoplasms, but accumulation of massive amounts of lipid is a characteristic of the folliculome lipidique. The "sex cord tumor with annular tubules" (SCTAT), which may be asso-

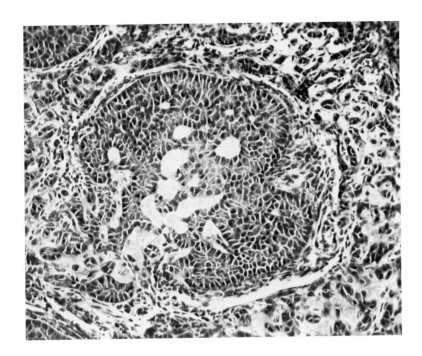

FIG. 59-45. Sertoli tumor. Complex tubular pattern with focal loss of tubular differentiation and infiltration of stroma. This neoplasm recurred twice. (×160) (Tavassoli FA, Norris HJ: Sertoli tumors of the ovary. A clinicopathologic study of 28 cases with ultrastructural observations. Cancer 46:2281, 1980. Reproduced with permission)

ciated with the Peutz–Jegher syndrome when it is small and bilateral, is a complex tubular variant of the Sertoli tumor.

Prognosis and Treatment

Most Sertoli tumors are benign, but a few recur or metastasize. The complex tubular pattern is the one most frequently associated with malignant behavior. Infiltration of the stroma by individual tumor cells or irregular clusters of cells is an ominous finding. Mitotic activity in the range of 4 to 8 per 10 high-power fields can be observed in tumors of children and adolescents but is not associated with an unfavorable prognosis.

Hysterectomy and bilateral salpingo-oophorectomy are the standard treatment. Unilateral salpingo-oophorectomy is adequate treatment for stage-Ia tumors in young women in whom preservation of reproductive function is important.

Sertoli–Leydig Tumors

Sertoli–Leydig tumors are relatively rare, accounting for less than 0.2% of all ovarian neoplasms. Most occur in young women of reproductive age; the average age is 24 years. Fewer than 5% of Sertoli–Leydig tumors occur in prepubertal girls; about 10% occur in women over the age of 45.

Sertoli–Leydig tumors are characteristically androgenic, and virilization has been noted in one half to three fourths of patients. Oligomenorrhea develops initially and is followed by amenorrhea, breast atrophy, acne, hirsutism, deepening of the voice, and enlargement of the clitoris. The most frequent combination of findings in virilized patients is amenorrhea, deepening of the voice, and hirsutism. After removal of the tumor, menstrual cycles return to normal within four to six weeks, but some changes, such as hirsutism, regress at a slower rate and often incompletely. Clitoral enlargement and deepening of the voice may not be altered by removal of the tumor. In prepubertal girls, Sertoli–Leydig tumors may be associated with isosexual precocity. Estrogenic manifestations may be due either to production of estrogen by the Sertoli cell component of the tumor or to peripheral conversion of androgenic hormones. Sertoli–Leydig tumors are not always associated with virilization; some tumors fail to produce hormones or produce them at a level insufficient to cause symptoms. Conversely, not all virilizing ovarian tumors are Sertoli–Leydig tumors.

Gross Pathology

Sertoli–Leydig tumors have an average diameter of 12 cm to 15 cm. They have a smooth external surface and are well circumscribed. The cut surfaces are soft and tan or yellow.

Microscopic Pathology

Sertoli–Leydig tumors are characterized by an admixture of Sertoli, Leydig, and undifferentiated gonadal stromal cells in varying proportions and degrees of differentiation. Columnar or cuboidal Sertoli cells line tubules or are arranged in cords. Clusters of polygonal Leydig cells with eosinophilic or foamy cytoplasm are scattered haphazardly within the stroma of the tumor. Undifferentiated gonadal stromal cells are present in intermediate and poorly differentiated Sertoli–Leydig tumors, and when they are the dominant cellular element, the neoplasm is classified as being poorly differentiated. Heterologous elements such as cartilage, mucinous epithelium, and skeletal muscle are found in 25% of Sertoli–Leydig tumors.

Prognosis and Treatment

The overall prognosis is favorable; the five- and ten-year actuarial survival rates of patients with stage-Ia neoplasms exceed 90%. Unfavorable prognostic indicators include extraovarian spread or rupture, poor differentiation, more than 5 mitotic figures per 10 high-power fields, and the presence of heterologous mesenchymal elements. The stage at diagnosis is the most important prognostic indicator.

Unilateral salpingo-oophorectomy is usually adequate treatment for young women who wish to preserve their fertility, since bilaterality and extraovarian spread are rare. Hysterectomy and bilateral salpingo-oophorectomy are the appropriate treatment when fertility is no longer an issue or when unfavorable prognostic features are present. Chemotherapy is administered to patients with extraovarian spread and to those whose neoplasms contain heterologous mesenchymal elements.

Lipid Cell Tumors

Lipid cell tumors account for less than 0.1% of all ovarian neoplasms. Most patients are adults; only a few cases have been reported in prepubertal children. Lipid cell tumors are frequently small and are therefore difficult to palpate on pelvic examination. Androgenic effects, including virilization, are the major functional manifestations of lipid cell tumors, occurring in 75% to 90% of patients. The majority of women present with progressive virilization over a five- to ten-year period. Typically, the tumor is manifested by hirsutism, amenorrhea, deepening of the voice, and clitoral enlargement. Cushing's syndrome is present in 5% to 10% of patients. A variety of hormones are produced by lipid cell tumors, including testosterone, androstenedione, dihydrotestosterone, 17-hydroxyprogesterone, progesterone, and, less frequently, estrogen. Curiously, there is evidence of estrogenic activity in nearly a quarter of patients. Although in some instances this may be due to the synthesis of estrogen by the tumor, in most cases it is the result of peripheral aromatization of androstenedione and testosterone to estradiol in adipose tissue. Removal of the tumor results in rapid regression of the hormonal effects, although some stigmata, such as deepening of the voice and clitoromegaly, usually persist.

Gross Pathology

Lipid cell tumors almost always have a smooth exterior and are lobulated and soft on the cut surface. Their color varies from yellow to orange tan or brown. Areas of hemorrhage and necrosis may be present. The size varies greatly, but the average diameter is 5 cm to 7 cm.

Microscopic Pathology

Lipid cell tumors are circumscribed and have expansile margins. Two cell types are present in varying proportions. One, the Leydig, or hilar, cell, is cuboidal or polyhedral with a round eccentric nucleus and granular eosinophilic cytoplasm, which may contain lipochrome pigment or Reinke crystals. The other cell type resembles an adrenal cortical cell; it is larger than the Leydig cell and has a rounded contour and abundant foamy or clear cytoplasm. Considerable intracytoplasmic lipid is present in both cell types. There is no correlation between the cell type and the functional manifestations. Cytologic atypia is present in 10% to 15% of tumors.

Prognosis and Treatment

Lipid cell tumors are generally benign, but 10% to 15% recur or metastasize. Tumors of the Leydig cell type are rarely malignant. Adverse prognostic features include extraovarian spread at the time of initial operation, size greater than 8 cm in diameter, nuclear atypia, and high level of mitotic activity.

Unilateral salpingo-oophorectomy is generally curative and is the treatment of choice for young women with stage-Ia neoplasms. Older women and those with advanced disease are treated by hysterectomy, bilateral salpingo-oophorectomy, and excision of all extraovarian tumor.

REFERENCES AND RECOMMENDED READING

Aure JC, Høeg K, Kolstad P: Clinical and histologic studies of ovarian carcinoma. Long-term follow-up of 990 cases. Obstet Gynecol 37:1–9, 1971

Berek JS, Hacker NF, Lagasse LD et al: Survival of patients following secondary cytoreductive surgery in ovarian cancer. Obstet Gynecol 61:189–193, 1983

Berek JS, Hacker NF, Lagasse LD et al: Second-look laparotomy in stage III epithelial ovarian cancer: Clinical variables associated with disease status. Obstet Gynecol 64:207–212, 1984

Bjorkholm E, Petterson F: Granulosa cell and theca cell tumors. The clinical picture and long-term outcome for the Radiumhemmet series. Acta Obstet Gynecol Scand 59:361–365, 1980

Centers for Disease Control: Oral contraceptive use and the risk of ovarian cancer: The Centers for Disease Control cancer and steroid hormone study. JAMA 249:1596–1599, 1983

Cohen CJ, Goldberg JD, Holland JF et al: Improved therapy cisplatin regimes for patients with ovarian carcinoma (FIGO stages III and IV) as measured by surgical end-staging (second-look operation). Am J Obstet Gynecol 145:955–965, 1983

Colgan TJ, Norris HJ: Ovarian epithelial tumors of low malignant potential: A review. Int J Gynecol Pathol 1:367–382, 1983

Cramer DW, Welch WR, Hutchison GB et al: Dietary animal fat in relation to ovarian cancer risk. Obstet Gynecol 63:833–838, 1984

Creasman WT, Park R, Norris HJ et al: Stage I borderline ovarian tumors. Obstet Gynecol 59:93–96, 1982

Curry SL, Smith JP, Gallagher HS: Malignant teratoma of the ovary: Prognostic factors and treatment. Am J Obstet Gynecol 131:845–849, 1978

Czernobilsky B: Endometrioid neoplasia of the ovary: A reappraisal. Int J Gynecol Pathol 1:203–210, 1982

Eifel P, Hendrickson M, Ross J et al: Simultaneous presentation of carcinoma involving the ovary and the uterine corpus. Cancer 50:163–170, 1982

Evans AT III, Gaffey TA, Malkasian GD Jr., Annegers JF: Clinicopathologic review of 118 granulosa and 82 theca cell tumors. Obstet Gynecol 55:231–238, 1980

Feldman GB, Knapp RC: Lymphatic drainage of the peritoneal cavity and its significance in ovarian cancer. Am J Obstet Gynecol 119:991–994, 1974

Genadry R, Parmley, T, Woodruff JD: Secondary malignancies in benign cystic teratomas. Gynecol Oncol 8:246–251, 1979

Gershenson DM, Del Junco G, Copeland LJ, Rutledge FN: Mixed germ cell tumors of the ovary. Obstet Gynecol 64:200–207, 1984

Gershenson DM, Del Junco G, Herson J, Rutledge FN: Endodermal sinus tumor of the ovary: The MD Anderson experience. Obstet Gynecol 61:194–202, 1983

Gordon A, Lipton D, Woodruff JD: Dysgerminoma: A review of 158 cases from the Emil Novak Ovarian Tumor Registry. Obstet Gynecol 58:497–504, 1981

Greene MH, Boice JD Jr., Greer BE et al: Acute nonlymphocytic leukemia after therapy with alkylating agents for ovarian cancer. A study of five randomized clinical trials. N Engl J Med 307:1416–1421, 1982

Hallgrimsson J, Scully RE: Borderline and malignant Brenner tumours of the ovary. A report of 15 cases. Acta Pathol Microbiol Scand Sect A (Suppl 233)80:56–66, 1972

Hart WR, Norris HJ: Borderline and malignant mucinous tumors of the ovary. Histologic criteria and clinical behavior. Cancer 31:1031–1045, 1973

Holtz F, Hart WR: Krukenberg tumors of the ovary. A clinicopathologic analysis of 27 cases. Cancer 50:2438–2447, 1982

Katsube Y, Berg JW, Silverberg SG: Epidemiologic pathology of ovarian tumors: A histopathologic review of primary ovarian neoplasms diagnosed in the Denver Standard Metropolitan statistical area, 1 July–31 December 1969 and 1 July–31 December 1979. Int J Gynecol Pathol 1:3–16, 1982

Katzenstein AL, Mazur MT, Morgan TE, Kao MS: Proliferative serous tumors of the ovary. Histologic features and prognosis. Am J Surg Pathol 2:339–355, 1978

Kurman RJ, Goebelsmann U, Taylor CR: Localization of steroid hormones in functional ovarian tumors. In DeLellis RA (ed): Diagnostic Immunohistochemistry, pp 137–148. New York, Masson Publishing, 1981

Kurman RJ, Petrilli ES: Germ cell tumors of the ovary: Pathology, behavior and treatment. In Griffiths CT, Fuller AF (eds): Gynecologic Oncology, pp 103–153. Boston, Martinus Nyhoff Publishers, 1983

Lurain JR: Newer diagnostic approaches to the evaluation of gynecologic malignancies. Obstet Gynecol Surv 37:437–448, 1982

Mazur MT, Hsueh S, Gersell DJ: Metastases to the female genital tract: Analysis of 325 cases. Cancer 53:1978–1984, 1984

McCaughey WTE, Kirk ME, Lester W, Dardick I: Peritoneal epithelial lesions associated with proliferating serous tumors of the ovary. Histopathology 8:195–208, 1984

Morrow CP, d'Ablaing G, Brady LW et al: A clinical and pathologic study of 30 cases of malignant mixed mullerian epithelial and mesenchymal ovarian tumors: A Gynecologic Oncology Group Study. Gynecol Oncol 18:278–292, 1984

Norris HJ, Zirkin HJ, Benson WL: Immature (malignant) teratoma of the ovary. A clinical and pathologic study of 58 cases. Cancer 37:2359–2372, 1976

Osborne BM, Robboy SJ: Lymphomas or leukemia presenting as ovarian tumors: An analysis of 42 cases. Cancer 52:1933–1943, 1983

Ozols RF, Garvin AJ, Costa J et al: Advanced ovarian cancer: Correlation of histologic grade with response to therapy and survival. Cancer 45:572–581, 1980

Piver MS, Barlow JJ, Lele SB: Incidence of subclinical metastasis in stage I and II ovarian carcinoma. Obstet Gynecol 52:100–104, 1978

Piver MS, Mettlin CJ, Tsukada Y et al: Familial ovarian cancer registry. Obstet Gynecol 64:195–199, 1984

Russell P: The pathological assessment of ovarian neoplasms. I. Introduction to the common "epithelial" tumours and analysis of benign "epithelial" tumours. Pathology 11:5–26, 1979

Russell P, Merkur H: Proliferating ovarian "epithelial" tumours: A clinico-pathological analysis of 144 cases. Aust NZ J Obstet Gynaecol 19:45–51, 1979

Serov SF, Scully RE: Histological typing of ovarian tumors. International Histological Classification of Tumors, No. 9. Geneva, World Health Organization, 1973

Shevchuk MM, Winkler-Monsanto B, Fenoglio CM, Richard RM: Clear cell carcinoma of the ovary: A clinicopathologic study with a review of the literature. Cancer 47:1344–1351, 1981

Slayton RE, Hreshchyshyn MM, Silverberg SG, Shingleton HM: Treatment of malignant ovarian germ cell tumors: Response to vincristine, dactinomycin and cyclophosphamide (preliminary report). Cancer 42:390–398, 1978

Smith JP, Day TG Jr.: Review of ovarian cancer at the University of Texas Systems Cancer Center, MD Anderson Hospital and Tumor Institute. Am J Obstet Gynecol 135:984–990, 1979

Stenwig JT, Hazekamp JT, Beecham JB: Granulosa cell tumors of the ovary. A clinicopathological study of 118 cases with long-term follow-up. Gynecol Oncol 7:136–152, 1979

Talerman A, Haije WG, Baggerman L: Serum alphafetoprotein (AFP) in patients with germ cell tumors of the gonads and extragonadal sites: Correlation between endodermal sinus (yolk sac) tumor and raised serum AFP. Cancer 46:380–385, 1980

Tavassoli FA, Norris HJ: Sertoli tumors of the ovary. A clinicopathologic study of 28 cases with ultrastructural observations. Cancer 46:2281–2297, 1980

Taylor HB, Norris HJ: Lipid cell tumors of the ovary. Cancer 20:1953–1962, 1967

Ulbright TM, Roth LM, Stehman FB: Secondary ovarian neoplasia: A clinicopathologic study of 35 cases. Cancer 53:1164–1174, 1984

Woodruff JD, Perry H, Genadry R, Parmley TH: Mucinous cystadenocarcinoma of the ovary. Obstet Gynecol 51:483–489, 1978

Young RH, Dickersin GR, Scully RE: Juvenile granulosa cell tumor of the ovary: A clinicopathological analysis of 125 cases. Am J Surg Pathol 8:575–596, 1984

Young RH, Scully RE: Ovarian sex cord–stromal tumors: Recent progress. Int J Gynecol Pathol 1:101–123, 1982

Zaloudek C, Kurman RJ: Recent advances in the pathology of ovarian cancer. Clin Obstet Gynaecol 10:155–186, 1983

Zaloudek C, Norris HJ: Sertoli–Leydig tumors of the ovary: A clinicopathologic study of 64 intermediate and poorly differentiated neoplasms. Am J Surg Pathol 8:405–418, 1984

Diseases of the Breast   *William L. Donegan*

60

Cancer is preeminent among diseases of the female breast. It is more likely to be responsible for the death of women 40 to 55 years of age than any other cause and causes more female deaths after age 15 than any other cancer. The total annual mortality from childbearing (320 in 1978) and all gynecologic neoplasms (22,800) falls far short of the 38,400 deaths that now result from cancer of the breast in the United States each year. In 1985 an estimated 119,000 new cases were expected, and the incidence—now 76 per 100,000 female population per year—is gradually rising. Breast cancer accounts for 27% of cancers in women and 20% of deaths from cancer.

Approximately 1 of every 11 women can be expected to develop cancer of the breast at some time during her life. Three percent of the cases will be coincident with a pregnancy. Most occur in the decade prior to menopause and in the two decades that follow (40–70 years of age), but risk climbs relentlessly with age, so there is no respite for the elderly, and only the declining number of the latter maintains the average age of all patients as low as 59 years.

Obstetricians and gynecologists examine several million women on a regular basis and have the opportunity to detect cancer of the breast in its earliest clinical stages. This opportunity is emphasized by the American College of Obstetricians and Gynecologists, which recommends that (1) examination of the breast be an integral part of the gynecologic examination, (2) patients be instructed in the importance and technique of breast self-examination (BSE), (3) use be made of mammography and needle aspiration as effective techniques for early detection, (4) ambulatory facilities for breast biopsy be encouraged, (5) breast biopsies be performed by properly trained persons, (6) women at high risk for breast cancer be recognized and innovative detection programs initiated for them, and (7) training for obstetricians and gynecologists include instruction in early diagnosis and treatment options.

Emphasis on early detection of breast cancer stems from the striking improvement in the prospects for cure when tumors are small and confined to the breast. Noninvasive or minimally invasive cancers can be cured in over 95% of cases. Although early detection is an opportunity for all physicians, the obstetrician–gynecologist is in a position to play a particularly important role in the diagnosis of breast disease.

WOMEN AT HIGH RISK FOR BREAST CANCER

Development of breast cancer is not a random event; certain demographic and personal characteristics confer greater than average risk. Appreciating these characteristics, which are summarized below, serves to focus attention on persons at greater than usual risk and to improve the efficiency of screening efforts.

Factors Leading to High Risk for Breast Cancer
Age > 40 years
Caucasian race
Obesity
Urban residence
High socioeconomic group
Jewish
Mother or sister with breast cancer
Previous surgery for benign breast disease
Previous cancer of one breast
Previous cancer of the endometrium or ovary
Excessive irradiation of the breast
Cowden's disease (multiple hamartoma syndrome)
Postmenopausal exogenous estrogen exposure
Early menarche (<12 years of age)
Late menopause (>55 years of age)

Aggregate lifetime menstrual cycles > 30 years
Nulliparity
First full-term pregnancy after the age of 30 years

Factors Leading to Low Risk for Breast Cancer
Surgical castration before the age of 37 years
Oriental race
First full-term pregnancy before 18 years of age
Age < 30 years

Most importantly, the disease is sex and age related. Ninety-nine percent of breast cancers occur in women. Breast cancer is unusual below the age of 30 years (<1.5% of cases) but steadily climbs in frequency thereafter. Almost 85% of patients are 40 years of age or older. Western women are considerably more likely to develop the disease than are Oriental women, and Danish women have greater mortality risk than any other nationality; breast cancer is uncommon in Japan, less than five times the incidence in the United States. In the United States, Jews and women of high socioeconomic status are notably susceptible.

Mortality from breast cancer in the United States has an uneven geographic distribution, the highest death rates being confined almost entirely to the northeastern part of the country and centered in urban and highly industralized areas.

The exceptionally high frequency of breast cancer in men with Klinefelter's syndrome (XXY sex chromosomes) and in women with Cowden's disease (multiple hamartoma syndrome, Fig. 60-1) and with the allele for wet ear wax, as well as the tendency of breast cancer to occur in some families, all suggest a genetic predisposition. Close relatives of breast cancer patients are 3 times more likely than expected to develop the disease, with daughters, sisters, and mothers conferring risk in ascending order of magnitude. If the disease involves both breasts, the risk to relatives increases to fivefold and to 9 times the expected risk if the patient is also premenopausal. Curiously, familial risk is not as great if the patient is postmenopausal.

Environmental factors associated with increased risk include high fat consumption, obesity, and carcinogen exposure. Women whose breasts were exposed to excessive fluoroscopy or were irradiated for postpartum mastitis or by atomic explosions are at excess risk. The fact that viruses (mouse mammary tumor virus [MMTV]) transmit breast cancer in mice and that certain polycyclic hydrocarbons, such as dimethybenzanthracine, can regularly cause breast cancer in rats after a small single dose makes both viruses and chemicals candidates for human carcinogens.

Although excess risk associated with the ingestion of estrogens has not been proven, considerable suspicion is justified. In 1976 Hoover found that women treated with conjugated estrogens for natural or surgical menopause developed an excess frequency of breast cancer after a latent period of ten years and had twice

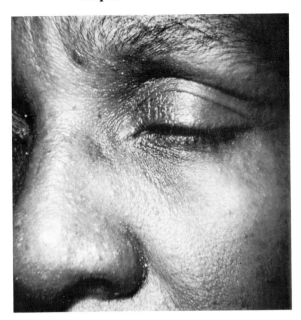

FIG. 60-1. Characteristic facial skin lesions of Cowden's syndrome. Small raised tumors (tricholimomas) are distributed on the face and hands, but in other cases occur also in the oral cavity. This patient had a mastectomy for carcinoma of breast and also had a thyroidectomy and a hysterectomy for tumors in these organs. An upper gastrointestinal series showed polypoid lesions of gastric mucosa. Women with Cowden's disease (multiple hamartomas) frequently have symptomatic fibrocystic disease of the breast and are at high risk for mammary carcinoma. Ten of the 21 cases reported through September 1977, as well as this patient, have had cancer of the breast. (Brownstein MH, Wolf M, Bikowski JB: Cowden's disease: A cutaneous marker of breast cancer. Cancer, 41:2393, 1978)

the expected risk after 15 years. Cyclic use, high doses, and development of fibrocystic disease while on estrogens increased the risk. No excess risk has been associated with oral contraceptives, and they may possibly prevent fibrocystic disease. Gambrell and co-workers, in 1983, emphasized that if estrogens are deemed desirable for postmenopausal replacement, the potential hazard should be made clear to the patient in advance, and combined estrogen and progesterone may be safer than estrogens alone.

The increased frequency of breast cancer in Japanese women who move to the United States is further evidence for the potential role of environmental carcinogens in this disease.

A consistent finding in several reports is the predisposition of patients treated for cancer of the endometrium to a subsequent cancer of the breast, both perhaps being related to a particular hormonal milieu or common stimulus. It is not clear that women with an initial breast cancer are more susceptible than usual to cancer at another site, although ovarian cancer is a possibility.

Among the most potent predispositions for the development of a new breast cancer is having been treated for cancer of the opposite breast. The frequency varies from 2 to 5 times the expected rate and makes the remaining breast deserving of special attention on follow-up examinations. This liability is concentrated in women whose first cancer was noninvasive multifocal, or of lobular type, and in those under 50 years of age or with a family history of breast cancer.

Symptomatic fibrocystic disease of the breast may place a woman at risk. Those who have had gross cysts or a biopsy showing fibrocystic disease, particularly epithelial proliferative changes, are from 3 to 5 times more likely than others to develop mammary carcinoma. Cellular atypia is particularly ominous. The relationship between mammographic tissue patterns and risk is controversial at present.

Other personal characteristics associated with increased risk of breast cancer implicate endocrine function: an early menarche (under 12 years of age), 30 or more years of active menstrual activity, a late menopause, two or fewer pregnancies, and a late initial full-term pregnancy. Women who give birth to their first child after the age of 35 years have a twofold higher risk than women who do so when under 20 years of age. Nulliparous women are at less risk than primiparas 35 years of age or older. This is a potentially important consideration in family planning and counseling. The important relationship between ovarian function and breast cancer is further illustrated by the fact that castration before the age of 40 years reduces the incidence of breast cancer by 75% regardless of previous parity. Subsequent to the fourth decade, when ovarian function has begun to decline, oophorectomy or irradiation castration no longer provides protection. Biochemical features of high risk include a low ratio of urinary estriol to total estrogens and a subnormal excretion of androgen metabolites, both suggesting an overbalance of estrogenic influences.

Contrary to earlier beliefs, epidemiologic studies fail to confirm protection against breast cancer attributable to breastfeeding; therefore, this can no longer be included among its virtues. Since virus particles similar to those of the MMTV can be found in human milk and human cancers, one might question the advisability of breastfeeding by women in high-risk groups.

Epitomizing high risk for breast cancer would be an elderly, obese, Caucasian women on long-term estrogen replacement who had been successfully treated for an endometrial carcinoma and cancer of one breast. Her risk would be further increased if her menarche had been early and her menopause later; if she had delivered her first and only child after the age of 35 years; if her remaining breast had been irradiated for postpartum mastitis and a biopsy subsequently performed, with a diagnosis of fibrocystic disease featuring ductal epithelial proliferation with atypia; and if urinary hormone excretion showed a low estriol ratio and was consistent with subnormal androgen production. Such patients are few, leading to the important point that most women who develop breast cancer have no distinguishing characteristics. For this reason it is not possible to exempt any from surveillance.

Factors of risk are additive, but to what ultimate extent is uncertain. In 1977, Farewell and associates considered the factors of family history, early age at menarche, and late first childbirth and found that the probability of breast cancer progressively doubled with the addition of each.

SIGNS AND SYMPTOMS OF BREAST CANCER

With few exceptions, breast cancers develop from the epithelial tissues of the breast; fewer than 1% are of connective tissue origin. More than 90% arise from the ductal system and the remainder from within the lobules. Hyperplasia of ductal cells, either those of the collecting ducts or those within the lobules, increasing cellular atypia, and progression to carcinoma *in situ* and finally to stromal invasion represent the course by which carcinomas evolve. These changes frequently occur simultaneously within many ducts; on careful examination, multiple sites of microscopic invasive or noninvasive cancer can be found in 50% of breasts removed for what appears clinically to be a single focus of cancer. The microscopic, asymptomatic growth phase is probably of protracted duration. Based on observed gross doubling times (the period required for an exponentially growing tumor to double its volume), a cancer that evolves from a single cell may require an average of seven years to become large enough to feel on palpatory examination (*i.e.,* a mass 1 cm in diameter). At this modest size 20% of cancers have already produced nodal metastases. If cancers can be detected and treated while "minimal" (*i.e.,* less than 5 mm in diameter) or while still noninvasive, metastasis is unlikely and cure is highly probable.

In almost 80% of cases the initial sign of cancer is a mass, and it is usually (70% of cases) discovered by the patient. The mass is characteristically nontender but may be associated with discomfort, tenderness, or a drawing sensation. Attachment to or dimpling of the overlying skin is highly suggestive of malignancy, although fat necrosis and plasma cell mastitis can also produce this change. Cancer can arise at any location within the breast, but the upper outer quadrant is most often the site, probably because tissue is concentrated in this location. The left breast is involved slightly more often than the right.

Nipple discharge is second only to a mass as the first sign of cancer; it can be bloody, nonbloody, clear, or of any color. Some discharge can be expressed from the breasts of most nonlactating women, but it is ordinarily obtainable from both sides, is nonbloody and small in quantity, and issues from more than one ductal orifice. Occasionally blood-tinged discharge can be expressed from the breasts of pregnant women, and persistent milky discharge is not unusual in parous women or those taking antidepressant medications. Bilateral discharge from multiple ducts in otherwise normal breasts is drug induced, physiologic, or secondary to a diffuse process such as fibrocystic disease. Cytology is rarely helpful in these instances. Unilateral discharge from a single orifice, particularly if spontaneous, is highly suggestive of a local lesion. Bloody fluid suggests a duct papilloma or carcinoma. The probability that cancer is the cause increases with age and in the presence of a mass.

Less frequent initial signs of malignancy include nipple retraction, localized edema of the skin, erythema, ulceration of the breast, pain, and ecchymoses.

Persistent erosion or crusting of the nipple may be a sign of Paget's disease, that is, intraepithelial carcinoma associated with cancer in the underlying ducts (Fig. 60-2). Biopsy should be performed on any lesion of the nipple that is suspicious or that does not respond rapidly to topical treatment within two weeks. Paget's disease of the nipple may or may not be accompanied by a palpable mass.

"Inflammatory" carcinoma mimics, in all respects, an acute infection with erythema, edema of the skin, enlargement of the breast, and discomfort. Too often it is mistaken for an infection and treated unsuccessfully

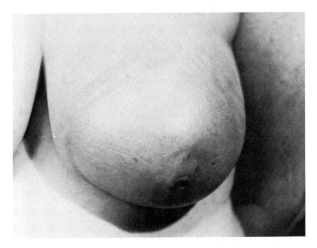

FIG. 60-3. Inflammatory carcinoma of this breast demonstrates characteristic features, including diffuse swelling without a distinct mass, erythema, and cutaneous edema. It can be confused with nonneoplastic inflammatory processes.

FIG. 60-2. The lesion on this nipple represents Paget's disease, intraepithelial cancer associated with underlying malignancy. Paget's disease can have several appearances but characteristically presents as a moist, nonhealing ulcer. In this instance it has destroyed the nipple and extended beyond it.

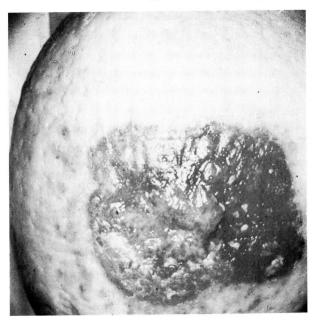

for prolonged periods with antibiotics and local heat (Fig. 60-3).

Occasionally an enlarged axillary lymph node due to metastasis is the only sign of occult carcinoma within the breast. The latter may be detectable only by mammography. Adenocarcinoma in the axillary nodes of a woman is more likely to be from a breast primary tumor than from any other site.

An increasing number of cancers are detected by routine mammograms in the absence of physical signs or symptoms. The radiographic changes that betray these early lesions include clusters of fine calcifications, small stellate densities, and focal architectural disturbances of the mammary parenchyma.

As cancer advances, other signs appear: nipple retraction, ulceration of the skin, retraction of the entire breast, pink satellite nodules within the skin, extensive edema and erythema of the skin, fixation to the chest wall, swelling of the arm due to extensive involvement of the axilla, and enlarged supraclavicular and parasternal lymph nodes (Fig. 60-4). Beyond the breast and its regional lymph nodes, mammary cancer can spread to any site in the body. Favored sites are distant lymph nodes, bones of the axial skeleton, the pleura, and the lungs. The liver is often eventually involved, and intracranial metastases are not unusual. Pleural effusions produce respiratory difficulties, and retroperitoneal involvement can obstruct the ureters. Additional spread within the skin is frequent, sometimes surrounding the chest like a constrictive breast plate, so-called carcinoma *en cuirasse.* Involvement of bones with lytic, sometimes blastic, metastases leads to pain, pathologic fractures, and potentially lethal hypercalcemia.

Cancer may appear in the opposite breast as a component of generalized dissemination, but it should also

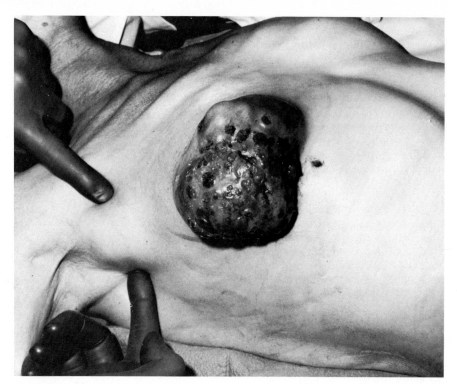

FIG. 60-4. Natural progression of untreated breast cancer is demonstrated by this large tumor that permeates and ulcerates overlying skin, is attached to underlying pectoralis major muscle, and is associated with enlarged tumor-bearing axillary lymph nodes. Cure is unlikely when disease has reached this extent.

be appreciated that approximately 5% of patients treated for one cancer develop an independent second cancer in the remaining breast. This may be discovered simultaneously with the first, but more often it is a subsequent development and, in the absence of dissemination, it also may be curable with vigorous treatment.

DIFFERENTIAL DIAGNOSIS

Several diseases of the breast present with signs or symptoms similar to those of cancer and must be distinguished from it; some are far more common. A biopsy is often necessary for diagnosis.

Fibrocystic Disease

Symptomatic fibrocystic disease of the breasts is a condition of the reproductive years, probably originating in hormonal imbalance. A relative estrogen excess or a progesterone deficiency in the luteal phase of the menstrual cycle may be responsible. Symptoms often become more prominent as menopause approaches. Characteristic symptoms are cyclic swelling, pain, and tenderness of one or both breasts, more prominent immediately before menses. Signs include irregular firmness and granularity of the breast tissue, masses, and expressible nipple discharge. These changes often wax and wane, paralleling symptoms.

A variety of histologic changes are involved, including gross and microscopic cysts, epithelial proliferation within ducts, sometimes to the point of diffuse papillomatosis or papilloma formation, proliferation of ducts (adenosis) associated with a varying degree of sclerosis (sclerosing adenosis), focal sclerosis (fibrous disease), and apocrine metaplasia of epithelium. Any or all of these changes can result clinically in masses, dominant nodules, and nipple discharge. Masses and cysts are often transient, and cysts can usually be identified with fine-needle aspiration, but persistent masses raise the possibility of cancer.

Symptomatic measures such as firm support with a well-fitting brassiere, mild analgesics, and local heat can provide relief. According to a theory described by Minton in 1979, the problem is aggravated by ingestion of foods and drinks containing methylxanthines (*e.g.,* caffeine, theophylline, and theobromine), and improvement often can be obtained by eliminating tea, coffee, cola drinks, and chocolate from the diet. Methylxanthines stimulate cyclic adenosine monophosphate (AMP) and increase metabolic activity in the breast. Nicotine and tyramines exacerbate the problem, so elimination of tobacco use and omission of cheese, wine, nuts, mushrooms, and bananas from the diet can also help. Hormonal therapy with progesterone during the second half of the menstrual cycle, and administration of gonadotropin inhibitors (danazol), androgens, thyroid substances, or prolactin inhibitors have been used with mixed success. Administration of tamoxifen has helped some women, as has discontinuing oral contraceptives. Danazol is currently the drug of choice when hormonal intervention is necessary. Women may become incapacitated by pain and require multiple diagnostic biopsies for suspected cancer. Difficult cases occasionally require subcutaneous mastectomy with prosthetic implants for relief.

Of all complaints related to the breast, fibrocystic disease continues to be the one encountered most commonly in clinical practice. It is important to appreciate that fibrocystic disease may be a precursor of malignant change, with atypical epithelial hyperplasia conferring the greatest risk. Women with histologically proven fibrocystic disease have 3 times the general risk of developing breast cancer. They are a well-defined group with a difficult problem: any abnormality is most likely to be further fibrocystic changes but is also more likely than usual to be breast cancer (Fig. 60-5).

Benign Neoplasms

Fibroadenomas

Fibroadenomas are the most common benign neoplasms of the breast, with a peak incidence in the third and fourth decades of life. Nevertheless, they also are found in the breasts of elderly women.

The physical findings are characteristic. Fibroadenomas are spherical, firm, and well defined, and they convey a palpatory sensation of easy mobility (Fig. 60-6). They occur most frequently in black women and are bilateral and multiple in approximately 15% of cases. Some are soft, demonstrate continued progressive growth, and can reach large size.

While the physical features of fibroadenomas are distinctive, they can be duplicated by the rare and treacherous cystosarcoma phyllodes, a fibrosarcoma mixed with benign ductal elements, and by granular cell myoblastomas. Mammographically, fibroadenomas have the same round shape and smooth borders as cysts, but some contain large, distinctive calcifications. Fibroadenomas are best removed, both for definitive diagnosis and to avoid progressive growth.

Lipomas

Benign lipomas of the breast are frequent and vary considerably in size. Differential diagnosis is not usually a problem, since large tumors are typically superficial, soft, and lobulated, but small lipomas can be deceptively firm. These tumors are usually in the subcutaneous tissues and may be located in any quadrant of the breast. The contour of the breast may be distorted, albeit smoothly so, and cutaneous or deep attachment is not usually a feature (Fig. 60-7). The mass transilluminates easily, and a mammogram is characteristic, showing a radiolucent tumor compressing breast tissue at its periphery.

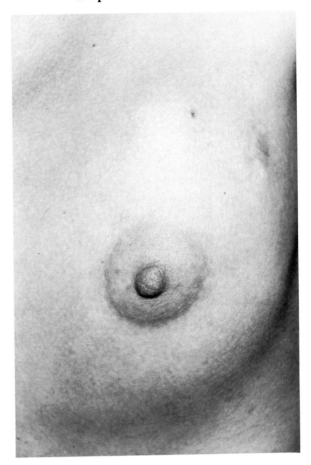

FIG. 60-5. Association between fibrocystic disease and carcinoma is illustrated by this young patient who presented with a mass in the upper midline of the breast, which subsequently proved to be cancerous. Scar in the upper outer quadrant marks site of previous biopsy that revealed fibrocystic disease.

Adenoma of the Nipple

An unusual benign neoplasm of both men and women, adenoma of the nipple produces firmness and soreness of the papilla of the nipple, often with crusting and a bloody discharge. Grossly, it mimics Paget's disease and, microscopically, has occasionally been mistaken for carcinoma. A biopsy is diagnostic, and local excision is curative.

Inflammations

Abscesses

Typical bacterial infections and abscesses are found most often in the postpartum period and are attributed to cracked nipples. They respond to appropriate antibiotics and to incision and drainage of pus when it is present. Abscesses in the breast of postmenopausal

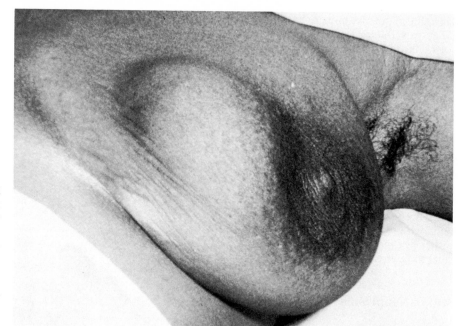

FIG. 60-6. This well-marginated tumor is a fibroadenoma, the most frequent benign neoplasm of the breast. Fibroadenomas predominate in the third and fourth decades of life and present as nontender, firm, round, highly mobile masses. Clefts are found on cut surface and represent distorted mammary ducts. Elective removal is appropriate.

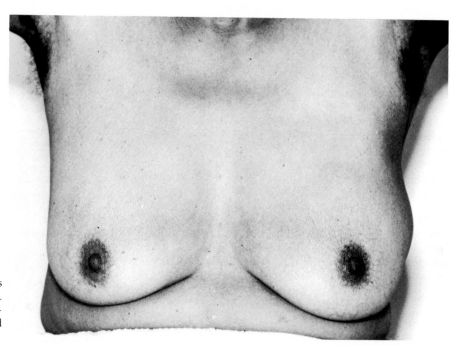

FIG. 60-7. Benign lipoma distorts lateral contour of the right breast. These neoplasms are generally identifiable by characteristic physical and mammographic features.

women are uncommon, are usually in the subareolar area, and result from ductal ectasia.

Squamous metaplasia within major lactiferous ducts of both the young and old can lead to repeated peri-areolar abscesses that drain at the areolar margin and to chronic sinuses communicating with the ductal system (Fig. 60-8). Patients have a characteristic history of repeated infections and multiple incisions for drainage.

Complete removal of the abnormal ducts, ordinarily the entire major duct system, is necessary for relief of the problem.

Carcinoma of the breast should not be missed in the differential diagnosis of inflammations or abscesses. Erythema, edema, tenderness, and swelling are characteristic features of inflammatory carcinoma. Fortunately, this virulent form of the disease accounts for

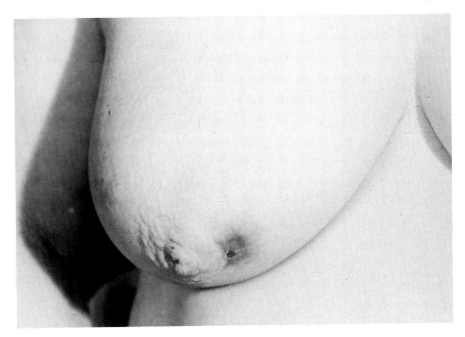

FIG. 60-8. Chronic sinus at the margin of the areola and a history of multiple abscesses in this area are typical of complications associated with ductal ectasia. Resection of major lactiferous ducts is usually necessary for cure.

only 2% of all cases. Diffuse induration rather than a discrete mass is the rule, and a mammogram provides no clue to set it apart from other sources of inflammation. Diagnosis depends on suspicion and a specimen of tissue and skin for microscopic examination. The histologic hallmark is cancer in dermal lymphatics. Failure of a postpartum infection to resolve promptly and infections in the breasts of postmenopausal women are suspicious of cancer and warrant biopsy. An incision and drainage for abscesses should be routinely accompanied by a tissue specimen.

Fat Necrosis and Plasma Cell Mastitis

Fat necrosis and plasma cell mastitis can mimic almost all signs of breast cancer; they are able to produce a mass and cause nipple retraction and skin dimpling. Mammograms are also highly suggestive of cancer with spiculated density and clustered calcification.

Fat necrosis is usually a sequel of direct trauma. The history is suggestive and a bruise may have been noted by the patient. Prominent histologic features are fibrosis intermixed with foamy macrophages, histiocytic giant cells, fat droplets, and necrotic debris. Microcalcification may be present.

Plasma cell mastitis, an inflammatory mass characterized by prominent infiltration of plasma cells, probably has its origin in ductal ectasia, a process in which squamous metaplasia within lactiferous ducts results in an accumulation of keratinous debris. This inspissated material eventually erodes the ductal wall, thereby inciting the characteristic tissue response.

Excisional biopsy is necessary for diagnosis of both of these lesions.

Mondor's Disease

Thrombosis of the thoracoepigastric vein, which courses lateral to or across the breast, Mondor's disease can present clinically either as an asymptomatic or tender subcutaneous fibrotic cord. The cord may attach to the dermis to produce a cutaneous furrow on the breast with retraction of the skin, most prominent when the arm is abducted. It is often associated with operations on the breast or thorax and is self-limited, resolving completely with time. The clinical features are characteristic but can sometimes be confused with cancer. In situations of uncertainty, a biopsy is necessary. If the cord traverses the axilla (Fig. 60-9), it can cause limitation of shoulder motion and may require transection, but this is unusual.

DETECTION AND DIAGNOSIS

Medical History

Evaluation of the patient for breast disease begins with a clinical history and a complete physical examination relevant to breast disease. After defining the presenting problem, the physician should inquire about previous breast disease, known risk factors, and current medications, particularly oral contraceptives and other hormones. A history of oophorectomy is noteworthy as well as previous treatment for cancers that may increase the risk of breast cancer, including carcinoma of the endometrium and of the ovary. The age of menarche, the number of pregnancies and live births, the age at first childbirth, and the date of last menses are important information. If previous operations included a hyster-

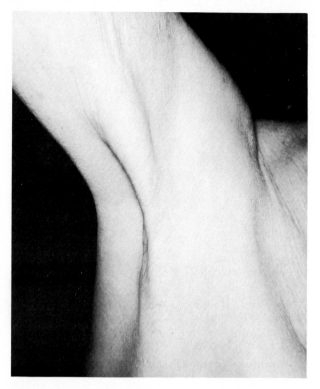

FIG. 60-9. Firm subcutaneous band crossing the axilla represents a form of Mondor's disease. Thrombophlebitis, usually of the thoracoepigastric vein, is responsible and sometimes has been confused clinically with infiltrating mammary carcinoma.

ectomy, pertinent information includes the indications for the surgery, whether the ovaries were removed and, if not, whether symptoms suggestive of menopause have been experienced subsequently. Inquiry should be made about breast cancer in other family members.

Visual Examination

General physical features of pertinence are signs of Cowden's disease, a previous mastectomy, or, in males, features of Klinefelter's syndrome. The breasts are examined visually and with palpation, and attention is given to the regional nodes in the axilla and the supraclavicular and infraclavicular areas.

No special equipment is necessary to perform an adequate examination. The examination is begun with the patient seated comfortably and disrobed to the waist. If the patient has a complaint specifically related to the breast such as a lump or point of tenderness, it is useful at this point for her to indicate the site so that it can receive special attention during the examination, the details of which are shown in Figure 60-10.

Considerable variation exists among patients with respect to the size of breasts and their general configuration, but outlines are normally curvilinear. These constitutional differences are all subject to change with age, pregnancy, and hormonal stimulation. Perfect symmetry is rarely found, and one must have an appreciation for the range of normal. Attention is given to unusual asymmetry in size or shape, color of the skin and its venous pattern, skin changes, and nipple excoriations, deviation, or inversion. Enlarged nodes may be visible in the supraclavicular areas.

The patient is instructed, in turn, to fully extend both arms above her head and then to place the hands on her hips and press inward, tightening the pectoralis major muscles. These positions change the relationship between the breasts and both the deep pectoral fascia and the skin; if abnormal attachments are present they will produce signs of retraction or dimpling.

Palpation

With the patient still seated, the supraclavicular, infraclavicular, and axillary areas are palpated for lymph nodes. Infraclavicular (actually apical axillary) lymph nodes can be felt in the deltopectoral triangle if they are enlarged. The coracoid process of the scapula, which may be prominent at this site, can mimic a hard, fixed lymph node but betrays its true nature by being present on both sides. The axilla is best examined with the patient's arm relaxed at her side, only slightly abducted, a position that loosens the axillary fascia and facilitates palpation. The left axilla is examined with the right hand while the examiner's left hand is placed on the patient's shoulder to prevent upward motion. The fingertips are

FIG. 60-10. (*1*) Examination of breasts begins with inspection; patient is disrobed to waist and comfortably seated facing examiner. Asymmetry, prominent veins, and skin changes may be signs of disease. (*2*) Patient raises arms above head, thereby altering position of breasts. Immobility or abnormal cutaneous attachments may become evident. (*3*) Inward pressure on hips tenses pectoralis major muscle. Abnormal attachments to its overlying fascia and skin can produce retraction or dimpling of skin. (*4*) Palpatory examination is performed of supraclavicular lymph nodes. (*5*) Deltopectoral triangle is palpated for evidence of infraclavicular nodal enlargement. (*6*) Each axilla is examined for nodal enlargement. Proper placement of examiner's hands and of patient's arm is important. (*7*) Thorough palpatory examination of entire breast for masses is performed with patient in supine position. A fine rotational movement of the hands is useful to apprecite the consistency of underlying tissues. (*8*) Nipple is compressed to elicit discharge.

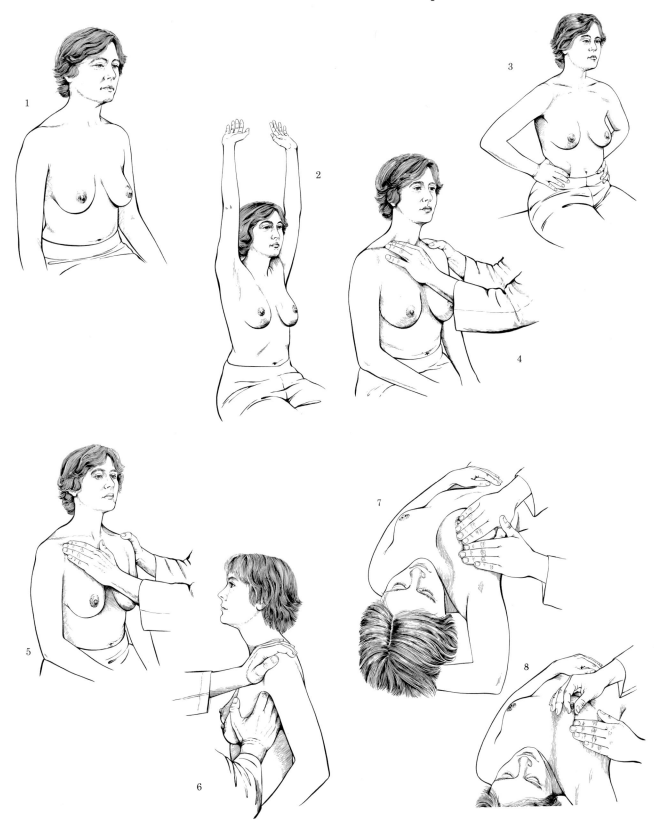

inserted high but gently into the axilla in a slightly cupped position and then withdrawn downward along the chest wall. This maneuver traps axillary lymph nodes so that they can be readily appreciated as they escape from beneath the fingers. If the heel of the hand that is on the shoulder is pressed gently upon the pectoralis major, the axillary contents are centralized for a better examination. Nevertheless, both the anterior and the posterior portions of the axilla should be explored. The right axilla is examined by reversing the position of the hands. The size, number, consistency, location, tenderness, and mobility of nodes are important to note.

The examination is continued with the patient in the supine position and ideally with a small pad or pillow beneath the back to elevate the side being examined. This flattens and distributes the breast evenly on the chest wall and thins the parenchyma. The arm should be abducted. All portions of the breast are examined using the volar surfaces of the fingertips. The examiner should appreciate that breast tissue can reach to the costal margin inferiorly, to the clavicle superiorly, to the midline of the chest, and to the posterior axillary line as well as into the lower axilla. A systematic palpation is best, using the fingers of both hands and proceeding progressively around the breast from center to periphery as if examining each spoke of a wheel. Some examiners prefer to begin peripherally and palpate in diminishing concentric circles centered on the areola. Fine rotating motions of the fingers serve to displace the underlying glandular tissue back and forth beneath the skin and permit a better appreciation of its consistency, which may vary from soft and lobular to finely or coarsely granular. The axillary extension of the breast should not be forgotten.

Masses or dominant nodules are described in detail and measured with a tape or caliper. The breast may be conceptualized as four quadrants—the upper outer, upper inner, lower outer, and lower inner—as well as a central portion beneath the areola. Masses are described in terms of their location in these quadrants, their size, shape, consistency, mobility, sensitivity, and attachment to skin or deep tissues. Fixation of an otherwise mobile mass when the patient presses her hand on her hip is a sign of attachment to the deep pectoral fascia or to the pectoralis major muscle itself. Dimpling or inability to move the skin independently of the mass connotes skin attachment. Complete immobility of a mass implies fixation to ribs and intercostal muscles, namely, the chest wall.

Simultaneous palpation of corresponding quadrants of the breasts is sometimes of value in deciding whether an abnormality is present. A significant asymmetry can be made more obvious with this technique.

Finally, the nipple and areola are examined for underlying masses, inversion, or discharge. A persistent excoriation or "dermatitis" may be a sign of Paget's disease of the nipple and an underlying carcinoma. Not infrequently women report a long history of nipple inversion; however, if this is a recent change and the nipple cannot be everted at least temporarily, it is a serious omen. Finally, the nipple is gently squeezed to elicit discharge. The characteristics of a discharge and the number of ducts involved are important observations.

Fine-Needle Aspiration

Since cysts of the breasts are frequent and breast cancers are rarely cystic, a reliable distinction between a solid mass and a cyst has considerable value. The distinction cannot be made reliably with palpation, transillumination, or mammograms. Fine-needle aspiration provides a rapid and relatively painless method of distinguishing between solid masses and cysts and can be performed at the time of a physical examination with readily available materials and without anesthesia. A 5-ml or 10-ml syringe, a 1.5-inch sharp 20-gauge needle, and an antiseptic solution such as 70% alcohol or an iodophor are sufficient (Fig. 60-11).

With the patient in the supine position and advised as to the nature of the procedure, the skin over the mass is prepared with the antiseptic solution. The mass is stabilized with the free hand, and with the other the

FIG. 60-11. (*1*) Aspiration of masses is a useful and simple office procedure. After preparing the skin with antiseptic solution, the mass is stabilized using the index and middle fingers of the left hand, and a No. 20 needle fitted to a syringe is introduced into it with one motion. No local anesthesia is necessary because discomfort is minimal. (*2*) With needle and syringe stabilized, aspiration is performed. All fluid that can be obtained is withdrawn. After the needle is removed, the site is reexamined to determine if the mass is persistent.

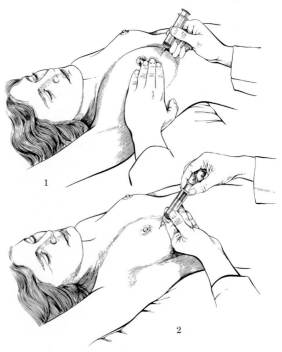

needle is passed into the mass and it is aspirated. Increased resistance to passage of the needle ordinarily indicates a solid mass and reduced resistance a cyst. Simple cysts will produce nonbloody fluid that may be thick or thin and vary from colorless to white, yellow, brown, or green. Milk is obtained from galactoceles. On aspiration of all fluid the cyst wall collapses and the mass disappears. If a mammogram is normal and reexamination in two to three weeks reveals no recurrence of the cyst, no further intervention is necessary.

A biopsy is indicated if no fluid is obtained on aspiration, the mass does not disappear completely after all fluid is removed, the fluid obtained is bloody, the mammogram is suspicious of cancer, or the cyst reappears after two apparently successful aspirations. These signs suggest a solid tumor (which may be cancer) or an intracystic or partially cystic cancer. It is not necessary routinely to examine the cytology of an innocent-appearing cyst aspirate; rarely is this useful.

Ultrasound

Ultrasound can distinguish cystic from solid masses, but it is more time consuming and expensive than needle aspiration and does not have the therapeutic benefit of the latter. The examination is painless, involves no ionizing irradiation, and can identify masses even within dense breast tissue (a distinct advantage in young women). Its limitations are such that it is not a substitute for mammography in screening or evaluation of complaints. It is most useful for determining the solid or cystic nature of small masses deep within the breast that cannot be felt or aspirated. There is no evidence that ultrasound damages tissues or facilitates the spread of cancer.

Cytology

The cytologic examination of nipple discharges, cyst aspirations, and tissue fluid from solid masses is of limited value. Although morphologically malignant cells from nipple discharge cannot be ignored and serve as an impetus for further diagnostic measures, false-positives are not infrequent, and false-negatives in the presence of cancer are common. Therefore, cytology cannot be considered diagnostic, and the absence of malignant cells should not lead to complacency. A positive cytologic examination of cyst fluid in the absence of other indications for biopsy is sufficiently rare that the examination can hardly be justified as routine.

Indisputably malignant cells seen in the tiny amount of tissue fluid obtained from aspiration of a solid mass is a reliable indicator of cancer, but failure to identify malignant cells in the aspirate does not rule out cancer. It is not possible to determine from the aspirate whether a cancer is invasive or not, making difficult the selection of a proper surgical procedure. Thus, while the finding of malignant cells may expedite an evaluation and justify staging, it still does not obviate a biopsy.

Mammography

Mammograms, soft-tissue radiographs of the breast, deserve special attention in early detection of breast cancer because they offer several unique capabilities. Cancer too small to be felt (*e.g.,* 0.2 cm in diameter) can be detected with mammography, making this a logical extension of the physical examination. Furthermore, mammograms can reveal signs of cancer in the absence of symptoms and therefore are useful for screening asymptomatic, apparently healthy women. Finally, the probable nature of a palpable mass can be determined by mammography with considerable, but not absolute, accuracy.

Mammograms are most useful for older women whose breasts are largely fatty and less dense than those of young women. Radiographically dense cancers are more easily visualized against this background.

Two views of each breast at right angles to one another (mediolateral and craniocaudal views) are a standard examination. Together they entail a total radiation exposure to each breast of less than 1 rad. Either of two techniques may be used: film mammograms, which have the appearance of radiographs, and xerograms, opaque blue and white images produced on paper backing. Both involve low radiation exposure. Examples of normal and abnormal xeromammograms are shown in Figures 61-13, 61-14, and 61-15. Interpretation of the films is discussed in Chapter 61.

It is important to understand that mammograms are an important complement to physical examination but are not a substitute for it. Approximately 15% of early cancers are detected by physical examination alone and are not visualized by mammograms; thus, a normal mammogram provides no assurance that cancer is absent. The images depend on differing radiographic densities within the breasts, and some tumors that are easily palpable can escape detection by mammography, presumably because of insufficient difference in radiographic density from the surrounding breast tissue. In other instances proximity to the chest wall or location at the periphery of the breast may place them outside the standard image of a routine examination. It is also important to appreciate that mammograms are not sufficiently precise to diagnose the nature of a palpable mass. Radiographic lesions judged "radiographically suspicious for cancer" by trained radiologists prove benign in 10% to 12% of cases, and about 5% of radiographically benign lesions prove on biopsy to be cancers. Subclinical lesions judged suspicious of cancer prove to be malignant neoplasms in one of six instances. Inaccuracy stems from the fact that slowly growing malignancies can appear well circumscribed and mimic the characteristics of fibroadenomas, cysts, and other innocent lesions, while a number of benign processes, such as fat necrosis, sclerosing adenosis, and biopsy scars, mimic to perfection the radiographic signs of cancer. Since the fibrosis of previous surgery and common skin lesions such as nevi can be misleading on mammograms, the accuracy of the examination is improved if a physical examination is performed by the radiologist and if pertinent information from the patient's history and physical examination is furnished by the clinician.

Indications for mammography are well established. Symptomatic adults should have mammograms in conjunction with a physical examination whenever a complaint is related to the breast, regardless of whether an abnormality is visible or palpable. Mammograms should be performed prior to biopsy or any other operation on the breast. They are also indicated, even if cancer in one breast is clinically obvious, as a check for subclinical cancer in the opposite breast.

Asymptomatic adults, according to the National Cancer Institute, should have mammograms performed annually in conjunction with a physical examination if they are 50 years of age or older; if they are 40 to 49 years of age with a history of cancer in a mother, sister, or daughter; and if they are any age and have had one breast removed for cancer. Recommendations of the American Cancer Society and the American College of Radiology vary from these only in recommending a baseline mammogram for all asymptomatic women between the ages of 35 to 40 and a mammogram every one to two years in women between ages 40 and 50, depending on personal risk.

Among the indications for mammography must be included the localization of nonpalpable lesions for biopsy. The localization technique permits accurate removal of nonpalpable lesions. With the two mammographic views, two topographic coordinates can be established for any subclinical lesion. A drop of visible and radiographically opaque dye (Evans blue and iothalamate meglumine 60%) previously mixed is injected at the junction of the coordinates, after which a second mammogram is performed. The relationship of the radiopaque "spot" to the lesion is observed, and the visible blue dye then serves to guide the surgeon. The occult lesion can be removed cosmetically with minimal sacrifice of normal tissue, an important point considering that most biopsies prove benign and that some women require multiple biopsies. If suspicious calcifications are the target of a biopsy, a specimen radiograph (*e.g.,* a roentgenogram of the tissue removed) can serve to ensure that all suspicious calcifications are present in the specimen and have been removed. Other techniques of localization include introducing a needle or a fine wire with a hook at its tip into the lesion under mammographic control to guide the surgeon's biopsy.

Mammography is also useful in conjunction with a physical examination of the breasts in search for the source of metastatic adenocarcinoma when the breasts are among the possible sites of an occult primary. The most frequent source of metastatic adenocarcinoma in axillary nodes of women is the breast.

The following should not be considered candidates for mammography: women under 25 years of age; pregnant women—radiation exposure is undesirable during pregnancy, and the breasts are dense and unlikely to provide satisfactory contrast; and asymptomatic women under 35 years of age who have no personal history of breast cancer.

The carcinogenic potential of mammograms due to irradiation of the breast cannot be ignored but should not be exaggerated. The value of mammography as a detection device is indisputable; the carcinogenic potential is still theoretic. Breslow and co-workers estimate that mammograms might result in six cancers per 1,000,000 women per year per rad of exposure after a latent period of ten years. This risk, although small, serves to emphasize that the indications for mammography should remain well defined.

Biopsy

Physical signs or mammographic lesions suggestive of cancer provide the indications for biopsy. Most frequently these indications are a persistent mass or a suggestive nipple discharge, but with current efforts for early detection and screening, asymptomatic lesions found with mammography are an increasingly common indication.

Biopsy must be performed on a persistent mass or dominant nodule despite a normal or "negative" mammogram. In the premenopausal breast, an equivocal mass or one of recent origin may be observed through one menstrual cycle to determine if it persists despite hormonal change. A brief trial off oral contraceptives is also worthwhile, and fine-needle aspiration can be employed immediately to identify a benign cyst; otherwise, a histologic diagnosis must be made.

The traditional one-stage procedure, that is, hospital admission with biopsy under general anesthesia, immediate diagnosis with frozen section, and mastectomy if indicated, is being replaced by a two-stage procedure with a deliberate interval between biopsy and treatment. In response to economic pressures and the evidence that a short delay between biopsy and surgical treatment does not compromise chances for cure, many biopsies are now performed as an outpatient procedure, often with the patient under local anesthesia. Since only one of four biopsies reveals cancer, this is expedient and spares the time and expense of many needless hospitalizations. It also permits the diagnosis to be made securely on the basis of thorough histologic examination of permanent sections rather than of frozen sections, an advantage when one considers that a distinction between hyperplasia and early cancer is sometimes difficult. With a diagnosis firmly established, consideration can be given to staging and to the options for treatment. If the patient is interested, the possibilities for future reconstruction of the breast can be discussed.

Biopsies should be performed by a surgeon who is

well informed about the management of breast diseases and skilled in the technique of biopsy and mastectomy. Biopsies must be performed with proper indications, with due consideration given to cosmetics, and with accuracy, so that a correct diagnosis is obtained. Infection or hematoma can delay further treatment, and misplaced or unnecessarily extensive biopsies can compromise the options for treatment or lead to suboptimal results.

Only microscopic analysis of a tissue specimen provides a definitive diagnosis of mammary cancer. No other procedure provides sufficient diagnostic assurance to permit treatment for cancer of the breast. A suitable tissue specimen can be obtained with a biopsy needle, an incisional biopsy, or an excisional biopsy. Several types of needles permit a core of tissue to be removed from suspicious masses with the patient under local anesthesia in an office or clinic. This is useful for large tumors that are easy targets or for women in whom a mastectomy or tumor removal is not anticipated. A negative result is not diagnostic, since cancer may have been missed.

An "open" biopsy can be performed under local or general anesthesia. Small masses are removed completely (excisional biopsy); a small specimen from a large mass (incisional biopsy) will usually identify it as cancer. In many instances it is possible to use a cosmetic para-areolar incision for biopsies.

Estrogen- and Progesterone-Receptor Protein

An important consideration at the time of biopsy in the patient in whom the entire tumor is removed or in whom no mastectomy is contemplated is special care of the specimen so that estrogen-receptor (ER) protein and progesterone-receptor (PR) protein analysis can be performed on the fresh or frozen tumor tissue. An adequate amount of tissue (usually >500 mg) and immediate cooling are necessary. The presence of ER in concentrations greater than 10 femtomoles per milligram of protein identifies the tumor as being hormonally dependent (*i.e.,* having a 67% probability of responding to hormone or endocrine therapy), and the probability of hormone responsiveness increases with the concentration of ER. More importantly, its absence signifies that such therapy will almost certainly be of no value (<8% chance of a response). This information is of considerable importance if adjuvant therapy or palliative therapy for recurrence is being considered. Since recurrent tumors after mastectomy may prove inaccessible, routine assay of primary tumors at the time they are removed is a wise precaution. If tumor tissue contains PR as well as ER, the likelihood of a response to hormonal or endocrine therapy is raised to almost 90%. Of additional importance is that the presence of ER signifies a relatively favorable prognosis. In a 1979 review by Degenshein and associates, analysis of tumor tissue for hormone-receptor proteins is described as a routine procedure in the management of patients with cancer of the breast.

Investigational Techniques of Detection

Still under investigation for detection of breast disease are computed tomography (CT), thermography, and diaphanoscopy. CT can be performed with acceptable levels of radiation exposure but is a cumbersome and lengthy procedure. Its advantage over mammography is perhaps in the evaluation of very dense breasts. However, in one study, 35% of subsequently proved carcinomas were missed by this technique; difficulties included failure to detect microcalcifications.

Thermography, which provides a visual pattern of heat from the skin of the breast, depends for detection on the fact that many cancers have a high metabolic rate and are therefore hotter than surrounding tissues. It has the advantage of involving no radiation exposure, but interpretation is subjective, false-positive rates are high, and many cancers produce no abnormalities. Twelve percent of examinations are falsely positive and up to 67% of cancers are missed. Consequently, it has found little place in clinical practice.

Diaphanoscopy refers to transillumination of the breast with yellow light. The examination is performed in a darkened room using a hand-held illuminator and is capable of revealing dense masses within the tissues of the breast. Lipomas and cysts transilluminate well, in contrast to solid tumors, which produce dark images. The examination has little value in detecting unsuspected cancers and is not widely used.

Breast Self-Examination

Most cancers (70% in a survey of tumor registries by the American College of Surgeons) continue to be found by patients themselves as a lump or nipple discharge. Yet few women perform routine BSE, a practice that should be encouraged. The objective is to detect tumors at the smallest possible size, when they are most likely to be localized and curable. Many neglect this examination for fear of making an unwanted discovery, but most are willing to do so if instructed properly (Fig. 60-12). Women expect their obstetrician–gynecologists to be informed on this subject, and the initial office visit is an opportune time at which to provide instruction. Supplementary literature on BSE is available from the American Cancer Society and the U.S. Department of Health and Human Services.

Self-examination should begin when a woman reaches adulthood. The examination is performed monthly, an interval generally sanctioned as convenient and not unduly repetitious; the best time for premenopausal women is immediately after each menstruation. Most women's breasts are least tender and swollen at this time, permitting a thorough examination without dis-

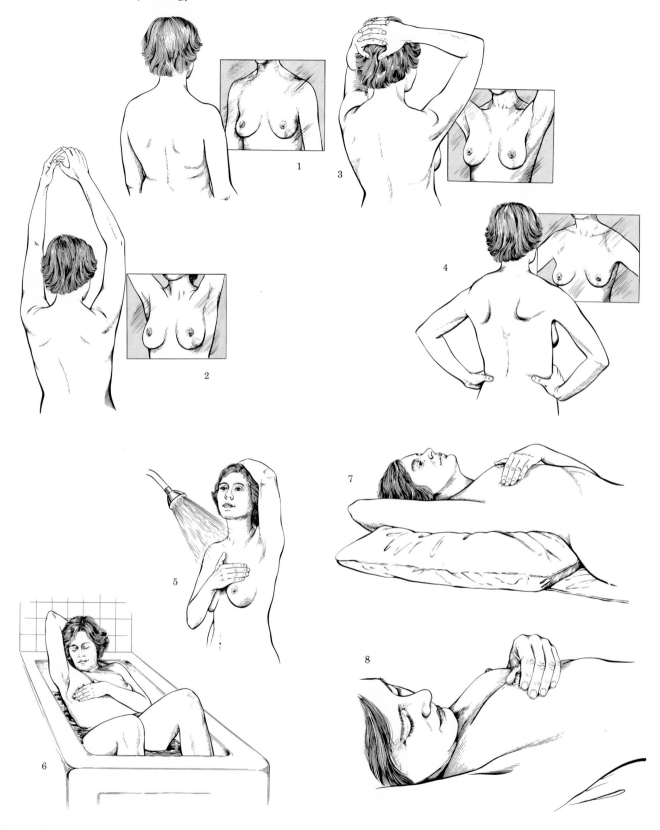

comfort. Inconsequential changes are also least likely to be present at this time. After menopause timing is not critical, and since menses no longer serve as a reminder, any regular time such as the first day of the month may be chosen for the examination. The time of bathing provides several conveniences: privacy, freedom from clothing confinements, and the opportunity to examine the breast with the skin wet and soapy, which seems to aid palpation by providing additional sensitivity.

The breasts are both viewed and manually examined. While standing before a mirror, the woman should view her breasts first facing forward with the arms relaxed at the sides and then alternately turning the torso to each side. Notable are asymmetry (some is normally present, since the breasts are seldom of equal size), unusually prominent veins, nipple deviation or inversion, and prominences or skin changes. Dimpling of the skin is particularly noteworthy. The arms are moved in various positions to elicit dimpling that may not be obvious otherwise. These positions include fully extending the arms above the head, placing them on top of the head, and, finally, placing the hands on the hips and pressing inward to tighten the pectoral muscles.

The palpatory examination should be performed thoroughly and systematically, including the entire breast from clavicle to costal margin and from midline to lateral chest. Ideally, the examination is performed in the supine position; raising the side to be examined by placing a pillow under the back facilitates palpation by flattening and distributing the breasts more evenly on the chest wall. The flats of the fingers, not the tips, are used, pressing firmly with a fine rotating motion. Palpation proceeds from the periphery in a diminishing spiral toward the nipple. Alternatively, the breast may be considered a wheel with radiating spokes, and each spoke is examined, in turn, from nipple to periphery.

This portion of the examination can also be done effectively in the shower or in the bathtub, when one has the advantage of wet and soapy skin. The axillary extension of the breasts should not be missed, and an axillary examination can be added. Attention is also given to the nipple, which is palpated, and a gentle squeeze can elicit discharge if it is present.

As a woman becomes familiar with her breasts through repeated examinations, she is better able to appreciate significant changes. She should be aware that most lumps are not cancers, but that persistent masses, discharge, or skin changes should prompt medical consultation.

Women who practice BSE discover breast cancers that are smaller and less often metastatic to axillary nodes than women who do not practice it, and this confers a survival advantage.

STAGING OF BREAST CANCER

The choice of treatment for cancer of the breast is guided by the stage, the apparent extent of the tumor. The "clinical" stage is determined by physical examination, radiographs, blood tests, and isotopic scans. Examples of current clinical classifications are the Columbia Clinical Classification and the TNM systems of The American Joint Committee for Cancer Staging (Fig. 60-13) and of the International Union Against Cancer. Tumors localized to the breast (stage I) and those with limited spread to axillary lymph nodes (stage II and many of stage III) are generally treated by mastectomy. Localized cancers are highly curable by mastectomy and almost uniformly so if the tumor is still noninvasive. The expectation of surgical cure is less in patients with clinically involved axillary nodes, but cure still can be obtained in a substantial number of cases. Locally unresectable and disseminated cases (stages IIIb and IV) are treated for palliation by irradiation to the breast and regional nodes, sometimes a limited mastectomy, and with hormonal, endocrine, or chemotherapy.

The extent of disease determined from resected tissues constitutes the "pathologic" stage. The pathologic stage of cases treated surgically is based primarily on the absence (stage I) or presence (stage II) of metastases in axillary lymph nodes. This is the single most

FIG. 60-12. (*1*) Breast self-examination is begun with inspection using a mirror. Attention is given to contours of breast and to skin. (*2*) Arms are extended high above the head, watching for abnormal motion or skin retraction. (*3*) Pressure is placed on back of head to tense the pectoralis major muscles that underlie mammary tissues. (*4*) Inward pressure on hips serves to tense pectoralis major muscles. Retraction of skin is a sign of abnormality. (*5*) Wet soapy skin facilitates manual examination of breast for lumps. (*6*) Tub bathing provides an optimal time for discovering lumps. Wet skin permits easy motion of the examining hand, and a reclining position flattens breast tissues upon the chest wall. (*7*) Palpatory examination is best performed in supine position with the side to be examined elevated on a pillow or blanket. Lumps are most evident when the breast is flattened and evenly distributed upon the chest wall. As a women gains familiarity with the appearance and feel of her breast through repeated examinations, she becomes more capable of appreciating changes. (*8*) Self-examination is completed with a squeeze of the nipple to detect abnormal discharge.

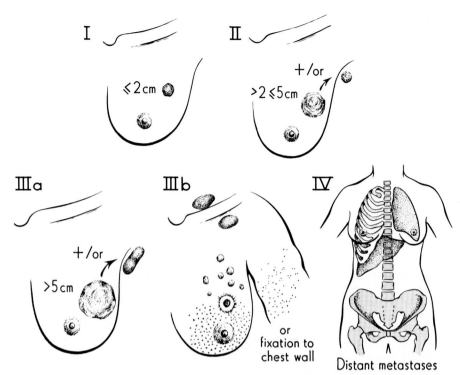

FIG. 60-13. The International Union Against Cancer and The American Joint Committee on Cancer recognize four clinical stages of invasive mammary carcinoma. Stage I includes tumors confined to the breast and no more than 2 cm in diameter. Stage II includes larger tumors localized to the breast but not exceeding 5 cm in diameter or smaller cancers with small, mobile, clinically involved axillary lymph nodes. Stage IIIa consists of large tumors exceeding 5 cm in diameter or cancers that have produced clinically enlarged axillary lymph nodes fixed to one another or to adjacent tissues. Stage IIIb designates more advanced, but still undisseminated cancers with evidence of direct involvement of the skin as edema, ulceration, or satellite nodules and those with fixation to the chest wall (ribs, intercostal muscles), or with clinically evident supraclavicular or infraclavicular nodal metastases. Cases with edema of the ipsilateral arm are also stage IIIb cancers as are inflammatory cancers, but the latter are designated separately. All cancers with distant metastases are stage IV. Noninvasive cancers are classified separately as stage TIS (tumor *in situ*), not pictured here. The same scheme applies to pathologic staging based on biopsies or mastectomies.

important prognosticator, and cure becomes progressively less likely with the presence and the extent of nodal involvement. The importance of this information for prognosis and the reason further treatment is usually considered for patients with metastases are evident from Table 60-1. When metastases are present in nodes, surgical treatment is often supplemented by systemic chemotherapy or irradiation to the thorax, or both, in order to reduce or delay recurrence.

Staging is also useful for estimating the prognosis after treatment and for comparing the results of different treatments. The prognoses of white and black women according to the Cancer Surveillance, Epidemiology, and End Results (SEER) program of the U.S. Department of Health and Social Services are shown in Table 60-2. This four-stage system, formerly used by the American Col-

Table 60-1

Survival of Patients Treated with Radical Mastectomy According to Axillary Nodal Status

Category	No.	Percent Survival	
		5 Years	10 Years
All cases	406	63.5	45.9
Negative axillary nodes	207	78.1	64.9
Positive axillary nodes	207	46.5	24.9
1–3 positive nodes	107	62.2	37.5
≥4 positive nodes	100	32.0	13.4

(Fisher B, Slack N, Katrych D et al: Ten-year follow-up results of patients with carcinoma of the breast in a cooperative clinical trial evaluating surgical adjuvant chemotherapy. Surg Gynecol Obstet 140:528, 1975)

Table 60-2
Stage of Breast Cancer Versus Prognosis

	Relative Survival (%)*			
	5-Year		10-Year	
Stage	White	Black	White	Black
All stages	64	46	52	41
Localized	84	77	74	77
Regional	54	44	39	34
Disseminated	7	6	2	4

* Survival after correcting for deaths unrelated to breast cancer.
(Cancer Patient Survival, Report No. 5, 1978)

lege of Surgeons, is based on both clinical and histologic information to categorize cases as being (1) *in situ,* (2) localized to the breast, (3) regionalized (direct involvement of adjacent tissues or signs of early axillary nodal involvement), and (4) disseminated. Prognosis after treatment according to the TNM system is shown in Table 60-3. These data are from patients treated at the Medical College of Wisconsin-affiliated hospitals.

TREATMENT OF BREAST CANCER

Surgical removal of the breast or local tumor excision followed by irradiation of the breast are alternative treatments for potentially curable cases of breast cancer. Removal or irradiation of the entire organ is predicated on the fact that cancer is often multifocal in the breast (28–74%) rather than confined to a single site. The knowledge that regional lymph nodes in the axilla contain metastases in at least 40% of cases whether or not they appear clinically involved has provided the rationale for routinely removing them. An axillary dissection, therefore, provides an estimate of prognosis and the basis for deciding on adjuvant therapy. Furthermore, a thorough axillary dissection almost eliminates risk of recurrence in the axilla and obviates any need for irradiation to this site. It is not demonstrated that axillary dissection in the absence of clinical adenopathy improves the chances of cure.

Radical Mastectomy

Until 1979 en bloc removal of the entire breast, the underlying pectoralis major and pectoralis minor muscles, and the entire axillary contents—the radical mastectomy (of Halsted)—was the standard treatment for operable breast cancer. This operation has now been supplanted by the less extensive modified radical mastectomy, a procedure that is equally effective and is less deforming. Approximately 60% of all women treated with radical or modified mastectomy survive for at least five years. The results by axillary node status are shown in Table 60-1.

Modified Radical Mastectomy (Total Mastectomy and Axillary Dissection)

Modified radical mastectomy is presently the operation most widely used for carcinoma of the breast. This surgical procedure consists of removal of the entire breast and all or most of the axillary tissue but spares the pectoralis major muscle, thereby preventing deformity of the anterior chest wall and facilitating reconstruction of the breast should the patient desire it. The Patey version of the modified radical mastectomy entails removal of the entire axillary contents, including the pectoralis minor muscle; the Auchincloss version spares the pectoralis minor muscle while removing lymph nodes from the low and middle-axilla. The latter is frequently employed when limited involvement of axillary lymph nodes is suspected.

Total Mastectomy with Low Axillary Dissection

In total mastectomy with low axillary dissection, the surgeon removes the entire breast and all lymph nodes lateral to the pectoralis minor muscles (*i.e.,* the low axillary lymph nodes). Its major indication is noninvasive carcinoma of the breast, and it has the primary ob-

Table 60-3
*Prognosis for TNM Clinical Stages of Breast Carcinoma**

	TIS	I	II	IIIa	IIIb	IV
Total cases	43	287	388	61	51	38
5-Year survival	96%	72%	58%	49%	27%	4%
3-Year local/regional recurrence	0%	5%	9%	11%	25%	

* Medical College of Wisconsin, 1967–1979.

jective of removing all mammary parenchyma, including the axillary tail of Spence, and providing a limited sampling of axillary lymph nodes.

Extended Radical Mastectomy

Extended radical mastectomy adds en bloc removal of the internal mammary lymph nodes to the radical mastectomy. Although these lymph nodes contain metastases in approximately 25% of surgical cases, their removal is technically difficult and results are not significantly improved. In general, metastases at this site can be controlled equally well with irradiation.

Partial Mastectomy (Local Tumor Excision and Irradiation)

Surgical removal of less than the entire breast has obvious cosmetic advantages but relies on high-dose irradiation to control cancer in the remaining breast. This approach is an acceptable alternative to modified mastectomy for selected patients who are motivated to avoid mastectomy. The extent of surgical resection varies from lumpectomy (removal of only the tumor) to segmental resection (wide tumor removal with overlying skin) or quadrantectomy (removal of a quarter of the breast), all in conjunction with removal or sampling of axillary lymph nodes for staging purposes. This is followed by high doses of irradiation (5000–6000 rad) to the breast and residual lymph nodes. Patients with subareolar tumors, large tumors with respect to breast size, multiple tumor masses, or large pendulous breasts are not good candidates for this approach. Survival rates approximate those associated with mastectomy. Two controlled randomized studies have demonstrated the success of this approach. One in Milan, Italy, by Veronesi involved 701 women with small tumors (<2 cm) and a clinically negative axilla. In this study quadrantectomy of the breast with complete axillary dissection followed by irradiation confined to the breast produced survival and local–regional tumor control comparable to those of radical mastectomy after ten years of observation. Cosmetic results were good in 70% of cases. The second, by Fisher and co-workers, involved more than 1800 women with tumors up to 4 cm in diameter and clinically involved axillary nodes. Wide tumor and axillary dissection followed by irradiation to the breast produced five-year survival and local tumor control comparable to that of modified radical mastectomy. Complications relate to intensive irradiation and can include fibrosis and contraction of the breast, rib fractures, pleural effusions, and rarely pericarditis. The possibility of long-term carcinogenesis has not been excluded.

Irradiation

Irradiation to the breast and regional lymphatics provides the best method for local control of unresectable advanced breast cancers. When it is technically feasible, limited mastectomy to eliminate gross tumor seems to improve the chances for effective palliation.

Postoperative irradiation to the mastectomy site and the axillary, supraclavicular, and internal mammary lymph nodes is sometimes employed when metastases are found in the axillary lymph nodes removed with mastectomy, or when cancers are located medially in the breast. This supplemental treatment reduces the frequency of recurrence in the irradiated areas but does not improve the prospects for cure; its use is declining in favor of systemic adjuvant chemotherapy.

Preoperative irradiation to the breasts and regional lymph nodes is used for locally advanced tumors prior to mastectomy and has theoretic advantages over postoperative irradiation, but benefits in terms of improved cure are difficult to demonstrate.

Localized irradiation of painful bony metastases can relieve pain and promote osseous repair. It is often employed for this purpose in conjunction with other therapy in patients with disseminated cancer. Irradiation is the treatment of choice for isolated local or regional recurrence after mastectomy. Whole-brain irradiation is particularly useful for controlling symptomatic intracranial metastases.

Chemotherapy

Many cytotoxic agents provide effective palliation for breast cancer and are often used in three- to five-drug combinations. Adriamycin, cyclophosphamide (Cytoxan), methotrexate, and fluorouracil are the most successful. Systemic chemotherapy has two roles in management: (1) systemic adjuvant therapy, designed to improve the results of mastectomy, and (2) palliative treatment of advanced disease. Prolonged treatment with chemotherapy after mastectomy is justified when lymph nodes contain metastases, since these patients are at high risk for recurrence. Adjuvant chemotherapy results in definite prolongation of disease-free survival as well as reduction in local recurrence of tumor. The most impressive benefits are achieved with combinations of drugs and are seen in premenopausal women.

Systemic chemotherapy has a well-established place in the treatment of patients with disseminated breast cancers. In response to treatment, 40% to 60% of cancers regress, about 20% completely, and regressions are associated with extended survival. Chemotherapy is, in fact, the initial management of patients who are unlikely to respond to hormone or endocrine therapy, that is, those whose tumors contain no ER protein or those who have predominantly visceral metastases.

Endocrine and Hormone Therapy

Approximately one third of patients with disseminated breast cancer derive benefit from endocrine or hormone therapy, including oophorectomy, adrenalectomy, or hypophysectomy, or the administration of estrogens, androgens, progesterones, or antiestrogens. Knowledge of the ER content of the patient's tumor considerably improves selection for therapy. The presence of ER increases the likelihood of a beneficial response to greater than 60%. If ER is lacking, fewer than 10% will respond. It has therefore become routine to perform the assay on primary tumors in order to identify patients for adjuvant hormone therapy or to have this information in case inaccessible metastases appear later. Adjuvant therapy with the antiestrogen tamoxifen is now standard for postmenopausal women with involved axillary nodes and ER-positive tumors. In advanced cases, biopsy of primaries or metastases is performed not only for diagnosis but also to obtain tissue for assay.

BREAST CANCER DURING PREGNANCY

Special problems are posed when breast cancer occurs in conjunction with pregnancy. This subject is discussed on page 568.

REFERENCES AND RECOMMENDED READING

American Joint Committee for Cancer Staging and End-results Reporting: Manual for Staging of Cancer, pp 101–107. Chicago, Whiting Press, 1978

Anderson DE: A genetic study of human breast cancer. J Natl Cancer Inst 48:1029, 1974

Bandeian J, Horton CE, Rosato FE: Evaluation of patients after augmentation mammoplasty. Surg Gynecol Obstet 147:596, 1978

Bassett LW, Gold RH, Cove HC: Mammographic spectrum of traumatic fat necrosis: The fallibility of "pathognomonic" signs of carcinoma. AJR 130:119, 1978

Bedwinek JM, Perez CA, Kramer S et al: Irradiation as the primary management of stage I and II adenocarcinoma of the breast. Cancer Clinical Trials 3:11, 1980

Best JJK, Asbury DL, George WD et al: Computed tomography (CT) of the breast. Clin Oncol 3, No. 4:394, 1977

Breslow L, Thomas LB, Upton AC: Final reports of the National Cancer Institute ad hoc working groups on mammography in screening for breast cancer and a summary report of their joint findings and recommendations. J Natl Cancer Inst 59, No. 2:468, 1977

British Breast Group: Steroid-receptor assays in human breast cancer: A statement by the British Breast Group and colleagues. Lancet 1:298, 1980

Brownstein MH, Wolf M, Bikowski JB: Cowden's disease: A cutaneous marker of breast cancer. Cancer 41:2393, 1978

Byrd BF Jr, Bayer DS, Robertson JC et al: Treatment of breast tumors associated with pregnancy and lactation. Ann Surg 155:940, 1962

Centers for Disease Control: Cancer and Steroid Hormone Study: Long-term oral contraceptive use. JAMA 249, No. 12:1591, 1983

Coombs LJ, Lilienfield AM, Bross IDJ et al: A prospective study of the relationship between benign breast diseases and breast carcinoma. Prev Med 8:40, 1979

Degenshein GA, Ceccarelli F, Bloom ND et al: Hormone relationships in breast cancer: The role of receptor-binding proteins. In Ravitch MM (ed): Current Problems in Surgery, vol 16, No. 6, pp 1–59. Chicago, Year Book Medical Publishers, 1979

Donegan WL: Breast cancer and pregnancy. Obstet Gynecol 59, No. 2:244, 1977

Farewell VT, Math B, Math M: The combined effect of breast cancer risk factors. Cancer 40:931, 1977

Fisher B, Bauer M, Margolese R et al: Five-year results of a randomized clinical trial comparing mastectomy with or without radiation in the treatment of breast cancer. N Engl J Med 312:665, 1985

Fisher B, Slack N, Katrych D et al: Ten-year follow-up results of patients with carcinoma of the breast in a cooperative clinical trial evaluating surgical adjuvant chemotherapy. Surg Gynecol Obstet 140:528, 1975

Gambrell RD, Maier RC, Sanders BI: Decreased incidence of breast cancer in postmenopausal estrogen-progestogen users. Obstet Gynecol 62, No. 4:435, 1983

Gapinski PV, Donegan WL: Estrogen receptors and breast cancer: Prognostic and therapeutic implications. Surgery 88:386, 1980

Golinger RC: Hormones and the pathophysiology of fibrocystic mastopathy. Surg Gynecol Obstet 146:273, 1978

Gray LA Sr: Breast pain: Causes, workup, and treatment. Consultant, 1976

Harmer MH (ed): TNM Classification of Malignant Tumors, 3rd ed, pp 47–56. Geneva, International Union Against Cancer, 1978

Harris JR, Levene MB, Hellman S: Results of treating stage I and II carcinoma of the breast with primary irradiation therapy. Cancer Treat Rep 62:985, 1978

Hoover R, Gray LA Sr, Cole P et al: Menopausal estrogens and breast cancer. N Engl J Med 295, No. 8:401, 1976

Hubay CA, Barry FM, Marr CC: Pregnancy and breast cancer. Surg Clin North Am 58, No. 4:819, 1978

Leavitt T Jr: The role of the obstetrician-gynecologist in the diagnosis and treatment of breast cancer. Breast 4, No. 3:19, 1978

Leis HP Jr: The diagnosis of breast cancer. CA 27, No. 4:209, 1977

Lipsett MB: Estrogen use and cancer risk. JAMA 237, No. 11:1112, 1977

Lipsett MB: Postoperative radiation for women with cancer of the breast and positive axillary nodes: Should it continue? N Engl J Med 304:112, 1981

Margolese RG: Current concepts in the management of primary breast cancer. Can J Surg 20, No. 3:199, 1977

Minton JP, Foecking MK, Webster DJT et al: Caffeine, cyclic nucleotides, and breast disease. Surgery 86, No. 1:105, 1979

Nemoto T: Changing treatment for breast cancer: A survey of surgeons. Breast 4, No. 1:16, 1978

Perry S: Recommendations of the Consensus Development Panel on Breast Cancer Screening. Cancer Res 38:476, 1978

Peters TG, Donegan WL, Burg EA: Minimal breast cancer: A clinical appraisal. Ann Surg 186, 6:704, 1977

Prosnitz LR, Goldenberg IS, Harris JR et al: Radiotherapy for carcinoma of the breast instead of mastectomy: An update. Front Radiat Ther Oncol 17:69, 1983

Rosemond GP, Maier WP, Brobyn TJ: Needle aspiration of breast cysts. Surg Gynecol Obstet 128:351, 1969

Sitruk–Ware R, Sterkers N, Mauvaris–Jarvis P: Benign breast disease: I. Hormonal investigation. Obstet Gynecol 53:457, 1979

Urban JA, Egeli RA: Non-lactational nipple discharge. CA 28, No. 3:130, 1978

Veronesi U: Quadrantectomy for carcinoma of the breast. Surg Rounds, Sept, 1984.

Wolfe JN: Breast patterns as an index of risk for developing breast cancer. AJR 126:1130, 1976

Imaging in Gynecology

Bruce D. Doust
Nita J. Durham

61

PLAIN ROENTGENOGRAPHY

Abdomen

In gynecology, the most important contribution of plain roentgenography of the abdomen is the incidental identification of pelvic masses in the course of investigation of other abnormalities. For example, uterine myomas are often detected for the first time during an intravenous urogram (Fig. 61-1). The myoma may indent the superior aspect of the contrast-filled bladder and may contain calcification, which is characteristically coarse and patchy.

A pelvic mass may also displace gas-filled bowel loops out of the pelvis and obstruct the ureters to produce hydronephrosis.

Certain conditions demonstrate characteristic calcification that may be diagnostic on plain radiographs. In addition to the coarse, patchy calcification of uterine myomas noted above, cystadenocarcinomas of the ovary may contain fine, granular calcification, which may also be seen in their omental, peritoneal, and liver metastases. Tuberculous pyosalpinx may contain amorphous calcification. Rarely, pseudomyxoma peritonei produces ringlike intra-abdominal calcification.

The identification of teeth or tooth remnants, possibly with associated areas of diminished radiographic density due to fat, is strongly suggestive of dermoid (ovarian teratoma) (Fig. 61-2).

Ultrasound (which is considered in Chap. 15) is much more sensitive in detecting small amounts of ascites, especially in the pelvis and around the liver, than are plain films. Large amounts of ascitic fluid cause bulging of the flanks, medial displacement of the ascending and descending colon from the fat stripes lying immediately outside the peritoneum, and loss of the outlines of intra-abdominal structures such as kidneys, psoas muscles, and liver. A large cystic ovarian tumor, which may be difficult to distinguish from ascites clinically, displaces bowel loops cranially rather than medially and because of its anterior intraperitoneal position does not obscure the renal and psoas outlines.

Bony metastases involving the lumbar spine and pelvis may be detected on plain abdominal radiographs. Most bony metastases, especially in women, are osteolytic; that is, they cause bone destruction only. Sclerotic metastases, most commonly from carcinoma of the breast and bladder, are occasionally seen. Radionuclide bone scanning is a much more sensitive means of detecting metastases than plain radiography of the bony skeleton.

Plain radiographs of the abdomen are sometimes requested to aid in localization of an intrauterine device (IUD). Ultrasound is more useful in determining whether the IUD is in the uterine cavity. If the IUD is not detected within the uterus on ultrasound examination and the patient is not pregnant, a plain film is a useful next step, since an IUD lying outside the uterus may be difficult to identify ultrasonically.

Chest

In the investigation of gynecologic disease, chest radiographs are usually obtained to exclude pulmonary metastases, particularly in cases of ovarian carcinoma, uterine carcinoma, and choriocarcinoma. Pleural effusions may be detected, for example, in association with ovarian fibromas (Meigs' syndrome).

Skull

In gynecologic practice, plain radiographs of the skull are usually obtained to demonstrate osseous metastases or to demonstrate the pituitary fossa as part of the in-

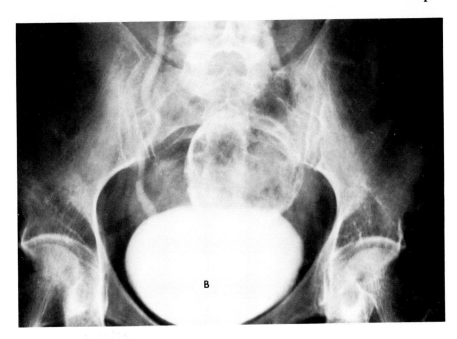

FIG. 61-1. Anteroposterior film of the pelvis taken as part of intravenous pyelography shows uterine myoma. The bladder (*B*) and right ureter are opacified. A large, rounded, calcified myoma is immediately cranial to the bladder.

FIG. 61-2. Anteroposterior film of the pelvis shows soft tissue mass in the left side of the pelvis, partly outlined by arrows. Within this mass are two well-formed teeth, making the diagnosis of ovarian dermoid virtually certain.

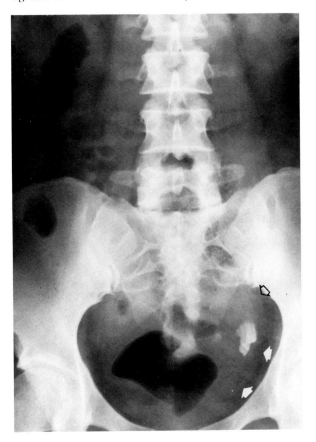

vestigation of infertility. Infertility may be secondary to pituitary or suprasellar tumors, which may expand the bony pituitary fossa and erode the dorsum sellae.

However, pituitary microadenomas, which may secrete prolactin and cause galactorrhea, often do not cause enlargement of the pituitary fossa. Computed tomography (CT) of the pituitary fossa is much more useful in these cases, since it can demonstrate the pituitary gland and small defects within it, as well as large pituitary tumors.

Where microadenoma is the most probable diagnosis, it is worth considering whether a CT scan would change patient management. In many cases, bromocriptine is tried regardless of the results of the CT scan.

Intravenous Urography

In intravenous urography, the kidneys, pelvicaliceal systems, ureters, and bladder are opacified by the excretion of an intravenously administered, iodine-containing, water-soluble contrast material. This widely used examination depends for its success on adequate renal function, that is, on the kidneys' ability to concentrate the contrast agent. In general, it is not worth attempting intravenous urography if the patient's blood urea nitrogen (BUN) is in excess of 10 mg/dl.

Intravenous urography is associated with low mortality (about 1 death in every 20,000 examinations) and significant morbidity. About 1 patient in 500 suffers a serious, nonfatal reaction to the injected contrast agent. Pretesting with a small dose of contrast agent is not helpful in preventing fatal reactions.

The indications for intravenous urography in gynecologic diseases are the following:

The demonstration of distortion, deviation, or obstruction of the ureters by pelvic masses

The demonstration of associated hydronephrosis

Preoperative evaluation of the urinary tract, including the position of the ureters, possible duplex ureters, pelvic kidney, and the separate evaluation of the functional status of each kidney

The demonstration of complications of hysterectomy, including partial or complete ureteric occlusion by a suture, division of a ureter, vesicovaginal fistula, and hematoma or lymphocele

Cystography

A water-soluble contrast medium is introduced into the bladder by means of a catheter inserted through the urethra. Cystography may be used, in association with urodynamic studies that determine flow during voiding, to investigate stress incontinence. It may also be used to demonstrate vesicoureteric reflux and vesicovaginal fistula.

Barium Enema

A barium enema is performed by introducing a tube into the rectum and allowing an aqueous suspension of barium sulfate, followed by air, to flow around the large bowel until it fills the appendix or refluxes into the terminal ileum. The barium sulfate suspension coats the mucosa while the air distends the bowel. Mucosal detail stands out with great clarity. Thorough cleansing of the colon with purgatives and low-residue diet prior to the study is essential. This preparation can be very unpleasant, especially for fragile, elderly patients. Nonetheless, the barium enema is a very safe examination and was once the best initial investigation for the detection of colonic lesions proximal to the rectum, although endoscopic visualization of the colon using fiberoptic sigmoidoscopy and colonoscopy has now become the initial form of investigation in many centers.

In gynecologic diagnosis, barium enema examinations are valuable in demonstrating displacement of the rectosigmoid colon by an extrinsic mass and involvement of the colon by endometriosis or gynecologic cancer, and in determining the origin of a pelvic mass (colonic rather than gynecologic). Complications of treatment, such as irradiation colitis and rectovaginal fistulas, may also be demonstrated.

Hysterosalpingography

In hysterosalpingography a radiopaque contrast agent is instilled through the cervix. It fills the cervical canal and body of the uterus and then flows on, through the fallopian tubes, to spill into the peritoneal cavity (Fig. 61-3).

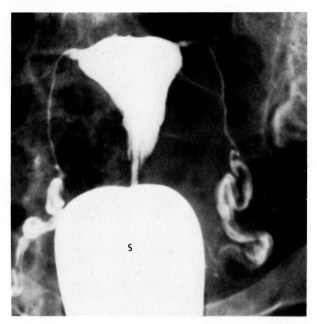

FIG. 61-3. Hysterosalpingogram shows normal uterus and tubes. The uterine cavity is of normal shape. The fundus extends slightly cranial to a line joining the fallopian tubes. The fallopian tubes are patent, and spillage of contrast agent into the peritoneal cavity can be seen bilaterally. A metal speculum (S) has been used. A plastic speculum is more satisfactory because it does not block the x-ray beam.

Indications

Indications for hysterosalpingography include the following:

Investigation of infertility, to determine whether the infertility is caused by an anatomic, surgically remediable defect such as tubal occlusion

Recurrent abortion, to demonstrate congenital uterine anomalies or cervical incompetence

Confirmation of interruption of fallopian tubes in elective sterilization

Contraindications

Contraindications to hysterosalpingography include the following:

Acute or simmering pelvic inflammatory disease
Severe renal or cardiac disease
Sensitivity to contrast media
Recent dilatation and curettage
Pregnancy
The week before menstruation

In recent times, laparoscopic evaluation of the fallopian tubes has replaced hysterosalpingography to some extent. Laparoscopy appears to be superior in the evaluation of peritubal adhesions.

Technique

The examination should be performed on a fluoroscopy table equipped with a spot-film device. The cannula, which should have a soft rubber tip, and the syringe should be entirely filled with contrast medium, since air bubbles can cause difficulty in interpretation. Water-soluble medium is preferred to oily medium because it is safer if extravasation into the uterine vasculature occurs.

The cannula is inserted into the cervical os through a plastic speculum. Contrast is then injected slowly and gently under fluoroscopic control. Usually 5 ml to 6 ml is required.

Spot films should be taken during the filling phase to demonstrate the cervix and uterus. Once the uterus and fallopian tubes have been filled, anteroposterior (AP) and both oblique films should be taken.

Failure of the fallopian tubes to fill immediately may be due to spasm. Antispasmodics are useful in distinguishing between spasm and true obstruction. After approximately 30 minutes another AP film should be taken to distinguish between intraperitoneal (spilled) contrast and contrast in the distal portion of an obstructed fallopian tube, conditions that may appear similar early in the examination.

Interpretation

In patients with an incompetent cervix, the cervical canal may appear widened. Abnormalities of uterine position, including retroversion and lateral deviation, can be readily diagnosed. It is important to distinguish between a laterally deviated uterus and the single horn of a bicornuate uterus. The latter is generally smaller and more markedly deviated from the midline.

Arcuate and bicornuate uteri are manifestations of differing degrees of failure of the two müllerian systems to fuse. The fundus of the normal uterine cavity is convex or only slightly concave. In an arcuate uterus, the fundus is indented caudally more than 1 cm. A bicornuate uterus represents a more severe failure of fusion. In a bicornuate uterus, indentation is deep and the angulation between the cornua wide. Each horn is fusiform and convex on its lateral aspect. (The lateral aspect of a normal uterus is slightly concave.)

Filling defects (such as polyps and subserous myomas) may also be identified. These must be differentiated from air bubbles.

Adenomyosis or endometriosis may produce small diverticular out-pouchings along the borders of the uterine cavity and the fallopian tubes, occlusion or narrowing of the fallopian tubes, or generalized thickening of the uterine wall.

The presence of intrauterine adhesions, caused by trauma such as repeated curettage, is known as the *Asherman syndrome.* It is characterized roentgenographically by irregular intrauterine filling defects that are not obliterated by increased amounts of contrast agent.

Abnormalities of the fallopian tubes are probably better examined by hysterosalpingography than by any other method. Tubal patency is proven if contrast agent spills into the peritoneal cavity. Absence of spill can be due to incomplete filling of the tubes as well as to tubal occlusion; thus, a special effort should be made to fill the tubes during injection and to document on film the extent of filling achieved during injection.

If the tubes appear occluded, a repeat examination performed after an antispasmodic has been given is advisable to eliminate tubal spasm as the cause (Fig. 61-4).

Pyosalpinx is readily diagnosed by hysterosalpingography and is commonly associated with tubal obstruction. The tube enlarges and becomes irregular in caliber. Dilatation may be generalized or localized principally to one section of the tube. Hysterosalpingography should not be performed in the presence of pelvic infection.

Lymphangiography

Bipedal lymphangiography is the only direct radiologic method of visualizing the lymphatic vessels and nodes of the pelvic and para-aortic region. It is therefore useful in detecting metastatic spread from carcinoma involving the genital tract. (It is also widely used to demonstrate other diseases involving primarily the lymph nodes, *e.g.,* lymphoma.)

Technique

Lymphangiography is a lengthy procedure. The time required varies widely, depending heavily on the experience of the operator, but is usually between one and two hours. The patient must be able to remain still for a prolonged period; there is no point in attempting the study on a disturbed or uncooperative patient.

A blue dye is injected subcutaneously into the web spaces between the toes of both feet. This dye is taken up by the lymphatic vessels and makes them visible through the skin.

A suitable lymphatic vessel is selected and a small incision made. The lymphatic is isolated, and a specially designed small needle (about 28 gauge) is introduced and tied into place.

Oily contrast medium (iodized poppy seed oil) is injected slowly; up to 8 ml of contrast is required on each side.

Films of the leg are taken during injection. At the end of the injection, AP, lateral, and oblique views of the abdomen and pelvis are taken. More films are taken 24 hours later, when glandular filling is more complete.

The contrast material passes through the lymphatics of the leg to the external iliac, common iliac, and para-aortic nodes. It then passes through the cisterna chyli and the thoracic duct to drain into the venous system, usually through the left brachiocephalic vein. Thus, oily

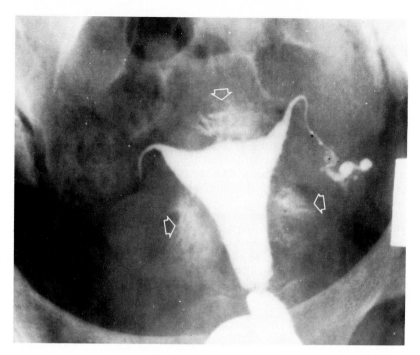

FIG. 61-4. Hysterosalpingogram shows tubal obstruction and extravasation of contrast agent into the myometrium. Intramural contrast is present bilaterally and in the fundus (*arrows*). The left fallopian tube is almost completely filled. The right tube is filled only in its juxtauterine part. Subsequent films showed no further filling of tubes and no evidence of spillage of contrast into the peritoneal cavity.

contrast that is not taken up by the lymph nodes eventually enters the pulmonary capillary bed as myriad minute oil emboli.

Bipedal lymphangiography opacifies only the lymph nodes in the inguinal, external, and common iliac chains and the paracaval and para-aortic nodes. Internal iliac, hypogastric, and presacral nodes are not opacified, nor are mesenteric nodes nor nodes in the porta hepatis.

Thus, many of the nodes commonly involved by metastatic pelvic malignancies are not opacified.

Contraindications

Contraindications to lymphangiography include the following:

Sensitivity to iodine
A definite history of allergy
Severe pulmonary disease (Embolization of oily contrast medium into the lungs always occurs. When the pulmonary capillary bed is severely compromised by preexisting pulmonary disease, the oil emboli may produce a critical fall in pulmonary perfusion.)

Interpretation

The normal lymph node is oval and regular in outline, with a granular mottled appearance (Fig. 61-5). Filling defects often occur normally, especially in the inguinal nodes, where they are thought to represent the residua of previous infection in the feet and legs. Abnormal findings include the following:

FIG. 61-5. Lymphangiogram shows normal node chains—AP film taken 24 hours after injection of contrast into lymphatics of both feet. Lymph node chains are symmetric. Para-aortic node chains have filled up to the level of L1. Minor irregularities of nodes of both external iliac chains are within normal limits.

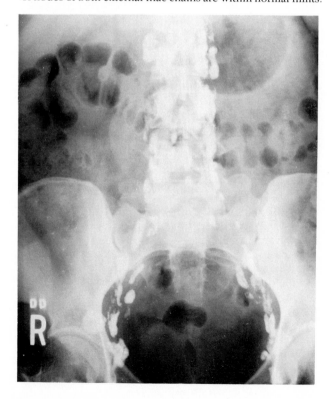

Filling defects. Defects due to metastases usually have sharply defined margins. They may be peripheral or central. Except in the inguinal region, these pathologic filling defects can usually be distinguished from normally occurring filling defects (Fig. 61-6).

Diffuse enlargement of nodes, a change usually seen in lymphoma

Abnormal texture of nodes. Lymphomatous nodes often have a typical "soap-bubble" appearance.

Obstruction of lymphatics by tumor, resulting in
  Failure to fill whole areas of the lymphatic system
  Filling of collateral channels
  Lymphaticovenous communication

FIG. 61-6. Lymphangiogram shows lymphatic spread of carcinoma of the uterus—oblique film taken 24 hours after injection. Note large, sharply marginated filling defect in left external iliac node (*thin black arrow*). Almost no filling of the left common iliac chain has occurred, suggesting extensive involvement by metastatic malignancy. Contrast agent can be seen in the right common iliac lymphatic vessels (*open arrow*). This is abnormal in a 24-hour film and suggests obstruction by metastatic involvement.

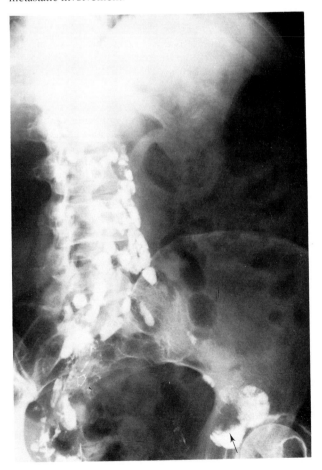

Computed Tomography Versus Lymphangiography in the Demonstration of Metastatic Spread

CT demonstrates the full extent of the neoplastic disease; that is, it demonstrates the entirety of lymph node masses, including nodes in those areas inaccessible to lymphangiography. It also demonstrates extranodal sites of disease, such as liver metastases.

CT is relatively noninvasive and requires less operator expertise than lymphangiography because lymphatic cannulation is not required.

On the other hand, CT cannot detect metastases in normal-sized nodes. Nodes must be enlarged to be recognized as abnormal. Thus, CT examination may produce false-negative results, especially in carcinomas of the female genital tract, where metastases are often found in normal-sized nodes.

Because CT cannot demonstrate the internal architecture of nodes, false-positive results may be produced when nodes are enlarged by benign conditions such as lymphoid hyperplasia, conditions that can be recognized by lymphangiography.

In summary, CT is more sensitive but less specific than lymphangiography. Therefore, pelvic malignancies are best evaluated by performance of a CT scan initially to assess the extent of local and metastatic disease. If the CT scan fails to show lymph node involvement *and* the presence of lymph node metastases would significantly change the patient's management, lymphangiography should be performed.

COMPUTED TOMOGRAPHY

CT is a radiographic technique of obtaining cross-sectional images of the body. CT images have proven to be valuable, principally because they enhance the slight differences in the densities of adjacent tissues to produce a clear demonstration of cross-sectional anatomy. A detailed description of the technology of CT is beyond the scope of this chapter; however, a brief outline of principles is appropriate.

An x-ray tube and an array of electronic detectors are mounted on opposite sides of a circular gantry in which the patient lies. Both the x-ray tube and the detectors travel in a circle around the patient while numerous x-ray exposures are made. As a result, a series of density readings taken from innumerable angles are obtained. All of the electronic signals generated by these multiple x-ray exposures, together with signals representing the position of the gantry at the time of each exposure, are stored in a computed memory.

This colossal mass of raw electronic data is then processed mathematically, or *reconstructed*. The object of the processing is to determine the attenuation coefficient of each tissue element in the body section under examination and to display this data as a useful image.

Reconstruction is possible because every structure in the slice of tissue is evaluated from many angles as the gantry rotates; thus, each tissue element makes a contribution to numerous detector readings.

Calculations are also required to allow for overlapping and incomplete sampling of tissue elements, to locate each element in its proper position in the image, to compensate for unevenness of x-ray output and instability in the x-ray detectors, to improve resolution, to eliminate artifacts, and so forth. Programs of mathematic manipulation, called *algorithms,* that are used to accomplish all of these operations have been the subject of intense research by the manufacturers of CT equipment, and striking improvements in image quality and speed of reconstruction have been achieved by refinement of the algorithms. The latest CT scanners can complete the radiographic exposure in less than 5 seconds, although longer exposures are also used in some circumstances. The calculations take between 5 and 45 seconds to complete.

The principal advantages of CT over other forms of radiographic examinations are the following:

Apart from the administration of contrast agents, the procedure is noninvasive

Much anatomic detail can be demonstrated, even without the use of contrast agents. The intrinsic differences in radiographic density between fat and other body tissues are enough to allow clear demonstration of most structures. (In patients who have little body fat [*e.g.,* neonates] CT images are less satisfactory.) Intravenous administration of a contrast agent allows vessels to be positively identified and tumor vascularity to be assessed. Orally and occasionally rectally administered contrast medium aids in distinguishing bowel from other pelvic organs. In some examinations, particularly those of the pelvis, the patient receives contrast by all three of the above routes.

The display is in the form of a cross-section through the body, a format that shows anatomic relationships that might otherwise be obscured.

The contrast and the density of the image can be manipulated after the examination has been completed to maximize the diagnostic value of the images without further irradiation of the patient.

The radiographic density of organs or masses can be estimated. These density values, called *attenuation coefficients,* are sometimes helpful in determining the nature of the structure being examined. However, dissimilar pathologic processes may have very similar density values.

The examination is unaffected by bowel gas, colostomies, and surgical dressings; however, metallic clips do cause troublesome artifacts.

Computed Radiographs

In addition to producing cross-sectional images, modern CT scanners produce pictures that resemble conventional radiographs. At present, computed radiographs are generally inferior to those produced conventionally because they have a lower spatial resolution. They are valuable for determining and recording the levels at which CT sections should be performed to ensure a complete examination of an organ or region and thus allow extremely accurate planning and rapid performance of each CT study.

Applications of Computed Tomography in Gynecologic Diagnosis

CT is primarily useful to the gynecologist for demonstrating the nature and extent of pelvic masses; examining the pelvic and para-aortic lymph node chains as part of the examination for metastatic deposits from gynecologic cancer; and examining liver, lungs, and brain for metastases.

Pelvic Masses

CT allows demonstration of the mass itself; the relationship of the mass to loops of bowel, the bladder, and the ureters; and the extent of tumor invasion of the pelvic side wall and the fascial planes around the rectum (Fig. 61-7). It does not demonstrate mucosal involvement of the bowel as well or as inexpensively as the barium enema examination, and it appears inferior to ultrasound in the delineation of normal ovaries and small ovarian cysts and the characterization of internal uterine architecture. It is the best method available for demonstrating soft tissue infiltration, lymphadenopathy, and areas of tumor necrosis (Figs. 61-8, and 61-9). It is

FIG. 61-7. CT demonstrating a large, multiloculated soft tissue mass containing extensive linear calcification (*arrowhead*), displacing bowel to the left. There are soft tissue strands of tumor (*arrow*), also partially calcified, extending posteriorly to invade the pararectal areas bilaterally. The dense material anteriorly is contrast agent in loops of bowel. The calcification is of much finer texture than the opacified bowel loops, and confusion between the two is therefore unlikely.

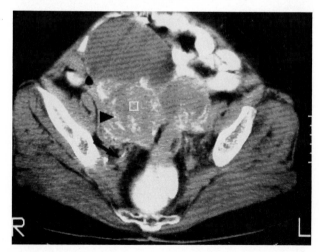

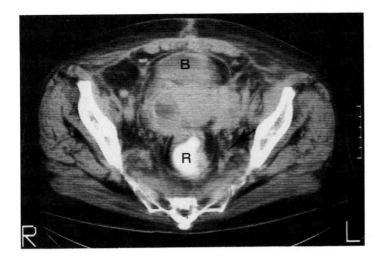

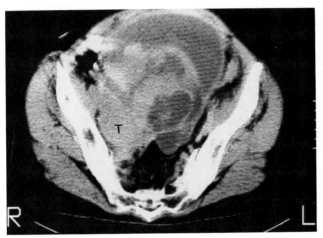

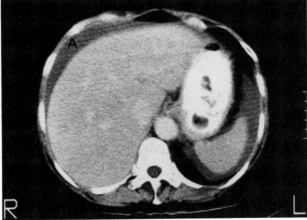

FIG. 61-8. Carcinoma of the ovary demonstrating necrosis and spread to pelvic lymph nodes. This CT slice was taken through the midpelvis. It shows an irregular soft tissue mass situated between the bladder (*B*) and rectum (*R*). The low-density areas in the right side of the mass indicate necrosis. Adjacent to and behind the left side of the mass are several smaller soft tissue masses (*arrow*), which are probably enlarged pelvic lymph nodes.

FIG. 61-9. (*Left*) CT demonstrating pseudomucinous cystadenocarcinoma of the ovary. This slice, taken through the pelvis, shows a large, multiloculated mass, with thick, irregular septa. The septa appear light, the enclosed fluid dark. Note extension of the tumor (*T*) to the right pelvic side wall with loss of the normal fat planes, indicating local invasion. (*Right*) Ascites in pseudomucinous cystadenocarcinoma of the ovary. The ascitic fluid (*A*), which has an attenuation coefficient between that of fat and liver, can be seen around the liver and spleen. The liver is normal, with no evidence of metastases. The presence of ascites suggests peritoneal involvement by the tumor. Peritoneal seeding is only occasionally visible on CT images.

probably less sensitive than the radionuclide bone scan in the detection of early bone involvement. It seems to be particularly valuable in demonstrating invasion of the tissue planes around the urinary bladder by bladder or uterine cancer and in evaluating tumor response to therapy, and it is unique in its ability to delineate tumors that have spread through the sciatic notches to the gluteal region.

Detection of Lymph Node Metastases

CT has proven useful in demonstrating the internal iliac lymph node chain, the para-aortic nodes of the upper abdomen (Fig. 61-10), including those above the cisterna chyli, the retrocrural nodes, the mesenteric nodes, and the nodes of the pelvic side wall, areas that are not usually opacified by lymphangiography. CT can also show omental involvement (Fig. 61-11). It demonstrates lymph node enlargement without the need for added contrast. Unfortunately, metastases that do not enlarge the lymph nodes are undetectable by CT.

Detection of Metastases Elsewhere in the Body

The radiographic density of metastases is often different from that of the normal tissue that surrounds them, and this difference frequently can be enhanced by an intravenous injection of contrast agent. In the case of

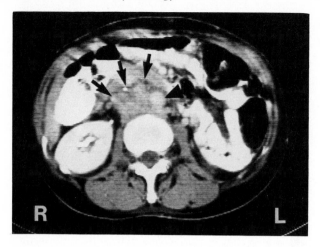

FIG. 61-10. CT demonstrates retroperitoneal nodes secondary to carcinoma of the ovary. There is a lobulated soft tissue mass (*arrows*), consistent with enlarged lymph nodes, adjacent to the right side of the aorta (*arrowhead*). The aorta has been displaced anteriorly, and the inferior vena cava has been obscured completely by the mass of lymph nodes. Opacification of vessels by intravenous contrast and of bowel by oral contrast is necessary for accurate delineation of mass lesions in the abdomen.

liver metastases, intravenous contrast usually increases the radiographic density of the normal parenchyma; thus, the normal tissue becomes more dense than the metastases. Rarely, dense metastases are obscured by the administration of intravenous contrast.

Hepatic metastases are probably better demonstrated by CT than by any other method; its overall accuracy is about 92%. Radionuclide scans and ultrasound are the only other atraumatic methods, but overall both appear to be less sensitive.

CT is the best means of seeking cerebral metastases. Pulmonary metastases may be resected if it is probable that all of them can be removed and there are no other deposits. Customarily, the patient is examined initially by means of plain films and conventional laminograms because these methods of examination are less expensive; if no lesions that would make resection impractical are demonstrated, CT is used as a final check. CT is particularly useful in identifying subpleural metastases. CT also provides the only noninvasive means of demonstrating the mediastinum.

Computed Tomography in Radiation Therapy Planning

CT has made significant changes in the techniques for planning radiation therapy fields. For instance, in lung cancer, a CT scan provides information that significantly modifies the radiation fields in about 30% of patients,

principally by demonstrating previously unsuspected abnormal tissue outside the radiation fields. CT also provides precise definition of body contours and chest wall thickness. Additionally, it allows measurement of the absorption coefficient of the various tissues in the fields to be irradiated, and this information allows accurate computation of depth doses. Furthermore, CT provides localization of vulnerable structures, such as the kidneys and spinal cord, allowing accurate placement of shields over these organs.

The clinician should be aware of the following special requirements for the performance of good radiation therapy–planning scans:

The patient should be scanned in precisely the position in which she will be irradiated. Minor changes, such as in arm position, may render the field outlines marked on the skin inaccurate.

The scanner couch should be of the same shape as the couch of the therapy machine (generally flat).

Computed radiographs documenting the precise level at which each slice was taken are very important, especially where the overall cross-sectional shape of the body changes suddenly, as at the cervicothoracic junction.

The clinician should make it clear to the radiologist beforehand whether the study is purely diagnostic, primarily a diagnostic study from which therapy-planning information will be derived incidentally, or purely a therapy-planning study, since there are significant differences in the way these studies are performed.

FIG. 61-11. CT demonstrates omental cake, secondary to carcinoma of the ovary. There is an extensive sheet of soft tissue of mottled density (*O*) situated immediately behind the anterior abdominal wall and lying in front of the opacified loops of bowel. This sheet represents a mass of omentum thickened by metastatic deposits and is a manifestation of transperitoneal spread of ovarian carcinoma.

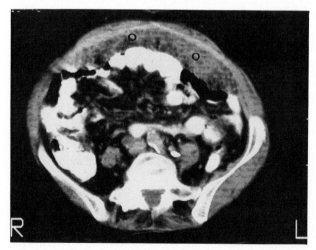

The Relative Roles of Computed Tomography, Ultrasound, and Radionuclide Imaging in the Management of Gynecologic Disease

The following comments are offered to assist referring clinicians in minimizing cost and delay in the use of the three most widely used high-technology imaging techniques. It is rare that any imaging technique can provide an exact diagnosis of the nature of a tumor. There are a few exceptions, such as dermoid, but a clinician who expects a histologically certain diagnosis from an imaging procedure will often be disappointed and sometimes frankly misled.

Ultrasonic imaging, which is discussed in Chapter 15, should be used when there is a realistic chance that the patient is pregnant and when fluid-filled structures such as ovarian tumors, ascites, or hydronephrosis are being sought. When the patient is thin, ultrasound is preferred over CT, since absence of body fat improves ultrasonic images but obscures outlines on CT. The pelvis is particularly suitable for ultrasonic examination. Nonetheless, the appearances of many pelvic abnormalities overlap, and a specific histologic diagnosis generally is not possible. Ultrasound should be avoided when the patient is obese, when solid lesions that are likely to have poorly defined margins (such as many liver metastases) are being sought, when much bowel gas is present, and when a skilled ultrasonologist is not available.

Radionuclide scans are an effective initial means of screening the liver for focal defects but give nonspecific images and are incapable of providing an overall view of the abdominal contents. Even in the liver, they are slightly less accurate than CT and considerably less specific but also much less expensive. The degree of obesity is not of great importance. If the patient is unable to lie still for several minutes at a time, neither CT nor radionuclide studies are likely to give much useful information.

Expense makes *CT* less desirable as an initial examination, but it is useful when a high-quality image of the entire abdominal or pelvic contents is desired. Loops of unopacified bowel are a common source of confusion in CT studies, since they may be misidentified as mesenteric or retroperitoneal lymphadenopathy. The administration of large amounts of a dilute contrast agent solution to opacify the bowel minimizes this problem. If a patient cannot take the oral contrast agent, the diagnostic value of a CT examination of the abdomen is considerably lessened. CT appears superior to ultrasound in outlining the lymph nodes of the pelvic side wall and in detecting infiltration of the pelvic fat planes by malignancy.

Evaluation of the Response to Therapy

Because tumors vary widely in their sensitivity to chemotherapeutic agents and the side-effects of these drugs are commonly unpleasant, it is desirable to determine objectively that a tumor is indeed responding to chemotherapy or radiation. Many gynecologic tumors produce macroscopically demonstrable masses, hydronephrosis, or ascites, and in these cases it is convenient to follow their progress by means of CT or ultrasound.

Because ultrasound examinations are less expensive than CT and it is often difficult to predict which of the two modalities will be the more useful, it has been our practice to perform a baseline ultrasound study before commencing a course of radiation or chemotherapy. If the ultrasound examination fails to show a readily measurable mass, a CT scan is performed.

It is desirable, when assessing the pelvis by any imaging method, to know in advance whether the patient has undergone a hysterectomy. Masses of recurrent tumor might otherwise be mistaken for a normal uterus.

Unless they are associated with ascites, peritoneal seedings are rarely recognizable by means of ultrasound or CT. CT is, however, capable of demonstrating omental involvement due to transperitoneal spread of malignancy (Fig. 61-11).

Unless there is reason to believe that a tumor has involved the liver or the bones, radionuclide studies are rarely useful in following gynecologic malignancy.

ANGIOGRAPHY

Diagnostic

Arteriography is used in gynecology to demonstrate the blood supply to a pelvic mass as an aid in planning the surgical approach to the lesion. It may also be used to assess the spread of vascular malignancies to the pelvic wall and to demonstrate vascular metastases to the liver. Avascular metastases, even if large, may produce little change in the hepatic arteriogram, and generally CT is preferred.

Therapeutic

When a patient is bleeding intractably from a pelvic malignancy, arteriography may be used to determine the site of bleeding. The arteries supplying the bleeding area can then be selectively catheterized and small pieces of solid material injected through the catheter until the artery is obstructed and the bleeding stopped. Gelfoam, Ivalon, and small spiral fragments of stainless steel wire to which fibers have been attached (to promote thrombosis) have been described as embolizing agents.

This technique can also be used to infarct inoperable tumors or to reduce tumor vascularity prior to surgical resection. Embolization of the hepatic artery offers improved survival in patients with inoperable hepatic metastases, particularly in those with carcinoid deposits. In other tumors, the improvement is statistically significant but of small extent, providing an increase in survival of a few months.

Infusion of chemotherapeutic agents intra-arterially is designed to improve the therapeutic efficiency of these toxic drugs; however, the place of this technique has not been fully determined. Some agents are just as effective when administered intravenously, while others seem to be more effective when administered intra-arterially, as close to the tumor as possible. Intra-arterial infusion requires that the tip of the catheter be positioned so that toxic agents are not infused into vulnerable organs.

Catheter positioning is sometimes difficult. The catheter is usually inserted through the axillary or femoral arteries and remains in place throughout the course of therapy, sometimes for weeks. During this time, the arterial puncture site is kept carefully dressed, and the patient is allowed to move about more or less normally. Some debilitated patients have difficulty maintaining cleanliness of a femoral entry site, and for this reason some angiographers prefer the axillary approach, although it is often more difficult technically.

Several variations on this technique have been described, including the following:

Prior occlusion of all alternative arterial blood supplies to the tumor-containing organ so that the agent infused through the one remaining artery of supply reaches the whole tumor

Open operation to insert a catheter and an implantable slow-infusion reservoir. The reservoir is placed beneath the skin of the anterior abdominal wall and is filled by injection of the drug through a rubber window lying beneath the skin. This technique avoids the problem of sepsis, allows maximum patient mobility, and provides an interrupted infusion of the agent 24 hours a day. Unfortunately, these reservoirs are expensive.

DIGITAL SUBTRACTION ANGIOGRAPHY

Digital subtraction angiography is a technique in which computers are used to enhance angiographic images.

Immediately before the injection of contrast agent, a plain image of the area of interest is taken, passed through a television camera, and digitized, that is, converted to an array of numbers that is stored in the computed memory. A series of images is then taken during the injection of contrast agent. These images are also digitized and stored. The first (precontrast) image is then subtracted from all succeeding images. Provided the patient has not moved, the images of bone and overlying soft tissue are removed, leaving a series of images of the injected contrast agent alone, that is, images of the vessel lumina.

Computer techniques are then used to enhance image contrast so that very slight differences in radiographic density are accentuated to produce clear images of the vessels; such images are not available with older techniques.

Useful images can be obtained even when the concentration of contrast agent in the artery is low. As a result, satisfactory images of most parts of the arterial system can be obtained from intravenous injections, thus avoiding the hazards of arterial puncture and catheterization. Economically, this change is highly significant because it makes it possible to perform extensive arteriographic procedures on outpatients. Since the contrast is given intravenously and there is no need to puncture the artery, there is no need for the patient to remain in the hospital after the study.

Inevitably there is a price for this added convenience. The new equipment is expensive, and the subtracted images are significantly compromised if the patient moves during the study. Furthermore, the subtracted image is rather grainy and may not possess sufficient detail for some purposes. In order to overcome these problems, there has been a tendency to revert to intra-arterial injection in special cases. When intra-arterial injection must be used, the digital subtraction technique is still beneficial because it allows the use of very fine catheters and small volumes and low concentrations of contrast and still produces superb pictures.

At present, the principal use of digital subtraction angiography is in the diagnosis of extracranial carotid artery disease. For the gynecologist, the impact of digital subtraction angiography at present is small, since most gynecologic tumors are not particularly vascular. Digital subtraction angiography provides a relatively atraumatic means of demonstrating vascular anatomy before surgery and should be considered when the information sought is thought not to be of sufficient importance to justify the risks of a conventional arteriogram. Digital subtraction angiography also provides a simple means of following the response of vascular tumors, such as choriocarcinoma, to chemotherapy. It is used occasionally as a prelude to transsphenoidal surgery if there is any possibility of aneurysm.

GENITOGRAPHY

In genitography, the contrast agent is injected into all of the perineal openings so that the internal genital passages are displayed. This technique is confined to pediatric radiology and is sometimes helpful in assigning sex in cases of ambiguous external genitalia.

RADIONUCLIDE IMAGING

Images that are produced by x-rays and ultrasound result from energy that originates outside the patient. Radionuclide imaging is fundamentally different in that the radiation that forms the image originates inside the body. The radiation is emitted by pharmaceuticals containing elements that are radioactive.

A radioactive atom is one that has an unstable nucleus. As the nucleus undergoes internal rearrangement, radiation is emitted. The only useful form of radiation for medical imaging purposes is gamma-rays, a form of electromagnetic radiation that is closely related to x-rays. Gamma-rays, with a photon energy in the range of 75 keV to 200 keV, are the best for imaging, although positron imaging systems that use gamma-rays with a photon energy of about 500 keV are gaining popularity.

By far the most useful radionuclide is Technetium 99m (^{99m}Tc). This radionuclide has a short half-life (6 hours) and emits only gamma-rays, two properties that keep the dose of radiation to the patient low and so allow large doses of the radionuclide to be given without undue irradiation risk. (It is desirable to give a large dose of radionuclide, because the larger the dose, the easier and quicker it is to obtain a high-quality image). Technetium 99m is easily obtained from commercially available generators containing molybdenum 99. The ^{99m}Tc is periodically eluted from the generator by flushing with saline.

The technetium is given the desired biologic properties by incorporation into a suitable molecule or particle. For instance, if one wishes to obtain a radionuclide image of the skeleton, the ^{99m}Tc is incorporated into a molecule, such as methylene diphosphonate, that is taken up by osteoblasts.

When a plain film or CT scan is performed, the patient is irradiated only during the time of image formation. The x-ray tube is energized only after the patient and film are set in position, and irradiation ceases as soon as image formation is completed.

With nuclear studies, the radiation comes from within the body and cannot be turned on and off at will. Thus, almost all the radiation is emitted either before or after the image is taken and thus contributes to radiation dose but not to image formation.

This enormous and unavoidable wastage of radiation means that the total number of photons that are collected to form an image must be severely limited if the dose of radiation to the patient is to be kept low and scanning time is to remain acceptably short. The sharpness of an image depends on the number of photons used in its formation, so that radionuclide images, which are necessarily photon poor, are grainy and blurred compared with ordinary plain-film or ultrasound images. Use of long imaging times increases the number of photons and thus improves the images unless patient movement becomes a problem. For instance, respiratory movement always causes degradation of liver scan images. Efficient gamma cameras and highly specific radiopharmaceuticals containing short half-life radionuclides that are purely gamma emitters, such as technetium, all help improve the image while keeping radiation dose acceptably low, but nonetheless radionuclide images are, and probably will remain, of much lower resolution than conventional radiographic images.

Although radionuclide images have a much lower spatial resolution than plain-film or ultrasonic images, their value lies in their sensitivity to alterations in physiologic processes (*e.g.,* osteoblastic activity) that are not easily detected by other methods. However, because alterations in a physiologic process may be due to many causes, radionuclide studies tend to be sensitive but nonspecific. It is especially important to interpret radionuclide studies in the light of clinical and other data. For instance, areas of increased osteoblastic activity may be due to metastases, healing fractures, osteoporosis with unusual bone stress, osteomyelitis, or arthritis. Although each may impart some distinctive feature to the radionuclide image, there are many similarities. In such instances, the precise pathologic diagnosis must usually be determined by other means.

Apart from the intravenous injection and minimal radiation dose, radionuclide examinations are painless and free from hazard. There is an unavoidable delay between the injection of the radionuclide and the commencement of imaging owing to the time needed for the radionuclide to clear from the blood and to concentrate in the tissue of interest. With modern radiopharmaceuticals (other than gallium), this delay ranges from a few seconds to two hours; gallium requires at least six hours. Several minutes are usually required to collect the data needed to form a good image, during which time the patient must remain motionless. The dose of radiation received by the patient from most modern radionuclide studies is low, and repeated studies can safely be performed in all but pregnant patients. Unless the thyroid itself is being examined, studies using iodine-containing radiopharmaceuticals require a preliminary dose of nonradioactive iodine to prevent thyroid uptake.

Radionuclide Detection of Metastases

Bone

Radionuclide bone scanning is a much more sensitive means of detecting bony metastases than plain films. The radiopharmaceutical, most commonly ^{99m}Tc methylene diphosphonate, is taken up in an amount depending on the osteoblastic activity and blood supply of the lesion. Most bone lesions, whether blastic or lytic, cause some osteoblastic activity. An area of increased osteoblastic activity, however, does not necessarily indicate a metastasis, and thus a plain film of the suspicious area should be taken to exclude lesions such as fractures and osteophytes. Conversely, a lesion that provokes no osteoblastic reaction is not detectable by bone scanning. Myeloma and rarely a metastasis from carcinoma of the breast fail to produce any osteoblastic reaction.

Normal bone takes up more radionuclide around the joints than elsewhere, but these areas of increase are symmetric. Metastases appear as areas of increased radioactivity that are asymmetric or located away from joints.

A clinician who suspects bony metastases should use the radionuclide bone scan as the initial test, particularly when seeking asymptomatic metastases. (A series of plain films of asymptomatic areas of the skeleton to seek metastases, a study known as a skeletal survey, has a low yield and should not be used.)

Liver

Liver metastases can be detected by scanning after intravenous injection of ^{99m}Tc-labeled colloidal sulfur. The colloidal particles are taken up by the reticuloendothelial phagocytes within the liver, spleen, and marrow. Imaging may commence immediately after the injection. Metastases usually appear as multiple round areas of diminished radioactivity. Hepatic metastases smaller than 2 cm in diameter cannot be routinely detected by radionuclide scanning, even with the best equipment. The margins of normal liver images are often irregular, and these irregularities are sometimes difficult to distinguish from defects due to subcapsular metastases. In spite of these difficulties, the radionuclide liver scan remains a useful first test for liver metastases. It is more accurate than ultrasound and slightly less accurate than modern high-resolution CT but is also less costly.

Brain

Abnormalities in cerebral radionuclide images are due to changes in the blood–brain barrier. Metastases disrupt the blood–brain barrier and thus appear as areas of abnormally increased radioactivity. The popularity of radionuclide brain scanning has declined greatly since the introduction of CT.

Gallium Scanning

The radionuclide gallium is taken up by actively proliferating tissue. Thus, most (85%) rapidly growing tumors, lymphoma, and abscesses take up the radionuclide. The gallium scan is useful when a patient is ill but there are no localizing signs.

Radionuclide Lymphography

If a radionuclide-labeled colloid of appropriate particle size is injected subcutaneously, it is taken up by lymphatics and transported to the regional nodes, and images of the draining lymph nodes can be obtained. This technique is generally inferior to conventional lymphangiography because, when compared with radiographic images, the resolution of a radionuclide image is poor. Its principal application is in the delineation of the internal mammary lymph node chain in patients with carcinoma of the breast.

Lesion Vascularity

The vascularity of a lesion can be simply determined by giving the dose of radionuclide as a concentrated intravenous bolus and placing the gamma camera over the lesion while the bolus of radioactive blood passes through the lesion. Occasionally this technique is of value to the gynecologist in determining vascularity before performing a biopsy.

Localization of Bleeding

Technetium labeling of red cells is now a simple routine procedure. This technique is a much more sensitive means of detecting bleeding than angiography. A positive study localizes the bleeding point only approximately, and arteriography may then be necessary to provide more accurate localization. Nonetheless, the radionuclide scan is the initial study of choice when low-volume or intermittent bleeding is suspected.

COMPUTED-EMISSION TOMOGRAPHY

CT techniques developed to identify the attenuation coefficient of each tissue element in a slice of tissue can also be applied to determine the source of gamma-rays emerging from the body. This technique improves the spatial resolution of radionuclide images.

INTERVENTIONAL RADIOLOGY

A number of invasive techniques have recently been developed, including dilatation of arterial stenoses (percutaneous transluminal angioplasty), fine-needle aspiration biopsy in both the chest and abdomen, percutaneous nephrostomy, percutaneous biliary drainage, and percutaneous drainage of abscesses, pseudocysts, lymphoceles, and other fluid collections. Of these, fine-needle aspiration biopsy, drainage of fluid collections, and percutaneous nephrostomy are the three procedures most likely to be of interest to gynecologists. All of these procedures can be performed without the need for general anesthesia or open surgery, provided satisfactory images of the target lesion are available. CT, ultrasound, and fluoroscopy are the three most commonly used imaging techniques. The high cost of the necessary imaging equipment has resulted in its centralization in departments of radiology, and thus most of these procedures are performed by radiologists.

Fine-Needle Aspiration Biopsy

Needles of 22 gauge or less may be safely passed through hollow viscera, since the puncture hole is so small that there is no risk of leakage of bowel contents. There is a theoretic risk that the passage of the needle through bowel on its way into a fluid collection could contaminate the needle and thus infect fluid such as a hematoma or pseudocyst, but this risk appears slight.

Because tumor cells lack the intercellular bridges of normal cells, agitation of a fine needle within a tumor dislodges a significant number of cells, which can then be aspirated and examined cytologically. Newer 22-gauge needles with a small slot cut in the side of the bore about 1 cm back from the tip can sometimes be used to produce specimens adequate for histologic as well as cytologic analysis. Generally, if a specimen from a solid lesion does not show malignant cells or a specific organism, it is not helpful, since it may not be a representative sample. Positive diagnoses appear reliable. The overall accuracy of the procedure depends, among other things, on the adequacy of fixation and staining, and it is our practice to have a cytotechnologist present during the procedure. The slides are then prepared and examined on the spot.

Drainage of Fluid Collections

Before a drainage procedure is undertaken, the nature of the fluid should be determined by means of fine-needle aspiration, with microscopy and culture of the sample. This procedure helps avoid the useless trauma of attempted drainage of fluid that is too thick to drain through a catheter. In general, hematomas containing solid clot and pseudocysts containing large amounts of solid debris are not suitable for percutaneous drainage. Also, some lymphoceles contain large numbers of small loculi separated by numerous fine septa, and these prevent drainage. Catheter drainage of fluid-filled tumors should not be undertaken.

Because drainage tubes and large needles cannot be passed safely through the bowel, it is necessary to plan the approach to a fluid collection along a line that avoids the hollow viscera, avoids crossing the pleura, and minimizes the extent of invasion of the peritoneum.

Percutaneous drainage of abscesses (Fig. 61-12) is generally superior to the traditional open surgical approach because general anesthesia is not required, the tissue plains confining the infection are not significantly disrupted, and there is less tendency to loculation, probably because of the smaller amount of tissue disruption.

RADIATION HAZARDS

X-rays, which are a form of ionizing radiation, produce chemical changes in the cells through which they pass. Chemical changes in the cytoplasm may so disorganize the biochemistry of the cell that it dies. Even if it does not die, changes in the cell's genetic material may alter it permanently, a change called *mutation*. These radiation-induced mutations are similar to those occurring naturally and are dose related: the more x-rays, the more mutations.

Injury due to small doses of radiation such as those used in medical imaging is manifested in two principal ways: an increase in the incidence of malignant tumors, and an increased risk of genetically determined disease in subsequent generations when the gonads are irradiated. This added risk makes it particularly desirable to avoid unnecessary irradiation of the gonads. Thus, it is desirable to keep the dose of ionizing radiation (x-rays, gamma-rays) to the minimum consistent with obtaining clinically necessary information; this is particularly important in the case of young patients, who are more

FIG. 61-12. Interventional radiology: liver abscesses have been treated by percutaneous drainage. (*Left*) Before drainage. There are two large well-defined lesions of relatively low density situated in the right lobe of the liver. The lesions are consistent with abscesses, although neoplasms, either primary or secondary, cannot be excluded by CT appearances alone. Multiple calcified granulomatous lesions are noted incidentally in the spleen. (*Right*) After drainage. Catheters, which show as dense curvilinear structures, have been inserted into both the anterior and posterior lesions. The low-density areas (seen in *A*) have almost completely resolved.

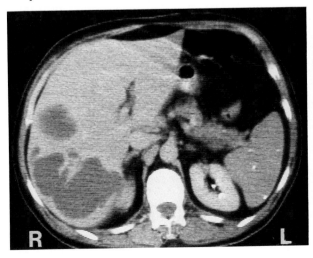
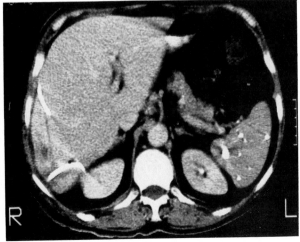

likely to reproduce subsequent to the radiographic examination than are the elderly. Nonetheless, the risks from a small dose of radiation are small, while the consequences of missed or delayed diagnosis are sometimes most unfortunate. A rational balance must be struck. The following general rules are offered as a guide to the clinician to allow him to play a part in minimizing radiation dose:

1. X-ray examinations should be avoided if at all possible during pregnancy. Since pregnancy is a common condition, the possibility of pregnancy should always be considered when requesting radiographic studies on any woman of childbearing age. When a radiographic procedure is necessary during pregnancy, a lead apron should be used to shield the fetus during the procedure, unless shielding would obscure diagnostically vital areas.
2. Any radiographic procedure that places the gonads in the x-ray beam gives a larger genetically significant dose than studies of other parts of the body. Studies that put the ovaries in the primary beam include barium enema, intravenous pyelogram, plain films of the pelvis or the lumbosacral spine, and CT scans of the pelvis.
3. The use of lead shields to cover the ovaries is of dubious value. The shield usually obscures a substantial area of the pelvis, an area that may contain significant disease. In addition, incorrect positioning of the shields is not rare, so that the ovaries are left unprotected.
4. There is no measurable advantage to performing a radiographic study at a particular time in the menstrual cycle.
5. CT scanners use a narrow, slitlike beam; thus, the dose of x-rays to the ovaries is very small unless slices are taken directly through or very near the ovaries.
6. A radiographic examination should be performed only for the patient's benefit.
7. In the absence of special risk factors, routine preoperative chest films should not be performed in asymptomatic patients under 30 years of age.
8. When several clinicians share responsibility for a patient's management, efforts should be made by both clinicians and radiologists to avoid duplication of radiographic procedures.
9. Ultrasonic and nuclear magnetic resonance studies are presently believed to be free of radiation hazard.
10. The taking of a clinical history and performance of a physical examination carry no radiation hazards whatsoever.

MAGNETIC RESONANCE IMAGING

Although the technique is relatively new, and also expensive, nevertheless it seems clear that magnetic resonance imaging may be uniquely valuable in the diagnosis of certain gynecologic problems. In carcinoma of the endometrium, magnetic resonance imaging may be important in FIGO staging by disclosing the depth of myometrial invasion, the presence or absence of cervical involvement, and, in some cases, the presence of pelvic and nodal extension. Magnetic resonance can localize adnexal cysts, and can distinguish serous from hemorrhagic fluid. (This technique appears also to have usefulness in obstetrics, especially in evaluation of the fetal lungs and in diagnosis of fetal anomalies when the amounts of amniotic fluid are too small to permit satisfactory sonographic examination.)

Physical Principles

Certain atoms in the body, the most abundant of which is hydrogen, behave as minute magnets. If the patient is placed in a powerful magnetic field, the spinning atoms of hydrogen line up, with their magnetic axes lying more or less parallel or antiparallel to the magnetic field. The action of the magnetic field on the spinning nucleus is rather like that of gravity on a spinning top, and as a result the magnetic axis wobbles, that is, it precesses around the axis of the magnetic field. If a pulse of radiofrequency energy of appropriate frequency is transmitted into the patient, the atoms of hydrogen rotate their magnetic axes by an amount that depends on the duration of the pulse and synchronize the wobbling of their magnetic axes. That is, they all precess together, in phase, a phenomenon called *coherent precession.* In so doing, they absorb energy from the radio pulse. When the pulse is turned off, the hydrogen atoms revert over time to their original alignment and lose their coherence of precession. In so doing, they give back the energy they absorbed from the radio pulse as minute radio signals.

The time hydrogen atoms take to revert to their resting state is expressed as a pair of constants known as T1 and T2, or alternatively the longitudinal and transverse relaxation times. These times depend upon the chemical and physical environment of the hydrogen atoms. That is, a hydrogen atom incorporated into a complex organic molecule has relaxation times different from those of a hydrogen atom located in a molecule of water. Both of these have relaxation times that are different from those of hydrogen atoms located in solids, such as bone. That is, the relaxation times act as tissue labels, each tissue having a relaxation time that is more or less characteristic.

In addition, the frequency of the radio signals given out by the hydrogen atoms depends on the strength of the magnetic field. If the magnetic field is not uniform but varies in a systematic way, the frequency of the radio energy given out by the hydrogen atoms varies, depending on where in the magnetic field the hydrogen atom is located. Thus, frequency can be used to determine the location in the body of hydrogen atoms with particular relaxation times. It is therefore possible to derive from the magnetic resonance signal the three types of information needed to build an image:

The relaxation times, which characterize the type of tissue and allow distinction of one tissue from another

The frequency of the signal, which allows determination of the location of each tissue element

The strength of the signal, which, all other things being equal, indicates the number of hydrogen atoms at each location.

Mathematical techniques very similar to those used in CT are applied to localize the hydrogen atoms from which particular signals emanate.

However, the picture that results has aspects that are unfamiliar to persons used to dealing with conventional radiographic and CT images, since the appearance of each tissue depends on multiple factors. The repetition rate, length, and sequence of the radio pulses and the chemical composition and physical state of the tissue all affect the images. Thus, stationary blood appears different from flowing blood. Adipose tissue gives a strong signal, while bone gives a very weak signal. These variations produce images that are unfamiliar and correspondingly difficult to interpret until an entirely new set of ground rules has been mastered.

Advantages and Disadvantages

At present the principal advantages appear to be the following:

There is no radiation hazard associated with magnetic resonance imaging.

Certain disease states such as multiple sclerosis and syringomyelia are more easily and clearly shown by magnetic resonance imaging than by any other technique. Differentiation of normal from diseased tissue is often more apparent than in CT images.

Images in any plane through the body have the same resolution, a considerable advantage over CT, in which views other than the standard axial views have lower spatial resolution.

Provided a sufficiently powerful magnetic field is used (1.5 Tesla or more), *in vivo* chemical analysis of tissue is theoretically possible.

The disadvantages appear to be the following:

Very strong, extremely uniform magnetic fields are needed to provide useful magnetic resonance images. These fields require large magnets that may be any one of three types: permanent, resistive, or superconducting. Unfortunately use of all three types is associated with considerable technical problems.

Resistive and superconductive magnets require specially designed shields to prevent nearby iron and steel (such as steel reinforcing in the floors and walls of the building) from interfering with field uniformity.

The magnetic fields are so strong that nearby steel objects such as metal pins or oxygen cylinders can be drawn forcefully into the machine with disastrous results, particularly if someone is in the way.

All magnetic resonance devices require substantial time (minutes) to produce an image.

Magnetic resonance imaging devices are at present very expensive, approximately twice as expensive as CT scanners.

Overall then, magnetic resonance imaging is likely to be an important imaging technique, particularly in the head and pelvis, where motion is not a problem. It is likely to be confined to large medical centers and will probably remain expensive for some time to come.

MAMMOGRAPHY

Mammography provides detailed radiographic images of intramammary structures. Two forms of mammography are currently in use: film mammography and xeromammography. The clinical use of these techniques is discussed in Chapter 60.

Xeromammography

When x-rays strike a charged, selenium-coated plate, they dissipate some of the charge. The amount of charge dissipated is in proportion to the amount of x-rays striking the plate. Thus, a latent image in the form of a pattern of varying electrical charges is created on the surface of the plate.

If the plate is then placed in a chamber into which charged pigment particles are blown, some particles are attracted by the charge on the plate and settle on its surface. The amount of pigment at each point on the plate depends upon the charge at that point. The resultant image is then transferred to a piece of plastic-coated paper by pressing the plate and the paper together and exposing the paper to heat. The entire process is performed automatically in a commercially available processor.

At the boundary between two differently charged areas, the electric field is distorted, causing an excessive amount of pigment to be deposited on the denser side of the boundary, while a disproportionately small amount of pigment is deposited on the less dense side. Thus, edges are sharply displayed, even though the difference in radiographic density between adjacent structures may be very slightly. Apart from this strong edge-enhancement effect, xeroradiography provides a low-contrast image that satisfactorily demonstrates the entire breast and the retromammary structures, all in one exposure (Fig. 61-13).

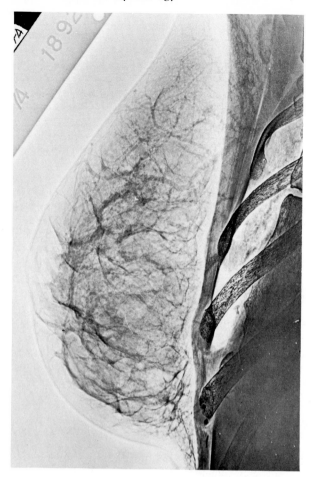

FIG. 61-13. Xeromammogram shows normal breast, mediolateral view. Nipple, skin, vasculature, ductal structures, and retromammary tissues are all clearly seen. No masses are present.

Film Mammography

The differences in radiographic density between the components of the breast are slight. Low-energy x-rays and high-contrast film must be used to display these slight differences in density.

To maximize the contrast of the image and to provide the sharp detail necessary for useful interpretation, special high-contrast film that has emulsion on one side only (conventional x-ray film has an emulsion on both sides) is used in combination with special cassettes containing a single, fine-grain intensifying screen.

To enhance the visibility of intramammary detail, the breast is drawn over a plate or film holder and compressed with a plastic cone or a balloon so that the breast tissue is spread out. Mediolateral, craniocaudal, axillary, and often lateromedial views of each breast are taken.

In xeromammography the dose of radiation to the skin of the breast is less than 1 rad per image. Film mammography using modern film-screen combinations

requires a slightly lower dose. These figures are only approximate, since reported values vary. With both xeromammography and film mammography, the radiation exposure to the gonads and the eyes is negligible, so that the only hazard from the examination is the direct effect of radiation on the breast tissue itself.

Interpretation

Malignancy is suggested by the following:

An increase in the vasculature of one breast (Unfortunately, increased vascularity can occur with inflammatory disease as well as malignancy.)
A mass, the borders of which are not sharp
Strands of tissue running from a mass to the skin, the nipple, or the chest wall (Fig. 61-14)
Thickening due to edema of the skin of the breast

FIG. 61-14. Xeromammogram shows carcinoma of breast, craniocaudal view. Carcinoma (*CA*) is about 2 cm in diameter and has poorly defined border. Note strands of dense tissue running forward from the mass to the subareolar region. Increased breast vascularity, skin thickening, and calcification (features often seen in malignancy) are not seen in this example.

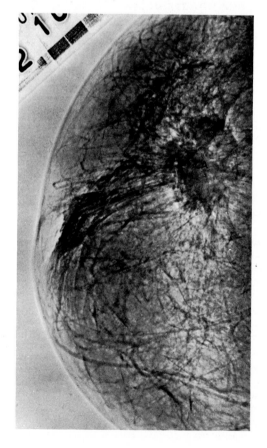

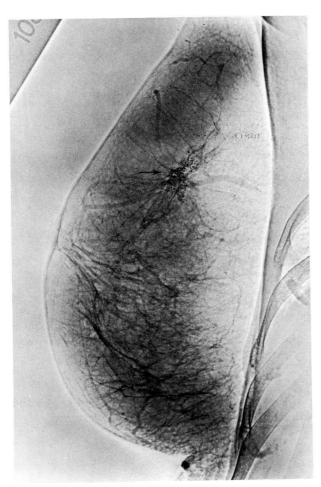

FIG. 61-15. Xeromammogram shows malignant calcification in carcinoma of breast. Calcified carcinoma (*arrow*) can be seen in upper part of breast. Malignant calcification is typically very fine and may be much more difficult to see than in this example.

Very fine punctate calcifications within a mass (Fig. 61-15)

Calcification may be so fine that it can be detected on the mammogram only with the aid of a magnifying glass. Malignant calcification must be distinguished from vascular calcification, which follows the course of blood vessels. Other benign forms of calcification are, in general, coarser than the calcification of malignancy. Comedocarcinoma (a form of intraductal carcinoma) also calcifies. Its calcification is often widespread and consists of fine, short, linear flecks. Secretory disease may also be associated with calcification that is similar to but, in general, coarser than that of comedocarcinoma.

Benign breast masses (*e.g.,* fibroadenoma) have sharply defined margins and do not show skin thickening or stranding. Increased vasculature is commonly seen with inflammatory disease, and benign masses may

be calcified. Hyperplastic cystic disease appears as a series of homogeneous densities (representing retention cysts) together with accentuation of the ductal pattern. Calcification may be present; benign calcification is, in general, coarser than malignant calcification.

In many cases the distinction between a benign and a malignant mass is straightforward; however, difficult and borderline cases are not rare, and carcinoma may be present in a breast that is roentgenographically normal. Therefore, mammographic normalcy does not guarantee absence of breast cancer; when any doubt exists, tissues should be excised for histologic analysis, or a follow-up examination should be performed in three months. Mammography should not be the sole diagnostic modality. Palpable carcinomas do occur in the presence of normal mammograms, although they are rare. (Fuller accounts of mammography are available in work published by Wolfe.)

REFERENCES AND RECOMMENDED READING

Amatuzzi R: Hazards to the human fetus from ionizing radiation at diagnostic dose levels: Review of the literature. Perinatol Neonatol 4:23, 1980

Brill AB, Masanobu T, Heyssel RM: Leukemia in man following exposure to ionizing radiation. Ann Intern Med 56:590, 1962

Brown WM, Doll R, Hill AB: Incidence of leukemia after exposure to diagnostic radiation in utero. Br Med J 2:1539, 1960

Chuang VP, Wallace S: Arterial infusion and occlusion in cancer patients. Semin Roentgenol 16:13, 1981

Dawson LL, Mueller PR, Ferrucci JL Jr.: Mucomyst for abscesses: A clinical comment. Radiology 151:342, 1984

Duff DE, Fried AM, Wilson EA et al: Hysterosalpingography and laparoscopy: A comparative study. AJR 141:761, 1983

Ferrucci T Jr., Wittenberg J: Interventional radiology of the abdomen. Baltimore, Williams & Wilkins, 1981

Gedgaudas RK, Kelvin FM, Thompson WM et al: The value of the pre-operative barium enema examination in the assessment of pelvic masses. Radiology 146:609, 1983

Ginaldi S, Wallace S, Jing BS et al: Carcinoma of the cervix: Lymphangiography and computed tomography. AJR 136:1087, 1981

Gross BH, Moss AA, Mihara K et al: Computed tomography of gynecologic diseases. AJR 141:765, 1983

Hricak H, Lacey C, Shriock E et al: Gynecologic masses: Value of magnetic resonance imaging. Am J Obstet Gynecol 153:31, 1985

Kruger RA, Riedener LJ: Basic concepts of digital subtraction angiography. Boston, GK Hall Medical Publishers, 1984

Lee JKT, Sagel SS, Stanley RJ: Computed body tomography. New York, Raven Press, 1983

Lee KR, Mansfield CM, Dwyer SS et al: CT for intracavitary radiotherapy planning. AJR 135:809, 1980

Lewis E, Zornoza J, Jing BS et al: Radiologic contribution to the diagnosis and management of gynecologic neoplasms. Semin Roentgenol 17:251, 1982

Mettler FA, Christie JH, Garcia JF et al: Radionuclide liver and bone scanning in the evaluation of patients with endometrial carcinoma. Radiology 141:777, 1981

Moss AA, Gamsu G, Genant HK: Computed tomography of the body. Philadelphia, WB Saunders, 1983

Mueller PR, van Sonnenberg E, Ferrucci T Jr.: Percutaneous drainage of 250 abdominal abscesses and fluid collections. Radiology 151:343, 1984

National Council on Radiation Protection: Critical Issues in Setting Radiation Dose Limits: Proceedings of the Seventeenth Annual Meeting of the National Council on Radiation Protection and Measurements 1982. Bethesda, National Council on Radiation Protection and Measurement, 1982

Partain CL, James AE, Rollo FD et al: Nuclear magnetic resonance imaging. Philadelphia, WB Saunders, 1983

Pizzarello DJ, Witcofski RL: Medical Radiation Biology, 2nd ed. Philadelphia, Lea & Febiger, 1982

Prasad SC, Pilepich MV, Perez CA: Contribution of CT to quantitative radiation therapy planning. AJR 136:123, 1981

Price RR, Rollo FD, Monahan WG et al: Digital radiography: A focus on clinical utility. New York, Grune & Stratton, 1982

Reuter SR, Redman HC: Gastrointestinal Angiography, 2nd ed Philadelphia, WB Saunders, 1977

Ring EJ, McLean GK: Interventional Radiology: Principles and Techniques. Boston, Little, Brown & Co, 1981

Sanders RC, McNeil BJ, Finberg HJ et al: A prospective study of computed tomography and ultrasound in the detection and staging of pelvic masses. Radiology 146:439, 1983

Swartz HM, Reichling BA: The safety of x-ray examination or radioisotope scan. JAMA 239:2031, 1978

U.S. Department of Health and Human Services: The selection of patients for x-ray examinations: The pelvimetry examination. HHS Publication (FDA) 80-8128, 1980

van Sonnenberg E, Mueller PR, Ferrucci T Jr.: Percutaneous drainage of 250 abdominal abscesses and fluid collections. Radiology 151:337, 1984

Young SW: Nuclear Magnetic Resonance Imaging: Basic Principles. New York, Raven Press, 1984

Weinreb JC, Lowe TW, Santos-Ramos R et al: Magnetic resonance imaging in obstetric diagnosis. Radiology 154:157, 1985

Zornoza J: Percutaneous Needle Biopsy. Baltimore, Williams & Wilkins, 1981

PART VIII

Radiation and Surgery in Gynecology

Radiation Therapy in Gynecology

Philip J. DiSaia

62

All life on this planet has evolved in a milieu in which the major source of energy essential for most biologic processes is in the form of radiant energy (*radiation*). Various forms of radiation influence living material in a variety of ways: sunlight provides heat, light, and energy for plant photosynthesis; radio waves provide a means of communication. These radiations are not harmful in ordinary quantities, but actually benefit life processes. However, certain types of high-energy (*ionizing*) radiations are not so harmless, but provide useful tools in gynecology for both diagnostic and therapeutic purposes. These high-energy radiations can be traumatic to biologic material, and their use in oncology stems from their ability to inflict an injury from which normal tissue recovers more effectively than malignant tissue. They are known to produce deleterious effects on all forms of life from the relatively simple unicellular plants and animals to the complex higher organisms.

The change produced by ionizing radiations is sometimes grossly apparent and may be visible soon after exposure of the living organism, but more often the radiation does not appear (on cursory examination) to have affected the organism at all. It may produce small changes that can be detected only by careful chemical or microscopic study and that may not become apparent for many years or, indeed, may manifest themselves only in the offspring of the irradiated organism. The attitude concerning radiation exposure should always be that diagnostic tests, therapeutic radiation, or radiation acquired incidentally from the environment may all be detrimental. Although in many instances the chance of injury is slight, the possibility of damage from a known exposure must always be weighed against the importance of the information to be gained or effect desired. Certainly, incidental exposure must be avoided through control of environmental hazards wherever possible.

NATURE AND EFFECTS OF IONIZING RADIATION

The radiation emitted by radioactive isotopes (*e.g.,* radium, cesium, iridium, etc.) is used in the treatment of a wide variety of malignancies. In addition, over the past four decades, machines capable of producing radiant energy of high intensity (supervoltage, megavoltage) have become available and are used extensively in the treatment of malignancies. Those machines that emit energies greater than 1 million electron volts (1 mev) are the most commonly used at the present time. Among these pieces of equipment are cobalt generators, betatrons, and linear accelerators (Table 62-1).

Physical and Chemical Nature

The physical forces of concern here are called *ionizing radiations* because of their characteristic ability to transfer their energy to matter by separating orbital electrons from their atoms and thus forming physical ion pairs. The term is an inclusive one, since the phenomenon may be caused by particulate radiations as well as electromagnetic waves. This discussion is limited to electromagnetic radiations with wavelengths in the range of 10^{-7} to 10^{-10} cm (10 to 10^{-3}Å). Radiations that originate from decay of an atomic nucleus are termed γ-rays (*gamma rays*); those that originate outside the atomic nucleus are termed *x-rays* and are produced when high-energy charged particles (electrons) bombard a suitable target such as tungsten. When these fast-moving electrons approach the fields around the nuclei of the atoms of the target material, they are deflected from their path and energy is emitted in the form of electromagnetic radiation. These emitted x-rays may

Table 62-1
Modalities of External Radiation

Modality	Voltage	Source
Low voltage (superficial)	85–150 kv	X-ray
Medium voltage (orthovoltage)	180–400 kv	X-ray
Supervoltage	500 kv–8 mv	X-ray ^{60}Co ^{137}Cs ^{226}Ra
Megavoltage	Above supervoltage energy	Betatron Synchrotron Linear accelerator

have any energy from zero to a maximum as determined by the kinetic energy of the impinging electrons. Machines such as the betatron are capable of generating electrons at high accelerations and, therefore, the x-rays generated by these machines are quite high in energy. A continuous spectrum of x-rays of various energies can be produced when a large number of impinging electrons is involved. Other x-rays are produced when a high-speed electron impinging on the target material knocks out an orbital electron (ionization) from a target atom. When this electron is from an inner shell, its place is immediately taken by an electron from an outer shell, and during this latter transition an x-ray is given off. The photon energy of that x-ray represents the difference in energies of the inner and outer orbital electron levels. It should be remembered that γ-rays and x-rays can be

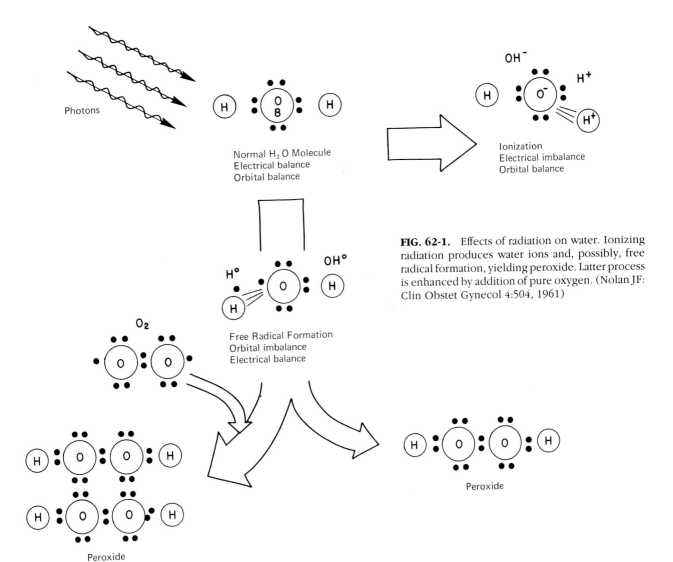

FIG. 62-1. Effects of radiation on water. Ionizing radiation produces water ions and, possibly, free radical formation, yielding peroxide. Latter process is enhanced by addition of pure oxygen. (Nolan JF: Clin Obstet Gynecol 4:504, 1961)

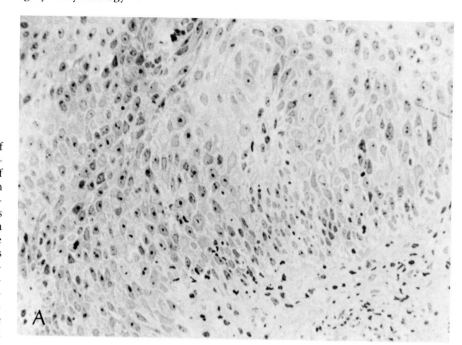

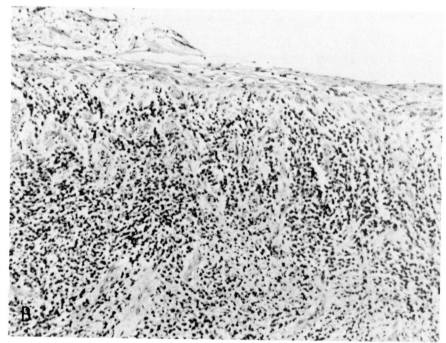

FIG. 62-2. (*A*) Photomicrograph of benign cervical squamous epithelium immediately after removal of intracavitary radiation applicator. An estimated 15,000 rad had been absorbed in this area at the time of this biopsy. Note the intercellular edema and general acute necrosis. The basement membrane area appears smudged. Thick section was embedded in Epon after glutaraldehyde fixation (×298). (*B*) The cervical squamous epithelium six weeks after radiation (intracavitary radioactive source) is thin and still coated with exudate in focal areas (*left*). Epithelial cells are vacuolated. The underlying stroma is densely infiltrated by plasma cells and lymphocytes. Capillary endothelial cells appear swollen; some capillaries are occluded by fibrin thrombi. Estimated dose to epithelium in this area is approximately 30,000 rad. The patient had endometrial adenocarcinoma that did not involve this area prior to treatment (×128). (*C*) Epidermoid carcinoma of cervix immediately after removal of intracavitary radiation source. The most dramatic morphologic change is in cells undergoing mitosis. Note the swelling and disruption of mitotic spindles (*arrow*). Cytoplasm and nuclei of interphase cells are vacuolated; cytoplasm generally appeared swollen when compared to tumor pattern prior to radiation (×255). (Kraus KT: Irradiation changes in the uterus. In Norris HJ, Hertig AT, Abell MR [eds]: The Uterus. Baltimore, Williams & Wilkins, 1973)

collectively termed *photons,* and it is the energy of the photon, not its source, that is important in terms of its biologic effects.

The interaction of photons with matter takes place primarily through three mechanisms: the photoelectric effect, Compton scattering, and pair production. All of these processes result in either ionization of molecules

within the target or free radical formation. Free hydrogen atoms and free hydroxyl radicals commonly result from the bombardment of water by high-energy photons (Fig. 62-1).

About half of the H atoms encounter OH radicals and form H_2O_2. In the irradiation of water by electrons or photons, very few of the H atoms or OH radicals are

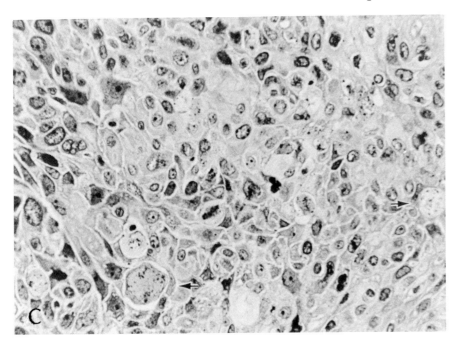

formed close enough to one another to react quickly before they diffuse. The addition of O_2, however, causes the H atoms to react to form the radical HO_2. This is less reactive than the OH radical and permits the decomposition of water to H_2O_2 to proceed. These excited and ionized molecules are very unstable and react with proteins and other key substances within the cell. Many other events may occur with photon bombardment: longchain molecules may be split and regrouped, aggregates may be produced, and ring forms may be disrupted indiscriminately. Certain chemical bonds may be vulnerable to inactivation by oxidation, resulting in loss of functional capacity. All of these chemical changes may ultimately be translated into biologic injury at the cellular level.

Biologic Effects

The mechanism of cell injury from radiation is varied, and the effects may become manifest at different time intervals after the primary event depending on the type of intracellular target affected and the time in which certain chemical constituents are called upon to perform. Thus, following some injury by ionization, a mature cell in a state of low metabolic activity may be grossly unaffected while an actively growing cell may be destroyed. Cells in the act of dividing are more vulnerable than those resting between mitoses. Low oxygen tension, dehydration, freezing, and the presence of chemical reducing agents may significantly protect cells from radiation injury. Radiation injury manifests itself as swelling of the cell, vacuolization of the cytoplasm, giant-cell formation, and fragmentation or partial separation of the chromosomes at the time of division. There occurs, after a latent period, evidence of cell death with loss of nuclear and cytoplasmic structure. Response is the typical inflammatory reaction—edema, capillary dilatation and proliferation, infiltration of round cells, and a fibroblastic response (Fig. 62-2). This immediate reaction is followed by gradual fibrosis, avascularity, and a walling off of the injured area. Very late changes are scarification and contracture, with occasional inelastic dilated blood vessels pinched off by essentially avascular stroma.

The selective destruction of tissues forms the basis of therapeutic radiology. Neoplastic cells are always more easily killed by radiation than are their parent cells of the surrounding normal tissues. The magnitude of the difference in radiovulnerability between normal and cancerous tissues determines, in large part, whether the particular portion of the disease considered for radiation can be eradicated. This relative difference in local radiovulnerability is referred to as a difference in *radiosensitivity*. Radiosensitivity and radiocurability are not identical in meaning. Relatively radioresistant tumors accessible to high-dose local radiotherapy are curable, whereas radiosensitive tumors that at the start of therapy or shortly thereafter are widely metastasized can only be controlled locally. An excellent example of a relatively radioresistant tumor is squamous cell carcinoma of the cervix. Yet this malignancy remains one of the most curable tumors because of its accessibility to high-dose radiation and the relatively radioresistant nature of the hosting normal tissues (cervix and vagina). The ability to place in juxtaposition to the malignancy a dose of radium that is tolerated by the surrounding normal tissue contributes to success.

As a result of the chemical changes described above, very large molecules (common in biologic systems) undergo a variety of structural changes that may lead to altered function. *Degradation,* or breaking into smaller units, has been shown to occur when large molecules are irradiated. *Cross-linking* is another common structural change. A long molecule that is somewhat flexible in structure can undergo intramolecular cross-linking when a chemically active locus is produced on it and when this spot can come in contact with another reactive area. If the cross-linking is extensive, not only are the molecules incapable of normal function, but they may no longer be soluble in the system. Many macromolecules are held in a rigid configuration by intramolecular cross-linking bonds, *i.e.,* specific chemical groups are linked together, frequently by hydrogen atoms, to form a three-dimensional structure. The hydrogen bonds are among the weakest in the molecule and, thus, are the first to be broken by radiation. Such structural changes can lead to severe alterations in the biochemical properties of the molecule.

In this manner, radiation effects on molecules such as proteins, enzymes, nucleic acids, and certain lipids can profoundly affect the cell, which in turn can alter the organ and organism. The initial chemical change occurs in but a fraction of a second and is rarely detected directly. Some of these chemical changes are repaired almost immediately; others that occur within less important structures may result in alterations that are rarely recognizable. In the majority, the transition between a chemical change in a system and the biologic manifestation of this change is complicated and often obscure. Absorption and utilization of energy by a cell is a complex chain of events in which many proteins are involved; radiation damage to these vital proteins can result in loss of cell membrane integrity and even cell death.

Although a variety of morphologic and functional changes have been described in irradiated cells, the bulk of both direct and inferential evidence suggests that the cell nucleus is the major site of radiation damage leading to cell death. For example, it has been calculated that 1 million rad is required to damage a cell membrane.* In contrast, chromosomal aberrations and mutations can be produced by low radiation doses. Since only a few hundred rad are needed to kill most proliferating cells in tissue culture, it seems most logical that the nuclear

---

* Quantity of radiation is expressed in roentgens (R) or rad. The roentgen is the unit of exposure, the rad the unit of absorbed dose. In the case of *x*- or γ-rays, exposure to 1 R results in an absorbed dose in soft tissue that is equivalent to 1 rad.

changes produced by the low doses are responsible for cell death.

Genetic Effects

It is not possible to assign a specific mutation rate to a specific radiation dose. Gene loci differ markedly in their mutability, and the rather random damage exerted by radiation on any particular chromosome makes predictability exceedingly difficult. Certainly mitotic stage, cell type, sex, species, and dose rate all influence the rate of mutation production in lower animals and bacteria. Data accumulated in lower animals are difficult to extrapolate to man and, therefore, predictions about mutation rates cannot be expected on the basis of the evidence accumulated from various types of radiation exposure; direct evidence of radiation-induced mutation in man is lacking. The largest group of humans available for study are descendants of those exposed to radiation in Hiroshima and Nagasaki, and while there has been no detectable effect on the frequency of prenatal or neonatal deaths or on the frequency of malformations in the offspring of these persons, this does not mean that no hereditary effects have been produced by the radiation. The number of exposed parents was small and doses were so low that it would be surprising if an increase in mutation had been detected to date. Several generations are needed to reveal recessive damage.

It is, however, logical to expect that radiation exposure will increase the mutation rate in humans. This expectation is based largely upon experiments on mice. It is estimated that the dose that will double the spontaneous mutation rate for man lies between 10 and 100 rad. For an acute exposure to radiation the probable value is between 15 and 30 rad and for chronic irradiation it is probably around 100 rad. The Committee of Genetics of the Atomic Energy Commission has recommended that no individual from conception to the age of 30 years be subjected to more than 10 rad. With appropriate shielding to prevent scatter, improved x-ray film, image intensifiers, and the like, it is possible to attain satisfactory roentgenographic visualization of internal structures with reduced exposure. The average radiation doses to a developing fetus and to the maternal gonads inflicted by some common diagnostic techniques are shown in Table 62-2.

Effects on the Fetus

The classic effects of radiation on the mammalian embryo are (1) intrauterine and extrauterine growth retardation, (2) embryonic, fetal, or neonatal death, and (3) gross congenital malformations. The structure most readily and consistently affected by radiation is the central nervous system. If the *in utero* absorbed dose is

Table 62-2
Average Radiation Dose to Fetus and to Maternal Gonads from Various Diagnostic Examinations

Examination	Dose to Fetus and Maternal Gonads (millirad)
Lower extremity roentgenography	1
Cervical spine roentgenography	2
Skull roentgenography	4
Chest roentgenography	8
Pelvimetry	750
Chest fluoroscopy	70
Cholecystography	300
Lumbar spinal roentgenography	275
Abdominal roentgenography	185/film
Hip roentgenography	100
Intravenous or retrograde pyelography	585
Upper gastrointestinal roentgenography	330
Lower gastrointestinal roentgenography	465

below 25 rad, these classic effects of radiation are never observed together in experimental animals or, in all likelihood, in the human. Not only are the absorbed dose and the stage of gestation important in determining the effect of radiation on a mammalian embryo, but the dose rate must also be considered. Embryonic damage can be reduced significantly by decreasing the dose rate to allow recovery processes to function. Gross malformations occur most often when the fetus is irradiated during the early organogenic period, although cell, tissue, and organ hypoplasia can be produced by radiation throughout organogenic, fetal, and neonatal periods, if the dose is high enough. There is no stage of gestation during which exposure to 50 rad is not associated with significant probability of observable embryonic defect: death during the preimplantation period, malformations during the early organogenic stage, and cell deletions and tissue hypoplasia during the fetal stages. Animal experiments indicate that all embryos exposed to 100 rad or more after implantation exhibit some degree of growth retardation. Finding and recognizing radiation-induced deleterious effects in offspring irradiated *in utero* becomes increasingly difficult with decreasing doses (less than 10 rad) because such small doses are unlikely to produce such defects and because the natural incidence of defects is high. From the clinical point of view, an absorbed dose of 10 rad to the fetus at any time during gestation can be considered a practical threshold for the induction of congenital defects, below which the probability of producing adverse effects becomes exceedingly small. Diagnostic x-ray procedures (see Table 62-2) should be avoided in the pregnant woman unless there is overwhelming urgency. In women of

childbearing age, possible damage to an early conceptus may be prevented by performing such tests immediately after the commencement of a normal menstrual period.

GENERAL CONCEPTS OF RADIATION THERAPY

The technical modalities used in modern radiation therapy may be classified as external irradiation and local irradiation. *External irradiation* refers to radiant energy from sources at a distance from the body (*e.g.,* therapy with ^{60}Co, linear accelerator, betatron, or standard orthovoltage x-ray machines). *Local irradiation* refers to radiant energy from sources in direct proximity to the tumor. Examples are intracavitary irradiation by means of applicators loaded with radioactive material such as radium or cesium (vaginal ovoids, vaginal cylinder, or Heyman capsules), interstitial irradiation usually delivered in the form of removable needles containing radium, cesium, or iridium, and direct therapy (*e.g.,* transvaginal) usually delivered by means of cones from an orthovoltage machine.

External Irradiation

The energy and penetrating power of ionizing radiation increase as the photon wavelength decreases. Thus, differences in the physical characteristics of the radiation utilized are of great importance in therapeutic radiology (Table 62-3). The clinically important changes occur with radiation generated in the range of 400 to 800 kv (see Table 62-1). Above this energy, the advantages are reduced absorption of radiation in bone, less damage to the skin at the portal of entry, better tolerance by the vasculoconnective tissue, greater radiation at the depth relative to the surface dose, and reduced lateral scatter of radiation in the tissues.

Table 62-3
The Electromagnetic Spectrum

Type of Wave	Wave Energy	Wavelength
Radio	10^{-10}–10^{-4} ev	3×10^5–1 cm
Infrared	0.01–1 ev	0.01–10^{-4} cm
Visible	2–3 ev	7000–4000 Å
Ultraviolet	3–124 ev	4000–100 Å
X-ray	124 ev–124 mev	100–0.0001 Å

An electron volt (ev) is the energy of motion acquired by an electron accelerated through a potential difference of 1 volt; 1 kiloelectron volt (kev) = 1000 ev; 1 millielectron volt (mev) = 1 million ev; 1 angstrom (Å) = 10^{-8} cm.

The reduced skin effect of supervoltage radiation as compared with orthovoltage radiation is a result of the fact that with higher energy radiation, forward scattering (in the direction of the primary beam) of radiation in the absorber is greater and lateral scattering less. With supervoltage radiation the maximal ionization occurs below the level of the epidermis. For example, with ^{60}Co teletherapy, maximal ionization occurs about 5 mm below the surface, while the surface dose may be only 40% of this maximum (Fig. 62-3). As the energy of radiation increases, it becomes more penetrating; as photons and resultant electrons become more energetic, they travel a greater distance into absorbing material. Therefore, the percentage of radiation at any specific depth, compared with the surface dose, increases as the energy increases. This advantage of supervoltage and megavoltage is of clinical importance in the treatment of tumors located deep within the organism (*e.g.,* carcinoma of the bladder and endometrium) where the introduction of a sufficiently high dose with orthovoltage radiation is difficult or impossible.

In the supervoltage range, absorption of radiation in bone approximates that in water or soft tissue per unit density, whereas with orthovoltage absorption of radiation is considerably greater in bone than in soft tissue. The vasculoconnective tissue immediately adjacent to the bone around the haversian canals receives a higher dose because of static irradiation. This higher dose increases the risk of bone necrosis by destruction of the osteoblastic elements and damage to the vascular system. Furthermore, preferential absorption by bone leads to a reduction in the dose at the point of interest when the radiation must traverse thick bone. In addition, it has been observed clinically that, as radiation energy increases, similar tumor effects can be produced with less damage to important adjacent normal structures. The incidence of mucosal and skin reactions is reduced and apparently there is less damage to the vasculoconnective tissue. This greater tolerance of vasculoconnective tissue to a higher dose of properly protracted supervoltage radiation therapy is one of the factors that permits the planned combination of preoperative radiation and surgery without appreciably increasing the surgical risks beyond those associated with surgery alone.

Local Irradiation

Local application of radiation permits delivery of very high doses to restricted tissue volumes. In this situation the physical principle that the intensity of irradiation

FIG. 62-3.   Three isodose curves showing differences in tissue penetration by same radiation dose generated by orthovoltage (250 kv), supervoltage (^{60}Co), and megavoltage (22 mev). CuHVL, copper half-value layer; FSD, focal skin distance; SSD, source skin distance; TSD, tumor source distance.

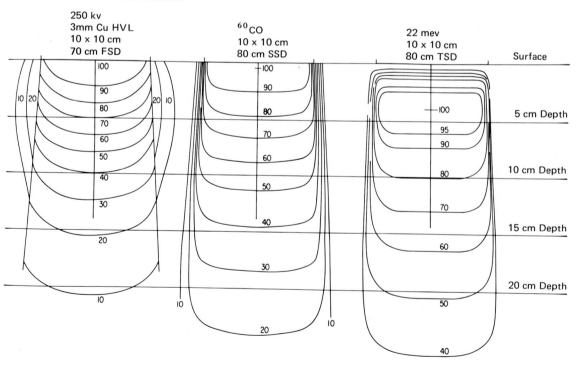

rapidly decreases with distance from the radiation source (inverse square law) is used to advantage. Local irradiation is suitable for a small tumor with well-defined limits and a clinical situation in which it is desirable to restrict the volume of tissue irradiated. A larger volume of tissue is best treated with external irradiation. In the past, radium was the element most frequently used for local application, both in tubes and needles. With the other materials (Table 62-4) now available for local application, the major disadvantage is an appreciably shorter half-life. Several, however, have an advantage in that they can be incorporated into a solid material such as ceramic or various metals and need not be used as a powder or gas, as is the case with radium. Radium tubes and needles contain radium powder, and many of its decay products are in gas form within the same container. In the past [198]Au was used as a permanent tumor implant. It had the disadvantages of difficulty in preparation, a rather rapid radioactive decay, and difficulty in obtaining homogeneity of dose. [125]I is now used instead of [198]Au for permanent implants.

Dosimetry is the measurement or calculation of the dose the patient receives. If the radiation intensity decreases rapidly with increasing depth in tissue, as is the case with local irradiation, the tissue adjacent to the radiation source may theoretically be treated adequately without damage to the underlying structures. The effectiveness of this distribution of radiation is, of course, dependent upon careful application of the source. Interstitial application of a radioactive source is a great deal more difficult than intracavitary application. A system of multiple discrete sources often results in a less homogeneous isodose pattern than irradiation from an external source or from a well-placed intracavitary source.

Some of the high cure rates possible in gynecologic cancer are due to the accessibility of vaginal and uterine cancer to local irradiation. This accessibility allows relatively high doses of radiation to be delivered to the neoplasm with relatively safe amounts of normal tissue exposure.

Another form of local irradiation that has value in the treatment of some vaginal and cervical malignancies is transvaginal radiation therapy. Utilizing a 140-kv to 250-kv unit and vaginal cones constructed of metal or Bakelite, an orthovoltage beam can be directed topically to the lesion. When these low-energy photons, there is a fast falloff of the depth dose so that almost all of the energy is absorbed in the central tumor mass, giving an effect quite similar to that achieved with radium therapy.

The Concept of Nominal Standard Dose

The work of Ellis has introduced a new expression of the biologic effect of radiation—*rad equivalent therapy* (RET). From a consideration of isoeffect relations in clinical radiotherapy, Ellis proposed that the tolerance dose of normal tissue (*D*) could be related to the overall treatment time (*T*) and the number of fractions (*N*) by the expression

$$D = (NSD) \times T^{0.11} \times N^{0.24}$$

This expression, which has come to be known as the Ellis *nominal standard dose* (NSD) equation, is based specifically on the isoeffect curve for skin, the overall slope of which is 0.33. In the Ellis equation this slope has been allocated partly to overall time, with an index of 0.11, and partly to the number of fractions, with an index of 0.24. The suggested dependence on time is close to that observed experimentally for pigskin by other investigators and appears to be a valid deduction on a theoretic basis. The concept of the NSD has the obvious advantage of providing a simple basis for comparison of techniques in the same Center and among Centers, and a further advantage of allowing the therapist to total the effect of two different types of treatment such as intracavitary application of radium and external beam irradiation. Thus, one can calculate the nominal single dose for any radiation treatment plan and express it in standard units. In day-to-day use, the NSD concept is most helpful in the comparison of two treatment regimens that differ in total dose, overall time, and fractionation pattern.

That this equation accurately assesses the normal tissue tolerance is yet to be proved in a wide spectrum of tissues. In addition, one of the principal weaknesses of the NSD system is that it does not include a systematic allowance for field size.

USE OF IONIZING RADIATION IN GYNECOLOGY

For practical purposes modern use of ionizing radiation in gynecology is limited to the treatment of malignant

Table 62-4
Isotopes Commonly Used in Radiation Therapy

Isotope	Energy (mev)	Half-Life
[137]Cs	0.662	30 years
[60]Co	1.173, 1,332	5.3 years
[125]I	0.027–0.035	60 days
[192]Ir	0.47	74 days
[226]Ra	0.8	1620 years
[222]Rn	0.8	3.83 days
[182]Ta	1.18	115 days

[226]Ra, ^{137}Cs, ^{192}Ir, and [182]Ta are suitable for temporary implants; and [222]Rn is suitable for permanent implants which remain in the patient; ^{60}Co has some uses in intracavitary therapy.

diseases. The student should understand, however, that in the recent past radiation was used for sterilization, in the treatment of dysfunctional or climacteric bleeding, to produce ovulation in cases of infertility, and in the treatment of eczematoid and other benign diseases of the vulva. A single dose of 400 to 500 rad is often sufficient to permanently arrest menses in a premenopausal woman. However, a dose of 1200 to 2000 rad in 10 days to 2 weeks is often required to produce complete arrest of ovarian steroidogenesis in younger patients. This technique for producing cessation of menses still has applicability in some women with severe menorrhagia who are not good surgical candidates, *e.g.,* a premenopausal, acutely leukemic woman with thrombocytopenia and menorrhagia. However, with this possible exception, all of these benign conditions are now managed by other means.

Tolerance of Pelvic Organs

The tolerance to radiation of the pelvic organs varies slightly from patient to patient and is, of course, subject to the factors mentioned above, such as volume, fractionation, and energy of radiation received. The administration of radium by different techniques may also result in different dose distributions and considerable differences in tolerance. The more advanced the lesion, the greater the dose necessary for eradication and the greater the likelihood of morbidity. With advanced disease, higher risks of injury are not only present but justified. In advanced cervical, vaginal, or corpus cancer the integrity of the bladder and rectum may be already compromised, with the result that serious sequelae may follow radiation of such lesions.

The cervix and corpus of the uterus can tolerate very high doses of radiation. In fact, they withstand higher doses than any other comparable volume of tissues in the body; doses of 20,000 to 30,000 rad in about two weeks are routinely tolerated. This remarkable tolerance level permits a large dose and allows a very high percentage of control of cervical cancer. The unusual tolerance of the uterus and the vagina to radiation accounts for the success of radium in the treatment of cervical lesions. In addition to the tissue tolerance, the epithelium of the uterus and vagina appears to have unusual ability to recover from radiation injury.

The sigmoid, rectosigmoid, and rectum are more susceptible to radiation injury than other pelvic organs. The frequency of injury to large bowel often depends on its relation to the distribution of radium as well as to the total dose administered by both external beam and intracavitary radium sources. With external beam alone the large bowel is the most sensitive of pelvic structures to radiation. An acute early reaction is heralded by diarrhea and tenesmus. A later manifestation of injury (usually occurring 6 to 12 months after treat-

ment) is chronic pelvic pain associated with constriction of the bowel lumen and partial bowel obstruction. The maximal dose that the rectum will tolerate depends upon many factors, including the time–dose relation of both external beam and local radium source. Kottmeier calculated that the dose to the bladder and rectum from the Stockholm technique of intracavitary application of radium is about 4000 rad/3 cm² of rectum and bladder.

The bladder tolerates slightly more radiation than the rectum according to most calculations. A convenient rule of thumb proposed by Fletcher gives upper limits of radiation and indirectly estimates the tolerance of the bladder and rectum: the sum of the central dose by external beam plus the number of milligram-hours of radium administered by intracavitary techniques should never exceed the number 10,000. (This rule of thumb may not be valid unless the Fletcher–Suit radium system is used.) Thus, if a heavy dose of intracavitary radium is applied centrally for a small lesion, the amount of external beam applied centrally must be kept to a minimum. Conversely, if the lesion is large and the vaginal geometry poor, a minimal intracavitary dose can be given and the dose administered centrally by external beam may be quite high (6000–7000 rad).

Since irradiation for carcinoma of the cervix is primarily directed to the pelvic contents, only limited portions of small bowel are included. The small bowel is normally in constant motion, and this tends to prevent any one segment from receiving an excessive dose. If loops of small bowel are immobilized as the result of adhesions from previous pelvic surgery, they may be held directly in the path of the radiation beam and thus be injured. The resultant injury usually becomes symptomatic a year or more after the completion of radiation and is manifest as a narrowed lumen with or without associated mucosal ulceration.

It is important for students of this subject to understand the concept of permanent injury to normal tissue. When any area of the body is subjected to tumoricidal doses of radiation, the normal tissues of that area suffer an injury that is only partially repaired, even if the individual survives several decades following treatment. Radiobiologists estimate that in the case of injury to normal tissues, only 5% to 20% of the damage is repaired. Thus, the normal tissues in the irradiated area can retain a very considerable handicap. Should a second malignant neoplasm arise in that same area many years later additional tumoricidal radiation would result in a normal tissue injury level that could be unacceptable. Thus, the same area must not be subjected to tumoricidal radiation on more than one occasion; the result will inevitably be massive loss of normal tissue.

Cancer of the Vagina and Vulva

Squamous cell carcinoma of the vagina usually occurs in elderly women who are not good candidates for surgery. Thus, the role of radiation in this disease is quite prominent. Most lesions are treated by whole pelvis irradiation, which effectively treats the pelvic lymph nodes and also markedly reduces the size of the central lesion. The central lesion is then additionally treated by local irradiation delivered by a transvaginal cone or by interstitial implantation of radium, cesium or iridium within the lesion. Overall cure rates of 40% to 50% with radiation therapy have been reported from some institutions. Indeed, about 80% of stage-I lesions are effectively eradicated.

Although some very large squamous cell cancers of the vulva have responded dramatically to radiation therapy, it is generally considered that ionizing radiation is not the treatment of choice for this lesion. Whereas the normal tissues of the cervix and vagina can tolerate large doses of radiation, the vulva is exquisitely sensitive to ionizing radiation. Some radiobiologists explain this on the basis that this area contains a disproportionately large number of end arteries, in which damage by radiation results in vasculitis and radiation necrosis. Radiation to the vulva is inevitably associated with severe vulvitis that almost invariably requires interruption of therapy. Thus, surgical excision of the vulvar lesion by means of a radical vulvectomy remains the treatment of choice. The rationale for a combination of wide local surgery followed by radiation to the regional nodes has some merit, especially in patients who are unable to undergo surgical removal of these regional nodes (see also Chapter 55).

Cancer of the Cervix

The justification for external pelvic irradiation in cervical cancer can be summarized in the following manner. First, as noted previously, intracavitary radium obeys the inverse square law of all radiation that emanates from radioactive isotopes (Fig. 62-4) and, therefore, it cannot safely deliver a cancericidal dose beyond 3 cm from the external cervical os. Second, structures other than the uterus, upper part of the vagina, and medial portions of the broad ligament (lateral portions of the broad ligament, uterosacral ligaments, uterovesical ligaments, and pelvic lymph nodes) also must be considered within the spread pattern of uterine cancer and, therefore, within the field to be treated. Third, the amount of intracavitary radium that can be safely applied is limited by the sensitivity of neighboring structures such as the bowel and bladder. Although the normal tissue of the uterus and vagina is extremely radioresistant, certain limits to the quantity of intracavitary radium must be set. External pelvic irradiation remains the only method capable of delivering an effective dose homogeneously throughout the large volume of tissue at risk.

In the treatment of cervical cancer the careful combination of external irradiation and intracavitary application of radium (many institutions now use cesium) is crucial. In early stage-Ib lesions, in which regional metastases are unlikely, intracavitary radium may be used alone, delivering a total of 10,000 mg-hour in two applications by the Fletcher technique. Conversely, for

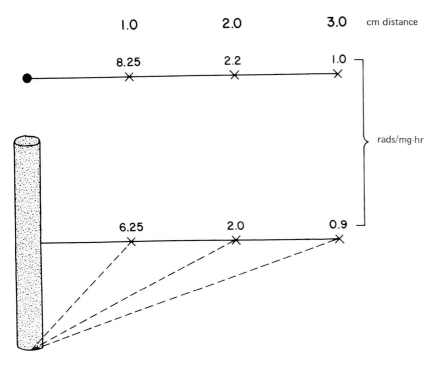

FIG. 62-4. Radiation effects at various distances from 1-mg point source of radium and 1-mg 2-cm-long tubular source of radium.

stage-III lesions (especially with poor vaginal geometry for radium) external beam irradiation may be the major component of the treatment plan and whole pelvis irradiation can be 6000 to 7000 rad. The distribution of disease must be carefully assessed by palpation and diagnostic techniques, and intracavitary application of radium and external beam irradiation must be applied judiciously to direct the greatest dose to the tumor that is compatible with acceptable morbidity.

The objective of treatment is twofold: (1) to sterilize the central lesion and (2) to destroy any islands of neoplasm in the paracervical tissues and regional lymph nodes. Almost always, external irradiation is used first to destroy metastases to the lateral lymph nodes and to reduce the size of the central lesion. Reduction in the size of the central lesion is desirable, since the lateral effect of a radium source diminishes according to the square of the distance (the inverse square law); hence, the smaller the cervix the greater the radium effect lateral to the cervix. The use of external irradiation initially prior to local radium therapy also allows resolution of badly infected cervical lesions and shrinkage of fungating exophytic lesions that interfere with the accurate placement of radium.

In order to quantitate the amount of radiation reaching certain areas in the pelvis, concomitant with the development of the Manchester system (see below), British workers suggested specific landmarks designated as Point A and Point B. They defined a point 2 cm above the mucosa at the lateral vaginal fornix and 2 cm lateral to the uterine canal as Point A and another point 5 cm lateral using the same landmarks as Point B (Fig. 62-5). This enables calculation of the dose (of both radium and x-ray) delivered and of the dose absorbed in the paracervical triangle (Point A) and in the region of the pelvic nodes (Point B). It was suggested that to control squamous cell carcinoma of the cervix, a tumor dose of 7000 to 8000 rad was necessary, and most followers of the Manchester system attempted to administer a minimum of 7000 rad to Point A. This precipitated concern for positioning of the radium, since it was desirable to keep the rectal dose at 6000 rad to Point A. Careful placement of radium makes this possible.

Application of Radium

STOCKHOLM TECHNIQUE. The Stockholm technique (Fig. 62-6A) usually employs two intracavitary applications of radium three weeks apart. Each application is approximately 25 to 28 hours in duration and the intrauterine applicator contains between 50 mg and 75 mg of radium. In an attempt to reduce the chance of overdose to the cervix and adjacent midline structures, the lower 2 cm of the uterine tandem contains no radium; the uterine applicator is otherwise evenly distributed with sources. The vaginal applicator consists of boxes or cylinders in series. In this manner, two to four rows of sources can be utilized to cover the cervical lesion; a total of 60 mg to 80 mg radium is commonly

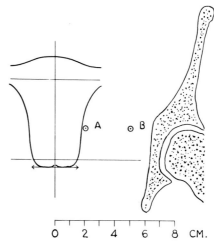

FIG. 62-5. Technique for determining radiation dose to various areas of pelvis. *Point A* is 2 cm lateral to cervical canal and 2 cm superior to lateral vaginal vault. *Point B* is 3 cm lateral to Point A. Calculation of radiation dose to Point A indicates radiation delivered to paracervical structures that may be involved by cervical cancer; calculation of radiation dose at Point B indicates radiation delivered to pelvic lymph glands draining cervix.

used. This technique utilizes a rather "hot loading" of radium over a relatively brief period. In the Stockholm technique the dose at Point A averages slightly less than 6000 rad; the dose at Point B is usually about 1900 rad.

PARIS TECHNIQUE. This technique (Fig. 62-6B) was initiated by the Curie Foundation and also employs a uterine tandem and vaginal sources. The tandem extends the length of the uterine cavity and in a typical case contains 6.6 mg radium in the cervical canal and two sources of 13.3 mg cephalad for a total of three sources within the tandem. A 10-mg or 15-mg source can be substituted for the 13.3-mg source. In the typical case, two cork cylinders containing 13.3 or 15 mg radium are pushed into the lateral vaginal fornices by a connecting spring. A third cork containing 6.6 mg is placed directly against the external os. With the Paris technique the dose at Point A is similar to that delivered by the Manchester technique. When equivalent milligram-hours are used, this dose is in the neighborhood of 5700 rad in six days. One treatment period of 96 to 200 hours is the rule for the Paris technique.

MANCHESTER TECHNIQUE. The Manchester technique (Fig. 62-6C), a convenient and popular modification of the Paris system, differs from the Paris technique in that the source placed in the neighborhood of the cervical canal is considered as unit strength and the remaining sources in the corpus and vagina are applied as multiples of this unit and are selected and arranged to produce the equivalent isodose curves in each case

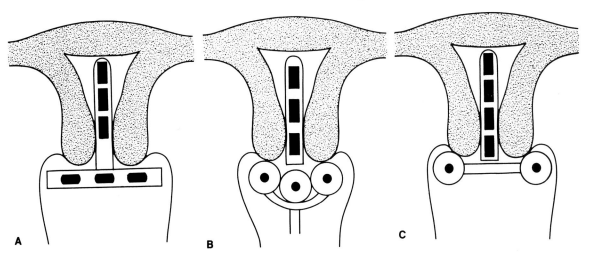

FIG. 62-6. Application of radium in treatment of cervical cancer. (*A*) Stockholm technique. (*B*) Paris technique. (*C*) Manchester technique.

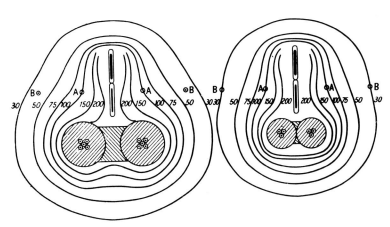

FIG. 62-7. Isodose curves showing dose delivered by Manchester technique to different depths in two cases in which differing amounts of radium could be used. In each, dose is calculated as 100% at Point A, or χ number of rads. Other numbers show percentage of this dose delivered at other depths. (*A*) Standard applicators for large vagina. (*B*) Standard applicators for small vagina. Note: the dose at Points A and B is considerably improved by utilizing larger vaginal ovoids. Thus, with the larger ovoids, the same maximal normal tissue tolerance of the bladder, rectum, and vaginal mucosa is arrived at, with more radiation being delivered to the parametria as represented by Point A and Point B. (Paterson R: The Treatment of Malignant Disease by Radiotherapy. London, Arnold, 1963)

and an optimal dose to preselected points in the pelvis (Points A and B). Thus, the Manchester system is designed to yield constant isodose patterns regardless of the size of the uterus and vagina (Fig. 62-7). A modification that has gained wide popularity because of its ability to accommodate to after-loading is the Fletcher–Suit radium system (Fig. 62-8).

External Pelvic Irradiation

Whole pelvis irradiation is usually administered through an anterior and posterior field approximately 15 to 18 cm² (Fig. 62-9). When the lesion is central and small, it may be judicious to conserve the tolerance of the bladder and rectum for radium and use a 4-cm lead block in the midline of the field. This technique, called *parametrial irradiation* (Fig. 62-10), allows the para-

metrium and pelvic wall to be irradiated homogeneously and conserves the tolerance of the midline structures for future intracavitary techniques. Supervoltage or megavoltage radiation has the advantages mentioned earlier, and whenever possible should be utilized for whole pelvis or parametrial irradiation.

Individualized therapy with judicious use of both external-beam and intracavitary irradiation can result in gratifying survival rates (Table 62-5).

Other considerations with regard to the treatment of cancer of the cervix are discussed in Chapter 56.

Carcinoma of the Endometrium

The most common malignant lesion of the uterine corpus is endometrial carcinoma, and this lesion often in-

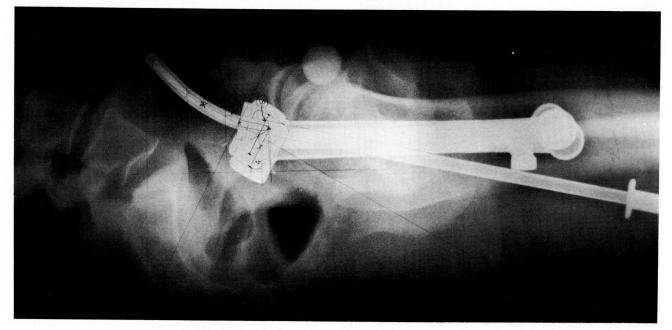

FIG. 62-8.   Fletcher–Suit after-loading radium system. All radium is placed into hollow tandem, and ovoids after placement films (similar to that seen here) are inspected and approved. Metal seed in posterior lip of cervix can be seen above ovoids, marking cervical tissue on film.

FIG. 62-9.   Whole pelvis irradiation for cervical cancer extending to involve upper part of vagina. Lower margin of 18-cm × 18-cm field is well below pubic symphysis. Lead tapes (*white strips*) show technique of excluding corners of a square field and thus reducing volume irradiated by roughly 10%.

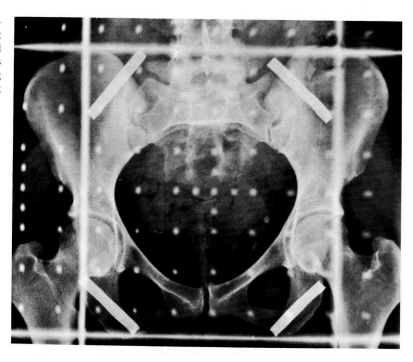

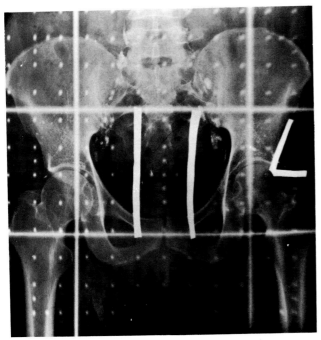

FIG. 62-10. Parametrial irradiation for cervical cancer. A 4-cm lead block is placed between strips of lead tape, sparing midline. Note that height of field is considerably reduced compared with that in Figure 62-9. Only a 10-cm height needs to be blocked in midline, and in larger field, top center portion should not be spared because this represents node-bearing areas.

Table 62-5
Survival Rates for Squamous Cell Carcinoma of Cervix Treated by Radiation Only, September 1954 Through December 1967, M. D. Anderson Hospital and Tumor Institute

Stage	5-Year Survival Rate* (%)	10-Year Survival Rate* (%)
Cervical carcinoma, intact uterus (1705 patients†)		
Ib	91.5	90.0
IIa	83.5	79.0
IIb	66.5	57.0
IIIa	45.0	39.5
IIIb	36.0	30.0
IV	14.0	14.0
Carcinoma of cervical stump (189 patients)		
Ib	97.0	97.0
IIa	93.0	89.0
IIb	67.0	67.0
IIIa	61.0	61.0
IIIb	32.0	32.0
IV	0	0

* Modified life table method. Patients dying from intercurrent disease are excluded.

† Includes patients treated incompletely or for palliation.

(Fletcher GH: Cancer of the uterine cervix. Am J Roentgenol Radium Ther Nucl Med 111:225, 1971)

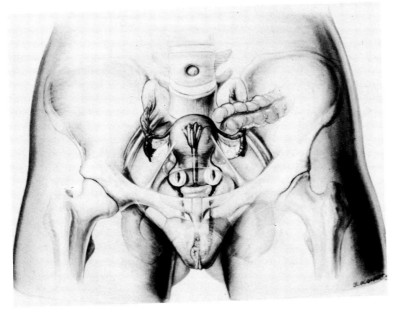

FIG. 62-11. Preoperative application of radium for uterine cancer. Heyman capsule packing can be seen in endometrial cavity and ovoids in vaginal fornices. (Costolow WE et al: Am J Roentgenol Radium Ther Nucl Med 71:669, 1954)

vades deeply into the myometrium. Thus, placing radium sources in close proximity to the disease so as to deliver optimal radiation to all the central lesion is usually not possible. As noted in Chapter 57, removal of the uterus along with both adnexa has proved essential for optimal results; when large series of patients are analyzed, it is apparent that the addition of hysterectomy to the treatment plan for endometrial cancer improves survival by at least 20%, even when the data are corrected for death due to intercurrent disease. Thus, unlike cervical cancer, treatment of endometrial cancer by irradiation alone is not advisable. Some institutions believe that radiation alone constitutes adequate treatment of stage-II endometrial cancer that has extended to involve the endocervical canal. However, this remains controversial. Currently, a very controversial issue is whether adjuvant radiation therapy should be used pre- or postoperatively in stage-I disease. Those who advocate postoperative therapy feel that selection of patients for radiation therapy can be made on the basis of pathologic findings (*e.g.,* deep myometrial invasion, involvement of the endocervix, or adnexal metastases).

Preoperative Application of Radium

The basic treatment for uterine corpus cancer is hysterectomy. However, the pelvic recurrence rate and incidence of cuff metastases can be lowered and the overall survival rate improved by the use of adjunctive radiation therapy, especially in a patient who harbors an anaplastic lesion in an enlarged uterus. Although external irradiation is often utilized, radium implantation either with or without external beam irradiation is effective and preferred by some. The simple tandem or string of radium sources is rarely adequate to irradiate uniformly the enlarged and irregular uterus so often associated with corpus cancer. Instead, a packing technique is used in which small radium sources in uniformly sized capsules are individually introduced and firmly packed to fill the uterine cavity (Fig. 62-11). It is important also to irradiate the endocervical canal and the vaginal fornices, and this is usually accomplished by a placement of short uterine tandem and the usual vaginal ovoids. Intrauterine radium is usually delivered in two applications of 2500 mg-hour each separated by a two-week to three-week interval, or as a single application of 3500 mg-hour if necessary. The value of radiation preoperatively lies in its ability to shrink the uterus and partially debilitate the malignant cells, leaving them less suitable for implantation. It is also thought that preoperative irradiation minimizes the possibility of dissemination of viable cancer at the time of the surgical procedure.

Preoperative External Radiation

The contribution of intrauterine radium to the parametrium and pelvic nodes is minimal and where these are at risk as possible sites of viable malignant cells (as when the cancer has extended to involve the cervix), appropriate therapy must be instituted. The parametrium and pelvic nodes must be treated in a manner similar to that utilized for cervical cancer. Data so far collected suggest that cervical or isthmic involvement, deep myometrial invasion, or anaplastic histology significantly increase the possibility of pelvic dissemination and mandate whole pelvis irradiation (preferably with an external beam). The customary dose is 4000 to 5000 rad if pelvic wall disease is suspected. This is often followed by one radium application delivering approximately 2500 mg-hour and then a simple extrafascial hysterectomy in four to six weeks. External therapy will usually shrink the uterus significantly, allowing safe use of a simple intrauterine tandem instead of the more difficult packing of capsules.

If the patient with endometrial cancer is elderly and unable to tolerate several anesthetics, one anesthetic can be eliminated by substituting external irradiation for intracavitary radium application. It is hoped, then, that the patient will be able to tolerate a single anesthetic so that hysterectomy and bilateral salpingo-oophorectomy can be performed.

Timing of Hysterectomy after Radiation

The interval between the completion of radiation and the performance of hysterectomy is the subject of controversy. Classically, a six-week interval following completion of radiation therapy is advised prior to hysterectomy, but several studies suggest that it is not necessary. The six-week treatment-free interval does, however, allow maximal shrinkage of the uterus and resolution of most of the acute inflammatory process associated with radiation therapy. If whole pelvis irradiation has been utilized, the treatment-free interval also allows recovery from the side effects of this therapy, such as diarrhea, crampy abdominal pain, and often a state of negative nitrogen balance. On the other hand, if radium alone has been used in the preoperative treatment, it may be advisable to do the hysterectomy as quickly as possible thereafter to prevent the distortion that results from radiation. As stated previously, patients with deep myometrial invasion or occult involvement of the cervix or isthmus often have pelvic node metastases. During a six-week waiting period, shrinkage of the uterine tumor occurs and these pathologic findings may be obscured. Immediate hysterectomy allows them to be revealed and may influence the decision for further treatment in the form of whole pelvis irradiation that would include the pelvic nodes.

Postoperative Radioisotopes

The intraperitoneal instillation of colloidal ^{32}P is recommended for stage-I patients in whom positive peritoneal washings are the only evidence of extrauterine disease (see later, under Carcinoma of the Ovary).

Postoperative Application of Radium to Vaginal Vault

Several recent studies have suggested strongly that postoperative adjunctive radiation therapy for endometrial carcinoma is as effective as preoperative radiation in the prevention of vaginal cuff recurrence. Indeed, some institutions advocate primary hysterectomy with bilateral salpingo-oophorectomy when there is no indication of cervical involvement or anaplastic histology. The specimens are then carefully reviewed by the pathologist and if an occult area of undifferentiated disease, occult involvement of the cervix or isthmus, deep myometrial invasion, or adnexal metastases is found, postoperative whole pelvis irradiation is applied. If none of these indicators of nodal involvement is found, the postoperative radiation therapy may be avoided or take the form of cuff irradiation delivered by a variety of radium applicators as soon as one week after hysterectomy. This cuff irradiation, which may also be delivered by transvaginal cone, is relatively simple and usually can be accomplished without an additional anesthetic.

Radiation Treatment of Recurrent Cancer

The development of a pelvic mass in a patient previously treated for endometrial carcinoma may indicate a pelvic sidewall recurrence. Laparotomy should be performed, if possible, to confirm the diagnosis and delineate the extent of the disease. Patients with an unresectable localized recurrence are candidates for a permanent implant with ^{125}I seeds. If whole pelvis irradiation has not already been utilized, consideration should be given to outlining the recurrence with metal clips and delivering external irradiation to the affected area after the operation. If the recurrence is at the apex of the vaginal vault, treatment depends on the size of the lesion. External irradiation should be considered if normal tissue tolerance has not been approached by previous radiation therapy. For vaginal recurrence external irradiation is usually supplemented by an interstitial implant or the use of a transvaginal cone. Unfortunately, these pelvic recurrences are often in a field of fibrosis and avascularity secondary to previous radiation therapy, and it is for this reason that the response of pelvic recurrence to systemic progestin therapy is much less favorable than that for distant recurrences.

Carcinoma of the Ovary

Some 80% of primary ovarian carcinomas arise from germinal epithelium, and this histogenesis is associated with limited radiosensitivity. In general, except for dysgerminoma, ovarian carcinomas are not easily treated with radiation. Although the adenocarcinomas have limited radiosensitivity, other ovarian tumors, such as malignant teratoma or embryonal carcinoma, are notoriously poor in their response to radiation. In addition to the limited radiovulnerability of these lesions, radiation therapy is severely handicapped by the fact that the disease is often widely distributed within the peritoneal cavity. Complete surgical extirpation of all grossly visible tumor considerably enhances the response to radiation therapy. Although bulky ovarian cancer within the pelvis may respond satisfactorily to standard pelvic irradiation, large residual areas of disease in the upper abdomen present a difficult problem for the radiotherapist. Indeed, the difficulty arises whenever the entire abdomen is at risk, since tolerance for whole abdomen irradiation is quite low and the dose that can be safely delivered is well below a tumoricidal dose. The abdomen tolerates a dose above 2500 rad very poorly. Fletcher has proposed that the peritoneal cavity be irradiated by "moving strip technique" in which small segments of the abdomen are systematically irradiated at high intensity. This technique theoretically keeps the morbidity at an acceptable level and permits radiobiologically greater effective doses to be delivered. Many institutions have been unable to adopt this technique successfully and its value remains uncertain. Several studies have found chemotherapy to be at least as effective as radiotherapy in the postoperative treatment of patients with advanced ovarian cancer (see Chapter 59). Certainly chemotherapy should be seriously considered when bulky residual disease remains in the upper abdomen following radiation therapy. Several current, prospective, randomized studies may settle the issue of whether chemotherapy is also equally valuable in patients with minimal residual disease following surgery. Two studies recently concluded suggest that single-agent (Alkeran) chemotherapy is indeed as effective as full-dose radiation therapy, even for patients with minimal residual disease.

There is much current interest in a treatment technique for stage-I and stage-II ovarian cancer that requires the postoperative intraperitoneal instillation of colloidal ^{32}P. This technique has considerable theoretic merit, if all gross disease is removed following hysterectomy and bilateral salpingo-oophorectomy and there remain only microscopic implants or cellular spill for postoperative therapy. ^{32}P emits β rays, which penetrate only to a depth of 1 mm to 4 mm. The colloidal substances have been shown to adhere to or be phagocytized by peritoneal surfaces and thus can discharge their ionizing radiation to malignant cells *in situ*.

NEW THERAPEUTIC STRATEGIES

Radiation therapy is an integral part of curative cancer therapy; however, the tolerance of normal tissues traversed by radiation and the resistance that tumor cell populations can develop have limited the curability of certain tumors, especially those in higher clinical stages. Research in radiobiology and radiation physics may provide methods to increase cure while decreasing morbidity. Computer-controlled dynamic treatment radioprotector drugs, hyperbaric oxygen, carbogen breathing during irradiation, particle irradiation, and hypoxic cell-sensitizing drugs are at this time undergoing clinical evaluation in various studies with some preliminary but encouraging results. The reader is referred to the article by Kinsella and Bluma for reviews of this material.

REFERENCES AND RECOMMENDED READING

Arneson AM, Nolan JF: Radiation therapy. Clin Obstet Gynecol 4:443, 1961

Brown GR, Fletcher GH, Rutledge FN: Irradiation of "in situ" and invasive squamous cell carcinomas of the vagina. Cancer 28:1278, 1971

Deeley TJ: Modern Radiotherapy: Gynecologic Cancer. New York, Appleton, 1971

Delclos L, Quinlan ET: Malignant tumors of the ovary treated with megavoltage postoperative irradiation. Radiology 93: 659, 1969

DiSaia PJ, Morrow CP, Townsend DE: Synopsis of Gynecologic Oncology. New York, Wiley & Son, 1975

Ellis F: The relationship of biological to dose-time fractionation factor: Radiotherapy. Curr Top Radiation Res 4:359, 1968

Fletcher GH: Correlated Seminar, Part II, Radiation Therapy of Cancer of the Cervix. Twelfth Annual Clinical Meeting, American College of Obstetrics and Gynecologists, 1964

Fletcher GH: Cancer of the uterine cervix. Am J Roentgenol Radium Ther Nucl Med 111:225, 1971

Fletcher GH: Textbook of Radiotherapy, 2nd ed. Philadelphia, Lea & Febiger, 1973

Fletcher GH, Rutledge FN, Chau PM: Policies of treatment in cancer of the cervix uteri. Am J Roentgenol Radium Ther Nucl Med 87:6, 1962

Fletcher GH, Rutledge FN, Delclos L: Adenocarcinoma of the uterus. In Vaeth JM (ed): Frontiers of Radiation Therapy and Oncology. White Plains, NY, Karger, 1970

Glasser O, Quimby EH, Taylor LS et al: Physical Foundations of Radiology, 3rd ed. New York, Hoeber, 1961

Hall EJ: Radiobiology for the Radiologist. Hagerstown, Harper & Row, 1973

Kinsella PJ, Bluma WD: New therapeutic strategies in radiation therapy. JAMA 245:169, 1981

Rosenshein NB, Leichner PK, Vogelsang G: Radiocolloids in the treatment of ovarian cancer. Obstet Gynecol Surv 34: 708, 1979

Swartz HM: Hazards of radiation exposure for pregnant women. JAMA 239:1907, 1978

Gynecologic Operations*

Harold M. M. Tovell

63

The intent of this chapter is to provide the student with a familiarity with the technical aspects of a number of frequently performed elective gynecologic operations. During a clinical clerkship the student will have an opportunity to observe or actually assist at a variety of major and minor gynecologic procedures, which are reviewed in one or more of the standard texts listed at the end of this discussion.

Once in the operating room with the patient, the student will be absorbed in correlating the clinical history and the findings of preoperative pelvic examination. He will observe directly the pathology involved when the abdomen is opened and the methodical way the surgeon proceeds through each step of the operation until its completion. The student should have some knowledge of the pathology and anatomy of the area so that he may understand and follow intelligently the reasons for each step of the operation.

Preoperative and Postoperative Investigation: General Considerations

While obtaining the gynecologic history and performing the preoperative workup, the student will learn that he is dealing with a shy, often inhibited patient. Even in these enlightened times, some patients are unwilling to discuss their genital tract disorders, and they protect themselves from their most private and intimate thoughts by devious subterfuge and obscure irrelevance that often confuse the unsuspecting student physician. Psychosomatic disorders are frequently encountered in

gynecologic practice and may further confuse the student in understanding the problem at hand. The student will have to be something of a psychiatrist to recognize these intercurrent disorders affecting the patient and to distinguish them from the obvious genital tract disease or disorder. He must have the patience to listen carefully as well as the sympathy and integrity of a confessor to gain the confidence of the patient that is necessary throughout her preoperative and postoperative period.

Because the gynecologist-obstetrician serves as the primary physician for the female patient, he will be knowledgeable of the patient's general physical and emotional health, her significant past health and illnesses, and medical problems, if any, including her previous operations, allergies, and sensitivities to drugs and medications, as well as the role she assumes within her famiy and her social and occupational milieus.

The extent of any preoperative investigation and evaluation will depend on the patient's age, her general present health and significant past health problems, the nature of the gynecologic problem, and the operation that is to be performed. If she is over 40 years of age or has a history or finding suggestive of cardiac or pulmonary disease, a chest film and electrocardiogram (ECG) are recommended, as well as blood studies, including a complete hemogram and cardiac, renal, and hepatic profiles. A complete urinalysis, including cultures and sensitivities as baseline studies, are important if the bladder is to be involved in the operation or postoperative catheterizations might be required.

If a medical problem exists or the patient is of advanced age and a major operation with prolonged anesthesia is to be performed, the assistance of a qualified internist for both the preoperative evaluation and postoperative supervisory management of the patient should be obtained to reassure both the patient and her gynecologist.

* The illustrations and portions of the text in this chapter are reproduced with permission of the publisher and authors from Tovell HMM, Dank LD: Gynecologic Operations. Hagerstown, Harper & Row, 1978.

Specific Preoperative Studies

All gynecologic patients undergoing an elective and sometimes even emergency procedure should have a Papanicolaou smear if one has not been performed recently. Some states have a law that requires such a smear in pregnancy and one every three years in all hospital admissions.

Patients with large pelvic masses, whether benign, malignant, or inflammatory in nature, should have an intravenous pyelogram to determine if any anatomic or functional disturbances in the upper or lower urinary excretory system exist. When a pelvic malignancy is present or suspected, intravenous pyelography, cystoscopy, and proctosigmoidoscopy should be routinely performed. Pelvic sonography is useful to distinguish between a solid and cystic or multicystic ovarian neoplasm, to determine the size and locations of myomata, and to diagnose an unruptured ectopic pregnancy.

Radiologic studies of the upper and lower gastrointestinal tract should be considered in patients with a suspected ovarian malignancy, and mammograms are indicated in patients with endometrial cancer.

In patients with advanced malignancy or in those receiving chemotherapy for malignant disease, special isotope scans of the liver, lung, kidneys, and bones may also be useful to determine the extent of the disease and its response to treatment.

Informed Operative Consent

The gynecologic patient who is to undergo an operation on her reproductive tract wants to be informed, within the limits of her comprehension, what the effects and benefits of the operation will be in terms of her physical well-being, her reproductive capabilities, and her sexual functions. Pictorial or graphic descriptions of the female reproductive tract, including its functional and physiologic aspects, will frequently clarify many of her previously held misconceptions. Simple explanations and assurances will help her to understand the operative procedures and will give her the confidence and reassurance she requires for an emotionally smooth postoperative course and recovery.

The patient should be informed of the type of incision to be used; other procedures that she will experience both before, during, and after the operation, such as enemas, shaving, premedication, type of anesthesia, intravenous infusions, and the possible use of transfusions, catheterizations, and drains should be described and the reasons for performing them explained.

Not always can the precise limits or extent of the operation be predicted. Alternative possibilities must be carefully explained so that she understands why the gynecologist requires some flexibility to do whatever he believes to be in her best interest in terms of correcting a situation and eradicating disease.

Time spent in listening to the patient and answering her questions with a compassionate understanding will invariably help to alleviate her fears and anxieties and will reward the student with her confidence.

The Role of the Anesthesiologist

The anesthesiologist shares with the surgeon the responsibility for the care of the patient through her operation and the immediate postoperative period. He must be fully aware of any medical conditions, and particularly of any cardiac or pulmonary problems the patient may have or has experienced in the past, as well as any other anesthetic experiences and how she reacted to them. He should be fully informed of the type of operation that is to be performed so that he can plan with the surgeon and the patient the best type of anesthesia and its method of administration for her particular operation. The patient will be told about the preoperative medication and what to expect in the operating room before the surgery and in the recovery room after the surgery.

Pelvic Examination Under Anesthesia

The student should never miss the opportunity to reexamine his patient when she is fully relaxed under anesthesia and the bladder has been catheterized. Not infrequently his findings will differ considerably from his previous examination performed when she was awake and somewhat reluctant and tense. When a pelvic malignancy exists, the opportunity to learn some of the subtleties of clinical staging of malignant disease can be learned under appropriate guidance.

The Role of the Student During the Operation

The primary purpose of the student in the operating room will be to correlate pertinent points in the patient's history and his findings at time of pelvic examination with the pathology seen *in situ*. While serving as a second assistant, he may be asked to hold a retractor in place, to cut sutures, and to occasionally sponge when requested by the surgeon or his first assistant. The teaching surgeon will offer the interested student the opportunity to refresh his memory of the gross anatomy of the involved area, such as the various pelvic ligaments, locations and identification of the pelvic ureters, and the major blood vessels of the pelvis and pelvic organs.

On opening the abdomen, the surgeon will prepare the operative field and the student will observe a variety of surgical techniques depending upon the problems at hand and the area in the pelvis immediately involved. Bacterial cultures may be taken if an infection is encountered, peritoneal fluid samples may be obtained for cell block studies, or peritoneal washings may be taken for cytologic studies if a malignancy is suspected or is known to exist. A complete manual exploration of the abdomen should be performed and the student instructed in the palpation of the liver, gallbladder, spleen, kidney, stomach, head of the pancreas, omentum, and bowel. If a cancer of the ovary, uterus, or cervix is present, palpation of the para-aortic lymph nodes should be done and biopsies taken if any are suspiciously involved or a precise staging of the disease is required.

Following the abdominal exploration, the surgeon will prepare the exposure of the pelvic organs and proceed with the planned procedure. Should the uterus or a cystic or solid ovarian mass be removed, it should be opened in the operating room. This is performed mostly as a teaching exercise for all concerned but may, on occasion, reveal unsuspected disease that may require the opinion of a pathologist as well as a different operative procedure than was planned originally.

The Role of the Student in the Postoperative Management

Once the operation has been completed, the student may be asked, as part of his learning experience, to write a brief operative note and postoperative orders on the patient's chart with the guidance of the surgeon or the first assistant. The operative note should list the surgeon and his assistants and the precise name of the operation performed, including what was removed and what pelvic organs were left in the patient. The pathology found and diagnosis, an estimate of the blood loss, the amount and type of fluid and blood, if any, that was given during the procedure, whether or not any drains were left in the patient, and the type of anesthesia should also be listed, along with a brief statement of the patient's general condition when she left the operating room.

Postoperative orders for both the recovery room and floor nurses include instructions concerning observation and recording of vital signs during the immediate post-anesthetic period, intravenous fluid therapy and its rate of flow, medications for sedation and pain, fluid intake and urinary output to be recorded, instructions for catheterization if necessary, and antibiotics, either for prophylaxis or therapy, if necessary. If bleeding from a wound is a possibility, an order should be written to alert the nurses.

Special orders that pertain to any preexisting medical problem may be required, such as those regarding diabetes; circulatory, cardiac, renal, or pulmonary conditions; or potential problems related to age or physical disability that might impair the patient's ability to manage herself during the initial postoperative period.

As the student makes his daily rounds he will observe the recorded fluid intake and output, pulse, respiration rate, and temperature and will read the nurses' notes on the patient's progress. His examination should include oscultation of the lungs for possible atelectasis, palpation of the abdomen for signs of distention, auscultation for bowel sounds, and inspection of the wound if necessary during the first two to three postoperative days. Ambulation may be started slowly, commencing

with assistance on the first postoperative day if there are no contraindications or complications.

Palpation of the calf muscles for evidence of phlebitis, particularly in obese or elderly patients, and a personal inspection of the perineal pad, or bed, for evidence of any unusual bleeding are also important. Any undue rise in temperature in the early postoperative days demands a careful search for the source of infection, which may be in the wound, urinary tract, or lungs, or which may indicate a deep leg or pelvic phlebitis or thromboembolic phenomenon. A delayed or persisting rise in temperature postoperatively indicates a pelvic abscess or wound infection.

Usually by the second or third day after surgery, narcotic pain-relieving medication can be discontinued, and a milder analgesic and appropriate sleeping medication can be prescribed.

Once the bowel sounds have returned and the patient has passed gas per rectum, usually by the third postoperative day, the intravenous fluid therapy can be discontinued and clear fluids taken by mouth. The diet can be progressed daily and laxatives or rectal suppositories ordered on the third or fourth postoperative day in lieu of enemas.

If a vaginal plastic operation has been performed and an indwelling Foley bag catheter left in to gravity drainage, it may be removed by the fifth day after surgery. Hopefully the patient will void, but she may not empty her bladder completely. Residual urine measurements should be taken until at least two are below 100 ml. Some gynecologists prefer the use of a suprapubic catheter over the transurethral catheter following vaginal plastic surgery, since it reduces the incidence of urinary tract infections and is more acceptable to the patient and the nursing staff. On the fifth postoperative day the catheter may be clamped, and it is hoped that the patient will void spontaneously. Residual urines are easily measured by releasing the catheter clamp and recording the output in a measuring beaker.

REFERENCES AND RECOMMENDED READING

Greenhill JP: Surgical Gynecology. Chicago, Year Book Medical Publishers, 1963

Howkins J, Hudson CN: Shaw's Textbook of Gynecologic Surgery. London, Churchill Livingston, 1977

Käser O, Iklé FA: Gynecologic Operations. New York, Grune & Stratton, 1965

Mattingly RF, Thompson JD: TeLinde's Operative Gynecology, 6th ed. Philadelphia, JB Lippincott, 1985

Nichols DH, Randall CL: Vaginal Surgery, 2nd ed. Baltimore, Williams & Wilkins, 1983

Parsons L, Ulfelder H: An Atlas of Pelvic Operations. Philadelphia, WB Saunders, 1968

Ridley JH (ed): Gynecologic Surgery: Errors, Safeguards and Salvage. Baltimore, Williams & Wilkins, 1974

Schaefer G, Graber EA (ed): Complications in Obstetric and Gynecologic Surgery. Hagerstown, Harper & Row, 1981

Tovell HMM, Dank LD: Gynecologic Operations. Hagerstown, Harper & Row, 1978

THE PFANNENSTIEL INCISION

Most elective gynecologic operations performed through the abdomen for benign disease and for elective cesarean section may be performed through a low transverse non–muscle cutting incision. The Pfannenstiel incision has the following physiological advantages over any vertical incision: (1) It is less painful because of reduced tension on the incision line, resulting in less inhibition of respiratory movements, all of which reduces the incidence of postoperative pulmonary complications and permits earlier ambulation, which is more comfortable to the patient. (2) Wound disruption, evisceration, and incisional hernias are rarely seen, probably because of the undisturbed apposition of tissue layers and improved wound healing. (3) Cosmetic results are superior because the incision is carried out in a natural skin line.

Should the incision prove to be too small to permit removal of a large, benign tumor or intact cyst, or if a malignancy is found unexpectedly, requiring an exploration of the epigastrium, the incision may be enlarged by extending the skin incision on both sides and cutting either partially or completely the tendinous attachments of the rectus muscles off the symphysis pubis. This procedure converts the Pfannenstiel incision to a Cherney incision.

FIGURE 1
The Skin Incision
A gently curved incision is made in the hairline or skin fold passing 2 cm to 3 cm above the upper border of the symphysis pubis and extending to the lateral borders of the rectus muscle on either side.

FIGURE 2
Incising the Subcutaneous Fat
Small bleeders are found in the depths between the fat globules and are clamped and tied, or cauterized. The superficial epigastric artery and vein on both sides are the major vessels found in this layer and have been ligated.

FIGURES 3 & 4
Opening the Rectus Sheath
A technique for opening and incising the rectus sheath and separating the fascia from the underlying rectus muscle is illustrated.

FIGURES 5 & 6
Separating the Lower Rectus Sheath Off the Rectus Muscles
Both finger and sharp dissection are required to separate the lower rectus sheath off the rectus and pyramidalis muscles down to the superior border of the symphysis pubis. The dissection is bloodless.

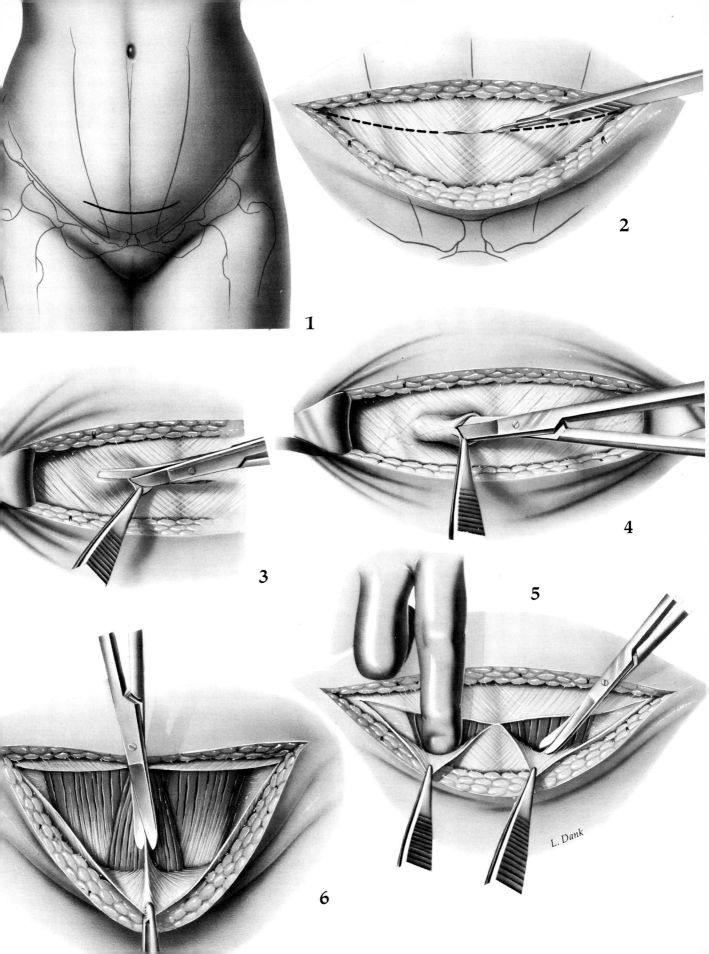

1

2

3

4

5

6

L. Dank

FIGURE 7

Separating the Upper Rectus Sheath Off the Rectus Muscle

The upper flap of the rectus sheath is separated off the rectus muscles. Perforating branches of the inferior epigastric vessels are identified and carefully tied as encountered to prevent a subsequent subfascial hematoma. The midline dissection is extended upward to the umbilicus to achieve a maximum midline longitudinal incision.

FIGURES 8 & 9

Opening the Peritoneal Cavity

The bellies of the rectus muscles have been digitally separated. The parietal peritoneum and the loosely adherent properitoneal fat are elevated away from the underlying bowel with smooth forceps as the surgeon carefully incises the tissues between the forceps to enter the peritoneal cavity. The peritoneal incision is extended superiorly to the umbilicus and inferiorly to the dome of the bladder. Additional length is achieved by extending the peritoneal incision to either the left or right side of the bladder.

FIGURE 10

The Self-Retaining Retractor

A systematic palpation of the abdominal viscera and organs for any abnormalities has been performed. A suitable self-retaining retractor is then placed in the incision and the operating table is tilted into the Trendelenburg position. The intestines are packed out of the pelvis to expose the pelvic organs.

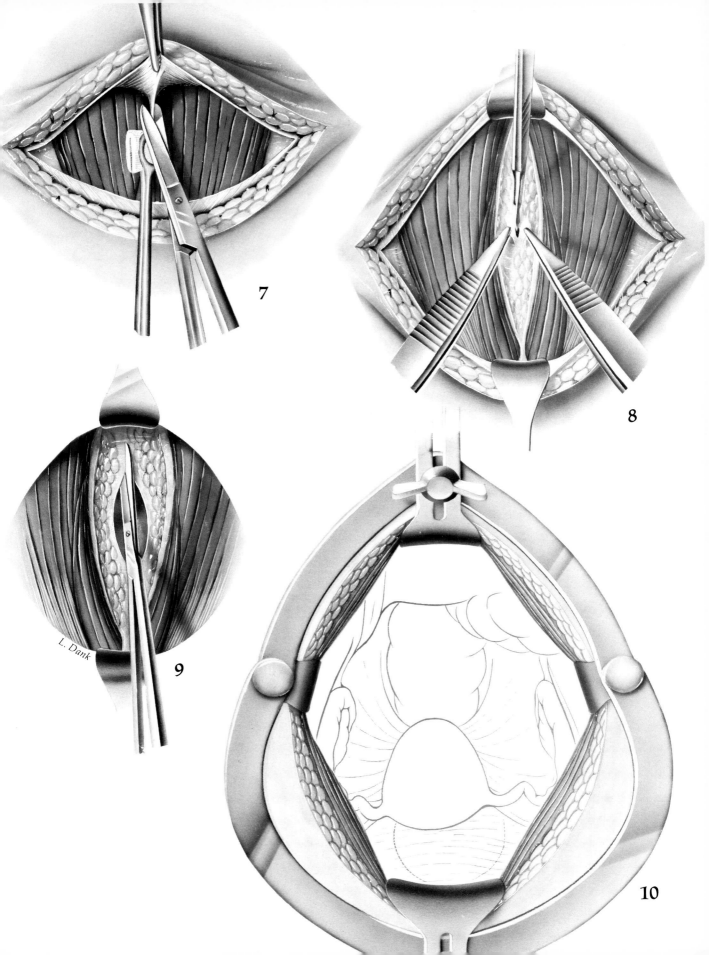

7

8

9

L. Dank

10

LAPAROSCOPIC EXAMINATION AND STERILIZATION BY ELECTROCAUTERIZATION OF THE FALLOPIAN TUBES

The indications for a laparoscopic examination can be either diagnostic or surgical. Diagnostic uses are in problems related to infertility, in which a direct inspection of the pelvic viscera, particularly of the fallopian tubes and their patency, is required and the status of the ovaries is of concern. Other uses include the diagnosing of suspected unruptured ectopic pregnancies, pelvic endometriosis, or tuberculosis; identifying causes, if any, of unexplained pelvic pain; and differentiating small pelvic or adnexal masses. Surgical procedures performed laparoscopically include tubal sterilization, lysis of small pelvic adhesions, biopsy of the ovaries or other tissues, aspiration of benign ovarian cysts, retrieval of eggs for *in vitro* fertilization, and removal of intrauterine devices located in the pelvic cavity.

In a cooperative patient the examination may be performed under suitable sedation and local anesthesia. However, it may be performed best in an operating room situation under general anesthesia with endotracheal intubation.

FIGURE 1

Positioning and Preparation of the Patient

The patient's legs have been placed in stirrups and the table declined to a moderate Trendelenburg position. The bladder has been catheterized and a dilatation and curettage may have been performed if indicated. A cervical tenaculum or cannula (not shown) may be placed to manipulate the uterus during the laparoscopic examination.

FIGURES 2 & 3

Creating the Pneumoperitoneum

A 1-cm skin incision is made in the lower aspect of the umbilical fold. The Verres needle is inserted and passed between the rectus fascia and fat for about 1 inch or more in the midline towards the pubic bone. It is then redirected toward the pelvic axis and firmly passed through the rectus fascia into the peritoneal cavity with a determined thrust to avoid separating the parietal peritoneum from abdominal wall muscles.

FIGURES 4 & 5

The Pneumoperitoneum

The Verres needle, shown in detail, is a double-barreled insufflation cannula with a spring-loaded blunt tip. It is now connected to the CO_2 source and 2 to 3 liters of gas are allowed to flow into the peritoneal cavity. When the abdomen is percussed a tympanic resonance can be heard as the peritoneal cavity is distended.

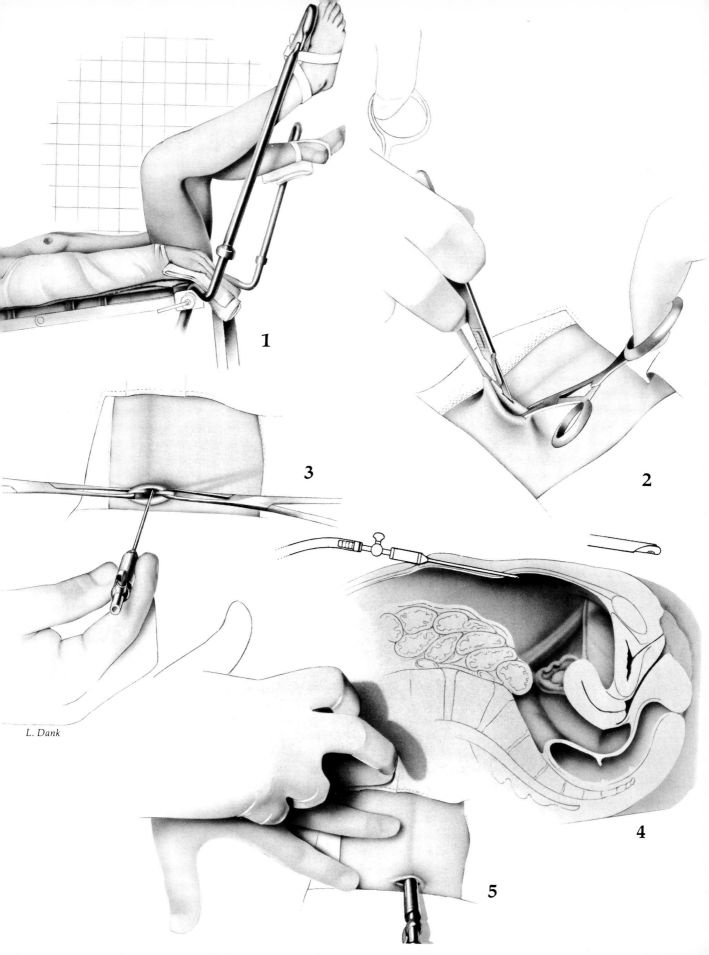

1

2

3

4

5

L. Dank

FIGURES 6 & 7
Insertion of the Laparoscopic Trochar and Cannula

The Verres needle has been removed and the trochar and cannula have been inserted through the same incision and firmly pushed through the subcutaneous fat for about 1½ inches. At this point the abdominal wall below the trochar is raised with the other hand. With a quick jabbing thrust the trochar and cannula are inserted into the peritoneal cavity at right angles to the pelvic inlet.

FIGURE 8
Inspection of the Pelvic Organs

The trochar has been removed and replaced by the laparoscope, which is already attached to the light source, and the pelvic organs are now inspected. The procedure is facilitated by gently manipulating the tenaculum or cannula previously attached to the cervix.

FIGURES 9 & 10
Insertion of Probe or Ancillary Trochar and Cannula

At a point halfway between the right anterior iliac spine and the symphysis pubis, a small incision is made to pass a probe or an ancillary cannulated trochar. The incisional site must be determined by transilluminating the abdominal wall with the laparoscope in a darkened room to avoid injuring the epigastric vessels.

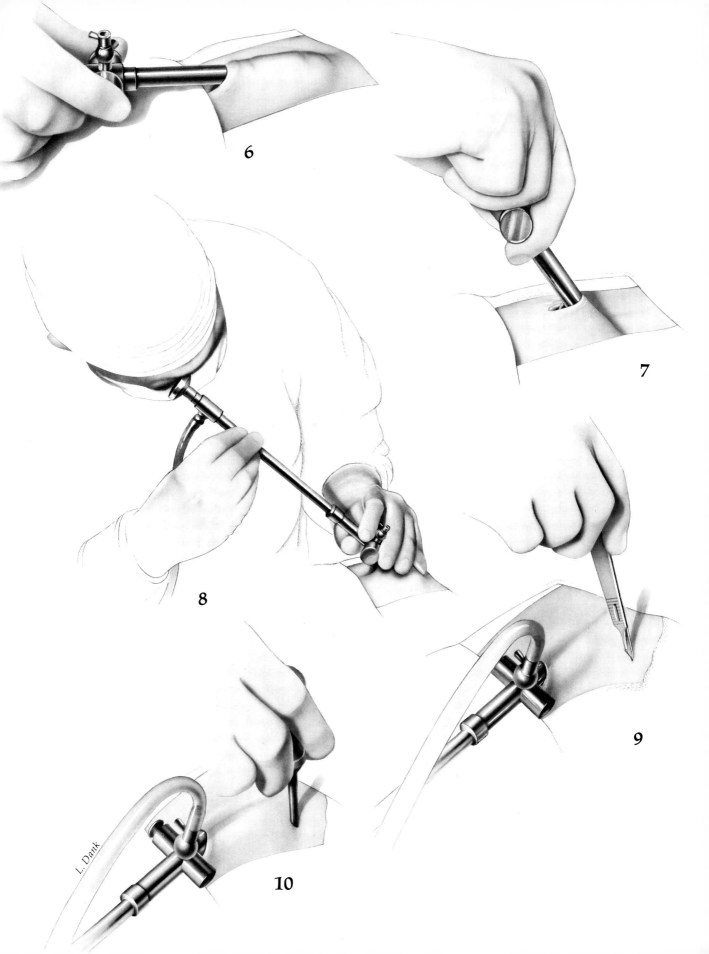

6

7

8

9

10

L. Dank

FIGURE 11

Passing the Probe or Cannulated Trocar into the Abdomen

The cannulated trocar is being observed through the laparoscope as the tip of the advancing point depresses the abdominal wall fascia and the underlying peritoneum. With a quick, determined thrust the trocar and cannula will be seen as they enter the peritoneal cavity.

Electrocauterization of the Fallopian Tubes

FIGURE 12

Placement of the Palmer Biopsy Cauterizing Forceps

The trocar has been removed and the Palmer biopsy cauterizing forceps has been inserted through the cannula and attached to the cautery unit.

FIGURE 13

Cauterization of the Fallopian Tube

A segment of tube 1½ inches to 2 inches from the cornual end is grasped with the Palmer forceps and pulled up. Great care must be taken to ensure that no other pelvic structure or loop of bowel is near the fallopian tube or touches the cauterizing forceps. Cauterization is performed, blanching a 1-inch segment of the fallopian tube.

FIGURES 14 & 15

Transection of Tube and Removal of Specimen

The Palmer forceps sleeve, with its serrated cutting edge, is pushed down and the blanched segment of tube is transected. The segment may be discarded or saved for pathologic analysis.

After the other tube has been treated in a similar manner, careful inspection will confirm that both tubes have been divided and that no bleeding points exist. All instruments are removed from their cannulas after the CO_2 has been allowed to escape. The cutaneous incisions are then closed with interrupted absorbable sutures and covered with an adhesive strip.

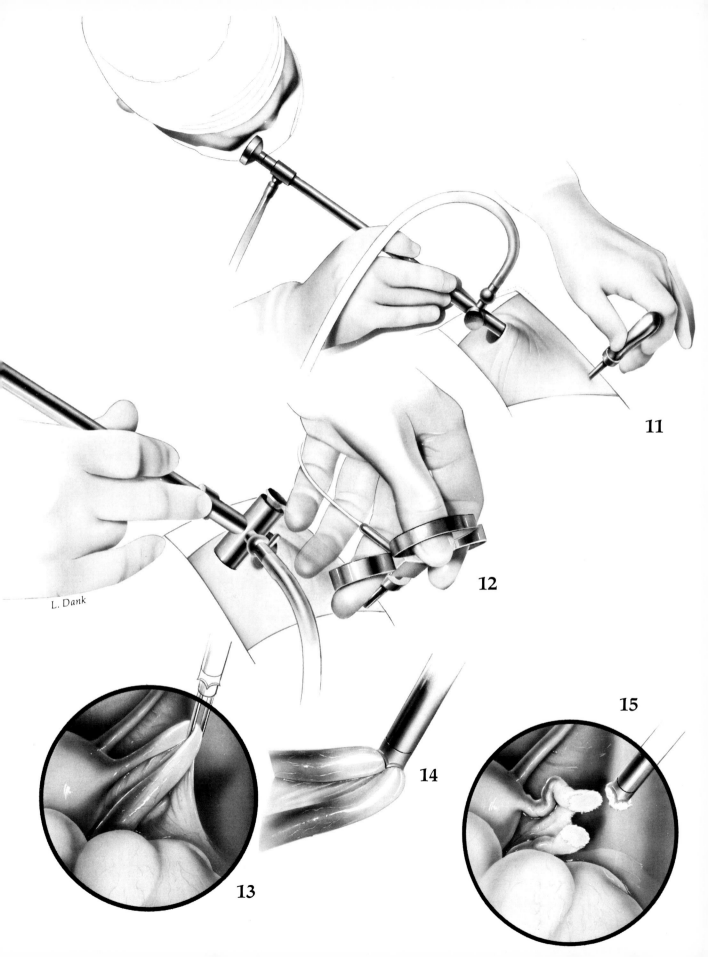

L. Dank

11

12

13

14

15

STERILIZATION BY TUBAL OCCLUSION WITH THE FALOPE RING

The use of a silicone band, the Falope ring, to occlude the tubes laparoscopically was developed as an alternative method to the cauterization technique and thereby avoids the danger of accidental burns to the bowel. Only a limited section of the tube is damaged with the Falope ring, making reversal of the procedure theoretically possible.

The method is contraindicated if the tubes are swollen or thickened by a recent pregnancy or old infection. Pain may be experienced for two to three days after surgery, presumably because of the ischemia produced in the occluded segment of the tube.

A double-puncture laparoscopic technique is used to provide a wider exposure and better sense of relative distances than can be achieved with a single-puncture laparoscopic technique.

FIGURE 1
Loading the Falope Ring Onto the Applicator

Under sterile conditions the Falope ring is placed on the tip of the cone of the applicator. With the aid of the guide it is advanced to the base of the cone, onto the inner cylinder of the applicator.

FIGURE 2
Grasping the Fallopian Tube

The ring applicator has been passed through the sleeve of the trochar inserted through the right lower quadrant of the abdomen. The grasping forceps has been advanced out of the inner cylinder of the ring applicator and has grasped the *whole* circumference of a segment of the tube in its midportion. It is gently drawn back to the opening of the inner sleeve of the ring applicator.

FIGURE 3
Applying the Falope Ring

The knuckle of tube is drawn gently into the inner cylinder of the applicator, while the applicator is simultaneously advanced over the tube to avoid tearing and bleeding in the mesosalpinx.

Once a sufficient loop of tube is in the inner cylinder, the inner cylinder is drawn into the outer cylinder forcing the ring onto the loop of tube.

FIGURES 4 & 5
Releasing the Fallopian Tube and Final Inspection

The spring action of the device has restored the inner cylinder to its original position. Any laceration or bleeding is carefully looked for before releasing the tube from the forceps. The same procedure is then repeated on the opposite tube.

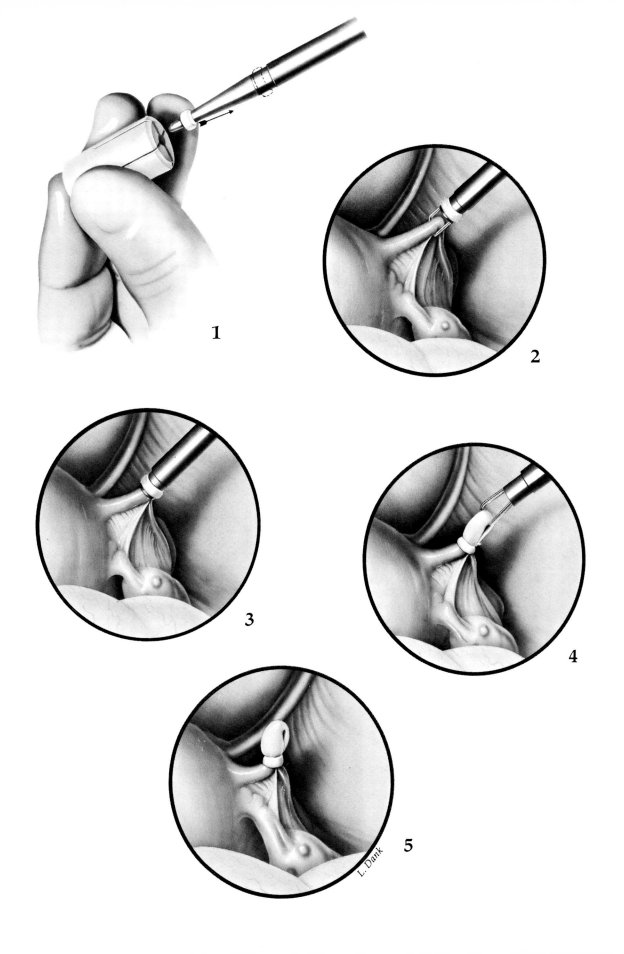

1

2

3

4

5

L. Dank

OVARIAN CYSTECTOMY

An ovarian cystectomy is a procedure designed to remove diseased ovarian tissue and to salvage as much normal ovarian tissue as possible in the same ovary. The decision when to operate and when to resect or not resect and to remove the whole ovary requires both the clinical and surgical judgment of the gynecologist. His decision will depend on the patient's symptoms, if any, her age, and the nature and size of the cyst. Once the pathology has been exposed, the gynecologist will recognize it as a simple enlargement of a physiologic cyst or as a benign or potentially or definite malignant neoplastic process. Should there be any question as to the true nature of the cyst, the opinion of the pathologist should be obtained. Encapsulated cysts such as simple serous cysts, benign cystic teratomas, and endometriotic cysts of small to moderate size can be easily excised without sacrificing the entire ovary. Multiple cysts may occur in a single ovary, and certain ovarian cysts have a bilateral incidence and require careful inspection and possible bivalving of the other ovary.

FIGURE 1
Exposure of the Involved Ovarian Cyst

The uterus is held in traction toward the opposite side and the involved ovary is stabilized with suitably placed Babcock clamps or held between the surgeon's thumb and fingers. An incision is made to establish a cleavage plane around the ovary at the junction of the cyst wall or its capsule and normal ovarian tissue.

FIGURES 2 & 3
Enucleating the Intact Cyst

A knife handle or blunt-pointed scissors are used to further develop the cleavage plane between the cyst wall and ovarian stroma. Once the cyst has been excised, its nature must be determined.

FIGURES 4, 5, & 6
Repair of the Defect

A continuous absorbable suture material is used to close the defect. It is important that the suture be passed deeply into the base of the defect to ensure the approximation of the walls to prevent a hematoma from developing in the repaired ovary.

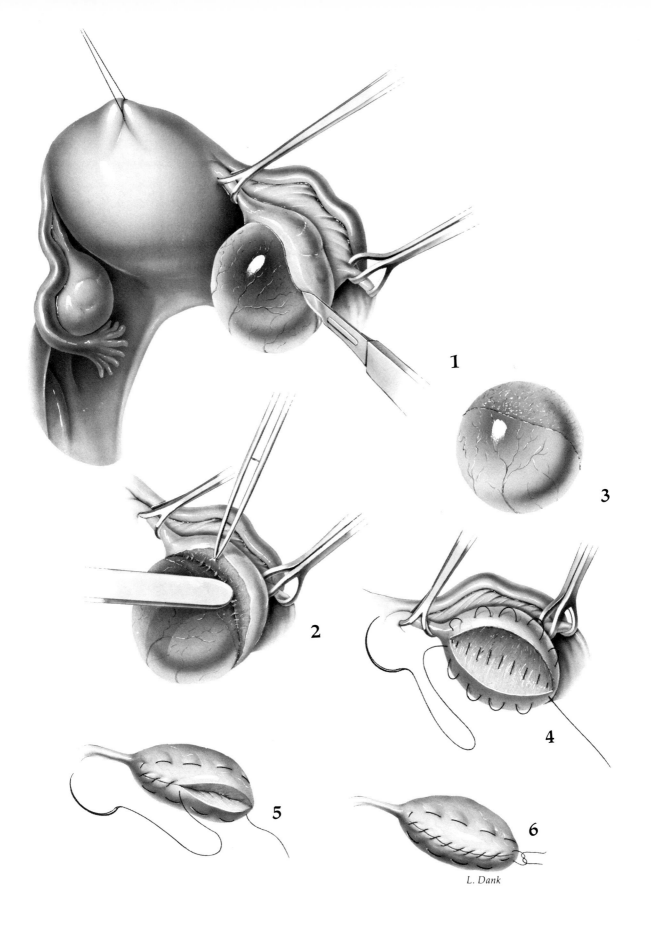

1

2

3

4

5

6

L. Dank

TOTAL ABDOMINAL HYSTERECTOMY: EXTRAFASCIAL TECHNIQUE

There are three techniques for removing the uterus abdominally: intrafascial, extrafascial, and radical. The intrafascial technique develops the pubocervical fascia surrounding the cervix to allow the uterine and paracervical vessels to be clamped deep to the fascia, thus ensuring no injury to the ureters. In the extrafascial technique, as shown here, the uterine and paracervical vessels are clamped externally to the pubocervical fascia, thus putting the ureter at a slightly increased risk of injury. However, this technique permits the removal of a large segment of the upper vagina attached to the cervix, which is believed to be important when operating for cervical dysplasia, carcinoma in situ, microinvasive cervical cancer, or endometrial carcinoma. A radical hysterectomy performed for early invasive cervical cancer is an en bloc removal of the cardinal and uterosacral ligaments dissected off their respective pelvic wall attachments and the upper paracolpos, leaving them attached to the uterine cervix and upper vagina.

My technique of an extrafascial hysterectomy, as illustrated here, uses silk sutures and avoids any unnecessary clamping or crushing of tissue that is to be left in the patient.

FIGURE 1
Incising the Vesical Peritoneal Fold

The uterus is held upward over the sacral promontory by two clamps placed at the junction of the broad ligaments and the cornual angles. The vesicouterine peritoneal fold is tented up with forceps just below its firm attachment to the anterior uterine surface and incised in both directions toward the round ligaments. The space between the bladder and uterus has been exposed.

FIGURE 2
Reflecting the Bladder Off the Uterus

The lower flap of the vesicoperitoneal fold is elevated. Both sharp and finger dissection are used and the bladder is easily pushed off the anterior aspect of the cervix, in a bloodless midline plane, to the level of the external cervical os. The uterine and paracervical vessels are seen on the lateral sides of the cervix. Injury to them should be avoided at this stage.

FIGURE 3
Preservation of the Ovary and Fallopian Tube

If the ovary is to be preserved, double sutures are placed through a bloodless area in the broad ligament around the ovarian ligament and proximal part of the fallopian tube. The structures are then cut between clamp and ligatures, and the broad ligament is opened.

FIGURE 4
Removal of the Ovary and Fallopian Tube

If the ovary and tube are to be removed, double ligatures are placed around the infundibulopelvic ligament containing the ovarian blood supply at the level of the pelvic brim. The ureter should be observed at this level as it crosses the pelvic brim deep to the ligament. A third suture is placed 1 inch distally toward the uterus and ligated. It prevents reflex bleeding when the ligament is cut and the broad ligament is opened.

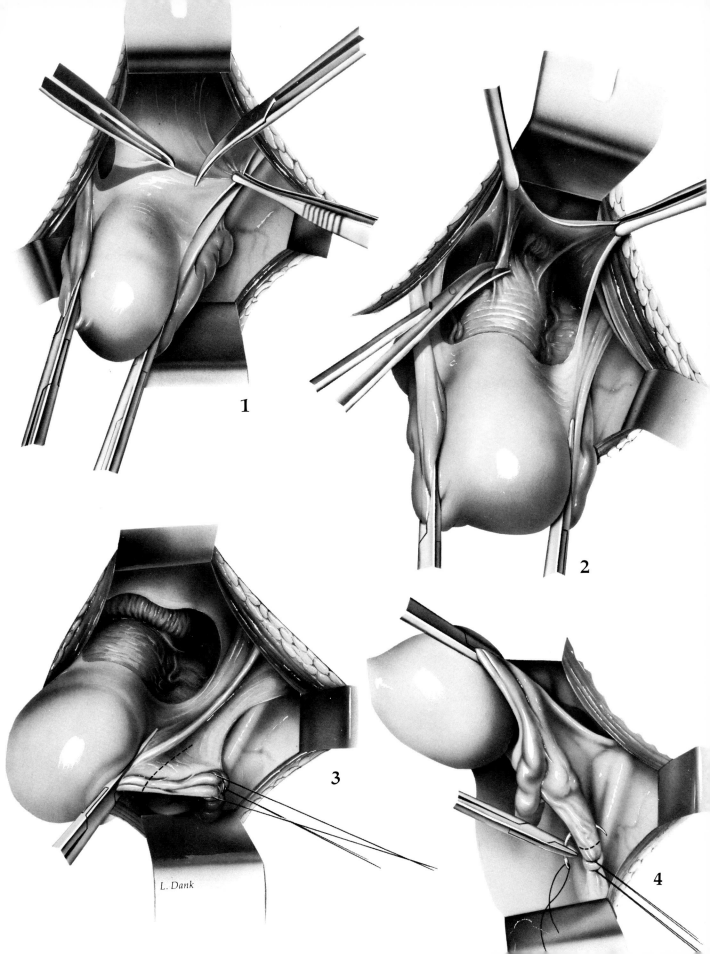

1

2

3

4

L. Dank

FIGURES 5, 6, & 7
Cutting the Round Ligament and Further Opening of the Broad Ligament

The round ligament is ligated at its midpoint and pulled laterally as the anterior layer of the broad ligament is completely cut, thus opening up the bloodless parauterine space filled with loose areolar tissue. While lateral tension is maintained on the round ligament and the uterus is pulled slightly to the opposite side, the posterior sheath of the broad ligament is cut down to the uterine vessels and posteriorly to a point where the uterosacral ligament is attached to the cervix. The dissection to this point is now carried out on the opposite side in a similar manner.

FIGURES 8 & 9
Ligating the Uterosacral Ligaments

The densely adherent peritoneum overlying the posterior surface of the cervix and upper vagina between the attachments of the uterosacral ligament is cut and shaved off the back of the cervix as the uterus is held upward toward the symphysis pubis.

The attachments of the uterosacral ligaments are ligated and held for subsequent identification during the repair stage of the operation.

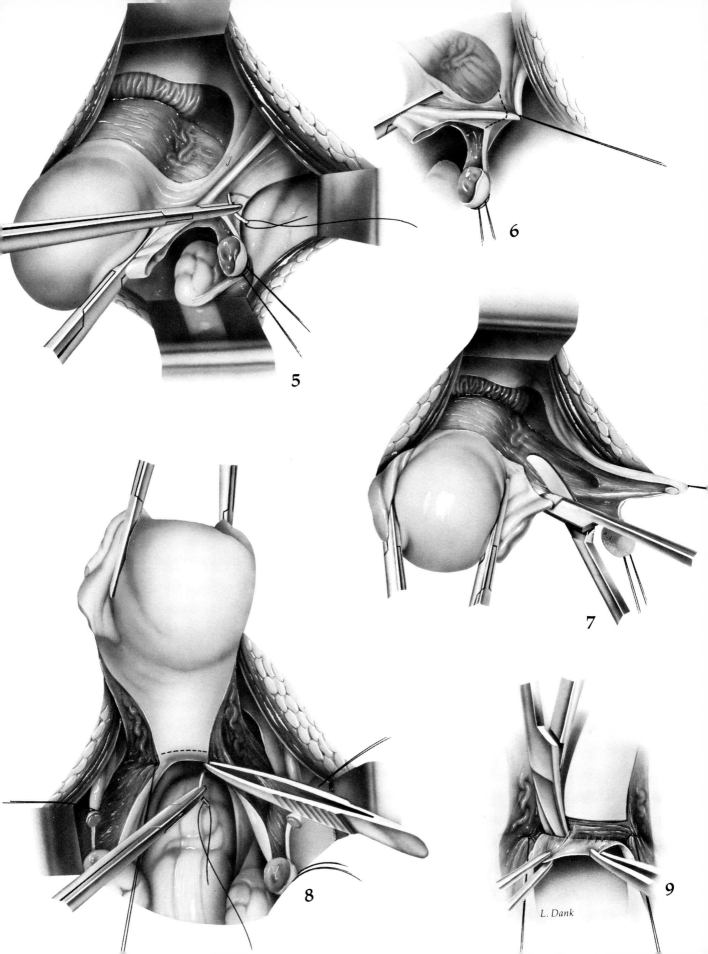

5

6

7

8

9

L. Dank

FIGURES 10 & 11

Clamping and Ligating the Uterine Vessels

The uterine vessels have been cleaned of their loosely attached connective tissue covering and a Kocher clamp has been applied. A Babcock clamp may be used to pull the vascular bundle gently away from the cervix below the Kocher clamp as a suture ligature is passed between the vessels and the cervix. The Babcock clamp is then removed, and the suture ligature is tied and gently pulled laterally as the vessels are cut away from the clamp. A second suture is customarily placed around the uterine vessels.

FIGURES 12 & 13

Clamping and Ligating the Paracervical Vessels

The tip of a Kocher clamp is placed approximately 1 inch to 1½ inches down on the lateral wall of the cervix incorporating the paracervical tissues (cardinal ligament attachments) between the cervix and stump of the cut uterine vessels. It is eased off the cervix as the clamp is firmly secured. The paracervical tissue is cut away from the cervix and a suture ligature passed between the tip of the clamp and the stump of the uterine vessels and tied. The process may need to be repeated two or more times depending on the length of the cervix or the amount of vaginal cuff that is to be removed.

Throughout each step of ligating the paracervical vessels the bladder must be kept well below the operative site and the uterus must be held in traction toward the sacral promontory.

The vessels on the opposite side are treated in the same way.

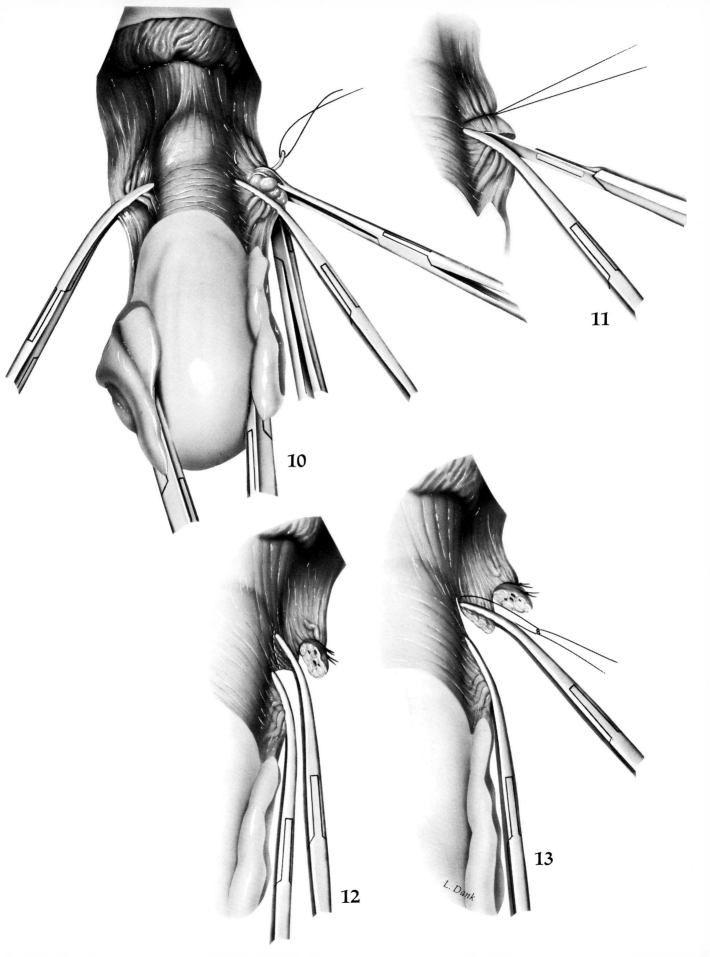

10

11

12

L. Dank

13

FIGURE 14
Incising the Vagina and Removal of the Uterus

With the uterus pulled upward under tension and the bladder retracted down on the vagina, a quick stab wound into the vagina is made below the level of the external cervical os. As the vagina is cut around, the assistant grasps the lower cut edge with four Allis clamps to prevent its retraction.

FIGURE 15
The Vaginal Vault Angle Sutures

A figure-of-eight absorbable suture is placed through each of the vaginal angles into the paracolpos (cardinal ligaments) and back through the vaginal wall and tied. Their purpose is for added hemostasis and support of the vagina, and they are held for traction during the closing of the vaginal vault.

FIGURE 16
Closing the Vaginal Vault

Either an interrupted or continuous running absorbable suture material is used. It is important to obtain wide bites on each edge to secure hemostasis and to prevent granulation tissue formation in the repaired vaginal vault. If bleeding throughout the operation has been a problem, or if any infection has been present, a small Penrose drain may be left in the vaginal vault and removed in two or three days.

FIGURE 17
Resupporting the Vaginal Vault

The supporting structures of the vaginal vault, namely the cardinal and uterosacral ligaments and pubocervical fascia, have been cut away, and it is now necessary to reattach them to the vagina to prevent a future vaginal vault prolapse. Using a silk suture a solid bite is taken in the substance of the uterosacral ligament, previously tagged but not shown here, and passed into the cardinal ligaments, avoiding the uterine vessels, and subsequently into the pubocervical fascia between the vaginal wall and bladder. The suture is tied and held. A similar suture is placed in the opposite side. The retroperitoneal dead space between the uterosacral ligaments and the posterior vaginal wall is closed with two or three additional sutures and attached over the closed vaginal vault to the pubocervical fascia anteriorly. The vaginal vault has now been resuspended by the fascial shelf that extends from the symphysis pubis to the pelvic sidewalls and to the sacrum.

FIGURE 18
Peritonizing the Pelvis

After hemostasis has been ensured, interrupted silk sutures are used to reapproximate the visceral and parietal peritoneum. All ligamentous stumps are buried to avoid any raw surfaces to which a loop of small bowel could become attached. The position of the ureters is constantly noted to avoid their injury.

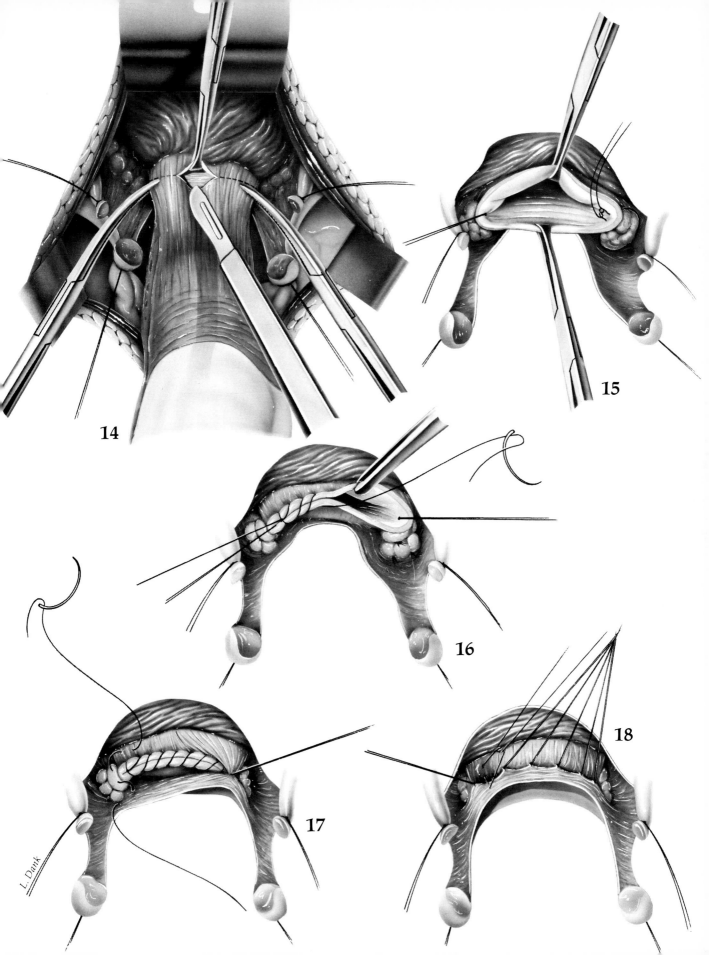

14

15

16

17

18

L. Dank

VAGINAL HYSTERECTOMY AND COLPOPERINEOPLASTY

The removal of the uterus through the vagina, with or without the adnexae, requires the experience of a trained gynecologic surgeon. It is frequently performed in association with a repair of cystocele, urethrocele, and rectocele. An early enterocele may also coexist and will require correction. The complete operation described here requires a thorough knowledge and understanding of the anatomy and function of the pelvic supporting structures as described in Chapter 51.

Many techniques have been described and discussed at length since the first operation of its kind was performed over 120 years ago. Modifications and improved techniques have been developed as our knowledge of the structure and functions of the pelvic supporting fascia and ligaments has increased.

A vaginal hysterectomy may be performed in the absence of any uterine or vaginal prolapse or when procidentia exists. The fundamental principles in the vaginal removal of the uterus, either alone without prolapse or with the repair of coexisting vaginal relaxation or hernia, are the same, and the repair must ensure the resupporting of the vagina and the prevention of any future or recurrent vaginal hernia.

Vaginal Hysterectomy

FIGURE 1
Preparing the Operative Field

A dilatation and curettage has been performed and a Foley catheter placed in the bladder (not shown). The labia minora are sutured laterally for better exposure of the operative field. The cervix is grasped and pulled down through the introitus and silk marking sutures are placed in the vaginal skin at points identifying the lower portion of the cardinal ligament attachments to the cervix. The vaginal wall overlying the cervicovaginal junction below the bladder is raised.

FIGURE 2
Opening the Anterior Vaginal Wall

With scissors or scalpel a transverse incision is made in the vaginal skin in the vesicovaginal layer of fascia. It is extended laterally on both sides passing below the marking sutures. The space between the vaginal wall and cervix is now opened.

FIGURES 3 & 4
Mobilizing and Dividing the Anterior Vaginal Wall

While downward traction is maintained on the cervix, closed blunt-pointed scissors are inserted into the space and advanced in the midline. While being maintained against the undersurface of the vaginal skin, the points of the scissors are sequentially spread, withdrawn, then closed and reinserted to a higher level in the midline. Tension is maintained on the loosened skin flaps as the sequence is repeated until a point below the external urethral meatus has been reached. To achieve this end point of dissection the vaginal skin is incised in the midline and a series of Allis clamps carefully placed on the cut edges are used for lateral retraction and further exposure of the developed space.

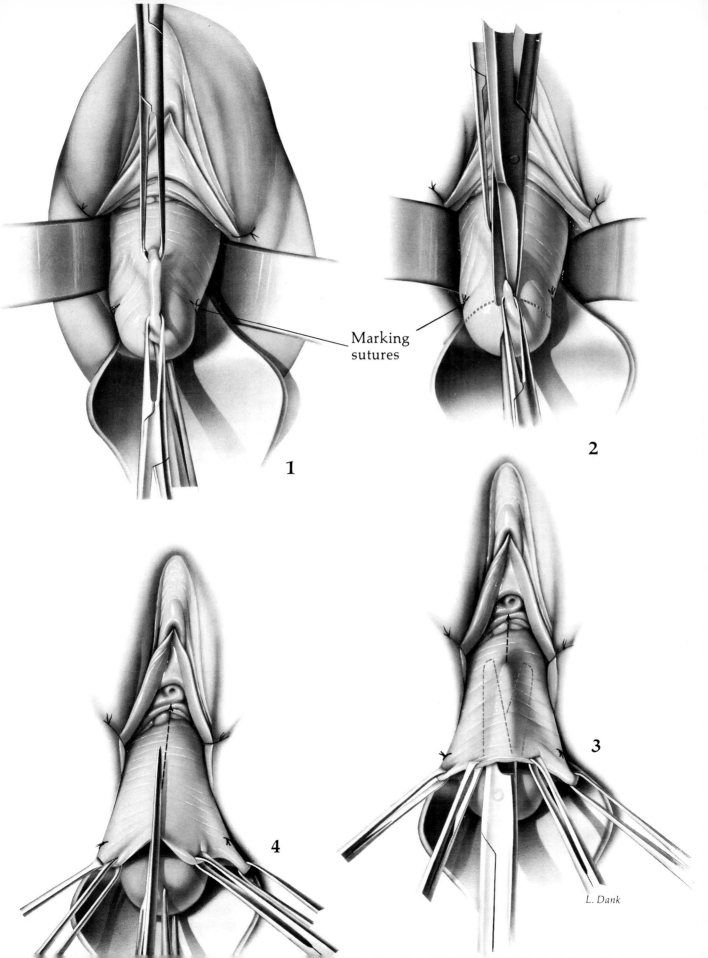

Marking
sutures

1

2

3

4

L. Dank

FIGURE 5
Mobilizing the Bladder

The bladder capsule is now exposed as the cut edges of the vaginal wall are retracted laterally. The loose capsular fibers are cut away from the vaginal skin in a bloodless plane extending from the urethra to the cervix on both sides. The dissection, which may be performed with a knife handle or gauze-covered finger, is extended laterally on each side to a level just above the inferior border of the pubic ramus. It is continued until the bladder and urethra are separated from all lateral vaginal wall attachments.

FIGURE 6
Dividing the Uterovesical Ligaments

The bladder and its capsule are separated off the cervix and lower uterine segment anteriorly as firm downward traction on the cervix is maintained. While the lower border of the bladder is elevated in the midline the ligamentous fibers attaching it to the cervix are cut.

FIGURE 7
Advancement of the Bladder on the Cervix

Once a bloodless cleavage plane between the bladder and cervix has been identified and developed in the midline and laterally, the bladder can be advanced easily on the uterus by being gently pushed upward against the cervix with a gauze-covered index finger. It is advanced to the point where the vesicouterine peritoneal fold is seen. The uterine vessels and their branches are seen on the anterolateral side of the cervix.

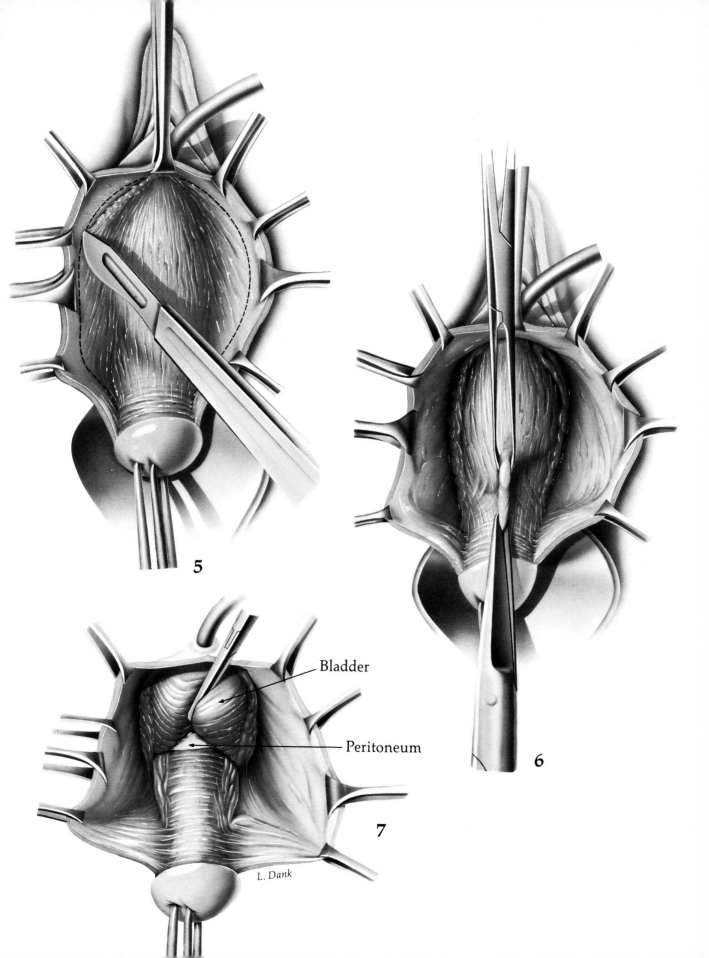

5

6

Bladder

Peritoneum

7

L. Dank

FIGURE 8
Mobilizing the Posterior Vaginal Wall Off the Cervix

The cervix is held upward toward the symphysis and a silk marking suture has been placed in the midline at the same level as the two previously placed lateral marking sutures. The anterior transverse vaginal skin incision has been extended posteriorly to encircle the cervix completely. The same bloodless areolar tissue plane that was seen between the bladder and cervix anteriorly has been exposed posteriorly.

FIGURE 9
Exposure of the Cardinal Ligaments

A gauze-covered finger pressed firmly against the cervix has further developed the bloodless space between vagina and cervix. Laterally the space is limited by the uterosacral and cardinal ligaments, which fuse at this level of their attachment to the cervix. The space is developed all the way to the peritoneal reflection of the cul-de-sac.

FIGURES 10 & 11
Clamping and Ligating the Cardinal Ligaments

The vaginal wall has been dissected off both cardinal ligaments as far laterally as is necessary to shorten them. The ligaments are clamped with two Kocher clamps on each side, with their tips placed against the cervix immediately below the uterine vessels and fanned out laterally at the base to shorten them to the extent indicated by their length.

The ligaments are cut and ligated with double sutures. One suture on each side is held in a clamp for later identification.

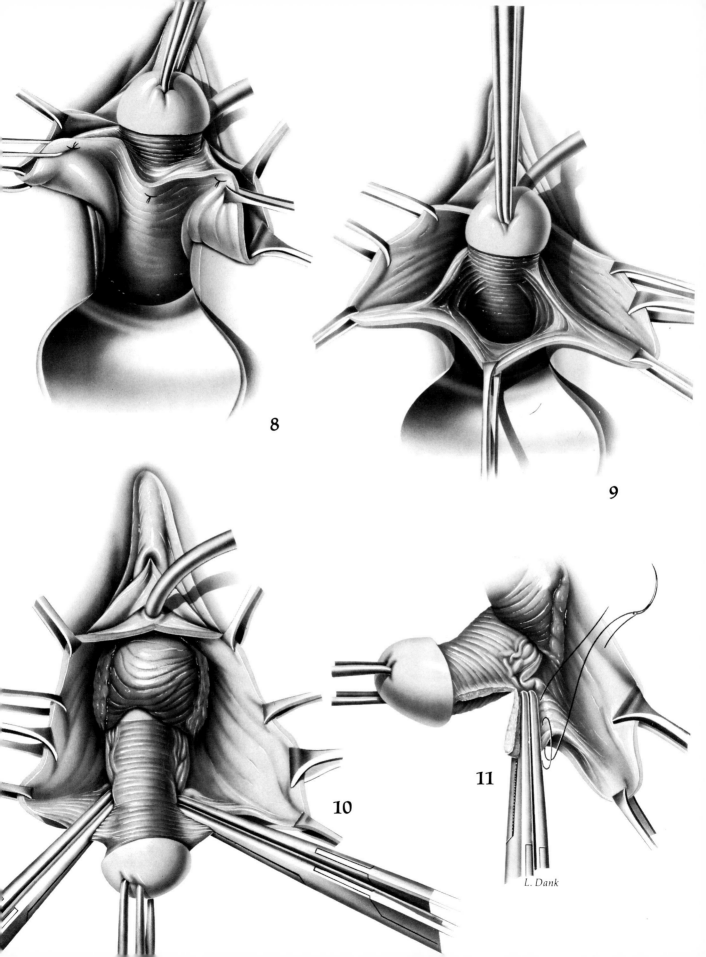

8

9

10

11

L. Dank

FIGURES 12 & 13
Clamping and Ligating the Uterine Vessels

While continuous traction is maintained on the cervix the uterine vessels are doubly clamped. The clamps are placed close to the cervix to avoid injury to the ureters should the bladder not be completely advanced on the uterus.

The uterine vessels have been cut between the cervix and clamps and ligated with double sutures lateral to the clamps. Additional vessels may require separate clamping and ligation.

FIGURE 14
Opening the Peritoneal Cavity Anteriorly

With the bladder retracted upward and the cervix pulled downward, the peritoneal cavity has been opened and the uterine body grasped with a tenaculum. A marking suture is placed on the peritoneum for identification.

FIGURE 15
Delivery of the Uterine Body and Ligation of the Broad Ligaments

The peritoneal incision has been extended laterally on both sides. With successive tenaculum bites applied to the anterior surface of the uterine body in a stepladder fashion and pulling downward with each bite, the uterus is delivered through the anterior fornix.

The bladder retractor is placed intraperitoneally and the ovaries and tubes are palpated and inspected for any disease; a decision is made to remove them or leave them in place. An iodoform gauze is placed in the peritoneal cavity to keep the intestines out of the operative field.

The depth of the cul-de-sac is explored for any real or potential enterocele between the exposed uterosacral ligaments.

It has been decided to leave the adnexa. Accordingly the round ligament, ovarian ligament, fallopian tube, and intervening broad ligament are doubly clamped down to but not including the uterosacral ligaments. They are cut between the clamp and uterus and ligated with double sutures lateral to the clamps. One suture is held long on each side for identification.

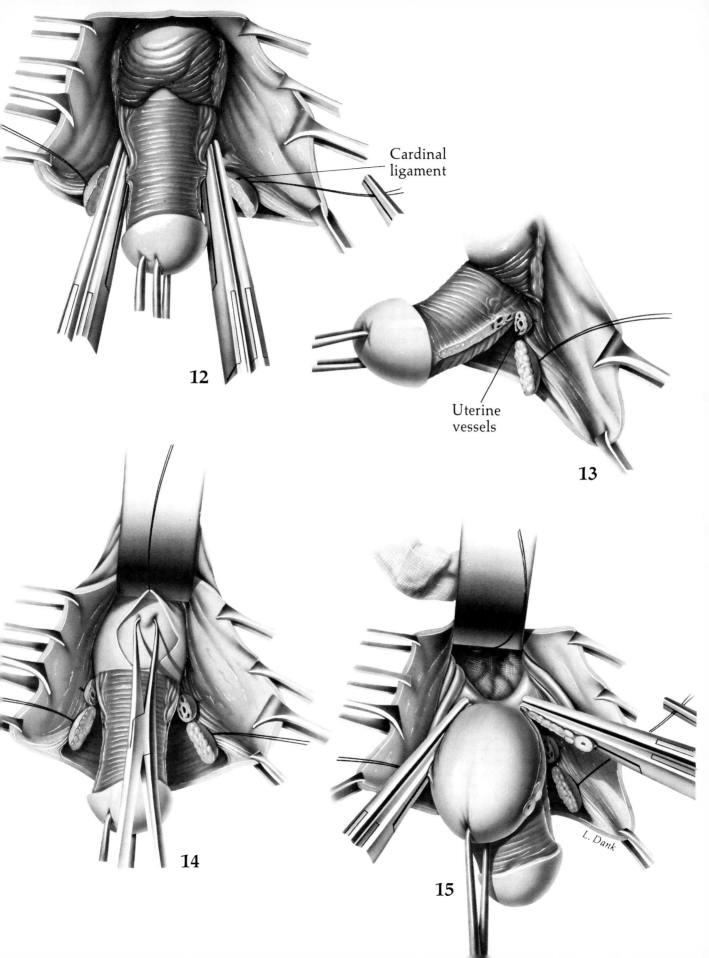

Cardinal
ligament

12

Uterine
vessels

13

14

L. Dank

15

FIGURES 16 & 17

Ligation, Clamping, and Cutting of Uterosacral Ligaments

The uterosacral ligaments are held with Allis clamps as deep sutures are placed in them close to the cervix, ligated, and held long. The uterus is pulled downward and clamps are placed on the uterosacral ligaments at their point of attachment to the posterior aspect of the cervix.

FIGURE 18

Removal of the Uterus and Further Ligation of the Uterosacral Ligaments

The uterus has been removed and an additional ligature has been placed in each stump of the uterosacral ligaments incorporating the intervening fascia to control bleeding. The ligaments are then cut.

FIGURES 19 & 20

Prevention or Correction of an Enterocele

The iodoform pack has been removed and the cul-de-sac exposed. If the cul-de-sac is abnormally deep or an enterocele exists, the peritoneum is cut and dissected off the underlying tissues to a point in front of the rectum. Excess peritoneum is excised and the cut edges are approximated in the midline.

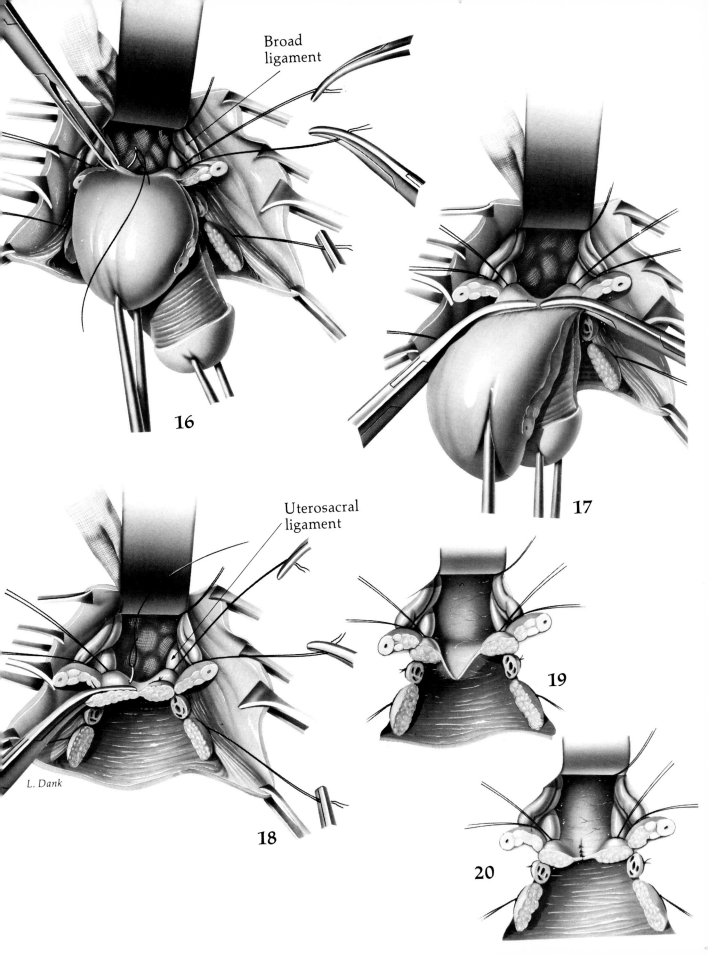

Broad
ligament

16

17

Uterosacral
ligament

L. Dank

18

19

20

FIGURE 21
Obliteration of the Cul-De-Sac

The cul-de-sac is further obliterated and the uterosacral ligaments are further shortened, with three or four interrupted silk sutures approximating them to each other to a point just anterior to the rectum. The purpose here is to prevent the development of an enterocele and to provide added strength to the support of the vaginal vault.

FIGURES 22 & 23
Closing of the Peritoneal Cavity

The peritoneal cavity is closed with a purse-string suture incorporating free peritoneum overlying the tubes, ovarian and round ligaments, and the approximated uterosacral ligaments. All raw surfaces of stumps are extraperitonealized. The suture, held here in a clamp with the broad ligament sutures, may be held for identification or cut. The vaginal hysterectomy has been completed. The marking sutures attached to the uterosacral ligaments are now held together for later attachment to the vaginal vault.

Repair of Cystocele

FIGURE 24
Reapproximation of Bladder Fascia

The pubocervical or paravesical fascia previously separated off the vaginal wall is now approximated to resupport the anterior vaginal wall and bladder and to correct any cystocele that may be present.

Starting at the level of the stumps of the uterosacral ligaments, a series of interrupted imbricated sutures is placed transversely and progressively upward to the urethrovesical angle.

FIGURE 25
Preventing or Correcting Urinary Stress Incontinence

The transverse fascial fold at the urethrovesical angle is readily identified by gentle traction on the Foley catheter. An additional supporting silk suture may be placed in this area to prevent or correct any urinary stress incontinence. One or two additional mattress sutures may be placed through the fascia 1 cm lateral to the previous suture on each side.

The paraurethral fascia is approximated with a series of interrupted sutures to the urethral meatus.

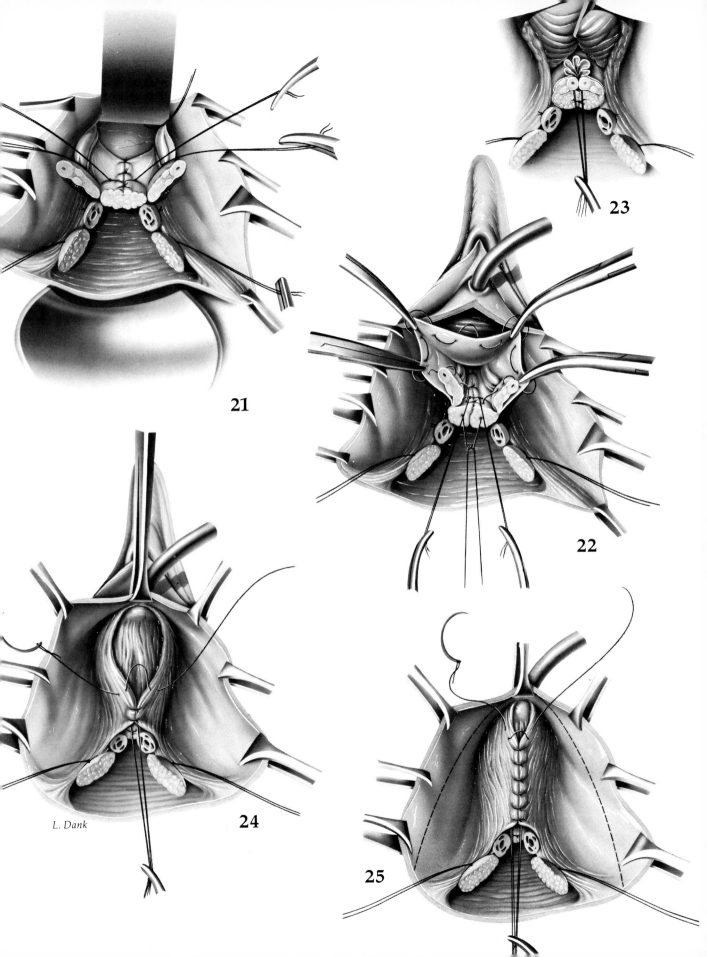

21

22

23

24

25

L. Dank

FIGURE 26
Excision of Excess Vaginal Skin

Excess vaginal skin is excised on both sides extending from 1 inch medial to the lateral silk marking sutures to the urethra. Care must be taken not to remove too much skin.

FIGURE 27
Closure of the Vaginal Wall and Resupporting the Vaginal Vault to the Uterosacral and Cardinal Ligaments

Starting at the level of the urethra the vaginal wall is closed by a series of interrupted sutures. Before complete closure the uterosacral ligaments are attached by their long marking sutures to the vaginal vault on either side of the single posterior marking suture previously placed in the midline. The long marking sutures of the cardinal ligaments are placed through the stump of the opposite cardinal ligament and attached to the vaginal vault at the site of the lateral marking silk suture on the opposite side.

The bladder and vaginal vault have been resupported by a greatly strengthened fascial layer that extends from the symphysis pubis anteriorly to the sacrum posteriorly.

FIGURE 28
Closure and Drainage of the Vaginal Vault

A strip of iodoform gauze is inserted under the vaginal skin in the midline for drainage purposes. It is removed on the fourth day after surgery. Redundant vaginal skin may be excised to close the vaginal vault neatly.

Repair of Rectocele and Perineorraphy

FIGURE 29
Excision of Perineal Scar

The perineum is exposed by traction on the tenacula placed on each side of the vaginal opening at a point that will become the midpoint of the vaginal introitus. The intervening scarred mucocutaneous tissue of the fourchette area is excised to gain access to the perineum and prerectal space. A transverse or triangular piece of scarred redundant tissue may be removed easily with scissors.

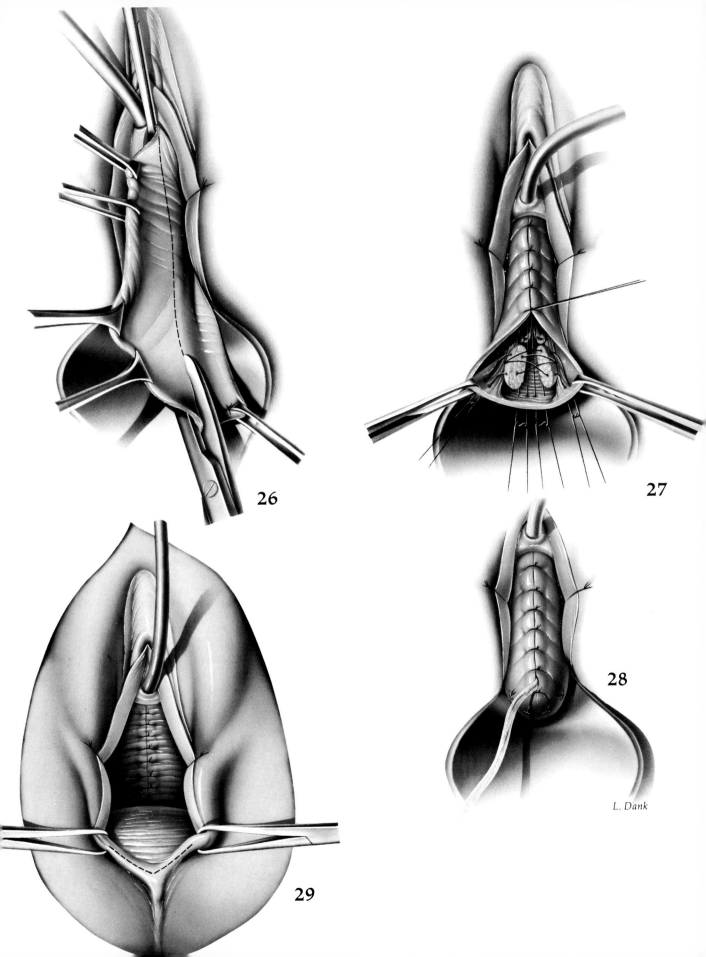

26

27

28

29

L. Dank

FIGURE 30

Opening the Prerectal Space

The space between the perineal body, posterior vaginal wall, and prerectal fascia is developed by both sharp and blunt scissor dissection. As the dissection proceeds upward, a gauze-covered finger will easily separate the rectum away from the vaginal wall in the midline to well above the rectocele—to the level of the vaginal vault if necessary. Bisection of the posterior vaginal wall in the midline will be necessary to obtain greater exposure.

The vagina is then freed laterally on both sides by sharp dissection to a point where the inferior borders of the levator ani muscles are exposed. The procedure can frequently produce more bleeding than in any other step in the entire operation.

FIGURE 31

Repair of Rectocele

The attenuated prerectal fascia overlying the rectocele is repaired by plication with several transversely placed imbricated sutures starting from well above the rectocele and proceeding downward to the perineal body. An initial purse-string suture may be placed in the prerectal fascia to assist in the obliteration of a large enterocele.

FIGURES 32 & 33

Excision of Vaginal Skin, Closure of the Vaginal Wall, and Repair of the Pelvic Floor

Redundant posterior wall vaginal skin is trimmed. A suture is placed at the apex of the vaginal incision and held upward as three or four "levator sutures" are placed in the substance of the lower border of these muscles and held. The posterior vaginal wall is then closed down to the introitus with either a continuous or an interrupted suture and held. Care must be taken to tack the vaginal wall sutures to the underlying fascia and the approximated levator muscles to obliterate dead space and prevent the formation of a hematoma. The levator sutures are progressively tied as the prerectal space and vaginal wall closure progresses down to the introitus.

FIGURE 34

Repair of the Perineum

The pelvic floor has been reconstructed with interrupted sutures placed in the substance of the perineal body. The subcutaneous fascia in the perineum is approximated with a continuous stitch (not shown) extending from the introitus to the lower angle of the perineal incision. It is then reversed and, using a cutting needle, carried upward as a subcuticular stitch and tied to the vaginal wall suture at the introitus.

The vagina may be packed with iodoform gauze to control oozing and to ensure approximation of the vaginal walls to the underlying structures. It is removed on the fourth day after surgery.

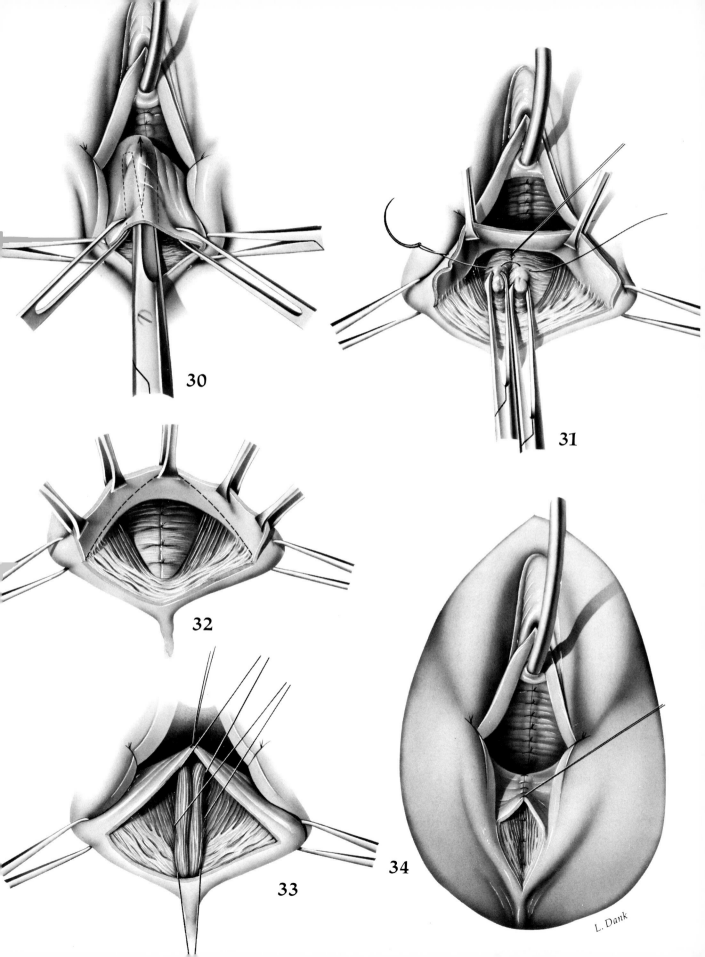

30

31

32

33

34

L. Dank

Index

Numbers followed by an *f* indicate a figure; *t* following a page number indicates tabular material.

DEPARTMENT OF FAMILY MEDICINE
COLLEGE OF OSTEOPATHIC MEDICINE
MICHIGAN STATE UNIVERSITY
EAST LANSING, MICHIGAN 48824